DIAGNOSTIC IMAGING OF FETAL ANOMALIES

DIAGNOSTIC IMAGING OF FETAL ANOMALIES

Edited by

DAVID A. NYBERG, M.D.

Director, OB/GYN Imaging
Scottsdale Medical Imaging
Scottsdale, Arizona

JOHN P. McGAHAN, M.D.

Professor
Director of Abdominal Imaging and Ultrasound
Department of Radiology
University of California, Davis, School of Medicine
Davis Medical Center
Davis, California

DOLORES H. PRETORIUS, M.D.

Professor of Radiology
Department of Radiology
University of California, San Diego, School of Medicine
La Jolla, California

GIANLUIGI PILU, M.D.

Consultant in Obstetrics and Gynecology
Clinica Ginecologica e Ostetrica
Policlinico S. Orsola-Malpighi
Università degli Studi di Bologna
Bologna, Italy

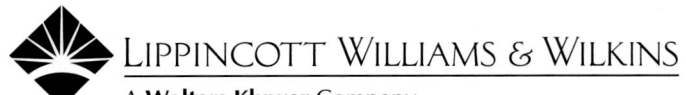

LIPPINCOTT WILLIAMS & WILKINS
A **Wolters Kluwer** Company
Philadelphia • Baltimore • New York • London
Buenos Aires • Hong Kong • Sydney • Tokyo

Acquisitions Editor: Joyce-Rachel John
Developmental Editor: Pamela Sutton/Tanya Lazar
Supervising Editor: Penny Bice
Production Editor: Brooke Begin, Silverchair Science + Communications
Manufacturing Manager: Ben Rivera
Cover Designer: Karen Quigley
Compositor: Silverchair Science + Communications
Printer: Walsworth Publishers

The publisher gratefully acknowledges contributions by Philippe Jeanty, M.D., Ph.D, of various tables, figures, and text to Chapters 5, 15, and 18. Dr. Jeanty retains the copyright of these contributions.

Library of Congress Cataloging-in-Publication Data

Diagnostic imaging of fetal anomalies / edited by David A. Nyberg ... [et al.].
    p. ; cm.
  Includes bibliographical references and index.
  ISBN 0-7817-3211-5
    1. Fetus--Abnormalities--Ultrasonic imaging. 2. Magnetic resonance imaging. 3.
Fetus--Diseases--Imaging. I. Nyberg, David A., 1952-
  [DNLM: 1. Fetus--abnormalities. 2. Ultrasonography, Prenatal--methods. 3. Fetal
Diseases--ultrasonography. 4. Magnetic Resonance Imaging--methods. WQ 209 D5354 2002]
RG628.3.U58 D63 2002
618.3'2--dc21

                                                              2002040638

Care has been taken to confirm the accuracy of the information presented and to describe generally accepted practices. However, the authors, editors, and publisher are not responsible for errors or omissions or for any consequences from application of the information in this book and make no warranty, expressed or implied, with respect to the currency, completeness, or accuracy of the contents of the publication. Application of this information in a particular situation remains the professional responsibility of the practitioner.

The authors, editors, and publisher have exerted every effort to ensure that drug selection and dosage set forth in this text are in accordance with current recommendations and practice at the time of publication. However, in view of ongoing research, changes in government regulations, and the constant flow of information relating to drug therapy and drug reactions, the reader is urged to check the package insert for each drug for any change in indications and dosage and for added warnings and precautions. This is particularly important when the recommended agent is a new or infrequently employed drug.

Some drugs and medical devices presented in this publication have Food and Drug Administration (FDA) clearance for limited use in restricted research settings. It is the responsibility of health care providers to ascertain the FDA status of each drug or device planned for use in their clinical practice.

10 9 8 7 6 5 4 3 2 1

To all those who have contributed, or will contribute,
toward prenatal diagnosis and treatment of fetal anomalies

CONTENTS

CONTRIBUTING AUTHORS

N. Scott Adzick, M.D.
C. Everett Koop Professor of Pediatric Surgery
Surgeon-in-Chief
Department of Surgery
Children's Hospital of Philadelphia
Philadelphia, Pennsylvania

Beryl R. Benacerraf, M.D.
Professor of Radiology and Obstetrics
    and Gynecology
Harvard Medical School
Boston, Massachusetts

Diana W. Bianchi, M.D.
Natalie V. Zucker Professor of Pediatrics and
    Obstetrics and Gynecology
Tufts University School of Medicine
Boston, Massachusetts

Ana Maria Bircher, M.D.
Women's Health Alliance
Nashville, Tennessee
Sanatorio General Sarmiento y Clinica y Maternidad
    Suizo Argentina
Buenos Aires, Argentina

Richard A. Bowerman, M.D.
Associate Professor
Department of Radiology
University of Michigan Medical School
Ann Arbor, Michigan

Rabih Chaoui, M.D.
Professor
Department of Obstetrics and Gynecology
Charité–University Hospital
Berlin, Germany

Ricardo Garcia Cavazos, M.D.
Genetics Institute
Mexico City, Mexico

Greggory R. DeVore, M.D.
Director
Fetal Diagnostic Center
Pasadena, California

Ian Glass, M.D., F.R.C.P., F.R.A.C.P., F.A.C.M.G.
Associate Professor of Pediatrics and Medicine
    (Medical Genetics)
University of Washington School of Medicine
Director
Department of Medical Genetics
Children's Hospital Regional Medical Center
Seattle, Washington

Ruth B. Goldstein, M.D.
Professor of Radiology, Obstetrics, Gynecology, and
    Reproductive Sciences
Department of Radiology
University of California, San Francisco, School of Medicine
San Francisco, California

Andree Gruslin, M.D., F.R.C.S.
Assistant Professor—GFT
Perinatologist
Department of Obstetrics, Gynecology, and Newborn Care
University of Ottawa
Ottawa, Ontario, Canada

Robert Harris, M.D.
Associate Professor of Radiology and Obstetrics
    and Gynecology
Director of Ultrasound
Dartmouth-Hitchcock Medical Center
Lebanon, New Hampshire

Barbara S. Hertzberg, M.D.
Professor of Radiology
Associate Professor of Obstetrics and Gynecology
Co-Director, Fetal Diagnostic Center
Duke University Medical Center
Durham, North Carolina

Lyndon M. Hill, M.D.
Professor of Obstetrics and Gynecology
Department of Ultrasound
Magee-Womens Hospital of UPMC Health System
Pittsburgh, Pennsylvania

Jonathan A. Hyett, M.D., M.R.C.O.G.
Lecturer in Fetal Medicine
Academic Department of Obstetrics
  and Gynecology
University College London
London, United Kingdom

Gina James, R.D.M.S.
Department of Radiology
University of California, San Diego,
  School of Medicine
La Jolla, California

Philippe Jeanty, M.D., Ph.D.
Chief Fetustician
Department of Ultrasound
Women's Health Alliance
Nashville, Tennessee

Deborah Levine, M.D.
Associate Professor of Radiology
Department of Radiology
Harvard Medical School
Beth Israel Deaconess Medical Center
Boston, Massachusetts

Nyree van Maarseveen
California Teratogen Information Service
Department of Pediatrics
University of California, San Diego,
  Medical Center
La Jolla, California

Tippi C. MacKenzie, M.D.
The Center for Fetal Diagnosis and Treatment
Children's Hospital of Philadelphia
Philadelphia, Pennsylvania

Fergal D. Malone, M.D.
Assistant Professor of Obstetrics and Gynecology
Department of Obstetrics and Gynecology
Columbia University College of Physicians
  and Surgeons
New York, New York

Robert W. McDonald, R.C.V.T., R.D.C.S.
Senior Cardiac Sonographer
Fetal Diagnostic Center
Pasadena, California

John P. McGahan, M.D.
Professor
Director of Abdominal Imaging and Ultrasound
Department of Radiology
University of California, Davis, School of Medicine
Davis Medical Center
Davis, California

Ana Monteagudo, M.D.
Professor of Obstetrics and Gynecology
Department of Obstetrics and Gynecology
New York University School of Medicine
Bellevue Hospital
Tisch Hospital
New York, New York

Ian R. Neilson, M.D., F.A.C.S.
Director of Pediatric Surgery
Swedish Medical Center
Seattle, Washington

Thomas R. Nelson, Ph.D.
Professor of Radiology
University of California, San Diego,
  School of Medicine
La Jolla, California

Kypros H. Nicolaides, M.D., M.R.C.O.G.
Professor of Fetal Medicine
Harris Birthright Research Centre for Fetal Medicine
King's College School of Medicine and Dentistry
London, United Kingdom

Cynthia G. Nodell, M.D.
Virginia Mason Medical Center
Seattle, Washington

David A. Nyberg, M.D.
Director, OB/GYN Imaging
Scottsdale Medical Imaging
Scottsdale, Arizona

Mary K. O'Boyle, M.D.
Associate Professor of Radiology
Department of Radiology
University of California, San Diego, School of Medicine
La Jolla, California

Gianluigi Pilu, M.D.
Consultant in Obstetrics and Gynecology
Clinica Ginecologica e Ostetrica
Policlinico S. Orsola-Malpighi
Università degli Studi di Bologna
Bologna, Italy

Dolores H. Pretorius, M.D.
Professor of Radiology
Department of Radiology
University of California, San Diego,
*   School of Medicine*
La Jolla, California

Laura A. Ribas
Certified Genetic Counselor
GeneTests-GeneClinics
Seattle, Washington

Mary Jo Rice, M.D., F.A.C.C.
Associate Professor of Pediatrics (Cardiology)
Fetal Diagnostic Center
Pasadena, California

Neil J. Sebire, M.D.
Pediatric and Perinatal Pathologist
Great Ormond Street Hospital for Children
London, United Kingdom

Waldo Sepulveda, M.D.
Consultant in Obstetrics and Fetal Medicine
Centre for Fetal Care
Queen Charlotte's and Chelsea Hospital
Hammersmith Hospitals NHS Trust
London, United Kingdom

Roya Sohaey, M.D.
Associate Professor of Radiology
Medical Director, Ultrasound
Oregon Health Sciences University
*   School of Medicine*
Portland, Oregon

Vivienne L. Souter, M.D.
Department of Obstetrics and Gynecology
Good Samaritan Hospital
Phoenix, Arizona

Kevin Spencer, B.Sc., M.Sc., D.Sc., Eur.Clin.Chem.,
**   C.Chem., C.Biol., M.I.Biol., F.R.S.C., F.R.C.Path.**
Consultant Biochemist
Department of Clinical Biochemistry
Harold Wood Hospital
Romford, Essex, United Kingdom
Director of Biochemical Screening
Fetal Medicine Foundation
London, United Kingdom

Ilan E. Timor-Tritsch, M.D.
Professor of Obstetrics and Gynecology
New York University School of Medicine
New York, New York

Dena Towner, M.D.
Associate Professor and Director of Prenatal Diagnosis
Department of Obstetrics and Gynecology
University of California, Davis, School of Medicine
Sacramento, California

Peter Twining, B.Sc., M.B., B.S., F.R.C.R.
Department of Radiology
Queen's Medical Centre Nottingham
University Hospital NHS Trust
Nottingham, United Kingdom

Susan Ulreich, M.B.B.S., F.R.A.N.Z.C.R.
Radiologist
SKG Radiology
West Perth, Western Australia, Australia

Gloria Valero, M.D.
Magdalena Sonora, Mexico

Yves Ville, M.D.
Professor of Obstetrics and Gynecology
Université de Paris-Ouest
CH de Poissy St. Germain
Poissy, France

PREFACE

Birth defects are common in human development. Approximately 3% of newborns have a recognizable major anomaly, and at least 5% will ultimately be diagnosed with a congenital defect. Because of improvements in other areas of prenatal care, birth defects are the single most common cause of perinatal mortality in developed countries.

Despite dramatic improvements in our understanding of birth defects, especially in the field of molecular genetics, the underlying cause remains uncertain in the majority of cases. Because most anomalies occur in the absence of family history or known risk factors, every pregnancy must be considered at risk for a significant birth defect. Therefore, it is clear that initial *detection* of fetal anomalies requires systematic screening of all pregnancies at an appropriate gestational age.

Integration of a systematic fetal survey as part of a properly performed obstetric ultrasound has led to significant improvement in detection of fetal anomalies over the last two decades. This concept of fetal ultrasound as a screening test, although controversial in some countries, has gained widespread acceptance in many others. Continued improvements in, and acceptance of, screening ultrasound can be expected.

For initial detection of fetal anomalies, sonographers need only be familiar with normal fetal anatomy and common variants in relation to gestational age (Chapter 1). Reflecting the importance of detecting cardiac abnormalities, a separate chapter addresses normal cardiac anatomy (Chapter 10). Abnormalities of fetal growth (Chapter 2), amniotic fluid (Chapter 3), or the placenta/umbilical cord (Chapter 4) can also provide important clues about possible underlying fetal anomalies.

Maternal biochemical screening (Chapter 22) is the most common alternative method for screening of fetal anomalies. Biochemical screening can identify patients at higher risk for certain anomalies but, with the arguable exception of screening for fetal aneuploidy, should not be considered a substitute for prenatal imaging in the detection of fetal anomalies. Serologic testing may also help to screen for fetal anomalies related to *in utero* infection (Chapter 17).

Accurate *diagnosis* of fetal anomalies requires definitive testing. The diagnosis of a fetal anomaly should include an assessment of its severity; differential diagnoses; and,

ideally, an understanding of its pathologic and embryologic basis, recurrence risks, and usual management. Accordingly, individual anomalies are discussed in detail throughout this book and are grouped by anatomic areas of interest.

Characterization of a fetal anomaly is not the final diagnostic step, because it is equally important to detect and diagnose important associated anomalies. The presence of multiple anomalies increases the likelihood of an underlying syndromic condition or chromosome abnormality. These conditions have received particular attention in this book because of the importance of associated anomalies to the underlying prognosis and management. Syndromes are addressed in Chapter 5, and chromosomal abnormalities are discussed in Chapter 21, in addition to sections of related chapters.

Two-dimensional real-time ultrasound remains the primary means of detecting and diagnosing birth defects. However, the title of this book also reflects the growing role of complementary imaging modalities such as three-dimensional ultrasound and magnetic resonance imaging. These modalities are presented throughout the book and are further highlighted in dedicated chapters (Chapters 24 and 25). Further improvements in these imaging techniques can be anticipated in the future.

In addition to prenatal imaging, other important methods of fetal diagnosis include cytogenetic testing for chromosome abnormalities and DNA or metabolic testing. These methods can provide a definitive diagnosis, although they may not always be able to determine the severity of the condition. A growing number of genetic markers are available for detecting specific malformations or syndromic conditions, and this is one of the most rapidly advancing areas of prenatal diagnoses. Although not meant to be exhaustive, genetic testing is presented, when known, in sections of specific anomalies throughout the book, and the techniques available are discussed with prenatal diagnostic techniques (Chapter 23).

Early, as well as reliable, diagnoses of fetal anomalies are beneficial and desirable. Accordingly, there has been a clear trend toward earlier detection of fetal anomalies. Indeed, early diagnoses of fetal anomalies have dramatically improved during the last two decades for detection of aneuploidy (Chapter 20) and anatomic anomalies (Chapter 19).

The ultimate aim is to provide the most accurate information possible to parents of an affected fetus with a serious anomaly. This information is essential for appropriate counseling and treatment. Although corrective prenatal management of fetal anomalies is still limited, the possibility of prenatal surgical correction or other treatment options continues to expand (Chapter 26).

In the end, it was not difficult to determine what to include in this book but, rather, what not to include. To be useful, however, we were naturally limited in content. For additional information, we direct the reader to other references and resources. In addition to other textbooks on fetal anomalies and birth defects, these resources include a number of Web sites dedicated to improved diagnosis and understanding of fetal anomalies. Although the number of Web sites are too numerous to list, important ones include Fetus (http://www.thefetus.net), Online Mendelian Inheritance in Man (http://www.ncbi.nlm.nih.gov/Omim), GeneClinics (http://www.geneclinics.com), and a Web site designed for this book (http://www.fetalanomalies.org) on which we plan to include updates, links, and other information.

David A. Nyberg, M.D.

FOREWORD

In 1901, Joseph Ballantyne, a professor of midwifery in Edinburgh, Scotland, proposed that the goals of prenatal care should be the prevention of seizures (eclampsia), treatment of maternal medical complications such as diabetes and hypertension, and antenatal diagnosis of congenital anomalies. Obstetrics and medicine have since made eclampsia and maternal death from medical complication rare occurrences in developed countries. The third goal of prenatal care—the detection of congenital anomalies—seemingly unattainable 100 years ago, is now a reality.

Congenital anomalies are frequent, complex, and heterogeneous disorders. The mechanisms of disease responsible for these conditions are still poorly understood. Yet, parents have a fundamental—perhaps even biologic—desire to know whether their unborn child will be healthy and, if not, to be informed of the precise nature of the congenital anomaly and its consequences.

The mainstay of anatomic diagnosis has been, and remains, sonographic imaging. Other modalities, such as magnetic resonance imaging and endoscopic examination of the embryo and fetus, are contributing to the improvement of diagnostic accuracy. However, the challenge of prenatal diagnosis of congenital anomalies has increased over the past 15 years; as technologic developments allow for more precise delineation of anatomy, prenatal and postnatal treatment options have broadened.

With *Diagnostic Imaging of Fetal Anomalies*, David Nyberg has assembled in a single source the wealth of information necessary to meet the clinical challenge of prenatal diagnosis of anatomic congenital anomalies. This exceptional book brings together the leaders of the field in an extraordinary compendium of knowledge and expertise accumulated to date. Illustrations of exceptional quality, accompanied by learned discussions of the epidemiology, genetics, differential diagnosis, and proposed management, are a great resource for clinicians and their patients.

David and his collaborators have made not only a major contribution to the practice of prenatal medicine but also justified the continued interest in this ever-growing medical field.

Roberto Romero, M.D.
Chief
Perinatology Research Branch
Intramural Division
National Institute of Child Health
and Human Development
National Institutes of Health
Bethesda, Maryland

ACKNOWLEDGMENTS

We would like to thank the many contributors to this book and the combined experience they provided. We would like to give special thanks to our families who have supported us in this endeavor.

NORMAL FETAL ANATOMIC SURVEY

Although there are many indications for performing obstetric ultrasonography (Table 1) as outlined by the National Institutes of Health Consensus Development Conference[1] and adopted by the American College of Obstetrics and Gynecology,[2] We believe that being pregnant is reason enough. Because most anomalies are sporadic and occur in otherwise low-risk women, a properly performed fetal anatomic survey is an essential part of obstetric screening. Indeed, the concept of a screening fetal anatomic survey during the second trimester has been widely adopted around the world by parents and physicians. This ultrasound can provide reassurance of a normal pregnancy in the vast majority of cases, and a systematic fetal survey can now detect the majority of fetal malformations.[3] A second-trimester scan is desired by most prospective parents and has been found to be cost-effective, at least at centers that have reasonable accuracy for detection of fetal anomalies.[4] In addition to a fetal survey, this examination can provide important information regarding other aspects of pregnancy, including fetal growth (see Chapter 2), placenta previa or other placental abnormalities (see Chapter 4), amniotic fluid (see Chapter 3), and the cervix.

GUIDELINES

Guidelines for a complete obstetric ultrasound have been published by various organizations.[2,5] These guidelines can be divided into two general components. First, measurements of several specific anatomic structures are made to establish gestational age, to evaluate fetal growth, and to assess the size of certain structures. Second, specific representative anatomic landmarks within organ systems or anatomic regions throughout the body are surveyed for the presence of major anomalies.

The published guidelines for fetal evaluation should be considered minimum standards. Most centers now routinely include documentation of other anatomic structures beyond those suggested by society guidelines. We have further modified the guidelines to reflect the complete fetal survey as it is performed at most obstetric centers (Table 2). Centers that adhere to these guidelines, when performed

systematically and by trained personnel, should identify most major detectable anomalies.

Detection of anomalies does not necessarily require a detailed understanding of fetal pathology; rather it requires thorough familiarity with normal fetal anatomy, sonographic landmarks, and normal variants. Even sonologists qualified to perform only the basic or minimum examination need a thorough understanding of the pertinent normal anatomy,[7] so that variances from normal are recognized. Deviations from normal or suspected anomalies can then be referred to a high-risk center for a more detailed fetal ultrasound examination and clinical consultation.

TECHNIQUE

A fetal anatomic survey requires a systematic approach. The fetus is examined quite literally from head to toe. In the vast majority of cases, the fetus appears normal and parents can be reassured regarding the health of their baby. The highest frequency probe possible should be used, to maximize resolution of targeted anatomy. Initial transverse and longitudinal scanning of the entire uterine cavity allows assessment of amniotic fluid volume, placental localization, and determination of fetal position. Noting the relationship of the head and spine makes the right and left sides of the fetus apparent. With this groundwork, subsequent scanning through contiguous parts of the fetus allows imaging of any desired anatomic component. Changes in maternal position or probe orientation are often necessary to expedite such a fetal survey.

Several circumstances require a more extensive evaluation of the fetus, commonly called a *targeted* or *level 2* ultrasound examination. A targeted ultrasound may include assessment of other structures not included in a fetal screening examination (Table 3). Detection of any abnormality on the basic examination necessitates a comprehensive and targeted anatomic survey to seek further information on the nature of the underlying abnormalities. In addition to patients with an abnormal basic or routine ultrasound examination, a directed/targeted examination must be undertaken when the routine examination will not survey all of the pertinent anat-

TABLE 1. POSSIBLE INDICATIONS FOR ULTRASOUND DURING PREGNANCY

Estimation of gestational age
Evaluation of fetal growth
Vaginal bleeding
Determination of fetal presentation late in pregnancy
Suspected multiple gestation
Adjunct to amniocentesis
Uterine size/clinical dates discrepancy
Pelvic mass
Suspected hydatidiform mole
Adjunct to cerclage placement
Suspected ectopic pregnancy
Possible placenta previa
Adjunct to interventional procedures
Suspected fetal death
Suspected uterine anomaly
Intrauterine device localization
Biophysical profile for fetal well being
Observation of intrapartum events
Suspected polyhydramnios or oligohydramnios
Suspected abruption
Adjunct to external version from breech to vertex
Estimation of fetal weight with premature ruptured membranes/labor
Abnormal serum biochemical screening test
Follow-up of anomalous fetus
History of previous congenital anomaly
Serial evaluation of fetal growth in multiple gestation
Evaluation of fetal condition in late presentation patients

Adapted from U.S. Department of Health and Human Services. Diagnostic ultrasound in pregnancy. National Institutes of Health publication no. 84-667, Bethesda, MD, 1984; and Technical Bulletin. Ultrasound in pregnancy. American College of Obstetrics and Gynecology, no. 187, 1993.

omy in a given patient. This includes patients, for instance, with an abnormal biochemical test (triple screen), abnormal amniotic fluid volume, or a family history of a syndrome or heritable disorder that might manifest morphologic changes that are detectable with ultrasound.

TIMING

The timing of the second-trimester ultrasound varies among centers. Although later scans permit improved anatomic detail and greater sensitivity for many structural defects, earlier scans can both provide useful information earlier and also provide information about the risk of fetal chromosomal abnormality. Thus, fetal surveys may be performed earlier, at 15 to 18 weeks, coinciding with the time of genetic amniocentesis or the second-trimester maternal serum screen. At our own center, patients obtain a scan at 15 to 18 weeks if they are considering genetic amniocentesis or 18 to 22 weeks if they are considered low risk. This approach supports other studies that suggest that, at least among low-risk women, a later scan will provide more

TABLE 2. COMPONENTS OF FETAL ANATOMIC SURVEY AT 18 TO 22 WEEKS[a]

Head and brain
  Calvaria: shape
  Brain—documentation of thalami, lateral ventricles, cerebellum, vermis, cisterna magna, and cavum septum pellucidum includes the following views:
    Transthalamic
    Transventricular
    Transcerebellar
Face/neck
  Face: lips, anterior maxilla, nose, orbits/globes, and profile view for mandible
  Neck: nuchal fold
Spine: longitudinal and transverse views
Thorax
  Heart
    Four-chamber view
    Views of outflow tracts
  Lungs
Abdomen
  Stomach: presence, situs, and size
  Gut
  Anterior abdominal wall/cord insertion site
Genitourinary tract
  Kidneys or kidney regions
  Urinary bladder
  ± Genitalia
Extremities
  Upper extremities, including both hands
  Lower extremities, including both feet
Vessels: number of vessels in umbilical cord
Measurements
  Biparietal diameter
  Head circumference
  Abdominal circumference
  Femur
  Lateral ventricular atrium cisterna magna
  ± Humerus
Other
  Placenta
  Amniotic fluid
  Cervix

[a]Evaluation should also include estimation of dates (or evaluation of growth).
Modified from Guidelines for the Performance of the Antenatal Obstetrical Ultrasound Examination, American Institute of Ultrasound in Medicine, Bethesda, MD, 1994.

information and is less likely to result in a repeat scan.[8] Centers that perform a first-trimester (10 to 14 weeks) ultrasound that includes nuchal translucency measurements and early fetal evaluation usually also obtain a later scan at 18 to 22 weeks.

LIMITATIONS

The detection rate of fetal anomalies depends on many factors. Certainly equipment quality, the expertise of the examining sonographer/physician, and length of time

TABLE 3. ADDITIONAL COMPONENTS THAT MIGHT BE INCLUDED ON A TARGETED EXAMINATION

Skull: configuration, mineralization, contiguity
Brain: cerebral hemispheres, third ventricle, fourth ventricle
Transcerebellar diameter
Face: nasal bridge, oral cavity/tongue, ears
Outer orbital diameter
Neck soft tissues and external contours
Thorax: configuration of bony thorax
Thoracic circumference
Heart: orthogonal views of four-chamber heart, dynamic views of atrioventricular valves and atrioventricular septa
Abdominal cavity/bowel/liver/spleen: any mass, calcification, dilatation
Long bone lengths: multiple within all extremities with interest in severity and distribution of shortening; clavicles
Extremities: exhaustive survey for limb reductions, malalignment, demineralization, extra digits, deformations

spent on the study are important variables. Maternal obesity, incomplete bladder filling, and early gestational age may all compromise image quality. The fetus may be positioned such that osseous structures obscure underlying soft-tissue anatomy, particularly a problem late in gestation. Oligohydramnios often compresses body parts together and to the uterus, making identification of some structures difficult and certain fetal measurements inaccurate.

NORMAL FETAL ANATOMY

In the following sections, we describe normal fetal anatomy that can be routinely evaluated. This discussion exceeds the recommended guidelines (Table 2) but may be less exhaustive than required for certain targeted ultrasound examinations. We have included mention of three-dimensional ultrasound because it is also being incorporated into routine obstetric scanning in some centers and can provide images of fetal anatomy that cannot be obtained otherwise. A more detailed discussion of both three-dimensional ultrasound and fetal magnetic resonance imaging is presented in Chapters 24 and 25.

Head, Brain

Views of the brain and head are among the most important images the sonographer can obtain for exclusion of a wide variety of anomalies (see Chapter 6). The calvaria can be readily identified from the late first trimester until term, which provides an easy means for estimation of gestational age through measurement of the biparietal diameter, head circumference, or both. Both are obtained from axial images through the brain at the level of the thalami[9,10] (Fig. 1). Due to excessive variation in the biparietal diameter, when the fetal head configuration is either dolichocephalic or brachycephalic, the head circumference will be the preferred parameter.

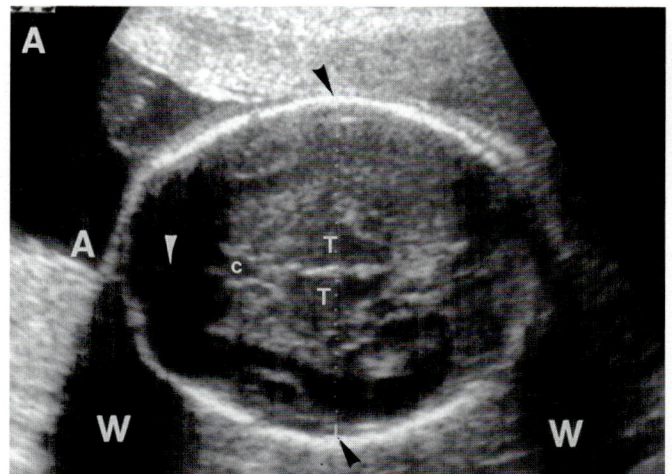
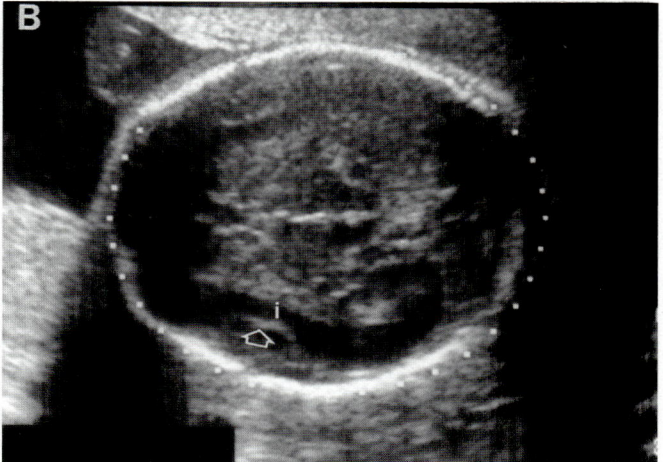
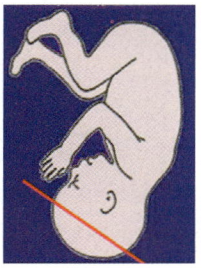

FIGURE 1. Biparietal diameter and head circumference at 21 weeks. **A:** An axial image shows the hypoechoic thalami (*T*), midline cavum septum pellucidum (*c*), and the echogenic falx/interhemispheric fissure (*white arrowhead*). The biparietal diameter is measured from the outer margin of the near calvarial echo to the inner margin of the deep calvarial echo (*black arrowheads*). A, anterior; W, refractive shadowing from the edges of the calvaria. **B:** Head circumference is measured circumferentially at the outer margin of the calvaria. The arrow indicates echogenic interface between the insular cortex (*i*) and the developing sylvian fissure.

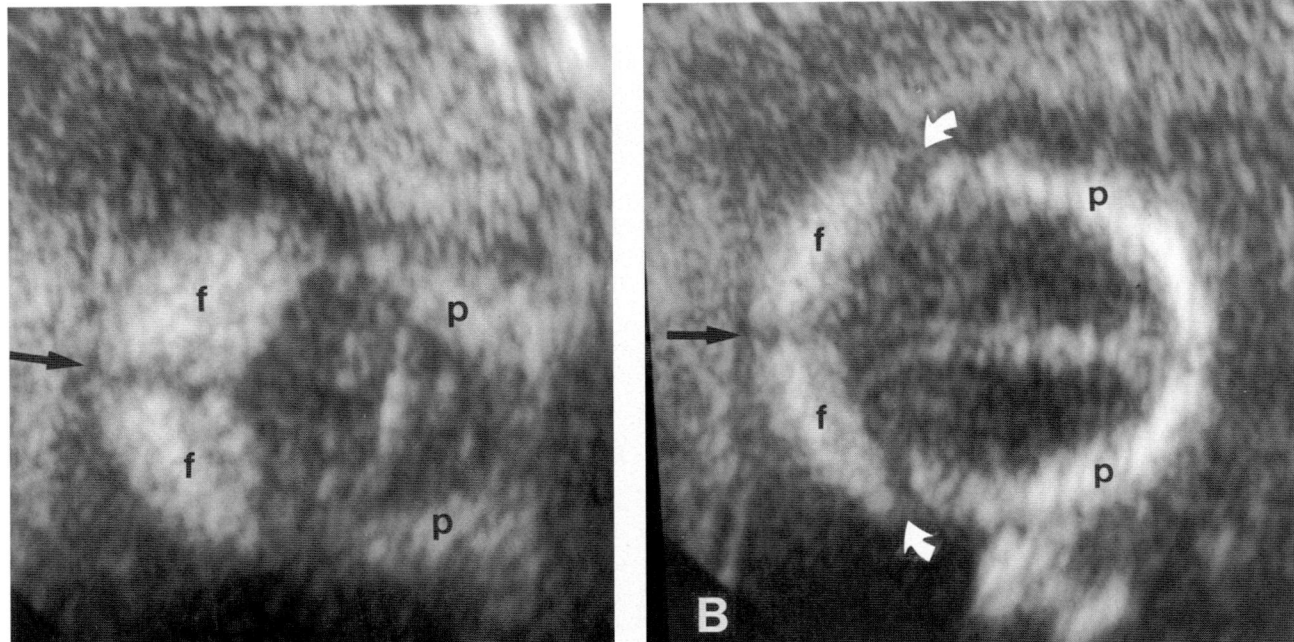

FIGURE 2. Cranial sutures at 15 weeks. **A:** A high, slightly angled axial image shows broad tangential sections of the frontal bones (*f*) separated by the metopic suture (*arrow*). Portions of the parietal bones (*p*) are noted posteriorly. **B:** An axial image high through the calvaria shows frontal (*f*) and parietal (*p*) bones. The lucent metopic (*black arrow*) and coronal (*white arrows*) sutures are noted between the echogenic bones.

A tangential image through the fetal calvaria creates a broader than usual echogenic appearance of the bones. Cranial sutures may be identified as hypoechoic spaces between bones, best seen early in gestation as ossification is progressing (Figs. 2 and 3). Normal cranial sutures are easier to assess using three-dimensional ultrasound with surface rendering compared to conventional two-dimensional scans. Premature closure of sutures may be seen with various syndromes and skeletal dys-

plasia [see Craniosynostosis Syndromes (Fibroblast Growth Factor Receptor–Related) in Chapters 5 and 15].

The lateral ventricles are complex anatomic structures that contain anechoic cerebrospinal fluid and lie deep within the cerebral hemispheres[11,12] (Fig. 4). Within the ventricular system lies the echogenic choroid plexus, best seen filling the body of the lateral ventricle from the medial to lateral wall and extending into the atrium (or trigone).

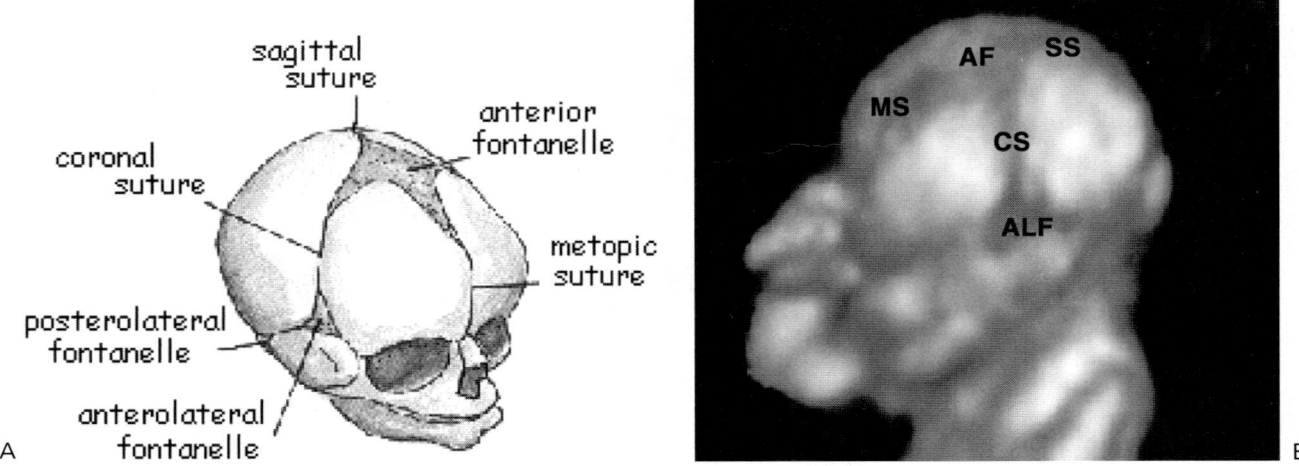

FIGURE 3. Cranial sutures. **A:** Normal sutures and fontanelles. **B:** Three-dimensional ultrasound at 12 weeks. AF, anterior fontanelle; ALF, anterolateral fontanelle; CS, coronal suture; MS, metopic suture; SS, sagittal suture.

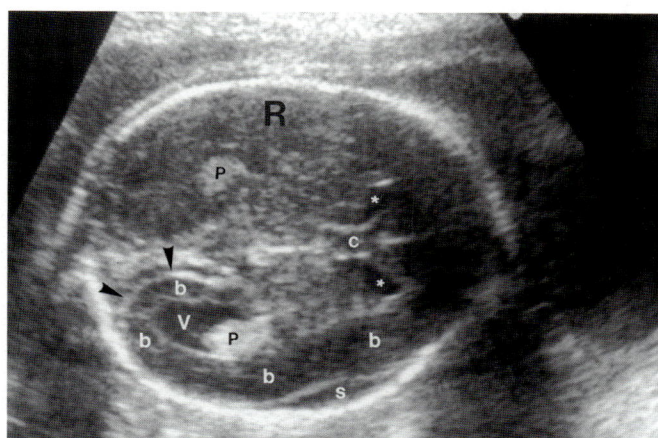

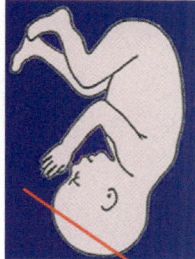

FIGURE 4. Lateral ventricle, cavum septum pellucidum, and subarachnoid spaces at 20 weeks. An axial image shows the cerebrospinal fluid–filled occipital horn (*V*) surrounded by the hypoechoic cerebral hemisphere (*b*). Echogenic choroid plexus (*p*) is seen within the ventricular atrium bilaterally, although anatomic detail is typically poor in the nearside hemisphere due to reverberation artifact (*R*) from the bone. The choroid plexus does not extend into the frontal horns (*asterisks*), which are well seen anterolateral to the midline cavum septum pellucidum (*c*). Arrowheads indicate cortical margins of the occipital lobe. Subarachnoid space (*s*) is noted lateral to the brain.

The choroid plexus does not extend into the frontal horns, and they are identified as prominent anechoic anterior components of the lateral ventricles. In contrast, the surrounding cerebral cortex is hypoechoic, with scarcely more echogenicity than the cerebrospinal fluid. The echogenic cortical margins of the cerebral hemispheres, surrounded by cerebrospinal fluid–containing subarachnoid spaces, should not be mistaken for the ventricular margins. The standard measurement of the cerebral ventricle is obtained in an axial plane through the atrium. The original work describing this measurement established a normal ventricular width of 7.6 mm ± 0.6 mm, with values over 10 mm indicative of ventriculomegaly.[13] Although subsequent investigators[14,15] determined the mean size of the ventricular atrium to be closer to 5.5 or 6.5 mm in their study populations, they still recommended a cutoff of 10 mm for separating normal subjects from abnormal subjects. In the late first and early second trimester the echogenic choroid plexus appears very prominent, whereas the cerebral hemispheres are quite diminutive (Fig. 5). Reverberation artifact from bone normally obscures the proximal hemisphere. Although absolute measurement of the nearside ventricle is usually impossible without a 180-degree change in fetal head position, alterations in probe orientation relative to the head may allow for subjective evaluation of intracranial anatomy within that hemisphere. A technique using an oblique scan plane angled superiorly through the temporal bone affords markedly improved visualization of the proximal hemisphere[16,17] (Fig. 6).

The cavum septum pellucidum, and its posterior extension the cavum vergae, is a fluid-filled midline structure located between the lateral ventricles. Sonographically it is usually identified as a fluid-filled structure anterior to the thalami on axial images (Figs. 1 and 4). Its presence suggests proper formation of the midline cerebral structures.

Examination of the posterior fossa is accomplished by angling the scan plane down posteriorly from the basic axial image for biparietal diameter determination until the cerebellum and cisterna magna (CM) are delineated. The hypo-

echoic cerebellar hemispheres can easily be seen on each side of the echogenic midline vermis, anterior to the CM. Identification of the CM and normal biconvex cerebellar hemispheres is important for exclusion of nearly all open spinal defects (see Chapter 7). The transcerebellar view is also useful for evaluating the nuchal soft-tissue thickness, which is important for assessment of fetal aneuploidy, especially trisomy 21 (see Chapter 21).

Standardized measurements of the CM, with a normal range of roughly 3 to 10 cm, are taken in the midline from the vermis to the occipital bone[18] (Fig. 7). Measured values

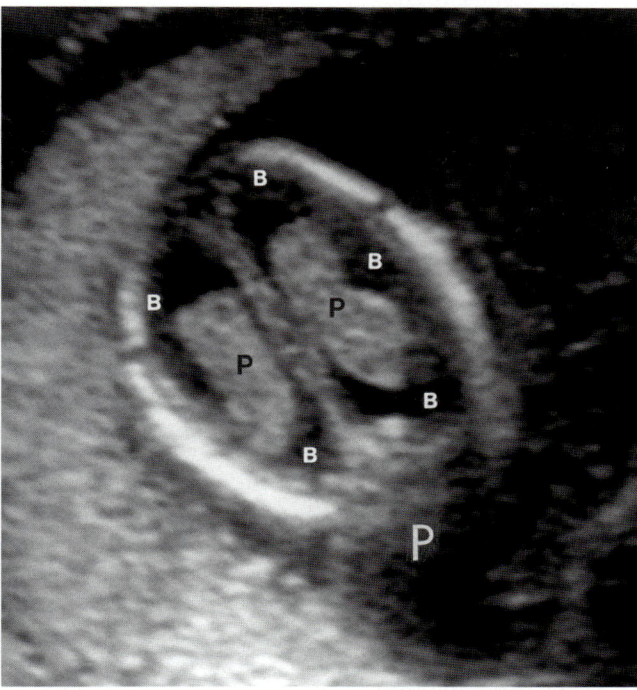

FIGURE 5. Brain at 13 weeks. An axial scan shows the prominent echogenic choroid plexus (*P*) filling the lateral ventricles. The diminutive hypoechoic cerebral cortex (*B*) should not be mistaken for fluid within the ventricular system.

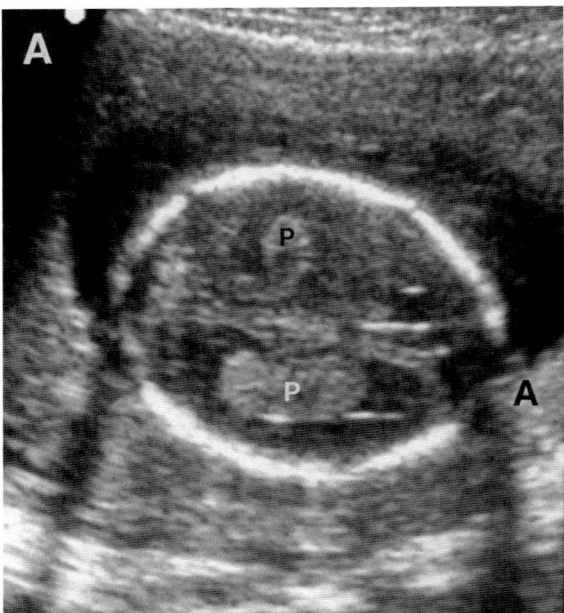
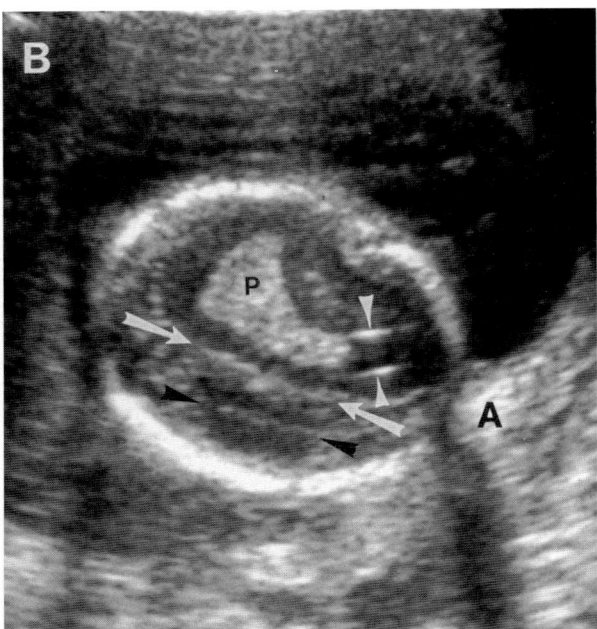

FIGURE 6. Cerebral ventricles at 16.5 weeks. **A:** An axial image shows the dependent hemisphere well, with choroid plexus (*white P*) filling the body of the lateral ventricle. Detail in the proximal hemisphere is poor, with only limited visualization of the choroid plexus (*black P*). **B:** The probe is positioned inferiorly over the temporal bone and angled steeply up to a high exit point on the opposite side of the skull. This reveals the choroid plexus filling the lateral ventricle in the proximal hemisphere (*P*). Note a small portion of the superior aspect of the dependent hemisphere (*arrowheads*) and an asymmetrically positioned midline echo (*arrows*). A, anterior.

at the lowest end of this range are expected only early in gestation, whereas a large CM is generally seen only in the third trimester. Occasionally a measurement exceeds these standards, which is usually still normal if the vermis is well seen and intact and the transverse cerebellar diameter is normal for gestational age. An inappropriate scan plane can also lead to an abnormally large measurement of the CM or even the appearance of a Dandy-Walker variant.[19] In most

fetuses, one to three linear echoes can be seen traversing the CM posteriorly from the cerebellum. These normal structures have been shown to be septa derived from or adjacent to the meninges.[20] Transverse cerebellar measurements may also be of value in the evaluation of some anomalous fetuses[21] (Fig. 7). Although the transverse cerebellar diameter can be measured quite early, definitive identification of the CM may be difficult in the early second trimester. Late

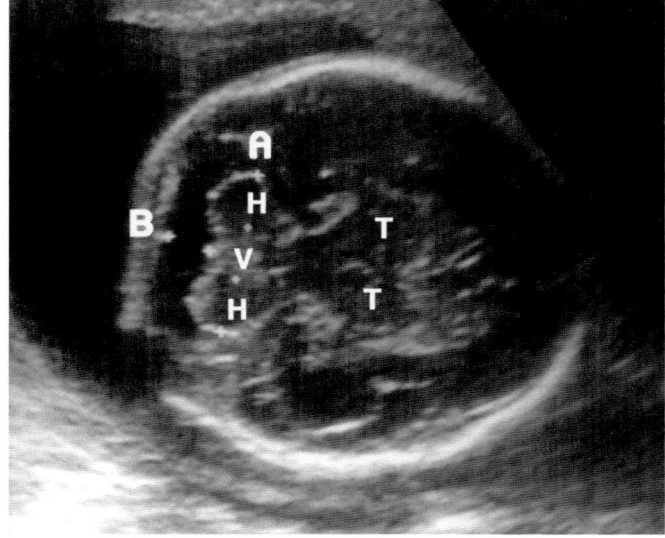

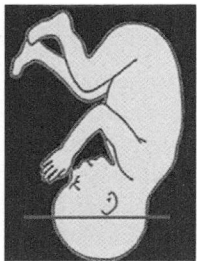

FIGURE 7. Posterior fossa measurements at 32 weeks. The cisterna magna is measured (*B*, calipers) from the posterior margin of the vermis (*V*) to the inner margin of the occipital bone. Calipers (*A*) indicate proper measurement for the transcerebellar diameter. H, cerebellar hemispheres; T, thalami.

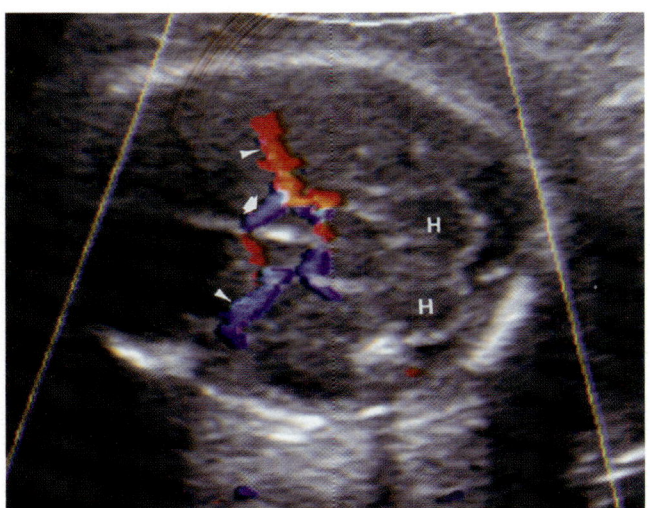

FIGURE 8. Circle of Willis at 20 weeks. An angled axial image through base of the brain with color-flow Doppler shows the circle of Willis and adjacent vessels. The vessels depicted in red are flowing toward the transducer, those in blue away. Arrowheads indicate the middle cerebral arteries passing to the sylvian fissures; the upside anterior cerebral artery is noted by the wide arrow. H, cerebellar hemispheres.

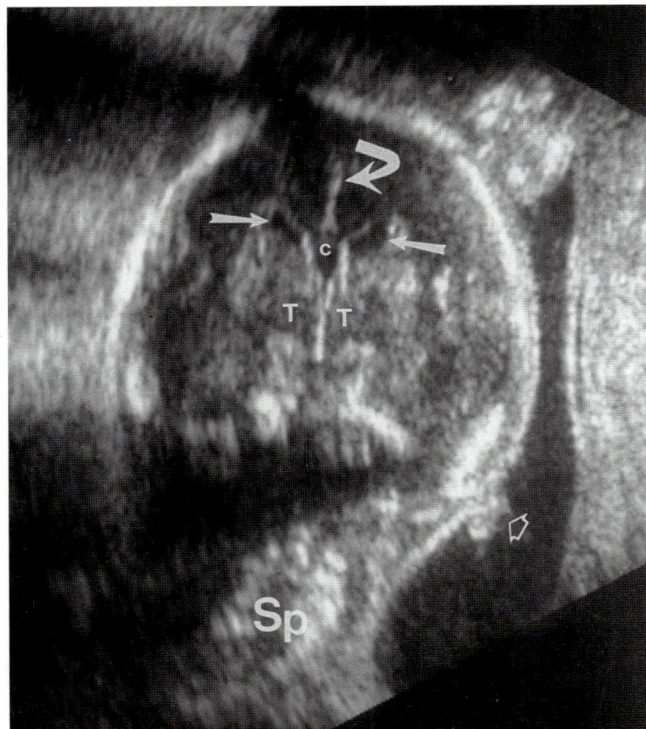

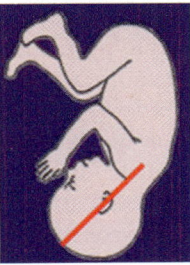

FIGURE 9. Coronal imaging of the fetal head at 21 weeks. This coronal sonogram of anterior brain shows thalami (*T*), cavum septum pellucidum (*c*), lateral ventricles (*straight arrows*), and falx (*curved arrow*). Open arrow, ear; Sp, cervical spine.

third-trimester imaging of posterior fossa structures may be inadequate due not only to fetal position but also to increased shadowing from osseous structures.

Major intracranial vessels can be identified with color or power Doppler imaging (Fig. 8). Localization of the middle cerebral artery is useful for duplex Doppler velocimetry, which can be helpful in assessment of intrauterine growth restriction (see Chapter 2) or fetal anemia (see Chapter 16).

Occasionally fetal head position prevents imaging in standard or angled axial planes. In such cases nonstandard imaging planes might be necessary for evaluating intracranial anatomy. In other circumstances these techniques may be useful to either confirm normalcy or to better evaluate anomalous structures suspected on routine imaging. Coronal (Fig. 9) and parasagittal (Fig. 10) images may nicely delineate the ventricles, cavum septum pellucidum, cerebral hemispheres, and posterior fossa.

Face

Examination of the face is not included in basic examination guidelines, however expertise in imaging these structures is useful in the complete examination of fetuses with suspected anomalies and when further information is needed to limit the differential diagnosis for an anomalous fetus.[22]

Imaging of the fetal face can be accomplished in coronal, sagittal, and axial planes (Figs. 11 through 13). Each

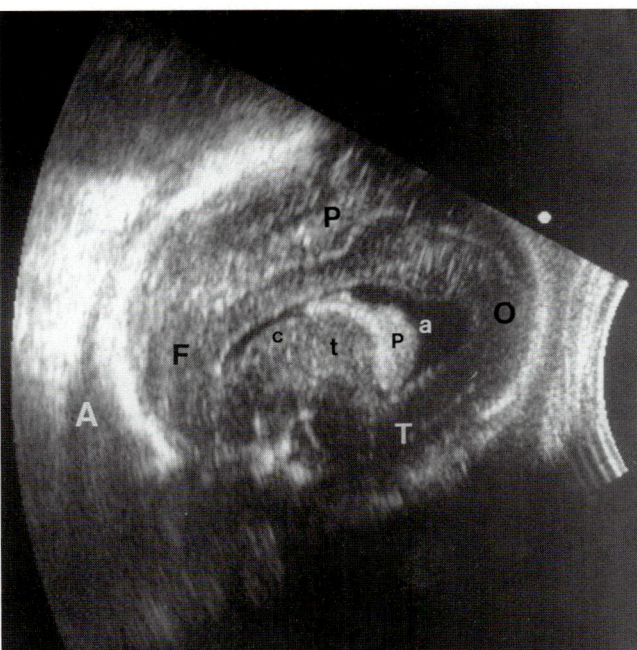

FIGURE 10. Parasagittal brain at 32 weeks. The fluid-filled lateral ventricle extends from the atrium (*a*) into the temporal (*T*), occipital (*O*), parietal (*P*), and frontal (*F*) lobes. Note the prominent glomus of the choroid plexus (*p*), the thalamus (*t*), and the slightly more echogenic head of the caudate nucleus (*c*). A, anterior.

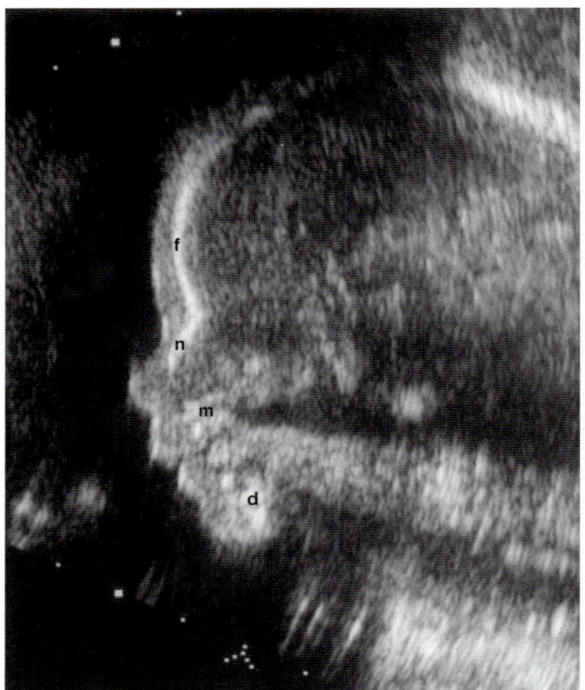

FIGURE 11. Facial profile at 22 weeks. A midline sagittal scan shows frontal bone (*f*), nasal bone (*n*), maxilla (*m*), and mandible (*d*), with the overlying soft tissues of the forehead, nose, lips, and chin, respectively.

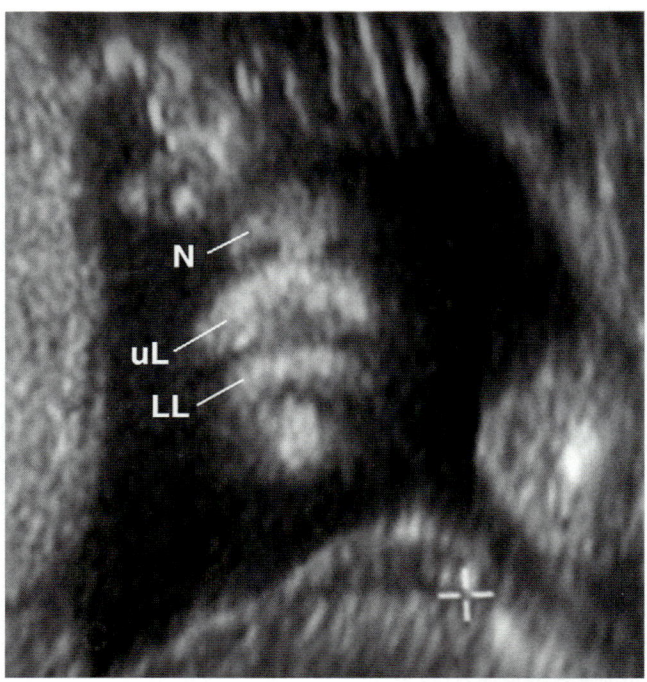

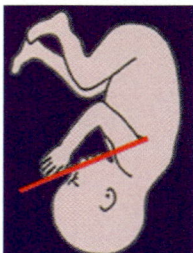

FIGURE 12. Lips and mouth. This oblique coronal view shows the nose (*N*), nares, upper lip (*uL*), and lower lip (*LL*). This is the single best image plane for evaluation of cleft lip.

scan plane has advantages and disadvantages, and a combination of scan planes is often desired, when positioning is favorable, to adequately delineate all anatomy. A midline sagittal scan, or profile view, is one of the most recognizable images of any fetus. It is useful for evaluation of size and position of the mandible (for exclusion of micrognathia), the nose and nasal bridge, and the tongue. The coronal view aligned along the anterior surface of the nose and upper lips (Fig. 12) is most useful for evaluation of possible cleft lip or palate (see Chapter 8).

Evaluation of the upper lip and anterior palate, or alveolar ridge of the maxilla, is important for exclusion of cleft lip/palate. The posterior or hard palate cannot be imaged sonographically, because it is obscured by overlying osseous structures. The upper lip and anterior maxilla can conveniently be imaged simultaneously in the axial plane (Fig. 13A). In this plane, the entire alveolar ridge is usually visible and the soft tissues of the upper lip can often be well seen. The oral cavity may also be nicely imaged in the axial plane (Fig. 13B).

Coronal imaging may also show easily identifiable features of the face, confirming in particular the integrity of the soft tissues of the nose and upper lip. Sections more posteriorly within the face may show the oral cavity and deep nasal structures (Fig. 14). The maxilla is difficult to image in a coronal section, but clefting of

the anterior maxilla does not occur without an overlying lip defect.

Unique and sometimes striking images of the face can also be obtained with three-dimensional ultrasound (see Chapter 24) (Fig. 15). Surface rendering appears to be particularly helpful for the display of complex shapes on the fetal surface.

The bony orbits are best imaged in the axial (Fig. 16) or coronal plane. Measurement of the outer orbital diameter, which correlates with gestational age,[23,24] allows detection of hypo-/hypertelorism. Intraorbital anatomy that can be identified includes the globe, lens, and hyaloid artery (Fig. 17).

The ears are not frequently targeted for imaging, but when necessary they are easily identified as complex soft-tissue protrusions external to the skull[25] (Fig. 18). This is another structure that is easier to assess with surface-rendered three-dimensional ultrasound (Fig. 18B). Evaluation of the ears may be helpful in assessment of multiple anomaly syndromes (see Chapter 5). Fetal hair may present an unusual picture in the third trimester, with multiple echoes seen close to the scalp in the expected distribution.[26]

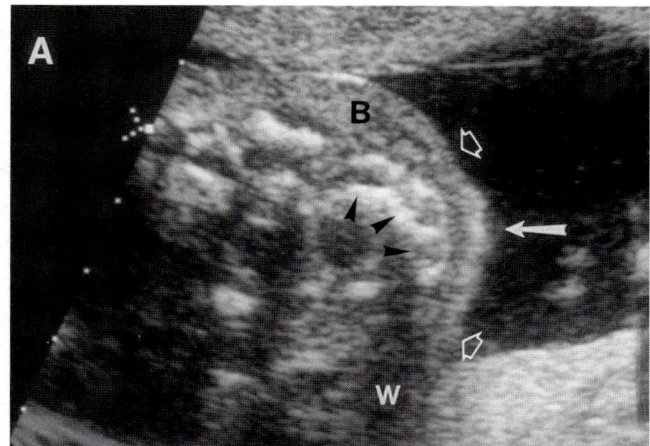

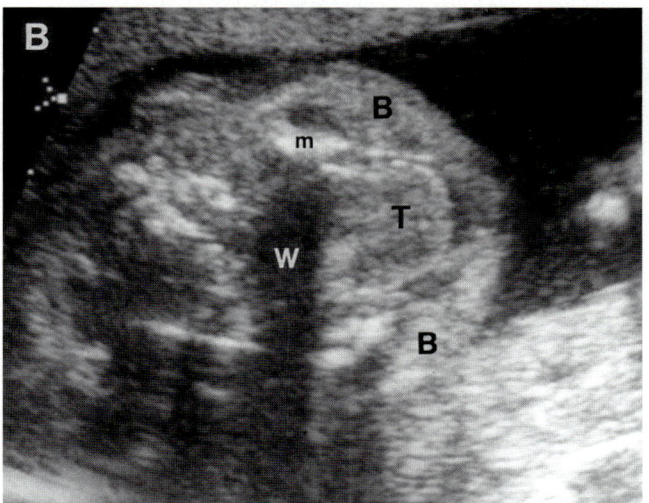

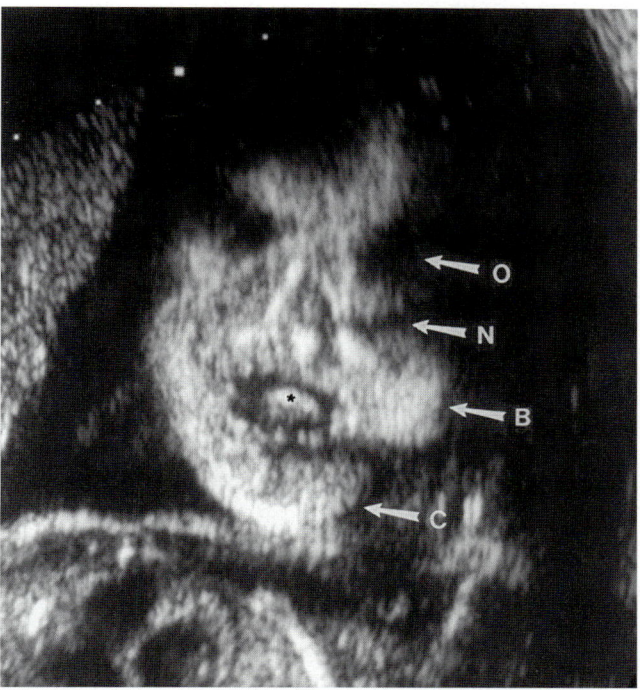

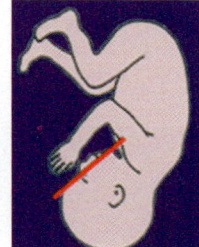

FIGURE 14. Oral cavity at 20 weeks. A coronal image deeper within the fetal face shows the anterior orbits (*O*), echogenic nasal bones (*N*), echogenic soft tissues of the cheeks bilaterally (*B*), and chin (*C*). The tongue (*asterisk*) can be seen surrounded by amniotic fluid within the oral cavity.

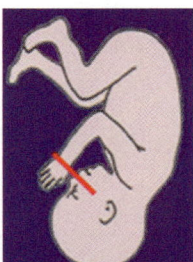

FIGURE 13. Maxilla, upper lip, and tongue at 21 weeks: axial images with the fetal face directed to the side and the probe positioned as far anteriorly over the fetal face as possible. **A:** The dependent aspect of the maxilla (*arrowheads*) is shadowed (*W*) by the nondependent portion. The midline is indicated with a long white arrow. The upper lip (*open arrows*) is still well imaged over the nonvisualized portion of the maxilla. **B:** Scanning just inferior to the alveolar ridge reveals the tongue (*T*) within the oral cavity. A portion of the mandible (*m*) causes a shadow (*W*) that obscures the posterior aspects of the oral cavity. Buccal tissues are noted (*B*).

The cervical region should be observed routinely to exclude abnormality of the spine or soft tissues. The nuchal thickness should be routinely assessed; this assessment is typically performed with the same view used to assess the cerebellum (transcerebellar view). Other structures that can be seen within the anterior neck include the thyroid and the fluid-filled trachea and hypopharynx[27] (Fig. 19).

Spine

Imaging of the fetal spine can be accomplished in three planes: parasagittal, coronal, and transverse. Generally only two of the three are possible in any particular fetus without intervening positional changes. The parasagittal and coronal images give the best overall views of the spine, whereas serial transverse scanning is generally believed most sensitive for detection of subtle defects. Transverse imaging is also the optimum means for evaluating the midline soft tissues, with parasagittal scanning second best.

Each vertebral segment is composed of three ossification centers, which appear echogenic sonographically.[28] The anterior center is the developing vertebral body, and the posterior centers are formed at the junction of the lamina and the pedicle on each side.[29] The ossification centers lie in a symmetric triangular configuration, with the posterior centers oriented toward the midline. In the second trimester, the spine ossification centers are more punctate than later in gestation as increasing ossification creates a more ringlike configuration. Any widening between the posterior centers or alteration in their orientation suggests a neural

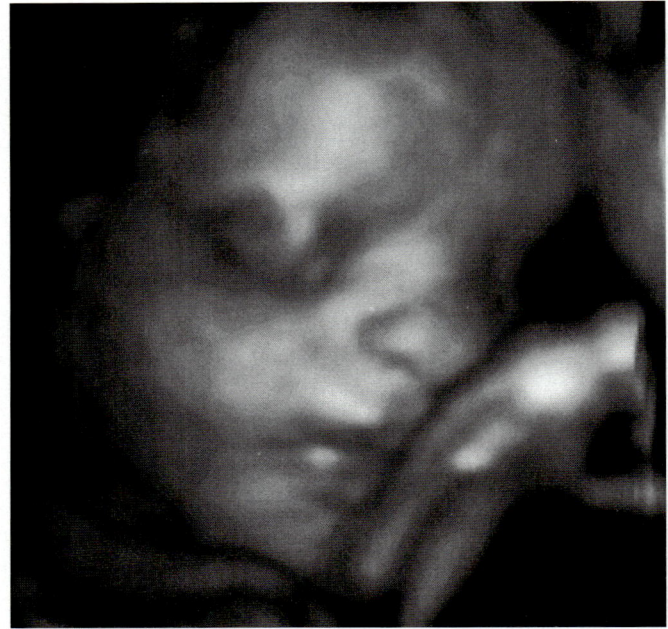

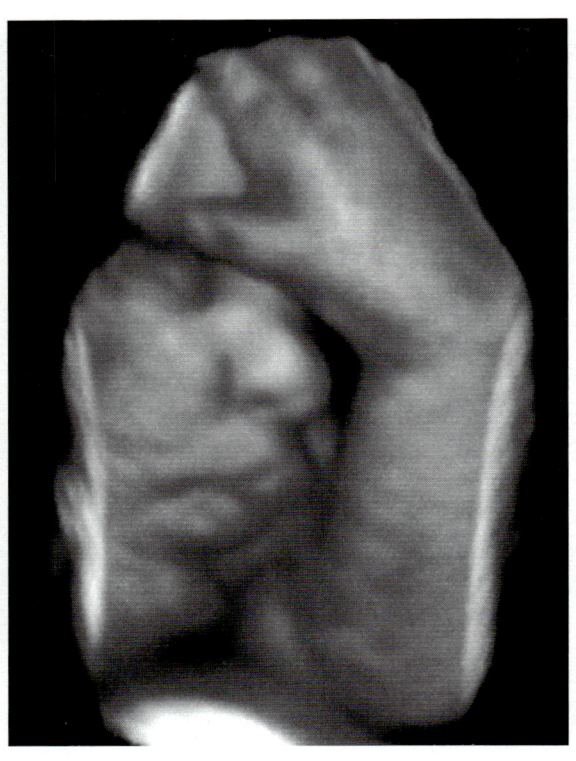

FIGURE 15. Three-dimensional ultrasound of the face and hand at 26 weeks **(A)** and 30 weeks **(B)**.

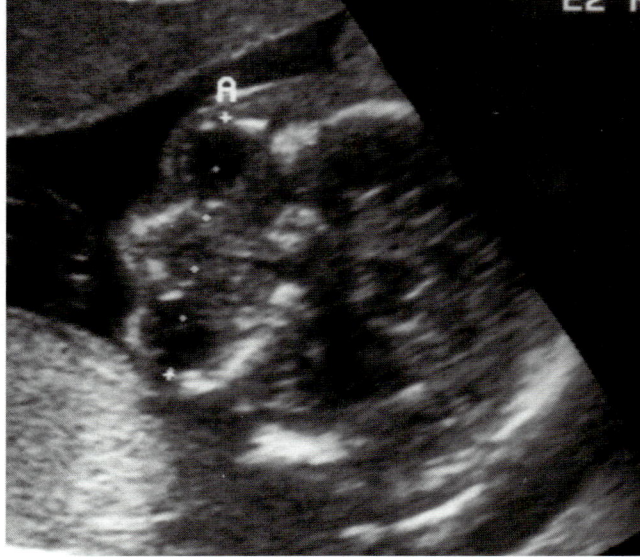

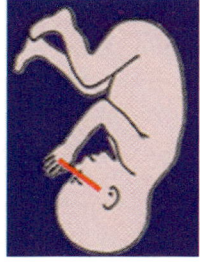

FIGURE 16. This coronal image shows calipers (*A*) positioned at the lateral margins of the bony orbits for outer orbital diameter measurement.

tube defect. The integrity of the overlying soft tissues should also be confirmed, which may be difficult if the scan plane is tangential to the spine.

Parasagittal imaging of the entire spine demonstrates two rows of roughly parallel ossification centers: the vertebral

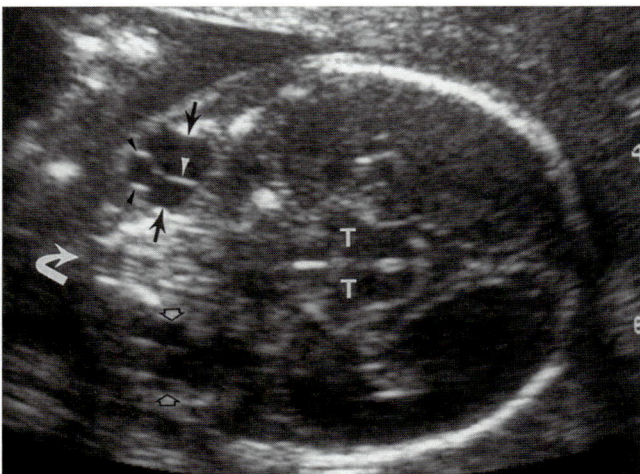

FIGURE 17. Eyes at 19 weeks. An axial image of the face and head includes the thalami (*T*) and a portion of the nose (*curved arrow*). Within the nearside globe (*long arrows*) are anterior echoes arising from the lens (*arrowheads*). A linear echo extending posteriorly from the lens to the retina represents the hyaloid artery, a nutrient vessel to the developing lens often visible in the latter half of the second trimester. The downside globe (*open arrows*) shows this anatomy with somewhat less detail.

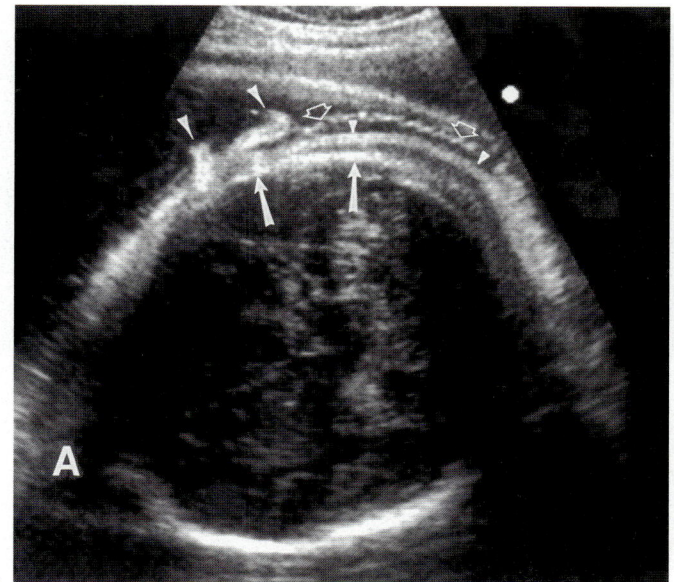

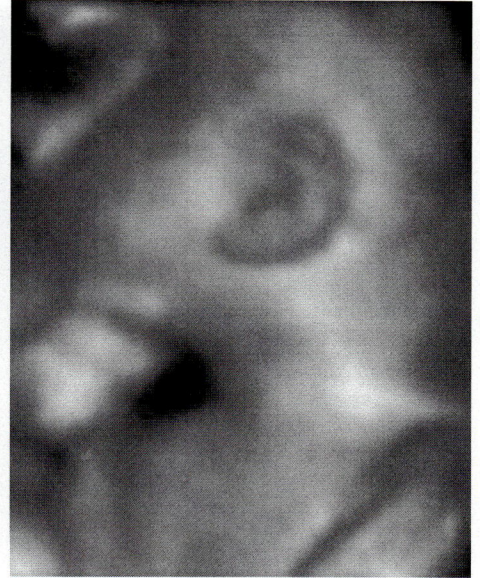

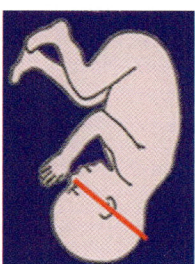

FIGURE 18. Ear, hair. **A:** An axial scan at 33 weeks shows portions of the fetal ear (*large arrowheads*) with an irregular curved line more posteriorly (*open arrows*) representing fetal hair. The underlying calvaria (*long arrows*) should not be mistaken for the relatively echogenic scalp (*small arrowheads*). A, anterior. **B:** Three-dimensional ultrasound of another fetus at 26 weeks better illustrates the normal ear.

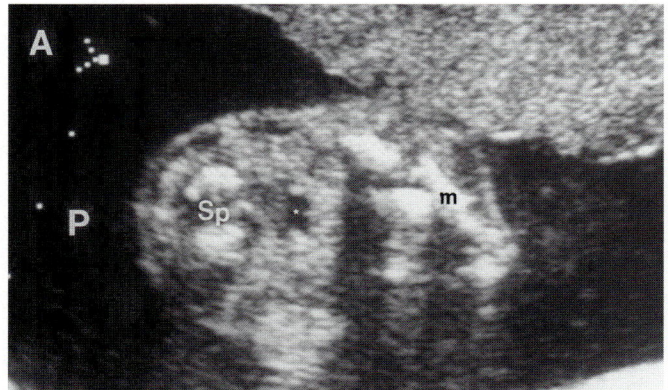

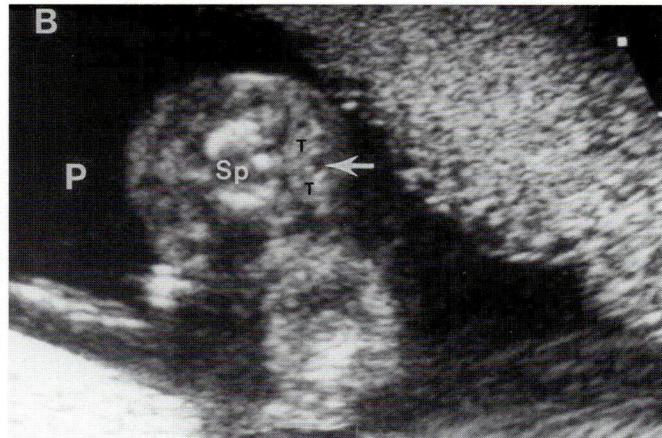

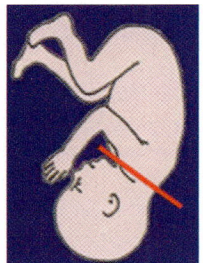

FIGURE 19. Hypopharynx and trachea at 18 weeks. **A:** An axial image through the craniocervical junction shows the fluid-filled hypopharynx (*asterisk*) anterior to the cervical spine (*Sp*) and posterior to the inferior oral cavity, shadowed by overlying bones, including the mandible (*m*). P, posterior. **B:** An axial image through the neck shows thick hypoechoic musculature posterior to the spine (*Sp*). The fluid-filled midline trachea (*arrow*) lies anterior to thyroid tissue (*T*). P, posterior.

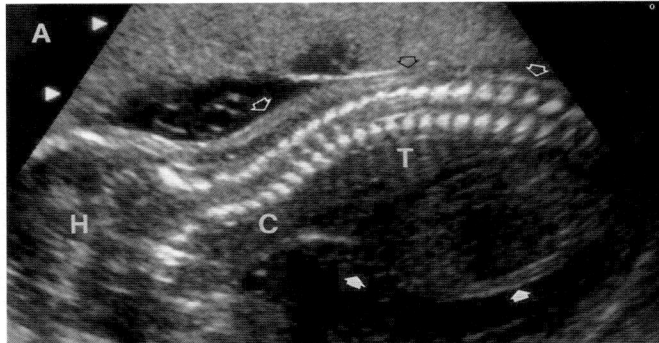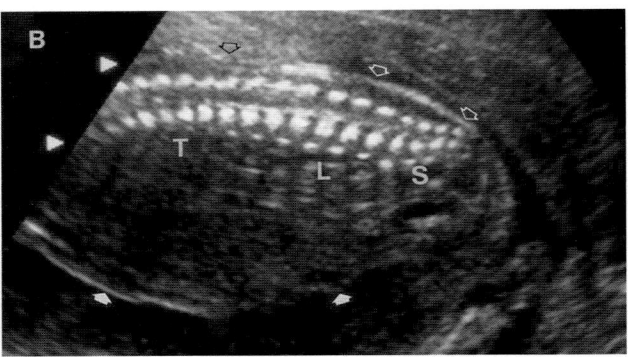

FIGURE 20. Complete spine at 17 weeks. **A, B:** Sequential parasagittal scanning through the sacral (*S*), lumbar (*L*), thoracic (*T*), and cervical (*C*) spine show the paired parallel ossification centers extending up to the head (*H*). The row of ossification centers closest to the skin surface (*open arrows*) is the posterior centers; the more anteriorly positioned centers are the vertebral bodies. The wide discrepancy between the minimal superficial soft tissues adjacent to the spine and the thicker deep tissues (*closed arrows* represent deep skin margin) indicates a parasagittal orientation to the scan. The gentle curvature of the sacrum should be visualized in each case to ensure a complete examination of the spine. In addition, the soft tissues posterior to the spine and inferiorly over the rump should be examined to exclude any discontinuous segments or protruding masses.

bodies and a row of posterior centers (Fig. 20). This plane of section nicely demonstrates the overall appearance of the spine and delineates the posterior soft tissues adjacent to the midline, but it might be less sensitive for subtle widening between the paired posterior ossification centers. Transverse imaging of the entire spine is the most sensitive means for excluding a spinal defect, allowing simultaneous evaluation of both the ossification centers and the overlying soft tissues (Fig. 21). The spinal cord can also sometimes be imaged within the spinal canal (Fig. 22).

Thorax and Heart

The osseous components of the thorax are readily identified due to their inherent subject contrast with the adjacent soft-tissue structures. The ribs can be visualized on coronal views (Fig. 23) with evaluation of the thoracic spine. The scapula can also be assessed (Fig. 24). Due to their complex shape, these structures may be better assessed with three-dimensional ultrasound (Fig. 25). Three-dimensional ultrasound can also assess the spine (Fig. 25). The clavicles (Fig. 26) can also be evaluated.[30] Evaluation of the ribs, clavicles, and scapula may be important in assessment of some types of skeletal dysplasia (see Chapter 15).

The intrathoracic structures are usually evaluated on axial images during evaluation of the heart. Measurement of the thoracic circumference (Fig. 27) may be of value in detecting pulmonary hyperplasia[31,32] (see Chapter 13.)

The heart is a complex structure and should be evaluated in multiple planes for evaluation of possible cardiac defects[33,34] (see Chapters 10 and 11). Cardiac rate and rhythm should be noted, with a normal range of 120 to 160 beats per minute from the second trimester to term. Cardiac position and axis within the thorax must be deter-

mined. The heart lies anteriorly within the thorax, slightly to the left of midline such that a line drawn posteriorly from the spine to the midline anteriorly passes through the right ventricle, the most anterior chamber. The cardiac apex, as determined by a line through the ventricular septum, is directed to the left side of the hemithorax at about a 45-degree angle from the midline, or roughly equidistant from the anterior and lateral aspects of the chest[35] (Fig. 28). Alterations in position, axis, or both suggest intrinsic cardiac malposition or displacement by an intrathoracic mass.

Examination of the internal cardiac anatomy begins with a four-chamber view (Fig. 28). The ventricles should be of roughly equal size, with the right more anterior than left. The ventricular septum appears as a continuous thick muscular structure separating the ventricles, except for its short, thinner membranous portion near the atrioventricular valves. The mitral and tricuspid valves are clearly separate and open symmetrically into their respective ventricles. Ventricular walls are thick relative to those of the atria. In some scan planes the ventricular walls or interventricular septum may have a component that is quite hypoechoic relative to the remaining muscle. This is a normal variant secondary to the complex orientation of the cardiac muscle fibers interacting variably as the scan plane changes.[36] The left atrium is the most posterior chamber and is similar in size to the right atrium. The atrial septum is often difficult to image, but it appears as a continuous thin structure with the exception of a physiologic opening, the foramen ovale, through which blood flows in the fetus from right to left atrium.

The dynamic nature of the heart can readily be appreciated during real-time examination in the four-chamber projection. In fact, a single static four-chamber view is inadequate for complete cardiac evaluation. At real time the variations in

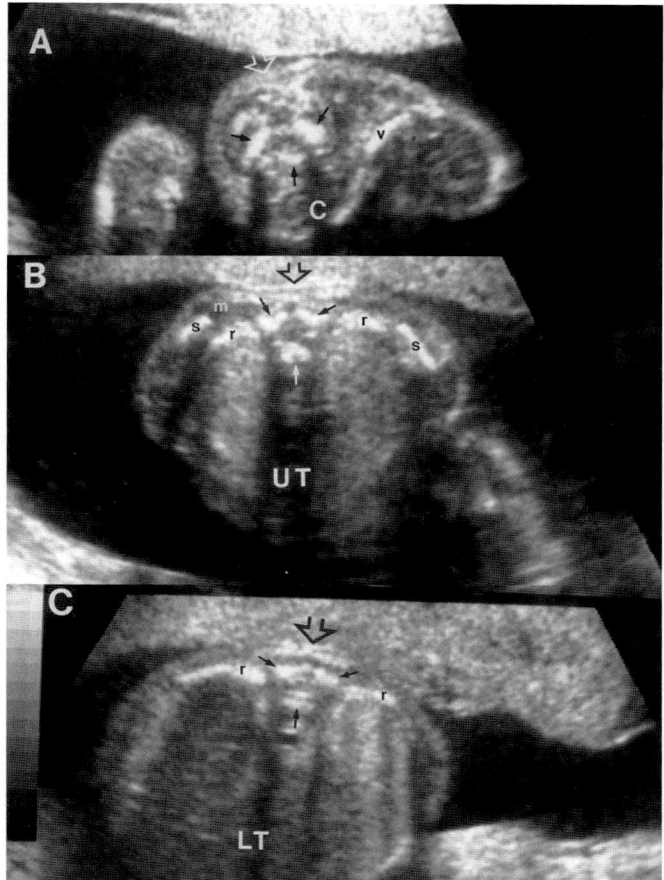

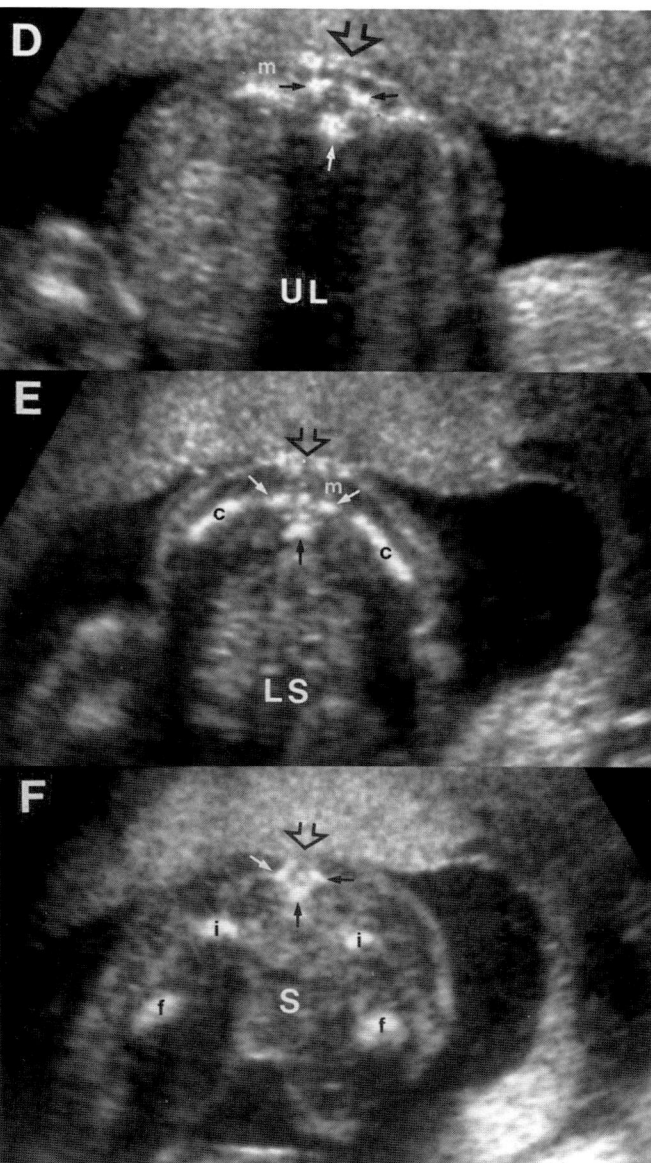

FIGURE 21. Spine at 21 weeks. **A–F:** Serial transverse scans show the three ossification centers (*small arrows*) in the cervical (*C*), upper thoracic (*UT*), lower thoracic (*LT*), upper lumbar (*UL*), lumbosacral (*LS*), and low sacral (*S*) spine. Note the posterior-medial orientation of the posterior elements at each level. Although the posterior skin surface (*open arrows*) is difficult to see at several levels because of close apposition with the placenta, at each level its intact nature can be determined by observing an echogenic cutaneous margin contiguous with adjacent skin surfaces overlying the hypoechoic paraspinal musculature (*m*). Other bony anatomy visualized includes a portion of the clavicle (*v*), ribs (*r*), the scapulae (*s*), the iliac crests (*c*), the ischial tuberosities within the deep pelvis (*i*), and portions of the proximal femoral shafts bilaterally (*f*).

chamber size and actual atrioventricular valve motion can be studied (Fig. 29). Minor variations in probe position and angulation slightly superiorly and inferiorly through the heart are necessary to fully evaluate the cardiac septa. Fetal rotation or probe position changes may dramatically alter the appearance and identification of some intracardiac structures, such as the ventricular septum, which can vary from appearing relatively thin to rather thick when imaging in orthogonal planes (Fig. 30). A commonly seen normal variant, usually within the left ventricle, is an echogenic focus caused by a specular reflection from the papillary muscles and chordae tendinae[37,38] (Fig. 31). A bright echogenic focus, usually in the left ventricle, has been termed an *echogenic intracardiac focus*. This finding is discussed in detail in Chapter 21.

Although examination of the heart in the four-chamber view has the potential to detect 60% to 70% of cardiac defects, additional views of the ventricular outflow tracts and great vessels further increase that sensitivity.[39–41] Appropriate views of the left ventricular outflow tract (Fig. 32) and right ventricular outflow tract (Fig. 33) require slight alterations in angle plane from the four-chamber view. The outflow tracts and great vessels of the heart should cross at roughly right angles to each other as they exit their respective ventricles. Long axis views may also be used to show the aortic and ductus arches arising from their respective ventricles.

While evaluating the heart, the lungs and diaphragm can also be assessed (Fig. 34). Coronal or parasagittal images are necessary to show the normal, thin diaphragm.

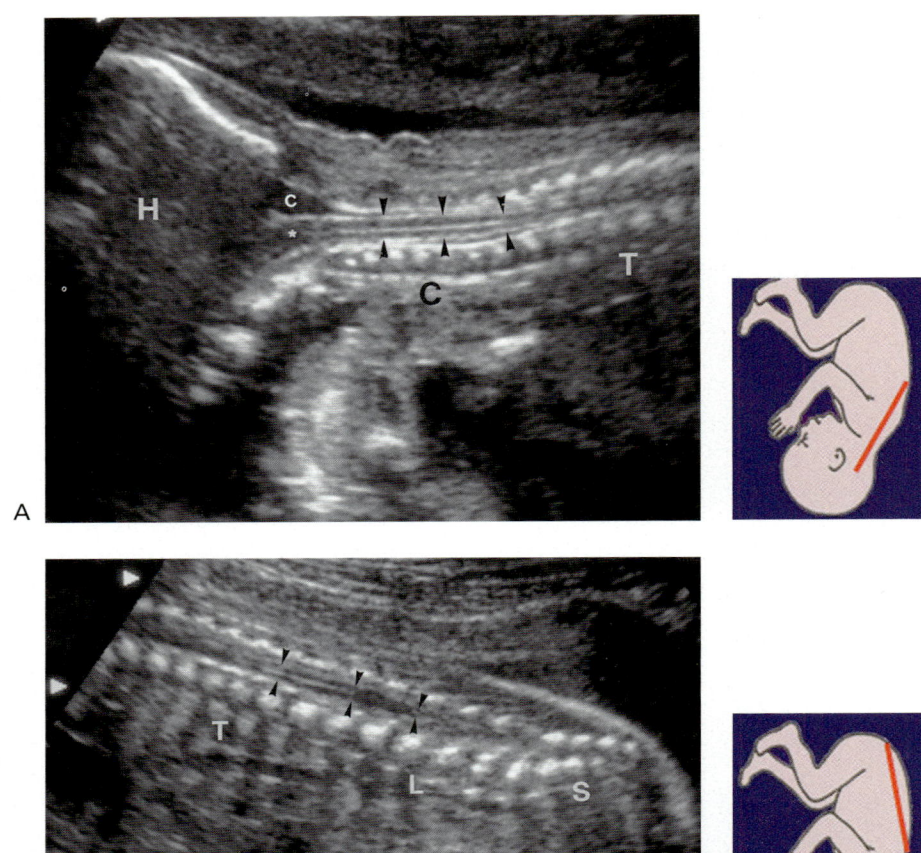

FIGURE 22. Spinal cord at 19 weeks. **A, B:** Parasagittal scans from the head (*H*) caudally through the cervical (*C*), thoracic (*T*), lumbar (*L*), and sacral (*S*) spine show the hypoechoic spinal cord (*arrowheads*) within the canal. The fine, echogenic linear structure positioned centrally within the cord is the central canal. The cord can be seen to taper inferiorly as the conus in the midlumbar region. Within the head, the medulla (*asterisk*) can be seen contiguous with the cervical spinal cord and just anterior to the fluid-filled cisterna magna (*c*).

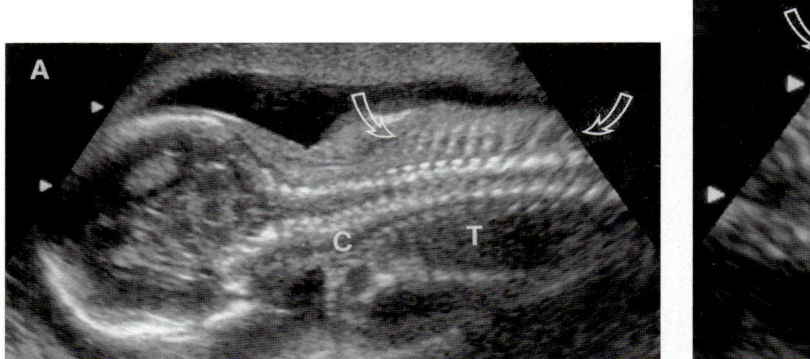

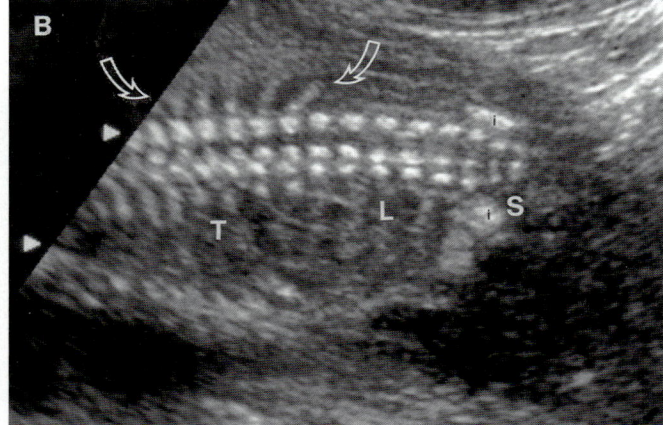

FIGURE 23. Spine and ribs. **A:** Coronal view of the cervical (*C*) and thoracic (*T*) spine. **B:** A coronal view of the lower thoracic (*T*), lumbar (*L*), and sacral (*S*) spine shows paired parallel ossification centers. Note paired ribs (*open arrows*) arising from the thoracic spine. i, iliac wings.

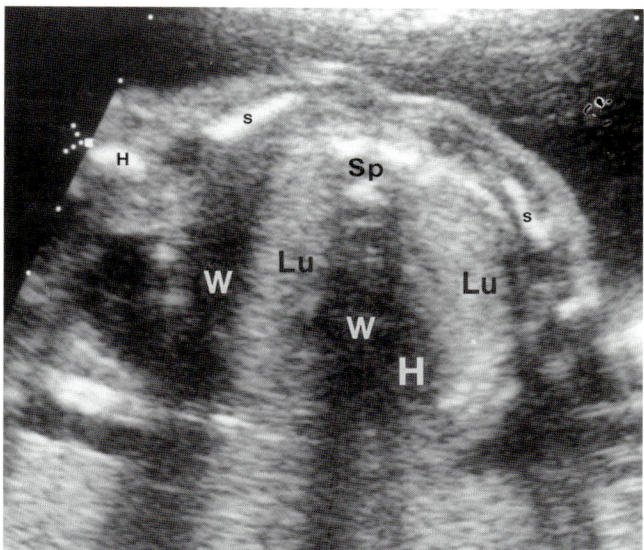

FIGURE 24. Scapulae and thorax at 22 weeks. An axial image through the upper thorax with the fetus in the prone position shows both scapulae (*s*) and the spine (*Sp*), with distal shadows (*W*) obscuring visualization of the underlying intrathoracic structures. Although portions of the lung (*Lu*) can be seen, the heart (*white H*) is only minimally visualized. Altering the scan plane allows determination of cardiac position and axis; however, optimum four-chamber views and outflow tracts are seldom adequately visualized with the fetus in this position. Black H, proximal humerus.

Abdomen

Intraabdominal organs that can easily be documented and measured include the liver,[42] spleen,[43] gallbladder,[44] kidneys, adrenals,[45] urinary bladder, and large and small bowel,[46,47] as well as major vascular structures. All of these

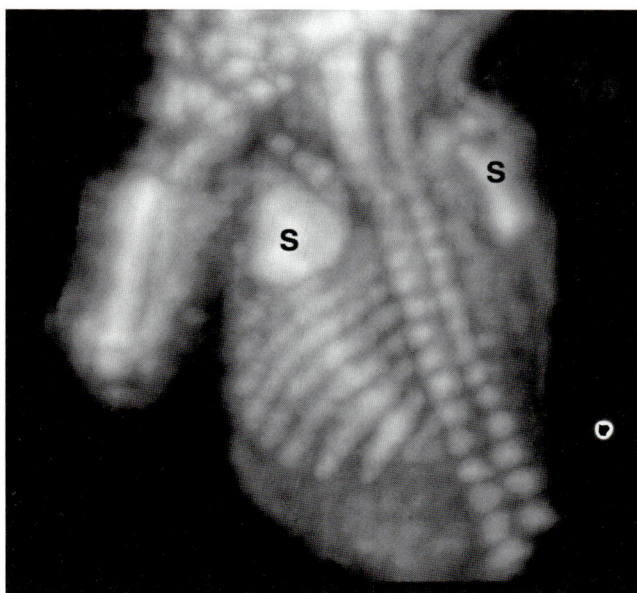

FIGURE 25. Three-dimensional ultrasound at 16 weeks shows cervical, thoracic, and lumbar spine as well as ribs and scapulae (*S*).

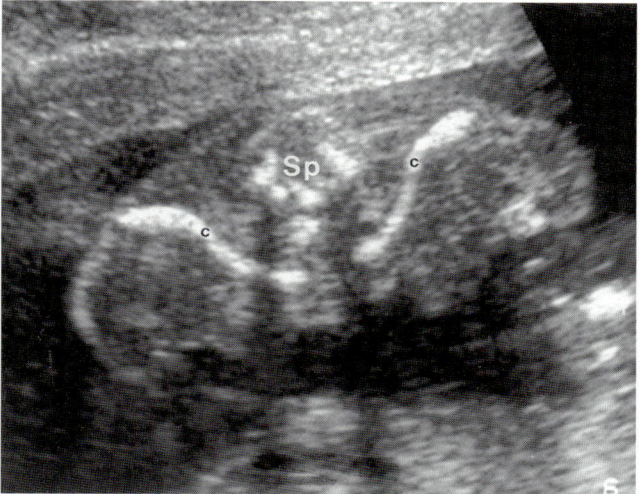

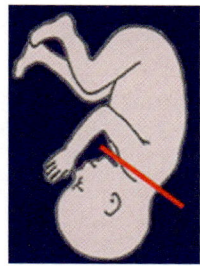

FIGURE 26. Clavicles at 18 weeks. An axial image through the high thorax shows the bilateral, curvilinear clavicles (*c*). Although portions of the clavicles are frequently visualized during routine scanning, mild angulation is necessary to visualize this bone in its entirety. When indicated, targeted examination for specific structures such as the clavicle can be performed readily due to the inherent subject contrast between bones and adjacent soft tissues. Sp, spine.

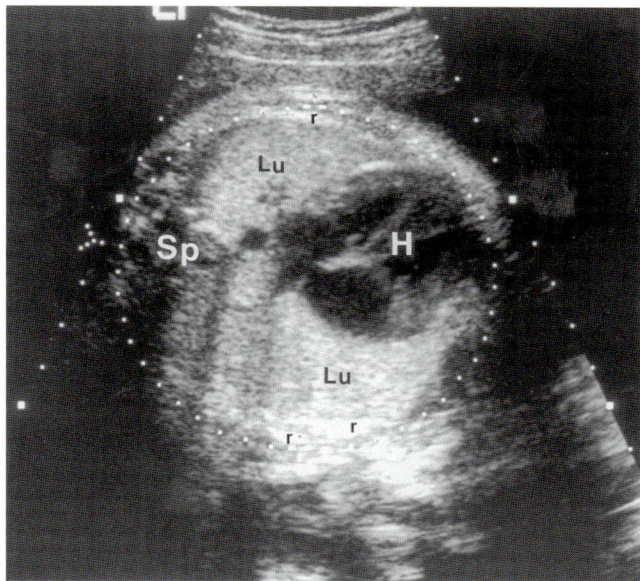

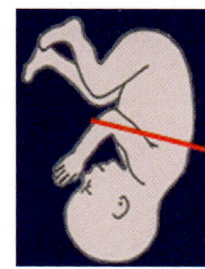

FIGURE 27. Thoracic circumference at 30 weeks. From an axial four-chamber view of the heart (*H*), the circumference measurement (electronic calipers) is generally taken at the outer margin of the rib cage, to exclude potentially edematous or thickened soft tissues. Ribs (*r*), spine (*Sp*), and lungs (*Lu*) are noted.

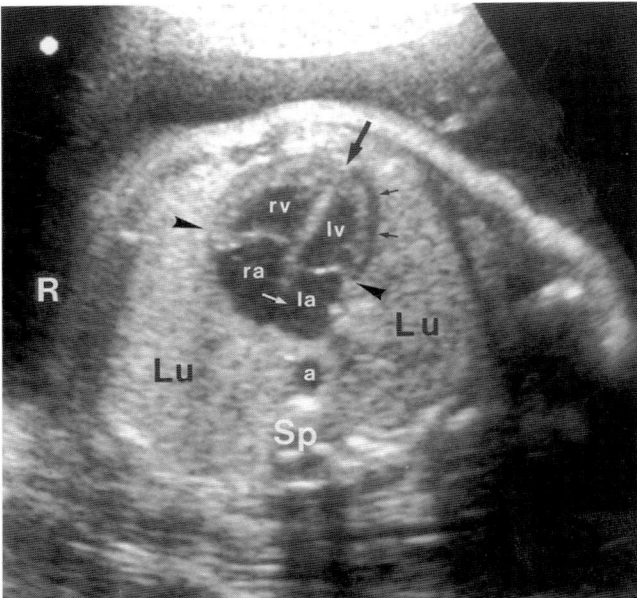

FIGURE 28. Four-chamber view of the heart at 26 weeks. An axial image shows the heart centrally positioned within the thorax, with its axis directed to the left side of the chest, as defined by the ventricular septum (*large arrow*) between the right ventricle (*rv*) and left ventricle (*lv*). The atrioventricular valves (*arrowheads*) are closed, separating the ventricles from the atria. The small white arrow indicates flow direction through the foramen ovale. A lucent band at the outer margin of left ventricle (*small arrows*) represents normal myocardium. Various portions of the myocardium, including the ventricular septum, may appear hypoechoic depending on the probe orientation relative to the heart muscle. The relatively echogenic lungs (*Lu*) are seen to fill the majority of the thorax. The descending thoracic aorta (*a*) is noted anterior to the spine (*Sp*). la, left atrium; R, right; ra, right atrium.

structures may be affected with various abnormalities (see Chapter 13). The basic ultrasound examination of the fetal abdomen and pelvis includes measurement of the abdominal circumference and identification of the stomach, kidneys, bladder, umbilical cord insertion, and adjacent anterior abdominal wall.

The abdominal circumference measurement, although useful as an adjunctive parameter for fetal dating, finds its greatest value in the evaluation of fetal growth in the latter part of pregnancy[48] (see Chapter 2) (Fig. 35). Deviations in abdominal circumference reflect changes in both the size of the liver and subcutaneous fat. On axial views only a short portion of the umbilical vein deep within the liver should be imaged, because visualization of the vein more anteriorly is only possible with oblique scans as it passes inferiorly towards the umbilicus.

The stomach is a variably sized fluid-filled structure in the left upper quadrant (Fig. 36). Usually imaged on transverse scans, longitudinal planes of section may also prove useful in confirming a normal relationship between the stomach and the diaphragm (Fig. 34). The stomach should be visualized on standard axial views of the abdominal circumference. Failure to visualize the stomach in the normal location after 14 weeks' gestational age is suggestive of pathology[49,50] (see Chapter 13).

The liver occupies the majority of the upper abdomen, with a prominent left lobe extending well into the left upper quadrant in the fetus (Figs. 35 and 36). Slight alterations in angulation can detect many of the other intraabdominal organs. The smaller spleen is identified as a solid organ posterior to the stomach. The fetal gallbladder is often seen at the inferior edge of the liver, within the right

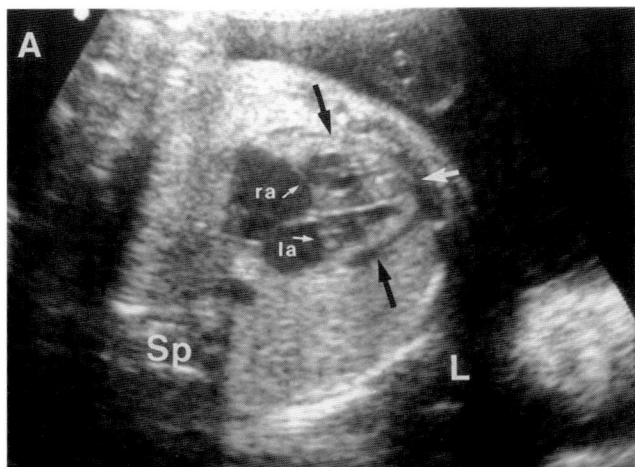
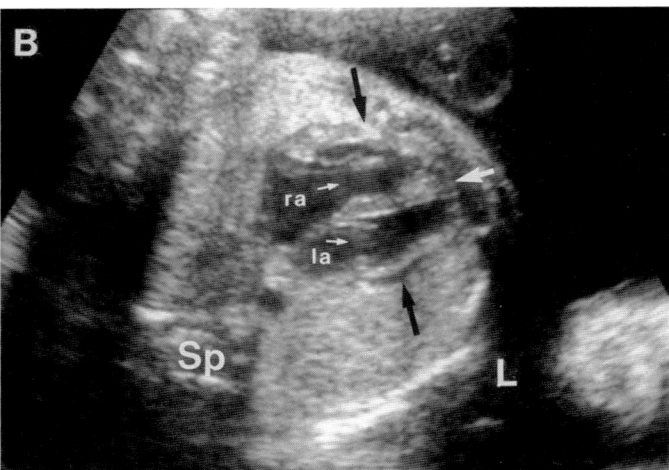

FIGURE 29. Heart, systole/diastole, at 26 weeks. **A:** Four-chamber view in ventricular systole with relatively small ventricular chambers (*black arrows*) and large left and right atria (*la, ra*). Small white arrows indicate the closed atrioventricular valves. Larger white arrow indicates ventricular septum and cardiac apex. L, left; Sp, spine. **B:** In diastole, the ventricular cavities (*black arrows*) are larger, atrioventricular valves (*small white arrows*) are open, and the left and right atria (*la, ra*) are smaller. Larger white arrow indicates ventricular septum and cardiac apex directed to the left (*L*).

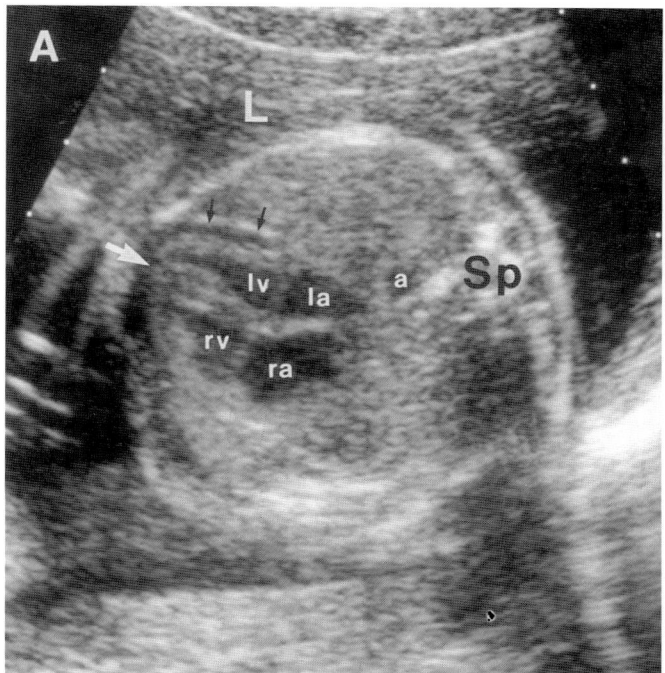
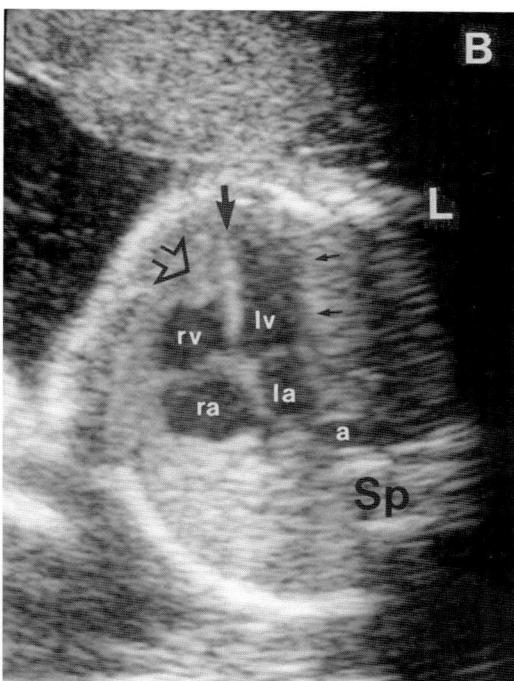

FIGURE 30. Heart, four-chamber views, with variable appearances at 24 weeks. **A:** An axial image with the cardiac axis perpendicular to the scan plane shows the right ventricle (*rv*), left ventricle (*lv*), right atrium (*ra*), and left atrium (*la*). The ventricular septum and apex (*white arrow*) are directed to the left (*L*). The ventricular septum appears thick, and sonolucent myocardium is noted in the wall of the left ventricle (*small black arrows*). The descending aorta (*a*) is seen anterior to the spine (*Sp*). **B:** With the scan plane directed parallel to the ventricular septum (*large black arrow*), the septum appears thinner, and the sonolucent myocardium in the left ventricular wall is no longer apparent (*small black arrows*). Thickening is noted in the right ventricular (*rv*) apex secondary to the moderator band (*open arrow*).

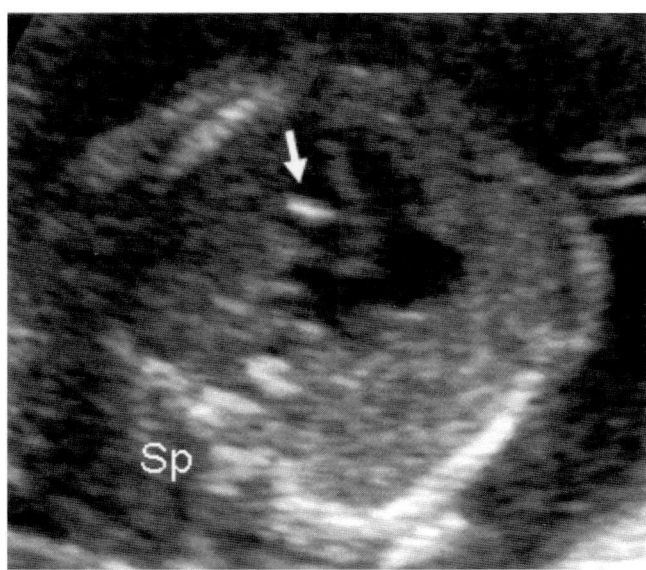

FIGURE 31. Heart with echogenic focus left ventricle at 18 weeks. On four-chamber view, a prominent echogenic focus (*arrow*) is present in the left ventricle. Occasionally, a similar finding is seen in the right ventricle. Sp, spine.

upper quadrant (Fig. 36). The gallbladder should be distinguished from the umbilical vein, to avoid incorrect measurement of the abdominal circumference. While both structures extend to the region of the porta hepatis, the umbilical vein is of uniform caliber, midline in position, and courses inferiorly to penetrate the abdominal wall; the gallbladder is clearly not midline, usually is somewhat teardrop shaped, and does not penetrate the abdominal wall.

The adrenal glands can be imaged cephalad to the kidneys. The hypoechoic cortex and echogenic medulla provide a distinctive appearance of the adrenal glands that becomes more obvious later in pregnancy. The right gland is positioned immediately posterior to the inferior vena cava, while the left gland lies lateral to the aorta (Fig. 37). The left adrenal gland is also more triangular and sits on the upper pole of the left kidney.

Aside from the organs described above, much of the remaining abdominal cavity is filled primarily with bowel (Fig. 38). The appearance of fetal bowel varies with gestational age. Early in the second trimester bowel appears as an area of midlevel to increased echogenicity filling the abdomen from the liver to the bladder. It is often mildly

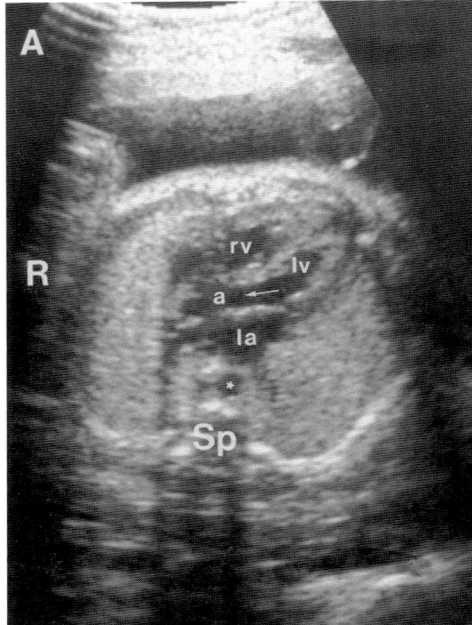

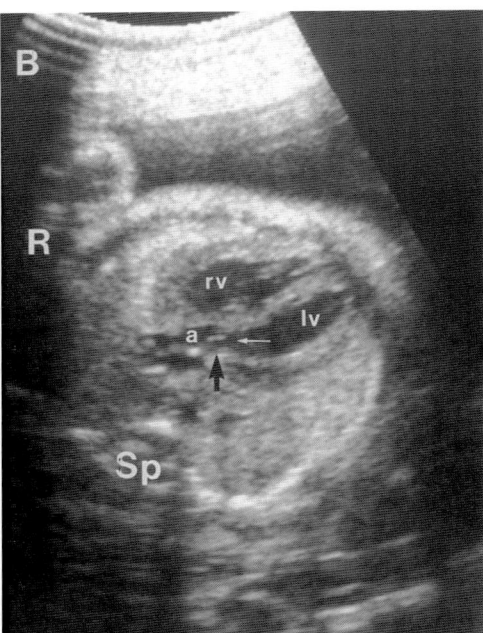

FIGURE 32. Heart, left ventricular outflow (LVO) tract, and aorta at 26 weeks: angled axial images of the same patient in Figure 29. **A:** The LVO tract (*arrow*) arises from the left ventricle (*lv*) and extends toward the right side of the thorax (*R*) as the ascending aorta (*a*). The LVO arises in close proximity to the mitral valve and left atrium (*la*). **B:** A slightly different angulation from the axial plane demonstrates the aortic valve as a bright echo (*black arrow*) between the LVO (*white arrow*) and the root of the ascending aorta. asterisk, descending aorta; R, right; rv, right ventricle; Sp, spine.

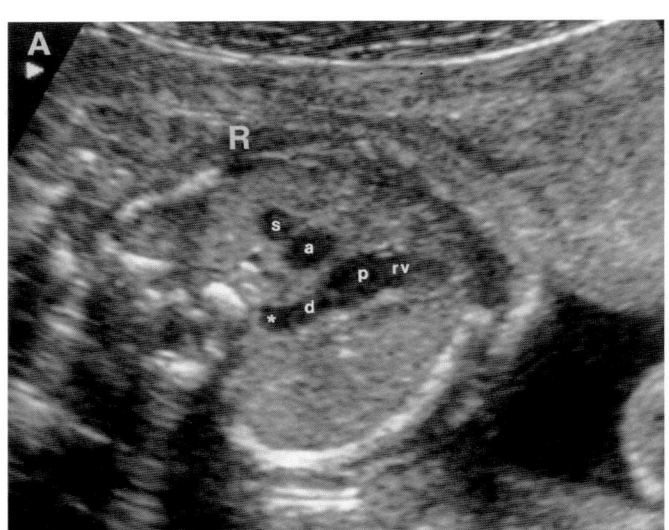

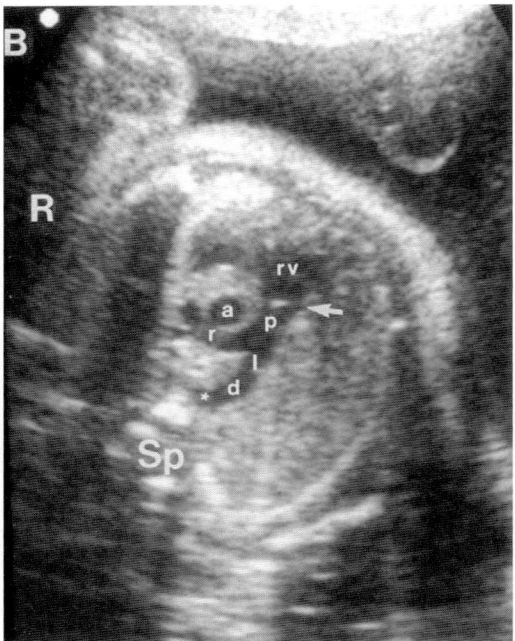

FIGURE 33. Heart, right ventricular outflow tract, pulmonary arteries, and ductus arteriosus at 26 weeks. **A:** A slightly angled axial view shows the very superior portion of the right ventricle/ right ventricular outflow tract (*rv*) contiguous with the pulmonary artery (*p*), ductus arteriosus (*d*), and descending aorta (*asterisk*). **B:** A slightly different axial angulation shows the superior aspect of the right ventricle/outflow tract, the echogenic pulmonary valve (*arrow*), and the main pulmonary artery, which divides into the right (*r*) and left (*l*) pulmonary arteries. The ductus arteriosus passes from the left pulmonary artery to the descending thoracic aorta (*asterisk*). The right pulmonary artery is seen curling posteriorly to the ascending aorta (*a*). R, right; s, superior vena cava; Sp, spine.

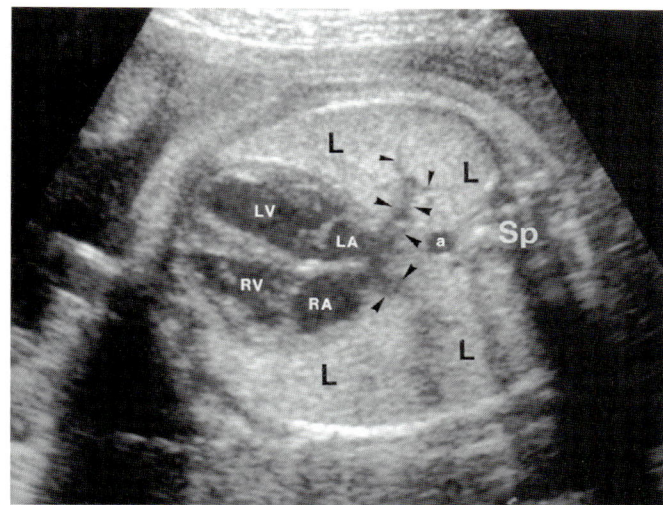

A

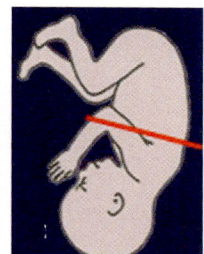

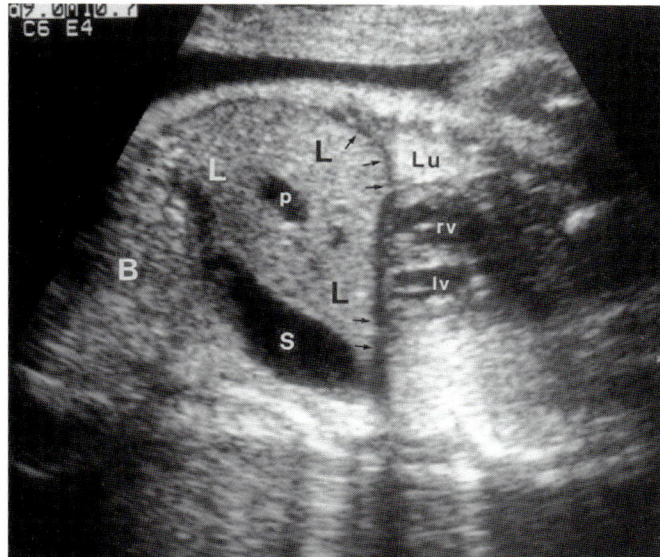

B

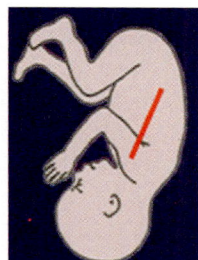

FIGURE 34. Lungs and diaphragm. **A:** A transverse view at 27 weeks shows lungs (*L*) surrounding the heart. Note the pulmonary veins (*arrowheads*) coursing to the posterior aspect of the left atrium (*LA*). a, aorta; LV, left ventricle; RA, right atrium; RV, right ventricle; Sp, spine. **B:** Coronal image shows lungs (*Lu*) and hypoechoic diaphragm (*arrows*). B, bowel; L, liver; lv, left ventricle; p, portal veins; rv, right ventricle; S, stomach.

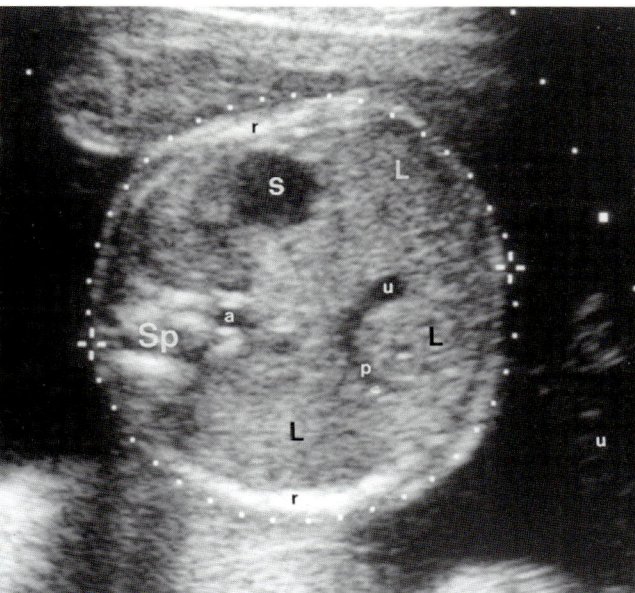

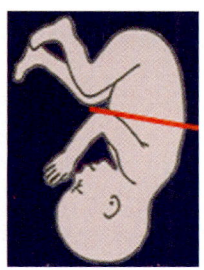

FIGURE 35. Abdominal circumference (AC) at 22 weeks. An axial image at the level where the umbilical vein (*u*) joins the portal venous system (*p*) deep within the liver (*L*) is the appropriate level for measuring an AC. The umbilical vein is identified in the midline, directly anterior from the spine (*Sp*). The measurement should be taken as close as possible to the skin surface (calipers). The AC can also be calculated by averaging the anteroposterior and transverse diameters of the abdomen, and multiplying that average diameter by *pi* (3.14). a, abdominal aorta; r, ribs; s, stomach.

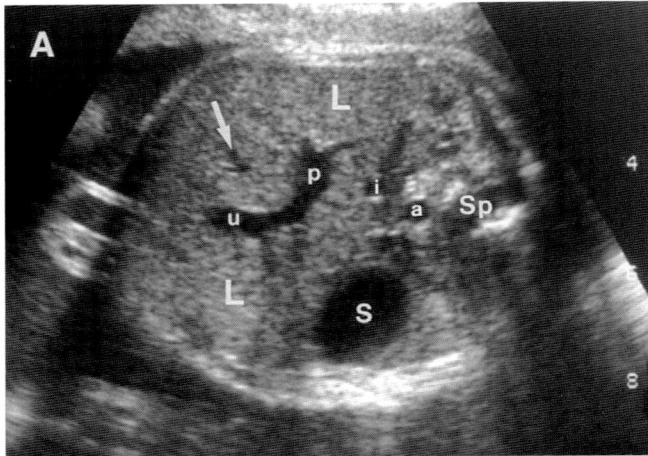
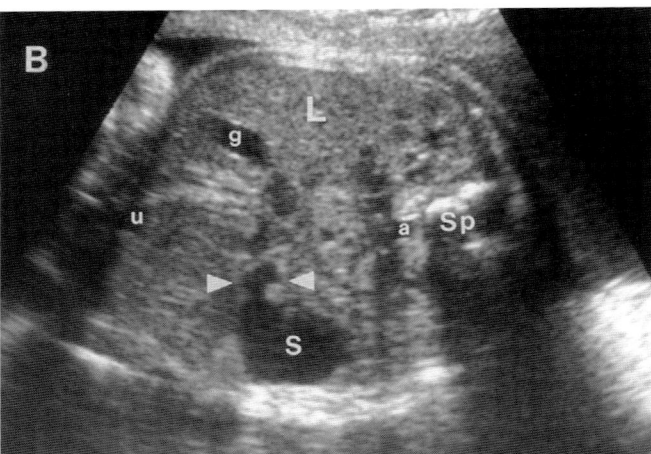

FIGURE 36. Stomach, liver, gallbladder, and liver at 28 weeks. **A:** An axial image through the upper abdomen shows the stomach (*S*) as a fluid-filled structure in the left upper quadrant. The liver (*L*) extends across the entire anterior abdomen. Within the liver, the midline umbilical vein (*u*) enters the portal venous system (*p*). The middle hepatic vein (*arrow*) is seen to the right of midline in a plane that will define the position of the gallbladder more inferiorly. The aorta (*a*) and inferior vena cava (*i*) are seen between the spine (*Sp*) and the liver. **B:** Lower within the abdomen, an axial image through the liver (*L*) shows the gallbladder (*g*) as a right-sided fluid-filled structure. The umbilical vein is in a very anterior position (*u*). The stomach (*S*) shows peristalsis within the antrum (*arrowheads*). a, aorta; Sp, spine.

echogenic compared to the echotexture of the liver, particularly using high-frequency transducers.[51] Unusually echogenic, or hyperechoic, bowel may be seen in normal fetuses.[52] However, it has also been associated with abnormalities including fetal aneuploidy, infection, and placental abnormalities.

In the third trimester the meconium-filled colon is readily discerned as prominent hypoechoic loops positioned around the more amorphous small bowel. At that same time, the normal small bowel may sometimes be seen to contain small quantities of fluid and to demonstrate peristalsis, particularly with higher resolution scanners.

Urinary Tract

Evaluation of the urinary tract is important because it is a common site of fetal anomalies[53] (see Chapter 14). The

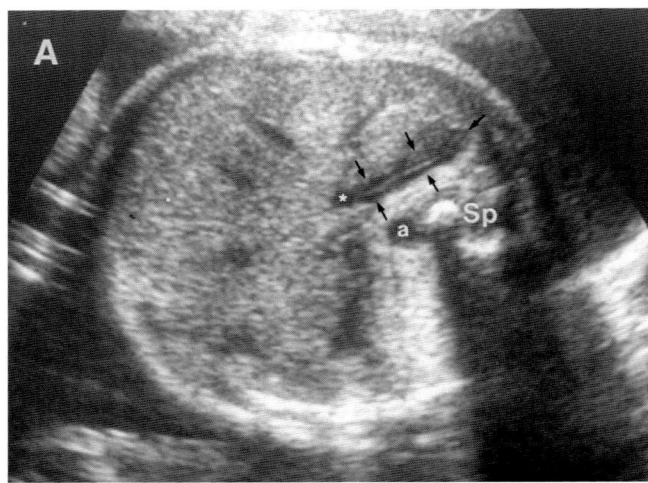
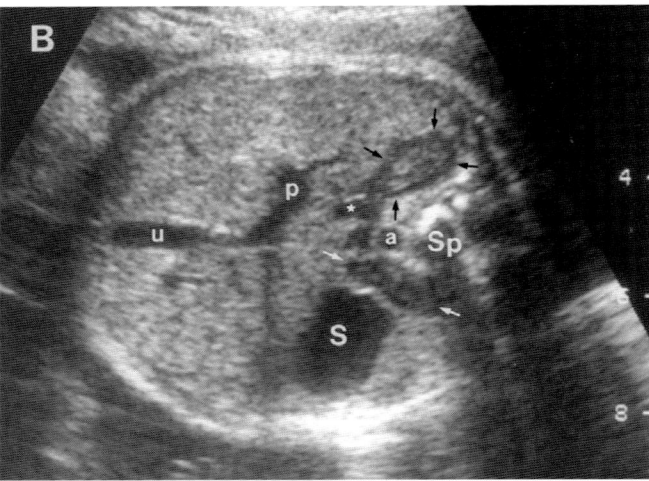

FIGURE 37. A: Adrenal glands at 28 weeks. **B:** A slightly lower axial image shows a more bulbous configuration of the right adrenal gland (*arrows*) as it enlarges caudally toward the underlying kidney. The right gland still is positioned posterior to the inferior vena cava (*asterisk*) whereas the left gland, less well seen, lies between the aorta (*a*) and stomach (*S*). Umbilical vein (*u*) and portal vein (*p*) can be seen within the liver. Sp, spine.

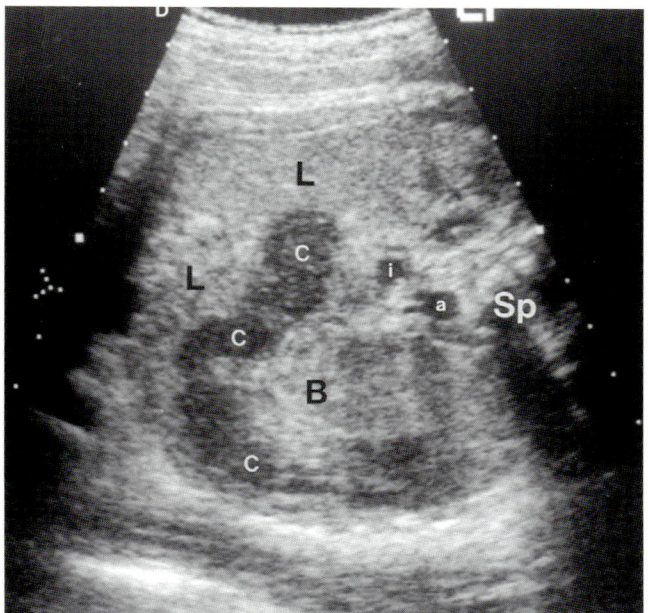

FIGURE 38. Bowel at 36 weeks. An axial image through midabdomen shows the ill-defined small bowel (*B*) located centrally. The tubular hypoechoic transverse colon (*C*) is located posterior to liver (*L*). Low-level echoes representing meconium fill the colon. a, aorta; i, inferior vena cava; Sp, spine.

kidneys appear as bilateral, hypoechoic, paraspinal structures with an echogenic central renal sinus that may be minimally separated by the fluid-containing renal pelvis[54,55] (Fig. 39). The fetal kidneys are often difficult to identify as discrete structures early in the second trimester (Fig. 36A), especially when no fluid is present in the renal pelvis.[56,57] Scans through the renal area are still useful at this time to screen for the presence of any renal masses or collecting system dilatation.[58,59] Later in pregnancy, the renal pyramids can be discerned separate from the cortex (Fig. 40). The renal arteries can also be evaluated with color or power Doppler imaging (Fig. 41).

The urinary bladder is a fluid-filled structure located low within the pelvis, in the midline anteriorly (Figs. 42 and 43). If there has been recent fetal voiding, further scanning for up to an hour or so may be needed to document the bladder. If the kidneys and fluid volume are normal, absence of bladder visualization is usually of little significance. However, abnormalities such as cloacal exstrophy should be considered (see Chapter 12).

Genitalia

Female and male genitalia are quite similar embryologically until late in the first trimester. The male penis is seen as a

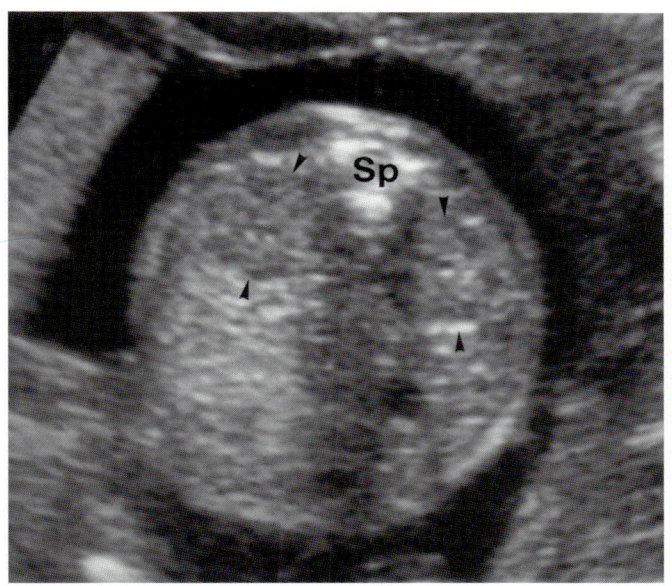

A

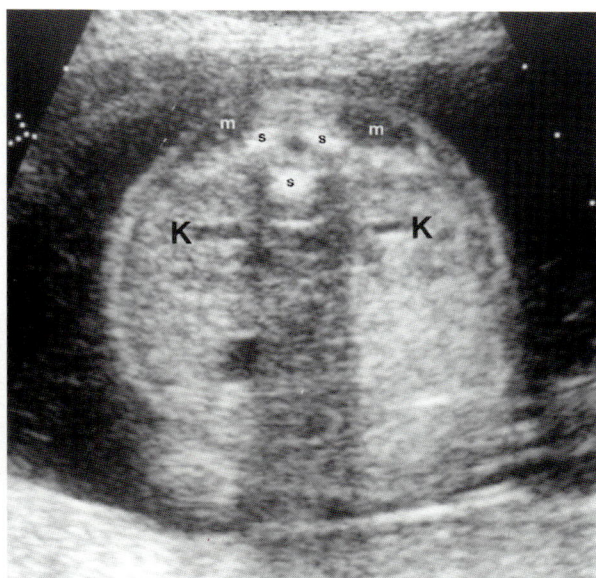

B

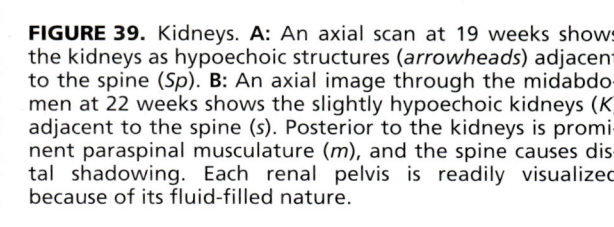

FIGURE 39. Kidneys. **A:** An axial scan at 19 weeks shows the kidneys as hypoechoic structures (*arrowheads*) adjacent to the spine (*Sp*). **B:** An axial image through the midabdomen at 22 weeks shows the slightly hypoechoic kidneys (*K*) adjacent to the spine (*s*). Posterior to the kidneys is prominent paraspinal musculature (*m*), and the spine causes distal shadowing. Each renal pelvis is readily visualized because of its fluid-filled nature.

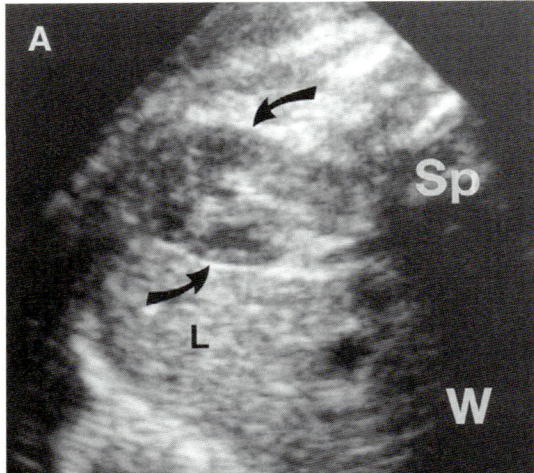

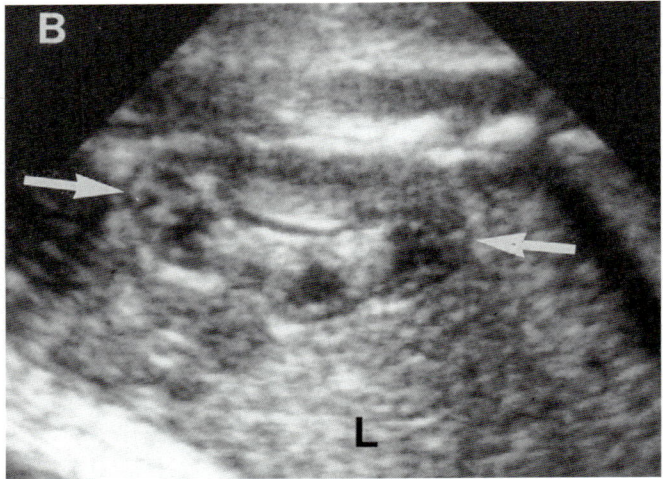

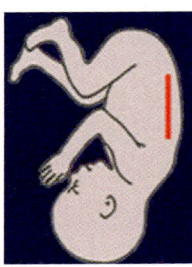

FIGURE 40. Kidney at 35 weeks. **A:** An axial image shows the right kidney (*arrows*) as less echogenic than the more anteriorly positioned liver (*L*). Focal hypoechoic regions within the renal parenchyma represent the pyramids. The spine (*Sp*) causes distal shadowing (*W*). **B:** A longitudinal image through the right kidney (*arrows*) shows the typical reniform appearance, with the renal parenchyma less echogenic than the central sinus and minimal collecting system present. Renal pyramids are seen as triangular hypoechoic regions within the parenchyma.

solid structure in contrast to the fluid-filled umbilical cord that may lie between the thighs. A prominent clitoris, seen during the early second trimester, may be confused for a penis by inexperienced sonographers. The scrotum is a bulbous soft-tissue structure that is increasingly apparent at the base of the penis as gestation progresses (Fig. 44). Echogenic testicles descend into the scrotum during the seventh month, and small hydroceles may often be seen normally.

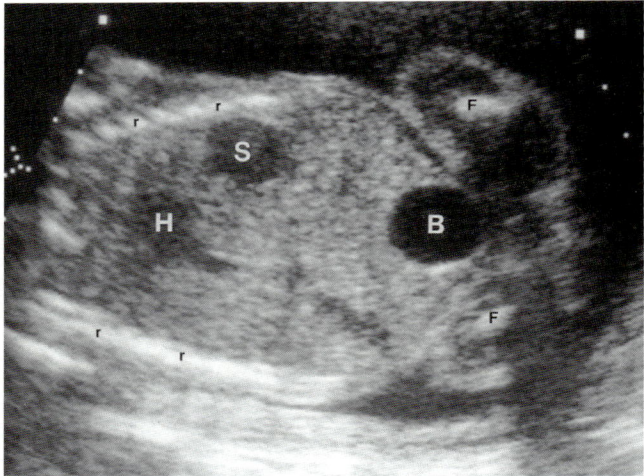

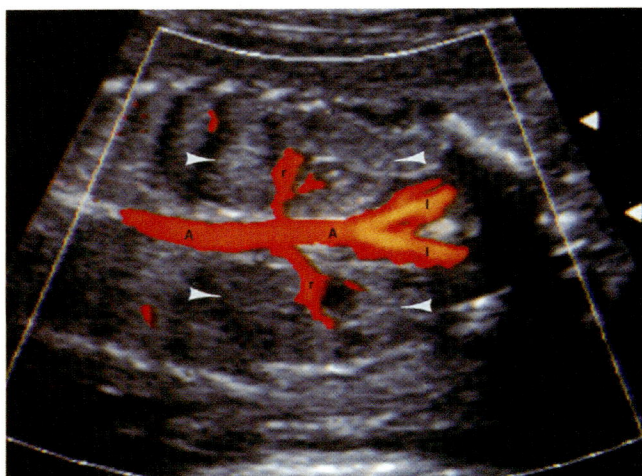

FIGURE 41. Renal arteries at 21 weeks. A coronal view through the kidneys (*arrowheads*) with power Doppler imaging clearly shows renal arteries (*r*) arising from the aorta (*A*). I, iliac arteries.

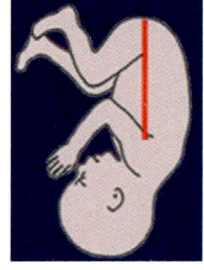

FIGURE 42. Bladder at 22 weeks. A coronal sonogram through the trunk shows the rib cage (*r*), heart (*H*), and stomach (*S*) within the left upper quadrant and the bladder (*B*) low within the pelvis. The femurs (*F*) can be seen within the hypoechoic musculature of the proximal thighs.

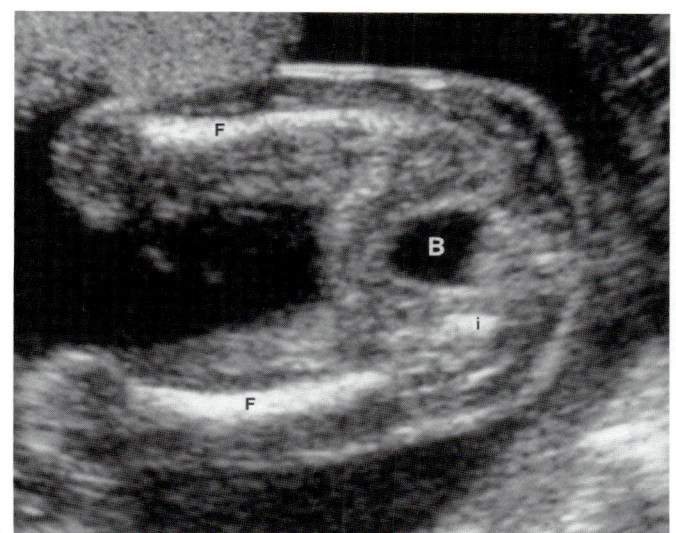
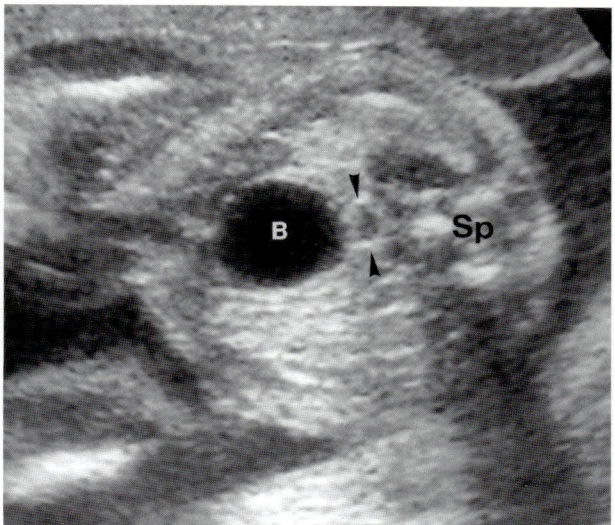

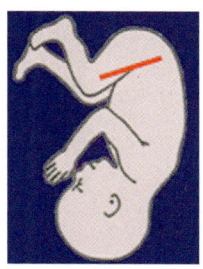

FIGURE 43. Bladder and rectum at 24 weeks. **A:** An axial image of the pelvis through the iliac crests (*i*) shows the anterior, midline, partially filled urinary bladder (*B*). The proximal thighs containing the femurs (*F*) are seen anteriorly. **B:** A second hypoechoic structure representing the rectum (*arrowheads*) is seen just posterior to the bladder (*B*). Sp, spine.

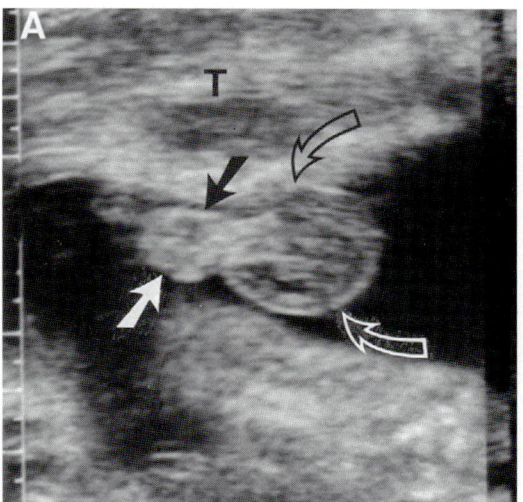
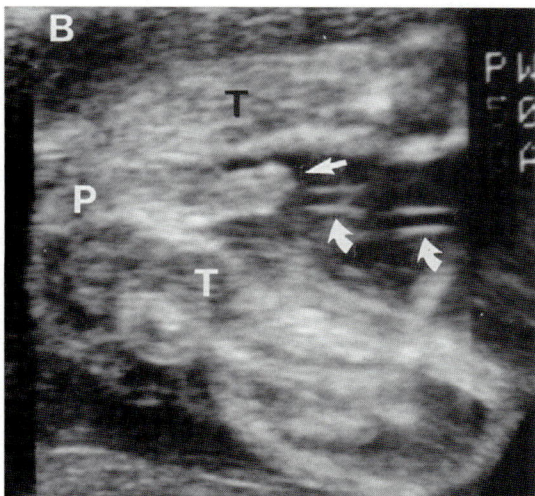

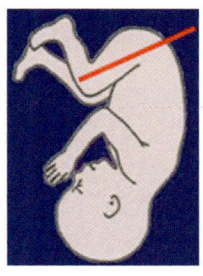

FIGURE 44. Male genitalia. **A:** Curved arrows show the scrotum with a small hydrocele on one side. Straight arrows show a cross-sectional image through the penis, adjacent to the soft tissues of the thigh (*T*). **B:** An angled axial image through the pelvis (*P*) and proximal thighs shows the echogenic penis (*straight arrow*) in contrast to fluid-filled loops of cord (*curved arrows*) that are often seen between the legs.

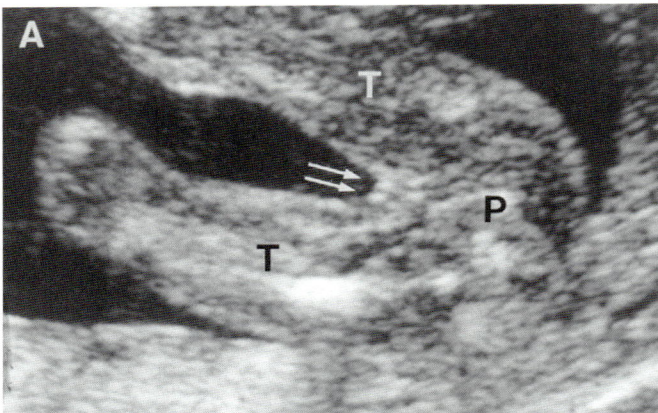
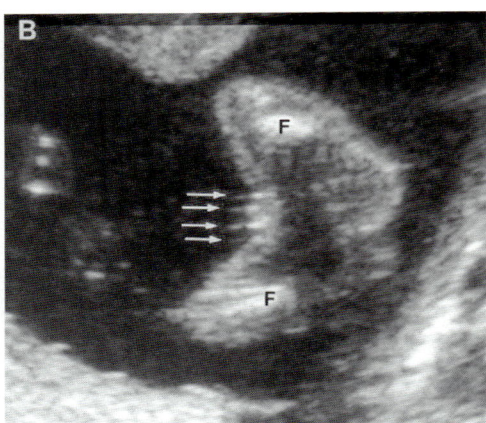

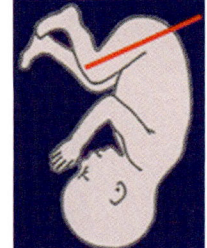

FIGURE 45. Female genitalia at 17 weeks. **A:** An axial image through the pelvis (*P*) and thighs (*T*) shows linear echoes arising from labia (*arrows*). **B:** An angled axial view shows parallel linear echoes (*arrows*) representing the labia. F, proximal femurs.

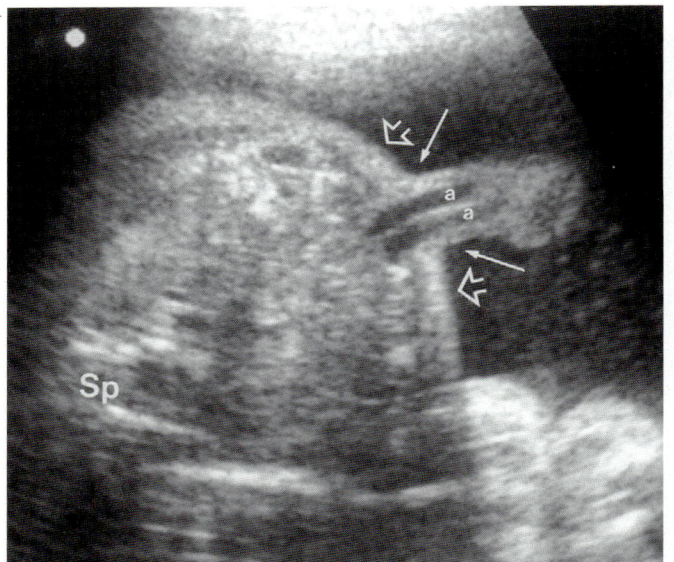
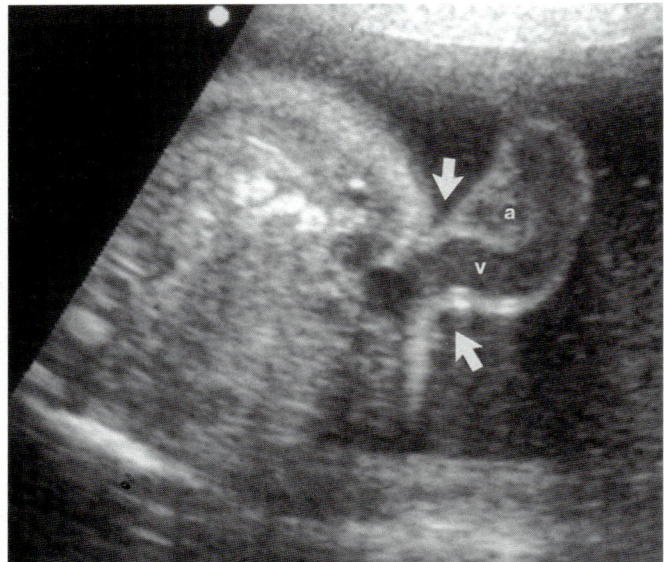

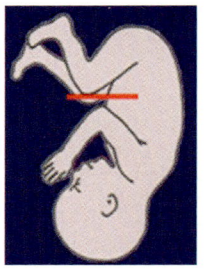

FIGURE 46. Anterior abdominal wall and cord insertion at 26 weeks. **A:** An axial image shows the umbilical cord entering the abdomen (*long arrows*). Two umbilical arteries (*a*) and no extraneous tissues are seen in the cord. Note the adjacent intact abdominal wall (*open arrows*). Sp, spine. **B:** Slight alteration of scan plane shows a portion of cord containing umbilical vein (*V*) within the cord.

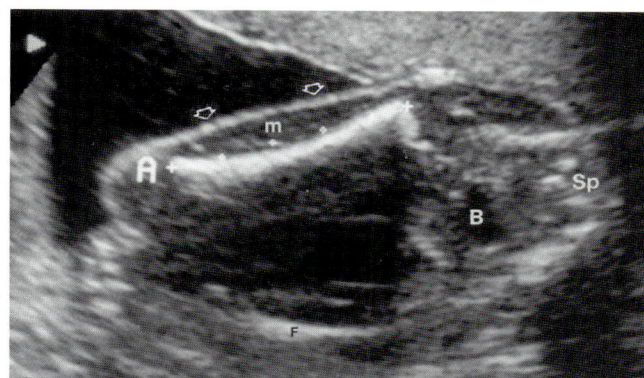

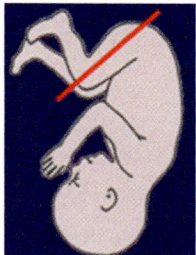

FIGURE 47. Femur at 21 weeks. The femur is measured (*A*, calipers) from its proximal end near the femoral neck to the distal metaphysis, including only the ossified portions. The musculature (*m*) of the thigh lies deep to the overlying skin and subcutaneous tissues (*arrows*). B, urinary bladder; F, portion of opposite femur; Sp, spine.

Female genitalia are confirmed early in gestation via identification of several parallel linear echoes representing the margins of the labia (Fig. 45). In the third trimester the prominent soft tissues of the labia majora border the linear echoes of the labia minora.

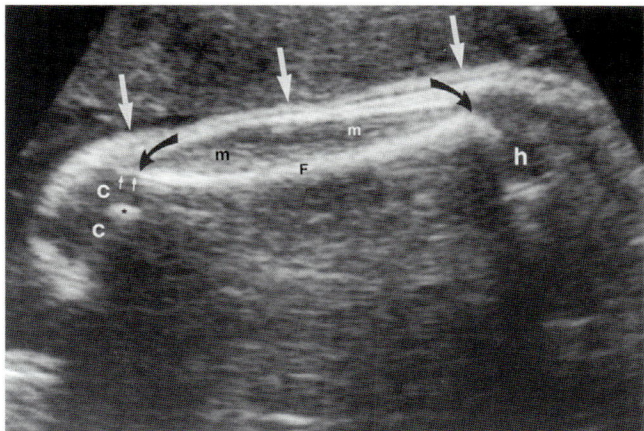

FIGURE 48. Femur at 35 weeks. The echogenic fetal femur (*F*) represents only the ossified component of the bone. The cartilaginous femoral head (*h*) and femoral condyles (*C*) are noted at their respective ends of the bone. Within the distal femoral epiphysis, an ossification center (*asterisk*) is generally present from 33 weeks' gestation onward. A thin echogenic "spike" extends from the distal end of the femoral shaft (*small white arrows*), representing an interface between soft tissues and underlying cartilage. This femoral spike should not be included in femoral length measurements. Appropriate points for femoral measurement are indicated with curved black arrows. The echogenic lateral skin margin (*large white arrows*) is noted overlying the hypoechoic musculature of the thigh (*m*).

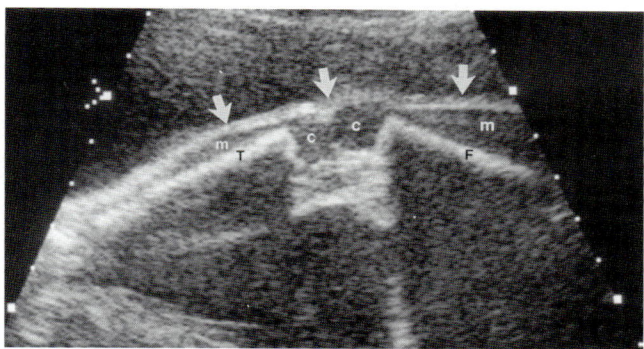

FIGURE 49. Knee at 28 weeks. A longitudinal image through the knee shows distal femur (*F*) and tibia (*T*) and their respective hypoechoic articular cartilage (*c*). The echogenic skin surface (*arrows*) can be seen overlying the musculature (*m*) of the thigh and leg.

Anterior Abdominal Wall

The site of the umbilical cord insertion into the abdominal wall must be evaluated to confirm a normal-sized cord penetrating the abdomen (Fig. 46). The adjacent abdominal wall must also be examined to confirm its integrity. Visualization of normal cord insertion and an adjacent anterior abdominal wall excludes the majority of ventral wall defects (see Chapter 12).

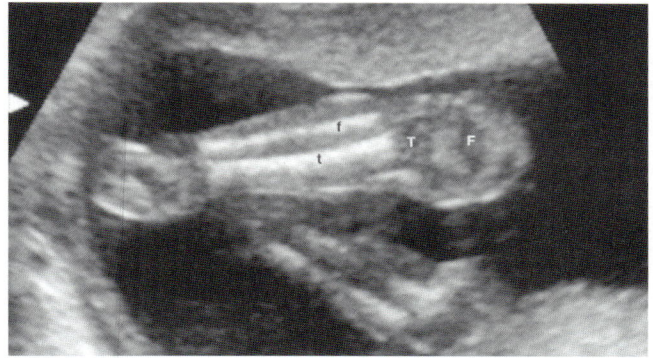

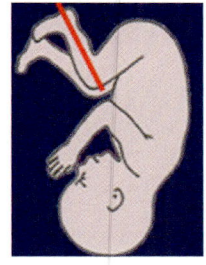

FIGURE 50. Tibia and fibula at 24 weeks. Long axis image of the leg shows the ossified portions of the fibula (*f*) and tibia (*t*). The hypoechoic, cartilaginous epiphyseal centers of the tibia (*T*) and femur (*F*) are faintly seen.

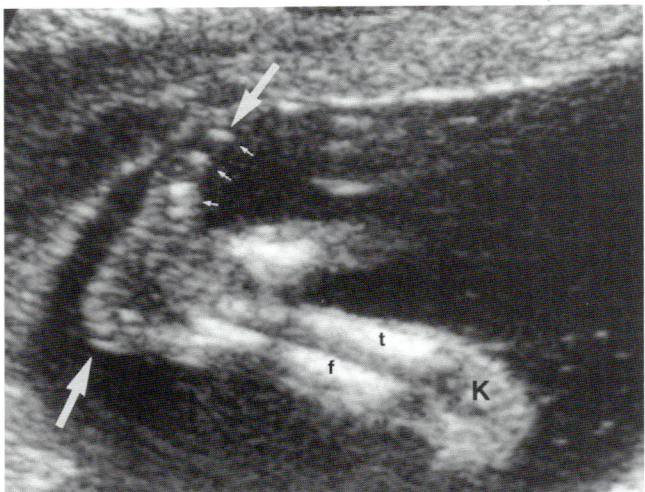

FIGURE 51. Leg and foot at 17 weeks A longitudinal image through the tibia (*t*) and fibula (*f*) shows the leg extending down to the foot (*large arrows*). The ossification centers within a single ray, including two phalanges and a metatarsal, are noted (*small arrows*). K, knee.

Extremities

The bones of the extremities are readily identifiable due to their inherent subject contrast with the surrounding soft tissues, from the late first trimester to term. The femur is the only long bone that is routinely measured, however (Fig. 47), being a primary parameter for fetal dating as well as a screen for skeletal dysplasias.[60] Mild contour variation in the normal femoral shaft is often apparent, with a

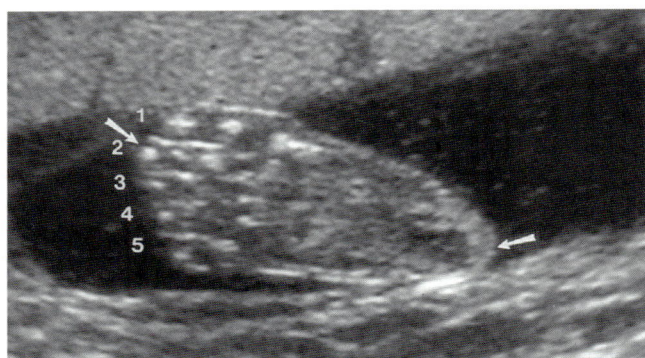

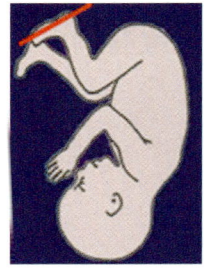

FIGURE 52. Foot at 18 weeks. A heel to toe distance (*arrows*) can be readily obtained on directed scanning. When the scan plane is oriented perpendicular to the digits (*1 to 5*), as in this case, multiple interfaces make identification of individual digits difficult to accomplish, particularly early in gestation.

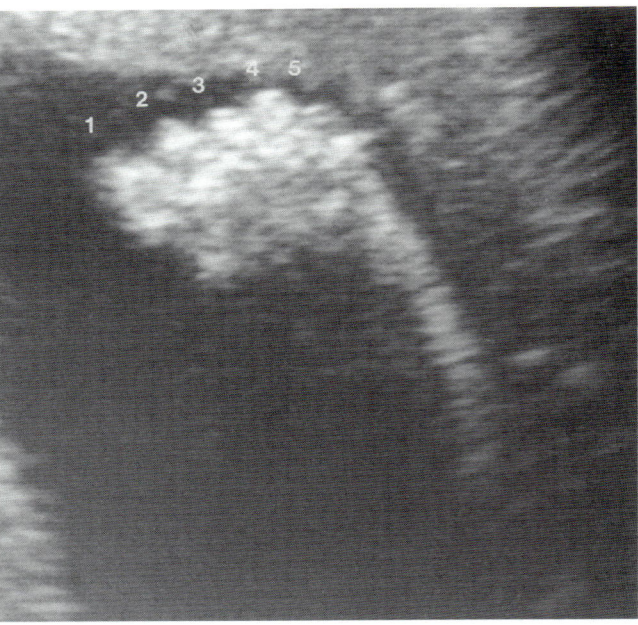

FIGURE 53. Toes at 32 weeks. The digits of the foot (*1 to 5*) may best be discriminated as individual structures when the scan plane is directed toward the anterior aspect of the foot. Increased soft tissue in the third trimester is also a factor in better visualization.

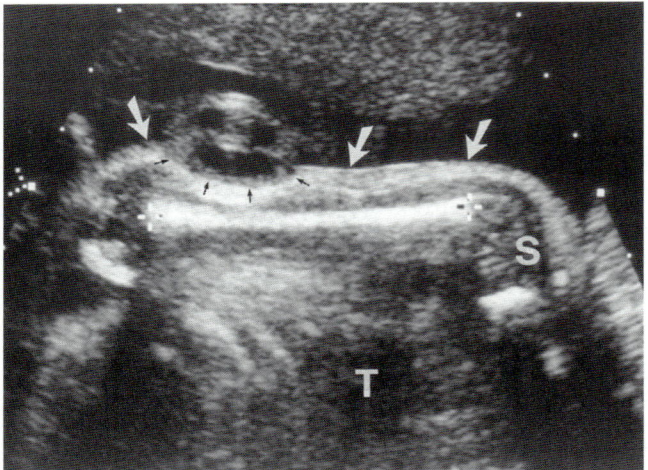

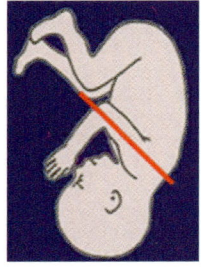

FIGURE 54. Humerus at 20 weeks. As the humerus may resemble the femur, care must be taken to scan from the adjacent bony thorax, through the shoulder (*S*) and into the arm to properly identify the humerus for measurement (calipers). Note that the humerus is positioned adjacent to the thorax (*T*). The echogenic lateral skin surface (*white arrows*) is indented distally by a loop of cord (*black arrows*).

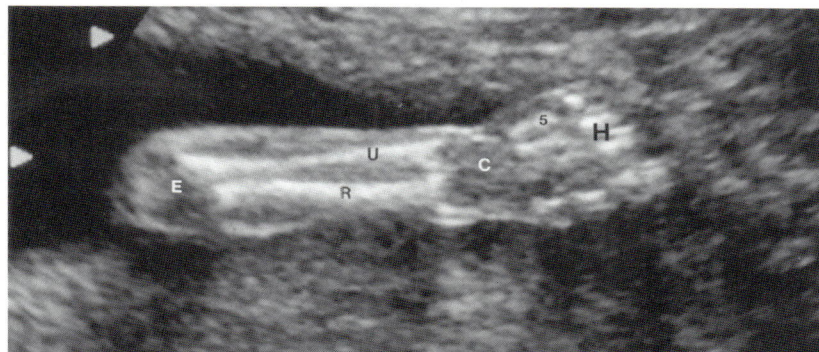

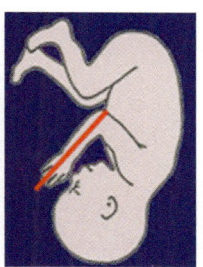

FIGURE 55. Forearm at 19 weeks. While the ulna (*U*) extends farther into the elbow (*E*) than the radius (*R*), both bones end at approximately the same level at the wrist (*C*). The wrist bone is nonossified in the fetus, appearing hypoechoic in contrast to the ossification centers, including the fifth metacarpal (*5*), visualized within the hand (*H*).

straighter appearance on the lateral aspect, and a mild bowed appearance medially.[61] Only the ossified portions of the bone are measured, excluding the hypoechoic cartilaginous epiphyses of the femoral head and condyles distally[62,63] (Fig. 48).

Although routine documentation of the extremities is not a component of the basic obstetrical ultrasound guidelines from many societies, brief survey of all extremities is recommended to confirm a grossly normal appearance of the bones and soft tissues to the level of the feet and hands.[64] Imaging of specific bones is accomplished by careful progression from one known structure to the next, adjusting probe position as needed to obtain the desired images. Scanning beyond the

femur will outline the hypoechoic cartilages of the distal femur and proximal tibia (Fig. 49). Subsequently the tibia and fibula (Fig. 50) and lower leg and foot (Fig. 51) can be shown. Measurement of foot length[65,66] (Fig. 52) and documentation of digits (Fig. 53) are possible with appropriate fetal positioning and careful scanning. Similar scanning through the upper extremities can detail the humerus (Fig. 54), radius and ulna (Fig. 55), and hand (Fig. 56). Three-dimensional ultrasound of the feet and hands also depicts these complex structures (Figs. 57 and 58).

Umbilical Vessels

Confirmation of a normal three-vessel cord may be made by direct imaging of the cord to delineate the two smaller umbilical arteries and the larger umbilical vein. Alternately, the paired umbilical arteries can be imaged within the fetus, extending along the anterior abdominal wall from the umbilicus to a position lateral to the fetal bladder (Fig. 59A). This can easily be confirmed with color flow Doppler, a valuable

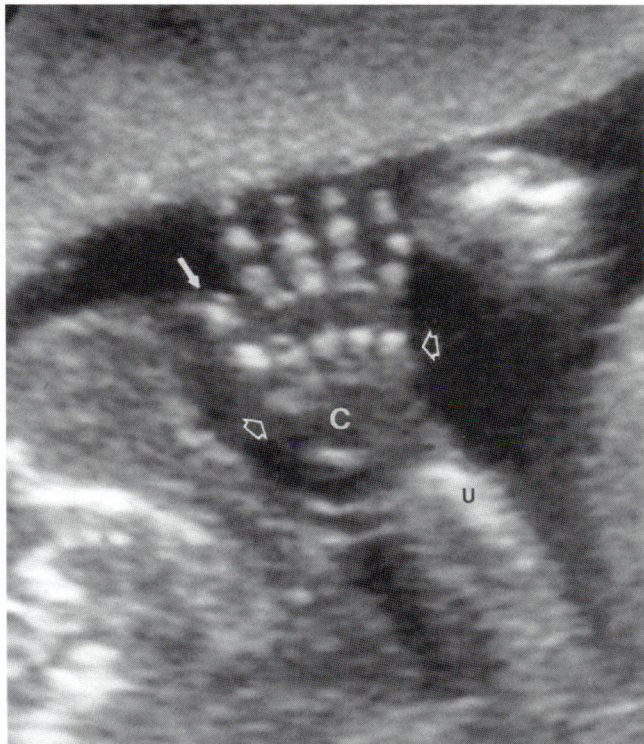

FIGURE 56. Hand at 19 weeks. A longitudinal image of the hand shows all five metacarpals (*open arrows*) and phalanges of the fingers and thumb (*white arrow*) in all five digits. C, carpus; U, ulna.

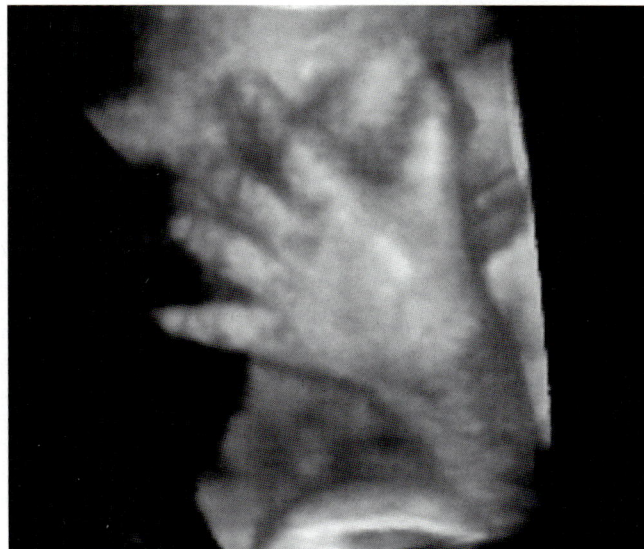

FIGURE 57. Three-dimensional ultrasound of the hand at 30 weeks.

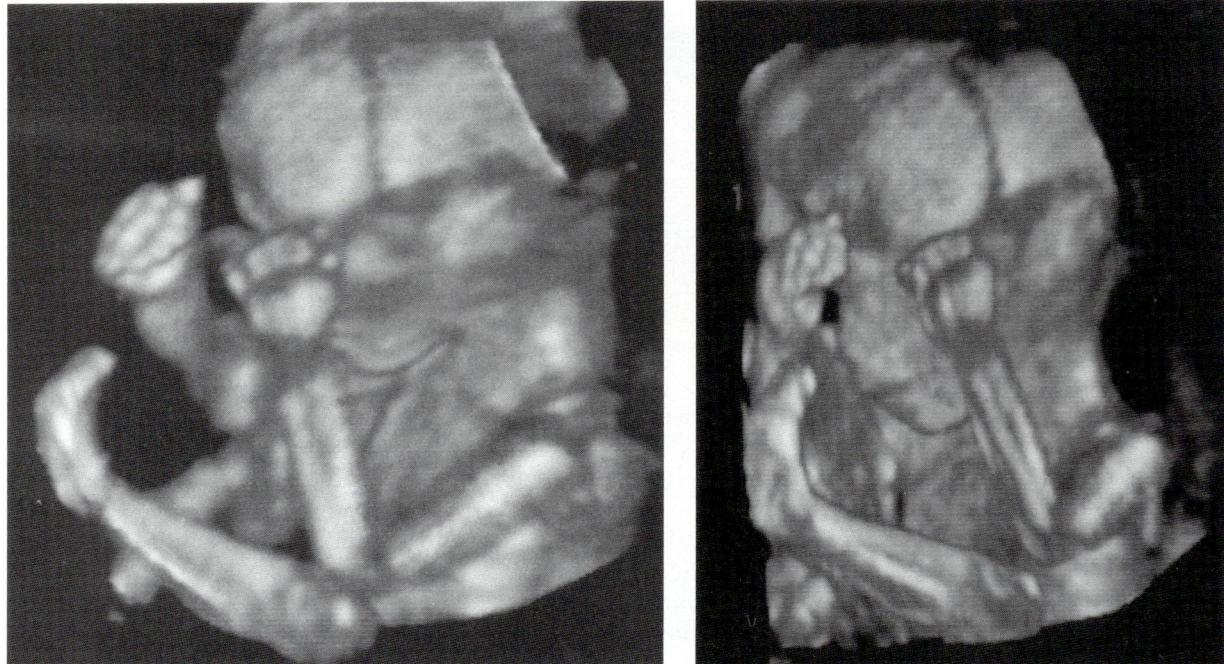

FIGURE 58. Two views of three-dimensional ultrasound at 20 weeks show normal extremities.

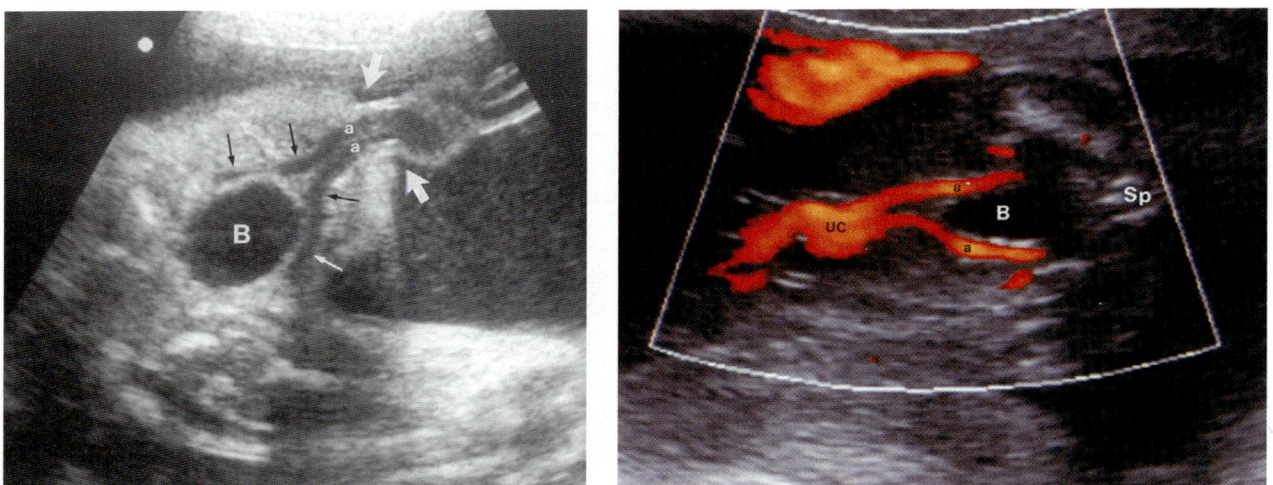

A   B

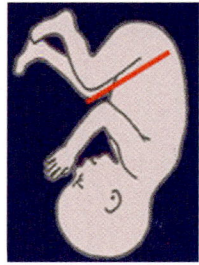

FIGURE 59. Umbilical arteries. **A:** An oblique view at 19 weeks from the cord insertion site (*large arrows*) to the pelvis shows paired umbilical arteries (*a, small arrows*) coursing lateral to the urinary bladder (*B*). **B:** A color-flow image shows two arteries (*a*) extending from the umbilical cord insertion site (*uc*) into the pelvis lateral to the bladder (*B*). Documentation of two umbilical arteries within the fetus can be substituted for visualizing three vessels within the umbilical cord. Sp, spine.

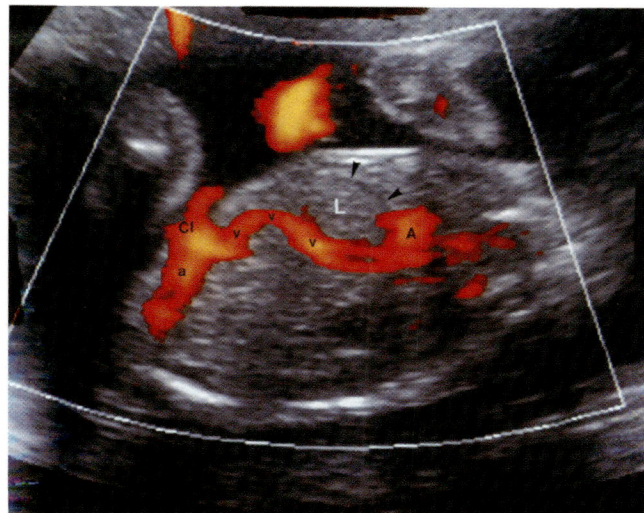

FIGURE 60. Umbilical vein at 23 weeks. Power Doppler in longitudinal view of abdomen shows the umbilical vein (*v*) extending from cord insertion (*CI*) to the liver (*L*), where it is directed posteriorly to join the ductus venosus and the right atrium (*A*) of the heart. Arrows indicate diaphragm. An umbilical artery (*a*) courses into the pelvis.

technique early in gestation when direct visualization of the arteries within the cord may be difficult (Fig. 59B).

The umbilical vein can also be visualized throughout its course (Fig. 60). Immediately after entering the umbilical insertion site, it turns superiorly and separates from the umbilical arteries. The umbilical vein remains anterior in the abdomen until it enters the liver, and then it courses posteriorly to communicate with the portal vein. Returning blood may then course through either the portal veins or continue superiorly and posteriorly into the ductus venosus and then the inferior vena cava and right atrium.

On transverse views of the abdomen, at the same level as the stomach, the umbilical vein should be seen entering the liver with its major branch, the right portal vein, curving toward the right side, opposite the side of the stomach (Fig. 36A). A relatively normal common variant is persistent left umbilical vein, in which case the major branch curves towards the side of the stomach. In this situation, the gallbladder will also be located between the umbilical vein and the stomach rather than in its normal position to the right of the umbilical vein.

Other

A complete obstetric ultrasound also includes assessment of fetal growth (see Chapter 2), the placenta (see Chapter 4), amniotic fluid (see Chapter 3), and the cervix.

REFERENCES

1. U.S. Department of Health and Human Services. Diagnostic ultrasound in pregnancy. National Institutes of Health publication no. 84-667, Bethesda, MD, 1984.

2. Technical Bulletin. Ultrasound in Pregnancy. American College of Obstetrics and Gynecology, No. 187, 1993.

3. Grandjean H, Larroque D, Levi S. The performance of routine ultrasonographic screening of pregnancies in the Eurofetus Study. *Am J Obstet Gynecol* 1999;181(2):446–454.

4. Vintzileos AM, Ananth CV, Smulian JC, Beazoglou T, Knuppel RA. Routine second-trimester ultrasonography in the United States: a cost-benefit analysis. *Am J Obstet Gynecol* 2000;182(3):655–660.

5. Guidelines for Performance of the Antepartum Obstetrical Ultrasound Examination. American Institute of Ultrasound in Medicine, Laurel, Maryland, 1994.

6. Reference deleted by author.

7. Bowerman RA. *Atlas of normal fetal ultrasonographic anatomy.* Chicago: Year Book Medical Publishers, 1992.

8. Schwarzler P, Senat MV, Holden D, Bernard JP, Masroor T, Ville Y. Feasibility of the second-trimester fetal ultrasound examination in an unselected population at 18, 20 or 22 weeks of pregnancy: a randomized trial. *Ultrasound Obstet Gynecol* 1999;14(2):92–97.

9. Hadlock FP, Harrist RB, Deter RJ, et al. Fetal head circumference: relation to menstrual age. *AJR Am J Roentgenol* 1982;138:649–653.

10. Shepard M, Filly RA. A standardized plane for biparietal diameter measurement. *J Ultrasound Med* 1982;1:145–150.

11. Chinn DH, Callen PW, Filly RA. The lateral cerebral ventricle in early second trimester. *Radiology* 1983;148:529–531.

12. Nyberg DA. Recommendations for obstetric sonography in the evaluation of the fetal cranium. *Radiology* 1989;1972:309–311.

13. Cardoza JD, Goldstein RB, Filly RA. Exclusion of fetal ventriculomegaly with a single measurement: the width of the lateral ventricular atrium. *Radiology* 1988;169:711–714.

14. Alagappan R, Browning PD, Laorr A, et al. Distal lateral ventricular atrium: reevaluation of normal range. *Radiology* 1994;193:405–408.

15. Farrell TA, Hertzberg BS, Kliewer MA, et al. Fetal lateral ventricles: reassessment of normal values for atrial diameter at US. *Radiology* 1994;193:409–411.

16. Browning PD, Laorr A, McGahan JP, et al. Proximal fetal cerebral ventricle: description of US technique and initial results. *Radiology* 1994;192:337–341.

17. Cronan MS, McGahan JP. A new ultrasound technique to visualize the proximal fetal cerebral ventricle. *J Diagn Med Sonography* 1991;6:333–335.

18. Mahony BS, Callen PW, Filly RA, et al. The fetal cisterna magna. *Radiology* 1984;153:173–176.

19. Laing FC, Frates MC, Brown DL, et al. Sonography of the fetal posterior fossa: false appearance of mega-cisterna magna and Dandy-Walker variant. *Radiology* 1994;192:247–251.

20. Knutzon R, McGahan JP, Salamat MS, Brant WB. Fetal cisterna magna septa: a normal anatomic finding. *Radiology* 1991;180:799–801.

21. McLeary RD, Kuhns LR, Barr M Jr. Ultrasonography of the fetal cerebellum. *Radiology* 1984;151:439–442.

22. Bowerman RA. Ultrasound of the fetal face. *Ultrasound Q* 1993;11:211–258.

23. Jeanty P, Cantraine F, Cousaert E, et al. The binocular distance: a new way to estimate fetal age. *J Ultrasound Med* 1984;3:241–243.

24. Mayden KL, Tortora M, Berkowitz RL, et al. Orbital diameters: a new parameter for prenatal diagnosis and dating. *Am J Obstet Gynecol* 1982;144:289–297.

25. Birnholz JC. The fetal external ear. *Radiology* 1983;147:819–821.

26. Petrikovsky BM, Vintzileos AM, Rodis JF. Sonographic appearance of occipital fetal hair. *J Clin Ultrasound* 1989;17:425–427.

27. Cooper C, Mahony BS, Bowie JD, et al. Ultrasound evaluation of the normal fetal upper airway and esophagus. *J Ultrasound Med* 1985;4:343–346.

28. Filly RA, Simpson GF, Linkowski G. Fetal spine morphology and maturation during the second trimester. *J Ultrasound Med* 1987;6:631–636.

29. Gray DL, Crane JP, Rudloff MA. Prenatal diagnosis of neural tube defects: origin of midtrimester vertebral ossification centers as determined by sonographic water-bath studies. *J Ultrasound Med* 1988;7:421–427.

30. Yarkoni S, Schmidt W, Jeanty P, et al. Clavicular measurement: a new biometric parameter for fetal evaluation. *J Ultrasound Med* 1985;4:467–470.

31. Fong K, Ohlsson A, Zalev A. Fetal thoracic circumference: a prospective cross-sectional study with real-time ultrasound. *Am J Obstet Gynecol* 1988;158:1154–1160.

32. Nimrod C, Davies D, Iwanicki S, et al. Ultrasound prediction of pulmonary hypoplasia. *Obstet Gynecol* 1986;68:495–497.

33. McGahan JP. Sonography of the fetal heart: findings on the four-chamber view. *AJR Am J Roentgenol* 1991;156:547–553.

34. Hess LW, Hess DB, McCaul JF, et al. Fetal echocardiography. *Obstet Gynecol Clin North Am* 1990;17:41–79.

35. Comstock CH. Normal fetal heart axis and position. *Obstet Gynecol* 1987;70:255–259.

36. Brown DL, Cartier MS, Emerson DS, et al. The peripheral hypoechoic rim of the fetal heart. *J Ultrasound Med* 1989;8:603–608.

37. Levy DW, Mintz MC. The left ventricular echogenic focus: a normal finding. *AJR Am J Roentgenol* 1988;150:85–86.

38. Petrikovsky BM, Challenger M, Wyse LJ. Natural history of echogenic foci within ventricles of the fetal heart. *Ultrasound Obstet Gynecol* 1995;5:92–94.

39. Bromley B, Estroff JA, Sanders SP. Fetal echocardiography: accuracy and limitations in a population at high and low risk for heart defects. *Am J Obstet Gynecol* 1992;166:1473–1481.

40. DeVore GR. The aortic and pulmonary outflow tract screening examination in the human fetus. *J Ultrasound Med* 1992;11:345–348.

41. DeVore GR. Color Doppler examination of the outflow tracts of the fetal heart: a technique for identification of cardiovascular malformations. *Ultrasound Obstet Gynecol* 1994;4:463–471.

42. Vintzileos AM, Neckles S, Campbell WA, et al. Fetal liver ultrasound measurements during normal pregnancy. *Obstet Gynecol* 1985;66:477–480.

43. Schmidt W, Yarkoni S, Jeanty P, et al. Sonographic measurements of the fetal spleen: clinical implications. *J Ultrasound Med* 1985;4:667–672.

44. Hata K, Aoki S, Hata T, et al. Ultrasonographic identification of the human fetal gall bladder in utero. *Gynecol Obstet Invest* 1987;23:79–83.

45. Rosenberg ER, Bowie JD, Andreotti RF, et al. Sonographic evaluation of the fetal adrenal glands. *AJR Am J Roentgenol* 1982;139:1145–1147.

46. Nyberg DA, Mack LA, Pattern RM, et al. Fetal bowel: normal sonographic findings. *J Ultrasound Med* 1987;6:3–6.

47. Parulekar SG. Sonography of normal fetal bowel. *J Ultrasound Med* 1991;10:211–220.

48. Hadlock FP, Harrist RB, Deter RJ, et al. Fetal abdominal circumference as a predictor of menstrual age. *AJR Am J Roentgenol* 1982;139:367–370.

49. Millener PB, Anderson NG, Chisholm RJ. Prognostic significance of non-visualization of the fetal stomach by sonography. *AJR Am J Roentgenol* 1993;160:827–830.

50. Pretorius DH, Gosink BB, Clautice-Engle T, et al. Sonographic evaluation of the fetal stomach: significance of non-visualization. *AJR Am J Roentgenol* 1988;151:987–989.

51. Vincoff NS, Callen PW, Smith-Bindman R, Goldstein RB. Effect of ultrasound transducer frequency on the appearance of the fetal bowel. *J Ultrasound Med* 1999;18(12):799–803.

52. Fakhry J, Reiser M, Shapiro LR, et al. Increased echogenicity in the lower fetal abdomen: a common normal variant in the second trimester. *J Ultrasound Med* 1986;5:489–492.

53. Mandell J, Blyth BR, Peters CA, et al. Structural genitourinary defects detected in utero. *Radiology* 1991;178:193–196.

54. Cohen HL, Cooper J, Eisenberg P, et al. Normal length of fetal kidneys: sonographic study in 397 obstetric patients. *AJR Am J Roentgenol* 1991;157:545–548.

55. Grannum P, Bracken M, Silverman R, et al. Assessment of fetal kidney size in normal gestation by comparison of ratio of kidney circumference to abdominal circumference. *Am J Obstet Gynecol* 1980;136:249–254.

56. Bowie JD, Rosenberg ER, Andreotti MD, et al. The changing sonographic appearance of fetal kidneys during pregnancy. *J Ultrasound Med* 1983;2:505–507.

57. Lawson TL, Foley WD, Berland LL, et al. Ultrasonic evaluation of fetal kidneys: analysis of normal size and frequency of visualization as related to stage of pregnancy. *Radiology* 1981;138:153–156.

58. Anderson N, Clautice-Engle T, Allan R, et al. Detection of obstructive uropathy in the fetus: predictive value of sonographic measurements of renal pelvic diameter at various gestational ages. *AJR Am J Roentgenol* 1995;164:719–723.

59. Corteville JE, Gray DL, Crane JP. Congenital hydronephrosis: correlation of fetal ultrasonographic findings with infant outcome. *Am J Obstet Gynecol* 1991;165:384–388.

60. Hadlock FP, Harrist RB, Deter RJ, et al. Fetal femur length as a predictor of menstrual age: sonographically measured. *AJR Am J Roentgenol* 1982;138:875–878.

61. Abrams SL, Filly RA. Curvature of the fetal femur: a normal sonographic finding. *Radiology* 1985;156:490.

62. Goldstein RB, Filly RA, Simpson G. Pitfalls in femur length measurements. *J Ultrasound Med* 1987;6:203–207.

63. Lessoway VA, Schulzer M, Wittmann BK. Sonographic measurement of the fetal femur: factors affecting accuracy. *J Clin Ultrasound* 1990;18:471–476.

64. Mahony BS, Filly RA. High resolution sonographic assessment of the fetal extremities. *J Ultrasound Med* 1984;3:489–498.

65. Goldstein I, Reece A, Hobbins JC. Sonographic appearance of the fetal heel ossification centers and foot length measurements provide independent markers for gestational age assessment. *Am J Obstet Gynecol* 1988;159:923–926.

66. Mercer BM, Sklar S, Shariatmadar A. Fetal foot length as a predictor of gestational age. *Am J Obstet Gynecol* 1987;156:350–355.

2

GROWTH, DOPPLER, AND FETAL ASSESSMENT

This chapter discusses sonographic evaluation of normal and abnormal fetal growth and fetal Doppler as well as other methods of fetal assessment. Because assessment of growth first requires establishing the correct gestational age (GA), methods of dating the pregnancy are initially discussed. These two tasks—establishing correct GA and assessing fetal growth—should be considered separately although the same biometric measurements may be used for both.

The gestational period is characterized by extraordinary fetal growth (Fig. 1). During the first trimester, the embryo grows approximately 1 mm per day. Fetal length continues in a predictable way, growing approximately 0.5 cm per week throughout pregnancy. By the end of the first half of pregnancy, the fetus is about one-half its eventual length but only about one-seventh of its ultimate weight. The fetus adds much of its weight during the third trimester of pregnancy, adding approximately 0.5 lb per week during the third trimester. At term, fetuses are relatively standard in length: the mean length is 51 cm (20 in.), with more than 95% of infants falling within 10% of the mean.[1] On the other hand, normal birth weight (BW) is much more variable at term. Variability in newborn weight is reflected more by variations in girth than in length.

SONOGRAPHIC DATING AND ASSESSMENT OF FETAL GROWTH

Dating

Accurate dating of the pregnancy is a cornerstone of obstetrical management of both normal and abnormal pregnancies. Dating by menstrual history is often unreliable. Up to 40% of women are not certain of their menstrual dates, and, even when they are certain, their wide distribution tends to overestimate GA when compared with ultrasound (US).[2] Overestimation of GA reflects a preponderance of misdated pregnancies owing to delayed ovulation in the conception cycle.

Overestimation of true GA by menstrual history results in an underestimate of the rate of preterm deliveries[3] and an overestimate of postdated pregnancies. In a routinely scan-dated population, Gardosi et al.[4] found that 72% of inductions carried out for postterm pregnancy (more than 294 days) calculated according to menstrual dates were not actually postterm according to US dating.

US has proved better than calculations based on the menstrual dates for both systematic and random errors of measurement. Systematic errors relate to the modal length of gestation, which is based on 283 days by the last menstrual period and 281 days by routine second trimester US using different dating formulas.[5] A study of the basal body temperature shift in 1,408 conception cycles also concluded that the average gestation of term pregnancies is 281 days.[6] This systematic error is important to consider in the decision of elective delivery for fetal or maternal disease.

Random error assesses how consistently the measure is performing within the population. US error appears to have a normal distribution and a narrow error margin. Studies in assisted conception pregnancies showed random errors of 2.4 and 3.8 days standard deviation (SD) for femur length (FL) and head circumference (HC), respectively.[7,8]

Comparative studies in large data sets revealed considerable discrepancies between even certain menstrual dates and US dates based on a scan in the first half of the pregnancy.[9–11] US dates are also better able to predict the date of delivery than menstrual dates alone or when adjusted to US dates according to 7-, 10-, or 14-day "rules."[12]

Although many embryonic and fetal structures can be measured, only a few measurements have proved to be necessary for assessment of dates and evaluation of fetal growth. In general, the earlier the US is performed, the more accurate the assessment of dates. This is logical because all fetuses begin at the same size yet may vary dramatically in size by term. The earlier the embryo/fetus can be measured, the more accurate the dating. Dating during the second trimester is also reliable because acceleration of normal fetal growth does not begin until the third trimester. Dating during the third trimester is less predictive because of differences in fetal growth and should be avoided.

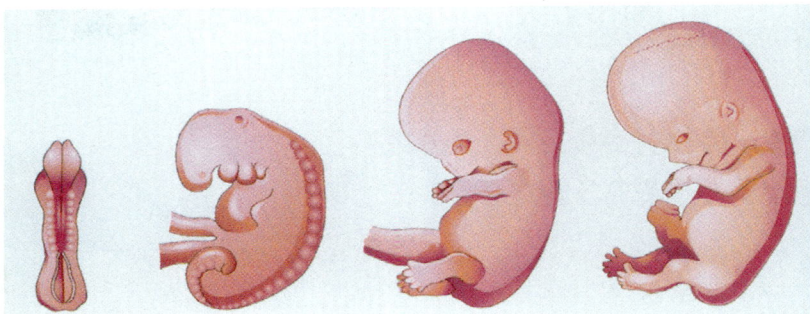

FIGURE 1. Rapid fetal growth and embryonic development occur between 6 and 10 weeks gestational age. The fetus continues to rapidly grow in size and length throughout pregnancy. (Reproduced with permission from Moore KL, Persaud TVN. *The developing human: clinically oriented embryology*, 6th ed. Philadelphia: WB Saunders, 1998.)

First Trimester

Dating by US in the first half of pregnancy has become a routine part of antenatal care in many institutions around the world. The first half of gestation is a period of rapid cell division, and GA is by far the strongest variable affecting fetal size in singletons as well as in multiple pregnancies.

Before 6 weeks, dating can be done by description and measurements of the gestational sac.[13] The gestational sac is visible at 4.5 weeks, and the yolk sac is present in 95% of the cases at 5 weeks and in nearly all cases by 6 weeks. Fetal heart is seen beating in 86% of the cases by 6 weeks and always by 7 weeks. The size of the gestational sac can be correlated to GA (Appendix 1, Tables 1 and 2).[14]

Among all measurements, maximum embryo's length at 6 to 10 weeks and crown rump length (CRL) measurement up to 14 weeks are the most accurate at determining GA (Fig. 2). The random error is in the range of 4 to 8 days SD at the ninety-fifth percentile.[15–20] The largest study using a strict methodology is that of Wisser et al.[20] The authors highlight potential pitfalls of previous studies and show a predictivity interval of 4.7 days SD on 160 *in vitro* fertilization patients, including 21 multiple pregnancies.

The technique may vary slightly, however the maximal embryo/fetal length is usually measured excluding the inferior limbs and without any correction of the body's flexion (Fig. 2). All the charts are concordant before 60 mm (predictivity interval of 3 days SD) but differ significantly thereafter.

To change the dates is questionable if the discrepancy between the last menstrual period and CRL measurement is less than 7 days. A discrepancy of more than 1 week suggests inaccurate menstrual dates. However, one study revealed a higher risk of preterm delivery in this patient group; 23% of women delivered before 37 weeks by spontaneous or iatrogenic delivery.[21]

Second and Third Trimesters

When the CRL is more than 60 mm, other biometric parameters have proven useful for dating the pregnancy optimally up to 20 weeks.[22] These other biometric parameters routinely include head measurements of biparietal diameter (BPD),

HC, FL, and abdominal circumference (AC). Normal values of the HC, FL, and AC are shown in Figure 3. The humerus length is also frequently obtained during the second trimester. Virtually any other bone or organ can be measured and compared with GA. Transcerebellar diameter in millimeters provides an accurate estimate of GA in weeks up to 30 mm for 25 weeks and becomes less accurate thereafter.[23]

Clavicles have a linear growth throughout the second and third trimesters also expressing GA in weeks when measured in mm.[24] Normal values are included in Appendix 1, Table 20.

Up to 18 weeks of gestation, the best predictive interval is given by the HC (7 days SD) whereas BPD, FL, and AC are less accurate (8 days SD).[25] Among standard measurements, AC is the most variable whereas bony measurements are the most reliable. Interobserver variation increases with GA and maternal size, reflected by the thickness of the anterior abdominal wall.[26]

Head Measurements

The BPD and HC reflect head size, which in turn reflects brain growth. Although head measurements primarily reflect the calcified calvaria, they are subject to variation based on compression of the calvaria.

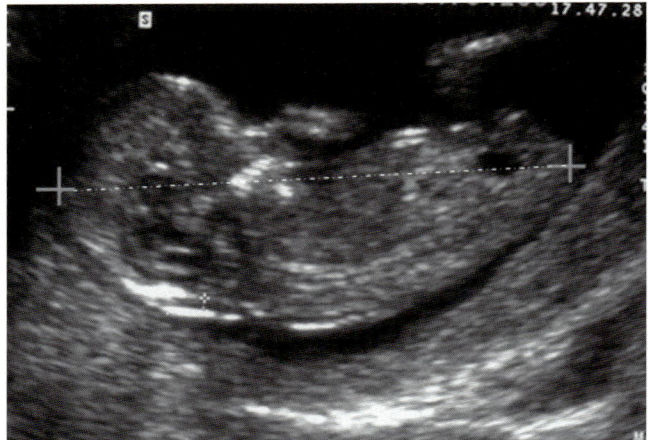

FIGURE 2. Crown-rump length measurement is an accurate dating method during the first trimester.

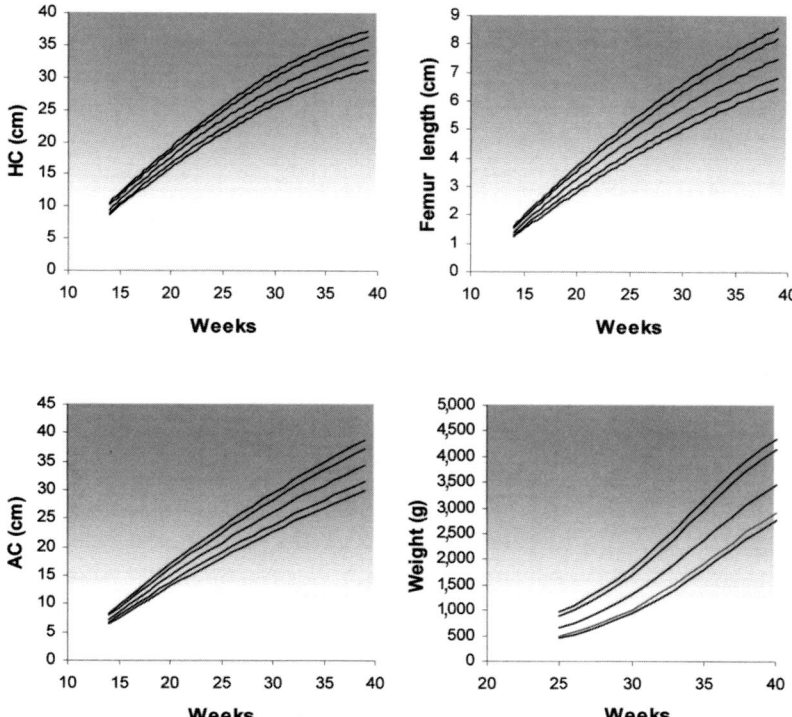

FIGURE 3. Normal fetal biometric charts. Range of head circumference (HC), femur length, and abdominal circumference (AC) measurements are shown between 14 and 40 weeks. Lines represent the third, tenth, fiftieth, ninetieth, and ninety-seventh percentiles. Range of fetal weight percentiles **(lower right)** illustrate the fifth, tenth, fiftieth, ninetieth, and ninety-fifth percentiles. (Data for HC, femur length, and AC measurements adapted from Hadlock FP, Deter RL, Harrist RB, et al. Estimating fetal age: computer-assisted analysis of multiple fetal growth parameters. *Radiology* 1984;152:497–501. Data for weight percentiles adapted from Doubilet PM, Benson CB, Nadel AS, et al. Improved birth weight table for neonates developed from gestations dated by early ultrasonography. *J Ultrasound Med* 1997;16:241–249.)

BPD and HC can be reliably measured from 13 weeks of gestation, when ossification of the parietal bones of the skull has occurred. BPD can be measured at the level of a plane defined by the frontal horns of the lateral ventricles and the cavum septi pellucidi anteriorly, the thalami and third ventricle centrally, and the occipital horns of the lateral ventricles, the sylvian fissure, the cisterna magna, and the insula posteriorly. Calipers should be placed where the skull is broader using a gain set up so that the thickness of the parietal bones is less than 3 mm. The measurement is taken from the outer table of the proximal skull with the cranial bones perpendicular to the US beam to the inner table of the distal skull (Fig. 4). The occipitofrontal diameter (OFD) is measured in the same plane as the BPD with the calipers placed on the outer skull table. The HC can be either directly measured or can be calculated from the BPD and OFD [HC = (BPD + OFD) × 1.57]. The direct method is less than 2% bigger than the calculated measurement. Fetal head shape variations (e.g., dolichocephaly, brachycephaly) and fetal position can affect head measurements, particularly the BPD in which case the HC is preferable. Normal measurements of the HC are shown in Figure 4 and are summarized in Appendix 1, Table 8.

Long Bone Measurements

FL is the most commonly obtained long bone measurement and is reproducibly measured from 13 weeks onward, although humerus length is also commonly obtained. FL is measured from the origin of the distal end of the shaft, from the greater trochanter to the lateral condyle. Femoral

diaphysis should be horizontal showing a homogeneous echogenicity (Fig. 5). The femoral head and distal epiphysis are not included in the measurement and this should be checked for in the methodology of the normal ranges used. Long bone measurements are purely "bony" in nature, and so tend to accurately reflect GA. The femur grows 3 mm per week from 14 to 27 weeks and 1 mm per week in the third trimester. Reported accuracy for pregnancy dating ranges from 1 week in the second trimester to 3 to 4 weeks at term.[24]

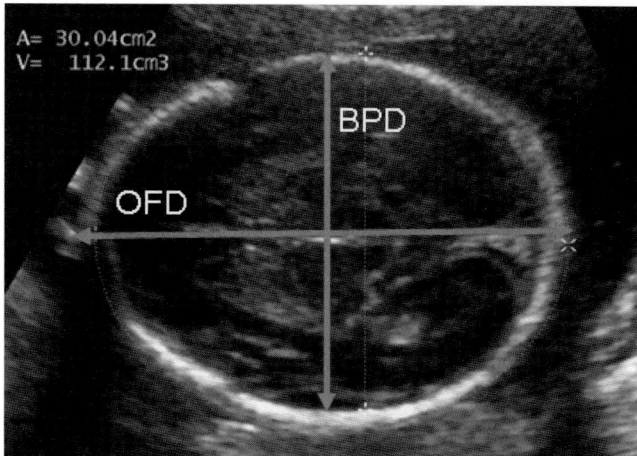

FIGURE 4. Cranial measurements. Normal measurements of the biparietal diameter (*BPD*) and occipitofrontal diameter (*OFD*) are shown. The head circumference can be measured directly or calculated from these two measurements.

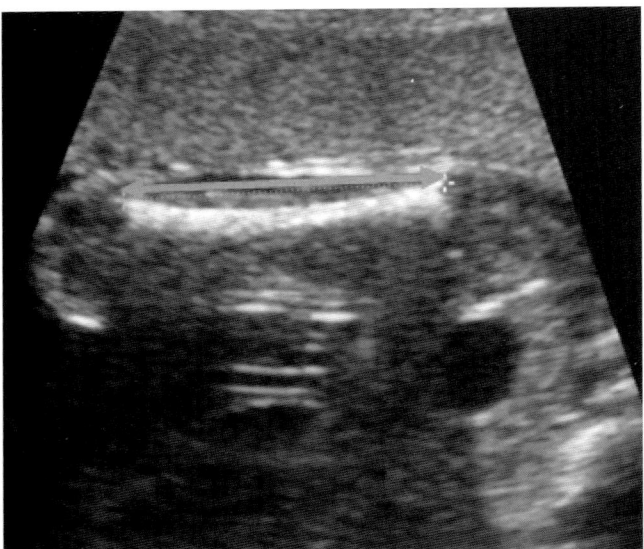

FIGURE 5. Femur length. Normal measurement of the femur length is shown.

Abdominal Circumference

The AC is a measure of fetal girth. It includes soft tissues of the abdominal wall as well as a measure of internal organs, primarily the liver. Unlike other commonly used fetal measurements, it is not influenced by bone. Not surprisingly, then, the AC is the single most sensitive measure of fetal growth.[27–29] Therefore, accurate and consistent measurement of the AC is particularly important whenever growth disturbances are suspected. Ensuring an accurate measure-

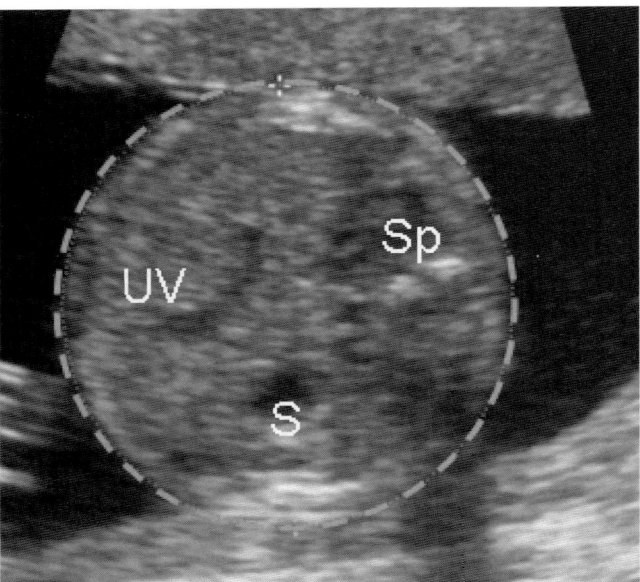

FIGURE 6. Abdominal circumference. Normal measurement of the abdominal circumference is shown. S, stomach; Sp, spine; UV, umbilical vein.

ment of the AC rather than adding other measurements of biometry is worthwhile.

The AC is measured on an axial plane at the level of the stomach and the bifurcation of the main portal vein into the right and left branches taking care of having a section as round as possible, not deformed by the pressure of the probe (Fig. 6). The most accurate is usually the smallest measurement obtained, as it should best approximate a perpendicular plane to the spine at the level of the hepatic vein. Ribs should show a symmetric covering of the AC contours.

Abdominal circumference measurements demonstrate linear growth with a mean of 11 to 12 mm per week throughout gestation (Fig. 6, Appendix 1, Table 7).[24]

Normal Fetal Growth

Sonographic assessment of growth is an important part of evaluating overall fetal wellness. Normal growth is influenced by genetic predisposition, parental influence, ethnic differences,[30] environment (e.g., altitude), and fetal gender. Despite these variables, fetal growth is relatively predictable, particularly during the first half of pregnancy.

An overall assessment of fetal size is possible by estimating fetal weight from US biometry. Numerous formulas for estimating fetal weight have been described and used.[31–33] Some formulas use head measurements and AC, others use long bone measurements and AC, and others use all four measurements. The AC is included in all commonly used formulas of estimated fetal weight (EFW), and AC also strongly influences fetal weight estimates.[34] Weight estimates based on AC alone have been reported.[35,36] Weight estimates based on other parameters, such as thigh circumference and soft tissues, have also been proposed, although these methods have not been found to be more accurate than standard biometry. Three-dimensional US assessment of normal fetal growth has also been performed.[37]

Weight formulas that include BPD, HC, AC, and FL result in a mean absolute error of around 10%.[38,39] Fetal weight formulas by Hadlock,[25] Dudley,[32] Coombs,[33] and Rose[40] seem to be the most accurate to estimate fetal weight in premature babies[41] and are often based on volumetric models. Some formulas have been specifically designed for premature babies.[42,43]

Once sonographic measurements are obtained and fetal weight is estimated, assessment of fetal growth is a simple matter of comparing the sonographic measurements to the expected size for GA. Comparison of EFW with expected weight is the best overall measure of fetal growth. When compared against standardized curves, the weight percentile can then be derived (Fig. 3 and Table 1). These expected weight standards have been generated either by weighing babies at birth or using sonographic estimates of fetal weight.[44]

Earlier weight charts showed a false flattening of BW curves at term in contrast to curves derived from US-based

TABLE 1. FETAL WEIGHT PERCENTILES

	Percentiles						
Weeks	5th	10th	25th	50th	75th	90th	95th
25	450	490	564	660	772	889	968
26	523	568	652	760	885	1,016	1,103
27	609	660	754	875	1,015	1,160	1,257
28	707	765	870	1,005	1,162	1,322	1,430
29	820	884	1,003	1,153	1,327	1,504	1,623
30	947	1,020	1,151	1,319	1,511	1,706	1,836
31	1,090	1,171	1,317	1,502	1,713	1,928	2,070
32	1,249	1,338	1,499	1,702	1,933	2,167	2,321
33	1,422	1,519	1,696	1,918	2,169	2,421	2,587
34	1,608	1,714	1,906	2,146	2,416	2,687	2,865
35	1,804	1,919	2,125	2,383	2,671	2,959	3,148
36	2,006	2,129	2,349	2,622	2,927	3,230	3,428
37	2,210	2,340	2,572	2,859	3,177	3,493	3,698
38	2,409	2,544	2,786	3,083	3,412	3,736	3,947
39	2,595	2,735	2,984	3,288	3,622	3,952	4,164
40	2,762	2,904	3,155	3,462	3,798	4,127	4,340
41	2,900	3,042	3,293	3,597	3,930	4,254	4,462
42	3,002	3,142	3,388	3,685	4,008	4,322	4,523
43	2,061	3,195	3,432	3,717	4,026	4,324	4,515

Note: Gestational age was established by early sonogram instead of menstrual dates.
Data from Doubilet PM, Benson CB, Nadel AS, et al. Improved birth weight table for neonates developed from gestations dated by early ultrasonography. *J Ultrasound Med* 1997;16:241–249.

estimation of GA.[45] This can be explained by overestimation of GA based on the menstrual history. Another problem with BW charts based on BWs is that premature births or stillbirths tend to be small for GA (SGA).[46] More accurate neonatal charts have been derived from neonates with accurate US dating.[44,47]

Expected fetal weights vary between published series.[48] These differences, however, are difficult to compare because of the prevalence of small figures and the wide heterogeneity in ethnic composition, physical characteristics, and socioeconomic status of the populations studied. Limitations of such standards should be recognized and have been reviewed by Altmann and Chitty.[49]

In clinical practice, when abnormal growth is suspected, serial US estimates may be more helpful than a single point on the growth curve. Growth arrest in a high-risk fetus is an important sign of chronic fetal distress, and dynamic evaluation of fetal growth is generally admitted as being more relevant than the actual biometry when fetal measurements are below the tenth percentile. This is true irrespective of the methods used, including cross-sectional or longitudinal growth charts, customized growth charts, or predicted fetal growth. The optimal measurement interval in small fetuses to combine an acceptable technical error and useful clinical data seems to be around 10 days to overcome intra- and inter-observer variabilities.[50] However, longer time intervals more accurately reflect fetal growth in low-risk patients.[51]

Different methods of quantifying and expressing serial changes in fetal size have been described, including the use of conditional percentiles[52,53] (Fig. 7). The use of serial measurements as indicators of abnormal fetal growth and subsequent predictors of adverse perinatal outcome are limited,[54,55] and most studies have used reference ranges either based on or presented as cross-sectional data. Cross-sectional data is limited for quantification of fetal growth.[56] Standards based on serial measurements seem a more appropriate technique for quantifying fetal growth, as these serial measurements account for fetal size earlier in gestation, which is an important determinant of subsequent fetal growth and correct for the mathematical phenomenon of "regression towards the mean."[53,54] Re-doing measure-

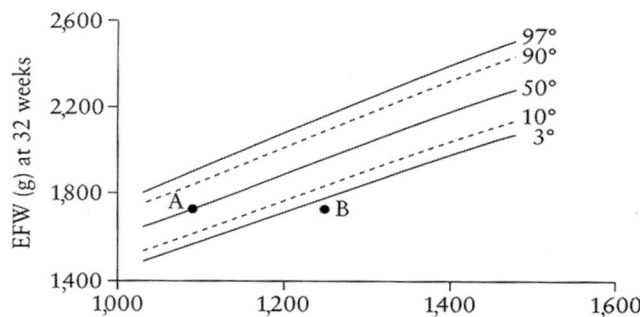

FIGURE 7. Illustration of conditional growth based on two ultrasound estimates of fetal weight (EFW) for two different fetuses (A and B). The second measurement is compared with the first to assess fetal growth. (Adapted from Owen P, Burton K, Ogston S, et al. Using unconditional and conditional standard deviation scores of fetal abdominal area measurements in the prediction of intrauterine growth restriction. *Ultrasound Obstet Gynecol* 2000;16:439–444.)

ments has proved moderately useful to predict infants with a low ponderal index using serial measurements of the AC, especially in late pregnancy.[55]

OTHER METHODS OF FETAL ASSESSMENT

Because fetal growth is only one measure of overall fetal health, other methods of fetal assessment are also discussed. These other methods include assessment of amniotic fluid (discussed in Chapter 3), Doppler studies, biophysical profile, and cardiotocography (i.e., electronic fetal monitoring). These methods may be used to assess fetal health in the setting of suspected growth disturbance, postdates, or maternal condition (e.g., hypertension or decreased fetal movements). Assessment of fetal growth is an integral part of fetal assessment in these situations. Indeed at postterm, small size for GA is the strongest risk factor for perinatal mortality.[57]

Amniotic Fluid Volume

Consideration of amniotic fluid volume is important whenever assessing fetal growth because, as a rough rule, amniotic fluid tends to reflect fetal size. Chronic fetal hypoxemia often produces oligohydramnios in addition to growth restriction, and this combination supports the diagnosis of intrauterine growth restriction (IUGR). Amniotic fluid can be normal in some cases of IUGR, although more often normal fluid indicates that the fetus is not compromised. Polyhydramnios is distinctly unusual in the setting of IUGR unless fetal anomalies are present. In contrast, polyhydramnios frequently accompanies a large-for-GA (LGA) fetus and adds confidence to that diagnosis. Normal amniotic fluid may also be present with an LGA fetus, although oligohydramnios is unusual (see Macrosomia).

Doppler Studies of Placental and Fetal Hemodynamics

To understand obstetric Doppler methods, it is important to first be aware of normal and adaptive circulations in the fetus.

Normal Circulation

The normal circulation of the fetus is remarkably different from that after birth because oxygenation takes place in the placenta rather than the lungs. Figure 8 illustrates the normal fetal circulation. The role of specific fetal "shunts" including foramen ovale, ductus venosus, and ductus arteriosus is of critical importance for normal brain and myocardial oxygenation. Oxygenated blood from the umbilical vein must pass through the foramen ovale to reach the ascending aorta without losing too much oxygen in the

hepatic circulation; around 40% of the total cardiac output contributes to this when the fetus is not hypoxic and when the placental resistances are normal.

The right ventricle is dominant *in utero*, contributing to 60% of the total cardiac output. The primary purpose of right ventricular outflow is to bring desaturated blood back to the placenta. This is made possible by the ductus arteriosus, which shunts much of the right ventricular output to the descending aorta. The right atrium plays an important role by directing desaturated blood from the superior vena cava and the coronary sinus through the tricuspid valve and to the right ventricle. In contrast, the inferior vena cava carries both desaturated blood from the iliac, hepatic, mesenteric, and hepatic circulations and oxygenated blood returning from the placenta through the ductus venosus. This oxygenated blood is preferentially shunted through the foramen ovale to the left atrium and left ventricle, owing to the direction and velocity of flow through the ductus venosus.

In basal conditions, more than 50% of the total umbilical vein output passes through the ductus venosus with an oxygen saturation of 83%. Oxygen saturation in the left atrium and ventricle is 73%, which is around 10% higher than in the right ventricle. This gradient can only be maintained because of the high pulmonary resistance, which receives only 13% of the right ventricular output. The remaining 87% of right ventricular outflow is directed through the ductus arteriosus and continues down the descending aorta. Two-thirds of aortic blood flow is pumped through the umbilical arteries to the placenta and one-third supplies various fetal organs.

Left ventricular output is pumped into the ascending aorta, allowing more oxygenated blood returning to the placenta to reach the fetal brain and myocardium. Approximately 70% of left ventricular outflow supplies the great vessels of the aortic arch; only 30% reaches the descending aorta, delivering 10% to the fetal organs and 20% to the placenta.

Partial oxygen pressure in fetal arterial blood is around 20 to 25 mm Hg. Fetal hemoglobin, however, has a higher affinity for oxygen than adult hemoglobin. Fetal oxygen requirements are low, as the oxygen costs for breathing and temperature adjustment are left to the mother. This allows for optimal oxygen capture at the placental level.

Adaptative Circulation

The fetal circulation is also remarkably adaptive in responding to hypoxia and preserving vital organs. Hypoxia can be of maternal (e.g., respiratory and cardiovascular diseases, high altitude), umbilical/placental (e.g., abruption, thrombosis, cord knots), or fetal (e.g., anemia) origin. Increasing cardiac output by increasing heart rate is of little help to the fetus in this situation. Rather, the distribution of oxygenated blood is altered to preferentially supply the

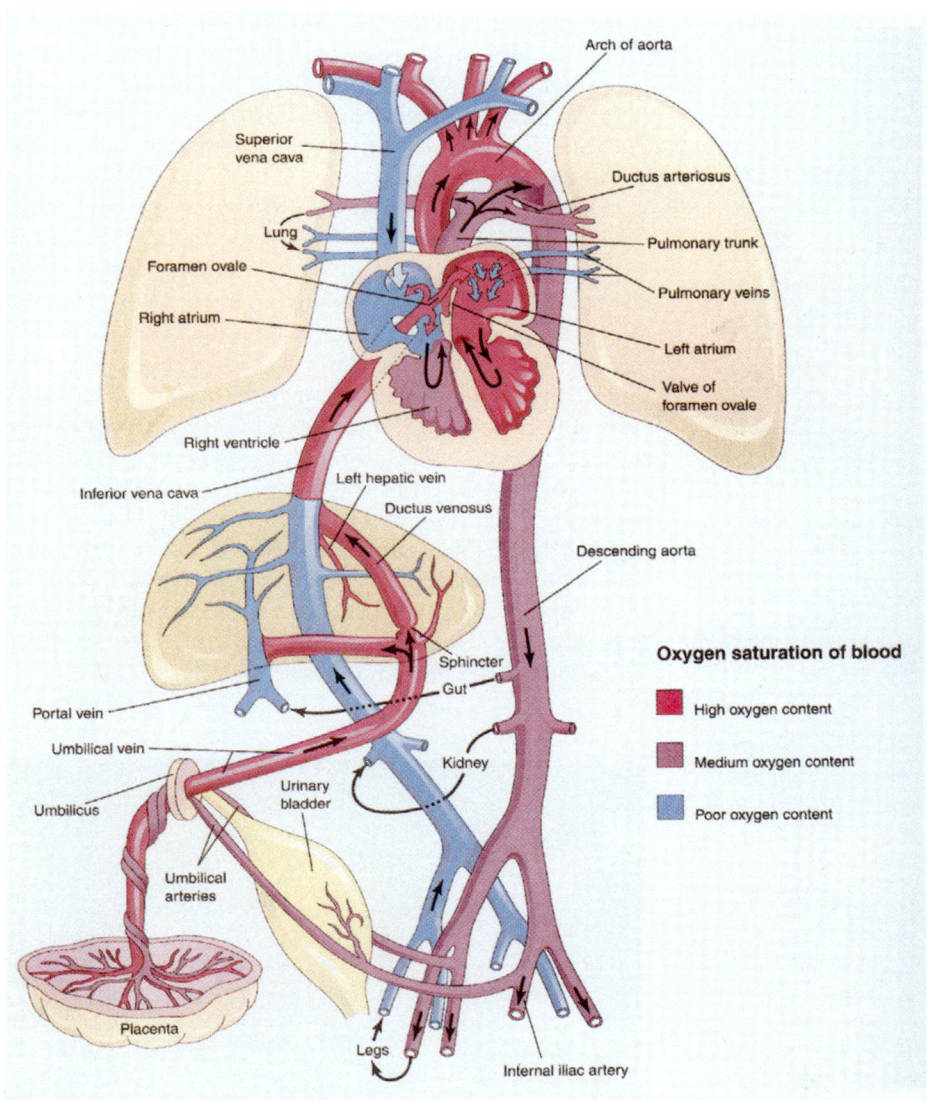

Oxygen saturation of blood

■ High oxygen content

■ Medium oxygen content

■ Poor oxygen content

FIGURE 8. Illustration of the normal fetal circulation. Specific fetal shunts include the foramen ovale, ductus venosus, and ductus arteriosus. These shunts are of critical importance for normal brain and myocardial oxygenation. (Reproduced with permission from Moore KL, Persaud TVN. *The developing human: clinically oriented embryology*, 6th ed. Philadelphia: WB Saunders, 1998.)

brain and heart. This phenomenon of "redistribution" or "centralization" has venous and arterial components.[58]

The venous redistribution is achieved by a larger part of the blood coming from the umbilical vein to enter the ductus venosus at the expense of the portal circulation to speed the oxygenated blood up to the heart. This is only possible because the ductus venosus has even lower resistance to flow that is oxygen mediated.

In response to hypoxia, arterial redistribution results from vasodilatation to cerebral and coronary arteries. Increased flow to the brain and myocardium come at the expense of decreased flow to other systemic arterial systems including the renal and mesenteric arteries. This is mediated by vasoconstriction. Thus, the consequences of fetal hypoxemia result in a "brain sparing" effect with more blood shunted toward the brain and away from other organs. This may produce other sonographic findings. For example, shunting of flow away from the kidneys produces smaller kidneys and

decreases urine production[59,60] although the relative proportion of the kidney to the abdomen may not be significantly different from normal. Shunting of blood away from the gut may result in hyperechoic bowel.

This redistribution and centralization phenomenon is a normal adaptive response to fetal hypoxemia and anemia. These dynamic circulatory changes can be detected and measured by Doppler methods for fetuses with growth restriction and fetal anemia.[61,62] Indeed in the former, there is little therapeutic alternative but to deliver a small and hypoxemic fetus while its vital and developmental potential are maintained, avoiding unnecessary iatrogenic preterm delivery. In the latter, noninvasive indicators of fetal anemia are useful in recognizing anemic fetuses and help in deciding on a diagnostic and therapeutic invasive procedure, avoiding subjecting nonanemic fetuses to the risk of procedure-related perinatal death.

Adaptive responses with cerebral redistribution do not mean neurologic dysfunction nor does it lead to neurologic

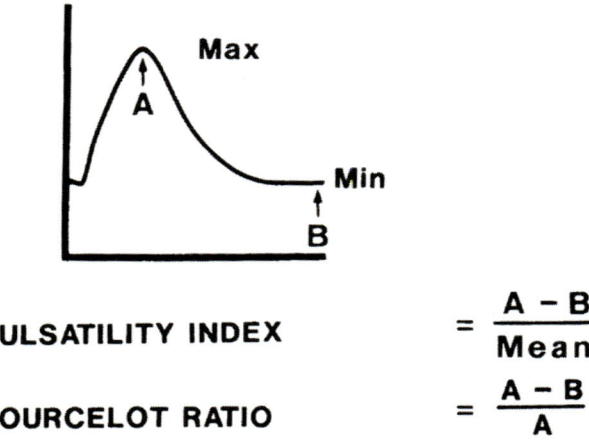

PULSATILITY INDEX $= \dfrac{A - B}{Mean}$

POURCELOT RATIO $= \dfrac{A - B}{A}$

SYSTOLIC/DIASTOLIC RATIO $= A/B$

FIGURE 9. Illustration of commonly used indices of Doppler waveform. (Reproduced with permission from Trudinger B. Doppler ultrasonography and fetal well-being. In: Reece EA, Hobbins JC, Mahoney MJ, Petrie RH, eds. *Medicine of the fetus and mother.* Philadelphia: JB Lippincott, 1992:704.)

impairment. In one series, Chan reported that this phenomenon was not predictive of long-term neurologic morbidity in 74 high-risk fetuses with growth restriction and Doppler evidence of cerebral redistribution.[63]

Doppler Studies

Doppler studies are not generally used to screen for IUGR, with the possible exception of uterine artery Doppler. Rather, Doppler studies provide greater specificity after identifying a fetus with suspected IUGR or fetal compromise. Although techniques such as Doppler velocimetry have improved the assessment of high-risk fetuses, the challenge that has not been adequately addressed is how to identify those pregnancies that need to be referred for investigation and closer surveillance.

Blood flow in arterial vessels, mainly the umbilical arteries, the middle cerebral artery (MCA), and the fetal thoracic descending aorta, can be assessed using various indices (Fig. 9). These indices include the systolic (S) to diastolic (D) ratio, pulsatility index (PI) (PI = S − D/Vm, where Vm is the mean of maximal velocities throughout the cardiac cycle), or resistive index (RI) (RI = S − D/S). The PI has the advantage of values even when the diastolic flow component is absent.

Impedance to flow into the ductus venosus or into the inferior vena cava can also be measured by calculating PI, referred to as PI for veins (PIV).[64]

Uterine Artery Doppler

Doppler US provides a noninvasive method for the study of the uteroplacental circulation. In normal pregnancy, impedance to flow in the uterine arteries decreases with gestation, which may be the consequence of trophoblastic invasion of the spiral arteries and their conversion into low-resistance vessels. Preeclampsia and IUGR are associated with failure of trophoblastic invasion of spiral arteries, and Doppler has then shown that impedance to flow in the uterine arteries is increased.

Doppler sampling can be performed at the level of the main uterine arteries at the level of the arcuate arteries[65] or as a combined approach of both sampling sites.[66] Color Doppler visualization of the uterine artery at the crossover with the external iliac artery is now the sampling site of choice. The normal waveform pattern shows a low resistance, high-flow pattern throughout diastole (Fig. 10A). The abnormal waveform patterns show high resistance and postsystolic notch (Fig. 10B).

GA at sampling is usually 16 to 20 weeks and 22 to 24 weeks in a one-stage or two-stage screening. High impedance to flow is generally assessed by RI or PI with cutoff values of 0.55 to 0.58 and 1.85, respectively, at these GAs. Early diastolic notch when bilateral is another and more stringent way of describing abnormal results. Notch quantification has not proven to be useful.

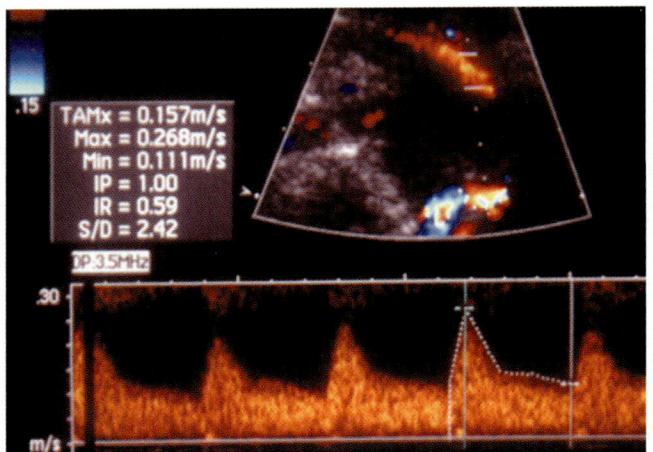

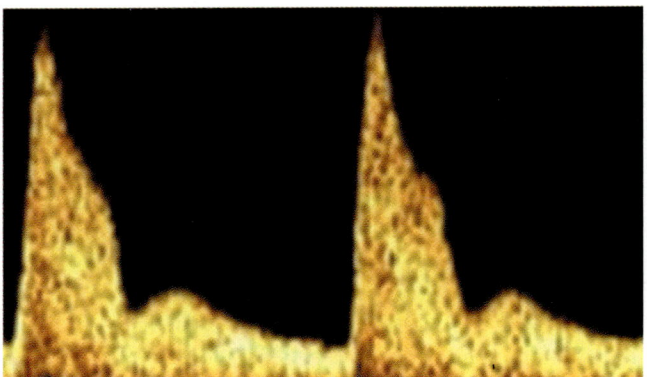

FIGURE 10. Uterine artery Doppler. **A:** Normal uterine artery Doppler sampled at the level of the crossover with the external iliac artery shows a normal flow pattern. **B:** Abnormal waveform shows high impedance to flow and postsystolic notch.

TABLE 2. SCREENING FOR INTRAUTERINE GROWTH RESTRICTION (LESS THAN THE FIFTH PERCENTILE) AND PREECLAMPSIA USING UTERINE ARTERY DOPPLER

Authors	Positive likelihood ratio	Test 95% confidence interval	Negative likelihood ratio	Test 95% confidence interval
Campbell et al.[65]	1.76	1.01–2.60	0.56	0.26–0.99
Hanretty et al.[210]	1.13	0.43–2.86	0.99	0.90–1.06
Steel et al.[75]	5.93	3.73–8.17	0.41	0.21–0.66
Bewley et al.[66]	5.08	2.69–9.03	0.80	0.64–0.91
Bower et al.[68]	5.19	4.17–6.14	0.29	0.18–0.45
Valensise et al.[69]	12.99	7.16–20.99	0.12	0.02–0.47
North et al.[70]	2.35	0.93–4.88	0.83	0.54–1.01
Harrington et al.[77]	11.79	8.84–15.28	0.24	0.14–0.40
Irion et al.[72]	2.14	1.19–3.51	0.84	0.66–0.97
Frusca et al.[78]	6.42	2.62–11.71	0.54	0.23–0.85
Kurdi et al.[73]	5.51	3.52–7.59	0.43	0.23–0.67
Albaiges et al.[74]	7.63	5.38–10.42	0.59	0.46–0.71
Pooled likelihood ratio	4.89	4.33–5.48	0.55	0.50–0.61

A series of screening studies involving assessment of impedance to flow in the uterine arteries have examined the potential value of Doppler in identifying pregnancies at risk of the complications of impaired placentation. Papageorgiou et al.[67] in a review article identified 15 studies[68–78] that followed a heterogeneous methodology. Nevertheless, the results of the overall analysis are that increased impedance to flow in the uterine arteries is associated with an increased risk of developing preeclampsia, IUGR, and perinatal death (Tables 2 and 3). In addition, women with normal impedance to flow in the uterine arteries constitute a group at low risk of developing such impaired placentation-related complications. Increased impedance to flow identified approximately 50% of pregnancies that will develop preeclampsia and around 30% of those that will develop IUGR subsequently. Abnormal Doppler is better at predicting severe rather than mild disease. The sensitivity for severe disease requiring premature delivery was approximately 80% for preeclampsia and 60% for IUGR. In the pooled data from all studies, the likelihood ratio for the subsequent delivery of a growth-restricted infant, occurrence of preeclampsia, and perinatal death in women with an abnormal result was 3.7, 5, and 2.4, respectively, and the likelihood ratio was 0.7, 0.5, and 0.8, respectively, for women with normal Doppler results. The incidence of complications varied from 2% to 24%; predictive values increased with the prevalence, and the false-positive rates decreased with gestation. Bilateral notches are found in 20% to 30% of pregnancies at 12 weeks, through to 10% to 20% at 16 weeks, around 10% at 20 to 22 weeks of gestation, and less than 5% at 23 to 24 weeks of gestation.[66]

Umbilical Artery Doppler

Decreased resistance to flow in the umbilical artery is normally seen between the fetal bladder and the placental cord insertion, and due to the reservoir effect of the placenta on impedance to flow along the umbilical cord. This will, however, remain within normal limits in normoxemic fetuses with normal placental resistance (Fig. 11A). The flow in the umbilical artery is a reflection of the placental resistance mainly and, to a certain extent, of the fetal systemic resistance. However, when the diastolic component is absent (Fig. 11B) or mainly reversed (Fig. 12), ominous fetal cardiac decompensation is likely.

Metaanalyses suggest a 36% to 50% decrease in perinatal mortality when considering one umbilical Doppler mea-

TABLE 3. STUDIES OF UTERINE ARTERY DOPPLER IN PREDICTING INTRAUTERINE GROWTH RESTRICTION LESS THAN THE FIFTH PERCENTILE

Authors	Positive likelihood ratio	Test 95% confidence interval	Negative likelihood ratio	Test 95% confidence interval
Hanretty et al.[210]	0.95	0.16–4.68	1	0.77–1.07
Steel et al.[75]	4.26	2.86–6.02	0.64	0.48–0.78
Bewley et al.[66]	3.84	1.74–7.67	0.84	0.66–0.96
Bower et al.[76]	3.22	2.52–4.01	0.63	0.52–0.74
Kurdi et al.[73]	3.41	2.26–4.90	0.71	0.56–0.84
Pooled likelihood ratio	3.38	2.82–4.00	0.71	0.65–0.77

Adapted from Papageorgiou AT, Cicero S, Yu CKH, et al. Screening for placental insufficiency by uterine artery Doppler. *Prenatal Neonatal Med* 2001;1:27–38.

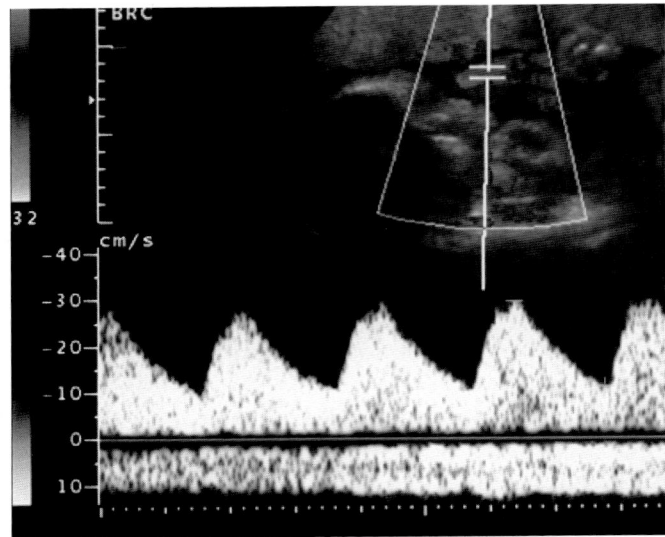

FIGURE 11. Umbilical artery Doppler waveform. **A:** Normal waveform pattern. The systolic to diastolic ratio is 2.6. **B:** Abnormal waveform pattern with absent diastolic flow (resistance index is 1.0).

surement in high-risk fetuses[79] as shown in Tables 4 and 5. This impressive effect of umbilical artery Doppler is mainly due to the high positive predictive value of absent/reversed end-diastolic flow on perinatal mortality (Table 5).[80] Absence, and especially reversal (Fig. 12), of end-diastolic flow of the umbilical artery Doppler is a worrisome finding associated with increased risk of perinatal and neonatal death as well as other complications (Table 5). Elevation of umbilical artery Doppler resistance with diastolic flow is less predictive. Normal values of umbilical artery Doppler are shown in Figure 13.

Fetal Thoracic Aorta Doppler

Recordings must be taken just above the fetal diaphragm with an insonation angle with the long axis of the aorta of less than 30 degrees. High PI correlates with fetal hypoxemia (Fig. 14). Doppler measurement in the descending fetal thoracic aorta seems to be a less effective screening procedure for fetal hypoxemia than umbilical artery Doppler, essentially because of the technical difficulty in getting reproducible results with an appropriate angle. However, evidence suggests that the fetal thoracic aorta Doppler better correlates with fetal blood gases.[81–83]

Middle Cerebral Artery Doppler

The easiest sampling site is at the level of the MCA along the sphenoid wing at the internal third of the vessel. Indeed, this vessel often presents with an ideal angle of insonation (Fig. 15). Special attention should be paid to not press on the transducer, which could result in a significant decrease in diastolic flow in the MCA.[84] PI in the MCA decreases with gestation[82] (Fig. 16). Doppler easily shows vascular redistribution. This redistribution includes a decrease in resistance to flow in the MCA together with an increase in resistance to flow in the fetal thoracic aorta. Ratios of PI in these vessels define and quantify redistribution with GA.[82]

TABLE 4. PERINATAL OUTCOME WITH ABSENT OR REVERSED END-DIASTOLIC FLOW IN UMBILICAL ARTERY DOPPLER

Outcome (n)	Doppler n (%)	Control n (%)	Odds ratio (confidence interval 95%)
Perinatal deaths (13)	75/4,512 (1.66)	123/4,602 (2.67)	0.64 (0.47; 0.86)[a]
Perinatal deaths excluding malformations (13)	57/4,512 (1.26)	97/4,602 (2.11)	0.62 (0.45; 0.86)[a]
Intrauterine deaths excluding lethal malformations (13)	23/4,512 (0.51)	45/4,602 (0.98)	0.54 (0.29; 0.91)[a]
Neonatal death excluding lethal malformations (13)	34/4,512 (0.75)	52/4,602 (1.13)	0.68 (0.40; 1.05)

n, number of trials.
[a]Odds ratio significantly different from 1 (*p* <.05).
Reproduced with permission from Goffinet F, Paris J, Nisand I, et al. Utilité clinique du Doppler ombilical: résultats des essais contrôlés en population à haut risque et à bas risque. *J Gynecol Obstet Biol Reprod* 1997;26:16–26.

TABLE 5. ASSOCIATIONS OF ABSENT AND REVERSED END-DIASTOLIC FLOW OF UMBILICAL ARTERY DOPPLER AND ADVERSE OUTCOME

Criteria	Positive end-diastolic flow (n = 214)	Absent end-diastolic flow (n = 178)	Reverse end-diastolic flow (n = 67)
Intrauterine death	3%	14%	24%
Neonatal death	1%	27%	51%
Birth weight	2,204 g	1,209 g	769 g
Transfer in neonatal intensive care unit	60%	96%	98%
Respiratory distress syndrome	3%	17%	41%
Intraventricular hemorrhage grade III or IV	1%	9%	35%

n, number of trials.
Adapted from Karsdorp VHM, Van Vugt JMG, Van Geijn HP, et al. Clinical significance of absent or reversed end diastolic velocity waveforms in umbilical artery. *Lancet* 1994;344:1664–1668.

The resistance pattern of the middle cerebral artery Doppler should always be greater than the umbilical artery Doppler resistance before birth. In the setting of fetal hypoxia, blood is preferentially shunted to the brain as the "brain sparing" adaptive response. A middle cerebral artery Doppler waveform showing less resistance (lower S/D ratio, PI, or RI) than the umbilical artery Doppler is the reverse of the normal relationship and is diagnostic of the brain sparing effect. Sterne et al.[85] found that this redistribution is associated with low birth weight and acidemia, and the severity of the abnormal Doppler pattern correlated with a shorter interval to delivery and the need for emergency delivery.

The middle cerebral artery Doppler may be more sensitive than umbilical artery Doppler for identifying fetuses at risk. Severi et al.[86] found that SGA fetuses with normal umbilical artery Doppler waveforms but abnormal uterine and middle cerebral artery waveforms have an increased risk of developing distress and being delivered by emergency cesarean section. Furthermore, abnormal velocimetry of the uterine and middle cerebral arteries was independently correlated with this risk.

Venous Doppler

Doppler examination of fetal veins is feasible and concerns mainly the ductus venosus and the inferior vena cava. The advantage of ductus venosus over the inferior vena cava in the assessment of IUGR fetuses is that the a wave in the ductus venosus gets reversed only in severely compromised fetuses, thus acting as a sign of ominous fetal demise.[61] Normal ranges for PI have been published.[86]

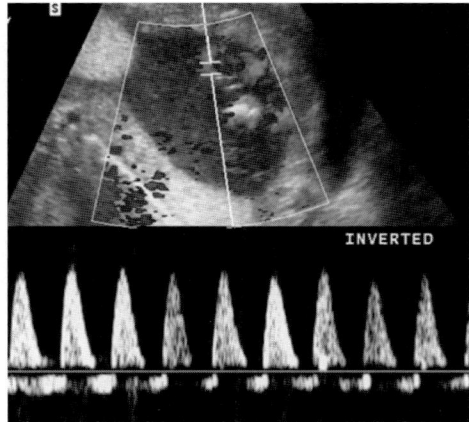

FIGURE 12. Umbilical artery Doppler shows reversal of diastolic signal, a worrisome finding associated with significant risk of perinatal and neonatal complications.

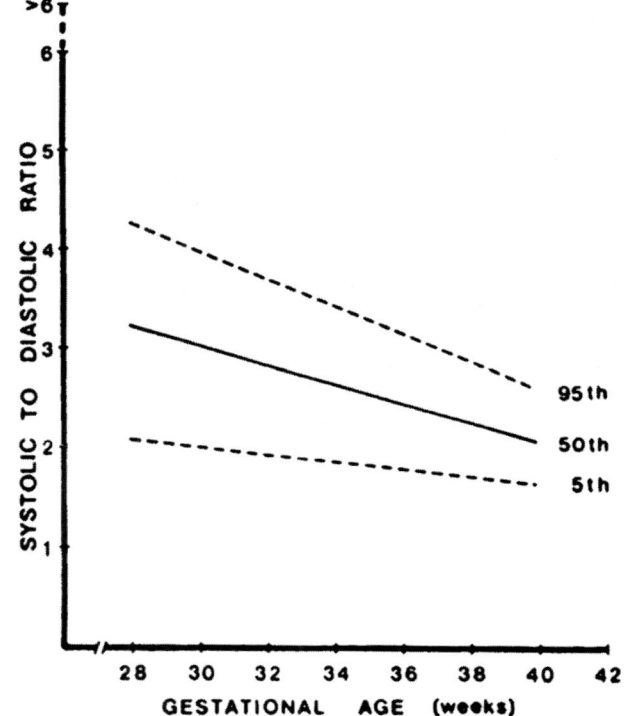

FIGURE 13. Normal systolic to diastolic ratio for umbilical artery Doppler from 28 to 42 weeks of gestation. (Adapted from Hendricks SK, Sorensen TK, Wang KY, et al. Doppler umbilical artery waveform indices—normal values from fourteen to forty-two weeks. *Am J Obstet Gynecol* 1989;161:761–765.)

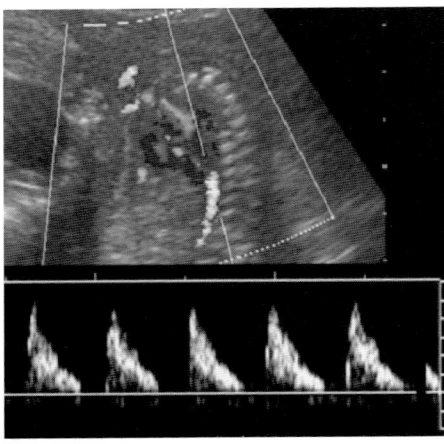

FIGURE 14. Abnormal thoracic Doppler waveforms show absent diastolic flow.

The ductus venosus can be identified with color flow imaging and duplex Doppler (Figs. 17 and 18). Imaging is performed either in sagittal or an oblique transverse section of the fetal abdomen to visualize the communication between the umbilical vein (i.e., portal sinus) and the inferior vena cava. Presence of characteristic high-velocity signals in the color Doppler mode ensures identification. Recording is taken in the inlet of the ductus venosus with an insonation angle as near to the long axis of the vessel as possible.[87]

Blood flow patterns merely reflect changes in pressure between the vessel and the right atrium throughout the cardiac cycle. Velocities, therefore, are maximal during ventricular systole (S wave) in relation with a rapid filling of the atria; the second peak (D wave) corresponds to the early ventricular diastole, and flow velocity is minimal during atrial contraction (A wave). As with fetal arteries, various indices can be used to describe the waveform pattern of the ductus venosus or other veins. These indices include the S/A ratio, the peak velocity index for veins [PVIV = (S − A)/D], and the PIV [PIV = (S − A)/time-averaged maximum velocity].

Various pathologic situations can influence the normal flow pattern:

1. A decrease in myocardial contractility, which can be seen in heart compression by pericardial or pleural effusion but also in subendocardial ischemia in severely acidotic fetuses
2. An increase in cardiac afterload, which can be seen with high placental resistance or in pulmonary stenosis with intact septum
3. An increase in cardiac preload, which impairs complete auricular emptying seen in hypervolemia in a recipient in twin-to-twin transfusion syndrome, and other situations with increased cardiac output

The potential role of ductus venosus Doppler, as well as Doppler of other sites, is discussed further in the Intrauterine Growth Restriction section.

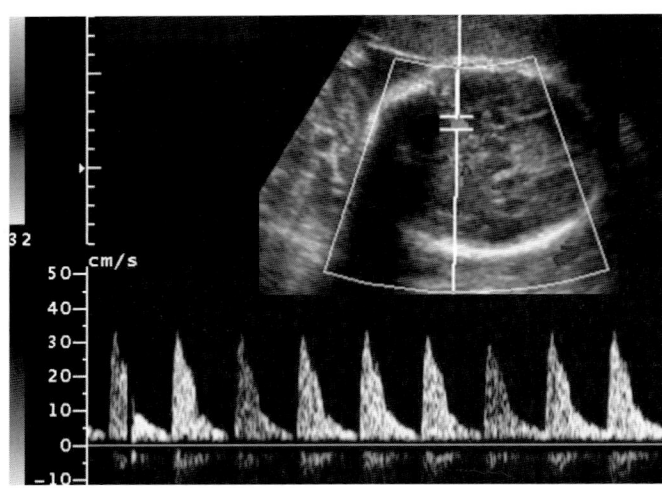

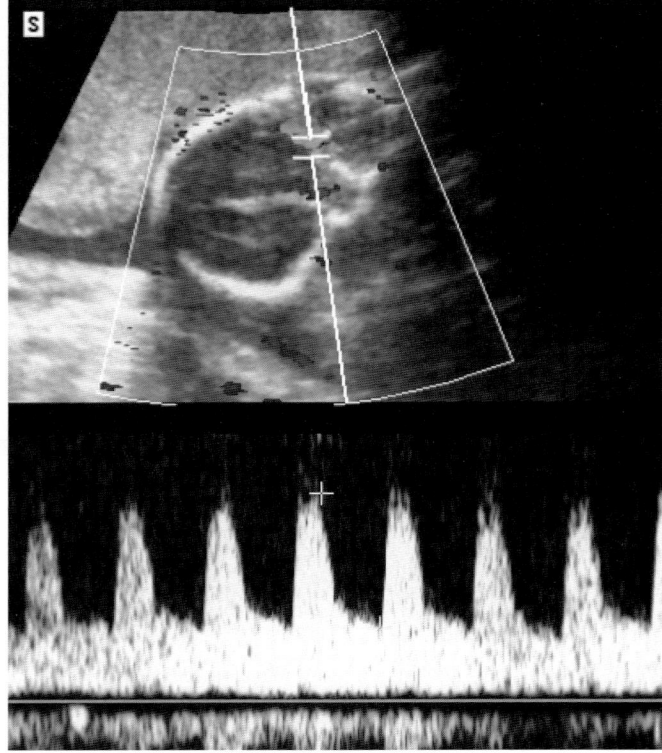

FIGURE 15. Middle cerebral artery Doppler waveforms. **A:** Normal waveform with high-resistance pattern. **B:** Abnormal waveform pattern with increased diastolic flow.

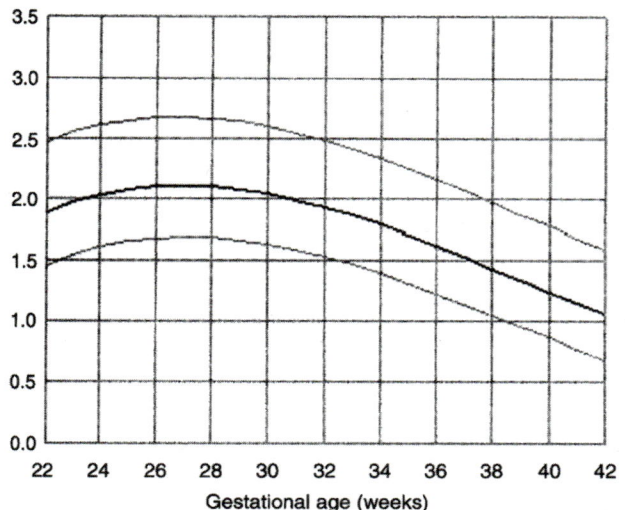

FIGURE 16. Reference range (mean, fifth, and ninety-fifth percentiles) for middle cerebral artery Doppler pulsatility index. (Reproduced with permission from Harrington K, Carpenter RG, Nguyen M, et al. Changes observed in Doppler studies of the fetal circulation in pregnancies complicated by pre-eclampsia or the delivery of a small-for-gestational-age baby. I. Cross-sectional analysis. *Ultrasound Obstet Gynecol* 1995;6:19–28.)

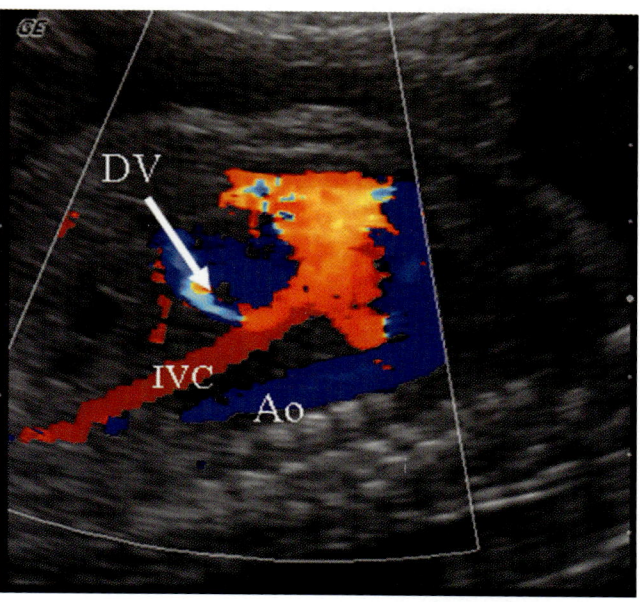

FIGURE 17. Normal ductus venosus. Color-flow imaging shows normal high-velocity jet of the ductus venosus (*DV*). Ao, aorta; IVC, inferior vena cava. (Courtesy of Martin Necas, New Zealand.)

Biophysical Profile

The biophysical profile attempts to test for fetal hypoxia. The oldest biophysical profile score was published by Manning et al.[88,89] and modified by Vintzileos et al.[90] as shown in Table 6. The complete biophysical profile includes electronic fetal monitoring (nonstress test or cardiotocography), although in clinical practice this is often considered separately. Amniotic

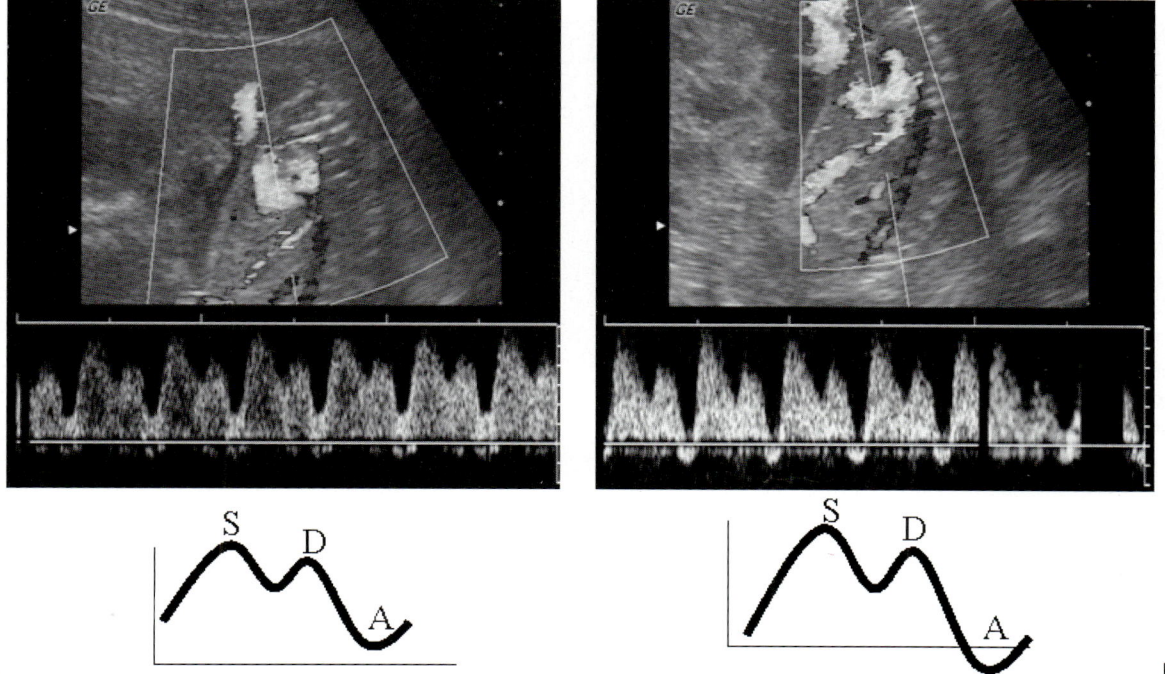

A   B

FIGURE 18. Ductus venosus flow patterns. **A:** Normal waveform pattern. Normal systole consists of two peaks, with the first corresponding to ventricular systole (*S*) and the second to ventricular diastole (*D*). Reduced velocity is observed during atrial diastole (*A*) but flow is always continuous, above the baseline. **B:** Abnormal waveform pattern with reversal of A wave.

TABLE 6. CRITERIA FOR BIOPHYSICAL PROFILE SCORE

Criteria	Conditions for a normal score (score = 2)[a] during a 30-min examination
Thoracic movements	At least one episode of at least 30 sec.
Active movements	At least three movements of fetal trunk or limbs.
Fetal tone	At least one episode of active extension and back inflexion of one limb, or one hand opening and closing.
Amniotic fluid volume	At least one vertical pool greater than 2 cm in two perpendicular planes.
Fetal monitor (cardiotocography)[a]	At least two accelerations (more than 15 beats per min and more than 15 sec) together with one fetal movement.

[a]May be combined with biophysical profile (10 points possible) or considered separately.
Adapted from Manning FA. Dynamic ultrasound-based fetal assessment: the fetal biophysical profile score. *Clin Obstet Gynecol* 1995;38:26–44.

fluid volume reflects chronic hypoxia, probably secondary to shunting of blood away from the kidneys, whereas the other components correlate with acute hypoxia.

A definite negative correlation exists between fetal hypoxemia and fetal movements. Cessation of movements follows a predictable sequence. Thoracic movements, inappropriately called *breathing movements*, disappear first, followed by the movements of fetal extremities, limb girdles, and finally fetal trunk and spine; the latter being best correlated with fetal acidemia.[91] These movements, however, can also be decreased after antenatal corticosteroids administration for fetal lung maturation.[92]

The minimal examination time for a suspicious or abnormal score is 30 minutes. A low biophysical profile score is strongly predictive of intrauterine death within a week. Its recognition helped reduce perinatal mortality from 7.7% to 1.9% in one high-risk population, with a low false-negative rate of less than 1% and a strong negative correlation with the occurrence of fetal distress in labor.[88,89] However, owing to the influence of antenatal steroids,[92] this becomes very time-consuming to repeat the assessment once the score is dubious or abnormal.

Two randomized studies compared biophysical profile score and fetal cardiotocography in the prediction of perinatal mortality and fetal distress; neither of them could show a benefit to biophysical profile score, even when both studies were analyzed within a metaanalysis.[93] However, neither of these studies considered the value of Doppler, GA, or BW. The combined experience suggests that although the biophysical profile is helpful in some settings, it should be correlated with other methods of fetal assessment when deciding the time of delivery.

Fetal Cardiotocography

Fetal cardiotocography (i.e., nonstress test) may be included in a biophysical profile score or considered separately. Car-

diac reactivity as defined by having at least one acceleration over 5 bpm for 30 seconds in 20 minutes is a rough component of fetal biophysical activity. The occurrence of late decelerations in high-risk fetuses is a sign of severe distress. The high-risk fetuses should benefit from computerized cardiotocographic assessment.[94] The best parameter to be monitored is the short-term variability, which is closely related to fetal hypoxemia when it falls below 3 milliseconds. However, false-positive results have been reported with antenatal corticosteroids administration for fetal lung maturation for a mean of 3 days following the first injection, whereas Doppler results were unchanged.[95]

ABNORMAL GROWTH

Abnormal growth may represent subnormal growth (i.e., growth restriction) or abnormally accelerated growth. Of the two, growth restriction is more strongly related to fetal abnormalities and adverse outcome. Various chromosome abnormalities and even abnormalities confined to the placenta (e.g., confined placental mosaicism) may exhibit delayed growth as a prominent feature. Abnormal growth and development have also been associated with disturbed genomic imprinting (i.e., expression of genes depending on whether they are located on the maternal or on the paternal chromosome). This association has led to the suggestion that the genomic imprinting has evolved as a mechanism to regulate embryonic and fetal growth.[96]

Various metabolic analytes have been associated with normal and abnormal fetal growth. Of these, the association between fetal leptin concentrations and fetal weight appear to be the strongest.[97]

Intrauterine Growth Restriction

Definition

The description *small for gestational age* is commonly used for all fetuses that are small. SGA fetuses represent a heterogeneous group of normal and *growth-restricted* fetuses. Although IUGR has also been defined by fetal size, this definition is not satisfactory because many small fetuses are not restricted at all, but rather have reached their full growth potential. For this reason, the term IUGR is appropriately applied to fetuses that are SGA and that show other evidence of chronic hypoxia or malnutrition. The terms SGA and IUGR, nevertheless, are frequently used interchangeably.

The most common definition of SGA is a fetus whose weight is below the tenth percentile for GA. This definition, however, is not universally accepted. Some authors may define it as fetal weight below the fifth or third percentile; AC below the tenth, fifth, or third percentile; or lack of normal growth of the AC on serial examinations. Others may categorize growth disturbance based on absolute weight at birth, such as less than 2,500 g or less than 1,500 g. However, this obscures the distinction between smallness owing to prematurity and that owing to growth restriction.

Risk Factors

Causes and associations for IUGR are shown in Table 7. Once underlying fetal anomaly or aneuploidy is excluded, the most common associations are with maternal hypertension and a history of IUGR in previous pregnancies. Conversely, a history of SGA fetuses is a risk factor for preeclampsia.[98] Fetus size also tends to reflect maternal and paternal BWs. Magnus et al.[99] found the mean maternal BW was significantly less among those who had experienced two SGA births compared to those with no SGA births (3,127 ± 54 g vs. 3,424 ± 22 g). Interestingly, the mean paternal BW was also lower (3,497 ± 88 g vs. 3,665 ± 24 g) from affected pregnancies with two SGA births.

Pathology

A variety of biochemical abnormalities have been associated with SGA fetuses. The abnormalities include lower mean glucose and cholesterol ester concentrations,[100] higher nitrous oxide and total nitrite levels in fetal plasma,[101] and higher serum levels of inhibin and human chorionic gonadotropin.[102] Other studies have found alterations in parathyroid hormone–related protein,[103] prothrombin gene mutation,[104] insulin-like growth factor-I, placental growth hormone,[105] and leptin.[97]

Underlying uterine-placental dysfunction is a commonly evoked cause for otherwise unexplained fetal IUGR. Uterine-placental dysfunction has been correlated with a range of pathologic findings, including smaller placentas, increase in the thickness of tertiary-stem villi vessel wall, and decrease in lumen circumference. Also, confined placental mosaicism has been found to carry a higher risk of IUGR and adverse outcome including fetal death.[106] Uterine-placental dysfunction produces fetal hypoxia, which results in subnormal growth, oligohydramnios, and alterations in blood flow.[107]

Diagnosis

Clinical methods of diagnosis detect only approximately one-fourth of SGA (i.e., BW less than tenth percentile) babies, some of whom may be growth restricted.[108] The rate of detection is even lower (16%) for those pregnancies considered low risk.[109] Adjusting for maternal physiologic characteristics may improve the clinical performance of IUGR screening, for single as well as for serial assessments. This applies to US measurements[110] and the measurement of symphysis-fundus height.[111]

The strong association of growth restriction with stillbirth supports the need for early recognition of growth

TABLE 7. CAUSES AND ASSOCIATIONS WITH INTRAUTERINE GROWTH RESTRICTION

Maternal
Pregnancy-induced hypertension/preeclampsia
Severe chronic hypertension
Severe maternal diabetes mellitus
Collagen vascular disease
Heart disease
Smoking[209]
Poor nutrition
Renal disease
Lung disease/hypoxia
Environmental agents
Endocrine disorders
Previous history of intrauterine growth restriction
Uterine-placental
Uterine-placental dysfunction
Placental infarct
Chronic abruption
Multiple gestation/twin transfusion syndrome
Confined placental mosaicism
Fetal
Chromosome abnormalities
Confined placental mosaicism
Anomalies
Skeletal dysplasias
Multiple anomaly syndromes
Aarskog
Ataxia-telangiectasia
Bloom
Brachmann-de Lange
Charge
Coffin-Siris
Dubowitz
Fanconi
Johanson-Blizzard
Neu-Laxova
Noonan
Pena-Shokeir
Roberts
Russell-Silver
Seckel
Smith-Lemli-Opitz
Williams (Catch 22)
Infection
Teratogens

restriction. Up to 85% of a subgroup of unexplained stillbirths in a large series of stillbirths occurred after 31 weeks, and 60% of these could be classified as growth restricted on *customized* growth charts but did not appear as such on *standard* growth charts.[112]

The primary means of detecting SGA fetuses is demonstration of EFW to be less than the tenth percentile. The predictive value of true IUGR is further increased in association with oligohydramnios or abnormal Doppler studies. Scoring systems that incorporate sonographic estimates of fetal weight, amniotic fluid assessment, and clinical parameters have also been devised.[113,114]

Small AC percentiles have been found to be a sensitive marker for IUGR. The small AC measurement may reflect a reduction in size of the liver or other intraabdominal organs, reduced amounts of fat, or possibly an elevated diaphragm because of poor lung growth.[115] In low-risk and high-risk subjects, AC below the tenth percentile has the highest sensitivity, and EFW has the highest odds ratio.

Symmetric versus Asymmetric Intrauterine Growth Restriction

Symmetric IUGR has been used to describe a growth pattern when all biometric measurements appear affected to the same degree, whereas *asymmetric* IUGR has been used to characterize a smaller AC compared to other growth parameters. Asymmetric IUGR would then show abnormal ratios such as the HC/AC ratio or FL/AC ratio.[116]

When first introduced, the term *symmetric IUGR* was suggested as more likely to reflect underlying fetal condition including aneuploidy, whereas *asymmetric IUGR* supposedly reflected underlying uterine-placental dysfunction. These assumptions, however, have proved to be largely false. Asymmetric IUGR may just as likely reflect underlying fetal condition,[117] aneuploidy (e.g., triploidy), and present as early as symmetric IUGR.[118] Fetuses with symmetric and asymmetric IUGR also show a similar degree of acid-base impairment.[119] Various ratios have also not been found to be useful.[120] The distinction, therefore, between symmetric versus asymmetric IUGR is usually not helpful.

Despite these arguments, comparing the pattern of fetal biometry is worthwhile. Low weight-to-length ratio is correlated with perinatal morbidity, even in infants not SGA.[121] This may reflect fetuses who are compromised but whose weight does not fall below the tenth percentile.

Disproportionately small HC is also important to identify and, when severe, may indicate microcephaly. Newborns exposed to high levels of cocaine exhibit asymmetric growth restriction in which the HC is disproportionately smaller than would be predicted from the BW (i.e., head wasting). The deficit in head size associated with cocaine exposure may reflect the effects of a specific central nervous system insult that interferes with prenatal brain growth.[122]

Other Measures of Intrauterine Growth Restriction

Other measures can help identify compromised fetuses. These measures include amniotic fluid, Doppler studies, biophysical profile, and cardiotocography (discussed previously). In prediction of SGA infants at birth, morphometric measurements are, not surprisingly, more accurate than Doppler studies.[123] In prediction of adverse outcome among SGA fetuses, however, US assessment of fetal growth and Doppler studies have been found to be useful.[124] Uterine artery Doppler (discussed previously) may help to identify patients at risk for IUGR before it develops, particularly in women who develop hypertension.

In a multicentric longitudinal study,[61] amniotic fluid index and umbilical artery PI were the first parameters to become abnormal, and they were followed by the middle cerebral artery, aorta, short-term variability, ductus venosus, and inferior vena cava. All parameters showed a trend toward an increase in abnormal findings close to delivery for fetal distress or fetal death. Changes in venous Doppler waveforms, therefore, were observed after fetal arterial blood flow redistribution from the descending thoracic aorta to the middle cerebral artery was established.

Abnormal Doppler findings correlate with the onset of abnormal fetal heart rate (FHR) patterns. Reduced FHR variation and the occurrence of FHR decelerations have been associated with fetal hypoxemia,[125–128] whereas extremely low values of short-term variation were found to be a reliable predictor of metabolic acidemia at delivery or intrauterine death.[129–131] Before 32 weeks, the increase in ductus venosus PI (Fig. 19) and the decrease in short-term variation were steeper than all the other parameters, and they became abnormal on average only a few days before delivery. These two parameters indicate more acute changes in the degree of abnormality. Based on a longitudinal study considering multiple variables, Hecher et al.[61] concluded that venosus PI and short-term variation of FHR are important indicators for the optimal timing of delivery before 32 weeks of gestation, and delivery should be considered if one of these parameters is persistently abnormal.

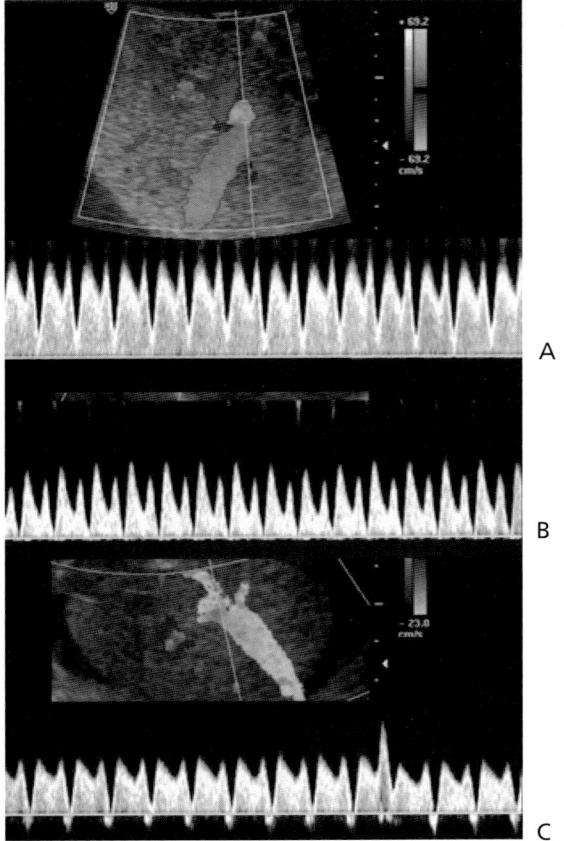

FIGURE 19. Ductus venosus flow patterns. **A:** Normal. **B:** Absent A wave. **C:** Reversed A wave.

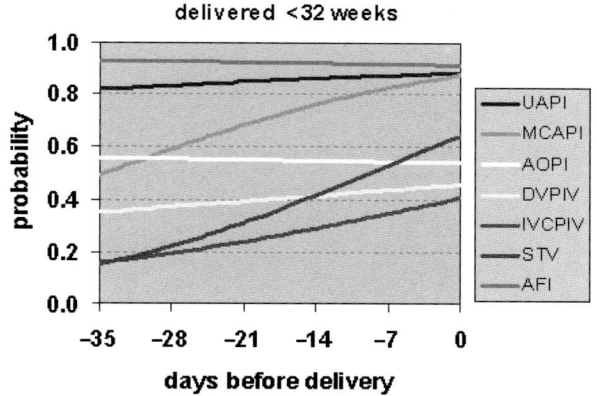

A

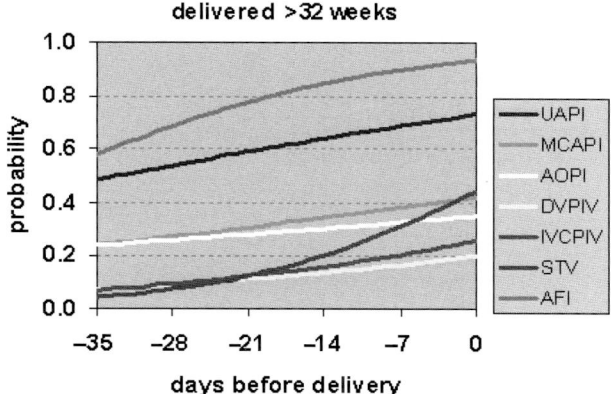

B

FIGURE 20. Probability for a test to be abnormal between inclusion and delivery (in days) before **(A)** and after **(B)** 32 weeks of gestation. AFI, amniotic fluid index; AOPI, aortic pulsatility index; DVPIV, ductus venosus pulsatility index for veins; IVCPIV, inferior vena cava pulsatility index for veins; MCAPI, middle cerebral artery pulsatility index; STV, abnormal short-term variability on electronic monitoring; UAPI, umbilical artery pulsatility index. (Reproduced with permission from Hecher K, Bilardo CM, Stigter RH, et al. Monitoring of fetuses with intrauterine growth restriction: a longitudinal study. *Ultrasound Obstet Gynaecol* 2001;18:564–570.)

Only analysis of trends of monitoring parameters in each individual fetus gives reliable information regarding the optimal timing of delivery, and each fetus should serve as its own control. Different probabilities for the presence of fetal distress can be derived from abnormal findings in the assessment of different parameters (Fig. 20). Single measurements of isolated parameters may be misleading. GA plays a crucial role in the sequence of events of fetal deterioration and regarding neonatal mortality and morbidity. GA, therefore, has a major influence on the interpretation of fetal monitoring parameters and on the decision to deliver a growth-restricted fetus.

Associated Anomalies

Many fetuses with chromosomal anomalies or other genetic syndromes may exhibit growth delay as a dominant feature.

Growth delay may be such a dominant feature that it may be considered an anomaly by itself. Growth delay may be the primary or, in some cases, the only sonographic evidence of underlying fetal anomalies. Early onset IUGR is a common manifestation of major chromosome abnormalities, particularly trisomy 13 syndrome, trisomy 18 syndrome, and triploidy.[132]

Whereas the overall frequency of chromosome abnormalities is low in fetuses with IUGR, this risk increases with the degree of growth restriction and early onset GA. Dicke and Crane[133] reported that midtrimester onset growth delay was evident in 43% of fetuses with trisomy 13 syndrome and in 59% of fetuses with trisomy 18 syndrome. In cases of early onset or severe IUGR and normal fetal karyotype, confined placental mosaicism should also be considered.

The combination of IUGR and polyhydramnios has been strongly associated with underlying fetal aneuploidy or other anomaly during the third trimester.[134–136] Sohaey et al.[137] found that BW among 156 fetuses with polyhydramnios and congenital anomalies was 3,003 g compared to 3,771 g among normal fetuses with polyhydramnios.

Prognosis

Fetuses with IUGR are at greater risk of death, preterm delivery, sepsis, and prolonged hospitalization.[138–140] Mortality and morbidity based on Apgar score, intubation at birth, sepsis, and seizures are significantly higher in infants born at term below the third percentile for their gestation.[141] However, limited information exists concerning other BW thresholds (fifteenth, tenth, fifth, or third percentile) for a given GA at which mortality and morbidity increase significantly.[142–145]

Abnormal Doppler velocimetry further increases the risk of adverse outcome. Among SGA infants, Gaziano et al.[146] also found that those with abnormal antenatal Doppler had lower BWs (1,379 g vs. 1,714 g), intraventricular hemorrhage (20% vs. 6%), prolonged hospitalization, mean intensive care days (31 vs. 14), and special care nursery days (25 vs. 9). Fetuses with IUGR and abnormal umbilical artery Doppler studies are more likely to present with abdominal problems with delayed meconium passage, abdominal distention, bilious vomiting, and a delay in tolerating enteral feeding within the first days of life.[147] Hyperechoic bowel and IUGR has also been found to be associated with abnormal bowel function.

Identification of fetuses at risk may be less reliable for preterm fetuses, especially before 34 weeks of gestation.[148] Stratifying infants in this GA group as SGA by BW or ponderal index into symmetrically or asymmetrically growth retarded showed no difference in neonatal outcome parameters. Stratification by maternal risk factors, however, did show a difference[149] (Table 8).

Long-term studies are now available among infants born with IUGR. Leitner et al. found that children with IUGR demonstrated a specific profile of neurodevelop-

TABLE 8. RISK FACTORS FOR THE DEVELOPMENT OF INTRAUTERINE GROWTH RESTRICTION: PERCENT DIFFERENCE IN ESTIMATED FETAL WEIGHT AND BIRTH WEIGHT ASSOCIATED WITH VARIOUS MATERNAL AND FETAL CHARACTERISTICS BY GESTATIONAL AGE

Characteristics	Mean gestational age				
	18 wk	25 wk	31 wk	36 wk	40 wk (birth)
Black vs. white	NS	NS	NS	−4.3[a]	−4.9[a]
Female vs. male	−9.2	−2.6	−1.4	−3.2[a]	−4.6[a]
Cigarettes, more than 20 vs. none	NS	NS	NS	−5.1[a]	−6.2[a]
Previous low-birth-weight vs. none	NS	NS	NS	−2.8	−3.6[a]
Height, less than 157 cm vs. greater than 167 cm	NS	NS	−3.3	−4.4[a]	−5.9[a]
Body mass index, less than 19.5 vs. more than 26.0	NS	−3.6	−3.8	−6.7[a]	−8.8[a]
Weight gain, less than 8 kg vs. more than 16 kg	NS	−3.6	−3.8	−5.0[a]	−7.5[a]
Hypertension vs. none	NS	NS	NS	NS	−4.3

NS, not significant.
[a]$p \leq .0001$.
Adapted from Goldenberg RL, Davis RO, Cliver SP, et al. Maternal risk factors and their influence on fetal anthropometric measurements. *Am J Obstet Gynecol* 1993;168:1197–1205.

mental disabilities at preschool age.[150] Affected children had difficulties in coordination, lateralization, and spatial and graphomotor skills. At 6-year follow-up, those infants with IUGR and neonatal complications had lower neurodevelopmental scores than the controls but no difference in IQ.

Ley et al.[151] found an association between abnormal fetal aortic velocity waveform and impaired intellectual outcome at 7-year follow-up. Logistic regression analysis showed only SGA versus non-SGA status and the mothers' education were found to be significant contributions to intellectual outcome, although these factors accounted for only 6% of the variance.[152] Another study found that SGA infants at term do not show intellectual impairment, although they show slightly lower intelligence test scores at age 17 years.[153]

Growing concern exists over other long-term outcomes in association with subnormal fetal growth, including ischemic heart disease, hypertension, and diabetes. Experimental studies in animals show that some of these outcomes can readily be induced by restriction of fetal growth.[154]

Management

Management includes

1. Exclusion of associated anomalies such as infection, anatomical defects, and chromosomal abnormalities. Chromosome analysis should be considered, especially when IUGR is severe, is early onset, or when IUGR is combined with polyhydramnios. Fluorescence *in situ* hybridization has been found to be helpful for obtaining a rapid result in this situation.[155] Snijders et al.[156] found that the risk of aneuploidy increased with a higher mean HC to AC ratio, normal or increased amniotic fluid volume, and normal waveforms from the uterine or umbilical arteries or both. The yield of workup for toxoplasmosis, other agents, rubella, cytomegalovirus, and herpes simplex infection among infants with IUGR is poor.[157]

2. Control of maternal factors such as hypertension.

3. Delivery.

Most patients exhibiting fetal IUGR can be monitored as outpatients. Those patients, however, showing absence or reversal of diastolic flow on umbilical artery Doppler should probably be hospitalized and closely monitored. Patients whose fetus shows cessation of growth and severe oligohydramnios should probably be hospitalized.

The optimal timing of delivery in pregnancies complicated by IUGR is still an issue to be resolved. Clinicians have to balance the risks of prematurity against the risks of prolonged fetal exposure to hypoxemia and acidemia, possibly resulting in fetal damage or death. GA and BW are the main components of parents' counseling and of the decision making process to deliver IUGR fetuses.

Table 9 lists survival by week of gestation and 100 g of BW steps. These survival rates are constantly underestimated by obstetricians,[158] which may have a negative influence on survival. In a study of low-birth-weight infants weighing between 800 and 1,000 g at birth (after exclusion of fetal anomalies), Bottoms et al.[159] reported survival without serious morbidity of 59% when cesarean section was readily considered and performed but only 28% survival when the obstetricians were reluctant to perform a cesarean section. The authors conclude that for fetuses weighing more than 800 g or at 26 weeks the obstetrician should usually be willing to perform cesarean delivery for fetal indications. Between 22 and 25 weeks, the outcome is generally poor secondary to complications of prematurity. Intervention at these ages results in greater likelihood of survival but at the cost of serious morbidity.

TABLE 9. OUTCOME BY WEEK OF BIRTH AND BIRTHWEIGHT, INCLUDING INTACT SURVIVAL (WITHOUT MAJOR HANDICAP), SEVERE MORBIDITY, NEONATAL DEATH, AND PERIPARTUM DEATH

	Intact survival at 120 d (%)	Severe morbidity at 120 d (%)	Neonatal death	Death peripartum
Gestational age (wk)				
21 (n = 41)	0	2.4	78.0	19.5
22 (n = 69)	2.9	11.6	71.0	14.5
23 (n = 91)	9.9	16.5	61.5	12.1
24 (n = 118)	15.3	33.0	50.0	16.9
25 (n = 124)	33.9	34.7	30.6	0.8
26 (n = 102)	40.2	34.3	25.5	0
27 (n = 76)	50.0	28.9	18.4	2.6
28 (n = 41)	53.7	34.1	12.2	0
29 (n = 21)	71.4	23.8	4.8	0
≥30 (n = 30)	86.7	10.0	3.3	0
Total	29.9	25.9	39.4	4.8
Weight (g)				
<400 (n = 31)	0	0	80.6	19.4
400–450 (n = 27)	3.7	0	81.5	14.8
450–500 (n = 45)	2.2	6.7	75.6	15.6
500–550 (n = 54)	1.9	14.8	74.1	9.3
550–600 (n = 59)	10.2	23.7	61.0	5.1
600–650 (n = 78)	16.7	26.9	50.0	6.4
650–700 (n = 58)	19.0	43.1	36.2	1.7
700–750 (n = 54)	25.9	51.9	22.2	0
750–800 (n = 65)	36.9	38.5	21.5	3.1
800–850 (n = 66)	56.1	21.2	21.2	1.5
850–900 (n = 59)	59.3	32.2	8.5	0
900–950 (n = 58)	55.2	27.6	17.2	0
950–1,000 (n = 59)	64.4	20.3	15.3	0

Newborn survival by week of gestation adapted from Copper RL, Goldenberg RL, Creasy RK, et al. A multicenter study of preterm birth weight and gestational age-specific neonatal mortality. *Am J Obstet Gynecol* 1993;168:78–84; and weight at birth adapted from Bottoms SF, Paul RH, Iams JD, et al. Obstetric determinant of neonatal survival: influence of willingness to perform cesarean delivery on survival of extremely low-birth-weight infants. *Am J Obst Gynecol* 1997;176:960–966.

The decision-making process should also avoid unnecessary and iatrogenic aggressive management. Indeed, a referral neonatal intensive care unit reported that 42% of these neonates did not require any intensive postnatal treatment.[160] Good knowledge of fetal physiology and pathophysiologic processes to use the various components of fetal assessment accurately and appropriately is clearly required.

Macrosomia

Definition

Large for gestational age is defined by an EFW greater than the ninetieth percentile. Neonatal macrosomia is defined in absolute terms as BW more than 4,500 g; old charts used 4,000 g, but physiologic BWs have increased over the years. As expected, the prevalence of macrosomia varies widely between countries.

Because of fetal mortality and morbidity (see Prognosis, later), prediction of macrosomia is a public health problem and the answer partly relies on fetal US examination. Three problems, however, exist in screening for macrosomia: the sonographic diagnosis of macrosomia is not reliable; 90% of macrosomic babies do not experience any complication;

and prevention of perinatal morbidity and mortality implies a 10% increase in the cesarean section rate and its maternal morbidity.

Risk Factors

Risk factors are well established (Table 10) with a good sensitivity but are not specific because most women at risk will deliver babies of normal weight. The main risk factors are grouped under the acronym DOPE (i.e., *d*iabetes, *o*besity, *p*ostdates, *e*xcessive fetal weight, or maternal weight gain sequence).

TABLE 10. RISK FACTORS FOR FETAL MACROSOMIA

Previous history	Current pregnancy
Maternal birth weight	Gestational diabetes
Shoulder dystocia	Excessive weight gain
Macrosomia	Suspicion of macrosomia
Preexisting diabetes	Postterm pregnancy
Gestational diabetes	Polyhydramnios
Obesity	Ultrasound-based estimated weight greater than ninetieth percentile
Multiparity	—
Maternal age older than 35 yr	—

TABLE 11. ASSOCIATIONS WITH EXCESSIVE FETAL GROWTH (MACROSOMIA)

Pertinent features in early overgrowth syndromes	Weaver	Sotos	Marshall-Smith	Beckwith-Wiedemann	Simpson-Golabi-Behmel
Excessive growth of prenatal onset	+++	++	+	++	+++
Accelerated osseous maturation	+++	+++	++	+++	++
Developmental delay	++	++	+++	+	++
Mental retardation	+	++	+++	+	++
Poor coordination	++	+++	+++	+	+
Learning difficulties	++	+++	+++	+	+
Hoarse, abnormal cry	+++	+	—	—	+
Dysarthric speech	—	—	No speech	—	—
Dilated ventricles and cavum septi pellucidi	+++	++	+	—	+
Craniofacial features	—	—	—	—	—
Macrocephaly	++	++	—	+	++
Hypertelorism	+++	++	—	—	++
Large ears	+++	—	—	+	—
Down-slanting palpebral fissures	+++	++	—	+	++
Relative micrognathia	+++	—	+	—	—
Limbs	—	—	—	—	—
Campto(clino)-dactyly	+++	+	+	—	—
Prominent finger pads	—	—	—	—	—
Flared metaphases	—	—	—	—	—
Increased risk for malignancy	—	++	—	++	+
Gene locus	?	5q35	?	11p15.5	Xp26

+, a feature of this condition.
Adapted from Schwartzler P, Homfray T, Campbell S, et al. Prenatal findings on ultrasound and x-ray in a case of overgrowth syndrome associated with increased nuchal translucency. *Prenat Diagn* 2001;21:341–5.

Pathology

Biochemical analytes have been correlated with macrosomia. Umbilical cord leptin concentration has been shown to be an independent risk factor for fetal macrosomia.[161]

Genetically driven excessive growth can be seen in a number of conditions (Table 11). An excessive prenatal growth rate is usually maintained throughout the pregnancy. Precise diagnosis is often difficult to ascertain and relies on subtle differences; the prognosis is also extremely difficult to ascertain antenatally and in the neonatal period.[162]

Diagnosis

Clinical symphysis to fundal height has a 500 g accuracy in the diagnosis of macrosomia in 82.5% of the cases but in only 35.3% of the cases when the BW is more than 4,500 g.[163,164]

Ultrasound Examination
Measurement of AC alone may help to identify macrosomic fetuses. Gilby et al.[165] found that if the AC is less than 35 cm, the risk of infant BWs to be more than 4,500 g is less than 1%. On the other hand, if the AC is 38 cm or more, the risk is 37% (37/99), and greater than 50% of these infants were identified (37/69 or 53.6%).

Numerous mathematical formulas and indices exist to predict fetal macrosomia.[166–172] Simple formulas for estimating fetal weight may do just as well as complex ones,[173,174] although formulas, including FL and AC, appear to be most accurate.

The mean sonographic error in estimating fetal weight is higher with macrosomic fetuses, reaching 15% at term compared to less than 10% for normal size fetuses. Diabetes, however, does not change the accuracy of the measurements. Field et al.[170] found that, regardless of maternal size, almost one-half of the weight predictions were within 5% of the actual BW. Approximately 50% to 70% of estimated weights fall within 10% of the actual BW, encompassing the cut-off of 4,000 g in 95% of the cases when the estimated birth weight is equal to or more than 4,000 g.[168–172] Repeating the measurements does not seem to increase their accuracy.[171] The predictive value of an LGA fetus is further increased when polyhydramnios is also present. Sohaey et al.[137] reported that 28% of fetuses with polyhydramnios had BWs at the ninetieth percentile or greater (Fig. 21). Conversely, the combination of oligohydramnios and a fetal weight estimate below the ninetieth percentile virtually excludes the possibility of LGA.[175]

The etiology for polyhydramnios among LGA fetuses remains unclear. Maternal diabetes is not independently associated with polyhydramnios, after accounting for macrosomia.[176] Some have suggested polyhydramnios may reflect increased renal vascular flow, whereas others suggest it is secondary to bulk flow of water across the surface of the fetus, umbilical cord, placenta, and membranes. Larger fetuses with larger lung volumes and placental surface areas are expected to produce greater amounts of amniotic fluid. Although one might also expect a relationship between the severity of polyhydramnios and BW, no direct correlation has been found.[176]

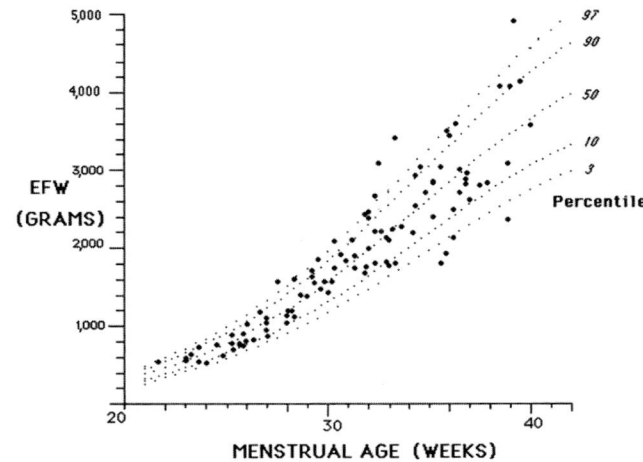

A

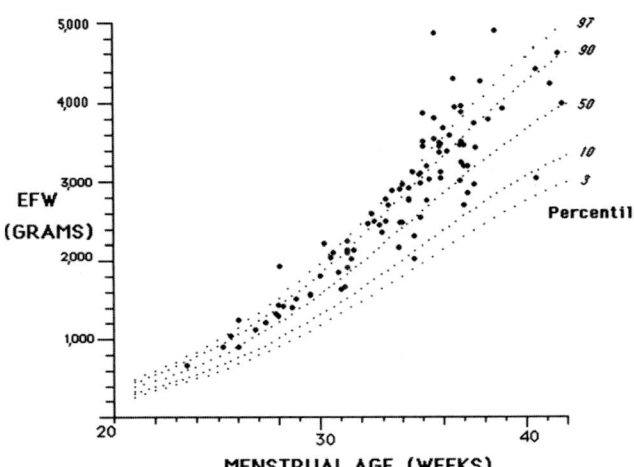

B

FIGURE 21. Idiopathic polyhydramnios and macrosomia in normal fetuses of nondiabetic mothers. Graph **A** represents the control group with normal amniotic fluid, and graph **B** represents consecutive fetuses with polyhydramnios in nondiabetic mothers. The estimated fetal weight (EFW) percentiles (plotted against Hadlock percentiles) of the study group are significantly higher than the control group. In this study, fetuses with polyhydramnios were three times more likely to have a birth weight at or more than the ninetieth percentile (relative risk is 2.7). (Reproduced with permission from Sohaey R, Nyberg DA, Sickler GK, et al. Idiopathic polyhydramnios: association with fetal macrosomia. *Radiology* 1994;190:393–396.)

US is not considered to be specific enough to predict shoulder dystocia. A few studies using US or even magnetic resonance imaging, however, have been encouraging.[177–179] The sensitivity and specificity of ultrasound are unlikely to be more than 40% and 75%, respectively, which would indicate the need to perform a cesarean section in 25% of the patients to avoid only 40% of all shoulder dystocias.[180]

Comparison of Clinical and Ultrasound Prediction
Most studies conclude that clinical examination works just as well as US to predict BW at term, especially when it is

more than 4,500 g.[181–185] Inclusion of soft-tissue measurement in the US EBW is unconvincing.[164] A two-step clinical and sonographic approach does not perform better because the sensitivity is 17% and the positive predictive value is only 36% for EBW more than 4,000 g.[181]

Prognosis

Primary potential complications of fetal macrosomia are related to the birth itself. These may include birth trauma, asphyxia, and shoulder dystocia. The incidence of cesarean deliveries, elective and in labor; perineal damage; postpartum hemorrhage; and infection are higher.

Shoulder dystocia occurs in 10% of macrosomia cases,[186] and this may lead to damage to the brachial plexus. Other perinatal complications resulting from shoulder dystocia include fractures of the clavicles and humerus, asphyxia, hypoglycemia, and low calcium plasma levels, when this is associated with gestational diabetes. The incidence of these complications is directly correlated to the degree of macrosomia.[187] Perinatal mortality associated with shoulder dystocia is around 2 per 100,000 births, accounting for 0.5% of all perinatal deaths.[188] However, 40% to 50% of all cases of shoulder dystocia occur in non-macrosomic neonates, and 30% to 50% of all brachial plexus damage occurs without shoulder dystocia and in non-macrosomic infants.[181]

Fetal and neonatal obesity in diabetes affects mainly the fetal trunk and gives a 1.5- to 4-fold increase in the incidence of shoulder dystocia in all BW subgroups between 4,000 and 5,000 g.[186,189] Other risk factors include previous history of shoulder dystocia (relative risk ×17), high maternal weight gain, multiparity, long labor, and forceps delivery.[180,190,191]

Management

Retrospective analyses of large series of macrosomic infants accounting for prenatal estimate or its absence report more inductions of labor, more failed inductions, and more cesarean sections in the group diagnosed antenatally as being macrosomic; and the mean BW was identical in both groups. No valid estimate existed on perinatal mortality and morbidity over the study periods.[192,193]

In cases in which the BW was more than 4,500 g with or without maternal diabetes, a large retrospective study showed that elective cesarean section when EBW is more than 4,250 g led to a 50% (2.8% vs. 1.5%) reduction in the incidence of shoulder dystocia for a moderate increase in cesarean section rate (21.7% vs. 25.1%).[194]

GROWTH ASSESSMENT IN TWIN PREGNANCIES

Epidemiologic studies in twins in the United States have clearly shown that SGA is more prevalent in primiparous women, with a previous history of IUGR, with cigarette consumption and in black Americans, especially after 32 weeks of gestation. BW varies with maternal characteristics as in singletons. Preeclampsia is 5 to 6 times more frequent in twins than in singletons. The incidence of velamentous insertion of the umbilical cord of at least one twin and that of single umbilical arteries is 10 times higher than in singletons. Monochorionic twins are smaller than dichorionic ones at all gestations, which is likely to happen because of an abnormal and unique type of placentation even when the pregnancy is not complicated by twin-to-twin transfusion.[195]

Fetal growth in twins follows a rather specific pattern, and specific growth charts have been established.[196] The charts show a growth pattern similar to that of singletons in the first two trimesters of pregnancy up to 28 to 30 weeks,[197,198] and the curve of singletons crosses over that of twins at 31 to 32 weeks.[199] These data from the US natality data files between 1991 and 1995 thus show that a 330 g difference exists between the fiftieth percentiles of twins and singletons at 32 weeks. This difference increases up to 507 g at 38 weeks and 570 g at 39 weeks of gestation. At 38 weeks, the tenth percentile in singletons equals the fiftieth percentile in twins.

Growth Restriction in Twin Pregnancies

Twin pregnancies are 2% of all pregnancies but account for 20% of perinatal mortality and morbidity, mainly as a result of prematurity and growth restriction, which accounts for 30% to 50% of perinatal mortality in twins.[199] A tenfold increase exists in the incidence of SGA in twins when compared with singletons[198] and when plotted on singleton BW charts; 12% to 47% of twins are below the tenth percentile for gestation.[200] Accurate diagnosis and management depends on GA, chorionicity, and placental and fetal hemodynamics.

Although the use of specific charts to screen for and manage IUGR in twins seems logical, the false-negative rate might be deleterious in such a high-risk population, and singleton charts should be used in clinical management of twin pregnancies. This has been substantiated using the tenth percentile for singletons,[201] especially when growth discordance between the twins exists.[202] Irrespective of GA, twins of less than 2,000 g have a tenfold increased perinatal morbidity over twins weighing more than 2,000 g.

Growth Discordance in Twins

Discordant growth is seen in 15% to 25% of twin pregnancies. Biometric discordance on CRL in the first trimester of pregnancy is usually confirmed in the second and third trimester of pregnancy. This discordance should also call for a detailed anatomic examination of the smaller twin, as the risk of congenital malformation is increased.[203]

Although growth discordance does not always imply growth restriction, the more severe the discordance the more likely growth restriction exists in one or both twins. The degree of growth discordance is assessed by EFW of each twin and by an index expressed as the difference between EFW of each twin as a proportion of the EFW of the bigger twin. Discordancy of 15% to 20% is usually considered to be significant.[204] Perinatal morbidity for the small twin in dichorionic pregnancies and in both twins in monochorionic pregnancies is increasing with the degree of discordance.[205]

The most reliable parameter to screen for discordance seems to be the AC, with a difference of 20 mm accounting for a 20% discordance with a sensitivity and a predictive value of 80% when compared to EFW with a sensitivity of 93% and a predictive value of 70%.[206] Umbilical Doppler measurement increases the sensitivity of the diagnosis of IUGR and growth discordance to up to 85% and the negative predictive value to around 90%.[207]

Once IUGR is suspected in one or both twins, the management is similar to that in singletons for fetal surveillance in dichorionic pregnancies. A dilemma may occur when a severely growth-restricted twin presents with terminal chronic fetal distress and the other twin is doing well at an early gestation. In dichorionic pregnancies, intrauterine death of one twin only exposes the other twin to an increased rate of prematurity, whereas in monochorionic twins, the death of one twin increases the risk of severe hemodynamic changes in the co-twin with a 20% to 30% risk of perinatal mortality and morbidity in the survivor. The risks are even higher in twin-to-twin transfusion syndrome.[208]

REFERENCES

1. Jones KL. *Smith's recognizable patterns of human malformation*, 5th ed. Philadelphia: WB Saunders, 1997.
2. Campbell S, Warsof SL, Little D, et al. Routine ultrasound screening for the prediction of gestational age. *Obstet Gynecol* 1985;65:613–620.
3. Goldenberg RL, Davis RO, Cutter GR, et al. Prematurity, postdates, and growth retardation: the influence of use of ultrasonography on reported gestational age. *Am J Obstet Gynecol* 1989;160:462–470.
4. Gardosi J, Vanner T, Francis A. Gestational age and induction of labour for prolonged pregnancy. *Br J Obstet Gynaecol* 1997;104:792–797.
5. Kramer MS, McLean FH, Boyd ME, Usher RH. The validity of gestational age estimation by menstrual dating in term, preterm, and postterm gestations. *JAMA* 1988;260:3306–3308.
6. Guerrero R, Florez PE. The duration of pregnancy. *Lancet* 1969;2:268–269.
7. Persson PH, Weldner BM. Reliability of ultrasound fetometry in estimating gestational age in the second trimester. *Acta Obstet Gynecol Scand* 1986;65:481.
8. Geirsson RT, Have G. Comparison of actual and ultrasound estimated second trimester gestational length in IVF pregnancies. *Acta Obstet Gynecol Scand* 1993;72:344–346.

9. Waldenstrom U, Axelsson O, Nilsson S. A comparison of the ability of a sonographically measured biparietal diameter and the last menstrual period to predict the spontaneous onset of labor. *Obstet Gynecol* 1990;76:336–338.

10. Wilcox M, Gardosi J, Mongelli M, et al. Birth weight from pregnancies dated by ultrasound in a multicultural British population. *BMJ* 1993;307:588–591.

11. Gardosi J, Mongelli M. Risk assessment adjusted for gestational age in maternal serum screening for Down's syndrome. *BMJ* 1993;306:1509.

12. Mongelli M, Wilcox M, Gardosi J. Estimating the date of confinement: ultrasonographic biometry versus certain menstrual dates. *Am J Obstet Gynecol* 1996;174:278–281.

13. Warren WB, Peisner DB, Raju S, et al. Dating the early pregnancy by sequential appearance of embryonic structures. *Am J Obstet Gynecol* 1989;161:747.

14. Daya S. Accuracy of gestational age estimation by means of fetal crown-rump length measurement. *Am J Obstet Gynecol* 1987;168:903–908.

15. Robinson HP, Fleming JE. A critical evaluation of sonar "crown-rump length" measurement. *Br J Obstet Gynaecol* 1975;82:702–710.

16. Drumm JE, Clinch J, McKenzie G. The ultrasonic measurement of fetal crown rump length as a method of assessing gestational age. *Br J Obstet Gynaecol* 1976;83: 417–421.

17. Daya S, Woods S, Ward S, et al. Early pregnancy assessment with transvaginal ultrasound scanning. *Can Med Assoc J* 1991;144:441–446.

18. Lasser DM, Peisner DB, Wollenbergh J, et al. First trimester fetal biometry using transvaginal sonography. *Ultrasound Obstet Gynecol* 1993;3:104–108.

19. McGregor SN, Tamura RK, Sabbagha RE, et al. Underestimation of gestational age by conventional crown rump length dating curves. *Am J Obstet Gynecol* 1987;70:344–348.

20. Wisser J, Dirscheld P. Estimation of gestational age by transvaginal sonographic measurement of greatest embryonic length in dated human embryos. *Ultrasound Obstet Gynecol* 1994;4:457–462.

21. Hall MH, Carr-Hill RA. The significance of uncertain gestation for obstetric outcome. *Br J Obstet Gynaecol* 1985;92:452–460.

22. Hadlock FP. Sonographic estimation of fetal age and weight. *Radiol Clin North Am* 1990;28:39–50.

23. Altman DG, Chitty LS. New charts for ultrasound dating of pregnancy. *Ultrasound Obstet Gynecol* 1997;10(3):174–191.

24. Stebbins B, Jaffe R. Fetal biometry and gestational age estimation. In: Jaffe R, Bui TH, eds. *Textbook of fetal ultrasound*. Parthenon Publishing, 1999:47–57.

25. Hadlock FP, Harrist RB, Shah YP, et al. Estimating fetal age using multiple parameters: a prospective evaluation in a racially mixed population. *Am J Obstet Gynecol* 1987;156:955–957.

26. Harstad TW, Little BB. Ultrasound anthropometric reliability. *J Clin Ultrasound* 1994;22:531–534.

27. Kurjak A, Kirkinen P, Latin V. Biometric and dynamic ultrasound assessment of small-for-dates infants: report of 260 cases. *Obstet Gynecol* 1980;56(3):281–284.

28. Landon MB, Mintz MC, Gabbe SG. Sonographic evaluation of fetal abdominal growth: predictor of the large for gestational age infant in pregnancies complicated by diabetes mellitus. *Am J Obstet Gynecol* 1989;160:115–121.

29. Basel D, Lederer R, Diamant YZ. Longitudinal ultrasonic biometry of various parameters in fetuses with abnormal growth rate. *Acta Obstet Gynecol Scand* 1987;66:143–149.

30. Alexander GR, Kogan MD, Himes JH, et al. Racial differences in birthweight for gestational age and infant mortality in extremely-low-risk US populations. *Paediatr Perinat Epidemiol* 1999;13(2):205–217.

31. Hadlock FP. Ultrasound evaluation of fetal growth. In: Callen PW, ed. *Ultrasonography in obstetrics and gynecology*. Philadelphia: WB Saunders, 1994:129–143.

32. Dudley NJ. Selection of appropriate ultrasound methods for estimation of fetal weight. *Br J Radiol* 1995;68:385–388.

33. Coombs CA, Jaekle RK, Rosenn B, et al. Sonographic estimation of fetal weight based on a model of fetal volume. *Obstet Gynecol* 1993;82:365–370.

34. Hadlock FP, Harrist RB, Carpenter RJ, et al. Sonographic estimation of fetal weight. *Radiology* 1984;150:535–540.

35. Smith GCS, Smith MFS, McNay MB, et al. The relation between fetal abdominal circumference and birthweight: findings in 3512 pregnancies. *Br J Obstet Gynaecol* 1997; 104:186–190.

36. Gore D, Williams M, O'Brien W, et al. Fetal abdominal circumference for prediction of intrauterine growth restriction. *Obstet Gynecol* 2000;95[4 Suppl 1]:S78–S79.

37. Zelop CM. Prediction of fetal weight with the use of three-dimensional ultrasonography. *Clin Obstet Gynecol* 2000; 43(2):321–325.

38. Robson SC, Gallivan S, Walkinshaw SA, et al. Ultrasonic estimation of fetal weight: use of targeted formulas in small for gestational age fetuses. *Obstet Gynecol* 1993;82:359–64.

39. Sabbagha RE, Minogue J, Tamura RK, et al. Estimation of birth weight by use of ultrasonographic formulas targeted to large-, appropriate-, and small-for-gestational-age fetuses. *Am J Obstet Gynecol* 1989;160:854–862.

40. Rose BI, McCallum WD. A simplified method for estimating fetal weight using ultrasound measurements. *Obstet Gynecol* 1987;69:671–675.

41. Medchill MT, Peterson CM, Garbaciak J. Prediction of estimated fetal weight in extremely low birth weight neonates (500–1000 g). *Obstet Gynecol* 1991;78:286–290.

42. Scott F, Beeby P, Abbott J, et al. New formula for estimating fetal weight below 1000 g: comparison with existing formulas. *J Ultrasound Med* 1996;15:669–672.

43. Weiner CP, Sabbagha RE, Vaisrub N, et al. Ultrasonographic fetal weight prediction: role of head circumference and femur length. *Obstet Gynecol* 1985;65:812–817.

44. Hadlock FP, Harrist RB, Martinez-Poyer J. In utero analysis of fetal growth: a sonographic weight standard. *Radiology* 1991;181(1):129–133.

45. Marsal K, Persson PH, Larsen T, et al. Intrauterine growth curves based on ultrasonographically estimated fetal weights. *Acta Paediatr Scand* 1996;85:843–848.

46. Singer DB, Sung CJ, Wigglesworth JS. Fetal growth and maturation with standards for body and organ development. In: Wigglesworth JS, Singer DB, eds. *Textbook of fetal and perinatal pathology*. Boston: Blackwell Science, 1991: 11–47.

47. Doubilet PM, Benson CB, Nadel AS, et al. Improved birth weight table for neonates developed from gestations dated by early ultrasonography. *J Ultrasound Med* 1997;16(4):241–249.

48. Goldenberg RL, Cutter GR, Hoffman HJ, et al. Intrauterine growth retardation: standards for diagnosis. *Am J Obstet Gynecol* 1989;161:271–277.

49. Altman DG, Chitty LS. Charts of fetal size. 1. Methodology. *Br J Obstet Gynaecol* 1994;101:29–34.

50. Divon M, Chamberlain P, Sipos L, et al. Identification of the small for gestational age independent indices of fetal growth. *Am J Obstet Gynecol* 1986;155:1197–2003.

51. Owen P, Maharaj S, Khan KS, et al. Interval between fetal measurements in predicting growth restriction. *Obstet Gynecol* 2001;97(4):499–504.

52. Chang TC, Robson SC, Spencer JAD, et al. Identification of fetal growth retardation: comparison of Doppler waveform indices and serial ultrasound measurements of abdominal circumference and fetal weight. *Obstet Gynecol* 1993;82:230–236.

53. Owen P, Ogston S. Conditional centiles for the quantification of fetal growth. *Ultrasound Obstet Gynecol* 1998;11:110–117.

54. Cole TJ. Conditional reference charts to assess weight gain in British infants. *Arch Dis Childhood* 1995;6:307–312.

55. Owen P, Burton K, Ogston S, et al. Using unconditional and conditional standard deviation scores of fetal abdominal area measurements in the prediction of intrauterine growth restriction. *Ultrasound Obstet Gynecol* 2000;16:439–444.

56. Royston P, Altman DG. Design and analysis of longitudinal studies of fetal size. *Ultrasound Obstet Gynecol* 1995;6:307–312.

57. Campbell MK, Ostbye T, Irgens L. Post term birth: risk factors and outcomes in a 10-year cohort of Norwegian births. *Obstet Gynecol* 1997;89:543–548.

58. Peters LL, Sheldon RE, et al. Blood flow to fetal organs as a function of arterial oxygen content. *Am J Obstet Gynecol* 1979;135:637–642.

59. Sato A, Yamaguchi Y, Liou SM, et al. Growth of the fetal kidney assessed by real-time ultrasound. *Gynecol Obstet Invest* 1985;20:1–5.

60. Bassan H, Trejo LL, Kariv N, et al. Experimental intrauterine growth retardation alters renal development. *Pediatr Nephrol* 2000;15(3–4):192–195.

61. Hecher K, Bilardo CM, Stigter RH, et al. Monitoring of fetuses with intrauterine growth restriction: a longitudinal study. *Ultrasound Obstet Gynaecol* 2001;18:564–570.

62. Mari GC, Deter RL, Carpenter RL, et al. Noninvasive diagnosis by Doppler ultrasonography of fetal anemia due to maternal red-cell alloimmunization. *N Engl J Med* 2000;342:9–14.

63. Chan FY, Pun TC, Lam C, et al. Fetal cerebral Doppler studies as a predictor of perinatal outcome and subsequent neurologic handicap. *Obstet Gynecol* 1996;87:981–988.

64. Hecher K, Snijders RJM, Campbell S, et al. Fetal venous, intracardiac and arterial blood flow measurements in intrauterine growth retardation: relationship with fetal blood gases. *Am J Obstet Gynecol* 1995;173:10–15.

65. Campbell S, Pearce JM, Hackett G, et al. Qualitative assessment of uteroplacental blood flow: early screening test for high-risk pregnancies. *Obstet Gynecol* 1986;68:649–653.

66. Bewley S, Cooper D, Campbell S. Doppler investigation of uteroplacental blood flow resistance in the second trimester: a screening study for pre-eclampsia and intrauterine growth retardation. *Br J Obstet Gynaecol* 1991;98:871–879.

67. Papageorgiou AT, Cicero S, Yu CKH, et al. Screening for placental insufficiency by uterine artery Doppler. *Prenatal Neonatal Med* 2001;1:27–38.

68. Bower S, Schuchter K, Campbell S. Doppler ultrasound screening as part of routine antenatal scanning: prediction of preeclampsia and intrauterine growth retardation. *Br J Obstet Gynaecol* 1993;100:989–994.

69. Valensise H, Bezzeccheri V, Rizzo G, et al. Doppler velocimetry of the uterine artery as a screening test for gestational hypertension. *Ultrasound Obstet Gynecol* 1993;3:18–22.

70. North RA, Ferrier C, Long D, et al. Uterine artery Doppler flow velocity waveforms in the second trimester for the prediction of preeclampsia and fetal growth retardation. *Obstet Gynecol* 1994;83:378–386.

71. Todros T, Ferrazzi E, Arduini D, et al. Performance of Doppler ultrasonography as a screening test in low risk pregnancies: results of a multicentric study. *J Ultrasound Med* 1995;14:343–348.

72. Irion O, Masse, Forest C, et al. Prediction of pre-eclampsia, low birthweight for gestation and prematurity by uterine artery blood flow velocity waveforms analysis in low risk nulliparous women. *Br J Obstet Gynaecol* 1998;105:422–429.

73. Kurdi W, Campbell S, Aquilina J, et al. The role of color Doppler imaging of the uterine arteries at 20 weeks' gestation in stratifying antenatal care. *Ultrasound Obstet Gynecol* 1998;12:339–345.

74. Albaiges G, Missfelder-Lobos H, Lees C, et al. One-stage screening for pregnancy complications by color Doppler assessment of the uterine arteries at 23 weeks' gestation. *Obstet Gynecol* 2000;96:559–564.

75. Steel SA, Pearce JM, McParland P, et al. Early Doppler ultrasound screening in prediction of hypertensive disorders of pregnancy. *Lancet* 1990;335:1548–51.

76. Bower S, Bewley S, Campbell S. Improved prediction of pre-eclampsia by two-stage screening of uterine arteries using the early diastolic notch and color Doppler imaging. *Obstet Gynecol* 1993;82:78–83.

77. Harrington K, Cooper D, Lees C, et al. Doppler ultrasound of the uterine arteries: the importance of bilateral notching in the prediction of pre-eclampsia, placental abruption or delivery of a small-for-gestational-age baby. *Ultrasound Obstet Gynecol* 1996;7:182–188.

78. Frusca T, Soregaroli M, Valcamonico A, et al. Doppler velocimetry of the uterine arteries in nulliparous women. *Early Hum Dev* 1997;48:177–185.

79. Goffinet F, Paris J, Nisand I, et al. Utilité clinique du Doppler ombilical: résultats des essais controlés en population à haut risque et à bas risque. *J Gynecol Obstet Biol Reprod* 1997;26:16–26.

80. Karsdorp VHM, Van Vugt JMG, Van Geijn HP, et al. Clinical significance of absent or reversed end diastolic velocity waveforms in umbilical artery. *Lancet* 1994;344:1664–1668.

81. Akalin-Sel T, Nicolaides KH, Peacock J, et al. Doppler dynamics and their complex interrelation with fetal oxygen

pressure, carbon dioxide pressure, and pH in growth-retarded fetuses. *Obstet Gynecol* 1994;84:439–444.

82. Bilardo CM, Nicolaides KH, Campbell S. Doppler measurement of fetal and uteroplacental circulations: relationship with umbilical venous blood gases measured at cordocentesis. *Am J Obstet Gynecol* 1990;162:115–120.

83. Rizzo G, Capponi A, Talone PE, et al. Doppler indices from the inferior vena cava and ductus venosus in predicting pH and oxygen tension in umbilical blood at cordocentesis I growth-retarded fetuses. *Ultrasound Obstet Gynecol* 1996;7:401–410.

84. Viyas S, Campbell S, Bower S, et al. Maternal abdominal pressure alters fetal cerebral blood flows. *Br J Obstet Gynaecol* 1990;97:740–747.

85. Sterne G, Shields LE, Dubinsky TJ. Abnormal fetal cerebral and umbilical Doppler measurements in fetuses with intrauterine growth restriction predicts the severity of perinatal morbidity. *J Clin Ultrasound* 2001;29:146–151.

86. Severi FM, Bocchi C, Visentin A, et al. Uterine and fetal cerebral Doppler predict the outcome of third-trimester small-for-gestational age fetuses with normal umbilical artery Doppler. *Ultrasound Obstet Gynecol* 2002;19(3):225–228.

87. Hecher K, Campbell S. Characteristics of fetal venous blood flow under normal circumstances and during fetal disease. *Ultrasound Obstet Gynecol* 1996;7:68–83.

88. Manning FA, Morrison I, Lange IR, et al. Fetal assessment based on fetal biophysical scoring: experience in 12,620 referred high-risk pregnancies. I. Perinatal mortality by frequency and etiology. *Am J Obstet Gynecol* 1985;151:343.

89. Manning FA. Dynamic ultrasound-based fetal assessment: the fetal biophysical profile score. *Clin Obstet Gynecol* 1995;38:26–44.

90. Vintzileos AM, Fleming AD, Scorza WE, et al. Relationship between fetal biophysical activities and umbilical cord blood gas values. *Am J Obstet Gynecol* 1991;165:707–713.

91. Vintzileos AM, Knuppel RA. Multiple parameter biophysical testing in the prediction of fetal acid-base status. *Clin Perinatol* 1994;21(4):823–848.

92. Multon O, Senat MV, Minoui S, et al. Effect of antenatal betamethasone and dexamethasone administration on fetal heart rate variability in growth retarded fetuses. *Fetal Diagn Ther* 1997;12:170–177.

93. Neilson J, Alfirevic Z. Biophysical profile for antepartum fetal assessment. In: *Cochrane Database of Systematic Reviews*. 1995, The Cochrane Collaboration, P.O. Box 777, Oxford, England.

94. Ribbert LSM, Snijders RJM, Nicolaides KH, et al. Relation of fetal blood gases and data from computer-assisted analysis of fetal heart rate patterns in small for gestation fetuses. *Br J Obstet Gynaecol* 1991;98:820–823.

95. Senat MV, Schwärzler P, Alcais A, et al. Longitudinal changes in the ductus venosus, cerebral transverse sinus and cardiotocogram in fetal growth restriction. *Ultrasound Obstet Gynecol* 2000;16:19–24.

96. Devriendt K. Genetic control of intra-uterine growth. *Eur J Obstet Gynecol Reprod Biol* 2000;92(1):29–34.

97. Cetin I, Morpurgo PS, Radaelli T, et al. Fetal plasma leptin concentrations: relationship with different intrauterine growth patterns from 19 weeks to term. *Pediatr Res* 2000;48(5):646–651.

98. Rasmussen S, Irgens LM, Albrechtsen S, et al. Predicting preeclampsia in the second pregnancy from low birth weight in the first pregnancy. *Obstet Gynecol* 2000;96(5 Pt 1):696–700.

99. Magnus P, Bakketeig LS, Hoffman H. Birth weight of relatives by maternal tendency to repeat small-for-gestational-age (SGA) births in successive pregnancies. *Acta Obstet Gynecol Scand Suppl* 1997;165:35–38.

100. Spencer JA, Chang TC, Crook D, et al. Third trimester fetal growth and measures of carbohydrate and lipid metabolism in umbilical venous blood at term. *Arch Dis Child Fetal Neonatal Ed* 1997;76(1):F21–F25.

101. Lyall F, Young A, Greer IA. Nitric oxide concentrations are increased in the fetoplacental circulation in preeclampsia. *Am J Obstet Gynecol* 1995;173(3 Pt 1):714–718.

102. Hamasaki T, Masuzaki H, Miyamura T, et al. High concentrations of serum inhibin in pre-eclampsia. *Int J Gynaecol Obstet* 2000;71(1):7–11.

103. Curtis NE, King RG, Moseley JM, et al. Preterm fetal growth restriction is associated with increased parathyroid hormone-related protein expression in the fetal membranes. *Am J Obstet Gynecol* 2000;183(3):700–705.

104. Kupferminc MJ, Peri H, Zwang E, et al. High prevalence of the prothrombin gene mutation in women with intrauterine growth retardation, abruptio placentae and second trimester loss. *Acta Obstet Gynecol Scand* 2000;79(11):963–967.

105. Sheikh S, Satoskar P, Bhartiya D. Expression of insulin-like growth factor-I and placental growth hormone mRNA in placentae: a comparison between normal and intrauterine growth retardation pregnancies. *Mol Hum Reprod* 2001;7(3):287–292.

106. Stipoljev F, Latin V, Kos M, et al. Correlation of confined placental mosaicism with fetal intrauterine growth retardation. A case control study of placentas at delivery. *Fetal Diagn Ther* 2001;16(1):4–9.

107. Mitra SC, Seshan SV, Riachi LE. Placental vessel morphometry in growth retardation and increased resistance of the umbilical artery Doppler flow. *J Matern Fetal Med* 2000;9(5):282–286.

108. Hepburn M, Rosenberg K. An audit of the detection and management of small-for-gestational age babies. *Br J Obstet Gynaecol* 1986;93:212–216.

109. Kean LH, Liu DT. Antenatal care as a screening tool for the detection of small for gestational age babies in the low-risk population. *J Obstet Gynecol* 1996;16:77–82.

110. Mongelli M, Gardosi J. Reduction of false-positive diagnosis of fetal growth restriction by application of customized fetal growth standards. *Obstet Gynecol* 1996;88:844–848.

111. Gardosi J, Francis A. Controlled trial of fundal height measurement plotted on customized antenatal growth charts. *Br J Obstet Gynaecol* 1999;106:309–17.

112. Gardosi J, Mul T, Mongelli M. Application of a fetal weight standard to study association between growth retardation and stillbirth. *Ultrasound Obstet Gynecol* 1995;6:66.

113. Benson CB, Belville JS, Lentini JF, et al. Intrauterine growth retardation: diagnosis based on multiple parameters—a prospective study. *Radiology* 1990;177(2):499–502.

114. Benson CB, Boswell SB, Brown DL, et al. Improved prediction of intrauterine growth retardation with use of multiple parameters. *Radiology* 1988;168(1):7–12.

115. Roberts AB, Mitchell JM, McCowan LM, et al. Ultrasonographic measurement of liver length in the small-for-gestational-age fetus. *Am J Obstet Gynecol* 1999;180(3 Pt 1):634–638.

116. David C, Gabrielli S, Pilu G, et al. The head-to-abdomen circumference ratio: a reappraisal. *Ultrasound Obstet Gynecol* 1995;5(4):256–259.

117. Dashe JS, McIntire DD, Lucas MJ, et al. Effects of symmetric and asymmetric fetal growth on pregnancy outcomes. *Obstet Gynecol* 2000;96(3):321–327.

118. Vik T, Vatten L, Jacobsen G, et al. Prenatal growth in symmetric and asymmetric small-for-gestational-age infants. *Early Hum Dev* 1997;48(1–2):167–176.

119. Blackwell SC, Moldenhauer J, Redman M, et al. Relationship between the sonographic pattern of intrauterine growth restriction and acid-base status at the time of cordocentesis. *Arch Gynecol Obstet* 2001;264(4):191–193.

120. Benson CB, Doubilet PM, Saltzman DH, et al. FL/AC ratio: poor predictor of intrauterine growth retardation. *Invest Radiol* 1985;20(7):727–730.

121. Williams MC, O'Brien WF. A comparison of birth weight and weight/length ratio for gestation as correlates of perinatal morbidity. *J Perinatol* 1997;17(5):346–350.

122. Bateman DA, Chiriboga CA. Dose-response effect of cocaine on newborn head circumference. *Pediatrics* 2000;106(3):E33.

123. Chang TC, Robson SC, Boys RJ, et al. Prediction of the small for gestational age infant: which ultrasonic measurement is best? *Obstet Gynecol* 1992;80:1030–1038.

124. Chang TC, Robson SC, Spencer JA, et al. Prediction of perinatal morbidity at term in small fetuses: comparison of fetal growth and Doppler ultrasound. *Br J Obstet Gynaecol* 1994;101(5):422–427.

125. Bekedam DJ, Visser GHA, Mulder EJH, et al. Heart rate variation and movement incidence in growth-retarded fetuses: the significance of antenatal late heart rate decelerations. *Am J Obstet Gynecol* 1987;157:126–133.

126. Visser GHA, Sadovsky G, Nicolaides KH. Antepartum heart rate patterns in small-for-gestational-age third-trimester fetuses: correlations with blood gas values obtained at cordocentesis. *Am J Obstet Gynecol* 1990;162:698–703.

127. Snijders RJM, Ribbert LSM, Visser GHA, et al. Numeric analysis of heart rate variation in intrauterine growth-retarded fetuses: a longitudinal study. *Am J Obstet Gynecol* 1992;166:22–27.

128. Pardi G, Cetin I, Marconi AM, et al. Diagnostic value of blood sampling in fetuses with growth retardation. *N Engl J Med* 1993;328:692–696.

129. Street P, Dawes GS, Moulden M, et al. Short-term variation in abnormal antenatal fetal heart rate records. *Am J Obstet Gynecol* 1991;165:515–523.

130. Dawes GS, Moulden M, Redman CWG. Short-term fetal heart rate variation, decelerations, and umbilical flow velocity waveforms before labor. *Obstet Gynecol* 1992;80:673–678.

131. Guzman ER, Vintzileos AM, Martins M, et al. The efficacy of individual computer heart rate indices in detecting acidemia at birth in growth-restricted fetuses. *Obstet Gynecol* 1996;87:969–974.

132. Snijders RJ, Sherrod C, Gosden CM, et al. Fetal growth retardation: associated malformations and chromosomal abnormalities. *Am J Obstet Gynecol* 1993;168(2):547–555.

133. Dicke JM, Crane JP. Sonographic recognition of major malformations and aberrant fetal growth in trisomic fetuses. *J Ultrasound Med* 1991;10(8):433–438.

134. Sickler GK, Nyberg DA, Sohaey R, et al. Polyhydramnios and fetal intrauterine growth restriction: ominous combination. *J Ultrasound Med* 1997;16(9):609–614.

135. Furman B, Erez O, Senior L, et al. Hydramnios and small for gestational age: prevalence and clinical significance. *Acta Obstet et Gynecol Scand* 2000;79(1):31–36.

136. Lazebnik N, Many A. The severity of polyhydramnios, estimated fetal weight and preterm delivery are independent risk factors for the presence of congenital malformations. *Gynecol Obstet Invest* 1999;48(1):28–32.

137. Sohaey R, Nyberg DA, Sickler GK, et al. Idiopathic polyhydramnios: association with fetal macrosomia. *Radiology* 1994;190(2):393–396.

138. Wennergren M, Wennergren G, Vilbergsson G. Obstetric characteristics and neonatal performance in a four-year small for gestational age population. *Obstet Gynecol* 1988;72(4):615–620.

139. Kramer MS, Olivier M, McLean FH, et al. Impact of intrauterine growth retardation and body proportionality on fetal and neonatal outcome. *Pediatrics* 1990;86:707–713.

140. Spinillo A, Capuzzo E, Egbe TO, et al. Pregnancies complicated by idiopathic intrauterine growth retardation: severity of growth failure, neonatal morbidity and two-year infant neurodevelopmental outcome. *J Reprod Med* 1995;40:209–215.

141. McIntire DD, Bloom SL, Casey BM, et al. Birth weight in relation to morbidity and mortality among newborn infants. *N Engl J Med* 1999;340:1234–1238.

142. Battaglia FC, Lubchenko LO. A practical classification of newborn infants by weight and gestational age. *J Pediatr* 1967;71:159–163.

143. Bréart G, Rabarison Y, Plouin PF, et al. Risk of fetal growth retardation as a result of maternal hypertension: preparation to a trial on antihypertensive drugs. *Dev Pharmacol Ther* 1982;4[Suppl]:116–123.

144. Usher R, McLean F. Intrauterine growth of live-born Caucasian infants at sea level: standards obtained from measurements in 7 dimensions of infants born between 25 and 44 weeks of gestation. *J Pediatr* 1969;74:901–910.

145. Seeds JW, Peng T. Impaired growth and risk of fetal death: is the tenth percentile the appropriate standard? *Am J Obstet Gynecol* 1998;178:658–669.

146. Gaziano EP, Knox H, Ferrera B, et al. Is it time to reassess the risk for the growth-retarded fetus with normal Doppler velocimetry of the umbilical artery? *Am J Obstet Gynecol* 1994;170(6):1734–1741; discussion 1741–1743.

147. Robel-Tillig E, Vogtmann C, Faber R. Postnatal intestinal disturbances in small-for-gestational-age premature infants after prenatal haemodynamic disturbances. *Acta Paediatr* 2000;89(3):324–330.

148. Ott WJ. Small for gestational age fetus and neonatal outcome: reevaluation of the relationship. *Am J Perinatol* 1995;12:396–400.

149. Goldenberg RL, Davis RO, Cliver SP, et al. Maternal risk factors and their influence on fetal anthropometric measurements. *Am J Obstet Gynecol* 1993;168:1197–1205.

150. Leitner Y, Fattal-Valevski A, Geva R, et al. Six-year follow-up of children with intrauterine growth retardation: long-term, prospective study. *J Child Neurol* 2000;15(12):781–786.

151. Ley D, Tideman E, Laurin J, et al. Abnormal fetal aortic velocity waveform and intellectual function at 7 years of age. *Ultrasound Obstet Gynecol* 1996;8(3):160–165.

152. Markestad T, Vik T, Ahlsten G, et al. Small-for-gestational-age (SGA) infants born at term: growth and development during the first year of life. *Acta Obstet Gynecol Scand Suppl* 1997;165:93–101.

153. Paz I, Laor A, Gale R, et al. Term infants with fetal growth restriction are not at increased risk for low intelligence scores at age 17 years. *J Pediatr* 2001;138(1):87–91.

154. Robinson JS, Moore VM, Owens JA, et al. Origins of fetal growth restriction. *Eur J Obstet Gynecol Reprod Biol* 2000;92(1):13–19.

155. Aviram-Goldring A, Daniely M, Dorf H, et al. Use of interphase fluorescence in situ hybridization in third trimester fetuses with anomalies and growth retardation. *Am J Med Genet* 1999;87(3):203–206.

156. Snijders RJ, Sherrod C, Gosden CM, et al. Fetal growth retardation: associated malformations and chromosomal abnormalities. *Am J Obstet Gynecol* 1993;168(2):547–555.

157. Khan NA, Kazzi SN. Yield and costs of screening growth-retarded infants for torch infections. *Am J Perinatol* 2000;17(3):131–135.

158. Stevens SM, Richardson DK, Gray JE, et al. Estimating neonatal mortality risk: an analysis of clinicians' judgments. *Pediatrics* 1994;93:945–950.

159. Bottoms SF, Paul RH, Iams JD, et al. Obstetric determinant of neonatal survival: influence of willingness to perform cesarean delivery on survival of extremely low-birth-weight infants. *Am J Obst Gynecol* 1997;176:960–966.

160. Pollack MM, Getson PR. Pediatric critical care cost containment: combined actuarial and clinical program. *Crit Care Med* 1991;19:12–20.

161. Wiznitzer A, Furman B, Zuili I, et al. Cord leptin level and fetal macrosomia. *Obstet Gynecol* 2000;96(5 Pt 1):707–713.

162. Schwartzler P, Homfray T, Campbell S, et al. Prenatal findings on ultrasound and x-ray in a case of overgrowth syndrome associated with increased nuchal translucency. *Prenat Diagn* 2001;21:341–345.

163. Ong HC, Sen DK. Clinical estimation of fetal weight. *Am J Obstet Gynecol* 1972;112:877–880.

164. Chauhan SP, West DJ, Scardo JA, et al. Antepartum detection of macrosomic fetus: clinical versus sonographic, including soft-tissue measurements. *Obstet Gynecol* 2000;95:639–642.

165. Gilby JR, Williams MC, Spellacy WN. Fetal abdominal circumference measurements of 35 and 38 cm as predictors of macrosomia. A risk factor for shoulder dystocia. *J Reprod Med* 2000;45(11):936–938.

166. Hirata GI, Medearis AL, Horenstein J, et al. Ultrasonographic estimation of fetal weight in the clinically macrosomic fetus. *Am J Obstet Gynecol* 1990;162:238–242.

167. Elliott JP, Garite TJ, Freeman RK, et al. Ultrasound prediction of fetal macrosomia in diabetic patients. *Obstet Gynecol* 1982;60:159–162.

168. Alsulyman OM, Ouzounian JG, Kjos SL. The accuracy of intrapartum ultrasonographic fetal weight estimation in diabetic pregnancies. *Am J Obstet Gynecol* 1997;177:503–506.

169. Benacerraf BR, Gelman R, Frigoletto FD. Sonographically estimated fetal weights: accuracy and limitations. *Am J Obstet Gynecol* 1988;159:1118–1121.

170. Field NT, Piper JM, Langer O. The effect of maternal obesity on the accuracy of fetal weight estimation. *Obstet Gynecol* 1995;86:102–107.

171. Hedriana HL, Moore TR. A comparison of single versus multiple growth ultrasonographic examinations in predicting birth weight. *Am J Obstet Gynecol* 1994;170:1600–1604; discussion 1604–1606.

172. Platek DN, Divon MY, Anyeagbunam A, et al. Intrapartum ultrasonographic estimates of fetal weight by the house staff. *Am J Obstet Gynecol* 1991;165:842–845.

173. Shepard MJ, Richards VA, Berkowitz RL. An evaluation of 2 equations for predicting fetal weight by ultrasound. *Am J Obstet Gynecol* 1982;142:47–51.

174. Coombs CA, Rosenn B, Miodovnik M, et al. Sonographic EFW and macrosomia: is there an optimum formula to predict diabetic fetal macrosomia? *J Matern Fetal Med* 2000;9:55–61.

175. Benson CB, Coughlin BF, Doubilet PM. Amniotic fluid volume in large-for-gestational age fetuses of nondiabetic mothers. *J Ultrasound Med* 1991;10:149–151.

176. Lazebnik N, Hill LM, Guzick D, et al. Severity of polyhydramnios does not affect the prevalence of large-for-gestational-age newborn infants. *J Ultrasound Med* 1996;15:385–388.

177. Winn HN, Holcomb W, Shumway JB, et al. The neonatal bisacromial diameter: a prenatal sonographic evaluation. *J Perinat Med* 1997;25:484–487.

178. Riska A, Laine H, Voutilainen P, et al. Estimation of fetal shoulder width by measurement of humerospinous distance by ultrasound. *Ultrasound Obstet Gynecol* 1996;7:272–274.

179. Kastler B, Gangi A, Mathelin C, et al. Fetal shoulder measurements with MRI. *J Comput Assist Tomogr* 1993;17:777–780.

180. Verspyck E, Goffinet F, Hellot M, et al. Newborn shoulder width: a prospective study of 2222 consecutive measurements. *Br J Obstet Gynaecol* 1999;106:589–593.

181. Gonen R, Spiegel D, Abend M. Is macrosomia predictable and are shoulder dystocia and birth trauma preventable? *Obstet Gynecol* 1996;88:526–529.

182. Watson WJ, Soisson AP, Harlass FE. Estimated weight of the term fetus. Accuracy of ultrasound vs. clinical examination. *J Reprod Med* 1988;33:369–371.

183. Raman S, Urquhart R, Yusof M. Clinical versus ultrasound estimation of fetal weight. *Aust N Z J Obstet Gynaecol* 1992;32:196–199.

184. Chauhan SP, Lutton PM, Bailey KJ, et al. Intrapartum clinical, sonographic and parous patient's estimation of newborn birth weight. *Obstet Gynecol* 1992;79:956–958.

185. Chauhan SP, Hendrix NW, Magann EF, et al. Limitations of clinical and sonographic estimates of birth weight: experience with 1034 parturients. *Obstet Gynecol* 1998;91:72–77.

186. Langer O, Berkus M, Huff RW, et al. Shoulder dystocia: should the fetus weighing greater than or equal to 4000 g be delivered by cesarean section? *Am J Obstet Gynecol* 1991;165:831–837.

187. Berard J, Dufour P, Vinatier D, et al. Fetal macrosomia: risk factors and outcome. A study of the outcome concerning 100 cases >4500 g. *Eur J Obstet Gynecol Reprod Biol* 1998;77:51–59.

188. Hope P, Breslin S, Lamont L, et al. Fatal shoulder dystocia: a review of 56 cases reported to the Confidential Enquiry into Stillbirths and Deaths in Infancy. *Br J Obstet Gynaecol* 1998;105:1256–1261.

189. Nesbitt TS, Gilbert WM, Herrchern B. Shoulder dystocia and associated risk factors with macrosomic infants born in California. *Am J Obstet Gynecol* 1998;179:476–480.

190. Smith RB, Lane C, Pearson JF. Shoulder dystocia: what happens at the next delivery? *Br J Obstet Gynecol* 1994;101:713–715.

191. Geary M, McParland P, Johnson H, et al. Shoulder dystocia—is it predictable? *Eur J Obstet Gynecol Reprod Biol* 1995;62:15–18.

192. Weeks JW, Pitman T, Spinnato JA. Fetal macrosomia: does antenatal prediction affect delivery route and birth outcome? *Am J Obstet Gynecol* 1995;173:1215–1219.

193. Coombs CA, Singh NB, Khoury JC. Elective induction versus spontaneous labor after sonographic diagnosis of fetal macrosomia. *Obstet Gynecol* 1993;81:492–496.

194. Conway DL, Langer O. Elective delivery of infants with macrosomia in diabetic women: reduced shoulder dystocia versus increased cesarean deliveries. *Am J Obstet Gynecol* 1998;178:922–952.

195. Ananth CV, Vintzlileos AM, Shen-Schwartz S, et al. Standards of birth weight in twin gestations stratified by placental chorionicity. *Obstet Gynecol* 1998;91:917–924.

196. Alexander GR, Kogan M, Martin J, et al. What are the fetal growth pattern of singletons, twins and triplets in the United States? *Clin Obstet Gynecol* 1998;41:115–125.

197. Xu D, Deter RL, Milner LL, et al. Evaluation of twin growth status at birth using individualized growth assessment: comparison with conventional methods. *J Clin Ultrasound* 1995;23:277–286.

198. Luke B, Keith L. The contribution of singletons, twins and triplets to low birth weight, infant mortality and handicap in the United States. *J Reprod Med* 1992;37:661–666.

199. Cohen SB, Dulitsky M, Lipitz S, et al. New birth weight nomograms for twin gestations on the basis of accurate gestational age. *Am J Obstet Gynecol* 1997;177:1101–1104.

200. Chitkara U, Berkowitz R, Levine R, et al. Twin pregnancy: routine use of ultrasound examination in the prenatal diagnosis of intrauterine growth retardation and discordant growth. *Am J Perinatol* 1985;2:49–54.

201. Bronsteen G, Goyert S, Bottom SB. Classification of twins and neonatal morbidity. *Obstet Gynecol* 1989;74:98–100.

202. Fraser D, Picard R, Picard E, et al. Birth weight discordance, intrauterine growth retardation and perinatal outcome. *J Reprod Med* 1994;39:504–508.

203. Weissman A, Achiron R, Lipitz S, et al. The first trimester growth-discordant twin: an ominous prenatal finding. *Obstet Gynecol* 1994;84:110–114.

204. Sherer DM, Divon MY. Fetal growth in multifetal gestation. *Clin Obstet Gynecol* 1998;40:764–770.

205. Blickstein I. The definition, diagnosis and management of growth-discordant twins: an international consensus survey. *Acta Genet Med Gemellol* 1991;40:345–351.

206. Hill M, Guzick D, Cheveney P, et al. The sonographic assessment of twin growth discordance. *Obstet Gynecol* 1994;84:501–504.

207. Beattie RB, McDowell MJ, Ritchie JWK. Optimizing fetal surveillance in twin pregnancies. *J Maternal Fetal Invest* 1993;3:53–57.

208. Ville Y. Monochorionic twins, les liaisons dangereuses. *Ultrasound Obstet Gynecol* 1997;10:82–85.

209. Andres RL, Day MC. Perinatal complications associated with maternal tobacco use. *Semin Neonatol* 2000;5(3):231–241.

210. Hanretty KP, Primrose MH, Neilson JP, Whittle MJ. Pregnancy screening by Doppler uteroplacental and umbilical artery waveforms. *Br J Obstet Gynaecol* 1989;96:1163–1167.

3

ABNORMALITIES OF AMNIOTIC FLUID

Abnormalities of amniotic fluid, whether deficient (oligohydramnios) or excessive (polyhydramnios), are frequently the first clues to an underlying fetal or maternal disorder. Even when not associated with a fetal malformation, oligohydramnios or polyhydramnios is associated with increased rates of perinatal morbidity and mortality. For these reasons, the obstetric sonographer should have a basic understanding of normal amniotic fluid production.

This chapter discusses current concepts in the derivation of normal and abnormal amniotic fluid volume. Definitions and sonographic criteria for oligohydramnios and polyhydramnios, their possible causes, sequelae, and potential treatment are also discussed.

NORMAL AMNIOTIC FLUID VOLUME

Before the twentieth century, relatively little was known about the formation, maintenance, and volume of amniotic fluid. In a review of the literature, Brace and Wolf[1] compiled 705 measurements from the literature of amniotic fluid volume from 8 to 43 weeks' gestation. All of the measurements were either taken directly at hysterotomy or by a dye-dilution technique. Amniotic fluid volume was found to increase progressively until 33 weeks' gestation (Fig. 1). There was an 8% decline in amniotic fluid from 38 to 43 weeks' gestation. The mean amniotic fluid volume between 22 and 39 weeks' gestation ranged from 630 to 817 mL. Below and above the 95% confidence interval defined oligohydramnios and polyhydramnios, respectively. For example, at 30 weeks' gestation, oligohydramnios was an amniotic fluid volume less than 300 mL, and polyhydramnios was an amniotic fluid volume greater than 2,100 mL.

ROLE OF AMNIOTIC FLUID

Amniotic fluid provides a number of important functions for the developing fetus (Table 1). Indeed, it is impossible for normal fetal development in the absence of amniotic fluid. The fluid helps protect the fetus from trauma, including compression by the intrauterine environment. Normal fluid allows fetal activity in a near weightless environment, permitting development of the musculoskeletal system. Normal fluid is also important in development of the gastrointestinal and pulmonary systems.

A relationship between amniotic fluid and fetal weight has been observed for some time.[2] Good evidence exists that ingestion of fluid is important for normal fetal growth in human and animal studies.[3,4] Conversely, interruption of normal fluid ingestion early in gestation results in profound changes in the growth and development of the gastrointestinal tract. These effects can be reversed.[5] It is estimated that normal fluid ingestion may contribute to 10% to 15% of fetal weight.

AMNIOTIC FLUID VOLUME REGULATION

The amount of amniotic fluid present at any one time reflects a balance between amniotic fluid production and amniotic fluid removal (Figs. 2 and 3). Hence, maintenance of amniotic fluid volume is a dynamic process, with different contributing factors at different stages of pregnancy.

The six potential pathways for fluid movement into and out of the amniotic cavity include (Figs. 2 and 3) the following:

1. Fetal urine
2. Fetal swallowing
3. Oral secretions
4. Secretions from the respiratory tract
5. Transfer across the placenta, umbilical cord, and fetal skin (intramembranous flow)
6. Across the fetal membranes (transmembranous flow)

Amniotic fluid volume increases rapidly during the first trimester (Fig. 4). The sonographically estimated amniotic fluid volume at 7, 10, and 12 weeks' gestation is 1 mL, 25 mL, and 60 mL, respectively.[6] These values are consistent with direct measurements obtained at hysterotomy.[7]

Swallowed amniotic fluid is reabsorbed by the gastrointestinal tract and then recirculates through the kidneys. The exponential rise in amniotic fluid after 9 weeks'

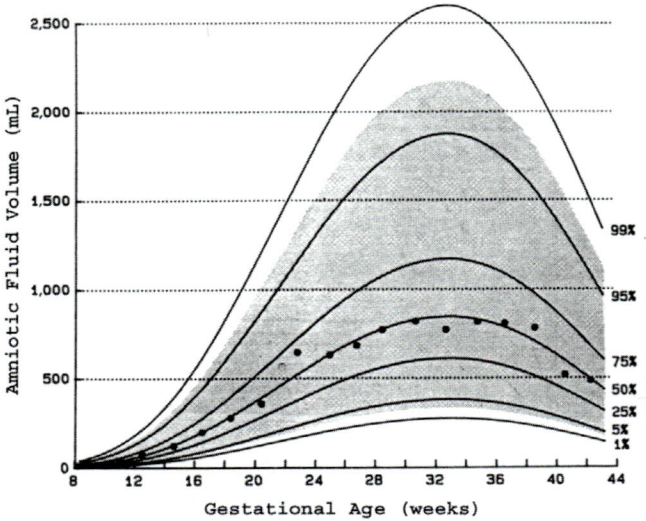

FIGURE 1. Normogram of normal amniotic fluid volume by gestational age. (Reproduced with permission from Brace RA. Normal amniotic fluid volume changes throughout pregnancy. *Am J Obstet Gynecol* 1989; 161:386.)

TABLE 1. ROLES OF AMNIOTIC FLUID

Protects the fetus from external trauma
Protects the umbilical cord from compression
Reduces the potential for infection through its bacteriostatic properties
Provides thermal stability
Permits fetal movement and allows development of the musculoskeletal system
Helps lung development
Helps gastrointestinal development
Nutritional effect

gestation[3] suggests that initiation of urine production begins in the first trimester.[8] By 18 weeks, the fetus excretes an estimated urine volume of 7 to 14 mL per 24 hours and swallows 4 to 11 mL per 24 hours.[9] During the latter stages of mid-pregnancy, the amniotic fluid volume increases by approximately 10 mL per day.[10] Because the amount of amniotic fluid produced by fetal urination only slightly exceeds the amount removed by fetal swallowing, more than 40% of the incremental increase in amniotic fluid originates from other sources.

In the third trimester, fetal swallowing and urination strongly influence the constitution and volume of amniotic fluid. Near term, the fetus swallows approximately 500 to 1,000 mL per hour and voids approximately 600 to 1,200 mL per hour.[11]

The intramembranous pathway includes the passive exchange that occurs across fetal skin, umbilical cord, and the fetal surface of the placenta. Because of the transcutaneous fluid loss, the postnatal treatment of the extremely preterm infant requires three times the fluid intake of the term neonate.[12] This higher water loss in preterm infants is due to a lack of keratin. This experience suggests that exchange across the skin also plays an important role in amniotic fluid regulation *in utero*. The equilibration between embryo and fetal plasma and amniotic fluid is secondary to diffusion across the skin.[13]

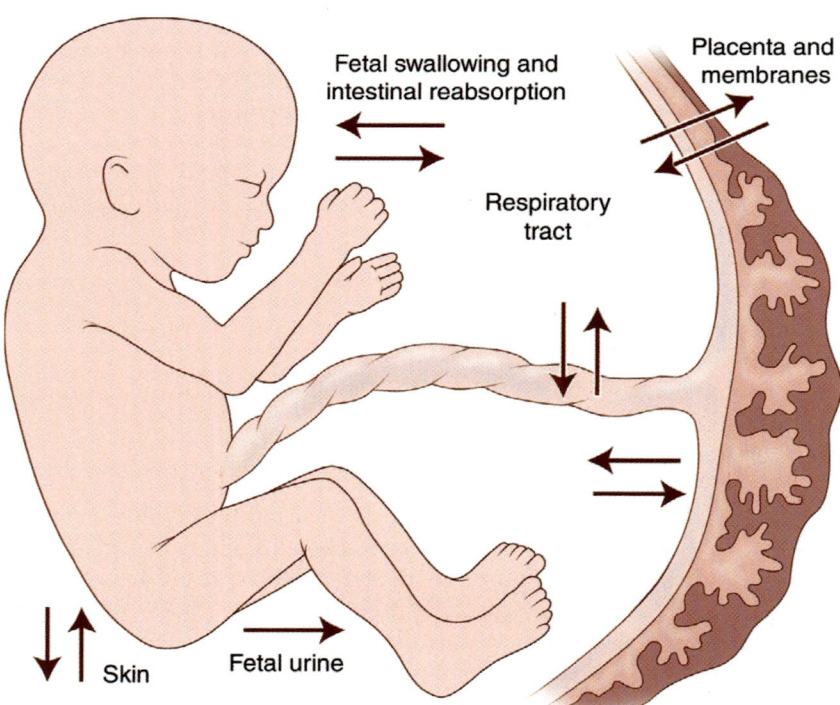

FIGURE 2. Normal amniotic fluid regulation.

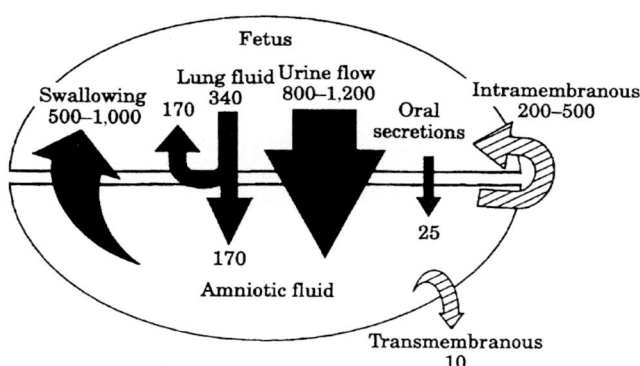

FIGURE 3. Best estimates of daily volume flows for the near-term fetus. (Reproduced with permission from Brace R. Progress toward understanding the regulation of amniotic fluid volume: water and solute fluxes in and through the fetal membranes. *Placenta* 1995;16:1.)

Estimates of intramembranous flow (400 mL per day) observed from the amniotic cavity have only been reported for the sheep model.[11] Small changes in daily intramembranous sodium flux may, therefore, result in large changes in amniotic fluid volume.[13] When the intramembranous pathway is functioning appropriately, a reduction in fetal urine production is countered by a reversal of the normal intramembranous flow from the amniotic fluid to the fetal plasma, resulting in a preservation of amniotic fluid volume.[14]

The fetal lungs normally secrete fluid into the amniotic cavity. Although fluid may enter the trachea during fetal breathing, it does not enter the fetal lungs. Approximately one-half of the fluid that exits the trachea enters the amniotic fluid, and the remaining 50% is swallowed[15]; 170 mL of lung fluid is swallowed and another 170 mL enters the amniotic fluid per day.[8,11]

The solute concentration rather than the volume of amniotic fluid is rigidly maintained. For example, Lingwood et al.[16] replaced 20% to 30% of the amniotic fluid volume in 17 pregnant ewes with isotonic saline, mannitol, or dextrose. Concentrations of sodium, potassium, and chloride returned to pre-infusion level by 6 hours. Amniotic fluid volume increased significantly with return of solute.

NORMAL AMNIOTIC FLUID VOLUME

The gold standard for determination of amniotic fluid volume is a dye-dilution technique, which requires amniocentesis, instillation of a dye, and then repeat measurement of the dye after diffusion throughout the amniotic fluid. This technique is obviously impractical on a clinical basis. Accepted sonographic methods for assessing amniotic fluid are subjective (visual criteria) or semiquantitative (measuring one or more pockets of amniotic fluid).

A simple way of assessing amniotic fluid is measurement of the single deepest vertical pocket of fluid, which is free of fetal extremities and umbilical cord (Fig. 5).[17] Another semiquantitative method for assessment of amniotic fluid volume using the largest pocket of amniotic fluid is the area of a two-diameter pocket[18] (Fig. 6). The horizontal and vertical dimensions of the maximum vertical pocket are multiplied together to obtain a single value. A two-diameter pocket of 15.1 to 50 cm² is considered normal.

In an attempt to more fully assess the amount of amniotic fluid within the entire uterine cavity, Phelan[19,20] initially described the amniotic fluid index (AFI) as the sum of the maximum vertical pocket in each of the four quadrants of the uterus (Fig. 7). Normal amniotic fluid was originally defined as AFI less than 5 cm and greater than 20 cm, respectively, and this was subsequently refined to correlate

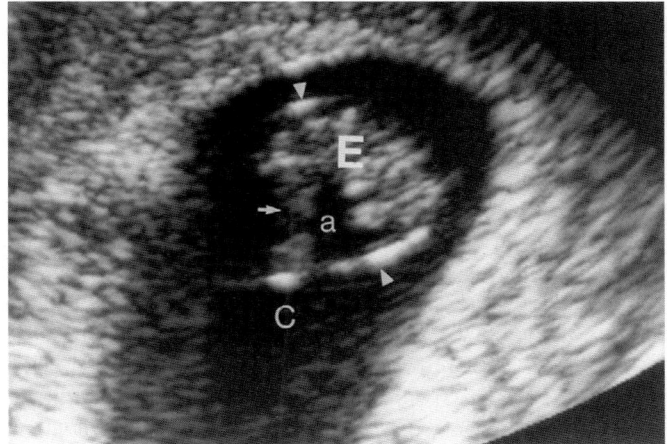

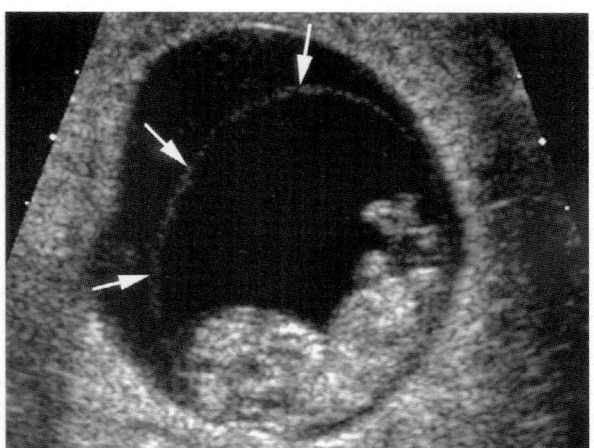

FIGURE 4. First-trimester amniotic fluid. **A:** Eight-week embryo (*E*). The amniotic cavity is relatively small (*a*) compared to the chorionic cavity (*C*). The amnion is visible (*arrowheads*) as is the early umbilical cord (*arrow*). **B:** Ten-week fetus. There is a dramatic rise in amniotic fluid volume after 9 weeks' gestation. Arrows point to amnion.

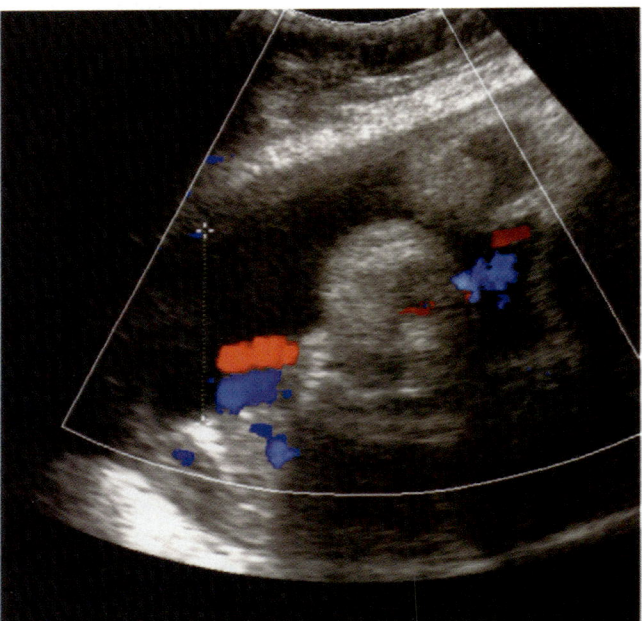

FIGURE 5. Normal single pocket measurement of amniotic fluid (calipers). The maximum vertical pocket measurement of 6 cm at 26 weeks' gestation is considered normal.

with gestational age. Moore[21] defined normal amniotic fluid as AFI between the 5th percentile and the 95th percentile (Table 2, Fig. 8).

There is good correlation between subjective assessment and semiquantitative measurements among experienced sonographers.[22] There is also fair correlation between the various semiquantitative measurements. As a general rule, although exceptions are common, the AFI is approximately three times the largest pocket of amniotic fluid.

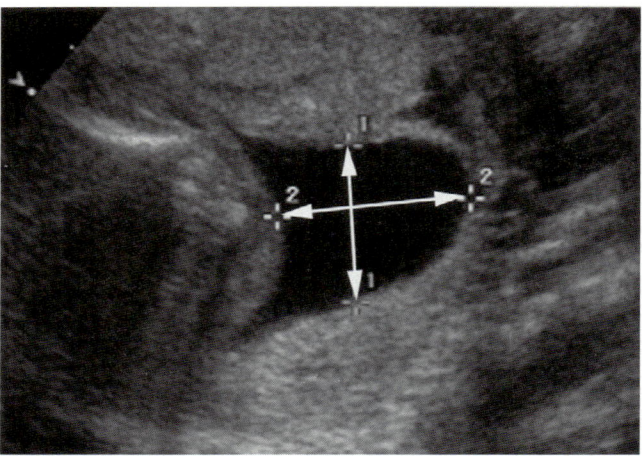

FIGURE 6. Two-diameter pocket measurement. The horizontal and vertical dimensions of the maximum vertical pocket are multiplied together to obtain a single value. In this case, the two-diameter pocket measurement is 9 cm², indicating oligohydramnios.

Semiquantitative measurements are useful for following amniotic fluid volume on serial examinations. However, it is less reliable for accurate determination of amniotic fluid volume on a single examination. Therefore, although the AFI is proportional to the amount of amniotic fluid, it cannot accurately measure the amniotic fluid volume.[18,23,24] The AFI tends to overestimate the actual volume at lower volumes and underestimate the volume at high volumes.[23]

Approximate normal and abnormal values of amniotic fluid during the third trimester are shown in Table 3. These values are relatively stable after 20 weeks until the end of the third trimester. Subjective assessment of normal amniotic fluid correlates with AFI of 10 to 20, with borderline values of 5 to 10 for low fluid and 20 to 24 for increased fluid. Definite oligohydramnios correlates with AFI of 0 to 5 and largest vertical pocket measuring 2 cm or less; definite polyhydramnios correlates with AFI of 24 or more and largest vertical pocket of 8 or more.

Amniotic fluid varies with gestational age during the mid-second trimester. Gramellini et al.[25] have published normal reference values of amniotic fluid during the second trimester, between 12 and 24 weeks (Fig. 9). They found good intra- and interoperative reproducibility for four methods of amniotic fluid assessment: the largest vertical pocket and largest transverse pocket measured on the same image, the two-diameter pocket (product of the vertical and transverse pocket), and the mean amniotic fluid diameter.

In comparing values, it should also be noted that the use of color Doppler imaging (Fig. 10) results in a lower AFI measurement[26] but has a more consistent result with reduction of intraobserver variation.

Three-dimensional ultrasound offers the promise of more accurately quantifying the volume of amniotic fluid.[27] It remains to be determined, however, if the improved accuracy of three-dimensional ultrasound also improves subsequent neonatal outcome.

AMNIOTIC FLUID IN TWIN PREGNANCIES

Initially, the amniotic fluid volume in twins was assessed without regard to the intervening membrane, although it is obvious that each sac should be measured separately.[28] Like singleton pregnancies, each sac can be assessed by subjective and semiquantitative methods, and there is good general agreement among experienced sonographers. Semiquantitative methods used to assess twin pregnancies include the single largest pocket of fluid, the two-diameter pocket, or the AFI (Fig. 11).[29,30] Although twin pregnancies have a slightly lower median AFI value than singleton pregnancies, the difference is not statistically significant.[29] In comparison with a dye-dilution technique, Magann et al.[31] found that the two-diameter pocket was a better predictor of oligohydramnios than the AFI or the largest vertical pocket.

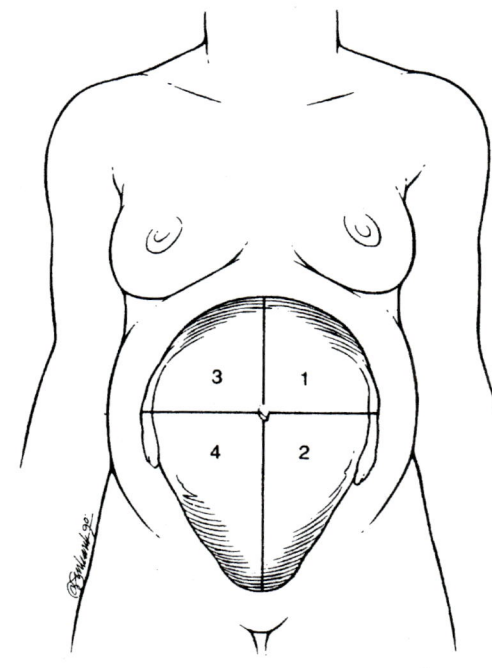

FIGURE 7. Amniotic fluid index. **A:** The uterus is divided into four equal quadrants (1, 2, 3, 4). The maximum vertical pocket of fluid void of fetal parts and umbilical cord is measured, and the sum of these measurements is calculated. Amniotic fluid index = 1 + 2 + 3 + 4. **B:** Ultrasound images from four quadrants of a 30-week pregnancy. The four-quadrant amniotic fluid index is 15. LLQ, left lower quadrant; LUQ, left upper quadrant; RLQ, right lower quadrant; RUQ, right upper quadrant. (Part **A** reproduced with permission from Gabbe SG, Nebyl JR, Simpson JL. *Obstetrics: normal and problem pregnancies*, 2nd ed. New York: Churchill Livingstone, 1991.)

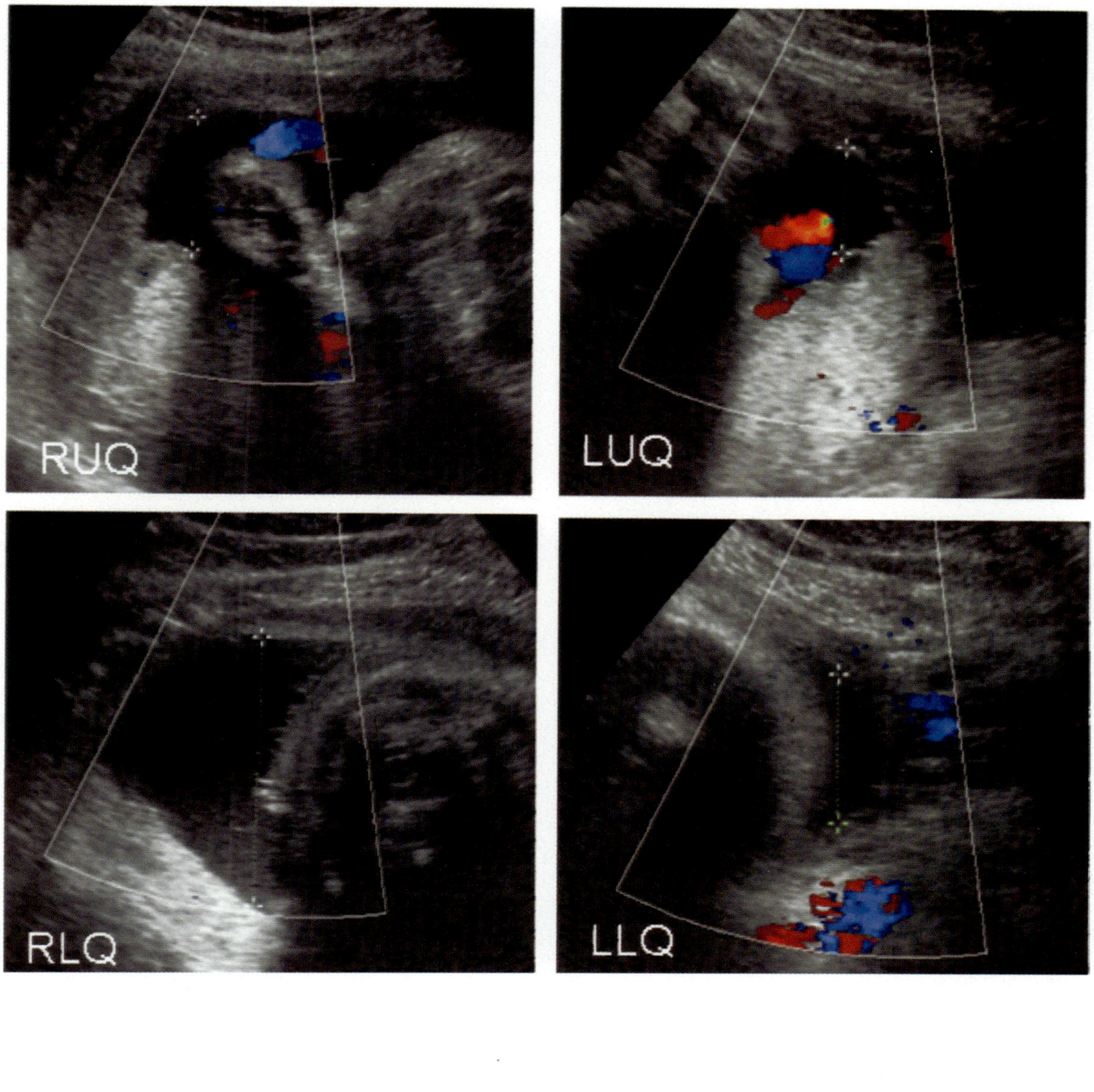

A

RUQ

LUQ

RLQ

LLQ

B

TABLE 2. COMPARISON OF AMNIOTIC FLUID INDEX VALUES WITH GESTATIONAL AGE

Gestational age (wk)	Amniotic fluid index values					
	2.5th percentile	5th percentile	50th percentile	95th percentile	97.5th percentile	n
16	73	79	121	185	201	32
17	77	83	127	194	211	26
18	80	87	133	202	220	17
19	83	90	137	207	225	14
20	86	93	141	212	230	25
21	88	95	143	214	233	14
22	89	97	145	216	235	14
23	90	98	146	218	237	14
24	90	98	147	219	238	23
25	89	97	147	221	240	12
26	89	97	147	223	242	11
27	85	95	146	226	245	17
28	86	94	146	228	249	25
29	84	92	145	231	254	12
30	82	90	145	234	258	17
31	79	88	144	238	263	26
32	77	86	144	242	269	25
33	64	83	143	245	274	30
34	72	81	142	248	278	31
35	70	79	140	249	279	27
36	68	77	138	249	279	39
37	66	75	135	244	275	36
38	65	73	132	239	269	27
39	64	72	127	226	255	12
40	63	71	123	214	240	64
41	63	70	116	194	216	162
42	63	69	110	175	192	30

Modified from Moore TR, Gayle JE. The amniotic fluid index in normal human pregnancy. *Am J Obstet Gynecol* 1990;162:1168–1173.

They conclude that the extremes of volume (low or high) are poorly identified by the subjective or objective assessment of volume.

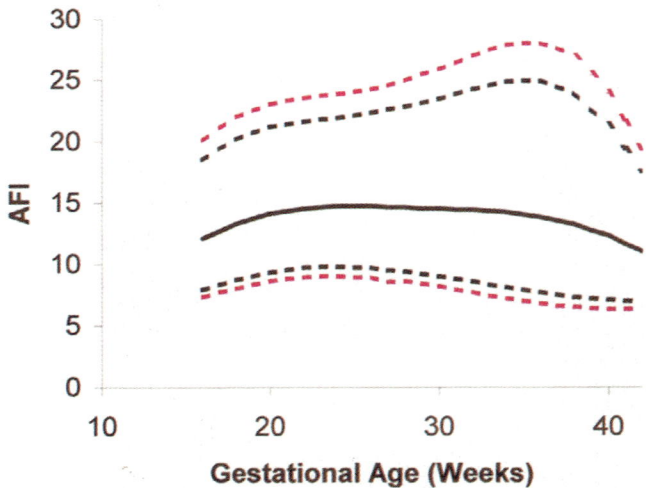

FIGURE 8. Normal amniotic fluid index (AFI) compared with gestational age. The mean (*black line*), ninety-fifth percentiles (*dashed black lines*), and ninety-seventh percentiles (*dashed red lines*) are shown.

OLIGOHYDRAMNIOS

Definition and Sonographic Criteria

Visual criteria for oligohydramnios include evidence of fetal crowding and an obvious lack of fluid (Fig. 12).[32]

Using the single largest pocket of amniotic fluid, oligohydramnios has been variously defined as a single pocket with a depth of less than or equal to 0.5 cm,[33] less than 1 and 2 cm,[34] and less than or equal to 3 cm.[35] Comparing

TABLE 3. APPROXIMATE VALUES FOR NORMAL FLUID, OLIGOHYDRAMNIOS, AND POLYHYDRAMNIOS DURING THE THIRD TRIMESTER

	Largest vertical pocket	Amniotic fluid index	Two-diameter pocket
Oligohydramnios	0–2	0–5	0–15
Normal range	2.1–8.0	5.1–24.0[a]	15.1–50.0
Polyhydramnios	>8	>24	>50

[a]Borderline decreased fluid may be considered 5.1 to 10.0. Borderline increased fluid may be considered 20 to 24.

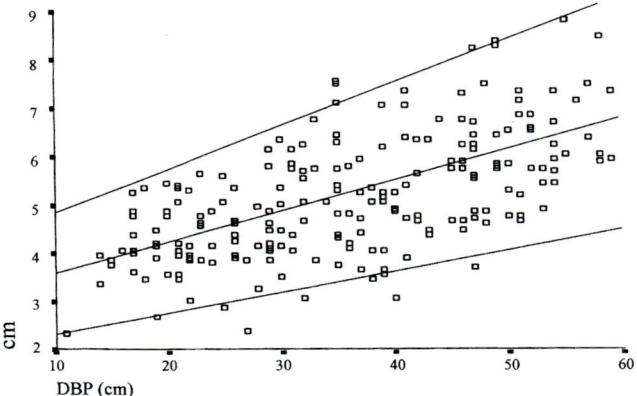

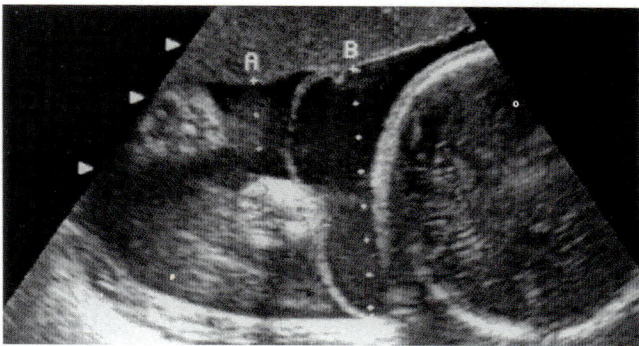

FIGURE 11. Measurement of the inner upper pockets of amniotic fluid (*A* and *B*) in a twin pregnancy at 29 weeks' gestation.

FIGURE 9. Normal amniotic fluid reference values between 12 and 24 weeks. Mean amniotic fluid diameter is the mean of maximum transverse and vertical pocket of amniotic fluid on the same image, and the two-diameter pocket is the product of these two measurements. Values are plotted against diameter of biparietal (DBP) head measurement. (Reproduced with permission from Gramellini D, Chiaie D, Piantelli G, Sansebastiano L, Fieni S, et al. Sonographic assessment of amniotic fluid volume between 11 and 24 weeks of gestation: construction of reference intervals related to gestational age. *Ultrasound Obstet Gynecol* 2001;17:410–415.)

criteria of AFI less than 5 cm, single deepest pocket less than 2 cm, and a two-diameter pocket less than 15 cm^2 resulted in widely different prevalence rates for oligohydramnios of 8%, 1%, and 30%, respectively.[36] The single deepest pocket showed the lowest false-positive rate, but also resulted in the lowest detection rates.

Moore[21] defined oligohydramnios as an AFI below the 5th percentile. This corresponds to AFI less than 7 cm near term. However, a more common definition for oligohydramnios is AFI less than 5 cm. This would incorporate less than 1% of term gestations. Criteria of AFI less than 5 cm

or largest pocket of fluid of less than 2 cm are highly specific for oligohydramnios but not sensitive when compared against the dye-dilution technique.[37,38] On the other hand, these more strict criteria for oligohydramnios are more likely to correlate with adverse clinical outcomes.

A wider intraobserver variation in the AFI has been observed when oligohydramnios is present. Therefore, averaging three AFI measurements is recommended when a low value is obtained.[21] Not unexpectedly, there is some degree of correlation between AFI and volume. In patients with oligohydramnios, infusion of 250 mL of saline into the amniotic cavity results in an increase of the AFI between 4 cm[39] and 6 cm.[40]

Etiology of Oligohydramnios

Oligohydramnios can usually be attributed to one of five etiologies (Table 4). These are discussed in this section. Infection is a less likely cause of oligohydramnios.

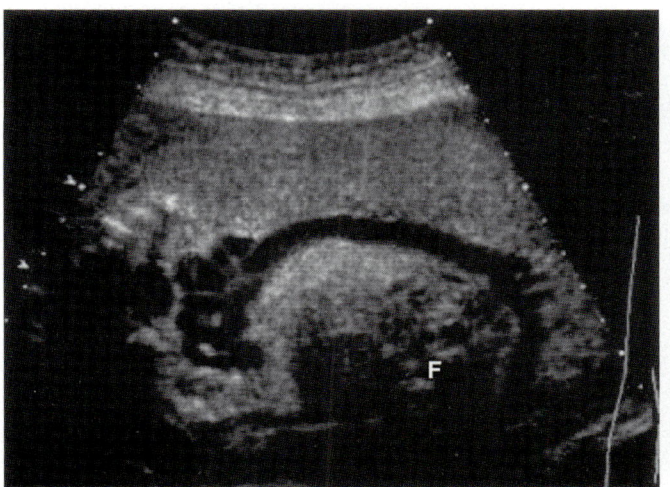

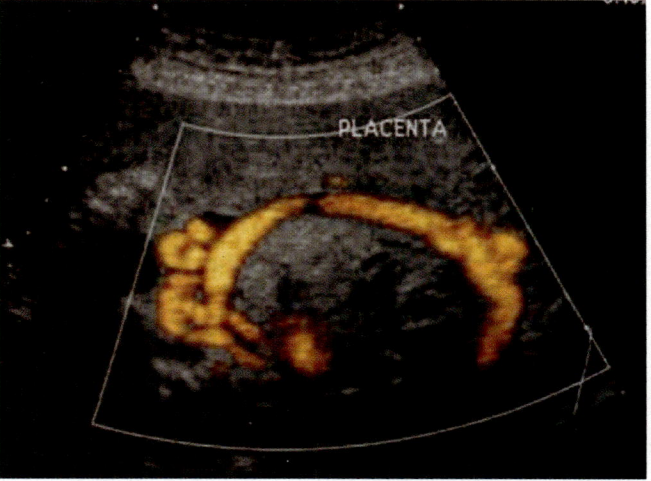

FIGURE 10. A: Sonolucent area surrounding fetus (*F*) could be mistaken for amniotic fluid. **B:** Color-flow imaging shows that the amniotic space is filled with umbilical cord, and little amniotic fluid is visible.

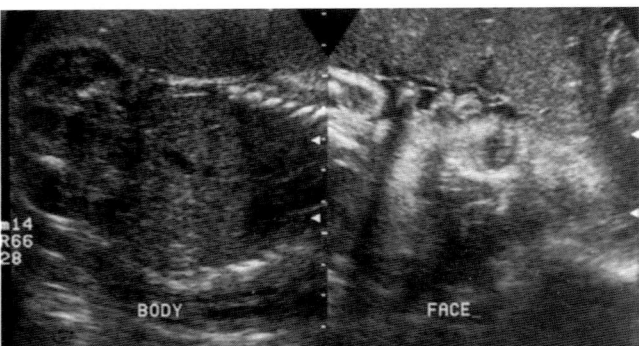

FIGURE 12. Oligohydramnios at 27 weeks' gestation. There is fetal crowding with an absence of visible amniotic fluid.

Fetal Anomalies and Aneuploidies

The prevalence of congenital anomalies (4.5% to 37.0%) and aneuploidy (0.0% to 4.4%) in fetuses with oligohydramnios is based on the size of the population under investigation and the mix of high- and low-risk patients.[41–47] The majority of fetal anomalies that result in oligohydramnios involve the urinary tract, although anomalies of virtually every organ system have been reported (Table 5). Sonography can accurately show the vast majority of significant renal anomalies resulting in oligohydramnios, including bilateral renal agenesis (Fig. 13), bladder outlet obstruction (Fig. 14), multicystic dysplastic kidneys (Fig. 15), and infantile polycystic kidney disease (Fig. 16).

Although renal agenesis is frequently suspected when amniotic fluid is markedly decreased to absent, it is a difficult malformation to confirm. Fetal anatomy is poorly visualized transabdominally because of the absence of amniotic fluid. Also, demonstrating the absence of normal structures is more difficult than showing the presence of a particular malformation. Hypertrophied adrenal glands may be confused with normal kidneys.

TABLE 4. CAUSES AND ASSOCIATIONS WITH OLIGOHYDRAMNIOS

Anomalies and/or chromosome abnormalities
Intrauterine growth restriction
Post-term pregnancies
Ruptured membranes
Iatrogenic

Transvaginal sonography may be used in the second trimester to more accurately assess the renal fossae. The documentation of a *lying down adrenal* (Fig. 13A) confirms that a kidney is not appropriately positioned in the renal fossa.[48] Color or power Doppler may be used to confirm the presence or absence of the renal arteries (Fig. 13B). The distance from the aortic branching of the external iliac arteries to the renal arteries has been determined sonographically.[49] Failure to detect the renal arteries at the appropriate distance confirms the diagnosis of bilateral renal agenesis.

Spontaneous filling and emptying of the urinary bladder virtually excludes a diagnosis of bilateral renal agenesis and should suggest alternative diagnoses, including less severe renal malformations, structural anomalies of other organ systems, severe intrauterine growth restriction (IUGR), or occult rupture of the membranes.

Demonstration of early symmetric IUGR with marked oligohydramnios should suggest the possibility of an underlying chromosomal disorder, notably trisomy 18 or triploidy. Generally, those fetuses with a karyotypic abnormality and oligohydramnios have one or more structural malformations.

Intrauterine Growth Restriction

Fetal hypoxemia may produce growth restriction and oligohydramnios. This association has historically been attributed to a decrease in fetal urine production secondary to a redistribution of blood flow away from the kid-

TABLE 5. TYPE AND PREVALENCE OF CONGENITAL MALFORMATIONS ASSOCIATED WITH OLIGOHYDRAMNIOS

Study	Year	Cases	Anomalies (%)	Anomalies by organ system						
				Renal	Central nervous	Skeletal	Cardiovascular	Other	Multiple	Aneuploidy
Chamberlain[85]	1984	223	4.5	7	1	—	1	—	—	1
Mercer[33]	1984	247	7.0	5	2	4	3	1	2	—
Sivit[186]	1986	16	56.0	9	—	—	—	—	—	—
Bastide[44]	1986	113	13.3	5	1	—	—	2	7	—
Shenker[45]	1991	80	13.8	9	—	—	—	—	2	—
Los[168]	1992	26	34.6	9	—	—	—	—	—	—
Golan[187]	1994	145	11.0	6	2	7	4	7	—	—
Shipp[47]	1996	250	37.0	68	3	1	—	3	6	11
Total		1,100	17.2	118 (62.4)[a]	9 (4.8)[a]	12 (6.3)[a]	8 (4.2)[a]	13 (7.0)[a]	17 (9.0)[a]	12 (6.3)[a]

[a]Percent of 189 reported anomalies.

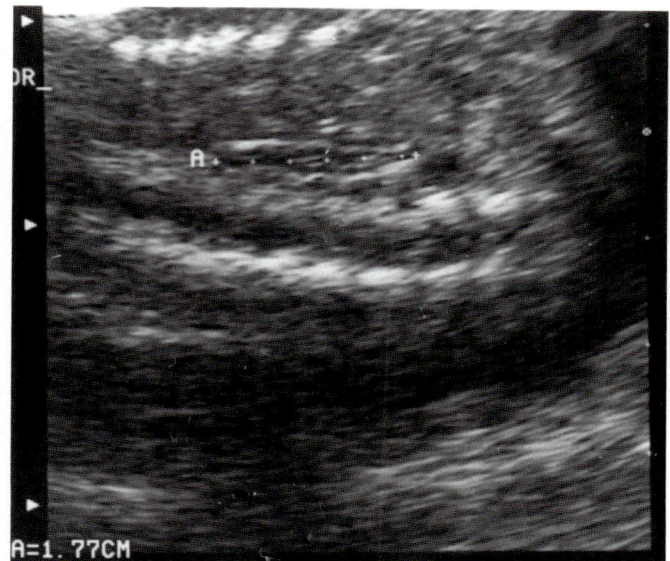

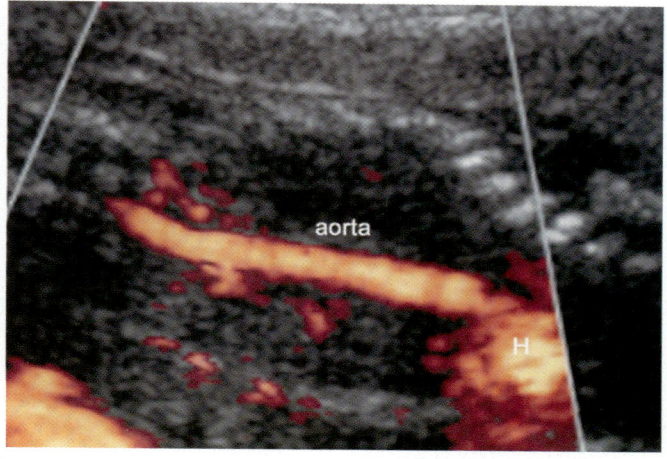

FIGURE 13. Bilateral renal agenesis. **A:** Laying-down adrenal (*A*) associated with renal agenesis. **B:** Power Doppler of the aorta in a 21-week fetus with bilateral renal agenesis. The renal arteries are not present. H, heart.

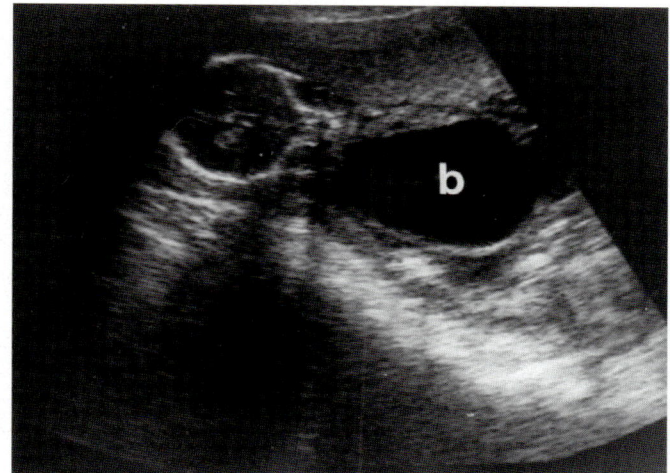

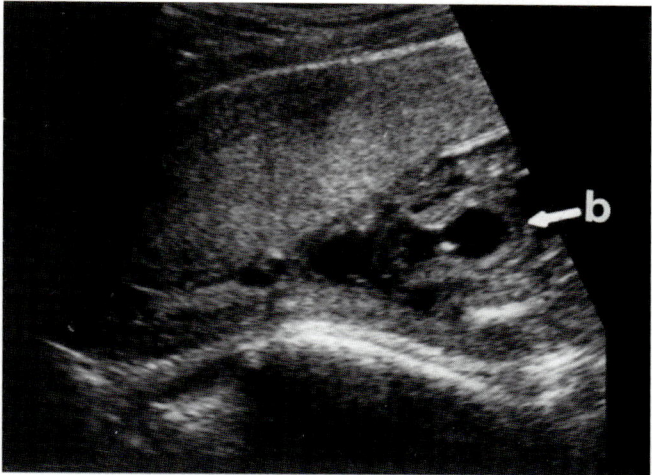

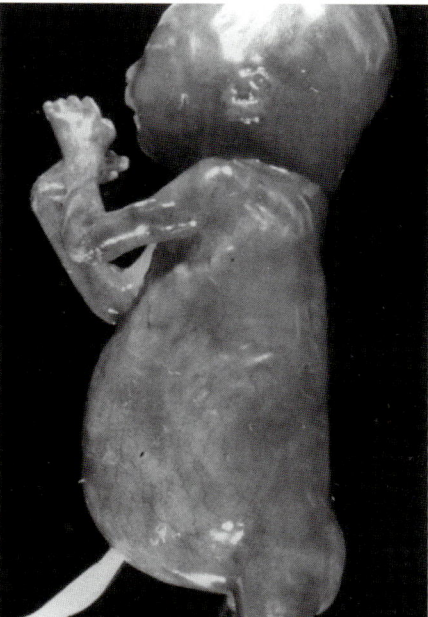

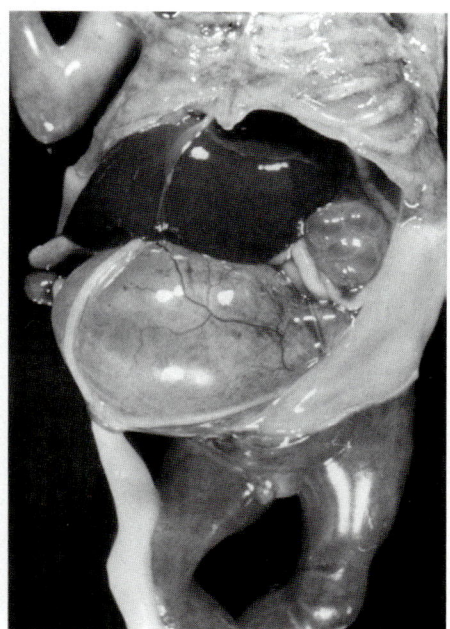

FIGURE 14. Posterior urethral valves at 18 weeks' gestation. **A:** There is oligohydramnios with an enlarged bladder (*b*). The fetus is in breech presentation. **B:** Completion of bladder (*b*) tap. Note the thickened bladder wall. **C:** Postmortem fetus with distended abdomen due to bladder obstruction. **D:** Postmortem distended bladder.

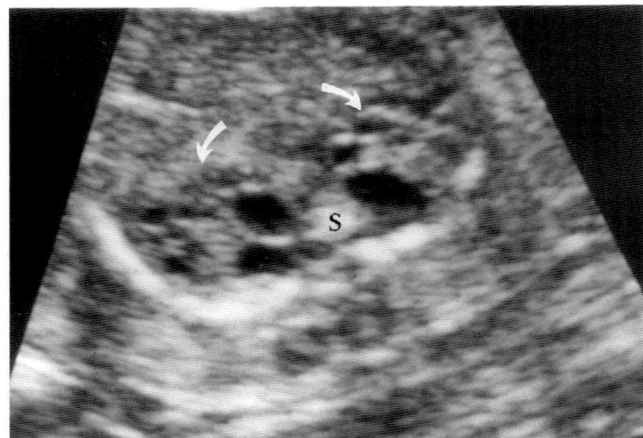
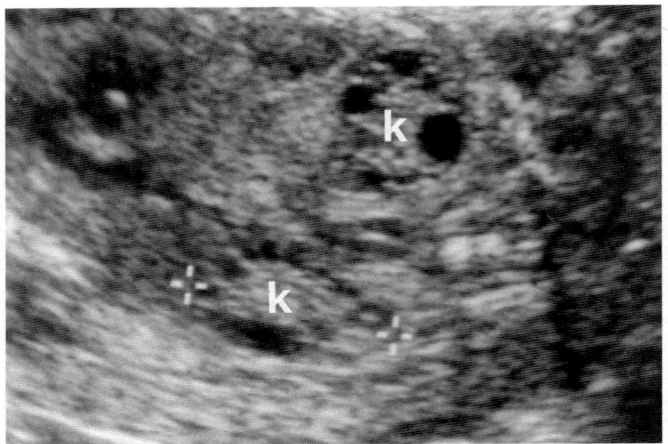

FIGURE 15. Bilateral renal cystic dysplasia and oligohydramnios at 18 weeks' gestation. **A:** Transverse view of the kidneys showing multiple cysts of varying sizes (*arrows*). S, spine. **B:** Coronal view of the cystic kidneys (*k*).

neys. However, this is not supported by an animal model (ewe) of induced hypoxemia,[50,51] suggesting a possible alternative of decreased intramembranous flow as the cause of oligohydramnios.

In general, IUGR is suspected when the estimated fetal weight falls below the 10th percentile for the expected gestational age (see Chapter 2). No single criterion can confidently diagnose IUGR, but multiple parameters can be used to help suggest the presence of IUGR.

In the setting of oligohydramnios, IUGR is more likely to be present even at higher estimated weight measurements. Chamberlain[43] found a 5% incidence of IUGR with a single amniotic fluid pocket dimension of greater than 2 cm. When the single largest pocket of amniotic fluid was less than or equal to 2 cm and less than or equal to 1 cm, the rate of IUGR was 20% and 39%, respectively.

Post-Term Pregnancies

Post-term pregnancies, defined by a gestational age of 42 weeks or more, occurs in approximately 5.7% of pregnancies.[52] Oligohydramnios is a common complication of postdate pregnancies, and it is associated with diminished placental function.[53] It also is associated with arterial redistribution of fetal blood flow with the *brain sparing* effect.[54] Because oligohydramnios is associated with adverse outcome, including fetal and neonatal death,[55,56] it is important to monitor amniotic fluid in post-term pregnancies.

In a randomized, controlled trial[57] of 500 women with post-term pregnancies, oligohydramnios was diagnosed by means of an AFI less than 7.3 cm or a single vertical pocket of less than 1.8 cm in 10% and 2% of cases, respectively. As a result, more inductions of labor occurred in the AFI group. Whereas there was no evidence that the increased induction rate improved perinatal outcome, this study was underpowered.

Ruptured Membranes

Premature rupture of the membranes occurs in approximately 10% of pregnancies.[58] This is usually diagnosed clinically although evaluation of amniotic fluid by ultrasound complements the clinical assessment. If the diagnosis is still in question after ultrasound and clinical assessment, amniocentesis with instillation of indigo carmine dye can be performed. The subsequent presence of the blue dye on a perineal pad confirms the diagnosis.

Persistent oligohydramnios in the second trimester carries a poor prognosis regardless of the etiology, and the patient should be counseled appropriately.

Severe oligohydramnios (single pocket less than 1 cm) lasting for 14 days or more after spontaneous premature rupture of the membranes at less than 25 weeks' gestation is associated with a 90% neonatal mortality.[59] On the other

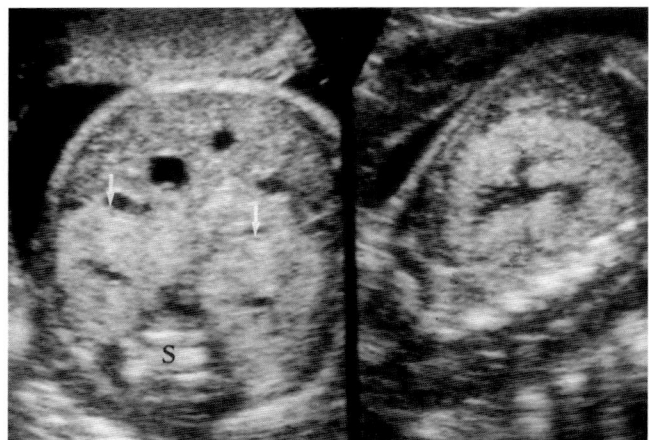

FIGURE 16. Autosomal recessive polycystic kidneys. Oligohydramnios and enlarged echogenic kidneys (*arrows*) at 31 weeks. S, spine.

TABLE 6. OUTCOME OF STRUCTURALLY NORMAL SECOND-TRIMESTER FETUSES WITH OLIGOHYDRAMNIOS AND AN ELEVATED MATERNAL SERUM ALPHA-FETOPROTEIN

Study	Cases	Living child	Intrauterine demise or neonatal death	Elective abortion
Seller[163]	4	1	1	2
Koontz[164]	1	0	1	2
Dyer[165]	21	1	16	4
Richards[166]	13	4	4	5
Hickok[167]	3	0	1	2
Bronshtein[63]	1	0	1	0
Los[168]	15	1	12	2
Total	58	17 (12.1%)	36 (62.1%)	15 (25.8%)

hand, iatrogenically ruptured membranes after genetic amniocentesis have a much more favorable prognosis. Survival rates of up to 91% have been reported in this patient group.[60] In these cases, leakage of fluid and oligohydramnios is transient and improves with time. Therefore, serial ultrasound examinations are suggested in the setting of second-trimester oligohydramnios from uncertain etiology.

Iatrogenic

Iatrogenic causes of oligohydramnios include medications, insensible fluid loss[61] and maternal intravascular fluid depletion,[62] and prior procedures such as chorionic villus sampling.[63]

Medications associated with oligohydramnios include nonsteroidal anti-inflammatory drugs, angiotensin-converting enzyme inhibitors, calcium channel blockers, and nitrous oxide. The nonsteroidal drugs are prostaglandin synthetase inhibitors that inhibit renal vascular flow and decrease glomerular filtration.[64] The angiotensin-converting enzyme inhibitors reduce fetal blood pressure, decrease renal perfusion, and subsequently result in oligohydramnios.[65]

Prognosis and Sequelae of Oligohydramnios

Potential complications that may occur as a result of oligohydramnios include fetal demise, pulmonary hypoplasia, and various skeletal and facial deformities. The prognosis is associated with

Underlying etiology
Severity of oligohydramnios
Gestational age (younger than 25 weeks)
Duration (greater than 14 days)

Those patients presenting in the second, in contrast to the third, trimester have a higher prevalence of structural malformations (50.7% vs. 22.1%) and a lower survival rate (10.2% vs. 85.3%). Isolated oligohydramnios during the third trimester is not necessarily associated with poor perinatal outcome.[66,67]

The presence or absence of structural malformations or aneuploidy is obviously important in assessing the progno-

sis in pregnancies with oligohydramnios. Demonstration of IUGR or other risk factors of placental dysfunction also puts fetuses at high risk of hypoxia and adverse outcome. For example, second-trimester fetuses with an elevated maternal serum alpha fetoprotein and oligohydramnios have a poor prognosis (Table 6).[68,69]

Marked oligohydramnios is associated with adverse outcome including preterm delivery, low-birth-weight, cesarean delivery, neonatal intensive care, and perinatal death.[56] Chamberlain[43] found the corrected perinatal mortality for a single pocket of amniotic fluid measuring less than 1 cm, between 1 cm and 2 cm, and from 2 cm to 8 cm is 1.97, 37.7, and 109.4, respectively (Table 7). Fetal hypoxia and deaths may occur, in part, from compression of the umbilical cord, which is accentuated during uterine contractions.

Disparate results have been reported when amniotic fluid is only mildly decreased or borderline. In a study of borderline oligohydramnios, defined as AFI between 5 and 10, Banks and Miller found a fourfold increase in the incidence of IUGR.[70] Other studies have found that, among normal-size fetuses, an AFI of less than 5 was associated with premature delivery but not with an increased risk of intrauterine death, or birth asphyxia.[66,71,72]

Pulmonary hypoplasia is a serious complication of oligohydramnios during the second trimester (Fig. 17). Pulmonary hypoplasia probably results from loss of the normal internal stenting force provided by pulmonary fluid[73] rather than thoracic compression.[74] Pulmonary hypoplasia is discussed in greater detail in Chapter 9.

TABLE 7. SINGLE POCKET MEASUREMENT OF AMNIOTIC FLUID VOLUME AND CORRECTED PERINATAL MORTALITY

Group	Pocket of amniotic fluid (cm)	Corrected perinatal mortality
Normal	2–8	1.97
Marginal	1–2	37.74
Decreased	<1	109.4

Modified from Chamberlain PF, Manning FA, Morrison I, Harman CR, Lange IR. Ultrasound evaluation of amniotic fluid volume. I. The relationship of marginal and decreased amniotic fluid volumes to perinatal outcome. *Am J Obstet Gynecol* 1984;150:245.

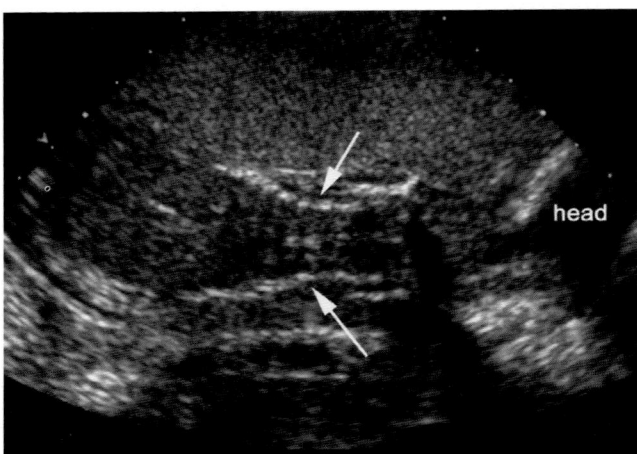

FIGURE 17. Pulmonary hypoplasia. Severe chronic oligohydramnios is associated with markedly decreased lung volumes and hypoplastic thorax (*arrows*).

The incidence of skeletal deformities (i.e., talipes equinovarus and craniofacial deformities) is also significantly higher in fetuses with prolonged oligohydramnios. As one would expect, there is an association between severe skeletal dysplasia and pulmonary hypoplasia. Neonates with deformities associated with oligohydramnios have a lower radial alveolar count (clinical evidence for pulmonary hypoplasia) than those without such deformities. In addition, those infants with skeletal deformities had more severe pulmonary hypoplasia, reflected by higher mortality, than those without skeletal deformities.[69]

In addition to preterm delivery and increased perinatal mortality, premature rupture of the membranes has been associated with fetal and maternal sepsis.[75] An AFI less than 5 cm is a significant independent risk factor for chorioamnionitis and early onset neonatal sepsis in women with ruptured membranes.[76]

Management

Maternal hydration has been shown to improve amniotic fluid in patients with oligohydramnios[77,78] as well as in women with normal amniotic fluid volumes.[79] However, maternal hydration would not be expected to alter amniotic fluid in patients with fetal anomalies or premature rupture of membranes. Also, none of the studies on maternal hydration has assessed clinically relevant outcomes or potential complications of this therapy. Therefore, further clinical trials are required.

Bed rest is commonly used in an effort to improve amniotic fluid in the U.S., particularly when the underlying etiology is poor placental perfusion. However, this option has not undergone carefully controlled studies.

Amnioinfusion may be advantageous in women with oligohydramnios who are in active labor and have evidence of umbilical cord compression.[80] It may reduce the occurrence of variable heart rate decelerations and decrease the use of cesarean section.[81] Although some studies suggest a role for amnioinfusion in women with ruptured membranes,[82] a meta-analysis study concluded that there are insufficient data to indicate whether this is of value.[83]

POLYHYDRAMNIOS

Definition and Sonographic Criteria

Polyhydramnios is generally defined as an amniotic fluid volume greater than 2,000 mL.[84] The reported prevalence of polyhydramnios is between 0.4% and 3.3%.[85–87] The frequency with which polyhydramnios is reported at an institution is determined by

1. The definition of polyhydramnios
2. The mix of high- and low-risk patients
3. The frequency with which ultrasound examinations are obtained in low- and high-risk pregnancies

Quite often, mild polyhydramnios is diagnosed sonographically when it has not been suspected clinically. Chronic polyhydramnios characteristically develops between 28 weeks' gestation and term with delivery occurring between 32 and 40 weeks. Neonatal outcome is primarily determined by the etiology of polyhydramnios.

Polyhydramnios may also develop acutely over a few days or chronically over weeks. Acute polyhydramnios occurs in the second trimester and accounts for approximately 2% of cases. Whereas the most common etiology of acute polyhydramnios is twin-to-twin transfusion syndrome, congenital anomalies may also be responsible.[88] Prolactin has been shown to stimulate fluid transport out of the amniotic cavity.[89] It has, therefore, been proposed that idiopathic acute polyhydramnios may, in some cases, be due to a functional deficit in the chorionic receptors for prolactin.[90] The etiology in some cases is still not determined.

Because the production and disposal of amniotic fluid is a dynamic process, it is reasonable to assume that changing maternal, fetal, or placental conditions may affect the amniotic fluid volume. Occasionally, documented polyhydramnios gradually resolves over serial ultrasound examinations.[91] Recurrent polyhydramnios in subsequent pregnancies occurs in less than 5% of cases. Approximately 25% of cases of recurrent polyhydramnios are associated with diabetes mellitus.

Sonographic Assessment

Subjective

Visual criteria for polyhydramnios include an obvious discrepancy between the size of the fetus and the amount of amniotic fluid. In the latter part of the third trimester the fetal abdomen approximates the anterior and posterior

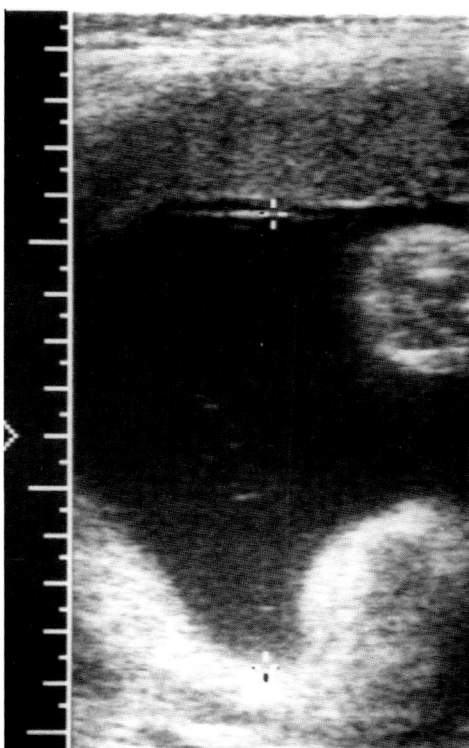

FIGURE 18. Polyhydramnios. A single pocket of amniotic fluid measures 10 cm, indicating polyhydramnios.

TABLE 8. NUMBER OF CORRECT ULTRASOUND ESTIMATES OF POLYHYDRAMNIOS AS DETERMINED BY DYE-DILUTION MEASUREMENTS

Study	Subjective assessment	Single pocket	Amniotic fluid index
Magann[22]	—	—	6/7
Magann[169]	6/10	2/10	3/10
Chauhan[170]	—	—	4/13
Magann[30]	—	—	6/7
Total	6/10 (60%)	5/16 (31.3%)	18/36 (50%)

hydramnios. The clinical relevance of the sonographic assessment of amniotic fluid volume as a marker of fetal, maternal, or placental disease should, therefore, distinguish the ability to accurately measure amniotic fluid.

Etiology

The most common etiologies of polyhydramnios are shown in Table 9.

Advances in maternal-fetal medicine have significantly altered not only the overall prevalence but also the types of cases seen with polyhydramnios. For example, Rh immune globulin has markedly reduced the incidence of erythroblastosis fetalis. Rigidly maintaining euglycemia in the pregnant diabetic has significantly reduced the frequency with which hydramnios is seen with this disease entity, and the first- or second-trimester detection of congenital anomalies has reduced the number of fetuses, particularly with central nervous anomalies, that reach the third trimester when polyhydramnios usually develops.[97,98]

As the severity of polyhydramnios increases, so does the likelihood of determining an underlying etiology (Table 10). In one study, 66 of 80 patients (82.5%) with mild polyhydramnios were categorized as idiopathic, whereas 20 of 22 patients (90.9%) with moderate or severe polyhydramnios had a maternal or fetal condition known to be associated with polyhydramnios.[92] The data in Table 10 also indicates that the likelihood of a congenital anomaly increases with the severity of polyhydramnios.[99]

Congenital Malformations

A wide variety of congenital malformations have been associated with polyhydramnios (Table 11). The fact that not

TABLE 9. COMMON ASSOCIATIONS WITH POLYHYDRAMNIOS

Macrosomia, with or without maternal diabetes
Fetal malformations and chromosome abnormalities
Twin-to-twin transfusion syndrome
Rhesus disease
Congenital infection
Idiopathic

uterine walls. When there is an ample amount of amniotic fluid between the fetus and the anterior and posterior uterine walls, significant polyhydramnios is generally present (Fig. 18). Sonographic recognition of mild polyhydramnios has more intraobserver variability than does the recognition of moderate to marked polyhydramnios. A false impression of polyhydramnios may occur during the second trimester when the fetus takes up proportionally less of the amniotic cavity than in the third trimester.

Semiquantitative

Using the single largest pocket of amniotic fluid, an amniotic fluid pocket greater than 8 cm, greater than 12 cm, and greater than 16 cm has been defined as mild, moderate, and severe polyhydramnios, respectively.[92] The definition of polyhydramnios using the AFI has been reported as greater than 20 cm,[20] greater than 24 cm,[93,94] and greater than 25 cm.[95,96] An AFI greater than 25 cm has been associated with a higher incidence of macrosomia and a higher congenital anomaly rate.[95]

There has been a limited number of small series comparing various sonographic measurements of polyhydramnios to the actual volume as determined by dye-dilution technique (Table 8). These studies concur that all of the semiquantitative sonographic methods for detecting polyhydramnios are relatively poor and tend to underestimate the degree of poly-

TABLE 10. SEVERITY OF POLYHYDRAMNIOS AND ETIOLOGY OF POLYHYDRAMNIOS

Etiology	Mild	Moderate	Severe	Total
Idiopathic	66	2	—	68
Congenital anomalies	2	9	2	13
Insulin-dependent diabetes mellitus	3	5	—	8
Gestational diabetes mellitus	7	—	—	7
Twins	1	2	2	5
Other	1	—	—	1
Total	80	18	4	102

Modified from Hill LM, Breckle R, Thomas ML, Fries JK. Polyhydramnios: ultrasonically detected prevalence and neonatal outcome. *Obstet Gynecol* 1987;69:21.

all fetuses with any of the congenital anomalies mentioned will have polyhydramnios is, in part, due to the severity of the impairment in a given case, as well as the ability of the maternal-fetal unit to compensate by using other pathways for fluid removal from the amniotic cavity.

In the past, central nervous system malformations were the most common anomalies associated with polyhydramnios.[100] More recent literature favors gastrointestinal malformations (39%), followed by central nervous system (26%), circulatory (22%), and urinary tract (13%) anomalies.[97]

Gastrointestinal Tract

Obstruction of the gastrointestinal tract is a relatively common fetal cause of polyhydramnios[101] reflecting the role of swallowing and fluid absorption by the fetal intestinal tract in the regulation of amniotic fluid. Proximal obstructions are particularly likely to produce polyhydramnios. This may include esophageal atresia, duodenal atresia, or jejunoileal atresia.[102] There is a progressive decrease in the prevalence of polyhydramnios with more distal obstruction (Fig. 19): proximal jejunal (32%); distal jejunal (24%); and ileal (17%).[101,103] Large bowel obstruction alone does not usually produce polyhydramnios. These observations support the importance of fetal swallowing with absorption of amniotic fluid by the gastrointestinal tract in the regulation of amniotic fluid volume.

Other gastrointestinal disorders that may cause partial bowel obstruction include intestinal volvulus, meconium ileus, abdominal wall defects, and meconium peritonitis.[104] In these cases, polyhydramnios presumably develops when the amount of swallowed amniotic fluid exceeds the absorptive capacity of the stomach and the bowel proximal to the site of obstruction.

Nonobstructive bowel disorders that may be associated with polyhydramnios include congenital chloridorrhea[105] and megacystis-microcolon intestinal hypoperistalsis syndrome[106] (see Chapter 13).

Central Nervous System

A wide variety of central nervous system abnormalities may produce polyhydramnios, probably by depression of fetal swallowing. As with other anomalies, central nervous system anomalies may produce polyhydramnios during the third trimester, but usually not before 25 weeks.[107]

Head and Neck

Facial clefts and neck masses, such as goiters and teratomas, have been associated with polyhydramnios. Neck masses cause mechanical obstruction to fetal swallowing, whereas facial clefts probably cause ineffective fetal swallowing.

Respiratory and Thoracic Abnormalities

Upper airway obstruction and cystic adenomatoid malformation can give rise to hydrops. Polyhydramnios may be due to either esophageal or cardiac compression.[108,109] Polyhydramnios often accompanies diaphragmatic hernia by producing partial obstruction of the gastrointestinal tract.

Genitourinary Anomalies

Unilateral renal anomalies (ureteropelvic obstruction, multicystic dysplasia, and renal tumors), as well as bilateral malformations, have been associated with polyhydramnios.[100,110,111]

Polyhydramnios also develops in 10% of cases of ovarian cysts, presumably from compression on the adjacent bowel.

Skeletal Dysplasias

Skeletal dysplasias most frequently associated with polyhydramnios include thanatophoric dysplasia (58%) and achondroplasia (27%).[112] The combination of skeletal dysplasia and polyhydramnios is associated with a poor prognosis and a high probability of pulmonary hypoplasia. In one series,[112] the only survivors with skeletal dysplasias and polyhydramnios were cases of heterozygous achondroplasia.

Cardiovascular Anomalies

Structural cardiac malformations that result in right atrial overload (i.e., pulmonary or tricuspid atresia) are most

TABLE 11. CONGENITAL ANOMALIES ASSOCIATED WITH POLYHYDRAMNIOS

Cardiovascular system
  Arrhythmias
  Congenital anomalies
  Cardiac tumors
  Ectopic cordis
  Agenesis of the ductus venosus[171]
Central nervous system
  Anencephaly
  Hydrocephaly
  Microcephaly
  Encephalocele
  Spina bifida
  Dandy-Walker malformation
  Cerebral arteriovenous malformation
  Iniencephaly
Head and neck
  Goiter
  Cleft palate
  Cystic hygroma
Respiratory system
  Tracheal agenesis
  Cystic adenomatoid malformation
  Hydrothorax
  Bronchopulmonary sequestration
  Asphyxiating thoracic dystrophy
  Primary pulmonary hypoplasia
  Congenital pulmonary lymphangiectasia
Gastrointestinal system
  Esophageal atresia
  Duodenal atresia
  Jejunoileal atresia
  Meconium peritonitis
  Annular pancreas
  Gastroschisis
  Omphalocele
  Diaphragmatic hernia
  Congenital megacolon[172]
Genitourinary system
  Hydronephrosis
  Ureteropelvic junction obstruction
  Ovarian cyst
  Bartter's syndrome[173]
Skeletal system
  Chondrodysplasia punctata
  Short-rib polydactyly syndrome
  Hypophosphatasia
  Thanatophoric dysplasia
  Camptomelia dysplasia
  Achondroplasia
  Osteogenesis imperfecta
  Arthrogryposis

commonly associated with fetal hydrops and polyhydramnios.[113] Because the ductus arteriosus can divert flow from the left ventricle, left-sided obstructive lesions (aortic or mitral stenosis) are less likely to result in hydrops. Fetal tachyarrhythmias more commonly cause fetal hydrops[114] than bradyarrhythmias.[115] Cardiac tumors (i.e., rhabdomyomas) may rarely cause fetal hydrops, but obstruct one or both outflow tracts.[116]

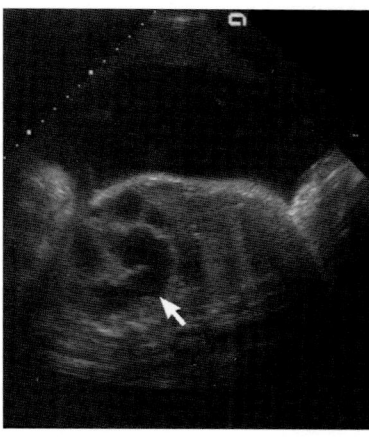

FIGURE 19. Gastrointestinal obstruction and polyhydramnios. Polyhydramnios is evident with fluid overlying the fetus. Enlarged loops of small bowel *(arrow)* were secondary to jejunal atresia.

Fetal Hydrops

Approximately 30% of fetuses with nonimmune hydrops have polyhydramnios.[117] Given the diverse etiologies of nonimmune hydrops, the underlying mechanism for polyhydramnios undoubtedly differs from case to case.

Fetal and Placental Tumors

Fetal and placental tumors are rare causes of polyhydramnios (Table 12) that are, for the most part, case reports. The etiology of polyhydramnios varies with the type of tumor.

Chromosome Abnormalities

Alterations in amniotic fluid (oligohydramnios, polyhydramnios) have been associated with an increased prevalence of karyotypic abnormalities.[118] Because the vast majority of fetuses with a major chromosomal abnormality have associated structural anomalies, the risk of chromosome abnormality in the setting of isolated polyhydramnios is very low (Table 13). Even assuming a 1% risk of aneuploidy, it is estimated that 4,700 patients with isolated

TABLE 12. FETAL AND PLACENTAL TUMORS ASSOCIATED WITH POLYHYDRAMNIOS

Sacrococcygeal teratoma
Intracranial tumors
Cervical teratoma
Cavernosus hemangioma
Congenital mesoblastic nephroma
Adrenal neuroblastoma
Epignathus
Mediastinal teratoma
Placental chorioangioma
Metastatic neuroblastoma

TABLE 13. KARYOTYPIC ABNORMALITIES DETECTED WITH ISOLATED POLYHYDRAMNIOS

Author	Isolated polyhydramnios	Abnormal karyotype
Zahn[174]	45	1
Brady[175]	125	2
Carlson[176]	49	0
Barnhard[119]	49	0
Hill[92]	68	0
Golan[177]	97	0
Hendricks[178]	138	0
Biggio[96]	267	1[a]
Total	838	4

[a]Details whether diagnosed antenatally not provided.

polyhydramnios are required to determine the need for genetic amniocentesis.[119] Factors to consider in deciding whether amniocentesis is indicated include maternal age and history, the skill of the sonologist in detecting anomalies, and the size of the fetus (see Idiopathic Polyhydramnios section later).

Twin Oligohydramnios-Polyhydramnios Sequence

The twin oligohydramnios-polyhydramnios sequence[120] is a heterogeneous group of disorders associated with discrepancy in amniotic fluid with polyhydramnios of one sac and oligohydramnios of the other. Etiologies may include fetal anomalies, IUGR affecting one fetus, infection, or twin-to-twin transfusion syndrome (Fig. 20).[121] The latter condition, particularly when it begins in the second trimester, produces some of the most severe cases of polyhydramnios.

Sonographic criteria for the presumptive antenatal diagnosis of twin-to-twin transfusion syndrome include

1. Monochorionic placentation
2. Growth discordancy that eventually results in one fetus being growth restricted
3. Discrepant amniotic fluid with oligohydramnios of the growth-restricted twin and polyhydramnios of the larger twin
4. An enlarged urinary bladder of the larger twin and absent or small bladder of the smaller twin

Congenital Infections

Cytomegalovirus, toxoplasmosis, varicella, parvovirus, and syphilis may all give rise to nonimmune hydrops and polyhydramnios.[122–125]

Macrosomia and Large-for-Gestational-Age Fetuses

The most common condition associated with polyhydramnios is undoubtedly macrosomia and large-for-gestational-age fetuses. Chamberlain[85] first reported macrosomia in 37% of cases with polyhydramnios compared to 8.7% of fetuses with normal amniotic fluid volume. Other studies

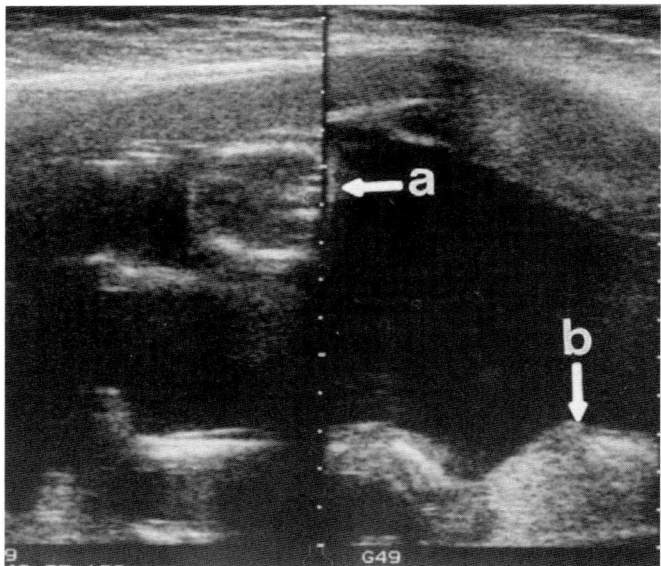
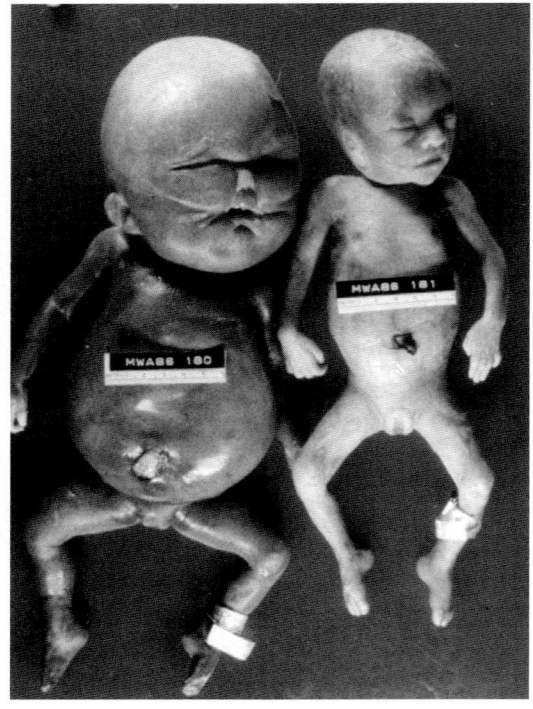

FIGURE 20. Twin oligohydramnios/polyhydramnios sequence secondary to twin-to-twin transfusion syndrome. **A:** Ultrasound (*a*, stuck twin due to oligohydramnios; *b*, twin with polyhydramnios). **B:** Postmortem photograph. The donor twin is growth restricted. The recipient twin is macrosomic and hydropic.

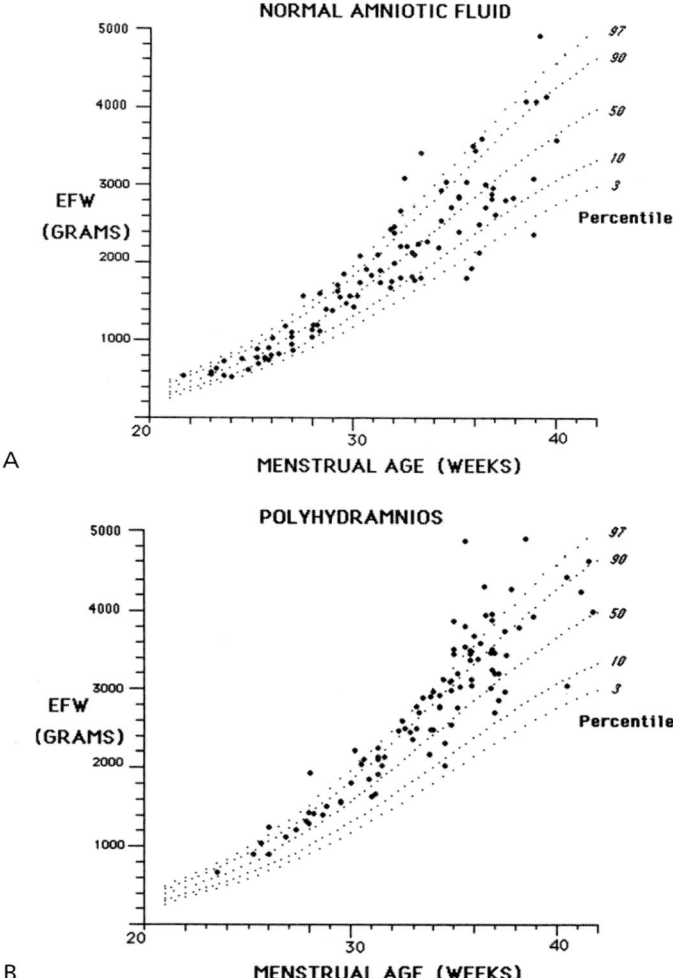

NORMAL AMNIOTIC FLUID

POLYHYDRAMNIOS

FIGURE 21. Idiopathic polyhydramnios and macrosomia in normal fetuses of nondiabetic mothers. **A:** Represents the control group with normal fluid and **(B)** represents consecutive fetuses with polyhydramnios in nondiabetic mothers. The estimated fetal weight percentile of the study group is significantly higher than the control group. In this study, fetuses with polyhydramnios were three times more likely to have a birth weight at or above the ninetieth percentile (relative risk, 2.7). (Reproduced with permission from Sohaey R, Nyberg DA, Sickler GK, Williams MA. Idiopathic polyhydramnios: association with fetal macrosomia. *Radiology* 1994;190:393–396.)

have found a 27% to 37% prevalence of macrosomia with polyhydramnios (Fig. 21).[126–128] Lazebnik et al.[128] found that polyhydramnios increased the risk of macrosomia by 2.7-fold.

In the setting of a suspected large-for-gestational-age fetus, the presence of polyhydramnios also adds further support to this diagnosis and increases the risk of macrosomia. Although there is a clear association between macrosomia and polyhydramnios, this relationship is not linear.[127,128]

The well-known association between polyhydramnios and maternal diabetes appears to be related to the higher frequency of macrosomia and large-for-gestational-age fetuses in this patient group and not to diabetes per se.[96,129,130] Lazebnik[128] reported diabetes more often among patients with polyhydramnios than controls (17.7% vs. 7.0%), but no relation was found after accounting for fetal weight. Therefore, polyhydramnios is present in an equivalent number of diabetic and nondiabetic women with macrosomic fetuses.

The cause of polyhydramnios with large-for-gestational-age fetuses is unknown. It has been suggested that the polyhydramnios may be due to

1. Increased renal vascular flow
2. A reversal of intramembranous flow (i.e., *from* the fetal circulation *to* the amniotic fluid)
3. An increase in the volume of fluid excreted by the fetal lungs

Idiopathic Polyhydramnios

Idiopathic polyhydramnios has been suggested when there is no identifiable cause. Although it has been listed as one of the most common associations with polyhydramnios in the older literature, true idiopathic polyhydramnios is unusual in our experience. Most cases can be accounted for by the association of large-for-gestational-age fetuses. At Swedish Medical Center, the mean birth weight among fetuses with idiopathic polyhydramnios was greater than fetuses with normal amniotic fluid (3,771 g vs. 3,476 g), which, in turn, was greater than observed for fetuses with polyhydramnios and anomalies (3,003 g).[127,131] Therefore, fetal size is an important determination in assessing the underlying etiology of idiopathic polyhydramnios.

Unusual Causes of Polyhydramnios

A number of rare and unusual maternal and fetal conditions have been associated with polyhydramnios (Table 14). Fetal cerebral dysfunction associated with nonketotic hyperglycinemia[132] and the abnormal renal concentrating ability in pseudohypoaldosteronism[133] explains the polyhydramnios in these conditions. Fetuses with arthrogryposis

TABLE 14. UNUSUAL CAUSES OF POLYHYDRAMNIOS

Fetal pseudohypoaldosteronism[133]
Fetal acetaminophen toxicity[179]
Myotonic dystrophy[180]
Nonketotic hyperglycinemia[132]
Beckwith-Wiedemann syndrome[181]
Intrahepatic arteriovenous shunt[182]
Retroperitoneal fibrosis[183]
DiGeorge syndrome[184]
Arthrogryposis[185]

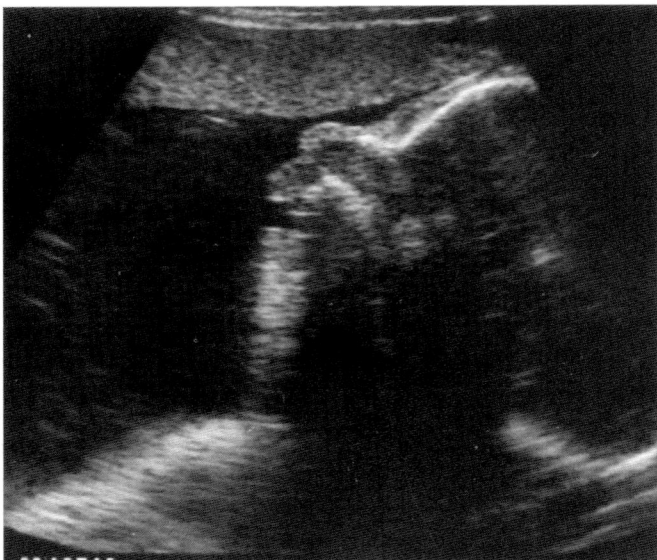

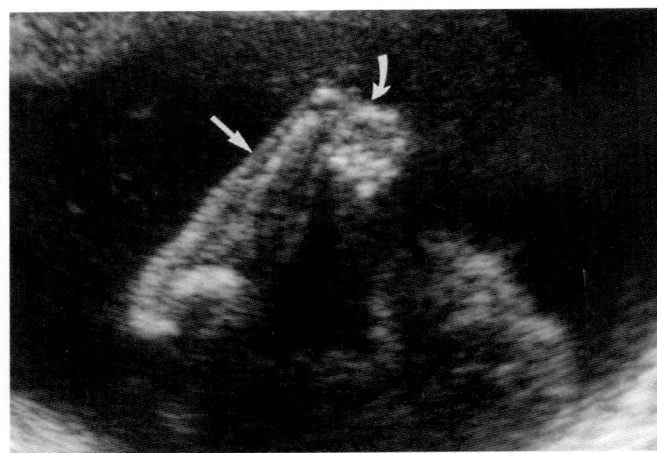

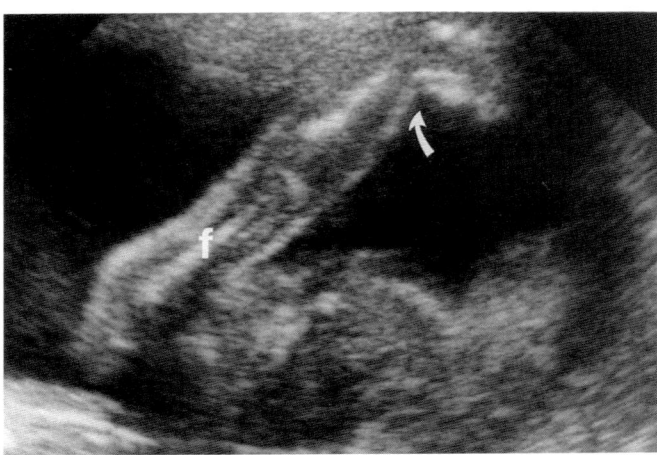

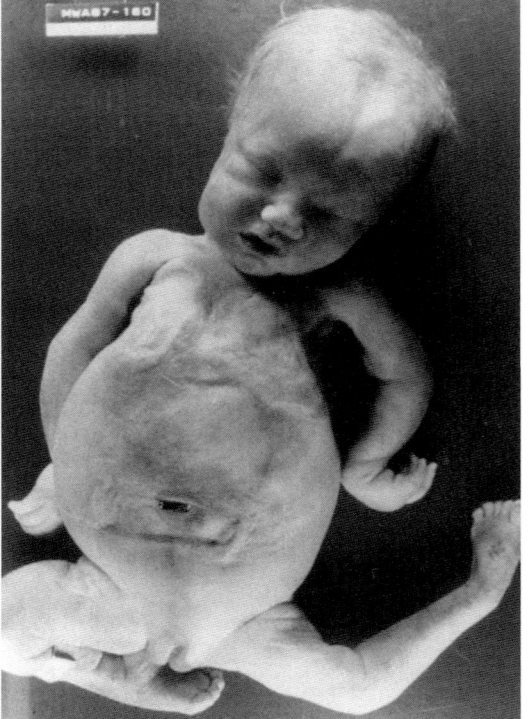

FIGURE 22. Arthrogryposis multiplex congenita and polyhydramnios. **A:** The fetal mouth remained open during the examination. There is micrognathia and polyhydramnios. **B:** Contractures of the extremities are present. The hand (*curved arrow*) is persistently flexed. The straight arrow indicates the forearm. **C:** Contracture of the ankle is present (*arrow*). f, femur. **D:** Postmortem photograph of arthrogryposis.

(Fig. 22) have contractures, significantly reduced movement, and an inhibition of swallowing.

Prognosis

The prognosis is directly related to the underlying condition. In the absence of fetal anomalies, the clinical significance of polyhydramnios at term remains controversial.[130,134,135] Only two studies used a multiple logistic regression to assess a multitude of variables associated with polyhydramnios.[130,134] They both found that isolated polyhydramnios either at term or preterm was associated with increased perinatal mortality, neonatal morbidity, and maternal mor-

bidity. The mechanism or mechanisms for the reported perinatal morbidity in these cases remain to be elucidated. It has been suggested that the raised amniotic fluid pressure may impair uteroplacental perfusion.[136–138]

Prematurity accounts for some of the excess neonatal morbidity associated with polyhydramnios. The risk of preterm delivery may not be secondary to excess fluid alone, but rather related to the underlying cause of polyhydramnios. For example, the prevalence of preterm delivery is highest among women with fetuses who have a congenital malformation, followed by pregnancies complicated by insulin-dependent diabetes mellitus. The incidence of preterm delivery is much lower in women with gestational diabetes mellitus or with unexplained polyhydramnios.[139,140]

Transient polyhydramnios is not usually associated with adverse outcome. However, one study[141] found that the prevalence of glucose intolerance and fetal macrosomia was significantly increased. Case reports have also documented karyotypical abnormalities in fetuses with growth restriction after resolution of polyhydramnios. Hence, growth restriction, even when polyhydramnios resolves, is of concern and warrants a thorough ultrasound examination for structural malformations, dysmorphologic features, and possible karyotyping.[119]

Treatment of Polyhydramnios

Prenatal treatment of polyhydramnios is desirable to decrease the risk of potential complications, such as preterm labor, rupture of membranes, and placental abruption. However, an effective treatment plan for polyhydramnios must take into consideration the underlying etiology. Treatment may address either a maternal (e.g., poor diabetic control) or fetal cause (e.g., anemia or arrhythmia).

Therapeutic Amniocentesis

Therapeutic amniocentesis has been used to treat symptomatic polyhydramnios. The most common indication has been in the setting of twin-to-twin transfusion syndrome or a major anomaly, whereas isolated polyhydramnios is usually not sufficiently severe to require therapy. Potential complications of the procedure include initiation of preterm labor, premature rupture of the membranes, chorioamnionitis, and placental abruption.[142] The overall complication rate with this procedure is 1.5%.[143] In series of twin-to-twin transfusion syndrome patients treated with reduction amniocentesis, the overall survival rate is 49% (range 17% to 79%).[142] The survival rate in historical controls of severe twin-to-twin transfusion syndrome without intervention was less than 5%.[144,145]

The gradual reduction in amniotic fluid pressure with a correction of baseline hypoxemia produces an increase in the pulsatility index of the middle cerebral artery (i.e., a reduction in diastolic flow to normal). The removal of too much amniotic fluid results in acute fetal hemodynamic compromise and a decrease in the pulsatility index of the middle cerebral artery.[146]

Medical Treatment

Indomethacin had been used for a number of years in the medical treatment of polyhydramnios. It is a nonsteroidal anti-inflammatory agent in which the mechanism of action involves inhibition of prostaglandin synthesis.[147] Indomethacin is rapidly absorbed from the gastrointestinal tract. It appears in plasma 30 minutes after oral administration,

peaks at 90 minutes, and has a half-life of 2.6 to 11.2 hours.[148] There is a rapid transplacental passage of the drug to the fetus.[149]

Indomethacin affects the amniotic fluid volume by impairing lung liquid production or enhancing the resorption of lung liquid and decreasing fetal urinary output. Because the amnion and chorion are rich in prostaglandins, it has been hypothesized that indomethacin may also affect transmembrane fluid movement.

Indomethacin has been shown to be most effective in the treatment of idiopathic polyhydramnios or polyhydramnios associated with either distal fetal gastrointestinal obstruction or maternal diabetes mellitus.[148] In patients with polyhydramnios, a marked reduction in amniotic fluid volume has been observed within one week of initiating indomethacin therapy.[150] Indomethacin is effective in reducing amniotic fluid volume as early as 21 weeks' gestation.[151] A dose of 25 mg every 6 hours has been shown to effectively reduce the amniotic fluid volume.

In a study of 57 patients with polyhydramnios, indomethacin reduced amniotic fluid in more than 90% of cases,[152] and pregnancies were prolonged an average of 8.4 weeks. To date, however, randomized controlled trials are lacking.

The maternal side effects of indomethacin are usually mild and, therefore, rarely necessitate a discontinuation of therapy (Table 15). The potential fetal effects of indomethacin (Table 15) are more significant.[148] There is a dose- and gestational age–related constriction effect of indomethacin on the ductus arteriosus.[153] With indomethacin therapy, ductal constriction has been observed as early as 24 weeks' gestation. In general, the risk of ductal constriction is 5% between 26 and 27 weeks' gestation and increases to 50% by 32 weeks.[154] With ductal constriction,

TABLE 15. SIDE EFFECTS OF INDOMETHACIN THERAPY

Maternal side effects
  Nausea
  Heartburn
  Vertigo
  Tinnitus
  Antagonizes antihypertensive medication
  Decreased urinary output
  Pulmonary edema
  Cholestatic jaundice
Fetal side effects
  Constriction of ductus arteriosus that may result in
    Pulmonary hypertension
    Pleural effusions
    Hydrops
    Persistent fetal circulation
  Intraventricular hemorrhage
  Necrotizing enterocolitis
  Transient neonatal renal failure
  Altered platelet function
  Prolonged bleeding time
  Neonatal death

TABLE 16. ABNORMALITIES OF FETAL GROWTH AND FLUID: COMMON PATTERNS AND ETIOLOGIES

Amniotic fluid findings	Fetal size	Common etiologies
Polyhydramnios	Large for gestational age	Macrosomia (with or without diabetes)
Polyhydramnios	Small for gestational age	Fetal anomaly or syndrome Chromosome abnormality
Early oligohydramnios	Small for gestational age	Fetal anomaly or syndrome Chromosome abnormality Infection Premature rupture of membranes Severe placental insufficiency Confined placental mosaicism
Late oligohydramnios or gradually decreasing fluid	Small for gestational age	Placental insufficiency Premature rupture of membranes
Oligohydramnios	Large for gestational age	Post-term pregnancy

blood is diverted into the constricted pulmonary circulation. The increase in right ventricular afterload pressure results in right ventricular dilatation and tricuspid regurgitation. The development of fetal pleural effusions and frank hydrops has been attributed to persistent ductal constriction from continued indomethacin use. Ductal constriction resolves within 24 hours of discontinuing indomethacin.[148]

Oligohydramnios is an additional complication associated with indomethacin therapy. Serial ultrasound examinations should, therefore, be performed to assess amniotic fluid volume. When indomethacin is discontinued, the amniotic fluid volume gradually reaccumulates.[64,151] Persistent neonatal anuria after antenatal indomethacin therapy for polyhydramnios has resulted in acute renal failure and death.[155]

There have been some reports suggesting an increased risk for intracranial hemorrhage and necrotizing enterocolitis with indomethacin therapy.[156–158] However, retrospective studies[156,157,159,160] have reached different conclusions regarding the safety of indomethacin. Until a randomized controlled trial is conducted, this issue cannot be resolved.

AMNIOTIC FLUID AND GROWTH PATTERNS

Assessment of amniotic fluid in conjunction with fetal growth is important for detection of fetal abnormalities. As discussed in detail throughout this chapter, fetal growth and amniotic fluid production are strongly related, and abnormalities of amniotic fluid often indicate abnormalities of growth. The timing of the finding is also important because early amniotic fluid abnormalities suggest a more serious etiology.

At the risk of oversimplification, Table 16 summarizes patterns of amniotic fluid finding, fetal size, and common etiologies. For example, polyhydramnios seen in the setting of a large-for-gestational-age fetus is more likely explained by macrosomia than by an undetectable fetal anomaly. Late oligohydramnios and a normal-sized fetus are more likely

from placental insufficiency or prematurely ruptured membranes than a chromosome anomaly or IUGR. Conversely, minimal oligohydramnios and a small fetus suggest IUGR.

Fetuses with multiple anomalies have a high incidence of IUGR. Whereas polyhydramnios is commonly associated with large-for-gestational-age fetuses, the combination of polyhydramnios and IUGR is unusual[161] and indicates a high risk of underlying anomalies (Figs. 23 and 24). In one study, 92% of fetuses with IUGR and polyhydramnios had other major anomalies at birth, though they were not visible sonographically in most cases.[131] Chromosome abnormalities, particularly trisomy 18, are also commonly encountered in this group of patients.[131,162]

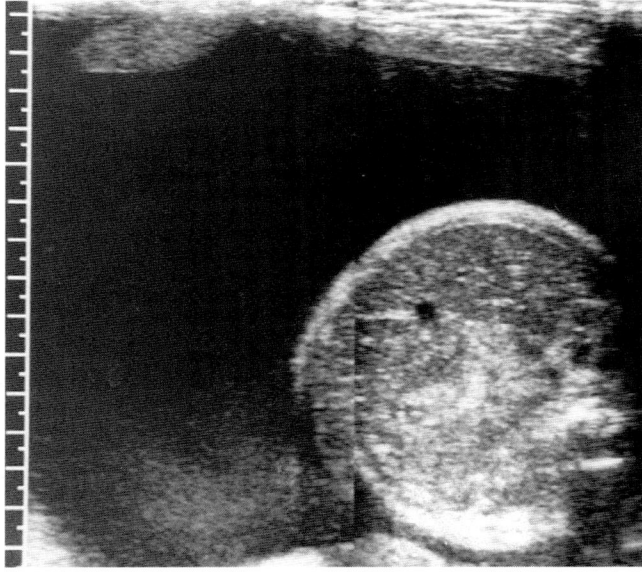

FIGURE 23. Polyhydramnios and trisomy 18. Obvious polyhydramnios is present, and estimated weight was less than the tenth percentile. The combination of polyhydramnios and intrauterine growth restriction is an ominous finding associated with a high rate of underlying anomalies and adverse outcome. In this case, large cisterna magna and cerebellar hypoplasia were also evident.

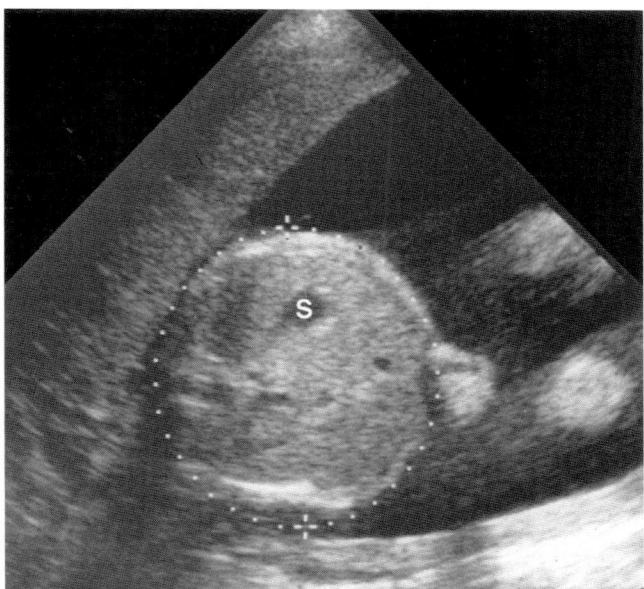

FIGURE 24. Esophageal atresia and polyhydramnios. Scan at 34 weeks shows polyhydramnios. A fluid-filled stomach is visible (S). However, the abdominal circumference was less than expected, and estimated fetal weight was less than the tenth percentile. Esophageal atresia was found at birth.

REFERENCES

1. Brace RA, Wolf EJ. Normal amniotic fluid volume changes throughout pregnancy. *Am J Obstet Gynecol* 1989;161:382–388.
2. Lind T, Hytten FE. Relation of amniotic fluid volume to fetal weight in the first half of pregnancy. *Lancet* 1970;1:1147–1149.
3. Trahair JF, Harding R. Ultrastructural anomalies in the fetal small intestine indicate that fetal swallowing is important for normal development: an experimental study. *Virchows Arch A Pathol Anat Histopathol* 1992;420:305–312.
4. Blakelock R, Upadhyay V, Kimble R, Pease P, Kolbe A, et al. Is a normally functioning gastrointestinal tract necessary for normal growth in late gestation? *Pediatr Surg Int* 1998;13:17–20.
5. Trahair JF, Harding R. Restitution of fetal swallowing in the fetal sheep restores intestinal growth after midgestation on esophageal obstruction. *J Pediatr Gastroenterol Nutr* 1995; 20:156–161.
6. Weissman A, Itskovitz-Eldor J, Jakobi P. Sonographic measurement of amniotic fluid volume in the first trimester of pregnancy. *J Ultrasound Med* 1996;15:771–774.
7. Wagner G, Fuchs F. The volume of amniotic fluid in the first half of human pregnancy. *J Obstet Gynaecol Br Commonw* 1962;69:131–136.
8. Mann SE, Nijland MJM, Ross MG. Mathematic modeling of human amniotic fluid dynamics. *Am J Obstet Gynecol* 1996;175:937–944.
9. Abramovich DR. The volume of amniotic fluid and its regulating factors. In: Fairweather DVE, Eskes TKAB, eds. *Amniotic fluid—research and clinical application*, 2nd ed. Amsterdam: Excerpta Medica, 1978:31–49.
10. Abramovich DR, Garden A, Jandial L, Page KR. Fetal swallowing and voiding in relation to hydramnios. *Obstet Gynecol* 1979;54:15–20.
11. Brace RA. Physiology of amniotic fluid volume regulation. *Clin Obstet Gynecol* 1997;40:280–289.
12. Sedin G, Hammarlund K, Nilsson GE, Oberg PA, Stromberg B. Water transport through the skin of newborn infants. *Ups J Med Sci* 1981;86:27–31.
13. Curran MA, Nijland MJM, Mann SE, Ross MG. Human amniotic fluid mathematical model: determination and effect of intramembranous sodium flux. *Am J Obstet Gynecol* 1998;178:484–490.
14. Mann SE, Nijland MJM, Ross MG. Ovine fetal adaptations to chronically reduced urine flow: preservation of amniotic fluid volume. *J Appl Physiol* 1996;81:2588–2594.
15. Brace RA, Wlodek ME, Cook ML, Harding R. Swallowing of lung liquid and amniotic fluid by the ovine fetus under normoxic and hypoxic conditions. *Am J Obstet Gynecol* 1994;171:764–770.
16. Lingwood BE, Hardy KJ, Long JG, et al. Amniotic fluid volume and composition following experimental manipulations in sheep. *Obstet Gynecol* 1980;56:451–458.
17. Manning FA, Platt LD. Antepartum fetal evaluation: development of a fetal biophysical profile score. *Am J Obstet Gynecol* 1980;136:787–795.
18. Magann EF, Nolan TE, Hess LW, Martin RW, Whitworth NS, et al. Measurement of amniotic fluid volume: accuracy of ultrasonography technique. *Am J Obstet Gynecol* 1992; 167:1533–1537.
19. Phelan JP, Ahn MO, Smith CV, Rutherford SE, Anderson E. Amniotic fluid index measurements during pregnancy. *J Reprod Med* 1987;32:601–604.
20. Phelan JP, Smith CV, Broussard P, Small M. Amniotic fluid volume assessment with the four-quadrant technique at 36–42 weeks' gestation. *J Reprod Med* 1987;32:540–542.
21. Moore TR, Cayle JE. The amniotic fluid index in normal human pregnancy. *Am J Obstet Gynecol* 1990;162:1168–1173.
22. Magann EF, Martin JN Jr. Amniotic fluid assessment in singleton and twin pregnancies. *Obstet Gynecol Clin North Am* 1999;26:579–593.
23. Dildy GA, Lira N, Moise KJ Jr, Ridle GD, Deter RL. Amniotic fluid volume assessment: comparison of ultrasonographic estimates versus direct measurements with a dye-dilution technique in human pregnancy. *Am J Obstet Gynecol* 1992;167:986–994.
24. Croom CS, Banias BB, Ramos-Santos E. Do semiquantitative amniotic fluid indexes reflect actual volume? *Am J Obstet Gynecol* 1992;167:995–999.
25. Gramellini D, Chiaie D, Piantelli G, Sansebastiano L, Fieni S, et al. Sonographic assessment of amniotic fluid volume between 11 and 24 weeks of gestation: construction of reference intervals related to gestational age. *Ultrasound Obstet Gynecol* 2001;17:410–5.
26. Bianco A, Rosen T, Kuczynski E, Tetrokalashvili M, Lockwood CJ. Measurement of the amniotic fluid index with and without color Doppler. *J Perinat Med* 1999;27:245–249.
27. Grover J, Mentakis A, Ross MG. Three-dimensional method for determination of amniotic fluid volume in intrauterine pockets. *Obstet Gynecol* 1997;90:1007–1010.

28. Chau AC, Kjas SL, Kovacs BW. Ultrasonographic measurement of amniotic fluid volume in normal twin pregnancies. *Am J Obstet Gynecol* 1996;174:1003–1007.

29. Hill LM, Krohn M, Lazebnik N, Tush B, Boyles D, et al. The amniotic fluid index in normal twin pregnancies. *Am J Obstet Gynecol* 2000;182:950–954.

30. Magann EF, Chauhan SP, Martin JN Jr, Whitworth NS, Morrison JC. Ultrasonic assessment of the amniotic fluid volume in diamniotic twin. *J Soc Gynecol Investig* 1995;2:609–613.

31. Magann EF, Chauhan SP, Whitworth NS, Anfanger P, Rinehart BK, et al. Determination of amniotic fluid volume in twin pregnancies: ultrasonographic evaluation versus operator estimation. *Am J Obstet Gynecol* 2000;182:1606–1609.

32. Philipson EH, Sokol RJ, Williams T. Oligohydramnios clinical associations and predictive value for intrauterine growth retardation. *Am J Obstet Gynecol* 1983;146:271–278.

33. Mercer LJ, Brown LG, Petres RE, Messer RH. A survey of pregnancies complicated by decreased amniotic fluid. *Am J Obstet Gynecol* 1984;149:355–361.

34. Manning FA, Harman CR, Morrison I, Menticoglous SM, Lange IR, et al. Fetal assessment based on fetal biophysical profile scoring IV. An analysis of perinatal morbidity and mortality. *Am J Obstet Gynecol* 1990;162:703–709.

35. Halpern ME, Fong KW, Zalev AH, et al. Reliability of amniotic fluid volume estimation from ultrasonograms: intraobserver and interobserver variation before and after the establishment of criteria. *Am J Obstet Gynecol* 1985;153:264–267.

36. Magann EF, Sanderson M, Martin JN, Chauhan S. The amniotic fluid index, single deepest pocket, and two-diameter pocket in normal human pregnancy. *Am J Obstet Gynecol* 2000;182:1581–1588.

37. Magann EF, Chauhan SP, Barrilleaux PS, Whitworth NS, Martin JN. Amniotic fluid index and single deepest pocket: weak indicators of abnormal amniotic volumes. *Obstet Gynecol* 2000 Nov;96:737–740.

38. Horsager R, Nathan L, Leveno KJ. Correlation of measured amniotic fluid volume and sonographic predictions of oligohydramnios. *Obstet Gynecol* 1994;83:955–958.

39. Strong TH, Hetzler G, Paul RH. Amniotic fluid volume increase after amnioinfusion of a fixed volume. *Am J Obstet Gynecol* 1990;162:746–748.

40. Chauhan SP. Amniotic fluid index before and after amnioinfusion of a fixed volume of normal saline. *J Reprod Med* 1991;36:801–802.

41. Manning FA, Hill LM, Platt LD. Qualitative amniotic fluid volume determination by ultrasound: antepartum detection of intrauterine growth retardation. *Am J Obstet Gynecol* 1981;139:254–258.

42. Hill LM, Breckle R, Wolfram KR, O'Brien PC. Oligohydramnios: ultrasonically detected incidence and subsequent fetal outcome. *Am J Obstet Gynecol* 1983;147:407–410.

43. Chamberlain PF, Manning FA, Morrison I, Harman CR, Lange IR. Ultrasound evaluation of amniotic fluid volume. I. The relationship of marginal and decreased amniotic fluid volume to perinatal outcome. *Am J Obstet Gynecol* 1984;150:245–249.

44. Bastide A, Manning F, Harman C, Lange I, Morrison I. Ultrasound evaluation of amniotic fluid: outcome of pregnancies with severe oligohydramnios. *Am J Obstet Gynecol* 1986;154:895–900.

45. Shenker L, Reed KL, Anderson CF, Borjon NA. Significance of oligohydramnios complicating pregnancy. *Am J Obstet Gynecol* 1991;164:1597–1600.

46. Nicolaides KH, Snijder RJM, Noble P. Cordocentesis in the study of growth-retarded fetuses. In: Divon MY, ed. *Abnormal fetal growth.* New York: Elsevier, 1991:166.

47. Shipp TD, Bromley B, Pauker S, Frigoletto FD Jr, Benacerraf BR. Outcomes of singleton pregnancies with severe oligohydramnios in the second and third trimester. *Ultrasound Obstet Gynecol* 1996;7:108–113.

48. Benacerraf BR. Examination of the second trimester fetus with severe oligohydramnios using transvaginal scanning. *Obstet Gynecol* 1990;75:491–493.

49. DeVore GR. The value of color Doppler sonography in the diagnosis of renal agenesis. *J Ultrasound Med* 1995;14:443–449.

50. Cock ML, McCrabb GJ, Wlodek ME, Handing R. Effects of prolonged hypoxemia on fetal renal function and amniotic fluid volume in sheep. *Am J Obstet Gynecol* 1997;176:320–6.

51. Herbertson RM, Hammond EM, Bryson MJ. Amniotic epithelial ultrastructure in normal, polyhydramnic and oligohydramnic pregnancies. *Obstet Gynecol* 1986;68:74–79.

52. Eden RD, Seifert LS, Winegar A, Spellacy WN. Perinatal characteristics of uncomplicated postdate pregnancies. *Obstet Gynecol* 1987;67:290–299.

53. Elliot PM, Inman WHW. Volume of amniotic fluid in normal and abnormal pregnancy. *Lancet* 1961;2:835–840.

54. Selam B, Koksal R, Ozcan T. Fetal arterial and venous Doppler parameters in the interpretation of oligohydramnios in postterm pregnancies. *Ultrasound Obstet Gynecol* 2000;15:403–406.

55. Hsieh TT, Hung TH, Chen KC, Hsieh CC, Lo LM, et al. Perinatal outcome of oligohydramnios without associated premature rupture of membranes and fetal anomalies. *Gynecol Obstet Invest* 1998;45:232–236.

56. Tongsong T, Srisomboon J. Amniotic fluid volume as a predictor of fetal distress in postterm pregnancy. *Int J Gynaecol Obstet* 1993 Mar;40:213–217.

57. Alfirevic Z, Luckas M, Walkinshaw SA, McFarlane M, Curran R. A randomized comparison between amniotic fluid index and maximum pool depth in the monitoring of postterm pregnancy. *Br J Obstet Gynaecol* 1997;104:207–211.

58. Mead PB. Management of the patient with premature rupture of the membranes. *Clin Perinatol* 1980;7:243–255.

59. Kilbride HW, Yeast J, Thibeault DW. Defining limits of survival: lethal pulmonary hypoplasia after midtrimester premature rupture of membranes. *Am J Obstet Gynecol* 1996;175:675–681.

60. Borgida AF, Mills A, Feldman DM, Rodis JF, Egan JFX. Outcome of pregnancies complicated by ruptured membranes after genetic amniocentesis. *Am J Obstet Gynecol* 2000;183:937–939.

61. Sciscione AC, Costigan KA, Johnson TRB. Increase in ambient temperature may explain decrease in amniotic fluid index. *Am J Perinatol* 1997;14:249–251.

62. Goodlin RC, Anderson JC, Gallagher TF. Relationship between amniotic fluid volume and maternal plasma volume expansion. *Am J Obstet Gynecol* 1983;146:505–511.

63. Bronshtein M, Blumenfeld Z. First and early second-trimester oligohydramnios—a predictor of poor fetal outcome except in iatrogenic oligohydramnios post chorionic villus sampling. *Ultrasound Obstet Gynecol* 1991;1:245–249.

64. Hill LM, Lazebnik N, Many A. Effect of indomethacin on individual amniotic fluid indices in multiple gestations. *J Ultrasound Med* 1996;15:395–399.

65. Piper JM, Ray WA, Rosa FW. Pregnancy outcome following exposure to angiotensin-converting enzyme inhibitors. *Obstet Gynecol* 1992;80:429–432.

66. Garmel SH, Chelmow D, Sha SJ, Roan JT, D'Alton ME. Oligohydramnios and the appropriately grown fetus. *Am J Perinatol* 1997;14:359–363.

67. Magann EF, Morton ML, Nolan TE, Martin JN, Whitworth NS, et al. Comparative efficacy of two sonographic measurements for the detection of aberrations in the amniotic fluid volume and the effect of amniotic fluid volume on pregnancy outcome. *Obstet Gynecol* 1994;83:959–962.

68. Nimrod C, Varela-Gittings F, Machin G, Campbell D, Wesenberg R. The effect of very prolonged membrane rupture on fetal development. *Am J Obstet Gynecol* 1984;148:540–543.

69. Thibeault DW, Beatty EC, Hall RT, et al. Neonatal pulmonary hypoplasia with premature rupture of fetal membranes and oligohydramnios. *J Pediatr* 1985;107:273–277.

70. Banks EH, Miller DA. Perinatal risks associated with borderline amniotic fluid index. *Am J Obstet Gynecol* 1999;180:1461–1463.

71. Conway DL, Adkins WB, Schroeder B, Langer O. Isolated oligohydramnios in the term pregnancy: is it a clinical entity? *J Matern Fetal Med* 1998;7:197–200.

72. Magann EF, Kinsella MJ, Chauhan SP, McNamara MF, Gehring BW, et al. Does amniotic fluid index <5 cm necessitate delivery in high risk pregnancies? A case control study. *Am J Obstet Gynecol* 1999;180:1354–1359.

73. Adzick NS, Harrision MJR, Glick PL, et al. Experimental pulmonary hypoplasia and oligohydramnios: relative contributions of lung fluid and fetal breathing movements. *J Pediatr Surg* 1984;19:658–665.

74. Chitkara U, Rosenberg J, Chervenak FA, et al. Prenatal sonographic assessment of the fetal thorax: normal values. *Am J Obstet Gynecol* 1987;156:1069–1074.

75. Vintzileos AM, Campbell WA, Nochimson DJ, Weinbaum PJ. Degree of oligohydramnios and pregnancy outcome in patients with premature rupture of the membranes. *Obstet Gynecol* 1985;66:162–167.

76. Vermillion ST, Kooba AM, Super DE. Amniotic fluid index values after preterm premature rupture of the membranes and subsequent perinatal infection. *Am J Obstet Gynecol* 2000;183:271–276.

77. Hofmeyr GJ, Gulmezoglu AM. Maternal hydration for increasing amniotic fluid volume in oligohydramnios and normal amniotic fluid volume. *Cochrane Database Syst Rev* 2000;(2):CD000134.

78. Doi S, Osada H, Seki K, Sekiya S. Effect of maternal hydration on oligohydramnios: a comparison of three volume expansion methods. *Obstet Gynecol* 1998;92:525–529.

79. Kilpatrick SJ, Safford SJ. Maternal hydration increases amniotic fluid index in women with normal amniotic fluid. *Obstet Gynecol* 1993;81:49–52.

80. Gramellini D, Piantelli G, Delle Chiaie L, Rutolo S, Vadora E. Amnioinfusion in the management of oligohydramnios. *J Perinat Med* 1998;26:293–301.

81. Hofmeyr GJ. Amnioinfusion for umbilical cord compression in labour. *Cochrane Database Syst Rev* 2000;(2): CD000013.

82. Locatelli A, Vergani P, DiPivo G, Doria V, Biffi A, et al. Role of amnioinfusion in the management of premature rupture of the membranes at <26 weeks' gestation. *Am J Obstet Gynecol* 2000;183:878–882.

83. Hofmeyr GJ. Amnioinfusion for preterm rupture of membranes. *Cochrane Database Syst Rev* 2000;(2):CD000942.

84. Queenan JT, Thompson W, Whitfield CR, Shah SI. Amniotic fluid volumes in normal pregnancy. *Am J Obstet Gynecol* 1972;114:34–38.

85. Chamberlain PF, Manning FA, Morrison I, Harmon CR, Lange IR. Ultrasound evaluation of amniotic fluid volume. II. The relationship of increased amniotic fluid volume to perinatal outcome. *Am J Obstet Gynecol* 1984;150:250–254.

86. Queenan JT, Gadow EC. Polyhydramnios: chronic versus acute. *Am J Obstet Gynecol* 1970;108:349–355.

87. Wallenburg HCS, Wladimiroff JW. The amniotic fluid. II. Polyhydramnios and oligohydramnios. *J Perinat Med* 1977; 5:233–243.

88. Broecker BH, Redwire FO, Petres RE. Reversal of acute polyhydramnios after fetal renal decompression. *Urology* 1998;31:60–62.

89. Josimovich JB, Mensko K, Bucella L. Amniotic prolactin control over amniotic and fetal extracellular fluid water and electrolytes in the rhesus monkey. *Endocrinology* 1977;100: 564–570.

90. DeSantis M, Cavaliere AF, Noia G, Masini L, Menini E, et al. Acute recurrent polyhydramnios and amniotic prolactin. *Prenat Diagn* 2000;20:347–348.

91. Glantz JC, Abramowicz JS, Sherer DM. Significance of idiopathic mid-trimester polyhydramnios. *Am J Perinatol* 1994;11:305–308.

92. Hill LM, Breckle R, Thomas ML, Fries JK. Polyhydramnios: ultrasonically detected prevalence and neonatal outcome. *Obstet Gynecol* 1987;69:21–25.

93. Smith CV, Plambeck RD, Rayburn WF, Albaugh KJ. Relation of mild idiopathic polyhydramnios to perinatal outcome. *Obstet Gynecol* 1992;79:387–389.

94. Panting-Kemp A, Nquyen T, Chang E, Quillen E, Castro L. Idiopathic polyhydramnios and perinatal outcome. *Am J Obstet Gynecol* 1999;181:1079–82.

95. Phelan JP, Park YW, Ahn MO, Rutherford SE. Polyhydramnios and perinatal outcome. *J Perinatol* 1990;10:347–350.

96. Biggio JR, Wenstrom KD, Dubard MB, Cliver SP. Hydramnios prediction of adverse perinatal outcome. *Obstet Gynecol* 1999;94:773–777.

97. Ben-Chetrit A, Hochner-Celnikier D, Ron M, et al. Hydramnios in the third trimester of pregnancy: a change in the distribution of accompanying fetal anomalies as a result of early ultrasonographic prenatal diagnosis. *Am J Obstet Gynecol* 1990;162:1344–1345.

98. Thompson O, Brown R, Gunnarson G, Harrington K. Prevalence of polyhydramnios in the third trimester in a population screened by first and second trimester ultrasonography. *J Perinat Med* 1998;26:371–377.

99. Damato N, Filly RA, Goldstein RB, Callen PW, Goldberg J, et al. Frequency of fetal anomalies in sonographically detected polyhydramnios. *J Ultrasound Med* 1993;12:11–15.

100. Barkin SZ, Pretorius DH, Beckett MK, Manchester DK, Nelson TR, et al. Severe polyhydramnios: incidence of anomalies. *AJR Am J Roentgenol* 1987;148:155–159.

101. Kimble RM, Harding JE, Kolbe A. Does gut atresia cause polyhydramnios? *Pediatr Surg Int* 1998;13:115–117.

102. Lloyd JR, Clatworthy HWS. Hydramnios as an aid to the diagnosis of congenital obstruction of the alimentary tract: a study of the maternal and fetal factors. *Pediatric* 1958;21:903–909.

103. DeLorimier AA, Funkalsrud EW, Hays AM. Congenital atresia and stenosis of the jejunum and ileum. *Surgery* 1969;65:819–827.

104. Foster MA, Nyberg DA, Mahony BS, Mack LA, Marks WM, et al. Meconium peritonitis: prenatal sonographic findings and clinical significance. *Radiology* 1987;165:661–665.

105. Langer JC, Winthrop AL, Burrows RF, Issenman RM, Caco CC. False diagnosis of intestinal obstruction in a fetus with congenital chloride diarrhea. *J Pediatr Surg* 1991;26:1282–1284.

106. Chen CP, Wang TY, Chuang CY. Sonographic findings in a fetus with megacystis-microcolon-intestinal hypoperistalsis syndrome. *J Clin Ultrasound* 1998;26:217–220.

107. Goldstein RB, Filly RA. Prenatal diagnosis of anencephaly: spectrum of sonographic appearances and distinction from the amniotic band syndrome. *AJR Am J Roentgenol* 1988;151:547–550.

108. de Hullu JA, Kornman LH, Beekhuis JR, Nikkels PGJ. The hyperechogenic lungs of laryngotracheal obstruction. *Ultrasound Obstet Gynecol* 1995;5:271–274.

109. Thorpe-Beeston JG, Nicolaides KH. Cystic adenomatoid malformation of the lung: prenatal diagnosis and outcome. *Prenat Diagn* 1994;14:677–688.

110. Mahony BS, Filly RA, Callen PW, Chinn DH, Golbus MS. Severe non-immune hydrops fetalis: sonographic evaluation. *Radiology* 1984;151:757–761.

111. Kleiner B, Callen PW, Filly RA. Sonographic analysis of the fetus with ureteropelvic junction obstruction. *AJR Am J Roentgenol* 1987;148:359–363.

112. Thomas RL, Hess LW, Johnson TRB. Prepartum diagnosis of limb-shortening defects with associated hydramnios. *Am J Perinatol* 1987;4:295–299.

113. Knilans TK. Cardiac abnormalities associated with hydrops fetalis. *Semin Perinatol* 1995;19:483–492.

114. Maxwell DJ, Crawford DC, Curry PV, Tynan MJ, Allan LD. Obstetric importance, diagnosis, and management of fetal tachycardias. *BMJ* 1988;297:107–110.

115. Machin GA. Hydrops revisited: literature review of 1,414 cases published in the 1980's. *Am J Med Genet* 1989;34:366–390.

116. DeVore GR, Harkin S, Kleinman CS, Hobbins JC. The in-utero diagnosis of an interventricular septal cardiac rhabdomyoma by means of real-time directed, m-mode echocardiography. *Am J Obstet Gynecol* 1982;143:967–969.

117. McCoy MC, Katz VL, Gould N, Kuller JA. Non-immune hydrops after 20 weeks' gestation: review of 10 years' experience with suggestions for management. *Obstet Gynecol* 1995;85:578–582.

118. Stoll CG, Alembik Y, Dott B. Study of 156 cases of polyhydramnios and congenital malformations in a series of 118,265 consecutive births. *Am J Obstet Gynecol* 1991;165:586–590.

119. Barnhard Y, Bar-Hava I, Divon MY. Is polyhydramnios in an ultrasonographically normal fetus an indication for genetic evaluation? *Am J Obstet Gynecol* 1995;173:1523–1527.

120. Bruner JP, Anderson TL, Rosemond RL. Placental pathophysiology of the twin oligohydramnios-polyhydramnios sequence and the twin-twin transfusion syndrome. *Placenta* 1998;19:81–86.

121. Bajoria R, Wigglesworth J, Fisk NM. Angioarchitecture of monochorionic placentas in relation to the twin-twin transfusion syndrome. *Am J Obstet Gynecol* 1995;172:856–863.

122. Drose JA, Dennis MA, Thickman D. Infection in-utero: ultrasound findings in 19 cases. *Radiology* 1991;178:369–374.

123. Nathan L, Twickler DM, Peters MT, Sánchez PJ, Wendel GD Jr. Fetal syphilis: correlation of sonographic findings and rabbit infectivity testing of amniotic fluid. *J Ultrasound Med* 1993;2:97–101.

124. Nikkari S, Ekblad U. A rapid and safe method to detect fetal parvovirus B-19 infection in amniotic fluid by polymerase chain reaction: report of a case. *Am J Perinatol* 1995;12:447–449.

125. Hohlfeld P, MacAleese J, Capella-Pavlovski M, Giovangrardi Y, Thalliez P, et al. Fetal toxoplasmosis: ultrasonographic signs. *Ultrasound Obstet Gynecol* 1991;1:241–244.

126. Rochelson B, Coury A, Schulman H, Dery C, Klotz M, et al. Doppler umbilical artery velocimetry in fetuses with polyhydramnios. *Am J Perinatol* 1990;7:340–2.

127. Sohaey R, Nyberg D, Sickler GK, Williams MA. Idiopathic polyhydramnios: association with fetal macrosomia. *Radiology* 1994;190:393–396.

128. Lazebnik N, Hill LM, Guzick D, Martin JG, Many A. Severity of polyhydramnios does not affect the prevalence of large-for-gestational-age newborn infants. *J Ultrasound Med* 1996;15:385–388.

129. Benson CB, Coughlin BF, Doubilet PM. Amniotic fluid volume in large-for-gestational-age fetuses of nondiabetic mothers. *J Ultrasound Med* 1991;10:149–151.

130. Maymon E, Ghezzi F, Shoham-Vardi I, Franchi M, Silberstein T, et al. Isolated hydramnios at term gestation and the occurrence of peripartum complications. *Eur J Obstet Gynecol Reprod Biol* 1998;77:157–161.

131. Sickler GK, Nyberg DA, Sohaey R, Luthy DA. Polyhydramnios and fetal intrauterine growth restriction: ominous combination. *J Ultrasound Med* 1997;16:609–614.

132. Sterniste W, Urban G, Stukler-ipsiroglu S, Mick R, Sacher M. Polyhydramnios as a first prenatal symptom of nonketotic hyperglycinaemia [Letter]. *Prenatal Diagn* 1998;18:863–864.

133. Narchi H, Santos M, Kulaylat N. Polyhydramnios as a sign of fetal pseudohypoaldosteronism. *Int J Gynecol Obstet* 2000;69:53–54.

134. Mazor M, Ghezzi F, Maymon E, Shoham-Vardi I, Vardi H, et al. Polyhydramnios is an independent risk factor for peri-

natal mortality and intrapartum morbidity in preterm delivery. *Eur J Obstet Gynecol Reprod Biol* 1996;70:41–47.

135. Chauhan SP, Martin RW, Morrison JC. Intrapartum hydramnios at term and perinatal outcome. *J Perinatol* 1993;13:186–189.

136. Fisk NM, Tarnirandorn Y, Nicolini U, Talbert DG, Rodeck CH. Amniotic pressure in disorders of amniotic fluid volume. *Obstet Gynecol* 1990;76:210–214.

137. Tabor B, Majer JA. Hydramnios and elevated intrauterine pressures during amnioinfusion. *Am J Obstet Gynecol* 1987;156:130–131.

138. Fisk NM, Vaughan J, Talbert D. Impaired fetal blood gas status in polyhydramnios and its relation to raised amniotic pressure. *Fetal Diagn Ther* 1994;9:7–13.

139. Many A, Hill LM, Lazebnik N, Martin JG. The association between polyhydramnios and preterm delivery. *Obstet Gynecol* 1995;86:389–391.

140. Many A, Lazebnik N, Hill LM. The underlying cause of polyhydramnios determines prematurity. *Prenat Diagn* 1996;16:55–57.

141. Hill LM, Lazebnik W, Many A, Martin JG. Resolving polyhydramnios: clinical significance and subsequent neonatal outcome. *Ultrasound Obstet Gynecol* 1995;6:421–424.

142. Moise KJ Jr. Polyhydramnios: problems and treatment. *Semin Perinatol* 1993;17:197–209.

143. Elliott JP, Sawyer AT, Radin T, Strong RE. Large-volume therapeutic amniocentesis in the treatment of hydramnios. *Obstet Gynecol* 1994;84:1025–1027.

144. Saunders NJ, Snijders RJ, Nicolaides KH. Therapeutic amniocentesis in twin-twin transfusion syndrome appearing in the second trimester of pregnancy. *Am J Obstet Gynecol* 1992;166:820–824.

145. Elliott JP, Urig MA, Clewell WH. Aggressive therapeutic amniocentesis for treatment of twin-twin transfusion syndrome. *Obstet Gynecol* 1991;77:537–540.

146. Mari G, Wasserstrum N, Kirshon B. Reduction in the middle cerebral artery pulsatility index after decompression of polyhydramnios in twin gestation. *Am J Perinatol* 1992;9:381–384.

147. Cabrol D, Jannet D, Pannier E. Treatment of symptomatic polyhydramnios with indomethacin. *Eur J Obstet Gynecol Reprod Biol* 1996;66:11–15.

148. Kramer WB, Van Der Veyver I, Kirshon B. Treatment of polyhydramnios with indomethacin. *Clin Perinatol* 1994;21:615–630.

149. Moise KJ, Ou C-N, Kirshon B, Cano LE, Rognerud C, et al. Placental transfer of indomethacin in the human pregnancy. *Am J Obstet Gynecol* 1990;162:549–554.

150. Mamopoulos M, Assimakopoulos E, Reece EA, et al. Maternal indomethacin therapy in the treatment of polyhydramnios. *Am J Obstet Gynecol* 1990;162:1225–1229.

151. Goldenberg RL, Davis RO, Baker RC. Indomethacin-induced oligohydramnios. *Am J Obstet Gynecol* 1989;160:1196–1197.

152. Moise KJ Jr. Polyhydramnios. *Clin Obstet Gynecol* 1997;40:266–279.

153. Moise KL, Huhta JC, Sharif DS, et al. Indomethacin in the treatment of premature labor. Effect on the fetal ductus arteriosis. *N Engl J Med* 1988;319:327–331.

154. Moise KL Jr. Indomethacin therapy in the treatment of

155. symptomatic polyhydramnios. *Clin Obstet Gynecol* 1991;34:310–318.

155. Gerson A, Roberts N, Colmorgen G, et al. Treatment of polyhydramnios with indomethacin. *Am J Perinatol* 1991;8:97–98.

156. Norton ME, Merrill J, Cooper BAB, Kuller JA, Clyman RI. Neonatal complications after the administration of indomethacin for preterm labor. *N Engl J Med* 1993;329:1602–1607.

157. Major CA, Lewis DF, Harding JA, et al. Tocolysis with indomethacin increases the incidence of necrotizing enterocolitis in the low-birth-weight neonate. *Am J Obstet Gynecol* 1994;170:102–6.

158. Eronen M, Pesonen E, Kurki T, et al. Increased incidence of bronchopulmonary dysplasia after antenatal administration of indomethacin to prevent preterm labor. *J Pediatr* 1994;124:782–788.

159. Dudley DKL, Hardie MJ. Fetal and neonatal effects of indomethacin used as a tocolytic agent. *Am J Obstet Gynecol* 1985;151:181–184.

160. Niebyl JR, Witter FR. Neonatal outcome after indomethacin treatment of preterm labor. *Am J Obstet Gynecol* 1986;155:747–749.

161. Snijders RJ, Sherrod C, Gosden CM, Nicolaides KH. Fetal growth retardation: associated malformations and chromosomal abnormalities. *Am J Obstet Gynecol* 1993;168:547–555.

162. Carlson DE, Platt LD, Medearis AL. The ultrasound triad of fetal hydramnios, abnormal hand posturing, and any other anomaly predicts autosomal trisomy. *Obstet Gynecol* 1992;79:731–734.

163. Seller MJ, Child AH. Raised maternal serum alphafetoprotein, oligohydramnios and the fetus. *Lancet* 1980;1:317–318.

164. Koontz WL, Seeds JW, Adams NJ, et al. Elevated maternal serum alpha-fetoprotein, second-trimester oligohydramnios and pregnancy outcome. *Obstet Gynecol* 1983;62:301–304.

165. Dyer SN, Burton BK, Nelson LH. Elevated maternal serum alpha-fetoprotein levels and oligohydramnios: poor prognosis for pregnancy outcome. *Am J Obstet Gynecol* 1987;157:336–339.

166. Richards DS, Seeds JW, Katz UL, Lingley LH, Albright SG, et al. Elevated maternal serum alpha-fetoprotein with oligohydramnios: ultrasound evaluation and outcome. *Obstet Gynecol* 1988;72:337–341.

167. Hickok DE, McClean J, Shepard TH, Hendrichs S. Unexplained second trimester oligohydramnios: a clinical-pathologic study. *Am J Perinatol* 1989;6:8–13.

168. Los FJ, Hagonaars AM, Marrink J, Cohen-Overbeek TE, Gaillard JLJ, et al. Maternal serum alpha-fetoprotein levels and fetal outcome in early second-trimester oligohydramnios. *Prenat Diagn* 1992;12:285–292.

169. Magann EF, Chauhan SP, Whitworth NS, Klausen JH, Saltzman AK, et al. Do multiple measurements employing different ultrasonic techniques improve the accuracy of amniotic fluid volume assessment? *Aust N Z J Obstet Gynecol* 1998;38:172–175.

170. Chauhan SP, Magann EF, Morrison JC, Whitworth NS, Hendrix NW, et al. Ultrasonographic assessment of amniotic fluid does not reflect actual amniotic fluid volume. *Am J Obstet Gynecol* 1997;177:291–297.

171. Hoppen T, Hofstatter C, Plath H, Kau N, Bratman P. Agenesis of the ductus venosus and its correlation to hydrops fetalis. *J Perinat Med* 2000;28:69–73.

172. Jacoby HE, Charles D. Clinical conditions associated with hydramnios. *Am J Obstet Gynecol* 1966;94:910–919.

173. Sieck U, Ohlsson A. Fetal polyuria and hydramnios associated with Bartter's syndrome. *Obstet Gynecol* 1984;63[Suppl]:22–24.

174. Zahn C, Hankins GBV, Yeomans ER. Karyotypic abnormalities and hydramnios. Role of amniocentesis. *J Reprod Med* 1993;38:599–602.

175. Brady K, Polzin WJ, Kopelman JN, Read JA. Risk of chromosomal abnormalities in patients with idiopathic polyhydramnios. *Obstet Gynecol* 1992;79:234–238.

176. Carlson DE, Platt LD, Medearis AL, Horenstein J. Quantifiable polyhydramnios: diagnosis and management. *Obstet Gynecol* 1990;75:989–992.

177. Golan A, Wolman I, Sall ER, David MP. Hydramnios in singleton pregnancy: sonographic prevalence and etiology. *Gynecol Obstet Invest* 1993;35:91–93.

178. Hendricks SK, Conway L, Wang K, Komarniski C, Mack LA, et al. Diagnosis of polyhydramnios in early gestation: indications for prenatal diagnosis? *Prenat Diagn* 1991;11:649–654.

179. Char VC, Chandra R, Fletcher AB, Avery GB. Polyhydramnios and neonatal renal failure—a possible association with maternal acetaminophen ingestion. *J Pediatr* 1975;86:638–639.

180. Dunn LJ, Dierker LJ. Recurrent hydramnios in association with myotonia dystrophica. *Obstet Gynecol* 1973;42:104–106.

181. Ranzini AC, Day-Salvatore D, Turner T, Smulian JC, Vintzileos AM. Intrauterine growth and ultrasound findings in fetuses with Beckwith-Wiedemann syndrome. *Obstet Gynecol* 1997;89:538–542.

182. Tseng JJ, Chou MM, Lee YH, Ho ESC. Prenatal diagnosis of intrahepatic arteriovenous shunts. *Ultrasound Obstet Gynecol* 2000;15:441–444.

183. Duffy SL. Fetal retroperitoneal fibrosis associated with hydramnios. *JAMA* 1966;198:993–996.

184. Devriendt K, Van Schoubroeck D, Eyskens B, et al. Polyhydramnios as a prenatal symptom of the DiGeorge/Velo-cardio-facial syndrome. *Prenat Diagn* 1998;18:68–72.

185. Goldberg JD, Chervenak FA, Lipman RA, Berkowitz RL. Antenatal sonographic diagnosis of arthrogryposis multiple congenita. *Prenat Diagn* 1986;6:45–49.

186. Sivit CJ, Hill MC, Larsen JW, Kent SG, Lande IM. The sonographic evaluation of fetal anomalies in oligohydramnios between 16 and 30 weeks gestation. *AJR Am J Roentgenol* 1986;146:1277–1281.

187. Golan A, Lin G, Evron S, Ariele S, Niv D, David MP. Oligohydramnios: maternal complications and fetal outcome in 145 cases. *Gynecol Obstet Invest* 1994;37:91–95.

4

THE PLACENTA, UMBILICAL CORD, AND MEMBRANES

Ultrasound examination of the placenta and umbilical cord is an integral part of all antenatal ultrasound scans, providing information on placental localization, which dictates future management; placental appearance that may aid diagnosis of intrauterine growth restriction (IUGR); abnormalities associated with fetal compromise; morphologic defects of the placenta; and assessment of fetoplacental and uteroplacental blood flow to direct antenatal management. This chapter examines the issues pertinent to ultrasound examination of the placenta, umbilical cord, and placental membranes.

Extensive pathologic literature exists relating to many aspects of placental development and specific conditions that may affect the placenta and umbilical cord,[1-3] but this chapter will limit its content to those major conditions that are clinically significant and have been reported by prenatal ultrasound. Similarly, the basic pathophysiology and clinical features of many of the conditions included are not repeated here and can be found in any obstetric textbook; only the features specifically relevant to ultrasound diagnosis and management are included for the most part.

EMBRYOLOGY

By menstrual day 20, the zygote has formed the blastocyst, a fluid-filled cystic cavity composed of an inner cell mass and an outer trophoblastic layer.[4] The inner cell mass eventually forms the fetus, yolk sac, and allantois; the trophoblasts form the placenta, chorion, and amnion (Fig. 1).

Implantation of the blastocyst in the endometrium begins approximately 1 week after ovulation and is completed by menstrual day 28 (end of the second week).[4] During implantation, trophoblasts erode adjacent maternal capillaries so that maternal blood comes into direct contact with the conceptus. This contact establishes an intercommunicating lacunar network, which becomes the intervillous space of the placenta. The endometrium also undergoes a decidual reaction that helps support and con-

trol trophoblastic invasion. Frond-like chorionic villi arise from the trophoblast. After menstrual day 29, blood vessels enter primary villi to form true or tertiary villi.

Chorionic villi initially cover the entire surface of the chorionic sac. After 8 weeks, those villi aligned toward the uterine cavity become compressed and their blood supply becomes restricted. Degeneration of these villi forms the chorion laeve (i.e., smooth chorion). Simultaneously, chorionic villi associated with the decidua basalis rapidly proliferate to form the chorion frondosum, which becomes the definitive placenta. As pregnancy progresses, the chorionic villi branch and gradually develop into a complex system of 50 to 60 subunits or cotyledons, each of which arises from a primary stem villus and is supplied by primary branches of the umbilical vessels. Each cotyledon is further subdivided into one to five lobules.

The mature placenta weighs 450 to 550 g and has a diameter of 16 to 20 cm. The fetal surface, which is continuous with the surrounding chorion, is termed the *chorionic plate*. The maternal surface of the placenta, which lies contiguous with the decidua basalis, is termed the *basal plate*.

Fetal-Placental-Uterine Circulation

The fetal-umbilical circulation originates with deoxygenated blood pumped by the fetal heart through the ductus arteriosus and into the descending aorta. Fetal blood continues through the hypogastric arteries to the umbilical arteries and into the umbilical cord. By term, approximately 40% of the fetal cardiac output (300 to 350 cc per minute) is directed through the umbilical circulation. Within the placenta, the umbilical arteries freely divide into multiple capillary branches that course through the tertiary villi (Fig. 2). This division produces a rich vascular network emanating from the umbilical cord (Fig. 3).

Oxygenated maternal blood is delivered to the placenta through 80 to 100 end branches of the uterine arteries, called *spiral arteries*.[4] Maternal blood enters the intervillous

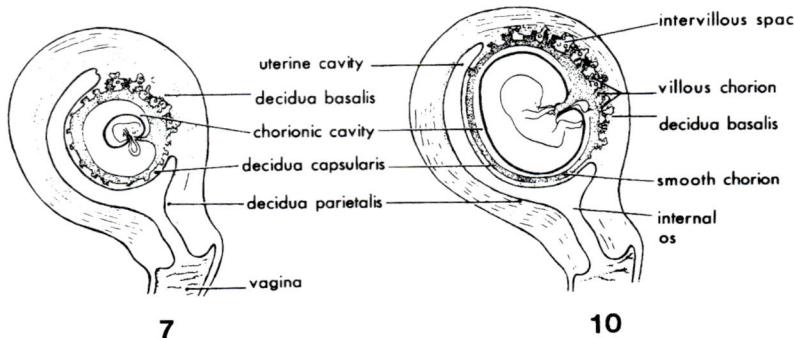

FIGURE 1. Development of chorionic villi and fetal membranes at 7 menstrual weeks (5 fetal weeks) and 10 menstrual weeks. (Reproduced with permission from Moore KL. *The developing human*, 4th ed. Philadelphia: WB Saunders, 1988.)

space near the central part of each placental lobule where it flows around and over the surface of the villi. This process permits exchange of oxygen and nutrients with fetal blood flowing in villous capillaries. Maternal blood then returns through a network of basilar, subchorial, interlobular, and marginal veins. The rate of uteroplacental flow increases from approximately 50 cc per min at 10 weeks to 500 to 600 cc per min at term. By term, the intervillous space of 150 cc is replaced three to four times per minute.[4]

As a result of changes in the trophoblast, only a thin layer normally separates fetal blood from maternal blood. This layer is composed of the capillary wall, the trophoblastic basement membrane, and a thin rim of cytoplasm of the syncytiotrophoblast.

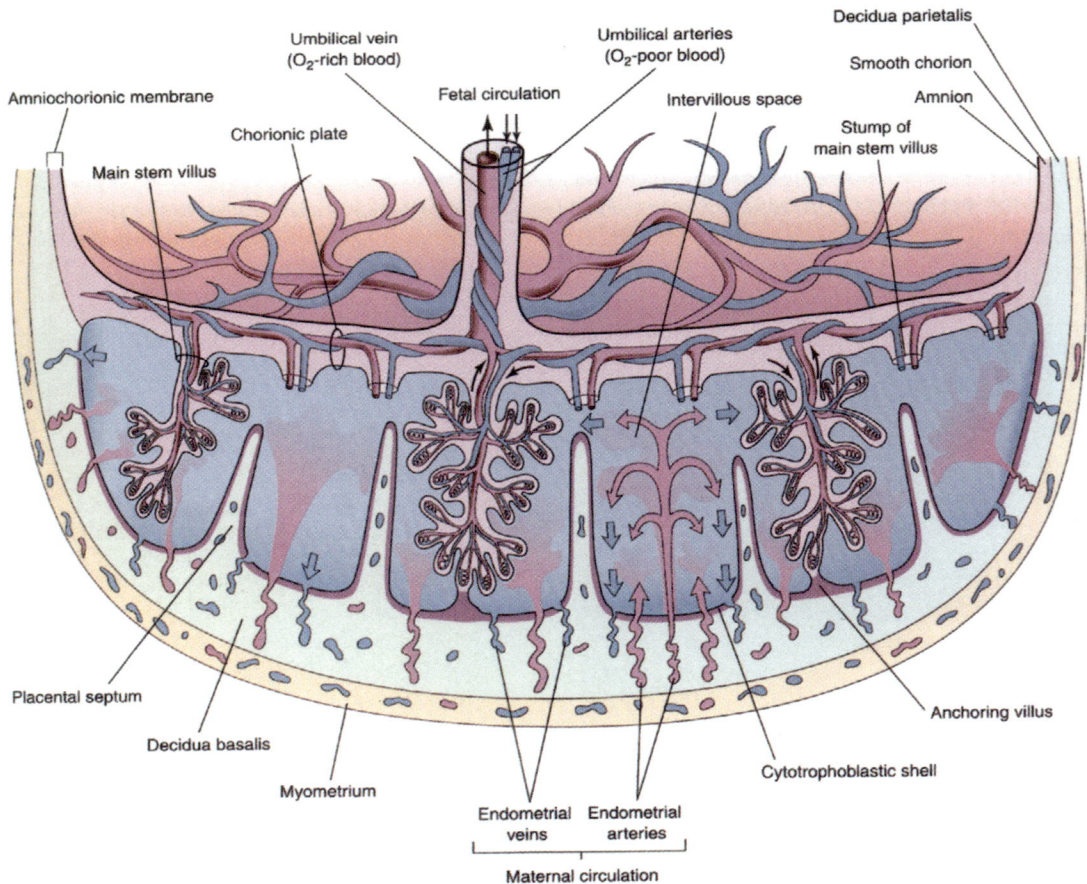

FIGURE 2. Schematic drawing of placental circulation during the third trimester. Maternal blood supplied by the spiral arteries circulates in the intervillous space, bathes the placental villi, and then egresses through periplacental veins. Fetal blood from the umbilical artery supplies the villi and returns via the umbilical vein. (Reproduced with permission from Moore KL, Persaud TW. *The developing human*, 8th ed. Philadelphia: WB Saunders, 1999.)

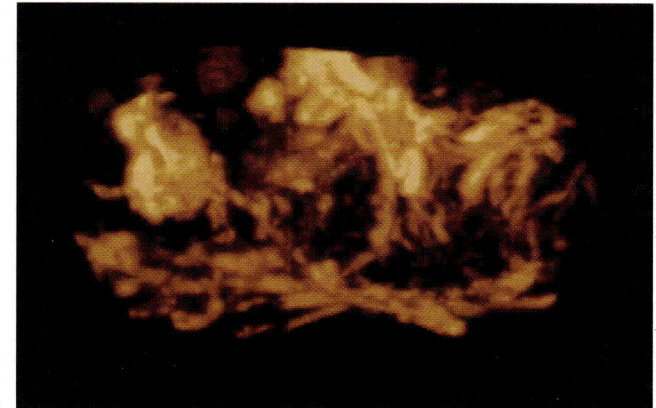

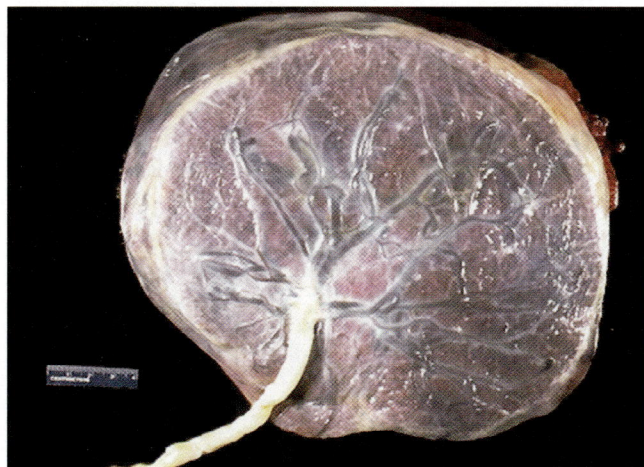

FIGURE 3. Placental circulation. **A:** Three-dimensional ultrasound with color-flow imaging shows rich vascular network of the placenta. **B:** Pathologic specimen of normal placenta. Multiple arteries and veins branch from the umbilical cord on the surface of the placenta. (Part **A** courtesy of Siemens Corporation; and Part **B** courtesy of Edward C. Klatt, MD, Department of Pathology, Florida State University, College of Medicine.)

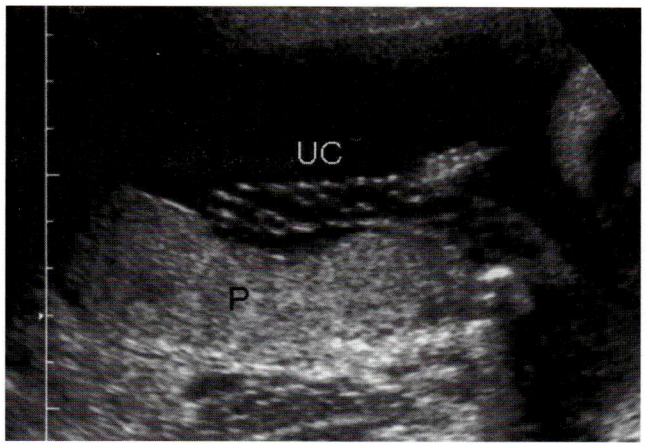

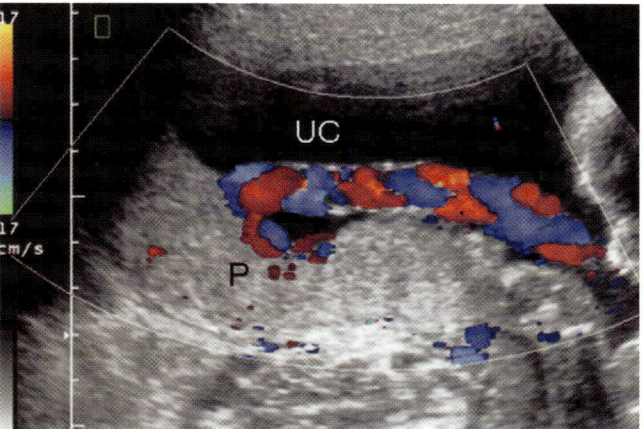

FIGURE 4. Normal placenta (*P*), 17 weeks. **A, B:** During the second trimester, the placenta is typically homogenous in echotexture. Normal insertion of the umbilical cord (*UC*) is also shown.

NORMAL SONOGRAPHIC FINDINGS OF THE PLACENTA

The placenta (i.e., chorion frondosum) can be identified on sonography as early as 8 menstrual weeks. Between 8 and 20 weeks, the placenta normally appears uniform in echotexture and thickness, measuring less than 2 to 3 cm (Fig. 4).

Many pathologic lesions may affect the placenta, especially during the third trimester (Fig. 5). After 20 weeks, intraplacental sonolucencies (e.g., venous lakes or intervillous thrombi) and placental calcification may begin to appear, and the placenta can measure 4 to 5 cm in thickness (Fig. 6).[5-7] Focal sonolucent areas within the placenta may have many various etiologies and are usually of no clinical significance. Prominent intraplacental sonolucencies during the second trimester are unusual but usually result in a normal outcome (Fig. 7). A heterogenous placenta may be more commonly observed in women with elevated maternal serum alpha-

fetoprotein (AFP) or a history of first-trimester bleeding (Fig. 8).[8,9] Intraplacental sonolucencies usually represent venous "lakes," and these may be seen to change dramatically during the course of the ultrasound exam. Blood flow is too slow usually to be detected with Doppler techniques. At delivery, these areas correspond to fibrin deposition or no abnormalities.

Jauniaux et al.[10] examined 20 cases in which placental sonolucencies were associated with increased AFP and reported several different types of sonolucency in addition to "placental lakes." These different types included gigantic enlargement of the whole placenta with multiple sonolucent spaces of different size and shape (i.e., "swiss cheese" placenta), which corresponded to mesenchymal dysplasia of the stem villi or *pseudomoles* (see Gestational Trophoblastic Neoplasia, Differential Diagnosis), and diffuse placental enlargement with patchy areas of decreased echogenicity (i.e., "jelly-like" placenta) corresponded to subchorial thromboses or massive fibrin deposition. Other focal sonolucent lesions include subchorionic cysts (subchorionic fibrin plaques pathologically)[11] and septal cysts.[12,13]

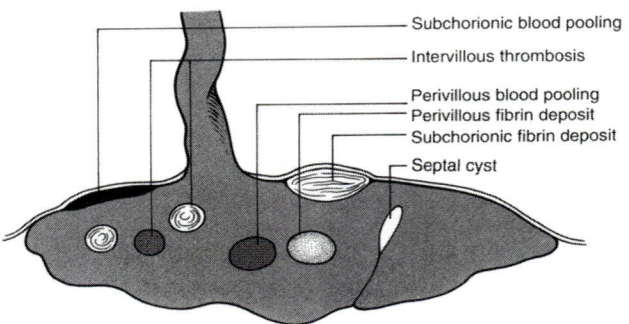

Subchorionic blood pooling
Intervillous thrombosis
Perivillous blood pooling
Perivillous fibrin deposit
Subchorionic fibrin deposit
Septal cyst

FIGURE 5. Schematic showing various pathologic lesions of the placenta. These are more common during the third trimester. (Reproduced with permission from McGahan JP, Proto M. *Diagnostic obstetrical ultrasound.* Philadelphia: JB Lippincott Co, 1994.)

The placental location is usually in the mid to fundal portion of the uterus, reflecting the site of implantation. The apparent location of the placenta, however, can change markedly with distention of the urinary bladder and development of focal uterine contractions. These factors can also produce a false-positive impression of a placenta previa by compressing the lower uterine walls together.

The placenta is separated from the myometrium by a subplacental venous complex (i.e., basilar and marginal veins).[14] These veins can become quite prominent, particularly for lateral and posterior placentas, and should not be mistaken for retroplacental or marginal hemorrhage. The myometrium can usually be identified as a thin, hypoechoic layer beneath the basilar veins. Together, the basilar veins and myometrium (i.e., subplacental complex) mea-

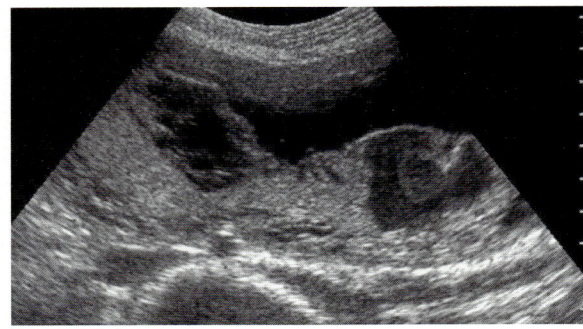

A

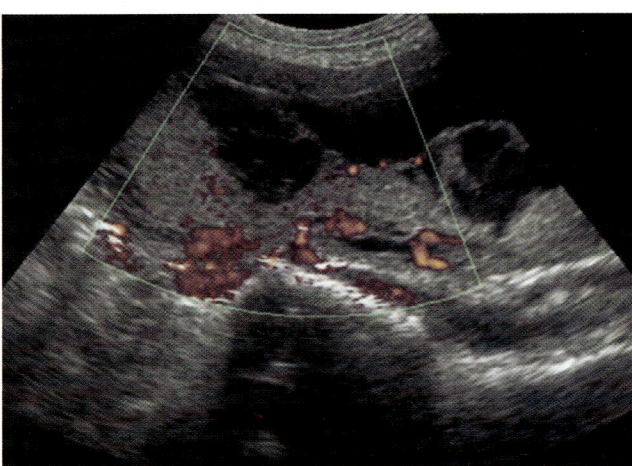

B

FIGURE 7. Sonolucent areas of placenta during the second trimester. **A:** Prominent placental sonolucent areas are disconcerting but are usually an incidental finding without clinical significance. These represent fibrin deposition or venous *lakes*, which may be observed to change dramatically during the course of the ultrasound examination. **B:** Color-flow imaging shows no detectable flow, owing to low sinus flow and fibrin deposition.

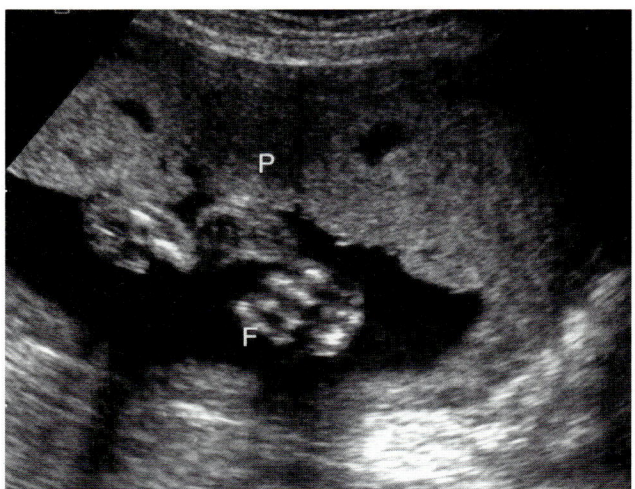

FIGURE 6. Normal placenta, 36 weeks. The third-trimester placenta (*P*) is typically heterogenous with intraplacental sonolucencies. Placental calcification may or may not be evident during the third trimester. F, fetus.

sure 9 to 10 mm in average thickness, which is better appreciated for posterior placentas than anterior placentas.

The placenta increases in thickness and volume with advancing gestation, and, in normal pregnancies, the maximum sonographically measured thickness usually remains less than 4 cm (Fig. 9).[6,15–17] Although a thickened placenta is nonspecific and usually results in a normal outcome,[18] placentomegaly may be associated with a variety of conditions (Table 1). One study of 561 singleton pregnancies showed that a sonographic placental thickness measurement above the ninetieth percentile of the normal range for gestation in the second half of pregnancy was associated with a significantly higher perinatal mortality rate and higher rates of small-for-gestational-age and large-for-gestational-age infants at term,[17] raising the possibility of potential clinical usefulness of such a measurement. Certainly, a very thickened placenta early in pregnancy appears to carry a greater risk of IUGR and placenta insufficiency (Fig. 10). Also, in cases of fetal anemia, placenta thickness may provide a clue to

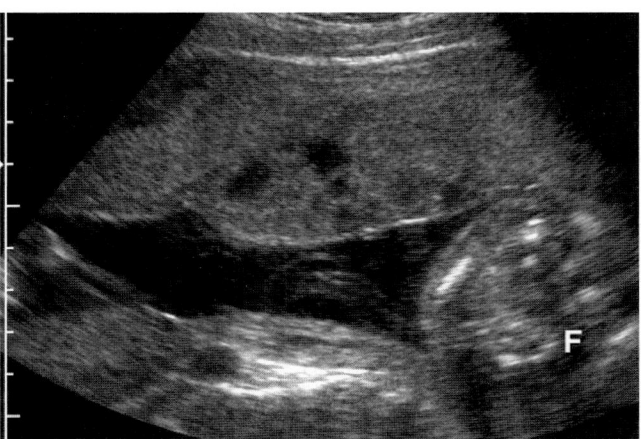

FIGURE 8. Heterogenous placenta. Prominent hypoechoic areas (*F*) that represent subchorionic and intervillous fibrin deposits in a woman who presented with elevated maternal serum alpha-fetoprotein. The outcome was normal.

TABLE 1. DISORDERS ASSOCIATED WITH PLACENTAL THICKENING OR PLACENTOMEGALY

Uterine placental insufficiency
Maternal diabetes
Maternal anemia
Fetal anemia
Hydrops of any cause
Placental hemorrhage
Intrauterine infection
Congenital neoplasms
Beckwith-Wiedemann syndrome
Hydatidiform mole
Chromosomal abnormalities
Confined placenta mosaicism

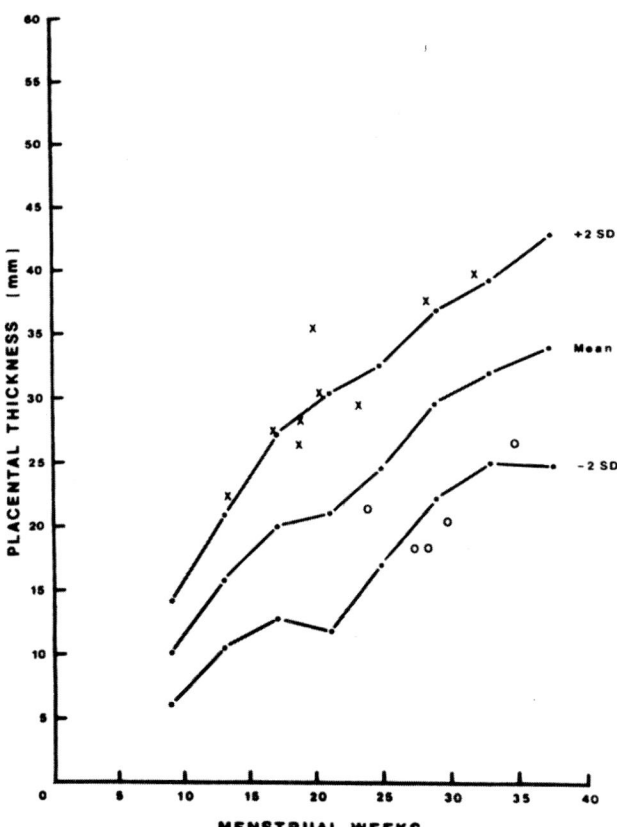

FIGURE 9. Graph showing that placental thickness progressively increases with menstrual age but rarely exceeds 4 to 5 cm at any age. Note that placentas with smaller surface area of attachment of the uterus (x) tend to be thicker than placentas with a larger area of attachment (o). (Reproduced with permission from Hoddick WK, Mahony BS, Callen PW, et al. Placental thickness. *J Ultrasound Med* 1985;4:479–482.)

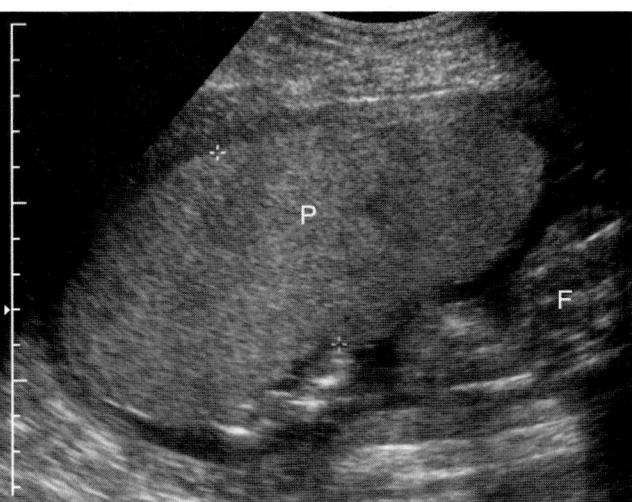

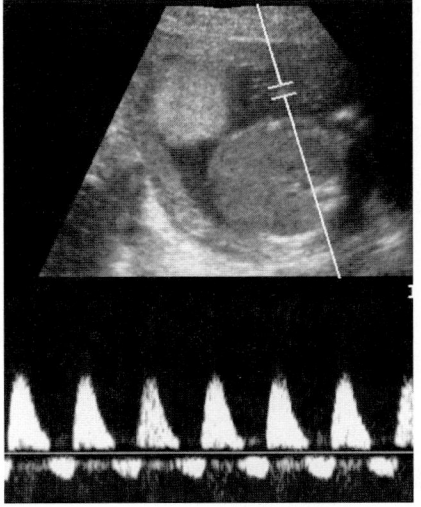

FIGURE 10. Placentomegaly, 25 weeks. **A:** The placenta (*P*) is abnormally thickened, measuring 6.3 cm in thickness. F, fetus. **B:** Umbilical artery Doppler shows reversal of diastolic flow. Hyperechoic fetal bowel was also present. The fetus died 1 week later.

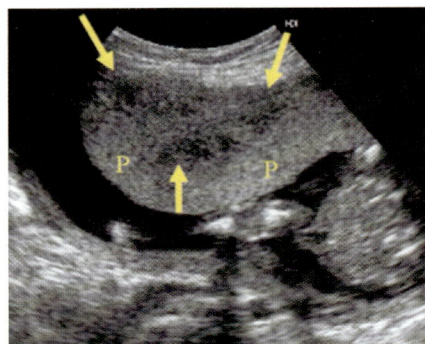
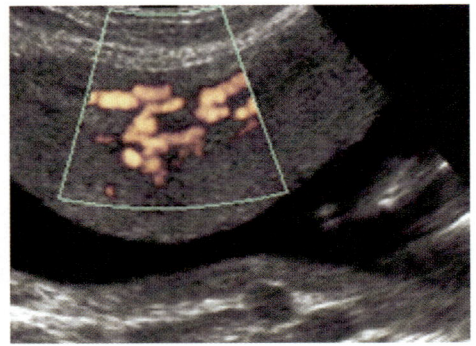

FIGURE 11. Focal uterine contraction. **A:** Uterine contraction (*arrows*) behind the placenta (*P*) at 18 weeks. **B:** Power Doppler shows hypervascular nature of uterine contraction. A hemorrhage would appear avascular and a fibroid would be hypovascular or isovascular compared to adjacent endometrium.

affected pregnancies. In the case of alpha thalassemia, placental thickness greater than 3 cm, or above the ninety-fifth percentile of the normal range, in late mid-trimester, is present in approximately 90% of affected cases, and thickness above the ninety-fifth percentile is present in approximately 75% of cases in the first trimester.[19–21]

Focal uterine contractions are common, especially during the second trimester (Fig. 11). These contractions are usually asymptomatic although the patient may experience some discomfort. The contractions can be confused for retroplacental hemorrhage or produce a false-positive appearance of placenta previa.

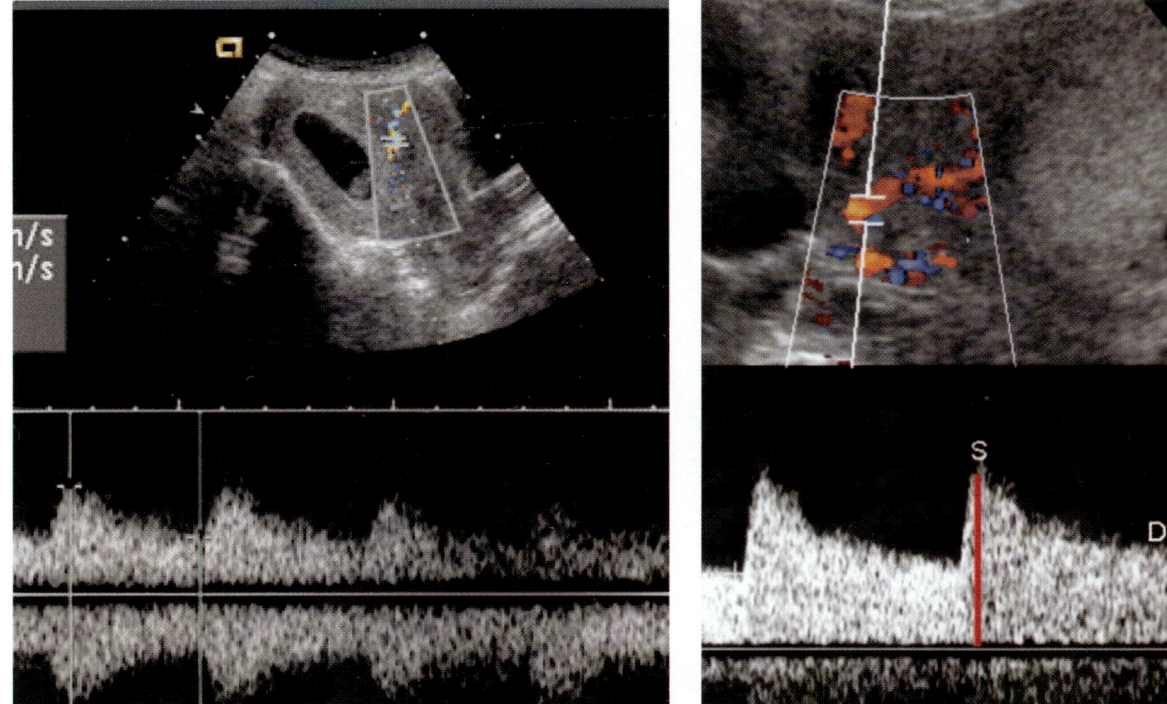

FIGURE 12. Normal flow pattern of the uterine and spiral arteries. **A:** At 9 weeks, Doppler of the spiral artery reveals a low resistive index (0.47) containing a high diastolic component (20 cm per second). **B:** At 22 weeks, Doppler of the right main uterine artery shows typical low resistance pattern with prominent end-diastole (*D*) and no post-systole (*S*) notch.

UTEROPLACENTAL DOPPLER BLOOD FLOW EXAMINATION

The study of uteroplacental Doppler flow velocity waveforms to predict adverse pregnancy outcome has become an increasingly important aspect of antenatal care, and extensive literature is available in this area. This section aims to simply summarize the important aspects of uteroplacental Doppler blood flow examination, with interested readers encouraged to consult the detailed review articles available. Also, see further discussion of Doppler techniques in Chapter 2.

Normal trophoblastic invasion of the spiral arteries produces a low resistance Doppler pattern (Fig. 12). Doppler signals of the uterine arteries are variable, depending on gestational age and location of the placenta. In early pregnancy, the flow velocity waveform from the uterine artery shows a notched appearance in diastole, but, with increasing gestation and normal trophoblastic invasion, the notch usually disappears. The lowest resistance pattern is seen on the side of the placenta. Before 20 weeks, uterine artery Doppler typically shows a high flow, low-resistance pattern, particularly for the uterine artery on the same side as the placenta. Patients who show a postsystolic notch may normalize by 22 to 24 weeks. Quantitative measures of impedance to flow, such as the resistance index and pulsatility index, fall with gestational age.

Abnormal trophoblastic invasion of the spiral arteries of the maternal uteroplacental circulation is associated with a range of pregnancy complications, including IUGR, preeclampsia, and placental abruption. Studies in high-risk populations of patients at increased risk for preeclampsia reported sensitivities for preeclampsia of around 40% to 60%, using a high resistance index as the criteria for detection at 18 to 24 weeks. Subsequently, studies in unselected populations were carried out, and sensitivities of approximately 60% for preeclampsia and specificities of more than 90% were reported.[22] The criteria used were either resistance index above the ninety-fifth percentile or uterine artery waveform notching. Detection rates for IUGR are lower, at around 40%. Although the false-positive rate is high before 20 weeks, the rate falls to only around 5% by 24 weeks with similar detection rates, hence improved positive predictive values if examination is carried out at this time rather than 20 weeks. The findings of abnormal uterine artery Doppler flow velocity waveforms allow appropriate pregnancy surveillance to be commenced in addition to allowing identification of high-risk groups for recruitment into intervention studies for these conditions.

PLACENTAL ABNORMALITIES

Circumvallate/Circummarginate Placenta

Extrachorial placenta (e.g., circummarginate placenta and circumvallate placenta) is defined as attachment of the placental membranes to the fetal surface of the placenta rather than to the underlying villous placental margin.[23]

Incidence

Circummarginate placenta can be found to some degree in up to 20% of placentas, but these are not usually of clinical significance.[3] By contrast, circumvallate placenta occurs in 1% to 2% of pregnancies, but these are usually partial, with no clinical significance.

Pathology

Circumvallate and circummarginate placentation is a result of discrepancies between the sizes of the chorionic and basal plates of the developing placenta. Circumvallate placenta is diagnosed when the placental margin also is folded, thickened, or elevated with underlying fibrin and often hemorrhage; circummarginate placenta is diagnosed when the placental margin is not deformed.[3]

Diagnosis

Prenatal ultrasound diagnosis has been reported, mainly of circumvallate rather than circummarginate cases, with main findings being an infolding of fetal membranes with an associated echogenic rim of tissue at the placental periphery, with or without a larger ridge or shelf (Fig. 13).[24–26] Although the diagnosis has been described, the diagnostic accuracy of these criteria may be low. Harris et al.[27] reported that up to 35% of normal placentas may appear focally circumvallate whereas less than 10% of true circumvallate placentas were identified by ultrasound.

Differential Diagnosis

When a placental shelf is identified, other considerations include intrauterine synechiae and subchorionic hemorrhage.

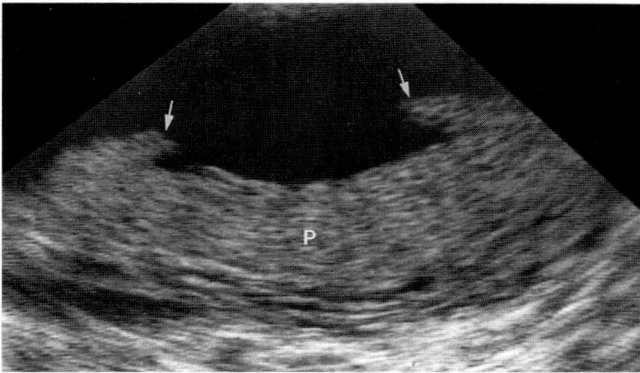

FIGURE 13. Circumvallate placenta. Scan shows infolding margins (*arrows*) of placenta (*P*) consistent with circummarginate placenta.

Prognosis and Management

Circumvallate placenta may be associated with increased risk for antepartum bleeding, preterm delivery, and IUGR.[3,24,28,29] Obstetric management should not be altered.

Succenturiate Placenta

Succenturiate placenta is defined as the presence of one or more accessory lobes separated from the body of the placenta.

Incidence

Succenturiate placenta is relatively common, reported in 3% to 6% of pregnancies.[3]

Pathology

Succenturiate placenta occurs from selective loss of parts of the placenta and growth of other parts. This phenomenon of trophoblastic *trophotropism*[31] also helps to explain other placental conditions such as velamentous insertion of the umbilical cord and placental *migration*. This phenomenon presumably occurs because the placenta preferentially grows where there is good decidua and vascular supply, and atrophies where these are insufficient.

Diagnosis

The sonographic antenatal diagnosis of placenta succenturiate has been well reported, with or without the use of Doppler examination to visualize the fetal vessels.[30–33] Succenturiate lobe (Fig. 14) is distinguished from a *bilobate* placenta, which shows communication of placental tissue between the lobes and central cord insertion.

When succenturiate lobe is identified, both the cord insertion of the umbilical cord and communicating vessels should be identified. The umbilical cord insertion marks the original implantation site of the placenta. The umbilical cord occasionally inserts between the two lobes in a vela-

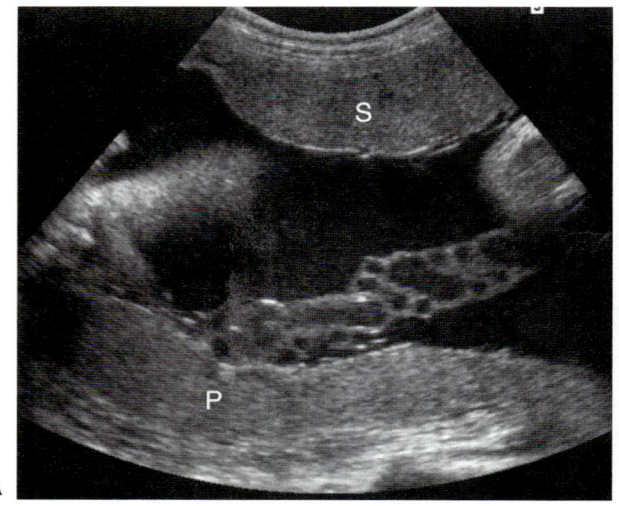

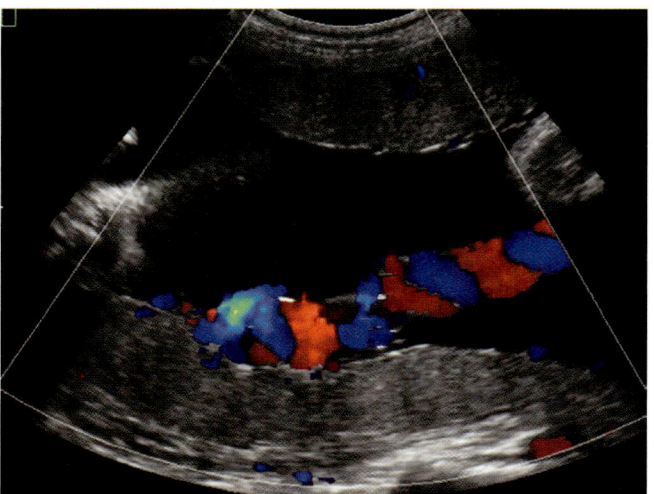

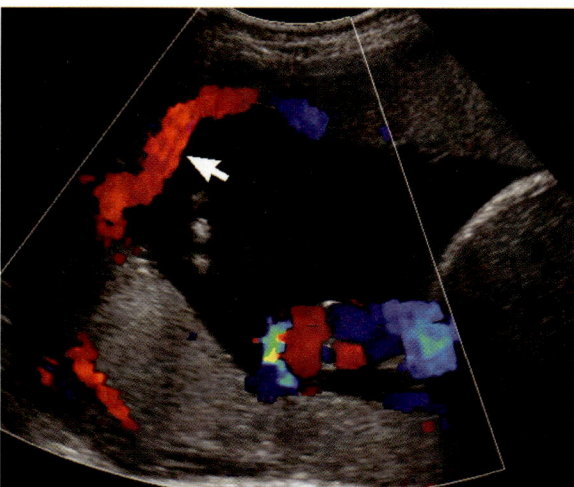

FIGURE 14. Succenturiate placentation. **A:** Sonogram demonstrates a succenturiate lobe (*S*) separate from the anterior placenta (*P*). **B:** The umbilical cord inserts normally into the anterior lobe. **C:** Anastomotic vessels (*arrows*) shown with color-flow imaging supply the succenturiate lobe.

mentous or marginal location. Identification of the communicating vessels is also important to ensure that they do not cover the cervix to form a vasa previa.

Differential Diagnosis

An accessory lobe may be simulated by a subchorionic hemorrhage or, less likely, from a myometrial contraction or uterine myoma.

Prognosis and Management

Retention of a succenturiate lobe at delivery may result in postpartum hemorrhage and infection. Rarely, rupture of the connecting vessels may occur during delivery, resulting in fetal hemorrhage and demise. This rupture is most likely when the vessels cover the cervix to form a vasa previa.

Placenta Previa

Placenta previa is defined as implantation of the placenta in the lower uterine segment in advance of the fetus. This implantation varies with amount of placenta covering the cervix (Fig. 15) and may be categorized as follows.

Complete Previa

In complete previa, the placenta covers the internal cervical os completely. A subcategory is central or symmetric complete previa when the placenta is concentrically located over the os. Asymmetric complete previa is when the placenta is eccentrically positioned over the os.

Marginal or Partial Previa

Marginal previa extends over the cervix but not to the level of the internal os, whereas partial previa extends partially over the internal os. These conditions are considered together because it is often difficult to distinguish a partial from a marginal previa, and the clinical distinction is not important.

Marginal or partial previa is defined as a low-lying placenta that extends to within 2 to 3 cm of the internal cervical os.

Incidence

The incidence of placenta previa varies greatly with gestational age at diagnosis and the criteria used. The incidence at term of clinically significant placenta previa is approximately 0.5%. Placenta previa is diagnosed in approximately 5% of second-trimester pregnancies before genetic amniocentesis (15 to 16 weeks).[34,35] At least 90% of placenta previa, therefore, resolve to a normal position by term.[36–40] Possible reasons for this improvement are discussed in the following Pathology section.

Pathology

Placenta previa results from implantation of the blastocyst in the lower uterine segment. A number of factors appear to increase the risk of this occurrence, including advancing age, multiparity, smoking, cocaine use, prior placenta previa, previous cesarean births, and prior suction curettage related to pregnancy.[39] The strong association between placenta previa and parity, previous cesarean delivery, and suction curettage suggests that endometrial damage is an etiologic factor. Subsequent pregnancies are more likely to implant in the lower uterine segment by a process of elimination. Multiple pregnancies are at higher risk because of the reduced surface area of the endometrium available.

Improvement in placenta previa with gestational age primarily reflects marked growth of the lower uterine segment during pregnancy, which pulls the placenta superiorly. At 20 weeks, the placenta covers approximately one-fourth of the myometrium surface area, but near term the placenta

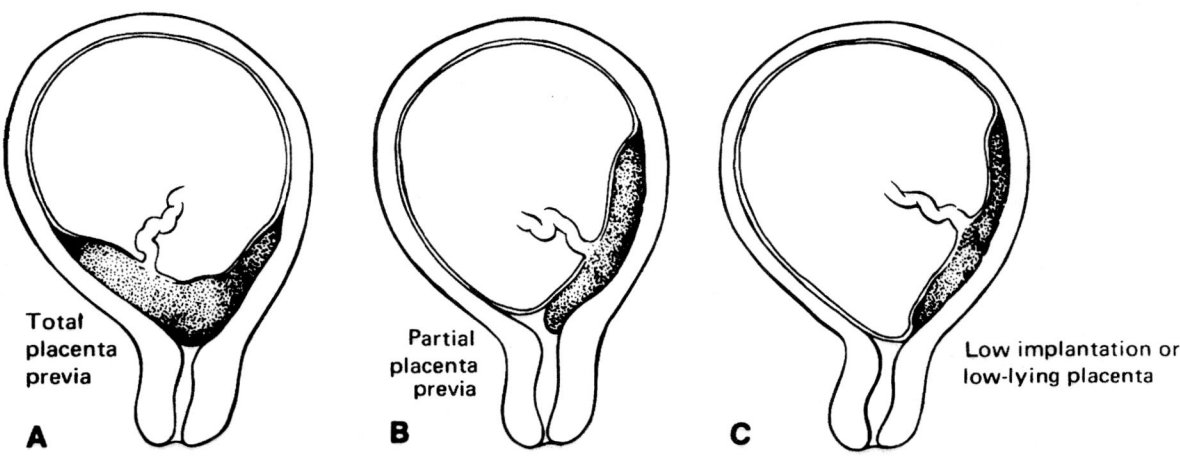

FIGURE 15. Classification of placental location. **A:** Complete placenta previa. **B:** Partial or marginal previa. **C:** Low-lying placenta. (Reproduced with permission from Goplerud CP. Bleeding in later pregnancy. In: Danforth DN, ed. *Obstetrics and gynecology,* 5th ed. New York: Harper & Row, 1986.)

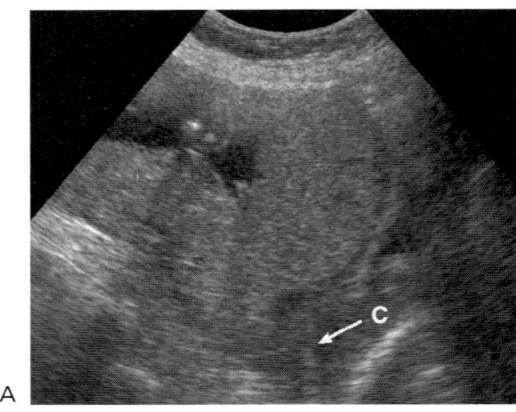
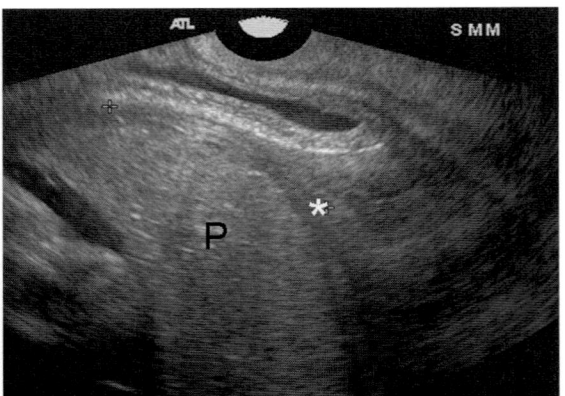

FIGURE 16. Complete placenta previa. **A:** Transabdominal scan with empty urinary bladder shows complete previa with placenta overlying the cervix (*C*). **B:** Transvaginal of another patient shows placenta (*P*) overlying internal os (*asterisk*).

covers one-eighth the myometrial surface.[40] Improvement may also be partly secondary to *trophotropism*, in which the placenta atrophies at suboptimal sites of implantation and hypertrophies at more optimal sites.

Diagnosis

One of the first, and most important, indications for ultrasonography of the placenta was accurate placental localization, with particular regard to the differential diagnosis of antepartum hemorrhage.[41] Accurate localization of the placenta remains one of the most important contributions to prenatal sonography.

In general, prenatal ultrasound is highly sensitive but not specific in diagnosis of placenta previa. Therefore, while false-negative diagnoses are rare, false-positive diagnoses are common depending on the gestational age, the sonographic technique used, the type of previa (complete vs. partial), and the indications for sonography.[42–45] This is especially true before the third trimester because of differential growth of the lower segment of the uterus in the second half of pregnancy.[46–50]

Placenta previa is readily diagnosed by the location of the placenta over the cervix (Figs. 16 through 19). Placental localization by transvaginal or translabial examination complements transabdominal scans and provides good visualization of the internal os and its relationship to the location of the

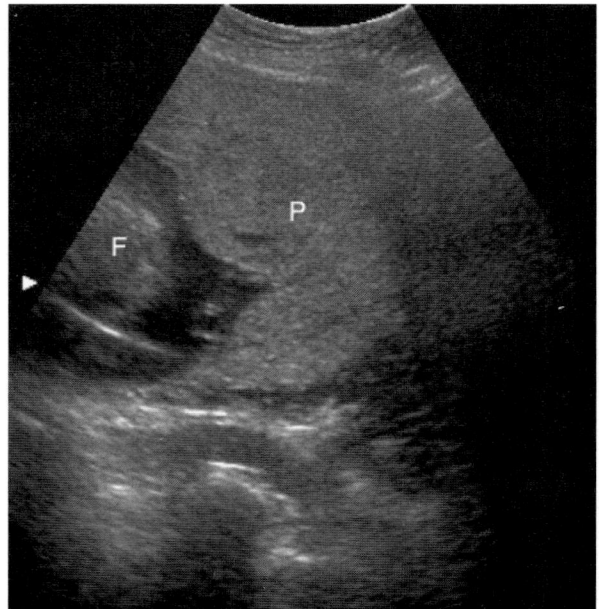
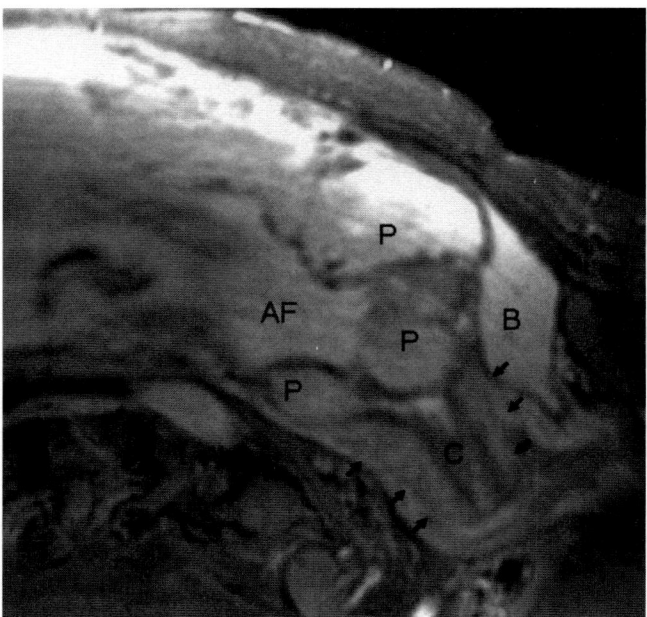

FIGURE 17. Complete placenta previa. **A:** Longitudinal scan shows the placenta (*P*) fills the lower uterine segment. F, fetus. **B:** Magnetic resonance image of same case shows placenta (*P*) overlying the cervix (*C, arrows*). Placenta accreta was also present in this case. Note thin myometrium between placenta and urinary bladder (*B*). AF, amniotic fluid.

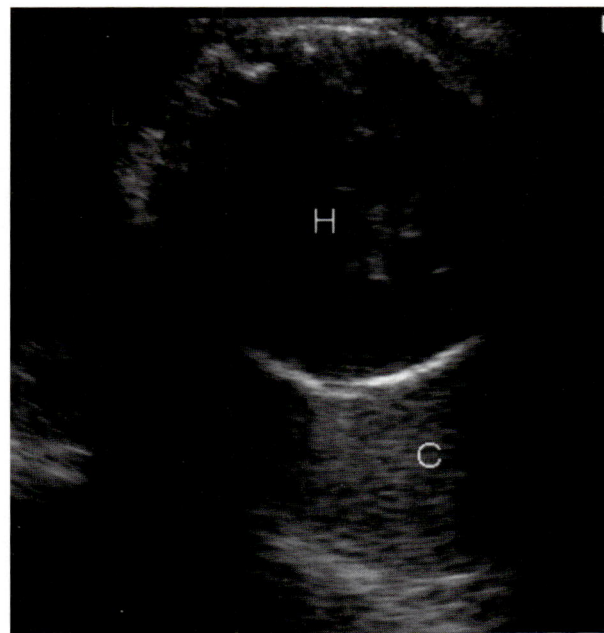

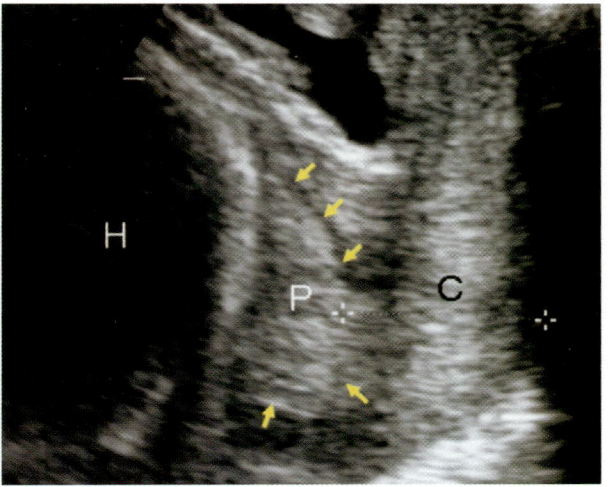

FIGURE 18. Placenta previa on translabial scan. **A:** Transabdominal scan at 32 weeks shows the fetal head (*H*) obscures the cervix (*C*). **B:** Translabial scan shows placenta (*P, arrows*) overlying the cervix (*C*) to form a complete previa. H, fetal head.

placenta.[51–53] This may help to decrease the number of false-positive diagnoses of placenta previa during early pregnancy.[54]

Ghourab[55] found that a low-lying placenta with a thick lower edge of the placenta was much less likely to resolve compared to placentas with a thin lower edge and were more likely to result in antepartum hemorrhage and surgery. He suggests that evaluation of the thickness of the lower placenta margin should also be considered when evaluating potential placenta previa.

Differential Diagnosis

False-positive diagnoses of placenta previa are common, particularly before 20 weeks. This is because differential growth of the lower uterine segment tends to pull the placenta upward, away from the cervix, with increasing gestational age. This phenomenon of *placental migration* is most pronounced during the second and early third trimesters and is unlikely after 34 weeks. Other factors contributing to false-positive diagnoses of placenta previa include an overly distended urinary bladder, focal uterine contractions involving the lower uterine segment (Fig. 20), fibroids, and placental hemorrhage.

Prognosis and Management

Patients with a low-lying placenta identified at midtrimester should be observed with further ultrasound examina-

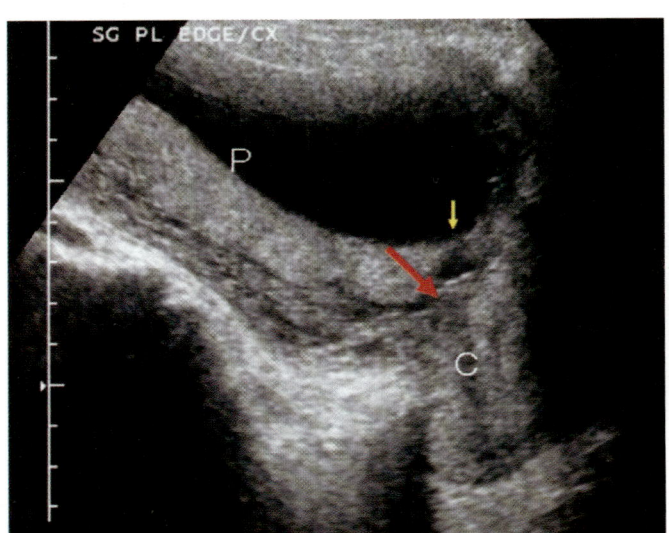

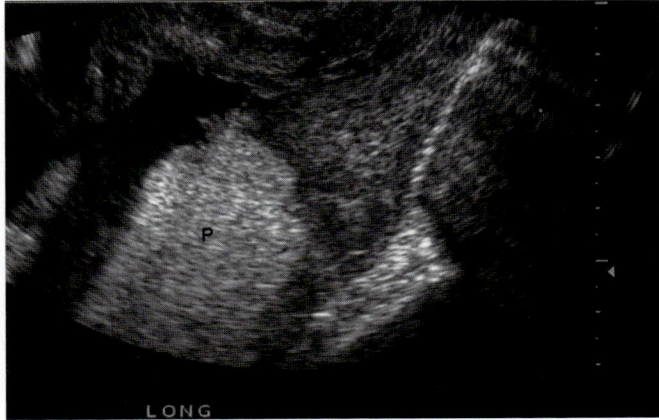

FIGURE 19. Partial placenta previa at 19 weeks. **A:** Transabdominal scan shows the lower margin (*yellow arrow*) of the placenta (*P*) partly covers the cervix (*C*) and internal cervical os (*red arrow*). **B:** Transvaginal scan shows the placenta (*P*) extending to cervical os (*arrow*).

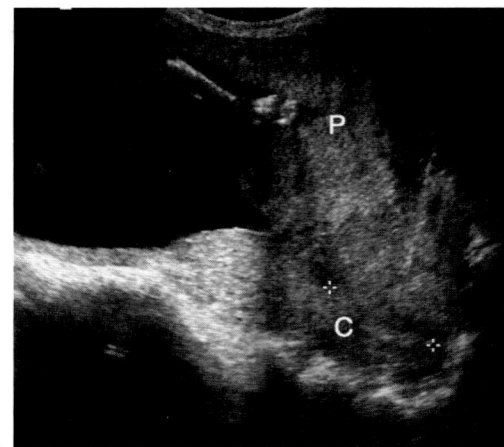
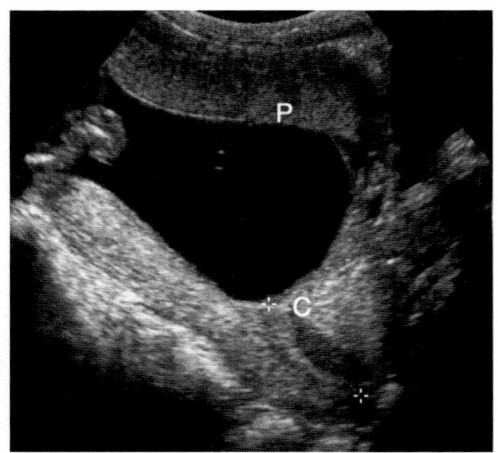

FIGURE 20. Focal uterine contraction simulating placenta previa. **A:** Longitudinal scan suggests that the placenta (*P*) overlies the cervix (*C*) to form a previa. However, note the thickened myometrium suggesting the presence of a focal uterine contraction. Calibers indicate approximate extent of true cervix. **B:** Repeat scan 20 minutes later shows normal relation of placenta (*P*) with cervix (*C*) and resolution of focal contraction.

tions until at least 34 weeks or unequivocal conversion has occurred.

Perinatal mortality from placenta previa is less than 5% currently, although it was as high as 40% in the 1950s.[36] Other potential complications of placenta previa include premature delivery and IUGR.[23,43] These complications occur more frequently from complete previa than marginal previa and are thought to be secondary to premature detachment of the placenta from the lower uterine segment.

Women with elevated maternal serum AFP (MSAFP) appear to be at greater risk among women with placenta previa. Butler et al.[58] reported elevated MSAFP in 14% of women with placenta previa. These women were significantly more likely to have antepartum bleeding before 30 weeks' gestation (50% vs. 15%) and preterm delivery before 30 weeks' gestation (29% vs. 5%).

Ghourab suggests that placentas that are low lying with a thick lower edge have a significantly higher rate of antepartum hemorrhage, cesarean delivery, abnormally adherent placenta, and low birth weight than those in whom the placental edge is thin.[55]

Vasa Previa

Vasa previa is a potentially life-threatening fetal complication of placentation in which relatively large fetal vessels run in the fetal membranes across the cervical os, thus placing them at risk of rupture and catastrophic hemorrhage.

Incidence

Vasa previa occurs in approximately 1 in 2,500 deliveries.[59]

Pathology

Vasa previa may occur in one of two situations: (a) when there is velamentous insertion of the umbilical cord into placental membranes, which then course over the cervix or (b) when succenturiate lobe is present and the connecting vessels course over the cervix. The unsupported fetal vessels are prone to rupture as the cervix dilates, which can quickly result in exsanguination of the fetus. Even when not torn, the fetal parts can compress these vessels during delivery, resulting in fetal hypoxia.

Diagnosis

Before the advent of ultrasound, a timely diagnosis was notoriously difficult. The diagnosis is occasionally made based by palpation of fetal vessels within intact membranes at the time of vaginal examination and can also be made by amnioscopy.[60]

Vasa previa is diagnosed by ultrasound when implanted fetal umbilical vessels are seen overlying the cervix (Figs. 21 through 23).[61,62] Introduction of color Doppler imaging, often combined with transvaginal sonography, has led to many reports describing the prenatal sonographic diagnosis.[63–79] Lee et al.[74] contributed 15 cases and Catanzarite et al.[81] contributed 10 confirmed cases of vasa previa. Three-dimensional ultrasound may further help to illustrate the complex anatomy.[82]

Demonstration of a normal umbilical cord insertion into the placenta excludes the typical situation of vasa previa associated with velamentous insertion of the umbilical cord. However, it does not exclude the possibility of communicating vessels crossing the cervix in cases of succenturiate lobe. For this reason, the course of communicating vessels should be sought in cases of succenturiate placenta.

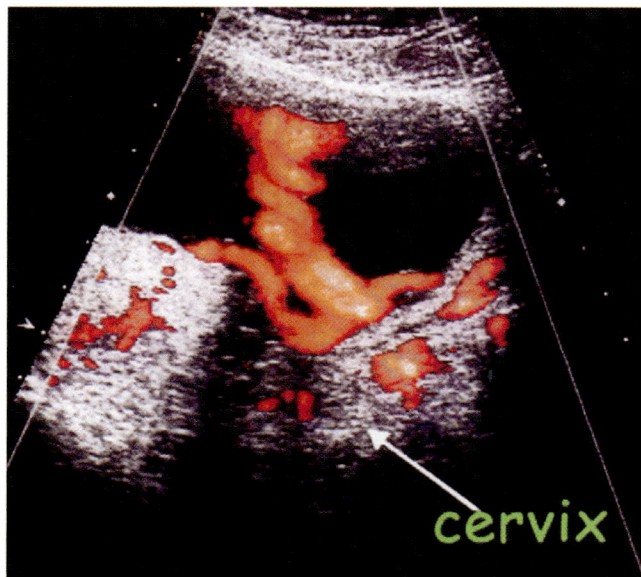

FIGURE 21. Vasa previa. Color-flow image shows velamentous insertion of the umbilical cord over the cervix. (Reproduced with permission from Catanzarite V, Maida C, Thomas W, et al. Prenatal sonographic diagnosis of vasa previa: ultrasound findings and obstetric outcome in ten cases. *Ultrasound Obstet Gynecol* 2001;18:109–115.)

In reviewing previous reports, Catanzarite et al.[81] suggest that placenta previa itself may be a risk factor for vasa previa. They also describe a case of apparent placenta previa that evolved into a bilobate placenta with communicating vessels overlying the cervix. They suggest this could be explained by either initial misinterpretation of a bilobate

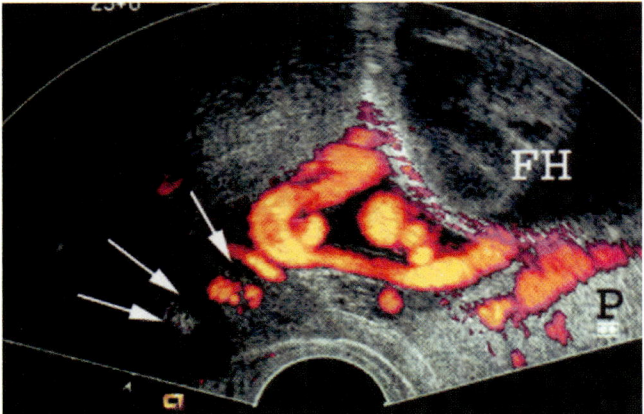

FIGURE 22. Vasa previa. Color-flow image with transvaginal scan at 23 weeks shows umbilical vessels overlying the cervix (*arrows*). Orientation is such that cervix is on the left of the screen. FH, fetal head; P, placenta. (Reproduced with permission from Becker RH, Vonk R, Mende BC, et al. The relevance of placental location at 20–23 gestational weeks for prediction of placenta previa at delivery: evaluation of 8,650 cases. *Ultrasound Obstet Gynecol* 2001;17:496–501.)

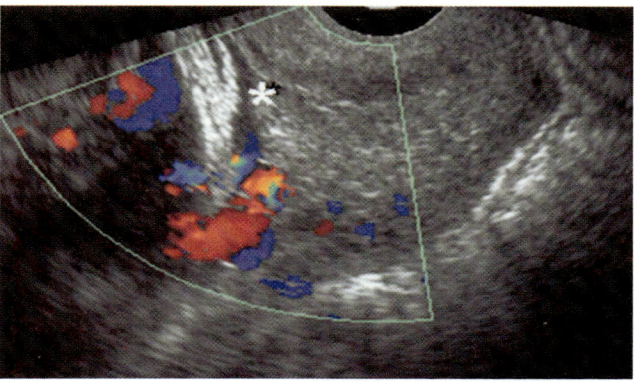

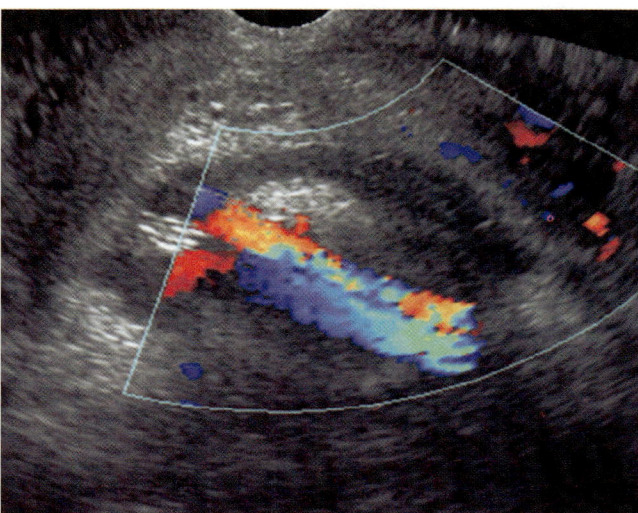

FIGURE 23. Vasa previa at 37 weeks. **A:** Sagittal transvaginal scan shows umbilical vessels near the internal os (*asterisk*). **B:** Transverse view of the same patient demonstrates the umbilical vessels crossing over the cervix. Vasa previa was proven at delivery and by pathology.

placenta for placenta previa or development of focal placental atrophy overlying the cervix (i.e., trophotropism) so that velamentous vessels remained over the cervix.

Differential Diagnosis

Marginal veins of a low-lying placenta or placental previa should not be mistaken for true vasa previa. Only vessels carrying fetal blood should be considered in evaluation of vasa previa.

Prognosis and Management

The outcome is fatal in at least 22% of cases when vasa previa is not diagnosed before delivery.[83] If recognized, a normal outcome can be expected, following cesarean delivery planned before the onset of labor.[83] Serial ultrasound exams are recommended, not only for assessment of vasa previa

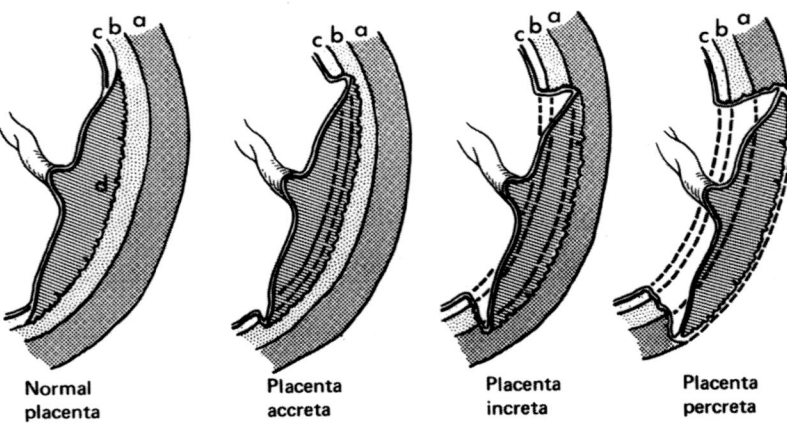

Normal placenta   Placenta accreta   Placenta increta   Placenta percreta

FIGURE 24. Classification of placenta accreta, increta, and percreta. a, myometrium; b, decidua basalis; c, decidua spongiosa; d, placenta. (Reproduced with permission from Newton M. Other complications of labor. In: Danforth DN, ed. *Obstetrics and gynecology*, 5th ed. New York: Harper & Row, 1986.)

but also for monitoring of cervical effacement. For complete vasa previa with vessels overlying the cervix, the accepted management is amniocentesis to confirm lung maturity followed by elective cesarean delivery before the onset of labor. Some obstetricians in the United States also advise hospitalization after the age of fetal viability. For patients with succenturiate lobe and small fetal vessels coursing near the cervix, Catanzarite et al.[81] suggest that vaginal delivery might be considered, with preparations for immediate intervention, if necessary.

Placenta Accreta/Increta/Percreta

Placenta accreta/increta/percreta describe an abnormally adherent placenta in which the chorionic villi grow directly into the myometrium without intervening decidua. Extension through the myometrium is termed *placenta increta*, and penetration of the uterine serosa is termed *placenta percreta* (Fig. 24). This is a theoretical classification, however, because all three conditions may be present in a single pregnancy; the term *placenta increta* is used here to refer to all three conditions.

Incidence

Placenta accreta/increta/percreta may be as high as 1 in 1,000[84] for mild cases. The most common predisposing factors are placenta previa and uterine scar from previous cesarean section. The risk of increta is 10% to 25% in women with one previous cesarean delivery when the placenta is implanted over the scar and exceeds 50% in women with placenta previa and multiple cesarean deliveries.

Pathology

Placenta increta results from underdeveloped decidualization of the endometrium. The underlying pathogenesis is undetermined although decidual inadequacy is supported

by the increased prevalence in pregnancies from women who have undergone previous lower-segment cesarean section. The association with placenta previa reflects the thin, poorly formed decidua of the lower uterine segment that offers little resistance to deeper invasion by the trophoblast. The scar of previous cesarean deliveries also permits trophoblastic invasion.

Diagnosis

Accurate prenatal detection of placenta increta/percreta is particularly important because of the high maternal mortality and morbidity associated with deeper invasion. The sensitivity of ultrasound for diagnosing this placental invasion may be 50% or less.[85] Ultrasound, however, is expected to be more sensitive for more severe cases of placental invasion.

The sonographic diagnosis of placenta increta has been well described. The primary initial finding is placenta previa, typically in an anterior location, in a woman with a previous history of cesarean deliveries (Figs. 25 and 26). The placenta is often thickened and heterogeneous (Fig. 25A). Focal outpouching of the placenta may be seen. The normal hypoechoic interface of the placenta and myometrium is obscured.[86–91] Uterine vessels beneath the abnormal placental insertion site often appear prominent with color-flow imaging (Fig. 26B) and duplex Doppler may show high velocity signals.[92,93]

After delivery, normal placental separation can be identified by cessation of blood flow between the basal placenta and myometrium whereas persistence of flow in this area, demonstrated by color Doppler examination, may suggest placenta accreta.[94]

Magnetic resonance imaging (MRI) may be helpful in the diagnosis of placenta invasion in some cases.[95–97] Although MRI may be more sensitive than ultrasound for showing invasion, it can also result in false-positive diagnoses. Therefore, it's role compared to ultrasound remains uncertain.

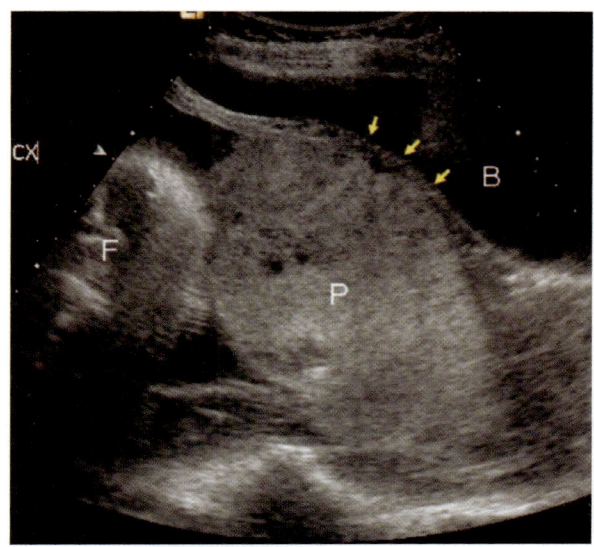
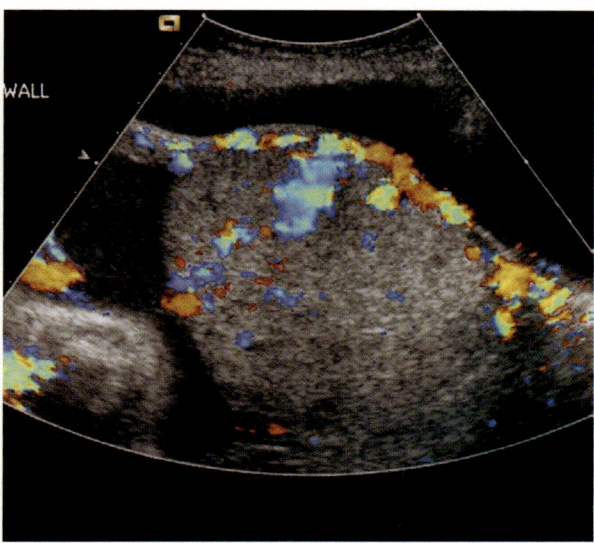

FIGURE 25. Placenta increta. **A:** Longitudinal sonogram in a woman with two previous cesarean deliveries demonstrates a thickened heterogeneous placenta forming a complete previa. Also note the loss of the normal hypoechoic boundary (*arrows*) between the placenta (*P*) and urinary bladder (*B*). F, fetus. **B:** Color Doppler scan shows prominent vascularity to the placenta and placental margin, which is highly suggestive of placental invasion. This patient required emergency hysterectomy after cesarean delivery for continued vaginal bleeding.

Differential Diagnosis

When the myometrial interface is not visualized, other considerations include a thin but normal myometrium, focal uterine contraction, and placental hemorrhage.

Prognosis

Prognosis varies with the depth and surface area of placental invasion. Placenta increta/percreta is a life-threatening condition and must be managed appropriately. Even when placenta increta/percreta is known to be present, the mother may still exsanguinate from uncontrolled hemorrhage.

Placenta percreta may present with spontaneous uterine rupture or hemoperitoneum throughout pregnancy.[98,99] Some patients may present with acute pain and signs of hemoperitoneum well before eventual delivery from tears through the myometrium that spontaneously seal.

Management

The management varies dramatically with the severity of the condition. Thorough ultrasound with color and duplex Doppler should be performed. MRI should also be considered.

Mild cases of placenta accreta may be treated with hemostatic sutures and removal of the placenta, or observation alone.[100] Patients may also be treated with methotrexate.[101] For more classic, severe cases the usual treatment is hysterectomy at the time of delivery. If the placenta also invades the urinary bladder, however, this may be insufficient to control the hemorrhage. Adequate blood for transfusion must be available at the time of delivery. The goal is to deliver a live, healthy baby and maintain the health of the mother. If both goals cannot be achieved, the mother's health is a priority.

In view of the rapid resolution of vascular invasion of the bladder, methotrexate may have an important role in the management of placenta percreta with bladder invasion. Arterial embolization of the hypogastric arteries may be a helpful adjunct for controlling the hemorrhage at the time of cesarean hysterectomy.[102–104]

Placental Hemorrhage/Abruption

Hemorrhage may occur at various sites in and around the placenta (Fig. 27). Placental abruption refers to separation of a normally implanted placenta before the birth of the fetus. Placental hemorrhage refers to hemorrhage originating from the placenta from any cause. Categories of placental hemorrhage based on location include retroplacental, subchorionic, subchorial (i.e., preplacental), subamniotic, and intraplacental sites.[105]

Incidence

Clinically apparent abruptions occur in at least 1% of pregnancies.[23] Placental hemorrhage is much more common. Approximately 20% of women experience vaginal bleeding during pregnancy and the placenta is the presumed source in the vast majority of cases.

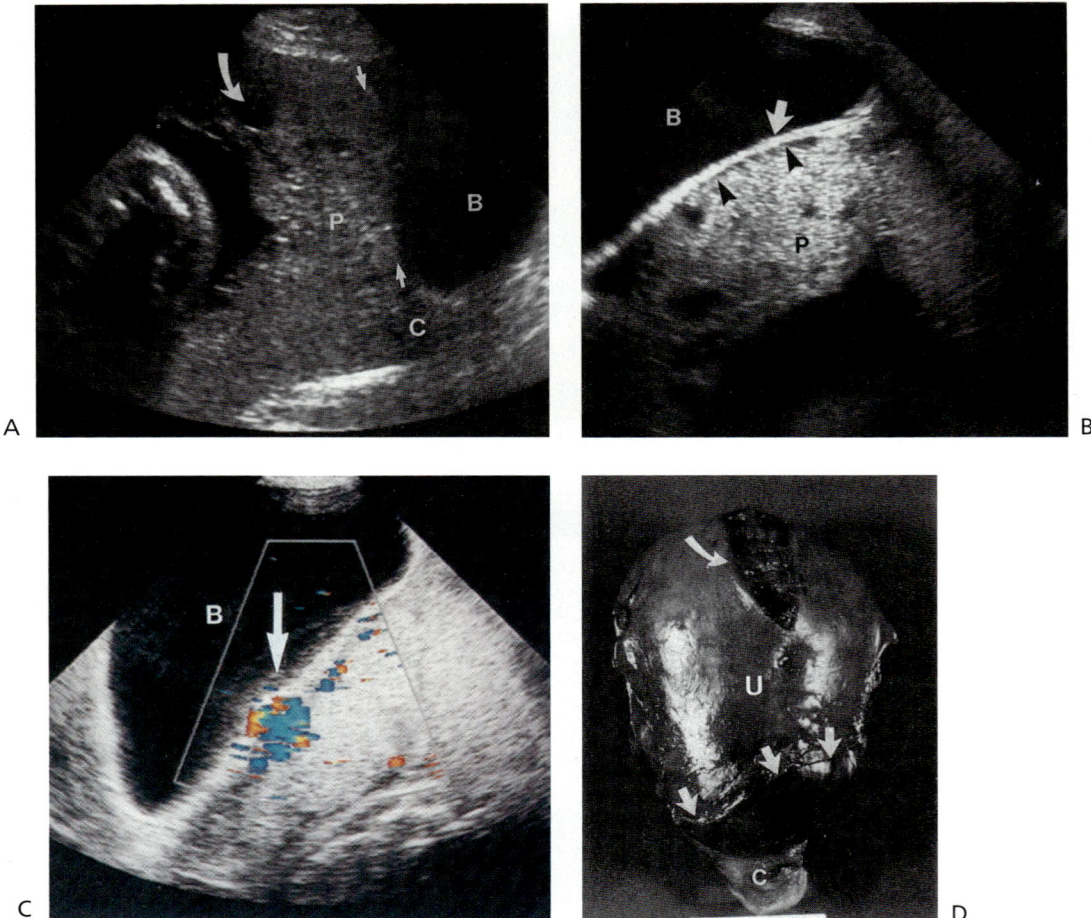

FIGURE 26. Placenta percreta. **A:** Transabdominal ultrasound showing anterior placenta (*P*) forming complete previa with prominent cystic regions (*curved arrow*). Thinning of the normal hypoechoic region of myometrium is suggested (*arrows*). B, bladder; C, cervix. **B:** Endovaginal scan shows loss of normal hypoechoic myometrium (*arrowheads*) between the placenta (*P*) and urinary bladder (*B*). Arrow points to urinary bladder wall. **C:** Color-flow image shows focal prominent vascularity (*arrow*) extending through myometrium into posterior bladder (*B*) wall. **D:** Gross specimen of uterus (*U*) after cesarean section and hysterectomy shows the placenta (*arrows*) bulging through serosa into lower uterine segment. C, cervix. Curved arrow indicates cesarean section scar. (Courtesy of Janelle Rasi, MD.)

Pathology

Placental hemorrhage and abruption appears to reflect underlying pathology of the decidual-placental relationship. A history of previous placental-related complications is one of the strongest risk factors; the risk of recurrent abruption is as much as 30 times the general population.[39] Other risk factors include maternal hypertension, cigarette smoking, cocaine, increased parity, and trauma.

Abruption is initiated by bleeding into the decidua basalis. The expanding hematoma can compress and elevate the overlying placenta. Resultant hypoxia can result in fetal death. Because of the natural placental reserve, however, fetal death does not usually occur from detachments involving less than 30% of the placenta.[3,106] Subchorial hemorrhages can also cause fetal death by compression of the umbilical cord.

Intraplacental hemorrhage (i.e., intervillous thrombosis) is caused by breaks in villous capillaries. This is a frequently encountered pathologic finding, seen in 36% of term placentas.[3] Pathologically, these lesions are composed of coagulated blood originating from the maternal and fetal system. As the lesions age, blood is replaced by fibrin, resulting in a white, laminated lesion. Adjacent villi are compressed and they may be associated with villous infarction.

Diagnosis

The diagnosis of placental abruption during the third trimester is usually apparent clinically with onset of vaginal bleeding and uterine contractions. Because the blood may not accumulate to form a hematoma, a negative ultrasound examination cannot exclude the diagnosis of placental abruption.

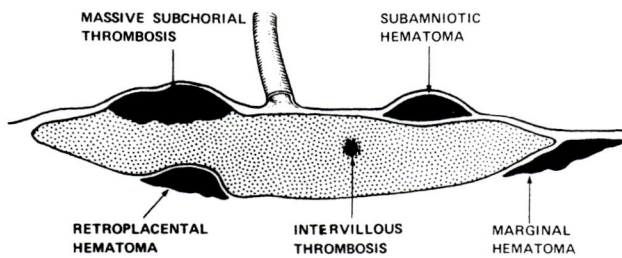

FIGURE 27. Sites of hemorrhage in and around the placenta that have been described pathologically. Retroplacental hematoma and marginal hematoma correspond to retroplacental and marginal abruptions, respectively. (Reproduced with permission from Fox H. *Pathology of the placenta.* Philadelphia: WB Saunders, 1978:107–157.)

The sonographic appearance of placental hemorrhage varies greatly with the location, size, and age of onset of hemorrhage (Figs. 28 and 29). Acute hemorrhage is hyperechoic and may be difficult to distinguish from the placenta. Resolving hemorrhage becomes hypoechoic and then sonolucent.

Subchorionic hemorrhage is by far the most common site of placental hemorrhage seen on sonography.[105,107–109] Of 57 periplacental hemorrhages detected on prenatal sonography, Nyberg et al. reported that subchorionic hemorrhage comprised 91% of cases before 20 weeks and 67% of cases after 20 weeks.[105] While it is thought that nearly all subchorionic hematomas arise from marginal abruptions, in only approximately one-half of the cases is placental detachment actually demonstrated.

Because retroplacental hemorrhage also typically extends into the placenta, sonographic findings of retroplacental

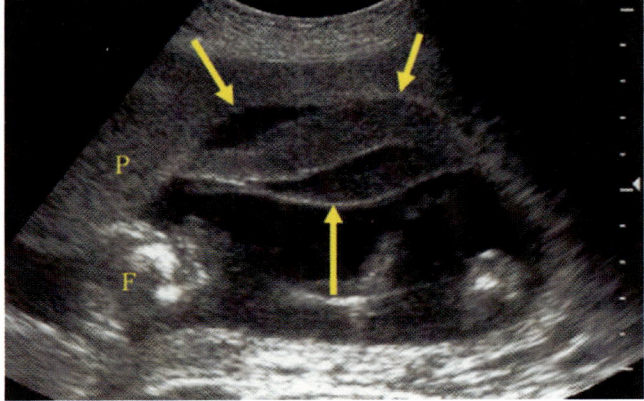

FIGURE 28. Subchorionic hemorrhage. Midtrimester sonogram shows large subchorionic hemorrhage (*arrows*). The blood is of mixed echogenicity, reflecting various ages of recurrent hemorrhage. P, placenta; F, fetus.

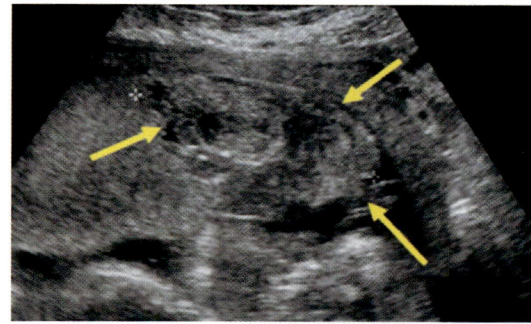

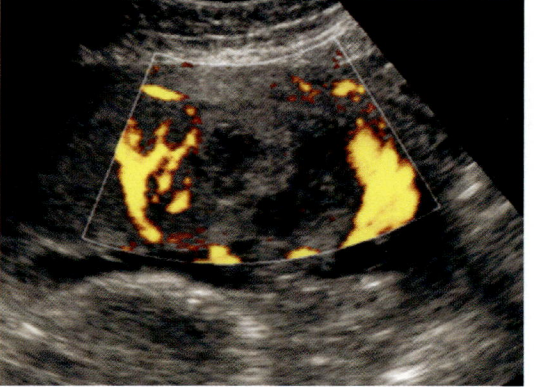

FIGURE 29. Acute subchorionic hemorrhage. **A:** Sonogram at 23 weeks shows hyperechoic hemorrhage (*arrows*), indicating recent onset. This was consistent with onset of bleeding within 48 hours. **B:** Power Doppler shows typical absent vascularity within clot.

placental hemorrhage include thickening of the placenta and occasionally retroplacental clot.[110] Subchorial hemorrhage is rare, appearing as hemorrhage along the amniotic surface of the placenta. Subchorial hemorrhage has been diagnosed by ultrasound and MRI.[111] Intermembranous placental abruption, a rare complication of twin pregnancy, has also been described with the sonographic appearance of a hypoechogenic blood-filled area within the intertwin membrane.[112,113] If intraamniotic hemorrhage has occurred, echogenic blood may be detected in the fetal intestinal tract.[114]

Sonographic-pathologic correlation has shown that intervillous thrombi may be seen as intraplacental sonolucencies.[115,116] The increasing number of intraplacental sonolucencies observed in normal placentas with advancing gestational age also is consistent with the frequency of intervillous thrombi seen pathologically. The association of maternal lakes with other intraplacental sonolucencies suggests that some may represent sites of prior hemorrhage that have resolved and now communicate with the intervillous space.

Hemorrhages observed during the first trimester are common and do not appear to carry the same risk as hemorrhages observed during the third trimester. Although first-trimester hemorrhages may also be associated with an increased risk of placental-related complications later, they are more likely to resolve spontaneously without clinical sequelae.

Differential Diagnosis

Other mass lesions that may simulate placental hemorrhage include a myoma, succenturiate lobe, chorioangioma, placenta previa, or coexisting molar pregnancy.[117–120]

Elevation of the chorioamnionic membranes from hemorrhage should be distinguished from chorioamnionic separation where the membrane (i.e., amnion) can be followed over the fetal surface of the placenta to the umbilical cord insertion and amniotic sheets.

Prognosis and Management

Sonographically detectable subchorionic hemorrhages after the first trimester have been associated with an increased risk of miscarriage, stillbirth, abruptio placentae, and preterm labor.[121]

Management is usually dictated by the clinical condition, not by the hemorrhage itself, although occasionally large hemorrhages can be identified before the onset of clinical symptoms. Acute abruptions during the third trimester may require hospitalization, fetal monitoring, and delivery. On the other hand, mild cases of placental abruption with small hematomas are common and can be managed expectantly.[122–125]

Placental Infarction

Placental infarction is a focal lesion caused by ischemic necrosis.

Incidence

Placental infarcts are found at pathology in up to 25% of normal placentas from clinically uncomplicated pregnancies at term. However, these usually are small and are of no clinical significance.[3] Large infarcts or infarcts that occur during early pregnancy usually reflect underlying maternal vascular disease. In some cases, an underlying myoma can contribute to placental infarction.

Pathology

Placental infarction is a focal lesion caused by ischemic necrosis of villus tissue secondary to focally impaired uteroplacental circulation. Infarcts within the placenta, as in other tissues, evolve through acute, subacute, and chronic stages.

Diagnosis

Placental infarcts have been identified by ultrasonography, but the features are not consistent and depend on the size and degree of maturation.[126,127] The majority of infarcts are hypoechoic in the acute stage and, therefore, difficult to detect with ultrasound. Harris et al.[128] reported that only 14% of placental infarcts were detected sonographically, and those that were identified were hypoechoic or anechoic foci with fibrin deposition or hemorrhage. Calcification may occur over time, aiding sonographic detection.[129]

Differential Diagnosis

Similar placental abnormalities may be seen with fibrin deposition as the placenta matures and placental hemorrhage occurs.

Prognosis and Management

The prognosis of placental infarction depends on the extent of infarction. Small infarcts are common and do not alter outcome, whereas large infarcts may result in fetal demise. Management should be based on the clinical condition.

Maternal Floor Infarction

Maternal floor infarction is a complication of the third trimester in which large amounts of fibrin are deposited in and around the maternal plate with extension into the intervillous space and entrapment of chorionic villi.

Incidence

Maternal floor infarction is rare, however, it may recur in subsequent pregnancies.

Pathology

The macroscopic pathologic features are those of thickened maternal floor with massive fibrin deposition involving the decidua basalis and the contiguous villi. Prominent placental septae with or without cystic parenchymal lesions are present.

The etiology is unknown, but several cases have been reported in association with maternal autoimmune diseases.[3] Matern et al.[130] suggested an association between maternal floor infarction and long-chain 3-hydroxyacyl-CoA dehydrogenase deficiency in one case.

Diagnosis

Sonographic diagnosis of this condition has been reported with fetal growth restriction, oligohydramnios, and increased placental echogenicity in pregnancies at risk.[131] Maternal floor infarction has also been associated with elevated MSAFP levels.[132]

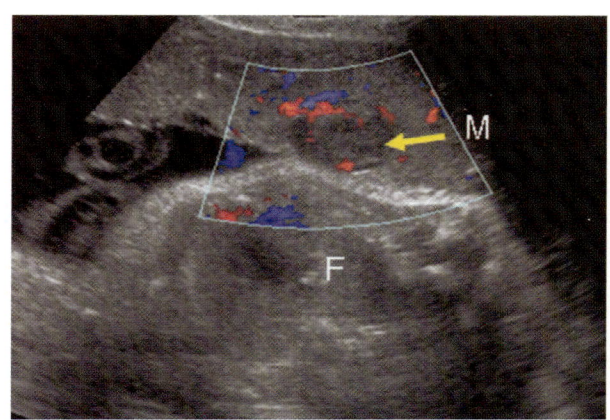
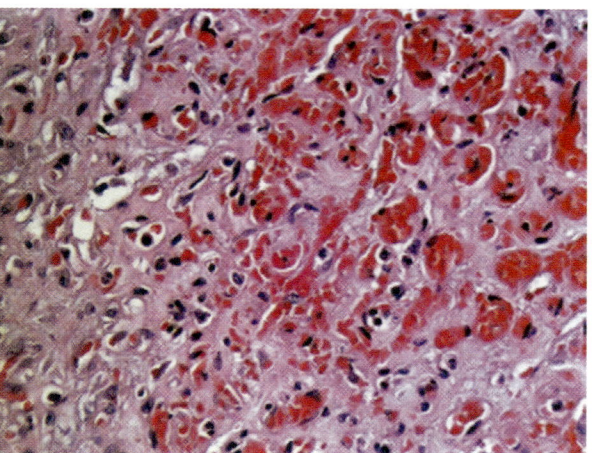

A   B

FIGURE 30. Chorioangioma. **A:** Small (2.4 cm) hypoechoic mass (*M, arrow*) is demonstrated within the placenta. Color-flow imaging shows some vascularity to the margin and some internal vascularity, confirming a solid lesion. F, fetus. **B:** Pathology confirms chorioangioma. Multiple dilated capillaries are seen in a fibrous background.

Differential Diagnosis

Placental dysfunction from other cause may produce a similar appearance.

Prognosis and Management

Maternal floor infarction is associated with complications including intrauterine death or growth restriction. Among 60 cases reported by Andres et al.,[133] fetal deaths occurred in 40%, preterm birth in 58%, and intrauterine growth restriction in 54% of live births.

Chorioangiomas

Chorioangiomas are benign tumors of the placenta.

Incidence

Small chorioangiomas can be identified in 1% of placentas, but these are usually microscopic in size. Tumors that are large enough to produce clinical symptoms and that can be visualized on sonography are uncommon, occurring in 1 in 8,000 to 1 in 50,000 pregnancies.[3]

Pathology

Chorioangiomas are pathologically benign tumors of small blood vessels that may be composed of predominantly vascular or associated solid stromal areas.[134,135] Two main histopathologic types of chorioangiomas exist: angiomatous, which are formed of numerous blood vessels, and cellular, which consist of loose mesenchymal tissue and few ill-formed vessels.

Large chorioangiomas are of variable shape, contain fibrous septa, and most commonly protrude from the fetal surface of the placenta near the cord insertion. Degenerative changes with necrosis, calcification, hyalinization, or myxoid changes are frequently present in large tumors.[3]

Diagnosis

Chorioangiomas are usually noted incidentally as discrete placental lesions. They may also present with increased levels of AFP in the amniotic fluid or maternal serum, especially from vascular tumors.

The prenatal sonographic diagnosis of chorioangiomas has been well described (Figs. 30 through 32).[136–139] The

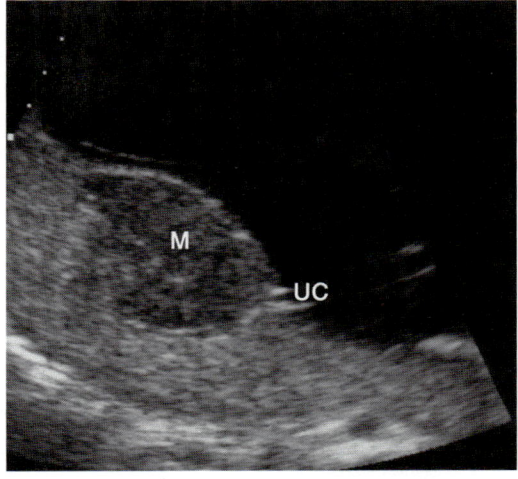

FIGURE 31. Chorioangioma. Hypoechoic mass (*M*) arises from placental surface near the umbilical cord (*UC*) insertion. The outcome was normal.

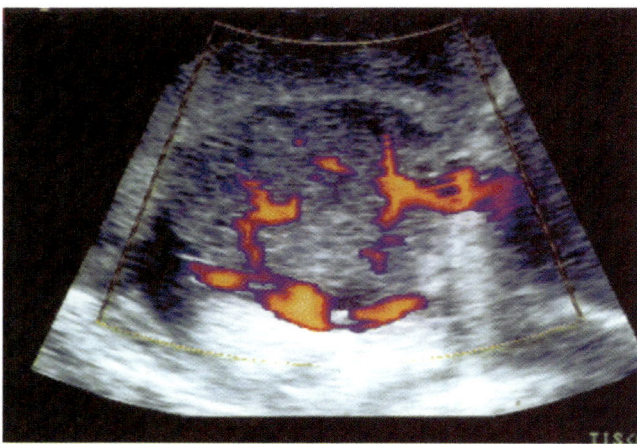

FIGURE 32. Chorioangioma. Color-flow imaging shows prominent vascularity to mass arising from placenta.

tumors appear as circumscribed solid (hyperechoic or hypoechoic) masses or complex masses that often protrude from the fetal surface of the placenta. Most reported tumors have been located near the umbilical cord insertion site; intraplacental tumors are more difficult to recognize. The size of the tumor usually remains constant throughout the second half of pregnancy,[140] although rapid growth of vascular tumors has been reported.[141]

Polyhydramnios has been reported in up to 33% of cases of detectable chorioangiomas.[140] Although a majority of such tumors are large (greater than 5 cm), the vascularity of the tumor may be more important than the size in development of polyhydramnios. Excess amniotic fluid probably occurs as a result of transudation through the wall of abnormal tumor vessels.

Chorioangiomas have also been assessed with MRI.[142,143]

Differential Diagnosis

The primary differential diagnosis is hematoma. This distinction can occasionally be difficult, because both lesions may be associated with vaginal bleeding and elevated MSAFP. Doppler ultrasound aids in distinction because hemorrhage does not show interval vascularity.[140,141,144] Conversely, most chorioangiomas show internal hemorrhage. Occasional chorioangiomas, however, do not show blood flow with color-flow imaging so that absence of flow should not be used as definitive evidence against a chorioangioma.[140] In questionable cases, MRI should be able to distinguish hemorrhage from chorioangioma although this should rarely be necessary.

Other differential diagnoses for solid placental masses include placental teratoma, partial hydatidiform mole, and maternal tumor metastatic to the placenta.[145] An unusual case of vascular aneurysm was mistaken for a chorioangioma.[146]

Associated Anomalies

An association has been noted between chorioangiomata and fetal hemangiomata, twinning, a single umbilical artery (SUA), and velamentous insertion.[135] This cluster of anomalies shares anomalies of blood vessels. A female predominance also has been observed among such anomalies.[135,147,148] Fetal hydrops is a poor prognostic finding that may be seen in association with large tumors involving the placenta or umbilical cord.[149,150]

Prognosis and Management

The clinical course is usually unremarkable but potential fetal complications include polyhydramnios, fetal hydrops, fetal growth restriction, and fetal demise.[151–153] Potential maternal complications include premature labor, toxemia of pregnancy, maternal thrombocytopenia, and maternal coagulopathy.[154]

Several studies suggest that complications are related to increased vascularity of the tumor rather than size alone.[140,155,156] Development of fetal hydrops probably requires a large tumor and increased vascularity owing to shunting of fetal blood through the tumor. Fetal growth restriction may occur from chronic shunting of lesser degree.

Jauniaux et al.[140] suggest that a good prognosis can be expected from even large tumors that are avascular. This is consistent with other reports showing spontaneous resolution of polyhydramnios and hydrops in some cases when the tumor degenerates, resulting in reduced shunting of fetal blood through the tumor.[157,158] For this reason, an increase in the echogenicity of the tumor on serial ultrasound exams is considered a favorable prognostic finding, as this appearance is related to fibrotic degeneration of the lesion.[140]

Several fetal therapies have been attempted with variable results. These therapies have included fetal blood transfusion[159] and endoscopic-guided ligation of communicating vessels to the tumor.[160] Ultrasound-guided thermocoagulation of communicating vessels is also a potential option.[140]

Gestational Trophoblastic Neoplasia

Gestational trophoblastic neoplasia represents autonomous and potentially malignant growth of trophoblastic tissue.

Incidence

The prevalence of gestational trophoblastic diseases is approximately 1 in 1,200 pregnancies in the United States; a much greater frequency is observed in other parts of the world (e.g., the Far East).

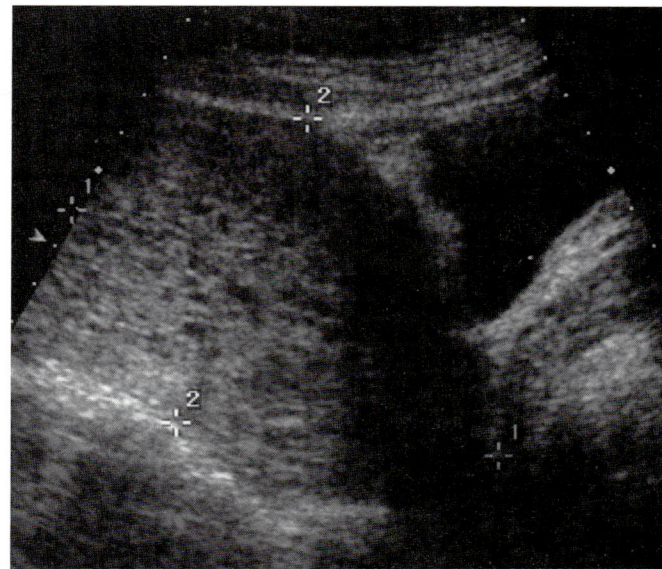

A

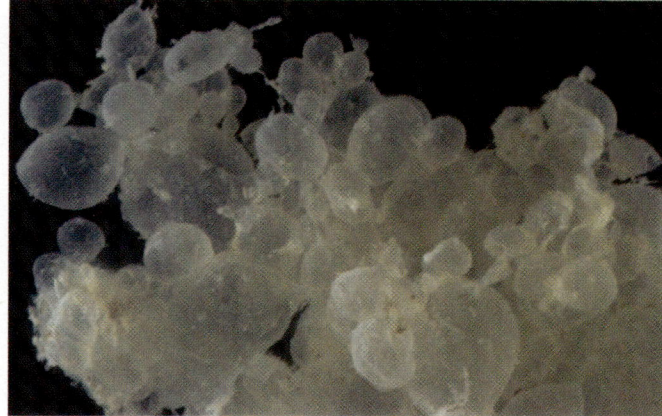

B

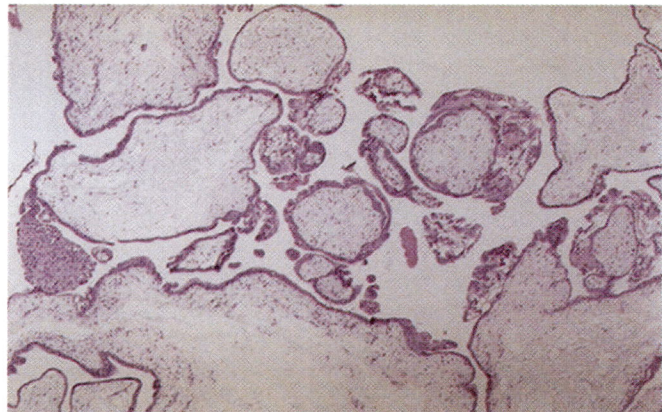

C

FIGURE 33. Complete molar pregnancy. **A:** Scan at 12 weeks shows thickened placenta containing multiple scattered tiny cysts. **B:** Pathology shows cystic villi. **C:** Histology shows hydropic villi and trophoblastic hyperplasia.

Pathology

Gestational trophoblastic disease can be categorized into three major groups: (a) classical or complete mole, (b) partial or incomplete mole, or (c) coexistent mole and fetus.[161] Invasive mole and metastatic trophoblastic disease can be considered as complications of a complete mole and rarely of a partial mole. Approximately 15% to 25% of women with complete mole develop persistent gestational trophoblastic disease.

Complete moles are unique in that they contain only paternal chromosomes.[162–164] Histologic features of the classic mole include trophoblastic hyperplasia, hydropic villi, and absence of fetal tissue.

Partial hydatidiform moles usually are associated with a fetus or fetal tissue and, unlike complete moles, carry a lower malignant potential.[165] Histologic features include focal trophoblastic hyperplasia. Partial moles are frequently associated with fetal anomalies and chromosome abnormalities, usually triploidy.[162–164] Hydatidiform degeneration or hydropic change is present in nearly all cases in which the extra haploid set of chromosomes is paternal in origin but is much less common with a maternal origin.[166]

Coexistent true trophoblastic disease and a living fetus are exceedingly rare.[165,167] Some of the reported cases appear to represent a partial mole or hydropic degeneration. Instances of a classic mole and coexisting fetus have been reported, however, and such moles carry malignant potential.[168,169] The presumed mechanism for this situation is hydatidiform degeneration arising from a co-twin.[162]

Diagnosis

Ultrasonography has long been used to diagnose gestational trophoblastic disease, most commonly complete or partial hydatidiform mole. The classic appearance of complete mole is multiple variable-sized cysts replacing the placental substance (Fig. 33).[170–173] The size of the cysts varies with gestational age.

Sonographic findings of partial hydatidiform mole (Fig. 34) may include reduced amniotic fluid and a thickened placenta with intraplacental cystic areas. However, the sonographic appearance varies. A living fetus may not be evident if early demise has occurred. When present, the fetus should show features of triploidy (see Chapter 21).

A coexisting mole and living embryo may be difficult to distinguish from a partial mole. In the case of partial mole, however, fetal triploidy is present, and anomalies should be evident by ultrasound.

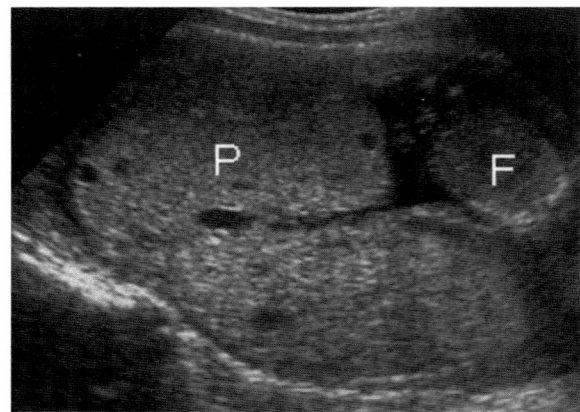

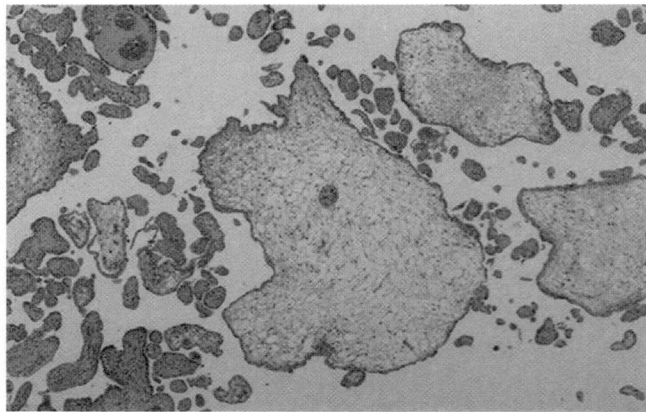

FIGURE 34. Partial mole and triploidy. **A:** Scan at 14 weeks shows thickened placenta (*P*) containing scattered cysts. A living fetus (*F*) has triploidy and is severely growth restricted. Oligohydramnios is also evident. **B:** Histology shows focal hydropic villi and trophoblastic hyperplasia.

Because of routine use of first-trimester ultrasound and serum human chorionic gonadotropin (hCG), most cases of molar pregnancy now present during the first trimester.[174,175] The ultrasound findings and clinical presentation are correspondingly different and variable. First-trimester ultrasound findings are considered diagnostic in only approximately 80% of cases, and theca lutein cysts are usually absent.[176–179] Benson et al.[179] found that the most common sonographic appearance of a complete molar pregnancy during the first trimester is a complex, echogenic mass containing many small (less than 1 cm) cystic areas and occasional larger cystic areas. The ability to detect ultrasound findings appears to be related to hCG levels. At lower levels of hCG (less than 700 mIU per mL), intramyometrial lesions may not be visualized by either ultrasound or MRI.[180]

In addition to early diagnosis of hydatidiform moles, ultrasonography plays a role in further management and follow-up. Adequate surgical uterine evacuation can be visualized, and areas of increased intrauterine echoes in the uterus may signal a developing invasive mole or choriocarcinoma.[181] In cases of invasive mole or choriocarcinoma, transvaginal sonography may show an echogenic uterine mass with myometrial invasion, and color Doppler examination shows a low impedance circulation at the periphery of the mass.[182] Sonographic monitoring of such lesions may be used to monitor treatment response.[183,184] It is difficult, however, to discriminate choriocarcinoma from invasive mole using the ultrasound findings alone.[185] Doppler examination may also provide some information, because invasive moles and choriocarcinoma show significantly increased peak systolic velocities.[186] Although sonography may allow diagnosis of trophoblastic disease, no ultrasound parameters allow accurate prediction of persistent trophoblastic disease, which requires detection by serial maternal hCG measurements.[187]

Differential Diagnosis

Other placental abnormalities that should be considered when molar pregnancy is suspected include intraplacental or periplacental hemorrhage, degenerating uterine leiomyomas, demise of a co-twin, or prominent maternal venous lakes.

If there is a living fetus and the placenta shows findings suggestive of molar pregnancy with multiple cysts, the possibilities include a triploid conceptus (partial mole), especially if detected in early pregnancy; a twin pregnancy with a complete mole and a normal fetus; and a group of conditions described as *pseudomoles* or mesenchymal dysplasia or the placenta. In this latter condition, the underlying pathogenesis is unknown, but the placenta shows marked stem villous hydrops with or without angiomatoid change. Some cases may apparently resolve, others may persist and be associated with a preeclampsia and a phenotypically normal infant at birth, while others may be associated with clinical features of Beckwith-Wiedemann syndrome.[188–192]

Simple hydropic degeneration seen with first-trimester pregnancy losses should be distinguished from trophoblastic disease. hCG levels are typically low in this situation.

Prognosis

The prognosis for gestational trophoblastic neoplasia is excellent, even for metastatic gestational trophoblastic disease. Symptoms of molar pregnancies include vaginal bleeding, preeclampsia, and signs of hormonal hyperstimulation (nausea, vomiting, and even hyperthyroidism).[167]

Management

Management of gestational trophoblastic disease is beyond the scope of this book and the reader is referred elsewhere for details.[193]

Confined Placental Mosaicism

Confined placental mosaicism is mosaic aneuploidy confined to placental tissues.

Incidence

The incidence of confined placental mosaicism is uncertain and undoubtedly underdiagnosed. Confined placental mosaicism has been seen with increased frequency with the development of chorionic villous sampling.[194,195] Confined placental mosaicism may account for some of the false-positive diagnoses by chorionic villous sampling.

Pathology

Commonly involved chromosome abnormalities are trisomies 16, 7, 8, and 17. Confined placental mosaicism may be associated with uniparental disomy of the fetus in some cases.

Diagnosis

Ultrasound
Sonographic findings of confined placental mosaicism are nonspecific. The most prominent is fetal growth restriction, which may be evident early in the second trimester. The placenta may be thickened and may show intraplacental cysts (Fig. 35).[196]

Laboratory
Atypical elevation of hCG and AFP may be an indication for confined placental mosaicism, especially in combination with early onset growth restriction.[197] Definitive diagnosis requires demonstration of placental mosaicism by sampling of the placenta. Genetic amniocentesis is not helpful. When evaluating the placenta, standard cytogenetic techniques may be used. Alternatively, comparative genomic hybridization using fluorescent in situ hybridization may be the most effective method for screening placentas for confined placental mosaicism.[198]

Associated Anomalies

In some cases, the fetus has uniparental disomy, which is associated with fetal anomalies. Fetal abnormalities have also been described in which no evidence existed for uniparental disomy. These cases presumably represent low levels of mosaicism.

Prognosis

Confined placental mosaicism has variable outcomes. Some fetuses result in early or late unexplained fetal demise.[199] Survivors may be small but are otherwise normal except for cases of uniparental disomy or fetal mosaicism.

Management

When confined placental mosaicism is suspected, placental biopsy should be performed. Patients with known or suspected confined placental mosaicism should be monitored closely because of the increased risk for spontaneous fetal death.

Recurrence Risk

No known recurrence risk exists for confined placental mosaicism.

UMBILICAL CORD AND FETAL CIRCULATION

The umbilical cord, as the supply line for the developing fetus, is one of the most important organs during prenatal life. Despite the umbilical cord's importance, it is a relatively simple structure, containing two arteries and one vein surrounded by a gelatinous stroma, the Wharton's jelly, and covered by a single layer of amnion. It must be flexible and long enough to allow free mobility of the fetus but strong enough to resist compression.

Excellent pathologic reviews of the placenta and umbilical cord are available.[1-3,200,201] Sonographic attention to the umbilical cord has intensified during the last decade so that nearly all pathologic diagnoses can now be made prenatally. The umbilical cord can be visualized from the eighth menstrual week onward, and this evaluation has been aided

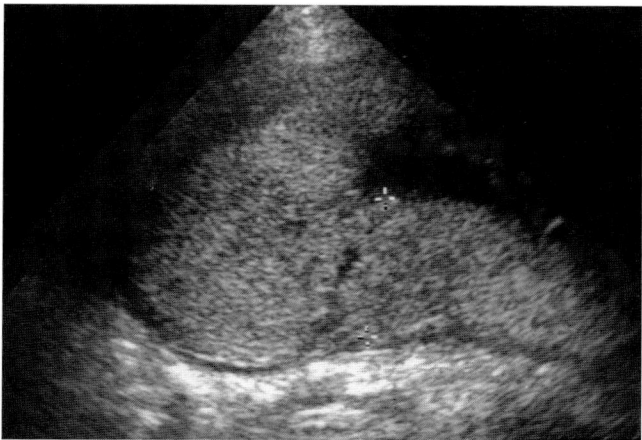

FIGURE 35. Confined placental mosaicism. Scan at 26 weeks shows nonspecific mildly thickened placenta, measuring 4 cm. The fetus was growth restricted and spontaneously died *in utero.* Placental analysis shows confined placental mosaicism for trisomy 7.

into the connecting stalk to form the allantois. The allantoic vessels become the definitive umbilical vessels.

Growth of the umbilical cord parallels growth of the fetus until 28 weeks, when the umbilical cord has attained its final length of 50 to 60 cm (range, 22 to 130 cm).[207] At term, the umbilical cord length is approximately 60 cm with a mean circumference of 3.6 cm.

The normal circulation through the umbilical cord is shown in Figure 37. The arteries transport deoxygenated blood from the fetus to the placenta and are branches of the internal iliac artery. Within the fetus, they run alongside the fetal bladder becoming adjacent at the umbilicus; course along the entire length of the cord, usually in a helicoidal fashion surrounding the vein; and branch along the chorionic plate of the placenta. The umbilical vein is formed by a confluence of the chorionic veins of the placenta and transports oxygenated blood back to the fetus. In the fetal abdomen, the umbilical vein courses

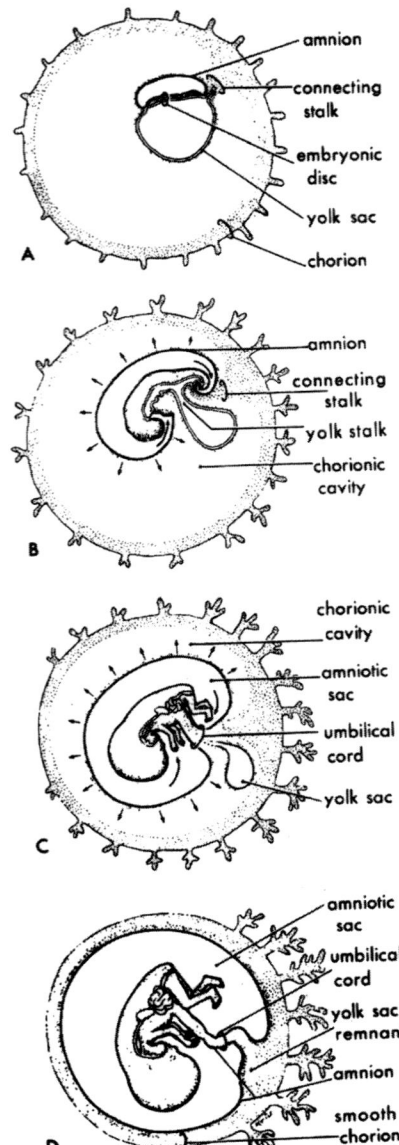

FIGURE 36. Formation of placental membranes, yolk sac, and fetus at 5 menstrual weeks **(A)** (3 fetal weeks); 6 menstrual weeks **(B)**; 12 menstrual weeks **(C)**; and 22 menstrual weeks **(D)**. (Reproduced with permission from Moore KL. *The developing human*, 4th ed. Philadelphia: WB Saunders, 1988.)

with the development of transvaginal ultrasound, color Doppler, and three-dimensional imaging techniques.[202–206]

Embryology

The umbilical cord derives from the stalk of the yolk sac (Fig. 36). As the result of expansion of the amniotic sac, the connecting stalk becomes covered by amniotic epithelium and fuses with the omphalomesenteric duct to form the umbilical cord at approximately 7 weeks. An outpouching from the urinary bladder forms the urachus, which projects

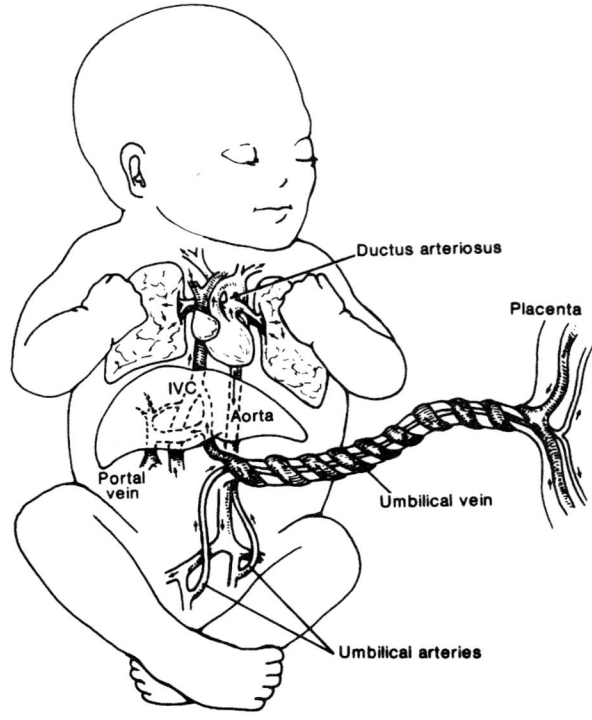

FIGURE 37. Normal fetal circulation. Oxygenated blood returns from the placenta through the umbilical vein. Some blood goes through the portal vein and liver, but the majority continues through the ductus venosus where it joins the inferior vena cava (*IVC*). Oxygenated blood from the ductus venosus is preferentially diverted to the left heart through the foramen ovale and is then pumped into the ascending aorta where it supplies the brain. Deoxygenated blood returning from the superior vena cava is preferentially shunted through the right atrium into the right ventricle where most of it continues through the ductus arteriosus into the descending aorta and then through the paired umbilical arteries where it returns to the placenta. (Reproduced with permission from Hill MC, Lande M, Grossman JH III. Obstetric Doppler. In: Grant EG, White EM, eds. *Duplex sonography*. New York: Springer-Verlag, 1987.)

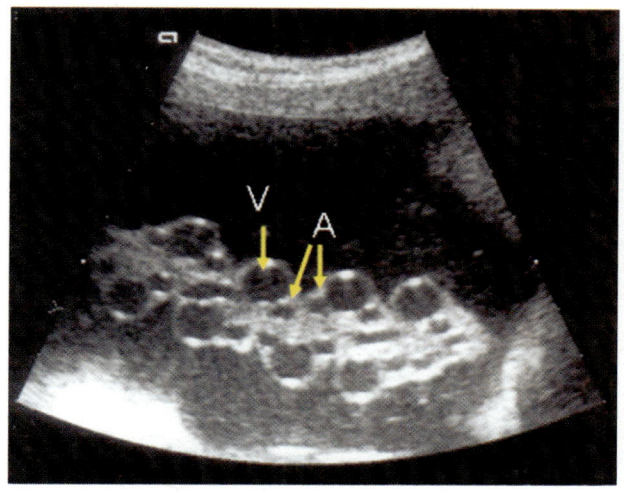
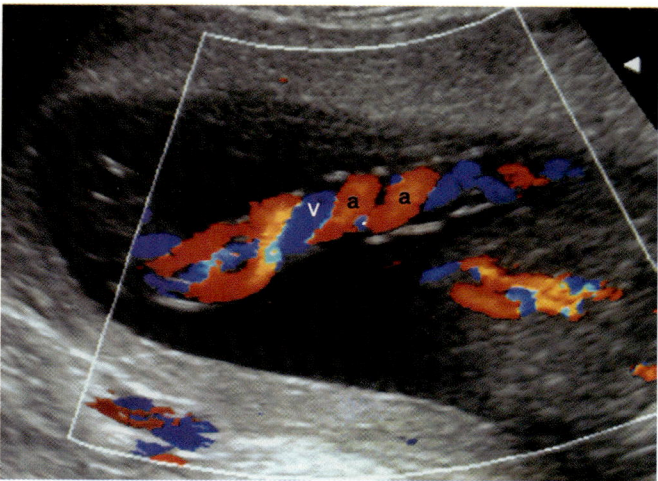

FIGURE 38. Normal three-vessel umbilical cord. Grey-scale **(A)** and color-flow **(B)** images from two patients show single umbilical vein (*V*) and two paired smaller arteries (*A, a*) coiled within umbilical cord.

cephalad from the cord insertion, enters the liver, and anastomoses with the portal vein. The intraabdominal portions of the umbilical vessels degenerate after birth; the umbilical arteries become the lateral ligaments of the bladder, and the umbilical vein becomes the round ligament of the liver.

NORMAL ULTRASOUND ANATOMY OF THE UMBILICAL VESSELS

The ability of ultrasound to evaluate the umbilical cord and number of vessels[208] has dramatically improved since the original sonographic description of the umbilical cord.[209]

Because it is bathed by amniotic fluid, the umbilical cord can be readily visualized as early as 8 menstrual weeks. In the first trimester, the length is approximately the same as the crown-rump length.[210]

In the second and third trimesters, the two arteries and the vein can be clearly seen (Fig. 38). The number of umbilical arteries can also be determined reliably at an early gestational age by assessing the umbilical arteries adjacent to the urinary bladder with color-flow imaging or power Doppler techniques (Fig. 39).

The placental and fetal insertions can also be visualized. Routine visualization of the placental insertion is essential in the diagnosis of marginal and velamentous insertion of the cord and can also help in the assessment of succenturi-

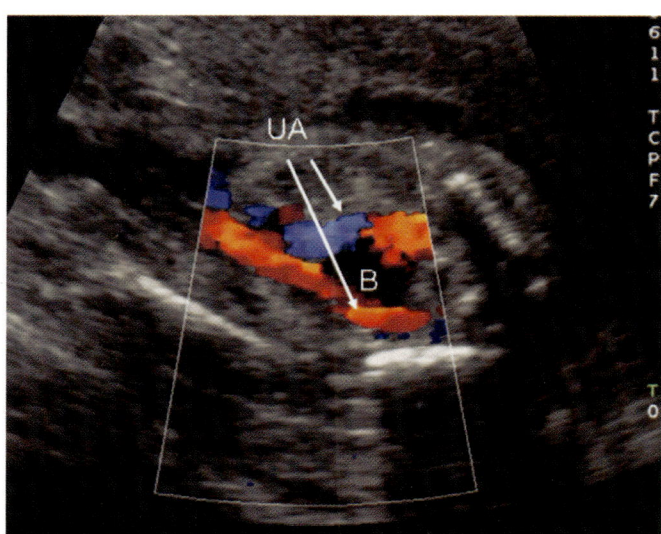
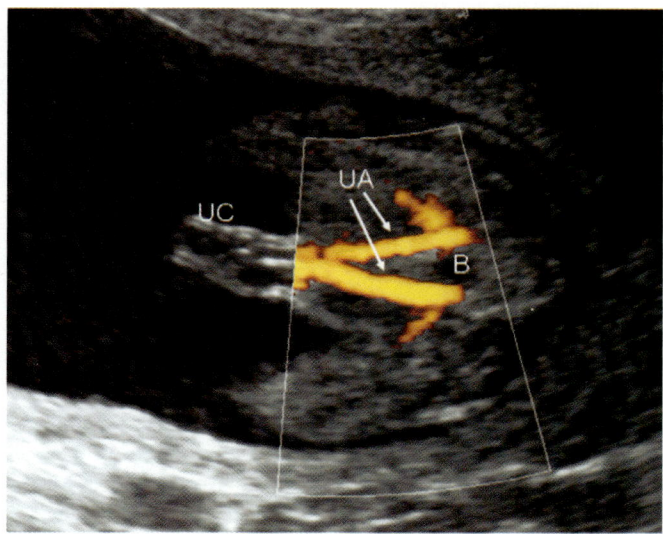

FIGURE 39. Normal paired umbilical arteries (*UA*) are confirmed adjacent to the urinary bladder (*B*) with color-flow imaging **(A)** or power Doppler **(B)**. UC, umbilical cord.

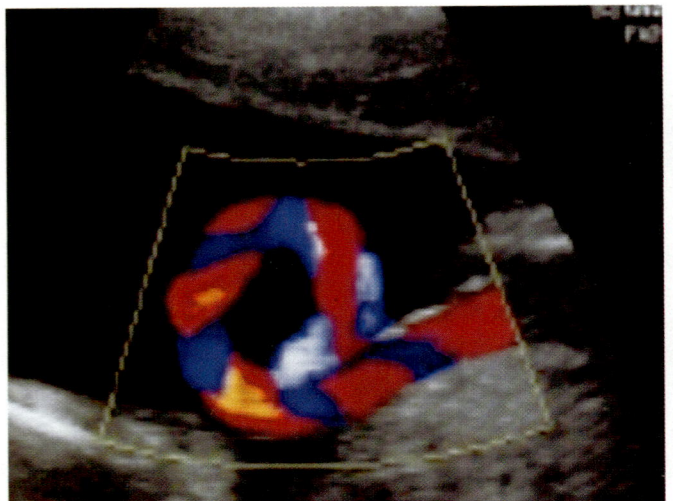
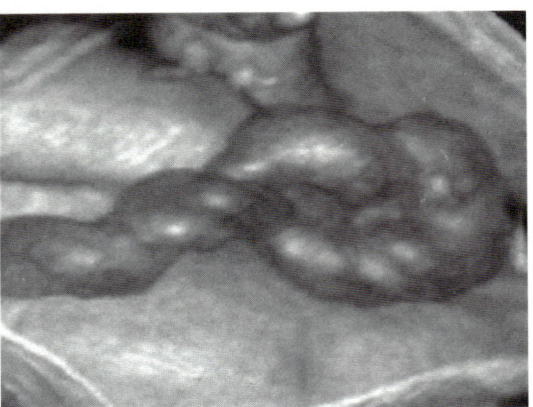

A   B

FIGURE 40. Normal umbilical cord. **A:** The circuitous course of the umbilical cord is greatly aided with color-flow imaging. **B:** Three-dimensional view of the umbilical cord. The complex course of the umbilical cord is shown. (Part **B** Courtesy of Martin Necas, New Zealand.)

ate placenta.[211,212] Color-flow imaging greatly aids in following the circuitous course of the umbilical cord and in identification of the umbilical cord insertion (Fig. 40A). Three-dimensional ultrasound can also display the complex course of the umbilical cord (Fig. 40B).

Coiling is an obvious characteristic of the umbilical cord that is established by 9 menstrual weeks.[213] The number of twists is usually between 0 and 40, with more twists present near the fetal insertion site. For unknown reasons, a predominance of left-sided twists (i.e., sinistral) has been observed compared to right-sided twists (i.e., dextral). In a series of 271 cords, Nakari observed that the spiral was left-sided in 87.5%, right-sided in 11.9%, and neither in 0.6%.[214]

The umbilical vessels can be followed after insertion of the umbilical cord into the umbilicus. The arteries course inferiorly around the urinary bladder while the umbilical vein courses superiorly in the free, inferior margin of the falciform ligament. On entering the liver, the umbilical vein becomes the umbilical portion of the left portal vein, which turns posteriorly and is continuous with the main portal vein and anterior and posterior divisions of the right portal vein. The ductus venosus courses superiorly from the transverse portion of the left portal vein to end in the inferior vena cava near the confluence of the hepatic veins.

ANOMALIES OF THE UMBILICAL CORD

Abnormalities of the umbilical cord are common (Table 2). These may affect the length, size, number, insertion, or course of the umbilical vessels. Short cords may be associated with decreased fetal movement, for example, by oligohydramnios.[215] Unusually long cords may prolapse and are associated with nuchal cords and true knots. The umbilical cord may

also be too thick or too thin, and coiling may be excessive or absent. Abnormal insertion of the umbilical cord may result in velamentous cord insertion or vasa previa. Umbilical veins may form aneurysms or strictures.[1] Umbilical cord enlargement may occur from edema in association with hydrops, rhesus sensitization, twin-twin transfusion syndrome, hematoma, and umbilical cord tumor (i.e., hemangioma).

In the following sections, abnormalities of the umbilical cord can be classified into vascular anomalies, cystic lesions, and solid lesions or tumors (Table 2).

Vascular Anomalies

Absent/Hypoplastic Umbilical Artery

Description
Congenital absence of one artery is a condition widely known as *single umbilical artery*. A hypoplastic umbilical artery is present but small.

TABLE 2. ANOMALIES OF THE UMBILICAL CORD

Abnormalities of insertion
  Marginal/velamentous umbilical cord insertion of the placenta
Vascular anomalies
  Single/hypoplastic umbilical artery
  Supernumerary vessels
  Umbilical artery aneurysm
  Umbilical vein varix
Cystic lesions
  True cysts
    Omphalomesenteric cyst
    Allantoic cyst
  Pseudocyst
Tumors
  Angiomyxoma
  Teratoma

Incidence

SUA is by far the most common anomaly of the umbilical cord and among the most common anomalies seen in newborn infants. In prospective series, the prevalence of SUA ranges from 0.08% to 1.9%, with an average of 0.63%.[216] SUA occurs more frequently in twins and in association with velamentous insertion.[217] SUA is invariably present in the twin reverse arterial perfusion sequence (see Chapter 18) and in sirenomelia (see Chapter 15).[217] Caucasians have a higher frequency of SUA than blacks or Japanese.[218] Monozygotic twins are usually discordant for SUA, suggesting that environmental factors are important.

The incidence of hypoplastic umbilical artery depends on the criterion used. A discrepancy of 2 mm in size of umbilical arteries was first reported in 6 of 310 (1.9%) high-risk pregnancies scanned after 20 weeks of gestation.[219] Another study of 444 pregnancies between 24 and 32 weeks showed three (0.7%) with discordant umbilical arteries.[220] Although these authors did not provide a clear definition for discordancy, differences in arterial diameter in their study were between 1 and 3 mm. Another prospective study using a criterion of 1 mm or more showed discordant arteries in 1.4% (14 of 1,012) consecutive pregnancies scanned in the second half of pregnancy.[221] However, using a more strict criterion of size difference of more than 50%, Petrikovsky and Schneider[222] showed discordant arteries in only 0.04% (12 of 31,000) consecutive second- and third-trimester scans. Before 20 weeks of gestation, the detection of marked discordancy between umbilical arteries seems difficult to document owing to the small size of the arteries.

Pathology and Embryology

It has been suggested that SUA results from the persistence of the normally transient SUA present in early stages of development.[223] Other possible etiologies include primary agenesis or secondary atrophy of a previously normal umbilical artery. The latter mechanism is probably the most common, which is strongly supported by the detection of muscular remnants in approximately 40% of umbilical cords from cases of SUA undergoing microscopic examination.[224] Not all cases of SUA necessarily share the same embryogenesis. For example, a SUA associated with sirenomelia arises from the abdominal aorta directly and probably represents persistence of the vitelline artery.

Diagnosis

SUA has been increasingly recognized in the second and third trimesters as the result of routine assessment of the umbilical cord to document the number of vessels. Several characteristic features exist that can be used in the prenatal detection of this condition:

1. One characteristic feature is the identification of a two-vessel cord. The basic screening technique to identify

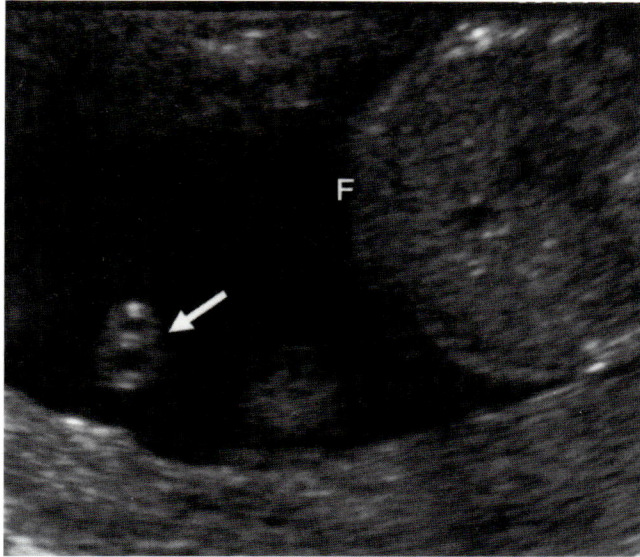

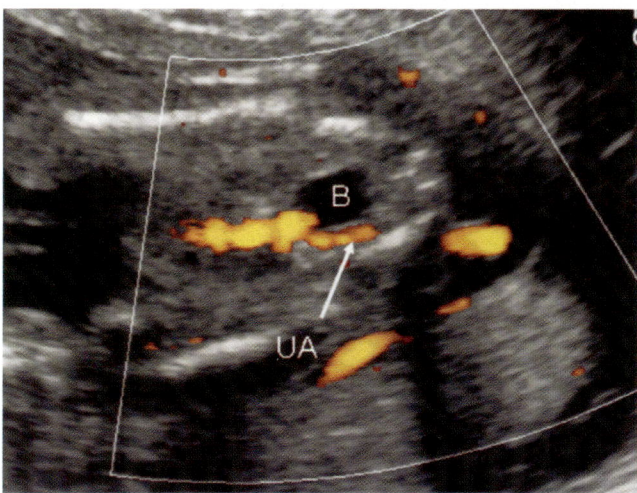

FIGURE 41. Single umbilical artery. **A:** Cross section of umbilical cord (*arrow*) shows two vessels instead of the normal three. F, fetus. **B:** Power Doppler confirms a single umbilical artery (*UA*) coursing around the urinary bladder (*B*).

the normal three-vessel cord consists of a detailed examination of transverse and longitudinal views of a free loop of the cord with adequate magnification (Fig. 41). In SUA, only two vessels are identified, of which the larger vessel is the vein and the smaller is the artery.[225–228] In the longitudinal view, the two-vessel cord frequently appears straight and noncoiled (Fig. 42), although occasionally the single artery may loop around the vein. The use of color-flow imaging enhances the diagnosis by better visualization of the umbilical vessels. In some cases, however, the clear identification of the number of vessels is limited by gestational age and in cases of maternal obesity, oligo-

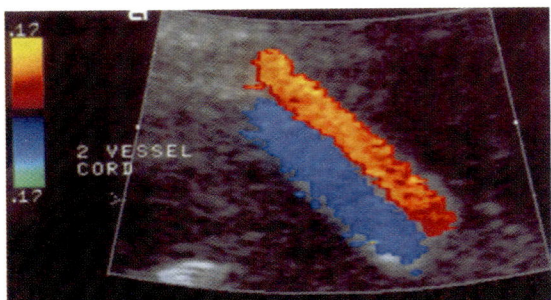

FIGURE 42. Single umbilical artery. Color-flow imaging shows a two-vessel umbilical cord, representing a single umbilical artery and vein. Also note the unusual straight course of the vessels.

hydramnios, twins, or when multiple loops of cord lie in close proximity to each other. Difficulties in establishing the diagnosis of SUA in hypercoiled cords have also been noted.

2. Another characteristic feature is increased diameter of the single artery. In the normal three-vessel cord, the blood to the placenta is approximately equally distributed through both arteries. In the two-vessel cord, the entire fetoplacental circulation is transported through only one artery, resulting in a compensatory increase of the arterial diameter.[229,230] In SUA, the diameter of the single artery usually measures more than 50% of the diameter of the vein, resulting in a vein-to-artery ratio less than 2. In contrast, the arteries in a three-vessel cord usually measure less than 50% of the diameter of the vein. In one study, artery and vein diameters were obtained prenatally in 55 fetuses with SUA, and the umbilical vein to artery ratio was less than 2 in 54 of 55 fetuses (98%) but greater than 4 mm in only 6 cases (11%).[230] With current ultrasound equipment and good scanning technique, the compensatory increase in the single artery diameter is evident even during the early second trimester.[230,231]

3. Demonstration of absent intraabdominal segment of the missing umbilical artery is a third characteristic feature that can be used in the prenatal detection of SUA. Absence of one umbilical artery necessarily implies the absence of the corresponding intraabdominal umbilical artery, which can be detected prenatally by examining the vessels running alongside the bladder in a transverse view of the fetal pelvis.[232] This feature is greatly enhanced with the use of color-flow imaging or power Doppler (Fig. 41B) and indeed appears to be the best screening technique for SUA. Furthermore, this site should also be examined if the diagnosis of SUA is suspected at the level of the cord, to confirm the diagnosis.

Hypoplastic umbilical artery has been frequently detected.[233–236] Diagnosis of a hypoplastic artery is made by the detection of size discordancy between umbilical arteries after detailed examination of a magnified cross-sectional view of the umbilical cord, usually after suspicion of SUA.

Hemodynamic Considerations

The absence of one artery in the cord is associated with hemodynamic alterations within the fetal circulation. In normal fetuses, the arterial blood flow to the placenta is equally or nearly equally distributed along both umbilical artery territories, including common iliac arteries, internal iliac arteries, and intraabdominal umbilical arteries. In SUA fetuses, the entire blood flow volume to the placenta is transported through the common and internal iliac artery of one side only, whereas the iliac vessels from the side of the missing artery do not participate in the fetomaternal circulation.[237] In this setting, the iliac artery from the side of the missing umbilical artery only transports the blood volume to the leg, a high-resistance territory. In contrast, the side of the single artery perfuses mainly the placenta, a territory characterized by decreasing resistance to blood flow throughout pregnancy. Using high-resolution color Doppler ultrasound, significant differences in both the size and the impedance indices in the pelvic circulation of fetuses with SUA have been demonstrated.[238,239] This discordant intraluminal blood flow between common iliac arteries is more marked as pregnancy progresses, which may be caused by the decrease in resistance in the placental circulation and the increase in resistance in femoral arteries.

Discordant umbilical arteries also show discordant blood flow with umbilical artery Doppler.[233,234] The resistance index is almost always higher in the smaller artery, and there may be absent end-diastolic flow. The adjunctive use of color Doppler ultrasound is required to confirm the presence of flow within the hypoplastic artery, thus ruling out the possibility of an atrophic nonfunctional artery.

Differential Diagnosis

A potential pitfall in the diagnosis of SUA is the visualization of the cord close to the placental insertion. In normal conditions, the umbilical arteries may fuse close to the placental insertion in a segment not longer than 3 cm.[1] Occasionally, the arteries are fused for a longer distance, resulting in the identification of an umbilical cord with a distal segment containing two vessels and a proximal segment with three vessels.[240,241]

Associated Anomalies

Large neonatal series have clearly demonstrated an association between the presence of SUA and congenital anomalies, chromosomal defects, IUGR, prematurity, and perinatal death.[201,242–245] Prenatal ultrasound has played an important role in the detection of associated anomalies.[246] One study comparing the prenatal and postnatal findings in 118 fetuses with SUA showed that prenatal findings were present in 31 of 37 fetuses with SUA, and 7% of apparently otherwise normal fetuses had structural anomalies at birth.[247] Therefore, a comprehensive ultrasound anatomic survey should be mandatory in those cases in which an SUA is detected prenatally. Even if no other associated anomalies are detected, a detailed examination of the neonate is suggested to exclude minor or internal organ anomalies.

The incidence of IUGR is significantly elevated among fetuses with an SUA and may be present without any other congenital anomalies in 15% to 20% of the cases. SUA has also been associated with chromosomal defects, specifically trisomy 13 and trisomy 18.[248,249] Prenatal karyotyping, therefore, should be considered when multiple malformations or IUGR are detected in association with SUA.

The use of fetal blood sampling is not contraindicated for rapid karyotyping with SUA. However, vasospasm or tamponade of the cord vessels, which can occur during fetal blood sampling, could have more serious consequences on the SUA fetus. The safety of cordocentesis has been addressed in a prospective study of 14 fetuses with SUA undergoing fetal blood sampling for karyotyping.[250] In all cases, associated structural anomalies existed. There were no procedure-related complications, and no fetal deaths occurred 2 weeks after the procedure. However, a higher incidence of complications, such as bleeding and fetal bradycardia, was noted with the transamniotic compared with the transplacental approach.[250]

Whether hypoplastic umbilical artery carries the same significance as SUA is uncertain. Although several studies suggest a higher frequency of association anomalies,[220–222,235] these have been diagnosed in high-risk populations. An association may exist between atrophy of one umbilical artery and other abnormalities of the placenta or abnormal insertion of the umbilical cord.[221,251]

Prognosis

Several investigators have attempted to identify factors associated with poor outcome in fetuses with SUA. In one series, the left umbilical artery was missing in 73% of 77 fetuses with SUA assessed with color Doppler ultrasound, and all complex malformations and chromosomal defects occurred in this group.[252] In contrast, in another series of 44 cases of SUA, the left umbilical artery was missing in only 46% of cases, with no association between the side missing and the occurrence of fetal anomalies.[253] This was confirmed by a larger series of 102 fetuses with SUA,[254] which demonstrated a higher prevalence of the left side missing (70%), but similar frequency of perinatally identified associated structural anomalies in both groups (42%). One study of fetuses with SUA calculated the area of the cord and subtracted the area of the vessels, and suggested that the amount of Wharton's jelly in fetuses with SUA is less than in normal three-vessel umbilical cords, raising the possibility that reduced Wharton's jelly content may play a role in the association with antepartum deaths in otherwise normal infants.[255]

Management

Whenever SUA is identified prenatally, a complete survey of the fetal anatomy should be performed to rule out associated anomalies,[256–258] and, if associated anomalies are found, prenatal karyotyping should be discussed. In cases of isolated SUA, follow-up for fetal well-being and fetal growth should be considered.[256–258] Some authors have recommended neonatal renal ultrasound whenever SUA is detected at birth, mainly because of the increased association between SUA and renal abnormalities.[259] If isolated SUA is detected prenatally, however, this step is not necessary if a thorough examination of the fetal urogenital system was performed before delivery.[260]

Supernumerary Vessels

Description
Supernumerary vessels are the presence of more than three vessels in the umbilical cord.

Incidence
Supernumerary vessels are an exceedingly rare condition, virtually always associated with conjoined twinning.

Embryology
Supernumerary vessels are thought to represent an abnormal splitting of the umbilical vessels between the third and the fifth week of development.

Diagnosis
Since the first description of a four-vessel umbilical cord in thoracoomphalopagus twins at 33 weeks of gestation,[261] the prenatal detection of a solitary umbilical cord with more than three vessels became an important ultrasonographic landmark for the prenatal diagnosis of conjoined twins (Fig. 43).[262–265] In the only case prenatally detected

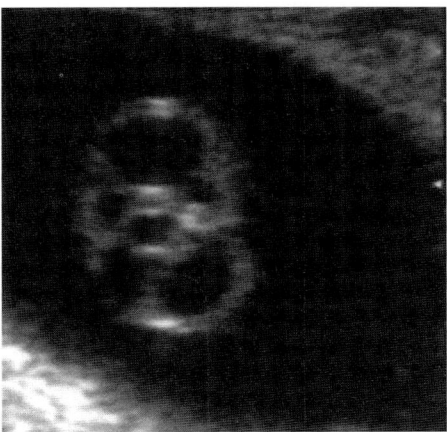

FIGURE 43. Supernumerary vessels. Cross section of umbilical cord shows supernumerary vessels from a case of conjoined twinning.

in a singleton, a four-vessel cord was reported in association with holoprosencephaly and polyhydramnios.[202]

Differential Diagnosis

Occasionally, a false impression of multivessel cord can be obtained when the transverse view of the cord through a false knot includes multiple loops of the same vessel.

Associated Anomalies

A four-vessel cord has been incidentally found in normal neonates[266,267] but also has been noted in association with multiple congenital anomalies.[268] In one case, a double umbilical vein was found in the cord of a macerated stillborn with multiple anomalies including ectopia cordis, bifid liver, and bilateral cleft lip and palate.[269]

Prognosis and Management

Prognosis and management of supernumerary vessels depend mainly on the underlying condition (see Chapter 18).

Varix of the Umbilical Vein

Description

Aneurysm and varix are focal dilatation of the umbilical vessels affecting the umbilical artery or vein, respectively.[270,271] Focal dilatation (varix) of the umbilical vein is nearly always intraabdominal but extrahepatic in location.

Incidence

These conditions were initially diagnosed by postpartum examination of the umbilical cord in stillborn infants and, therefore, recognized as a cause of fetal death.[1,201] Indeed, varix of the umbilical vein was found in 3.8% of 184 malformations of the cord noted in association with perinatal death,[270] but, because series are primarily obtained from autopsy cases, the incidence in an unselected population remains unknown.

Pathology

The pathologic origin of umbilical vein varix is uncertain. An acquired etiology is more likely than a congenital origin. The extrahepatic, intraabdominal portion of the umbilical vein has the weakest supporting structure of any part of the umbilical circulation. Therefore, any condition that increases venous pressure could potentially dilate the umbilical vein, resulting in an umbilical vein varix. It is of interest in this regard that umbilical vein varix has been seen in association with cardiomegaly and subsequent hydrops.

Diagnosis

Varix of the umbilical vein is usually seen as a dilated intraabdominal, extrahepatic portion of the umbilical vein (Figs. 44 and 45).[232,272–275] Rarely, it may show as a large mass.[276] Color-flow imaging and its continuity with the umbilical vein permits definite diagnosis of umbilical vein varix (Fig.

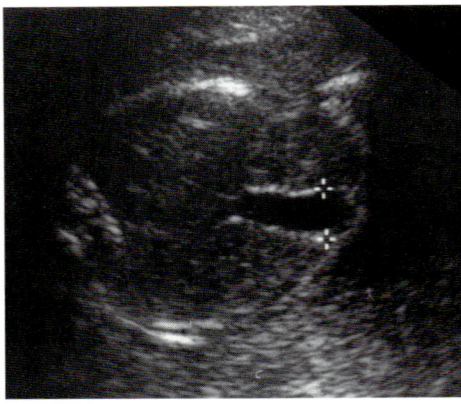

FIGURE 44. Umbilical vein varix. Axial view of abdomen at 26 weeks shows dilatation of extrahepatic portion of the umbilical vein, measuring 12 mm in diameter. Although most cases of umbilical vein varix have a normal outcome, this fetus showed early-onset growth restriction and died *in utero.*

45). Diagnostic criteria include an umbilical vein diameter greater than 9 mm[277] or an enlargement of the varix of at least 50% larger than the diameter of the intrahepatic umbilical vein.[278]

Varix of a persistent right umbilical vein has also been reported.[279] Aneurysm of the extrafetal portion of the umbilical vein has been rarely reported.[280]

Differential Diagnosis

Differential diagnosis of umbilical vein varix includes normal structures (e.g., stomach, gallbladder) as well as cystic masses (e.g., duplication or mesenteric cyst, ovarian cyst) and all types of cystic masses of the cord, including pseudocyst or true cyst (see Cystic Lesions of the Umbilical

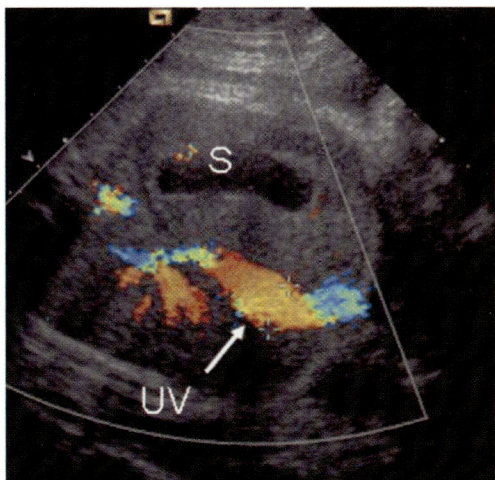

FIGURE 45. Umbilical vein varix. Color-flow imaging shows dilated extrahepatic, intraabdominal portion of umbilical vein (*UV*). The fetus had a normal outcome. S, stomach. (Courtesy of Martin Necas, New Zealand.)

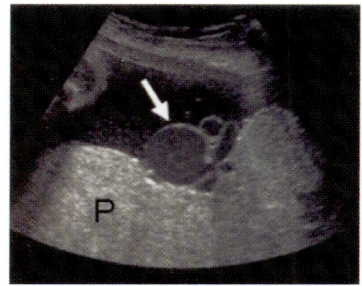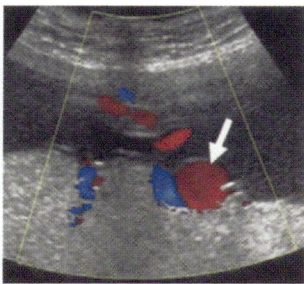

A,B

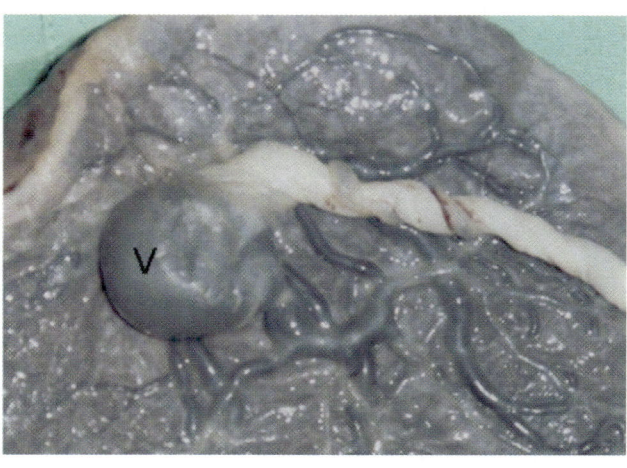

C

FIGURE 46. Varix of extraabdominal portion of umbilical vein. Grey-scale **(A)** and color-flow **(B)** images show dilated umbilical vein (*arrow*) near the insertion of the umbilical cord into the placenta (*P*). **C:** Pathologic correlation shows varix (*V*) of umbilical vein.

Cord). Color Doppler and color-flow imaging can easily assist in the prenatal diagnosis by the demonstration of arterial, continuous, or turbulent flow within the mass.

At least two cases of umbilical artery aneurysm have been reported prenatally: one in association with SUA[281] and the other in a trisomy 18 fetus.[282] A further case has been diagnosed by our group in a trisomy 18 fetus with multiple anomalies including SUA (Fig. 46) (*unpublished*).

Associated Anomalies

Umbilical vein varix has been associated with other anomalies, aneuploidy, and hydrops.[278] Among 42 cases of umbilical vein varix, Sepulveda et al.[278] noted that 12% had a chromosomal abnormality, and 5% developed hydrops. Batton et al.[283] reported an unusual case associated with fetal anemia secondary to schistocytic hemolysis.

Prognosis

In most cases, umbilical vein varix is associated with a normal outcome.[284] However, reports have documented an increased prevalence of perinatal death, karyotypic abnormalities, and hydrops.[273,285,286] Mahony et al.[272] reported that 44% (four of nine) fetuses with umbilical vein varix subsequently died, including one with trisomy 21, and a fifth fetus subsequently developed hydrops. They suggested that earlier diagnosis in the second trimester might be a poor prognostic factor. In a series of ten cases, Sepulveda et al.[278] reported that three fetuses with associated anomalies died, whereas six of the remaining seven fetuses had normal outcome. Combined with previous reports, these authors report that 24% of 42 affected fetuses died, 12% had a chromosomal abnormality, and 5% developed hydrops. Another series of 25 cases confirmed an increased risk of adverse outcome.[286] Most authors conclude that umbilical vein varix increases the risk for adverse outcome, but the prognosis is generally good as an isolated finding.[274,275]

Reasons for fetal demise are uncertain. Thrombosis of the varix, however, has been reported, and this could contribute to fetal demise in some cases.[285,287,288] Varix of the intraamni-

otic segment of the umbilical vein has also been reported to cause intraamniotic hemorrhage through the amniotic sheath, fetal exsanguination, and thrombosis leading to fetal death.[289]

Management

No data exist to support altered obstetric management based on umbilical vein varix alone. Follow-up ultrasound exams may be performed, although these are more useful for evaluation of fetal growth than re-evaluation of the varix.

Persistent Intrahepatic Right Portal Vein

Description

Persistence of right portal vein rather than normal left-sided portal vein is called persistent intrahepatic right portal vein.

Incidence

The incidence of persistent intrahepatic right portal vein is approximately 0.2%. Blazer et al.[290] reported this finding in 1 per 438 among 30,240 low and high-risk consecutive pregnancies, and Hill et al.[291] found it in 1 per 476 among 15,237 consecutive pregnancies.

Pathology and Embryology

Development of the normal venous drainage is complex. At 4 weeks fetal age (6 weeks menstrual age), paired umbilical veins carry blood from the developing placenta to the primitive heart. At 5 weeks (7 menstrual weeks), they join an anastomotic venous network formed by the omphalomesenteric veins in the developing liver thereby establishing the umbilical-portal venous connection. By 6 weeks, the right umbilical vein regresses, and the left umbilical vein enlarges to accommodate the increasing flow. The umbilical vein now enters the left portal vein directly. The vast majority of blood flows through branches of the left and right portal veins, through the liver sinusoids, and eventually to the inferior vena cava via the hepatic veins. Development of the ductus venosus, however, permits a portion of returning blood to flow directly from the left portal vein to the sys-

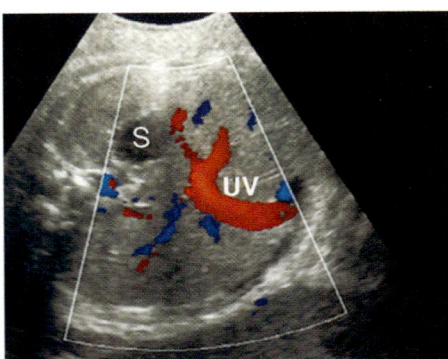

FIGURE 47. Persistent right umbilical vein. Transverse view of abdomen at 22 weeks shows the umbilical vein (*UV*) curving toward the stomach (*S*) rather than the liver. This is a relatively common vascular variant.

temic venous system. After birth, the intracorporeal umbilical vein obliterates to form the ligamentum teres within the falciform ligament, and the ductus venosus obliterates as part of the fissure for the ligamentum venosum.

Diagnosis

The diagnosis is not difficult, but can be easily overlooked (Fig. 47). The umbilical vein curves toward the left-sided stomach rather than toward the liver.[292] Also, the gallbladder is visualized medial to the umbilical vein rather than its normal lateral position.

Differential Diagnosis

No differential diagnosis exists for persistent intrahepatic right portal vein.

Associated Anomalies

Persistent intrahepatic right portal vein is usually an isolated finding but may have an increased association with other anomalies, similar to an SUA. Jeanty[292] first called attention to the increased risk of anomalies, and others have also observed a higher association of anomalies including cardiac anomalies.[293] Others have not observed other anomalies when it is an isolated finding.[294,295] Among 69 cases reported by Blazer et al.,[290] 60 had no additional sonographic abnormalities, four had transient nuchal findings, and four had minor anomalies or anatomic variants.

Prognosis and Management

The prognosis for persistent intrahepatic right portal vein is a normal outcome if no other anomalies are identified. Obstetric management should not be altered.

Velamentous Umbilical Cord Insertion

Description

Velamentous insertion is defined as insertion of the umbilical cord into the membranes before entering the placental tissue.

Incidence

Velamentous umbilical cord insertion occurs in approximately 1% of pregnancies. In comparison, marginal insertion of the umbilical cord into the periphery of the placenta has been reported in 2% to 10% of pregnancies.

Embryology and Pathology

Velamentous cord insertion may result from atrophy of parts of the placenta, because the umbilical cord insertion site marks the original site of implantation. Risk factors for velamentous insertion include abnormalities that may affect alignment of the embryonic body stalk at implantation. Such factors include uterine enlargement, multiple gestations, uterine anomalies, and pregnancies with an intrauterine device.

Diagnosis

The diagnosis can be established by showing insertion of the umbilical cord into membranes or margin of the placenta (Fig. 48). The sensitivity of diagnosing velamentous cord insertion has dramatically improved during the last decade, with routine use of color imaging and with increased awareness of the potential problems associated with it. Hence, the sensitivity has ranged from 0% in 1992[296] to 100% in 1998 with routine, systematic search for umbilical cord insertion using color-flow imaging.[77] The specificity is high.

Differential Diagnosis

Care should be taken to distinguish marginal/velamentous insertion of the umbilical cord from an adjacent free loop of the umbilical cord. Branching of vessels after insertion helps to confirm the correct diagnosis.

Associated Anomalies

Velamentous cord insertion has a higher frequency of twin-twin transfusion syndrome. Fries and colleagues[297] found velamentous cord insertion in 64% of those affected with twin-twin transfusion compared to 19% without twin-twin transfusion. Velamentous cord insertion also has a higher rate of other placental abnormalities and is an essential feature of vasa previa.

Prognosis and Management

Velamentous cord insertion is associated with higher risk of low birth weight, small for gestational age, preterm delivery, and lower Apgar scores.[298] Thrombosis is more common,[1] and cord rupture during traction of the cord may require manual extraction of the placenta. Velamentous cord insertion may be particularly important in monochorionic gestations. Monochorionic twins with velamentous cord insertion had a significantly higher rate of fetal twin-twin transfusion syndrome, perinatal mortality, and preterm delivery.[299] Those twin-twin transfusion syndrome pregnancies with velamentous insertions also deliver at a significantly earlier gestational age, and they had fewer surviving infants.[297] Monochorionic pregnancies with velamentous insertion should be carefully monitored for signs of twin-twin transfusion syndrome.

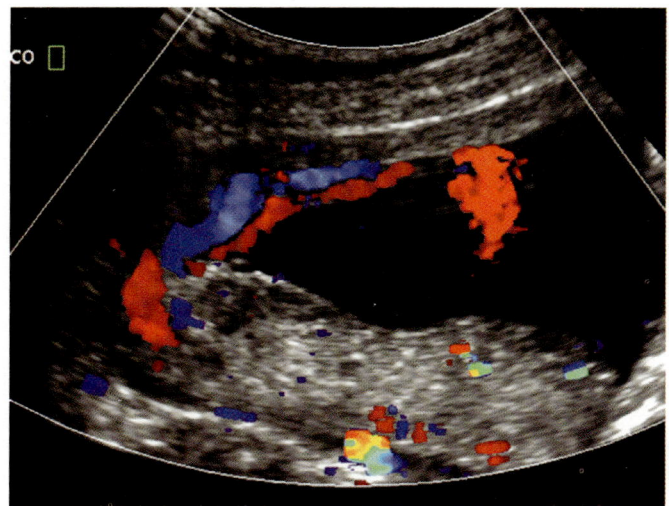

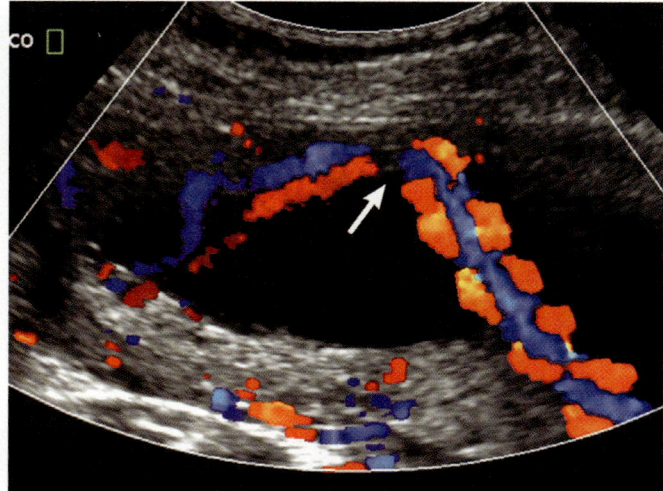

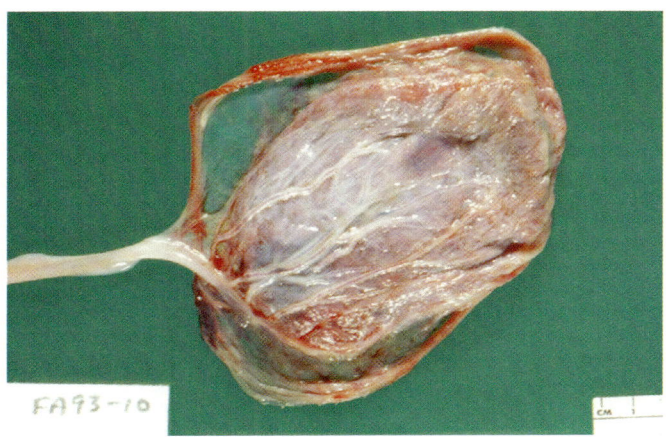

FIGURE 48. Velametous insertion of the umbilical cord. **A:** Right image shows the umbilical cord inserting into a velamentous site (*arrow*), separate from the posterior placenta. Left image shows umbilical vessels continuing in a submembranous location to the posterior placenta. **B:** Pathologic correlation confirms velamentous umbilical cord.

Whether management should be altered for singleton pregnancies with velamentous cord insertion is uncertain.

Masses of the Umbilical Cord

A variety of masses may be seen in association with the umbilical cord, especially at the fetal insertion site (Table 3). These may be subcategorized as cystic and solid lesions.

Cystic Lesions of the Umbilical Cord

Description
Umbilical cord cystic lesions may represent true cysts or pseudocysts, which can only be differentiated by histologic examination after delivery.

Incidence
The incidence for umbilical cord cystic lesions is unknown, but umbilical cord pseudocysts are far more common than true cysts.

Pathology and Embryology
True cysts are epithelial lined, whereas pseudocysts are caused by local degeneration or focal edema of the Wharton's jelly and, therefore, lack an epithelial lining. True umbilical cord cysts originate from embryonic remnants such as the allantois or omphalomesenteric duct.[1,2] Omphalomesenteric cysts originate from the vitelline duct.

TABLE 3. CAUSES OF UMBILICAL OR PARAUMBILICAL CORD MASS

Edema
Mucoid degeneration of Wharton's jelly
Allantoic duct cyst
Omphalomesenteric duct cyst
Urachal cyst
Hemangioma
Hematoma
Varix of umbilical vein
Omphalocele
Gastroschisis
Umbilical hernia

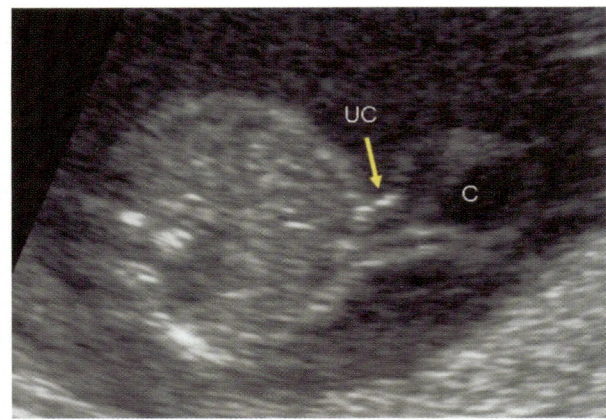 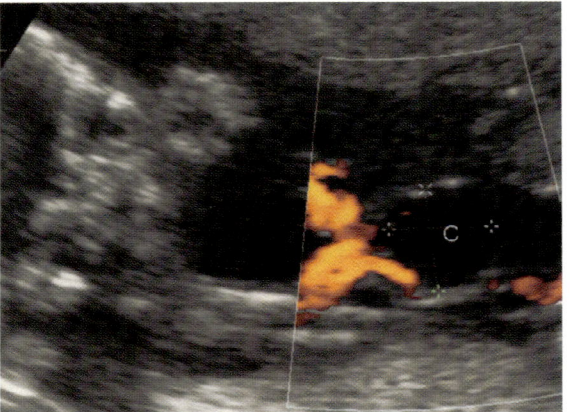

FIGURE 49. Umbilical cord cyst and trisomy 13. **A:** Transverse view of fetal cord insertion at 16 weeks shows a cystic area (*C*) associated with the umbilical cord (*UC*) consistent with a pseudocyst. **B:** Power Doppler confirms the cyst (*C*) is not a vascular structure. Other anomalies identified were a cardiac defect and echogenic intracardiac foci on the left and right ventricles of the heart.

The reason for the formation of umbilical cord pseudocyst is unknown. Factors such as an increased vascular pressure within the umbilicoplacental circulation leading to raised hydrostatic umbilical cord pressure favoring transfer of fluid into the Wharton's jelly have been suggested,[300] perhaps operative in cases of IUGR and abdominal wall defects. Focal degeneration, either cystic or mucoid, of Wharton's jelly in association with a local pathologic process of the umbilical cord is also associated with the formation of umbilical cord pseudocysts.[301] Pseudocysts are frequently associated with angiomyxoma of the cord, suggesting that exudation of plasma from the tumor is another etiologic factor in cyst formation.

Diagnosis
Most umbilical cord cystic lesions are discovered incidentally during ultrasound assessment. Most are located at either end of the umbilical cord—near the placenta or near the cord insertion into the fetus (Figs. 49 through 51). They can be overlooked because they are fluid-filled and so blend in with the amniotic fluid. The wall of the cyst is seen as a rounded structure of varying size. The cyst may contain internal echoes.

Prenatal diagnosis of allantoic cysts has been reported by several authors, usually in association with urachal anomalies.[302–308] In this condition, persistence of the communication between the bladder and the umbilical cord, known as *patent urachus*, allows extravasation of urine from the bladder into the base of the cord, resulting in cystic dilatation of the extraembryonic portion of the allantois. Less frequently, the urine may leak into the Wharton's jelly, resulting in a giant umbilical cord.[309,310] Although the differential diagnosis between allantoic cyst and other umbilical cord cystic masses is difficult, several ultrasound features may assist in the prenatal differential diagnosis. In cases of allantoic cysts, the umbilical cord cystic mass is always in close relationship with the fetal anterior abdominal wall, and, indeed, they are usually mistaken for anterior abdominal wall defects. Although not a true abdominal wall defect, allantoic cysts can, however, coexist with an omphalocele.[311] Careful examination of the umbilical cord insertion in the fetal abdomen can easily establish the diagnosis. A prenatal feature of allantoic cyst due to patent urachus is the identification of a communication between the cyst and the fetal bladder. This is not always present, however.

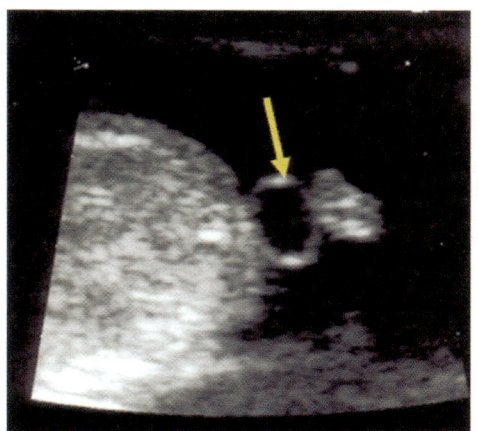 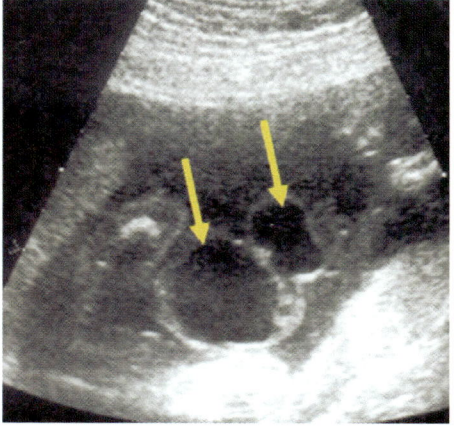

FIGURE 50. Variable size and appearance of umbilical cord cysts/pseudocysts. **A:** A small cyst (*arrow*) is present near the fetal insertion of the umbilical cord. **B:** Two adjacent cysts (*arrows*).

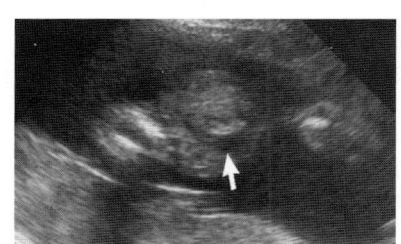
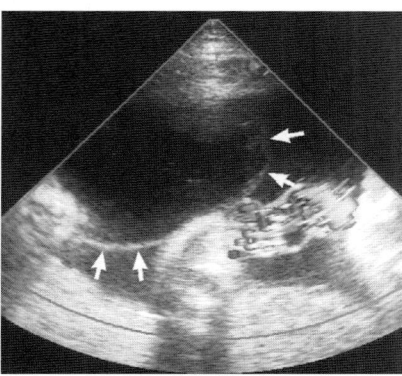

A,B

FIGURE 51. Pseudocyst associated with umbilical cord hemangioma (angiomyxoma). **A:** An echogenic mass *(arrow)* is seen of the umbilical cord. **B:** A large 9-cm pseudocyst *(arrows)* arises from the umbilical cord adjacent to the mass. Though the mass is large, it is difficult to visualize because it blends in with the amniotic fluid. Cystic areas are commonly demonstrated in association with umbilical cord hemangiomas and probably develop from transudation of fluid.

Color Doppler ultrasound allows the detection of another characteristic feature of allantoic cyst.[306] Embryologically, the allantois is the only vestigial remnant located at the center of the umbilical cord and surrounded by the umbilical vessels. If an allantoic cyst develops owing to retrograde micturition into the umbilical cord, progressive separation of the umbilical vessels occurs. By using color-flow imaging, it is then possible to identify umbilical vessels surrounding the cyst.[306,307] With other cystic lesions, the cyst is expected to push the vessels away altogether, and the umbilical vessels are seen in only one side of the cyst wall.

Prenatal documentation of resolution of allantoic cysts has been reported,[304] which does not necessarily mean that the urachus became obliterated, and, therefore, pediatric urology consultation is advised even in these cases. Once an allantoic cyst is diagnosed, it is advisable to perform regular follow-up examinations to monitor the size of the cyst. Color Doppler velocimetry of umbilical artery is also important because rapidly increasing cyst size has been reported to produce progressive obliteration of the blood flow within the cord, requiring immediate delivery.[312] In view of the high association with urachal anomalies, pediatric urology consultation is recommended.

Umbilical cord pseudocysts appear as a cystic lesion of variable size in association with the umbilical cord. The pseudocysts are usually located near the fetal insertion or in a free loop of the cord. Occasionally more than one cystic mass is detected, most often close to each other. In the case of angiomyxoma (see Solid Masses of the Umbilical Cord), the pseudocyst is always located close to the tumor and may be large (Fig. 51). Multiple small cysts seldom are detected in close relation to a localized thickening of Wharton's jelly; these cases have been noted in association with aneuploidies, mainly trisomy 18 and trisomy 13.[300]

First-Trimester Cysts

Prenatal diagnosis of umbilical cord cysts in the first trimester by means of transvaginal ultrasound has been reported.[313–316] These cysts usually resolve by the second trimester. The cyst must be clearly distinguished from the yolk sac, which has a more echoic wall and is extraamniotic in location. Color Doppler imaging is useful to exclude the possibility of a prominent umbilical vessel or an aneurysm and to document the relation with the umbilical vessels.

The origin of first-trimester umbilical cord cysts is still unknown. Current theories suggest that they probably represent embryonic remnants such as allantoic or omphalomesenteric cysts, amniotic inclusion cyst, or mucoid degeneration or edema of the Wharton's jelly (pseudocysts). In the only case in which sonographic-histopathologic correlation is available, an amniotic inclusion cyst and adjacent mucoid degeneration of the Wharton's jelly were found,[314] suggesting that first-trimester umbilical cord cysts could represent either entity. The rapid resolution of the cysts may favor that they represent pseudocysts rather than true cysts. Because the formation of cysts is coincidental with the onset of umbilical cord coiling and formation of the physiologic midgut hernia, these developmental phenomena could increase hydrostatic pressure within the umbilical vessels, favoring exudation of water into the Wharton's jelly and formation of pseudocysts.[315]

Differential Diagnosis

Intraamniotic membranes should be distinguished from umbilical cord cysts. Other umbilical abnormalities that can appear cystic on sonography include focal accumulation of Wharton's jelly with mucoid degeneration, resolving hematoma, focal dilatation of umbilical vessels, and umbilical cord hemangiomas. Abdominal wall defects should be readily distinguished.

Associated Anomalies

Allantoic cysts are frequently seen in association with urachal anomalies. In addition to cysts and polyps of the umbilical cord, omphalomesenteric duct remnants may give rise to Meckel's diverticula, intraabdominal mesenteric cysts, and anomalies of the umbilicus (e.g., fistulas, polyps, cysts). Other anomalies that have been associated with a patent omphalomesenteric duct include omphalocele, hernias, cardiac defects, trisomy 21, spina bifida, and cleft lip.

Initial reports described first-trimester umbilical cord cysts as transient and having no effect on pregnancy outcome,[313,314] but associated fetal structural anomalies and chromosomal defects in around 25% of cases have been reported in a high-risk population.[315] Most first-trimester umbilical cord cysts are, however, no longer present at the second-trimester follow-up scan, and they are usually associated with a normal pregnancy outcome.[316]

Pseudocysts have been associated with chromosomal defects and other congenital anomalies.[317–319] Of the 13 prenatally diagnosed umbilical cord cystic lesion pseudocysts reviewed by Smith et al.,[319] eight were associated with aneuploidy and two with other anomalies. Most reports, however, have been limited to isolated or small numbers of cases, thus precluding overall evaluation and limiting information for counseling. In the largest series of umbilical cord pseudocysts in a high-risk population,[300] chromosomal abnormalities were noted in 7 of 13 cases, and three additional euploid fetuses had structural defects. All cases of isolated umbilical cord pseudocyst were associated with a normal outcome.

Prognosis and Management

The prognosis and management varies with associated anomalies. Isolated cysts have a good prognosis and do not require alteration in obstetric management.

Solid Masses of the Umbilical Cord

Description

Solid masses of the umbilical cord may represent hemangioma (angiomyxoma),[320] hematoma,[321] or the rare teratoma.

Incidence

True tumors of the umbilical cord are rare.

Pathology and Embryology

Angiomyxomas, also known as *hemangiomas of the cord*, are hamartoma that arises from proliferation of the primitive angiogenic mesenchyme of the cord.[1–3] Hemangiomas of the umbilical cord are similar to hemangiomas of the placenta (i.e., chorioangiomas) in origin and significance. Benirschke and Dodds[251] have called these angiomyxomas because of the prominence of myxoid material.

Teratomas of the cord derive from germ cells.[1–3] Some controversy regarding its etiology exits basically because some investigators consider this entity to represent small acardiac twins rather than a true neoplasm.[322–325]

Diagnosis

Prenatal diagnosis of angiomyxomas (Figs. 51 and 52) has been made by a number of authors.[326–329] This tumor usually presents as a hyperechogenic mass in close relation to the umbilical vessels and is invariably associated with a pseudocyst of variable size. Sometimes the cyst is the most

prominent finding,[328,329] with one case reporting a 16-cm cyst that required prenatal aspiration to achieve vaginal delivery.[329] A very similar case, with the pseudocysts containing 400 mL of fluid, has been seen by the authors. Angiomyxomas of the cord can be considered the counterpart of chorioangioma of the placenta, a condition frequently associated with pregnancy complications. Most cases of angiomyxomas are incidental findings. Hemangiomas and angiomyxomas have been associated with elevated MSAFP levels.[328]

Teratoma of the umbilical cord has been observed in several cases.[330] These tumors have a variable presentation. Among ten cases reviewed by Satge et al.,[330] four fetuses and infants died.

Differential Diagnosis

Other masses of the umbilical cord, including omphalocele,[331] should be considered when the mass is at the insertion site of the fetus.

Associated Anomalies

Satge et al.[330] reported a large umbilical cord teratoma associated with an omphalocele.

Prognosis and Management

The possibility of compression of the adjacent umbilical vessels and fetal hydrops leading to fetal death should prompt fetal surveillance on serial ultrasound exams. Like placental chorioangiomas, umbilical cord hemangiomas may be associated with fetal hydrops and elevated MSAFP.[332] Fetal demise occasionally has been reported from umbilical cord hemangioma, possibly secondary to umbilical cord compression.

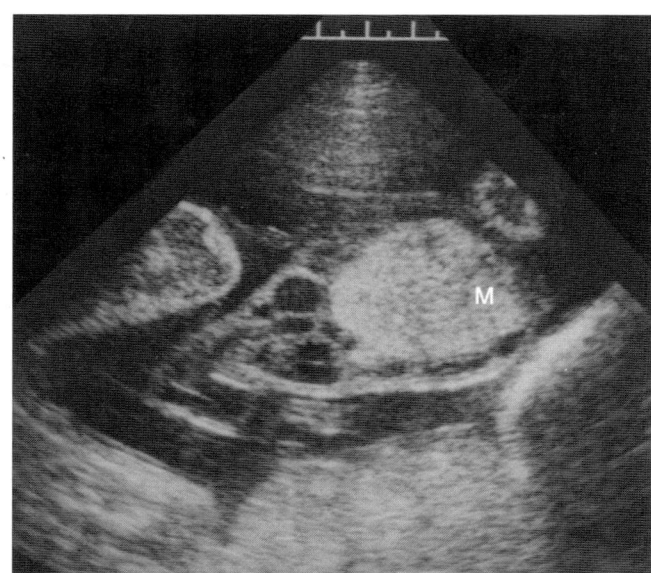

FIGURE 52. Angiomyxoma. Large echogenic mass (*M*) arises from the umbilical cord.

TABLE 4. TYPES OF INTRAUTERINE MEMBRANES

Chorioamnionic separation
Chorioamnionic elevation (subchorionic hemorrhage)
Multiple gestations
  Dichorionic
  Monochorionic, diamniotic
Intrauterine synechiae
Amniotic bands (rare)
Uterine septum

MEMBRANES

Various intrauterine membranes, septations, and bands have been described in and about the amniotic cavity (Table 4). The most common include chorioamnionic separation, chorioamnionic elevation, membranes of twins and blighted ova, and amniotic sheet (synechiae) in addition to umbilical cord cysts and pseudocysts. Oblique scans of circumvallate placenta or prominent marginal sinuses of the placenta may also simulate a membrane. Recognition of these common, *benign* types of membranes is important so they are not confused with amniotic bands.

Embryogenesis

The fetal membranes are composed of the chorion, amnion, allantois, and yolk sac. The chorion originates from trophoblastic cells and remains intimately in contact with trophoblasts throughout pregnancy. The amnion develops at approximately the twenty-eighth menstrual day from cytotrophoblasts immediately adjacent to the dorsal aspect of the bilaminar embryonic disk. Initially, the amnion is attached to the margins of the embryonic disk. By 16 menstrual weeks, the amnion fuses with the chorion, thereby obliterating the space between them (extraembryonic coelom).

Amniotic Sheets

Synonyms include intrauterine *synechiae*, amniotic *sheets*, or *pillars*. Amniotic sheets are linear, extraamniotic tissue that projects into the amniotic cavity.

Incidence

The incidence of amniotic sheets is approximately 1 per 200. An amniotic sheet was identified in 0.45% of 17,553 pregnancies between 12 and 28 weeks' gestation[333] and 0.47% of 29,543 pregnancies in another series.[334]

Pathology

Mahony et al. first described the sonographic appearance of such membranes in a series of seven patients.[335] The

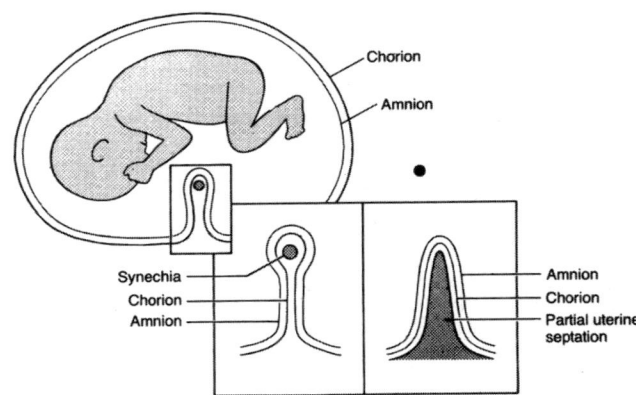

FIGURE 53. Schematic drawing of intrauterine amniotic sheet (synechia). A layer of amnion and chorion is draped over an intrauterine synechia or septum. There is no restriction of fetal motion. (Reproduced with permission from Mahony BS, Filly RA, Callen PW, et al. The amniotic band syndrome: antenatal sonographic diagnosis and potential pitfalls. *Am J Obstet Gynecol* 1985;152:63–68.)

authors suggested that these structures represent intrauterine synechiae covered by a layer of amnion and chorion. Others have also found a higher frequency of uterine procedures.[336] Although the synechiae appear to be within the amniotic fluid, they are anatomically external to the amniotic sac (Fig. 53).[335]

Diagnosis

Amniotic sheets are diagnosed prenatally, almost always as an incidental finding. Characteristically, the membrane demonstrates a broad base that probably represents the synechia itself; the placental margin occasionally may attach to this base (Figs. 54 and 55). The placenta is contiguous with, is indented by, or extends along the synechia in up to two-thirds of cases. The placenta appeared implanted on the amniotic sheet in 41 (26.1%) of 157 patients.[337] The membrane causes no fetal entrapment and does not adhere to the fetus. No associated fetal deformities exist, and fetal parts move freely around the membrane.

In the late third trimester, the membrane no longer may be visualized as it becomes obliterated or compressed. Amniotic sheets caused by preexisting uterine synechiae may be recognized in pregnancy by presence of a bulbous free edge containing a hypoechoic zone and Y-shaped splitting of the sheet at the endometrial margin. Previous curettage had been done in the majority of these patients.[338]

Differential Diagnosis

Septated uterus should be considered when the membrane courses in an anterior-posterior direction and is located at the fundal aspect of the uterus. Circumvallate placenta shows a

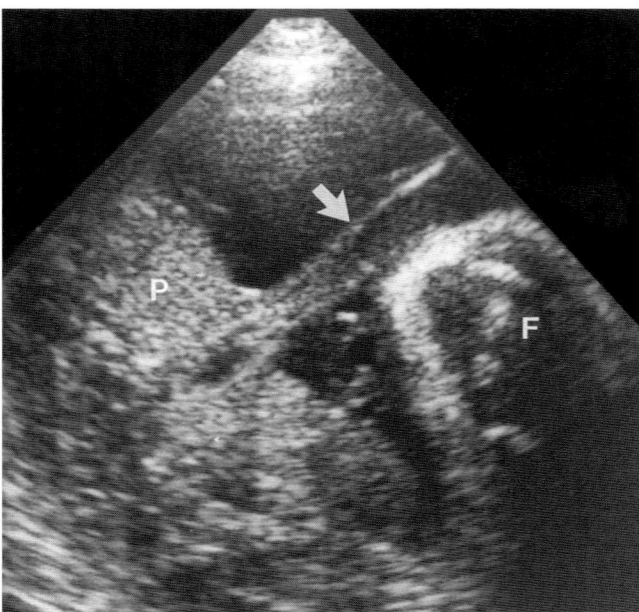

FIGURE 54. Amniotic sheet. Scan shows intrauterine membrane (*arrow*) representing amniotic sheet or synechia. The fetus (*F*) is freely mobile around the membrane. P, placenta.

ridge or shelf of placental tissue, and this may simulate a synechiae when seen in parallel with the placental rim. Amniotic band syndrome rarely shows the actual bands, and the fetal defects dominate the sonographic picture.

Associated Anomalies

No associated anomalies exist for amniotic sheets.

Prognosis

Amniotic sheets do not cause fetal damage, but can occasionally compartmentalize a large component of the amniotic fluid, thereby limiting fetal mobility. For this reason, an association exists between amniotic sheets and abnormal fetal presentation (i.e., breech or transverse).

Although others have observed this association, it may depend on the course of the sheet. Sheets orientated perpendicular to the placental surface were more likely to be associated with an abnormal presentation at delivery compared to nonperpendicular sheets, seen either oblique or parallel in orientation to the placental surface.[333]

Management

Obstetric management depends on orientation of the fetus at term. No change in management is required for amniotic sheets alone.

Chorion-Amniotic Membrane Separation

Description

Chorioamnionic separation is defined as separation of the amnion and chorion.

Incidence

The incidence of chorion-amniotic membrane separation varies with gestational age. This finding is normal until normal fusion at approximately 14 to 16 menstrual weeks.

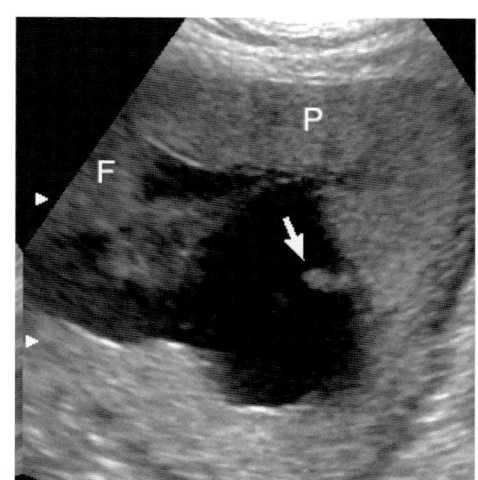
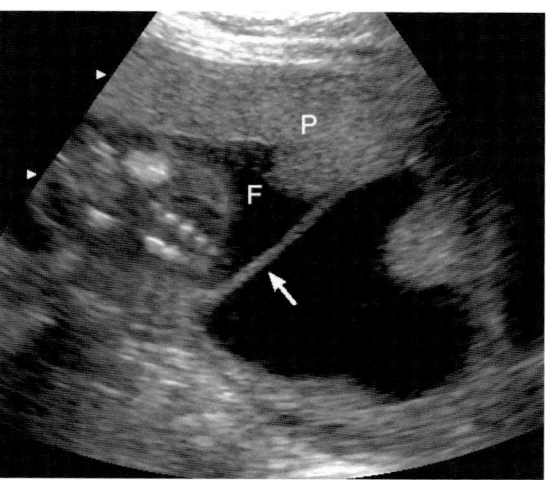

FIGURE 55. Amniotic sheet. **A:** A small wedge of tissue (*arrow*) is seen. F, fetus; P, placenta. **B:** Scan just lateral to image **(A)** shows characteristic amniotic sheet (*arrow*) attaching to the anterior and posterior walls. Note that the placenta (*P*) is characteristically contiguous to the synechia and may partly extend onto it. Also note the fetus (*F*) is above the sheet. Sheets orientated perpendicular to the placental surface, as in this case, are more likely to be associated with an abnormal presentation at delivery compared to nonperpendicular sheets seen in oblique or parallel orientation relative to the placental surface.

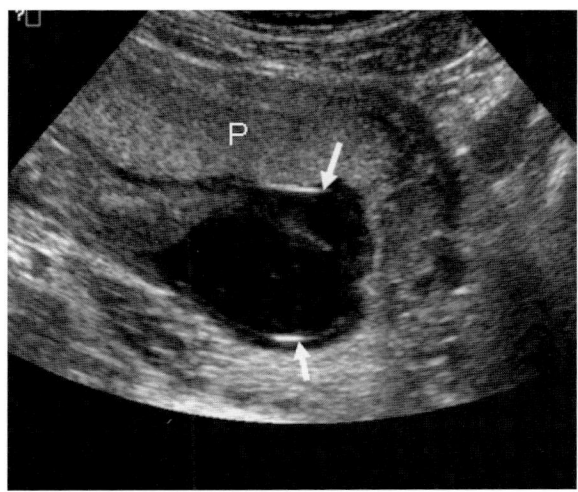
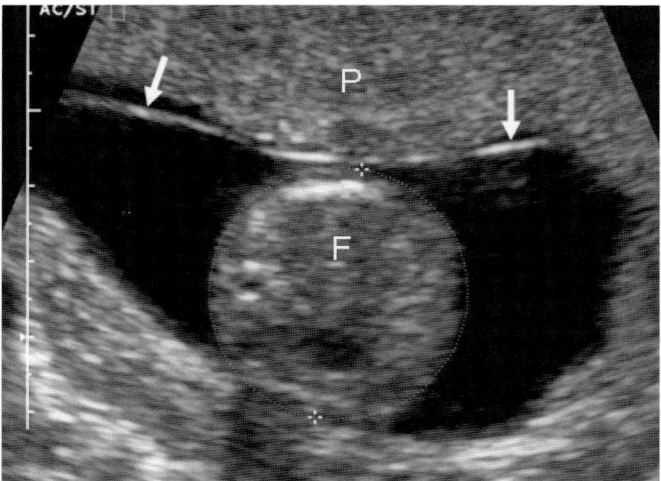

FIGURE 56. Chorioamnionic separation. **A:** Scan at 16 weeks shows detachment of the amnion (*arrows*) from the chorion. P, placenta. **B:** Unfused amnion (*arrows*) extends on surface of placenta (*P*). F, fetus.

Levine et al.[339] found some degree of separation in 25% of 388 women who underwent genetic amniocentesis.

Pathology

Chorioamnionic separation may represent primary nonfusion of the amnion or chorion, or secondary separation. Nonfusion represents persistence of the extraembryonic coelomic space. Secondary separation is usually iatrogenic from amniocentesis but can also result from polyhydramnios.

Diagnosis

The sonographic diagnosis of separation is possible when the amnion is visible as a discrete membrane separate from the chorion (Fig. 56). Because the amnion is a very thin, pliable membrane, it is usually seen only when it lies perpendicular to the ultrasound beam. Careful examination occasionally shows that the space between the amnion and chorion (i.e., extraembryonic coelom) demonstrates a different echo pattern than amniotic fluid. Unlike elevation, the membrane does not end at the placental margin but rather continues to the base of the umbilical cord. The yolk sac is always located between the amnion and chorion.

Differential Diagnosis

Chorioamnionic separation should be distinguished from chorioamnionic elevation (Fig. 57). Because the chorion is normally adherent to the myometrium and the chorionic plate

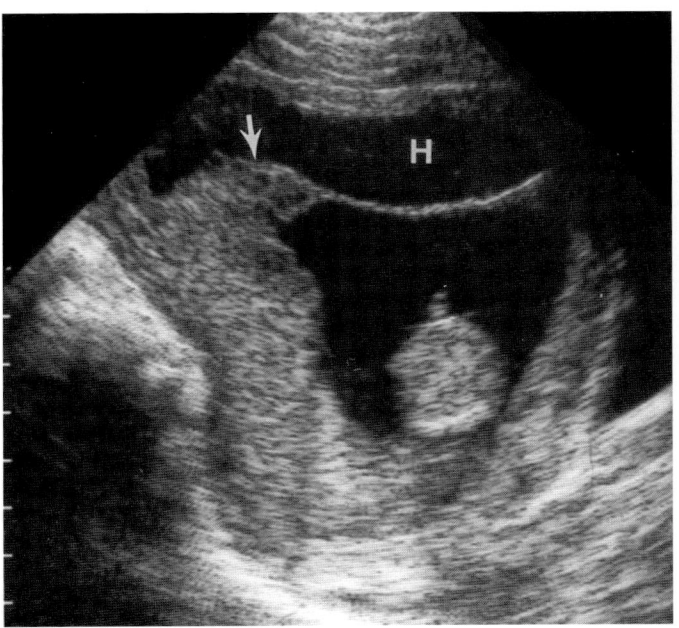
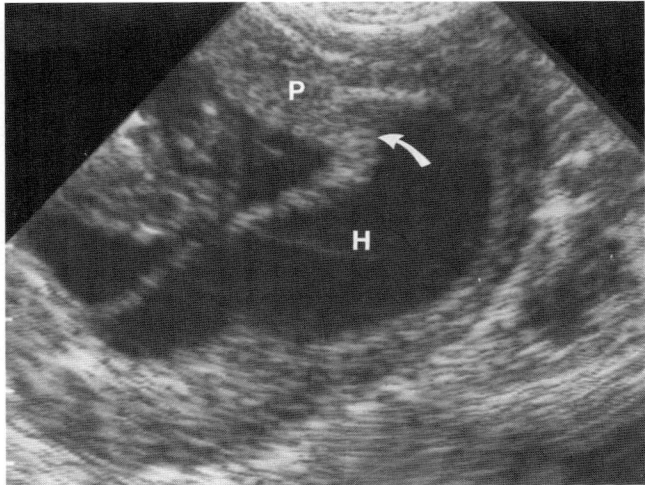

FIGURE 57. A, B: Subchorionic hemorrhage. Two examples of sonolucent hemorrhage (*H*) beneath the chorionic membranes. The margin (*arrows*) of the placenta (*P*) is elevated. Subchorionic hemorrhage with chorioamnionic elevation should be distinguished from other types of membranes.

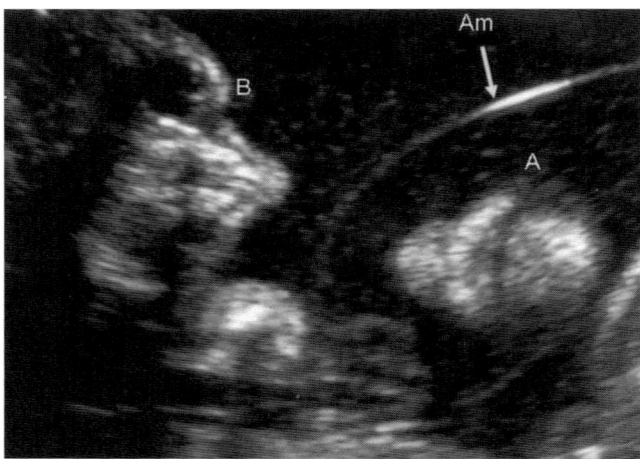

FIGURE 58. Amnion. Amniotic membrane in a monochorionic, diamniotic twin pregnancy represents two opposed layers of amnion. The thin amnionic membrane (*Am*) shows the highest amplitude where the membrane is perpendicular to the ultrasound beam and becomes difficult to visualize as it curves parallel to the ultrasound beam. A, twin A; B, twin B.

of the placenta, demonstration of chorioamnionic elevation implies the presence of underlying hemorrhage or other mass lesion. The amnion from a monochorionic, diamniotic twin gestation is identified by its separation of two fetuses (Fig. 58).

Associated Anomalies

Nonfusion of the amnion after 14 weeks has been associated with fetal aneuploidy in several studies (see Chapter 21).[340,341]

Prognosis and Management

Partial separation is usually a benign finding that resolves. Complete separation has been associated with adverse outcome including fetal distress and death.[339] Rupture of the amnion can result in entanglement of the umbilical cord or fetal parts, leading to fetal distress and death.[342] Management is observation alone.

REFERENCES

1. Benirschke K, Kaufmann P. *Pathology of the human placenta*, 4th ed. New York: Springer-Verlag, 2000.
2. Fox H. Pathology of the umbilical cord. In: Fox H, ed. *Pathology of the placenta*, 2nd ed. London: WB Saunders, 1997:418–452.
3. Fox H. *Pathology of the placenta*, 2nd ed. London: WB Saunders, 1997.
4. Moore KL. *The developing human*, 4th ed. Philadelphia: WB Saunders, 1988:104–130.
5. Nyberg DA, Finberg HF. The placenta. In: Nyberg DA, Mahony BS, Pretorius DH, eds. *Diagnostic ultrasound of fetal anomalies: text and atlas*. Chicago: Year Book Publishers, 1990.
6. Hoddick WK, Mahony BS, Callen PW, et al. Placental thickness. *J Ultrasound Med* 1985;4:479–482.
7. Harris RD, Alexander RD. Ultrasound of the placenta and umbilical cord. In: Callen PW, ed. *Ultrasonography in obstetrics and gynecology*, 4th ed. Philadelphia: WB Saunders, 2000:597–625.
8. Bernstein IM, Barth RA, Miller R, et al. Elevated maternal serum alpha-fetoprotein: association with placental sonolucencies, fetomaternal hemorrhage, vaginal bleeding, and pregnancy outcome in the absence of fetal anomalies. *Obstet Gynecol* 1992;79:71–74.
9. Kelly RB, Nyberg DA, Mack LA, et al. Sonography of placental abnormalities and oligohydramnios in women with elevated alpha-fetoprotein levels: comparison with control subjects. *AJR Am J Roentgenol* 1989;153(4):815–819.
10. Jauniaux E, Moscoso G, Campbell S, et al. Correlation of ultrasound and pathologic findings of placental anomalies in pregnancies with elevated maternal serum alpha-fetoprotein. *Eur J Obstet Gynecol Reprod Biol* 1990;37:219–230.
11. Raga F, Ballester MJ, Osborne NG, et al. Subchorionic placental cyst: a cause of fetal growth retardation-ultrasound and color-flow Doppler diagnosis and follow-up. *J Natl Med Assoc* 1996;88:285–288.
12. Ferrara N, Menditto C, Di Marino MP, et al. Subchorionic placental cyst: histopathological and clinical aspects in two cases. *Pathologica* 1996;88:439–443.
13. Jauniaux E, Avni FE, Elkhazen N, et al. Morphologic study of ultrasonic placental anomalies in the second half of pregnancy. *J Gynecol Obstet Biol Reprod* (Paris) 1989;18:601–613.
14. Callen P, Filly R. The placental subplacental complex: a specific indicator of placental position on ultrasound. *J Clin Ultrasound* 1980;8:21–26.
15. Geirsson RT, Ogston SA, Patel NB, et al. Growth of total intrauterine, intra-amniotic and placental volume in normal singleton pregnancy measured by ultrasound. *Br J Obstet Gynaecol* 1985;92:46–53.
16. Elchalal U, Ezra Y, Levi Y, et al. Sonographically thick placenta: a marker for increased perinatal risk—a prospective cross-sectional study. *Placenta* 2000;21:268–272.
17. Wolf H, Oosting H, Treffers PE. Second-trimester placental volume measurement by ultrasound: prediction of fetal outcome. *Am J Obstet Gynecol* 1989;160:121–126.
18. Hafner E, Philipp T, Schuchter K, et al. Second-trimester measurements of placental volume by three-dimensional ultrasound to predict small-for-gestational-age infants. *Ultrasound Obstet Gynecol* 1998;12:97–102.
19. Tongsong T, Wanapirak C, Sirichotiyakul S. Placental thickness at mid-pregnancy as a predictor of Hb Bart's disease. *Prenat Diagn* 1999;19:1027–1030.
20. Ko TM, Tseng LH, Hsu PM, et al. Ultrasonographic scanning of placental thickness and the prenatal diagnosis of homozygous alpha-thalassemia in the second trimester. *Prenat Diagn* 1995;15:7–10.
21. Ghosh A, Tang MH, Lam YH, et al. Ultrasound measurement of placental thickness to detect pregnancies affected by homozygous alpha-thalassaemia-1. *Lancet* 1994;344:988–989.
22. Nicolaides KH, Rizzo G, Hecher K. Screening for placental insufficiency by uterine artery Doppler. In: Nicolaides KH, Rizzo G, Hecher K, eds. *Placental and fetal Doppler*. Carnforth: Parthenon Press, 2000:89–104.

23. Goplerud CP. Bleeding in late pregnancy. In: Danforth DN, ed. *Obstetrics and gynecology*, 3rd ed. Hagerstown, MD: Harper & Row, 1977:378–384.

24. Jauniaux E, Auni FE, Conner C, et al. Ultrasonographic diagnosis and morphologic study of placenta circumvallate. *J Clin Ultrasound* 1989;17:126–131.

25. Bey M, Dott A, Miller JM. The sonographic diagnosis of circumvallate placenta. *Obstet Gynecol* 1991;78:515–517.

26. McCarthy J, Thurmond AS, Jones MK, et al. Circumvallate placenta: sonographic diagnosis. *J Ultrasound Med* 1995;14:21–26.

27. Harris RD, Wells WA, Black WC, et al. Accuracy of prenatal sonography for detecting circumvallate placenta. *AJR Am J Roentgenol* 1997;168:1603–1608.

28. Rolschau J. Circumvallate placenta and intrauterine growth retardation. *Acta Obstet Gynecol Scand Suppl* 1978;72:11–14.

29. Cutillo DP, Swayne LC, Schwartz JR, et al. Intra-amniotic hemorrhage secondary to placenta circumvallate. *J Ultrasound Med* 1989;8:399–401.

30. Nelson LH, Fishburne JI, Stearns BR. Ultrasonographic description of succentruiate placenta. *Obstet Gynecol* 1977;49:79–80.

31. Spirt BA, Kagan EH, Gordon LP, et al. Antepartum diagnosis of a succenturiate lobe: sonographic and pathologic correlation. *J Clin Ultrasound* 1981;9:139–140.

32. Hata K, Hata T, Aoki S, et al. Succenturiate placenta diagnosed by ultrasound. *Gynecol Obstet Invest* 1988;25:273–276.

33. Meizner I, Mashiach R, Shalev Y, et al. Blood flow velocimetry in the diagnosis of succenturiate placenta. *J Clin Ultrasound* 1998;26:55.

34. Artis AA III, Bowie JD, Rosenberg ER, et al. The fallacy of placental migration: effect of sonographic techniques. *AJR Am J Roentgenol* 1985;144:79–81.

35. Townsend RT, Laing FC, Nyberg DA, et al. Technical factors responsible for "placental migration:" sonographic assessment. *Radiology* 1986;160:105–108.

36. Khan AT, Stewart KS. Ultrasound placental localisation in early pregnancy. *Scotl Med J* 1987;32:19–21.

37. Green-Thompson RW. Antepartum hemorrhage. *Clin Obstet Gynecol* 1982;9:479–515.

38. Hibbard LT: Placenta praevia. *Am J Obstet Gynecol* 1969;104:172–176.

39. Clark SL. Placenta previa and abruptio placentae. In: Creasy RK, Resnik R, eds. *Maternal fetal medicine*, 4th ed. Philadelphia: WB Saunders, 1999:616–631.

40. Laing FC. Ultrasound evaluation of obstetric problems relating to the lower uterine segment and cervix. In: Sanders RC, James AE Jr, eds. *The principles and practice of ultrasonography in obstetrics and gynecology*, 3rd ed. Norwalk, CT: Apple-Century-Crofts, 1985:355–367.

41. Kobayashi M, Hellman LM, Fillisti L. Placental localization by ultrasound. *Am J Obstet Gynecol* 1970;106:279–285.

42. Mittelstaedt CA, Partain CL, Boyce IL Jr, et al. Placenta previa: significance in the second trimester. *Radiology* 1979;131:465–468.

43. Naeye RL. Placenta previa: predisposing factors and effects on the fetus and surviving infants. *Obstet Gynecol* 1978;52:521–525.

44. Newton ER, Barss V, Cetrulo CL. The epidemiology and clinical history of asymptomatic midtrimester placenta previa. *Am J Obstet Gynecol* 1984;148:743–748.

45. Scheer K. Ultrasonic diagnosis of placenta previa. *Obstet Gynecol* 1973;42:707–710.

46. Chapman MG, Furness ET, Jones WR, et al. Significance of the ultrasound location of placental site in early pregnancy. *Br J Obstet Gynaecol* 1979;86:846–848.

47. Rizos N, Doran TA, Miskin M, et al. Natural history of placenta previa ascertained by diagnostic ultrasound. *Am J Obstet Gynecol* 1979;133:287–291.

48. Comeau J, Shaw L, Marcell CC, et al. Early placenta previa and delivery outcome. *Obstet Gynecol* 1983;61:577–580.

49. Ancona S, Chatterjee M, Rhee I, et al. The mid-trimester placenta previa: a prospective follow-up. *Eur J Radiol* 1990;10:215–216.

50. Lauria MR, Smith RS, Treadwell MC, et al. The use of second-trimester transvaginal sonography to predict placenta previa. *Ultrasound Obstet Gynecol* 1996;8:337–340.

51. Farine D, Fox HE, Jakobson S, et al. Vaginal ultrasound for diagnosis of placenta previa. *Am J Obstet Gynecol* 1988;159:566–569.

52. Dawson WB, Dumas MD, Romano WM, et al. Translabial ultrasonography and placenta previa: does measurement of the os-placenta distance predict outcome? *J Ultrasound Med* 1996;15:441–446.

53. Smith RS, Lauria MR, Comstock CH, et al. Transvaginal ultrasonography for all placentas that appear to be low-lying or over the internal cervical os. *Ultrasound Obstet Gynecol* 1997;9:22–24.

54. Hill LM, DiNofrio DM, Chenevey P. Transvaginal sonographic evaluation of first-trimester placenta previa. *Ultrasound Obstet Gynecol* 1995;5:301–303.

55. Ghourab S. Third-trimester transvaginal ultrasonography in placenta previa: does the shape of the lower placental edge predict clinical outcome? *Ultrasound Obstet Gynecol* 2001;18:103–108.

56. Reference deleted.

57. Reference deleted.

58. Butler EL, Dashe JS, Ramus RM. Association between maternal serum alpha-fetoprotein and adverse outcomes in pregnancies with placenta previa. *Obstet Gynecol* 2001;97(1):35–38.

59. Oyelese KO, Turner M, Lees C, et al. Vasa previa: an avoidable obstetric tragedy. *Obstet Gynecol Surv* 1999;54(2):138–145.

60. Young M, Yu N, Barham K. The role of light and sound technologies in the detection of vasa praevia. *Reprod Fertil Dev* 1991;3:439–451.

61. Gianopoulos J, Carver T, Tomich PG, et al. Diagnosis of vasa previa with ultrasonography. *Obstet Gynecol* 1987;69:488–491.

62. Hurley VA. The antenatal diagnosis of vasa praevia: the role of ultrasound. *Aust N Z J Obstet Gynaecol* 1988;28:177–179.

63. Harding JA, Lewis DF, Major CA, et al. Color flow Doppler—a useful instrument in the diagnosis of vasa previa. *Am J Obstet Gynecol* 1990;163:1566–1568.

64. Nelson LH, Melone PJ, King M. Diagnosis of vasa previa with transvaginal and color flow Doppler ultrasound. *Obstet Gynecol* 1990;76:506–509.

65. Hsieh FJ, Chen HF, Ko TM, et al. Antenatal diagnosis of vasa previa by color-flow mapping. *J Ultrasound Med* 1991;10:397–399.

66. Hata K, Hata T, Fujiwaki R, et al. An accurate antenatal diagnosis of vasa previa with transvaginal color Doppler ultrasonography. *Am J Obstet Gynecol* 1994;171:265–267.

67. Meyer WJ, Blumenthal L, Cadkin A, et al. Vasa previa: prenatal diagnosis with transvaginal color Doppler flow imaging. *Am J Obstet Gynecol* 1993;169(6):1627–1629.

68. Daly Jones E, Hollingsworth J, Sepulveda W. Vasa praevia: second trimester diagnosis using colour flow imaging. *Br J Obstet Gynaecol* 1996;103:284–286.

69. Devesa R, Muñoz A, Torrents M, et al. Prenatal diagnosis of vasa previa with transvaginal color Doppler ultrasound. *Ultrasound Obstet Gynecol* 1996;8:139–141.

70. Clerici G, Burnelli L, Lauro V, et al. Prenatal diagnosis of vasa previa presenting as amniotic band. 'A not so innocent amniotic band.' *Ultrasound Obstet Gynecol* 1996;7: 61–63.

71. Baschat AA, Gembruch U. Ante- and intrapartum diagnosis of vasa praevia in singleton pregnancies by colour coded Doppler sonography. *Eur J Obstet Gynecol Reprod Biol* 1998;79:19–25.

72. Oyelese KO, Schwärzler P, Coates S, et al. A strategy for reducing the mortality rate from vasa previa using transvaginal sonography with color Doppler. *Ultrasound Obstet Gynecol* 1998;12:434–438.

73. Hertzberg BS, Kliewer MA. Vasa previa: prenatal diagnosis by transperineal sonography with Doppler evaluation. *J Clin Ultrasound* 1998;26:405–408.

74. Fleming AD, Johnson C, Targy M. Diagnosis of vasa previa with ultrasound and color flow Doppler. *Nebr Med J* 1996;81:191–193.

75. Megier P, Desroches A, Esperandieu O, et al. Prenatal diagnosis of vasa previa with velamentous cord insertion, using Doppler color echography. *J Gynecol Obstet Biol Reprod* (Paris) 1995;24:415–417.

76. Raga F, Ballester MJ, Osborne NG, et al. Role of color flow Doppler ultrasonography in diagnosing velamentous insertion of the umbilical cord and vasa previa. A report of two cases. *J Reprod Med* 1995;40:804–808.

77. Nomiyama M, Toyota Y, Kawano H. Antenatal diagnosis of velamentous umbilical cord insertion and vasa previa with color Doppler imaging. *Ultrasound Obstet Gynecol* 1998;12: 426–429.

78. Devesa R, Munoz A, Torrents M, et al. Prenatal diagnosis of vasa previa with transvaginal color Doppler ultrasound. *Ultrasound Obstet Gynecol* 1996;8(2):139–141.

79. Sauerbrei EE, Davies GL. Diagnosis of vasa previa with endovaginal color Doppler and power Doppler sonography: report of two cases. *J Ultrasound Med* 1998;17:393–398.

80. Reference deleted.

81. Catanzarite V, Maida C, Thomas W, et al. Prenatal sonographic diagnosis of vasa previa: ultrasound findings and obstetric outcome in ten cases. *Ultrasound Obstet Gynecol* 2001;18:109–115.

82. Lee W, Kirk JS, Comstock CH, et al. Vasa previa: prenatal detection by three-dimensional ultrasonography. *Ultrasound Obstet Gynecol* 2000;16(4):384–387.

83. Fung TY, Lau TK. Poor perinatal outcome associated with vasa previa: is it preventable? A report of three cases and review of the literature. *Ultrasound Obstet Gynecol* 1998;12:430–433.

84. Ota Y, Watanabe H, Fukasawa I, et al. Placenta accreta/ increta. Review of 10 cases and a case report. *Arch Gynecol Obstet* 1999;263(1–2):69–72.

85. Avila C, Devine P, Lowre C, et al. Accuracy of prenatal ultrasonography in the diagnosis of placenta accreta, increta or percreta. *Am J Obstet Gynecol* 2001;185(6):s256.

86. Pasto ME, Kurtz AB, Rifkin MD, et al. Ultrasonographic findings in placenta increta. *J Ultrasound Med* 1983;2:155–159.

87. Kerr de Mendonça L. Sonographic diagnosis of placenta accreta. Presentation of six cases. *J Ultrasound Med* 1988;7:211–215.

88. Finberg HJ, Williams JW. Placenta accreta: prospective sonographic diagnosis in patients with placenta previa and prior cesarean section. *J Ultrasound Med* 1992;11:333–343.

89. Hoffman-Tretin JC, Koenigsberg M, Rabin A, et al. Placenta accreta. Additional sonographic observations. *J Ultrasound Med* 1992;11:29–34.

90. Jauniaux E, Toplis PJ, Nicolaides KH. Sonographic diagnosis of a non-previa placenta accreta. *Ultrasound Obstet Gynecol* 1996;7:58–60.

91. Silver LE, Hobel CJ, Lagasse L, et al. Placenta previa percreta with bladder involvement: new considerations and review of the literature. *Ultrasound Obstet Gynecol* 1997;9:131–138.

92. Chou MM, Ho ES, Lee YH. Prenatal diagnosis of placenta previa accreta by transabdominal color Doppler ultrasound. *Ultrasound Obstet Gynecol* 2000;15:28–35.

93. Mégier P, Gorin V, Desroches A. Ultrasonography of placenta previa at the third trimester of pregnancy: research for signs of placenta accreta/percreta and vasa previa. Prospective color and pulsed Doppler ultrasonography study of 45 cases. *J Gynecol Obstet Biol Reprod* (Paris) 1999;28:239–244.

94. Krapp M, Baschat AA, Hankeln M, et al. Gray scale and color Doppler sonography in the third stage of labor for early detection of failed placental separation. *Ultrasound Obstet Gynecol* 2000;15:138–142.

95. Thorp JM Jr, Councell RB, Sandridge DA, et al. Antepartum diagnosis of placenta previa percreta by magnetic resonance imaging. *Obstet Gynecol* 1992;80(3 Pt 2):506–508.

96. Maldjian C, Adam R, Pelosi M, et al. MRI appearance of placenta percreta and placenta accreta. *Magn Reson Imaging* 1999;17(7):965–971.

97. Ha TP, Li KC. Placenta accreta: MRI antenatal diagnosis and surgical correlation. *J Magn Reson Imaging* 1998;8(3): 748–750.

98. Carlton SM, Zahn CM, Kendall BS, et al. Placenta increta/ percreta associated with uterine perforation during therapy for fetal death. A case report. *J Reprod Med* 2001;46(6):601–605.

99. Oral B, Guney M, Ozsoy M, et al. Placenta accreta associated with a ruptured pregnant rudimentary uterine horn. Case report and review of the literature. *Arch Gynecol Obstet* 2001;265(2):100–102.

100. Taylor AA, Sanusi FA, Riddle AF. Expectant management of placenta accreta following stillbirth at term: a case report. *Eur J Obstet Gynecol Reprod Biol* 2001;96(2):220–222.

101. Mussalli GM, Shah J, Berck DJ, et al. Placenta accreta and methotrexate therapy: three case reports. *J Perinatol* 2000; 20(5):331–334.

102. Levine AB, Kuhlman K, Bonn J. Placenta accreta: comparison of cases managed with and without pelvic artery balloon catheters. *J Matern Fetal Med* 1999;8(4):173–176.

103. Descargues G, Clavier E, Lemercier E, et al. Placenta percreta with bladder invasion managed by arterial emboliza-

tion and manual removal after cesarean. *Obstet Gynecol* 2000;96(5 Pt 2):840.

104. Kidney DD, Nguyen AM, Ahdoot D, et al. Prophylactic perioperative hypogastric artery balloon occlusion in abnormal placentation. *AJR Am J Roentgenol* 2001;176(6):1521–1524.

105. Nyberg DA, Cyr DR, Mack LA, et al. Sonographic spectrum of placental abruption. *AJR Am J Roentgenol* 1987; 148:161–164.

106. Douglas RG, Buchman ML, MacDonald FA. Premature separation of the normally implanted placenta. *J Obstet Gynecol* 1955;72:710–736.

107. Nyberg DA, Mack LA, Benedetti TJ, et al. Placental abruption and placental hemorrhage: correlation of sonographic findings with fetal outcome. *Radiology* 1987;164;357–361.

108. Odendaal HJ. The frequency of uterine contractions in abruptio placentae. *S Africa Med J* 1976;50:2129–2131.

109. Sauerbrei EE, Pham DH. Placental abruption and subchorionic hemorrhage in the first half of pregnancy: ultrasound appearance and clinical outcome. *Radiology* 1986;160:109–112.

110. Mintz MC, Kurtz AB, Arenson R, et al. Abruptio placentae: apparent thickening of the placenta caused by hyperechoic retroplacental clot. *J Ultrasound Med* 1986;5:411–413.

111. Kojima K, Suzuki Y, Makino A, et al. A case of massive subchorionic thrombohematoma diagnosed by ultrasonography and magnetic resonance imaging. *Fetal Diagn Ther* 2001;16(1):57–60.

112. Biskup I, Malinowski W. Ultrasound in abruptio placentae praecox of the second twin. 'Boomerang phenomenon.' *Acta Obstet Gynecol Scand* 1994;73:515–516.

113. Grisaru D, Jaffa AJ, Har Toov J, et al. Prenatal sonographic diagnosis of intermembranous abruptio placentae in a twin pregnancy. *J Ultrasound Med* 1994;13:807–808.

114. Walker JM, Ferguson DD. The sonographic appearance of blood in the fetal stomach and its association with placental abruption. *J Ultrasound Med* 1988;7:155–161.

115. Spirt BA, Gordon LP, Kagan EH. Intervillous thrombosis: sonographic and pathologic correlation. *Radiology* 1983; 147:197–200.

116. Wentworth P. A placental lesion to account for fetal haemorrhage into the maternal circulation. *Br J Obstet Gynecol* 1964;71:379–387.

117. Fleischer AC, Kurtz AB, Wapner RJ, et al. Elevated alpha-fetoprotein and a normal fetal sonogram: association with placental abnormalities. *AJR Am J Roentgenol* 1988;150:881–883.

118. McGahan JP, Phillips HE, Reid MH, et al. Sonographic spectrum of retroplacental hemorrhage. *Radiology* 1982;142:481–485.

119. Spirt BA, Kagan EH, Rozanski RM. Abruptio placenta: sonographic and pathologic correlation. *AJR Am J Roentgenol* 1979;133:877–881.

120. Williams CH, VanBergen WS, Prentice RL. Extraamniotic blood clot simulating placenta previa on ultrasound scan. *J Clin Ultrasound* 1976;5:45–47.

121. Ball RH, Ade CM, Schoenborn JA, et al. The clinical significance of ultrasonographically detected subchorionic hemorrhages. *Am J Obstet Gynecol* 1996;174(3):996–1002.

122. Sher G. A rational basis for the management of abruptio placentae. *J Reprod Med* 1978;31:123–129.

123. Sholl JS. Abruptio placentae: clinical management in non-acute cases. *Am J Obstet Gynecol* 1987;156:40–51.

124. Combs CA, Nyberg DA, Mack LA, et al. Expectant management after sonographic diagnosis of placental abruption. *Am J Perinatol* 1992;9(3):170–174.

125. Rivera-Alsina ME, Saldana LR, Maklad N, et al. The use of ultrasound in the expectant management of abruptio placentae. *Am J Obstet Gynecol* 1983;146:924–927.

126. Jauniaux E, Campbell S. Antenatal diagnosis of placental infarcts by ultrasonography. *J Clin Ultrasound* 1991;19:58–61.

127. Levine AB, Frieden FJ, Stein JL, et al. Prenatal sonographic diagnosis of placental infarction in association with elevated maternal serum alpha-fetoprotein. *J Ultrasound Med* 1993;12:169–171.

128. Harris RD, Simpson WA, Pet LR, et al. Placental hypoechoic-anechoic areas and infarction: sonographic-pathologic correlation. *Radiology* 1990;176:75–80.

129. Sherer DM, Allen TA, Metlay LA, et al. Linear calcification in a placental infarct causing complete distal sonographic shadowing. *J Clin Ultrasound* 1994;22:212–213.

130. Matern D, Schehata BM, Shekhawa P, et al. Placental floor infarction complicating the pregnancy of a fetus with long-chain 3-hydroxyacyl-CoA dehydrogenase (LCHAD) deficiency. *Mol Genet Metab* 2001;72(3):265–268.

131. Mandsager NT, Bendon R, Mostello D, et al. Maternal floor infarction of the placenta: prenatal diagnosis and clinical significance. *Obstet Gynecol* 1994;83:750–754.

132. Katz VL, Bowes WA Jr, Sierkh AE. Maternal floor infarction of the placenta associated with elevated second trimester serum alpha-fetoprotein. *Am J Perinatol* 1987;4(3):225–228.

133. Andres RL, Kuyper W, Resnik R, et al. The association of maternal floor infarction of the placenta with adverse perinatal outcome. *Am J Obstet Gynecol* 1990;163(3):935–938.

134. Benirschke K, Kaufmann P. *Pathology of the human placenta.* New York: Springer-Verlag New York, 1990:841–851.

135. Froehlich LA, Fujikura T, Fisher P. Chorioangiomas and their clinical implications. *Obstet Gynecol* 1971;37:51–59.

136. Willard DA, Moeschler JB. Placental chorioangioma: a rare cause of elevated amniotic fluid alpha-fetoprotein. *J Ultrasound Med* 1986;5:221–222.

137. Cardwell MS. Antenatal management of a large placental chorioangioma. A case report. *J Reprod Med* 1988;33:68–70.

138. Hirata GI, Masaki DI, O'Toole M, et al. Color flow mapping and Doppler velocimetry in the diagnosis and management of a placental chorioangioma associated with nonimmune fetal hydrops. *Obstet Gynecol* 1993;81:850–852.

139. Esen UI, Orife SU, Pollard K. Placental chorioangioma: a case report and literature review. *Br J Clin Pract* 1997;51: 181–182.

140. Jauniaux E, Ogle R. Color Doppler imaging in the diagnosis and management of chorioangiomas. *Ultrasound Obstet Gynecol* 2000;15:463–467.

141. Prapas N, Liang RI, Hunter D, et al. Color Doppler imaging of placental masses: differential diagnosis and fetal outcome. *Ultrasound Obstet Gynecol* 2000;16(6):559–563.

142. Mochizuki T, Nishiguchi T, Ito I, et al. Case report. Antenatal diagnosis of chorioangioma of the placenta: MR features. *J Comput Assist Tomogr* 1996;20(3):413–416.

143. Kawamotoa S, Ogawa F, Tanaka J, et al. Chorioangioma: antenatal diagnosis with fast MR imaging. *Magn Reson Imaging* 2000;18(7):911–914.

144. Sepulveda W, Aviles G, Carstens E, et al. Prenatal diagnosis

of solid placental masses: the value of color flow imaging. *Ultrasound Obstet Gynecol* 2000;16(6):554–558.

145. Wolfe BK, Wallace JHK. Pitfall to avoid: chorioangioma of the placenta simulating fetal tumor. *J Clin Ultrasound* 1987;15:405–408.

146. Reinhart RD, Wells WA, Harris RD. Focal aneurysmal dilatation of subchorionic vessels simulating chorioangioma. *Ultrasound Obstet Gynecol* 1999;13(2):147–149.

147. Asadourian LA, Taylor HB. Clinical significance of placental hemangiomas. *Obstet Gynecol* 1968;31:551–555.

148. De Costa EJ, Gerbie AB, Andresen RH, et al. Placental tumors: hemangiomas. *Obstet Gynecol* 1956;7:249.

149. Makino Y, Horiuchi S, Sonoda M, et al. A case of large placental chorioangioma with non-immunological hydrops fetalis. *J Perinat Med* 1999;27:128–131.

150. Haak MC, Oosterhof H, Mouw RJ, et al. Pathophysiology and treatment of fetal anemia due to placental chorioangioma. *Ultrasound Obstet Gynecol* 1999;14:68–70.

151. Hadi HA, Finley J, Strickland D. Placental chorioangioma: prenatal diagnosis and clinical significance. *Am J Perinatol* 1993;10:146–149.

152. Zoppini C, Acaia B, Lucci G, et al. Varying clinical course of large placental chorioangiomas. Report of 3 cases. *Fetal Diagn Ther* 1997;12:61–64.

153. van Wering JH, van der Slikke JW. Prenatal diagnosis of chorioangioma associated with polyhydramnios using ultrasound. *Eur J Obstet Gynecol Reprod Biol* 1985;19:255–259.

154. Wallenburg HCS. Chorioangioma of the placenta. *Obstet Gynecol Surv* 1971;26:411–425.

155. Sepulveda W, Aviles G, Carstens E, et al. Prenatal diagnosis of solid placental masses: the value of color flow imaging. *Ultrasound Obstet Gynecol* 2000;16:554–558.

156. Prapas N, Liang RI, Hunter D, et al. Color Doppler imaging of placental masses: differential diagnosis and fetal outcome. *Ultrasound Obstet Gynecol* 2000;16:559–563.

157. MacIntosh AM, Osborn RA. Chorioangioma of the placenta: report of a case associated with spontaneous reabsorption of an acute hydramnios. *Med J Austral* 1968;2:313–314.

158. Chazotte C, Girz B, Koenigsberg M, et al. Spontaneous infarction of placental chorioangioma and associated regression of hydrops fetalis. *Am J Obstet Gynecol* 1990;163:221–224.

159. Hubinont C, Bernard P, Khalil N, et al. Fetal liver hemangioma and chorioangioma: two unusual causes of severe fetal anemia and its perinatal management. *Ultrasound Obstet Gynecol* 1994;4:330–331.

160. Quintero RA, Reich H, Romero R, et al. In utero endoscopic devascularization of a large chorioangioma. *Ultrasound Obstet Gynecol* 1996;8:48–52.

161. Munyer TP, Callen PW, Filly RA, et al. Further observations on the sonographic spectrum of gestational trophoblastic disease. *J Clin Ultrasound* 1981;9:349–358.

162. Szulman AE, Surti U. The syndromes of hydatidiform mole. 1. Cytogenetic and morphologic correlations. *Am J Obstet Gynecol* 1978;131:665–671.

163. Szulman AE, Philippe E, Boue JG, et al. Human triploidy: association with partial hydatidiform moles and nonmolar conceptuses. *Hum Pathol* 1981;12:1016–1021.

164. Uchida JA, Freeman VCP. Triploidy and chromosomes. *Am J Obstet Gynecol* 1985;151:65–69.

165. Watson EJ, Hernandez E, Miyazawa K. Partial hydatidiform moles: a review. *Obstet Gynecol Surv* 1987;42:540–544.

166. Jacobs PA, Szulman AE, Funkhauser J, et al. Human triploidy: relationship between parenteral origin of the additional haploid complement and development of partial hydatidiform mole. *Ann Hum Genet* 1982;46:223–231.

167. Callen PW. Ultrasonography in evaluation of gestational trophoblastic disease. In: Callen PW, ed. *Ultrasonography in obstetrics and gynecology.* Philadelphia: WB Saunders, 1983:259–270.

168. Bree RL, Silver TM, Wicks JD, et al. Trophoblastic disease with coexistent fetus: a sonographic and clinical spectrum. *J Clin Ultrasound* 1978;6:310–314.

169. Sauerbrei EE, Salem S, Fayle B. Coexistent hydatidiform mole and live fetus in the second trimester. *Radiology* 1980;135:415–417.

170. Gottesfeld KR, Taylor ES, Thompson HE, et al. Diagnosis of hydatidiform mole by ultrasound. *Obstet Gynecol* 1967;30:163–171.

171. Jouppila P, Kolu U. Hydatidiform mole with a co-existent fetus diagnosed in advance by ultrasound. *Ann Chir Gynaecol Fenn* 1971;60:89–91.

172. Lamb GH, Oakley R. The ultrasound diagnosis of hydatidiform mole and coexistent fetus associated with elevated maternal serum alpha fetoprotein. *Br J Radiol* 1981;54:268.

173. Zaki ZM, Bahar AM. Ultrasound appearance of a developing mole. *Int J Gynaecol Obstet* 1996;55:67–70.

174. Jauniaux E. Ultrasound diagnosis and follow-up of gestational trophoblastic disease. *Ultrasound Obstet Gynecol* 1998;11:367–377.

175. Coukos G, Makrigiannakis A, Chung J, et al. Complete hydatidiform mole. A disease with a changing profile. *J Reprod Med* 1999;44(8):698–704.

176. Crade M, Weber PR. Appearance of molar pregnancy 9.5 weeks after conception. Use of transvaginal ultrasound for early diagnosis. *J Ultrasound Med* 1991;10:473–474.

177. Jauniaux E, Nicolaides KH. Early ultrasound diagnosis and follow-up of molar pregnancies. *Ultrasound Obstet Gynecol* 1997;9:17–21.

178. Lazarus E, Hulka C, Siewert B, et al. Sonographic appearance of early complete molar pregnancies. *J Ultrasound Med* 1999;18(9):589–594; quiz 595–596.

179. Benson CB, Genest DR, Bernstein MR, et al. Sonographic appearance of first trimester complete hydatidiform moles. *Ultrasound Obstet Gynecol* 2000;16(2):188–191.

180. Kohorn EI, McCarthy SM, Taylor KJ. Nonmetastatic gestational trophoblastic neoplasia. Role of ultrasonography and magnetic resonance imaging. *J Reprod Med* 1998;43(1):14–20.

181. Hönigl W, Reich O, Ranner G, et al. Choriocarcinoma of the uterus after term pregnancy: imaging by vaginal color Doppler ultrasound. *Ultraschall Med* 1997;18:165–168.

182. Schneider DF, Bukovsky I, Weinraub Z, et al. Transvaginal ultrasound diagnosis and treatment follow-up of invasive gestational trophoblastic disease. *J Clin Ultrasound* 1990;18;110–113.

183. Bidziński M, Lemieszczuk B, Drabik M. The assessment of value of transvaginal ultrasound for monitoring of gestational trophoblastic disease treatment. *Eur J Gynaecol Oncol* 1997;18:541–543.

184. Fukumoto S. A study on ultrasound imaging of invasive mole and choriocarcinoma with regard to clinical significance. *Nippon Sanka Fujinka Gakkai Zasshi* 1986;38:366–374.

185. Hsieh FJ, Wu CC, Lee CN, et al. Vascular patterns of gestational trophoblastic tumors by color Doppler ultrasound. *Cancer* 1994;74:2361–2365.

186. Requard CK, Mettler FA. The use of ultrasound in the evaluation of trophoblastic disease and its response to therapy. *Radiology* 1980;135:419–422.

187. Rubenstein JB, Swayne LC, Dise CA, et al. Placental changes in fetal triploidy syndrome. *J Ultrasound Med* 1986;5:545–550.

188. Moscoso G, Jauniaux E, Hustin J. Placental vascular anomaly with diffuse mesenchymal villous hyperplasia. A new clinicopathological entity? *Pathol Res Pract* 1991;187:324–328.

189. Pridmore BR, Khong TY, Wells WA. Ultrasound placental cysts associated with massive placental stem villous hydrops, diploid DNA content, and exomphalos. *Am J Perinatol* 1994;11:14–18.

190. McCowan LM, Becroft DM. Beckwith-Wiedemann syndrome, placental abnormalities, and gestational proteinuric hypertension. *Obstet Gynecol* 1994;83:813–817.

191. Hillstrom MM, Brown DL, Wilkins Haug L, et al. Sonographic appearance of placental villous hydrops associated with Beckwith-Wiedemann syndrome. *J Ultrasound Med* 1995;14:61–64.

192. Jauniaux E, Nicolaides KH, Hustin J. Perinatal features associated with placental mesenchymal dysplasia. *Placenta* 1997;18:701–706.

193. Berman ML, Di Saia PJ, Brewster WR. Pelvic malignancies, gestational trophoblastic neoplasia, and nonpelvic malignancies. In: Creasy RK, Resnik R, eds. *Maternal fetal medicine*, 4th ed. Philadelphia: WB Saunders, 1999:1128–1150.

194. Johnson MP, Childs MD, Robichaux AG III, et al. Viable pregnancies after diagnosis of trisomy 16 by CVS: lethal aneuploidy compartmentalized to the trophoblast. *Fetal Diagn Ther* 1993;8(2):102–108.

195. Williams J III, Wang BB, Rubin CH, et al. Apparent nonmosaic trisomy 16 in chorionic villi: diagnostic dilemma or clinically significant finding? *Prenat Diagn* 1992;12(3):163–168.

196. Astner A, Schwinger E, Caliebe A, et al. Sonographically detected fetal and placental abnormalities associated with trisomy 16 confined to the placenta. A case report and review of the literature. *Prenat Diagn* 1998;18(12):1308–1315.

197. Wolstenholme J, White I, Sturgiss S, et al. Maternal uniparental heterodisomy for chromosome 2: detection through 'atypical' maternal AFP/hCG levels, with an update on a previous case. *Prenat Diagn* 2001;21(10):813–817.

198. Lestou VS, Lomax BL, Barrett IJ, et al. Screening of human placentas for chromosomal mosaicism using comparative genomic hybridization. *Teratology* 1999;59(5):325–330.

199. Stipoljev F, Latin V, Kos M, et al. Correlation of confined placental mosaicism with fetal intrauterine growth retardation. A case control study of placentas at delivery. *Fetal Diagn Ther* 2001;16(1):4–9.

200. Benirschke K. Obstetrically important lesions of the umbilical cord. *J Reprod Med* 1994;39:262–272.

201. Heifetz SA. The umbilical cord: obstetrically important lesions. *Clin Obstet Gynecol* 1996;39:571–587.

202. Hill LM, Kislak S, Runco C. An ultrasonic view of the umbilical cord. *Obstet Gynecol Surv* 1987;42:82–88.

203. Dudiak CM, Salomon CG, Posniak HV, et al. Sonography of the umbilical cord. *Radiographics* 1995;15:1035–1050.

204. Sherer DM, Anyaegbunam A. Prenatal ultrasonographic morphologic assessment of the umbilical cord: a review. Part I. *Obstet Gynecol Surv* 1997;52:506–514.

205. Sherer DM, Anyaegbunam A. Prenatal ultrasonographic morphologic assessment of the umbilical cord: a review. Part II. *Obstet Gynecol Surv* 1997;52:515–523.

206. Sepulveda W. Time for a more detailed prenatal examination of the umbilical cord? *Ultrasound Obstet Gynecol* 1999;13:157–160.

207. Walker CW, Pye BG. The length of the human umbilical cord: a statistical report. *BMJ* 1960;1:546–548.

208. American Institute of Ultrasound in Medicine. *Guidelines for performance of the antepartum obstetrical ultrasound examination.* Laurel: AIUM, 1994.

209. Morin FR, Winsberg F. The ultrasonic appearance of the umbilical cord. *J Clin Ultrasound* 1978;6:324–326.

210. Hill LM, DiNofrio DM, Guzick D. Sonographic determination of first trimester umbilical cord length. *J Clin Ultrasound* 1994;22:435–438.

211. Pretorius DH, Chau C, Poeltler DM, et al. Placental cord insertion visualization with prenatal ultrasonography. *J Ultrasound Med* 1996;15:585–593.

212. Di Salvo DN, Benson CB, Laing FC, et al. Sonographic evaluation of the placental cord insertion site. *AJR Am J Roentgenol* 1998;170:1295–1298.

213. Lacro RV, Jones KL, Benirschke K. The umbilical cord twist: origin, direction, and relevance. *Am J Obstet Gynecol* 1987;157:833–838.

214. Nakari BG. Congenital anomalies of the human umbilical cord and their clinical significance: a light and microscopic study. *Ind J Med Res* 1969;57:1018–1025.

215. Miller ME, Higginbottom M, Smith DW. Short umbilical cord: its origin and relevance. *Pediatrics* 1981;67:618–621.

216. Heifetz SA. Single umbilical artery. A statistical analysis of 237 autopsy cases and review of the literature. *Perspect Pediatr Pathol* 1984;8:345–378.

217. Persutte WH, Hobbins J. Single umbilical artery: a clinical enigma in modern prenatal diagnosis. *Ultrasound Obstet Gynecol* 1995;6:216–229.

218. Peckham CH, Yerushalmy J. Aplasia of one umbilical artery: incidence by race and certain obstetric factors. *Obstet Gynecol* 1965;26:359–366.

219. Dolkart LA, Reimers FT, Kuonen CA. Discordant umbilical arteries: ultrasonographic and Doppler analysis. *Obstet Gynecol* 1992;79:59–63.

220. Aoki S, Hata T, Ariyuki Y, et al. Antenatal diagnosis of aberrant umbilical vessels. *Gynecol Obstet Invest* 1997;43:232–235.

221. Raio L, Ghezzi F, Di Naro E, et al. The clinical significance of antenatal detection of discordant umbilical arteries. *Obstet Gynecol* 1998;91:86–91.

222. Petrikovsky B, Schneider E. Prenatal diagnosis and clinical significance of hypoplastic umbilical artery. *Prenat Diagn* 1996;16:938–940.

223. Monie IW. Genesis of single umbilical artery. *Am J Obstet Gynecol* 1970;108:400–405.

224. Altshuler G, Tsang RC, Ermocilla R. Single umbilical artery. Correlation of clinical status and umbilical cord histology. *Am J Dis Child* 1975;129:697–700.

225. Jassani MN, Brennan JN, Merkatz IR. Prenatal diagnosis of single umbilical artery by ultrasound. *J Clin Ultrasound* 1982;8:447–448.

226. Tortora M, Chervenak FA, Mayden K, et al. Antenatal sonographic diagnosis of single umbilical artery. *Obstet Gynecol* 1984;63:693–696.

227. Herrmann UJ, Sidiropoulos D. Single umbilical artery: prenatal findings. *Prenat Diagn* 1988;8:275–280.

228. Sepulveda WH. Prenatal sonographic detection of single umbilical artery. *J Perinat Med* 1991;19:391–395.

229. Persutte WH, Lenke RR. Transverse umbilical arterial diameter: technique for the prenatal diagnosis of single umbilical artery. *J Ultrasound Med* 1994;13:763–766.

230. Sepulveda W, Peek MJ, Hassan J, et al. Umbilical vein to artery ratio in fetuses with single umbilical artery. *Ultrasound Obstet Gynecol* 1996;8:23–26.

231. De Catte L, Burrini D, Mares C, et al. Single umbilical artery: analysis of Doppler flow indices and arterial diameters in normal and small-for-gestational-age fetuses. *Ultrasound Obstet Gynecol* 1996;8:27–30.

232. Jeanty P. Fetal and funicular vascular anomalies: identification with prenatal US. *Radiology* 1989;173:367–370.

233. Dolkart LA, Reimers FT, Kuonen CA. Discordant umbilical arteries: ultrasonographic and Doppler analysis. *Obstet Gynecol* 1992;79:59–63.

234. Sepulveda W, Addis JR, Romero R, et al. Umbilical artery, hypoplasia. *Fetus* 1992;3:9–12.

235. Sepulveda W, Flack NJ, Bower S, et al. The value of color Doppler ultrasound in the prenatal diagnosis of hypoplastic umbilical artery. *Ultrasound Obstet Gynecol* 1994;4:143–146.

236. Sepulveda W, Reyes M, Goncalves LF. Two uncommon umbilical vessel anomalies in a fetus with trisomy 18. *Prenat Diagn* 1998;18:1098–1099.

237. Meyer WW, Lind J. Iliac arteries in children with a single umbilical artery. Structure, calcifications, and early atherosclerotic lesions. *Arch Dis Child* 1974;49:671–679.

238. Sepulveda W, Bower S, Flack NJ, et al. Discordant iliac and femoral artery flow velocity waveforms in fetuses with single umbilical artery. *Am J Obstet Gynecol* 1994;171:521–525.

239. Sepulveda W, Nicolaidis P, Bower S, et al. Common iliac artery flow velocity waveforms in fetuses with a single umbilical artery: a longitudinal study. *Br J Obstet Gynaecol* 1996;103:660–663.

240. Rosenak D, Meizner I. Prenatal sonographic detection of single and double umbilical artery in the same fetus. *J Ultrasound Med* 1994;13:995–996.

241. Sepulveda W, Dezerega V, Carstens E, et al. Fused umbilical arteries: prenatal sonographic diagnosis and clinical significance. *J Ultrasound Med* 2001;20:59–62.

242. Froehlich LA, Fujikura T. Follow-up of infants with single umbilical artery. *Pediatrics* 1973;52:22–29.

243. Bryan EM, Kohler HG. The missing umbilical artery. I. Prospective study based on a maternity unit. *Arch Dis Child* 1974;49:844–852.

244. Soma H. Single umbilical artery with congenital anomalies. *Curr Top Pathol* 1979;66:159–173.

245. Leung AK, Robson WL. Single umbilical artery. A report of 159 cases. *Am J Dis Child* 1989;143:108–111.

246. Nyberg DA, Mahony BS, Luthy D, et al. Single umbilical artery. Prenatal detection of concurrent anomalies. *J Ultrasound Med* 1991;10:247–253.

247. Chow JS, Benson CB, Doubilet PM. Frequency and nature of structural anomalies in fetuses with single umbilical arteries. *J Ultrasound Med* 1998;17:765–768.

248. Saller DN, Keene CL, Sun CC, et al. The association of single umbilical artery with cytogenetically abnormal pregnancies. *Am J Obstet Gynecol* 1990;163:922–925.

249. Khong TY, George K. Chromosomal abnormalities associated with a single umbilical artery. *Prenat Diagn* 1992;12:965–968.

250. Sepulveda W, Dezerega V, Carstens E, et al. Risks of funipuncture in fetuses with single umbilical arteries. *Obstet Gynecol* 2000;95:557–560.

251. Benirschke K, Dodds JP. Angiomyxoma of the umbilical cord with atrophy of an umbilical artery. *Obstet Gynecol* 1967;30:99–102.

252. Abuhamad AZ, Shaffer W, Mari G, et al. Single umbilical artery: does it matter which artery is missing? *Am J Obstet Gynecol* 1995;173:728–732.

253. Blazer S, Sujov P, Escholi Z, et al. Single umbilical artery—right or left? Does it matter? *Prenat Diagn* 1997;17:5–8.

254. Geipel A, Germer U, Welp T, et al. Prenatal diagnosis of single umbilical artery: determination of the absent side, associated anomalies, Doppler findings and perinatal outcome. *Ultrasound Obstet Gynecol* 2000;15:114–117.

255. Raio L, Ghezzi F, Di Naro E, et al. Prenatal assessment of Wharton's jelly in umbilical cords with single artery. *Ultrasound Obstet Gynecol* 1999;14:42–46.

256. Lee CN, Cheng WF, Lai HL, et al. Perinatal management and outcome of fetuses with single umbilical artery diagnosed prenatally. *J Matern Fetal Invest* 1998;8:156–159.

257. Catanzarite VA, Hendricks SK, Maida C, et al. Prenatal diagnosis of the two-vessel cord: implications for patient counseling and obstetric management. *Ultrasound Obstet Gynecol* 1995;5:98–105.

258. Parrilla BV, Tamura RK, MacGregor SN, et al. The clinical significance of single umbilical artery as an isolated finding on prenatal ultrasound. *Obstet Gynecol* 1995;85:570–572.

259. Bourke WG, Clarke TA, Mathews TG, et al. Isolated single umbilical artery—the case for routine renal screening. *Arch Dis Child* 1993;68:600–601.

260. Thummala MR, Raju TN, Langenberg P. Isolated single umbilical artery anomaly and the risk for congenital malformations: a meta-analysis. *J Pediatr Surg* 1998;33:580–585.

261. Gore RM, Filly RA, Parer JT. Sonographic antepartum diagnosis of conjoined twins. Its impact on obstetric management. *JAMA* 1982;247:3351–3353.

262. Koontz WL, Herbert WN, Seeds JW, et al. Ultrasonography in the antepartum diagnosis of conjoined twins. A report of two cases. *J Reprod Med* 1983;28:627–630.

263. Sepulveda WH, Quiroz VH, Mercado M, et al. Prenatal ultrasonographic diagnosis of thoracopagus conjoined twins. *J Perinat Med* 1989;17:297–303.

264. Cohen HL, Shapiro ML, Haller JO, et al. The multivessel umbilical cord: an antenatal indicator of possible conjoined twinning. *J Clin Ultrasound* 1992;20:278–282.

265. Van den Brand SF, Nijhuis JG, Van Dongen PW. Prenatal

ultrasound diagnosis of conjoined twins. *Obstet Gynecol Surv* 1994;49:656–662.

266. Murdoch DE. Umbilical cord doubling. Report of a case. *Obstet Gynecol* 1966;27:555–557.

267. Rodriguez MA. Four-vessel umbilical cord without congenital abnormalities. *South Med J* 1984;77:539.

268. Painter D, Russel O. Four-vessel umbilical cord associated with multiple congenital anomalies. *Obstet Gynecol* 1977;50:505–507.

269. Beck R, Naulty CM. A human umbilical cord with four arteries. *Clin Pediatr* 1985;24:118–119.

270. Konstantinova B. Malformations of the umbilical cord. *Acta Genet Med Gemellol* 1977;26:259–266.

271. Fortune DW, Ostor AG. Umbilical artery aneurysm. *Am J Obstet Gynecol* 1978;131:339–340.

272. Mahony BS, McGahan JP, Nyberg DA, et al. Varix of the fetal intra-abdominal umbilical vein: comparison with normal. *J Ultrasound Med* 1992;11(2):73–76.

273. Moore L, Toi A, Chitayat D. Abnormalities of the intra-abdominal fetal umbilical vein: reports of four cases and a review of the literature. *Ultrasound Obstet Gynecol* 1996;7(1):21–25.

274. Zalel Y, Lehavi O, Heifetz S, et al. Varix of the fetal intra-abdominal umbilical vein: prenatal sonographic diagnosis and suggested in utero management. *Ultrasound Obstet Gynecol* 2000;16(5):476–478.

275. Prefumo F, Thilaganathan B, Tekay A. Antenatal diagnosis of fetal intra-abdominal umbilical vein dilatation. *Ultrasound Obstet Gynecol* 2001;17(1):82–85.

276. Fuster JS, Benasco C, Saad I. Giant dilatation of the umbilical vein. *J Clin Ultrasound* 1985;13:363–365.

277. Challis D, Trudinger BJ, Moore L, et al. Intra-abdominal varix of the umbilical vein—is it an indication for fetal karyotyping? *Am J Obstet Gynecol* 1997;176[Suppl]:93(abst).

278. Sepulveda W, Mackenna A, Sanchez J, et al. Fetal prognosis in varix of the intrafetal umbilical vein. *J Ultrasound Med* 1998;17:171–175.

279. Ami MB, Perlitz Y, Matilsky M. Prenatal sonographic diagnosis of persistent right umbilical vein with varix. *J Clin Ultrasound* 1999;27(5):273–275.

280. Vandevijver N, Hermans RH, Schrander-Stumpel CC, et al. Aneurysm of the umbilical vein: case report and review of literature. *Eur J Obstet Gynecol Reprod Biol* 2000;89(1):85–87.

281. Siddiqi TA, Bendon R, Schultz DM, et al. Umbilical artery aneurysm: prenatal diagnosis and management. *Obstet Gynecol* 1992;80:530–533.

282. Berg C, Geipel A, Germer U, et al. Prenatal diagnosis of umbilical cord aneurysm in a fetus with trisomy 18. *Ultrasound Obstet Gynecol* 2001;17:79–81.

283. Batton DG, Amanullah A, Comstock C. Fetal schistocytic hemolytic anemia and umbilical vein varix. *J Pediatr Hematol Oncol* 2000;22(3):259–261.

284. Estroff JA, Benacerraf BR. Fetal umbilical vein varix: sonographic appearance and postnatal outcome. *J Ultrasound Med* 1992;11(3):69–73.

285. Allen SL, Bagnall C, Roberts AB, et al. Thrombosing umbilical vein varix. *J Ultrasound Med* 1998;17:189–192.

286. Rahemtullah A, Lieberman E, Benson C, et al. Outcome of pregnancy after prenatal diagnosis of umbilical vein varix. *J Ultrasound Med* 2001;20:135–139.

287. Schrocksnadel H, Holbock E, Mitterschiffthaler G, et al. Thrombotic occlusion of an umbilical vein varix causing fetal death. *Arch Gynecol Obstet* 1991;248(4):213–215.

288. Viora E, Sciarrone A, Bastonero S, et al. Thrombosis of umbilical vein varix. *Ultrasound Obstet Gynecol* 2002;19(2):212–213.

289. White SP, Kofinas A. Prenatal diagnosis and management of umbilical vein varix of the intra-amniotic portion of the umbilical vein. *J Ultrasound Med* 1994;13:992–994.

290. Blazer S, Zimmer EZ, Bronshtein M. Persistent intrahepatic right umbilical vein in the fetus: a benign anatomic variant. *Obstet Gynecol* 2000;95(3):433–436.

291. Hill LM, Mills A, Peterson C, et al. Persistent right umbilical vein: sonographic detection and subsequent neonatal outcome. *Obstet Gynecol* 1994;84(6):923–925.

292. Jeanty P. Persistent right umbilical vein: an ominous prenatal finding? *Radiology* 1990;177(3):735–738.

293. Lai WW. Prenatal diagnosis of abnormal persistence of the right or left umbilical vein: report of 4 cases and literature review. *J Am Soc Echocardiogr* 1998;11(9):905–909.

294. Kirsch CF, Feldstein VA, Goldstein RB, et al. Persistent intrahepatic right umbilical vein: a prenatal sonographic series without significant anomalies. *J Ultrasound Med* 1996;15(5):371–374.

295. Shen O, Tadmor OP, Yagel S. Prenatal diagnosis of persistent right umbilical vein. *Ultrasound Obstet Gynecol* 1996;8(1):31–33.

296. Eddleman KA, Lockwood CJ, Berkowitz GS, et al. Clinical significance and sonographic diagnosis of velamentous umbilical cord insertion. *Am J Perinatol* 1992;9(2):123–126.

297. Fries MH, Goldstein RB, Kilpatrick SJ, et al. The role of velamentous cord insertion in the etiology of twin-twin transfusion syndrome. *Obstet Gynecol* 1993;81(4):569–574.

298. Heinonen S, Ryynanen M, Kirkinen P, et al. Perinatal diagnostic evaluation of velamentous umbilical cord insertion: clinical, Doppler, and ultrasonic findings. *Obstet Gynecol* 1996;87(1):112–117.

299. Machin GA. Velamentous cord insertion in monochorionic twin gestation. An added risk factor. *J Reprod Med* 1997;42(12):785–789.

300. Sepulveda W, Gutierrez J, Sanchez J, et al. Pseudocyst of the umbilical cord: prenatal sonographic appearance and clinical significance. *Obstet Gynecol* 1999;93:377–381.

301. Iaccarino M, Baldi F, Persico O, et al. Ultrasonographic and pathologic study of mucoid degeneration of umbilical cord. *J Clin Ultrasound* 1986;14:127–129.

302. Persutte WH, Lenke RR, Kropp K, et al. Antenatal diagnosis of fetal patent urachus. *J Ultrasound Med* 1988;7:399–403.

303. Donnenfeld AE, Mennuti MT, Templeton JM, et al. Prenatal sonographic diagnosis of a vesico-allantoic abdominal wall defect. *J Ultrasound Med* 1989;8:43–45.

304. Persutte WH, Lenke RR. Disappearing fetal umbilical cord masses. Are these findings suggestive of urachal anomalies? *J Ultrasound Med* 1990;9;547–551.

305. Frazier HA, Guerrini JP, Thomas RL, et al. Detection of a patent urachus and allantoic cyst of the umbilical cord on prenatal ultrasonography. *J Ultrasound* 1992;11:117–120.

306. Sepulveda W, Bower S, Dhillon HK, et al. Prenatal diagnosis of congenital patent urachus and allantoic cyst: the value of color flow imaging. *J Ultrasound Med* 1995;14:47–51.

307. Tolaymat LL, Maher JE, Kleinman GE, et al. Persistent patent urachus with allantoic cyst: a case report. *Ultrasound Obstet Gynecol* 1997;10:366–368.

308. Yoo SJ, Lee YH, Ryu HM, et al. Unusual fate of vesicoallantoic cyst with non-visualization of fetal urinary bladder in a case of patent urachus. *Ultrasound Obstet Gynecol* 1997;9:422–424.

309. Chandler C, Baum JD, Wigglesworth JS, et al. Giant umbilical cord associated with a patent urachus and fused umbilical arteries. *J Obstet Gynaecol Br Commonw* 1969;76:273–274.

310. Ente G, Penzer PH, Kenigsberg K. Giant umbilical cord associated with patent urachus. An external clue to internal anomaly. *Am J Dis Child* 1970;120:82–83.

311. Fink IJ, Filly RA. Omphalocele associated with umbilical cord allantoic cyst: sonographic evaluation in utero. *Radiology* 1983;149:473–476.

312. Battaglia C, Artini PG, D'Ambrogio G, et al. Cord vessel compression by an expanding allantoic cyst: case report. *Ultrasound Obstet Gynecol* 1992;2:58–60.

313. Rempen A. Sonographic first-trimester diagnosis of umbilical cord cyst. *J Clin Ultrasound* 1989;17:53–55.

314. Skibo LK, Lyons EA, Levi CS. First-trimester umbilical cord cysts. *Radiology* 1992;182:719–722.

315. Ross JA, Jurkovic D, Zosmer N, et al. Umbilical cord cysts in early pregnancy. *Obstet Gynecol* 1997;89:442–445.

316. Sepulveda W, Leible S, Ulloa A, et al. Clinical significance of first trimester umbilical cord cysts. *J Ultrasound Med* 1999;18:95–99.

317. Jauniaux E, Donner C, Thomas Francotte J, et al. Umbilical cord pseudocyst in trisomy 18. Prenat Diagn 1988;8:557–563.

318. Sepulveda W, Pryde PG, Greb AE, et al. Prenatal diagnosis of umbilical cord pseudocyst. *Ultrasound Obstet Gynecol* 1994;4:147–150.

319. Smith GN, Walker M, Johnson S, et al. The sonographic finding of persistent umbilical cord cystic masses is associated with lethal aneuploidy and/or congenital anomalies. *Prenat Diagn* 1996;16:1141–1147.

320. Sondergaard G. Hemangioma of the umbilical cord. *Acta Obstet Gynecol Scand* 1994;73(5):434–436.

321. Clausen I, Thomsen SG. Pseudotumors of the umbilical cord and fetal membranes. *Acta Obstet Gynecol Scand* 1992;71(2):148–150.

322. Stephens TD, Spall R, Urfer AG, et al. Fetus amorphus or placental teratoma? *Teratology* 1989;40:1–10.

323. Kreyberg L. A teratoma-like swelling in the umbilical cord possibly of acardius nature. *J Pathol Bacteriol* 1958;75:109–112.

324. Smith D, Majmudar B. Teratoma of the umbilical cord. *Hum Pathol* 1985;16:190–193.

325. Kreczy A, Alge A, Menardi G, et al. Teratoma of the umbilical cord. Case report with review of the literature. *Arch Pathol Lab Med* 1994;118:934–937.

326. Ghidini A, Romero R, Eisen RN, et al. Umbilical cord hemangioma. Prenatal identification and review of the literature. *J Ultrasound Med* 1990;9:297–300.

327. Jauniaux E, Moscoso G, Chitty L, et al. An angiomyxoma involving the whole length of the umbilical cord. Prenatal diagnosis by ultrasonography. *J Ultrasound Med* 1990;9:419–422.

328. Yavner DL, Redline RW. Angiomyxoma of the umbilical cord with massive cystic degeneration of Wharton's jelly. *Arch Pathol Lab Med* 1989;113:935–937.

329. Wilson RD, Magee JF, Sorensen PHB, et al. In utero decompression of umbilical cord angiomyxoma followed by vaginal delivery. *Am J Obstet Gynecol* 1994;171:1383–1385.

330. Satge DC, Laumond MA, Desfarges F, et al. An umbilical cord teratoma in a 17-week-old fetus. *Prenat Diagn* 2001;21(4):284–288.

331. Miller KA, Gauderer MW. Hemangioma of the umbilical cord mimicking an omphalocele. *J Pediatr Surg* 1997;32(6):810–812.

332. Resta RG, Luthy DA, Mahony BS. Umbilical cord hemangioma associated with extremely high alphafetoprotein levels. *Obstet Gynecol* 1988;72:488–491.

333. Lazebnik N, Hill LM, Many A, et al. The effect of amniotic sheet orientation on subsequent maternal and fetal complications. *Ultrasound Obstet Gynecol* 1996;8(4):267–271.

334. Ball RH, Buchmeier SE, Longnecker M. Clinical significance of sonographically detected uterine synechiae in pregnant patients. *J Ultrasound Med* 1997;16(7):465–469.

335. Mahony BS, Filly RA, Callen PW, et al. The amniotic band syndrome: antenatal diagnosis and potential pitfalls. *Am J Obstet Gynecol* 1985;152:63–68.

336. Randel SB, Filly RA, Callen PW, et al. Amniotic sheets. *Radiology* 1988;166:633–636.

337. Korbin CD, Benson CB, Doubilet PM. Placental implantation on the amniotic sheet: effect on pregnancy outcome. *Radiology* 1998;206(3):773–775.

338. Finberg HJ. Uterine synechiae in pregnancy: expanded criteria for recognition and clinical significance in 28 cases. *J Ultrasound Med* 1991;10(10):547–555.

339. Levine D, Callen PW, Pender SG, et al. Chorioamnionic separation after second-trimester genetic amniocentesis: importance and frequency. *Radiology* 1998;209(1):175–181.

340. Ulm B, Ulm MR, Bernaschek G. Unfused amnion and chorion after 14 weeks of gestation: associated fetal structural and chromosomal abnormalities. *Ultrasound Obstet Gynecol* 1999;13(6):392–395.

341. Bromley B, Shipp TD, Benacerraf BR. Amnion-chorion separation after 17 weeks' gestation. *Obstet Gynecol* 1999;94(6):1024–1026.

342. Graf JL, Bealer JF, Gibbs DL, et al. Chorioamnionic membrane separation: a potentially lethal finding. *Fetal Diagn Ther* 1997;12(2):81–84.

SYNDROMES AND MULTIPLE ANOMALY CONDITIONS

EDITOR'S NOTE

This chapter discusses certain syndromes or multiple anomaly conditions. Determining which conditions to include was a difficult and arbitrary decision, but we tried to include those conditions that typically affect multiple organs and thus are referenced in more than one chapter. We have divided these conditions into nonchromosomal and chromosomal categories. This is by no means exhaustive, but we hope to give the reader an idea of the complexity of syndromic conditions. Excellent resources on specific conditions are available on the Internet at Online Mendelian Inheritance in Man,[1] GeneClinics,[2] and The Fetus[3] as well as in well-known textbooks.[4–6]

NONCHROMOSOMAL SYNDROMES

▶ AMNIOTIC BAND SYNDROME

Amniotic band syndrome is a set of congenital malformations ranging from minor constriction rings and lymphedema of the digits to complex, bizarre multiple congenital anomalies that are attributed to amniotic bands that stick, entangle, and disrupt fetal parts.[7]

Synonyms for amniotic band syndrome include *ADAM complex* (*a*mniotic *d*eformities, *a*dhesion, *m*utilation), *amniotic band sequence, amniotic disruption complex, annular grooves, congenital amputation, congenital constricting bands, Streeter bands, transverse terminal defects of limb,*[8] *aberrant tissue bands, amniochorionic mesoblastic fibrous strings,* and *amniotic bands.*[9,10]

Incidence

Amniotic band syndrome is rare but more common among spontaneous abortions.

Genetic Defect

The genetic basis is unknown.

Etiology

Rupture of the amnion leads to entrapment of fetal structures by "sticky" mesodermic bands that originate from the chorionic side of the amnion, followed by disruption.[11,12] Various teratogenic factors have been implicated.[13–15] Entrapment of fetal parts may cause amputation or slash defects in random sites, unrelated to embryologic development. The estimated date of insult ranges from 6 to 18 weeks after the last menstrual period.[9]

Pathologic and Clinical Features

The variable age of fetal entrapment can explain the spectrum of pathologic findings seen with the amniotic band syndrome. Early entrapment (28 to 45 days postconception) can lead to severe craniofacial defects and internal malformations as seen with the limb-body wall complex (LBWC), whereas late entrapment can lead to simple amputations or limb restrictions.[10,16–18] Rupture of the amnion does not, however, invariably result in fetal deformity and amniotic band syndrome.[19]

Craniofacial deformities occur in approximately one-third of cases and include asymmetric encephaloceles, microphthalmos, and bizarre facial clefts. Limb defects include constriction or amputation defects of the extremities. Clubfoot is found in up to one-third of cases, possibly due to transient oligohydramnios resulting from ruptured membranes. Like those in LBWC, karyotypes of the amniotic band syndrome have been reported to be normal.

The syndrome results in structural anomalies that vary from minor to lethal forms. The most common findings are constriction rings around the digits, arms, and legs; swelling of the extremities distal to the point of constriction; amputation of digits, arms, and legs; asymmetric face; facial clefts; cephalocele; anencephaly; multiple joint contractures; pterygium; clubfeet, clubhands, and pseudosyndactyly; microphthalmos; and ocular abnormalities.[20–22]

Diagnosis

The amniotic band syndrome can frequently be suspected based on prenatal sonography.[9,23–25] Malformations range

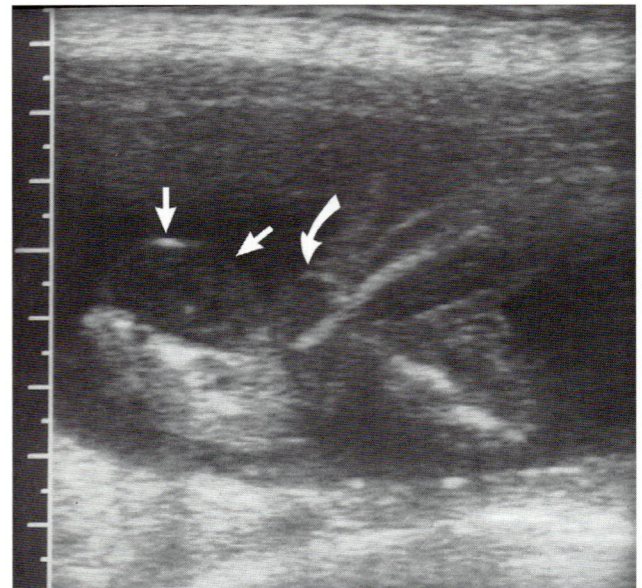
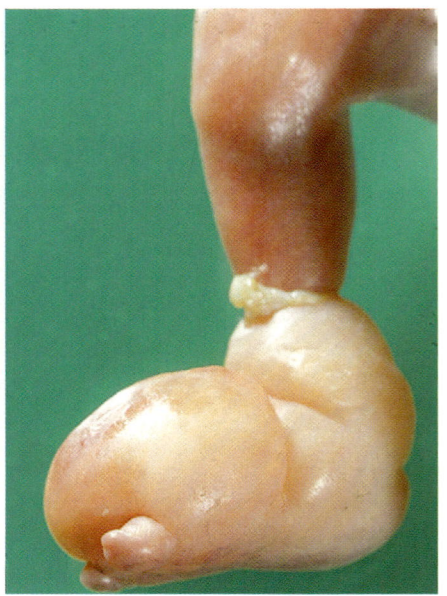

FIGURE 1. Amniotic band syndrome. **A:** Marked swelling and edema of the foot are evident (*arrows*). A constriction band of the leg is suggested (*curved arrow*). **B:** The pathologic photograph correlates with ultrasound findings, showing marked edema of the foot and lower leg secondary to constriction by amniotic band.

from mild, isolated constriction bands in an extremity (Fig. 1) to multiple severe anomalies incompatible with life (Fig. 2). When anomalies are multiple and severe, the sonographic appearance may not be distinguishable from LBWC.

Prenatal sonographic findings may include a wide variety of anomalies, including neural tube defect, unusual clefts of the lip/palate, abdominal wall defects, and amputation-type defects.[26] Constriction rings of the limbs have been observed, and these typically show edema distal to the constriction ring (Fig. 1). This may result in an amputation defect of the extremity.[7,27] It is the effect of the amniotic bands that is usually visualized; the amniotic bands themselves are rarely seen.

Differential Diagnosis

Various membranes should not be mistaken for amniotic bands, including amniotic sheets (or synechiae),[28] chorio-

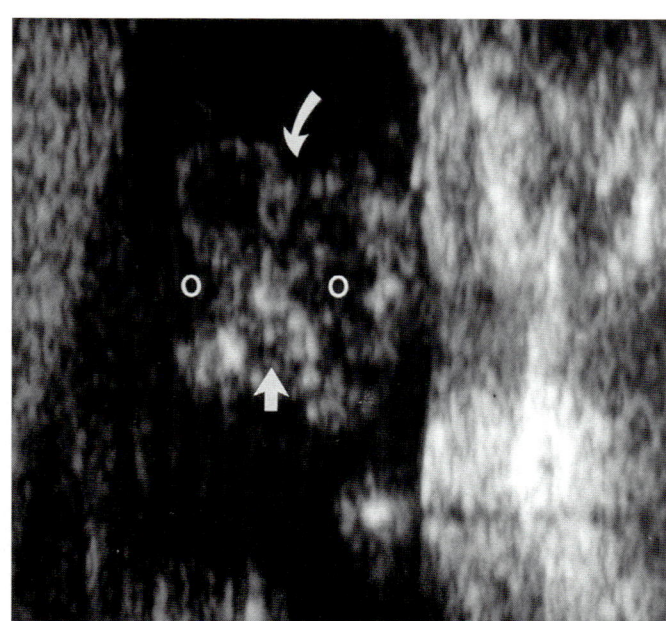
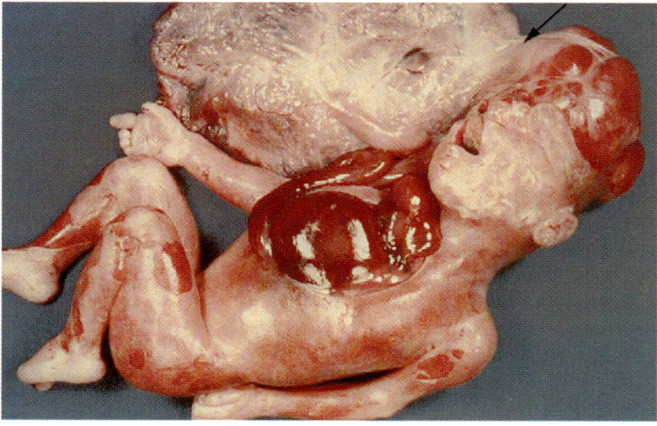

FIGURE 2. Amniotic band syndrome. **A:** A coronal scan of face and head shows exencephaly with eviscerated brain (*curved arrow*). A facial cleft (*straight arrow*) is also evident. O, orbits. **B:** A pathologic photograph of a similar case shows exencephaly, a ventral wall defect, and an amniotic band extending through the mouth.

amnionic separation of membranes, subchorionic hemorrhage, and cysts of the placenta or umbilical cord. Amniotic sheets are layered by amnion and are not sticky. They are commonly observed as incidental findings and may increase the risk of breech presentation at term but are otherwise not considered to be of significance.

The cranial appearance in some severely affected fetuses can resemble anencephaly.[29,30] In contrast to anencephaly, the cranial malformation in amniotic band syndrome is usually asymmetric and associated with other defects typical of the syndrome. It is also possible to confuse the septations in a large cystic hygroma with the bands in amniotic band syndrome.[31]

Similarities between the amniotic band syndrome and LBWC are obvious. Some investigators believe LBWC is simply a severe form of amniotic band syndrome. Others believe that LBWC is due to a primary vascular abnormality that subsequently ruptures the amnion.[13] Whether they represent distinct disorders or a continuum remains open to question.

Prognosis

The prognosis for fetuses with the amniotic band syndrome varies, depending on the severity and distribution of anomalies. Few infants with severe craniofacial deformities survive.[32] In comparison, the prognosis is good and life expectancy is normal for mildly affected infants with isolated limb defects.

Management

Management depends on the extent of the anomalies. Termination of pregnancy can be offered for the severe forms. Endoscopic release has been reported and may prove beneficial when an extremity is at risk for amputation.[33]

Recurrence Risk

No recurrence risk, except in rare sporadic familial cases, which have been reported in association with epidermolysis bullosa and Ehlers-Danlos syndrome.[34,35]

▶ APERT SYNDROME

Also called *acrocephalosyndactyly*, Apert syndrome is a rare developmental deformity, characterized by craniofacial and limb malformations accompanied by variable degrees of mental delay.[36] Although described earlier by Wheaton, Apert summarized the disorder in 1906, presenting nine cases.[37,38] See also the Craniosynostosis Syndromes (Fibroblast Growth Factor Receptor–Related) section, later in this chapter.

Incidence

The incidence of Apert syndrome and Crouzon syndrome is approximately 1 in 70,000. Apert syndrome accounts for approximately 4.5% of all cases of craniosynostosis. An association with advanced paternal age has been well established.[39]

Genetic Defect

The most common mutations associated with Apert syndrome are missense mutations (S252W and P253R) of the gene encoding the fibroblast growth factor receptor (FGFR) 2. These two mutations account for approximately 98% of affected patients. Mutations exclusive to sperm have been demonstrated.

Pathologic and Clinical Features

Typical findings in Apert syndrome are craniosynostosis secondary to synostosis of the coronal sutures, bilateral symmetric syndactyly of the limbs (mittenlike hands and feet), and midfacial hypoplasia (Table 1). Although pronounced syndactyly ("mitten hands") is considered diagnostic, some infants show only mild forms. Other skeletal abnormalities include high cranial vault (acrocephaly), prominent forehead (frontal bossing), hypertelorism and

TABLE 1. PATHOLOGIC AND CLINICAL FEATURES OF APERT SYNDROME

Central nervous system
　Craniosynostosis with acrocephaly/turricephaly
　Agenesis/hypoplasia of corpus callosum
　Hydrocephalus
　Cephalocele
　Spina bifida
　Cerebral atrophy/hypoplasia of the white matter
　Gyral abnormalities, heterotopic gray matter
Extremities
　Brachydactyly
　Broad thumbs
　Elbow joint/radiohumeral synostosis
　Hypoplastic or absent humerus
　Polysyndactyly of fingers (mitten hands)
　Polydactyly of toes
Facial
　Cleft palate
　Hypertelorism
　Prominent eyes/proptosis
　Prominent forehead (frontal bossing)
　Malar hypoplasia
　Depressed nasal bridge with parrot-beaked nose
Cardiac anomalies
　Pulmonic stenosis
　Overriding aorta
　Ventricular septal defects
Genitourinary: hydronephrosis

Reproduced with permission from McKusick VA, ed. Online mendelian inheritance in man. Available at: http://www.ncbi.nlm.nih.gov/omim/. McKusick-Nathans Institute for Genetic Medicine, Johns Hopkins University (Baltimore, MD) and National Center for Biotechnology Information, National Library of Medicine (Bethesda, MD), 2000.

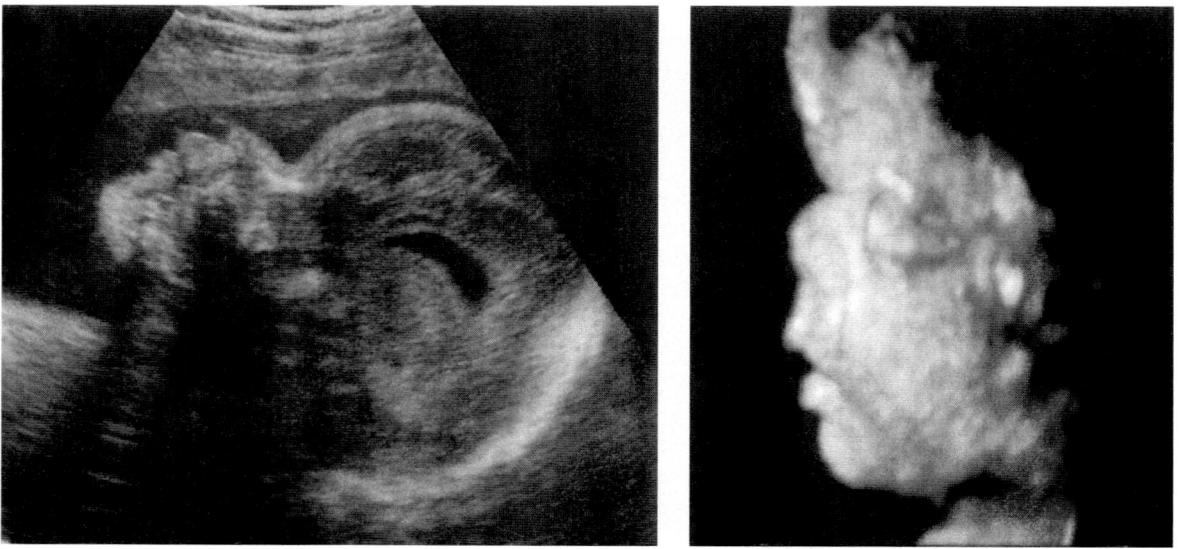

FIGURE 3. Apert syndrome. **A:** A third-trimester sagittal view shows typical facial abnormalities with deformity, acrocephaly, frontal bossing, and sunken nasal bridge. **B:** A third-trimester three-dimensional scan in the lateral view shows facial deformities. (Courtesy of Bernard Benoit, Nice, France.)

proptosis, and a depressed nasal bridge with parrot-beaked nose. The abnormalities are now known to be associated with abnormalities of the *FGFR2* gene.[40,41]

Diagnosis

Characteristic features of Apert syndrome include craniosynostosis (Fig. 3), midfacial hypoplasia, and bilateral symmetric syndactyly of the limbs[42,43] (Fig. 4). The earliest case of abnormal skull shape was reported at 19 weeks.[44] Sonographic demonstration is difficult before then and may even be absent pathologically,[45] which suggests that craniosynostosis develops after the midtrimester in most cases. Both normal and fused sutures of craniosynostosis can be best evaluated using three-dimensional ultrasound.[46] Prenatal three-dimensional computed tomography (CT) has also been used.[47] Characteristic mitten hands have been detected as early as 14 weeks[48] (Fig. 4) and have also been detected by fetoscopy.[49,50] Patients with the P253R mutation show a more severe syndactyly.[51]

Diaphragmatic hernia has been reported as the initial sonographic sign of Apert syndrome.[52] Increased nuchal fold at the first trimester might be a sonographic marker for the disorder.[42] In the third trimester, polyhydramnios may develop from decreased fetal swallowing related to central nervous system (CNS) abnormalities.[53]

Genetic Testing

Molecular testing is now available for affected families[54] and is usually done on chorionic villi. Suspicious ultrasound findings can also lead to definitive molecular testing.[55]

Differential Diagnosis

Similar facial and cranial features may be seen with all the craniosynostoses including Carpenter syndrome,[56,57] Pfeiffer syndrome,[58,59] and Crouzon syndrome.[60,61] Mutations of the *FGFR2* gene are also associated with Crouzon syndrome and Pfeiffer, Jackson-Weiss, and Beare-Stevenson cutis gyrata syndromes. Other clinical findings and diagnostic molecular genetic studies should distinguish these possibilities.

Prognosis

Airway obstruction is observed in 40% of patients with severe craniosynostotic syndromes.[62,63] Obstruction may be secondary to midface hypoplasia, lower airway obstruction, tonsillar and adenoid hypertrophy, or choanal atresia. Airway obstruction may result in apnea and cor pulmonale and may require tracheostomy.[63,64]

Mental delay or retardation may occur in approximately one-half of cases.[65] The frequency of increased intracranial hypertension and the risk of mental impairment depend on the age of the child and the type of craniosynostosis.[66]

Abnormalities of the extremities may be symptomatic. Foot and toe deformities may lead to foot problems and pain.[67,68]

Management

Facial surgery is performed for cosmetic and functional reasons. Treacher Collins syndrome, Crouzon syndrome, or

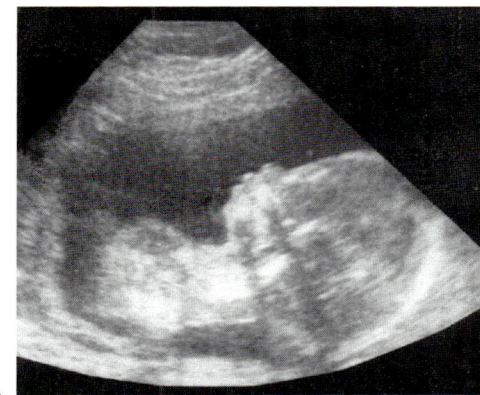

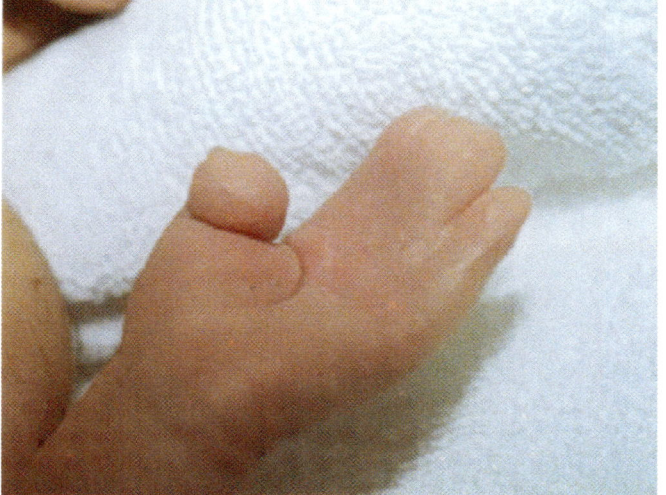

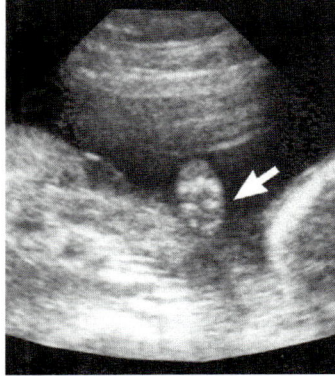

FIGURE 4. Apert syndrome. **A:** A second-trimester fetus with Apert syndrome shows subtle acrocephaly. **B:** The typical mitten hand (*arrow*), consistent with polysyndactyly, is seen in the same fetus. **C:** A photograph after birth of a similar case shows typical mitten hand.

Apert syndrome requires more than one operation to achieve maximum correction.[69,70] Surgical correction of the craniosynostosis may not alter the mental retardation.

Recurrence Risk

Apert syndrome is an autosomal disorder with dominant inheritance; the recurrence risk is 50% in affected parents. However, most cases are sporadic, resulting from new mutations.

▶ ARTHROGRYPOSIS/AKINESIA SEQUENCE

Arthrogryposis is a highly heterogeneous condition describing fixed contractures at multiple sites.[71] Generalized arthrogryposis may affect nearly all joints. The heterogeneous conditions associated with arthrogryposis have produced a confusing medical literature and terminology. Arthrogryposis usually results in other deformations because of absent or decreased movement.[72]

Synonyms for arthrogryposis include fetal akinesia/hypokinesia sequence and fetal akinesia deformation sequence. Conditions that may be categorized as arthrogryposis include Pena-Shokeir syndrome, lethal multiple pterygium syndrome, arthrogryposis multiplex congenita, Neu-Laxova syndrome, and congenital muscular dystrophies or myopathies.

Prevalence

The prevalence of arthrogryposis is unknown.

Genetic Defect

Myotonic dystrophy is caused by an increased number of CTG trinucleotide repeats in the DMPK gene (chromosomal locus 19q13). Expansions of the CTG trinucleotide repeat that are large enough to cause congenital myotonic dystrophy occur almost exclusively in maternal meiosis. This explains why congenital myotonic dystrophy is associated with maternal inheritance.

Pathologic and Clinical Features

A wide variety of conditions may include arthrogryposis as a primary feature (Table 2). The major features of some of the recognized conditions of arthrogryposis are summarized in Table 3.[73] The underlying abnormality has been reported as both neurogenic (central as well as peripheral)[74] and myogenic.[75] Absent or reduced fetal movement leads to stiff joints, contractures, pterygia, impaired growth, and abnormal bone morphology with decreased calcification. The bones may be slender and hypoplastic. Decreased fetal swallowing causes pulmonary hypoplasia and polyhydramnios. The classic form of

TABLE 2. SYNDROMES ASSOCIATED WITH ARTHROGRYPOSIS

Pena-Shokeir syndrome
Lethal multiple pterygium syndrome
Cerebro-oculo-facio-skeletal syndrome
Neu-Laxova syndrome
Arthrogryposis multiplex congenita (amyoplasia congenita)
Congenital myotonic dystrophy
Gaucher disease type 2
Alpers disease (progressive infantile poliodystrophy)
Restrictive dermopathy

arthrogryposis multiplex congenita, also called *amyoplasia congenita*, is characterized by different degrees of maldevelopment of the skeletal muscles, which are replaced by fibrous and fatty tissue. Although sporadic, it is more common among monozygotic twins and is the most common form of arthrogryposis seen in children. It may be associated with gastroschisis and bowel atresia, suggesting a vascular origin in some cases.[76,77]

Pena and Shokeir[78] first described Pena-Shokeir syndrome in 1974 as a recessive disorder characterized by arthrogryposis and pulmonary hypoplasia. Moerman et al.[79] suggested that Pena-Shokeir syndrome I is a primary motor neuropathy characterized by marked paucity of anterior horn cells in the spinal cord and diffuse muscle atrophy. Moessinger[72] suggested that the Pena-Shokeir I phenotype is not specific but rather the result of a deformation sequence caused by fetal akinesia.

Cerebro-oculo-facial-skeletal syndrome has also been called *Pena-Shokeir type II*, although this designation has been abandoned. It is a lethal condition characterized by contractures, dysmyelinization, and facial anomalies.

The lethal multiple pterygium syndrome, also autosomal recessive, shares similar features with the Pena-Shokeir phenotype.[80] Features include multiple contractures, pterygia of joints, cystic hygroma, and skeletal deformities. The pathogenesis is believed to be either early arrest in muscle development or replacement of muscle by fatty tissue.

Myotonic dystrophy is an autosomal dominant condition that results in continued active contraction of a muscle after ceasing voluntary activity. It is characterized by difficulty in releasing one's grip, masklike facies, cataracts, gonadal atrophy, and frontal balding in males. Congenital myotonic dystrophy is a severe form resulting in respiratory and feeding difficulties in association with severe neonatal hypotonia and mental retardation. Muscles of the lower extremities are generally more severely affected than the upper limbs.

Neu-Laxova syndrome is another autosomal recessive disorder associated with neurogenic akinesia. Features include exophthalmos, microcephaly, brain malforma-

TABLE 3. MAJOR FEATURES OF DISORDERS EXHIBITING EVIDENCE OF ARTHROGRYPOSIS

Disorder	Major features	Inheritance	Prognosis
Pena-Shokeir syndrome	Growth retardation, multiple joint contractures, facial anomalies, pulmonary hypoplasia, hypertelorism, abnormal bone morphology with decreased calcification, short umbilical cord	Autosomal recessive or sporadic	Usually lethal
Lethal multiple pterygium syndrome	Soft tissue webbing and flexion contractures of neck, axilla, antecubital, and popliteal regions; hypoplastic lungs; intrauterine growth restriction; cystic hygroma; hydrops	Usually autosomal recessive	Uniformly lethal
Arthrogryposis multiplex congenita	Fixed contractures, clubfeet, involvement of all four extremities in two-thirds of cases, normal intelligence	Sporadic	Variable, usually lethal when severe
Congenital myotonic dystrophy	Clubfoot (50%), hypotonia, facial muscle weakness, swallowing and speech difficulties, respiratory distress, occasional joint contractures, mental retardation	Autosomal dominant; affected infants are born only to mothers with myotonic dystrophy	Mental retardation and motor delay common
Restrictive dermopathy	Hyperkeratosis; flexion of knees, elbows, wrists, and ankles; camptodactyly; short umbilical cord; prematurity; hypertelorism; tight, rigid, shiny skin	Autosomal recessive	Lethal after birth
Cerebro-oculo-facial-skeletal syndrome	Microcephaly, microphthalmos, cataract, scoliosis, hip and pelvic defects, flexion contractures, sloping forehead, rockerbottom feet	Autosomal recessive	Survival typically <3 yr
Alpers disease (progressive infantile poliodystrophy)	Intrauterine growth restriction, microcephaly, retrognathia, joint contractures, seizures	Autosomal recessive	Survival typically <3 yr
Gaucher disease type 2	Multiple contractures, visceromegaly, pulmonary hypoplasia, ichthyosis	Autosomal recessive	Survival typically <1 yr

Modified from Hammond E, Donnenfield AE. Fetal akinesia. *Obstet Gynecol Surv* 1995;50:140–149.

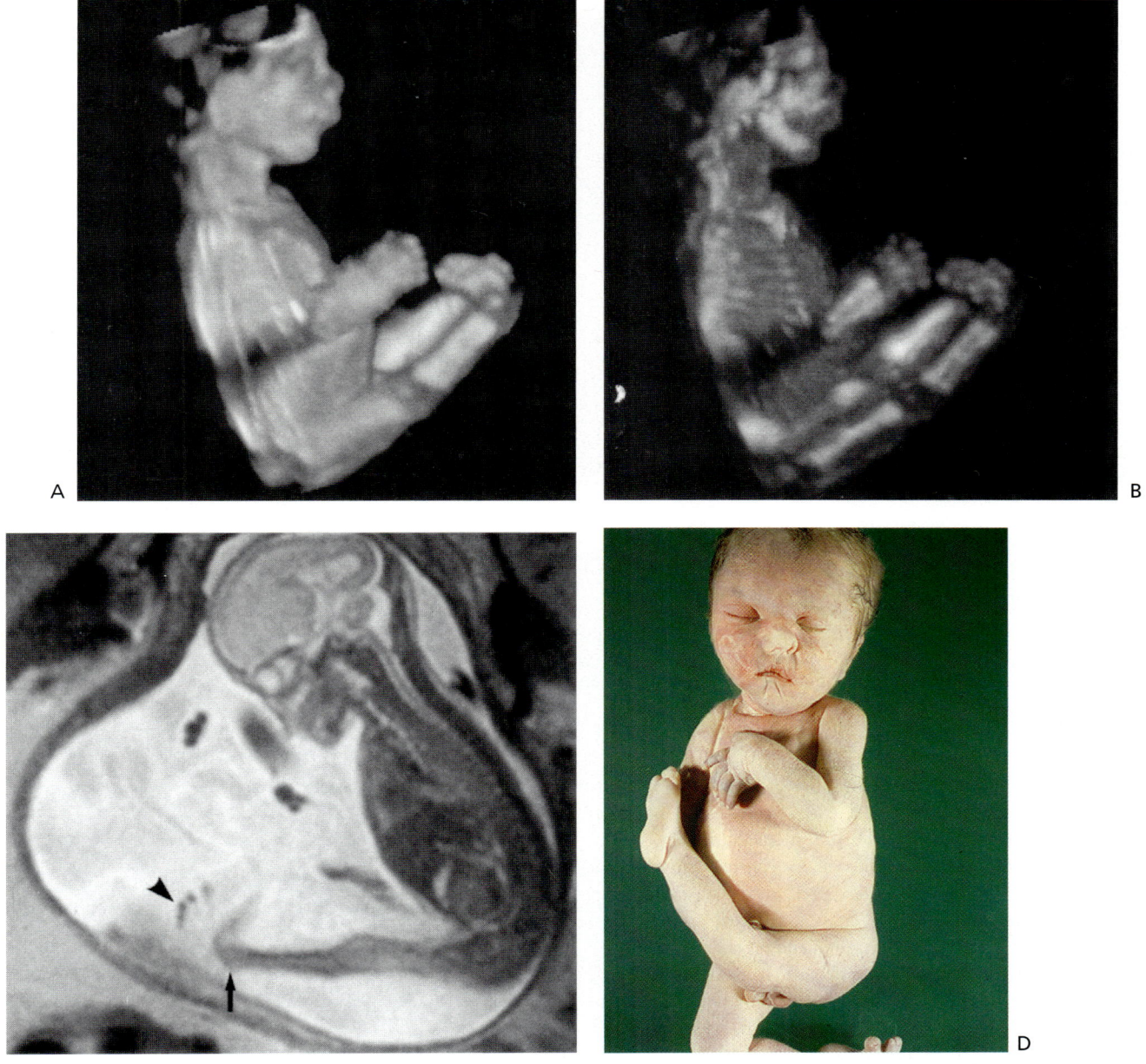

FIGURE 5. Arthrogryposis. Three-dimensional ultrasound in soft tissue **(A)** and skeletal **(B)** modes shows arthrogryposis with fixed contractures of the ankles and hips and fixed extension of the knees. (**A** courtesy of Raj Kapur, Pathology Department, Children's Hospital, Seattle, WA.) **C:** A magnetic resonance image of a similar case shows abnormal fetal positioning with flexed knees, extended knees, and clubfoot (*arrow*). Arrowhead points to toes. (Reproduced with permission from Huppert BJ, Brandt KR, Ramin KD, King BF. Single-shot fast spin-echo MR imaging of the fetus: a pictorial essay. *Radiographics* 1999;19:S215–S227.) **D:** A postmortem photograph of another case shows marked contraction deformities of the lower and upper extremities. (Courtesy of Joe Siebert, Pathology Department, Children's Hospital, Seattle, WA.)

tions, lymphedema, ichthyosis, an open gaping mouth, and severe intrauterine growth restriction (IUGR). CNS anomalies include lissencephaly, cerebellar hypoplasia, Dandy-Walker malformation, and agenesis of the corpus callosum.

Gaucher disease type 2 is a sphingolipid storage disorder resulting from decreased cerebrosidase. Features include

multiple contractures, visceromegaly, pulmonary hypoplasia, and ichthyosis.

Diagnosis

The major finding of arthrogryposis is abnormal limb position with restrictive fetal movement of more than one joint

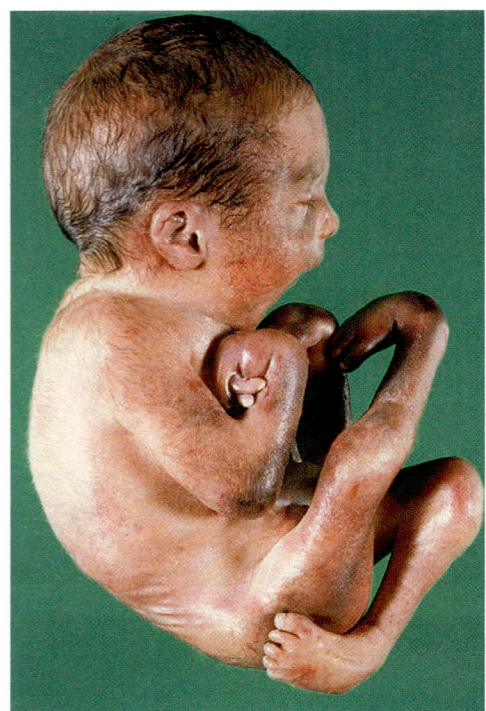
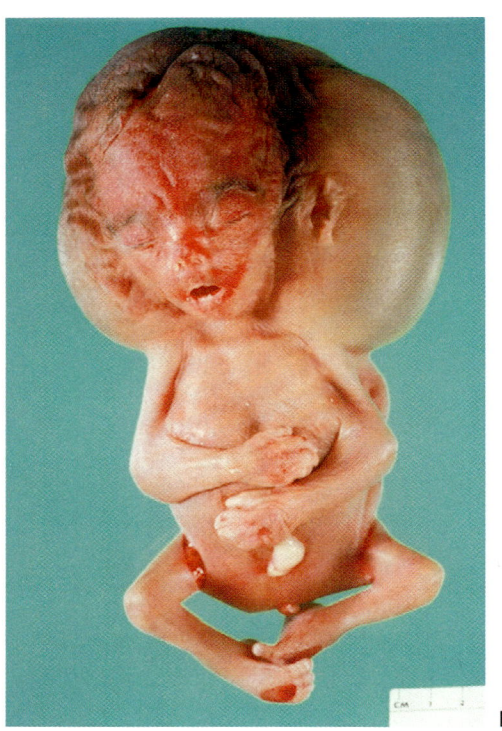

FIGURE 6. Arthrogryposis. Pathologic photographs of marked arthrogryposis multiplex congenita **(A)** and lethal multiple pterygium syndrome with contractures **(B)**. (Courtesy of Joe Siebert, Pathology Department, Children's Hospital, Seattle, WA.)

(Fig. 5). This may progress during pregnancy and have variable age of onset, although it is usually evident during the second trimester.[81] Polyhydramnios usually develops during the third trimester. IUGR and pulmonary hypoplasia also develop.[82] Low-set malformed ears, hypertelorism, short neck, cleft palate, scalp edema, thoracic deformities, camptodactyly, and micrognathia may also be found.[83] Anomalies less frequently described in association with Pena-Shokeir syndrome include diaphragmatic hernia, gastroschisis, and microcephaly.[84–86]

Contraction abnormalities may be severe and generalized (Fig. 6A). Cystic hygroma and hydrops are relatively common findings during the first and second trimesters in association with lethal multiple pterygium syndrome (Fig. 6B), in which case the contractures may not be recognized. Ocular abnormalities including microphthalmos may suggest a diagnosis of cerebro-oculo-facial-skeletal syndrome.[87] Gastroschisis and intestinal atresia may be seen with amyoplasia.

Prenatal findings of congenital myotonic dystrophy include contractures, which may initially present only as clubfoot.[88] Other findings may include polyhydramnios, hydrops, and hydrocephaly. In some cases, the presence of a fetus with congenital myotonic dystrophy has led to the identification of myotonic dystrophy in a previously undiagnosed mother.

Differential Diagnosis

Trisomy 18 may exhibit similar features, in particular craniofacial, limb, and intrathoracic abnormalities.[89] Teratogens and some infections may also result in similar findings. Any cause of severe oligohydramnios may result in contractures and pulmonary hypoplasia. Nonlethal forms of arthrogryposis show similar findings, except for pulmonary hypoplasia.

Prognosis

The prognosis is generally poor, especially for cases diagnosed prenatally. In its most severe form, Pena-Shokeir syndrome is lethal, with pulmonary complications as the primary cause of death. Fetuses who have conditions without pulmonary hypoplasia may survive. For congenital myotonic dystrophy, the severity of the clinical condition is related to the number of trinucleotide repeats.[90] Children with the congenital form of myotonic dystrophy show the most severe phenotype and have large expansions, usually more than 1,000 repeats. For arthrogryposis multiplex congenita, involvement can be mild and a favorable prognosis has been reported among some postnatal cases with physical therapy or orthopedic surgery.[91]

Management

Termination of pregnancy can be offered before viability. Occasional survivors require a multidisciplinary team including the primary physician, orthopedist, physical therapist, and plastic surgeon.

Recurrence Risk

Sporadic, X-L, AR, and AD forms of arthrogryposis have been reported, and the recurrence risk depends on the underlying etiology. For cases in which the etiology is unknown, an empiric recurrence risk of 5% has been suggested for unaffected couples with one previously affected pregnancy.[91a] For patients with a history of myotonic dystrophy, rapid prenatal diagnosis is available following chorionic villus sampling or amniocentesis.[92]

▶ BECKWITH-WIEDEMANN SYNDROME

Beckwith-Wiedemann syndrome (BWS) was first described by Beckwith in 1963[93] and Wiedemann in 1964.[94] It is characterized primarily by macrosomia, omphalocele, macroglossia, and a propensity to develop childhood tumors. Synonyms for BWS include *Wiedemann-Beckwith syndrome* and *exomphalos-macroglossia-gigantism syndrome*.

Incidence

The reported incidence of approximately 1 in 13,700[95] is probably an underestimate given the existence of milder, undiagnosed cases. BWS has been reported in a wide variety of ethnic populations with an equal incidence in males and females. The frequency may be higher in monozygotic twins.

Genetic Defect

The chromosomal locus is 11p15.5. A small number (1%) have cytogenetic abnormalities involving chromosome 11p15.[96–98] Ten percent to 20% of infants with nonfamilial BWS and a normal karyotype have uniparental (paternal) disomy. Mutations in the gene *p57^KIP2^* (also known as *CDKN1C*) are found in 5% to 10% of patients with normal chromosome studies. This gene helps regulate cyclin-dependent kinase inhibitor, which negatively regulates cell proliferation. This gene is both a tumor-suppressor gene and a potential negative regulator of fetal growth.[99]

Pathologic and Clinical Features

BWS is characterized by macrosomia, macroglossia, visceromegaly, embryonic tumors (i.e., Wilms tumor, hepatoblastoma, neuroblastoma, rhabdomyosarcoma), omphalocele,

TABLE 4. PATHOLOGIC AND CLINICAL FEATURES OF BECKWITH-WIEDEMANN SYNDROME

Growth
  Macrosomia
  Hemihypertrophy
Craniofacial
  Metopic ridge
  Large fontanelle
  Prominent occiput
  Coarse facial features
  Prominent eyes
  Linear earlobe creases
  Posterior helical indentations
  Macroglossia
Abdomen
  Omphalocele
  Hepatomegaly
  Pancreatic hyperplasia
  Hepatoblastoma
  Adrenal carcinoma
Metabolic: neonatal hypoglycemia
Hormonal
  Adrenocortical cytomegaly
  Pituitary amphophil hyperplasia
Genitourinary
  Renal medullary dysplasia
  Large kidneys
  Overgrowth of external genitalia
  Cryptorchidism
  Wilms tumor
  Gonadoblastoma
Cardiovascular
  Cardiomyopathy
  Cardiomegaly

Reproduced with permission from McKusick VA, ed. Online mendelian inheritance in man. Available at: http://www.ncbi.nlm.nih.gov/omim/. McKusick-Nathans Institute for Genetic Medicine, Johns Hopkins University (Baltimore, MD) and National Center for Biotechnology Information, National Library of Medicine (Bethesda, MD), 2000.

neonatal hypoglycemia, and ear creases/pits (Table 4). Hemihypertrophy is also common. Pancreatic cell hyperplasia may affect 30% to 50% of patients, causing hyperinsulinism, which can result in profound neonatal hypoglycemia.[100]

Diagnosis

Ultrasound

BWS should be suspected if antenatal ultrasound demonstrates any combination of omphalocele, growth acceleration, macroglossia, and visceromegaly (Fig. 7). A positive family history is obviously helpful but is usually absent. Polyhydramnios is common in fetuses with BWS during the third trimester. Early diagnosis is also possible. One case observed before 14 weeks' gestation showed increased nuchal translucency and omphalocele.[101]

BWS should be considered whenever the karyotype is normal and omphalocele is present, especially for omphaloceles with intracorporeal liver (Fig. 7A). Several studies sug-

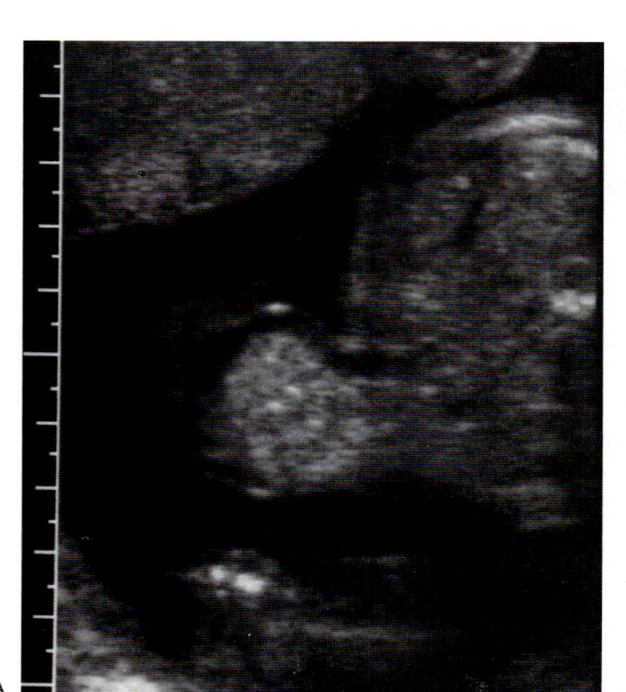

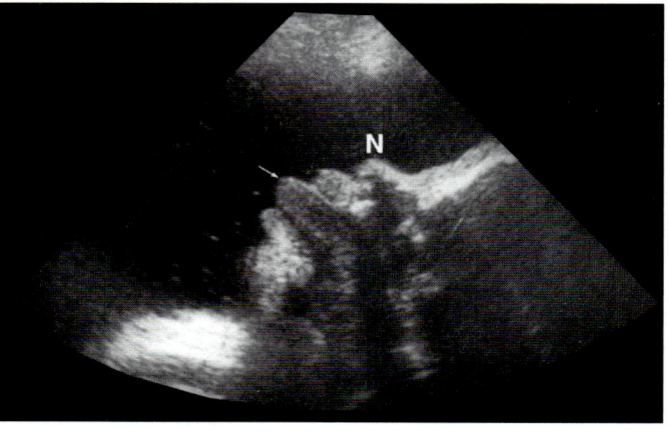

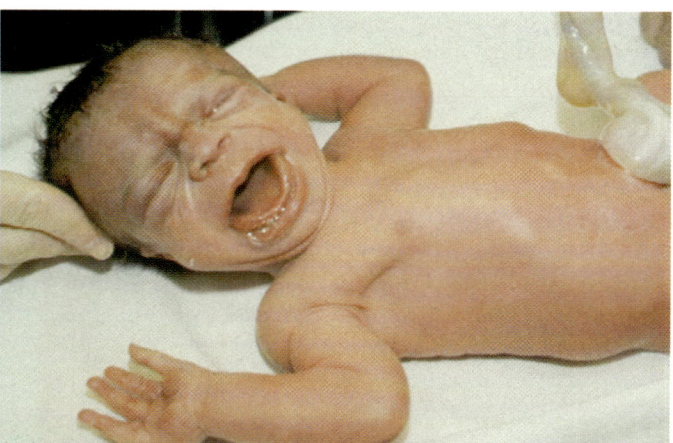

FIGURE 7. Beckwith-Wiedemann syndrome. **A:** Typical omphalocele with intracorporeal liver is seen on transverse view. **B:** A third-trimester sagittal view shows macroglossia (*arrow*) in a fetus who proved to have Beckwith-Wiedemann syndrome. N, nose. (Courtesy of Beryl Benacerraf, Boston, MA.) **C:** A photograph after birth of another infant with Beckwith-Wiedemann syndrome shows macroglossia and a small omphalocele with intracorporeal liver.

gest that patients with BWS and omphalocele are more likely to show *p57^KIP2* mutations[96] and less likely to exhibit uniparental disomy.[97] Furthermore, these patients may not be at risk for development of embryonic tumors.[98]

Genetic Testing

Cytogenetic testing is appropriate to look for translocations, inversions, and duplications involving 11p15. Molecular genetic testing for either uniparental disomy or *p57^KIP2* mutations can be offered if there is a high index of suspicion for BWS. Other biochemical tests are also available on a research basis.

Differential Diagnosis

Chromosome abnormalities must be excluded, especially when omphalocele with intracorporeal liver is observed. Down syndrome may also show macroglossia but does not usually exhibit macrosomia. Zellweger syndrome may show

liver and kidney enlargement and may be diagnosed prenatally by measuring fatty acid concentration and activity of marker enzymes.[102]

Simpson-Golabi-Behmel syndrome is an X-linked recessive condition that shares many features with BWS (e.g., macrosomia, visceromegaly, macroglossia, and renal anomalies). It is distinguished by the presence of distinctive facial features, cleft lip, and skeletal abnormalities including polydactyly.

Perlman syndrome is a rare autosomal recessive condition with macrosomia and a high incidence of Wilms tumor. Facial features are distinctive, neonatal mortality is high, and significant intellectual handicap is common. Perlman syndrome is thought to be genetically distinct from BWS, although the gene causing Perlman syndrome has not been identified.

Prognosis

Infants with BWS have a mortality rate of approximately 20%, mainly due to complications of prematurity associated with omphalocele, macroglossia, neonatal hypoglycemia, and, rarely, cardiomyopathy.[103] Other less common endocrine, metabolic, and hematologic findings include hypothyroidism, hyperlipidemia/hypercholesterolemia, and polycythemia.

Children with BWS have an increased risk of mortality associated with neoplasia, particularly Wilms tumor and hepatoblastoma, but also including neuroblastoma, adrenocortical carcinoma, and rhabdomyosarcoma. The estimated risk for tumor development in children with BWS is 7.5%. This increased risk for neoplasia seems to be concentrated in the first 8 years of life. An increased relative risk of cancer has been associated with hemihypertrophy[104] and, perhaps, nephromegaly.

Management

The omphalocele, when present, is repaired soon after birth. Management of a newborn in whom BWS is suspected includes early and close monitoring for hypoglycemia, especially in the first 7 days of life. Early treatment of hypoglycemia is necessary to reduce the risk of CNS complications. Occasionally, delayed onset of hypoglycemia occurs; parents should be informed of the symptoms of hypoglycemia so that they can seek appropriate medical attention. Treatment for hemihyperplasia and macroglossia may be necessary. Abdominal ultrasound is recommended every 3 months until 8 years of age for tumor surveillance.[105] A baseline magnetic resonance imaging (MRI) or CT examination of the abdomen may also be obtained.

Recurrence Risk

The mode of inheritance is complex. Approximately 85% of cases are sporadic and karyotypically normal; 10% to 15% of cases are associated with an autosomal dominant mode of inheritance with incomplete penetrance and preferential maternal transmission. Even with a negative family history, the recurrence risk is up to 50% if $p57^{KIP2}$ mutation is present in a parent.[99] In families in which the proband has paternal uniparental disomy for chromosome 11p15, the recurrence risk is empirically very low, because the uniparental disomy in this region appears to arise from a postzygotic somatic recombination. In familial cases, transmission is always through the mother.

▶ CHARGE ASSOCIATION

Hall[106] first reported a constellation of nonrandomly associated malformations occurring with choanal atresia. This was subsequently broadened by Pagon et al.[107] who first used the acronym *CHARGE*: *c*oloboma of the eye, *h*eart defects, *a*tresia of the choanae, *r*etarded mental and growth development, *g*enital anomalies, and *e*ar anomalies.

Incidence

The CHARGE association is rare.

Genetic Defect

The CHARGE association is heterogeneous. Although the *PAX2* gene has been found not to be the cause, it may be indirectly involved.[108] A significantly higher mean paternal age at conception together with concordance in monozygotic twins and the existence of rare familial cases supports the role of genetic factors such as *de novo* dominant mutation or submicroscopic chromosome rearrangement.

Pathologic and Clinical Features

For a thorough list of the pathologic and clinical features of the CHARGE association, see Table 5. Orofacial clefts and esophageal atresia are primary features. However,

TABLE 5. PATHOLOGIC AND CLINICAL FEATURES OF THE CHARGE ASSOCIATION

Growth
  Short stature
  Growth delay
Central nervous system/neurologic
  Dandy-Walker malformation
  Holoprosencephaly
  Mental retardation
  Deafness
Cardiovascular
  Tetralogy of Fallot
  Double-outlet right ventricle
  Atrial septal defect
Craniofacial
  Choanal atresia/stenosis
  Cleft lip/palate
  Ear abnormalities, deafness, abnormal auditory ossicles
  Vestibular dysfunction
  Temporal bone malformation
  Ocular abnormalities, colobomas
  Microcephaly
  Micrognathia
Gastrointestinal
  Esophageal atresia/stenosis
  Tracheoesophageal fistula
  Anal atresia, stenosis
  Omphalocele
Genitourinary
  Central hypogonadism
  Cryptorchidism
  Horseshoe kidney
  Hydronephrosis
Hormonal
  Hypopituitarism
  Hypothyroidism
  Parathyroid hypoplasia
  Growth hormone deficiency

CHARGE, *c*oloboma of the eye, *h*eart defects, *a*tresia of the choanae, *r*etarded mental and growth development, *g*enital anomalies, and *e*ar anomalies.
Reproduced with permission from McKusick VA, ed. Online mendelian inheritance in man. Available at: http://www.ncbi.nlm.nih.gov/omim/. McKusick-Nathans Institute for Genetic Medicine, Johns Hopkins University (Baltimore, MD) and National Center for Biotechnology Information, National Library of Medicine (Bethesda, MD), 2000.

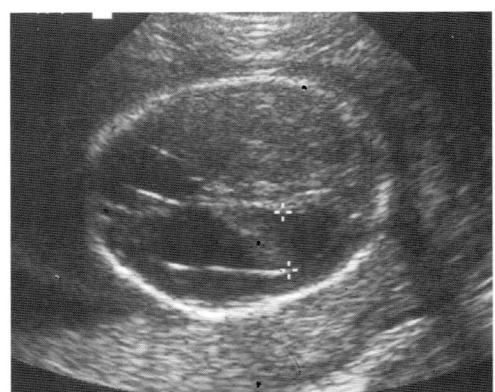 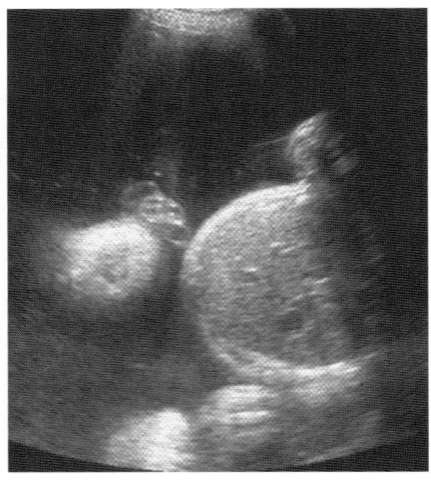

FIGURE 8. CHARGE (*c*oloboma of the eye, *h*eart defects, *a*tresia of the choanae, *r*etarded mental and *g*rowth development, *g*enital anomalies, and *e*ar anomalies) association. **A:** An axial scan of the head at 19 weeks shows mild cerebral ventricular dilatation (11 mm). **B:** In a follow-up scan at 36 weeks, ventricular dilatation is resolved, but marked polyhydramnios, nonvisible stomach, and growth restriction are shown. At birth, the infant was found to have the CHARGE association with choanal atresia, colobomas, and genital anomalies.

abnormalities of the ears appear to be even more common. Tetralogy of Fallot is the most frequent heart defect reported in the CHARGE association.[109] Tellier et al.[110] evaluated 47 CHARGE patients for the frequency of major anomalies: coloboma (79%), heart malformation (85%), choanal atresia growth and/or mental retardation (100%), genital anomalies (34%), ear anomalies (91%), and deafness (62%). In addition, they commented on anomalies observed frequently in neonates and infants with the CHARGE association, including minor facial anomalies, neonatal brainstem dysfunction with cranial nerve palsy, and internal ear anomalies, such as semicircular canal hypoplasia, which was found in each patient tested. The presence of CNS malformations has been associated with choanal atresia.[111] Forebrain anomalies, particularly arrhinencephalia and holoprosencephaly, are common.

Diagnosis

Affected fetuses have been rarely detected by prenatal sonography.[112] Findings may appear indistinguishable from cases of esophageal atresia with polyhydramnios and absent or small fluid-filled stomach (Fig. 8). Holoprosencephaly or other brain abnormalities may be evident. We have also seen an affected fetus who presented with increased nuchal translucency during the first trimester.

Because hypogonadotropic hypogonadism appears to be the usual cause of genital and pubertal abnormalities in the CHARGE association, measurement of serum luteinizing hormone and follicle-stimulating hormone

concentrations in infants up to 2 to 3 months of age in whom this disorder is suspected could help establish the diagnosis.[113]

Differential Diagnosis

Some phenotypic overlap is shown with the VATER complex. Similar features may also be seen with chromosome abnormalities including trisomy 13, trisomy 18, 4p– syndrome, and cat-eye syndrome.

Prognosis

Choanal atresia is a threat to life because young infants cannot establish the habit of mouth breathing. Airway instability can lead to cerebral hypoxia and developmental delay in some patients.

Management

Effective management requires early diagnosis and intervention as well as an interdisciplinary approach.[114] Surgical correction is required for choanal atresia,[115] although early tracheostomy rather than definitive repair has been recommended because of airway instability.[116] Deafness from inner ear malformations can be improved with implanted multichannel cochlear implants.[117]

Recurrence Risk

Risk of recurrence is low.

► CORNELIA DE LANGE SYNDROME

Also known as *Brachmann–de Lange* or *de Lange syndrome*, Cornelia de Lange syndrome is a developmental syndrome characterized by mental handicap, growth retardation, limb reduction abnormalities, and distinctive facial features.[118,119] It was first reported as a severe form in 1916. In 1933, Cornelia de Lange, a Dutch pediatrician, described two children with similar features.[120]

Incidence

The incidence of Cornelia de Lange syndrome is approximately 1 in 40,000.[121]

Genetic Defect

The chromosome locus for this syndrome is 3q26.3.[122] The genetic and biochemical basis is unknown. Suggested genetic abnormalities include anomalous human chordin gene, *THPO* (thrombopoietin), *CLCN2* (a voltage-gated chloride-channel gene), and *EIF4G1* (a eukaryotic translation-initiation-factor-gamma gene, which maps within a gene cluster at 3q27),[123] and *SHOT* (a homeobox gene).[124] Others have suggested mitochondrial DNA deletions,[125] which would support a more common maternal transmission of the disorder from the mother.[126]

Pathologic and Clinical Features

Pathologic and clinical features of Cornelia de Lange syndrome are summarized in Table 6. The syndrome is characterized by profound pre- and postnatal growth delay,

TABLE 6. PATHOLOGIC AND CLINICAL FEATURES OF CORNELIA DE LANGE SYNDROME

Growth: growth delay
Central nervous system/neurologic
   Mental retardation
   Feeding difficulties
Craniofacial
   Cleft palate
   Long curly eyelashes
   Long philtrum
   Microphthalmos
   Thin upper lip, down-turned angles of mouth
   Synophrys (eyebrows appear to meet in midline)
Skin: generalized hirsutism
Skeletal
   Micromelia
   Syndactyly of second and third toes
   Hypoplastic or absent ulna
   Split/cleft hand/forefoot/ectrodactyly
Gastrointestinal
   Intestinal malrotation
   Small bowel atresia
Cardiovascular: cardiac defects

microbrachycephaly, hirsutism, various visceral and limb anomalies, and a typical face.[127,128] Other finding include low hairline, synophrys (i.e., the eyebrows appear to meet in midline), ocular anomalies, high arched palate, brain malformations,[129] malrotation of the gut,[130] duplications, and occasional renal anomalies.[131] Although IQ is rarely normal,[132] developmental delay is typically borderline (10%), mild (8%), moderate (18%), severe (20%), or profound (43%).[133,134]

Diagnosis

Ultrasound

Prenatal sonographic diagnoses of Cornelia de Lange syndrome have been made. The primary feature is IUGR. Other findings may include microcephaly, brachycephaly, micrognathia, long eyelashes, hirsutism, cardiac anomalies, polycystic and ectopic kidneys, and limb anomalies (Fig. 9). More subtle anomalies that can occasionally be noted on three-dimensional ultrasound include unusual palpebral fissures, low-set ears, anteverted nostrils, prominent philtrum, thin upper lip, broad or depressed nasal bridge, and down-turned angles of the mouth. Cases have been reported showing increased nuchal translucency, early-onset IUGR, and limb abnormalities in the first trimester.[135]

Biochemistry

Aitken et al.[136] observed an association between Cornelia de Lange syndrome and lower levels of pregnancy-associated plasma protein A in maternal serum during the second trimester. For parents with a previously affected child, the pregnancy-associated plasma protein A test can give an estimate of the likelihood of recurrence in the current pregnancy (NTD Laboratories: http://www.ntdlaboratories.com).

Differential Diagnosis

Partial trisomy 3q,[137] IUGR, prominent philtrum, phocomelia, and syndactyly of the second and third toes are more frequent in Cornelia de Lange syndrome, whereas craniosynostosis, cleft palate, and urinary tract anomalies are more typical of dup(3q).

Prognosis

Affected patients have severe mental impairment with an estimated IQ under 60. Self-destructive behavior and orthopedic and respiratory complications may also occur. Gastrointestinal complications and postnatal growth deficiency are also common.

Management

Postnatal management requires a multidisciplinary approach.

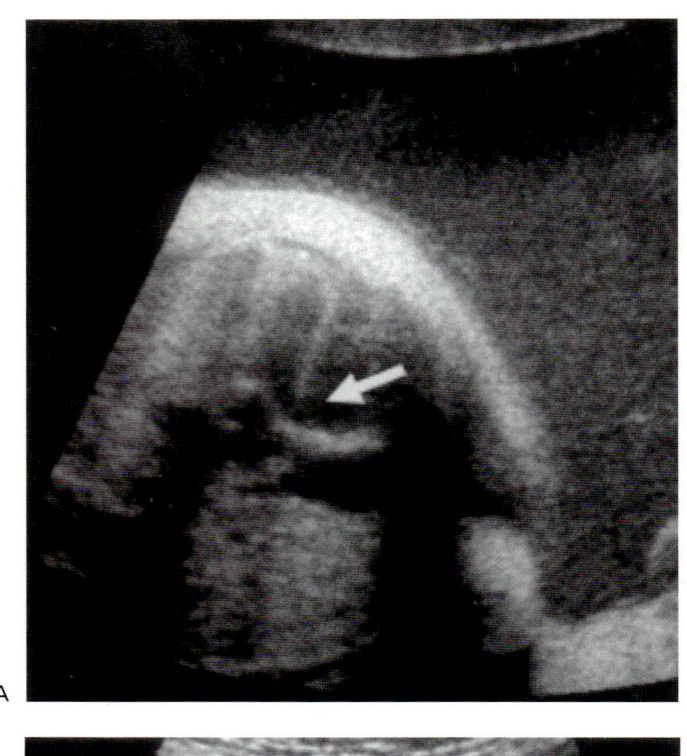

A

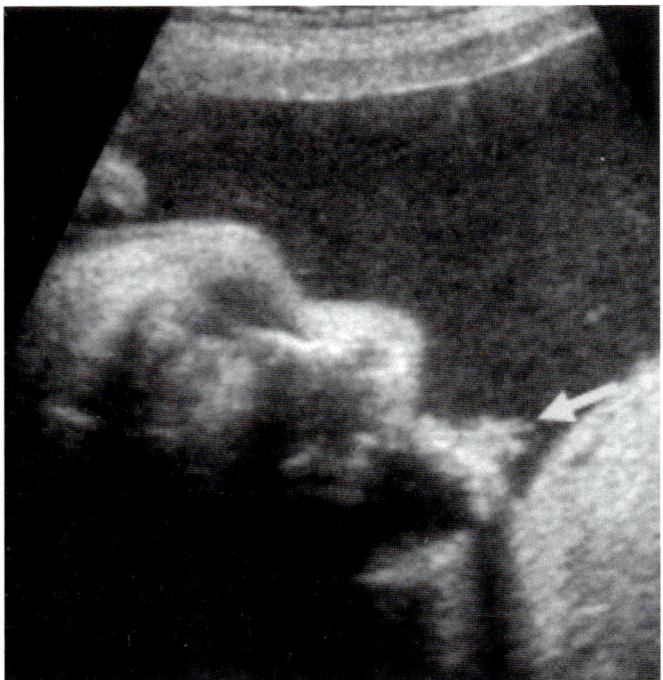

B

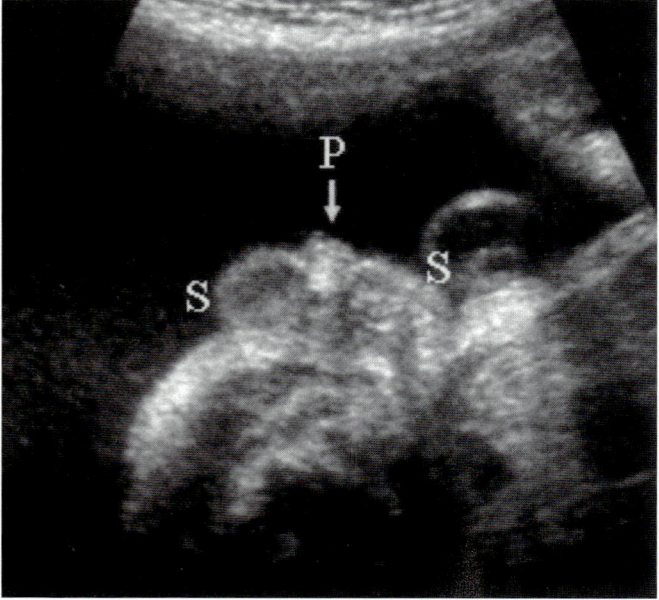

C

FIGURE 9. Cornelia de Lange syndrome. **A:** A transverse view of the thorax shows a high ventricular septal defect (*arrow*). A small pulmonary artery is also evident, suggesting pulmonary stenosis. **B:** An image of orbits shows long eyelashes (*arrow*). **C:** An image of the genitals shows ambiguous genitalia with a small penis (*P*). S, scrotum. (Courtesy of Gerald Mulligan, MD, Marshfield, WI, with permission from http://www.thefetus.net.)

Recurrence Risk

Risk of recurrence of this syndrome is less than 1%.[138] Several authors have suggested an autosomal dominant inheritance.[139] Discordant features have been shown in twin pregnancies including monozygotic twins.[140] There are other reports, however, of affected sibs with no parents affected.[141]

▶ CRANIOSYNOSTOSIS SYNDROMES (FIBROBLAST GROWTH FACTOR RECEPTOR–RELATED)*

The craniosynostosis syndromes include Muenke syndrome (*FGFR3*-associated craniosynostosis, *FGFR3*-associated coronal synostosis, Adelaide-type craniosynostosis), Crouzon syn-

*Modified from Robin NH. Craniosynostosis syndromes (FGFR-related). In: Pagon RA, ed. *GeneReviews* at GeneTests GeneClinics: medical genetics information resource (database online). Available at http://www.geneclinics.org/profiles/craniosynostosis. Copyright, University of Washington, Seattle, WA: Children's Health System and University of Washington, October 1998. Accessed October 2002.

drome, Jackson-Weiss syndrome, Apert syndrome, Pfeiffer syndrome, and Beare-Stevenson syndrome.

The craniosynostoses are etiologically and pathogenetically heterogeneous. More than 90 craniosynostosis syndromes have been delineated. Most cases of simple craniosynostosis are sporadic. Sagittal synostosis is most common, accounting for more than half the cases. The FGFR-related craniosynostosis syndromes are characterized by bicoronal craniosynostosis or cloverleaf skull, distinctive facial features, and variable hand and foot findings.

(See also the section on Apert syndrome, earlier in this chapter.)

Prevalence

The overall prevalence for all forms of craniosynostosis is 1 in 2,000 to 2,500 live births.[142] Sagittal synostosis is the most common, with an incidence of 1 in 5,250. Coronal synostosis is the second most common form of craniosynostosis, with an overall incidence of 1 in 16,000 in males and 1 in 8,000 in females. Approximately 5% of patients with isolated coronal synostosis have *FGFR3* mutations.[143]

The prevalence of Apert syndrome and Crouzon syndrome is approximately 1 in 70,000.[144,145] Apert syndrome accounts for approximately 4.5% of all cases of craniosynostosis. A suggested association with advanced paternal age has been confirmed for new mutations in Apert syndrome, Crouzon syndrome, and Beare-Stevenson syndrome.[8–19,39]

Genetic Defect

FGFRs are a family of four tyrosine kinase receptors that bind a group of 17 fibroblast growth factors (FGFs) in a nonspecific manner (any FGF can bind to any FGFR). The FGFs help regulate cell proliferation, differentiation, and migration through a variety of complex pathways.[146,147] They are important in angiogenesis, wound healing, limb development, malignant transformation, and spermatogenesis.[148]

Mutations in *FGFR1*, *FGFR2*, and *FGFR3* have been associated with a variety of clinical phenotypes. *FGFR* mutations are hypermorphic, causing the gene product to perform its normal function excessively. Gene map locus and corresponding syndromes for known FGFR-related conditions are shown in Table 7. The most common mutations associated with Apert syndrome are substitution S252W and P253R of the *FGFR2* gene. These two mutations account for approximately 98% of affected patients.[40,41]

To date there is no evidence that *FGFR4* is involved in craniofacial or skeletal disorders.

Pathologic and Clinical Features

Because the skull grows in planes perpendicular to the cranial sutures, premature suture closure causes skull growth

TABLE 7. GENE MAP LOCUS AND CORRESPONDING SYNDROMES FOR KNOWN FGFR-RELATED CONDITIONS

Gene	Chromosomal locus	Clinical phenotype
FGFR1	8p11	Pfeiffer syndrome
FGFR2	10q26	Apert syndrome
		Crouzon syndrome (95%)
		Pfeiffer syndrome
		Jackson-Weiss syndrome
		Beare-Stevenson syndrome
FGFR3	4p16	Muenke syndrome
		Crouzon syndrome (5%)
		Achondroplasia
		Hypochondroplasia
		Thanatophoric dysplasia

FGFR, fibroblast growth factor receptor.
Reproduced with permission from Robin NH. Craniosynostosis syndromes (FGFR-related). In: Pagon RA, ed. *Gene reviews*. Available at: http://www.geneclinics.org/profiles/ craniosynostosis. Seattle, WA: Children's Health System and University of Washington. Accessed October 1998.

to cease in the plane perpendicular to the closed suture and to proceed in a plane parallel to the affected suture. The skull shape becomes asymmetric, with the exact shape depending on which suture closes prematurely (Fig. 10). Coronal craniosynostosis causes the skull to be turricephalic, or "tower shaped." Occasionally, cloverleaf skull (or *Kleeblattschädel*) is seen. Cloverleaf skull involves a trilobar skull deformity usually caused by synostosis of the coronal, lambdoid, metopic, and sagittal sutures.

Clinical features of FGFR-related craniosynostosis syndromes are summarized in Table 8. Each shows bilateral coronal craniosynostosis or rarely cloverleaf skull, characteristic facial features, and variable hand and foot findings. Facial abnormalities include midfacial hypoplasia, a high cranial vault (acrocephaly), a prominent forehead (frontal bossing), hypertelorism and proptosis, and a depressed nasal bridge with parrot-beaked nose. A high arched palate is often present or, rarely, a cleft palate or choanal stenosis/atresia. Brain abnormalities, cardiac defects, diaphragmatic hernia, and genitourinary anomalies may also occur.

Diagnosis

FGFR-related craniosynostosis syndromes have been recognized prenatally with increasing frequency in recent years. Similar facial and cranial features may be seen with Apert syndrome (see Apert syndrome, earlier in this chapter), Carpenter syndrome,[56,57] Pfeiffer syndrome[46,58,149,150] (Fig. 11), and Crouzon syndrome.[60,61,151] A specific diagnosis of craniosynostosis is not usually appreciated until nearly 20 weeks or later, at least for new mutations.[44] Three-dimensional ultrasound has aided this diagnosis.

Characteristic facial abnormalities may be seen with craniosynostosis, including midfacial hypoplasia, acrocephaly,

TABLE 10. PATHOLOGIC AND CLINICAL FEATURES OF FRYNS SYNDROME

Central nervous system
  Hydrocephalus
  Holoprosencephaly
  Dandy-Walker malformation
  Mental retardation in survivors
Craniofacial
  Broad nasal bridge
  Micrognathia
  Abnormal ears
  Cleft palate
  Microphthalmos
  Loose skin in neck
  Facial hirsutism
  Flat nose
Gastrointestinal: duodenal atresia
Skeletal
  Distal digital hypoplasia
  Camptodactyly
  Hypoplastic nails
  Scoliosis
  Vertebral anomalies
  Extra ribs
  Osteochondrodysplasia
Thorax
  Lung hypoplasia/agenesis
  Diaphragmatic hernia
  Small thorax
  Chylothorax
Genitourinary
  Bicornuate uterus
  Renal cysts
Cardiovascular: cardiac defects

Reproduced with permission from McKusick VA, ed. Online mendelian inheritance in man. Available at: http://www.ncbi.nlm.nih.gov/omim/. McKusick-Nathans Institute for Genetic Medicine, Johns Hopkins University (Baltimore, MD) and National Center for Biotechnology Information, National Library of Medicine (Bethesda, MD), 2000.

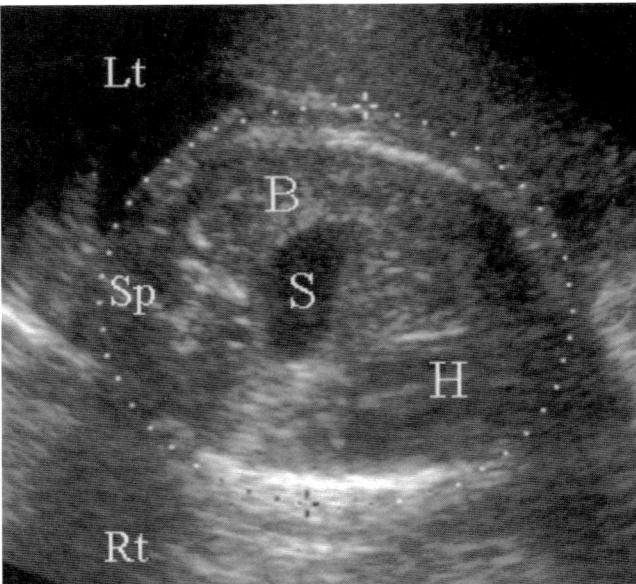

FIGURE 13. Fryns syndrome. A transverse view of the thorax shows a diaphragmatic hernia. The stomach (*S*) and bowel (*B*) are herniated into the left thorax and displace the heart (*H*) to the right (*Rt*) and anteriorly. Similar findings may be seen in fetuses with Fryns syndrome. Lt, left; Sp, spine.

central nervous, gastrointestinal, and genitourinary systems. Distal limb deficiencies include hypoplasia of the terminal phalanges and nails.

Diagnosis

The phenotypic variability makes the sonographic diagnosis of Fryns syndrome a challenge. It should be suspected when diaphragmatic hernia (Fig. 13) and other anomalies are identified with normal fetal karyotype. Development of polyhydramnios late in the second trimester and normal growth or overgrowth of the fetus are expected. The use of three-dimensional ultrasound may be helpful to precisely define the facial and extremity anomalies.[169] Cystic hygroma may be observed in the first trimester.[170]

Differential Diagnosis

The differential diagnosis includes trisomy 18 (which can be excluded by karyotype), Pallister-Killian syndrome (mosaic tetrasomy 12p), Zellweger syndrome (deficiency of peroxisomal enzyme), and Cornelia de Lange syndrome (usually associated with severe growth restriction). Overlap between Fryns syndrome and the Pallister-Killian syndrome has been noted.[171,172] The differential diagnosis between the two conditions depends on the demonstration of the 12p isochromosome in fibroblasts in the latter condition, although the karyotype of lymphocytes is normal.[173,174] Facial abnormalities of the Pallister-Killian syndrome can be identified prenatally.[175]

Prognosis

The majority of affected infants are stillborn or die in the early neonatal period. The few reported survivals have severe mental and developmental retardation.[176,177]

Management

When detected before viability, termination of pregnancy can be offered. After viability, standard prenatal care is not altered.

Recurrence Risk

Fryns syndrome is transmitted via autosomal recessive inheritance, with a 25% recurrence risk.[178] Phenotypic expression is variable[179]; discordance has been noted in a set of monozygotic twins.[180]

▶ GOLDENHAR SYNDROME

Goldenhar syndrome[181] is typically sporadic with classic features of unilateral deformity of the external ear, small ipsilateral half of the face, and vertebral anomalies. Gorlin et al.[182] suggested the designation *oculoauriculovertebral dysplasia*. Additional synonyms for Goldenhar syndrome include *oculoauriculovertebral spectrum*, *Goldenhar-Gorlin syndrome*, *facioauriculovertebral dysplasia*, and *hemifacial microsomia*.

Incidence

Goldenhar syndrome occurs in approximately 1 in 50,000 births.

Genetic Defect

The genetic basis is unknown. A case of Goldenhar syndrome has been associated with mosaic trisomy 22.[183]

Pathologic and Clinical Features

It has been proposed that Goldenhar syndrome may result from diminished unilateral embryonic vascular supply to the first and second branchial arches when the primary blood supply changes from the stapedial artery to the external carotid artery.[184] Although this could explain the facial anomalies, it does not satisfactorily explain the number of extrafacial anomalies associated with Goldenhar syndrome. Table 11 lists clinical and pathologic features of this syndrome.

Facial anomalies are characteristic and include a range of unilateral facial abnormalities including cleft lip/palate, ear deformities, and ocular abnormalities. Coloboma of the upper eyelid and epibulbar dermoids are frequent. Vertebral anomalies, especially of the cervical and upper thoracic regions, are common, and hydrosyringomyelia may occur. A number of other anomalies have been associated with Goldenhar syndrome.[185–188] Cardiac defects include tetralogy of Fallot,[189] double-outlet right ventricle, ventricular septal defect (VSD), and total anomalous pulmonary venous return.[190] In some cases, abnormalities of situs or heterotaxy appear to be associated.[191]

Diagnosis

Goldenhar syndrome should be suspected whenever unilateral cleft lip/palate is associated with other facial anomalies, such as facial asymmetry, unilateral orbital anomalies (microphthalmos or anophthalmia), and ear abnormalities, which may include absent ears[192–194] (Fig. 14). Extrafacial findings may include cardiac or urinary anomalies or lipoma of the corpus callosum.

A dichorionic pregnancy showing increased nuchal translucency proved to have Goldenhar syndrome.[195]

TABLE 11. PATHOLOGIC AND CLINICAL FEATURES OF GOLDENHAR SYNDROME

Craniofacial
  Unilateral ear abnormalities
  Unilateral cleft lip/palate
  Preauricular tags, sinuses
  External auditory canal atresia
  Microtia
  Facial asymmetry, hemifacial microsomia
  Epibulbar dermoid
  Upper eyelid coloboma
  Microphthalmos, anophthalmia
  Macrostomia
  Mandibular hypoplasia
Skeletal
  Vertebral anomalies
  Acroosteolysis of terminal phalanges
Cardiovascular: cardiac defects
Gastrointestinal
  Situs abnormalities
  Biliary atresia
  Anal atresia
  Esophageal atresia/tracheoesophageal fistula
Central nervous system
  Lipoma of the corpus callosum
  Hydrocephalus
Genitourinary
  Ectopic and/or fused kidneys
  Renal agenesis
  Ureteropelvic junction obstruction
  Multicystic kidney

Reproduced with permission from McKusick VA, ed. Online mendelian inheritance in man. Available at: http://www.ncbi.nlm.nih.gov/omim/. McKusick-Nathans Institute for Genetic Medicine, Johns Hopkins University (Baltimore, MD) and National Center for Biotechnology Information, National Library of Medicine (Bethesda, MD), 2000.

Differential Diagnosis

Kaufman syndrome (oculocerebrofacial syndrome), acrofacial dysostosis, the CHARGE association, Treacher Collins–Franceschetti syndrome (mandibulofacial dysostosis; generally referred to as Treacher Collins syndrome), Lambert syndrome (branchial dysplasia, mental deficiency, clubfoot, inguinal hernia, and cholestasis), and cardiosplenic syndrome should also be considered.[196]

Prognosis

Microphthalmos is often associated with mental retardation, and neurodevelopmental delay is common.[197] Aside from mental handicap, these patients may have respiratory, feeding, and vertebral complications.

Management

Chromosome analysis is recommended to exclude aneuploidy. If the condition is recognized early enough, termination of pregnancy is an option. Postnatal management involves both surgical and nonsurgical treatment of underlying disorders including respiratory and feeding difficulties.[198]

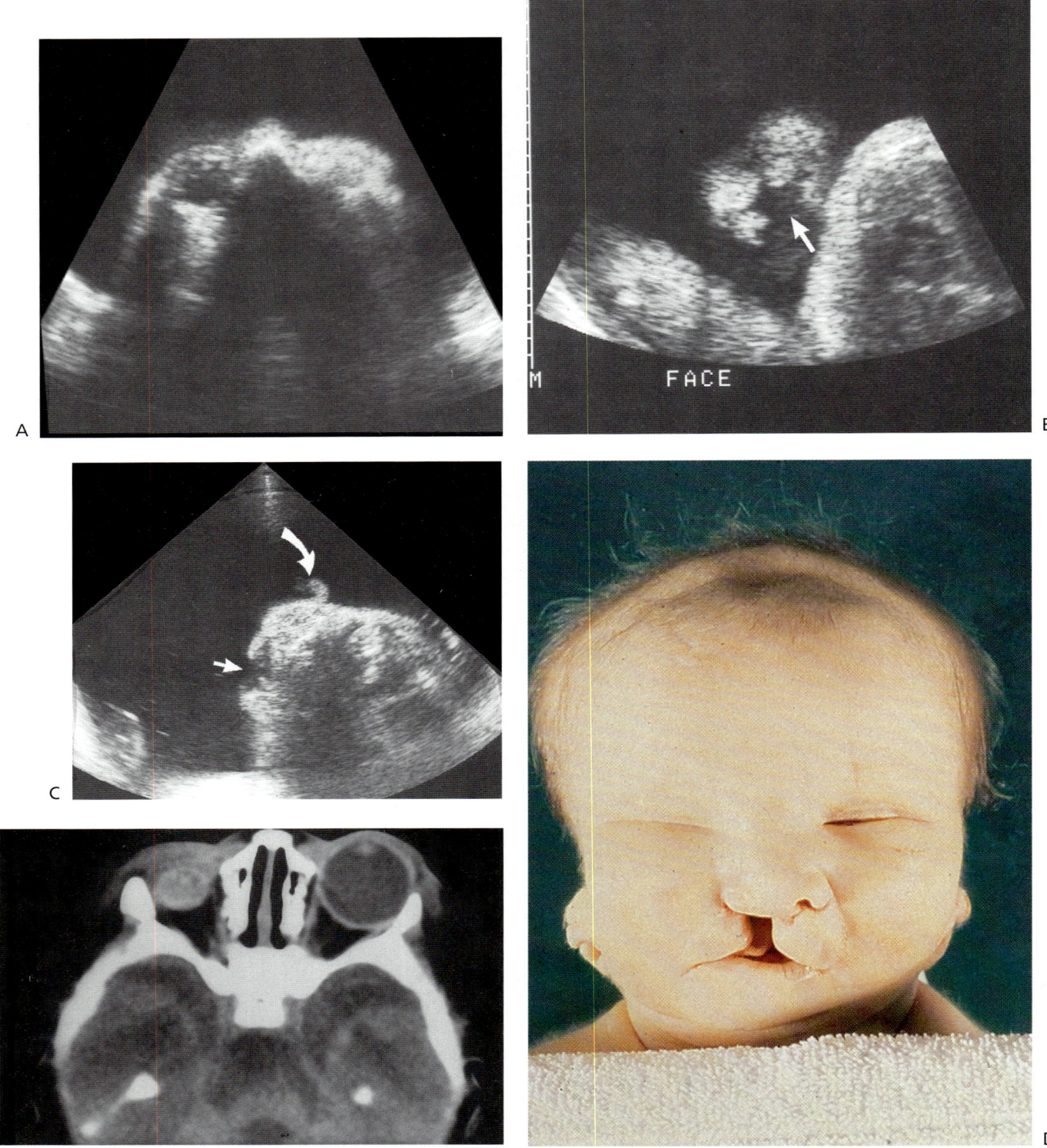

FIGURE 14. Goldenhar syndrome. **A:** An axial view through the orbits shows unilateral anophthalmia. **B:** A coronal view of the face shows unilateral cleft lip/palate (*arrow*). **C:** A transverse view of the face shows cleft (*arrow*) and ipsilateral abnormal ear (*curved arrow*). **D:** A postmortem photograph confirms the ultrasound findings. **E:** A postnatal computed tomographic scan of another infant with Goldenhar syndrome shows anophthalmia.

Recurrence Risk

Recurrence is usually sporadic with rare cases suggesting an autosomal recessive or dominant inheritance.

▶ HETEROTAXY SYNDROMES (CARDIOSPLENIC SYNDROMES, POLYSPLENIA/ASPLENIA)

Situs solitus is the usual arrangement of organs and vessels within the body. Variation from this normal arrangement results in heterotaxy, expressed either as complete reversal (*situs inversus*) of normal organ position or randomization (*situs ambiguus*). Situs ambiguus may be expressed in one of four conditions: asplenia syndrome, bilateral right-sidedness (also known as *right isomerism* and *Ivemark's syndrome*), polysplenia syndrome, or bilateral left-sidedness (also known as *left isomerism*). Together, these are termed the *cardiosplenic syndromes*.

Incidence

Heterotaxy syndromes are rare. Asplenia occurs in approximately 1 in 40,000 live births[199] and 1 in 1,750 autopsy examinations.[200] Polysplenia appears to occur with equal frequency in both sexes, whereas there is a male predominance for asplenia.

Genetic Defect

Heterotaxy syndromes are heterogeneous. No single genetic defect has been identified, and there is no recognized chromosome abnormality. However, a number of genes are asymmetrically expressed in early chick embryos well before the appearance of morphologic asymmetries. These genes regulate each other in a sequential cascade,[201] which independently determines the situs of the heart and other organs.[202] Several genes have been shown to be associated with some heterotaxy cases.

Pathologic and Clinical Features

Table 12 summarizes the pathologic and clinical features of the polysplenia and asplenia syndromes.[203] The incidence of congenital heart disease in patients with heterotaxy is very high, ranging from 50% to nearly 100%. Complex cardiac defects include atrioventricular septal defect (AVSD), univentricular heart, transposition of the great arteries, pulmonary stenosis or atresia, and persistent truncus arteriosus.[204] These may be associated with either the

TABLE 12. PATHOLOGIC AND CLINICAL FEATURES OF POLYSPLENIA AND ASPLENIA

System	Polysplenia (bilateral left-sidedness)	Asplenia (bilateral right-sidedness)
Pulmonary	Bilateral bilobed lungs	Bilateral trilobed lungs
Gastrointestinal	Transposed liver, spleen, and stomach (abdominal situs inversus)	Horizontal, midline liver
	Multiple spleens	Absent spleen
	Absent gallbladder	Midline gallbladder
	Biliary atresia	Duodenal atresia
	Duodenal atresia	Esophageal abnormalities
	Esophageal abnormalities	Malrotation of bowel
	Malrotation of bowel	
Cardiovascular	Atrioventricular septal defect	Anomalous pulmonary venous return
	Atrial and ventricular septal defects	Truncus arteriosus
	Anomalous pulmonary venous return	Atrioventricular septal defect
	Right ventricular outflow obstruction	Univentricle heart
	Transposition of the great arteries	Right ventricular outflow obstruction
	Interrupted inferior vena cava	Transposition of the great arteries
	Bradycardia	Inferior vena cava and aorta on the same side (left or right)
	Heart block	Bilateral superior vena cava
Genitourinary	—	—
Central nervous system	Spina bifida	Spina bifida
	Hydranencephaly	Hydranencephaly
	Hydrocephaly	Hydrocephaly
	Holoprosencephaly	Holoprosencephaly
	Cephalocele	Cephalocele
Facial	Anophthalmia	Anophthalmia
	Absent mandible	Absent mandible
Skeletal	—	—

Modified from Silva SR, Jeanty P. Asplenia-polysplenia syndromes. In: Jeanty P, ed. The fetus. Available at: http://www.thefetus.net/page.php?id=407. Accessed 1999.

polysplenia or asplenia syndrome, although they are usually more complex and more frequently are cyanotic with asplenia syndrome.

Visceral abnormalities are found in all the cardiosplenic syndromes. In polysplenia, the stomach is usually on the right or indeterminately located. Multiple splenic nodules, often clustered along the greater curvature of the stomach, are usually present and these may accompany one or more larger spleens. Other visceral abnormalities include malrotation of the bowel and mesentery, biliary atresia, genitourinary abnormalities, duodenal atresia, tracheal and esophageal abnormalities, and anomalies of the CNS and skeletal systems.[205]

Common anomalies of asplenia include anomalous pulmonary venous return, bilateral superior vena cavae, malpositioned inferior vena cava, midline liver, intestinal malrotation, and absence of the spleen.

An association of biliary atresia with splenic malformations, especially polysplenia, has been recognized.[206–208] These patients may first present in infancy with liver failure requiring a liver transplant.[209] In a series of 308 infants treated for biliary atresia, 23 (7.5%) had polysplenia and two had asplenia.[206]

Diagnosis

The diagnosis of heterotaxy may be made on the basis of the following:

1. Abdominal situs inversus with right-sided stomach (Fig. 15). Although theoretically this finding could reflect partial situs inversus without heterotaxy, nearly all cases observed prenatally are a reflection of the cardiosplenic syndromes. The stomach may be left- or right-sided with either asplenia or polysplenia.

2. Cardiac abnormalities. Cardiac and other anomalies usually dominate the appearance of the asplenic and polysplenic syndromes.[210–214] Therefore, the combination of a heart defect and right-sided stomach is virtually diagnostic of the cardiosplenic syndromes. AVSD is particularly common (Fig. 15). Although major cardiac anomalies, such as AVSD, might otherwise suggest a diagnosis of Down syndrome or other chromosome abnormality, the cardiosplenic syndromes are not associated with aneuploidy.[215] The cardiosplenic syndromes also tend to have more complex cardiac defects than AVSD associated with fetal Down syndrome. Congenital heart block has been associated with the polysplenia syndrome and may be the initial sign at presentation.[216,217]

3. Characteristic venous or arterial abnormalities. Abnormalities of the venous and arterial system are common with the cardiosplenic syndromes. Sheley et al.[218] describe a method for detecting azygous continuation of the interrupted inferior vena cava—a common characteristic of polysplenia syndrome (Fig. 15). In contrast to the normal azygos vein,[219] the abnormally dilated azygos vein is similar in diameter to the adjacent aorta and parallels its course behind the heart before the azygos vein empties into the superior vena cava. This "double vessel" sign was evident in nine cases, including all eight fetuses who proved to have the polysplenia syndrome and one fetus with asplenia. In combination with cardiac anomalies or situs abnormalities, interruption of the inferior vena cava with azygous continuation should suggest a specific diagnosis of a cardiosplenic syndrome, especially polysplenia.

Abuhamad et al.[220] suggested that identification of the splenic artery may be useful in distinguishing polysplenia from asplenia. The splenic artery was imaged in six of eight fetuses, all of whom had polysplenia and was not imaged in two fetuses with asplenia.

Differential Diagnosis

Partial situs inversus should be distinguished from complete situs inversus, in which the heart is also a mirror image with the apex oriented to the right. Complete situs inversus may be observed in 20% of patients with Kartagener's syndrome (i.e., total situs inversus, bronchiectasis, nasal polyposis)[221,222] and may also be found in normal, asymptomatic patients. The risk of cardiac malformation with complete situs inversus is less than 3%.

AVSD should suggest chromosome abnormality, particularly trisomy 21. However, when AVSD and abdominal situs inversus are present, the diagnosis is invariably polysplenia syndrome with normal karyotype.

Prognosis

Due to the severity of complex cardiovascular malformations, the mortality rate for cardiosplenic syndromes is high. Up to 95% of infants with asplenia die by the first year of life. Survivors with asplenia have an abnormal immune status and may not have a normally functional spleen. Polysplenia has a somewhat better prognosis than asplenia, because the cardiac anomalies are typically less complex. The 1-year mortality rate for polysplenia syndrome has been reported as 60% to 80%.[211] In a review of 146 cases, 50% died by 4 months, 25% survived to 5 years, and only 10% lived to adolescence.[211] The association of congenital complete heart block with polysplenia may have a worse prognosis.[216]

Management

The Fontan procedure remains the preferred palliative procedure for patients with heterotaxy syndrome and major cardiac defects. Culbertson et al.[223] found that a poorer surgical outcome was associated with atrioventricular valve regurgitation and hypoplastic pulmonary arteries.

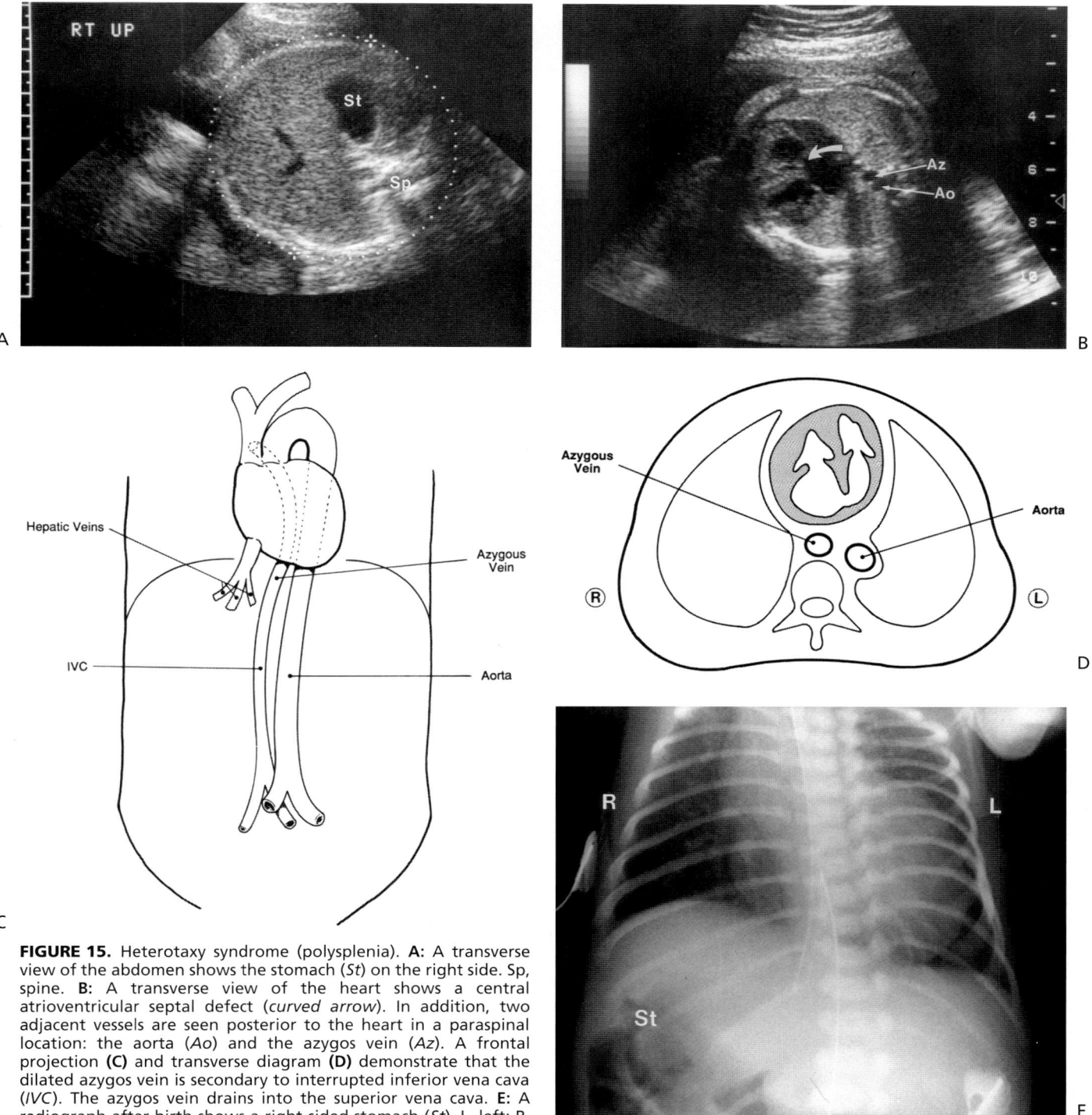

FIGURE 15. Heterotaxy syndrome (polysplenia). **A:** A transverse view of the abdomen shows the stomach (*St*) on the right side. Sp, spine. **B:** A transverse view of the heart shows a central atrioventricular septal defect (*curved arrow*). In addition, two adjacent vessels are seen posterior to the heart in a paraspinal location: the aorta (*Ao*) and the azygos vein (*Az*). A frontal projection (**C**) and transverse diagram (**D**) demonstrate that the dilated azygos vein is secondary to interrupted inferior vena cava (*IVC*). The azygos vein drains into the superior vena cava. **E:** A radiograph after birth shows a right-sided stomach (*St*). L, left; R, right. (Reproduced with permission from Sheley RC, Nyberg DA, Kapur R. Azygous continuation of the interrupted inferior vena cava: a clue to prenatal diagnosis of the cardiosplenic syndromes. *J Ultrasound Med* 1995;14:381–387.)

Recurrence Risk

Heterotaxy is usually a multifactorial disorder. However, a number of cases of familial heterotaxy have also been reported with autosomal dominant, recessive, and X-linked inheritance.[224] All possible situs variants—solitus, ambiguus, inversus—can appear among some heterotaxy families.[225]

▶ HOLT-ORAM SYNDROME*

The Holt-Oram syndrome, sometimes called *heart-hand syndrome* or *atriodigital dysplasia*, was first clearly described by Holt and Oram in 1960.[226]

Incidence

Holt-Oram syndrome occurs in 1 in 100,000 live births.

Genetic Defect

Mutations in the T-box genes (*TBX5* and *TBX3*) on chromosome 12q24.1[227] have been shown to be responsible for the congenital abnormalities associated with Holt-Oram syndrome.[228–230] *TBX5* is a transcription factor important for the development of the forelimb and heart.[231]

Pathologic and Clinical Features

Pathologic and clinical features of Holt-Oram syndrome are summarized in Table 13. The characteristic findings are thumb anomaly and atrial septal defect (ASD). The thumb may be absent or may be a triphalangeal, nonopposable, fingerlike digit. Other extremity abnormalities may also occur

*Modified with permission from Silva and Jeanty at http://www.TheFetus.net.

TABLE 13. PATHOLOGIC AND CLINICAL FEATURES OF HOLT-ORAM SYNDROME

Cardiovascular
Atrial septal defect
Ventricular septal defect
Hypoplastic left heart syndrome
Thorax
Absent pectoralis major muscle
Pectus excavatum or carinatum
Skeletal
Vertebral anomalies
Thoracic scoliosis
Absent thumb
Bifid thumb
Triphalangeal thumb
Carpal bone anomalies
Upper extremity phocomelia
Radial-ulnar anomalies
Asymmetric involvement

including upper limb phocomelia (4.5%), radial ray aplasia, and clinodactyly.[232]

Diagnosis

Cardiac defects that can be detected include ASD and VSD (Fig. 16), AVSD, hypoplasia of the left ventricle, and conduction disturbances, in addition to more complex anomalies.[233] Extremity abnormalities may include radial ray deformity[234] or absence of the thumb or carpal bones.[235]

Differential Diagnosis

The differential diagnosis usually includes radial ray aplasia and may include thrombocytopenia–absent radius syndrome, Fanconi

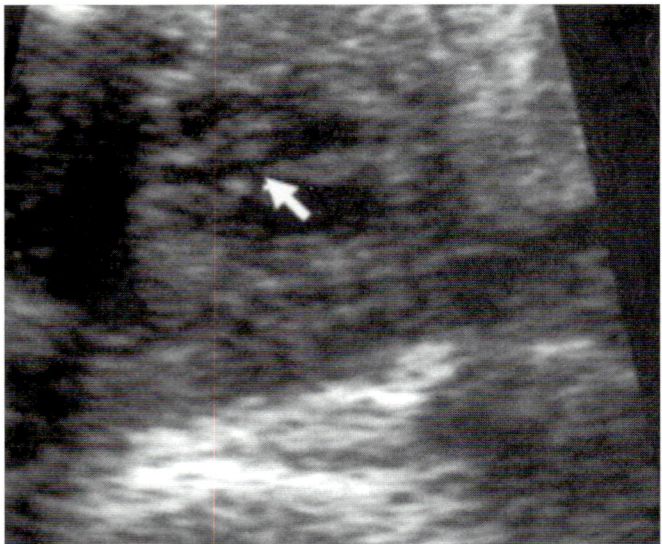
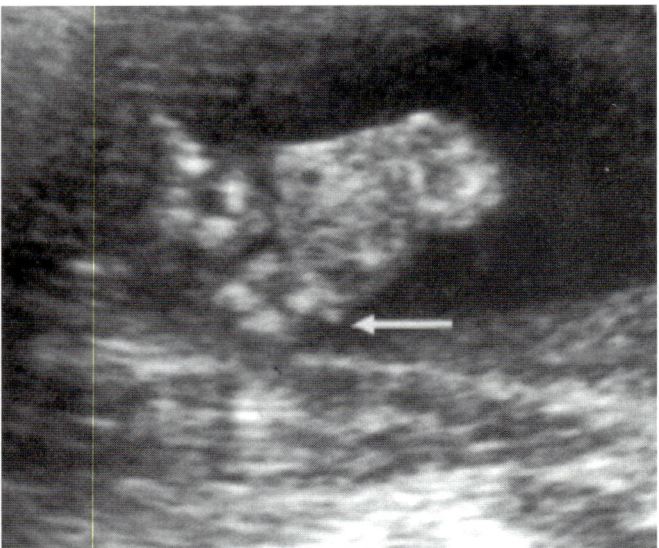

A   B

FIGURE 16. Holt-Oram syndrome. **A:** An axial view of the heart shows a small ventricular septal defect (*arrow*). **B:** A view of the hand shows only four digits with a small skin tag in place of the thumb (*arrow*).

anemia, and the VACTERL association (see Treacher Collins Syndrome, later in this chapter).

Prognosis

The prognosis mainly depends on the severity of the cardiac and orthopedic handicap.

Management

Management addresses both defects of the heart and the upper extremity. Orthopedic management allows opposition of the index finger.[236]

Recurrence Risk

Risk of recurrence is 50%. Transmission of Holt-Oram syndrome is autosomal dominant with 100% penetrance.

▶ JOUBERT SYNDROME

Marie Joubert et al.[237] described the syndrome in 1968 as a developmental defect of the cerebellar vermis. It may also

TABLE 14. PATHOLOGIC AND CLINICAL FEATURES OF JOUBERT SYNDROME

Facial
  Abnormal eye movements
  Coloboma of optic nerve
  Chorioretinal coloboma
  Retinal dystrophy
  Soft tissue tumors of tongue
  Colobomas
Neurologic
  Partial agenesis, cerebellar vermis
  Dandy-Walker malformation
  Hypoplasia of the corpus callosum
  Occipital meningoencephalocele
  Truncal ataxia
  Developmental delay
  Tongue protrusion
  Tremor
  Hypotonia
  Seizures
Renal: renal cysts

Reproduced with permission from references 239, 240, and McKusick VA, ed. Online mendelian inheritance in man. Available at: http://www.ncbi.nlm.nih.gov/omim/. McKusick-Nathans Institute for Genetic Medicine, Johns Hopkins University (Baltimore, MD) and National Center for Biotechnology Information, National Library of Medicine (Bethesda, MD), 2000.

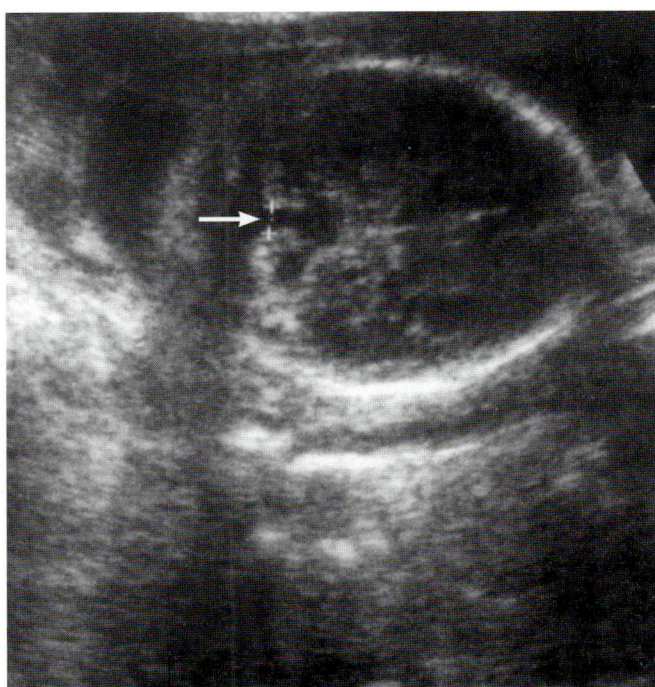

A

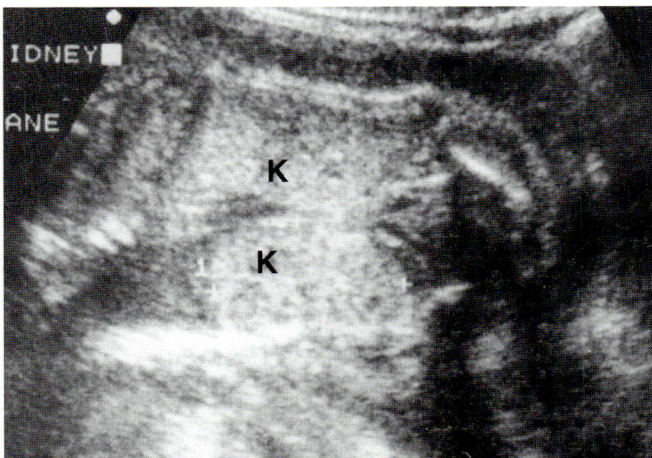

B

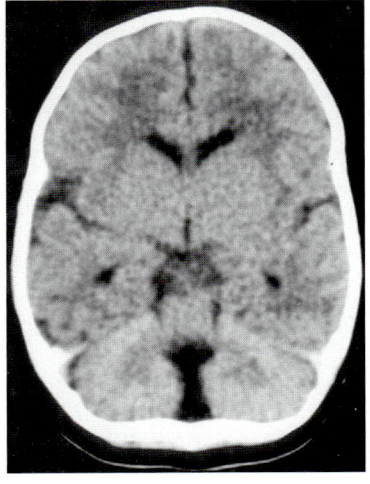

C

FIGURE 17. Joubert syndrome. **A:** A scan of the head at 28 weeks shows a discrete cleft of the cerebellar vermis (*arrow,* calipers) indicating at least partial vermian agenesis. **B:** The kidneys (*K*) are large and echogenic. **C:** A postnatal computed tomographic scan confirms the prenatal sonographic findings of vermian agenesis. (Reproduced with permission from Ni Scanaill S, Crowley P, Hogan M, Stuart B. Abnormal prenatal sonographic findings in the posterior fossa: a case of Joubert's syndrome. *Ultrasound Obstet Gynecol* 1999;13:71–74.)

include CNS, respiratory, renal, and eye anomalies. Synonyms for Joubert syndrome include cerebelloparenchymal disorder IV and Joubert-Boltshauser syndrome.

Incidence

Joubert syndrome is rare.

Genetic Defect

Joubert syndrome has been linked to the telomeric region of chromosome 9q in some families, although not in others.[238]

Pathologic and Clinical Features

Pathologic and clinical features of Joubert syndrome[239,240] are summarized in Table 14. In addition to vermian agenesis, Joubert syndrome may be associated with malformations of brainstem structures.[241,242] Other reported anomalies include ectodermal dysplasia,[243] Gaucher's disease,[244] multicystic kidney disease, and hepatic fibrosis.[245] Polydactyly has also been reported in some cases of Joubert syndrome.

Diagnosis

The first ultrasonic diagnosis was made by Campbell et al.[246] in 1984. A growing number of additional reports have described prenatal detection of Joubert syndrome.[247–250] The primary finding is vermian agenesis, which may be partial or complete. The vermian defect is usually subtle and usually not associated with hydrocephalus (Fig. 17). The postnatal diagnosis is based on the clinical findings and supported by the pathognomonic "molar tooth" sign on MRI (Fig. 18). This sign results from a combination of midbrain, vermian, and superior cerebellar peduncle abnormalities.[251] A number of other brain findings may be observed on postnatal MRI.[252,253]

Other abnormalities that may be seen include cephalocele, hydrocephalus, and renal anomalies. Increased nuchal translucency has also been reported during the first trimester.[254]

Differential Diagnosis

Vermian cleft without Joubert syndrome, the Dandy-Walker malformation, and the many conditions associated with Dandy-Walker variant must all be considered.[255]

Prognosis

A decreased life span has been reported in many patients.[256] A variety of deficits in cognition; verbal memory; and visuomotor, motor, and language-related tasks are described as well as problems in temperament, hyperactivity, aggres-

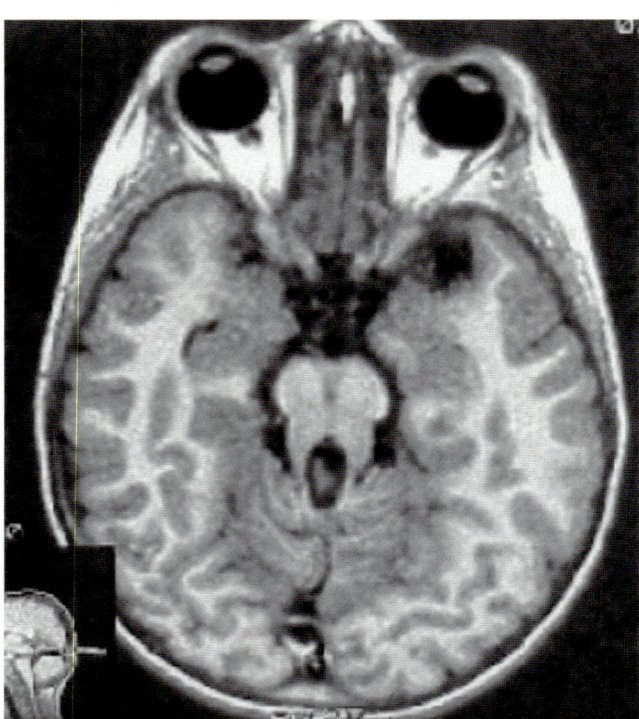

FIGURE 18. Joubert syndrome. A postnatal magnetic resonance image shows the "molar tooth" sign, composed of the midbrain and partial vermian agenesis. (From Bruck I, Antoniuk SA, Carvalho Neto AD, Spessatto A. Cerebellar vermis hypoplasia-nonprogressive congenital ataxia: clinical and radiologic findings in a pair of siblings. *Arq Neuropsiquiatr* 2000;58:897–900, with permission.)

siveness, and dependency.[257] The degree of developmental delay in Joubert syndrome and the severity of gross CNS malformations appear independent.[258]

The outcome is highly variable. Siblings from the same family and even monozygotic twins[259] with Joubert syndrome may present with phenotypes ranging from minimally to severely handicapped. The motor handicap varies from being wheelchair-bound to being able to walk and run.

Management

Obstetric management is usually not altered. Postnatal management varies with the severity and types of anomalies.

Recurrence Risk

Joubert syndrome is autosomal recessive; the recurrence risk is 25%.

▶ KLIPPEL-TRÉNAUNAY-WEBER SYNDROME

Described by Klippel and Trénaunay[260] and then Weber,[261] Klippel-Trénaunay-Weber syndrome is associated with large

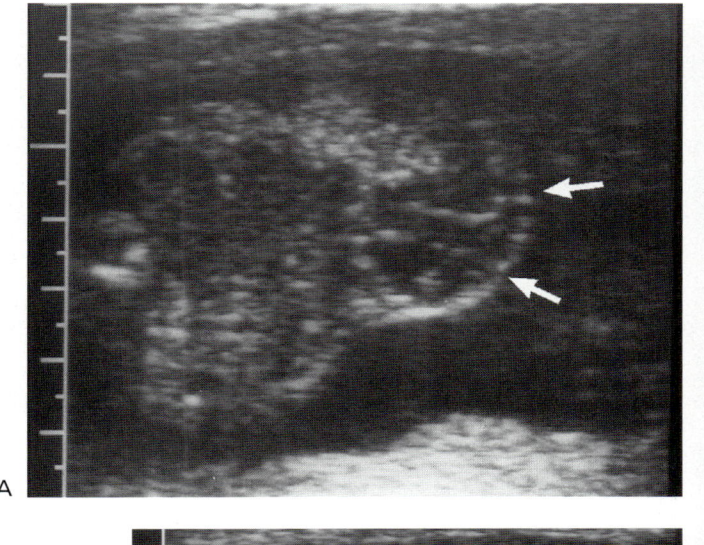

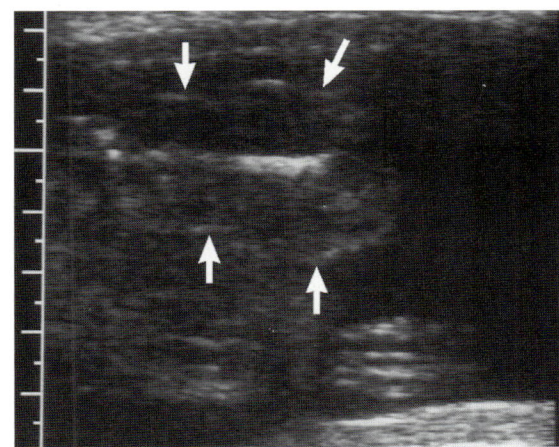

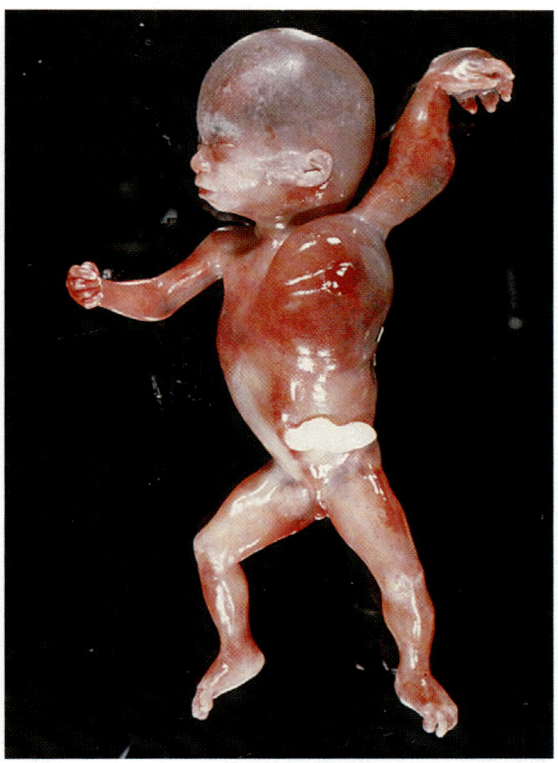

FIGURE 19. Klippel-Trénaunay-Weber syndrome. **A:** A transverse view of the upper chest shows soft tissue mass of axilla (*arrows*). **B:** View of arm shows marked soft tissue swelling (*arrows*). **C:** A pathologic photograph shows hemangiolymphangioma of the chest wall and arm with associated hypertrophy.

cutaneous hemangiomas with hypertrophy of the related bones and soft tissues.[262,263] It is sometimes called *Klippel-Trénaunay syndrome* or angioosteohypertrophy syndrome.

Incidence

Klippel-Trénaunay-Weber syndrome is rare.

Genetic Defect

No definite genetic defect has been identified.

Pathologic and Clinical Features

The features of Klippel-Trénaunay-Weber syndrome are large cutaneous hemangiomas with hypertrophy of the related bones and soft tissues. Capillary malformations,

atypical varicosities, and venous malformations leading to localized masses are also seen. The trait is only expressed when a somatic mutation occurs in the normal allele at an early stage of embryogenesis. The embryo is then a mosaic of homozygous or heterozygous cell lines for the mutation, which explains the patchy distribution of the defect.[264]

Diagnosis

The appearance is a soft tissue mass of an extremity, usually affecting the adjacent trunk (Figs. 19 and 20). Other findings may include hydrops fetalis (from high-output cardiac failure), ascites, abdominal hemangiomatous masses, and hepatomegaly.[265,266] The diagnosis has been made as early as 15 weeks.[267] Three-dimensional ultrasound and prenatal MRI may be used to better demonstrate the mass.[268]

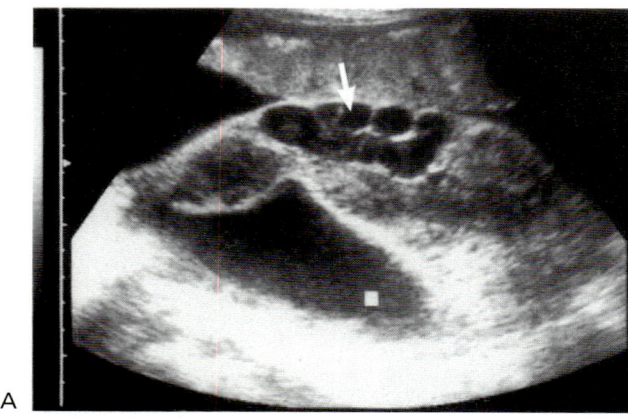

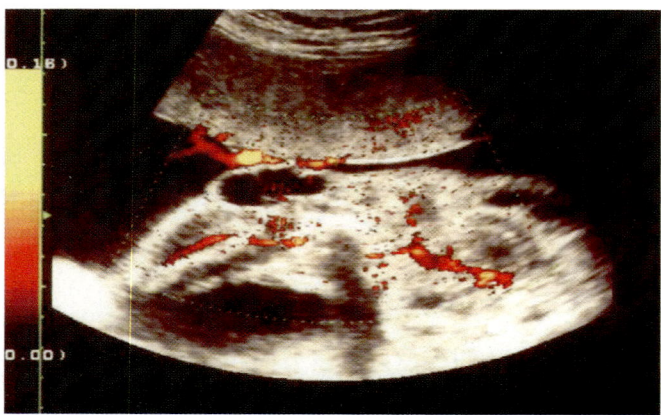

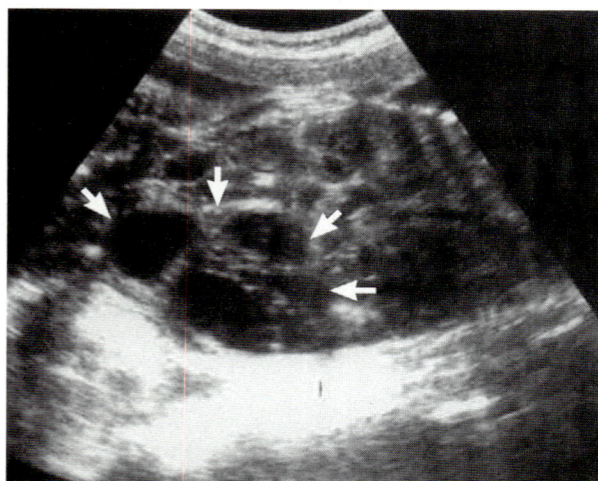

FIGURE 20. Klippel-Trénaunay-Weber syndrome. **A:** A scan of the right leg at 20 weeks shows soft tissue swelling with a sonolucent mass (*arrow*). **B:** A color-flow Doppler image shows increased vascularity to the leg. **C:** A coronal scan of the abdomen shows a multilocular cystic mass (*arrows*). Extensive hemangiolymphangioma was found at birth. (Reproduced with permission from Escobar CAM, Ramirez J, Medina O, Gómez J. Klippel-Trénaunay-Weber syndrome. In: The fetus. Available at: http://www.thefetus.net. Accessed September, 2002.)

Differential Diagnosis

Isolated lymphangioma, Sturge-Weber syndrome, and Proteus syndrome[269] should be considered. Cohen[270] believed that Joseph Merrick (the Elephant Man), the famous patient of Sir Frederick Treves, had Proteus syndrome and not neurofibromatosis.

Prognosis

When detected prenatally, the disorder may be severe. Thrombocytopenia due to platelet consumption within the hemangioma and high-output cardiac failure may complicate the outcome. Cerebral atrophy may occur in a minority of cases, presumably due to diversion of blood to the vascular anomaly.[271]

Management

Termination of pregnancy can be offered in the severe forms; otherwise no alteration of management is expected. The management of newborns is primarily nonoperative, but some patients may benefit from surgical intervention.[272]

Recurrence Risk

The risk of recurrence appears to be extremely low; however, occasional cases have been consistent with autosomal dominant inheritance.[273–275]

▶ LIMB-BODY WALL COMPLEX

LBWC comprises a number of complex defects commonly including abdominothoracic defects, craniofacial defects, scoliosis, and limb defects. Synonyms for this complex include *body-stalk anomaly* and *cyllosoma*.

Incidence

Reported incidence rates vary from 1 in 7,000 to 42,000.[276–278]

Genetic Defect

There is no known genetic defect. Three general pathogenic mechanisms have been proposed for this disorder: amnion rupture,[279,280] vascular disruption,[281] and embryonic malfor-

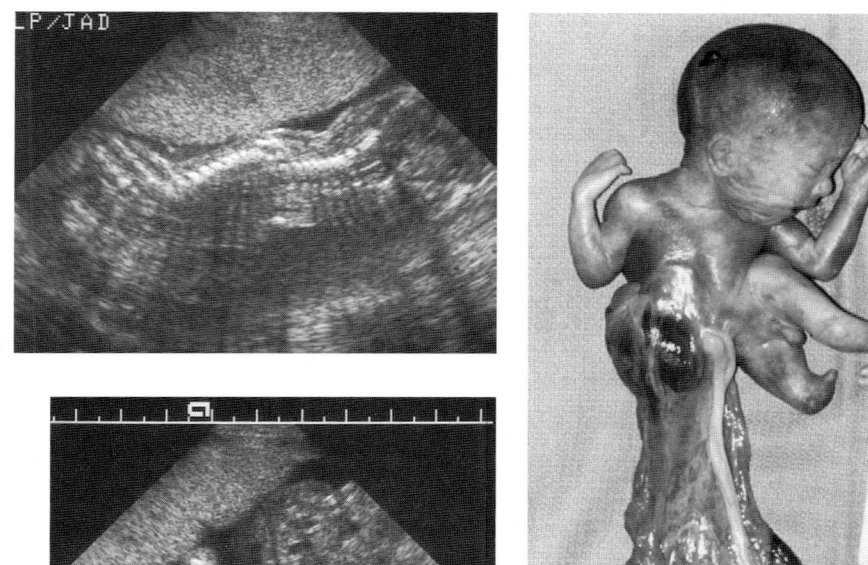

FIGURE 21. Limb-body wall complex. **A:** A scan at 15 weeks shows marked scoliosis. **B:** A transverse view of the abdomen shows a complex abdominal wall defect. The liver is eviscerated but is not midline or covered by a membrane. The amnion (*AM*) is seen posteriorly. **C:** A postnatal photograph of a similar fetus shows marked scoliosis and a complex abdominal wall defect that is fused with the placenta.

mation.[282] Craven et al.[282] propose that the pathogenesis is a primary malformation of body wall closure, with abnormal fusion of the amnion during the first month of development.

Pathologic and Clinical Features

A common feature is fusion of the body, including all or part of the chest, abdomen, and pelvis, with the placenta in association with a short or absent umbilical cord. The list of associated abnormalities is long and includes both external and internal defects. External defects include craniofacial defects, cloacal exstrophy, and limb defects.[277,283] Craniofacial defects may include facial cleft and encephalocele or exencephaly. Internal malformations, present in 95% of cases, include cardiac defects (56%), absent diaphragm (74%), bowel atresia (22%), and renal abnormalities including agenesis, hydronephrosis, or dysplasia (65%).

Russo et al.[281] recognize two distinguishable phenotypes of LBWC: the first shows craniofacial defects and amniotic bands, adhesion, or both, and the second presents with urogenital anomalies, anal atresia, abdominal-placental attachment, absent or short umbilical artery, and persistence of the extraembryonic

coelom but no craniofacial defects. They suggest the first type is related to an early vascular disruption, and the second one is attributable to an intrinsic embryonic abnormality.

Karyotypes have been reported to be normal in all cases of LBWC. A normal karyotype might be surprising considering the severity of malformations, supporting a disruptive defect rather than abnormal embryologic development.

Diagnosis

Ultrasound

Ventral wall defects, craniofacial defects, and scoliosis are the typical features of LBWC[284–286] (Fig. 21). Ventral wall defects are generally large, involving both the thorax and abdomen, and forming a complex mass.[284] Fusion of fetal parts with the placenta may be seen. If specifically sought, the umbilical cord may be visibly short or even absent and adherent to placental membranes.[287,288]

LBWC can be diagnosed during the first trimester and has been diagnosed as early as 10 weeks.[289–293] Among 14 cases diagnosed during the first trimester, Daskalakis et al.[290] indicate that the upper part of the fetal body was in the amniotic cavity, whereas the lower part was in the coelomic cavity. They suggest that early amnion rupture before obliteration of the coelomic cavity is a possible cause of the syndrome.

Three-dimensional ultrasound has been used.[294]

Laboratory

Many cases of LBWC produce elevated maternal serum alpha-fetoprotein (AFP) levels during the second trimester.[233,295]

Differential Diagnosis

Amniotic band syndrome may have very similar features, and some authorities do not distinguish these conditions. Some cases of LBWC have been initially misdiagnosed as omphalocele or gastroschisis.

Prognosis

The prognosis is uniformly fatal.

Recurrence Risk

There is no known recurrence risk of LBWC.

▶ MECKEL-GRUBER SYNDROME

Meckel made a clear description of the syndrome as early as 1822.[296] Synonyms include *Meckel syndrome*, *Gruber syndrome*, and *dysencephalia splanchnocystica*.

Prevalence

The reported prevalence is as high as 1 in 9,000 births.[297]

Genetic Defect

Meckel-Gruber syndrome has been mapped to chromosome 17q[298] and 11q.[299] However, as yet, a specific causative gene has not been identified.

Pathologic and Clinical Features

A large number of abnormalities may be seen with the Meckel-Gruber syndrome (Table 15). The classic triad is occipital encephalocele, polydactyly, and polycystic kidneys. Polydactyly is usually postaxial but may be occasionally preaxial.

Diagnosis

The triad of fetal occipital encephalocele, polycystic kidneys, and postaxial polydactyly can be detected by ultrasound as early as 13 weeks[300] (Fig. 22). Sepulveda et al.[301] correctly identified four of nine pregnancies at risk for

TABLE 15. PATHOLOGIC AND CLINICAL FEATURES OF THE MECKEL-GRUBER SYNDROME

Growth: variable growth deficiency
Central nervous system/neurologic
  Arnold-Chiari malformation
  Occipital encephalocele
  Hydrocephalus
  Dandy-Walker malformation
  Cerebral hypoplasia
  Cerebellar hypoplasia
  Anencephaly
  Absence of corpus callosum
  Optic tract agenesis
Craniofacial
  Microcephaly
  Sloping forehead
  Micrognathia
  Low-set ears
  Microphthalmos
  Hypotelorism, hypertelorism
  Iris coloboma
  Cleft lip/palate
  Lobulated tongue
  Macrostomia
  Short neck
  Webbed neck
Genitourinary
  Small, ambiguous genitalia
  Cryptorchidism
  Uterine abnormalities
  Polycystic kidneys
  Renal agenesis
  Duplicated ureters
  Hypoplastic bladder
Skeletal
  Postaxial polydactyly
  Syndactyly
  Clinodactyly
  Talipes
  Bowed long bones
Cardiovascular
  Septal defects
  Single umbilical artery
Respiratory: pulmonary hypoplasia
Gastrointestinal
  Bile duct proliferation, dilatation
  Splenomegaly
  Asplenia
  Accessory spleen
  Omphalocele
  Intestinal malrotation
  Imperforate anus

Reproduced with permission from McKusick VA, ed. Online mendelian inheritance in man. Available at: http://www.ncbi.nlm.nih.gov/omim/. McKusick-Nathans Institute for Genetic Medicine, Johns Hopkins University (Baltimore, MD) and National Center for Biotechnology Information, National Library of Medicine (Bethesda, MD), 2000.

recurrent Meckel-Gruber syndrome by 13 weeks. Dandy-Walker syndrome is a relatively frequent associated brain malformation.[302–305] Oligohydramnios is universal and may develop as early as 14 weeks.[306] Marked variation in phenotypic variation may be seen.[307]

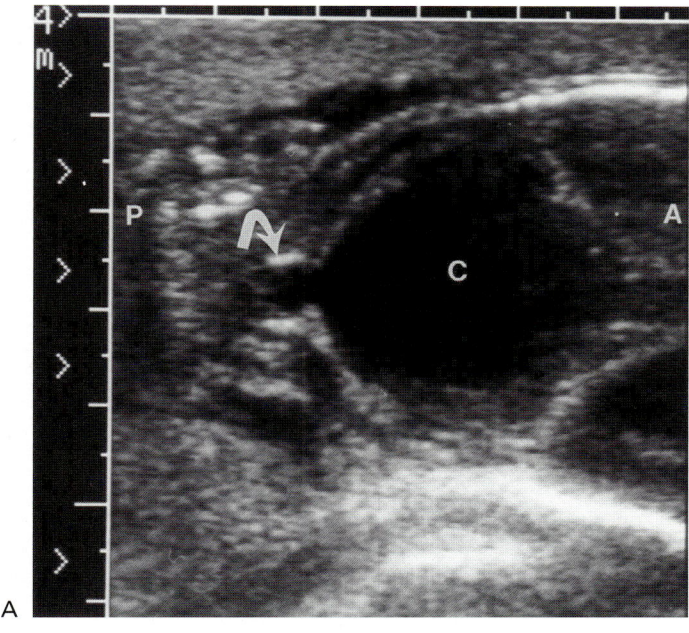

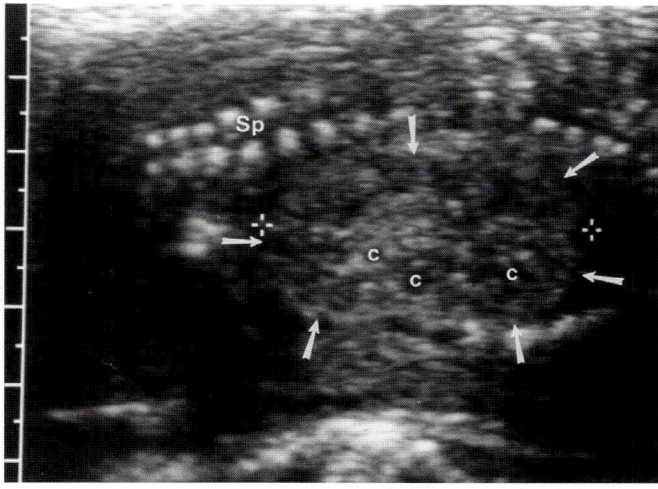

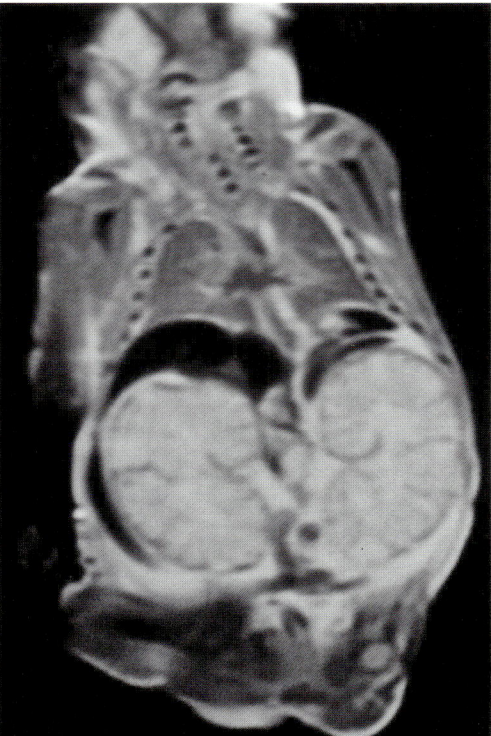

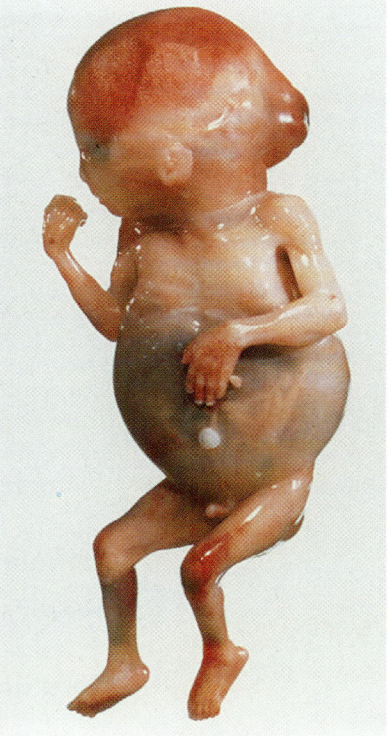

FIGURE 22. Meckel-Gruber syndrome. **A:** An axial view through the posterior fossa shows a small posterior cephalocele (*arrow*). A Dandy-Walker cyst (*C*) is also present. A, anterior; P, posterior. **B:** A longitudinal view of the abdomen shows an enlarged echogenic kidney (*arrows*) with multiple cysts (*c*). Sp, spine. **C:** A postnatal magnetic resonance image of a similar case shows enlarged dysplastic kidneys. **D:** A postmortem photograph shows typical features, including posterior cephalocele and postaxial polydactyly.

Differential Diagnosis

Trisomy 13 and other causes of polycystic kidney disease should be considered.

Prognosis

Meckel-Gruber syndrome is universally fatal when bilateral renal dysplasia is present.

Management

Termination of pregnancy may be offered. Early diagnosis permits termination of pregnancy during the first trimester.

Recurrence Risk

Meckel-Gruber syndrome is autosomal recessive with 25% recurrence risk.

TABLE 16. PATHOLOGIC AND CLINICAL FEATURES OF NAGER SYNDROME

Face
  Antimongoloid slant
  Ptosis of lower lids
  Hypoplasia of lower eyelashes
  Microtia
  Malar hypoplasia
  Micrognathia
  Mandibular hypoplasia
  Hearing loss
  Auricular tags
  Cleft lip/palate
Skeletal
  Radial hypoplasia or aplasia
  Fibular hypoplasia or aplasia
  Radioulnar synostosis
  Hypoplastic thumbs
  Absent metacarpals
  Syndactyly
Thorax: tracheal or laryngeal anomalies

Reproduced with permission from McKusick VA, ed. Online mendelian inheritance in man. Available at: http://www.ncbi.nlm.nih.gov/omim/. McKusick-Nathans Institute for Genetic Medicine, Johns Hopkins University (Baltimore, MD) and National Center for Biotechnology Information, National Library of Medicine (Bethesda, MD), 2000.

▶ NAGER SYNDROME (ACROFACIAL DYSOSTOSIS 1)*

Nager syndrome, also known as *mandibulofacial dysostosis, Treacher Collins type with limb anomalies*, and *Nager acrofacial dysostosis*, was recognized as a specific entity by Nager and de Reynier[308] but was probably first reported by Slingenberg.[309] It consists of limb anomalies including absence of the radius, synostosis of the radius and ulna, and hypoplasia or absence of the thumbs; severe micrognathia; and malar hypoplasia.[308]

Prevalence

Nager syndrome is uncommon. A paternal age effect has been observed.

Genetic Defect

Nager syndrome has been localized to 9q32.[310]

Pathologic and Clinical Features

The pathologic and clinical features of Nager syndrome are summarized in Table 16.

Diagnosis

Affected fetuses show severe micrognathia and the typical micromesomelia with abnormal hands (Fig. 23). Occasional cases have been detected by prenatal ultrasound.[311]

---

*Modified with permission from Silva and Jeanty at http://www.TheFetus.net.

Differential Diagnosis

Trisomy 18 should be considered. The Genée-Wiedemann syndrome (Miller syndrome) is characterized by mandibulofacial dysostosis and postaxial limb defects. Rodriguez lethal acrofacial dysostosis syndrome is a variant with preaxial limb deficiencies, postaxial limb anomalies, severe hypoplasia of the shoulder and pelvic girdles, and cardiac and CNS malformations.[312]

Prognosis

The prognosis is poor secondary to lung hypoplasia and airway obstruction.

Management

Termination of pregnancy can be offered before viability. For live births, airway obstruction is an immediate, emergent problem. The craniofacial anomalies make intubation difficult and often necessitate emergency tracheostomy.[63,313] For longer-term management, surgical treatment with mandibular distraction may help alleviate the airway obstruction.[314]

Recurrence Risk

Most reported cases of Nager syndrome have been sporadic. However, rare recurrences have suggested the possibility of autosomal dominant or recessive inheritance in some families.[315]

▶ NOONAN SYNDROME

First described by Jacqueline Noonan in 1968, Noonan syndrome is very similar to the disorder described by Turner.[316] Synonyms for Noonan syndrome include *Turner syndrome with normal XX, pseudo-Turner syndrome, male Turner syndrome*, and *Ullrich syndrome*.

Prevalence

Noonan syndrome occurs in 1 in 10,000 to 40,000 deliveries.

Genetic Defect

X-linked dominant inheritance of either a single mutant gene or a submicroscopic deletion was originally suspected,[317,318] but it is now known that one of the genes for Noonan syndrome is located on chromosome 12 in the 12q24.2-q24.31 region.[319–322]

Pathologic and Clinical Features

The pathologic and clinical features of Noonan syndrome are summarized in Table 17. There is some phenotypic overlap with Turner syndrome. Two major features are

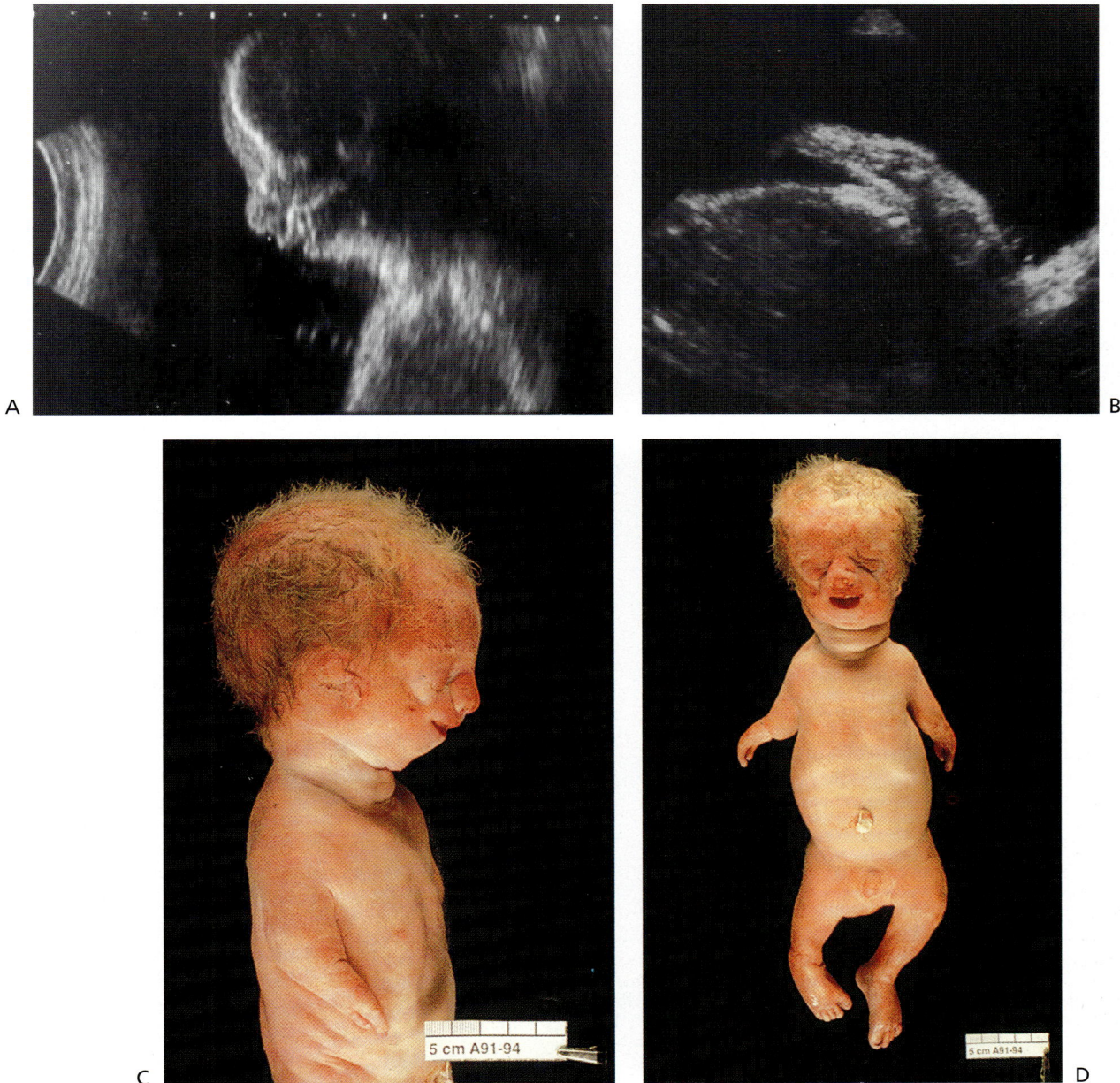

FIGURE 23. Nager acrofacial dysostosis syndrome. **A:** A profile view of the face shows marked micrognathia. **B:** In a longitudinal view of the arm, the forearm is markedly shortened, and the radius is absent. **C, D:** Postnatal photographs confirm the prenatal findings. (Reproduced with permission from Benson CB, Pober BR, Hirsh MP, Doubilet PM. Sonography of Nager acrofacial dysostosis syndrome *in utero*. *J Ultrasound Med* 1988;7:163–167.)

lymphedema and cystic hygroma. Infants may have thickening or pterygium colli at birth.[323,324]

Diagnosis

Ultrasound

Noonan syndrome may be one of many outcomes associated with increased nuchal translucency during the first trimester[325] (Fig. 24A). Increased nuchal thickening or cystic hygroma may be also demonstrated.[254] Other sonographic findings may include cardiac defects,[326] pleural effusions and hydrops,[327] renal abnormalities, and shortened extremities.[328] Various venous abnormalities have also been associated with Noonan syndrome, particularly abnormalities of the umbilical vein[329,330] (Fig. 24).

Laboratory

Some fetuses have been identified by triple-marker screening.[331]

TABLE 17. PATHOLOGIC AND CLINICAL FEATURES OF NOONAN SYNDROME

Growth
  Short stature
  Failure to thrive
Face
  Low-set, posteriorly rotated ears
  Nerve deafness
  Ptosis
  Hypertelorism
  Downward-slanting palpebral fissures
  Epicanthal folds
  Myopia
  Blue-green irides
  Deeply grooved philtrum
  High peaks of upper lip vermillion border
  High arched palate
  Micrognathia
  Low posterior hairline
  Webbed neck/cystic hygroma
Cardiovascular
  Cardiac defects
  Pulmonic stenosis
  Patent ductus arteriosus
  Venous anomalies
Chest
  Broad chest
  Widely spaced nipples
Genitourinary
  Occasional hypogonadism
  Cryptorchidism
Skeletal
  Vertebral abnormalities
  Cubitus valgus
  Clinodactyly
  Brachydactyly
Hematologic
  Amegakaryocytic thrombocytopenia
  von Willebrand disease
  Bleeding tendency

Reproduced with permission from McKusick VA, ed. Online mendelian inheritance in man. Available at: http://www.ncbi.nlm.nih.gov/omim/. McKusick-Nathans Institute for Genetic Medicine, Johns Hopkins University (Baltimore, MD) and National Center for Biotechnology Information, National Library of Medicine (Bethesda, MD), 2000.

Differential Diagnosis

Turner syndrome (excluded in boys or otherwise by karyotype) is unlikely to be familial, whereas Noonan syndrome has a strong familial predilection in approximately 30% of cases. Trisomy 21 should also be considered.

Prognosis

Life expectancy is fairly normal for those without major complications of heart disease. Hypertrophic cardiomyopathy, with myocardial fiber disarray, may occur in 20% to 25% of cases with Noonan syndrome.[332] Dilated cardiomyopathy may also occur.

Management

Standard prenatal care is not altered when continuing the pregnancy.

Recurrence Risk

Noonan syndrome is autosomal dominant with sporadic new mutations.

▶ ORAL-FACIAL-DIGITAL SYNDROME

The oral-facial-digital syndrome (OFDS) comprises four types (I through IV; type II is also known as *Mohr syndrome*) that share oral abnormalities, facial dysmorphism, and variable abnormalities of the hands and feet, including polydactyly. Gorlin et al.[333] first recognized this condition in the English literature.

Incidence

Incidence rates are uncertain.

Genetic Defect

OFDS type I is caused by mutations in the *CXORF*5 gene. The critical zone is Xp22.3.[334,335]

Pathologic and Clinical Features

Pathologic and clinical features of OFDS are summarized in Table 18. Facial abnormalities include tongue lobulation, tongue hamartomas, small nostrils, asymmetric clefts of the palate, aberrant hyperplastic oral frenula, alveolar anomalies, and clefts of the jaw and tongue. Cleft lip is typically a median cleft lip. Anomalies of the hands include syndactyly, clinodactyly, brachydactyly, and occasionally postaxial polydactyly. Anomalies of the kidneys and CNS are also common. The latter may include heterotopic gray matter, agenesis of the corpus callosum, vermian agenesis, and Dandy-Walker malformation. Mental retardation is typical.

Diagnosis

OFDS has been diagnosed prenatally.[336,337] A number of cases have shown brain abnormalities including Dandy-Walker malformation and vermian agenesis.[338–341]

The median cleft lip is usually too small to diagnose by prenatal ultrasound. However, other facial abnormalities such as micrognathia may be seen (Fig. 25). We have observed cystic hygroma in association with one case of OFDS in a monozygotic twin pregnancy.

DNA probes for Xp22 can be used for diagnosis of OFDS type I.

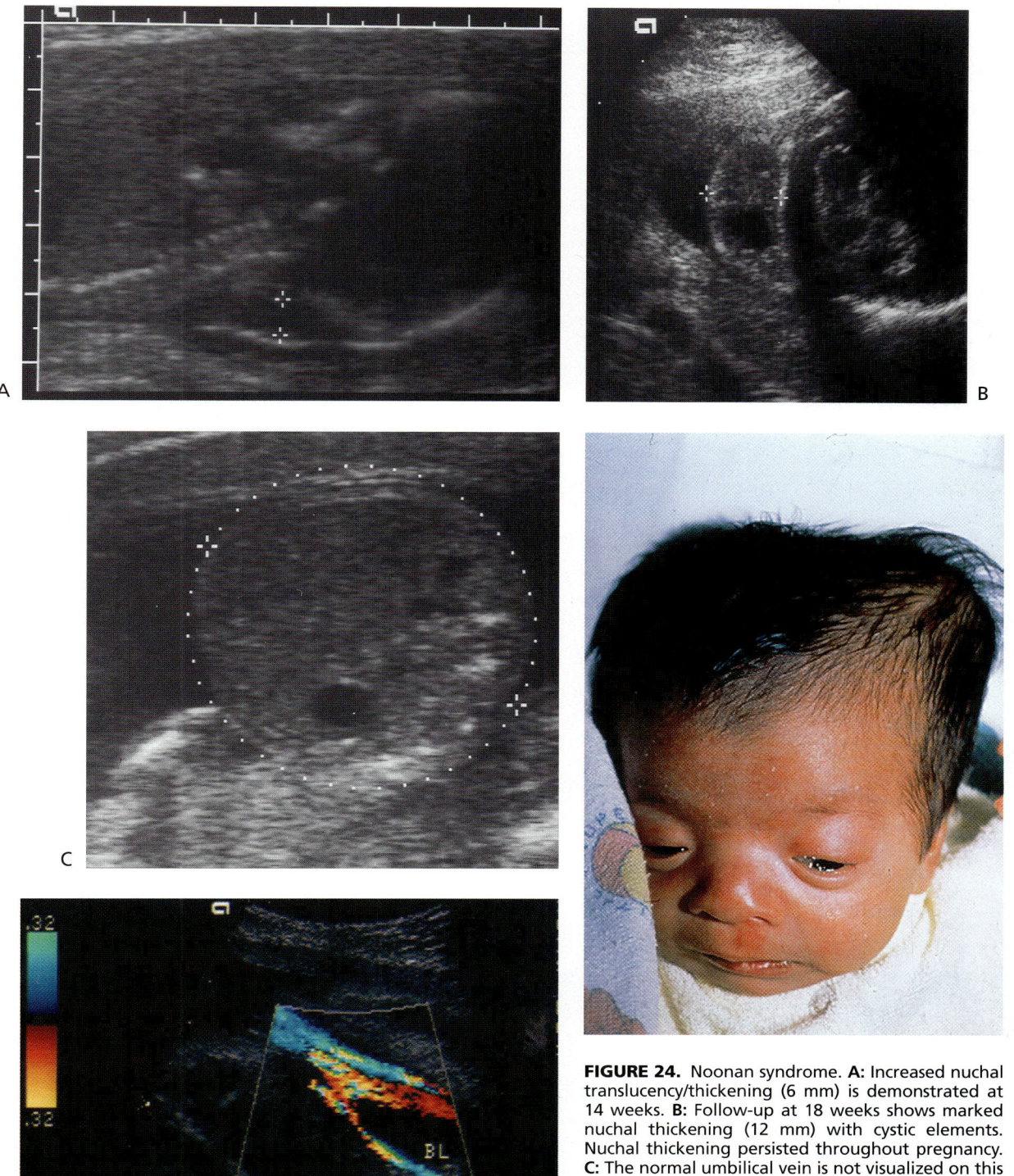

FIGURE 24. Noonan syndrome. **A:** Increased nuchal translucency/thickening (6 mm) is demonstrated at 14 weeks. **B:** Follow-up at 18 weeks shows marked nuchal thickening (12 mm) with cystic elements. Nuchal thickening persisted throughout pregnancy. **C:** The normal umbilical vein is not visualized on this transverse view of the abdomen. **D:** Color-flow imaging of the pelvis shows two umbilical arteries and umbilical vein draining into the right external iliac vein. **E:** A photograph at birth shows characteristic facial features of Noonan syndrome with drooping eyelids. BL, urinary bladder.

TABLE 18. PATHOLOGIC AND CLINICAL FEATURES OF ORAL-FACIAL-DIGITAL SYNDROME

Craniofacial
  Cleft jaw
  Broad nasal root
  Small nostrils
  Hypoplastic alar cartilage
  Cleft lip
  Irregular, asymmetric cleft palate
  Aberrant hyperplastic oral frenula
  Lobulate tongue
  Tongue hamartomas
Skeletal
  Syndactyly
  Brachydactyly
  Postaxial polydactyly
Central nervous system
  Mental retardation
  Agenesis of the corpus callosum
  Dandy-Walker malformation
  Heterotopic gray matter
Renal
  Polycystic kidneys
  Renal failure

Differential Diagnosis

OFDS shares features with Jeune syndrome.[342] Type III overlaps the Majewski type of short-rib polydactyly.

Prognosis

The prognosis varies with the specific condition and associated anomalies. Mental retardation is typical.

Management

Management varies with the specific anomalies.

Recurrence Risk

OFDS type I is inherited as an X-linked dominant trait that is lethal in male fetuses.[343] All cases have been female with the exception of a phenotypic male with an XXY karyotype. The other three types of OFDS appear to be autosomal recessive.

▶ ROBERTS SYNDROME

Roberts syndrome, or Roberts SC syndrome, is a rare developmental disorder characterized by multiple malformations, in particular symmetric limb reduction, craniofacial anomalies, and severe mental and growth retardation. It was initially described by Roberts in 1919[344] and more recently reviewed by Appelt et al.[345] In 1974, Herrmann et al.[346] described cases of a very similar entity called *pseudothalidomide* or *SC syndrome* (named for the initials of the two families originally described). Currently, Roberts syndrome and SC phocomelia are considered a single genetic entity, with a wide phenotypic variation.[347]

Incidence

Incidence rates are unknown.

Genetic Defect

This disorder has an autosomal recessive transmission with marked variability of phenotypic expression. The unique cytogenetic abnormality of premature centromere separation[348] is discussed further under Cytogenetic Testing.

Pathologic and Clinical Features

Pathologic and clinical features of the syndrome are summarized in Table 19. Roberts syndrome is characterized by

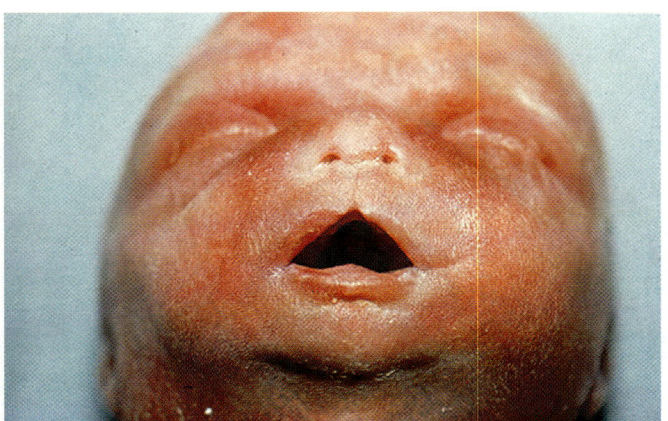

A   B

FIGURE 25. Oral-facial-digital syndrome. **A:** A facial profile shows micrognathia (*arrow*). (Courtesy of Beryl Benacerraf, Boston, MA.) **B:** A postmortem photograph from a similar case shows a small midline cleft lip, which was not detected prenatally.

TABLE 19. PATHOLOGIC AND CLINICAL FEATURES OF ROBERTS SYNDROME

Growth
  Short length
  Growth delay
Craniofacial
  Microcephaly
  Brachycephaly
  Micrognathia
  Malformed ears: low-set, posteriorly angulated
  Hypertelorism
  Prominent eyes
  Bluish sclerae
  Corneal clouding
  Microphthalmos
  Cataract
  Lid coloboma
  Thin nares
  Hypoplastic nasal alae
  Widened nasal bridge
  Cleft lip/palate
  Short neck
  Nuchal cystic hygroma
Cardiovascular
  Atrial septal defect
  Ventricular septal defect
Gastrointestinal
  Rudimentary gallbladder
  Accessory spleen
Genitourinary
  Hypospadias
  Prominent phallus
  Enlarged clitoris
  Enlarged labia minora
  Cryptorchidism
  Bicornuate uterus
  Polycystic kidney
  Horseshoe kidney
Skeletal
  Craniosynostosis
  Hypomelia (more severe in upper limbs)
  Tetraphocomelia
  Absence or reduced length of the humerus, radius, or ulna
  Contractures
  Absence or reduced length of femur, tibia, or fibula
  Syndactyly
  Clinodactyly
  Oligodactyly
  Talipes equinovalgus
  Reduced number of toes
Central nervous system/neurologic
  Mental retardation
  Encephalocele
  Hydrocephalus
  Cranial nerve paralysis
Laboratory: premature separation of centromeric heterochromatin

Reproduced with permission from McKusick VA, ed. Online mendelian inheritance in man. Available at: http://www.ncbi.nlm.nih.gov/omim/. McKusick-Nathans Institute for Genetic Medicine, Johns Hopkins University (Baltimore, MD) and National Center for Biotechnology Information, National Library of Medicine (Bethesda, MD), 2000.

upper and lower limb phocomelia, facial clefts, mental retardation, and severe pre- and postnatal growth retardation.[349,350] Microcephaly, craniosynostosis, anterior encephalocele, hydrocephalus, cardiac defects (mainly septal defects), cataracts or cloudy corneas, nose and ear anomalies, genital abnormalities, renal abnormalities (including multicystic kidneys), toe syndactyly, and silvery blonde hair have also been reported.[351–354] Dysmorphic facial features have also been described, including protuberant eyeballs, beaked nose, prominent philtrum, and hypertelorism. In a review of 100 cases of Roberts syndrome, 90% of cases were associated with tetraphocomelia, 10% with phocomelia affecting the upper limbs only, and 80% with facial clefts.[350]

Diagnosis

Ultrasound

Severe growth delay and skeletal abnormalities are the most prominent sonographic features. Tetraphocomelia is observed in 90% of cases, and phocomelia of the upper extremities alone is observed in 10%. Less common findings include oligodactyly, cryptorchidism, enlarged phallus compared to rest of the body, oligohydramnios, renal anomalies (polycystic or dysplastic kidneys), and heart defects.

In the first trimester, increased nuchal translucency has been observed with Roberts syndrome.[355]

Cytogenetic Testing

A characteristic cytogenetic feature described as premature centromere separation, heterochromatic repulsion or splaying, and centromere puffing[349,356] is observed in approximately 80% of postnatally diagnosed cases of Roberts syndrome and appears to be very specific for this condition.[357] The sensitivity in prenatal cases is uncertain, however, and cases have been reported of normal chromosome appearance on amniocytes but positive findings from lymphocytes or skin fibroblasts on postnatal analysis.

Centromere puffing particularly affects those chromosomes with a secondary constriction (i.e., 1, 9, and 16), the short arms of acrocentric chromosomes, and the distal long arm of the Y chromosome.[358,359] Affected siblings within the same family may be discordant for these cytogenetic findings, and the presence or absence of cytogenetic findings does not correlate with the severity of the abnormalities. Unaffected parents who are presumed heterozygotes do not exhibit these cytogenetic findings.[360]

Differential Diagnosis

There is wide overlap between thrombocytopenia–absent radius syndrome and Roberts syndrome. Roberts syndrome is more typically associated with cleft lip/palate. Premature separation of centromeric heterochromatin is characteristic of Roberts syndrome but may be observed less common prenatally than postnatally. Other considerations include Holt-Oram, craniofacial dysostosis, Fanconi anemia, and VATER syndrome (see Treacher Collins Syndrome, earlier in this chapter).

Prognosis

In most reported cases death occurs *in utero* or soon after birth. A better prognosis has been observed for those longer than 37 cm at birth and with less severe defects. Survival beyond infancy is uncommon, although rare survival into adulthood has been documented.[361]

Management

When detected before viability, termination of pregnancy can be offered. After viability, standard obstetric management is not altered. For those families previously affected, chorionic villous sampling during the first trimester can be offered.

Recurrence Risk

The recurrence risk for a couple with a previous affected pregnancy is 25%.

▶ SMITH-LEMLI-OPITZ SYNDROME

Recognition of the Smith-Lemli-Opitz syndrome (SLOS) represents a triumph of the combining of clinical, biochemical, and genetic observations. The clinical syndrome was first described in 1964 by David Smith, John Opitz, and Luc Lemli[362] in a report of three patients who had in common a distinctive facial appearance, microcephaly, broad alveolar ridges, hypospadias, a characteristic dermatoglyphic pattern, severe feeding disorder, and global developmental delay. A more complete description of SLOS was presented in 1969 as the RSH syndrome, an acronym of the first letters of the original patients' surnames.[363] Many new cases of SLOS over the next 20 years expanded the known characteristics of the syndrome. Defective synthesis of cholesterol was first observed in SLOS patients in 1993,[364] and shortly thereafter Natowicz and Evans[365] reported marked elevation of plasma levels of 7-dehydrocholesterol (7DHC). This observation correctly suggested a deficiency of 7DHC reductase (DHCR7).

Incidence

Although an incidence as high as 1 in 10,000 was suggested in one clinical study,[366] other clinical and biochemical data estimate the incidence of SLOS to be no more than 1 in 40,000 to 60,000.[367] The prevalence also varies among ethnic groups, with a higher incidence among those of European descent.

Genetic and Metabolic Defects

The human *DHCR7* gene was cloned and localized to chromosome 11q12-13 in 1998.[368] Numerous mutations have been identified in *DHCR7*, but seven individual mutations account for 67% of the total mutations reported in the literature.[369]

A defect in cholesterol synthesis (Fig. 26) is now recognized as the cause of SLOS. Even patient *S*, one of the three patients reported as RSH syndrome, proved to have the cholesterol defect of SLOS.[370] As such, SLOS is the first known genetic syndrome with a metabolic etiology.

Cholesterol is an important component of cell membranes, bile acid, and vitamin D and is the precursor of all steroid hormones.[371] Low levels of cholesterol prevent normal structural and neurologic development, and processes that require steroid hormones, such as masculinization of genitalia, are deficient. Accumulation of 7DHC may also interfere with proper membrane function.[372]

Cholesterol is a 27-carbon, monounsaturated sterol synthesized from lanosterol (Fig. 26) that is mostly limited to the endoplasmic reticulum. In contrast to many other small metabolites, very little cholesterol is transported from the mother after the first trimester and most cholesterol must be synthesized by the fetus. Furthermore, most if not all cholesterol in the brain is synthesized locally.[373] Development of holoprosencephaly has been linked to abnormal cholesterol metabolism at several levels.[374]

Pathologic and Clinical Features

SLOS may be associated with a wide variety of clinical and pathologic features[375,376] (Table 20). Typical features include microcephaly, ptosis, a small upturned nose with anteverted nares, micrognathia, postaxial polydactyly, second- and third-toe syndactyly, genital anomalies, growth failure, and mental retardation. Less frequent facial anomalies include hypertelorism, epicanthic folds, unusually long cilia, and low-set ears. The palate is usually highly arched, often with a midline cleft of the uvula, soft palate, or hard palate.

In addition to typical features of SLOS, associated anomalies are common but variable. Almost half of SLOS patients have a congenital heart defect, although when only biochemically confirmed patients are taken into consideration, this percentage is somewhat lower.[377,378] There is a strong predominance of AVSDs and hypoplastic left heart, whereas conotruncal defects are uncommon. Genitourinary anomalies are common and may include hypospadias, cryptorchidism, and ambiguous genitalia.

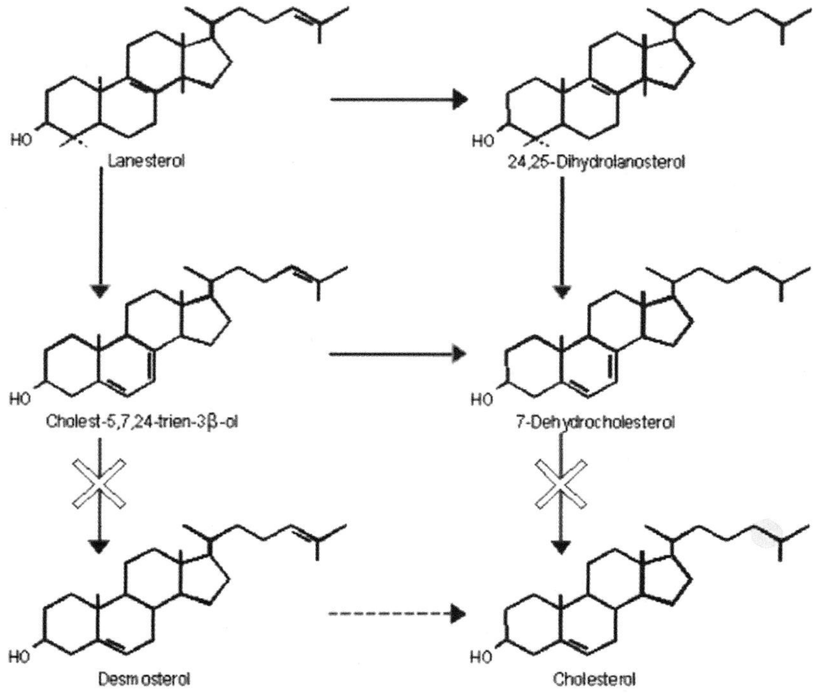

FIGURE 26. Smith-Lemli-Opitz syndrome. (Courtesy of Silva SR, Jeanty P. Prenatal ultrasound findings of Smith-Lemli-Opitz syndrome. Available at: http://www.thefetus.net/page.php?id=442. In: Jeanty P, ed. The fetus. Accessed 2000.)

Diagnosis

Ultrasound

Prenatal sonographic findings of SLOS are highly variable. Findings may include IUGR, microcephaly, facial anomalies, polydactyly, renal anomalies (including cystic kidneys), cardiac defects (Fig. 27), lung malformations, or other anomalies. Ambiguous genitalia are a common finding, and some fetuses may even exhibit phenotypically female genitalia with a known 46,XY karyotype. Affected fetuses may first present with nuchal edema[379,380] or nonimmune hydrops.

TABLE 20. PATHOLOGIC AND CLINICAL FEATURES OF SMITH-LEMLI-OPITZ SYNDROME

Growth	Hypoplastic left heart	Cataract
Pre- and postnatal growth restriction	Atrial septal defect	Hypertelorism
Hypotonia	Genitourinary	Prominent nasal bridge
Extremities	Hypospadias	Prominent epicanthal folds
Syndactyly (especially the second and third toes)	Cryptorchidism	Cleft palate
Postaxial polydactyly	Micropenis	Micrognathia
Short limbs	Bifidum scrotum	Short nose
Clinodactyly	Ambiguous genitalia	Anteverted nostrils
Valgus deformity	Hypoplastic labia	Low-set ears
Radial deviation of the hands	Rudimentary uterus	Ptosis
Ulnar deviation of the fingers	Ureteropelvic junction obstruction	Broad maxillary alveolar ridges
Rockerbottom feet	Renal hypoplasia	Increased nuchal translucency
Abnormal palmar creases	Urethral stenosis	Gastrointestinal
Central nervous system	Cystic renal dysplasia	Rectal atresia
Agenesis of the corpus callosum	Male pseudohermaphroditism	Abdominal calcifications
Demyelination	Hydronephrosis	Inguinal hernia
Hydrocephalus	Renal aplasia/agenesis	Hirschsprung disease
Holoprosencephaly	Renal cystic dysplasia	Pyloric stenosis
Cerebral hypoplasia	Renal duplication	Other
Cerebellar hypoplasia	Pulmonary: abnormal pulmonary lobation	Adrenal enlargement
Cardiac	Craniofacial	Moderate to severe mental retardation
Atrioventricular septal defect	Microcephaly	Hypoplasia of thymus
Ventricular septal defect	Trigonocephaly	Hydrops

Reproduced with permission from Silva SR, Jeanty P. Prenatal ultrasound findings of Smith-Lemli-Opitz syndrome. Available at: http://www.thefetus.net/page.php?id=442. In: Jeanty P, ed. The fetus. Accessed 2000; and Abuelo DN, Tint GS, Kelley R, Batta AK, Shefer S, Salen G. Prenatal detection of the cholesterol biosynthetic defect in the Smith-Lemli-Opitz syndrome by the analysis of amniotic fluid sterols. *Am J Med Genet* 1995;56:281–285.

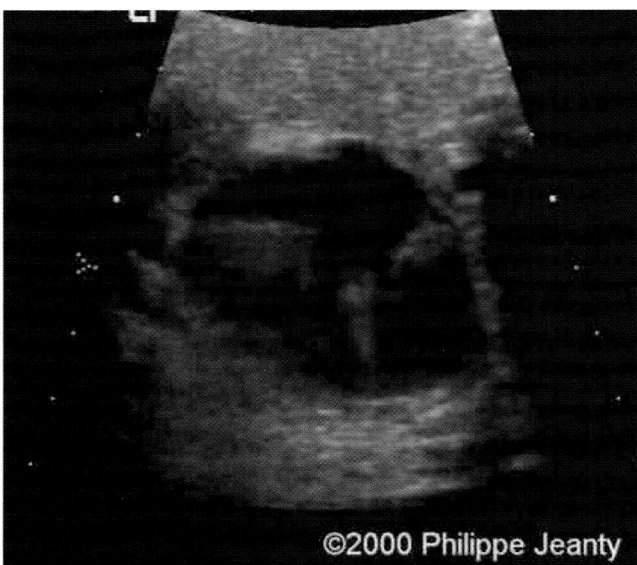

FIGURE 27. Smith-Lemli-Opitz syndrome. An axial view of the heart at 35 weeks shows a large central atrioventricular septal type of defect. Other anomalies seen included short extremities (all limbs below the fifth percentile), clubfeet, hypoplastic kidneys, and oligohydramnios. The fetal karyotype was normal. Biochemical analysis showed extremely low levels of cholesterol and elevated levels of 7-dehydrocholesterol. The infant died shortly after birth. Anomalies at pathology included bilateral cataracts, micrognathia, polydactyly of the right hand and syndactyly of the fourth and fifth digits on the left hand, shortened limbs, clubfeet, short webbed neck, partial agenesis of the corpus callosum, hypoplastic kidneys, severe hypospadias, and atrioventricular septal defect. (Reproduced with permission from Silva SR, Jeanty P. Prenatal ultrasound findings of Smith-Lemli-Opitz syndrome. Available at: http://www.thefetus.net/page.php?id=442. In: Jeanty P, ed. The fetus. Accessed 2000.)

Laboratory

Accurate diagnosis of SLOS can be made by detecting elevated 7DHC levels in the amniotic fluid, with typically a more than 500-fold increase in affected pregnancies.[378] Comparison of the 7DHC-to-cholesterol ratio can also be made. In some pregnancies, the amniotic fluid level of cholesterol is abnormally low, whereas in others the level is normal. Direct analysis of the sterol composition of chorionic villi at 10 weeks is also a reliable method for diagnosis of SLOS, although the relative increase in the 7DHC to cholesterol ratio is not as great as it is in amniotic fluid.[378]

Despite the feasibility of prenatal diagnosis by genetic testing of villus tissue or amniocytes, the simplicity and accuracy of biochemical testing obviate the need for genetic testing, except, perhaps, in a rare case with equivocal biochemical results.

Some fetuses with SLOS may first present with abnormally low maternal serum levels of unconjugated estriol.[381–383] However, this may be neither sensitive nor specific. Maymon et al.[380] identified 26 pregnancies with estriol levels of 0.25 MoM or lower from 12,141 pregnan-

cies screened for Down syndrome, and SLOS was not clinically diagnosed in any of the live-born infants. Maternal estriol levels may also be reduced in the maternal urine late in pregnancy.[384]

After birth, the diagnosis of SLOS may be made by measuring levels of 7DHC or 8DHC in the plasma. Because a minority of patients with SLOS has normal serum cholesterol levels at any age, a blood cholesterol level is not a reliable screening test for SLOS. In rare cases in which 7DHC and 8DHC levels are normal or fall in the heterozygote range, the diagnosis can be made by *DHCR7* mutational testing, *DHCR7* enzymatic assay, or analysis of sterol biosynthesis in cultured cells.[385]

Differential Diagnosis

The pattern of multisystem anomalies should suggest aneuploidy, including trisomies 21, 18, and 13. Before the era of biochemical diagnosis, SLOS was suspected or confirmed in some affected infants with acrodysgenital syndrome,[386] Gardner-Silengo-Wachtel syndrome, and holoprosencephaly-polydactyly syndrome.[387] Other considerations include Noonan syndrome, Opitz syndrome, Zellweger syndrome, and alpha-thalassemia–mental retardation syndrome. Other disorders that may resemble SLOS include Meckel syndrome, hydrolethalus syndrome, Pallister-Hall syndrome, and OFDS type VI. Occipital encephalocele and dysplastic kidneys favor a diagnosis of Meckel syndrome, whereas genital anomalies and syndactyly support SLOS.[388]

Prognosis

Clinical signs vary in severity, ranging from fetal loss or holoprosencephaly with multiple malformations to isolated syndactyly to variable degrees of mental and growth retardation.[389] Among newborns, 20% die within the first year of life, and the most common cause is pneumonia.[390] Severe hypotonia and global psychomotor retardation are characteristic of SLOS in infancy, although some patients have normal or borderline normal development.

The severity of the insult depends on the severity of the metabolic deficiency. Biochemical differences in the conversion of 7DHC to cholesterol have been correlated to severity of the syndrome.[391] SLOS patients with multiple internal anomalies and early death have had, in general, much lower total sterol levels and higher 7DHC-to-sterol ratios than surviving SLOS patients. A strong correlation has been shown between the predicted enzymatic effect of a patient's particular mutations and the clinical phenotype.[392]

Management

Cholesterol dietary supplementation after birth has been used successfully, reducing the growth retardation and recurrent infection. Supplementary cholesterol eliminates or ameliorates many of the feeding and growth problems of SLOS and has also been shown to reduce or even eliminate the autistic behaviors of children with SLOS.[393] Cholesterol supplementation can also lead to an objective improvement in the recently recognized photosensitivity of SLOS.[394] Although still uncertain, it is unlikely that long-term cholesterol supplementation significantly improves cognitive development because cholesterol does not cross the blood–brain barrier.[395] Even if cholesterol could reach brain cells and myelin, cognitive performance might not improve, since the mental retardation of SLOS appears to reflect early abnormalities of cerebral neuronal development.

Fetal cholesterol supplementation by multiple plasma transfusions has been performed prenatally in an attempt to improve clinical outcome.[396] Fetal cholesterol levels were shown to increase with therapy, although the possible clinical benefit of prenatal treatment remains uncertain.

Recurrence Risk

The recurrence risk is 25%.

▶ TREACHER COLLINS SYNDROME

British ophthalmologist Edward Treacher Collins (1862–1932) first described this syndrome—also known as *mandibulofacial dysostosis*—which is characterized by a variety of facial abnormalities.

Incidence

Treacher Collins syndrome occurs in approximately 1 in 50,000 live births.

Genetic Defect

Treacher Collins syndrome is caused by mutations in the Treacle (*TCOF1*) gene, which is located on chromosome 5q32-33.[397–399] At least 35 mutations in the *TCOF1* gene have been identified.[400] The gene encodes a protein that may be involved in nucleolar-cytoplasmic transport.[401]

Pathologic and Clinical Features

Pathologic and clinical features of Treacher Collins syndrome are summarized in Table 21. Multiple anomalies appear to reflect bilateral symmetric anomalies of the structures within the first and second branchial arches.[402] The clinical characteristics of the disease include (a) hypoplasia of the mandible and zygomatic complex; (b) abnormalities of the ears, often associated with atresia of the external auditory canals and anomalies of the middle ear ossicles and leading to a conductive hearing loss; (c) downward-slanting palpebral fissures with colobomas of the lower eye-

TABLE 21. PATHOLOGIC AND CLINICAL FEATURES OF TREACHER COLLINS SYNDROME

Craniofacial
Absent auditory canal
Auricular tags, pits, fistulas
Choanal atresia/stenosis
Dysplastic ears
Deafness
Cleft palate
Coloboma of eyelids
Flat malar region
Macrostomia
Microstomia
Downward-slanting palpebral fissures
Gastrointestinal
Anal atresia/stenosis
Tracheoesophageal fistula
Cardiovascular: cardiac defects

Reproduced with permission from McKusick VA, ed. Online mendelian inheritance in man. Available at: http://www.ncbi.nlm.nih.gov/omim/. McKusick-Nathans Institute for Genetic Medicine, Johns Hopkins University (Baltimore, MD) and National Center for Biotechnology Information, National Library of Medicine (Bethesda, MD), 2000.

lids; and (d) cleft palate. Associated anomalies include choanal atresia.

Diagnosis

The prenatal sonographic findings of Treacher Collins syndrome include polyhydramnios, microcephaly, abnormal fetal facial features (slanting forehead, microphthalmos, micrognathia), and abnormal fetal swallowing.[403–407] Evidence of hypertelorism (Fig. 28) may be present. The ears may be malformed, low set, and hypoplastic; skin tags may be seen in lieu of ears. The prenatal sonographic diagnosis of Treacher Collins syndrome has been made as early as 15 weeks in cases at risk for recurrence. Because the physical deformities are so variable, mildly affected parents can have a severely affected fetus.

Prenatal diagnosis has also been performed in families with a history of *TCOF1* using fetoscopy.[408,409] The diagnosis can be made by gene linkage.[410,411]

Differential Diagnosis

Goldenhar syndrome (hemifacial microsomia) is asymmetric. Nager acrofacial dysostosis shows some phenotypic overlap, although the latter is associated with reduction of the forearms. Administration of retinoic acid at a critical developmental period can lead to anomalies that are virtually identical to the Treacher Collins syndrome.[412]

Prognosis

Patients can develop respiratory problems as a result of a narrow airway and may occasionally require tracheostomy.

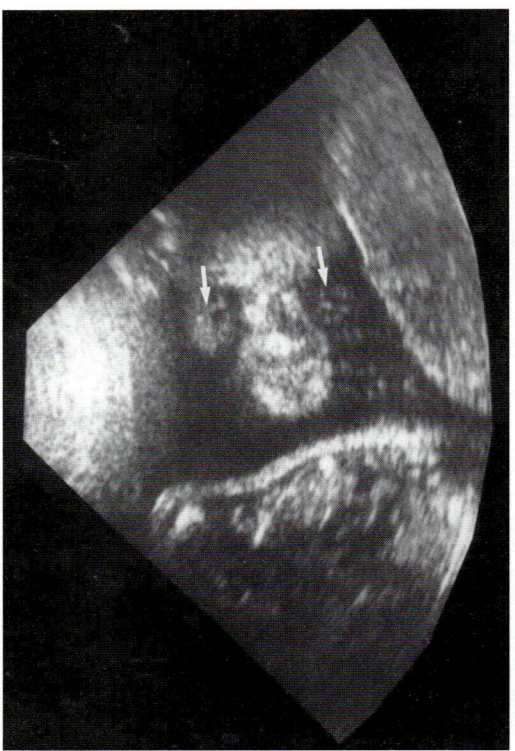
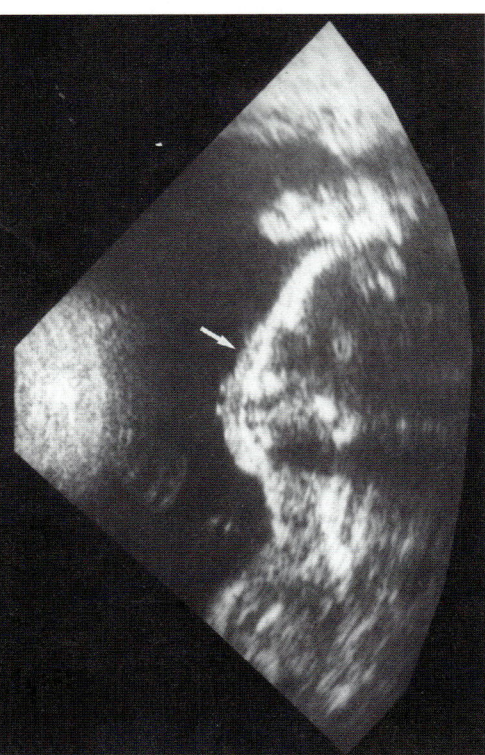

A,B

FIGURE 28. Treacher Collins syndrome. **A:** A coronal view shows hypertelorism and downward slanting of the orbits (*arrows*). **B:** A sagittal view shows a flattened nose (*arrow*). The infant had choanal atresia. (Courtesy of Beryl Benacerraf, Boston, MA.)

The great majority of patients are of normal intelligence. Deafness is common. Visual disturbances may occur.

Management

Growth of the facial bones during infancy and childhood results in improvement that may be further enhanced with surgical techniques. Surgical management is individualized depending on the severity of the abnormality.[413] Patients are typically treated in two to three operative sessions beginning early in the second decade of life. The first operation consists of chin advancement and malar osteotomies. In the second operation, the chin prominence is moved further forward. Some patients may require additional procedures.

Recurrence Risk

Treacher Collins is autosomal dominant, although approximately 60% of cases are sporadic, apparently new mutations. Expressivity and penetrance of this syndrome can vary widely, even within a single family. In general, there is complete penetrance and variable expressivity of the trait.

▶ TUBEROUS SCLEROSIS

Tuberous sclerosis, or Bourneville's disease, is an autosomal dominant condition characterized by hamartomas in multiple organs, primarily the skin, brain, kidneys, and heart.

Incidence

The prevalence of tuberous sclerosis is suggested to be as high as 1 in 5,800 live births.[414]

Genetic Defect

Two causative genes, *TSC1* (chromosomal locus 9q34) and *TSC2* (chromosomal locus 16p13), have been identified.[415,416] *TSC1* codes for hamartin, and *TSC2* codes for tuberin. Most new mutations are secondary to defects of *TSC2*.[417] More than 300 mutations have been identified with tuberous sclerosis, and only a handful of recurrent mutations have been observed.

Pathologic and Clinical Features

Pathologic and clinical features of tuberous sclerosis are summarized in Table 22. Tuberous sclerosis affects many organ systems including the skin (hypomelanotic macules, facial angiofibromas, shagreen patches, fibrous facial plaques, ungual fibromas), brain (cortical tubers, subependymal nodules, seizures, mental retardation/developmental delay), kidneys (angiomyolipomas, cysts), and heart (rhabdomyomas, arrhythmias).[418] Cutaneous manifestations are characteristic.[419] CNS manifestations of subependymal tubers are present in 95% of patients at birth. Brain tumors such as ependymoma of the third ventricle and astrocytoma may occur.

TABLE 22. PATHOLOGIC AND CLINICAL FEATURES OF TUBEROUS SCLEROSIS

Craniofacial
  Achromatic retinal patches
  Retinal astrocytoma
  Pitted dental enamel
  Gingival fibroma
Cardiovascular
  Cardiac rhabdomyoma
  Wolff-Parkinson-White syndrome
Respiratory: lymphangiomyomatosis
Genitourinary
  Renal cysts
  Renal angiomyolipoma
  Renal carcinoma
Skeletal: cystic areas of bone rarefaction, especially phalanges
Skin, hair, nails
  Facial angiofibroma
  White ash leaf–shaped macules
  Shagreen patch
  Subcutaneous nodules
  Café-au-lait spots
  Subungual fibromata
Neurologic/central nervous system
  Infantile spasms
  Seizures
  Mental retardation
  Intracranial calcification on radiographic or computed tomographic examination
  Subependymal nodules
  Ependymoma
  Giant cell astrocytoma
Endocrine
  Precocious puberty
  Hypothyroidism

Reproduced with permission from McKusick VA, ed. Online mendelian inheritance in man. Available at: http://www.ncbi.nlm.nih.gov/omim/. McKusick-Nathans Institute for Genetic Medicine, Johns Hopkins University (Baltimore, MD) and National Center for Biotechnology Information, National Library of Medicine (Bethesda, MD), 2000.

Diagnosis

Ultrasound

The prenatal diagnosis is usually suggested by the discovery of rhabdomyomas[420] (Fig. 29). They are typically multiple rather than solitary, although prenatal ultrasound may readily miss small lesions. Cardiac tumors are detectable as early as 22 weeks of gestation. It is estimated that up to half of all patients with tuberous sclerosis develop rhabdomyomas. Conversely, the majority of cardiac rhabdomyomas are associated with tuberous sclerosis,[421] and nearly all patients with multiple rhabdomyomas prove to have tuberous sclerosis. Occasionally, the finding of a rhabdomyoma during routine second-trimester ultrasound examination may lead to the discovery that the mother is affected.[422]

Brain abnormalities may also be seen prenatally. The subependymal tubers are difficult to detect by prenatal ultrasound but can be detected by MRI.[423–426] MRI is more

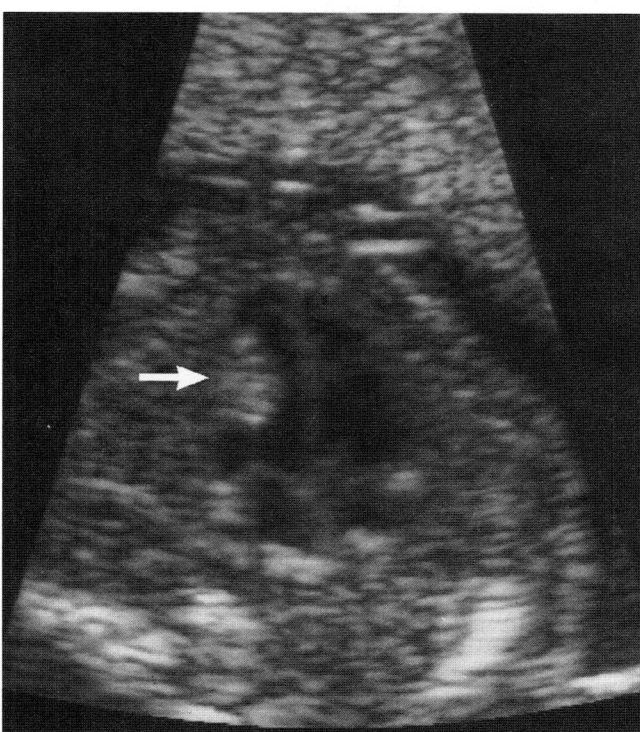

A

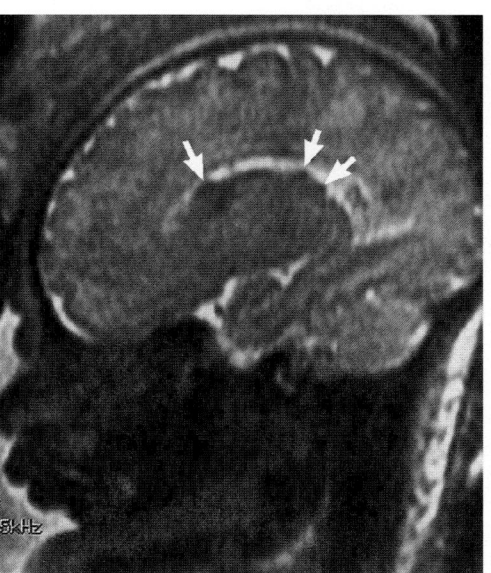

B

FIGURE 29. Tuberous sclerosis. **A:** A four-chamber view shows an echogenic mass (*arrow*) in the left ventricle of the heart at 23 weeks. The appearance is typical of a rhabdomyoma. **B:** A prenatal magnetic resonance image, T2-weighted in the parasagittal plane, shows several hypointense subependymal lesions (*arrows*). These were also bright on T1-weighted images. They are characteristic of subependymal tubers.

sensitive than ultrasound for detection of lesions (Fig. 30A). Several cases have found tuberous sclerosis in association with unilateral ventricular dilatation, presumably on the basis of unilateral obstruction of the foramen of Monro by a subependymal tuber.[427–429] One case was visualized as early as 14 weeks.[427]

Laboratory

Molecular diagnosis by mutation analysis of the *TSC1* and *TSC2* genes is available on a research basis only in affected families. Testing is difficult because of the large size of the two genes, the large number of disease-causing mutations, and the high rate of somatic mosaicism (10% to 25%).

Differential Diagnosis

Other cardiac tumors such as fibroma should also be considered when a single mass is identified. Unusually large echogenic intracardiac foci should not be mistaken for cardiac tumors.

Prognosis

Rhabdomyomas typically resolve postnatally,[430,431] remain unchanged during childhood, and then again regress in adolescence.[432] Rhabdomyomas may cause rhythm disruptions (Wolff-Parkinson-White syndrome, supraventricular tachycardia, paroxysmal arrhythmias), obstructions, or regurgitation. Patients are at risk for development of renal hemorrhage from angiomyolipomas and often develop seizures.

Management

Termination of the pregnancy may be offered before viability. Infants with tuberous sclerosis should be monitored clinically and with imaging studies: renal ultrasound for cysts and angiomyolipoma, CT and MRI for brain tumors, and echocardiography for rhabdomyomas.

Recurrence Risk

Tuberous sclerosis is inherited in an autosomal dominant fashion, so offspring have a 50% risk of being affected, although clinical manifestations are variable. Two-thirds of affected individuals have tuberous sclerosis as the result of a new gene mutation.

▶ VATER/VACTERL ASSOCIATION

VATER is an acronym, suggested in 1972,[433] for an association of *v*ertebral defects, *a*nal atresia, *t*racheo*e*sophageal fistula, and *r*enal anomalies. This was later modified to VACTERL (*v*ertebral anomalies, *a*norectal atresia, *c*ardiac anomalies, *t*racheo*e*sophageal fistula, *r*enal anomalies, and *l*imb anomalies).[434,435] An association with hydrocephalus (VACTERL-H) should probably be considered separately.[436]

Caudal regression syndrome/sirenomelia may represent a severe form of the VATER association.

Incidence

The VATER association is rare and sporadic. Associations with maternal diabetes[437] and high levels of lead exposure have been noted.[438]

TABLE 23. PATHOLOGIC AND CLINICAL FEATURES OF VATER (VACTERL) SYNDROME

Growth: growth delay
Central nervous system/neurologic
  Spinal dysraphia
  Occipital encephalocele
  Hydrocephalus
Craniofacial: cleft lip/palate
Cardiovascular
  Ventricular septal defect
  Patent ductus arteriosus
  Tetralogy of Fallot
  Transposition of the great arteries
  Single umbilical artery
Respiratory/chest
  Choanal atresia
  Laryngeal stenosis
  Tracheal agenesis
  Rib anomalies
  Sternal anomalies
Gastrointestinal
  Tracheoesophageal fistula
  Esophageal atresia
  Anal atresia
Genitourinary
  Hypospadias
  Renal aplasia
  Renal dysplasia
  Hydronephrosis
  Renal ectopia
  Vesicoureteral reflux
  Ureteropelvic junction obstruction
  Persistent urachus
Skeletal
  Vertebral anomalies
  Scoliosis
  Radial aplasia
  Radial hypoplasia
  Radioulnar synostosis
  Preaxial polydactyly
  Vertebral anomalies (fusion, hemivertebrae)
  Absent or hypoplastic thumbs
  Syndactyly
  Triphalangeal thumb

VACTERL, *v*ertebral anomalies, *a*norectal atresia, *c*ardiac anomalies, *t*racheoesophageal fistula, *r*enal anomalies, and *l*imb anomalies; VATER, *v*ertebral defects, *a*nal atresia, *t*racheoesophageal fistula, and *r*enal anomalies.
Reproduced with permission from McKusick VA, ed. Online mendelian inheritance in man. Available at: http://www.ncbi.nlm.nih.gov/omim/. McKusick-Nathans Institute for Genetic Medicine, Johns Hopkins University (Baltimore, MD) and National Center for Biotechnology Information, National Library of Medicine (Bethesda, MD), 2000.

Genetic Defect

The genetic basis is unknown. Defective mesodermal development of unknown origin, perhaps a mitochondrial disorder, has been suggested.[439]

Pathologic and Clinical Features

A wide variety of anomalies have been associated with the VACTERL syndrome (Table 23). The most suggestive features are any combination of the anomalies that make up its acronym: vertebral anomalies, anorectal atresia, cardiac anomalies, tracheoesophageal fistula, renal anomalies, and limb anomalies.

Diagnosis

The association of vertebral anomalies, renal, heart, and radial defects constitutes the classic manifestation of the VACTERL association (Figs. 30 and 31). However, the manifestations are variable. Important clues include radial aplasia, absent or collapsed stomach, and polyhydramnios.[440] The diagnosis can also be suspected in the presence of hemivertebrae, scoliosis, or other limb anomalies (club-

hand, reduction defects, and polydactyly). Nearly one-half of patients with tracheoesophageal fistulas exhibit other VACTERL malformations.[441]

Differential Diagnosis

Because VACTERL syndrome is characterized by anomalies of multiple systems, chromosomal disorders such as trisomies 18 and 13 must be excluded by karyotype study. Disorders characterized by the presence of vertebral, renal, or radial defects may include Fanconi anemia, MURCS association (*mü*llerian duct aplasia, *r*enal aplasia, and *c*ervicothoracic *s*omite dysplasia), and the Roberts, Holt-Oram, Nager, caudal regression, thrombocytopenia–absent radius, Jarcho-Levin, and ectrodactyly–ectodermal dysplasia–clefting syndromes.[442] Townes-Brocks syndrome (anal atresia, ear anomalies, triphalangeal thumbs) also shares some features.[443]

Prognosis

The overall prognosis depends on the type and severity of underlying defects. Anal atresia and esophageal atresia can

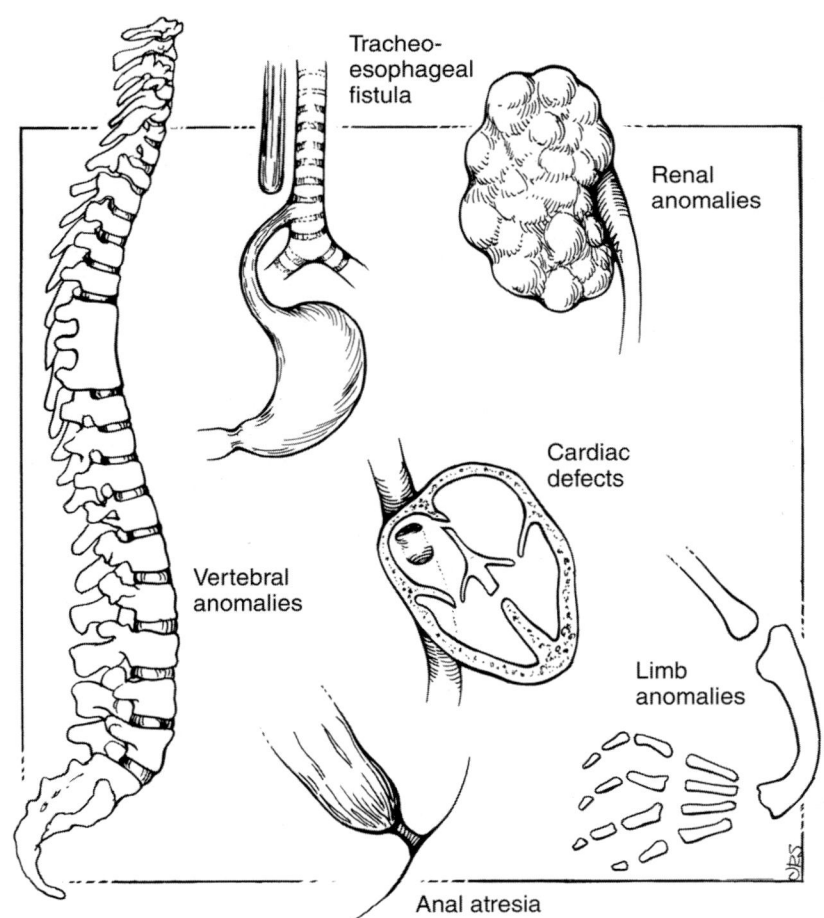

FIGURE 30. The VACTERL association: *v*ertebral anomalies, *a*nal atresia, *c*ardiac defects, *t*racheo-*e*sophageal fistula, *r*enal anomalies, and *l*imb anomalies.

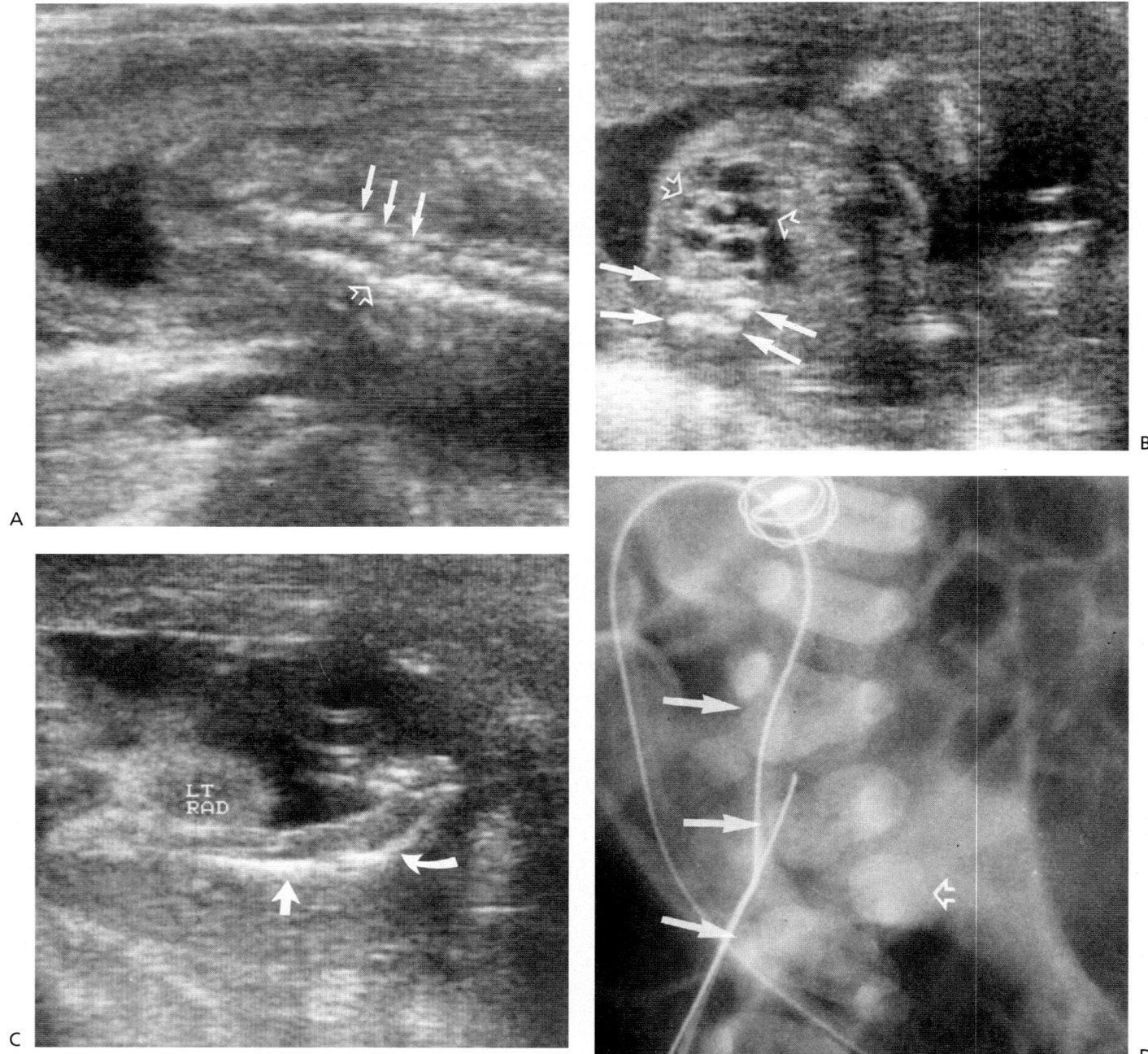

A

B

C

D

FIGURE 31. The VACTERL (*v*ertebral anomalies, *a*nal atresia, *c*ardiac defects, *t*racheoesophageal fistula, *r*enal anomalies, and *l*imb anomalies) association. **A:** Coronal ultrasound of the spine demonstrates asymmetric ossifications in the high lumbar spine (*solid* and *open arrows*). **B:** A transverse ultrasound demonstrates widely dispersed ossification centers of the lumbar spine (*solid arrows*) and multicystic renal disease (*open arrows*). **C:** A scan of the left upper extremity shows a normal humerus (*straight arrow*), absent radius, and a curved but otherwise normal ulna (*curved arrow*). **D:** A postnatal radiograph shows scoliosis secondary to hemivertebra in the lumbar spine (*solid* and *open arrows*). (*continued*)

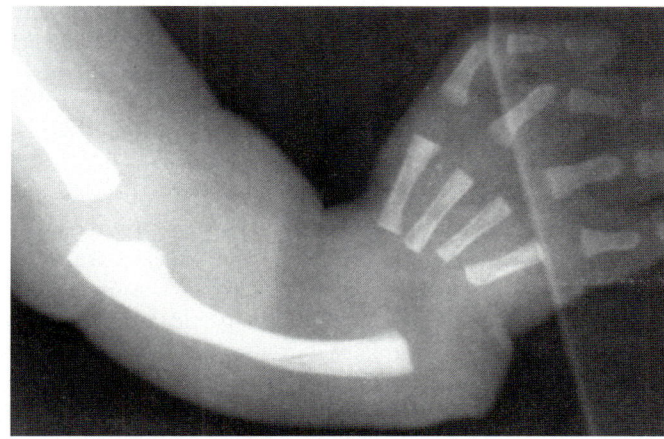

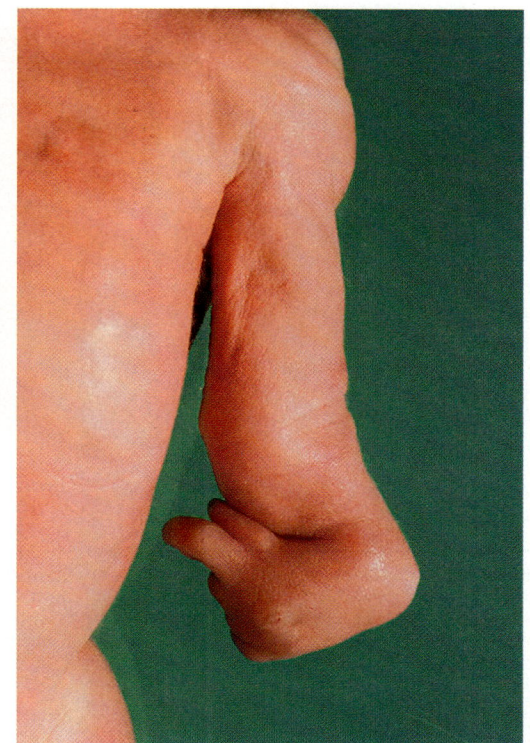

FIGURE 31. *Continued.* **E:** An upper-extremity radiograph shows radial agenesis and absence of the first metacarpal and thumb. **F:** A postmortem photograph from a similar case with the VATER (*v*ertebral defects, *a*nal atresia, *t*racheoesophageal fistula, and *r*enal anomalies) complex shows radial aplasia. (Reproduced with permission from McGahan JP, Leeba JM, Lindfors KK. Prenatal sonographic diagnosis of VATER association. *J Clin Ultrasound* 1988;16:588.)

be surgically repaired. Most surviving children with VATER association display normal development. Early postnatal growth delay may indicate a higher risk for developmental problems.[444]

Management

Termination of pregnancy can be offered before viability. Monthly sonographic monitoring of fetal growth and evaluation of the structural defects are recommended. Delivery in a tertiary center is required for prompt surgical repair and rehabilitation. If present, the esophageal atresia and anorectal malformations must be repaired.

Recurrence Risk

True VACTERL association is usually sporadic with a low recurrence risk. However, rare autosomal recessive and X-linked forms have also been described in association with hydrocephalus.[436]

▶ WALKER-WARBURG SYNDROME

Walker-Warburg syndrome (WWS) was first reported by Walker in 1942[445] and reviewed by Warburg in 1971.[446] Synonyms for this syndrome include *HARDE syndrome* (*h*ydrocephalus, *a*gyria, *r*etinal *d*ysplasia, and *e*ncephalocele), cerebrooculomuscular syndrome, cerebro-ocular dysplasia–muscular dystrophy, Warburg's syndrome, Walker's

lissencephaly, encephalo-ophthalmic dysplasia, and oculocerebral malformation.[447,448]

Incidence

The incidence of WWS is unknown.

Genetic Defect

WWS is autosomal recessive and maps to 9q31.

Pathologic and Clinical Features

Pathologic and clinical features of WWS are summarized in Table 24. WWS is one of a group of disorders that result in altered cell migration.[449] The clinical features include lissencephaly type II, brain malformations, retinal malformation, and congenital muscular dystrophy.[450] Brain abnormalities may include hydrocephalus, cephalocele, microcephaly, agenesis of the corpus callosum, and Dandy-Walker malformation. Ocular abnormalities are an essential feature of WWS and may include microphthalmos, buphthalmos, congenital glaucoma, cataract, optic nerve hypoplasia, and persistent hyaloid artery.

Type II lissencephaly, more recently known as *cobblestone dysplasia* or *cobblestone lissencephaly*, consists of cerebral and cerebellar cortex with a granular or pebbled surface; areas of atypical agyria, macrogyria, and polymicrogyria; and a thick fibroglial rind over the surface that often

TABLE 24. PATHOLOGIC AND CLINICAL FEATURES OF WALKER-WARBURG SYNDROME

Brain
   Agyria, micropolygyria, cortical disorganization, heterotopia
   Type II lissencephaly
   Hydrocephalus
   Encephalocele
   Cerebellar malformations, Dandy-Walker malformation
Muscle: myopathy
Face
   Retinal detachment, dysplasia
   Cataract
   Microphthalmos
   Persistent hyperplastic primary vitreous
   Optic nerve hypoplasia
   Coloboma
   Cleft lip/palate
   Microtia
   Absent auditory canals
Genitourinary anomalies

Reproduced with permission from McKusick VA, ed. Online mendelian inheritance in man. Available at: http://www.ncbi.nlm.nih.gov/omim/. McKusick-Nathans Institute for Genetic Medicine, Johns Hopkins University (Baltimore, MD) and National Center for Biotechnology Information, National Library of Medicine (Bethesda, MD), 2000.

obstructs the subarachnoid space. The abnormal cytoarchitecture results from gaps in the pial limiting membrane during embryogenesis, which allows migrating neurons and glia to extend past the true cortical plate and into the subarachnoid space.

Diagnosis

Monteagudo et al.[451] reviewed prenatal reports of WWS. Prenatal ultrasound findings may include ventricular dilatation, Dandy-Walker malformation, cephalocele, brain abnormalities including lissencephaly, ocular abnormalities, and occasionally renal abnormalities (Figs. 32 and 33). Ocular abnormalities include microphthalmos, retinal detachment, and cataracts[452,453] (Fig. 32). Detection of subtle ocular abnormalities is more likely in patients with a family history of this disorder.[454,455] Based on the wide spectrum of defects, the association of any type of eye abnormality with cerebral malformations should elicit suspicion of WWS.

Early diagnosis is possible in some cases at risk.[456] Transvaginal sonography may be helpful when the head is low in the maternal pelvis.[457] MRI is particularly helpful in diagnosis of lissencephaly, but this diagnosis is possible only during the third trimester, when gyri normally develop.

Differential Diagnosis

Meckel-Gruber syndrome may demonstrate cephalocele and kidney abnormalities (usually enlarged, cystic kidneys) in association with oligohydramnios. Other considerations include Fryns syndrome, trisomies 18 and 13, and maternal viral infections.

Similar brain abnormalities may be found in a spectrum of rare congenital syndromes characterized by migration disorders of the brain and muscular dystrophy. Along with WWS, these include Fukuyama type congenital muscular dystrophy and muscle-eye-brain disease, also known as *Haltia-Santavuori syndrome*.[458–460] Both Miller-Dieker and Neu-Laxova syndromes include lissencephaly and microcephaly, and the latter may also have Dandy-Walker malformation.[461]

Prognosis

Most newborns affected by WWS die within the first year of life. Of those few who survive until 5 years of age, most have severe mental and developmental retardation.

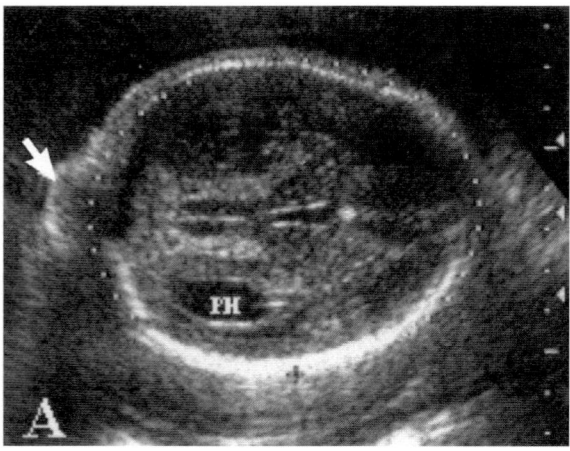
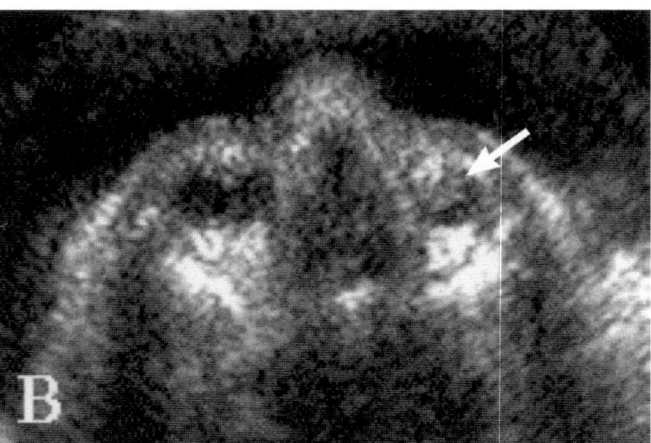

FIGURE 32. Walker-Warburg syndrome. **A:** A transabdominal scan shows a posterior cephalocele (*arrow*) at the level of the thalami. PH, posterior horn of ventricle. **B:** An axial view of the eyes shows a cataract of the left eye (*arrow*). (Reproduced with permission from Monteagudo A, Alayon A, Mayberry P. Walker-Warburg syndrome: case report and review of the literature. *J Ultrasound Med* 2001;20:419–426.)

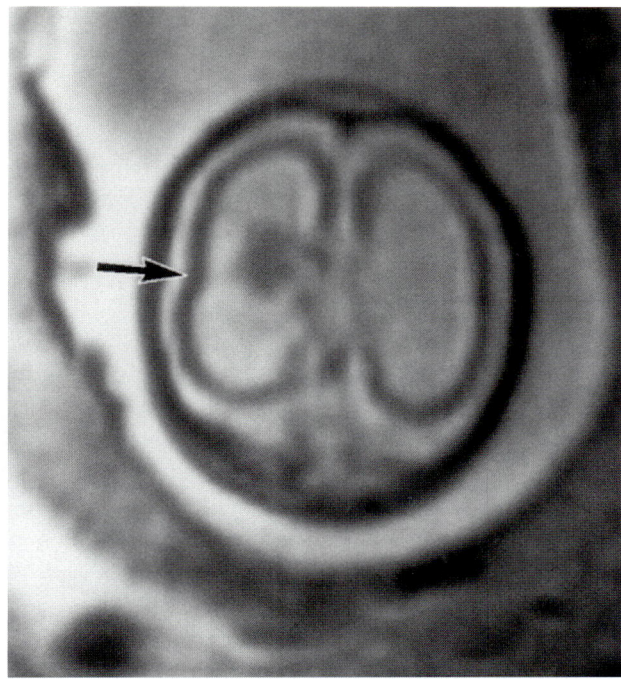

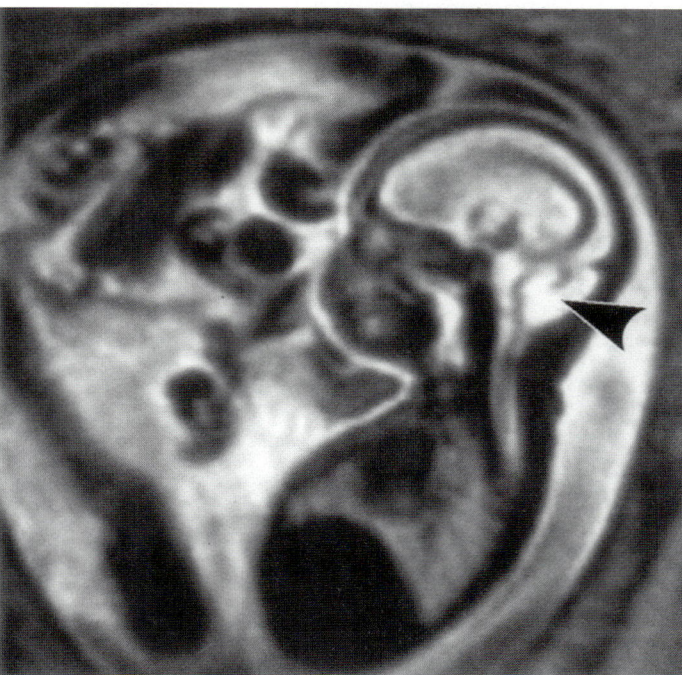

FIGURE 33. Walker-Warburg syndrome. **A:** An axial magnetic resonance image at 27 weeks shows ventricular dilatation with only a thin rim of smooth cerebral tissue (*arrow*) and no differentiation between gray and white matter. **B:** A sagittal magnetic resonance image shows a prominent, fluid-filled posterior fossa (*arrowhead*) with little cerebellar tissue. The brainstem appears abnormally small. Autopsy demonstrated microcephaly; thinned, lissencephalic cerebral hemispheres; cerebellar hypoplasia; and partial absence of the corpus callosum. (Reproduced with permission from Huppert BJ, Brandt KR, Ramin KD, King BF. Single-shot fast spin-echo MR imaging of the fetus: a pictorial essay. *Radiographics* 1999;19:S215–S227.)

Management

When detected before viability, termination of pregnancy can be offered. After viability, standard prenatal care is not altered.

Recurrence Risk

WWS is an autosomal recessive disorder. The recurrence risk for couples with previously affected children is 25%.

CHROMOSOMAL SYNDROMES

▶ DOWN SYNDROME (TRISOMY 21)

The characteristic clinical features of trisomy 21 were first described in 1866 by John Langdon Down,[462] well before the corresponding chromosome abnormality was discovered in 1959.[463]

Incidence

Down syndrome occurs in 1 in 504 pregnancies during the second trimester in the United States.[464] The prevalence varies significantly with maternal age.[465] It may also increase slightly with paternal age.[466]

Genetic Defect

Trisomy 21 is caused by triplicate state (trisomy) of all or a critical portion of chromosome 21. The critical zone for producing phenotypic features of Down syndrome appears to be 21q22.3. Most individuals (95%) with trisomy 21 have three copies of chromosome 21, and the remainder has mosaicism or a robertsonian translocation, most involving chromosome 14 or 21.

Pathologic and Clinical Features

Pathologic and clinical features of Down syndrome are summarized in Table 25. Clinical features during the neonatal period are often absent or poorly developed compared to the adult.[467,468] Hall[467] identified ten major clinical features of Down syndrome from a group of 48 newborns. Characteristic craniofacial features include brachycephaly; a relatively flat occiput and mild microcephaly; flat, small nose; low nasal bridge; protruding tongue; epicanthal folds; small, low-set ears that show overfolding of the upper helix; and excess skin on the back of a rather short neck. The hands are short and broad. The midphalanx of the fifth finger is hypoplastic and curved inward (clinodactyly) in 60% of cases. A single palmar crease is present in 30% of cases. There may be a wide gap between the first and second toes.

TABLE 25. PATHOLOGIC AND CLINICAL FEATURES OF TRISOMY 21

Growth
  Short stature
  Hypotonia
Central nervous system/neurologic
  Mental retardation
  Alzheimer's disease
  Conductive hearing loss
  Mild ventricular dilatation/hydrocephalus
  Shortened frontal lobes
Craniofacial
  Brachycephaly
  Flat, small nose
  Low nasal bridge
  Protruding tongue
  Epicanthal folds
  Small, low-set ears
  Short neck
  Upward-slanting palpebral fissures
  Nuchal thickening/increased nuchal translucency/cystic hygroma
Skeletal
  Hypoplastic, outward-flaring iliac wings
  Shallow acetabulum
  Atlantoaxial instability
  Short digits
  Short, broad hands
  Fifth-finger midphalanx hypoplasia (clinodactyly)
  Single transverse palmar (simian) crease
  Joint hypermobility
  "Sandal gap" between first and second toes
Cardiac
  Ventricular septal defect
  Endocardial cushion defect (atrioventricular septal defect)
  Mineralization of papillary muscle (echogenic intracardiac focus)
Gastrointestinal
  Duodenal stenosis/atresia
  Imperforate anus
  Hirschsprung disease
  Omphalocele
Endocrine: hypothyroidism
Hematologic: leukemoid reactions
Neoplasia
  Leukemia (acute lymphoblastic leukemia and acute myelogenous leukemia)
  Acute megakaryocytic leukemia

Reproduced with permission from McKusick VA, ed. Online mendelian inheritance in man. Available at: http://www.ncbi.nlm.nih.gov/omim/. McKusick-Nathans Institute for Genetic Medicine, Johns Hopkins University (Baltimore, MD) and National Center for Biotechnology Information, National Library of Medicine (Bethesda, MD), 2000.

The pelvis is hypoplastic with outward-flaring iliac wings and shallow acetabular angle ("elephant ear" shaped). Cardiac anomalies, primarily VSDs and endocardial cushion defects, are present in approximately 25% of infants with trisomy 21. A similar frequency has been found in fetal specimens.[469] Gastrointestinal anomalies include duodenal atresia or stenosis (8%) and tracheoesophageal fistula.

Morphologic features of trisomy 21 in fetuses are even less developed than in neonates and have been studied infrequently. Stephens and Shepard[470] examined 13 fetuses with trisomy 21 who were aborted during the second trimester and found few consistent features. The most common findings were a simian crease, clinodactyly (91%), and a cleft between the first and second toes. In another group of 26 fetuses with trisomy 21 who underwent autopsy, Keeling[469] reported the following anomalies: transverse palmar crease (65%), low-set ears (54%), VSD or AVSD (19%), short digits (8%), hydrops fetalis (8%), duodenal atresia (8%), and hydrocephalus (4%).

Diagnosis

A variety of sonographic findings may be seen in fetuses with trisomy 21 (Figs. 34 and 35). These can be considered as two types, structural or major anomalies and nonstructural markers. Structural or major anomalies include cardiac defects, nonimmune hydrops, hydrothorax, omphalocele, and (rarely before 20 weeks) duodenal atresia. Structural anomalies were detected by sonography in 16% to 17% of fetuses with trisomy 21 in two different prenatal series before 20 weeks.[471,472] Studies that do not omit patients referred for an abnormal ultrasound will show a higher rate of major abnormalities.

Higher detection rates of cardiac defects are expected at a later gestational age when the heart can be better visualized. Scanning at an optimal gestational age (24 weeks), under optimal conditions (dedicated fetal echocardiographic center), with inclusion of subtle VSDs and prior knowledge of the fetal karyotype, Paladini et al.[473] were able to detect heart defects in just over half of fetuses with Down syndrome. Using nonspecific cardiac findings, such as right-left disproportion, pericardial effusion, and tricuspid regurgitation, DeVore[474] reported cardiac findings in 76% of fetuses with trisomy 21, but just 9% showed an AVSD. The mean gestational age for ultrasound in that study was 18 weeks.

Although structural abnormalities are observed in the minority of cases of trisomy 21 before 20 weeks, a number of nonspecific markers of fetal Down syndrome have been described.[471,475–480] The most common sonographic markers evaluated include nuchal thickening, shortened limbs, hyperechoic bowel, and pyelectasis, because they can be easily sought during the course of a routine second-trimester sonogram (Figs. 34 and 35). Other potential markers include widened pelvic angle, shortened frontal lobes,[481,482] small ears, clinodactyly,[483] small or absent nasal bone,[484] pericardial effusion, and right-left disproportion of the heart. Another potential marker for trisomy 21, although not related to fetal anatomy, is unfused amnion and chorion after 14 weeks. The frequency of sonographic markers and associated risks are discussed in detail in Chapter 21.

Prognosis

The mean survival age is now 20 years. Early mortality rate reflects the severity of anomalies, especially cardiac malformations. Mental retardation is invariably present in adults,

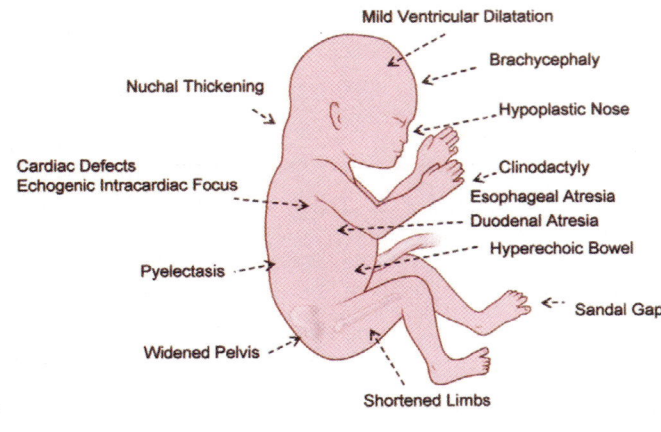

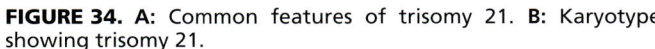

A

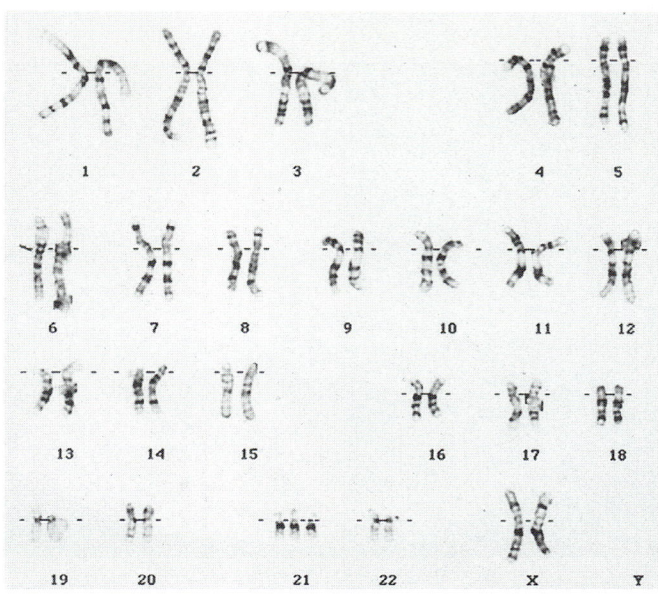

B

FIGURE 34. A: Common features of trisomy 21. **B:** Karyotype showing trisomy 21.

with a mean IQ of 50 to 60. The association with acute leukemia is 20-fold higher than normal.[485,486] Other medical problems include congestive heart failure, frequent respiratory infections, strabismus (20%), cataract formation, and premature aging. Ninety percent of all Down syndrome patients have a significant hearing loss, usually of the conductive type. Patients with Down syndrome also develop premature onset of Alzheimer's disease.

Management

For ongoing pregnancies, fetal echocardiography should be performed to exclude a major cardiac defect. Pregnancies should also be monitored during the third trimester for development of IUGR. After birth, immediate concerns are the presence and severity of cardiac or other major anomalies.

Recurrence Risk

The risk of recurrence is approximately 1.00%.

▶ EDWARDS SYNDROME (TRISOMY 18)

Also known as *trisomy E*, Edwards syndrome is a multiple malformation syndrome with a trisomy for all or a large part of chromosome 18.

Incidence

Edwards syndrome occurs in 1 in 3,000 to 6,000 births. Because intrauterine demise or stillbirth is common, the incidence varies with gestational age. It is estimated that 50% to 90% of fetuses alive at 16 weeks do not survive to live birth.[487] Males experience a higher mortality rate both during pregnancy and after birth, leading to a female-male preponderance among newborns. Like other major autosomal disorders, trisomy 18 is positively correlated with maternal age, although there also are a large number of age-independent cases.

Genetic Defect

Approximately 80% of the patients show typical trisomy for chromosome 18, another 10% are mosaics, and the remainder is either double trisomics for another chromosome or have a translocation. Pericentric inversion in chromosome 18 has been described to recombine during meiosis and cause unbalanced offspring phenotypically similar to those fetuses with trisomy.[487,488]

Pathologic and Clinical Features

Pathologic and clinical features of trisomy 18 are summarized in Table 26. Characteristic clinical findings of trisomy 18 include IUGR, loose skin, hypoplasia of skeletal muscle, and diminished fetal activity.[489,490] The head is dolichocephalic with a prominent occiput. Facial features include a small mouth, micrognathia, and low, pointed "pixie" ears. Cleft lip/palate is much less common (15%) than with trisomy 13. The hands often are clenched with overlapping fingers, most frequently with the index finger overlapping the middle finger and the fifth finger curving inward. Cardiovascular malformations, present in approximately 90% of cases, include VSD, ASD, double-outlet right ventricle, and bicuspid aortic and pulmonic valves.[469] The placenta is small, and a single umbilical artery is present in greater than 50% of cases.

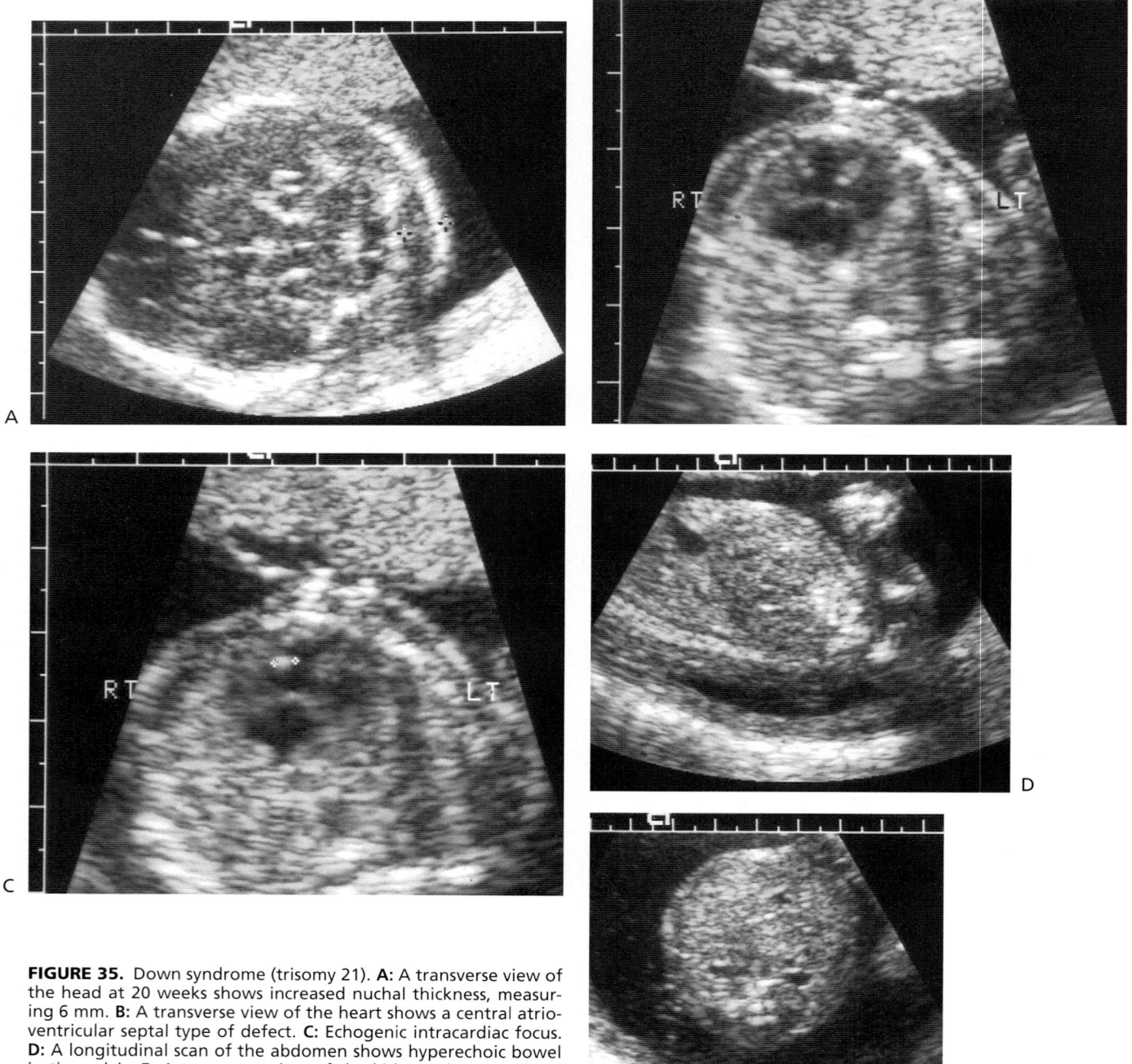

FIGURE 35. Down syndrome (trisomy 21). **A:** A transverse view of the head at 20 weeks shows increased nuchal thickness, measuring 6 mm. **B:** A transverse view of the heart shows a central atrioventricular septal type of defect. **C:** Echogenic intracardiac focus. **D:** A longitudinal scan of the abdomen shows hyperechoic bowel in the pelvis. **E:** A transverse view of the kidneys shows minimal pyelectasis, measuring 3.0 to 3.5 mm. LT, left; RT, right.

In addition to the common malformations noted above, more than 100 different abnormalities involving virtually every organ system have been noted in conjunction with trisomy 18.[4] These include diaphragmatic and inguinal hernias, omphalocele, umbilical hernia, genitourinary anomalies (hydronephrosis, hydroureter, bladder outlet obstruction, horseshoe kidney, and duplication abnormalities), and anomalies of the gastrointestinal tract (tracheoesophageal fistula, anorectal atresia). CNS anomalies may include hydrocephalus, cerebellar hypoplasia, agenesis of the corpus callosum, and spina bifida.[491] Limb reduction abnormalities have been noted in 16% of cases, equally divided between lower and upper extremities.[492] Other skeletal problems include prominent heels, rockerbottom feet, arthrogryposis, and short sternum.

The most common structural findings at postmortem examination in a series of 31 fetuses with trisomy 18 were congenital heart defects (87%), skeletal anomalies (39%),

TABLE 26. PATHOLOGIC AND CLINICAL FEATURES OF TRISOMY 18

Growth: growth delay
Craniofacial
  Micrognathia
  Low-set ears
  Microphthalmos
  Small, low-set ears
  Nuchal thickening/increased nuchal translucency/cystic hygroma
  Cleft lip/palate (rare)
Central nervous system/neurologic
  Profound mental retardation
  Brachycephaly (strawberry-shaped head)
  Choroid plexus cysts (second trimester)
  Myelomeningocele
  Cerebellar anomalies
  Mild ventricular dilatation
Skeletal
  Clenched hands, wrists
  Overlapping fingers
  Radial aplasia
  Clubfoot, rockerbottom feet
  Arthrogryposis
  Hemivertebrae
Cardiovascular
  Cardiac defects
  Polyvalvular dysplasia
  Left superior vena cava
  Single umbilical artery
  Umbilical cord cysts
Thoracic
  Diaphragmatic hernia
  Pulmonary hypoplasia
Genitourinary: genital abnormalities
Gastrointestinal
  Omphalocele
  Umbilical hernia
  Tracheoesophageal fistula
  Malrotation of intestine
  Meckel diverticulum
  Absent gallbladder

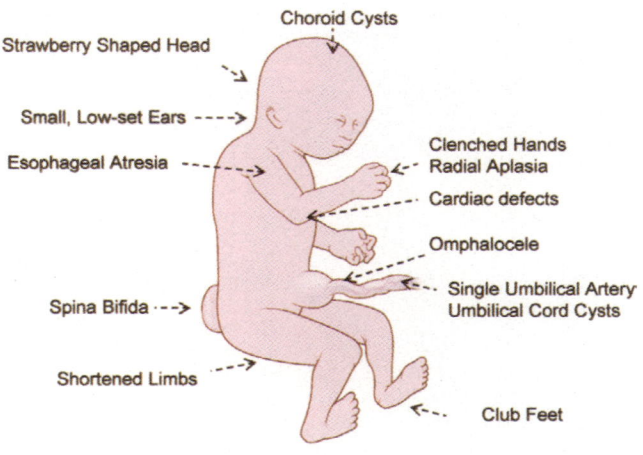

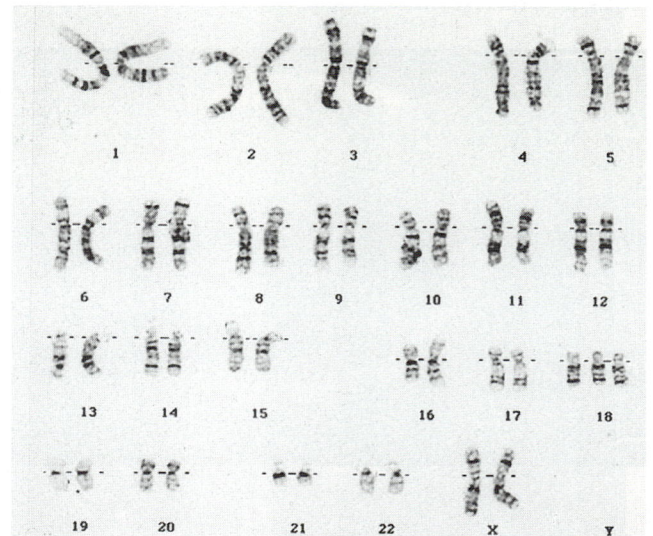

FIGURE 36. Trisomy 18. **A:** Common features. **B:** Karyotype showing trisomy 18.

urinary tract anomalies (35%), CNS anomalies (32%), and omphalocele (10%).[493]

Diagnosis

Ultrasound

The diversity of prenatal sonographic findings reported with trisomy 18 reflects the pathologic findings (Fig. 36). Some fetuses with trisomy 18 show no abnormalities or only subtle findings (Fig. 37), whereas others show multiple anomalies (Figs. 38 and 39). Also, no one feature dominates the phenotypic expression of trisomy 18[494–497] (Table 27).

Symmetric IUGR, often in association with polyhydramnios or oligohydramnios, may be the initial clue to the presence of trisomy 18, especially during the third trimester. Major anomalies may include cystic hygroma, nonimmune hydrops, hydrocephalus, spina bifida, diaphragmatic hernia, tracheoesophageal fistula, genitourinary anomalies, cardiovascular malformations, omphalocele, clubfoot, short extremities, and clenched hands, often with overlapping fingers. Subtle or nonstructural findings of trisomy 18 may include choroid plexus cysts, brachycephaly or strawberry-shaped head,[498] and single umbilical artery. Of these, choroid plexus cysts have been the most controversial and the subject of considerable interest (see section on Choroid Plexus Cysts in Chapter 21). Flexion abnormalities of the hands may be subtle and or unilateral and may develop with increasing gestational age.

A number of studies have reported the sensitivity of ultrasound for detection of trisomy 18.[494–496,499] Results from four studies are summarized in Table 27. Abnormalities have been detected in approximately 80% of fetuses

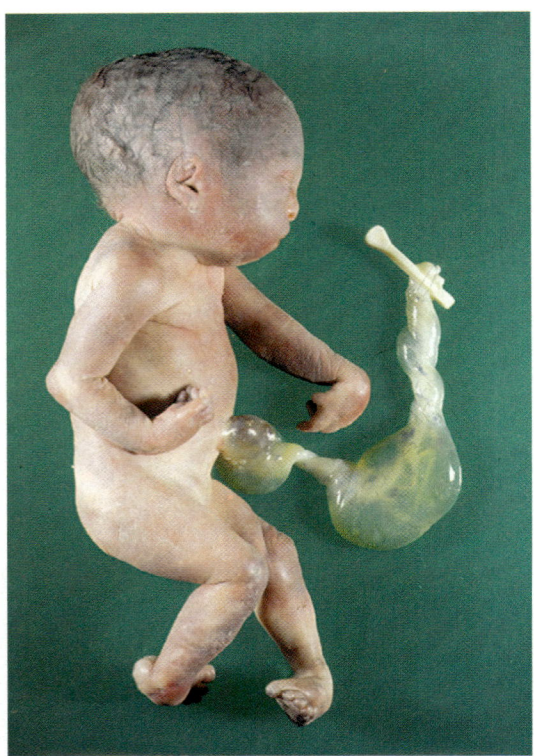

FIGURE 39. Trisomy 18. A postmortem photograph shows multiple anomalies, including flexed hands and wrists, clubfeet, brachycephaly, omphalocele, and umbilical cord pseudocyst, all of which were detected by prenatal ultrasound. A cardiac defect was also present and identified prenatally. (Courtesy of Raj Kapur, Pathology Department, Children's Hospital, Seattle, WA.)

ultrasound, of which the most common isolated finding was choroid plexus cyst. Eleven fetuses (37%) had positive biochemistry screen for trisomy 18, and two others had positive biochemistry screen for Down syndrome. Combining the two testing methods yielded the highest detection rate (80%).

It is clear that a careful search must be made of fetuses considered at risk for trisomy 18. Markers that are otherwise considered nonspecific, such as growth delay or choroid cysts, assume a much greater importance in this clinical setting. Awareness of the type of anomalies and the usual menstrual age of diagnosis in fetuses with trisomy 18 should improve patient counseling and prenatal detection of fetuses considered at risk for this disorder.

Differential Diagnosis

Other possibilities that should be considered include other chromosome abnormalities (trisomy 13 and triploidy) and multiple anomaly syndromes. Pena-Shokeir syndrome should be included in the differential diagnosis when the extremities are affected.

Prognosis

The prognosis of fetuses with trisomy 18 is uniformly poor. Approximately two-thirds of fetuses with an *in utero* diagnosis of trisomy 18 die before delivery. Intrauterine demise or stillbirth is common; it is estimated that 50% to 90% of fetuses alive at 16 weeks do not survive to live birth.[487] Males experience a higher mortality rate both during pregnancy and after birth.

Many undiagnosed cases are delivered prematurely and by cesarean section. The median survival for infants born with trisomy 18 is 5 days, with a mean of 48 days.[504] Only 5% to 6% of live-born trisomy 18 infants survive to the first year of life.[4] Survivors are profoundly mentally retarded.

TABLE 27. PREVALENCE (AS A PERCENTAGE OF ALL CASES) OF SOME OF THE COMMON PRENATAL ULTRASOUND FINDINGS IN FOUR STUDIES OF FETUSES WITH TRISOMY 18 IN THE SECOND TRIMESTER (14–24 WEEKS OF GESTATION)

Finding	Nyberg et al.[496]	Shields et al.[494]	DeVore[495]	Brumfield et al.[497]	Combined data[a]
Fetuses (N)	29	35	30	30	**124**
Intrauterine growth restriction	28%	29%	—	10%	22%
Polyhydramnios	3%	9%	3%	7%	6%
Choroid plexus cysts	38%	43%	53%	30%	41%
Nuchal translucency/cystic hygroma	31%	17%	17%	13%	19%
Clenched hands	17%	46%	3%	10%	20%
Abnormal feet	21%	—	—	—	21%
Abdominal wall defect	17%	14%	—	10%	14%
Cardiac defect	14%	37%	80%	13%	30%
Myelomeningocele	14%	9%	—	—	11%
Strawberry-shaped head	14%	34%	—	3%	18%
Posterior fossa abnormality	3%	3%	—	—	3%
Cleft lip/palate	3%	—	3%	—	3%
Urinary tract anomalies	17%	9%	—	7%	11%
Single umbilical artery	10%	40%	7%	3%	16%
≥1 ultrasound finding	72%	86%	97%	70%	82%

[a]Combined data consider only those studies reporting that feature.

Common neonatal problems include feeding difficulties, poor sucking reflex, hypotonia, and failure to thrive.

Management

When ultrasound findings are consistent with trisomy 18, prenatal karyotyping should be undertaken. Pregnancy termination should be considered. Tocolysis for preterm labor and cesarean section should be avoided.

Recurrence Risk

For trisomy 18, the recurrence risk is lower than the 1% for trisomy 21 syndrome. A carrier of pericentric inversion in chromosome 18 may produce affected offspring in 6% of pregnancies and carrier offspring in 53% of such pregnancies.[487,488] There is little information available about the recurrence risks for trisomy 13 and trisomy 18. An empiric risk of approximately 1% is frequently given to patients.[504a]

▶ TRISOMY 13

Also known as *Patau syndrome*, trisomy 13 and its association with certain congenital malformations were first described by Patau in 1960.[4]

Incidence

The prevalence of trisomy 13 is 1 in 6,000 births, but it accounts for approximately 1% of spontaneous first-trimester miscarriages. A bimodal distribution of maternal ages has been noted with peaks at 25 and 38 years, consistent with age-independent and -dependent subgroups.[505,506]

Genetic Defect

Trisomy for chromosome 13 is the genetic basis.

Pathologic and Clinical Features

Pathologic and clinical features of trisomy 13 are summarized in Table 28. The phenotype of trisomy 13 may be so striking that a diagnosis can often be made on the basis of clinical observations alone. Characteristic physical findings include microcephaly, anophthalmia, or microphthalmos; receding forehead; cleft lip and palate (60% to 70%); flexed and overlapping fingers; and postaxial polydactyly (75%). Limb deficiency may also occur.[507] Malformations of the CNS are among the most common and severe. These include holoprosencephaly, agenesis of the corpus callosum, cerebellar anomalies, and hydrocephalus.[505] However, CNS abnormalities may also be absent or subtle. Cardiovascular malformations are common (greater than 80%) and may include VSD, ASD, patent ductus arteriosus, mitral or aortic atresia, pulmonary stenosis, and anomalous venous return. Genitourinary anoma-

TABLE 28. PATHOLOGIC FEATURES OF TRISOMY 13

Growth: growth delay
Craniofacial
  Cleft lip/palate
  Microcephaly
  Anophthalmia or microphthalmos
  Receding forehead
  Micrognathia
  Capillary hemangioma
  Scalp defects over the parieto-occipital region
  Small, low-set ears
  Nuchal thickening/increased nuchal translucency/cystic hygroma
Central nervous system/neurologic
  Profound mental retardation
  Holoprosencephaly
  Agenesis of the corpus callosum
  Cerebellar anomalies
  Hydrocephalus
  Mild ventricular dilatation
Skeletal
  Polydactyly
  Clubfeet
  Rockerbottom feet
Cardiac
  Cardiac defects
  Mitral or aortic atresia
  Hypoplastic left heart
  Pulmonary stenosis
  Anomalous pulmonary venous return
  Mineralization of papillary muscle (echogenic intracardiac focus)
Genitourinary
  Cystic dysplasia
  Hydronephrosis
  Duplication abnormalities
Gastrointestinal
  Omphalocele
  Umbilical hernia
  "Dinosaur" appendix with multiple diverticula[a]
Umbilical: single umbilical artery

[a]Favara BE. Multiple congenital diverticula of the vermiform appendix. *Am J Clin Pathol* 1968;49:60–64.

lies include renal cystic dysplasia, hydronephrosis, and duplication abnormalities. Omphalocele or umbilical hernia is found in nearly one-third of cases. The calcaneus is often prominent, and the feet may be rockerbottom or clubbed. Other features of trisomy 13 that are not normally detected on sonograms include colobomas, capillary hemangioma of the forehead, and localized scalp defects over the parieto-occipital region.

Diagnosis

Ultrasound

Because of the severity of malformations usually present, the sensitivity of sonography for detecting trisomy 13 is high, with most studies reporting sensitivity greater than 90%[508–511] (Table 29). However, this is not a uniform experience, even in recent studies, and anomalies can be readily missed among low-risk patients unless a systematic survey is routinely performed.[510]

TABLE 29. PREVALENCE (AS A PERCENTAGE OF ALL CASES) OF SOME OF THE COMMON PRENATAL ULTRASOUND FINDINGS IN FOUR STUDIES OF FETUSES WITH TRISOMY 13

Finding	Nicolaides et al.[509]	Lehman et al.[508]		De Vigan et al.[510]	Tongsong et al.[511]	Combined data[a]
Fetuses (*N*)	31	18	15	85	15	**164**
Gestational age (wk)	15–44	12–20	20–32	All ages	16–22	—
Holoprosencephaly	35%	22%	60%	18%	47%	**28%**
Hypotelorism/cyclopia	—	28%	47%	—	40%	**40%**
Proboscis	—	—	—	—	27%	**27%**
Facial cleft	48%	17%	60%	18%	33%	**29%**
Abnormal extremities	68%	17%	53%	—	40%	**48%**
Cardiac defect	45%	44%	53%	20%	33%	**32%**
Urinary tract anomalies	65%	22%	47%	14%	27%	**29%**
Ventriculomegaly	10%	11%	7%	3%	20%	**7%**
Abdominal wall defect	23%	17%	13%	3%	13%	**6%**
Abnormal posterior fossa	19%	11%	20%	—	7%	**14%**
Intrauterine growth restriction	48%	22%	80%	—	27%	**44%**
Echogenic intracardiac foci	—	39%	20%	—	20%	**27%**
Nuchal translucency/cystic hygroma	23%	33%	7%	11%	7%	**15%**
Hyperechoic bowel	—	11%	0%	—	—	**6%**
Single umbilical artery	—	6%	47%	—	13%	**21%**
≥1 structural abnormality	100%	91%	91%	68%	93%	**81%**

[a]Combined data consider only those studies reporting that feature.

A number of characteristic features of trisomy 13 may be seen by ultrasound (Figs. 40 through 42). In a review of 36 cases of trisomy 13, Lehman et al.[508] reported one or more abnormalities in 91%. Major anomalies detected by ultrasound included holoprosencephaly (39%) or other CNS anomalies (58%), facial anomalies (48%), and renal (33%) and cardiac (48%) defects. IUGR was also present in 48%. Echogenic intracardiac foci were observed in 30%, including 39% of those examined before 20 weeks. Other findings included a large cisterna magna (18%), mild cerebral ventricular dilatation (9%), nuchal thickening or cystic hygroma (21%), and hypoplastic left heart (21%). The combination of echogenic intracardiac foci and small left ventricle is highly suggestive of trisomy 13 (Fig. 42C). Echogenic intracardiac foci may be the initial sonographic finding and rarely may be the only sonographic manifestation of trisomy 13.

Laboratory

Maternal serum screening does not appear to be of benefit in detection of trisomy 13.

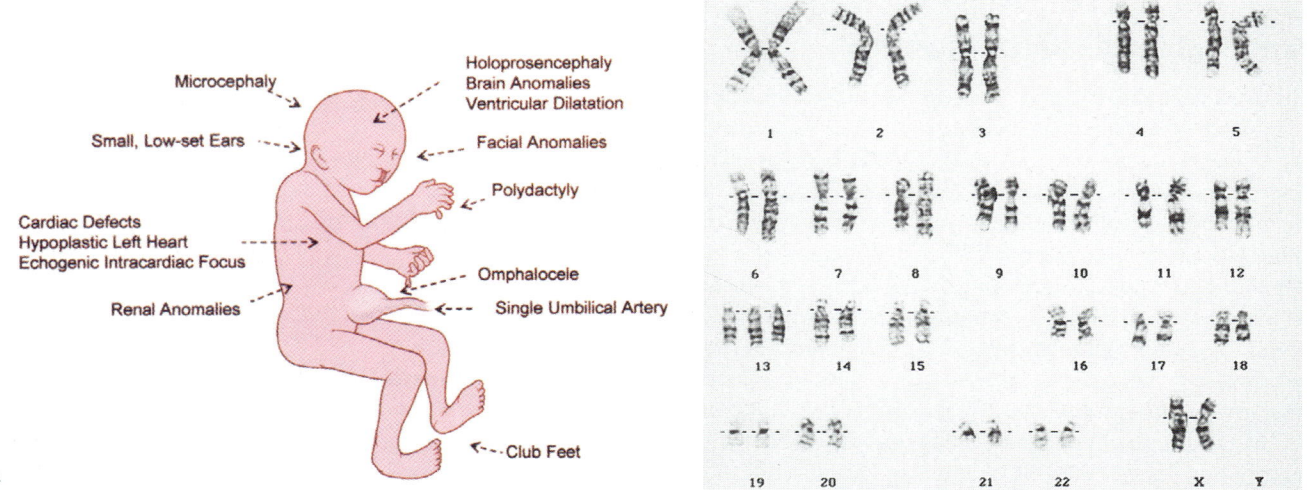

FIGURE 40. Trisomy 13. **A:** Common features. **B:** Karyotype showing trisomy 13.

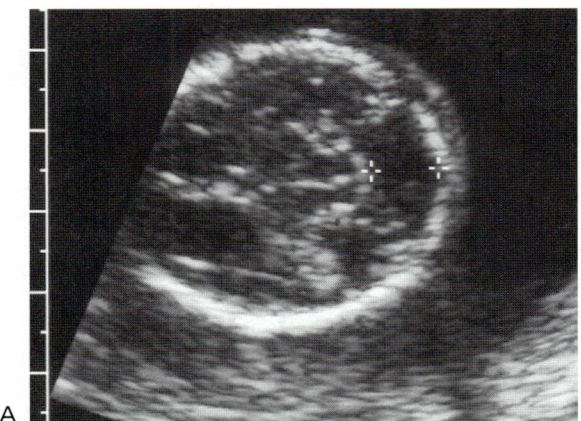
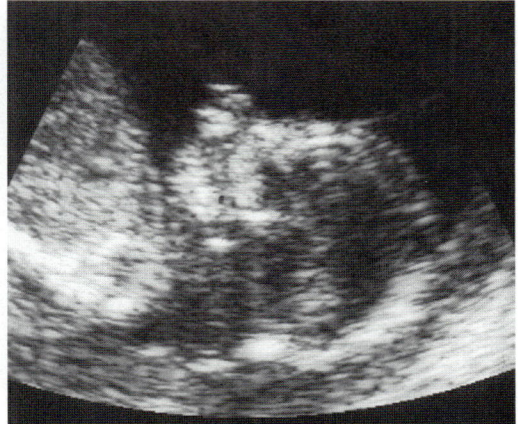

FIGURE 41. Trisomy 13. **A:** An axial view of the brain at 16 weeks shows an abnormal posterior fossa with absent vermis and visible cerebellum at this level. The cisterna magna is in direct contact with the midbrain. **B:** A facial profile shows an echogenic mass protruding beneath the nose, representing premaxillary protrusion of bilateral cleft lip and palate. **C:** A transverse view of the heart shows the markedly hypoplastic left atrium and ventricle and an echogenic intracardiac focus in the right ventricle. RT, right.

Differential Diagnosis

Certain sonographic findings of trisomy 13 are also found in the Meckel-Gruber syndrome, an autosomal recessive disorder characterized by cystic kidneys and one or more findings of polydactyly and a midline CNS malformation (occipital encephalocele, holoprosencephaly, or Dandy-Walker malformation).

Prognosis

The prognosis for infants with trisomy 13 is extremely poor. Approximately one-half die within the first month, 75% die by 6 months, and less than 5% survive more than 3 years. The mean survival for live-born infants is 130 days. Death usually occurs within the first month of life; long-term survivors rarely have been reported.[512] Common neonatal problems include hypotonia or hypertonia, seizures, apnea, feeding difficulties, and failure to thrive.

Management

Termination of pregnancy can be offered at any time because of the extremely poor prognosis and high natural mortality rate.

Recurrence Risk

There is little information available about the recurrence risks for trisomy 13 and trisomy 18. An empiric risk of approximately 1% is frequently given to patients.[504a]

▶ TURNER SYNDROME (45,X)

In 1938, Turner described a chromosomal disorder of female patients.[513] However, the syndrome was actually described by Ullrich 8 years earlier and was shown to be secondary to 45,X chromosome aberration in 1959.[514,515] Hence, it is also known as *Ullrich-Turner syndrome* or *monosomy X*. Wiedemann and Glatzl[515] studied Ullrich's original patient with Ullrich-Turner syndrome in 1987 when the patient was 66 years old and confirmed a 45,X karyotype.

Incidence

Turner syndrome (45,X) occurs in 1 in 2,500 to 5,000 live female births but as many as 9% of first-trimester abortuses. Advanced maternal age is not associated with this aneuploidy.

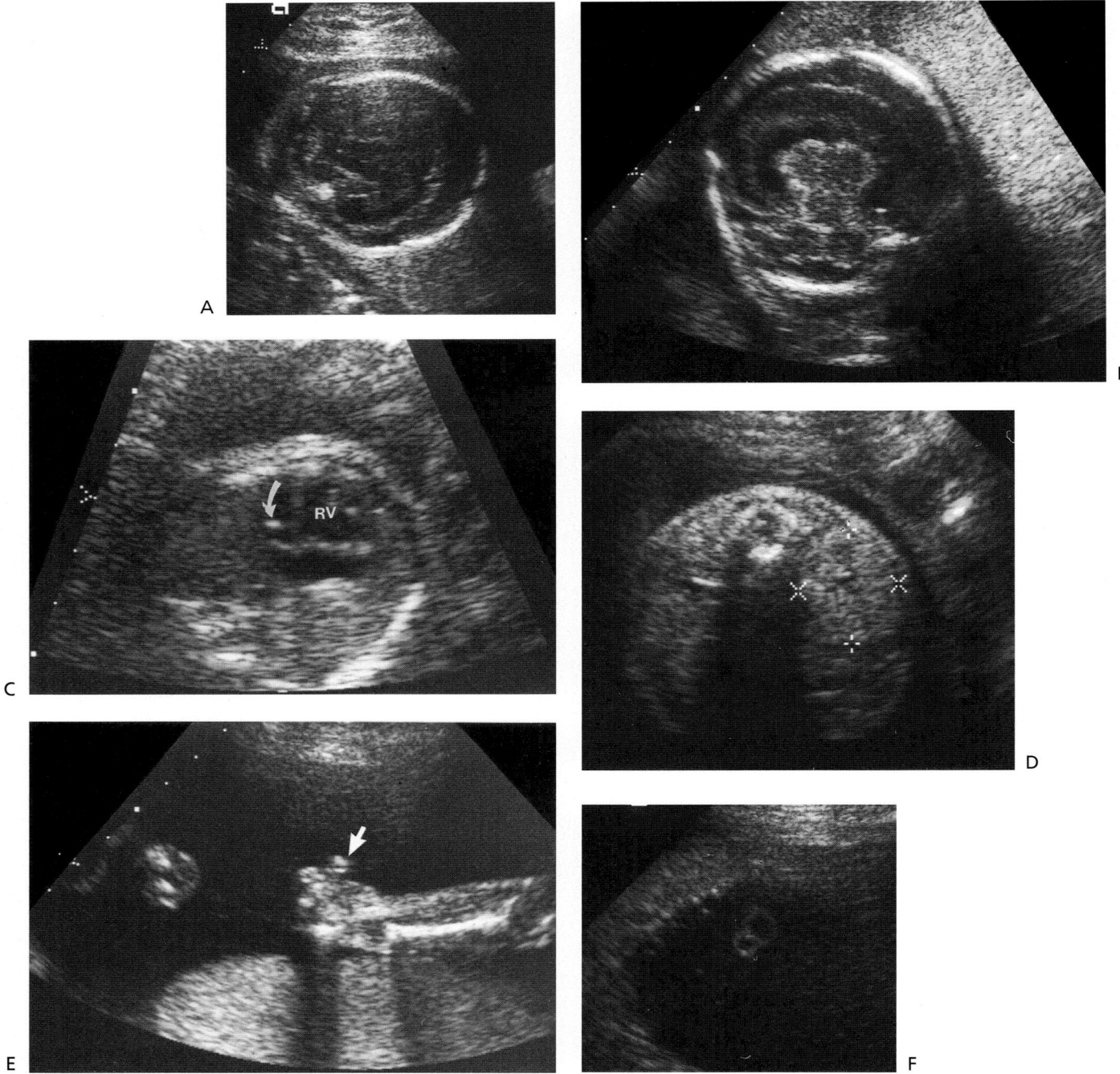

FIGURE 42. Trisomy 13. **A:** An axial view of the head shows an abnormal configuration of normal landmarks, suggesting monoventricle. **B:** A coronal view with transvaginal scanning confirms monoventricle and fused thalami, indicating alobar holoprosencenphaly. Midline cleft lip and palate were also seen. **C:** A transverse view of the heart shows the hypoplastic left atrium and ventricle and an echogenic intracardiac focus in the left ventricle (*arrow*). RV, right ventricle. **D:** Echogenic, enlarged kidneys are seen on a transverse plane. **E:** A view of the hand shows abnormal posturing with polydactyly (*arrow*). **F:** A single umbilical artery is seen as a two-vessel umbilical cord in cross section.

TABLE 30. PATHOLOGIC FEATURES OF TURNER SYNDROME

Lymphatic
  Cystic hygroma
  Lymphedema
  Hydrops
Growth
  Short stature
  Failure to thrive
Craniofacial
  Short neck
  Webbed neck
  Cystic hygroma
  Abnormal ears
  Narrow maxilla (palate)
  Small mandible
  Ptosis
Cardiac
  Cardiac defects
  Bicuspid aortic valve
  Coarctation of aorta
Skeletal
  Cubitus valgus
  Short fourth metacarpal/metatarsal
  Short limbs
Chest
  Broad chest
  Widely spaced nipples
Genitourinary
  Horseshoe kidney
  Ovarian dysgenesis

Reproduced with permission from McKusick VA, ed. Online mendelian inheritance in man. Available at: http://www.ncbi.nlm.nih.gov/omim/. McKusick-Nathans Institute for Genetic Medicine, Johns Hopkins University (Baltimore, MD) and National Center for Biotechnology Information, National Library of Medicine (Bethesda, MD), 2000.

Genetic Defect

Turner syndrome is due to absence of one sex chromosome, usually the paternal chromosome. Mosaic 45,X is found in 8% to 16% of cases. Structural abnormalities of the sex chromosomes can also result in Turner syndrome.[516,517]

Pathologic and Clinical Features

Pathologic and clinical features of Turner syndrome are summarized in Table 30. The most characteristic congenital malformation associated with Turner syndrome is cystic hygroma (Figs. 43 and 44). However, this anomaly is not specific for Turner syndrome and can be associated with other chromosome abnormalities as well as a normal karyotype. Other common abnormalities include nonimmune hydrops and cardiovascular malformations (25%), including coarctation of the aorta. Genitourinary anomalies may include ovarian dysgenesis, horseshoe kidney, hydronephrosis, renal agenesis, and renal hypoplasia.

Diagnosis

During the second trimester, Turner syndrome may show the typical appearance of cystic hygroma, usually with internal septation.[518–522] Other sonographic findings that have been reported with Turner syndrome include hydrothorax and nonimmune hydrops.

Saller et al.[523] reported that both hydropic and nonhydropic cases were associated with markedly decreased levels of estriol and slightly reduced levels of AFP. Human chorionic gonadotropin and inhibin levels are also elevated with hydrops but low in the absence of hydrops. Using the quadruple screen, Wenstrom et al.[524] reported detection of nine of 17 (53%) fetuses with Turner syndrome, 10 of 17

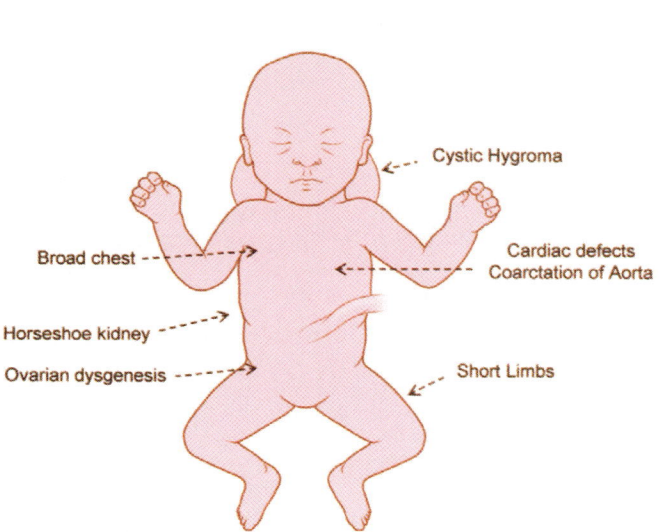

A

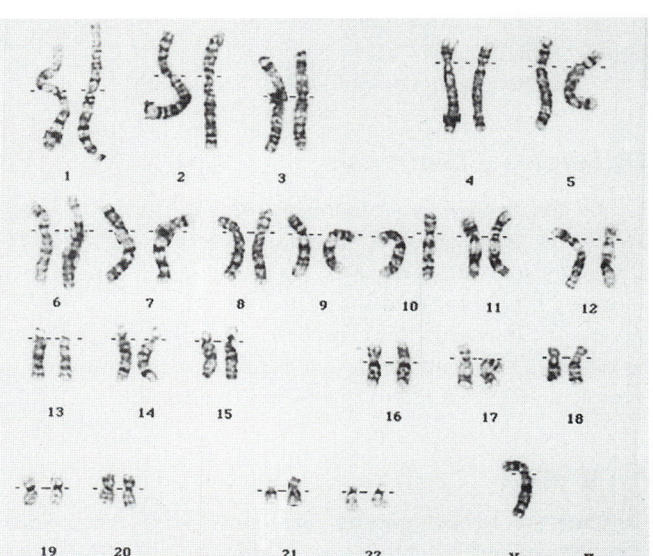

B

FIGURE 43. Turner syndrome (45,X). **A:** Common features. **B:** Karyotype showing 45,X.

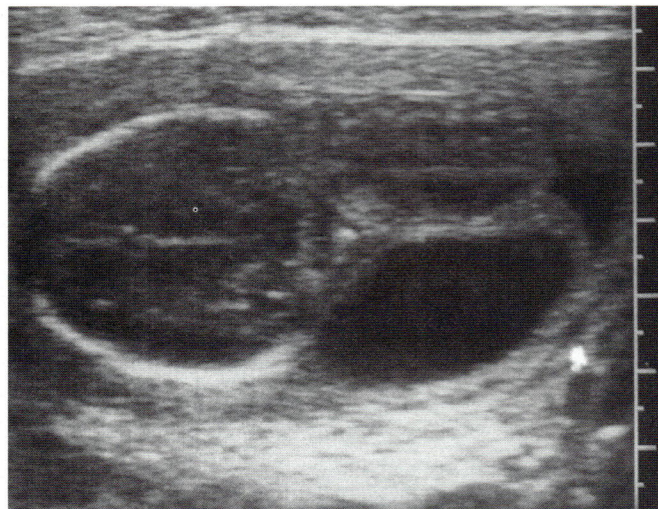

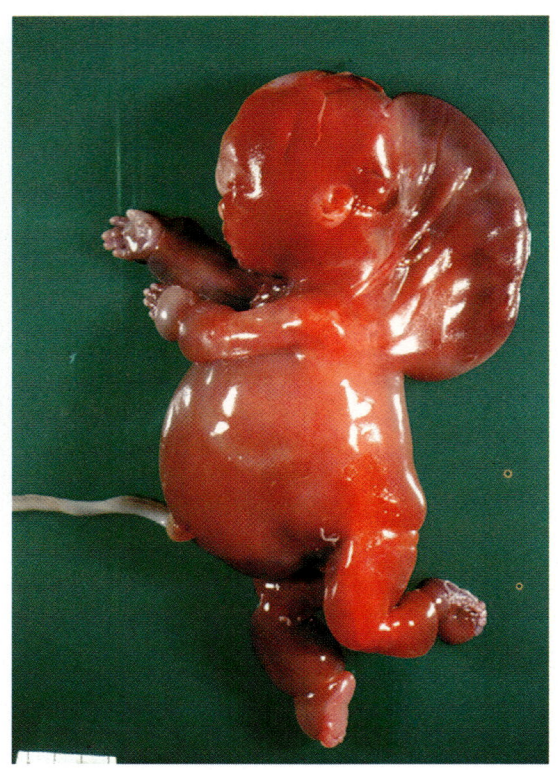

FIGURE 44. Turner syndrome. **A:** A large cystic hygroma with septations is identified. **B:** A postmortem photograph of another infant with Turner syndrome shows a large cystic hygroma.

(59%) with other sex chromosome aneuploidies, and one case of trisomy 22. Sex chromosome abnormalities may also be detected on the basis of elevated AFP.[525]

During the first trimester, Turner syndrome may show cystic hygroma or increased nuchal translucency. Using a combined first-trimester protocol of nuchal translucency, pregnancy-associated plasma protein A, free beta–human chorionic gonadotropin, and maternal age, Spencer et al.[526] estimated that 96% of fetuses with Turner syndrome and 62% of fetuses with other sex chromosomal anomalies could be identified.

Definitive diagnosis requires fetal karyotype.

Differential Diagnosis

Cystic hygroma may occasionally be present in Roberts syndrome and other autosomal recessive disorders.[522] Chromosomal analysis can exclude these conditions. Noonan syndrome shows features similar to Turner syndrome but the karyotype is normal and may occur in males or females. This is an autosomal dominant condition with a genetic defect localized to 12q24 in some families.

Prognosis

Turner syndrome accounts for one-fourth of the spontaneous abortions caused by chromosomal anomalies.[527] Intrauterine demise occurs in many cases, generally caused by hydrops, which is the major intrauterine complication. Cystic hygroma/

nuchal translucency typically resolves among fetuses who survive to term.[528] Among survivors, the prognosis usually varies with the severity of the associated anomalies. Mosaics tend to have a better prognosis, and in some cases the syndrome remains undiagnosed for years.[529] Early development is usually normal, although delays in motor skills are common.

If a fetus with Turner syndrome survives to a live birth, the long-term survival rate is good. Turner syndrome in adults is characterized by sexual infantilism, primary amenorrhea, webbed neck, and cubitus valgus. The verbal IQ usually is normal, but the motor IQ is lower than average. A distinctive difficulty with spatial relationships is present. Hearing loss is present in approximately 50% of cases.

Management

A karyotype is recommended when Turner syndrome is suspected. Termination of pregnancy can be offered before viability.

Recurrence Risk

Risk of recurrence is low.

▶ TRIPLOIDY AND TETRAPLOIDY

Triploidy is the presence of a complete extra set of chromosomes (for a total of 69). *Tetraploidy* refers to two extra sets of chromosomes (for a total of 92).

Incidence

Triploidy may be the most common chromosome abnormality, occurring in as many as 1% of all conceptions and 25% of chromosomally abnormal first-trimester miscarriages.[530,531] However, spontaneous demise occurs in the vast majority of cases, predominantly in the first trimester. The frequency of triploidy is greatly reduced by the time of delivery, when it is present in only 1 in 2,500 births. Unlike trisomies, the rate of triploidy does not increase with maternal age and may even decrease.

Tetraploidy is less common than triploidy, and most cases result in first-trimester spontaneous miscarriage. Among spontaneous abortions, the ratio of tetraploidy to triploidy was approximately 1 to 3. The live birth of apparently nonmosaic tetraploid infants has been reported in rare cases.[532,533]

Genetic Defect

Among abortuses, approximately 60% are 69,XXY, 37% are 69,XXX, and only 3% are XYY.[515] Those with 69,XYY manifest the least embryonic development. The extra set of chromosomes of triploidy may be either maternal in origin (digyny) or paternal (diandry). Maternally derived triploidy results from errors in meiosis with fertilization of a diploid oocyte. Paternally derived triploidy may result from fertilization of a haploid oocyte by a diploid sperm or, more commonly, by fertilization of a haploid oocyte by two haploid sperm. More complex mechanisms have also been proposed and are almost certainly at work in some cases.

Neuber et al.[530] reported a decrease in the rate of polyploidies with increasing maternal age and a reversal of the XXY-to-XXX ratio from 2 to 1 in younger mothers to 1 to 2 in older mothers. This suggests that digyny may be more common with increasing maternal age, whereas diandry is less common.[534]

There has been disagreement over whether triploidy is most commonly diandry or digyny in origin. Although earlier cytologic studies reported that the majority of cases were diandry,[535,536] this appears to reflect the gestational age at time of ascertainment. Because fetuses with triploidy of paternal origin are more likely to abort during early pregnancy, a maternal origin of triploidy may be more common by the time of sonographic diagnosis.[534,537,538] Hence, different studies may report disparate results depending on gestational age and degree of embryonic development.

Pathologic and Clinical Features

Pathologic and clinical features of triploidy are summarized in Table 31. The parental origin of the extra set of chromosomes affects the pathologic findings of triploidy. Hence, triploidy can be categorized into two distinct phenotypes depending on the parental origin (Table 32), although some exceptions invariably occur. This is an example of

TABLE 31. TYPICAL PATHOLOGIC AND CLINICAL FEATURES OF TRIPLOIDY

Growth
   Severe growth delay
   Head-abdomen discordance with small abdominal circumference
   Hypotonia
Craniofacial
   Microphthalmos
   Hypertelorism
   Colobomas
   Facial asymmetry
   Low-set, malformed ears
   Cleft lip/palate
   Micrognathia
   Nuchal thickening/increased nuchal translucency/cystic hygroma
Central nervous system
   Holoprosencephaly
   Hydrocephalus
   Agenesis of the corpus callosum
   Myelomeningocele
Skeletal
   Syndactyly, especially third and fourth digits
   Clubfeet
Cardiac: cardiac defects
Gastrointestinal
   Omphalocele
   Umbilical hernia
Genitourinary
   Cystic dysplasia
   Hydronephrosis
   Renal hypoplasia
   Adrenal hypoplasia
   Hypospadias
   Cryptorchidism

Reproduced with permission from McKusick VA, ed. Online mendelian inheritance in man. Available at: http://www.ncbi.nlm.nih.gov/omim/. McKusick-Nathans Institute for Genetic Medicine, Johns Hopkins University (Baltimore, MD) and National Center for Biotechnology Information, National Library of Medicine (Bethesda, MD), 2000.

genomic imprinting or the differential expression of genes depending on the maternal or paternal origin of the genetic material.

Type I is associated with a large cystic placenta, partial molar changes, and symmetric growth restriction of the fetus, and type II is associated with a small nonmolar preg-

TABLE 32. FEATURES ASSOCIATED WITH TRIPLOIDY TYPES I AND II

Type I	Type II
Large, cystic placenta (partial molar change)	Small, noncystic placenta
Symmetric growth restriction	Asymmetric growth restriction
Parental origin of extra set of chromosomes (diandry)	Maternal origin of the extra set of chromosomes (digyny)
Increased levels of maternal serum human chorionic gonadotropin, alpha-fetoprotein, and inhibin-A	Low levels of maternal serum human chorionic gonadotropin and estriol

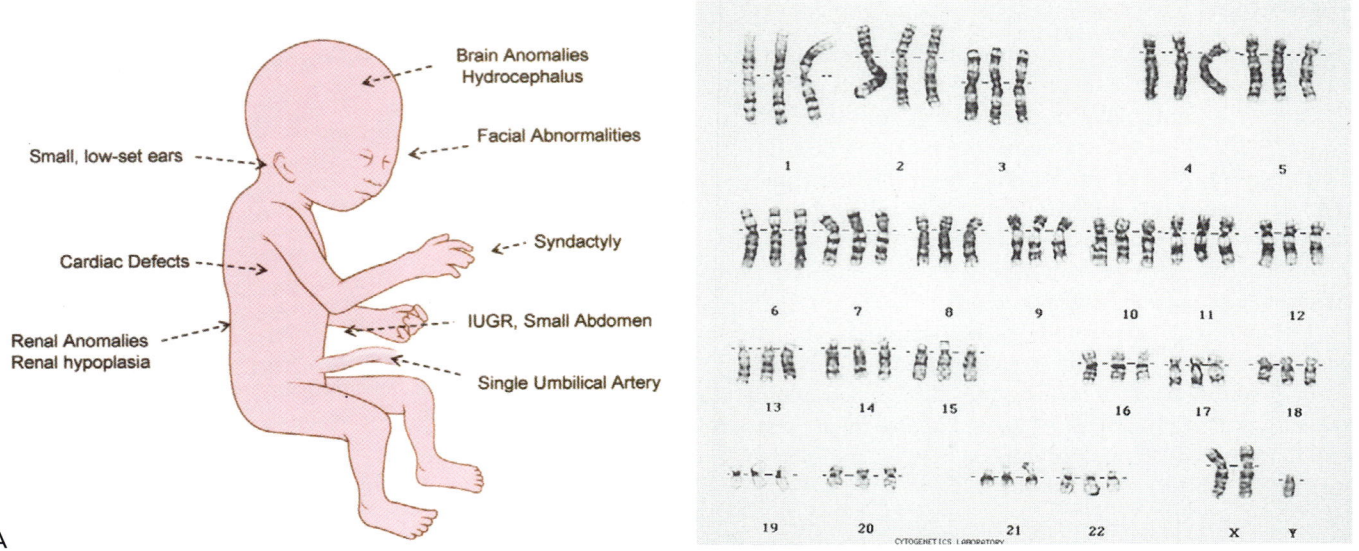

FIGURE 45. Triploidy. **A:** Common sonographic and pathologic features. IUGR, intrauterine growth restriction. **B:** Karyotype shows triploidy with 69 chromosomes.

nancy and a fetus with severe asymmetric growth restriction.[536] Most type I phenotypes are associated with paternal origin of triploidy (diandry) and earlier demise of the fetus than the type II phenotype, which is most often associated with maternal origin (digyny).[534,539,540] Although not all cases of diandry are partial moles, digyny does not appear to be associated with partial molar change.[539]

The histopathologic diagnosis of partial molar change is based on the presence of fetal tissue and a number of placental features including trophoblastic hyperplasia and the presence of two populations, one of which is composed of enlarged hydropic villi. However, histologic changes may be detected less commonly in triploidy among first-trimester miscarriages compared with later in pregnancy.[536]

Pathologic features of triploid fetuses include low birth weight and head-abdomen discordance. Common facial features include microphthalmos; hypertelorism; colobomas; facial asymmetry; low-set, malformed ears; cleft palate; micrognathia, syndactyly of the third and fourth fingers (greater than 50%), and talipes equinovarus. CNS malformations are common and include holoprosencephaly, hydrocephalus (50%), agenesis of the corpus callosum, and myelomeningocele (25%). Other anomalies include cardiovascular malformations (60%), omphalocele or umbilical hernia, adrenal hypoplasia, and genitourinary anomalies (cystic renal dysplasia, hydronephrosis, hypospadias, cryptorchidism).[541]

Diagnosis

Common features of triploidy are shown in Figure 45. IUGR is a prominent feature and universally present in

prenatally reported cases of triploidy (Fig. 46). IUGR is typically of the asymmetric type with small body relative to head size. Marked oligohydramnios also is nearly always demonstrated, although polyhydramnios occasionally has been reported.[537,542–544] Abnormalities of the face (Fig. 46) and CNS may also be detected.

Placental abnormalities of hydatidiform degeneration or hydropic changes are present in nearly all cases in which the extrahaploid set of chromosomes is paternal in origin but are much less common with a maternal origin.[545] The placenta may appear thickened or demonstrate cystic changes on sonography. However, these findings are variable.[546]

Sonographic identification of specific anomalies is often difficult in the presence of marked oligohydramnios. CNS malformations are the most frequent specific malformations identified and are present in most fetuses with triploidy who survive to term. Other anomalies that may be detected include spina bifida, omphalocele, and cardiovascular malformations.

Jauniaux et al.[547] reviewed 70 cases of triploidy presenting between 13 and 29 weeks' gestation over a 10-year period. Each fetus had at least one measurement below the normal range, and 50 cases (71%) presented with asymmetric growth restriction and normal placental appearance. All cases of triploidy associated with partial mole were diagnosed before 25 weeks. Structural defects were observed antenatally in 65 (93%) cases. The most common defects were abnormalities of the hands (52%), cerebral ventriculomegaly (37%), heart anomalies (34%), and micrognathia (26%). The most frequent combination of abnormalities was malformation of the hands and ventriculomegaly. The authors suggest triploidy should be

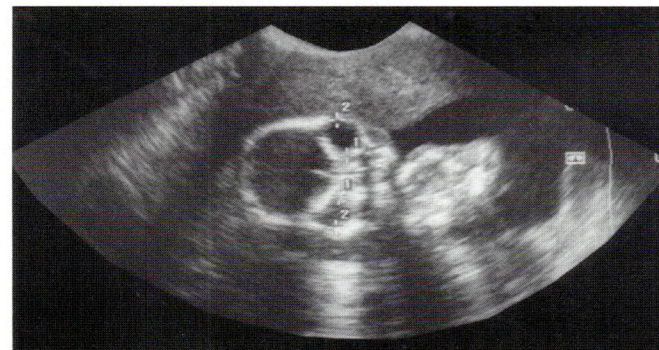

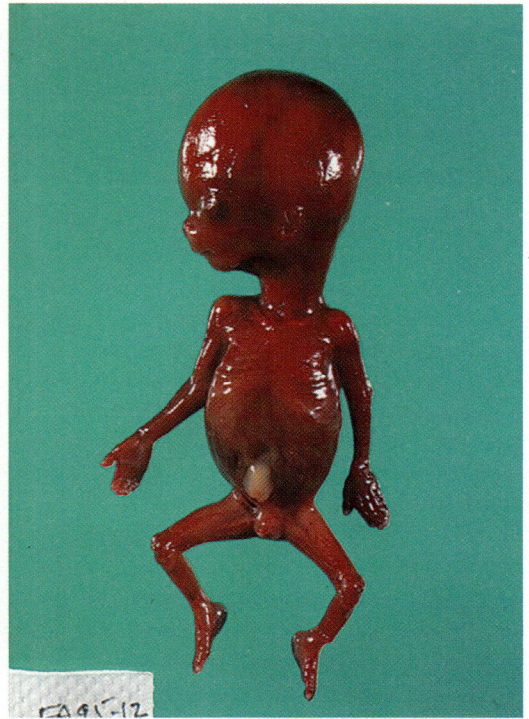

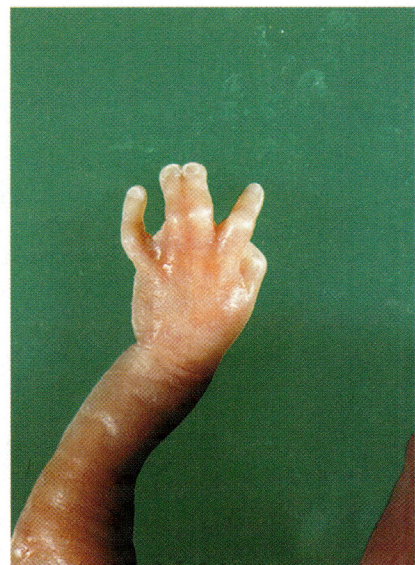

FIGURE 46. Triploidy. **A:** A coronal view of the face shows hypertelorism. A disproportionately small abdomen was also present. (Courtesy of Beryl Benacerraf, Boston, MA.) **B:** A pathologic photograph from a similar case shows head-body disproportion. **C:** A pathologic photograph shows characteristic syndactyly of the third and fourth fingers. (Courtesy of Joe Siebert, Pathology Department, Children's Hospital, Seattle, WA.)

suspected with partial molar changes or severe asymmetric fetal growth restriction in the presence of an apparently normal placenta.

In the first trimester (10- to 14-week period), features reported in association with triploidy include mildly increased median nuchal translucency, low fetal heart rate, holoprosencephaly, posterior fossa cyst, omphalocele, and cystic placental appearance.[548,549] Spencer et al.[550] reported the nuchal translucency to be increased in type I and low to normal in type II triploidy (median nuchal translucencies of 2.76 MoM and 0.88 MoM, respectively).

Several prenatal cases of tetraploidy have been reported in the second trimester.[532,551,552]

Differential Diagnosis

Conditions other than triploidy that may produce similar appearances to partial mole include BWS, placental angiomatous malformation, twin gestation with complete mole and existing fetus, early complete hydatidiform mole, and hydropic spontaneous abortion.[553]

Early-onset IUGR should suggest other conditions including trisomies 13 and 18 and, in some cases, confined placental mosaicism.

Prognosis

True triploidy is uniformly lethal, with most fetuses spontaneously aborted during early pregnancy. Most live-born infants die within a few hours of birth. However, rare cases have been reported to survive for weeks or months.[554,555] Mosaic individuals may live a normal life span.

Partial moles are associated with a high risk of severe preeclampsia, which may arise before 20 weeks' gestation and can be severe.[556,557] In addition, a small percentage of partial molar pregnancies progress to persistent trophoblastic tumor and even metastatic disease in rare cases.[558,559]

Management

Termination of pregnancy can be offered at any gestational age for a uniformly fatal condition.

Recurrence Risk

The risk for triploidy does not appear to be significantly increased in individuals with a previous affected pregnancy.

▶ VELOCARDIOFACIAL SYNDROME

Velocardiofacial syndrome (VCFS) was originally characterized as velopharyngeal incompetence, congenital heart disease, characteristic facial features, and developmental delay or learning difficulties,[560,561] whereas the DiGeorge syndrome was originally characterized as a major congenital heart defect, hypocalcemia, and aplasia or hypoplasia of the thymus gland. The acronym *CATCH 22* is used to refer to *c*ardiac defects, *a*bnormal facies, *t*hymic hypoplasia, *c*left palate, and *h*ypocalcemia resulting from 22q11 deletions.[562] It is now recognized that these clinical conditions are all represented by a hemizygous 22q11 deletion syndrome. Most patients with DiGeorge syndrome were identified in the neonatal period, whereas patients with VCFS were more often diagnosed in cleft palate or craniofacial centers when speech and learning difficulties became evident.[563]

Synonyms for VCFS include *Shprintzen syndrome, CATCH-22 syndrome, DiGeorge syndrome,* and *22q11 deletion syndrome.*

Incidence

The incidence is approximately 1 in 5,000. It is the most common microdeletion defect known.

Genetic Defect

VCFS is localized to 22q11 (Fig. 47). More than 90% of cases of VCFS are associated with a microdeletion of 22q11.2.[564] Chromosome 22q11.2 deletion has also been found in some patients classified on a clinical basis as having conotruncal anomaly face syndrome, Opitz G/BBB syndrome, Cayler cardiofacial syndrome, and sporadic or familial tetralogy of Fallot. VCFS and microdeletion of 22q11 have also been associated with giant platelets.[565] A number of gene products from within the deletion have been identified and are being further characterized.[566,567] One candidate (GNB1L) is highly expressed in the heart.[568]

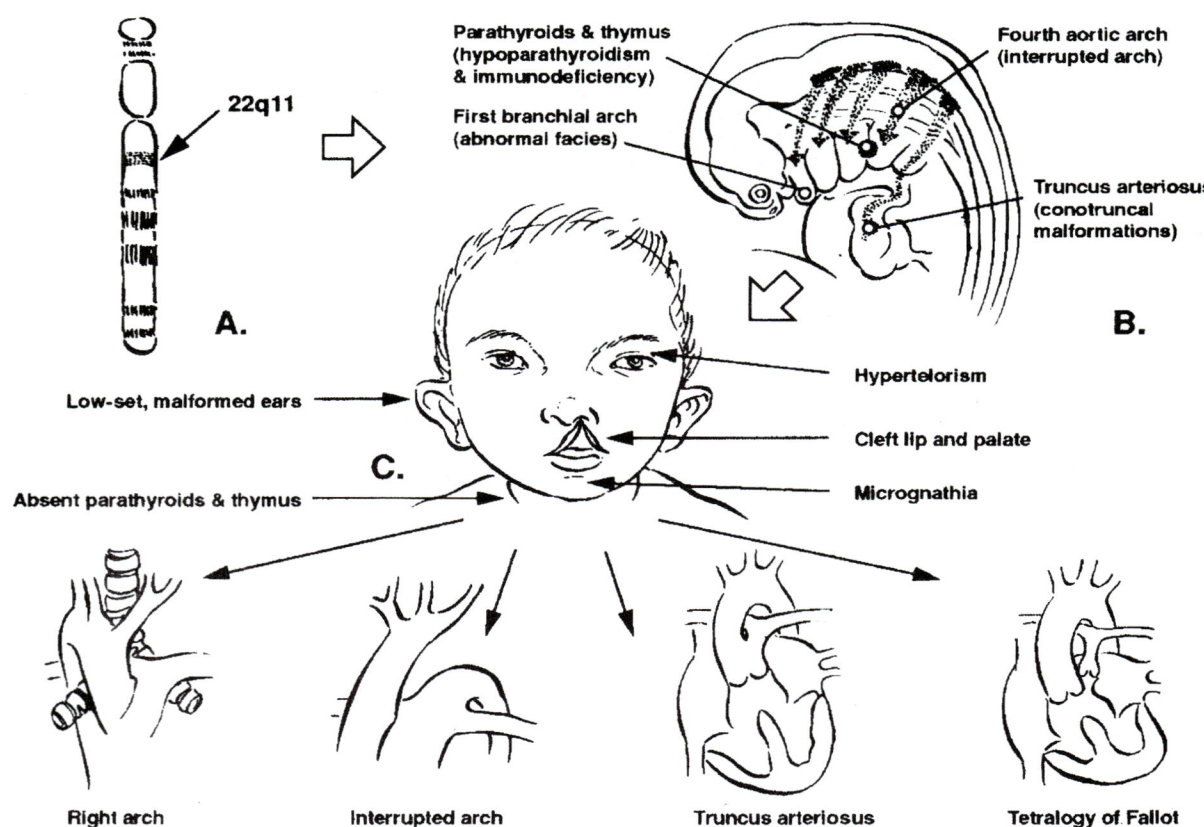

FIGURE 47. Velocardiofacial syndrome. Characteristic features. (Reproduced with permission from Sze RW, Yutzey KE. The molecular genetic revolution in congenital heart disease. *AJR Am J Roentgenol* 2001;176:575–581.)

TABLE 33. PATHOLOGIC AND CLINICAL FEATURES OF VELOCARDIOFACIAL SYNDROME

Craniofacial
  Cleft palate
  Velopharyngeal insufficiency
  Small mouth
  Pierre Robin syndrome
  Retrognathia
  Narrow palpebral fissures
  Flat malar region
  Prominent tubular nose
  Hypoplastic nasal alae
  Microcephaly
  Ocular abnormalities (colobomas, cataract, microphthalmos)
  Ptosis
  Minor auricular anomalies
Cardiovascular
  Ventricular septal defect
  Tetralogy of Fallot
  Right aortic arch
  Aberrant left subclavian artery
Central nervous system/neurologic
  Brain abnormalities
  Learning disability
  Blunt or inappropriate affect
  Mental retardation
  Psychotic illness
Growth: short stature
Skeletal
  Slender hands and digits
  Short stature
  Clubfoot
  Syndactyly
Gastrointestinal
  Inguinal hernia
  Umbilical hernia
Genitourinary
  Single kidney
  Echogenic kidney
  Multicystic dysplastic kidney
  Small kidneys
  Horseshoe kidney
  Renal duplication
Endocrine
  Parathyroid, absent/hypoparathyroidism, hypocalcemia
  Absent/hypoplastic thymus, T-cell deficiency

Reproduced with permission from McKusick VA, ed. Online mendelian inheritance in man. Available at: http://www.ncbi.nlm.nih.gov/omim/. McKusick-Nathans Institute for Genetic Medicine, Johns Hopkins University (Baltimore, MD) and National Center for Biotechnology Information, National Library of Medicine (Bethesda, MD), 2000.

Pathologic and Clinical Features

Pathologic and clinical features of VCFS are summarized in Table 33. Anomalies are highly variable.[564] Heart defects are present in the majority of patients.[569] The primary cardiac malformations are tetralogy of Fallot, interrupted aortic arch, truncus arteriosus, and VSD. Hypoplastic left ventricle, double-outlet right ventricle, and other cardiac defects may also occur. Renal abnormalities are common, present in approximately one-third of cases. This may include single kidney, echogenic kidney, multicystic dysplastic kidney, small kidneys, horseshoe kidney, and duplicated collecting system. Extremity abnormalities may include pre- and postaxial polydactyly, clubfoot, overfolded toes, and 2,3 syndactyly of the second and third toes.[570] Growth disturbances with short height and slender hands and digits are also observed.[571]

Diagnosis

Ultrasound

The phenotype of 22q11 deletion syndrome shows considerable variation (Figs. 48 and 49). Detection of a conotruncal cardiac defect is the ultrasound finding most likely to suggest VCFS (Fig. 48). However, it is estimated that less than 10% of prenatal cases of conotruncal defects are associated with VCFS.[572] Of cardiac defects, interruption of the aortic arch[573] or tetralogy of Fallot probably has the highest yield of VCFS. In one study, deletions were found in three of 26 pregnancies with cardiac defects tested.[574]

Polyhydramnios may occur during the third trimester, presumably because of the cleft palate or pharyngeal abnormality. Clefts are unlikely to be detected by ultrasound since these are usually cleft palate without cleft lip. Renal abnormalities are relatively common. The combination of cardiac defect and renal abnormality should suggest the possibility of VCFS.[575] It is possible that absence of the thymus can be diagnosed in some cases (R. Chaoui, *personal communication*, 2002). However, it is unlikely that this will be diagnosed before the third trimester.

Increased nuchal translucency at 12 weeks has been described as the initial finding in a fetus who proved to have cardiac defects, hypocalcemia at birth, and evidence of the DiGeorge syndrome.[576]

Laboratory

Given that these deletions are difficult to visualize at the light microscopic level, fluorescent *in situ* hybridization has been instrumental in the diagnosis of this disorder.[577]

Differential Diagnosis

The features of VCFS are protean, so the differential diagnosis is large. Possibilities include the VATER association, oculo-auriculo-vertebral (Goldenhar) syndrome, SLOS when polydactyly and cleft palate are present, and Alagille syndrome when butterfly vertebrae and heart defects are present. Similar features may be seen with other chromosome abnormalities including other microdeletions.[578]

Prognosis

The immediate prognosis depends largely on the presence and severity of the cardiac defect. Among a large European

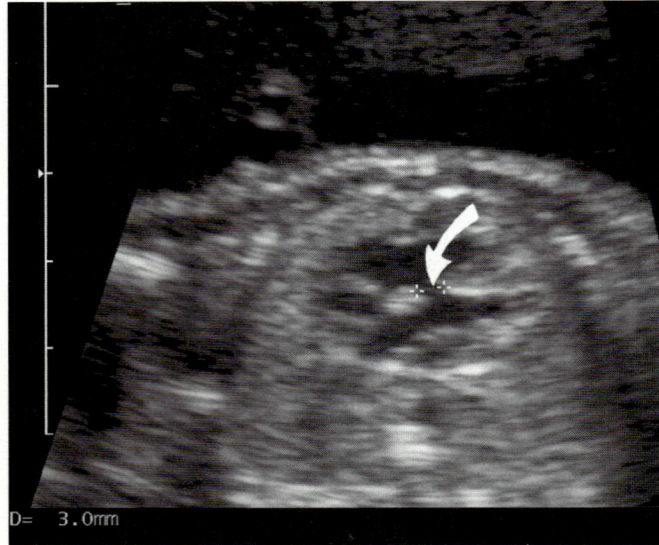

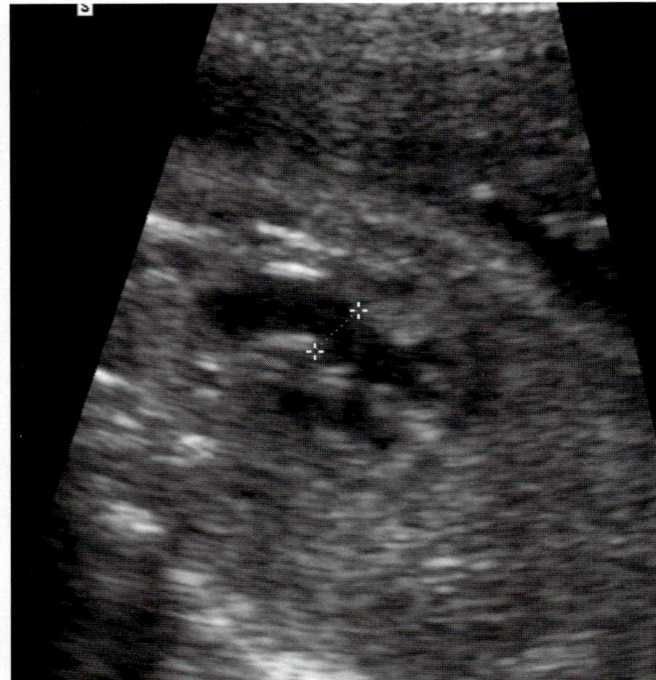

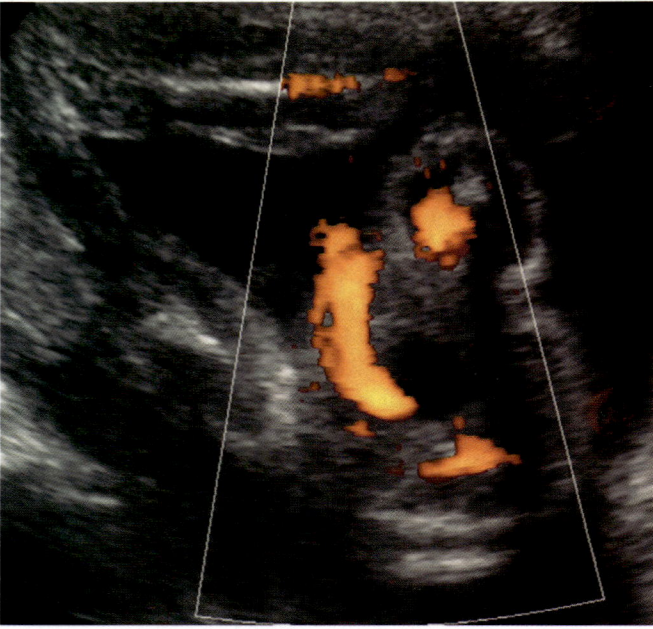

FIGURE 48. Velocardiofacial syndrome. **A:** A transverse view of the heart shows a ventricular septal defect (*arrow*) measuring 3 mm. **B:** A single great vessel trunk arises from the heart. **C:** Single umbilical artery is demonstrated with color-flow imaging of the pelvis. A single artery surrounds the urinary bladder. Fluorescent *in situ* hybridization analysis revealed a 22q deletion consistent with velocardiofacial syndrome.

collaborative study of 558 patients with deletions of 22q11, Ryan et al.[579] reported that 44 patients died, most commonly from heart disease. One patient also died from severe immune deficiency. The mortality rate is likely to be much higher among prenatal cases.

Hypocalcemia is common from hypoplasia of the parathyroid glands, and this may result in neonatal seizures.[579] Hypotonia and feeding disorders are common in infancy.

Learning and developmental problems are relatively common. Ryan et al.[579] noted that 231 patients among 338 affected individuals had abnormal development, including 102 with mild delay and 60 with moderate-severe learning difficulties. Of 107 cases with normal development, 37 had speech delay. In childhood testing, reading skills are much stronger than math skills.[580] Behavioral or psychiatric problems have been a subject of considerable interest but probably occur in less than 10% of cases.[579] Various brain abnormalities have been reported on CT and MRI[581,582] and may show similar features to some patients with schizophrenia. A neurodegenerative disorder has also been associated with VCFS.[583]

Other problems include delayed growth and height,[584] polyarticular juvenile rheumatoid arthritis,[585] and immunodeficiency, usually from impaired T-cell function.

Management

If VCFS is suspected, the diagnosis should be confirmed by fluorescent *in situ* hybridization on amniotic fluid or

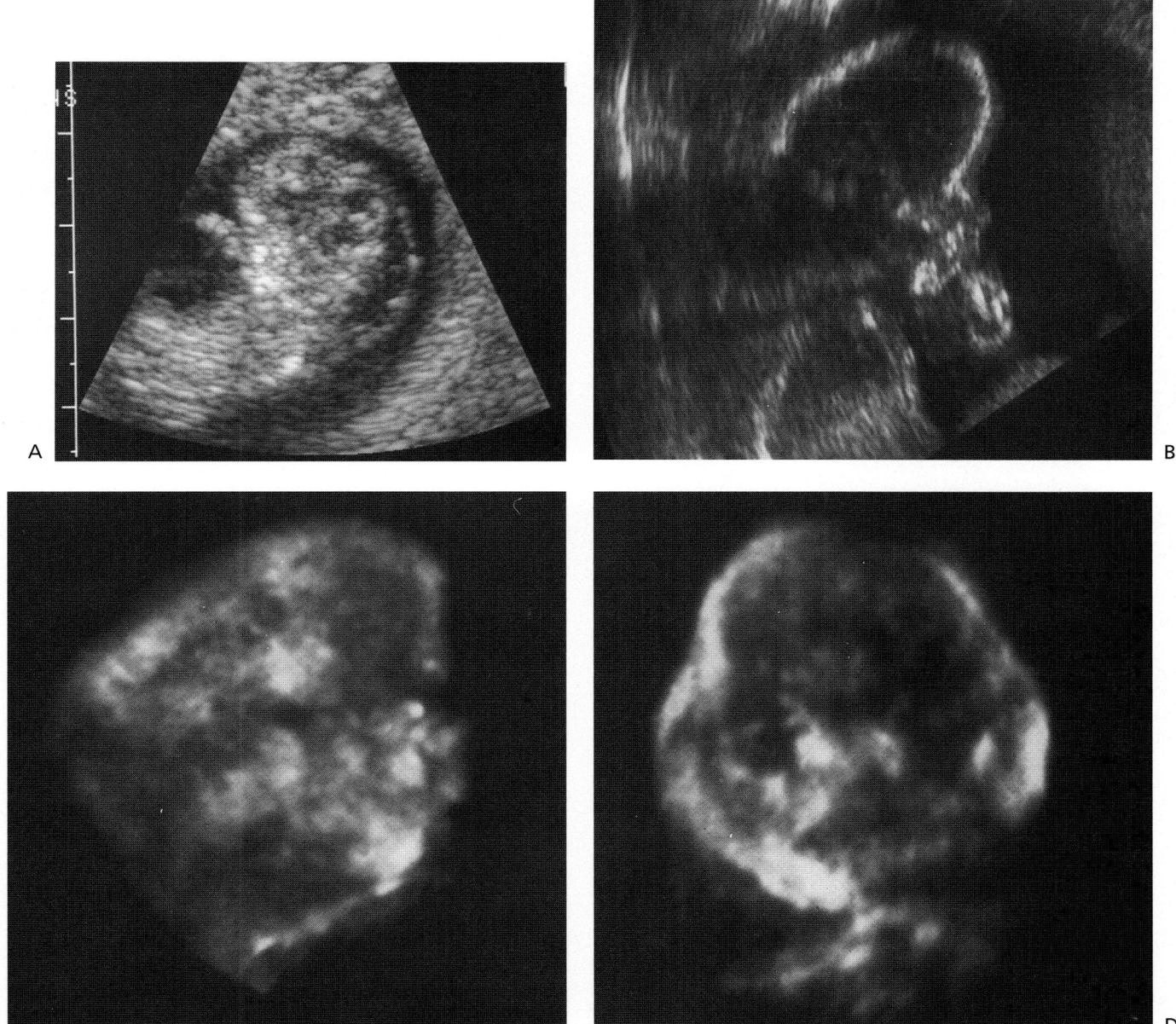

FIGURE 49. Velocardiofacial syndrome, unusual presentation. **A:** A scan at 12 weeks shows increased nuchal translucency. An echocardiogram at 20 weeks was normal but showed an unusual head shape. **B:** A sagittal view on follow-up at 22 weeks shows an unusual head shape with acrocephaly, frontal bossing, and a deep nasal bridge. **C:** A three-dimensional surface rendered image in lateral view shows craniosynostosis. **D:** A three-dimensional surface rendered image in frontal projection shows an unusual cranial shape. (*continued*)

other fetal specimen. Routine cytogenetic studies should be performed on all individuals in whom 22q11 deletion is suspected because they may have a chromosome abnormality involving some other chromosomal region including other microdeletions.[578] After birth, the immediate concerns are related to possible cardiac defects and hypocalcemia. A fetal echocardiogram and renal ultrasound are recommended.

After the newborn period, a multidisciplinary approach, which may include general pediatrics, genetics, plastic surgery, speech pathology, otolaryngology, audiology, dentistry, cardiology, immunology, child development, child psychology, and neurology, is necessary. Some patients also require evaluation by health care providers specializing in feeding, endocrinology, rheumatology, gastroenterology, neurosurgery, general surgery, orthopedics, urology, hema-

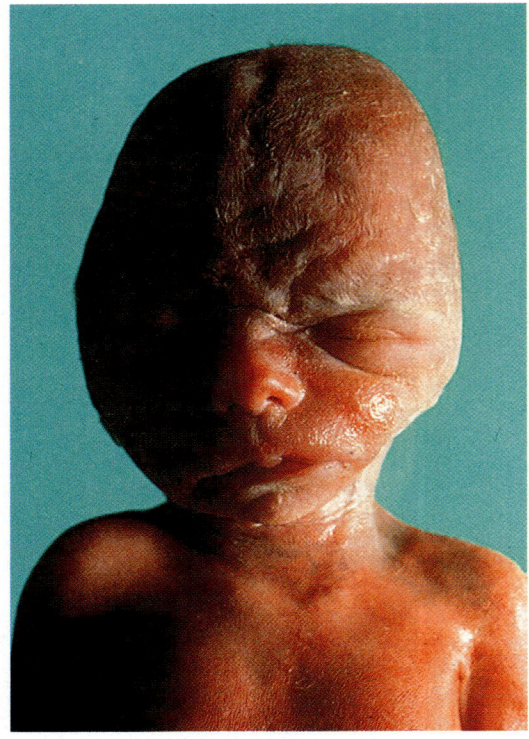

FIGURE 49. *Continued.* **E:** Pathologic correlation: Bilateral craniosynostosis was confirmed. The pathologic examination also showed absent thymus, which led to fluorescent *in situ* hybridization analysis, showing 22q11 deletion. (Part **E** courtesy of Joe Siebert, Pathology Department, Children's Hospital, Seattle, WA.)

tology, psychiatry, or ophthalmology. Children with growth failure should be evaluated by an endocrinologist for possible growth hormone deficiency.[584] Early educational intervention should include speech therapy, due to the incidence of speech and language delay, beginning at 1 year of age.

Recurrence Risk

Offspring of a carrier parent have a 50% chance of inheriting the deletion. It is not possible to predict the phenotype in children with the deletion.

REFERENCES

General

1. McKusick VA, ed. Online mendelian inheritance in man. Available at: http://www.ncbi.nlm.nih.gov/omim/. McKusick-Nathans Institute for Genetic Medicine, Johns Hopkins University (Baltimore, MD) and National Center for Biotechnology Information, National Library of Medicine (Bethesda, MD), 2000.
2. Pagon RA, ed. GeneClinics. Available at: http://www.geneclinics.org. Seattle, WA: Children's Health System and University of Washington, Accessed 1993–2002.
3. Jeanty P, ed. The fetus. Available at: http://www.thefetus.net. Accessed 1999–2001.
4. Jones KL. *Smith's recognizable patterns of human malformation*, 5th ed. Philadelphia: WB Saunders, 1997.
5. Rimoin DL, O'Connor JM, Pyeritz RE, Korf BR, eds. *Emery and Rimoin's principles and practice of medical genetics*. London: Churchill Livingstone, 2002.
6. Benacerraf BR. *Ultrasound of fetal syndromes*. New York: Churchill Livingstone, 1998.

Amniotic Band Syndrome

7. Higginbottom MC, Jones KL, Hall BD, Smith DW. The amniotic band disruption complex: timing of amniotic rupture and variable spectra of consequent defects. *J Pediatr* 1979;95:544–549.
8. Buyse ML. *Birth defects encyclopedia*. Cambridge, MA: Blackwell Science, 1990.
9. Seeds JW, Cefalo RC, Herbert WNP. Amniotic band syndrome. *Am J Obstet Gynecol* 1982;144:243.
10. Tadmor OP, Kreisberg GA, Achiron R, Porat S, Yagel S. Limb amputation in amniotic band syndrome: serial ultrasonographic and Doppler observations. *Ultrasound Obstet Gynecol* 1997;10:312–315.
11. Dimmick JE, Kalousek DK. *Developmental pathology of the embryo and fetus*. Philadelphia: JB Lippincott Co, 1992.
12. Torpin R. *Fetal malformations caused by amnion rupture during gestation*. Springfield, IL: Charles C Thomas, 1968:1–76.
13. Lockwood C, Ghidini A, Romero R. Amniotic band syndrome in monozygotic twins: prenatal diagnosis and pathogenesis. *Obstet Gynecol* 1988;71(6 Pt 2):1012–1016.
14. Lockwood C, Ghidini A, Romero R, Hobbins JC. Amniotic band syndrome: reevaluation of its pathogenesis. *Am J Obstet Gynecol* 1989;160(5 Pt 1):1030–1033.
15. Daly CA, Freeman J, Weston W, Kovar I, Phelan M. Prenatal diagnosis of amniotic band syndrome in a methadone user: review of the literature and a case report. *Ultrasound Obstet Gynecol* 1996;8:123–125.
16. Ashkenazy M, Borenstein R, Katz Z, Segal M. Constriction of the umbilical cord by an amniotic band after midtrimester amniocentesis. *Acta Obstet Gynecol Scand* 1982;61:89–91.
17. Baker CJ, Rudolph AJ. Congenital ring constrictions and intrauterine amputations. *Am J Dis Child* 1971;212:393–400.
18. Moessinger AC, Blanc WA, Byrne J, Andrews D, Warburton D, Bloom A. Amniotic band syndrome associated with amniocentesis. *Am J Obstet Gynecol* 1981;141:588–591.
19. Benacerraf BR, Frigoletto FD Jr. Sonographic observation of amniotic rupture without amniotic band syndrome. *J Ultrasound Med* 1992;11:109–111.
20. BenEzra D, Frucht Y. Uveal coloboma associated with amniotic band syndrome. *Can J Ophthalmol* 1983;18:136–138.
21. BenEzra D, Frucht Y, Paez JH, Zelikovitch A. Amniotic band syndrome and strabismus. *J Pediatr Ophthalmol Strabismus* 1982;19:33–36.
22. Hashemi K, Traboulsi E, Chavis R, Scribanu N, Chrousos GA. Chorioretinal lacuna in the amniotic band syndrome. *J Pediatr Ophthalmol Strabismus* 1991;28:238–239.

23. Fiske CE, Filly RA, Golbus MS. Prenatal ultrasound diagnosis of amniotic band syndrome. *J Ultrasound Med* 1982;1:45–47.

24. Mahony BS, Filly RA, Callen PW, Golbus MS. The amniotic band syndrome: antenatal sonographic diagnosis and potential pitfalls. *Am J Obstet Gynecol* 1985;152:63–68.

25. Burton DJ, Filly RA. Sonographic diagnosis of the amniotic band syndrome. *AJR Am J Roentgenol* 1991;156:555–558.

26. Goncalves LF, Jeanty P. Amniotic band syndrome. *Fetus* 1992;2(4):1–6.

27. Van Allen MI, Siegel-Bartelt J, Dixon J, Zuker RM, Clarke HM, Toi A. Constriction bands and limb reduction defects in two newborns with fetal ultrasound evidence for vascular disruption. *Am J Med Genet* 1992;44:598–604.

28. Randel SB, Filly RA, Callen PW, Anderson RL, Golbus MS. Amniotic sheets. *Radiology* 1988;166:633–636.

29. Goldstein RB, Filly RA. Prenatal diagnosis of anencephaly: spectrum of sonographic appearances and distinction from the amniotic band syndrome. *AJR Am J Roentgenol* 1988; 151:547–550.

30. Seidman JD, Abbondanzo SL, Watkin WG, Ragsdale B, Manz HJ. Amniotic band syndrome. Report of two cases and review of the literature. *Arch Pathol Lab Med* 1989;113:891–897.

31. Bracero LA, Rochelson BL, Kaplan C, Monheit A. Sonographic differentiation of a large fetal cystic hygroma from the amniotic band syndrome. *Am J Perinatol* 1990;7:94–96.

32. Ossipoff V, Hall BD. Etiologic factors in the amniotic band syndrome: a study of 24 patients. *Birth Defects* 1977;13: 117–132.

33. Quintero RA, Morales WJ, Phillips J, Kalter CS, Angel JL. *In utero* lysis of amniotic bands. *Ultrasound Obstet Gynecol* 1997;10:316–320.

34. Marras A, Dessi C, Macciotta A. Epidermolysis bullosa and amniotic bands. *Am J Med Genet* 1984;19:815.

35. Young ID, Lindenbaum RH, Thompson EM, Pembrey ME. Amniotic bands in connective tissue disorders. *Arch Dis Child* 1985;60:1061–1063.

Apert Syndrome

36. Parent P, Le Guern H, Munck MR, Thoma M. Apert syndrome, an antenatal ultrasound detected case. *Genet Couns* 1994;5:297–301.

37. Kaufmann K, Baldinger S, Pratt L. Ultrasound detection of Apert syndrome: a case report and literature review. *Am J Perinatol* 1997;14:427–430.

38. Jones KL. Apert syndrome. In: *Smith's recognizable patterns of human malformation.* Philadelphia: WB Saunders, 1997:418–419.

39. Erikson JD, Cohen MM Jr. A study of parental age effects on the occurrence of fresh mutations for the Apert syndrome. *Ann Hum Genet* 1974;38:89–96.

40. Wilkie AO, Slaney SF, Oldridge M, Poole MD, Ashworth GJ, et al. Apert syndrome results from localized mutations of *FGFR2* and is allelic with Crouzon syndrome. *Nat Genet* 1995;9:165–172.

41. Park WJ, Theda C, Maestri NE, Meyers GA, Frigurg JS, et al. Analysis of phenotypic features and *FGFR2* mutations in Apert syndrome. *Am J Hum Genet* 1995;57:321–328.

42. Chenoweth-Mitchell C, Cohen GR. Prenatal sonographic findings of Apert syndrome. *J Clin Ultrasound* 1994;22:510–514.

43. Hill LM, Thomas ML, Peterson CS. The ultrasonic detection of Apert syndrome. *J Ultrasound Med* 1987;6:601–604.

44. Pooh RK, Nakagawa Y, Pooh KH, Nakagawa Y, Nagamachi N. Fetal craniofacial structure and intracranial morphology in a case of Apert syndrome. *Ultrasound Obstet Gynecol* 1999;13:274–280.

45. Lyu KJ, Ko TM. Prenatal diagnosis of Apert syndrome with widely separated cranial sutures. *Prenat Diagn* 2000;20:254–256.

46. Benacerrraf BR, Spiro R, Mitchell A. Using three-dimensional ultrasound to detect craniosynostosis in a fetus with Pfeiffer syndrome. *Ultrasound Obstet Gynecol* 2000;16:391–394.

47. Mahieu-Caputo D, Sonigo P, Amiel J, Simon I, Aubry MC, et al. Prenatal diagnosis of sporadic Apert syndrome: a sequential diagnostic approach combining three-dimensional computed tomography and molecular biology. *Fetal Diagn Ther* 2001;16:10–12.

48. Filkins K, Russo JF, Boehmer S, Camous M, Przylepa KA, et al. Prenatal ultrasonographic and molecular diagnosis of Apert syndrome. *Prenat Diagn* 1997;17:1081–1084.

49. Narayan H, Scott IV. Prenatal diagnosis of Apert's syndrome. *Prenat Diagn* 1991;10:187–192.

50. Leonard CO, Daikoku NH, Winn K. Prenatal fetoscopic diagnosis of the Apert syndrome. *Am J Med Genet* 1982;11:5–9.

51. von Gernet S, Golla A, Ehrenfels Y, Schuffenhauer S, Fairley JD. Genotype-phenotype analysis in Apert syndrome suggests opposite effects of the two recurrent mutations on syndactyly and outcome of craniofacial surgery. *Clin Genet* 2000;57:137–139.

52. Witters I, Devriendt K, Moerman P, van Hole C, Fryns JP. Diaphragmatic hernia as the first echographic sign in Apert syndrome. *Prenat Diagn* 2000;20:404–406.

53. Cohen MM, Kreibord S. The central nervous system in the Apert syndrome. *Am J Med Genet* 1990;35:36–45.

54. Chang CC, Tsai FJ, Tsai HD, Tsai CH, Hseih YY, et al. Prenatal diagnosis of Apert syndrome. *Prenat Diagn* 1998;18:621–625.

55. Ferreira JC, Carter SM, Bernstein PS, Jabs EW, Glickstein JS, et al. Second-trimester molecular prenatal diagnosis of sporadic Apert syndrome following suspicious ultrasound findings. *Ultrasound Obstet Gynecol* 1999;14:426–430.

56. Balci S, Onol B, Eryilmaz M, Haytoglu T. A case of Carpenter syndrome diagnosed in a 20-week-old fetus with postmortem examination. *Clin Genet* 1997;51:412–416.

57. Ashby T, Rouse GA, De Lange M. Prenatal sonographic diagnosis of Carpenter syndrome. *J Ultrasound Med* 1994;13:905–909.

58. Bernstain PS, Gross SJ, Cohen DJ, Tiller GR, Shanske AL, et al. Prenatal diagnosis of type 2 Pfeiffer syndrome. *Ultrasound Obstet Gynecol* 1996;8:425–428.

59. Hill LM, Grzybek PC. Sonographic findings with Pfeiffer syndrome. *Prenat Diagn* 1994;14:47–49.

60. Gollin YG, Abuhamad AZ, Inati MN, Shaffer WK, Copel JA, Hobbins JC. Sonographic appearance of craniofacial dysostosis (Crouzon syndrome) in the second trimester. *J Ultrasound Med* 1993;12:625–628.

61. Menashe Y, Ben Baruch G, Rabinovitch O, Shalev Y, Katzenlson MB, Shalev E. Exophthalmus—prenatal ultrasonic features for diagnosis of Crouzon syndrome. *Prenat Diagn* 1989;9:805–808.

62. Lo LJ, Chen YR. Airway obstruction in severe syndromic craniosynostosis. *Ann Plast Surg* 1999;43:258–264.

63. Sculerati N, Gottlieb MD, Zimbler MS, Chibbaro PD, McCarthy JG. Airway management in children with major craniofacial anomalies. *Laryngoscope* 1998;108:1806–1812.

64. Perkins JA, Sie KC, Milczuk H, Richardson MA. Airway management in children with craniofacial anomalies. *Cleft Palate Craniofac J* 1997;34:135–140.

65. Sarimski K. Cognitive functioning of young children with Apert's syndrome. *Genet Couns* 1997;8:317–322.

66. Renier D, Lajeunie E, Arnaud E, Marchac D. Management of craniosynostoses. *Childs Nerv Syst* 2000;16:645–658.

67. Grayhack JJ, Wedge JH. Anatomy and management of the leg and foot in Apert syndrome. *Clin Plast Surg* 1991;18:399–405.

68. Mah J, Kasser J, Upton J. The foot in Apert syndrome. *Clin Plast Surg* 1991;18:391–397.

69. Munro IR, Sabatier RE. An analysis of 12 years of craniomaxillofacial surgery in Toronto. *Plast Reconstr Surg* 1985;76:29–35.

70. Kaplan LC. Clinical assessment and multispecialty management of Apert syndrome. *Clin Plast Surg* 1991;18:217–225.

Arthrogryposis/Akinesia Sequence

71. Hall JG, Reed SD, Greene G. The distal arthrogryposes: delineation of new entities—review and nosologic discussion. *Am J Med Genet* 1982;11:185–239.

72. Moessinger AC. Fetal akinesia deformation sequence: an animal model. *Pediatrics* 1983;72:857–863.

73. Hammond E, Donnenfield AE. Fetal akinesia. *Obstet Gynecol Surv* 1995;50:140–149.

74. Lavi E, Montone KT, Rorke LB, Kliman HJ. Fetal akinesia deformation sequence (Pena-Shokeir phenotype) associated with acquired intrauterine brain damage. *Neurology* 1991;41:1467–1468.

75. Reiser P, Briner J, Schinzel A. Skeletal muscular changes in Pena-Shokeir sequence. *J Perinat Med* 1990;18:267–274.

76. Robertson WL, Glinski LP, Kirkpatrick SJ, Pauli RM. Further evidence that arthrogryposis multiplex congenita in the human sometimes is caused by an intrauterine vascular accident. *Teratology* 1992;45:345–351.

77. Reid CO, Hall JG, Anderson C, Bocian M, Carey J, et al. Association of amyoplasia with gastroschisis, bowel atresia, and defects of the muscular layer of the trunk. *Am J Med Genet* 1986;24:701–710.

78. Pena SDJ, Shokeir MHK. Syndrome of camptodactyly, multiple ankyloses facial anomalies and pulmonary hypoplasia: a lethal condition. *J Pediatr* 1974;85:373–375.

79. Moerman P, Fryns JP, Goddeeris P, Lauweryns JM. Multiple ankyloses, facial anomalies, and pulmonary hypoplasia associated with severe antenatal spinal muscular atrophy. *J Pediatr* 1983;103:238–241.

80. Moerman P, Fryns JP. The fetal akinesia deformation sequence. A fetopathological approach. *Genet Couns* 1990;1:25–33.

81. Paladini D, Tartaglione A, Agangi A, Foglia S, Martinelli P,

Nappi C. Pena-Shokeir phenotype with variable onset in three consecutive pregnancies. *Ultrasound Obstet Gynecol* 2001;17:163–165.

82. Tongsong T, Chanprapaph P, Khunamornpong S. Prenatal ultrasound of regional akinesia with Pena-Shokeir phenotype. *Prenat Diagn* 2000;20:422–425.

83. Ohlsson A, Fong KW, Rose TH, Moore DC. Prenatal sonographic diagnosis of Pena-Shokeir syndrome type I, or fetal akinesia deformation sequence. *Am J Med Genet* 1988;29:59–65.

84. de Die-Smulders CE, Vonsee HJ, Zandvoort JA, Fryns JP. The lethal multiple pterygium syndrome: prenatal ultrasonographic and postmortem findings; a case report. *Eur J Obstet Gynecol Reprod Biol* 1990;35:283–289.

85. Azar GB, Snijders RJ, Gosden C, Nicolaides KH. Fetal nuchal cystic hygromata: associated malformations and chromosomal defects. *Fetal Diagn Ther* 1991;6:46–57.

86. Witters I, Moerman PH, Van Assche FA, Fryns JP. Cystic hygroma colli as the first echographic sign of the fetal akinesia sequence. *Genet Couns* 2001;12:91–94.

87. Paladini D, D'Armiento M, Ardovino I, Martinelli P. Prenatal diagnosis of the cerebro-oculo-facio-skeletal (COFS) syndrome. *Ultrasound Obstet Gynecol* 2000;16:91–93.

88. Esplin MS, Hallam S, Farrington PF, Nelson L, Byrne J, Ward K. Myotonic dystrophy is a significant cause of idiopathic polyhydramnios. *Am J Obstet Gynecol* 1998;179:974–977.

89. Muller LM, de Jong G. Prenatal ultrasonographic features of the Pena-Shokeir I syndrome and the trisomy 18 syndrome. *Am J Med Genet* 1986;25:119–129.

90. Redman JB, Fenwick RG Jr, Fu YH, Pizzuti A, Caskey CT. Relationship between parental trinucleotide GCT repeat length and severity of myotonic dystrophy in offspring. *JAMA* 1993;269:1960–1965.

91. Sells JM, Jaffe KM, Hall JG. Amyoplasia, the most common type of arthrogryposis: the potential for good outcome. *Pediatrics* 1996;97:225–231.

91a. Hall JG. Genetic aspects of arthrogryposis. *Clin Orthop* 1985;184:44–53.

92. Zuhlke C, Atici J, Martorell L, Gembruch U, Kohl M, et al. Rapid detection of expansions by PCR and non-radioactive hybridization: application for prenatal diagnosis of myotonic dystrophy. *Prenat Diagn* 2000;20:66–69.

Beckwith-Wiedemann Syndrome

93. Beckwith JB. Extreme cytomegaly of the adrenal fetal cortex, omphalocele, hyperplasia of kidneys and pancreas, and Leydig-cell hyperplasia. Another syndrome? Presented at: Annual meeting of Western Society for Pediatric Research; November 1963; Los Angeles.

94. Wiedemann HR. Complex malformatif. Familial avec hernie ombilicale et macroglossie—un "syndrome nouveau"? *J Hum Genet* 1964;13:223–232.

95. Thorburn MJ, Wright ES, Miller CG, Smith-Read EH. Exomphalos-macroglossia-gigantism syndrome in Jamaican infants. *Am J Dis Child* 1970;119:316–321.

96. Hatada I, Nabetani A, Morisaki H, Xin Z, Ohishi S, et al. New p57KIP2 mutations in Beckwith-Wiedemann syndrome. *Hum Genet* 1997;100:681–683.

97. Catchpoole D, Lam WW, Valler D, Temple IK, Joyce JA, et al. Epigenetic modification and uniparental inheritance of

H19 in Beckwith-Wiedemann syndrome. *J Med Genet* 1997;34:353–359.

98. Engel JR, Smallwood A, Harper A, Higgins MJ, Oshimura M, et al. Epigenotype-phenotype correlations in Beckwith-Wiedemann syndrome. *J Med Genet* 2000;37:921–926.

99. Shuman S, Weksberg R. Beckwith-Wiedemann syndrome. *GeneReviews* http://www.geneclinics.org/profiles/bws. March 2000.

100. Nyhan WL, Sakati NO. *Genetic and malformation syndromes in clinical medicine.* Chicago: Mosby–Year Book, 1976.

101. Souka AP, Snijders RJ, Novakov A, Soares W, Nicolaides KH. Defects and syndromes in chromosomally normal fetuses with increased nuchal translucency thickness at 10–14 weeks of gestation. *Ultrasound Obstet Gynecol* 1998;11:391–400.

102. Nowotny T, Bollmann R, Pfeifer L, Windt E. Beckwith-Wiedemann syndrome: difficulties with prenatal diagnosis. *Fetal Diagn Ther* 1994;9:256–260.

103. Pettenati MJ, Haines JL, Higgins RR, Wappner RS, Palmer CG, Weaver DD. Wiedemann-Beckwith syndrome: presentation of clinical and cytogenetic data on 22 new cases and review of the literature. *Hum Genet* 1986;74:143–154.

104. DeBaun MR, Tucker MA. Risk of cancer during the first four years of life in children from the Beckwith-Wiedemann Syndrome Registry. *J Pediatr* 1998;132:398–400.

105. Beckwith JB. Nephrogenic rests and the pathogenesis of Wilms' tumor: developmental and clinical considerations. *Am J Med Genet* 1998;79:268–273.

CHARGE Association

106. Hall BD. Choanal atresia and associated multiple anomalies. *J Pediatr* 1979;95:395.

107. Pagon RA, Graham JM Jr, Zonana J, Young SL. Coloboma, congenital heart disease, and choanal atresia with multiple anomalies: CHARGE association. *J Pediatr* 1981;99:223–227.

108. Tellier AL, Amiel J, Delezoide AL, Audollent S, Auge J, et al. Expression of the *PAX2* gene in human embryos and exclusion in the CHARGE syndrome. *Am J Med Genet* 2000;93:85–88.

109. Cyran SE, Martinez R, Daniels S, Dignan PS, Kaplan S. Spectrum of congenital heart disease in CHARGE association. *J Pediatr* 1987;110:576–578.

110. Tellier AL, Cormier-Daire V, Abadie V, Amiel J, Sigaudy S, et al. CHARGE syndrome: report of 47 cases and review. *Am J Med Genet* 1998;76:402–409.

111. Lin AE, Siebert JR, Graham JM Jr. Central nervous system malformations in the CHARGE association. *Am J Med Genet* 1990;37:304–310.

112. Hertzberg BS, Kliewer MA, Lile RL. Antenatal ultrasonographic findings in the CHARGE association. *J Ultrasound Med* 1994;13:238–242.

113. Wheeler PG, Quigley CA, Sadeghi-Nejad A, Weaver DD. Hypogonadism and CHARGE association. *Am J Med Genet* 2000;94:228–231.

114. Goldson E, Smith AC, Stewart JM. The CHARGE association. How well can they do? *Am J Dis Child* 1986;140:918–921.

115. Carinci F, Hassanipour A, Mandrioli S, Pastore A. Surgical treatment of choanal atresia in CHARGE association: case report with long-term follow-up. *J Craniomaxillofac Surg* 1999;27:321–326.

116. Asher BF, McGill TJ, Kaplan L, Friedman EM, Healy GB. Airway complications in CHARGE association. *Arch Otolaryngol Head Neck Surg* 1990;116:594–595.

117. Ishida K, Makoto S, Iida M, Takahashi M, Naito A, et al. [Cochlear implantation in children with inner ear malformation and postoperative performance.] *Nippon Jibiinkoka Gakkai Kaiho* 1999;102:1300–1310.

Cornelia de Lange Syndrome

118. Opitz JM. The Brachmann–de Lange syndrome. *Am J Med Genet* 1985;22:89–102.

119. Brachmann W. Ein fall von symmetrischer monodaktylie durch Ulnadefekt, mit symmetrischer flughautbildung in den ellenbeugen, sowie anderen abnormitaten (zwerghaftogkeit, halsrippen, behaarung). *Jarb Kinder Phys Erzie* 1916;84:225–235.

120. Wolland AM, Lindback T. Cornelia de Lange syndrome and the woman behind the syndrome. *Tidsskr Nor Laegeforen* 1995;115:3724–3726.

121. Ireland M, Donnai D, Burn J. Brachmann–de Lange syndrome. Delineation of the clinical phenotype. *Am J Med Genet* 1993;47:959–964.

122. Wilson GN, Hieber VC, Schmickel RD. The association of chromosome 3 duplication and the Cornelia de Lange syndrome. *J Pediatr* 1978;93:783.

123. Smith M, Herrell S, Lusher M, Lako L, Simpson C, et al. Genomic organisation of the human chordin gene and mutation screening of candidate Cornelia de Lange syndrome genes. *Hum Genet* 1999;105:104–111.

124. Blaschke RJ, Monaghan AP, Schiller S, Schechinger B, Rao E, et al. SHOT, a *SHOX*-related homeobox gene, is implicated in craniofacial, brain, heart, and limb development. *Proc Natl Acad Sci U S A* 1998;95:2406–2411.

125. Melegh B, Bock I, Gati I, Mehes K. Multiple mitochondrial DNA deletions and persistent hyperthermia in a patient with Brachmann-de Lange phenotype. *Am J Med Genet* 1996;65:82–88.

126. de Die–Smulders C, Schrander-Stumpel C, Fryns JP, Theunissen P. Exclusively maternal transmission of autosomal dominant Brachmann–de Lange syndrome. *Am J Med Genet* 1994;52:363.

127. Ackerman J, Gilbert-Barness E. Brachmann–de Lange syndrome. *Am J Med Genet* 1997;68:367–368.

128. Van Allen MI, Filippi G, Siegel-Bartelt J, Yong SL, McGillivray B, et al. Clinical variability within Brachmann–de Lange syndrome: a proposed classification system. *Am J Med Genet* 1993;47:947–958.

129. Hayashi M, Sakamoto K, Kurata K, Nagata J, Satoh J, Morimatsu Y. Septo-optic dysplasia with cerebellar hypoplasia in Cornelia de Lange syndrome. *Acta Neuropathol (Berl)* 1996;92:625–630.

130. Holthusen J, Rottingen JA. Cecal volvulus as a complication in Cornelia de Lange syndrome. A case report and literature review. *Tidsskr Nor Laegeforen* 1998;118:1559–1560.

131. Charles AK, Porter HJ, Sams V, Lunt P. Nephrogenic rests and renal abnormalities in Brachmann–de Lange syndrome. *Pediatr Pathol Lab Med* 1997;17:209–219.

132. Saal HM, Samango-Sprouse CA, Rodnan LA, Rosenbaum KN, Custer DA. Brachmann–de Lange syndrome with normal IQ. *Am J Med Genet* 1993;47:995–998.

133. Berney TP, Ireland M, Burn J. Behavioural phenotype of Cornelia de Lange syndrome. *Arch Dis Child* 1999;81:333–336.

134. Kousseff BG, Newkirk P, Root AW. Brachmann–de Lange syndrome. 1994 update. *Arch Pediatr Adolesc Med* 1994; 148:749–755.

135. Sekimoto H, Osada H, Kimura H, Kamiyama M, Arai K, Sekiya S. Prenatal findings in Brachmann–de Lange syndrome. *Arch Gynecol Obstet* 2000;263:182–184.

136. Aitken DA, Ireland M, Berry E, Crossley JA, Macri JN, et al. Second-trimester pregnancy associated plasma protein–A levels are reduced in Cornelia de Lange syndrome pregnancies. *Prenat Diagn* 1999;19:706–710.

137. Holder SE, Grimsley LM, Palmer RW, Butler LJ, Baraitser M. Partial trisomy 3q causing mild Cornelia de Lange phenotype. *J Med Genet* 1994;31:150–152.

138. Jackson L, Kline AD, Barr MA, Koch S. de Lange syndrome: a clinical review of 310 individuals. *Am J Med Genet* 1993;47:940–946.

139. McKenney RR, Elder FF, Garcia J, Northrup H. Brachmann–de Lange syndrome: autosomal dominant inheritance and male-to-male transmission. *Am J Med Genet* 1996;66:449–452.

140. Sheela SR. Cornelia de Lange syndrome: discordance in twins. *Indian Pediatr* 2000;37:458.

141. Krajewska-Walasek M, Chrzanowska K, Tylki-Szymanska A, Bialecka M. A further report of Brachmann–de Lange syndrome in two sibs with normal parents. *Clin Genet* 1995;47:324–327.

Craniosynostosis Syndromes (Fibroblast Growth Factor Receptor–Related)

142. Lajeunie E, Le Merrer M, Bonaiti-Pellie C, Marchac D, Renier D. Genetic study of nonsyndromic coronal craniosynostosis. *Am J Med Genet* 1995;55:500–504.

143. Gripp KW, McDonald-McGinn DM, Gaudenz K, Whitaker LA, Bartlett SP, et al. Identification of a genetic cause for isolated unilateral coronal synostosis: a unique mutation in the fibroblast growth factor receptor 3. *J Pediatr* 1998;132:714–716.

144. Blank CE. Apert's syndrome (a type of acrocephalosyndactyly). Observations on a British series of thirty-nine cases. *Ann Hum Genet* 1960;24:151–164.

145. Cohen MM Jr, Kreiborg S, Lammer EJ, Cordero JF, Mastroiacovo P, et al. Birth prevalence study of Apert syndrome. *Am J Med Genet* 1992;42:655–659.

146. Mason IJ. The ins and outs of fibroblast growth factors. *Cell* 1994;78:547–552.

147. Wilkie AO. Craniosynostosis: genes and mechanisms. *Hum Mol Genet* 1997;6:1647–1656.

148. Van Dissel-Emiliani FM, De Boer-Brouwer M, De Rooij DG. Effect of fibroblast growth factor-2 on Sertoli cells and gonocytes in coculture during the perinatal period. *Endocrinology* 1996;137:647–654.

149. Martinelli P, Paladini D, D'Armiento M, Scarano G. Prenatal diagnosis of cloverleaf skull in the subtype 2 Pfeiffer syndrome. *Clin Dysmorphol* 1997;6:89–90.

150. Hill LM, Grzybek PC. Sonographic findings with Pfeiffer syndrome. *Prenat Diagn* 1994;14:47–49.

151. Leo MV, Suslak L, Ganesh VL, Adhate A, Apuzzio JJ. Crouzon syndrome: prenatal ultrasound diagnosis by binocular diameters. *Obstet Gynecol* 1991;78:906–908.

152. Krakow D, Santulli T, Platt LD. Use of three-dimensional ultrasonography in differentiating craniosynostosis from severe fetal molding. *J Ultrasound Med* 2001;20:427–431.

Fraser Syndrome

153. Fraser GR. Our genetical "load": a review of some aspects of genetical variation. *Ann Hum Genet* 1962;25:387–415.

154. Thomas IT, Frias JL, Felix V, Sanchez de Leon L, Hernandez RA, Jones MC. Isolated and syndromic cryptophthalmos. *Am J Med Genet* 1986;25:85–98.

155. Karas DE, Respler DS. Fraser syndrome: a case report and review of the otolaryngologic manifestations. *Int J Pediatr Otorhinolaryngol* 1995;31:85–90.

156. Gattuso J, Patton MA, Baraitser M. The clinical spectrum of the Fraser syndrome: report of three new cases and review. *J Med Genet* 1987;24:549–555.

157. Fryns JP, van Schoubroeck D, Vandenberghe K, Nagels H, Klerckx P. Diagnostic echographic findings in cryptophthalmos syndrome (Fraser syndrome). *Prenat Diagn* 1997;17:582–584.

158. Stevens CA, McClanahan C, Steck A, Shiel FO, Carey JC. Pulmonary hyperplasia in the Fraser cryptophthalmos syndrome. *Am J Med Genet* 1994;52:427–431.

159. Feldman E, Shalev E, Weiner E, Cohen H, Zuckerman H. Microphthalmia—prenatal ultrasonic diagnosis: a case report. *Prenat Diagn* 1985;5:205–207.

160. King SJ, Pilling DW, Walkinshaw S. Fetal echogenic lung lesions: prenatal ultrasound diagnosis and outcome. *Pediatr Radiol* 1995;25:208–210.

161. Serville F, Carles D, Broussin B. Fraser syndrome: prenatal ultrasonic detection [Letter]. *Am J Med Genet* 1989;32:561–563.

162. Schauer GM, Dunn LK, Godmilow L, Eagle RC, Knisely AS. Prenatal diagnosis of Fraser syndrome at 18.5 weeks gestation, with autopsy findings at 19 weeks. *Am J Med Genet* 1990;37:583–591.

163. Lesniewicz R, Midro AT. Ultrasound diagnosis of four fetuses with Fraser syndrome during pregnancy. *Ginekol Pol* 1998;69:152.

164. Balci S, Altinok G, Ozaltin F, Aktas D, Niron EA, Onol B. Laryngeal atresia presenting as fetal ascites, olygohydramnios and lung appearance mimicking cystic adenomatoid malformation in a 25-week-old fetus with Fraser syndrome. *Prenat Diagn* 1999;19:856–858.

165. Dibben K, Rabinowitz YS, Shorr N, Graham JM Jr. Surgical correction of incomplete cryptophthalmos in Fraser syndrome. *Am J Ophthalmol* 1997;124:107–109.

166. Lurie IW, Cherstvoy ED. Renal agenesis as a diagnostic feature of the cryptophthalmos-syndactyly syndrome. *Clin Genet* 1984;25:528–532.

Fryns Syndrome

167. Fryns JP, Moerman F, Goddeeris P, Bossuyt C, van den Berghe H. A new lethal syndrome with cloudy cornea, dia-

phragmatic defects, and distal limb deformities. *Hum Genet* 1979;50:65–70.

168. Ayme S, Julian C, Gambarelli D, Mariotti B, Luciani A, et al. Fryns syndrome, report on 8 new cases. *Clin Genet* 1994;35:191–201.

169. Van Wymersch D, Favre R, Gasser B. Use of three-dimensional ultrasound to establish the prenatal diagnosis of Fryns syndrome. *Fetal Diagn Ther* 1996;11:355–340.

170. Hösli IM, Tercanli S, Rehder H, Holzgreve W. Cystic hygroma as an early first trimester ultrasound marker for recurrent Fryns syndrome. *Ultrasound Obstet Gynecol* 1997;10:422–424.

171. McPherson EW, Ketterer DM, Salsburey DJ. Pallister-Killian and Fryns syndromes: nosology. *Am J Med Genet* 1993;47:241–245.

172. Rodriguez JI, Garcia I, Alvarez J, Delicado A, Palacios J. Lethal Pallister-Killian syndrome: phenotypic similarity with Fryns syndrome. *Am J Med Genet* 1994;53:176–181.

173. Peltomaki P, Knuutila S, Ritvanen A, Kaitila I, de la Chapelle A. Pallister-Killian syndrome: cytogenetic and molecular studies. *Clin Genet* 1987;31:399–405.

174. Schinzel A. Tetrasomy 12p (Pallister-Killian syndrome). *J Med Genet* 1991;28:122–125.

175. Paladini D, Borghese A, Arienzo M, Teodoro A, Martinelli P, Nappi C. Prospective ultrasound diagnosis of Pallister-Killian syndrome in the second trimester of pregnancy: the importance of the fetal facial profile. *Prenat Diagn* 2000;20:996–998.

176. Jones KL. Fryns syndrome. In: *Smith's recognizable patterns of human malformation*. Philadelphia: WB Saunders, 1998:210–211.

177. Van Hove JL, Spiridigliozzi GA, Heinz R, McConkie-Rosell A, Iafolla AK, Kahler SG. Fryns syndrome survivors and neurologic outcome. *Am J Med Genet* 1995;59:334–340.

178. Meinecke P, Fryns JP. The Fryns syndrome: diaphragmatic defects, craniofacial dysmorphism, and distal digital hypoplasia. Further evidence for autosomal recessive inheritance. *Clin Genet* 1985;28:516–520.

179. Ramsing M, Gillessen-Kaesbach G, Holzgreve W, Fritz B, Rehder H. Variability in the phenotypic expression of Fryns syndrome: a report of two sibships. *Am J Med Genet* 2000;95:415–424.

180. Vargas JE, Cox GF, Korf BR. Discordant phenotype in monozygotic twins with Fryns syndrome. *Am J Med Genet* 2000;94:42–45.

Goldenhar Syndrome

181. Goldenhar M. Associations malformatives de l'oeil et de l'oreille: en particulier, le syndrome: dermoide epibulbaire–appendices auriculaires–fistula auris congenita et ses relations avec la dysostose mandibulo-faciale. *J Genet Hum* 1952;1:243–282.

182. Gorlin RJ, Jue KL, Jacobsen V, Goldschmidt E. Oculoauriculovertebral dysplasia. *J Pediatr* 1963;63:991–999.

183. Pridjian G, Gill WL, Shapira E. Goldenhar sequence and mosaic trisomy 22. *Am J Med Genet* 1995;59:411–413.

184. Ryan CA, Finer NN, Ives E. Discordance of signs in monozygotic twins concordant for the Goldenhar anomaly. *Am J Med Genet* 1988;29:755–761.

185. Ritchey ML, Norbeck J, Huang C, Keating MA, Bloom DA. Urologic manifestations of Goldenhar syndrome. *Urology* 1994;43:88–91.

186. Gustavson EE, Chen H. Goldenhar syndrome, anterior encephalocele, and aqueductal stenosis following fetal primidone exposure. *Teratology* 1985;32:13–17.

187. Jeanty P, Zaleski W, Fleischer AC. Prenatal sonographic diagnosis of lipoma of the corpus callosum in a fetus with Goldenhar syndrome. *Am J Perinatol* 1991;8:89–90.

188. Sutphen R, Galan-Gomez E, Cortada X, Newkirk PN, Kousseff BG. Tracheoesophageal anomalies in oculoauriculovertebral (Goldenhar) spectrum. *Clin Genet* 1995;48:66–71.

189. Sharma SN, Shrivastava S, Rao IM. Goldenhar syndrome with tetralogy of Fallot. *Indian Heart J* 1993;45:223.

190. Kumar A, Friedman JM, Taylor GP, Patterson MW. Pattern of cardiac malformation in oculoauriculovertebral spectrum. *Am J Med Genet* 1993;46:423–426.

191. Lin HJ, Owens TR, Sinow RM, Fu PC Jr, DeVito A, et al. Anomalous inferior and superior venae cavae with oculoauriculovertebral defect: review of Goldenhar complex and malformations of left-right asymmetry. *Am J Med Genet* 1998;75:88–94.

192. De Catte L, Laubach M, Legein J, Goossens A. Early prenatal diagnosis of oculoauriculovertebral dysplasia or the Goldenhar syndrome. *Ultrasound Obstet Gynecol* 1996;8:422–424.

193. Tamas DE, Mahony BS, Bowie JD, Woodruff WW 3d, Kay HH. Prenatal sonographic diagnosis of hemifacial microsomia (Goldenhar-Gorlin syndrome). *J Ultrasound Med* 1986;5:461–463.

194. Benacerraf BR, Frigoletto FD. Prenatal ultrasonographic recognition of Goldenhar's syndrome. *Am J Obstet Gynecol* 1988;159:950–952.

195. Monni G, Zoppi MA, Ibba RM, Putzolu M, Floris M. Nuchal translucency in multiple pregnancies. *Croat Med J* 2000;41:266–269.

196. Cohen J, Schanen NC. Branchial cleft anomaly, congenital heart disease, and biliary atresia: Goldenhar complex or Lambert syndrome? *Genet Couns* 2000;11:153–156.

197. Cohen MS, Samango-Sprouse CA, Stern HJ, Custer DA, Vaught DR, et al. Neurodevelopmental profile of infants and toddlers with oculo-auriculo-vertebral spectrum and the correlation of prognosis with physical findings. *Am J Med Genet* 1995;60:535–540.

198. Stellzig A, Basdra EK, Sontheimer D, Komposch G. Nonsurgical treatment of upper airway obstruction in oculoauriculovertebral dysplasia: a case report. *Eur J Orthod* 1998;20:111–114.

Heterotaxy Syndromes (Cardiosplenic Syndromes, Polysplenia/Asplenia)

199. Rose V, Izukawa T, Moes CAF. Syndromes of asplenia and polysplenia: a review of cardiac and non-cardiac malformations in 60 cases with special reference to diagnosis and prognosis. *Br Heart J* 1975;37:840–852.

200. Majeski JA, Upshur JK. Asplenia syndrome: a study of congenital anomalies in 16 cases. *JAMA* 1978;240:1508–1510.

201. Opitz JM, Gilbert EF. CNS anomalies and the midline as a "developmental field." *Am J Med Genet* 1982;12:443–455.

202. Fujinaga M. Development of sidedness of asymmetric body structures in vertebrates. *Int J Dev Biol* 1997;41:153–186.

203. Silva SR, Jeanty P. Asplenia-polysplenia syndromes. In: Jeanty P, ed. The fetus. Available at: http://www.thefetus.net/page.php?id=407. Accessed 1999.

204. Stanger P, Rudolph AM, Edwards JE. Cardiac malpositions: an overview based on study of sixty-five necropsy specimens. *Circulation* 1977;56:159–172.

205. Chandra RS. Biliary atresia and other structural anomalies in the congenital polysplenia syndrome. *J Pediatr* 1974;85: 649–655.

206. Karrer FM, Hall RJ, Lilly JR. Biliary atresia and the polysplenia syndrome. *J Pediatr Surg* 1991;26:524–527.

207. Davenport M, Savage M, Mowat AP, Howard ER. Biliary atresia splenic malformation syndrome: an etiologic and prognostic subgroup. *Surgery* 1993;113:662–668.

208. Tanano H, Hasegawa T, Kawahara H, Sasaki T, Okada A. Biliary atresia associated with congenital structural anomalies. *J Pediatr Surg* 1999;34:1687–1690.

209. Varela-Fascinetto G, Castaldo P, Fox IJ, Sudan D, Heffron TG, et al. Biliary atresia–polysplenia syndrome: surgical and clinical relevance in liver transplantation. *Ann Surg* 1998;227:583–589.

210. Anderson C, Devine WA, Anderson RH, Debich DE, Zuberbuhler JR. Abnormalities of the spleen in relation to congenital malformations of the heart: a survey of necropsy findings in children. *Br Heart J* 1990;63:122–128.

211. Peoples WM, Moller JH, Edwards JE. Polysplenia: a review of 146 cases. *Pediatr Cardiol* 1983;4:129–137.

212. Winer-Muram HT, Tonkin ILD. The spectrum of heterotaxic syndromes. *Radiol Clin North Am* 1989;27:1147–1170.

213. Moller JH, Nakib A, Anderson RC, Edwards RH. Congenital cardiac disease associated with polysplenia. A developmental complex of bilateral "left-sidedness." *Circulation* 1967;36:789–799.

214. Applegate KE, Goske MJ, Pierce G, Murphy D. Situs revisited: imaging of the heterotaxy syndrome. *Radiographics* 1999;19:837–852.

215. Brown DL, Emerson DS, Shulman LP, Doubilet PM, Felker RE, Van Praagh S. Predicting aneuploidy in fetuses with cardiac anomalies: significance of visceral situs and noncardiac anomalies. *J Ultrasound Med* 1993;3:153–161.

216. Garcia OL, Mehta AV, Pickoff AS, Tamer DF, Ferrer PL, et al. Left isomerism and complete atrioventricular block: a report of 6 cases. *Am J Cardiol* 1981;48:1103–1107.

217. Shaw CT. Polysplenia in a fetus with bradycardia from 26 to 36 weeks' gestation, complex cardiac malformations, and heart block. *J Am Osteopath Assoc* 1990;90:1100–1102.

218. Sheley RC, Nyberg DA, Kapur R. Azygous continuation of the interrupted inferior vena cava: a clue to prenatal diagnosis of the cardiosplenic syndromes. *J Ultrasound Med* 1995;14:381–387.

219. Belfar HL, Hill LM, Peterson CS, Young K, Hixson J, et al. Sonographic imaging of the fetal azygous vein. Normal and pathologic appearance. *J Ultrasound Med* 1990;9:569–573.

220. Abuhamad AZ, Robinson JN, Bogdan D, Tannous RJ. Color Doppler of the splenic artery in the prenatal diagnosis of heterotaxic syndromes. *Am J Perinatol* 1999;16:469–473.

221. Gray SW, Skandalakis JE. Body asymmetry and splenic anomalies. In: *Embryology for surgeons*. Philadelphia: WB Saunders, 1972:877–895.

222. Mayo CW, Rice RG. Situs inversus totalis: statistical review of data on seventy-six cases, with special reference to diseases of the biliary tract. *Arch Surg* 1949;58:724–730.

223. Culbertson CB, George BL, Day RW, Laks H, Williams RG. Factors influencing survival of patients with heterotaxy syndrome undergoing the Fontan procedure. *J Am Coll Cardiol* 1992;20:678–684.

224. Kosaki K, Casey B. Genetics of human left-right axis malformations. *Semin Cell Dev Biol* 1998;9:89–99.

225. Cesko I, Hajdu J, Marton T, Tarnai L, Papp Z. Polysplenia and situs inversus in siblings. Case reports. *Fetal Diagn Ther* 2001;16:1–3.

Holt-Oram Syndrome

226. Holt M, Oram S. Familial heart disease with skeletal malformations. *Br Heart J* 1990;22:236–242.

227. Bonnet D, Terrett J, Pequignot-Viegas E, Weissenbach J, Munnich A, et al. Gene localisation in 12q12 in Holt-Oram atriodigital syndrome. *Arch Mal Coeur Vaiss* 1995;88:661–666.

228. Campbell CE, Casey G, Goodrich K. Genomic structure of *TBX2* indicates conservation with distantly related T-box genes. *Mamm Genome* 1998;9:70–73.

229. Smith J. Brachyury and the T-box genes. *Curr Opin Genet Dev* 1997;7:474–480.

230. Li QY, Newbury-Ecob RA, Terrett JA, Wilson DI, Curtis AR, et al. Holt-Oram syndrome is caused by mutations in *TBX5*, a member of the Brachyury (T) gene family. *Nat Genet* 1997;15:21–29.

231. Basson CT, Huang T, Lin RC, Bachinsky DR, Weremowicz S, et al. Different *TBX5* interactions in heart and limb defined by Holt-Oram syndrome mutations. *Proc Natl Acad Sci U S A* 1999;96:2919–2924.

232. Newbury-Ecob RA, Leanage R, Raeburn JA, Young ID. Holt-Oram syndrome: a clinical genetic study. *J Med Genet* 1996;33:300–307.

233. Sletten LJ, Pierpont ME. Variation in severity of cardiac disease in Holt-Oram syndrome. *Am J Med Genet* 1996;65:128–132.

234. Brons JT, van Geijn HP, Wladimiroff JW, van der Harten JJ, Kwee ML, et al. Prenatal ultrasound diagnosis of the Holt-Oram syndrome. *Prenat Diagn* 1988;8:175–181.

235. Tongsong T, Chanprapaph P. Prenatal sonographic diagnosis of Holt-Oram syndrome. *J Clin Ultrasound* 2000;28:98–100.

236. Weber M, Wenz W, van Riel A, Kaufmann A, Graf J. The Holt-Oram syndrome. Review of the literature and current orthopedic treatment concepts. *Z Orthop Ihre Grenzgeb* 1997;135:368–375.

Joubert Syndrome

237. Joubert M, Eisenring JJ, Andermann F. Familial dysgenesis of the vermis: a syndrome of hyperventilation, abnormal eye movements and retardation. *Neurology* 1968;18:302–303.

238. Saar K, Al-Gazali L, Sztriha L, Rueschendorf F, Nur-E-Kamal M, et al. Homozygosity mapping in families with Joubert syndrome identifies a locus on chromosome 9q34.3

and evidence for genetic heterogeneity. *Am J Hum Genet* 1999;65:1666–1671.

239. Pellegrino JE, Lensch MW, Muenke M, Chance PF. Clinical and molecular analysis in Joubert syndrome. *Am J Med Genet* 1997;72:59–62.

240. Suzuki T, Hakozaki M, Kubo N, Kuroda K, Ogawa A. A case of cranial meningocele associated with Joubert syndrome. *Childs Nerv Syst* 1996;12:280–282.

241. Yachnis AT, Rorke LB. Neuropathology of Joubert syndrome. *J Child Neurol* 1999;14:655–659; discussion 669–672.

242. Yachnis AT, Rorke LB. Cerebellar and brainstem development: an overview in relation to Joubert syndrome. *J Child Neurol* 1999;14:570–573.

243. Nuri Sener R. A patient with ectodermal dysplasia, Joubert's syndrome, and brain cysts. *Comput Med Imaging Graph* 1998;22:349–351.

244. van Royen-Kerkhof A, Poll-The BT, Kleijer WJ, van Diggelen OP, Aerts JM, et al. Coexistence of Gaucher disease type 1 and Joubert syndrome. *J Med Genet* 1998;35:965–966.

245. Silverstein DM, Zacharowicz L, Edelman M, Lee SC, Greifer I, Rapin I. Joubert syndrome associated with multicystic kidney disease and hepatic fibrosis. *Pediatr Nephrol* 1997; 11:746–749.

246. Campbell S, Tsannatos C, Pearce JM. The prenatal diagnosis of Joubert's syndrome of familial agenesis of the cerebellar vermis. *Prenat Diagn* 1984;4:391–395.

247. Anderson JS, Gorey MT, Pasternak JF, Trommer BL. Joubert's syndrome and prenatal hydrocephalus. *Pediatr Neurol* 1999;20:403–405.

248. Wang P, Chang FM, Chang CH, Yu CH, Jung YC, Huang CC. Prenatal diagnosis of Joubert syndrome complicated with encephalocele using two-dimensional and three-dimensional ultrasound. *Ultrasound Obstet Gynecol* 1999;14:360–362.

249. Ni Scanaill S, Crowley P, Hogan M, Stuart B. Abnormal prenatal sonographic findings in the posterior cranial fossa: a case of Joubert's syndrome. *Ultrasound Obstet Gynecol* 1999;13:71–74.

250. Aslan H, Ulker V, Gulcan EM, Numanoglu C, Gul A, et al. Prenatal diagnosis of Joubert syndrome: a case report. *Prenat Diagn* 2002;22:13–16.

251. Maria BL, Hoang KB, Tusa RJ, Mancuso AA, Hamed LM, et al. "Joubert syndrome" revisited: key ocular motor signs with magnetic resonance imaging correlation. *J Child Neurol* 1997;12:423–430.

252. Shen WC, Shian WJ, Chen CC, Chi CS, Lee SK, Lee KR. MRI of Joubert's syndrome. *Eur J Radiol* 1994;18:30–33.

253. Quisling RG, Barkovich AJ, Maria BL. Magnetic resonance imaging features and classification of central nervous system malformations in Joubert syndrome. *J Child Neurol* 1999;14:628–635.

254. Reynders CS, Pauker SP, Benacerraf BR. First trimester isolated fetal nuchal lucency: significance and outcome. *J Ultrasound Med* 1997;16:101–105.

255. Keogan MT, DeAtkine AB, Hertzberg BS. Cerebellar vermian defects: antenatal sonographic appearance and clinical significance. *J Ultrasound Med* 1994;13:607–611.

256. Steinlin M, Schmid M, Landau K, Boltshauser E. Follow-up in children with Joubert syndrome. *Neuropediatrics* 1997;28:204–211.

257. Fennell EB, Gitten JC, Dede DE, Maria BL. Cognition, behavior, and development in Joubert syndrome. *J Child Neurol* 1999;14:592–596.

258. Gitten J, Dede D, Fennell E, Quisling R, Maria BL. Neurobehavioral development in Joubert syndrome. *J Child Neurol* 1998;13:391–397.

259. Raynes HR, Shanske A, Goldberg S, Burde R, Rapin I. Joubert syndrome: monozygotic twins with discordant phenotypes. *J Child Neurol* 1999;14:649–654.

Klippel-Trénaunay-Weber Syndrome

260. Klippel M, Trénaunay P. Du naevus variqueux osteo-hypertrophique. *Arch Gen Med* 1900;185:641–672.

261. Weber FP. Angioma formation in connection with hypertrophy of limbs and hemihypertrophy. *Br J Dermatol* 1907;19:231–235.

262. Berry SA, Peterson C, Mize W, Bloom K, Zachary C, et al. Klippel-Trénaunay syndrome. *Am J Med Genet* 1998;79: 319–326.

263. Jacob AG, Driscoll DJ, Shaughnessy WJ, Stanson AW, Clay RP, Gloviczki P. Klippel-Trénaunay syndrome: spectrum and management. *Mayo Clin Proc* 1998;73:28–36.

264. Happle R. Mosaicism in human skin. Understanding the patterns and mechanisms. *Arch Dermatol* 1993;129:1460–1470.

265. Christenson L, Yankowitz J, Robinson R. Prenatal diagnosis of Klippel-Trénaunay-Weber syndrome as a cause for *in utero* heart failure and severe postnatal sequelae. *Prenat Diagn* 1997;17:1176–1180.

266. Paladini D, Lamberti A, Teodoro A, Liguori M, D'Armiento M, et al. Prenatal diagnosis and hemodynamic evaluation of Klippel-Trénaunay-Weber syndrome. *Ultrasound Obstet Gynecol* 1998;12:215–217.

267. Shih JC, Shyu MK, Chang CY, Lee CN, Lin GJ, et al. Application of the surface rendering technique of three-dimensional ultrasound in prenatal diagnosis and counseling of Klippel-Trénaunay-Weber syndrome. *Prenat Diagn* 1998;18:298–302.

268. Martin WL, Ismail KM, Brace V, McPherson L, Chapman S, Kilby MD. Klippel-Trénaunay-Weber (KTW) syndrome: the use of *in utero* magnetic resonance imaging (MRI) in a prospective diagnosis. *Prenat Diagn* 2001;21:311–313.

269. Wiedemann HR, Burgio GR, Aldenhoff P, Kunze J, Kaufmann HJ, Schirg E. The Proteus syndrome: partial gigantism of the hands and/or feet, nevi, hemihypertrophy, subcutaneous tumors, macrocephaly or other skull anomalies and possible accelerated growth and visceral affections. *Eur J Pediatr* 1983;140:5–12.

270. Cohen MM Jr. Understanding Proteus syndrome, unmasking the Elephant Man, and stemming elephant fever. *Neurofibromatosis* 1988;1:260–280.

271. Torregrosa A, Marti-Bonmati L, Higueras V, Poyatos C, Sanchis A. Klippel-Trénaunay syndrome: frequency of cerebral and cerebellar hemihypertrophy on MRI. *Neuroradiology* 2000;42:420–423.

272. Noel AA, Gloviczki P, Cherry KJ Jr, Rooke TW, Stanson AW, Driscoll DJ. Surgical treatment of venous malformations in Klippel-Trénaunay syndrome. *J Vasc Surg* 2000;32: 840–847.

273. Lorda-Sanchez I, Prieto L, Rodriguez-Pinilla E, Martinez-Frias ML. Increased parental age and number of pregnancies in Klippel-Trénaunay-Weber syndrome. *Ann Hum Genet* 1998;62(Pt 3):235–239.

274. Ceballos-Quintal JM, Pinto-Escalante D, Castillo-Zapata I. A new case of Klippel-Trénaunay-Weber (KTW) syndrome: evidence of autosomal dominant inheritance. *Am J Med Genet* 1996;63:426–427.

275. Aelvoet GE, Jorens PG, Roelen LM. Genetic aspects of the Klippel-Trénaunay syndrome. *Br J Dermatol* 1992;126:603–607.

Limb-Body Wall Complex

276. Van Allen MI, Curry C, Gallagher L. Limb body wall complex: I. Pathogenesis. *Am J Med Genet* 1987;28:529–548.

277. Van Allen M, Curry C, Walden CE, Gallagher L, Patten RM. Limb-body wall complex: II. Limb and spine defects. *Am J Med Genet* 1987;28:549–565.

278. Kurosawa K, Imaizumi K, Masuno M, Kuroki Y. Epidemiology of limb-body wall complex in Japan. *Am J Med Genet* 1994;51:143–146.

279. Balentyne G, Moesinger AC, James LS, Blank WA. Short umbilical cord and multiple anomalies in experimental oligohydramnios. *Teratology* 1978;17[Suppl 2]:43A.

280. Miller ME, Higginbottom M, Smith DW. Short umbilical cord: its origin and relevance. *Pediatrics* 1981;67:618.

281. Russo R, D'Armiento M, Angrisani P, Vecchione R. Limb body wall complex: a critical review and a nosological proposal. *Am J Med Genet* 1993;47:893–900.

282. Craven CM, Carey JC, Ward K. Umbilical cord agenesis in limb body wall defect. *Am J Med Genet* 1997;71:97–105.

283. Goldstein I, Winn HN, Hobbins JC. Prenatal diagnosis criteria for body stalk anomaly. *Am J Perinatol* 1989;6:84.

284. Patten RM, Van Allen M, Mack LA, Wilson D, Nyberg D, et al. Limb-body wall complex: in utero sonographic diagnosis of a complicated fetal malformation. *AJR Am J Roentgenol* 1986;146:1019–1024.

285. Gorczyca DP, Lindfors KK, McGahan JP, Hanson FW. Limb-body-wall complex: another cause for elevated maternal serum alpha fetoprotein. *J Clin Ultrasound* 1990;18:198–201.

286. Nevils BG, Maciulla JE, Izquierdo LA, et al. Umbilical cord, short umbilical cord syndrome. *Fetus* 1993;7599:1–4.

287. Jauniaux E, Vyas S, Finlayson C, Moscoso G, Driver M, Campbell S. Early sonographic diagnosis of body stalk anomaly. *Prenat Diagn* 1990;10:127–132.

288. Giacoia GP. Body stalk anomaly: congenital absence of the umbilical cord. *Obstet Gynecol* 1992;80:527–529.

289. Shalev E, Eliyahu S, Battino S, Weiner E. First trimester transvaginal sonographic diagnosis of body stalk anomaly. *J Ultrasound Med* 1995;14:641–642.

290. Daskalakis G, Sebire NJ, Jurkovic D, Snijders RJ, Nicolaides KH. Body stalk anomaly at 10–14 weeks of gestation. *Ultrasound Obstet Gynecol* 1997;10:416–418.

291. Ginsberg NE, Cadkin A, Strom C. Prenatal diagnosis of body stalk anomaly in the first trimester of pregnancy. *Ultrasound Obstet Gynecol* 1997;10:419–421.

292. Becker R, Runkel S, Entezami M. Prenatal diagnosis of body stalk anomaly at 9 weeks of gestation. Case report. *Fetal Diagn Ther* 2000;15:301–303.

293. Paul C, Zosmer N, Jurkovic D, Nicolaides K. A case of body stalk anomaly at 10 weeks of gestation. *Ultrasound Obstet Gynecol* 2001;17:157–159.

294. Chen CP, Shih JC, Chan YJ. Prenatal diagnosis of limb-body wall complex using two- and three-dimensional ultrasound. *Prenat Diagn* 2000;20:1020.

295. Negishi H, Yaegashi M, Kato EH, Yamada H, Okuyama K, Fujimoto S. Prenatal diagnosis of limb-body wall complex. *J Reprod Med* 1998;43:659–664.

Meckel-Gruber Syndrome

296. Meckel JF. Beschreibung zweier, durch sehr aehnliche Bildungsabweichungen entstellter Geschwister. *Dtsch Arch Physiol* 1822;7:99–172.

297. Salonen R, Norio R. The Meckel syndrome in Finland: epidemiologic and genetic aspects. *Am J Med Genet* 1984;18:691–698.

298. Paavola P, Salonen R, Weissenbach U, Peltonen L. The locus for Meckel syndrome with multiple congenital anomalies maps to chromosome 17q21-q24. *Nat Genet* 1995;11:213–215.

299. Roume J, Genin E, Cormier-Daire V, Ma HW, Mehaye B, et al. A gene for Meckel syndrome maps to chromosome 11q13. *Am J Hum Genet* 1998;63:1095–1101.

300. Pachi A, Giancotti A, Torcia F, de Prosperi V, Maggi E. Meckel-Gruber syndrome: ultrasonographic diagnosis at 13 weeks' gestational age in an at-risk case. *Prenat Diagn* 1989;9:187–190.

301. Sepulveda W, Sebire NJ, Souka A, Snijders RJ, Nicolaides KH. Diagnosis of the Meckel-Gruber syndrome at eleven to fourteen weeks' gestation. *Am J Obstet Gynecol* 1997;176:316–319.

302. Al-Gazali LI, Abdel Raziq A, Al-Shather W, Shahzadi R, Azhar N. Meckel syndrome and Dandy Walker malformation. *Clin Dysmorphol* 1996;5:73–76.

303. Herriot R, Hallam LA, Gray ES. Dandy-Walker malformation in the Meckel syndrome. *Am J Med Genet* 1991;39:207–210.

304. Yapar EG, Ekici E, Dogan M, Gokmen O. Meckel-Gruber syndrome concomitant with Dandy-Walker malformation: prenatal sonographic diagnosis in two cases. *Clin Dysmorphol* 1996;5:357–362.

305. Cincinnati P, Neri ME, Valentini A. Dandy-Walker anomaly in Meckel-Gruber syndrome. *Clin Dysmorphol* 2000;9:35–38.

306. Nyberg DA, Hallesy D, Mahony BS, Hirsch JH, Luthy DA, Hickok D. Meckel-Gruber syndrome. Importance of prenatal diagnosis. *J Ultrasound Med* 1990;9:691–696.

307. Gallimore AP, Davies PF. Meckel syndrome: prenatal ultrasonographic diagnosis in two cases showing marked differences in phenotypic expression. *Aust Radiol* 1992;36:62–64.

Nager Syndrome (Acrofacial Dysostosis 1)

308. Nager FR, de Reynier JP. Das Gehoerorgan bei den Angeborenen Kopfmissbildungen. *Pract Otorhinolaryng* 1948;10 [Suppl 2]:1–128.

309. Slingenberg B. Misbildungen von Extremitaeten. *Virchows Arch Pathol Anat* 1908;193:1–92.

310. Zori RT, Gray BA, Bent-Williams A, Driscoll DJ, Williams CA, Zackowski JL. Preaxial acrofacial dysostosis (Nager syn-

drome) associated with an inherited and apparently balanced X;9 translocation: prenatal and postnatal late replication studies. *Am J Med Genet* 1993;46:379–383.

311. Benson CB, Pober BR, Hirsh MP, Doubilet PM. Sonography of Nager acrofacial dysostosis syndrome *in utero*. *J Ultrasound Med* 1988;7:163–167.

312. Rodríguez JL, Palacios J, Urioste M. New acrofacial dysostosis syndrome in 3 sibs. *Am J Med Genet* 1990;35:484–489.

313. Friedman RA, Wood E, Pransky SM, Seid AB, Kearns DB. Nager acrofacial dysostosis: management of a difficult airway. *Int J Pediatr Otorhinolaryngol* 1996;35:69–72.

314. Denny AD, Talisman R, Hanson PR, Recinos RF. Mandibular distraction osteogenesis in very young patients to correct airway obstruction. *Plast Reconstr Surg* 2001;108:302–311.

315. Hecht JT, Immken LL, Harris LF, Malini S, Scott CI Jr. The Nager syndrome. *Am J Med Genet* 1987;27:965–969.

Noonan Syndrome

316. Noonan JA. Hypertelorism with Turner phenotype. A new syndrome with associated congenital heart disease. *Am J Dis Child* 1968;116:373–380.

317. Nora JJ, Nora AH, Sinha AK, Spangler RD, Lubs HA Jr. The Ullrich-Noonan syndrome (Turner phenotype). *Am J Dis Child* 1974;127:48–55.

318. Bolton MR, Pugh DM, Mattioli LF, Dunn MI, Schimke RN. The Noonan syndrome: a family study. *Ann Intern Med* 1974;80:626–629.

319. van der Burgt I, Berends E, Lommen E, van Beersum S, Hamel B, Mariman E. Clinical and molecular studies in a large Dutch family with Noonan syndrome. *Am J Med Genet* 1994;53:187–191.

320. Brady AF, Jamieson CR, van der Burgt I, Crosby A, van Reen M, et al. Further delineation of the critical region for Noonan syndrome on the long arm of chromosome 12. *Eur J Hum Genet* 1997;5:336–337.

321. Legius E, Schollen E, Matthijs G, Fryns JP. Fine mapping of Noonan/cardio-facio cutaneous syndrome in a large family. *Eur J Hum Genet* 1998;6:32–37.

322. Lee L, Dowhanick-Morrissette J, Katz A, Jukofsky L, Krantz ID. Chromosomal localization, genomic characterization, and mapping to the Noonan syndrome critical region of the human Deltex (*DTX1*) gene. *Hum Genet* 2000;107:577–581.

323. Izquierdo L, Kushnir O, Sanchez D, Curet L, Olney P, et al. Prenatal diagnosis of Noonan's syndrome in a female infant with spontaneous resolution of cystic hygroma and hydrops. *West J Med* 1990;152:418–421.

324. Donnenfeld AE, Nazir MA, Sindoni F, Librizzi RJ. Prenatal sonographic documentation of cystic hygroma regression in Noonan syndrome. *Am J Med Genet* 1991;39:461–465.

325. Adekunle O, Gopee A, el-Sayed M, Thilaganathan B. Increased first trimester nuchal translucency: pregnancy and infant outcomes after routine screening for Down's syndrome in an unselected antenatal population. *Br J Radiol* 1999;72:457–460.

326. Sonesson SE, Fouron JC, Lessard M. Intrauterine diagnosis and evolution of a cardiomyopathy in a fetus with Noonan's syndrome. *Acta Paediatr* 1992;81:368–370.

327. Benacerraf BR, Greene MF, Holmes LB. The prenatal sonographic features of Noonan's syndrome. *J Ultrasound Med* 1989;8:59–63.

328. Nisbet DL, Griffin DR, Chitty LS. Prenatal features of Noonan syndrome. *Prenat Diagn* 1999;19:642–647.

329. Currarino G, Stannard MW, Kolni H. Umbilical vein draining into the inferior vena cava via the internal iliac vein, bypassing the liver. *Pediatr Radiol* 1991;21:265–266.

330. Bradley E, Kean L, Twining P, James D. Persistent right umbilical vein in a fetus with Noonan's syndrome: a case report. *Ultrasound Obstet Gynecol* 2001;17:76–78.

331. Aranguren G, Garcia-Minaur S, Loridan L, Uribarren A, Martin Vargas L, Rodriguez-Soriano J. Multiple-marker screen positive results in Noonan syndrome. *Prenat Diagn* 1996;16:183–184.

332. Yu CM, Chow LT, Sanderson JE. Dilated cardiomyopathy in Noonan's syndrome. *Int J Cardiol* 1996;56:83–85.

Oral-Facial-Digital Syndrome

333. Gorlin RJ, Anderson VE, Scott CR. Hypertrophied frenuli, oligophrenia, familial trembling and anomalies of the hand: report of four cases in one family and a forme fruste in another. *N Engl J Med* 1961;264:486–489.

334. Feather SA, Woolf AS, Donnai D, Malcolm S, Winter RM. The oral-facial-digital syndrome type 1 (OFD1), a cause of polycystic kidney disease and associated malformations, maps to Xp22.2–Xp22.3. *Hum Mol Genet* 1997;6:1163–1167.

335. Malcolm S, Feather SA, Woolf AS, Donnai D, Winter RM. Oral-facial-digital syndrome type 1 (OFD1), a male-lethal X linked disorder, maps to Xp22.2-Xp22.3 [Abstract]. *Am J Hum Genet* 1997;61(Suppl):A283.

336. Iaccarino M, Lonardo F, Giugliano M, Della Bruna MD. Prenatal diagnosis of Mohr syndrome by ultrasonography. *Prenat Diagn* 1985;5:415–418.

337. Shipp TD, Chu GC, Benacerraf B. Prenatal diagnosis of oral-facial-digital syndrome, type I. *J Ultrasound Med* 2000;19:491–494.

338. Leao MJ, Ribeiro-Silva ML. Orofaciodigital syndrome type I in a patient with severe CNS defects. *Pediatr Neurol* 1995;13:247–251.

339. Toriello HV, Lemire EG. Optic nerve coloboma, Dandy-Walker malformation, microglossia, tongue hamartomata, cleft palate and apneic spells: an existing oral-facial-digital syndrome or a new variant? *Clin Dysmorphol* 2002;11:19–23.

340. Haug K, Khan S, Fuchs S, Konig R. OFD II, OFD VI, and Joubert syndrome manifestations in 2 sibs. *Am J Med Genet* 2000;91:135–137.

341. Nagai K, Nagao M, Nagao M, Yanai S, Minagawa K, et al. Oral-facial-digital syndrome type IX in a patient with Dandy-Walker malformation. *J Med Genet* 1998;35:342–344.

342. Majewski E, Ozturk B, Gillessen-Kaesbach G. Jeune syndrome with tongue lobulation and preaxial polydactyly, and Jeune syndrome with situs inversus and asplenia: compound heterozygosity Jeune-Mohr and Jeune-Ivemark? *Am J Med Genet* 1996;63:74–79.

343. Krakow D, Hall JG. The dysostoses. In: Rimoin DL, Connor JM, Pyeritz RE, eds. *Emery and Rimoin's principles and*

practice of medical genetics, 3rd ed. London: Churchhill Livingstone, 1997.

Roberts Syndrome

344. Roberts JB. A child with double cleft of lip and palate, protrusion of the intermaxillary portion of the upper jaw and imperfect development of the bones of the four extremities. *Ann Surg* 1919;70:252.

345. Appelt H, Gerken H, Lenz W. Tetraphokomelie mit Lippen-Kiefer-Gaumenspalte und Clitorishypertrophie—Ein Syndrom. *Paediatr Paedol* 1966;2:119.

346. Herrmann J, et al. A familial dysmorphogenetic syndrome of limb deformities, characteristic facial appearance and associated anomalies: the pseudothalidomide or SC-syndrome. *Birth Defects* 1969;5:81.

347. Jones KL. Roberts–SC phocomelia. In: *Smith's recognizable patterns of human malformation*. Philadelphia: WB Saunders, 1997:298–299.

348. German J. Roberts syndrome 1. Cytological evidence for a disturbance in chromatid pairing. *Clin Genet* 1979;16:441–447.

349. Freeman MVR, Williams WW, Schimke N, Temtamy SA, Vachier E, German J. The Roberts syndrome. *Clin Genet* 1974;5:1–16.

350. Van Den Berg DJ, Francke U. Roberts syndrome: a review of 100 cases and a new rating system for severity. *Am J Med Genet* 1993;15:1104–1123.

351. Mann NP, Fitzsimmons J, Fitzsimmons E, Cooke P. Roberts syndrome: clinical and cytogenetic aspects. *J Med Genet* 1982;19:116–119.

352. Robins DB, Ladda RL, Thieme GA, Boal DK, Emanuel BS, Zackai EH. Prenatal detection of Roberts-SC phocomelia syndrome: report of 2 sibs with characteristic manifestations. *Am J Med Genet* 1989;32:390–394.

353. Stioui S, Privitera O, Brambati B, Zuliani G, Lalatta F, Simoni G. First-trimester prenatal diagnosis of Roberts syndrome. *Prenat Diagn* 1992;12:145–149.

354. Palladini D, Palmieri S, Lecora M, Perone L, Di Meglio A, et al. Prenatal ultrasound diagnosis of Roberts syndrome in a family with negative history. *Ultrasound Obstet Gynecol* 1996;7:208–210.

355. Souter V, Nyberg D, Gonzalez A, Siebert JR, Rutledge JC, Glass I. Upper limb phocomelia associated with increased nuchal translucency in a monochorionic twin pregnancy. *J Ultrasound Med* 2002;21:355–360.

356. Stanley WS, Pai GS, Horger E, Yan YS, McNeal KS. Incidental detection of premature centromere separation in amniocytes associated with a mild form of Roberts syndrome. *Prenat Diagn* 1988;8:565–569.

357. Tomkins DJ. Premature centromere separation and the prenatal diagnosis of Roberts syndrome [Letter]. *Prenat Diagn* 1989;9:450–452.

358. Louie E, German J. Robert's syndrome. II. Aberrant Y-chromosome behavior. *Clin Genet* 1981;19:71–74.

359. Benzacken B, Savary JB, Manouvrier S, Bucourt M, Gonzalez J. Prenatal diagnosis of Roberts syndrome: two new cases. *Prenat Diagn* 1996;16:125–130.

360. Parry DM, Mulvihill JJ, Tsai S, Kaiser-Kupfer MI, Cowan JM. SC phocomelia syndrome, premature centromere separation, and congenital cranial nerve paralysis in two sisters, one with malignant melanoma. *Am J Med Genet* 1986;24:653–672.

361. Maserati E, Pasquali F, Zuffardi O, Buttitta P, Cuoco C, et al. Roberts syndrome: phenotypic variation, cytogenetic definition and heterozygote detection. *Ann Genet* 1991;34:239–246.

Smith-Lemli-Opitz Syndrome

362. Smith DW, Lemli L, Opitz JM. A newly recognized syndrome of multiple congenital anomalies. *J Pediatr* 1964;64:210–217.

363. Opitz JM, Zellweger H, Shannon WR, Ptacek LJ. The RSH syndrome. *Birth Defects* 1969;V(2):43–52.

364. Irons M, Elias ER, Salen G, Tint GS, Batta AK. Defective cholesterol biosynthesis in Smith-Lemli-Opitz syndrome. *Lancet* 1993;341:1414.

365. Natowicz MR, Evans JE. Abnormal bile acids in the Smith-Lemli-Opitz syndrome. *Am J Med Genet* 1994;50:364–367.

366. Kelley RI. Editorial. A new face for an old syndrome. *Am J Med Genet* 1997;68:251–256.

367. Kelley R, Hennekam RC. The Smith-Lemli-Opitz syndrome. *J Med Genet* 2000;37:321–335.

368. Moebius FF, Fitzky BU, Lee JN, Paik YK, Glossmann H. Molecular cloning and expression of the human delta7-sterol reductase. *Proc Natl Acad Sci U S A* 1998;95:1899–1902.

369. Battaile KP, Steiner RD. Smith-Lemli-Opitz syndrome: the first malformation syndrome associated with defective cholesterol synthesis. *Mol Genet Metab* 2000;71:154–162.

370. Pauli RM, Williams MS, Josephson KD, Tint GS. Smith-Lemli-Opitz syndrome: thirty-year follow-up of "S" of "RSH" syndrome. *Am J Med Genet* 1997;68:260–262.

371. Opitz M, De La Cruz F. Cholesterol metabolism in the RSH/Smith-Lemli-Opitz syndrome: summary of NICHD conference. *Am J Med Genet* 1994;50:326–338.

372. Tint GS, Irons MB, Elias ER, Batta AK, Frieden R, et al. Defective cholesterol biosynthesis associated with the Smith-Lemli-Opitz syndrome. *N Engl J Med* 1994;330:107–113.

373. Tint GS, Seller M, Hughes-Benzie R, Batta AK, Shefer S, et al. Markedly increased tissue concentrations of 7–dehydrocholesterol combined with low levels of cholesterol are characteristic of the Smith-Lemli-Opitz syndrome. *J Lipid Res* 1995;36:89–95.

374. Roessler E, Belloni E, Gaudenz K, Jay B, Berta P, et al. Mutations in the human Sonic Hedgehog gene cause holoprosencephaly. *Nat Genet* 1996;14:357–360.

375. Silva SR, Jeanty P. Prenatal ultrasound findings of Smith-Lemli-Opitz syndrome. http://www.thefetus.net/page.php?id=442. In: Jeanty P, ed. The fetus. 2000.

376. Abuelo DN, Tint GS, Kelley R, Batta AK, Shefer S, Salen G. Prenatal detection of the cholesterol biosynthetic defect in the Smith-Lemli-Opitz syndrome by the analysis of amniotic fluid sterols. *Am J Med Genet* 1995;56:281–285.

377. Cunniff C, Kratz LE, Moser A, Natowicz MR, Kelley RI. Clinical and biochemical spectrum of patients with RSH/Smith-Lemli-Opitz syndrome and abnormal cholesterol metabolism. *Am J Med Genet* 1997;68:263–269.

378. Ryan AK, Bartlett K, Clayton P, et al. Smith-Lemli-Opitz syndrome; a variable clinical and biochemical phenotype. *J Med Genet* 1998;35:558–565.

379. Hyett JA, Clayton PT, Moscoso G, Nicolaides KH. Increased first trimester nuchal translucency as a prenatal manifestation of Smith-Lemli-Opitz syndrome. *Am J Med Genet* 1995;58:374–376.

380. Maymon R, Ogle RF, Chitty LS. Smith-Lemli-Opitz syndrome presenting with persisting nuchal oedema and non-immune hydrops. *Prenat Diagn* 1999;19:105–107.

381. Kratz LE, Kelley RI. Prenatal diagnosis of the RSH/Smith-Lemli-Opitz syndrome. *Am J Med Genet* 1999;82:376–381.

382. Canick JA, Abuelo DN, Bradley LA, Tint GS. Maternal serum marker levels in two pregnancies affected with Smith-Lemli-Opitz syndrome. *Prenat Diagn* 1997;17:187–189.

383. Bick DP, McCorkle D, Stanley WS, Stern HJ, Staszak P, et al. Prenatal diagnosis of Smith-Lemli-Opitz syndrome in a pregnancy with low maternal serum estriol and a sex-reversed fetus. *Prenat Diagn* 1999;19:68–71.

384. Donnai D, Young ID, Owen WG, Clark SA, Miller PFW, Knox, WF. The lethal congenital anomaly syndrome of polydactyly, sex reversal, renal hypoplasia and unilobar lungs. *J Med Genet* 1986;23:64–71.

385. Kelley RI. Diagnosis of Smith-Lemli-Opitz syndrome by gas chromatography/mass spectrometry of 7-dehydrocholesterol in plasma, amniotic fluid and cultured skin fibroblasts. *Clin Chim Acta* 1995;236:45–58.

386. Le Merrer M, Briard ML, Girard S, Mulliez N, Moraine C, Inibert MC. Lethal acrodysgenital dwarfism: a severe lethal condition resembling Smith-Lemli-Opitz syndrome. *J Med Genet* 1988;25:88–95.

387. Verloes A, Ayme S, Gambarelli D, Gonzales M, Le Merrer M, et al. Holoprosencephaly-polydactyly ("pseudotrisomy 13") syndrome: a syndrome with features of hydrolethalus and Smith-Lemli-Opitz syndromes. A collaborative multicentre study. *J Med Genet* 1991;28:297–303.

388. Lowry RB. Variability in the Smith-Lemli-Opitz syndrome: overlap with the Meckel syndrome. *Am J Med Genet* 1983;14:429–433.

389. Jeanty P, Delbeke D, Lemli L, Dorchy H. Smith-Lemli-Opitz syndrome without failure to thrive. *Acta Pediatr Belg* 1977;30:27–29.

390. Jones KL. Smith-Lemli-Opitz syndrome. In: *Smith's recognizable patterns of human malformation.* Philadelphia: WB Saunders, 1997.

391. Kelley RI, Moser A, Natowicz M. The clinical and biochemical spectrum of 7-dehydrocholesterolemia: Smith-Lemli-Opitz syndrome and its variants In: Cholesterol metabolism in the RSH/Smith-Lemli-Opitz syndrome: summary of an NICHD conference. *Am J Med Genet* 1994;50:335.

392. Witsch-Baumgartner M, Fitzky BU, Ogorelkova M, Kraft HG, Moebius FF, et al. Mutational spectrum and genotype-phenotype correlation in 84 patients with Smith-Lemli-Opitz syndrome. *Am J Hum Genet* 2000;66:402–412.

393. Kelley RI. Inborn errors of cholesterol biosynthesis. *Adv Pediatr* 2000;47:1–53.

394. Azurdia RM, Anstey AV, Rhodes LE. Cholesterol supplementation objectively reduces photosensitivity in the Smith-Lemli-Opitz syndrome. *Br J Dermatol* 2001;144:143–145.

395. Morell P, Jurevics H. Origin of cholesterol in myelin. *Neurochem Res* 1996;21:463–470.

396. Irons MB, Nores J, Stewart TL, Craigo SD, Bianchi DW, et al. Antenatal therapy of Smith-Lemli-Opitz syndrome. *Fetal Diagn Ther* 1999;14:133–137.

Treacher Collins Syndrome

397. Treacher Collins Syndrome Collaborative Group. Positional cloning of a gene involved in the pathogenesis of Treacher Collins syndrome. *Nat Genet* 1996;12:130–136.

398. Dixon MJ, Read AP, Donnai D, Colley A, Dixon J, Williamson R. The gene for Treacher Collins syndrome maps to the long arm of chromosome 5. *Am J Hum Genet* 1991;49:17–22.

399. Jabs EW, Li X, Coss CA, Taylor EW, Meyers DA, Weber JL. Mapping the Treacher Collins syndrome locus to 5q31.3–q33.3. *Genomics* 1991;11:193–198.

400. Edwards SJ, Gladwin AJ, Dixon MJ. The mutational spectrum in Treacher Collins syndrome reveals a predominance of mutations that create a premature-termination codon. *Am J Hum Genet* 1997;60:515–524.

401. Dixon J, Hovanes K, Shiang R, Dixon MJ. Sequence analysis, identification of evolutionary conserved motifs and expression analysis of murine tcof1 provide further evidence for a potential function for the gene and its human homologue, *TCOF1. Hum Mol Genet* 1997;6:727–737.

402. Winter RM. What's in a face? *Nat Genet* 1996;12:124–129.

403. Meizner I, Carmi R, Katz M. Prenatal ultrasonic diagnosis of mandibulofacial dysostosis (Treacher Collins syndrome). *J Clin Ultrasound* 1991;19:124–127.

404. Crane JP, Beaver HA. Midtrimester sonographic diagnosis of mandibulofacial dysostosis. *Am J Med Genet* 1986;25:251–255.

405. Milligan DA, Harlass FE, Duff P, Kopelman JN. Recurrence of Treacher Collins syndrome with sonographic findings. *Mil Med* 1994;159:250–252.

406. Cohen J, Ghezzi F, Goncalves L, Fuentes JD, Paulyson KJ, Sherer DM. Prenatal sonographic diagnosis of Treacher Collins syndrome: a case and review of the literature. *Am J Perinatol* 1995;12:416–419.

407. Ochi H, Matsubara K, Ito M, Kusanagi Y. Prenatal sonographic diagnosis of Treacher Collins syndrome. *Obstet Gynecol* 1998;91(5 Pt 2):862.

408. Nicolaides KH, Johansson D, Donnai D, Rodeck CH. Prenatal diagnosis of mandibulofacial dysostosis. *Prenat Diagn* 1984;4:201–205.

409. Behrents RG, McNamara JA, Avery JK. Prenatal mandibulofacial dysostosis (Treacher Collins syndrome). *Cleft Palate J* 1977;14:13–34.

410. Edwards SJ, Fowlie A, Cust MP, Liu DTY, Young ID, Dixon MJ. Prenatal diagnosis in Treacher Collins syndrome using combined linkage analysis and ultrasound imaging *J Med Genet* 1996;33:603–606.

411. Dixon MJ. Treacher Collins syndrome: from linkage to prenatal testing. *J Laryngol Otol* 1998;112:705–709.

412. Johnston MC, Bronsky PT. Prenatal craniofacial development: new insights on normal and abnormal mechanisms. *Crit Rev Oral Biol Med* 1995;6:25–79.

413. Freihofer HP. Variations in the correction of Treacher Collins syndrome. *Plast Reconstr Surg* 1997;99:647–657.

Tuberous Sclerosis

414. Osborne JP, Fryer A, Webb D. Epidemiology of tuberous sclerosis. *Ann N Y Acad Sci* 1991;615:125–127.

415. Northrup H, Kwiatkowski DJ, Roach ES, Dobyns WB, Lewis RA, et al. Evidence for genetic heterogeneity in tuberous sclerosis: one locus on chromosome 9 and at least one locus elsewhere. *Am J Hum Genet* 1992;51:709–720.

416. Haines JL, Short MP, Kwiatkowski DJ, Jewell A, Andermann E, et al. Localization of one gene for tuberous sclerosis within 9q32-9q34, and further evidence for heterogeneity. *Am J Hum Genet* 1991;49:764–772.

417. Jones AC, Shyamsundar MM, Thomas MW, Maynard J, Idziaszczyk S, et al. Comprehensive mutation analysis of *TSC1* and *TSC2*—and phenotypic correlations in 150 families with tuberous sclerosis. *Am J Hum Genet* 1999;64:1305–1315.

418. Cook JA, Oliver K, Mueller RF, Sampson J. A cross sectional study of renal involvement in tuberous sclerosis. *J Med Genet* 1996;33:480–484.

419. Webb DW, Clarke A, Fryer A, Osborne JP. The cutaneous features of tuberous sclerosis: a population study. *Br J Dermatol* 1996;135:1–5.

420. Gushiken BJ, Callen PW, Silverman NH. Prenatal diagnosis of tuberous sclerosis in monozygotic twins with cardiac masses. *J Ultrasound Med* 1999;18:165–168.

421. Harding CO, Pagon RA. Incidence of tuberous sclerosis in patients with cardiac rhabdomyoma. *Am J Med Genet* 1990;37:443–446.

422. Journel H, Roussey M, Plais MH, Milon J, Almange C, Le Marec B. Prenatal diagnosis of familial tuberous sclerosis following detection of cardiac rhabdomyoma by ultrasound. *Prenat Diagn* 1986;6:283–289.

423. Sgro M, Barozzino T, Toi A, Johnson J, Sermer M, Chitayat D. Prenatal detection of cerebral lesions in a fetus with tuberous sclerosis. *Ultrasound Obstet Gynecol* 1999;14:356–359.

424. Czechowski J, Langille EL, Varady E. Intracardiac tumour and brain lesions in tuberous sclerosis. A case report of antenatal diagnosis by ultrasonography. *Acta Radiol* 2000;41:371–374.

425. Axt-Fliedner R, Qush H, Hendrik HJ, Ertan K, Lindinger A, et al. Prenatal diagnosis of cerebral lesions and multiple intracardiac rhabdomyomas in a fetus with tuberous sclerosis. *J Ultrasound Med* 2001;20:63–67.

426. Levine D, Barnes P, Korf B, Edelman R. Tuberous sclerosis in the fetus: second-trimester diagnosis of subependymal tubers with ultrafast MR imaging. *AJR Am J Roentgenol* 2000;175:1067.

427. Brackley KJ, Farndon PA, Weaver JB, Dow DJ, Chapman S, Kilby MD. Prenatal diagnosis of tuberous sclerosis with intracerebral signs at 14 weeks' gestation. *Prenat Diagn* 1999;19:575–579.

428. Mitra AG, Dickerson C. Central nervous system tumor with associated unilateral ventriculomegaly: unusual prenatal presentation of subsequently diagnosed tuberous sclerosis. *J Ultrasound Med* 2000;19:651–654.

429. Durfee SM, Kim FM, Benson CB. Postnatal outcome of fetuses with the prenatal diagnosis of asymmetric hydrocephalus. *J Ultrasound Med* 2001;20:263–268.

430. Webb DW, Thomas RD, Osborne JP. Cardiac rhabdomyomas and their association with tuberous sclerosis. *Arch Dis Child* 1993;68:367–370.

431. Geipel A, Krapp M, Germer U, Becker R, Gembruch U. Perinatal diagnosis of cardiac tumors. *Ultrasound Obstet Gynecol* 2001;17:17–21.

432. Smith HC, Watson GH, Patel RG, Super M. Cardiac rhabdomyomata in tuberous sclerosis: their course and diagnostic value. *Arch Dis Child* 1989;64:196–200.

VATER/VACTERL Association

433. Quan L, Smith DW. The VATER association: vertebral defects, anal atresia, tracheoesophageal fistula with esophageal atresia, radial dysplasia. *Birth Defects* 1972;VIII:75–78.

434. Khoury MJ, Cordero JF, Greenberg F, James LM, Erickson JD. A population study of the VACTERL association: evidence for its etiologic heterogeneity. *Pediatrics* 1983;71:815–820.

435. Rittler M, Paz JE, Castilla EE. VACTERL association, epidemiologic definition and delineation. *Am J Med Genet* 1996;63:529–536.

436. Froster UG, Wallner SJ, Reusche E, Schwinger E, Rehder H. VACTERL with hydrocephalus and branchial arch defects: prenatal, clinical, and autopsy findings in two brothers. *Am J Med Genet* 1996;62:169–172.

437. Jones KL. VATER association. In: *Smith's recognizable patterns of human malformation.* Philadelphia: WB Saunders, 1998:664–665.

438. Levine F, Muenke M. VACTERL association with high prenatal lead exposure: similarities to animal models of lead teratogenicity. *Pediatrics* 1991;87:390–392.

439. Damian MS, Seibel P, Schachenmayr W, Reichmann H, Dorndorf W. VACTERL with the mitochondrial np 3243 point mutation. *Am J Med Genet* 1996;62:398–403.

440. Tongsong T, Wanapirak C, Piyamongkol W, Sudasana J. Prenatal sonographic diagnosis of VATER association. *J Clin Ultrasound* 1999;27:378–384.

441. McMullen KP, Karnes PS, Moir CR, Michels VV. Familial recurrence of tracheoesophageal fistula and associated malformations. *Am J Med Genet* 1996;63:525–528.

442. Benacerraf BR. *Ultrasound of fetal syndromes.* New York: Churchill Livingstone, 1998:285–287.

443. Townes PL, Brocks ER. Hereditary syndrome of imperforate anus with hand, foot, and ear anomalies. *J Pediatr* 1972;81:321–326.

444. Bull MJ, Bryson CQ, Grosfeld J, Schreiner RL. VATER association: analysis of growth and development. *Am J Perinatol* 1985;2:35–38.

Walker-Warburg Syndrome

445. Walker AE. Lissencephaly. *Arch Neurol Psychiatry* 1942;48:13.

446. Warburg M. The heterogeneity of microphthalmia in the mentally retarded. *Birth Defects* 1971;7:136–154.

447. Jones KL. Walker-Warburg syndrome. In: *Smith's recognizable patterns of human malformation.* Philadelphia: WB Saunders, 1997:192–193.

448. Chemke J, Czernobilsky B, Mundel G, Barishak YR. A familial syndrome of central nervous system and ocular malformations. *Clin Genet* 1975;7:1–7.

449. Miller G, Ladda RL, Towfighi J. Cerebro-ocular dysplasia–muscular dystrophy (Walker Warburg) syndrome. Findings in 20-week-old fetus. *Acta Neuropathol (Berl)* 1991;82:234–238.

450. Dobyns WB, Pagon RA, Armstrong D, Curry CJ, Greenberg F, et al. Diagnostic criteria for Walker-Warburg syndrome. *Am J Med Genet* 1989;32:195–210.

451. Monteagudo A, Alayon A, Mayberry P. Walker-Warburg syndrome: case report and review of the literature. *J Ultrasound Med* 2001;20:419–426.

452. Crowe C, Jassani M, Dickerman L. The prenatal diagnosis of the Walker-Warburg syndrome. *Prenat Diagn* 1986;6:177.

453. Chitayat D, Toi A, Babul R, Levin A, Michaud J, et al. Prenatal diagnosis of retinal nonattachment in the Walker-Warburg syndrome. *Am J Med Genet* 1995;56:351–358.

454. Gasser B, Lindner V, Dreyfus M, Feidt X, Leissner P, et al. Prenatal diagnosis of Walker-Warburg syndrome in three sibs. *Am J Med Genet* 1998;76:107–110.

455. Beinder EJ, Pfeiffer RA, Bornemann A, Wenkel H. Second-trimester diagnosis of fetal cataract in a fetus with Walker-Warburg syndrome. *Fetal Diagn Ther* 1997;12:197–199.

456. van Zalen-Sprock RM, van Vugt JM, van Geijn HP. First-trimester sonographic detection of neurodevelopmental abnormalities in some single-gene disorders. *Prenat Diagn* 1996;16:199–202.

457. Maynor CH, Hertzberg BS, Ellington KS. Antenatal sonographic features of Walker-Warburg syndrome. Value of endovaginal sonography. *J Ultrasound Med* 1992;11:301–303.

458. Leyten QH, Gabreels FJ, Renier WO, ter Laak HJ. Congenital muscular dystrophy: a review of the literature. *Clin Neurol Neurosurg* 1996;98:267–280.

459. Valanne L, Pihko H, Katevuo K, Karttunen P, Somer H, Santavuori P. MRI of the brain in muscle-eye-brain (MEB) disease. *Neuroradiology* 1994;36:473–476.

460. Gordon N. Muscle and brain disease: an update. *Child Care Health Dev* 1994;20:279–287.

461. Benacerraf BR. Walker-Warburg syndrome. In; *Ultrasound of fetal syndromes.* New York: Churchill Livingstone, 1998:134–137.

Down Syndrome (Trisomy 21)

462. Down JLH. Observations on an ethnic classification of idiots. *London Hosp Clin Lect Rep* 1866;3:259.

463. Lejeune J, Gautier M, Turpin R. Etude des chromosomes somatiques de neuf enfants mongoliens. *Coll Royal Acad Sci* 1959;248:1721–1722.

464. Egan JF, Benn P, Borgida AF, Rodis JF, Campbell WA, Vintzileos AM. Efficacy of screening for fetal down syndrome in the United States from 1974 to 1997. *Obstet Gynecol* 2000;96:979–985.

465. Penrose LS. The relative effects of paternal and maternal age in mongolism. *J Genet* 1933;27:219.

466. Jyothy A, Kumar KS, Mallikarjuna GN, Babu Rao V, Uma Devi B, et al. Parental age and the origin of extra chromosome 21 in Down syndrome. *J Hum Genet* 2001;46:347–350.

467. Hall B. Mongolism in newborn infants. *Clin Pediatr* 1966;5:12.

468. Rex AP, Preus M. A diagnostic index for Down syndrome. *J Pediatr* 1982;100:903–906.

469. Keeling JW. Examination of the fetus following prenatal suspicion of congenital abnormality. In: Keeling JW, ed. *Fetal and neonatal pathology.* New York: Springer-Verlag, 1987:99–122.

470. Stephens TD, Shepard TH. The Down syndrome in the fetus. *Teratology* 1980;22:37–41.

471. Sohl BD, Scioscia AL, Budorick NE, Moore TR. Utility of minor ultrasonographic markers in the prediction of abnormal fetal karyotype at a prenatal diagnostic center. *Am J Obstet Gynecol* 1999;181:898–903.

472. Nyberg DA, Souter VL, El-Bastawissi A, Young S, Luthardt F, Luthy DA. Isolated sonographic markers for detection of fetal Down syndrome during the second trimester. *J Ultrasound Med* 2001;20:1053–1063.

473. Paladini D, Tartaglioine A, Agangi A, Teodoro A, Forleo F, et al. The association between congenital heart disease and Down syndrome in prenatal life. *Ultrasound Obstet Gynecol* 2000;15:104–8.

474. DeVore GR. Trisomy 21: 91% detection rate using second-trimester ultrasound markers. *Ultrasound Obstet Gynecol* 2000;16:133–141.

475. Benacerraf BR, Neuberg D, Bromley B, Frigoletto FD Jr. Sonographic scoring index for prenatal detection of chromosomal abnormalities. *J Ultrasound Med* 1992;11:449–458.

476. Benacerraf BR, Nadel AS, Bromley B. Identification of second-trimester fetuses with autosomal trisomy by use of a sonographic scoring index. *Radiology* 1994;193:135–140.

477. Nyberg DA, Resta R, Luthy DA, Hickok DE, Mahony BS, Hirsch JH. Prenatal sonographic findings of Down syndrome: review of 94 cases. *Obstet Gynecol* 1990;76:370–377.

478. Nyberg DA, Luthy DA, Resta RG, Nyberg BC, Williams MA. Age-adjusted ultrasound risk assessment for fetal Down's syndrome during the second trimester: description of the method and analysis of 142 cases. *Ultrasound Obstet Gynecol* 1998;12:8–14.

479. Vintzileos AM, Campbell WA, Guzman ER, Smulian JC, McLean DA, Ananth CV. Second-trimester ultrasound markers for detection of trisomy 21: Which markers are best? *Obstet Gynecol* 1997;89:941–944.

480. Vergani P, Locatelli A, Piccoli MG, Ceruti P, Mariani E, et al. Best second trimester sonographic markers for the detection of trisomy 21. *J Ultrasound Med* 1999;18:469–473.

481. Winter TC, Reichman JA, Luna JA, Cheng EY, Doll AM, et al. Frontal lobe shortening in second-trimester fetuses with trisomy 21: usefulness as a US marker. *Radiology* 1998;207:215–222.

482. Winter TC, Ostrovsky AA, Komarniski CA, Uhrich SB. Cerebellar and frontal lobe hypoplasia in fetuses with trisomy 21: usefulness as combined US markers. *Radiology* 2000;214:533–538.

483. Benacerraf BR, Osathanondh R, Frigoletto FD. Sonographic demonstration of hypoplasia of the middle phalanx of the fifth digit: a finding associated with Down syndrome. *Am J Obstet Gynecol* 1988;159:181–183.

484. Cicero S, Curcio P, Papageorghiou A, Sonek J, Nicolaides K. Absence of nasal bone in fetuses with trisomy 21 at 11–

14 weeks of gestation: an observational study. *Lancet* 2001;358(9294):1665–1667.

485. Fong CT, Brodeur GM. Down's syndrome and leukemia: epidemiology, genetics, cytogenetics and mechanisms of leukemogenesis. *Cancer Genet Cytogenet* 1987;28:55–76.

486. Robinson LL. Down syndrome and leukemia. *Leukemia* 1992;6:5–7.

Edwards Syndrome (Trisomy 18)

487. Hook EB, Woodbury DF, Albright SG. Rates of trisomy 18 in livebirths, stillbirths, and at amniocentesis. *Birth Defects* 1979;XV:81–93.

488. Edwards JH, Harnden DG, Cameron AH, et al. A new trisomic syndrome. *Lancet* 1960;1:787–789.

489. Smith DW, Patau K, Therman E, et al. A new autosomal trisomy syndrome: multiple congenital anomalies caused by an extra chromosome. *J Pediatr* 1960;57:338–345.

490. Smith DW, Patau K, Therman E, et al. The no. 18 trisomy syndrome. *J Pediatr* 1962;57:338–345.

491. Flannery DB, Kahler SG. Neural tube defects in trisomy 18. *Prenat Diagn* 1986;6:97–99.

492. Christianson AL, Nelson MM. Four cases of trisomy 18 syndrome with limb reduction malformation. *J Med Genet* 1984;21:293.

493. Isaksen CV, Eik-Nes SH, Blaas HG, Torp SH, Van Der Hagem CB, Ormerod E. A correlative study of prenatal ultrasound and post-mortem findings in fetuses and infants with an abnormal karyotype. *Ultrasound Obstet Gynecol* 2000;16:37–45.

494. Shields LE, Carpenter LA, Smith KM, Nghiem HV. Ultrasonographic diagnosis of trisomy 18: Is it practical in the early second trimester? *J Ultrasound Med* 1998;17:327–331.

495. DeVore GR. Second trimester ultrasonography may identify 77% to 97% of fetuses with trisomy 18. *J Ultrasound Med* 2000;19:565–576.

496. Nyberg DA, Kramer D, Resta RG, Kapur R, Mahony BS, et al. Prenatal sonographic findings of trisomy 18: review of 47 cases. *J Ultrasound Med* 1993;12:103–113.

497. Brumfield CG, Wenstrom KD, Owen J, Davis RO. Ultrasound findings and multiple marker screening in trisomy 18. *Obstet Gynecol* 2000;95:51–54.

498. Nicolaides KH, Salvesen DR, Snijders RJ, Gosden CM. Strawberry-shaped skull in fetal trisomy 18. *Fetal Diagn Ther* 1992;7:132–137.

499. Bundy AL, Saltzman DH, Pober B, Fine C, Emerson D, Doubilet PM. Antenatal sonographic findings in trisomy 18. *J Ultrasound Med* 1986;5:361–364.

500. Benacerraf BR, Miller WA, Frigoletto FD Jr. Sonographic detection of fetuses with trisomies 13 and 18: accuracy and limitations. *Am J Obstet Gynecol* 1988;158:404–409.

501. Palomaki GE, Haddow JE, Knight GJ, Wald NJ, Kennard A, et al. Risk-based prenatal screening for trisomy 18 using alpha-fetoprotein, unconjugated oestriol and human chorionic gonadotropin. *Prenat Diagn* 1995;15:713–223.

502. Seppo H, Markku R, Marko N, Pertti K. Detection of trisomy 18 by double screening in a low-risk pregnant population. *Fetal Diagn Ther* 1999;14:15–19.

503. Feuchtbaum LB, Currier RJ, Lorey FW, Cunningham GC. Prenatal ultrasound findings in affected and unaffected pregnancies that are screen-positive for trisomy 18: the California experience. *Prenat Diagn* 2000;20:293–299.

504. Carter PE, Pearn JH, Bell J, Martin N, Anderson NG. Survival in trisomy 18. Life tables for use in genetic counselling and clinical paediatrics. *Clin Genet* 1985;27:59–61.

504a.Carey JC. Trisomy 18 and trisomy 13 syndromes. In: Cassidy SB, Allanson JE, eds. *Management of genetic syndromes*. New York: Wiley, 2001:419–420.

Trisomy 13

505. Warkany J. Syndromes of chromosomal abnormalities. In: *Congenital malformations*. Chicago: Year Book Medical Publishers, 1971:296–345.

506. Gilbert EF, Aryas Laxova R, Opitz JM. Pathology of chromosome abnormalities in the fetus—pathologic markers. *Birth Defects* 1987;23:293–296.

507. Martinez-Frias ML, Villa A, de Pablo RA, Ayala A, Calvo MJ, et al. Limb deficiencies in infants with trisomy 13. *Am J Med Genet* 2000;93:339–341.

508. Lehman CD, Nyberg DA, Winter TC III, Kapur R, Resta RG, Luthy DA. Trisomy 13 syndrome: prenatal US findings in a review of 33 cases. *Radiology* 1995;194:217–222.

509. Nicolaides KH, Snijders RJ, Gosden CM, Berry C, Campbell S. Ultrasonographically detectable markers of fetal chromosomal abnormalities. *Lancet* 1992;340(8821):704–707.

510. De Vigan C, Baena N, Cariati E, Clementi M, Stoll C. Contribution of ultrasonographic examination to the prenatal detection of chromosomal abnormalities in 19 centres across Europe. *Ann Genet* 2001;44:209–217.

511. Tongsong T, Sirichotiyakul S, Wanapirak C, Chanprapah P. Sonographic features of trisomy 13 at midpregnancy. *Int J Gynecol Obstet* 2002;76:143–148.

512. Redheendran R, Neu RL, Bannerman RM. Long survival in trisomy-13-syndrome: 21 cases including prolonged survival in two patients 11 and 19 years old. *Am J Med Genet* 1981;8:167–172.

Turner Syndrome (45,X)

513. Turner HH. A syndrome of infantilism, congenital webbed neck, and cubitus valgus. *Endocrinology* 1938;23:566.

514. Ford CE, Miller OJ, Polani PE, de Almeida JC, Briggs JH. A sex-chromosome anomaly in a case of gonadal dysgenesis (Turner's syndrome). *Lancet* 1959;1:711–713.

515. Wiedemann HR, Glatzl J. Follow-up of Ullrich's original patient with "Ullrich-Turner" syndrome. *Am J Med Genet* 1991;41:134–136.

516. Gravholt CH, Juul S, Naeraa RW, Hansen J. Prenatal and postnatal prevalence of Turner's syndrome: a registry study. *BMJ* 1996;312:16–21.

517. Blagowidow N, Page DC, Huff D, Mennuti MT. Ullrich-Turner syndrome in an XY female fetus with deletion of the sex-determining portion of the Y chromosome. *Am J Med Genet* 1989;34:159–162.

518. Phillips HE, McGahan JP. Intrauterine fetal cystic hygromas: sonographic detection. *AJR Am J Roentgenol* 1981;136:799–802.

519. Toftager-Larsen K, Benzie RJ, Doran TA, Miskin M, Allen LC, Becker L. Alpha-fetoprotein and ultrasound scanning

in the prenatal diagnosis of Turner's syndrome. *Prenat Diagn* 1983;3:35–40.

520. Chervenak FA, Isaacson G, Blakemore KJ, Breg WR, Hobbins JC, et al. Fetal cystic hygroma. Cause and natural history. *N Engl J Med* 1983;309:822–825.

521. Newman DE, Cooperberg PL. Genetics of sonographically detected intrauterine fetal cystic hygromas. *J Can Assoc Radiol* 1984;35:77–79.

522. Brown BSJ, Thompson DL. Ultrasonographic features of the fetal Turner syndrome. *J Can Assoc Radiol* 1984;35:40–46.

523. Saller DN Jr, Canick JA, Schwartz S, Blitzer MG. Multiple-marker screening in pregnancies with hydropic and nonhydropic Turner syndrome. *Am J Obstet Gynecol* 1992;167(4 Pt 1):1021–1024.

524. Wenstrom KD, Chu DC, Owen J, Boots L. Maternal serum alpha-fetoprotein and dimeric inhibin A detect aneuploidies other than Down syndrome. *Am J Obstet Gynecol* 1998;179:966–970.

525. Hiett AK, Callaghan CM, Brown HL, Golichowski AM, Heerema NA. The association of aneuploidy and unexplained elevated maternal serum alpha-fetoprotein. *J Perinatol* 1998;18:343–346.

526. Spencer K, Tul N, Nicolaides KH. Maternal serum free beta-hCG and PAPP-A in fetal sex chromosome defects in the first trimester. *Prenat Diagn* 2000;20:390–394.

527. Robinow M, Spisso K, Buschi AJ, Brenbridge ANAG. Turner syndrome: sonography showing fetal hydrops simulating hydramnios. *AJR Am J Roentgenol* 1980;135:846–848.

528. Chodirker BN, Harman CR, Greenberg CR. Spontaneous resolution of a cystic hygroma in a fetus with Turner syndrome. *Prenat Diagn* 1988;8:291–292.

529. Koeberl DD, McGillivray B, Sybert VP. Prenatal diagnosis of 45,X/46XX mosaicism and 45,X: implications for postnatal outcome. *Am J Hum Genet* 1995;57:661–666.

Triploidy and Tetraploidy

530. Neuber M, Rehder H, Zuther C, Lettau R, Schwinger E. Polyploidies in abortion material decrease with maternal age. *Hum Genet* 1993;91:563–566.

531. Jauniaux E, Kadri R, Hustin J. Partial mole and triploidy: screening patients with first-trimester spontaneous abortion. *Obstet Gynecol* 1996;88(4 Pt 1):616–619.

532. Coe SJ, Kapur R, Luthardt F, Rabinovitch P, Kramer D. Prenatal diagnosis of tetraploidy: a case report. *Am J Med Genet* 1993;45:378–382.

533. Lafer CZ, Neu RL. A liveborn infant with tetraploidy. *Am J Med Genet* 1988;31:375–378.

534. McFadden DE, Langlois S. Parental and meiotic origin of triploidy in the embryonic and fetal periods. *Clin Genet* 2000;58:192–200.

535. Uchida IA, Freeman VCP. Triploidy and chromosomes. *Am J Obstet Gynecol* 1985;151:65–69.

536. Jauniaux E. Partial moles: from postnatal to prenatal diagnosis. *Placenta* 1999;20:379–388.

537. Lockwood C, Scioscia A, Stiller R, Hobbins J. Sonographic features of the triploid fetus. *Am J Obstet Gynecol* 1987;157:285–287.

538. Zaragoza MV, Surti U, Redline RW, Millie E, Chakravarti A, Hassold TJ. Parental origin and phenotype of triploidy in spontaneous abortions: predominance of diandry and association with the partial hydatidiform mole. *Am J Hum Genet* 2000;66:1807–1820.

539. Redline RW, Hassold T, Zaragoza MV. Prevalence of the partial molar phenotype in triploidy of maternal and paternal origin. *Hum Pathol* 1998;29:505–511.

540. McFadden DE, Kwong LC, Yam IY, Langlois S. Parental origin of triploidy in human fetuses: evidence for genomic imprinting. *Hum Genet* 1993;92:465–469.

541. Blackburn WR, Miller WP, Superneau DW, Cooley NR Jr, Zellweger H, Wertelecki W. Comparative studies of infants with mosaic and complete triploidy: an analysis of 55 cases. *Birth Defects* 1982;18:251–274.

542. Chatterjee MS, Tejani NA, Verma UL, Weiss RR. Prenatal diagnosis of triploidy. *Int J Gynaecol Obstet* 1983;21:155–157.

543. Crane JP, Beaver HA, Cheung SW. Antenatal ultrasound findings in fetal triploidy syndrome. *J Ultrasound Med* 1985;4:519–524.

544. Benacerraf BR. Intrauterine growth retardation in the first trimester associated with triploidy. *J Ultrasound Med* 1988;7:153–154.

545. Jacobs PA, Szulman AE, Funkhouser J, Matsuura JS, Wilson CC. Human triploidy: relationship between parenteral origin of the additional haploid complement and development of partial hydatidiform mole. *Ann Hum Genet* 1982;46:223–231.

546. Rubenstein JB, Swayne LC, Dise CA, Gersen SL, Schwartz JR, Risk A. Placental changes in fetal triploidy syndrome. *J Ultrasound Med* 1986;4:545–550.

547. Jauniaux E, Brown R, Rodeck C, Nicolaides KH. Prenatal diagnosis of triploidy during the second trimester of pregnancy. *Obstet Gynecol* 1996;88:983–989.

548. Snijders RJ, Sebire NJ, Souka A, Santiago C, Nicolaides KH. Fetal exomphalos and chromosomal defects: relationship to maternal age and gestation. *Ultrasound Obstet Gynecol* 1995;6:250–255.

549. Jauniaux E, Brown R, Snijders RJ, Noble P, Nicolaides KH. Early prenatal diagnosis of triploidy. *Am J Obstet Gynecol* 1997;176:550–554.

550. Spencer K, Liao AW, Skentou H, Cicero S, Nicolaides KH. Screening for triploidy by fetal nuchal translucency and maternal serum free beta-hCG and PAPP-A at 10–14 weeks of gestation. *Prenat Diagn* 2000;6:495–499.

551. Meiner A, Holland H, Reichenbach H, Horn LC, Faber R, Froster UG. Tetraploidy in a growth-retarded fetus with a thick placenta. *Prenat Diagn* 1998;18:864–865.

552. Sagot P, Nomballais MF, David A, Yvinec M, Beaujard MP, et al. Prenatal diagnosis of tetraploidy. *Fetal Diagn Ther* 1993;8:182–186.

553. Genest DR. Partial hydatidiform mole: clinicopathological features, differential diagnosis, ploidy and molecular studies, and gold standards for diagnosis. *Int J Gynecol Pathol* 2001;20:315–322.

554. Sherard J, Bean C, Bove B, DelDuca V Jr, Esterly KL, et al. Long survival in a 69,XXY triploid male. *Am J Med Genet* 1986;25:307–312.

555. Niemann-Seyde SC, Rehder H, Zoll B. A case of full triploidy (69,XXX) of paternal origin with unusually long survival time. *Clin Genet* 1993;43:79–82.

556. Ramsey PS, Van Winter JT, Gaffey TA, Ramin KD. Eclampsia complicating hydatidiform molar pregnancy with a coexisting, viable fetus. A case report. *J Reprod Med* 1998;43:456–458.

557. Rahimpanah F, Smoleniec J. Partial mole, triploidy and proteinuric hypertension: two case reports. *Aust N Z J Obstet Gynaecol* 2000;40:215–218.

558. Lage JM, Berkowitz RS, Rice LW, Goldstein DP, Bernstein MR, Weinberg DS. Flow cytometric analysis of DNA content in partial hydatidiform moles with persistent gestational trophoblastic tumor. *Obstet Gynecol* 1991;77:111–115.

559. Zalel Y, Dgani R. Gestational trophoblastic disease following the evacuation of partial hydatidiform mole: a review of 66 cases. *Eur J Obstet Gynecol Reprod Biol* 1997;71:67–71.

Velocardiofacial Syndrome

560. Shprintzen RJ, Goldberg RB, Lewin ML, Sidoti EJ, Berkman MD, et al. A new syndrome involving cleft palate, cardiac anomalies, typical facies, and learning disabilities: velo-cardio-facial syndrome. *Cleft Palate J* 1978;15:56–62.

561. Shprintzen RJ, Goldberg RB, Young D, Wolford L. The velo-cardio-facial syndrome: a clinical and genetic analysis. *Pediatrics* 1981;67:167–172.

562. Wilson DI, Burn J, Scambler P, Goodship J. DiGeorge syndrome: part of CATCH 22. *J Med Genet* 1993;30:852–856.

563. Wulfsberg EA, Leana-Cox J, Neri G. What's in a name? Chromosome 22q abnormalities and the DiGeorge, velocardiofacial, and conotruncal anomalies face syndromes. *Am J Med Genet* 1996;65:317–319.

564. Pike AC, Super M. Velocardiofacial syndrome. *Postgrad Med J* 1997;73:771–775.

565. Van Geet C, Devriendt K, Eyskens B, Vermylen J, Hoylaerts MF. Velocardiofacial syndrome patients with a heterozygous chromosome 22q11 deletion have giant platelets. *Pediatr Res* 1998;44:607–611.

566. Sirotkin H, Morrow B, Saint-Jore B, Puech A, Das Gupta R, et al. Identification, characterization, and precise mapping of a human gene encoding a novel membrane-spanning protein from the 22q11 region deleted in velo-cardio-facial syndrome. *Genomics* 1997;42:245–251.

567. Scambler PJ. The 22q11 deletion syndromes. *Hum Mol Genet* 2000;9:2421–2426.

568. Gong L, Liu M, Jen J, Yeh ET. *GNB1L*, a gene deleted in the critical region for DiGeorge syndrome on 22q11, encodes a G-protein beta-subunit-like polypeptide. *Biochim Biophys Acta* 2000;1494:185–188.

569. McDonald-McGinn DM, LaRossa D, Goldmuntz E, Sullivan K, Eicher P, et al. The 22q11.2 deletion: screening, diagnostic workup, and outcome of results; report on 181 patients. *Genet Test* 1997;1:99–108.

570. Ming JE, McDonald-McGinn DM, Megerian TE, Driscoll DA, Elias ER, et al. Skeletal anomalies and deformities in patients with deletions of 22q11. *Am J Med Genet* 1997;72:210–215.

571. Goldberg R, Motzkin B, Marion R, Scambler PJ, Shprintzen RJ. Velo-cardio-facial syndrome: a review of 120 patients. *Am J Med Genet* 1993;45:313–319.

572. Alikasifoglu M, Malkoc N, Ceviz N, Ozme S, Uludogan S, Tuncbilek E. Microdeletion of 22q11 (CATCH 22) in children with conotruncal heart defect and extracardiac malformations. *Turk J Pediatr* 2000;42:215–218.

573. Davidson A, Khandelwal M, Punnett HH. Prenatal diagnosis of the 22q11 deletion syndrome. *Prenat Diagn* 1997;17:380–383.

574. Levy-Mozziconacci A, Piquet C, Heurtevin PC, Philip N. Prenatal diagnosis of 22q11 microdeletion. *Prenat Diagn* 1997;17:1033–1037.

575. Goodship J, Robson SC, Sturgiss S, Cross IE, Wright C. Renal abnormalities on obstetric ultrasound as a presentation of DiGeorge syndrome. *Prenat Diagn* 1997;17:867–870.

576. Lazanakis MS, Rodgers K, Economides DL. Increased nuchal translucency and CATCH 22. *Prenat Diagn* 1998;18:507–510.

577. Berend SA, Spikes AS, Kashork CD, Wu JM, Daw SC, et al. Dual-probe fluorescence in situ hybridization assay for detecting deletions associated with VCFS/DiGeorge syndrome I and DiGeorge syndrome II loci. *Am J Med Genet* 2000;91:313–317.

578. Tsai CH, Van Dyke DL, Feldman GL. Child with velocardiofacial syndrome and del (q34.2): another critical region associated with a velocardiofacial syndrome-like phenotype. *Am J Med Genet* 1999;82:336–339.

579. Ryan AK, Goodship JA, Wilson DI, Philip N, Levy A, et al. Spectrum of clinical features associated with interstitial chromosome 22q11 deletions: a European collaborative study. *J Med Genet* 1997;34:798–804.

580. Wang PP, Solot C, Moss EM, Gerdes M, McDonald-McGinn DM, et al. Developmental presentation of 22q11.2 deletion (DiGeorge/velocardiofacial syndrome). *J Dev Behav Pediatr* 1998;19:342–345.

581. Kraynack NC, Hostoffer RW, Robin NH. Agenesis of the corpus callosum associated with DiGeorge-velocardiofacial syndrome: a case report and review of the literature. *J Child Neurol* 1999;14:754–756.

582. Eliez S, Schmitt JE, White CD, Reiss AL. Children and adolescents with velocardiofacial syndrome: a volumetric MRI study. *Am J Psychiatry* 2000;157:409–415.

583. Lynch DR, McDonald-McGinn DM, Zackai EH, Emanuel BS, Driscoll DA, et al. Cerebellar atrophy in a patient with velocardiofacial syndrome. *J Med Genet* 1995;32:561–563.

584. Weinzimer SA, McDonald-McGinn DM, Driscoll DA, Emanuel BS, Zackai EH, Moshang T Jr. Growth hormone deficiency in patients with 22q11.2 deletion: expanding the phenotype. *Pediatrics* 1998;101:929–932.

585. Keenan GF, Sullivan KE, McDonald-McGinn DM, Zackai EH. Arthritis associated with deletion of 22q11.2: more common than previously suspected. *Am J Med Genet* 1997;71:488.

6

CEREBRAL MALFORMATIONS

Central nervous system (CNS) malformations are some of the most common yet devastating of all congenital abnormalities. The incidence of these malformations may be as high as one in 100 births.[1] Additionally, congenital CNS abnormalities are associated with an increased rate of spontaneous abortion, adding to their rate of *in utero* occurrence when compared to birth rate statistics.[2] Eventually, CNS malformations may be associated with a variety of genetic disorders and chromosomal abnormalities, which may be important for genetic counseling of the patients.[3]

Ultrasound has been used for nearly 30 years to help diagnose fetal CNS anomalies. Anencephaly is one of the first abnormalities detected by ultrasound in the early 1970s.[4] Modern equipment allows the diagnosis of many CNS malformations since early gestation. Yet a firm understanding of the sonographic appearance of normal and abnormal developmental anatomy of the CNS is required. This chapter reviews sonography of the normal CNS development and details specific cerebral abnormalities. Craniosynostosis is discussed separately (see Craniosynostosis, Chapter 5). Neural tube defects and spinal abnormalities are addressed in Chapter 7.

EMBRYOGENESIS AND NORMAL NEURAL ANATOMY

At approximately 4.5 menstrual weeks, the neural plate has developed. At this stage the coelomic cavity of the gestational sac can usually be identified as a hypoechoic region within the echogenic decidua. The primitive neural plate, which subsequently divides into the neural crest and the neural tube, cannot be identified at this time. The neural tube differentiates into the spinal cord and the primitive brain in approximately 6 menstrual weeks. The brain begins to segment into three primary vesicles: the forebrain (*prosencephalon*), the midbrain (*mesencephalon*), and the hindbrain (*rhombencephalon*). At 7 to 8 weeks, the primary vesicles can be identified. The rhombencephalon is identified in the posterior aspect of the fetal head as a cystic structure.[5] With further development, the *prosencephalon* differentiates into the *telencephalon* and the *diencephalon*. The diencephalon forms midline structures such as the thalami and also the third ventricle. The vesicles of the telencephalon appear as outgrowths that protrude from either side of the diencephalon. These vesicles form the future cerebral hemispheres and lateral ventricles. The choroid plexus invaginates into the lateral ventricles, and the ventricles grow to approach each other in the midline. Before 13 menstrual weeks, the choroid plexus fills nearly the entire lateral ventricles.[6] However, with normal development the choroid recedes to the posterior portion of the ventricles and no longer occupies the frontal horns of the lateral ventricles.

The *rhombencephalon* differentiates into the *metencephalon* and the *myelencephalon*. The metencephalon gives rise to the pons, cerebellum, and the upper portion of the fourth ventricle. The myelencephalon gives rise to the medulla and the lower portion of the fourth ventricle.

Transvaginal high-frequency, high-resolution sonography may give surprising detail of the intracerebral contents in the first trimester of pregnancy. Many of the structures, including the echogenic choroid occupying the entire lateral ventricles, are easily appreciated using transvaginal scanning.

Knowledge of this embryology is important from two standpoints. First, understanding the normal embryology is necessary to understanding CNS abnormalities that may be identified by sonography. Second and probably most important, inexperienced sonologists frequently interpret normal findings as cerebral anomalies, which may have unfortunate consequences. A few errors seem to account for the majority of this misdiagnosis. First, the normally large rhombencephalon is frequently interpreted as an abnormal CNS fluid collection. Second, the frontal horns of lateral ventricles normally large and devoid of choroid plexus at 14 to 15 weeks may give the erroneous impression of ventriculomegaly. Third, the development of the corpus callosum and cavum septum pellucidum is a late event in cerebral ontogenesis and failure to visualize these structures before 18 weeks does not indicate agenesis of the corpus callosum.[7] The cerebellar vermis does not close over the fourth ventricle until approximately as late

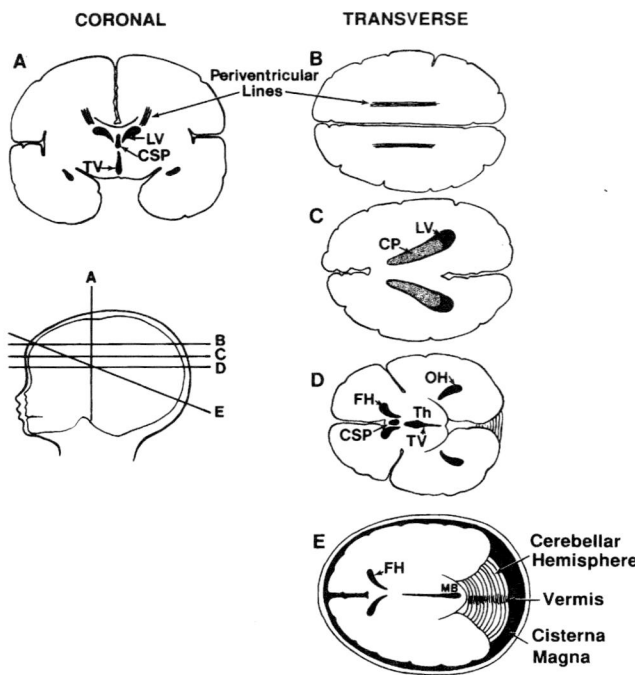

FIGURE 1. Schematic drawing of normal ventricles and intracranial anatomy of coronal view **(A)** and transverse view **(B)**. C–E: Recommended as a part of routine obstetric sonograms after the first trimester. CP, choroid plexus; CSP, cavum septum pellucidum; FH, frontal horn; LV, lateral ventricle; MB, midbrain; OH, occipital horn; Th, thalamus; TV, third ventricle. (Reproduced with permission from Nyberg DA, Pretorius PH. Cerebral malformations. Nyberg DA, Mahony BS, Pretorius DH, eds. *Diagnostic ultrasound of fetal anomalies: text and atlas.* Chicago: Year Book, 1990:83–145.)

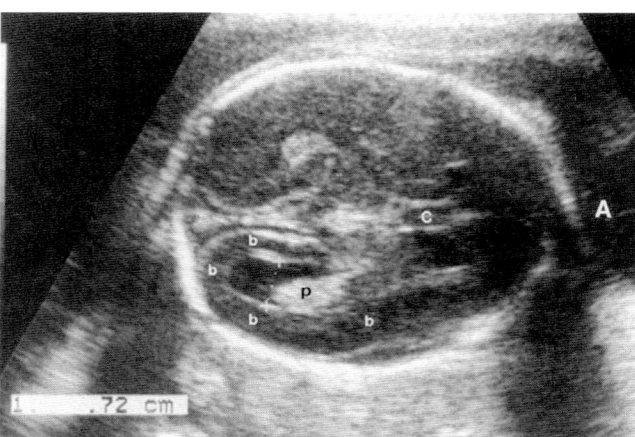

FIGURE 2. Normal lateral ventricles at 20 weeks. Axial scan angled slightly superiorly to level for biparietal diameter shows echogenic choroid plexus (*p*) in the trigone/atrium of the lateral ventricle. Calipers indicate measurement of the ventricle from medial to lateral wall. Note the normal hypoechoic cerebral hemisphere (*b*) surrounding the ventricle. A, anterior; C, cavum septum pellucidum.

as 18 menstrual weeks, and this may simulate the appearance of a Dandy-Walker malformation in a completely normal brain.[8,9]

ANTENATAL DIAGNOSIS

Transabdominal Sonography

In the second and third trimester of pregnancy, transabdominal sonography is the technique of choice to investigate the fetal CNS. Several anatomic planes are used to visualize the relevant cerebral structures (Fig. 1).[10,11] These include the *transventricular*, *transthalamic*, and *transcerebellar views*.

Transventricular View

The transventricular view is most cephalad and should include a view through the lateral cerebral ventricles and the echogenic choroid plexus (Fig. 2). Normally the choroid plexus should fill the bodies of the lateral ventricles from side to side. The atrium of lateral ventricles is measured at the level of the glomus of the choroid plexuses, perpendicular to

the cavity, positioning the calipers inside the echoes generated by the lateral walls. The measurement is stable in the second and early third trimester, with a mean diameter of 6 to 8 mm and is normally less than 10 mm.[12] In the standard transventricular plane only the downside atrium is usually clearly visualized, the hemisphere close to the transducer being usually obscured by artifacts. As ventriculomegaly may be unilateral, an attempt should be made to visualize the contralateral ventricle as well. This can be obtained with a variety of approaches, but a simple angle technique is adequate in the majority of cases.[13,14]

Transthalamic View

The transthalamic view is used for measurement of the biparietal diameter and head circumference. Biparietal diameter and head circumference have a positive correlation with gestational age (Table 1). This view includes visualization of the frontal horns and the interposed cavum septum pellucidum. The cavum septum pellucidum is a fluid-filled cavity situated between the membranes, which form the septum pellucidum. It develops relatively late in gestation and undergoes obliteration near term gestation. With transabdominal ultrasound, it should always be visualized between 18 and 37 weeks or with a biparietal diameter of 44 to 88 mm. Conversely, failure to visualize it before 18 weeks or later than 37 weeks is a normal finding.[7]

Transcerebellar Plane

The transcerebellar plane includes visualization of the midline thalamus, the cerebellar hemispheres, and the cisterna

TABLE 1. BIOMETRY OF THE FETAL HEAD THROUGHOUT GESTATION

Gestational Age (wk)	Biparietal diameter (mm)			Head circumference (mm)			Transverse cerebellar diameter (mm)		
	−2 SD	Mean	+2 SD	−2 SD	Mean	+2 SD	−2 SD	Mean	+2 SD
14	23	29	36	59	107	155	9	13	17
15	27	33	39	73	121	169	10	14	18
16	30	36	43	86	134	182	11	15	19
17	34	40	46	98	146	194	12	16	20
18	37	43	50	111	159	207	13	17	21
19	40	47	53	123	171	219	14	18	22
20	44	50	56	134	182	230	15	20	24
21	47	53	59	145	193	241	17	21	25
22	50	56	63	156	204	252	18	22	26
23	53	59	66	166	214	262	19	23	28
24	56	62	68	176	224	272	21	25	29
25	58	65	71	186	234	282	22	26	30
26	61	68	74	195	243	291	23	28	32
27	64	70	77	204	252	300	25	29	33
28	66	73	79	212	260	308	26	30	34
29	69	75	82	220	268	316	28	32	36
30	71	78	84	228	276	324	29	33	37
31	74	80	86	235	283	331	30	34	38
32	76	82	89	242	290	338	32	36	40
33	78	84	91	248	296	344	33	37	41
34	80	86	93	254	302	350	34	38	42
35	82	88	95	260	308	356	35	39	44
36	84	90	97	265	313	361	36	41	45
37	86	92	99	270	318	366	38	42	46
38	87	94	100	275	323	371	39	43	47
39	89	96	102	279	327	375	40	44	48
40	91	97	104	282	330	378	41	45	49

Courtesy of Ginaluigi Pilu, MD, Bologna, Italy.

magna (Fig. 3). Other planes of the brain and cerebellum including coronal planes can also be obtained (Fig. 4). The transverse cerebellar diameter increases by approximately 1 mm per week of pregnancy between 14 and 21 menstrual weeks. This measurement, along with the head circumfer-

ence and the biparietal diameter, is helpful to assess fetal growth. The transcerebellar diameter can be used to compare the growth of the cerebellum with other intracranial structures and is included in Table 1.[15] The depth of the cisterna magna measured between the cerebellar vermis and the inter-

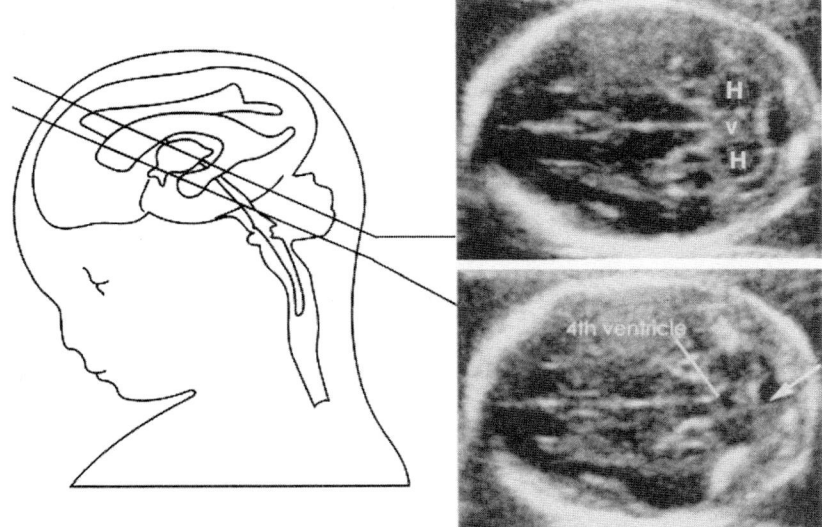

FIGURE 3. Normal posterior fossa. Schematic diagram shows oblique views through posterior fossa. Normal landmarks include the cisterna magna (*arrow*), cerebellar hemispheres (*H*), mid cerebellar vermis (*v*), and fourth ventricle.

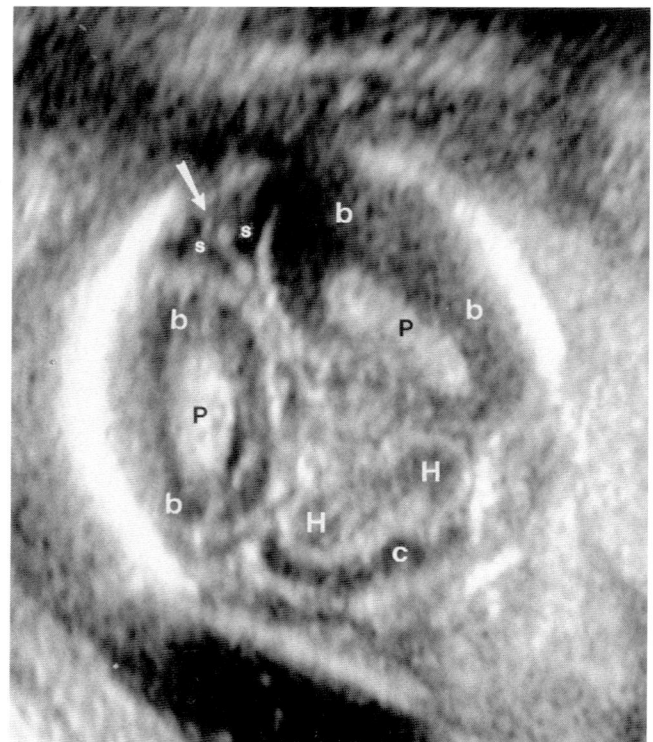

A

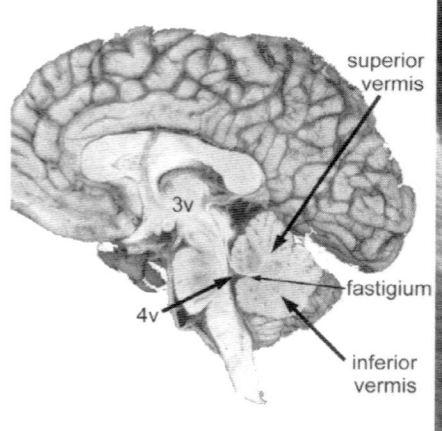

B

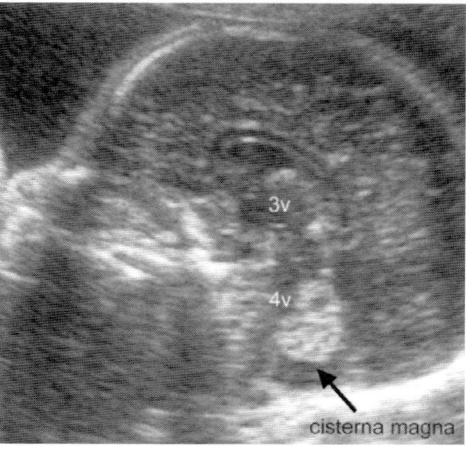

FIGURE 4. Normal posterior fossa. **A:** Posteriorly angled coronal scan shows choroid plexus (*P*) within the atrium/trigone of the lateral ventricles, cerebellar hemispheres (*H*), and cisterna magna (*c*). Superiorly, the echogenic falx (*arrow*) is bordered by subarachnoid spaces (*s*), adjacent to the hypoechoic cerebral hemispheres (*b*). **B:** Sagittal plane and corresponding pathologic specimen show third ventricle (*3v*), fourth ventricle (*4v*), cerebellar vermis, and cisterna magna. The ideal horizontal plane intersecting the fastigium of the fourth ventricle divides the cerebellar vermis into a superior and inferior portion that have about the same size.

nal side of the occipital bone should be no more than 10 mm in depth and no less than 2 mm.[16] Typically, septations are visualized within the cisterna magna. These are normal structures and should not be confused with vascular structures or cystic abnormalities in the cisterna magna.[17]

In the second and third trimesters, the vast majority of intracranial abnormalities can be identified with a systematic approach that includes these three views. At the same time, identification of (a) the ventricular atrium, (b) the cisterna magna, and (c) the cavum septi pellucidum allows exclusion of most intracranial abnormalities.[10] If the transventricular plane and the transcerebellar plane are satisfac-

torily obtained, the atrial width is less than 10 mm, and the cisterna magna width is between 2 and 10 mm, the risk of a CNS anomaly is exceedingly low.[10] Visualization of the cavum septum pellucidum may also be helpful to detect abnormalities such as the agenesis of the corpus callosum or forms of holoprosencephaly.[7]

Other Diagnostic Methods

In addition to conventional ultrasound, other commonly used diagnostic methods to evaluate the brain include color-flow Doppler, transvaginal ultrasound, three-dimen-

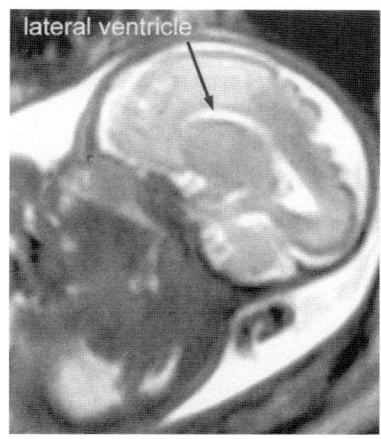 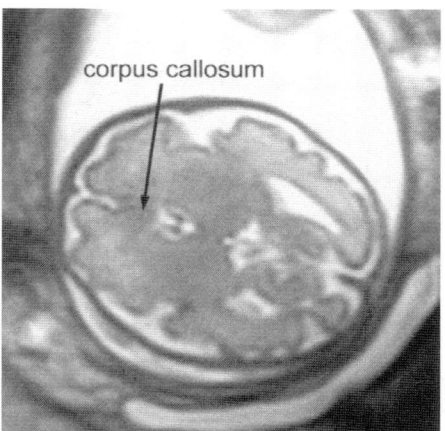 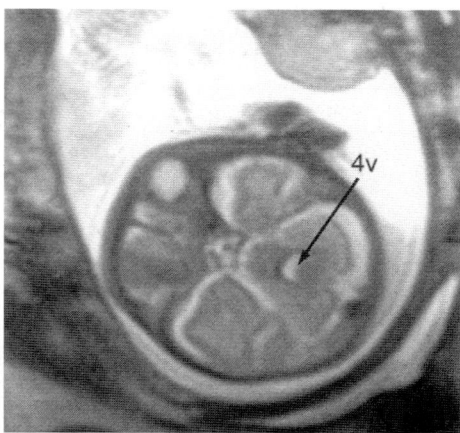

A–C

FIGURE 5. Normal anatomy, magnetic resonance imaging at 32 weeks. **A:** Parasagittal view shows lateral ventricle. **B:** Axial view corresponding to transthalamic view shows normal brain anatomy, including anterior genu of the corpus callosum. The cortex can be clearly distinguished from the surrounding subarachnoid space. The cerebral convolutions and ventricular system are easily recognized. **C:** Axial plane through posterior fossa showing cerebellum and fourth ventricle (*4v*).

sional ultrasound, and magnetic resonance imaging (MRI).[18–22]

Transvaginal sonography has been used mostly in early gestation. The images obtained closely match classic embryologic studies and have provided a new insight into the ontogenesis of the cerebrum, allowing longitudinal studies of healthy embryos.

Transvaginal sonography is also of value even in later gestation, especially in evaluations of the head and brain when the fetus is in vertex presentation. Vaginal probes have the advantage of operating at a higher frequency than abdominal probes and, therefore, allow a greater definition of anatomic details. Transvaginal neurosonography is particularly helpful in the evaluation of complex malformations. The obvious shortcoming of vaginal sonography of the fetal head is that a cephalic lie is required. However, in selected cases, an external version may be considered.

Monteagudo and Timor Tritsch[22] have described in depth the technique of transvaginal multiplanar neurosonography.

Magnetic resonance imaging (MRI) has been used in obstetric patients for the evaluation of fetal anatomy and in particular for the prediction of fetal cerebral anomalies. The MRI procedure is not believed to be hazardous to the fetus. Although the safety of MRI procedures during pregnancy has not been definitively proved,[23] MRI procedures are indicated for use in pregnant women when other nonionizing diagnostic imaging methods are inadequate or when the examination may provide important information that would otherwise require exposure to ionizing radiation [e.g., x-ray, computed tomography (CT)].[24] Early studies on the use of MRI in the evaluation of fetal morphology were hindered by fetal motion, as a long time was required for the acquisition of the images. New equipment

allows fast scanning at a reasonable level of resolution. In general, the anatomy is well depicted in fetuses older than 20 weeks' gestation.[25] Compared with ultrasound, MRI allows better discrimination between the cortex and the cerebrospinal fluid (CSF) (Fig. 5) and is not influenced by fetal position, skull calcification, and oligohydramnios. Most of the latest clinical studies tend to demonstrate that fast MRI provides additional information to the sonographic examination, which may have value in the presence of complex cerebral anomalies.[26] It may be particularly helpful in confirming or diagnosing brain abnormalities including agenesis of the corpus callosum, posterior fossa cysts, cerebral clefts, migrational disorders, and intracranial haemorrhage.[27–29] The use of MRI is discussed in greater detail in Chapter 25.

ABNORMALITIES

Ventriculomegaly

Ventriculomegaly in the strictest sense refers to enlargement of the cerebral ventricles without specifying a cause. The term *hydrocephalus* is usually reserved for more severe cases of ventriculomegaly, and this usually implies an obstructive etiology. Subsequent sections within this chapter discuss in more detail the specific disorders that may cause ventriculomegaly, whereas this section discusses more general concepts relating to ventriculomegaly.

Pathogenesis

Ventriculomegaly is frequently the consequence of a cranial or cerebral malformation or disruptive event, but may be secondary to a number of etiologies, and is frequently

TABLE 2. ANOMALIES MOST FREQUENTLY ASSOCIATED WITH VENTRICULOMEGALY AND DISTINGUISHING FEATURES

Anomaly	Feature
Spina bifida	Deformed cranium (*lemon* sign), usually disappears in third trimester
	Obliteration of cisterna magna (*banana* sign)
	Open spinal defect
Cephalocele	Open cranial defect, usually occipital skull base
	Obliteration of the cisterna magna
	Occasional *lemon* sign
Holoprosencephaly	Absent/incomplete midline
	Single ventricular cavity
	Facial anomalies
Dandy-Walker complex	Midline posterior fossa cyst
	Defect in cerebellar vermis
Agenesis of corpus callosum	Absent cavum septi pellucidi
	Elevated third ventricle
	Interhemispheric cyst/lipoma
Arachnoid/glioependymal cyst	Intracranial cyst with regular contours displacing/compressing cortex
Porencephaly	Intracranial cyst with jagged outline often communicating with lateral ventricles
	Destruction of brain tissue
Schizencephaly	Clefts in cortical mantle
Intracranial hemorrhage	Echogenic/complex mass in lateral ventricles/brain parenchyma
Microcephaly	Small head
Vascular malformations	Fluid-filled lesion with blood flow at Doppler examination
Craniostenosis	Abnormal skull shape
Lissencephaly	Absent/reduced cerebral convolutions
Infection	Intracranial/periventricular echogenicities

Modified from Nyberg et al. Cerebral malformations. In: Nyberg DA, Mahony BS, Pretorius DH, eds. *Diagnostic ultrasound of fetal anomalies: text and atlas.* Chicago: Year Book, 1990; and McGahan J, Thurmond A. The fetal head. In: McGahan J, Porto M, eds. *Diagnostic obstetrical ultrasound.* Philadelphia: JB Lippincott, 1994.

found in association with a number of fetal anomalies or fetal syndromes, including chromosomal aberrations and infections. A list of conditions that are most commonly found with fetal ventriculomegaly is in Table 2.

Excluding mild degrees of ventriculomegaly, which may be transient and normal, ventriculomegaly may be due to one of three broad categories: obstructive hydrocephalus, brain atrophy, and abnormal development of the brain. Obstructive hydrocephalus may be further categorized as noncommunicating when the blockage of flow of CSF is within the ventricles or communicating when the blockage of flow of the CSF is outside the ventricular system. In the fetus, obstructive hydrocephalus is usually noncommunicating.

In utero destruction of the cortex may result in brain atrophy and secondary ventriculomegaly from an *ex vacuo* phenomenon. Brain destruction may include *in utero* damage from a vascular accident or an infection. Maldevelopment of the brain may be associated with secondary ventricular dilatation secondary to decreased brain mass, similar to that from brain destruction. For example, agenesis of the corpus callosum is commonly associated with mild to moderate ventriculomegaly, which is nonobstructive and nonprogressive. This is presumably secondary to abnormal development of the white matter and decreased brain mass. Similarly, lissencephaly is associated with thinning of the cortex and ventriculomegaly, and this is probably also the basis for nonobstructive ventricular dilatation observed with many cases of fetal aneuploidy.

Diagnosis

The cerebral lateral ventricles have a complex three-dimensional architecture that furthermore undergoes major developmental changes throughout gestation. Sonographic assessment of these structures has been the object of many sonographic studies, and many different approaches to the definition and diagnosis of fetal ventriculomegaly have been suggested from time to time. Reference charts have been established for all the different portions of the lateral ventricles, measured both in standard axial planes[30,31] as well as with coronal and sagittal sections.[32]

Measurement of the transverse diameter of the ventricular atrium at the level of the glomus of the choroid plexus is the most commonly accepted method of assessing ventricular size.[10,12] The measurement is easily obtained and is reproducible.[33] Different studies yielded very similar results in the midtrimester, reporting a mean value of the atrial width of approximately 7 mm and a standard deviation of approximately 1 mm.[10,12,34–36] There is less agreement on the normal values in the third trimester, however. In two studies, the atrial width was found to remain constant between 15 weeks and term gestation.[10,31] However, these studies included relatively small numbers of third-trimester fetuses. Two larger reports were at variance with these results. One study of 503 fetuses demonstrated similar mean values in the second and third trimester but revealed an increase in the standard deviation throughout gestation. The mean +2 standard deviations increased from 9.2 at 16 weeks to 10.2 at term.[36] Another series of 838 cases described a slight increase throughout gestation, with mean values of approximately 6 mm and 8 mm at 14 and 40 weeks, respectively, and a 95% confidence interval that exceeded 10 mm from 34 weeks on.[35] Some degree of asymmetry of the lateral ventricles exists in the human fetal brain[37] and is detectable *in utero*.[38]

It is clear that there is no specific value of ventricular size that absolutely differentiates between a normal and an abnormal group. Ventriculomegaly is dynamic, and there is no doubt fetuses with a normal ventricular measurement early in pregnancy may become abnormal. Likewise, there are fetuses with mild ventriculomegaly that were later found to be normal. At present, however, clinical series indicate that a measurement of the ventricular atrium of less than 10 mm should be considered normal, whereas a measurement of 10 mm or more indicates an increased risk of cerebral malformations and extracranial anomalies and warrants the need for further investigation.

Other secondary signs that may be helpful to diagnose ventriculomegaly include choroid plexus separation from the ventricular wall. Because the choroid normally fills the ventricles from side-to-side, separation of the choroids from the ventricular wall is an easy subjective sign that may indicate ventricular dilatation. Separation of 4 mm or greater[39] or 3 mm or greater[40] has been used to identify fetuses' ventricular dilatation, even when the atrium was 10 mm or less.

Finally, the choroid plexus can be seen to *dangle* within the dilated ventricle when there is true ventriculomegaly or hydrocephalus. The intersection of the long axis of the downside of the choroid plexus and the long axis of the midline structures form the choroid angle, which is usually between 16 and 22 degrees. If the choroid angle is greater than 29 degrees, this is usually indicative of ventriculomegaly.[41] In most cases, this dangling choroid is easy to recognize and no specific measurement is made.

It is also important to note the location of the choroid plexus in all cases of possible ventriculomegaly. In the second trimester of pregnancy, the cerebral hemispheres may appear hypoechoic, falsely giving the appearance of hydrocephalus, which in fact is pseudo-hydrocephalus. However, with pseudo-hydrocephalus the choroid plexus never is dangling (as the ventricles are not enlarged). Thus, noting if the choroid plexus is not dangling is helpful in distinguishing true hydrocephalus from pseudo-hydrocephalus.[42,61]

Borderline Ventriculomegaly

Synonyms for borderline ventriculomegaly include mild hydrocephalus and mild ventriculomegaly.

Borderline ventriculomegaly is mild enlargement of the lateral ventricles in the absence of other sonographically demonstrable CNS anomalies. Ventriculomegaly is suspected when the atrial diameter reaches 10 mm[43] although separation of the dependent choroid from the medial ventricular wall may be visible evidence for early ventricular dilatation.[40]

Incidence

The incidence is uncertain. An atrial width of 10 mm is approximately 3 standard deviations above the mean.[12,31] The only two prospective series on low-risk patients had conflicting results, ranging from 1 per 50[36] to 1 per 1,600.[34] The reason for such a discrepancy is not obvious.

It may represent the consequence of a different technique for obtaining the measurement or of a discrepancy in the gestational age of the fetuses examined.

Etiology and Pathology

In most cases, borderline or mild ventriculomegaly is probably a normal variant, but in other cases it may be the only obvious sign of an underlying fetal anomaly. It is more likely to be seen as a normal variant later in the second trimester (after 20 weeks) in male fetuses and fetuses who are large for gestational age.

The observation that borderline or mild ventricular dilatation is more commonly seen in male fetuses is consistent with the observation that male fetuses have been shown to have slightly but significantly larger measurements of ventricular size than females.[44,45] Although this is unexplained, it might reflect a slightly but significantly larger size of the calvaria in male fetuses that has been observed compared to female fetuses.[46] Assuming the brain size is no bigger in males, the *extra* intracranial room is taken up by subarachnoid and ventricular volume. Whereas this is speculative, it does help explain two gender-specific observations.

Diagnosis

Ultrasound is highly sensitive for detecting borderline or mild cerebral ventricular dilatation but is nonspecific. As described with ventriculomegaly, recognition of ventricular dilatation may be made by subjective or objective criteria. The most widely accepted objective definition of ventricular dilatation is an atrial width of 10 mm or more (Fig. 6).[43] Some consider mild ventricular dilatation to include measurements of 10 mm to 15 mm, whereas others consider it as an atrial width of 10 mm to 12 mm.[47] Borderline ventriculomegaly may be unilateral.[48]

Whereas objective measurements of ventricular dilatation are most commonly accepted and are satisfactory in permitting comparison of measurements, it is clear that some cases of visible ventricular dilatation have measurements of lateral ventricles of less than 10 mm. For example, fetuses with spina bifida typically have only borderline or mild degrees of ventricular dilatation during the second trimester, and their ventricles may measure less than 10 mm, even when the ventricle appears subjectively increased and when ventricular dilatation is progressive on serial examinations.

Hertzberg et al.[40] defined a population in which the downside ventricular atrium was 10 mm or less, but there was a 3 mm or greater separation in the choroid plexus from the ventricular wall. The outcome was normal in 80% but abnormal in 20%. This is an interesting observation and worthwhile to consider. For lack of other distinguishing criteria, however, most authorities consider ventricles less than 10 mm in the second or third trimester to be normal.[5,10]

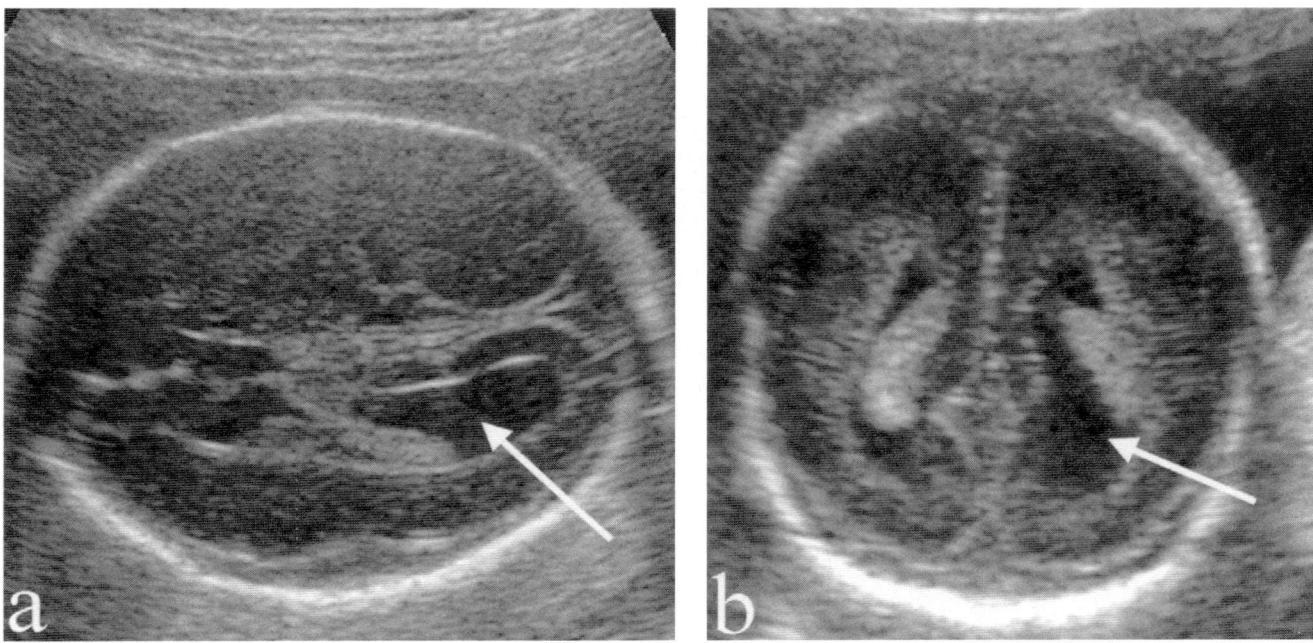

FIGURE 6. Borderline dilatation of the lateral ventricles. **A:** Axial scan shows borderline dilatation of the dependent lateral ventricle (*arrow*) with separation of the choroid from the medial wall of the ventricle. At the level of ventricular atrium, the ventricle measures 11 mm in diameter. **B:** Transvaginal scan shows mild dilatation only of the dependent ventricle (*arrow*).

Differential Diagnosis

Isolated borderline ventriculomegaly should be differentiated from more complex abnormalities of the fetal brain that have frequently a different prognosis (e.g., agenesis of the corpus callosum, spina bifida, and fetal infections).

Prognosis

Determining the prognosis in an individual case of fetal mild cerebral ventriculomegaly is a difficult task. Although the vast majority of fetuses have a normal outcome (Fig. 7), a variety of adverse outcomes have also been reported. A summary of these

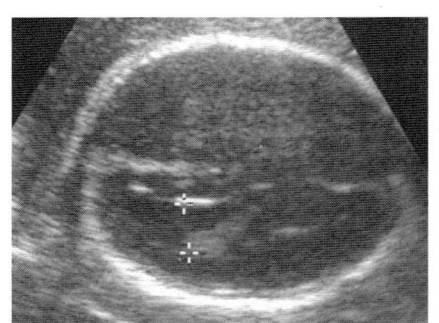
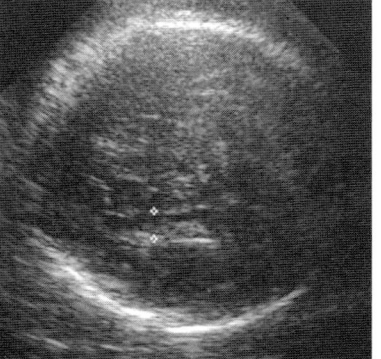

FIGURE 7. Borderline dilatation of the lateral cerebral ventricles in normal fetus. **A:** Axial scan at 19 weeks shows borderline dilatation of the dependent lateral ventricle, which measures 10 to 11 mm at the level of the ventricular atrium. **B:** Follow-up scan at 37 weeks shows normal ventricular size of 7 to 8 mm. This was a male fetus who was also large for gestational age.

TABLE 3. A SUMMARY OF THE OUTCOMES OF INFANTS WITH A PRENATAL DIAGNOSIS OF BORDERLINE CEREBRAL VENTRICULOMEGALY

Aneuploidies	9/234	3.8%
Cerebral anomalies undiagnosed *in utero*	9/221	4%
Malformations undiagnosed *in utero*, overall	19/221	8.6%
Perinatal deaths	8/209	3.7%
Abnormal development	24/209	11.5%
Abnormal outcome (overall)	43/219	19.6%

Modified from Pilu G, Falco P, Gabrielli S, Perolo A, Sandri F, et al. The clinical significance of fetal isolated cerebral borderline ventriculomegaly: report of 31 cases and review of the literature. *Ultrasound Obstet Gynecol* 1999;14:320–326.

studies[49] is demonstrated in Table 3. In 4% of cases, aneuploidies were present, and trisomy 21 was the most frequent one (Fig. 8). In 4% of cases, developmental malformations of the cerebrum were found in late gestation or after birth, including progressive hypertensive hydrocephalus and cystic brain lesions. Independently from the presence of aneuploidies or underlying malformations, most studies were consistent in indicating an excess of abnormal intellectual and motor development. This was predominantly of mild and moderate entity.

Males were found to have borderline ventriculomegaly more frequently than females and to have a lesser degree of abnormal outcomes (5% vs. 24%), and this is consistent with the observation that male fetuses tend to have a slightly greater atrial width than females.[44,45] Abnormal outcomes were also more frequent with an atrial width greater than 11 mm (9% vs. 24%). Intrauterine resolution of borderline-mild ventriculomegaly has been found to be a favorable prognostic finding.[40,44] It is uncertain whether the prognosis is better for fetuses with unilateral mild ventricular dilatation. In a report of 28 such fetuses, one had trisomy 21 and another developed seizures.[48]

Management

Detection of borderline-mild ventricular dilatation should initiate a search for associated congenital anomalies, and this may include fetal karyotyping. Some authorities might also recommend exclusion of fetal infections associated with hydrocephaly (i.e., toxoplasmosis, cytomegalovirus, rubella). MRI might also be considered, to help exclude an underlying brain abnormality. In continuing pregnancies, borderline cerebral ventriculomegaly is not an indication to modify standard obstetric care. Serial scans should be performed, as in a handful of cases ventriculomegaly and macrocrania may develop.

Because fetuses with isolated borderline cerebral ventriculomegaly are at increased risk for developmental delay, it has been suggested that this finding could represent an indication for early childhood intervention, as special educational programs maximize the developmental potential.[50]

Recurrence Risk

The recurrence risk is not known to be increased.

Isolated Moderate and Severe Lateral Ventriculomegaly/Aqueductal Stenosis

Synonyms for isolated moderate and severe lateral ventriculomegaly/aqueductal stenosis include ventriculomegaly, hydrocephalus, aqueductal stenosis, and communicating hydrocephalus.

Sonographic diagnosis of ventricular dilatation depends on subjective impression and objective measurement of the lateral ventricle obtained at the ventricular atrium. Moderate to severe ventriculomegaly is defined here as atrial width greater than 15 mm in the absence of other sonographically demonstrable CNS anomalies.[6,10]

Incidence

The incidence of congenital cerebral lateral ventriculomegaly ranges between 0.3 to 1.5 in 1,000 births in different series.[51] Isolated ventriculomegaly accounts for 30% to 60% of fetuses with enlarged lateral cerebral ventricles.[52]

Etiology

Congenital ventriculomegaly is a heterogeneous disease for which genetic, infectious, teratogenetic, and neoplastic causes have been implicated. X-linked hydrocephalus (MIM 307000)[53] comprises approximately 5% of all cases. This condition is caused by mutations in the gene at Xq28 encoding for L1, a cell surface glycoprotein implicated in migration of neurons and the signal transduction events that control axonal growth. Mutations in this gene are also responsible for

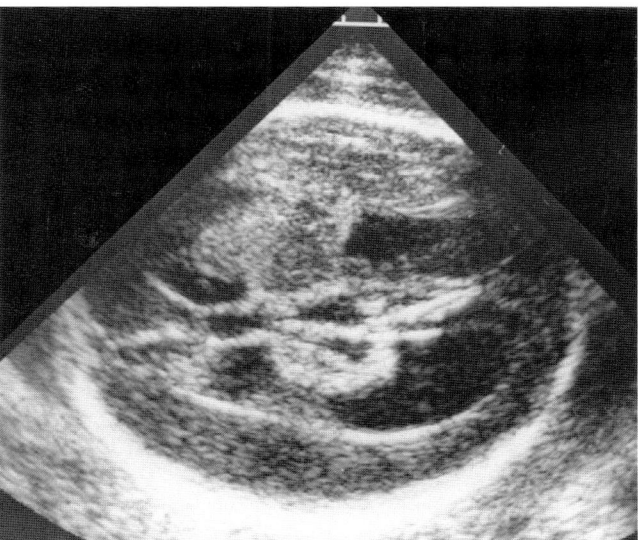

FIGURE 8. Mild dilatation of lateral ventricles, trisomy 21. Transvaginal scan at 20 weeks shows mild dilatation of lateral ventricles to 12 mm. Chromosome analysis yielded trisomy 21.

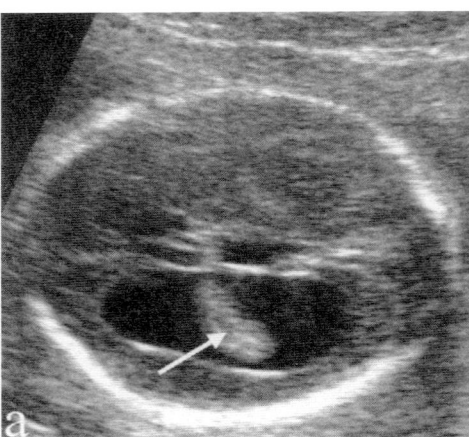 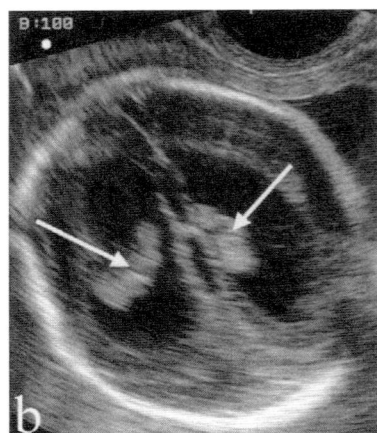 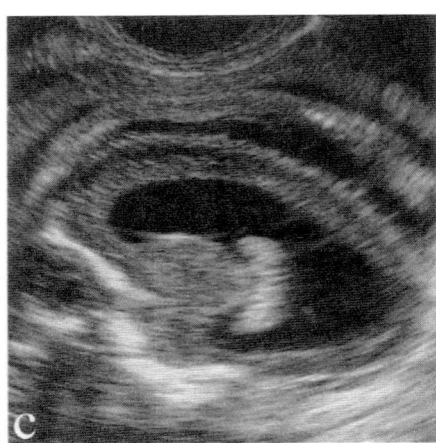

FIGURE 9. Moderate ventriculomegaly at midgestation. Axial **(A)**, coronal **(B)**, and parasagittal **(C)** images show overall enlargement of both lateral ventricles, with dangling choroid plexuses (*arrows*) and thinning of the cortex.

other syndromes with clinical overlap that are frequently referred to as the X-linked hydrocephalus spectrum or L1 spectrum and include mental retardation, aphasias, shuffling gait, adducted thumbs syndrome; complicated X-linked spastic paraplegia; X-linked mental retardation–clasped thumb syndrome; and some forms of X-linked agenesis of the corpus callosum.[54] Infections implicated in the determination of congenital ventriculomegaly include toxoplasmosis, syphilis, cytomegalovirus, mumps, and influenza virus.

Pathology

Moderate to severe lateral ventriculomegaly (Figs. 9 and 10) can result from different pathologic entities. Fetuses with isolated ventriculomegaly to this degree are usually found at

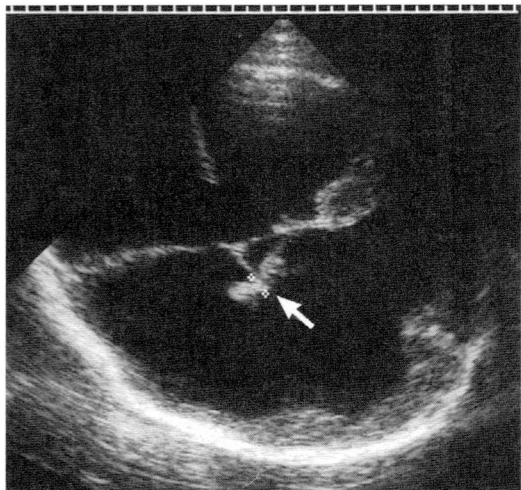

FIGURE 10. Marked hydrocephalus. Axial scan at term shows marked hydrocephalus. The choroid from the near ventricle is dangling into the dependent ventricle (*arrow*).

birth to have either aqueductal stenosis or communicating ventriculomegaly. Progression from communicating ventriculomegaly to aqueductal stenosis has been documented, and it is uncertain whether these two conditions are separate clinical entities. Communicating hydrocephalus may, however, derive from acute events such as subarachnoid hemorrhage or be caused by overproduction of CSF by a choroid plexus papilloma. The degree of ventricular enlargement is variable. Knowledge about the pathogenesis of congenital ventriculomegaly is largely incomplete. Thinning of the cortex, macrocrania, and symptoms of intracranial hypertension are frequently found. Studies performed in experimental animals and based on biopsies of brain tissue obtained in children at the time of shunting seem to demonstrate the following sequence of events: initially there is disruption of the ependymal lining followed by edema of the white matter. This phase has been considered reversible. Later, there is proliferation of astrocytes and fibrosis of the white matter. The gray matter seems to be spared during the initial stages of the process.

Diagnosis

Ultrasound
Sonographic diagnosis of ventricular dilatation depends on subjective impression and objective measurement of the lateral ventricle obtained at the ventricular atrium. Moderate to severe lateral cerebral ventriculomegaly has been defined by some as a ventricular measurement of 15 mm or more.[6,10] It has been our experience, and it has been reported in a handful of cases, that ventriculomegaly may develop only in late gestation or after birth, particularly with the X-linked hydrocephalus spectrum.[55] Therefore, patients at risk should be informed that a normal midtrimester sonogram does not rule out this condition.

Sonographic demonstration of abducted thumbs in combination with ventriculomegaly and other intracranial abnormalities should prompt the diagnosis of X-linked hydrocephalus spectrum.[56]

Laboratory

Couples with a previously affected child should receive genetic counseling because sometimes a generic diagnosis of congenital hydrocephalus may hinder a more complex anomaly with significant genetic implications. Patients at risk for X-linked hydrocephalus spectrum should be offered deoxyribonucleic acid analysis.[57]

Differential Diagnosis

Other disorders, such as holoprosencephaly, porencephaly, and agenesis of corpus callosum, should be identified by their specific intracranial abnormality. Intraventricular hemorrhage can be identified by the appearance of the ventricles with internal echoes and echogenic ventricular wall. Infectious etiology can be suggested by periventricular echogenicities in some cases.

Associated Anomalies

Extracranial abnormality occurs in 30%[60] of cases.[52] Chromosomal aberrations are found in 11% of cases, including 6% of fetuses with ventriculomegaly as the only antenatal finding, and 25% when multiple anomalies are present.[58] The X-linked hydrocephalus spectrum is frequently associated with abduction of the thumbs, abnormal facies, and absence of the septum pellucidum.[54]

Prognosis

X-linked hydrocephalus spectrum carries a severe prognosis, being usually associated with severe neurologic deficits and premature death.[54] In a large pediatric series (excluding cases with X-linked hydrocephalus and congenital toxoplasmosis), the survival rate was 62% at 10 years, and 50% of survivors had a low developmental quotient (less than 60). Only 29% of infants attending school reached a normal academic level. Macrocrania at birth, ventricular size, and age at surgery had no influence on the outcome.[59] In a review of hydrocephalus diagnosed prenatally, Gupta et al. suggested a 70% survival rate, and 59% of the survivors had normal developmental quotient at follow-up.[60] On the other hand, among 30 cases of moderate to severe hydrocephalus in which a more specific aqueductal stenosis was diagnosed *in utero* and the pregnancy was continued, Levitsky et al.[61] reported normal development in only 10% and moderate or severe developmental delay in 73%. The overall survival rate was 60% in that series.

In most, albeit not all, cases, intracranial hypertension develops after birth, and a shunting procedure is necessary.

Management

A search for associated congenital anomalies (including fetal karyotyping) and a workup for congenital infections associated with hydrocephaly (i.e., toxoplasmosis, cytomegalovirus, rubella) is indicated. MRI should be considered in any case of hydrocephalus to detect additional brain anomalies.

Little data exist to support any specific management plan in continuing pregnancies. Cesarean section should be reserved for standard obstetric indications.

Cephalocentesis and *in utero* shunting has been virtually abandoned in the United States. In a group of 39 fetuses treated with *in utero* shunting, the perinatal mortality rate was 18%, and 66% of the survivors was affected by moderate to severe handicaps.[62] However, the major shortcoming of this study was the poor selection of cases undergoing treatment. Many of these fetuses had malformations that were either untreatable or very severe (e.g., holoprosencephaly, Dandy-Walker malformation). A better selection of cases to treat as well as use of the new fetal endoscopic techniques may provide a different approach to the problem in the future.

Recurrence Risk

In a study of 261 prospectively ascertained pregnancies, Varadi et al. reported the overall recurrence risk is approximately 4%, and that, apart from the X-linked recessive cases, ventriculomegaly is mostly multifactorially determined.[63]

MIDLINE ANOMALIES

Midline anomalies of the brain include a heterogenous group of conditions with similarities in the etiology and pathogenetic mechanisms.[64] Table 4 reports the classification originally proposed by De Myer[65] and later revised by Fitz[66] that distinguishes two main categories: disorders of closure and disorders

TABLE 4. CLASSIFICATION OF MIDLINE ANOMALIES OF THE BRAIN

Disorders of diverticulation
Holoprosencephaly
Lobar
Semilobar
Alobar
Disorders of closure
Facial clefts
Cranioschisis
Corpus callosum
Agenesis
Lipoma
Chiari malformation
Dandy-Walker malformation

Modified from DeMyer W. Classification of cerebral malformations. *Birth Defects* 1971;7:78; and Fitz CR. Midline anomalies of the brain and spine. *Radiol Clin North Am* 1982;20:95.

TABLE 5. MIDLINE INTRACRANIAL CYSTS: DISTINGUISHING FEATURES

Cyst type	Location	Features
Dandy-Walker	Posterior fossa	Communication with fourth ventricle
		Concomitant hydrocephalus
Vein of Galen aneurysms	Supratentorial, posterior to corpus callosum	Doppler signal within cyst
		Arteriovenous shunting
Arachnoid cyst	Any location	Smooth wall
		Asymmetric location
		Mass effect
		With or without hydrocephalus (dependent on location)
Cystic neoplasm	Any location	Solid mass
		Cystic components
		Irregular outline
		Mass effect
Agenesis of the corpus callosum with interhemispheric cyst	Interhemispheric cyst between frontal horns of the lateral ventricles	Communication with cephalad displaced third ventricle
Alobar holoprosencephaly	Posterior, supratentorial	Typical features of alobar holoprosencephaly (see Table 2 and Fig. 12)

Reproduced with permission from McGahan J, Thurmond A. The fetal head. In: McGahan J, Porto M, eds. *Diagnostic obstetrical ultrasound*. Philadelphia: JB Lippincott, 1994.

of diverticulation. Disorders of closure include mostly neural tube defects that are considered in Chapter 7. Disorders of diverticulation include a series of conditions that are thought to derive from failure of cleavage of the cerebral hemispheres and formation of the midline structures. The ontogenesis of the cerebral midline is frequently referred to as the process of *ventral induction*. It takes place between the seventh week of amenorrhea and midgestation and is embryologically related to the development of the midface. Disorders of cerebral diverticulation are indeed often a part of malformative sequences that include typical craniofacial malformations.[67]

This section covers intracranial midline abnormalities, namely holoprosencephaly, septooptic dysplasia, agenesis of corpus callosum, and Dandy-Walker malformation. The rationale for grouping together these conditions is mostly clinical and is twofold. First, these disorders are very frequently found in association and are, therefore, most likely related embryologically and etiologically. Second, the approach to the sonographic diagnosis in the antenatal period requires a similar approach. Indeed, these anomalies result in complex rearrangements of the cerebral architecture. A meticulous scanning technique and the use of nonroutine views of the fetal brain, such as those obtained in coronal and sagittal planes, are frequently necessary for a specific recognition.

In addition to these midline abnormalities, other malformations may occur in the midline. For instance, Galen's vein aneurysms or Galen's vein malformation primarily appears as a supratentorial midline cyst. Pulsed Doppler, color Doppler, or power Doppler demonstrates this cyst has flow with arteriovenous shunting. In addition to this abnormality, arachnoid cysts may be located in a number of regions within the calvaria. Whereas a majority of these cysts are lateralizing cysts, some of the cysts may be midline in location. Thus, these should be considered when identifying a cystic midline structure. Finally, *in utero* intracranial

neoplasms are rare. They may be in a variety of the locations but may appear midline or close to the midline. Some of these distinguishing features of midline abnormalities are listed in Table 5. Many of these abnormalities are discussed in more detail elsewhere in this chapter.

Holoprosencephaly

Holoprosencephaly is a genetically and phenotypically heterogeneous disorder, involving the development of the forebrain and midface.

A synonym for holoprosencephaly is arrhinencephaly.

Incidence

Holoprosencephaly is rarely found at birth. An incidence of 1 per 16,000 neonates is commonly quoted.[68] This condition, however, is probably associated with a high intrauterine fatality rate, and it is likely that the obstetric sonographers encounter it more frequently than expected from epidemiologic surveys at birth. This concept is supported by one study on voluntary terminations of pregnancies in the first and second trimester, in which holoprosencephaly was found in 1 of 250 conceptuses[69] and by a considerable number of reports on cases diagnosed antenatally with ultrasound published in the 1980s and 1990s. Whereas the most severe forms of holoprosencephaly are probably associated with early pregnancy loss, it is also very likely that the minor forms are not recognized at birth, thus escaping epidemiologic surveys.

Etiology

Holoprosencephaly is a genetically heterogeneous condition involving at least 12 loci on 11 chromosomes.[70] The known holoprosencephaly-associated genes include (SHH) on 7q36 (MIM 600725); ZIC2 on 13q32 (MIM 603073); SIX3 on 2p21 (MIM 603714); and TG-interacting factor on 18p11.3 (MIM 602630). There are no environmental teratogens known to cause this malformation in humans, but in animals the condition can be induced by veratrum alkaloids and radiation. Ingestion of salicylates in pregnancy has also been reported in relation to holoprosencephaly.[68]

Pathology

Holoprosencephaly is commonly regarded as the result of a failure of cleavage of the prosencephalon (Fig. 11). The prosencephalon is the most rostrad of the three primitive cerebral vesicles and gives rise to the cerebral hemispheres and diencephalic structures (including neurohypophysis, thalami, third ventricle). This differentiation process is thought to be induced by the prechordal mesenchyma, which is probably also responsible for the differentiation of the median facial structures (forehead, nose, interorbital structures, premaxilla, and upper lip).

An interference with the activity of the prechordal mesenchyma leads to defects in both areas, brain and midface. The cerebral anomalies are due to varying degrees of failure of cleavage of the derivatives of the prosencephalon, with incomplete division of the cerebral hemispheres and underlying structures.

A widely accepted classification recognizes three major varieties of holoprosencephaly: the alobar, semilobar, and lobar type.[68] Alobar holoprosencephaly has been further subcategorized as three different configurations: the *pancake*, *cup*, and *ball* variations. This concept refers to the residual cerebral tissue that appears in these forms (Fig. 12).

In the alobar form of holoprosencephaly, the interhemispheric fissure and the falx cerebri are totally absent; there is a single primitive ventricle; the thalami are fused on the midline; and there is absence of the third ventricle, neuro-

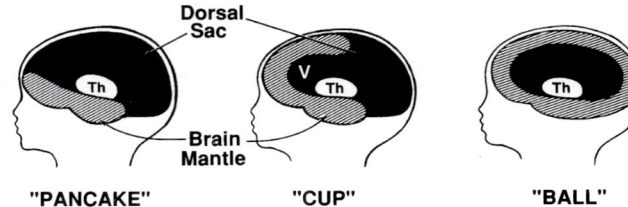

FIGURE 12. Diagram of three morphologic types of alobar holoprosencephaly (and semilobar holoprosencephaly) in sagittal view. Pancake type: The residual brain mantle is flattened at the base of the brain. The dorsal sac is correspondingly large. Cup type: More brain mantle is present, but it does not cover the monoventricle. The dorsal sac communicates widely with the monoventricle. Ball type: Brain mantle completely covers the monoventricle, and a dorsal sac may or may not be present. Th, thalami; V, ventricle. (Modified from McGahan JP, Ellis W, Lindfors KK, et al. Congenital cerebrospinal fluid–containing intracranial abnormalities: sonographic classification. *J Clin Ultrasound* 1988:16:531–544.)

hypophysis, olfactory bulbs, and tracts. In the semilobar variety, the two cerebral hemispheres are partially separated posteriorly, but there is still a single ventricular cavity. In the alobar and semilobar forms, the roof of the ventricular cavity, the tela choroidea, normally enfolded within the brain, may balloon out between the cerebral convexity and the skull to form a cyst of variable size, commonly referred to as the *dorsal sac*.

With lobar holoprosencephaly, the anatomic derangement is much more subtle. In pathologic studies, this condition is usually described as a brain almost completely divided into two distinct hemispheres, with the only exception of a variable degree of fusion at the level of the cingulate gyrus and frontal horns of lateral ventricles. The septum pellucidum is always absent. The olfactory bulbs and tracts and the corpus callosum may be absent, hypoplastic, or normal. An interesting aspect of lobar holoprosencephaly that has been recently described in studies using magnetic resonance is the fusion of the fornices, which are seen as a solid fascicle running in the midline in the upper portion of the third ventricle.[71]

Diagnosis

The most valuable clue to the diagnosis is the demonstration of the single primitive ventricle[72] and fused central thalami (Figs. 13 through 16). Dilatation of the monoventricle may be obvious later but is often subtle or mild during early pregnancy (Figs. 13 and 15). Therefore, it is important to be familiar with normal anatomic landmarks (see Chapter 1) to recognize abnormalities such as alobar and semilobar holoprosencephaly.[72,73]

When present, the dorsal sac can be recognized (Fig. 16), as well as facial anomalies such as cyclopia, hypotelorism, anophthalmia, arhinia, proboscis, and median cleft lip.[74] By using high-frequency transvaginal transducers, the diagnosis is easily made at the onset of the second trimester and may be possible as early as 10 weeks' gesta-

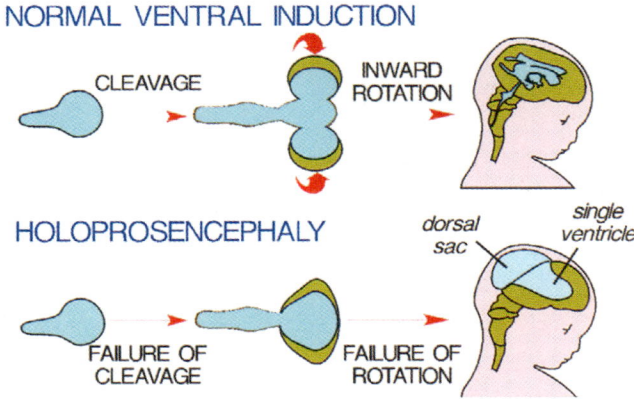

FIGURE 11. The process of ventral induction, in normal fetuses and in holoprosencephaly. In alobar holoprosencephaly, there is failure of brain cleavage and rotation, resulting in a monoventricular cavity.

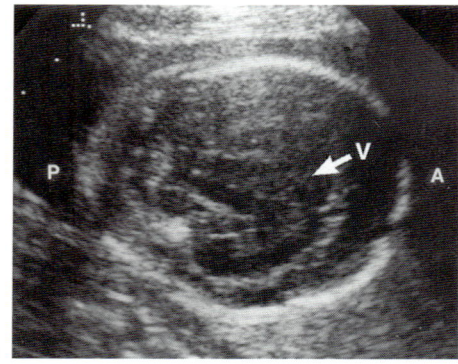
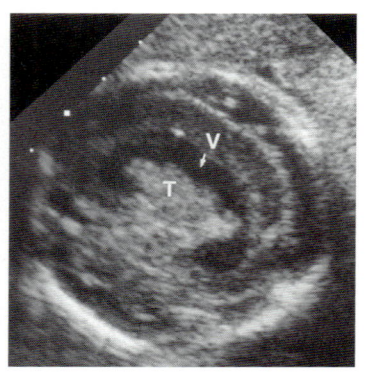
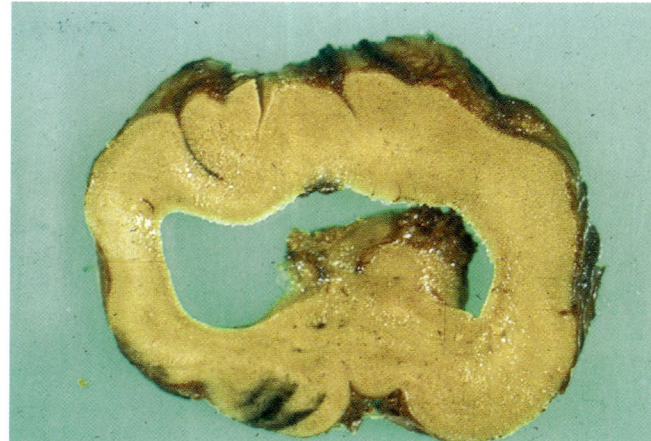

FIGURE 13. Alobar holoprosencephaly, *ball* type. **A:** Transverse view of head might superficially be considered to appear normal. However, normal bilateral choroids filling both ventricles were not demonstrated, and there is evidence of a monoventricular cavity (*V*). A, anterior; P, posterior. **B:** Transvaginal coronal scan better shows the monoventricular cavity (*V*) and fused thalami (*T*). Other views also showed a cleft lip and palate. **C:** Pathologic correlation of similar case shows monoventricle and fused central thalami. (Part **C** courtesy of Raj Kapur, MD, Department of Pathology, Children's Hospital, Seattle, WA.)

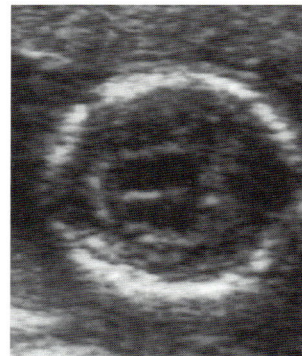
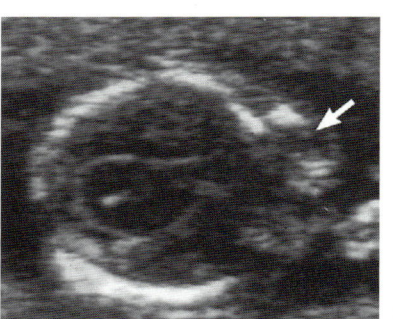

FIGURE 14. Alobar holoprosencephaly. **A:** Transverse view of head at 14 weeks shows prominent central fused thalami. Normal lateral ventricles were not demonstrated. **B:** View slightly inferior shows hypotelorism (*arrow*). Fetal karyotype was trisomy 13.

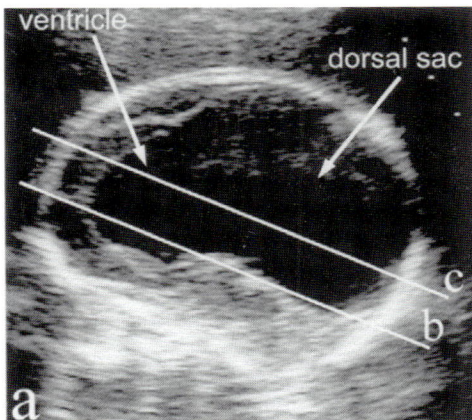
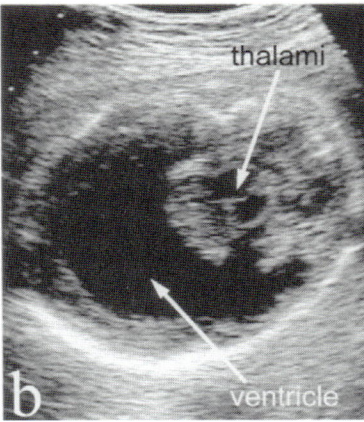
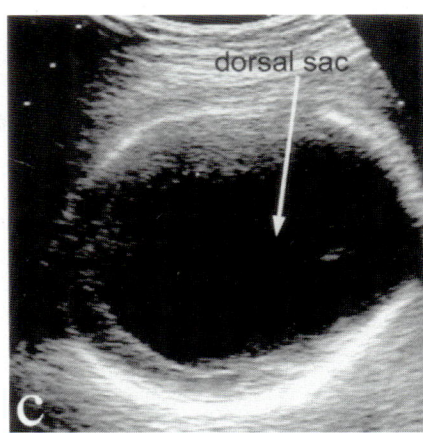

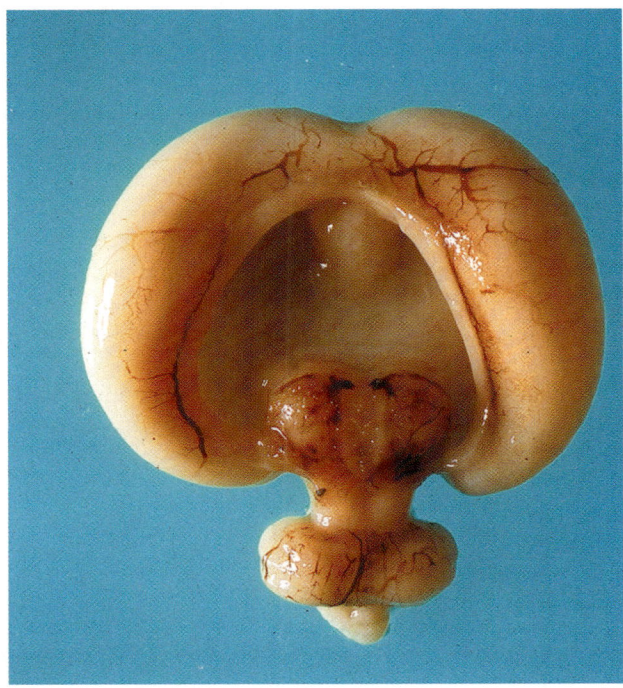

FIGURE 15. Alobar holoprosencephaly *cup* type. **A:** Sagittal plane demonstrating the single ventricular cavity that has a rim of cortex anteriorly and amply communicates posteriorly with a dorsal sac. b and c, axial scans corresponding to parts **A** and **B**. **B:** Axial scan at the level of the thalamus, demonstrating the crescent-shaped single ventricle, absence of midline structures in the anterior cortex, and fused thalami. **C:** At a slightly higher axial plane than the previous one, the communication between the ventricular cavity and the dorsal sac is demonstrated. **D:** Pathologic correlation shows monoventricle. Dorsal sac was also present. The karyotype was normal. (Courtesy of Joseph R. Siebert, PhD, Department of Pathology, Children's Hospital, Seattle, WA.)

tion.[75] All varieties of holoprosencephaly are often associated with microcephaly, and less frequently associated with macrocephaly, which is invariably due to internal obstructive hydrocephalus.

Prenatal recognition of the lobar type of holoprosencephaly may be difficult (Fig. 17). Findings include absence of the septum pellucidum and a wide communication between the frontal horns and the inferior third ventricle.[76] The lateral ventricles may or may not be enlarged. In some cases the fornices have an abnormal configuration, seen in the midline as a thick fascicle running from the anterior to the posterior commissure. In a midcoronal scan the abnormal fornices result in a peculiar image: a small round structure is seen in the midportion of the third ventricle.[71]

MRI can diagnose holoprosencephaly but is usually not required.

Differential Diagnosis

Hydranencephaly could be confused for alobar holoprosencephaly with a large ventricular cavity and dorsal sac but should be distinguished by absence of cerebral cortex and fusion of midline thalami seen with holoprosencephaly. Hydranencephaly should also show absence of facial and other anomalies. From a practical perspective, alobar holoprosencephaly and hydranencephaly share in common a poor prognosis, and a diagnostic error is uneventful.

Lobar holoprosencephaly must be distinguished from simple hydrocephalus, which is at times associated with sec-

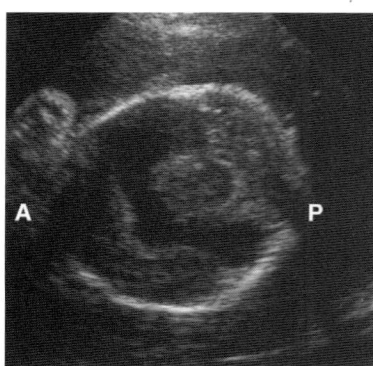

FIGURE 16. Semilobar holoprosencephaly. Transverse image shows partial separation of monoventricle. Cleft lip and palate were also identified. A, anterior; P, posterior.

ondary disruption of the septum pellucidum. A midcoronal scan of the fetal head is the most important view to differentiate between these two conditions, because it allows the identity of findings that are typical of lobar holoprosencephaly: the flat roof of the frontal horns and the possible presence of the fused fornices.

It may be impossible to distinguish lobar holoprosencephaly from septooptic dysplasia. With septooptic dysplasia, the cavum septi pellucidi is also absent, and the frontal horns are fused on the midline and have a typical squared roof (Fig. 18). The corpus callosum is usually present,

albeit is frequently described as thinned in postnatal studies. Ventriculomegaly may be present.[77]

Associated Anomalies

Pleomorphic facial anomalies are a part of the holoprosencephalic sequence (see Chapter 8).[78] Cyclopia and ethmocephaly are invariably associated with alobar holoprosencephaly. On the other hand, infants with any kind of holoprosencephaly may have a normal face.[68] In one prenatal series, facial abnormalities were present in 90% of cases.[79]

Chromosomal abnormalities are present in 50% to 60% of fetuses with alobar or semilobar holoprosencephaly. Trisomy 13 is the most common abnormality, found in approximately 50% to 75% of those with abnormal karyotype. Conversely, Lehman et al. reported holoprosencephaly in 39% of a prenatal series with trisomy 13.[80] Other aneuploidies associated with holoprosencephaly include trisomy 18, triploidy, 5p+, 13q–, 18p–, trisomy 22, and various other karyotypes.[81] The probability of an underlying chromosome abnormality is related primarily to extrafacial anomalies. Among 38 fetuses with holoprosencephaly reported by Berry et al.,[82] the karyotype was normal in all fetuses with isolated holoprosencephaly or holoprosencephaly and facial defects only, whereas 52% (11 of 21) fetuses with extrafacial malformations had a chromosomally abnormality.

Syndromes that include holoprosencephaly among their manifestations are DiGeorge, Meckel, Kallman, camptomelic dysplasia, Hall-Pallister, and Vasadi, among others.

A–C

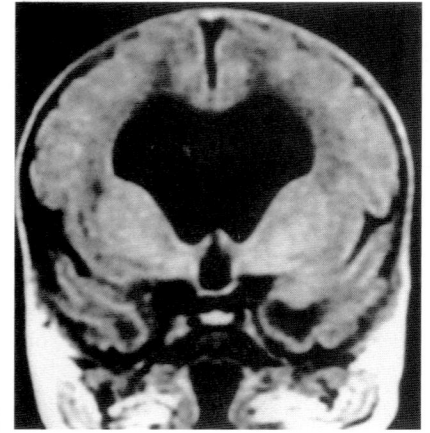
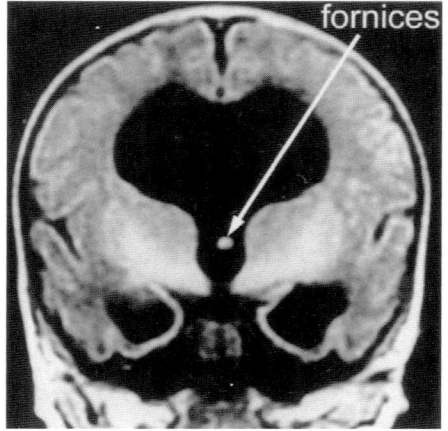
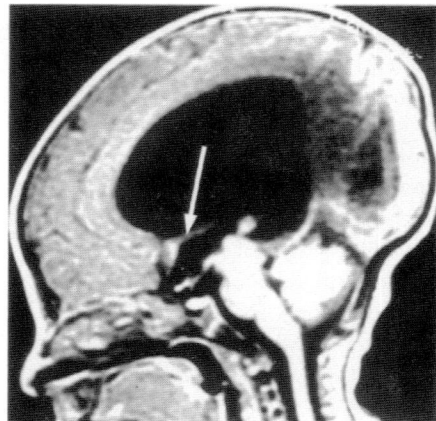

FIGURE 17. Lobar holoprosencephaly. **A–C:** Magnetic resonance imaging in a newborn shows fused frontal horns with a square-shaped roof. The fornices appear fused to form a solid fascicle that runs from anterior to posterior (*arrows*) at the border between the lateral ventricles and the third ventricle. (Reproduced with permission from Pilu G, Ambrosetto P, Sandri F, Tani G, Perolo A, et al. Intraventricular fused fornices: a specific sign of fetal lobar holoprosencephaly. *Ultrasound Obstet Gynecol* 1994;4:65.)

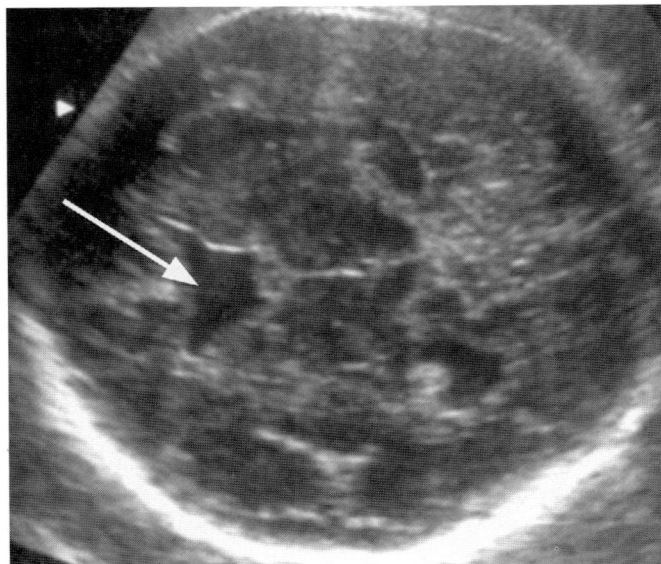
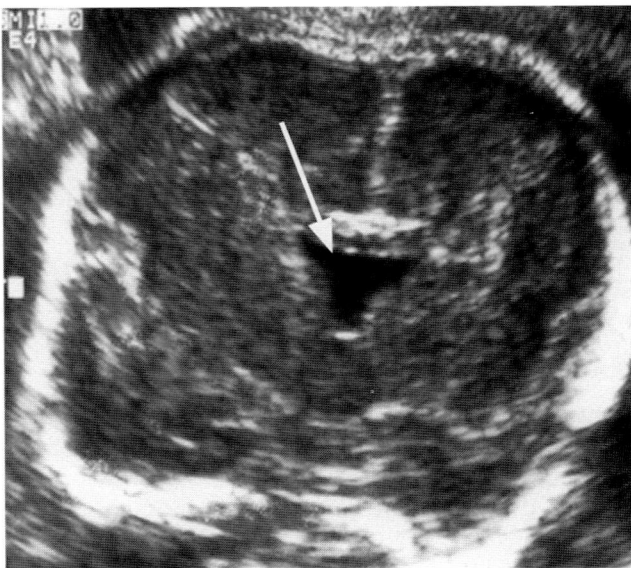

FIGURE 18. Septooptic dysplasia. Antenatal **(A)** and postnatal **(B)** coronal images. Notice absence of the septum pellucidum and fused frontal horns with inferior pointing horns (*arrows*).

Prognosis

Alobar holoprosencephaly is lethal, albeit occasional cases with long survival have been described. Semilobar holoprosencephaly is not necessarily lethal, but it is associated with extremely severe neurologic compromise.[68] When these conditions are identified *in utero*, termination of pregnancy could be offered before viability. A conservative management is recommended in continuing pregnancies.

The prognosis of lobar holoprosencephaly is uncertain. The available clinical data are limited. It has been reported that affected individuals may have a normal life span, but mental retardation and neurologic sequelae are common.[83] Dysplasia of the aqueduct of Sylvius is presumably present in many cases, leading to obstructive hydrocephalus. The only available antenatal series includes five infants that were followed after birth, and all had very abnormal developmental quotients.[76]

Management

Fetal karyotype is mandatory when holoprosencephaly is discovered by ultrasound. Termination of pregnancy should be offered to parents with previable fetuses. As alobar and semilobar holoprosencephaly are associated with a dismal prognosis, in the presence of severe hydrocephalus ultrasound-guided cephalocentesis could be considered to avoid the risk of dystocia.

Recurrence Risk

With absence of chromosomal abnormalities, the recurrence risk has been estimated to be 6% (but this includes truly sporadic events and hereditary conditions with 25% to 50% risk).[84] Hereditary holoprosencephaly has been reported with autosomal dominant inheritance with variable penetrance (MIM 142945); autosomal recessive (MIM 236100); and X-linked recessive (MIM 306990).

Dandy-Walker Complex

Synonyms for Dandy-Walker complex include Dandy-Walker syndrome and Dandy-Walker malformation. Related abnormalities are Dandy-Walker variant and mega cisterna magna.

The term *Dandy-Walker syndrome* was introduced to indicate the association of (a) ventriculomegaly of variable degree, (b) a large cisterna magna, and (c) a defect in the cerebellar vermis through which the cyst communicates with the fourth ventricle.[85]

In the 1970s and 1980s, different definitions have been suggested to indicate a group of posterior fossa abnormalities similar to the classic Dandy-Walker syndrome. Most of these definitions agree in including the following findings: (a) cystic dilatation of the fourth ventricle, (b) dysgenesis of the cerebellar vermis, and (c) a high position of the tentorium. At present, the term *Dandy-Walker complex* is used to indicate a spectrum of anomalies of the posterior fossa. By using axial CT scans these anomalies are categorized as follows: classic *Dandy-Walker malformation* (enlarged posterior fossa, complete or partial agenesis of the cerebellar vermis, elevated tentorium); *Dandy-Walker variant* (variable hypoplasia of the cerebellar vermis with or without enlargement of the posterior fossa); and *mega-cisterna magna* (enlarged cisterna magna with integrity of cerebellar vermis and fourth ventricle).[86]

Incidence

Dandy-Walker malformation has an estimated prevalence of approximately 1 per 30,000 births and is found in 4% to 12% of all cases of infantile hydrocephalus.[87] The incidence of minor varieties of the complex is unknown.

Etiology

Genetic factors have a major role in the etiology of this condition. Dandy-Walker malformation may occur as a part of mendelian disorders and chromosomal aberrations (Table 6).[88,89] Teratogens, including viral infections, alcohol, and diabetes, have also been suggested to play a role in the genesis of Dandy-Walker malformation, but the evidence is uncertain.

TABLE 6. ABNORMALITIES ASSOCIATED WITH DANDY-WALKER MALFORMATION

Mendelian
  Aase-Smith (autosomal dominant)
  Aicardi syndrome (X-linked dominant)
  Coffin-Siris syndrome (autosomal recessive)
  Ellis-van Creveld syndrome (autosomal recessive)
  Fraser cryptophthalmus syndrome (autosomal recessive)
  Joubert syndrome (autosomal recessive)
  Neu-Laxova
  Orofaciodigital syndrome, type II (autosomal recessive)
  Smith-Lemli-Opitz syndrome
  Meckel Gruber syndrome (autosomal recessive)
  Walker-Warburg syndrome (autosomal recessive)
Chromosomal
  Trisomy 18
  Trisomy 13
  45,X
  6p–
  9q+
  Duplication 5p
  Duplication 8p
  Duplication 8q
  Trisomy 9
  Triploidy
  Duplication 17q
Environmental
  Alcohol
  Cytomegalovirus
  Coumadin
  Diabetes
  Isotretinoin
  Rubella
Sporadic
  Cornelia de Lange syndrome
  Goldenhar syndrome
  Holoprosencephaly
  Klippel-Feil syndrome
  Polysyndactyly

Embryology and Pathology

According to the original theory of Dandy and Walker, atresia of the foramina of Luschka and Magendie leads to dilatation of the ventricular system. Benda[85] subsequently observed that the foramina of Luschka and Magendie are not always atretic. Gardner[90] has proposed that the malformation is due to an imbalance between the CSF production in the lateral and third ventricles and in the fourth ventricle. Overproduction of fluid in the fourth ventricle results in early dilatation and herniation of the rhombencephalic roof. Compression causes secondary hypoplasia of the cerebellar vermis, and the fourth ventricle then enlarges to form the cyst of the posterior fossa. Barkovich et al.[91] have suggested that the spectrum of Dandy-Walker complex is due to different degrees of abnormalities in the development of the roof of the fourth ventricle. Under normal conditions, at approximately 10 weeks' gestation, the roof of the fourth ventricle is divided by a ridge of developing choroid plexus into two portions, defined anterior and posterior membranous areas. Normally the anterior membranous area is incorporated into the developing choroid plexus, while the posterior area remains and eventually cavitates to form the central foramen of Magendie. In the Dandy-Walker complex, either the anterior membranous area is not incorporated into the choroid plexus or there is delayed opening of the foramen of Magendie. This causes posterior expansion of the fourth ventricle. In some cases, the insult is particularly diffuse and severe, and results in a large fourth ventricle cyst that expands the posterior fossa and marked hypoplasia of the cerebellar vermis or entire cerebellum (classic Dandy-Walker malformation). In other cases, the development of the cerebellum is compromised but the cisterna magna is of normal size (Dandy-Walker variant). Eventually, in other cases, the cerebellum may be intact but the cisterna magna is enlarged (mega cisterna magna).

The Dandy-Walker complex is a spectrum of posterior fossa abnormalities that are frequently difficult to differentiate. The most common classification is based on axial CT scans.[86] Classic Dandy-Walker malformation is characterized by the presence of a large cisterna magna communicating with the fourth ventricle through a defect in the cerebellar vermis, ranging from mild hypoplasia of the inferior lobules to complete aplasia. The entire cerebellum is small, and frequently the hemispheres are asymmetric. As a consequence of the large cisterna magna, the posterior fossa is expanded, with elevation of the tentorium and torcular Herophili. Although hydrocephalus has been classically considered to be an essential diagnostic element of this condition, more recent evidence suggests that it is not overtly present at birth in most patients, but it develops usually in the first months of life.[92]

The Dandy-Walker variant is characterized by a defect of variable size in the inferior cerebellar vermis with or without dilatation of the cisterna magna. Mega cisterna complex. Some degree of vermian dysgenesis can be found in all cases, even with mega cisterna magna, whereas classic Dandy-Walker malformation and Dandy-Walker variant have so many similarities that a clear-cut distinction is often impossible.[91]

Diagnosis

Dandy-Walker malformation has been frequently diagnosed prenatally[93–99] and has been reported as early as the first trimester.[100,101] The classic Dandy-Walker malformation (Figs. 19 through 21) is less commonly encountered than the Dandy-Walker variant (Figs. 22 through 24). Borderline to overt ventriculomegaly and other neural and extraneural malformations are frequently present with the classic Dandy-Walker malformation (Figs. 19 and 20), whereas in Dandy-Walker variant, ventricular dilatation is usually absent and careful scanning may be required to identify the defect (Fig. 23). In either condition, an enlarged cisterna magna communicates to the area of the fourth ventricle through a defect in the cerebellar vermis.

Caution is encouraged during the early second trimester in making the diagnosis of partial vermian agenesis because the incompletely formed inferior cerebellar vermis may give the false impression of a vermian defect.[8,9] This is especially common with a steep angle of section through the posterior fossa (Fig. 25). A follow-up scan at 18 weeks or later is recommended if only a defect of the vermis, especially the inferior vermis, is suspected. The normal measurements of

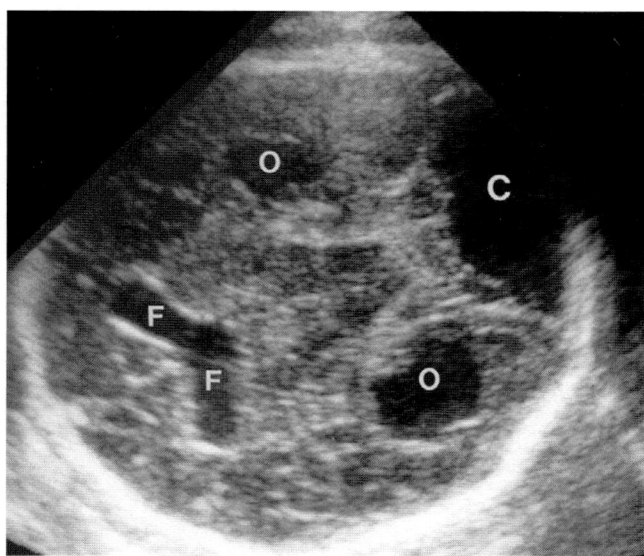

FIGURE 19. Dandy-Walker malformation. Transvaginal scan shows dilated frontal (*F*) and occipital (*O*) views of lateral ventricles and posterior fossa cyst (*C*).

magna is defined as a large cisterna magna with a normal fourth ventricle and inferior cerebellar vermis.

More recently, the excellent resolution of MRI in the sagittal planes has demonstrated that the classification based on CT axial planes is inadequate to describe anatomic derangement encountered in the Dandy-Walker

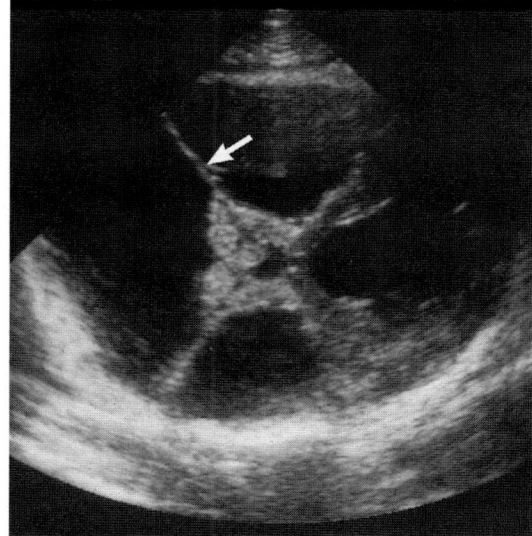

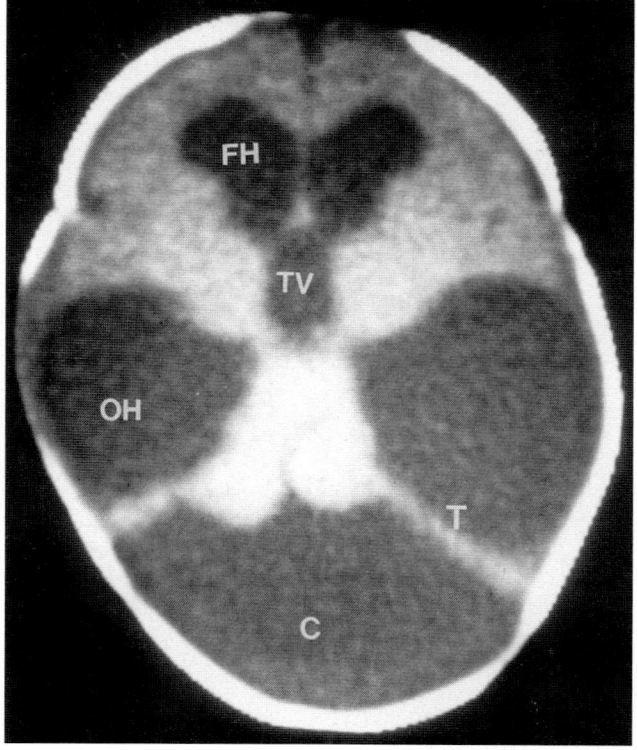

FIGURE 20. Dandy-Walker malformation. **A:** Transverse image shows moderate-marked dilatation of ventricles and large "cyst" of posterior fossa (*arrow*). **B:** Postnatal computed tomography scan shows dilatation of ventricles and posterior fossa cyst (*C*). FH, frontal horn; OH, occipital horn; T, tentorium; TV, third ventricle.

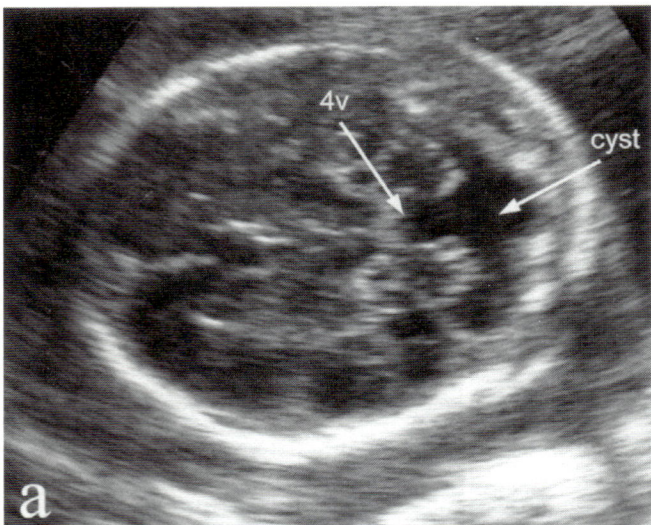

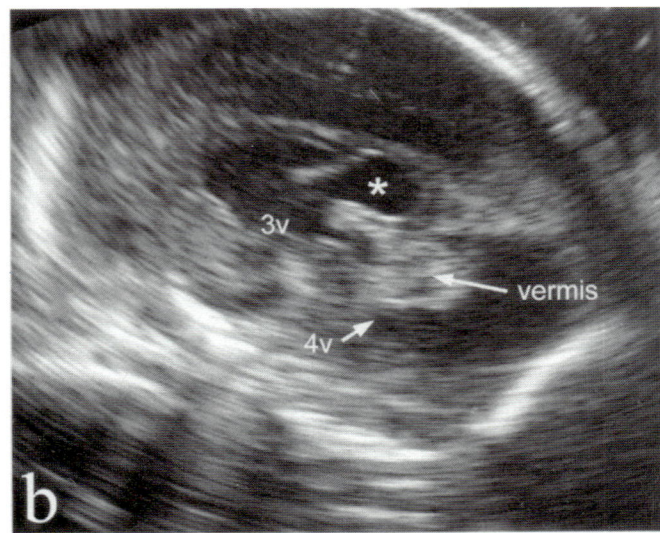

FIGURE 21. Dandy-Walker malformation. **A:** In the axial plane, the cisterna magna is obviously increased in size, and the cerebellum is V-shaped because of a large defect in the inferior vermis connecting the cystic cisterna magna to the area of the fourth ventricle (*4v*). **B:** Sagittal plane confirms that the cisterna magna is large and the vermis is smaller than normal because of the absence of the inferior portion; the fastigium of fourth ventricle (*4v*) is not recognized. After birth, Dandy-Walker malformation with obstructive hydrocephalus was diagnosed. 3v, third ventricle. *, small cyst in the quadrigeminal cistern.

the cerebellar vermis in the median plane have been described (see Appendix 1, Table 23).

Criteria for an enlarged cisterna magna have not been firmly established thus far. An enlarged cisterna magna typically measures greater than 10 mm[93] in anteroposterior dimension. However, this appearance is most commonly seen in normal fetuses, especially during the third trimester because the size of the cisterna magna varies slightly with gestational age. When an enlarged cisterna

magna is the only finding, especially during the third trimester, the overwhelming outcome is normal. However, an enlarged cisterna magna may be a primary clue to trisomy 18 (Fig. 26), although in this situation other subtle anomalies are often seen and the fetus is small for gestational age. Therefore, demonstration of an enlarged cisterna magna should stimulate a careful search for other anomalies, and this finding should be correlated with other risk factors.

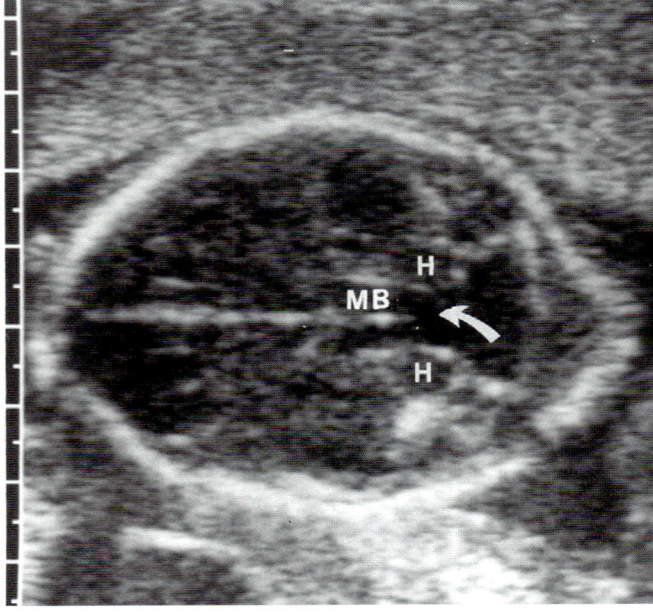

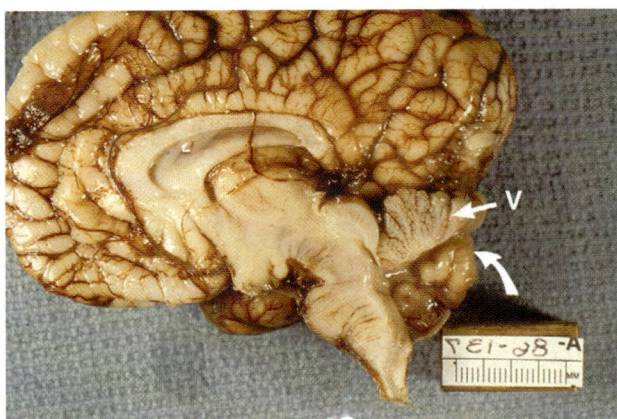

FIGURE 22. Dandy-Walker variant. **A:** Oblique plane though posterior fossa shows partial vermian agenesis with cisterna magna contiguous with posterior aspect of midbrain (*MB*), shown by the arrow. In the normal situation, the vermis intervenes at this level. H, cerebellar hemispheres. **B:** Pathologic photograph of similar case shows absence of inferior cerebellar vermis (*curved arrow*). Superior aspect of vermis (*V*) is present.

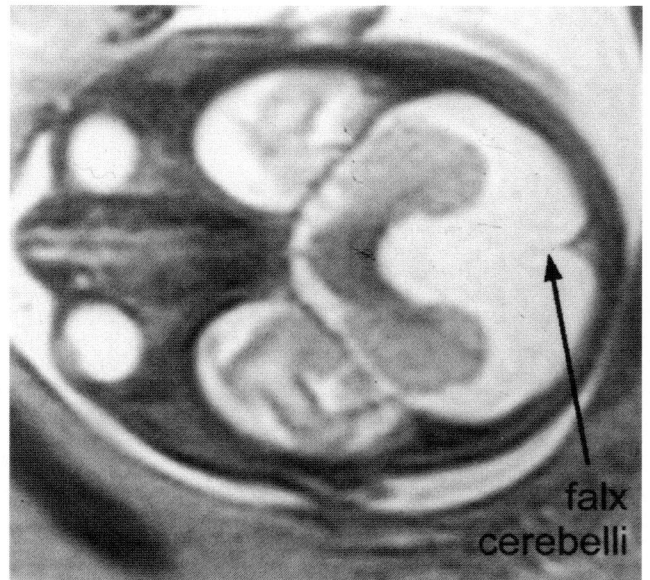
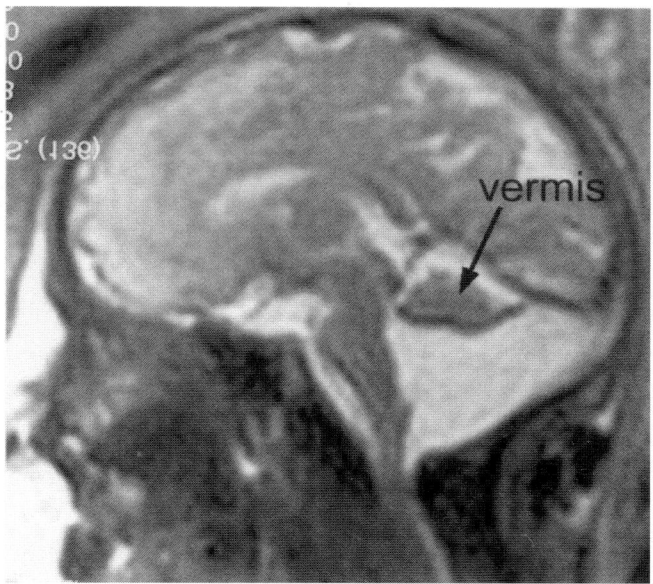

A

B

FIGURE 23. Dandy-Walker malformation on magnetic resonance imaging at 32 weeks. **A:** Axial scan demonstrating a large posterior fossa with a V-shaped cerebellum; the presence of the falx cerebelli (*arrow*) is a further finding suggesting that the cyst is a part of the Dandy-Walker type of malformation and is not a posterior fossa arachnoid cyst. **B:** Sagittal scan demonstrates that the vermis is present but obviously defective in the inferior portion. (Courtesy of Bruno Bernard, MD, Bologna, Italy.)

It is worth noting that in one large antenatal series, the Dandy-Walker malformation was frequently over- and under-diagnosed compared to pathology.[102] Whereas false-positive diagnoses are common, vermian defects can also be missed. One of the authors has been unable to demonstrate any cerebellar defect in a fetus that had a borderline cisterna magna, which was found at birth to have Dandy-Walker variant and overt ventriculomegaly requiring a shunt.[49]

As with other cerebral malformations, MRI can be useful in the assessment of Dandy-Walker malformation, particularly to evaluate the vermian defect as well as to identify associated anomalies, such as heterotopia (Figs. 23 and 24).[29]

Differential Diagnosis

The sonographic appearance of normal cerebellar development can resemble partial vermian agenesis during the early second trimester. This may give the false impression of a vermian defect. Even in the second and third trimester, however, a scanning angle too steep may create the impression of an excessive size of the cisterna magna and even of a vermian defect.[103] In doubtful cases, the median plane is

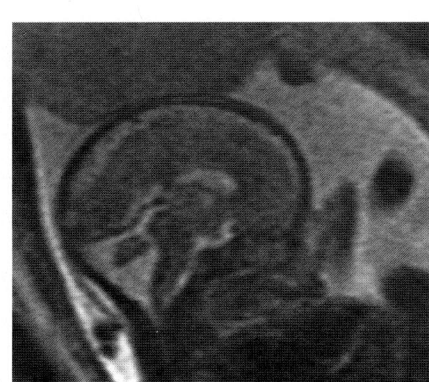
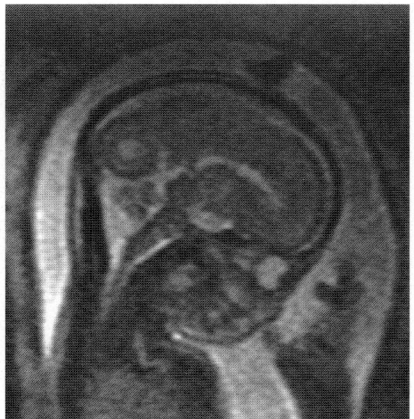

A

B

FIGURE 24. Dandy-Walker variant on magnetic resonance imaging at 23 weeks. **A:** Sagittal image of affected fetus in a twin pregnancy confirms ultrasound findings with absent or hypoplastic inferior vermis. **B:** Sagittal image of unaffected co-twin shows normal cerebellar vermis.

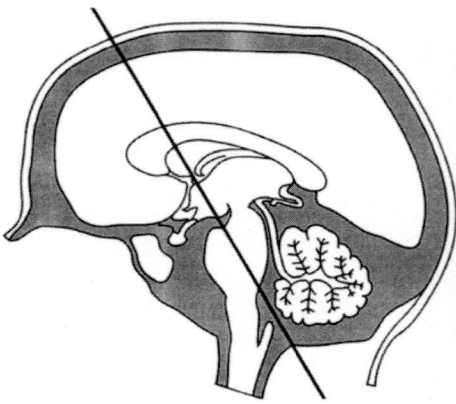
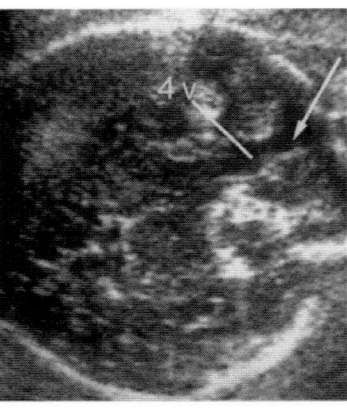

FIGURE 25. A too steeply angled plane can produce a false-positive impression of partial absence of cerebellar vermis as fluid in the cisterna magna (*arrow*) extends between cerebellar hemispheres through the foramen of Magendie to the fourth ventricle (*4v*).

certainly helpful, in that it allows the visualization of the vermis in the sagittal plane.

Associated Anomalies

Postnatal studies indicate a frequency of associated malformations ranging between 50% and 70%.[87,92,104] Other anomalies of the CNS include ventriculomegaly; other midline anomalies, such as agenesis of the corpus callosum and holoprosencephaly; and cephaloceles. Other deformities may include polycystic kidneys, cardiovascular defects, and cleft lip and palate.

Chromosome abnormalities, including trisomies 18, 13,[80,105] and Turner syndrome, are common and are even more likely in cases of partial vermian agenesis without ventricular dilatation.[93,97,106] Although chromosome abnormalities are unlikely when no other anomalies are identified, Dandy-Walker malformation and variant may still be associated with a variety of other syndromes and genetic conditions (Table 6). Among these, Joubert syndrome, an autosomal recessive condition,[107] has been reported in several cases (see Joubert Syndrome, Chapter 5).[108,109]

Prognosis

Classic Dandy-Walker malformation is usually clinically manifested within the first year of life, with symptoms of hydrocephalus and other neurologic symptoms. Mortality rates as high as 24% have been reported in the first neuro-

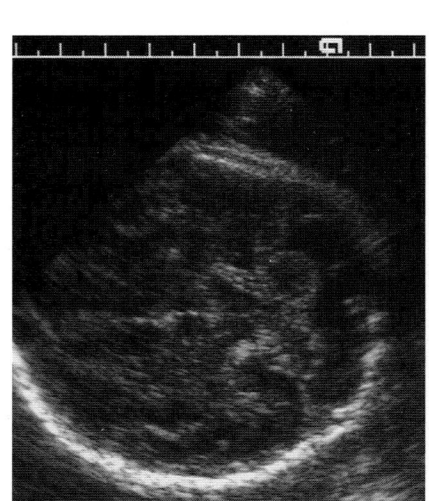
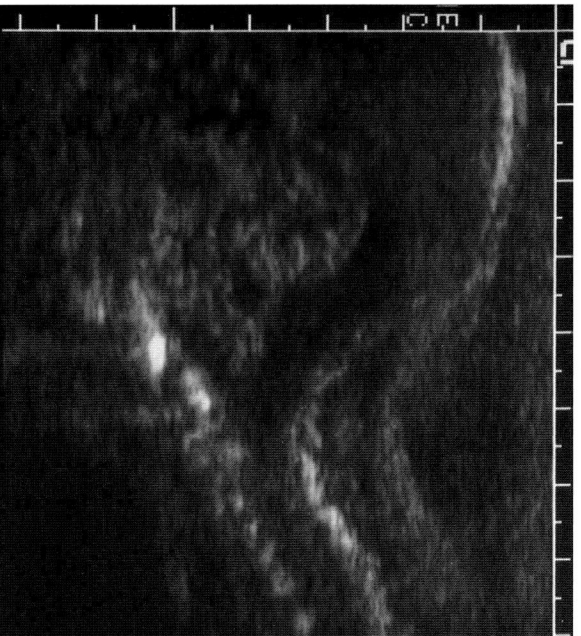

FIGURE 26. Enlarged cisterna magna as sign of trisomy 18. **A:** Axial scan through posterior fossa at 36 weeks shows enlargement of the cisterna magna. **B:** Sagittal scan of posterior fossa shows enlarged cisterna magna, but the cerebellar vermis appears intact. Intrauterine growth restriction and polyhydramnios were also present in this fetus, who proved to have trisomy 18 after birth. An enlarged cisterna magna is most commonly seen in normal fetuses, but, in these cases, the fetus typically is average size or large for dates.

surgical series, but because of advances in pediatric anesthesia and surgical techniques, deaths have certainly become less common. Intellectual development in survivors is controversial. Given the rarity of this condition, only limited series are available. Nevertheless, a subnormal intelligence is reported in 40% to 70% of cases.[87,92]

The clinical significance of Dandy-Walker variant and mega-cisterna magna is less certain. An isolated defect of the inferior vermis, in the absence of aneuploidy or other visible anomalies, appears to be associated with a favorable prognosis.[99,110]

Management

In continuing pregnancies, no modification of standard obstetric management is indicated. Cesarean delivery is indicated only if macrocrania is present. A careful search for associated malformation and postnatal follow-up is indicated in these cases as well as in the fetuses with either a suspicion of Dandy-Walker variant or with a cisterna magna depth greater than 10 mm.

Recurrence Risk

In the absence of a recognizable syndrome, a recurrence risk of 1% to 5% is suggested.[88]

Agenesis of the Corpus Callosum

Agenesis of the corpus callosum is complete or partial absence of the corpus callosum.

Incidence

The incidence varies in different studies, depending on the population investigated and the method of ascertainment. Estimates of 0.3% to 0.7% in the general population[111] and 2% to 3% in the developmentally disabled[112,113] are usually quoted.

Etiology

Agenesis of the corpus callosum is heterogenous. Genetic factors are probably predominant. The genetics of agenesis of the corpus callosum has been reviewed in depth by Young et al.[114] and by Dobyns.[115] Various teratogens have also been implicated as possible causes of agenesis of the corpus callosum, including alcohol,[116] valproate,[117] cocaine,[118] rubella,[119] and influenza virus.[120]

Embryology and Pathology

The corpus callosum is the largest commissure connecting the cerebral hemispheres (Figs. 27 and 28). It is a broad plate of dense myelinated fibers—located deep in the longi-tudinal fissure—that reciprocally interconnects regions of the cortex in all lobes with corresponding regions of the opposite hemispheres. It derives from the *massa commissuralis*, an embryologic structure formed by the fusion of the lateral margins of the groove that separates the primitive telencephalic vesicles. Formation of the corpus callosum is a late event in cerebral ontogenesis, which takes place between 12 and 18 weeks' gestation. The most anterior portion, the rostrum, develops first and is followed by the genu, body, and splenium. The corpus callosum is in close anatomic and embryologic relationship with the underlying septum pellucidum. Although there is no a priori evidence to suggest that the development of the septum pellucidum cannot proceed independently of the corpus callosum, most observers claim that there can be no septum pellucidum without a corpus callosum.[65]

At least two possible mechanisms have been recognized to cause this condition[115]:

1. Defects in which axons form but are unable to cross the midline because of the absence of the *massa commissuralis* and form aberrant longitudinal fiber bundles that run along the medial hemispheric walls (Probst bundles). This is probably the most common type. It may be either complete or partial. When partial, the caudad portion (splenium and body) is missing to varying degrees.

2. Defects in which the commissural axons or their parent cell bodies fail to form in the cerebral cortex. In these cases, the Probst bundles are usually not seen. This is the type of agenesis of the corpus callosum that occurs with several types of lissencephaly and X-linked hydrocephalus with stenosis of the aqueduct of Sylvius and the mental retardation, aphasias, shuffling gait, adducted thumbs syndrome.

Complete agenesis of the corpus callosum also occurs with major malformations of the embryonic forebrain before formation of the anlage of the corpus callosum, such as frontal encephaloceles and alobar holoprosencephaly. Eventually, degeneration or atrophy of the corpus callosum may result in thinning, a condition usually referred to as hypoplasia of the corpus callosum.[115]

Agenesis of the corpus callosum is typically associated with significant and variable distortion of the intracranial architecture (Fig. 28). The lateral ventricles tend to be larger than normal, particularly at the level of the atria and occipital horns. It has been postulated that the absence of the posterior portion of the corpus callosum results in distortion of the array of white matter tracts in the occipital lobes leading to caudad expansion of the ventricles.[121] Such ventricular enlargement tends per se to be stable and is not usually associated with intracranial hypertension. The frontal horns are usually normal in size but are more separated than normal from the midline. The third ventricle is often superiorly elongated, reaching the area normally occupied by the corpus callosum. At times, it may be found to com-

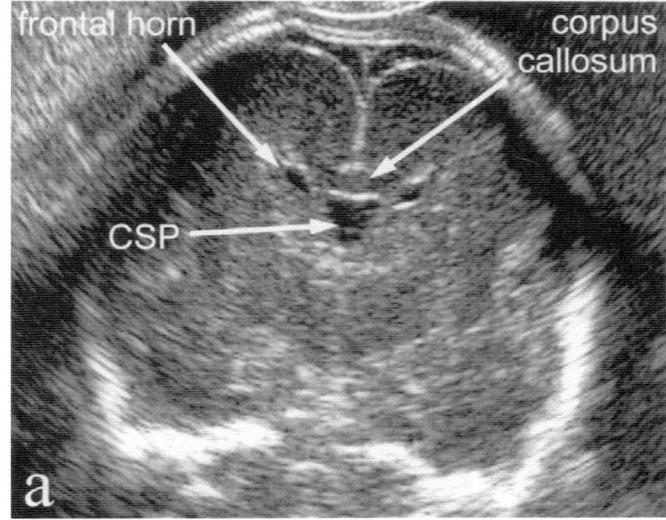

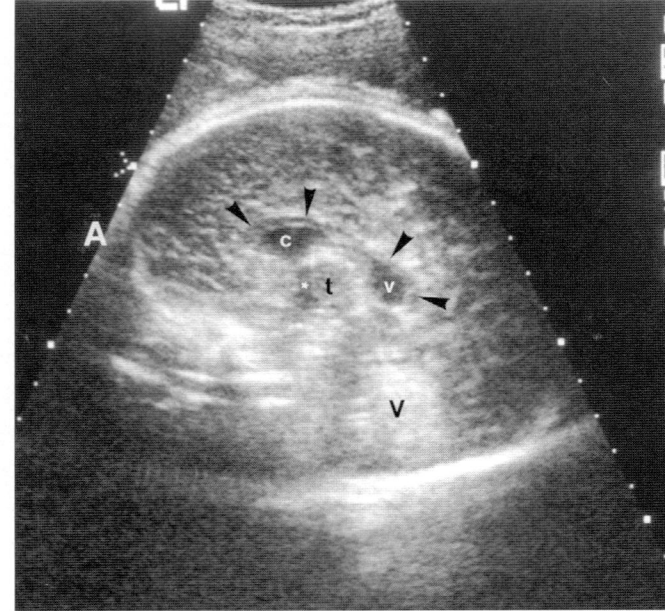

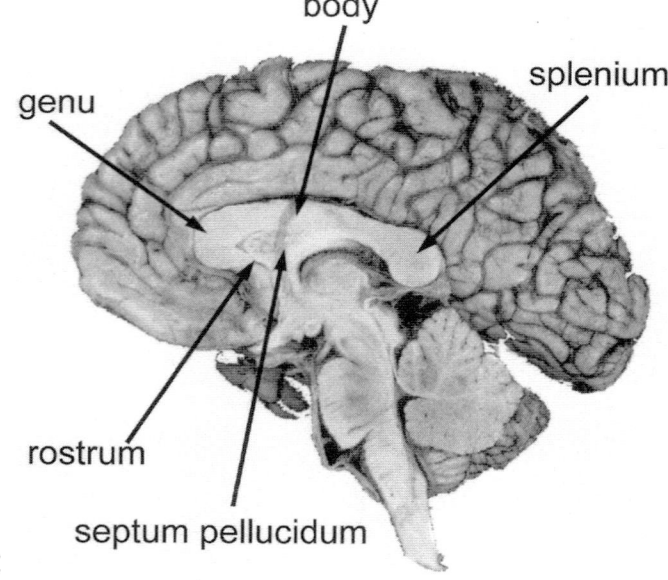

FIGURE 27. Normal corpus callosum. **A:** Normal coronal view at 20 weeks. The corpus callosum forms the roof over the cavum septum pellucidum (*CSP*) and ventricles. **B:** Normal midline sagittal plane in third trimester shows hypoechoic corpus callosum (*arrowheads*) overlying cavum septum pellucidum (*c*) and cavum vergae (*v*). A portion of the thalami (*t*) and the anterior third ventricle (*asterisk*) are also seen in the midline. The echogenic cerebellar vermis (*V*) is poorly seen in the posterior fossa. A, anterior. **C:** Corresponding fully formed corpus callosum with labeled parts.

municate with a large interhemispheric cyst.[122,123] Absence of the corpus callosum also results in abnormal induction of medial cerebral convolutions, determining a radiate arrangement of cerebral sulci around the roof of the third ventricle, extending through the zone normally occupied by the cingulate gyrus.

Diagnosis

Because development of the corpus callosum is a late event, complete only by 18 weeks, early diagnosis of its absence is difficult. In one antenatal series, 10 of 15 affected fetuses were found to have an unremarkable intracranial sonogram at 16 to 22 weeks' gestation.[124] However, agenesis of the corpus callosum can be diagnosed after 18 to 20 weeks, especially in expert hands.[125]

As agenesis of the corpus callosum is anatomically heterogeneous, the sonographic findings are variable (Figs. 29 through 31). Definitive diagnosis depends on showing absence of the complex formed by the corpus callosum and cavum septum pellucidum in median and coronal planes (Fig. 29). There are, however, a number of indirect clues on standard transverse views. Failure to visualize the cavum septum pellucidum, which under normal conditions is easily seen beyond 18 weeks, should raise the suspicion of agenesis of the corpus callosum. Other findings include

- Ventriculomegaly, typically mild. Prenatal studies suggest that agenesis of the corpus callosum is found in 3% of all fetuses with ventriculomegaly.[6]
- Disproportionate enlargement of the occipital horns (also referred to as *colpocephaly*). This may produce a

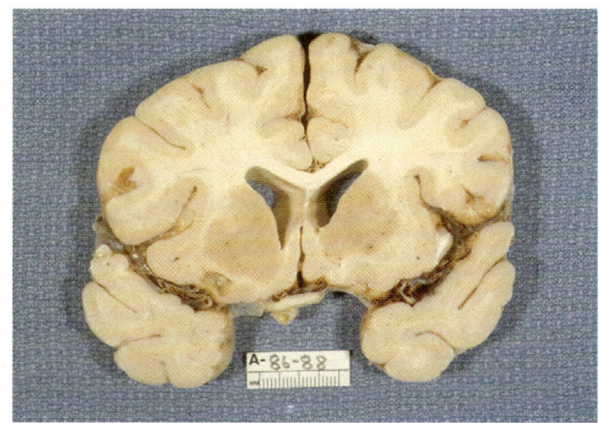

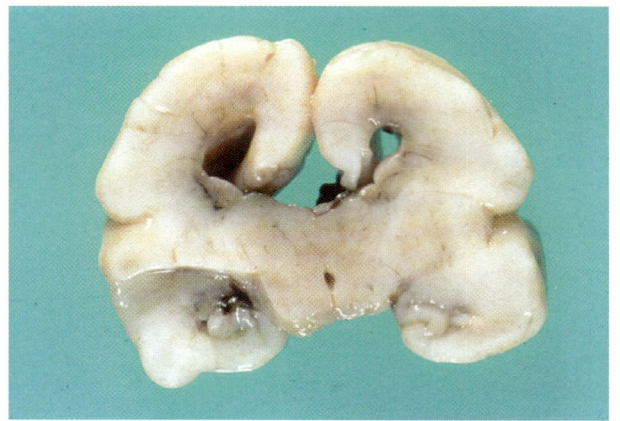

A · · · B

FIGURE 28. Coronal pathologic specimens show normal corpus callosum **(A)** and agenesis of the corpus callosum **(B)**. Note corresponding abnormalities of the adjacent ventricles with agenesis of the corpus callosum.

teardrop configuration of the lateral ventricles (Figs. 29 and 30A).

■ Increased separation of the hemispheres with a prominent interhemispheric fissure resulting from absence of the main cerebral commissure. Under such circumstances, sonography reveals three echogenic lines running parallel in the upper cranium, with the middle one representing the falx cerebri and the lateral ones representing the medial borders of the separated hemispheres (Fig. 31).

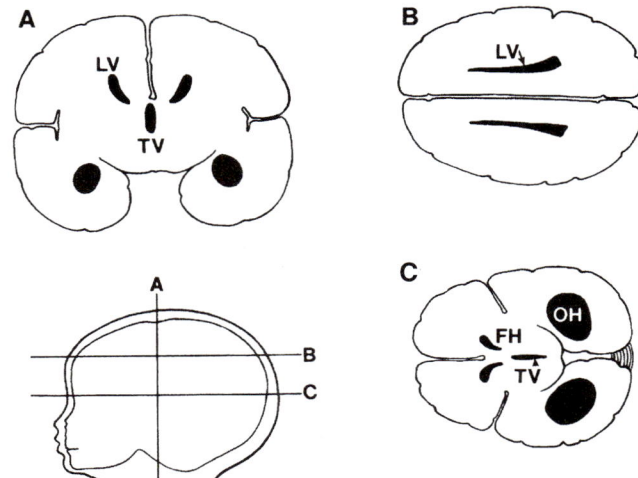

FIGURE 29. Schematic diagram of agenesis of the corpus callosum without interhemispheric cyst. Note the characteristic configuration of the lateral ventricles (*LVs*), which point superiorly on a coronal view **(A)**. **B:** Both walls of the LVs are identified where only periventricular lines are normally present. **C:** Also note characteristic dilatation of the occipital horns (colpocephaly). The third ventricle (*TV*) may or may not be dilated. FH, frontal horn; OH, occipital horn. (Reproduced with permission from Nyberg DA, Pretorius PH. Cerebral malformations. Nyberg DA, Mahony BS, Pretorius DH, eds. *Diagnostic ultrasound of fetal anomalies: text and atlas.* Chicago: Year Book, 1990:83–145.)

■ Upward displacement of the third ventricle, which can be identified by demonstrating that this structure reaches superiorly the level of lateral ventricles. This is a very specific sign but only occurs in approximately 50% of cases and requires a coronal or axial scan.

■ Abnormal midline lesions occur frequently, including cysts (Fig. 32) and lipomas (Fig. 33). Lipomas appear as brightly echogenic lesions. A lipoma in the anterior midline is associated with agenesis of the corpus callosum in 50% of cases.[126] It is worth noting, however, that lipomas are not usually demonstrable in the second trimester and tend to appear only in late gestation.[125]

■ Absence of the pericallosal artery, a branch of the anterior callosal artery that normally runs along the superior surface of the corpus callosum in a semicircular loop. When the corpus callosum is absent such loop is lost, and branches of the anterior cerebral artery are seen ascending linearly with a radiate arrangement (Fig. 34).[125]

Most of the experience with prenatal diagnosis is limited to complete agenesis of the corpus callosum, but a few cases of partial agenesis have been described as well.[125,127] The cerebral findings in these cases may be more subtle than with the complete form. The lateral ventricles may have a *teardrop* configuration, but the cavum septum pellucidum is usually present. The definitive diagnosis depends on a median scan demonstrating that the corpus callosum is small and does arch completely above the third ventricle later than 20 weeks' gestation. Nomograms of the length of the corpus callosum are also available.[128]

Magnetic resonance may be helpful for validating the diagnosis of agenesis of the corpus callosum (Fig. 35) and for identifying associated cerebral anomalies, such as heterotopia of the gray matter, which is very frequently associated with neurologic sequelae and seizures.[129]

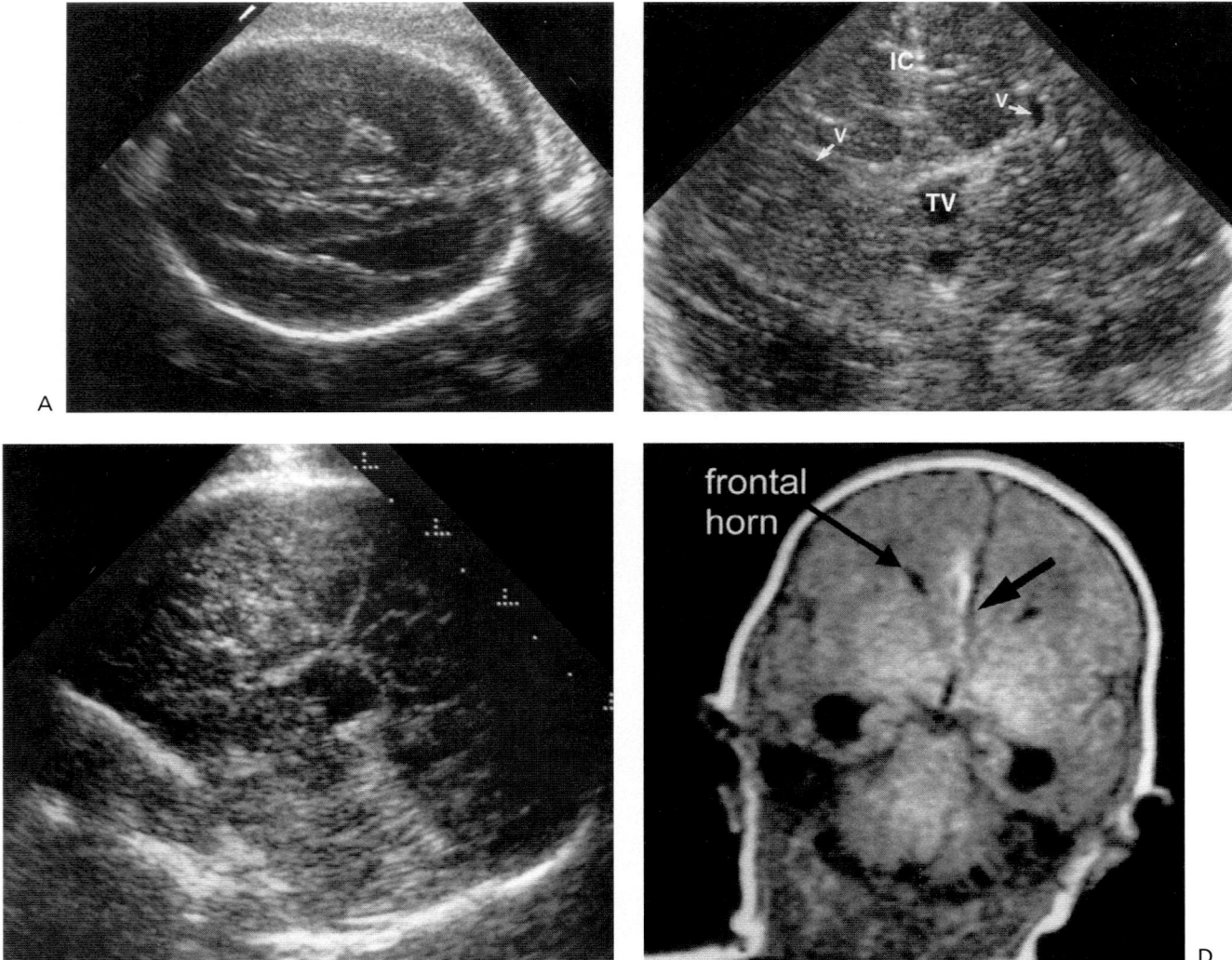

FIGURE 30. Agenesis of the corpus callosum without interhemispheric cyst. **A:** Axial scan through ventricles shows characteristic teardrop shape of lateral ventricles. **B:** Coronal scan shows that the lateral ventricles (*V*) are displaced laterally and point superiorly. The interhemispheric cisterna (*IC*) extends to the third ventricle (*TV*) without the intervening corpus callosum. **C:** Sagittal image shows radiating sulcal and gyral pattern without corpus callosum. **D:** Postnatal magnetic resonance image in coronal plane of similar fetus shows prominent interhemispheric cistern dividing the hemispheres without a connecting corpus callosum.

Differential Diagnosis

Agenesis of the corpus callosum must be distinguished from other causes of ventriculomegaly; agenesis of the corpus callosum with an interhemispheric cyst must be differentiated from other intracranial fluid-filled lesions, such as arachnoid cyst, porencephaly, or an aneurysm of the vein of Galen.

Associated Anomalies

The high frequency of associated malformations suggests that agenesis of the corpus callosum is frequently a part of a widespread developmental disturbance. In a large postnatal series,[130] CNS anomalies, including microcephaly, abnor-mal convolutional patterns, heterotopia, intracranial lipomas, interhemispheric cysts, neural tube defects, Dandy-Walker malformation (Fig. 36), aplasia, or hypoplasia of the pyramidal tracts, were found in 85% of the cases. In antenatal series, anatomic anomalies were found in 50% of cases. The anomaly most frequently encountered was Dandy-Walker malformation.

Systemic anomalies including a variety of musculoskeletal, cardiovascular, genitourinary, and gastrointestinal malformations were found in 62% of cases postnatally.[130] Cardiovascular anomalies include conotruncal malformations: tetralogy of Fallot, double outlet right ventricle.[125] Chromosomal anomalies are found in 20% of cases and mostly include trisomy 18, trisomy 8, and trisomy 13.[131]

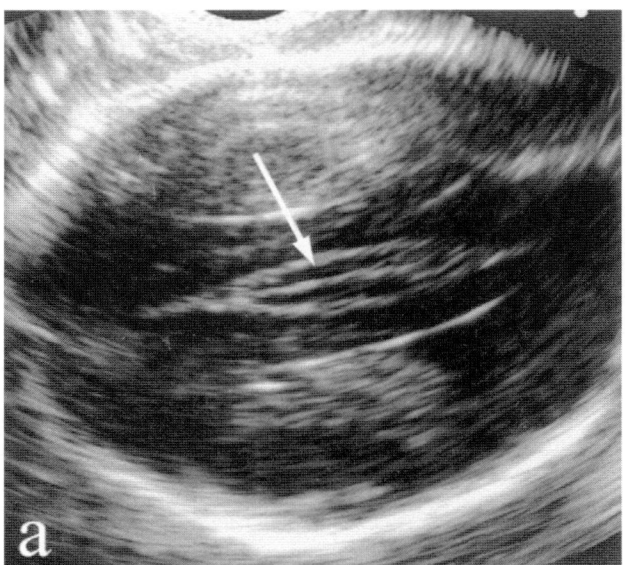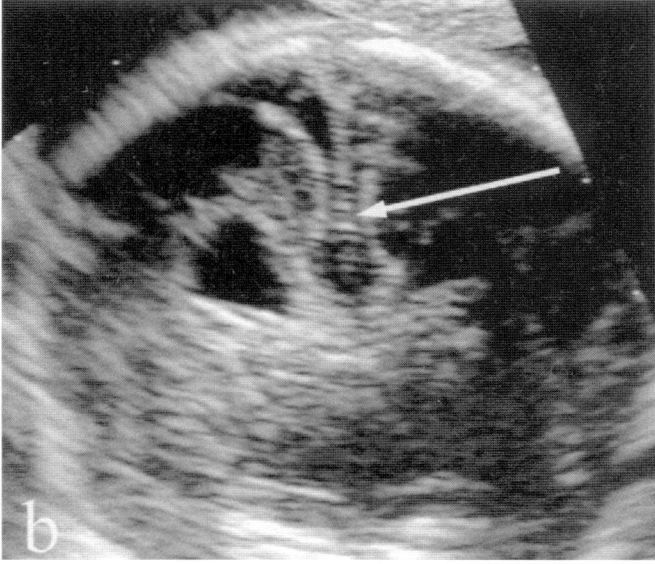

FIGURE 31. Agenesis of the corpus callosum. Axial **(A)** and midcoronal **(B)** views of the brain with agenesis of the corpus callosum demonstrating that the midline echo (*arrows*) has become a three-line complex due to distention of the interhemispheric fissure.

Agenesis of the corpus callosum is also a part of many genetic and nongenetic syndromes (Table 7). Some genetic conditions, such as Aicardi syndrome,[132] have sex-linked dominant etiology.

Prognosis

Isolated agenesis of the corpus callosum may be either a completely asymptomatic event or revealed during the course of a neurologic examination by subtle deficits, such as inability to match stimuli using both hands or to discriminate differences in temperature, shape, and weight in objects placed in both hands. However, individuals with agenesis of the corpus callosum may have severe neurologic

problems, including seizures, intellectual impairment, and psychosis. These conditions are believed to be caused by underlying cerebral anomalies rather than by the absence of the corpus callosum per se. The worst outcomes are found in the presence of migrational disorder with or without Dandy-Walker malformation.[133]

There is a lack of clinical data to counsel couples with fetuses with agenesis of the corpus callosum. Pediatric series are based on investigation of symptomatic individuals and are, therefore, presumably biased. A total of 37 infants with a prenatal diagnosis of isolated agenesis of the corpus callosum (no other malformations were demonstrable at sonography, and they had a normal karyotype) have been reported thus far.[125,134–137] The duration of postnatal follow-up studies

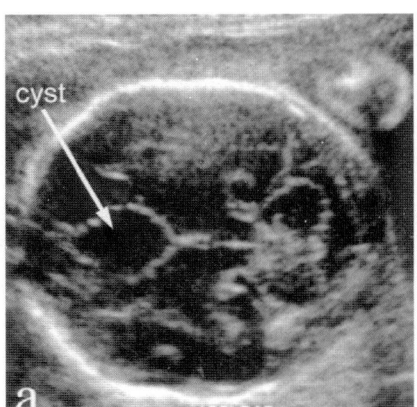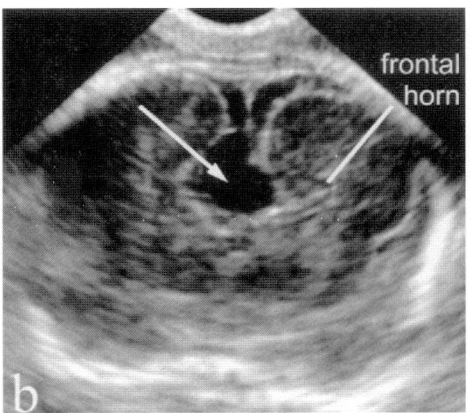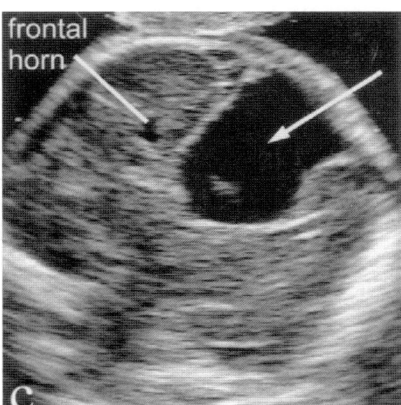

FIGURE 32. Axial and coronal views of agenesis of the corpus callosum with interhemispheric cyst. **A** and **B** are derived from the same fetus. Note the midline cyst (*arrows*), which splays the frontal horns from the midline. **C:** In another fetus, note the frontal horn that is displaced laterally and the large interhemispheric cyst (*arrow*) that extends to the cortex.

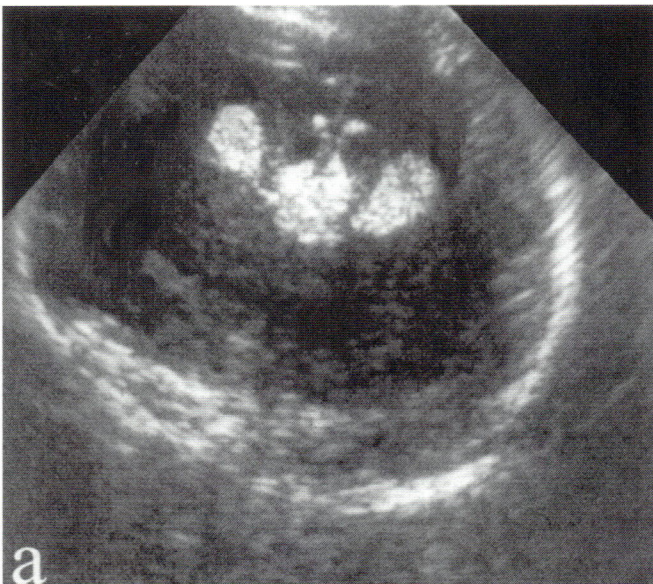
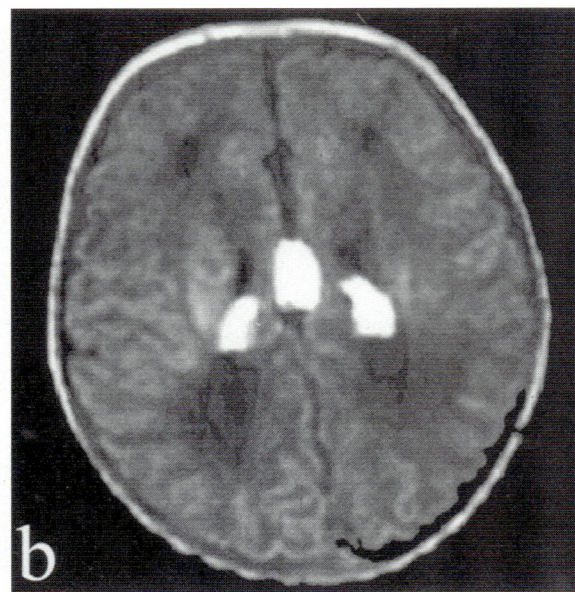

FIGURE 33. Lipoma with complete agenesis of the corpus callosum. **A:** Coronal scan shows symmetric lipomas are found within the bodies of lateral ventricles and midline lipoma replacing corpus callosum. **B:** Postnatal T1-weighted magnetic resonance imaging of similar case shows high signal intensity of fat from lipomas. (Reproduced with permission from Bromley B, Estroff JA, Scott MR, Benacerraf BR. Brain masses: differential diagnosis. *The Fetus* 3:219–222.)

ranges between a few months to 11 years. A normal or borderline development was present in 32, or 86%. In all cases with severe handicap, other anomalies were present, although they could not be demonstrated antenatally [one case each of ethmoidal cephalocele, CHARGE (*c*oloboma, *h*eart anomalies, *a*tresia choane, *r*etarded growth or development, *g*enital or hypogonadism, and *e*ar anomalies) association, and oral-facial-digital syndrome type I, and two cases of Aicardi syndrome].

Some intracranial findings have been found in excess in fetuses with a poor outcome and are presumed to have prognostic value, albeit the experience thus far is limited. In our experience, upward displacement of the third ventricle

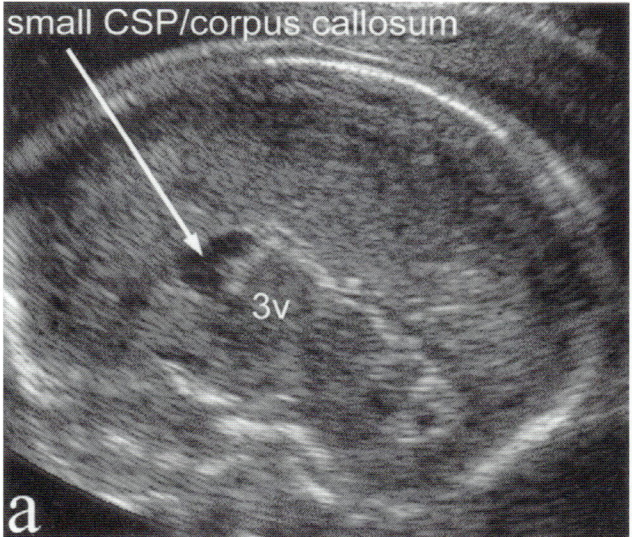
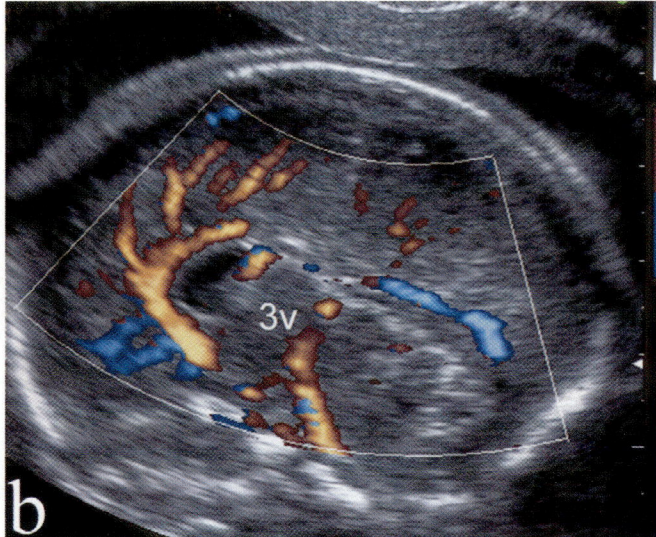

FIGURE 34. Partial agenesis of the corpus callosum. **A:** Sagittal scan at 20 weeks shows the corpus callosum/cavum septi pellucidi (*CSP*) complex is much smaller than normal; in fact, it does not entirely cover the third ventricle (*3v*), but only reaches about midway. **B:** The corpus callosum appears thin and barely discernible with grey-scale imaging and can be positively identified only when highlighted by the course of the pericallosal artery.

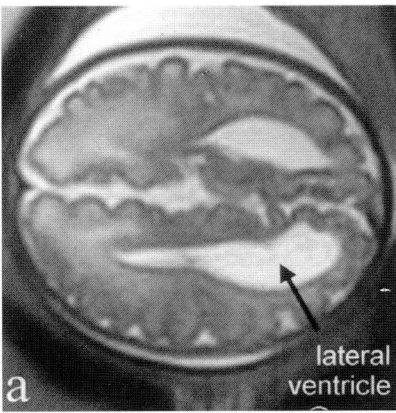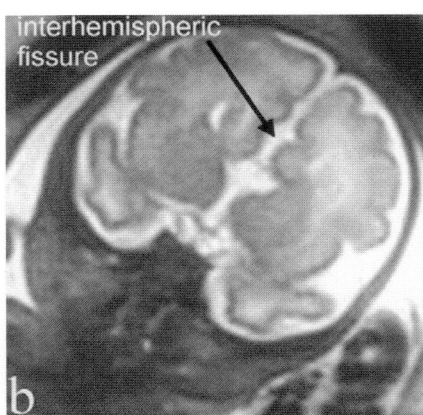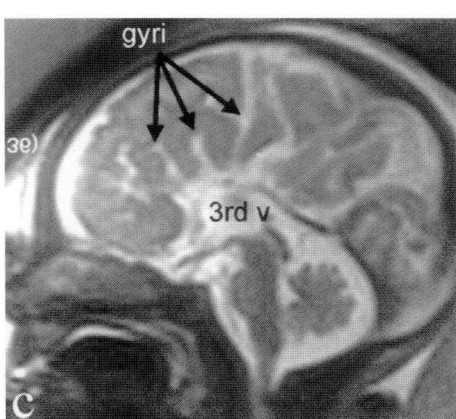

FIGURE 35. Antenatal magnetic resonance imaging in a third-trimester fetus with complete agenesis of the corpus callosum. **A:** Axial scan demonstrating ventriculomegaly and teardrop sign. **B:** Coronal scan demonstrating absence of the corpus callosum and a wide interhemispheric fissure. **C:** Median scan demonstrating absence of the corpus callosum with radiate distribution of the cerebral convolutions around the roof of the third ventricle (*3rd v*). Although a precise diagnosis of this condition had been made before with ultrasound, the symmetry of the hemispheres, the normal pattern of convolutions, and the normal distribution of the gray matter are reassuring in the absence of other intracerebral anomalies. (Courtesy of Dr. Bruno Bernardi, Bologna, Italy.)

and a distended interhemispheric fissure were most frequently associated with neurologic impairment, associated anomalies, or both. Interestingly enough, no correlation was found between the degree of ventricular enlargement and the outcome.[125] Similarly, the antenatal demonstration by MRI of heterotopia represents probably a poor prognostic factor.

It should be remembered that agenesis of the corpus callosum is a unique condition that even in the presence of a normal intelligence is associated with peculiar neurologic findings and subtle cognitive deficits. The interested reader is referred to specific works on this subject.[138–142] It has also been hypothesized that a possible relationship exists between agenesis of the corpus callosum and psychotic disorders.[143]

Management

Agenesis of the corpus callosum is associated with an excess of neural and extraneural malformations as well as with chromosomal aberrations. Antenatal identification of callosal agenesis dictates, therefore, the need of a careful survey of the entire fetal anatomy, including echocardiography and karyotype. In continuing pregnancies, the management depends on the sum of the different anomalies that are identified. Isolated agenesis of the

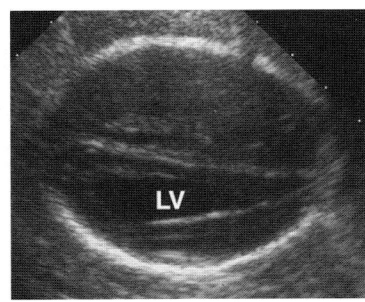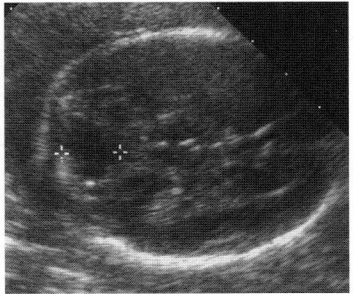

FIGURE 36. Agenesis of the corpus callosum with Dandy-Walker variant. **A:** Axial scan through ventricles shows characteristic teardrop configuration of lateral ventricles (*LV*). Other views confirmed agenesis of the corpus callosum. **B:** View of posterior fossa shows vermian agenesis (*calipers*).

TABLE 7. SYNDROMES FEATURING AGENESIS OF THE CORPUS CALLOSUM

Frequent in
  Acrocallosal syndrome (autosomal recessive)
  Aicardi syndrome (X-linked dominant)
  Andermann syndrome (autosomal recessive)
  Cerebro-oculo-facio-skeletal syndrome (autosomal recessive)
  Fryns syndrome (autosomal recessive)
  Marden-Walker syndrome (autosomal recessive)
  Meckel-Gruber syndrome (autosomal recessive)
  Microphthalmia-linear skin defects syndrome (X-linked dominant)
  Miller-Dieker syndrome (lissencephaly syndrome)
  Neu-Laxova syndrome (autosomal recessive)
  Septooptic dysplasia sequence
  Walker-Warburg syndrome (X-linked dominant)
  Zellweger syndrome (autosomal recessive)
  X-linked hydrocephalus (X-linked recessive)
Occasional in
  Apert syndrome (autosomal recessive)
  Baller-Gerold syndrome (autosomal recessive)
  Calloso-genital dysplasia syndrome (autosomal recessive)
  Coffin-Siris syndrome (?autosomal recessive)
  Congenital microgastria–limb reduction complex (unknown)
  Crouzon disease (autosomal dominant)
  Duplication 4p syndrome
  Fetal alcohol syndrome
  Fetal warfarin syndrome
  FG syndrome (X-linked recessive)
  Frontonasal dysplasia sequence (sporadic/autosomal dominant)
  Gorlin syndrome (autosomal dominant)
  Greig cephalopolysyndactyly syndrome (autosomal dominant)
  Hydrolethalis syndrome (autosomal recessive, X-linked dominant)
  Lens dysplasia (X-linked recessive)
  Marshall-Smith syndrome (unknown)
  Oculoauriculovertebral spectrum (unknown)
  Oculocerebrocutaneous syndrome (Delleman syndrome) (unknown)
  Opitz syndrome (autosomal dominant, X-linked recessive)
  Orofaciodigital syndrome, type 1 (X-linked dominant)
  Peters'-Plus syndrome (autosomal recessive)
  Radial aplasia-thrombocytopenia syndrome (autosomal recessive)
  Rubinstein-Taybi syndrome (sporadic)
  Shapiro syndrome (X-linked recessive)
  Simpson-Golabi-Behmel syndrome (X-linked recessive)
  Trisomy 8 syndrome
  Trisomy 13 syndrome
  Trisomy 18 syndrome
  X-linked hydrocephalus spectrum (X-linked recessive)
  XO syndrome
  XXXXY syndrome (hypoplastic)
  Yunis-Varon syndrome
  Metabolic disorders

Modified from Blum A, Andre M, Droulle P, Husson S, Leheup B. Prenatal echographic diagnosis of corpus callosum agenesis. *Genet Counsel* 1990;38:115–126.

corpus callosum does not require any modification of standard obstetric management. In one series,[125] failure to progress in labor requiring cesarean delivery occurred on several occasions, and this was speculated to be related to the high frequency of macrocrania in infants with callosal agenesis.

Recurrence Risk

The recurrence risk is dependent on the etiology in the specific case. Agenesis of the corpus callosum is frequently part of syndromes with mendelian transmission (Table 7). Autosomal dominant, autosomal recessive, and sex-linked transmission have all been documented.

Septooptic Dysplasia

A synonym for septooptic dysplasia is De Morsier syndrome.

Septooptic dysplasia is a cerebral anomaly featured by absence of the septum pellucidum and optic disc hypoplasia.

Etiology

The etiology is unknown. There is evidence that septooptic dysplasia can be caused by mutation in the homeobox gene HESX1.[144]

Pathology

Due to the association of midline defects of the brain and occasionally of the face, this anomaly has been regarded as part of the spectrum of the holoprosencephalies.[67] Agenesis or thinning of the septum pellucidum is found in most cases. The optic nerves and chiasm are affected by different degrees of hypoplasia, resulting in poor vision and nystagmus. A subset of these infants is blind but usually develops a modest degree of vision function in later life. The pituitary infundibulum may be absent.[65,145] Signs of anterior and posterior hypopituitarism are virtually always present. Deficiency of growth hormone and antidiuretic hormone may result in hypopituitary dwarfism[146] and diabetes insipidus, respectively.[147] Low levels of thyroid-stimulating hormone, luteinizing hormone, and follicle-stimulating hormone are usually present.[148]

Diagnosis

Septooptic dysplasia should be suspected when the cavum septi pellucidi is absent. The frontal horns are fused on the midline and have a typical squared roof (Fig. 18). The corpus callosum is usually present, although it is frequently described as thinned in postnatal studies. Ventriculomegaly may be present.[149]

Differential Diagnosis

The finding of an absent cavum septi pellucidi with central fusion and squaring of frontal horns is virtually identical to that encountered with lobar holoprosencephaly. The presence of fused fornices within the ventricular cavity favors the diagnosis of lobar holoprosencephaly.[71] The occasional presence of schizencephaly indicates a greater probability septooptic dysplasia. After birth, a definitive diagnosis of septooptic hypoplasia is made by the CT or MRI demonstration of optic tract hypoplasia, endocrine evaluation, and visual assessment.[150] It has been suggested that fetal blood sampling for the evaluation of pituitary hormones could be helpful in dubious cases, by demonstrating signs of hypopituitarism, but this approach is untested thus far.[149]

Associated Anomalies

Associated anomalies include ventriculomegaly, schizencephaly, agenesis of the corpus callosum, and craniofacial anomalies such as hypotelorism and clefting.[145,146]

Prognosis

The outcome of individuals affected by septooptic dysplasia is controversial. Visual impairment is usually present, but blindness is rare. Hypopituitarism is amenable to medical treatment. The developmental outcome is debated. Absence of the septum pellucidum[151] and optic nerve hypoplasia[152] are associated with an excess of cerebral palsy, mental retardation, and seizures. However, it has been pointed out that abnormal development is usually limited to those cases with coexistent cerebral hemispheric anomalies, such as schizencephaly. Of seven infants with isolated septooptic dysplasia, with no other brain abnormalities, only one was found to have moderate cognitive and language delays.[153]

Management

In continuing pregnancies no alteration of standard obstetric care is indicated.

Recurrence Risk

Standard counseling is that the risk of recurrence is low, although hereditary cases have been reported that were compatible with autosomal recessive and autosomal dominant transmission.[154,155]

NEURONAL MIGRATION ANOMALIES

The neuronal cells that form the gray matter originate internally to the brain, on the surface of the lateral ventricles, and only later migrate along radially aligned glial cells to the surface of the brain. Most of the process takes place between 8 weeks' and 16 weeks' gestation, but continues up to 25 weeks. Once the neuronal cells have reached their destination on the surface of the brain, they undergo a process of maturation and differen-

tiation, grow axons and dendrites, and develop synapses with other neurons, giving rise to a well-ordered cortex in which six different layers can be eventually recognized.[156] These six layers, from the cortex to the ventricle, are (a) a plexiform layer, (b) an outer granule layer, (c) a pyramidal layer, (d) an inner granular layer, (e) a ganglionic layer, and (f) a multiform layer.

The process of neuronal migration results in an increase in the surface of the cortex, leading to the formation of sulci and gyri. Whereas the surface of the hemispheres is smooth at 20 weeks' gestation, the dramatic increase in brain mass between 20 and 28 weeks results in folding of the cerebral cortex. At 27 weeks' gestation, the central, cingulate, parietooccipital, and calcarine sulci are usually evident. Secondary and tertiary gyration occurs later in gestation.

Migration abnormalities are characterized by the incomplete formation of the cortical layers, with abnormal locations of neurons that have failed to reach their final destination. In general, the cortex is thickened by a large, disorganized layer of neurons. Conversely, the white matter underneath the cortex is thinned by failure of production of axons by the disorganized neuronal cells. Macroscopically, the main finding is an alteration in the convolutional pattern of the brain, which may be associated with modifications in brain mass and size of the ventricles.

Failure of neuron migration includes a broad spectrum of anomalies: absence to severe reduction of convolutions (lissencephaly), increased number of small convolutions (polymicrogyria), unilateral megalencephaly, schizencephaly, and gray matter heterotopias.

The migrational process may be arrested by environmental factors (ischemia, teratogens), but a genetic predisposition is clearly present at least for some anomalies.

Postnatally, the technique of choice for the diagnosis of this condition is MRI, which allows clear discrimination between white and gray matter.[157] Sonographic detection of typical macroscopic abnormalities of brain anatomy (clefts in the cortex, gyral anomalies, and so forth), however, has led to suspicion and even diagnosis of these conditions antenatally, although usually only in late gestation.

Lissencephaly

Lissencephaly is derived from the Greek word for "smooth brain." It is a primary feature of a wide range of conditions in which the whole or parts of the surface of the brain appear smooth. In addition to agyria, these conditions may include a reduced number of broad gyri, termed *pachygyria*.

The classification of lissencephaly has undergone evolution in the last decade based on findings on MRI and autopsy. Four types of lissencephaly are now recognized, each with subtypes (Table 8). These are (a) the classic form of agyria-pachygyria and subcortical band heterotopia; (b) cobblestone dysplasia; (c) lissencephaly variants with agenesis of the corpus callosum, cerebellar hypoplasia, or other anomalies; and (d) microlissencephaly.

TABLE 8. CLASSIFICATION OF LISSENCEPHALY

I. Classic lissencephaly and subcortical band heterotopia
    X-linked lissencephaly
    17-linked lissencephaly
    Isolated 17-linked lissencephaly
    Miller-Dieker syndrome
    Baraitser-Winter syndrome
II. Cobblestone dysplasia
    Cobblestone lissencephaly without other anomalies
    Fukuyama muscular dystrophy
    Muscle-eye-brain disease
    Walker-Warburg syndrome
III. Lissencephaly variants with other anomalies
IV. Microlissencephaly
    Microcephaly with simplified gyral pattern
    Microlissencephaly I
    Microlissencephaly II
    Microlissencephaly III

Adapted from Dobyns WB. Available at: http://www.geneclinics.com. Accessed October 24, 1999.

Incidence

The incidence for lissencephaly is unknown but rare.

Pathogenesis and Pathology

Failure of migration of the neurons results in either a significant reduction (pachygyria) or absence (agyria) of cerebral convolutions. Histologically, abnormalities of the layering of the neocortex are found, from a reduction of the layers to a complete architectural disorganization.

Classic lissencephaly is characterized by agyria with or without pachygyria, a wide cortical mantle and minimal or no ventriculomegaly. Agyric and pachygyric regions have a four-layer cortex instead of the normal six layers: (a) a molecular layer, (b) an outer cellular layer (true cortex), (c) a cell sparse layer, and (d) a deep cellular layer composed of heterotopic incompletely migrated neurons.[156]

A less severe variant of lissencephaly is known as *subcortical band heterotopia*. Characteristic findings on MRI examination are a normal or mildly simplified gyral pattern with shallow sulci, a normal cortical layer, and a striking subcortical band of heterotopic gray matter.

Cobblestone dysplasia (also known as *type II lissencephaly*) shows a thickened, disorganized cortex without layering. It is associated with ventriculomegaly and other severe central nervous system defects and is usually part of a syndrome such as the Walker-Warburg syndrome (see Walker-Warburg Syndrome in Chapter 5).

Diagnosis

Postnatally and during the third trimester of pregnancy, the diagnosis of lissencephaly can be established by demonstrating a reduction or an absence of cerebral sulci.[159–162]

Incomplete opercularization of the insula is also a well-established postnatal finding. MRI is superior to ultrasound for detection of lissencephaly because of its ability to evaluate cerebral convolutions, as well as the cortical plate.

In addition to absence or reduction of cerebral convolutions, the diagnosis of lissencephaly may be suggested by ventriculomegaly, usually of the borderline type, and increased subarachnoid space (Figs. 37 and 38). Pilu et al. reported one fetus with borderline ventriculomegaly at 21 weeks that was found to have lissencephaly at birth.[49] Some forms of lissencephaly are also associated with microcephaly, which may be detected during the third trimester, and other brain anomalies.

Miller-Dieker syndrome is caused by cytogenetically visible or submicroscopic deletions of the Miller-Dieker syndrome critical region at chromosome locus 17p13.3. Among patients with a history of classical lissencephaly in whom standard cytogenetic analysis and FISH studies are normal, DNA-based testing by sequencing of the LIS1 and XLIS (also known as *DCX*) genes is now available.

Differential Diagnosis

The primary differential diagnosis of lissencephaly is immature gestational age when lack of gyri is a normal developmental finding. The developing brain is normally smooth until the onset of the third trimester, and the opercularization of the insula is not complete until 27 to 28 weeks.[163] Therefore, the diagnosis of lissencephaly based on imaging is not possible until the third trimester.

Associated Anomalies

Miller-Dieker syndrome is associated with facial dysmorphism, agenesis of the corpus callosum, ventriculomegaly, midline calcifications, microcephaly, congenital heart disease, omphalocele, kidney dysplasia, and genital anomalies. Transverse palmar creases and clinodactyly are common. Polyhydramnios and decreased fetal movements are also frequent.[164,165] Baraitser-Winter syndrome is associated with various facial abnormalities, including webbed neck.

Walker-Warburg syndrome (see Chapter 5) is an autosomal recessive lethal disorder that shows central nervous system malformations such as corpus callosum agenesis, cerebellar dysplasia with vermian agenesis/dysgenesis or Dandy-Walker malformation, and white brain atrophy. It is the most well-known subtype of type II lissencephaly.

Neu-Laxova syndrome is a lethal autosomal recessive disorder consisting of growth restriction, microcephaly, lissencephaly, corpus callosum agenesis, intracranial calcifications, cerebellar hypoplasia, facial dysmorphism, microphthalmia, exophthalmus, cataracts, absent eyelids, hydrops, ichthyosis, contractures of extremities,

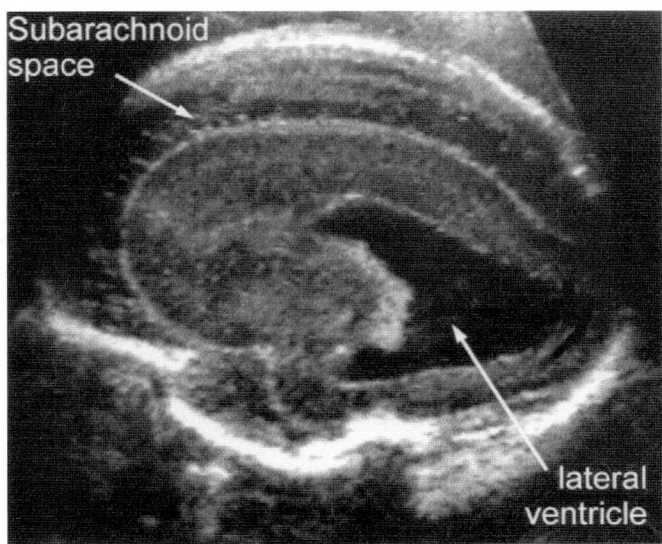

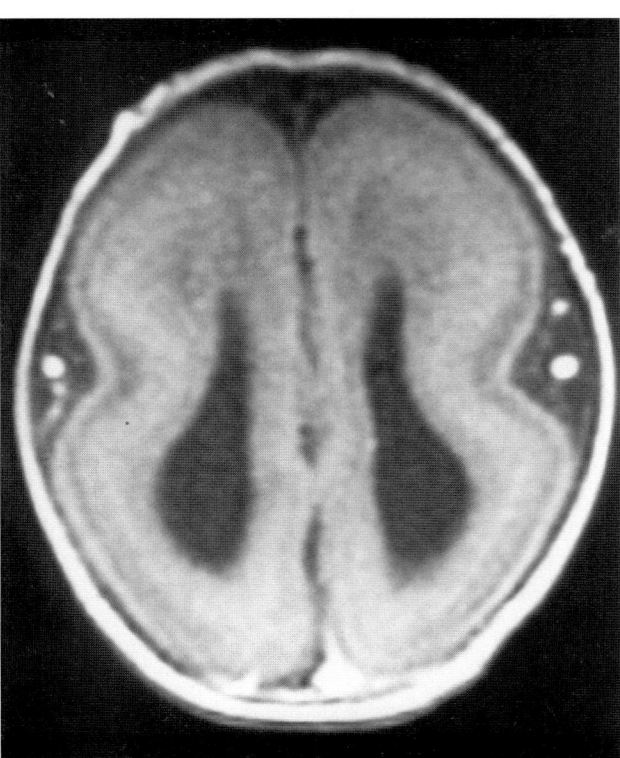

FIGURE 37. Lissencephaly. **A:** Parasagittal scan in third trimester shows mild dilation of the trigone and occipital horn of the lateral ventricle. The frontal horn was not dilated. **B:** Postnatal magnetic resonance image demonstrates smooth appearance of the brain surface with dilation of the trigone in the occipital horn in this infant with lissencephaly. (Reproduced with permission from McGahan JP, Thurmond AS. *Fetal head and brain in diagnostic ultrasound: a logical approach.* Philadelphia: Lippincott–Raven Publishers, 1997:231–270.)

and syndactyly. It has been classified as a type of type III lissencephaly.

Prognosis

The prognosis of lissencephaly is universally poor, regardless of etiologic type. Severe mental retardation is almost the rule. Failure to thrive, infantile spasms, and seizures are frequent. Death occurs usually within the first 6 years.

Management

Management is conservative. Usually the ultrasound diagnosis is made during the third trimester, and termination is not an option.

Recurrence Risk

The pattern of inheritance varies by the specific syndrome. Approximately 80% of patients with Miller-Dieker syndrome have *de novo* deletions, and approximately 20% have inherited a deletion from a parent who carries a balanced chromosome rearrangement. Other forms of lissencephaly may be inherited as an X-linked or autosomal recessive form.

Unilateral Megalencephaly

A synonym for unilateral megalencephaly is hemimegalencephaly.

Unilateral megalencephaly is a complex abnormality of the brain characterized by abnormal neuronal migration with hypertrophy of one hemisphere.[166]

Etiology

The etiology is unknown.

Pathology

Unilateral megalencephaly is characterized by overgrowth of one cerebral lobe or an entire hemisphere. It is considered part of the spectrum of abnormal neuronal cell migration.[157,166] Associated findings include ipsilateral ventriculomegaly, shift of the midline, and macrocephaly. Anatomic dissection demonstrates macroscopic and histologic abnormalities of the affected portion of the brain, including aberrant convolutional patterns (micropolygyria, pachygyria, agyria) and ectopic nodules of gray matter. The cortex is thickened, and there is disorganization of the cortical layers.[166]

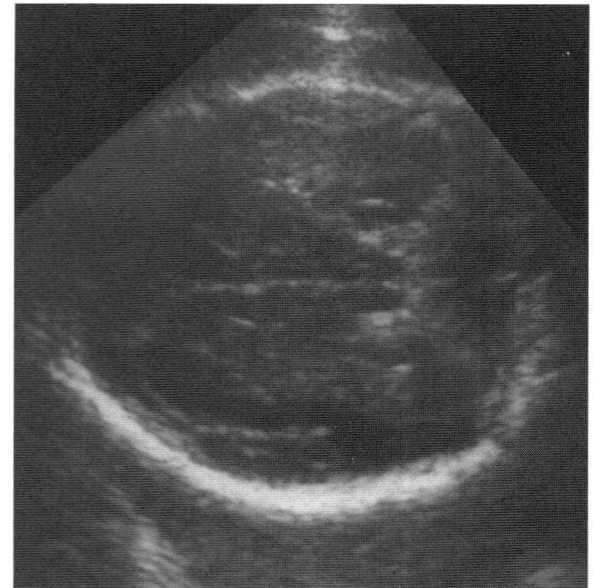

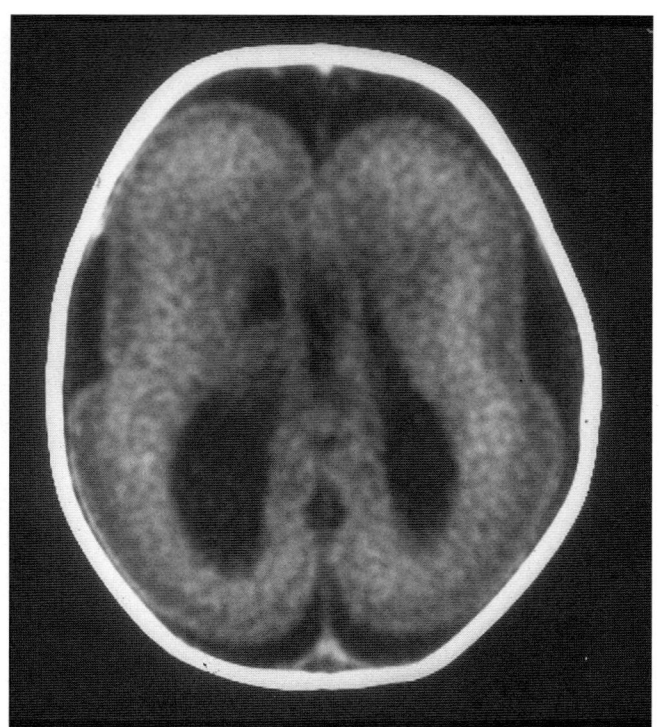

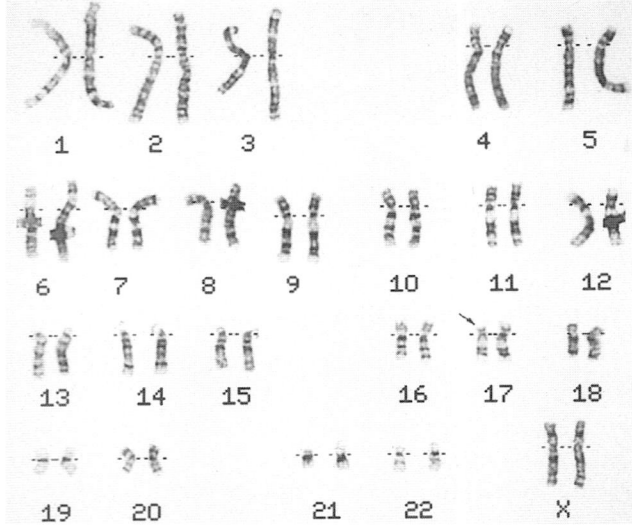

FIGURE 38. Lissencephaly, Miller-Dieker syndrome. **A:** Axial scan near term shows immature sulcal and gyral pattern. **B:** Postnatal computed tomography scan shows smooth cortex. **C:** Karyotype analysis showed 46 XX del(17 p13).

Diagnosis

Postnatal diagnostic imaging of unilateral megalencephaly demonstrates enlargement of one hemisphere in the absence of a mass effect, a shift in the midline, mild ipsilateral ventriculomegaly, and abnormal convolutions.[157,166] Similar findings have been described with sonography in three fetuses, two in the third trimester and one in the second trimester (Fig. 39).[167–169] In one case, fetal MRI was found to be useful by further demonstrating the overgrowth of one hemisphere.[168] In another case, three-dimensional ultrasound facilitated the demonstration of the asymmetry between the hemispheres.[169] We have experience with two further cases, in which multiplanar neurosonography allowed us to establish clearly the diagnosis. In the third trimester, apart from further defining abnormal macroscopic anatomy,

MRI may be useful to demonstrate gray matter heterotopia (Fig. 40).

Differential Diagnosis

Enlargement of one hemisphere with ventriculomegaly may be encountered with unilateral ventriculomegaly and brain tumors. Unilateral megalencephaly has the distinctive feature of a distorted, thickened cortex without mass effect. The presence of abnormal convolutions is a very specific sign, but it is expected to be present only in the third trimester.

Associated Anomalies

Although many publications describe an association between unilateral megalencephaly and hemigigantism, the increased mass of one hemisphere seen with this condition

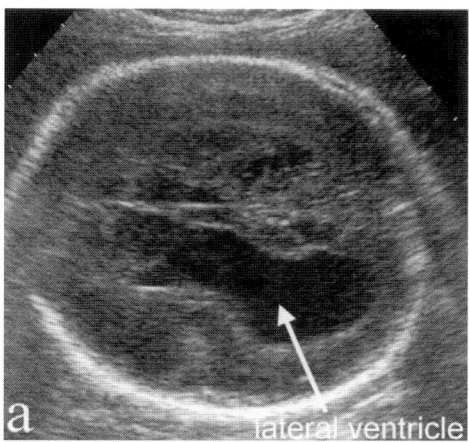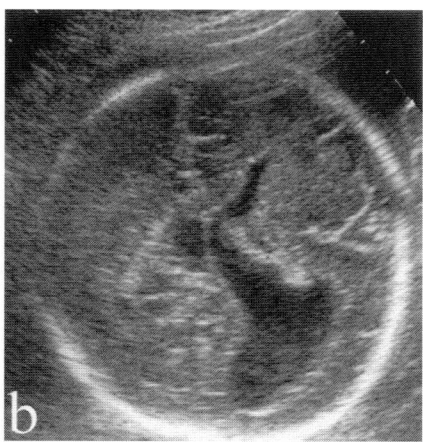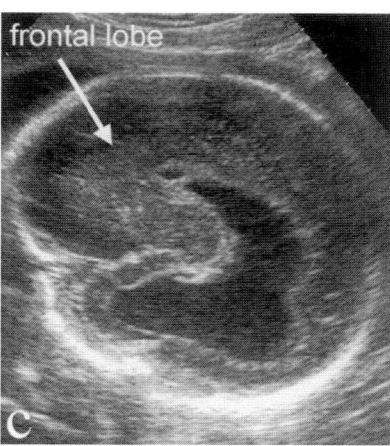

FIGURE 39. Unilateral megalencephaly in a third-trimester fetus. Axial **(A)**, coronal **(B)**, and parasagittal **(C)** views show a shift in the midline echo, with overgrowth of one hemisphere and ipsilateral ventriculomegaly, with large irregular convolutions. The parasagittal view shows lack of gyri consistent with lissencephaly (see Figs. 37 and 38).

is now considered a different entity. Several case reports suggest an association with linear sebaceous nevus syndrome, which is probably pathogenetically related.[170] The occurrence of Dandy-Walker complex[171] and tuberous sclerosis has also been documented.[172] Neonatal cardiac failure has also been described, probably as a consequence of increased blood flow through the enlarged dysplastic cerebral hemisphere.[173]

Prognosis

The prognosis is poor. There are variable degrees, but all infants have seizures, hemiplegia, and neurodevelop-

mental delay. Surgical removal of the involved lobe or hemisphere is the recommended therapy with intractable seizures.[174]

Management

Cesarean section may be necessary to avoid cephalopelvic disproportion.

Recurrence Risk

The recurrence risk is not increased. However, it has been suggested that unilateral megalencephaly is a part of the

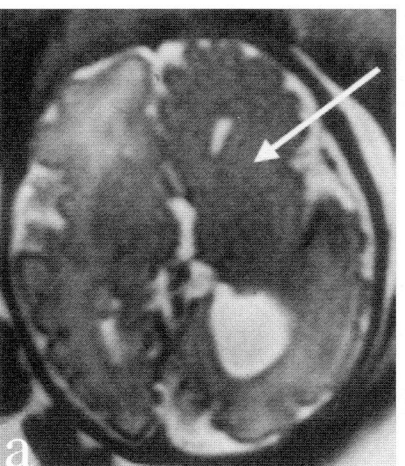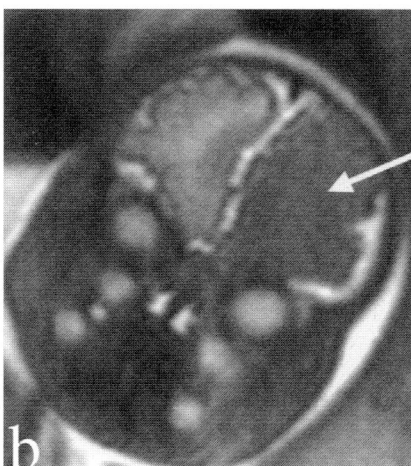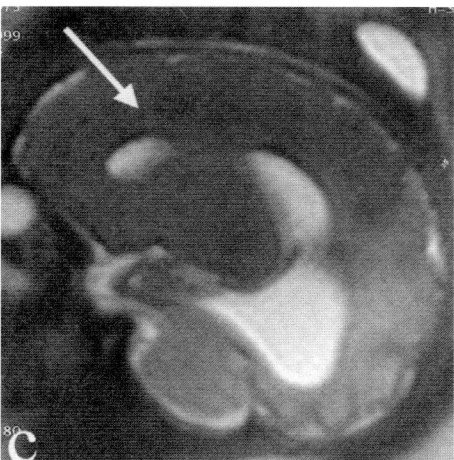

FIGURE 40. Magnetic resonance in the same case as in Figure 39 on axial **(A)**, coronal **(B)**, and parasagittal **(C)** views show overgrowth of one hemisphere (*arrows*), unilateral ventriculomegaly, and thickened convolutions. In the affected hemisphere, the cortical plate cannot be clearly demonstrated, and the cortex has an altered signal intensity from normal white matter, probably secondary to decreased myelination and increased water content. (Courtesy of Dr. A. Couture, Montpellier.)

spectrum of neuronal migration disorders. These conditions have been reported to be associated with a 5% to 20% chance of cerebral malformations in siblings.[163]

Schizencephaly

Schizencephaly is a disorder characterized by congenital full-thickness clefts of the cerebral mantle. The clefts can be either unilateral or, more frequently, bilateral and symmetric; are lined by pia-ependyma; and put into communication the cavity of the lateral ventricles with the subarachnoid space.

A synonym for schizencephaly is true porencephaly.

Prevalence

The prevalence is unknown. Schizencephaly is a rare congenital brain malformation with approximately 70 cases described in children, including six *in utero*.

Etiology

The etiology of schizencephaly is unknown.

Pathology

The precise pathogenesis of schizencephaly is debated. The original work of Yakovlev and Wadsworth[175,176] contends that a failure of normal migration of the primitive neuroblasts results in the cerebral cleft. Barkovich and Norman argue that schizencephaly is a part of a spectrum of encephaloclastic disorders due to vascular infarction[177] in an area of the germinal matrix during the seventh week of embryogenesis. Their theory is based on the demonstration of watershed zones in the gray matter along the lateral ventricles in the area of the germinal matrix.

The neuropathologic features of schizencephaly are as follows: (a) hemispheric clefts, lined with pia-ependyma, usually bilateral, in the area of the sylvian fissure; (b) communication of the subarachnoid space with the lateral ventricle medially, with infolding of gray matter along the cleft; and (c) multiple associated intracranial malformations, including polymicrogyria, gray matter heterotopias, absent septum pellucidum, optic nerve hypoplasia, and agenesis of the corpus callosum.[175–177] Two varieties of schizencephaly are commonly recognized: those with *fused* clefts in the cerebral mantle (type I) and those with separated clefts, usually in association with ventriculomegaly of varying degrees (type II).

Diagnosis

Prenatal diagnosis of schizencephaly has been reported in six cases, always of the type II variety.[178–182] In these cases, the most striking finding was the presence of clefts in the cortex in the area of the sylvian fissures, establishing a communication between the enlarged lateral ventricle medially

and the subarachnoid space laterally (Fig. 41). Agenesis of the septum pellucidum with fusion of the frontal horns was also noted in several cases.[183]

We anticipate that the type I variety is extremely difficult to diagnose antenatally. Fused clefts within the cortex can be identified by CT and MRI after birth, but it is uncertain whether they can be recognized by fetal sonography.[177]

Differential Diagnosis

The sonographic findings in fetal schizencephaly may be similar to those encountered with other intracranial abnormalities, such as encephaloclastic porencephaly, lobar holoprosencephaly, septooptic dysplasia, and intracranial cyst. Distinguishing a large porencephalic cyst in the area of the Sylvian fissure from schizencephaly may be impossible. However, large porencephalic cysts are unilateral, have a jagged contour, and may contain blood clots.

In lobar holoprosencephaly and septooptic dysplasia, the septum pellucidum is absent and the frontal horns are fused, similarly to most cases of schizencephaly. However, schizencephaly (at least, the type II variety) is featured by the presence of cortical clefts. Intracranial cysts (arachnoid cysts, glioependymal cysts) may occur in the area of the Sylvian fissure, however, they do not communicate with lateral ventricles. The largest available series thus far indicates that expert sonography is accurate in the diagnosis of schizencephaly. Multiplanar brain imaging and vaginal sonography of vertex fetuses are useful.[182]

Associated Anomalies

Ventriculomegaly, polymicrogyria, heterotopias, agenesis of the corpus callosum, and absent septum pellucidum are frequently found.[175–177] The incidence of an absent septum pellucidum is reported to be near 50%.[177] In addition to these well-known associations, optic nerve hypoplasia has been identified along with schizencephaly, simulating septooptic dysplasia.[184]

Prognosis

The prognosis is variable. Schizencephalic patients generally experience varying degrees of mental retardation and developmental delay, as well as seizures and various motor abnormalities.[175,176] In one small postnatal series, patients with bilateral schizencephaly had severe neurologic impairment (seizures, severe developmental delay) in the first years of life. Patients with unilateral schizencephaly usually had mild neurologic symptoms with onset in adulthood.[157]

Management

Termination of pregnancy can be offered when the diagnosis is made before viability. There is no indica-

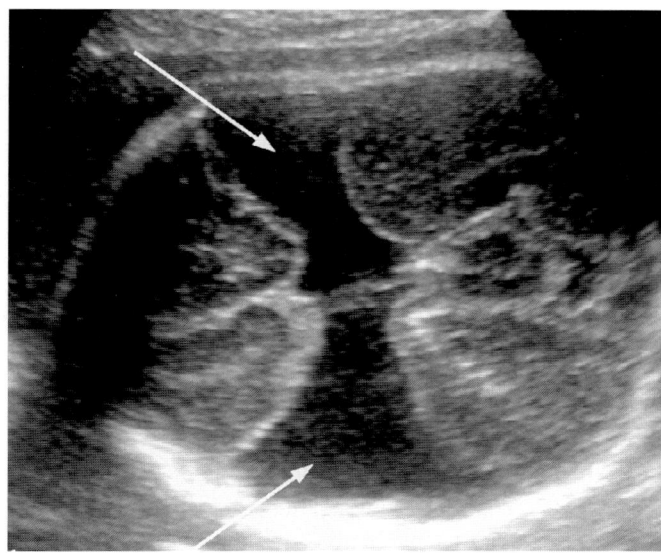
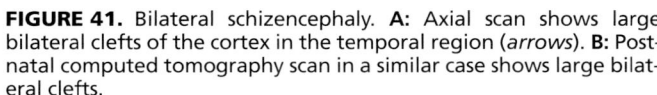
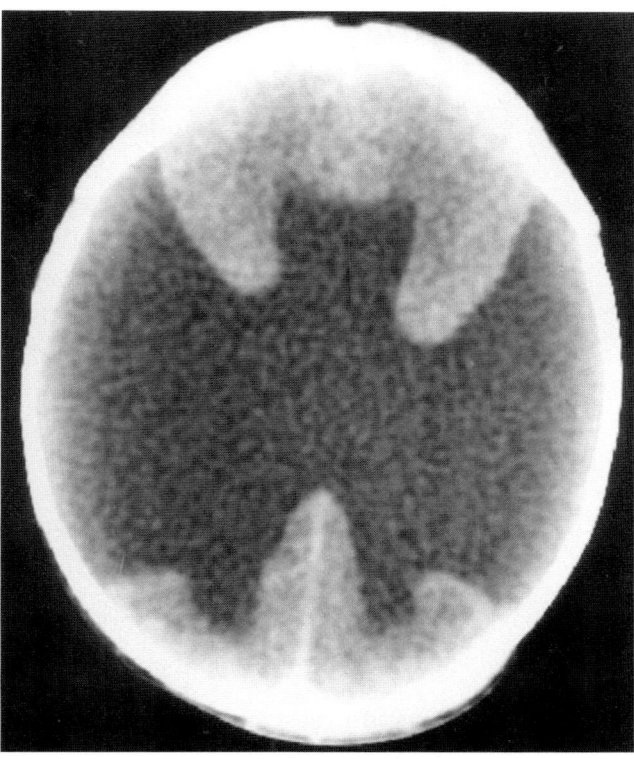

FIGURE 41. Bilateral schizencephaly. **A:** Axial scan shows large bilateral clefts of the cortex in the temporal region (*arrows*). **B:** Postnatal computed tomography scan in a similar case shows large bilateral clefts.

tion to alter standard obstetric management in continuing pregnancies.

Recurrence Risk

The recurrence risk is not increased. However, it has been suggested that schizencephaly be a part of the spectrum of neuronal migration disorders. These conditions have been reported to be associated with a 5% to 20% chance of cerebral malformations in siblings.[156]

Intracranial Cyst

The presence of a fluid-filled lesion is one of the most frequent abnormal findings of the fetal brain. The fluid collections may be due to enlargement of the ventricular system (ventriculomegaly) or are the consequence of a destructive lesion of the cortex (schizencephaly, porencephaly). As discussed in the section on midline anomalies, there are several cystic intercranial abnormalities that are typically midline.

Other cystic abnormalities may occur within the brain, and many of these abnormalities are lateralizing abnormalities (Tables 5 and 9). The most common cause of a lateralizing intracranial cyst is a choroid plexus cyst. This cyst is usually present within the choroid plexus of the lateral ventricles. It may be bilateral or unilateral and usually regresses before birth. Other cysts may occur in the midline or may be lateralizing. These can include arachnoid

cysts or glioependymal cysts. Arachnoid cysts are smooth-wall, asymmetrical cysts, which may have a mass effect. They may be associated with hydrocephalus depending on the location of the cyst. Glioependymal cysts may have a similar appearance to arachnoid cysts but are often midline. They are different from arachnoid cysts in that they usually have an epididymal lining as compared to the fibrous walls of arachnoid cysts and are often associated with agenesis of corpus callosum.

Other abnormalities that may appear cystic within the brain include porencephaly, schizencephaly, a cystic neoplasm, intracranial hemorrhage, or unilateral hydrocephalus. Porencephaly and schizencephaly may have a similar appearance on *in utero* ultrasound. These defects usually communicate with the ventricles. Porencephaly is usually unilateral, whereas schizencephaly may be bilateral.

Specific cysts including arachnoid cysts, glioependymal cyst, and choroid plexus cysts are considered in this section.

Arachnoid Cysts

Arachnoid cysts are the accumulation of cerebrospinal-like fluid between the cerebral meninges.

Incidence

Arachnoid cysts are rare. They represent 1% of all intracranial masses in newborns.[185] Only a few cases of this anomaly have been reported in the prenatal literature.[178,182,186]

TABLE 9. DISTINGUISHING FEATURES OF LATERAL INTRACRANIAL CYSTS

Abnormality	Features
Choroid plexus cyst	Cyst present within the choroid plexus of the lateral ventricle
	Bilateral or unilateral
Arachnoid cyst	Smooth wall
	Asymmetric
	Mass effect
	Possible hydrocephalus (dependent on location)
Porencephaly	Usually unilateral
	Communicates with ventricle
	Cavity size increases with distance from ventricle
	Decreased size of ipsilateral bony calvaria
	Cavity lined by white matter (postnatal magnetic resonance imaging)
Schizencephaly	Unilateral or bilateral
	May or may not communicate with ventricle
	Cavity size increases with distance from ventricle
	Defect lined by gray matter (postnatal magnetic resonance imaging)
Unilateral hydrocephalus	Unusual; check opposite ventricle after changing fetal position, or perform angled scanning (see text)
Cystic neoplasm	Mass effect
	Solid or irregular with cystic components
Intracranial hemorrhage	Initial echogenic clot in ventricle
	Later echogenic clot plus ventriculomegaly on side of hemorrhage

Adapted from McGahan J, Thurmond A. The fetal head. In: McGahan J, Porto M, eds. *Diagnostic obstetrical ultrasound.* Philadelphia: JB Lippincott, 1994.

Pathogenesis and Pathology

Arachnoid cysts may be primary (congenital) or secondary (acquired). Congenital types are believed to be formed by maldevelopment of the leptomeninges and do not freely communicate with the subarachnoid space. Acquired types are formed as the result of hemorrhage, trauma, and infection and often communicate with subarachnoid space.[185,187,188]

Arachnoid cysts have the potential to grow as the result of either some communication with the subarachnoid space from a ball valve mechanism or CSF production by a choroid plexus-like tissue contained within the cyst wall.[189]

Intracranial arachnoid cysts are accumulation of clear cerebrospinal-like fluid between the dura and the brain substance. They may occur (a) between the pia mater and the arachnoid membrane (subarachnoid cysts); (b) between the two leaves of the arachnoid (intraarachnoid cysts); or (c) between the outer arachnoid membrane and the dura mater. The precise location is often not easily discernible, and the term *arachnoid cyst* is frequently used independently from the histologic diagnosis to indicate any intracranial cyst located in the subarachnoid space.[188]

Arachnoid cysts have been found anywhere in the CNS, including the spinal canal. The most frequent locations are the surface of the cerebral hemispheres in the sites of the major fissures (sylvian, rolandic, and interhemispheric), the region of sella turcica, the anterior fossa, and the middle fossa. Less frequently, they are seen in the posterior fossa.[190] Arachnoid cysts may communicate with the subarachnoid space.[191]

Diagnosis

Ultrasound examination of arachnoid cysts demonstrates a well-defined anechoic lesion with adjacent mass effect, occasionally associated with hydrocephalus (Figs. 42 and 43). The overall majority of arachnoid cysts diagnosed *in utero* thus far have been recognized only in the third trimester. In a few cases, unremarkable sonograms had been obtained in the midtrimester. Most of the cases diagnosed antenatally involve supratentorial cysts, in the midline, sylvian fissure, and ambient cistern.

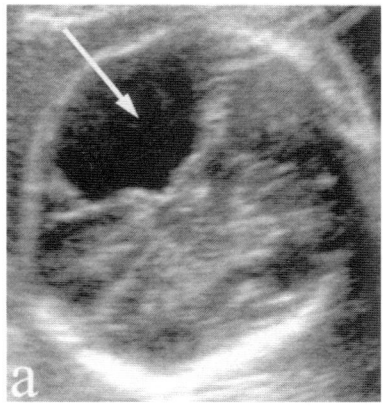 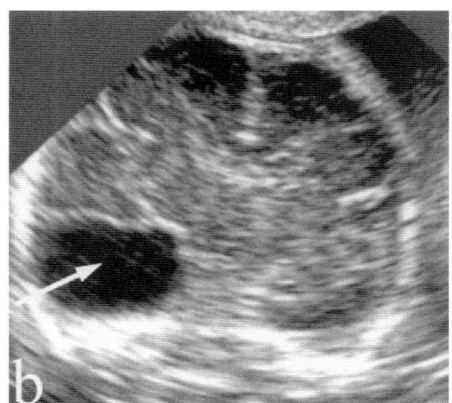 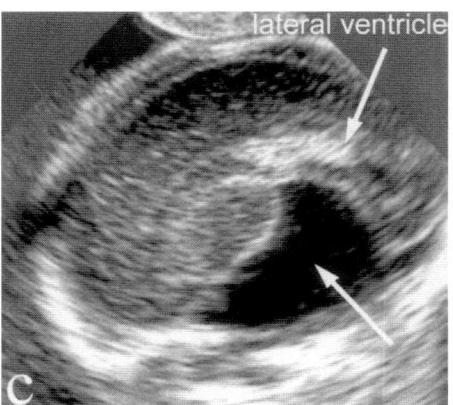

FIGURE 42. Arachnoid cyst. Axial **(A)**, coronal **(B)**, and parasagittal **(C)** scans show a large fluid collection (*arrows*) in the temporal fossa. The differential diagnosis is porencephalic cyst. The correct diagnosis is suggested by smooth contour and mass effect, which compresses rather than replaces the cortex. The cyst is seen separate from the ventricles. The presence of an arachnoid cyst was confirmed after delivery.

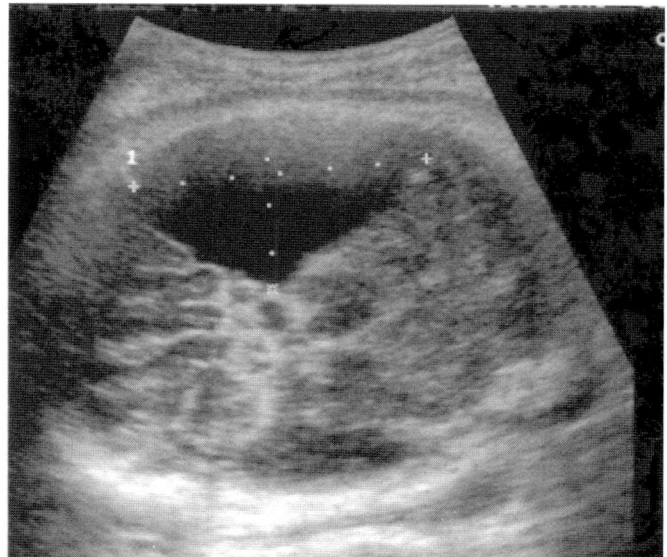 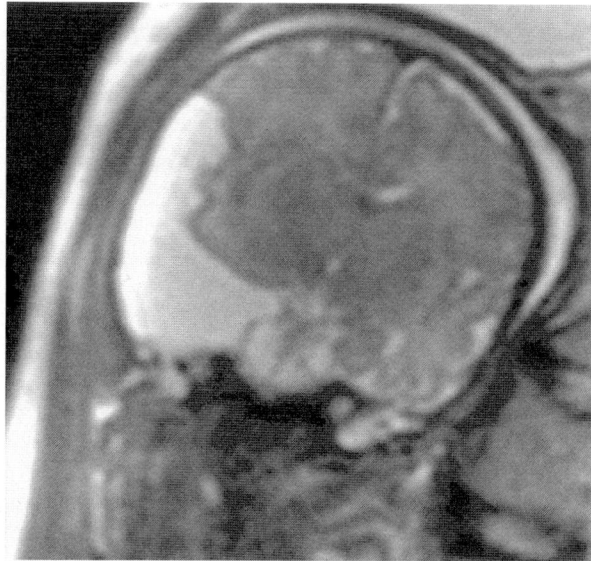

A   B

FIGURE 43. Arachnoid cyst. **A:** Scan at 39 weeks shows a well-defined cyst in the left parietal area. **B:** Magnetic resonance imaging shows extraaxial fluid collection in left-temporal position corresponding to a perisylvian arachnoidal cyst. No compression of adjacent brain is evident. (Courtesy of Dr. W. Blaicher, Department of Gynecology and Obstetrics, Division of Prenatal Diagnosis and Therapy, University Hospital, Vienna, Austria.)

MRI has also been used to evaluate arachnoid cysts.[192]

Differential Diagnosis

Porencephalic cysts are located inside the brain substance, whereas arachnoid cysts lie between the skull and brain surface. Furthermore, the majority of congenital porencephalic cysts communicates with the lateral ventricles. In schizencephaly, the fluid-filled collection connects the lateral ventricles to the subarachnoid space. Unilateral ventriculomegaly should be recognized by the location and shape of the cystic mass.

Demonstration that the corpus callosum is present allows to differentiate a midline arachnoid from dysgenesis of corpus callosum with an associated interhemispheric cyst.[125,185] A posterior fossa arachnoid cyst is distinguished from the Dandy-Walker complex by demonstrating the integrity of the cerebellar vermis. At times, however, the cerebellar defect may be small and difficult to demonstrate.

It may be difficult to distinguish arachnoid cysts from the more rare glioependymal cysts, although arachnoid cysts are more frequently located at the surface of the hemispheres. The distinction may not be clinically relevant, as it is uncertain whether these two entities have different prognostic implications. It may occasionally be difficult to differentiate the rare cystic tumor from arachnoid cyst.[193]

Associated Anomalies

Large arachnoid cysts can cause obstructive ventriculomegaly by compressing the foramen of Monro, the aqueduct posteriorly, or blocking the basal cisterns. Hydrocephalus

and macrocephaly are the most common presentations in the neonatal period.[194] Absence of the septum pellucidum and corpus callosum, cervical syringomyelia, Chiari malformation type I, and deficient cerebellar lobulation have been occasionally reported and may be derived from mechanical compression, at least in part.

Arachnoid cysts have been reported very rarely in association with other anomalies. The list includes trisomy 18, tetralogy of Fallot, sacrococcygeal tumor, and neurofibromatosis.[182,186]

Prognosis

In many cases, arachnoid cysts are asymptomatic, but they may cause epilepsy, mild motor or sensory abnormalities, or hydrocephalus. Hydrocephalus and macrocephaly are the most common presentations in the neonatal period. Later, the *midline syndrome* can develop, consisting of headaches, vomiting, bilateral papilledema, hyperreflexia, and ataxia. Subdural hygromas may develop when rupture of the outer membrane of the cyst occurs and fluid leaks into the subdural compartments. Depending on the location and extent, arachnoid cysts can be treated by resection or shunting.[195,196]

Neurosurgical series suggest a good prognosis. Out of 118 cases coming from two series,[196,197] 85 (72%) were reported to be free of symptoms or with only slight neurologic manifestations and 25 (21%) had variable degrees of disability. There were seven (6%) postoperative deaths. The location of the cyst has influence on the final outcome. In one series, the temporal cysts were found to have the best outcome, with 93% of patients recovering completely or with only slight deficits, and there were no deaths. The other locations were associated with a significantly lower success rate (handicap in 20% to 30% of cases, mortality in 10% to 20%). In particular, posterior fossa arachnoid cysts had the worst outcomes. The series contain probably many postnatal cases, and it is uncertain whether their favorable results apply to the large congenital cysts that are amenable to intrauterine diagnosis. However, antenatal series, though limited, do report a good outcome in most cases. Follow-up is available on nine cases that were diagnosed antenatally.[182,186,197,198] Surgery was performed in six cases. There was only one death in one infant with a posterior fossa cyst associated with hydrocephalus. Seven of the eight survivors were neurologically normal at the time of report. Developmental retardation was present only in one case, in which small arachnoid cysts of the ambient cistern were associated with agenesis of the corpus callosum.

Management

When the lesion strongly suggests an arachnoid cyst, the patient should be counseled on the rather benign prognosis of the lesion. It is uncertain whether a fetal karyotype should be obtained. Only one case of trisomy 18 was found among the 14 cases thus far diagnosed antenatally. When the head has a normal size there is no reason to modify the mode and time of delivery. Given the good outcome associated with intracranial cysts, intrauterine treatment by either needling or shunting is hard to justify. However, large cysts rapidly increasing in size may represent an exception. Whether cephalocentesis could be offered in cases with macrocrania to overcome cephalopelvic disproportion is uncertain. The traditional view is that cephalocentesis is associated with excessive perinatal mortality.[199] Careful aspiration with fine needles guided with high-resolution ultrasound equipment, trying to limit as much as possible damage to brain parenchyma and cerebral vessels, may cause however much less harm than these rather old data indicate.

Glioependymal Cysts

Synonyms for glioependymal cysts include ependymal cysts, neuroepithelial cysts, epithelial cysts, choroidal epithelial cysts, and agenesis of the corpus callosum with interhemispheric cyst.

Glioependymal cysts are intracranial cysts with an ependymal lining.

Incidence

The incidence is unknown. Glioependymal cysts are extremely rare.

Etiology

The etiology for glioependymal cysts is unknown.

Pathology

Glioependymal cysts are thought to derive from displaced neuroectodermal tissue.[200] The natural history of glioependymal cysts is uncertain. The histologic appearance of the cyst wall is heterogenous. It always comprises an ependymal lining with or without cilia and an outer layer of either basement membrane or glial tissue.

Glioependymal cysts are different from arachnoid cysts in that the latter have fibrous walls with no ependyma. Similarly to arachnoid cysts, glioependymal cysts may have different locations, although they are usually found deeply enfolded within the cerebrum. They may also be located within the cisterns, interhemispheric, intracerebellar, and intraspinal. They are commonly associated with other anomalies, especially agenesis of the corpus callosum.

Diagnosis

Glioependymal cysts appear similar to arachnoid cysts. However, they are more likely to be located within the brain parenchyma, multilocular, and associated with other brain abnormalities including agenesis of the corpus callosum.[183,201–203] They may have significant mass effect.

Differential Diagnosis

Other considerations include arachnoid cyst, porencephaly, and cystic tumors.

Associated Anomalies

Large glioependymal cysts can cause obstructive ventriculomegaly. Agenesis of the corpus callosum may be present, especially with interhemispheric cysts.[201,204] In these cases, it remains uncertain whether the absence of the corpus callosum is a part of a generalized maldevelopment of the midline structures that involves formation of the midline cyst, or it represents the consequence of mechanical compression operated by the cyst.

Prognosis

The experience so far is limited. It is likely that the available series on arachnoid cysts do include at least some glioependymal cysts. Indeed, there is no clear evidence that these two entities have different clinical implications.

Management

To our knowledge, no chromosomal aberrations have been reported thus far in these cases. Obstetric management does not differ from that outlined for arachnoid cysts.

Recurrence Risk

There is no known recurrence risk.

Choroid Plexus Cysts

A choroid plexus cyst is a round sonolucent in the context of the choroid plexus of lateral ventricles, with a diameter of greater than 2 mm.

Incidence

Choroid plexus cysts are frequently detected during the second trimester. A survey of low-risk pregnant patients indicates that the frequency of this finding in the midtrimester is in the range of 1%.[205] However, the real incidence is probably dependent on the resolution of the ultrasound equipment, the attention of the operator, and the definition of choroid plexus cyst that is used. Figures as high as 3.6% have been reported.[206]

Pathology

Cysts of the choroid plexuses are most frequently transient and benign findings, and, therefore, there is a lack of pathologic studies. The ultrasound appearance suggests that a collection of fluid surrounded by choroid plexus tissue exists.

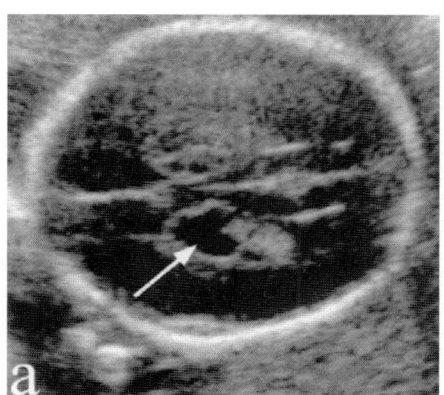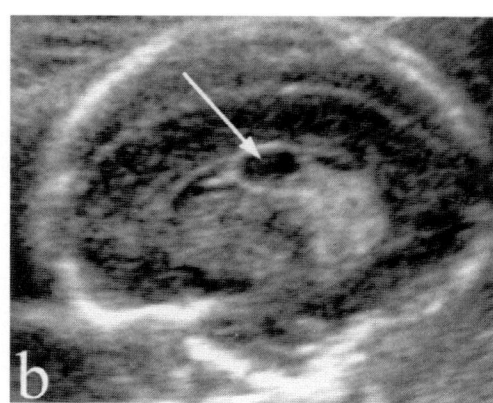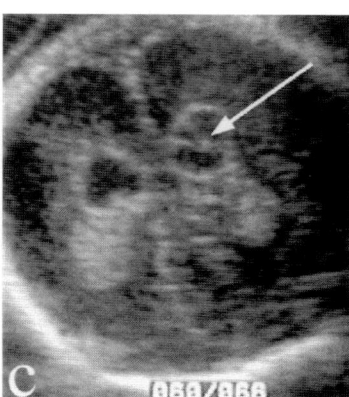

FIGURE 44. Choroid plexus cyst. Axial **(A)**, parasagittal **(B)**, and coronal **(C)** views show typical choroid plexus cyst (*arrows*).

Diagnosis

Choroid plexus cysts appear as sonolucent spaces within the choroid plexus, with well-defined walls (Fig. 44). The cysts may be unilateral or bilateral, and occasionally are multiple. They are typically found at the level of the atrium of lateral ventricles, less frequently within the bodies. When examined with high-resolution ultrasound equipment, the choroid plexus of lateral ventricle often appears slightly dishomogeneous. Choroid plexus cysts should measure at least 2 mm in diameters. Large cysts filling the ventricles are occasionally seen, and these appear to carry an increased risk for trisomy 18 (Fig. 45). Other sonographic features of trisomy 18 should be specifically sought when choroid plexus cysts are seen.

Differential Diagnosis

Large choroid plexus cysts could be mistaken for ventricular dilatation. However, choroid plexus cysts have a thick echogenic wall and may have internal septations. A localized intraventricular bleed may result in a blood clot resembling an abnormality of the choroid plexus. However, the clot is less regular than a choroid plexus cyst, and the surrounding ventricle is usually enlarged.

Associated Anomalies

The possible risk of abnormal karyotypes is discussed in detail in Chapter 21. There are no other known associations with choroid plexus cysts.

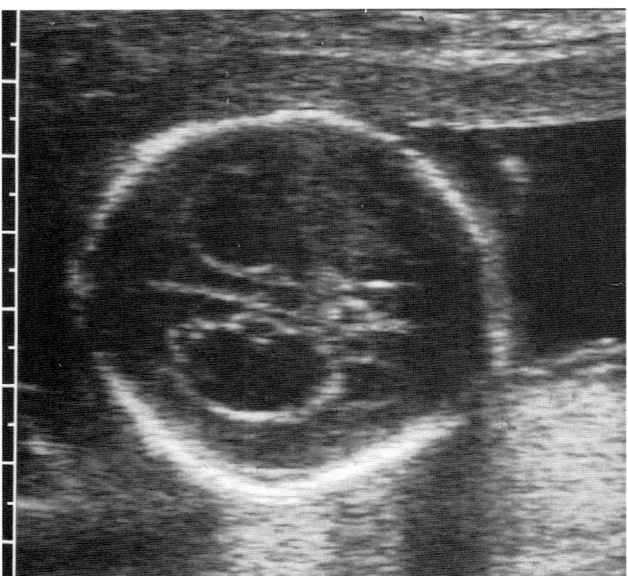

FIGURE 45. Large choroid plexus cyst and brachycephaly are noted. These were the only sonographic abnormalities. Fetal karyotype revealed trisomy 18.

Prognosis

In the absence of associated anomalies, choroid plexus cysts should be considered normal anatomic variants. They are typically seen around midgestation, decrease rapidly in size, and tend to disappear by the third trimester. Only rarely, remnants are detected by a scan performed after birth. We are not aware of any case in which a choroid plexus cyst detected antenatally has been associated *per se* with adverse outcome. A handful of very large cysts of the choroid plexuses causing intracranial hypertension has been described in the neurosurgical literature, but these represent probably a separate clinical entity.[207]

Management

Fetal choroid plexus cysts are benign, transient findings that are associated with an increased likelihood of trisomy 18. On the basis of available data, a prudent approach is to perform a thorough sonographic examination of the fetus when a choroid plexus cyst is identified. This examination should include evaluation of the hands and feet, and a thorough examination of the fetal heart. If an additional ultrasound abnormality is identified, chromosomal analysis should be offered to the patient. Additional reassurance can be obtained by correlating ultrasound findings with serum biochemical markers.[208] Isolated choroid plexus cysts do not modify standard obstetric management. As no deleterious effect on the fetus has been thus far reported with this finding, there is no need, in our opinion, for follow-up scans.

Recurrence Risk

The recurrence risk is not known to be increased.

INTRACRANIAL HEMORRHAGE AND DESTRUCTIVE LESIONS

This section includes several entities that may have different etiologies, but all result in brain destruction. Hydranencephaly and porencephaly may be a common entity. Hydranencephaly is derived from the combination of the words *hydrocephalus* and *anencephaly*. Hydranencephaly is thought to result from bilateral internal carotid artery occlusion and cerebral infarction. However, there may be different etiologies of hydranencephaly that are outlined within this section. Hydranencephaly is quite different than hydrocephalus and anencephaly in that, unlike anencephaly, there is bone, skin, and dura leptomeningeal covering. Unlike hydrocephalus, no ventricles are identified.

Porencephaly is thought to be secondary to a partial or complete middle artery occlusion and infarction. This results in an asymmetric cranial defect that appears cystic. The defect usually originates from the ventricle and increases in size toward the bony calvaria. *In utero* infections may cause brain destruction. This is discussed separately (see Chapter 17).

Intracranial hemorrhage usually occurs after birth but has been documented to occur *in utero*. It has been reported as early as the first trimester. Initially, the echogenic clot fills the entire ventricles and later hydrocephalus may occur.

Intracranial Hemorrhage

Synonyms for intracranial hemorrhage are germinal matrix hemorrhage, intraventricular hemorrhage, intraparenchymal hemorrhage, and subdural hematoma.

Intracranial hemorrhage refers to hemorrhage anywhere within the fetal cranium. It is most commonly identified prenatally as intraventricular hemorrhage, although hemorrhage can occur in other sites, including subarachnoid, subdural, and intraparenchymal locations.

It is, however, a common occurrence in the premature infant following delivery. In infants less than 1,500 g or less than 32 gestational weeks, intracranial hemorrhage occurs with an incidence as high as 40%.[209,210]

Incidence

The overall incidence has been estimated to be 1 per 10,000 pregnancies.[211]

Pathogenesis and Pathology

Antenatal fetal intracranial hemorrhage may occur spontaneously or occur in association with various maternal or fetal conditions. Predisposing maternal conditions at risk include platelet disorder, coagulation disorders, medications (warfarin) or drugs (cocaine), seizures, trauma, amniocentesis, and febrile disease. Predisposing fetal conditions include congenital factor-X and factor-V deficiencies, hemorrhage into various congenital tumors, twin-twin transfusion, demise of a co-twin, or fetomaternal hemorrhage.[212–219]

The most common risk factor for intracranial hemorrhage is a platelet disorder. Immune thrombocytopenic purpura (ITP), in rare cases, can produce fetal thrombocytopenia severe enough to cause fetal hemorrhage. Although rare, alloimmune thrombocytopenia is an even more predictable cause of fetal thrombocytopenia and has been linked to cases of fetal hemorrhage. It is estimated that in alloimmune thrombocytopenia, 20% of offspring can experience intracranial hemorrhage, one-half of which occurs *in utero*.[220–222] A case has also been reported of Bernard-Soulier syndrome, a rare autosomal recessive bleeding disorder characterized by platelet dysfunction.[223] Hidden maternal autoimmunity, in which antiplatelet antibodies are present in a patient with a normal platelet count, has also been reported as a predisposing condition to fetal hemorrhage.[224,225]

Intraventricular hemorrhage usually originates in the subependymal germinal matrix region because the germinal matrix contains thin-walled friable vessels supported by a delicate matrix.[214,226] The germinal matrix of the premature brain is particularly vulnerable and may bleed from hypoxia, coagulopathy, trauma, or alterations in cerebral blood pressure.

Germinal matrix hemorrhage commonly extends into lateral ventricles. Blood can then accumulate in both lateral ventricles and migrate into the third ventricle or into the aqueduct of Sylvius and result in hydrocephalus. In severe cases, hemorrhage may occur into the brain substance. Intracranial hemorrhage is eventually resorbed, although this may take many weeks. Ventricular blood results in a chemical ventriculitis with thickening of the subependymal lining of the ventricles.[227]

Germinal matrix or intraventricular hemorrhage is commonly classified in four grades (Fig. 46):

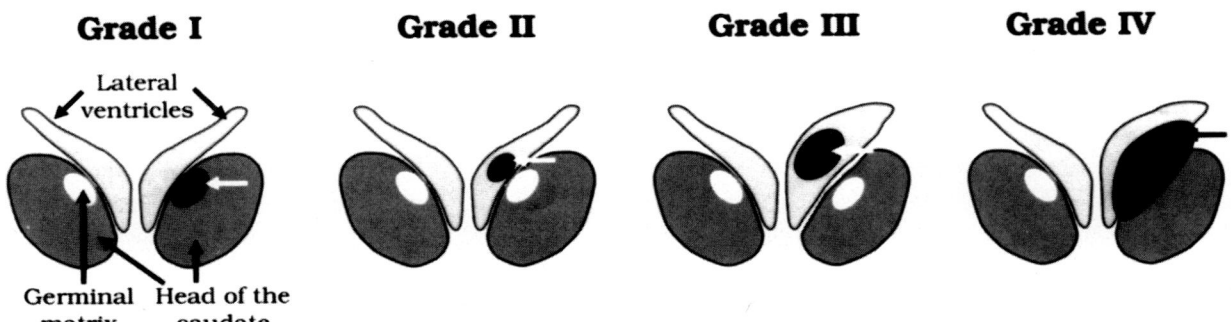

FIGURE 46. Grading of intracranial hemorrhage (indicated in black). Grade I, hemorrhage remains confined to the germinal matrix (*arrow*); grade II is intraventricular hemorrhage (*arrow*); grade III is intraventricular hemorrhage (*arrow*) and ventricular dilatation; and grade IV represents extension of the hemorrhage into brain parenchyma (*arrow*). (Modified from Malinger G, Katz R, Amsel S, Gewurtz G, Zakut H. Brain hemorrhage, germinal matrix. *The Fetus* 1992;1:1–4.)

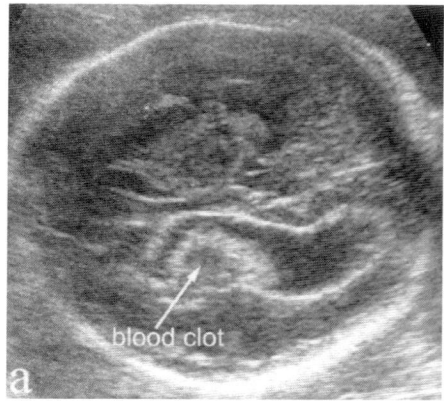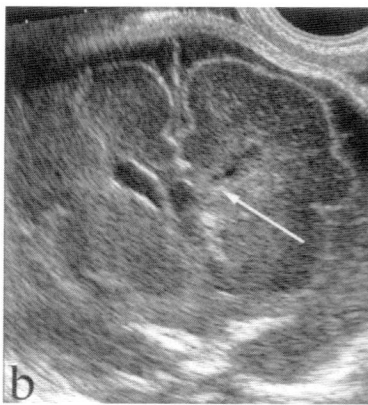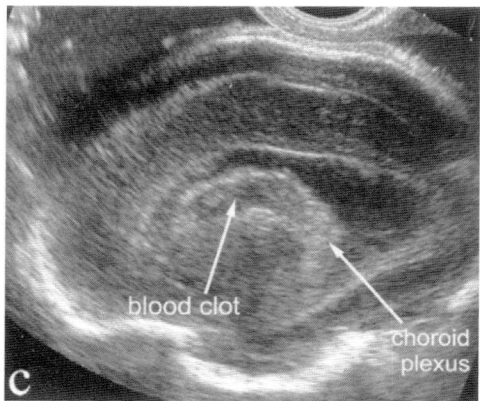

FIGURE 47. Intraventricular hemorrhage (grade III). **A–C:** Axial, coronal, and parasagittal scans at 28 weeks show hypoechoic clot (*arrow*) within ventricle originating from germinal matrix. The involved ventricle is mildly dilated. The ventricular wall is echogenic, which is characteristic of intraventricular hemorrhage, related to sterile ependymitis incited by the hemorrhage.

Grade I—Limited to subependal matrix

Grade II—Intraventricular extension, but without ventriculomegaly

Grade III—Intraventricular extension, with ventriculomegaly

Grade IV—Intraparenchymal extension

Diagnosis

Intracranial hemorrhages have been frequently reported prenatally.[27,182,209,228–236] The sonographic appearance varies with the size, location, and age of hemorrhage. Large hemorrhages can produce marked mass effect. On the other hand, small germinal matrix hemorrhages escape detection in most cases and may resolve or show a residual small cyst. Prenatal hemorrhages are most often detected during the third trimester but can be diagnosed as early as the second trimester in some cases.[27]

Acute hemorrhage appears as an echogenic collection. This echogenicity is similar to that of the choroid plexus and may be difficult to distinguish from it. Clots may be asymmetrically situated within the ventricles and, in time, become hypoechoic. Intraventricular hemorrhage often leads to dilatation of the lateral ventricles and the third ventricle (Figs. 47 and 48).[182,209,215,229,237] The ependymal wall becomes thickened, echogenic, and may appear *granular* from a chemical ventriculitis.

Once the hemorrhage resolves, only ventricular dilatation may be evident. The ventricular dilatation may resolve or even progress after the hemorrhage is no longer evident. This has suggested to several authors that undiagnosed intracranial hemorrhage may be a more common cause for hydrocephalus than generally thought.[234,238]

Grade IV hemorrhage (Fig. 49) may eventually evolve into a porencephalic cyst (Fig. 50)[182] or even hydranencephaly.[239] Subdural hematomas appear as echogenic or complex fluid collections just beneath the cranium, displacing and distorting the brain.[225,240–246]

Increased pulsatility of the middle cerebral artery with reverse diastolic flow may be seen from grade IV or subdural hemorrhages. This probably occurs as a consequence of acutely increased intracranial pressure.[182,214]

MRI is particularly sensitive to hemorrhage[238,247,248] and can detect some hemorrhages missed by ultrasound.[247] MRI imaging should include T1-weighted sequences, which show hemorrhage as an area of increased intensity.[24]

Differential Diagnosis

The differential diagnosis for intracranial hemorrhage seems limited. Certainly if the intracranial hemorrhage is large or involves a brain substance and has a mass effect, this may be mistaken for intracerebral neoplasm. Usually with intraventricular hemorrhage, hemorrhage is noted in both lateral ventricles, which should be a distinguishing feature. In dubious cases, fetal MRI should be performed and is usually diagnostic. Alternatively, serial sonograms could be performed. The appearance of an intraparenchymal hemorrhage changes with time. At first a purely echogenic lesion is found. In 1 to 2 weeks, the blood clots tend to develop a hypoechogenic core, while ventricles become enlarged and a porencephalic cyst may appear. The differential diagnosis for ventriculomegaly caused by intraventricular hemorrhage includes other etiologies of ventriculomegaly. Etiologies for ventriculomegaly could include hydrocephalus from a number of causes, developmental abnormalities of the brain, or destructive abnormalities of the brain. The presence of irregular echogenic areas within the ventricles is indicative of a hemorrhage.

Associated Anomalies

Usually, there are no associated fetal anomalies with *in utero* intracranial hemorrhage. Associated defects are secondary

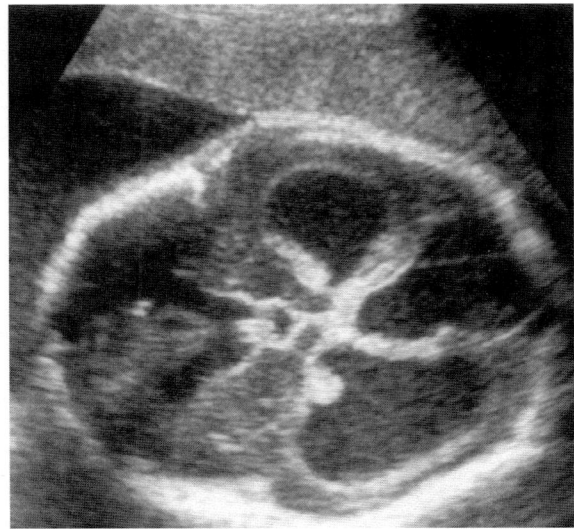

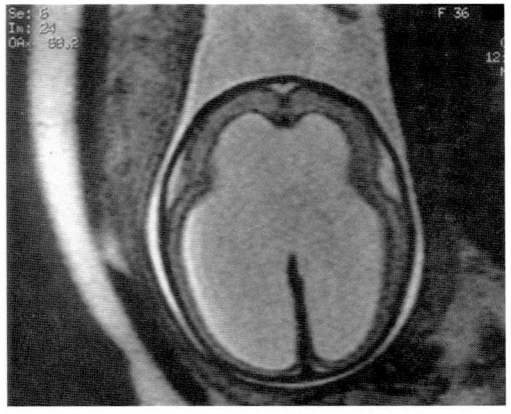

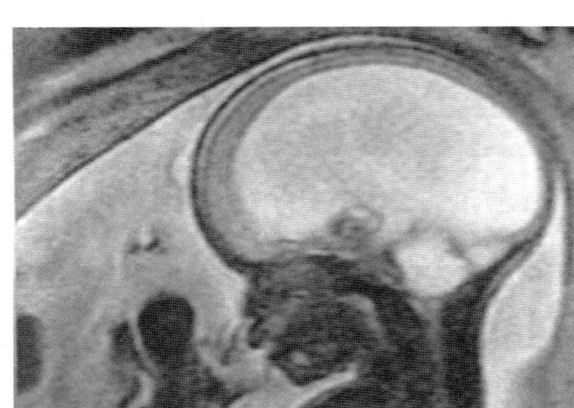

FIGURE 48. Intraventricular hemorrhage. Axial ultrasound **(A)** scan shows dilated ventricles, including fourth ventricle. The ventricles contained low-level echoes, characteristic of hemorrhage. The ventricular walls are also echogenic, characteristic of intraventricular hemorrhage and indicating a sterile ventriculitis. A thin septation is seen in the dilated fourth ventricle. Axial **(B)** and sagittal **(C)** magnetic resonance images show hydrocephalus and dilated fourth ventricle.

to underlying etiologies of the *in utero* hemorrhage such as growth restriction, hydrops, and so forth.

Prognosis

The prognosis for fetal germinal matrix or intraventricular hemorrhage spans from mild neurologic deficit to neonatal death. In neonates, the extent of the hemorrhage correlates with the final outcome. Grade I and grade II hemorrhages usually have little or no impact on the probability of survival or impairment; grade III hemorrhage is associated with an increased risk of post-hemorrhagic hydrocephalus; grade IV hemorrhage is associated with a mortality rate of 25% to 69% and adverse neurologic development in approximately one-half of survivors.[226,249] In general, the outcome of hemorrhage diagnosed *in utero* thus far has been disappointing. Vergani et al. reported a 92% inci-

dence of severe neurologic sequelae or perinatal death among 13 cases of fetal parenchymal bleeding.[211] Also, De Spirlet et al.[225] reviewed 14 cases of subdural hematoma diagnosed prenatally. The overall outcome was poor, with 50% resulting in fetal death *in utero* and the remaining 50% demonstrating postnatal sequelae.

It must be pointed out that ultrasound probably only detects more severe intracranial hemorrhage. It is likely that technologic improvements and the widespread use of high-resolution vaginal probes will allow in the future detection of less severe lesions, with a better outcome.

Management

Management should first focus on identifying the etiology of the intracranial hemorrhage. An interview should focus on obstetric history, drug use, or recent trauma (motor

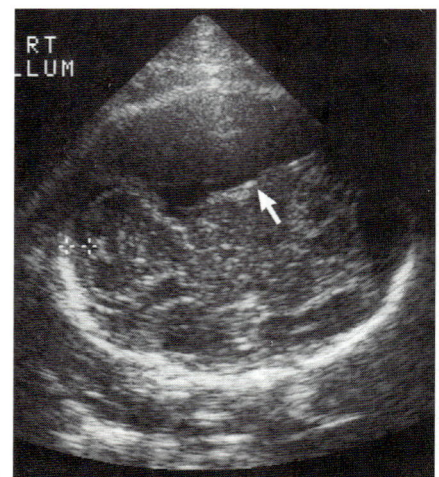
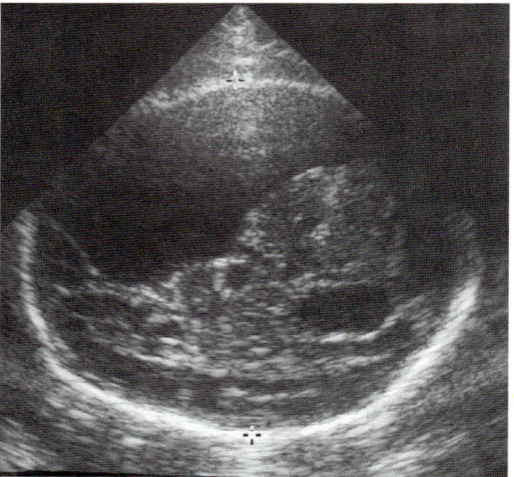

FIGURE 51. Porencephaly. **A:** Axial scan of twin pregnancy at 36 weeks, at level of cisterna magna and cerebellum, shows unilateral fluid collection (*arrow*). Note that the cerebellum is intact, and there is a normal cisterna magna (*calipers*). **B:** Scan at a more superior level shows large fluid collection replacing much of one hemisphere.

multiple cystic lesions replacing most of the cortex (multicystic encephalomalacia).[182]

Differential Diagnosis

Distinction from *unilateral schizencephaly* may be difficult but is practically not important. Fetal MRI could be helpful, at least in the third trimester, by demonstrating whether the defect is lined with white matter (porencephaly) or gray matter (schizencephaly).[29] *Arachnoid cysts* are usually smooth-walled; asymmetrical; do not communicate with the lateral ventricles; and, in contradistinction to porencephaly, have a mass effect. Hydrocephalus is variable depending on the location of the arachnoid cyst. *Cystic neoplasms* are rare. They usually have a mass effect with solid and cystic components. *Hydrocephalus* may occasionally be unilateral (Fig. 52) but should easily be distinguished from porencephaly by noting the distinguishing features of hydrocephalus.

Associated Anomalies

With the exception of ventriculomegaly, associated anomalies are rare. There may be amygdala-hippocampal atrophy as previously discussed (see Pathogenesis and Pathology). Most cases of porencephaly are isolated.[267]

Prognosis

Patients with porencephaly may have a variety of symptoms, including seizures, developmental delay, hemiparesis, and intellectual impairment. Occasionally, children with

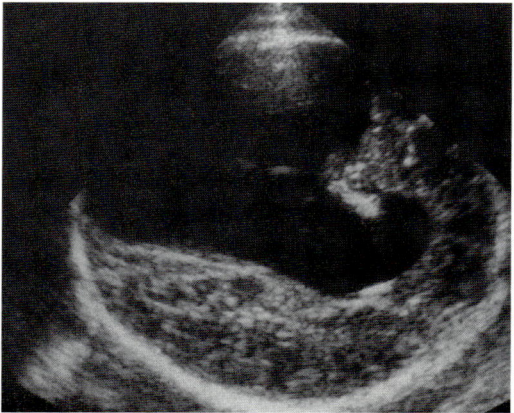

FIGURE 52. Unilateral ventriculomegaly. This unusual fluid collection represents unilateral ventricular dilatation secondary to stenosis at the level of the foramen of Monro. This produces mass effect, has well-formed margins, and corresponds in shape and course to the ventricle. It should not be confused with porencephaly.

porencephaly may have normal neurologic development.[268] There are no clear figures. Most cases diagnosed *in utero*, however, tend to have a poor outcome.[182]

Management

Most cases of fetal porencephaly are only seen in the third trimester so that pregnancy termination is not usually an available option. As porencephaly may be a consequence of a cerebral hemorrhage, a similar diagnostic workup is recommended. Conservative management should be offered, as many cases have a poor outcome. In cases with associated ventriculomegaly and macrocrania, cephalocentesis may be an option to overcome fetopelvic disproportion. Otherwise there is no reason to modify standard obstetric management.

Hydranencephaly

Synonyms for hydranencephaly include hydrocephalic anencephaly, hydroencephalodysplasia, and cystencephali.

Hydranencephaly is the absence of the cerebral hemispheres, which are replaced by a sac-like structure containing CSF.

Incidence

The incidence for hydranencephaly is 1.0 to 2.5 per 10,000 births.[269] As many as 1% of infants thought to have hydrocephalus by clinical examination are later found to have hydranencephaly.[267]

Pathogenesis and Pathology

Hydranencephaly is characterized by the absence of the cerebral hemispheres and an incomplete or absent falx. The leptomeninges form a sac that is filled with CSF and surrounds the brain stem and basal ganglia.[270,271]

Hydranencephaly is thought to derive from a destructive process that leads to the liquefaction of the cerebral hemispheres. In animal models, occlusion of the carotid arteries or the middle cerebral arteries lead to the transformation of the cerebral hemispheres, however, they were thin membranous sacs filled with CSF.[268] Fetal hypoxia due to maternal exposure to carbon monoxide or butane gas may result in massive tissue necrosis. Subsequent cavitation and resorption of necrotized tissue create the characteristic findings.[272] Congenital toxoplasmosis, cytomegalovirus, and herpes simplex infections have been associated with hydranencephaly, probably because of necrotizing vasculitis or local destruction of the brain tissue.[273–276] Intrauterine demise of one twin of a monochorionic pair is frequently associated with a variety of cerebral lesions in the surviving fetus, from destruction of the cortex to migrational abnormalities. The pathogenesis of brain damage in these cases is debated. It was traditionally believed to result from emboli or thromboplastic material originating from the macerated co-twin. According to a more recent hypothesis, the presence of large intraplacental shunts would lead to a passage of blood from the circulation of the live fetus to that of the dead fetus, and this would cause hypotension, hypoperfusion, and acute cerebral and visceral ischemia.[277]

Diagnosis

On ultrasound, fetal hydranencephaly presents as a large cystic mass filling the entire cranial cavity with absence or discontinuity of the cerebral cortex and of the midline echo (Fig. 53). The appearance of the thalami and brainstem protruding inside a cystic cavity is characteristic. The falx is often present. With extreme hydrocephaly, alobar holoprosencephaly, or porencephaly, these structures should still be surrounded by a rim of cortex, and the choroid plexuses should be normally visible. The initial diagnosis of hydranencephaly may be difficult when the infarction and hemorrhage is an evolving process. Recent hemorrhage is typically echogenic while an organizing clot assumes a more transonic texture. Layering of this debris may masquerade as cortical tissue. Finally, the clot lyses and becomes an anechoic liquid characteristic of hydranencephaly.[278]

Differential Diagnosis

The most common diagnostic problem is differentiation among hydranencephaly, extreme hydrocephalus, alobar holoprosencephaly, and porencephaly. Some spared cortical mantle should still be seen with porencephaly and alobar holoprosencephaly. Serial sonograms may be necessary to evaluate an evolving intracranial process. Extreme hydrocephalus may be difficult to differentiate from hydranencephaly if a falx remnant is present. The presence of even minimal frontal cerebral cortex, however, indicates extreme hydrocephalus instead of hydranencephaly.[279] Color Doppler could prove useful for a definitive diagnosis, because we expect that in hydranencephaly it fails to demonstrate the anterior and middle cerebral arteries, whereas the posterior cerebral arteries should appear normal. At autopsy, differentiation can be made by examining the lining of the cystic structures. Leptomeninges are found in hydranencephaly, whereas ependyma lines the ventricular system in hydrocephalus. MRI may serve as an additional means for confirming the ultrasound diagnosis.[280]

Associated Anomalies

Associated anomalies for hydranencephaly are renal aplastic dysplasia, polyvalvular developmental heart defect,[281] and trisomy.

Prognosis

The prognosis is universally dismal. Irritability, clonus, and hyperreflexia are common. Survival may last several months

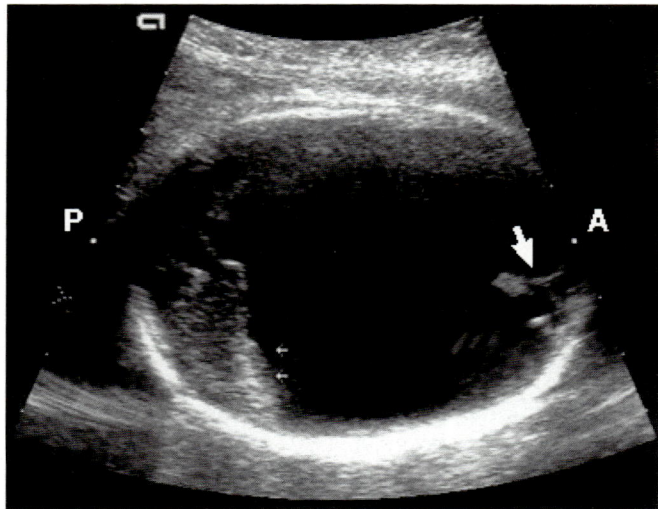

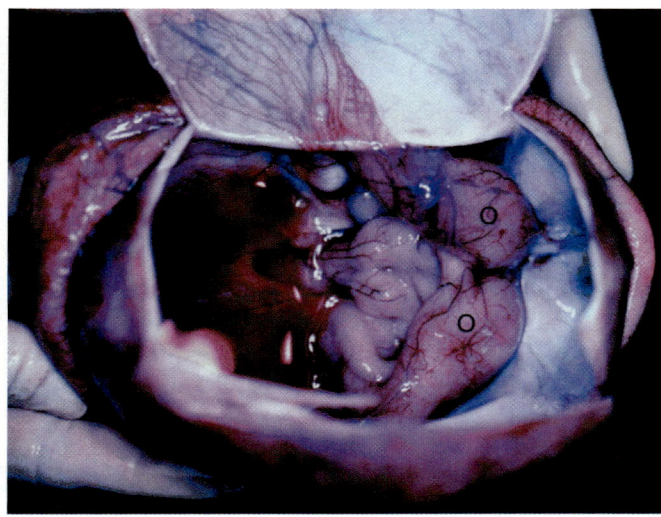

FIGURE 53. Hydranencephaly. **A:** Axial scan at 28 weeks shows typical features of hydranencephaly with no visible brain structure. A midline falx is present (*arrow*). A, anterior; P, posterior. **B:** Postmortem photograph after term delivery shows occipital horns (*O*) but no other brain tissue. The thalami, brain stem, and cerebellum were normal. (Reproduced with permission from Lam YH, Tang MH. Serial sonographic features of a fetus with hydranencephaly from 11 weeks to term. *Ultrasound Obstet Gynecol* 2000;16:77–79.)

if an intact hypothalamus permits thermoregulation, but most die in the first year of life. Occasional long-term survival has been reported.

Management

Termination of pregnancy should be offered before viability. Whether termination of pregnancy can be performed in the third trimester is debatable.

Recurrence Risk

The recurrence risk is not known to be increased. A persistent infectious disorder caused recurrent encephaloclastic damage in the same sibship.[282]

Intracranial Infections

A number of fetal infections may be associated with intracranial abnormalities. For instance, cytomegalovirus as well as toxoplasmosis is associated with ventriculomegaly and intracranial calcifications. Other fetal infections such as rubella and varicella have been associated with multiple fetal anomalies including microcephaly. These specific infections are dealt with in great detail in Chapter 17.

VASCULAR ANOMALIES

Vascular anomalies of the fetal brain are rare, and only a handful of cases have been described thus far. The majority of reports concentrate on the vein of Galen vascular malfor-

mations. More recently, thrombosis of the dural sinuses has been described. These conditions are considered in the same section, as the diagnosis largely depends on the use of Doppler ultrasound.

The arterial and venous sides of the circulation of the developing fetal brain have been the object of several studies. Color Doppler allows rapid identification of the relevant vessels.[283–285] The circle of Willis is rapidly imaged in an axial plane obtained at the level of the base of the skull. At the same level, the transverse dural sinuses can be imaged. Other vessels can be identified by using multiplanar neurosonography. The median plane allows the demonstration of the branching of the anterior cerebral artery into the pericallosal artery, the great vein of Galen connecting to the transverse sinus, and the superior sagittal sinus.

Nomograms of the pulsatility index of the waveforms derived with spectral Doppler from the major cerebral vessels are available.[286] The middle cerebral artery is particularly used in the assessment of small-for-gestational-age fetuses.[287]

Vein of Galen Aneurysm

Synonyms for vein of Galen aneurysm are ectasia, or varix of the vein of Galen.

Vein of Galen aneurysm is a rare arteriovenous malformation of the CNS characterized by a high venous flow.

Incidence

The incidence is unknown; the prenatal diagnosis has been reported with increasing frequency in the recent literature.

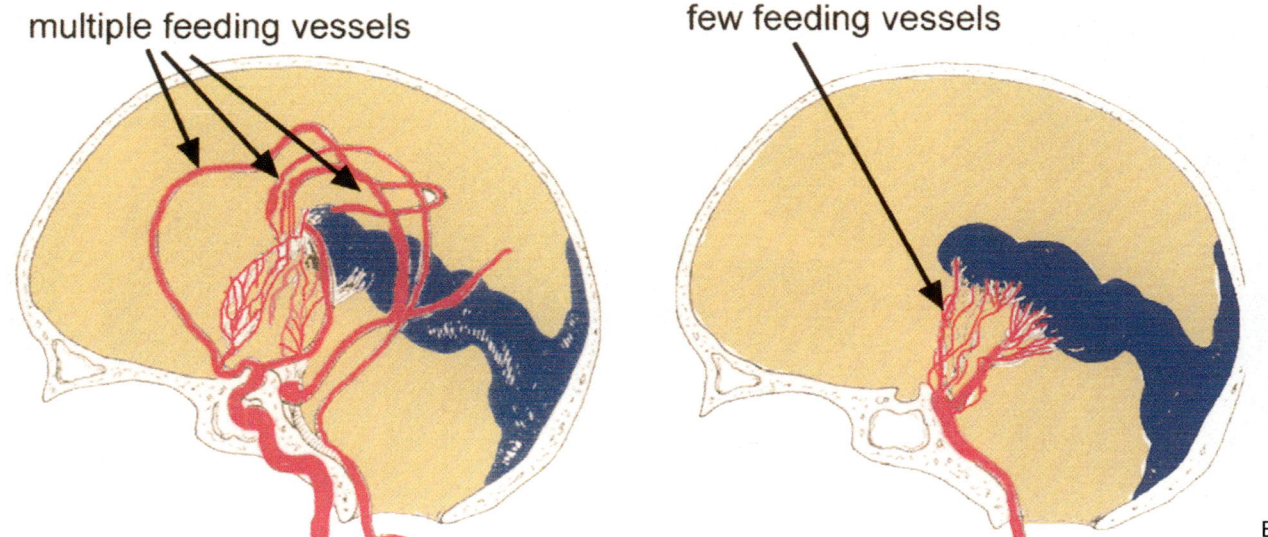

FIGURE 54. Vein of Galen malformation. The vein of Galen malformation comprises in reality a spectrum of vascular anomalies that share in common a dilatation of the vein of Galen. In this schematic drawing, the two ends of the spectrum are represented. **A:** A complex arteriovenous malformation with multiple anomalous arterial vessels arises from the circle of Willis. This condition is likely to result in significant vascular compromise, with stealing of blood from the cortex, infarction, hemorrhage, and high-output cardiac failure manifested during fetal life. **B:** A simple dilatation of the vein of Galen with few arterial vessels. This condition is unlikely to cause vascular compromise and may become symptomatic (excessive head growth, headache) only postnatally. (Adapted from Mori. *Neuroradiology and neurosurgery.* New York: Thieme-Stratton, 1985.)

Pathology

Aneurysmal enlargement of the vein of Galen is a rare and complex malformation, which involves several afferent branches of the vertebrobasilar system and carotid arteries draining into the great cerebral veins. These vessels are located in the brain deeply and posteriorly to the thalami, in the subarachnoid space called *cistern of the great cerebral vein of Galen.* The term *aneurysm of the vein of Galen* indicates a spectrum of arteriovenous malformations, ranging from a single large aneurysmal dilatation of the vein of Galen to multiple communications between the vein and the carotid and vertebrobasilar systems (Fig. 54).[288]

According to the traditional view, the aneurysm of the vein of Galen is thought to derive from maldevelopment of the Galenic system, which is formed from the choroidal veins. However, the observation that arteries of the velum interpositum and ambient cistern may be feeders of the fistula suggests that the abnormal system may derive rather from a persistent fetal vein: the median prosencephalic vein, which drains the large choroid plexuses of the developing fetal brain between 7 and 12 weeks' gestation.[289]

Three types of aneurysms are described: (a) arteriovenous fistula, (b) arteriovenous malformation with ectasia of the vein of Galen, and (c) varix of the vein of Galen.[290,291] The arteriovenous fistula frequently manifests in the neonatal period with cardiac failure. The ectasia and the varix tend to present later in life with bleeding episodes and are not associated with cardiac failure.[292] Arteriovenous fistulae associated with a varix are not part of the definition when they are located elsewhere in the brain.[292]

Diagnosis

The typical finding is an elongated anechoic area at the level of the cistern of the vein of Galen, with color and pulsed Doppler evidence of turbulent venous and arterial flow (Figs. 55 and 56).[182,289,293] Hyperechogenicity of the vascular malformation may ensue if a clot has formed within it. The cerebral architecture may be intact, or it may be distorted because of ventriculomegaly, porencephaly, and brain edema. The cortex may be heterogenous and echogenic. The dural sinuses and neck vessels are frequently enlarged, and signs of cardiac overload may be present, including cardiomegaly, hepatosplenomegaly, soft tissue edema, polyhydramnios, and overt hydrops (Fig. 56). Color Doppler may help in identifying the origin of the vessels feeding the lesion, an observation that may have practical implications for assessing the prognosis. Three-dimensional power Doppler has been used in several cases.[294,295] MRI may be also useful in these cases (Fig. 55C).[296]

Differential Diagnosis

When the combination of a fluid-filled lesion in the posterior third of the brain is found in association with hydrops, the diagnosis of vein of Galen aneurysm is rapidly established.

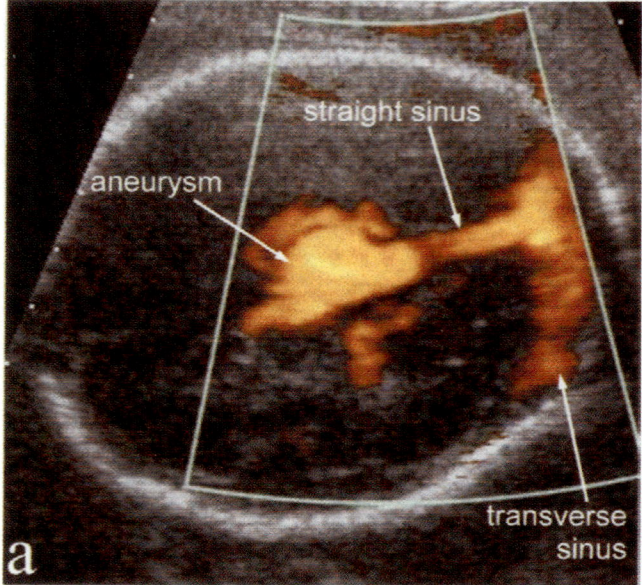

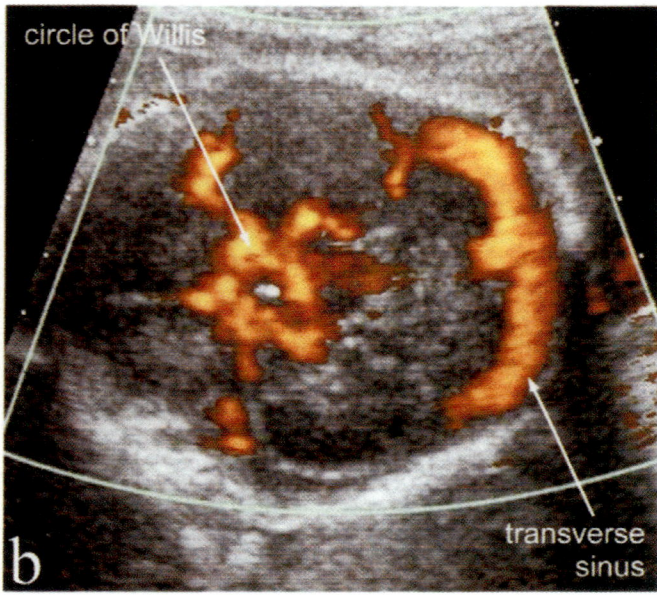

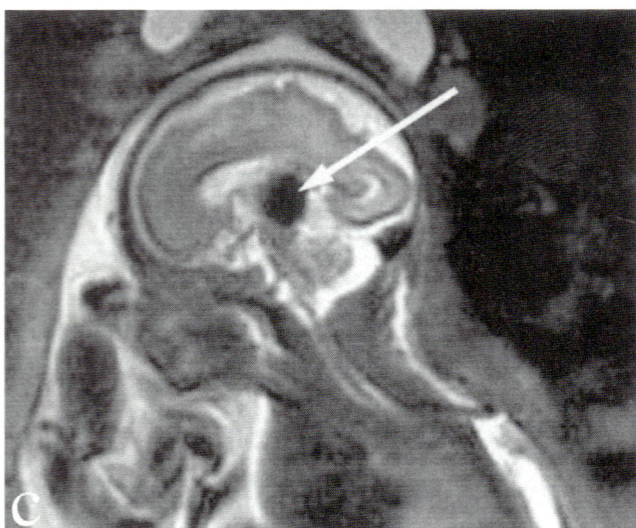

FIGURE 55. Vein of Galen aneurysm. **A, B:** Power Doppler shows dilatation of the aneurysm as well as the straight and transverse sinuses. **C:** T2-weighted magnetic resonance imaging in sagittal plane shows the aneurysm as a signal void (*arrow*). The brain structures otherwise appear unremarkable. (Courtesy of Renato Ximenes, Sao Paulo, Brazil.)

Color and pulsed Doppler are, however, required to differentiate small vein of Galen aneurysms not associated with hemodynamic perturbance from a midline arachnoid cyst.[182]

Associated Anomalies

Associated anomalies may include ventriculomegaly, porencephaly, hydrops, single umbilical artery, chorioangioma, and limb reduction defects.[297]

Prognosis

The common clinical features in the neonate are cardiomegaly with congestive heart failure and increased intracranial pressure with hydrocephaly or cranial bruit.[298,299] Focal neurologic deficit, seizure, and hemorrhages are less common findings. In older patients, a variety of symptoms have been reported, including headache,[300] visual defect,[301] syncope, subarachnoid hemorrhage, seizure,[302] mental retardation, and even psychiatric disorders.[303–305]

Information is available for intracranial arteriovenous malformations diagnosed *in utero*, mostly vein of Galen aneurysms.[182,289,306] The outcome is strongly dependent on the antenatal evidence of other intracranial abnormalities (hydrocephalus, brain edema, porencephaly) and hydrops. When any of these was found, the prognosis was always poor. In general, cases with a normal postnatal development had isolated vascular lesions, without cerebral or cardiovascular compromise *in utero*. More favorable outcomes have also been reported in neonatal series.[307]

Large arteriovenous malformations may lead to cardiac overload and high-output cardiac failure. Vein of Galen

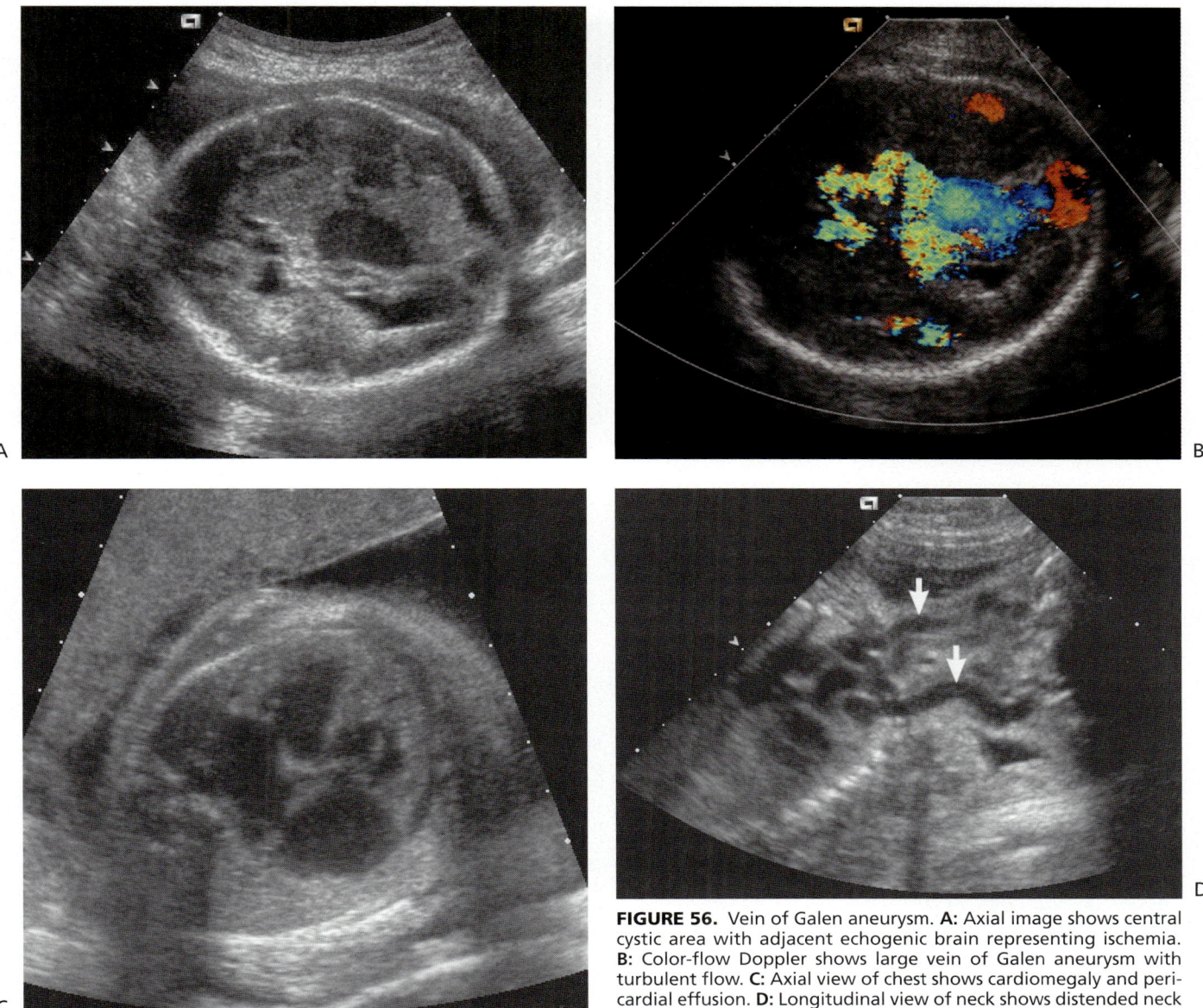

FIGURE 56. Vein of Galen aneurysm. **A:** Axial image shows central cystic area with adjacent echogenic brain representing ischemia. **B:** Color-flow Doppler shows large vein of Galen aneurysm with turbulent flow. **C:** Axial view of chest shows cardiomegaly and pericardial effusion. **D:** Longitudinal view of neck shows distended neck vessels (*arrows*) secondary to shunting through the vein of Galen aneurysm. (Courtesy of Martin Necas, New Zealand.)

aneurysm is indeed a well-recognized cause of nonimmune fetal hydrops.[289]

Management

Fetuses with isolated aneurysms of the vein of Galen, without hydrops or other intracranial abnormalities, are amenable to a successful postnatal treatment. Vaginal delivery is not contraindicated. Serial scans to monitor the cardiovascular conditions of the fetus and identify early signs of hydrops are recommended. Color Doppler mapping of the vessels feeding the lesion is possible, and we expect that it may help in identifying the cases with a higher probability of successful treatment.

Modern management of vascular anomalies includes a variety of endovascular techniques, including embolization. Multiple embolization sessions, novel approaches, and multiple embolic agents may be necessary.[307] This can lead to a good outcome, however, even in infants with high cardiac output failure.

Recurrence Risk

The recurrence risk is not known to be increased.

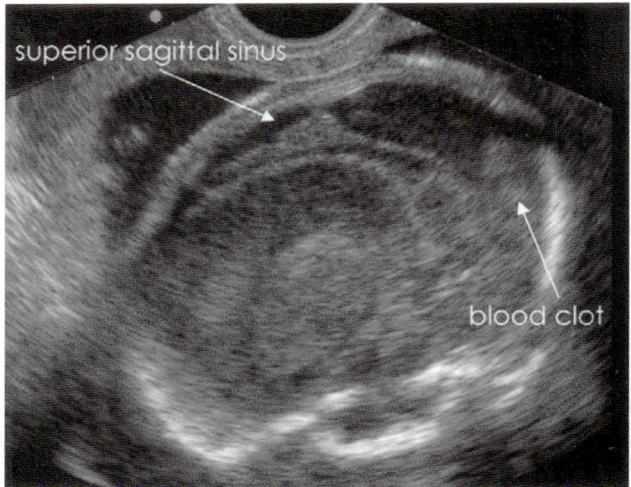

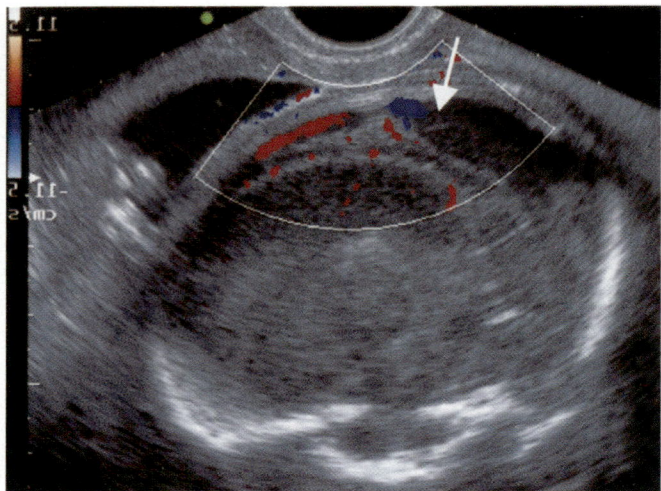

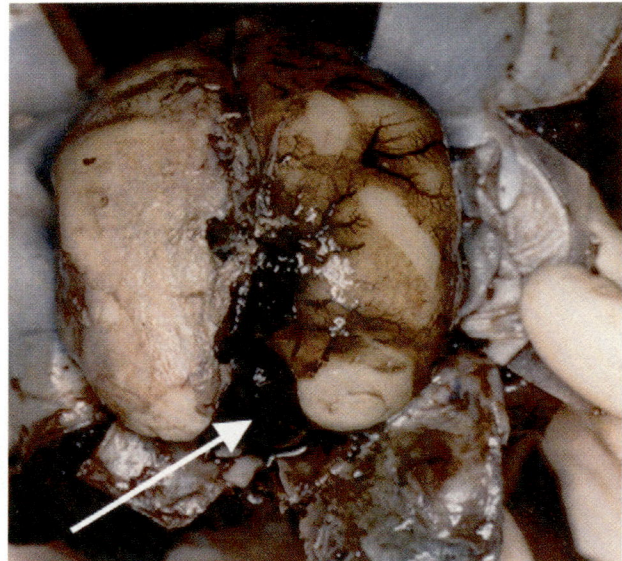

FIGURE 57. Sagittal vein thrombosis. Transvaginal scan without **(A)** and with **(B)** color Doppler shows blood clot within the expanded sagittal vein sinus (*arrow*). Normal blood flow within the sinus is abruptly terminated. **C:** Pathologic photograph of similar case shows large blood clot (*arrow*) within the superior sagittal sinus down from dilatation of collateral venous vessels. (Reproduced with permission from Visentin A, Falco P, Pilu G, Perolo A, Valeri B, et al. Prenatal diagnosis of thrombosis of the dural sinuses with real-time and color Doppler ultrasound. *Ultrasound Obstet Gynecol* 2001;17:322–325.)

Thrombosis of the Dural Sinuses

Incidence

The incidence is rare. Only three cases thus far have been described in fetuses.[308]

Etiology

Early reports of dural sinus thrombosis in neonates emphasized an association with trauma and underlying systemic conditions such as sepsis, meningitis, and dehydration. More recent studies have also focused on hypercoagulopathy caused by polycythemia[309,310] or deficiency of physiologic anticoagulants (antithrombin, protein C or protein S, factor V Leiden mutation).[311,312] Prematurity and perinatal asphyxia are considered predisposing factors.[310,313] A possible role of maternal preeclampsia has

also been suggested.[311] However, in up to 40% of cases the condition is idiopathic.[314–316]

Pathology

A blood clot is found, most frequently at the level of the torcular Herophili or sinus confluence. In the most severe cases, the thrombus may extend into the straight sinus and the great cerebral vein as well. The thrombus may obstruct blood flow, leading to enlargement of the tributary sinuses and vein. Cerebral circulation may be impaired, resulting in infarct of the cortex.[309–311]

Diagnosis

In the cases thus far diagnosed *in utero*, the dilated superior sagittal sinus was seen as a triangular sonolucent area in the occipital region (Fig. 57). In the most posterior aspect of the fluid collection, the thrombus was seen as a round echogenic mass. Transvaginal sonography may be helpful in identifying the dilated sinuses and to demonstrate, with color Doppler, interruption of blood flow at the level of the dilated sinuses.[309]

MRI and MRI angiography are the techniques of choice for the diagnosis after birth. In some cases, they could also be used prenatally.

Differential Diagnosis

Dilatation of the venous collecting system must be differentiated from intracranial cysts, and the thrombus must be distinguished from other echogenic masses, such as tumors.

Associated Anomalies

The only associated anomaly in the cases thus far described has been ventriculomegaly.

Prognosis

Symptoms in the newborn include seizures, unexplained irritability, macrocephaly, or a bulging fontanel. Postnatal studies reveal that in general thrombosis of the cerebral venous circulation is an important and under-recognized cause of seizures in term infants. The natural history is variable. In the absence of perinatal asphyxia, normal neurodevelopmental outcome is likely, and the risk of seizure recurrence is low. A poor outcome should be expected especially in preterm neonates and in cases of secondary cerebral sinus thrombosis. Associated imaging signs such as infarction or ventricular hemorrhage are correlated with poor prognosis. Sequelae may also depend on the location of the thrombus. In a recent study, all patients with permanent neurologic disability had thrombosis of the deep veins with an associated deep cerebral infarction; in contrast, all patients with thrombosis without infarction or with superficial cortical venous infarction had uniformly a good outcome.[316]

Management

Termination of pregnancy may be offered in the midtrimester. In continuing pregnancies, it has been speculated that cesarean delivery may avoid further compromise to the cerebral circulation of affected fetuses.[308] Postnatally, a conservative general medical and neurologic supportive care is the mainstay of treatment. The experience indicates that surgery is associated with significant risk and should be considered with extreme caution.

Recurrence Risk

The recurrence risk is not known to be increased; however, some of the thrombophilias that have been found in associ-

ation with neonatal thrombosis of the dural sinuses have mendelian transmission.

DISORDERS OF NERVE CELL PROLIFERATION

The relationship between head size and brain mass is well established, and disorders of nerve cell proliferation may result either in microcephaly or macrocephaly. However, either a small or a large head size does not necessarily imply an abnormality. The obstetric sonographer is not infrequently challenged with the finding of head measurements either too small or too large. In most cases, the ultrasound is normal, but neurologic abnormalities may be encountered when severe.

In the following section, the available experience is reviewed and a rational approach to these problems is proposed. Finally, we have included in the broad spectrum of disorders of nerve cell proliferation the intracranial tumors. While these tumors are exceedingly rare *in utero* and in the fetus, they do occur, and a relevant number of cases have been described thus far.

Microcephaly

Microencephaly is a synonym for microcephaly.

Microcephaly (small head) is not a specific condition but the end result of different pathologic entities. The diagnosis has been based on measurement of the head circumference at the level of the base of the skull. Different thresholds have been proposed. Some authors have used a head circumference 2 SD below the mean[317] as a diagnostic criterion, whereas most require 3 SD below the mean.[318–321] Although the head circumference of a normally shaped head correlates with brain weight (volume), this may not be true in cases of true microcephaly, since the cranial deficit is mostly above the base of the skull. This problem may explain the difficulties and pitfalls in diagnosing microcephaly purely on the basis of a head circumference.

Incidence

The incidence is estimated to be 1.6 per 1,000 single birth deliveries. Only 14% of all microcephalic infants diagnosed by the first year of age had been detected at birth.[322]

Pathogenesis and Pathology

Microcephaly can result from primary cerebral malformations or exposure to teratogens. It is often a part of a wide variety of syndromes. Table 10 presents a classification of microcephaly and associated entities.

When microcephaly is present, the most affected part is usually the forebrain. Cerebral maldevelopment is frequent and includes asymmetries, macrogyria, pachygyria, and atrophy of the basal ganglia. The lateral ventricles and subarachnoid space are enlarged due to the atrophy of the cortex. The

TABLE 10. CLASSIFICATION OF MICROCEPHALY

Microcephaly with associated malformations
Genetic
  Chromosomal aberrations
    Trisomy 13
    Trisomy 18
    Trisomy 22
    4p–
    Cat cry (5p–) syndrome
    18p– syndrome
    18q– syndrome
  Single gene defects
    Bloom syndrome (autosomal recessive)
    Börjeson-Forssman-Lehmann syndrome (X-linked recessive)
    Cockayne syndrome (autosomal recessive)
    De Sanctis-Cacchione syndrome (autosomal recessive)
    Dubowitz syndrome (autosomal recessive)
    Fanconi pancytopenia (autosomal recessive)
    Focal dermal hypoplasia (X-linked dominant)
    Incontinentia pigmenti (X-linked dominant)
    Lissencephaly syndrome (autosomal recessive)
    Meckel-Gruber syndrome (autosomal recessive)
    Menkes syndrome (X-linked recessive)
    Roberts syndrome (autosomal recessive)
    Seckel bird-headed dwarfism (autosomal recessive)
    Smith-Lemli-Opitz syndrome (autosomal recessive)
Environmental
  Prenatal infections
    Rubella syndrome
    Cytomegalovirus disease
    Herpesvirus hominis
    Toxoplasmosis
  Prenatal exposure to drugs or chemicals
    Fetal alcohol syndrome
    Aminopterin syndrome
    Hydantoin syndrome
  Maternal phenylketonuria
Unknown etiology
  Recognized syndromes
    Coffin-Siris syndrome
    Cornelia de Lange syndrome
    Johanson-Blizzard syndrome
    Langer-Giedion syndrome
    Neu-Laxova syndrome
    Rubinstein-Taybi syndrome
    Williams syndrome
  Undefined combinations
Microcephaly without associated malformations
Genetic
  Primary microcephaly (autosomal recessive)
  Paine syndrome (X-linked recessive)
  Alper disease (autosomal recessive)
  Inborn errors of metabolism
    Disorders of folic acid metabolism (autosomal recessive)
    Hyperlysinemia (autosomal recessive)
    Methylmalonic acidemia (autosomal recessive)
    Phenylketonuria (autosomal recessive)
Environmental
  Prenatal exposure to radiation
  Fetal malnutrition
  Perinatal trauma or hypoxia
  Postnatal infections
Unknown etiology
  Happy puppet syndrome

Adapted from Ross, Frias. In: Vinken, Bruyn, eds. *Handbook of clinical neurology*, vol. 30. Amsterdam: Elsevier Science, 1977:507–524.

---

basal ganglia appear disproportionately large. A decrease in dendritic arborization has also been described.[323]

Diagnosis

Severe cases of microcephaly can be visibly recognized by ultrasound (Fig. 58). Less severe cases can be suspected if the head perimeter is 3 SD below the mean for gestational age. Interpretation of the head perimeter assumes a precise knowledge of the gestational age. Because this information is not always available, an alternative is to use noncephalic biometric parameters instead of gestational age, such as the head to femur and abdominal circumference to head circumference ratio.[324]

Other clues to microcephaly include diminished size of the frontal lobe[325] and abnormal shape of the head. Microcephalic fetuses have a sloping forehead that can be demonstrated by ultrasound.[326] In severe microcephaly, normal intracranial contents may not be visible.[327] Affected fetuses with microcephaly have brains that are not only small, but dysmorphic as well, in about two-thirds of cases. A wide spectrum of abnormalities has been described, from malformations such as holoprosencephaly, porencephaly, and agenesis of the corpus callosum to more subtle degrees of maldevelopment, including undergrowth of selected areas and anomalous convolutions.[328,329] An additional finding demonstrated by postnatal imaging studies is the frequent enlargement of the subarachnoid spaces that is presumed to reflect cortical atrophy.[330,331]

Some cases of microcephaly cannot be diagnosed until the third trimester.[324,325] Also, false-positive and false-negative diagnoses of microcephaly have been reported prenatally.[332–334] Available experience suggests that even experts fail to diagnose fetal microcephaly before viability in some cases. As most microcephalic infants have different types of cerebral maldevelopment, attention should be focused not only on the cranial measurements but on the cerebral anatomy as well. In most cases of true microcephaly, abnormalities of the brain can be detected by ultrasound and MRI.

Differential Diagnosis

Craniosynostosis may result in a restriction of the fetal head that may affect the measurement of the head circumference. Craniosynostosis is further discussed in Chapter 5.

Prognosis

The prognosis is different for infants with or without associated anomalies (Table 10). For the latter group, the outlook is related to the severity of the associated anomalies. Trisomy 13, trisomy 18, Meckel's syndrome, and alobar holoprosencephaly are all fatal conditions.

For infants without associated malformations, the prognosis is dependent on head size. This information was obtained in the postnatal period, and it is not known if these figures are applicable to antenatally diagnosed cases. Avery et al.[335] have addressed the issue of the clinical relevance of biometrically diagnosed

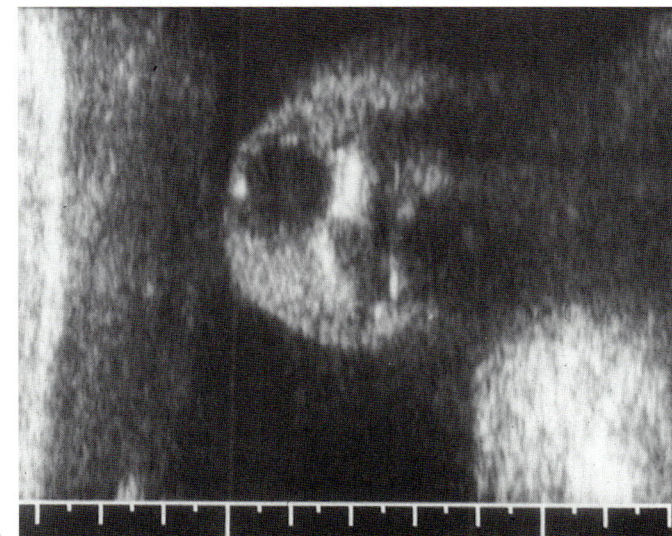

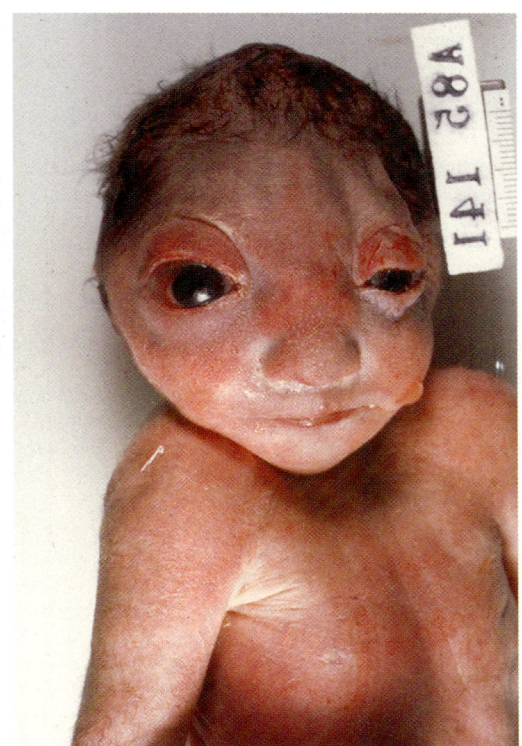

FIGURE 58. Microcephaly. **A:** Coronal sonogram shows microcephaly with relatively large orbits in comparison to the head. **B:** Corresponding photograph after birth shows similar findings. The infant was found to have Neu-Laxova syndrome.

microcephaly and found that infants with head circumferences between 2 and 3 SD below the mean had an incidence of moderate to severe mental retardation of 33%. The remaining infants were either normal or mildly retarded. Infants with head circumferences below 3 SD had a 62% incidence of moderate to severe mental retardation. These observations were made in infants diagnosed during the first year of life with a Bailey mental development index. Pryor and Thelander[317] reported that infants with head circumferences between 4 SD and 7 SD below the mean had a mean IQ of 35.6, and those with head circumferences below 7 SD had a mean IQ of 20.

Management

Microcephaly is not a treatable disease. An attempt should be made to identify associated congenital anomalies whenever microcephaly is suspected. A detailed ultrasound evaluation and an amniocentesis for fetal karyotype are mandatory. In the absence of associated anomalies, patients are counseled only on the basis of the head perimeter. If this is between 2 SD and 3 SD below the mean for gestational age, there is a very good chance that the infant is normal. Below 4 SD, the prognosis is guarded. If the diagnosis is made before viability, the option of termination of pregnancy should be considered.

Recurrence Risk

Microcephaly is associated with a large number of syndromes with mendelian transmission. A low recurrence risk can be anticipated in cases that are certainly due to teratogens.

Macrocephaly

Macrocephaly is a common feature of many cerebral abnormalities. Therefore, the demonstration of abnormally large head measurements (a reasonable cutoff is more than 2 SD above the mean expected from gestational age) should prompt a careful evaluation of the intracranial anatomy, with particular attention to a possible enlargement of the ventricular system, shift in the midline, and presence of a mass effect. The examination should be extended to the entire fetal anatomy as well, because there is a long list of syndromes that are associated with macrocrania, such as achondroplasia or thanatophoric dysplasia (Table 11).

Megalencephaly, an unusually large brain, is usually found in individuals of normal and even superior intelligence, albeit occasionally it may be associated with mental retardation and neurologic impairment.[336] Examination of the parents may be helpful because asymptomatic megalencephaly is frequently familial. In general, a good outcome is anticipated in cases in which no cerebral abnormalities are detected and the family history is negative for abnormal intellectual development.

Intracranial Tumors

A number of different intracranial tumors have been described (see Pathology).

TABLE 11. SYNDROMES AND MALFORMATIONS ASSOCIATED WITH MACROCEPHALY

Structural
  Hydrocephalus
  Tumors
Skeletal dysplasias
  Achondroplasia (autosomal dominant)
  Achondrogenesis
  Camptomelic dysplasia
  Hypochondrogenesis
  Thanatophoric dysplasia (sporadic, autosomal recessive)
Syndromes
  Bannayan-Riley-Ruvalcaba (lipomatosis, angiomatosis, micro-
    cephaly) (autosomal dominant)
  Beckwith-Wiedemann syndrome (sporadic, autosomal dominant)
  Benign familial megalencephaly (autosomal dominant)
  Megalencephaly with neurologic compromise, familial (?X-
    linked recessive)
  Neurofibromatosis (autosomal dominant)
  Perlman syndrome
  Proteus syndrome
  Unilateral megalencephaly (sporadic)

Incidence

Fetal intracranial tumors are rare. The incidence has been estimated at 0.34 per 1 million live births.[337]

Etiology

Embryonic tumors are thought to derive from embryologically displaced cells. Brain tumors have been produced in animals by the use of chemical and viral teratogens. The relevance of these experiments to human brain neoplasms is unclear.

Pathology

There are several classifications of congenital brain tumors (Table 12). Teratomas, by far the most frequent variety diagnosed antenatally, may contain well-differentiated structures, such as hair, bone, or muscle, or undifferentiated structures. In the latter case, they have a tendency toward malignancy. Teratomas usually occur in the pineal region, the suprasellar region, or the fourth ventricle. Most of the teratomas diagnosed antenatally are large and cause major distortion of the surrounding brain tissues and are often associated with macrocrania. Epidermoid tumors (also known as *cholesteatomas*) derive from epithelial cells and frequently appear as cystic lesions, containing a leaflike material, that originate from the desquamation of the internal epithelial lining. They are most commonly located at the level of the cerebellopontine angle, suprasellar region, and temporal lobe. Dermoid tumors are characterized by the presence of desquamated epithelium, sebaceous secretions, and hair. They are often connected with the skin surface by a dermal sinus and usually occur in the posterior fossa.

TABLE 12. CLASSIFICATION OF CONGENITAL INTRACRANIAL TUMORS

Embryonic tumors
  Teratoma
  Epidermoid
  Dermoid
Germinal tumors
  Germinoma
  Embryonal carcinoma
  Choriocarcinoma
  Endodermal sinus tumor
  Teratoma
Neuroblastic tumors
  Medulloblastoma
  Neuroblastoma
  Retinoblastoma
Tumors related to embryonal remnant tissues
  Craniopharyngioma
  Chordoma
Tumors of ependymal origin
  Ependymoma
  Subependymal mixed glioma
  Choroid plexus papilloma
  Glioblastoma multiforme
  Malignant astrocytoma
Tumors associated with genetic diseases
  Tuberous sclerosis (Bourneville disease)
  Neurofibromatosis (Von Recklinghausen disease)
  Systemic angiomatosis of the central nervous system and eye
    (von Hippel-Lindau disease)
Colloid cyst of the third ventricle
Heterotopia and hamartoma
Lipoma
Vascular tumors: hemangioblastoma

Adapted from Mori K. *Neuroradiology and neurosurgery.* New York: Thieme-Stratton, 1985; and Wilson, et al. In: Newton TH, Potts BG, eds. *Radiology of the skull and brain. Anatomy and pathology.* St. Louis: Mosby, 1977.

Germinomas originate from germ cells and are usually solid lesions occurring in the pineal and suprasellar regions. Tumors originating from differentiated germ cells include choriocarcinoma (trophoblastic cells), endodermal sinus tumor (yolk sac), embryonal carcinoma, and teratoma. Medulloblastoma only arises in the posterior fossa. It is a very malignant lesion that appears as a soft, friable mass often with internal necrosis.

Craniopharyngioma is the most frequent supratentorial tumor in children. It derives from remnants of the craniopharyngeal duct, consists of cystic and solid components, and occurs in the suprasellar region.

Tuberous sclerosis, neurofibromatosis, and systemic angiomatosis of the CNS and eye are autosomal dominant diseases that are characterized by the presence of intracranial tumors. In tuberous sclerosis, multiple neuroglial nodules occur in the cerebral cortex or ventricular system.

Neurofibromatosis is associated with brain tumors, such as acoustic neurinoma, multiple meningioma, and glioma. Systemic angiomatosis of the CNS and eye is characterized by the presence of cerebellar hemangioblastoma. The col-

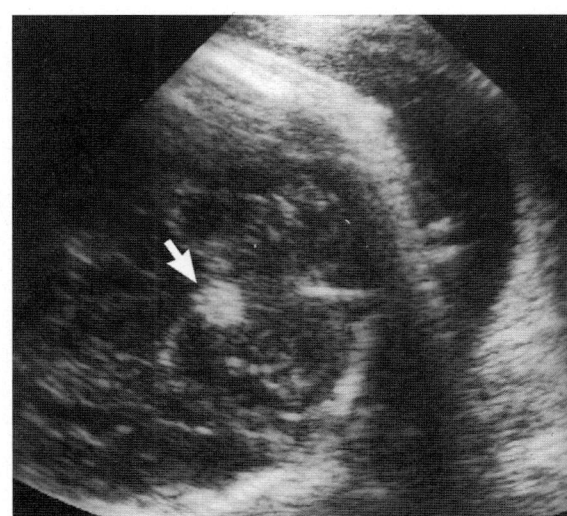
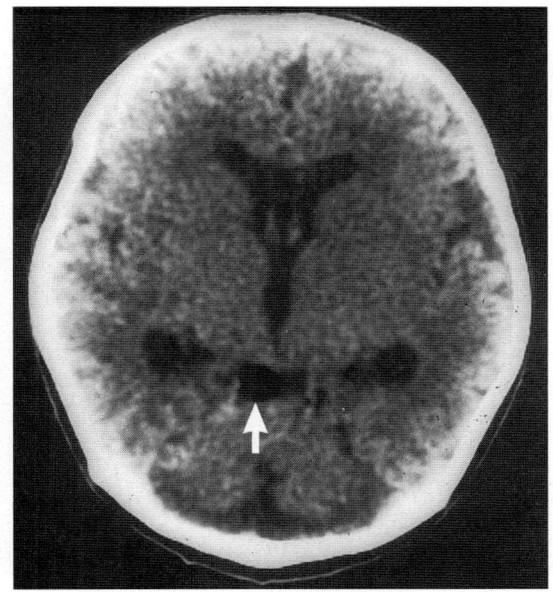

FIGURE 59. Lipoma of pontine cistern. **A:** Transverse scan of posterior fossa shows small midline echogenic nodule (*arrow*) just anterior to cerebellum. **B:** Postnatal computed tomography scan shows low-density lipoma (*arrow*). (Courtesy of Tom Winter, MD, Madison, WI.)

loid cyst of the third ventricle is thought to derive from the epithelium that forms the roof of the tela choroidea and is located in the anterior portion of the third ventricle.

Diagnosis

A number of cases of brain tumors have been described in the literature, and the subject has been extensively reviewed.[195,337–340] Most of the lesions are, however, supratentorial, in contrast to the more frequent infratentorial location of brain tumors occurring in older children. A brain tumor is suspected when mass-occupying lesions, cystic areas, or solid areas are seen within the fetal head or when there is a change in shape or size of the normal anatomic structures (e.g., a shift in the midline) (Figs. 59 through 62).

Intracranial lipomas show a characteristic appearance as well-defined echogenic areas. Lipomas of the corpus callosum are most common and are usually associated with agenesis of the corpus callosum (Fig. 33). Lipomas have also been rarely reported elsewhere (Fig. 59).[341]

Teratomas (Figs. 60 and 61) are the most common tumor seen prenatally, accounting for 62% of 48 cases reported by Sherer and Onyeije.[340] Neuroepithelial tumors were present in 15%, lipomas in 10%, and craniopharyngiomas in 6%. Schlembach et al.[338] have also extensively reviewed the antenatal literature and have found that fetal teratomas, astrocytomas, and craniopharyngiomas (Fig. 62) have a similar appearance, that is a complex mass distorting the brain architecture, possibly associated with macrocephaly, ventriculomegaly, and intracranial calcifications. Craniopharyngiomas may also appear as echogenic midline masses.[342] Brain tumors may grow rapidly during the third trimester so that second-trimester sonograms may appear completely normal.

Differential Diagnosis

The differential diagnosis of brain tumors includes other space-occupying intracranial lesions. At times, it may be particularly challenging to distinguish between a tumor and a fresh intraparenchymal hemorrhage. Cerebral hemorrhage usually lacks the mass effect that is found with tumors. In these cases, serial sonograms (in 2 to 3 weeks most severe intracranial hemorrhages are expected to result in cavitation, ventriculomegaly, and blood clot formation) or antenatal MRI usually solves the problem.

Associated Anomalies

Fetal intracranial tumors are frequently associated with macrocephaly, ventricular enlargement, intracranial calcifications, and hemorrhage. Ventriculomegaly is most frequently the cause of obstruction to CSF circulation. However, overproduction of fluid may occur with teratomas and choroid plexus papillomas. Polyhydramnios is present in 40% of cases. In most cases, the mechanism is probably related to failure of swallowing, whether this is neurologically induced or is the consequence of mechanical obstruction to the pharynx. Hydrops and high-output cardiac failure may develop as a consequence of arteriovenous shunting within the large tumoral mass. Facial dysmorphism is frequent with large tumors. There is well-established association between interhemispheric lipomas and

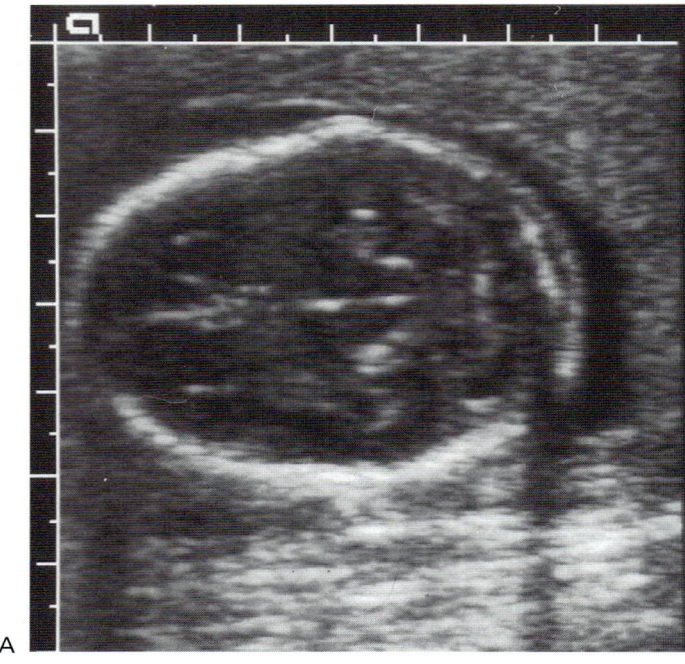

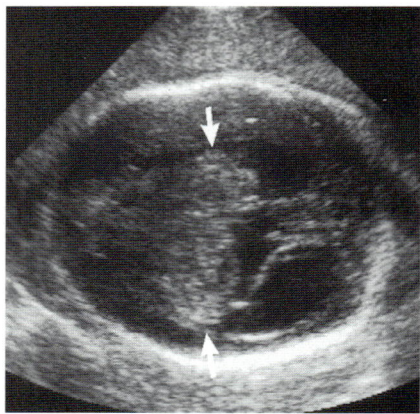

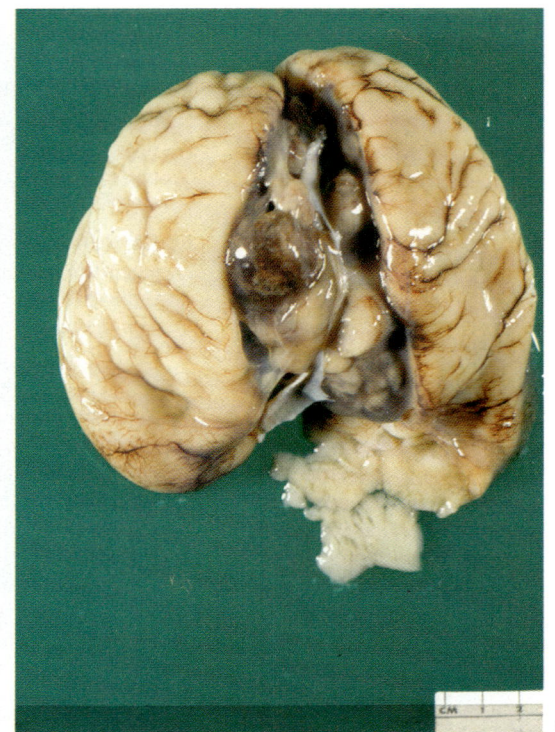

FIGURE 60. Brain tumor (teratoma). **A:** Transverse scan at 17 weeks shows normal brain anatomy. **B:** Follow-up scan at 30 weeks shows large solid, echogenic mass (*arrows*) replacing much of anterior brain. **C:** Postmortem photograph shows large mass growing in midline and displacing brain hemispheres.

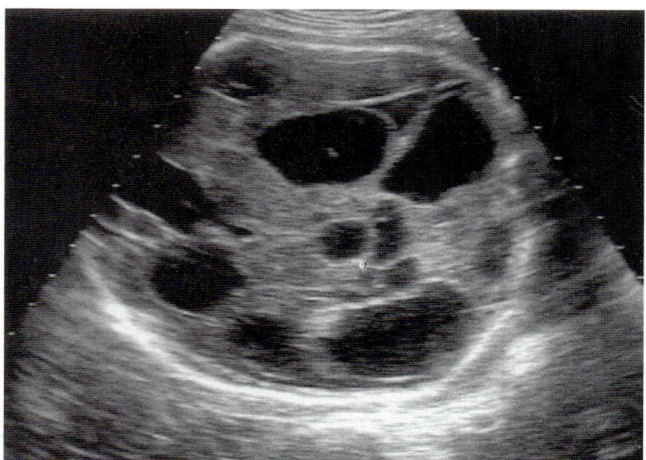

FIGURE 61. Intracranial teratoma in a third-trimester fetus. Cerebral anatomy is completely distorted. The intracranial cavity is occupied by a combination of cysts of variable size and echogenic areas.

agenesis of the corpus callosum. There is no established association between fetal and neonatal tumors and chromosomal aberrations.

Prognosis

In general, the prognosis of congenital tumors is poor. In a review of 48 cases, the overall mortality rate was 77%.[340] No clear data are available with regard to the degree of neurologic impairment in survivors, but this is expected to be high as well. The histologic type of the tumor is certainly a major factor. In a postnatal series,[343] the 1-year survival rate of teratomas was only 7%, compared with 44% of astrocytomas and 50% of choroid plexus papillomas. There are many limitations to the antenatal diagnosis of the specific type of tumor. However, large complex mass-distorting intracranial anatomy (usually teratomas, astrocytomas, or craniopharyngiomas) was found to have an overall survival

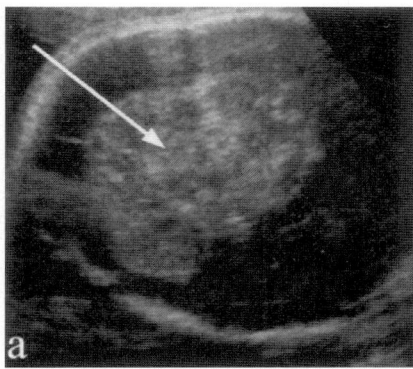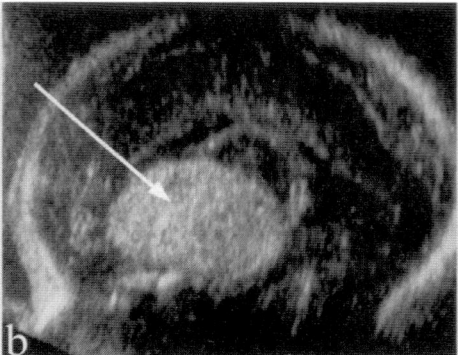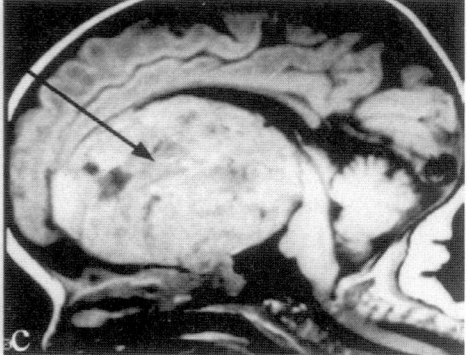

FIGURE 62. Brain tumor (craniopharyngioma). Transverse **(A)** and sagittal **(B)** scans show well-defined echogenic mass (*arrows*) in midline at base of brain. **C:** Postnatal magnetic resonance image in sagittal plane confirms the diagnosis. (Courtesy of Philippe Jeanty, MD, Nashville, TN.)

rate of only 14%. On the other hand, intracranial lipomas were associated with a survival rate of 100% and no developmental handicap.[340]

Management

Pregnancy termination can be offered to the parents before viability. Many cases, however, are diagnosed only in late gestation. In the presence of a large complex mass-distorting cerebral anatomy, the prognosis is generally poor and a conservative management can be offered to the couple. If the tumor is associated with severe macrocrania, vaginal delivery may not be possible. In these severe cases, a cephalocentesis might be considered in the attempt to decrease the size of the head.

Recurrence Risk

No known recurrence risk exists.

REFERENCES

1. McIntosh R, Merritt K, Richards M. The incidence of congenital anomalies. A study of 5,964 pregnancies. *Pediatrics* 1954;14:505.
2. Creasy MR, Alberman ED. Congenital malformations of the central nervous system: I. Spontaneous abortions. *J Med Genet* 1976;13:9.
3. Singh PR, Carr DH. Anatomic findings in human abortions of known chromosomal constitution. *Obstet Gynecol* 1967;29:806.
4. Campbell S, Johnstone FD, Holt EM, May P. Anencephaly: early ultrasonic diagnosis and active management. *Lancet* 1972;2:1226.
5. Cyr DR, Mack LA, Nyberg DA, Shepard TH, Shuman WP. Fetal rhombencephalon: normal ultrasound findings. *Radiology* 1988;166:691.
6. Filly RA, Goldstein RB, Callen PW. Fetal ventricle: importance in routine obstetric sonography. *Radiology* 1991;181:1.
7. Falco P, Gabrielli S, Visentin A, Perolo A, Pilu G, et al. Transabdominal sonography of the cavum septum pellucidum in normal fetuses in the second and third trimesters of pregnancy. *Ultrasound Obstet Gynecol* 2000;16:549.
8. Babcook CJ, Chong BW, Salamat MS, Ellis WG, Goldstein RB. Sonographic anatomy of the developing cerebellum: normal embryology can resemble pathology. *AJR Am J Roentgenol* 1996;166:427–433.
9. Bromley B, Nadel AS, Pauker S, et al. Closure of the cerebellar vermis: evaluation with second trimester US. *Radiology* 1994;193:761.
10. Filly RA, Cardoza JD, Goldstein RB, Barkovich AJ. Detection of fetal central nervous system anomalies: a practical level of effort for a routine sonogram. *Radiology* 1989;172:403.
11. Nyberg DA. Recommendations for obstetric sonography in the evaluation of the fetal cranium. *Radiology* 1989;172:309–311.
12. Cardoza JD, Goldstein RB, Filly RA. Exclusion of fetal ventriculomegaly with a single measurement: the width of the lateral ventricular atrium. *Radiology* 1988;169:711.
13. Cronan MS, McGahan JP. A new ultrasound technique to visualize the proximal fetal cerebral ventricle. *J Diagn Med Sonography* 1991;6:333.
14. Browning BP, Laorr A, McGahan JP, et al. Proximal fetal cerebral ventricle: description of US technique and initial results. *Radiology* 1994;192:337–341.
15. Goldstein I, Reece EA, Pilu G, Bovicelli L, Hobbins JC. Cerebellar measurements with ultrasonography in the evaluation of fetal growth and development. *Am J Obstet Gynecol* 1987;156:1065.
16. Mahony BS, Callen PW, Filly RA, Hoodick WK. The fetal cisterna magna. *Radiology* 1984;153:773.
17. Knutson R, McGahan JP, Salamat MS, Brant WB. Fetal cisterna magna septa: a normal anatomic finding. *Radiology* 1991;80:799.
18. Blaas HG, Eik-Nes SH, Kiserud T, Hellerik LR. Early development of the forebrain and midbrain: a longitudinal ultrasonographic study from 7 to 12 weeks of gestation. *Ultrasound Obstet Gynecol* 1994;4:183.
19. Blaas HG, Eik-Nes SH, Kiserud T, Hellerik LR. Early development of the hindbrain: a longitudinal ultrasono-

graphic study from 7 to 12 weeks of gestation. *Ultrasound Obstet Gynecol* 1995;5:151.

20. Blaas HG, Eik-Nes SH, Berg S, Torp H. In vivo three dimensional ultrasound reconstructions of embryos and early fetuses. *Lancet* 1998;352:1182.

21. Johnson SP, Sebire NJ, Snijders RJM, Tunkel S, Nicolaides KH. Ultrasound screening for anencephaly at 10–14 weeks. *Ultrasound Obstet Gynecol* 1997;9:14.

22. Timor Tritsch IE, Monteagudo A. Transvaginal neurosonography: standardization of the planes and sections by anatomic landmarks. *Ultrasound Obstet Gynecol* 1996;8:42.

23. U.S. Food and Drug Administration. *Guidance for content and review of a magnetic resonance diagnostic device 510 (k) application.* Washington, DC: U.S. Food and Drug Administration, 1988.

24. Shellock FG, Kanal E. Policies, guidelines, and recommendations for MR imaging safety and patient management: SMRI safety committee. *J Magn Reson Imaging* 1991;1:97.

25. Levine D, Barnes P, Sher S. Fetal fast MR imaging: reproducibility, technical quality, and conspicuity of anatomy. *Radiology* 1998;206:549.

26. Levine D, Barnes PD, Edelman R. State of the art: obstetric MR imaging. *Radiology* 1999;211:609.

27. Reiss I, Gortner L, Moller J, Gehl H, Baschat A, et al. Fetal intracerebral hemorrhage in the second trimester: diagnosis by sonography and magnetic resonance imaging. *Ultrasound Obstet Gynecol* 1996;7:49.

28. Greco P, Resta M, Vimercati A, Dicuonzo F, Loverro G, et al. Antenatal diagnosis of isolated lissencephaly by ultrasound and magnetic resonance imaging. *Ultrasound Obstet Gynecol* 1998;12:276.

29. Levine D, Barnes PD, Madsen JR, Abbot J, Tejas Mehta T, et al. Central nervous system abnormalities assessed with prenatal magnetic resonance. *Obstet Gynecol* 1999;94:1011.

30. Goldstein I, Reece EA, Pilu G, Hobbins JC, Bovicelli L. Sonographic development of the normal developmental anatomy of fetal cerebral ventricles: I. The frontal horns. *Obstet Gynecol* 1988;72:588.

31. Pilu G, Reece EA, Goldstein I, Hobbins JC, Bovicelli L. Sonographic evaluation of the normal developmental anatomy of the fetal cerebral ventricles: II. The atria. *Obstet Gynecol* 1989;73:250.

32. Monteagudo A, Timor Tritsch IE, Moomjy M. Nomograms of the lateral ventricles using transvaginal sonography. *J Ultrasound Med* 1993;12:265.

33. Heiserman J, Filly RA, Goldstein RB. The effect of measurement errors on the sonographic evaluation of ventriculomegaly. *J Ultrasound Med* 1991;10:121.

34. Achiron R, Schimmel M, Achiron A, Mashiach S. Fetal mild idiopathic lateral ventriculomegaly: is there a correlation with fetal trisomy? *Ultrasound Obstet Gynecol* 1993;3:89.

35. Snijders RJM, Nicolaides KH. Fetal biometry at 14–40 weeks' gestation. *Ultrasound Obstet Gynecol* 1994;4:34–48.

36. Alagappan R, Browning PD, Laorr A, McGahan JP. Distal lateral ventricular atrium: reevaluation of normal range. *Radiology* 1994;193:405.

37. Kier EL. The cerebral ventricles: a phylogenetic and ontogenetic study. In: Newton TH, Potts DG, eds. *Radiology of the skull and brain: anatomy and pathology.* St. Louis: Mosby, 1977:2787.

38. Achiron R, Yagel S, Rotstein Z, Inbar O, Mashiach S, et al. Cerebral lateral ventricular asymmetry: is this a normal ultrasonographic finding in the fetal brain? *Obstet Gynecol* 1997;89:233.

39. Mahony BS, Nyberg DA, Hirsch JH, Petty CN, Hendricks SK, et al. Mild idiopathic lateral cerebral ventricular dilatation in utero: sonographic evaluation. *Radiology* 1988; 169:715.

40. Hertzberg BS, Lile R, Foosaner DE, Kliewer MA, Paine SS, et al. Choroid plexus-ventricular wall separation in fetuses with normal-sized cerebral ventricles at sonography: postnatal outcome. *AJR Am J Roentgenol* 1994;163:405.

41. Cardoza JD, Filly RA, Podrasky AE. The dangling choroid plexus: a sonographic observation of value in excluding ventriculomegaly. *AJR Am J Roentgenol* 1988;151:767.

42. Laing F, Stamler C, Jeffrey B. Ultrasonography of the fetal subarachnoid space. *J Ultrasound Med* 1983;2:29.

43. Goldstein RB, La Pidus AS, Filly RA, Cardoza J. Mild lateral cerebral ventricular dilatation in utero: clinical significance and prognosis. *Radiology* 1990;176:237.

44. Patel MD, Goldstein RB, Tung S, Filly RA. Fetal cerebral ventricular atrium: difference in size according to sex. *Radiology* 1995;194:713.

45. Nadel AS, Benacerraf BR. Lateral ventricular atrium: larger in male than female fetuses. *Int J Gynecol Obstet* 1995;51:123.

46. Smulian JC, Campbell WA, Rodis JF, Feeney LD, Fabbri EL, et al. Gender-specific second-trimester biometry. *J Obstet Gynecol* 1995;173:1195–1201.

47. Bromley B, Frigoletto FD Jr, Benacerraf BR. Mild fetal lateral cerebral ventriculomegaly: clinical course and outcome. *Am J Obstet Gynecol* 1991;164:863.

48. Lipitz A, Malinger G, Meizner I, Zalel Y, Achiron R. Outcome of fetuses with isolated borderline unilateral ventriculomegaly diagnosed at mid-gestation. *Ultrasound Obstet Gynecol* 1998;12:23.

49. Pilu G, Falco P, Gabrielli S, Perolo A, Sandri F, et al. The clinical significance of fetal isolated cerebral borderline ventriculomegaly: report of 31 cases and review of the literature. *Ultrasound Obstet Gynecol* 1999;14:320.

50. Bloom SL, Bloom DD, Dellanebbia C, Martin LB, Lucas MJ, et al. The developmental outcome of children with antenatal mild isolated ventriculomegaly. *Obstet Gynecol* 1997;90:93.

51. Myrianthopoulos NC. Epidemiology of central nervous system malformations. In: Vinken PJ, Bruyn GW, eds. *Handbook of clinical neurology,* vol. 30. Amsterdam: Elsevier, 1977:139.

52. Chervenak FA, Berkowitz RL, Romero R, Tortora M, Mayden K, et al. The diagnosis of fetal hydrocephalus. *Am J Obstet Gynecol* 1983;147:703.

53. National Center for Biotechnology Information. Online Mendelian inheritance in man. Available at: http://www.ncbi.nlm.nih.gov/entrez/query.fcgi?db=OMIM.

54. Fransen E, Vits L, Van Camp G, Willems PJ. The clinical spectrum of mutations in L1, a neuronal cell adhesion molecule. *Am J Med Genet* 1996;64:73.

55. Schrander-Stumpel C, Fryns JP. Congenital hydrocephalus: nosology and guidelines for clinical approach and genetic counseling. *Eur J Pediatr* 1998;157:355.

56. Timor-Tritsch IE, Monteagudo A, Haratz-Rubinstein N, Levine RU. Transvaginal sonographic detection of adducted thumbs, hydrocephalus, and agenesis of the corpus callosum at 22 postmenstrual weeks: the masa spectrum or L1 spectrum. A case report and a review of the literature. *Prenat Diagn* 1996;16:543.

57. Jouet M, Kenwrick S. Gene analysis of L1 neural cell adhesion molecule in prenatal diagnosis of hydrocephalus. *Lancet* 1995;345;161.

58. Schwanitz G, Schuler H, Gembruch U, Zerres K. Chromosomal findings in fetuses with ultrasonographically diagnosed ventriculomegaly. *Ann Genet* 1993;36:150.

59. Renier D, Sainte-Rose C, Pierre-Kahn A, Hirsch JF. Prenatal hydrocephalus: outcome and prognosis. *Childs Nerv Syst* 1988;4:213.

60. Gupta JK, Bryce F, Lilford RJ. Management of apparently isolated fetal ventriculomegaly. *Obstet Gynecol Surv* 1994;49:716.

61. Levitsky DB, Mack LA, Nyberg DA, Shurtleff DB, Shields LA, et al. Fetal aqueductal stenosis diagnosed sonographically: how grave is the prognosis? *AJR Am J Roentgenol* 1995;164:725–730.

62. Manning FA, Harrison MR, Rodeck C. Catheter shunts for fetal hydronephrosis and hydrocephalus. Reports of the International Fetal Surgery Registry. *N Engl J Med* 1986;315:336.

63. Varadi V, Toth Z, Torok O, Papp Z. Heterogeneity and recurrence risk for congenital hydrocephalus (ventriculomegaly): a prospective study. *Am J Med Genet* 1998;29:305.

64. Pilu G, Perolo A, Falco P, Visentin A. Median anomalies of the brain. In: Timor Tritsch I, Monteagudo A, Cohen HL, eds. *Ultrasonography of the prenatal and neonatal brain*, 2nd ed. New York: McGraw-Hill, 2001:259.

65. De Myer W. Classification of cerebral malformations. *Birth Defects* 1971;7:78.

66. Fitz CR. Midline anomalies of the brain and spine. *Radiol Clin North Am* 1982;20:95.

67. Leech RW, Shuman RM. Holoprosencephaly and related midline cerebral anomalies. *J Child Neurol* 1986;1:3.

68. DeMyer W. Holoprosencephaly. In: Vinken PJ, Bruyn GW, eds. *Handbook of clinical neurology*, vol. 30. Amsterdam: Elsevier, 1977:431.

69. Matsunaga E, Shiota Y. Holoprosencephaly in human embryos: epidemiological studies of 150 cases. *Teratology* 1977;16:261.

70. Roessler E, Muenke M. Holoprosencephaly: a paradigm for the complex genetics of brain development. *J Inherit Metab Dis* 1998;21:481.

71. Pilu G, Ambrosetto P, Sandri F, et al. Intraventricular fused fornices: a specific sign of fetal lobar holoprosencephaly. *Ultrasound Obstet Gynecol* 1994;4:65.

72. Filly RA, Chinn DH, Callen PW. Alobar holoprosencephaly. Ultrasonographic prenatal diagnosis. *Radiology* 1984;151:455.

73. Cayea PD, Balcar I, Alberti O, et al. Prenatal diagnosis of semilobar holoprosencephaly. *AJR Am J Roentgenol* 1984;142:455.

74. Pilu G, Reece EA, Romero R, Bovicelli L, Hobbins JC. Prenatal diagnosis of cranio-facial malformations by sonography. *Am J Obstet Gynecol* 1986;155:45.

75. Blaas HG. Holoprosencephaly at 10 weeks 2 days (CRL 33 mm). *Ultrasound Obstet Gynecol* 2000;15:62.

76. Pilu G, Sandri F, Perolo A, et al. Prenatal diagnosis of lobar holoprosencephaly. *Ultrasound Obstet Gynecol* 1992;2:88.

77. Pilu G, Sandri F, Cerisoli M, Alvisi C, Salvioli GP, et al. Sonographic findings in septo-optic dysplasia in the fetus and newborn infant. *Am J Perinatol* 1990;7:337.

78. DeMyer W, Zeman W, Palmer CG. The face predicts the brain. Diagnostic significance of median facial anomalies for holoprosencephaly (arrhinencephaly). *Pediatrics* 1964;34:259.

79. McGahan JP, Nyberg DA, Mack LA. Sonography of facial features of alobar and semilobar holoprosencephaly. *AJR Am J Roentgenol* 1990 Jan;154:143–148.

80. Lehman CD, Nyberg DA, Winter TC 3rd, Kapur RP, Resta RG, et al. Trisomy 13 syndrome: prenatal US findings in a review of 33 cases. *Radiology* 1995 Jan;194:217–222.

81. Rizzo N, Pittalis MC, Pilu G, Orsini LF, Perolo A, et al. Prenatal karyotyping in malformed fetuses. *Prenat Diagn* 1990;10:17.

82. Berry SM, Gosden C, Snijders RJ, Nicolaides KH. Fetal holoprosencephaly: associated malformations and chromosomal defects. *Fetal Diagn Ther* 1990;5:92–99.

83. Osaka K, Matsumoto S. Holoprosencephaly in neurosurgical practice. *J Neurosurg* 1978;48:787.

84. Cohen MM. An update on the holoprosencephalic disorders. *J Pediatr* 1982;101:865.

85. Benda CE. The Dandy-Walker syndrome or the so-called atresia of the foramen Magendie. *J Neuropathol Exp Neurol* 1954;13:14.

86. Harwood Nash DC, Fitz CR. *Neuroradiology in infants and children*, vol. 3. St. Louis: Mosby, 1976:1014.

87. Osenbach RK, Menezes AH. Diagnosis and management of the Dandy-Walker malformation: 30 years of experience. *Pediatr Neurosurg* 1991;18:179.

88. Murray JC, Johnson JA, Bird TD. Dandy-Walker malformation: etiologic heterogeneity and empiric recurrence risk. *Clin Genet* 1985;28:272.

89. Chitayat D, Moore L, Del Bigio MR, et al. Familial Dandy-Walker malformation associated with macrocephaly, facial anomalies, developmental delay, and brain stem dysgenesis: prenatal diagnosis and postnatal outcome in brothers. A new syndrome? *Am J Med Genet* 1994;52:406.

90. Gardner E, O'Rahilly R, Prolo D. The Dandy-Walker and Arnold-Chiari malformations. Clinical, developmental and teratological considerations. *Arch Neurol* 1975;32:393.

91. Barkovich AJ, Kjos BO, Norman D, et al. Revised classification of the posterior fossa cysts and cystlike malformations based on the results of multiplanar MR imaging. *AJNR Am J Neuroradiol* 1989;10:977.

92. Hirsch JF, Pierre Kahn A, Reiner D, Sainte-Rose C, Hoppe-Hirsch E. The Dandy-Walker malformation. A review of 40 cases. *J Neurosurg* 1984;61:515.

93. Nyberg DA, Mahony BS, Hegge FN, Hickok D, Luthy DA, et al. Enlarged cisterna magna and the Dandy-Walker malformation: factors associated with chromosome abnormalities. *Obstet Gynecol* 1991;77:436.

94. Estroff JA, Scott MR, Benacerraf BR. Dandy-Walker variant: prenatal sonographic diagnosis and clinical outcome. *Radiology* 1992;185:755.

95. Pilu G, Visentin A, Valeri B. The Dandy-Walker complex and fetal sonography. *Ultrasound Obstet Gynecol* 2000;16:115.

96. Chang MC, Russell SA, Callen PW, Filly RA, Goldstein RB. Sonographic detection of inferior vermian agenesis in Dandy-Walker malformations: prognostic implications. *Radiology* 1994 Dec;193:765–770.

97. Ulm B, Ulm MR, Deutinger J, Bernaschek G. Dandy-Walker malformation diagnosed before 21 weeks of gestation: associated malformations and chromosomal abnormalities. *Ultrasound Obstet Gynecol* 1997 Sep;10:167–170.

98. Kolble N, Wisser J, Kurmanavicius J, Bolthauser E, Stallmach T, et al. Dandy-Walker malformation: prenatal diagnosis and outcome. *Prenat Diagn* 2000;20:318–327.

99. Ecker JL, Shipp TD, Bromley B, Benacerraf B. The sonographic diagnosis of Dandy-Walker and Dandy-Walker variant: associated findings and outcomes. *Prenat Diagn* 2000;20:328.

100. Achiron R, Achiron A. Transvaginal ultrasonic assessment of the early fetal brain. *Ultrasound Obstet Gynecol* 1991;1:336.

101. Achiron R, Achiron A, Yagel S. First trimester transvaginal sonographic diagnosis of Dandy-Walker malformation. *J Clin Ultrasound* 1993;21:62–64.

102. Carroll SGM, Porter H, Abdel-Fattah S, Kyle PM, Soothill P. Correlation of prenatal ultrasound diagnosis and pathologic findings in fetal brain abnormalities. *Ultrasound Obstet Gynecol* 2000;16:149.

103. Laing FC, Frates MC, Brown DL, Benson CB, DiSalvo DN, et al. Sonography of the fetal posterior fossa: false appearance of Mega-Cisterna Magna and Dandy-Walker variant. *Radiology* 1994;192:247.

104. Sawaya R, McLaurin RL. Dandy-Walker syndrome: clinical analysis of 23 cases. *J Neurosurg* 1981;55:89.

105. Blazer S, Berant M, Sujov PO, Zimmer EZ, Bronshtein M. Prenatal sonographic diagnosis of vermal agenesis. *Prenat Diagn* 1997;17:907–911.

106. Chang MC, Russell SA, Callen PW, Filly RA, Goldstein RB. Sonographic detection of inferior vermian agenesis in Dandy-Walker malformations: prognostic implications. *Radiology* 1994;193:765–770.

107. Joubert M, Eisenring JJ, Robb JP, Andermann F. Familial agenesis of the cerebellar vermis. A syndrome of episodic hyperpnea, abnormal eye movement, ataxia and retardation. *Neurology* 1969;19:813.

108. Ni Scanaill S, Crowley P, Hogan M, Stuart B. Abnormal prenatal sonographic findings in the posterior cranial fossa: a case of Joubert's syndrome. *Ultrasound Obstet Gynecol* 1999;13:71–74.

109. Wang P, Chang FM, Chang CH, Yu CH, Jung YC, et al. Prenatal diagnosis of Joubert syndrome complicated with encephalocele using two-dimensional and three-dimensional ultrasound. *Ultrasound Obstet Gynecol* 1999;14:360–362.

110. Keogan MT, DeAtkine AB, Hertzberg BS. Cerebellar vermian defects: antenatal sonographic appearance and clinical significance. *J Ultrasound Med* 1994;13:607–611.

111. Grogono JL. Children with agenesis of the corpus callosum. *Dev Med Child Neurol* 1968;10:613.

112. Han J, Benson JE, Kaufman B, et al. MR imaging of pediatric cerebral abnormalities. *J Computed Assist Tomogr* 1985; 9:103.

113. Jeret JS, Serur D, Wisniewski K, Fisch C. Frequency of agenesis of the corpus callosum in the developmentally disabled population as determined by computerized tomography. *Pediatr Neurosci* 1986;12:101.

114. Young ID, Trounce JQ, Levene MI, Fitzsimmons JS, Moore JR. Agenesis of the corpus callosum and macrocephaly in siblings. *Clin Genet* 1985;28:225.

115. Dobyns WB. Absence makes the search grow longer. *Am J Hum Genet* 1996;58:7.

116. Ettlinger G. Agenesis of the corpus callosum. In: Vinken P, Bruyn G, eds. *Handbook of clinical neurology*, vol. 30. New York: Elsevier Science, 1977:285.

117. Lindhout D, Omtzigt JG, Cornel MC. Spectrum of neural tube defects in 34 infants prenatally exposed to antiepileptic drugs. *Neurology* 1992;42:111.

118. Dominguez R, Villa Coro AA, Slopis JM, Bohan TP. Brain and ocular abnormalities in infants with in utero exposure to cocaine and other street drugs. *Am J Dis Child* 1991;145:688.

119. Friedman M, Cohen P. Agenesis of the corpus callosum as a possible sequel to maternal rubella during pregnancy. *Am J Dis Child* 1947;7:178.

120. Cornover PT, Roessmann U. Malformational complex in an infant with intrauterine influenza viral infection. *Arch Pathol Lab Med* 1990;114:535.

121. Barkovich AJ, Norman D. Anomalies of the corpus callosum. Correlation with further anomalies of the brain. *AJNR Am J Neuroradiol* 1988;9:493.

122. Swett HA, Nixon AW. Agenesis of the corpus callosum with interhemispheric cyst. *Radiology* 1975;114:641.

123. Barth PG, Uylings HBM, Stam FC. Interhemispheral neuroepithelial (glio-ependymal) cyst associated with agenesis of the corpus callosum and neocortical maldevelopment. A case study. *Child's Brain* 1984;11:312.

124. Bennet GL, Bromley B, Benacerraf BR. Agenesis of the corpus callosum: prenatal detection usually is not possible before 22 weeks of gestation. *Radiology* 1996;199:447.

125. Pilu G, Sandri F, Perolo A, et al. Sonography of fetal agenesis of the corpus callosum: a survey of 35 cases. *Ultrasound Obstet Gynecol* 1993;3:318.

126. Mulligan G, Meier P. Lipoma and agenesis of the corpus callosum with associated choroid plexus lipomas. In utero diagnosis. *J Ultrasound Med* 1989;8:583.

127. Lockwood CJ, Ghidini A, Aggarwal R, Hobbins JC. Antenatal diagnosis of partial agenesis of the corpus callosum. A benign cause of ventriculomegaly. *Am J Obstet Gynecol* 1988;159:184.

128. Malinger G, Zakut H. The corpus callosum: normal fetal development as shown by transvaginal sonography. *AJR Am J Roentgenol* 1993;161:1041.

129. D'Ercole C, Girard N, Cravello L, et al. Prenatal diagnosis of fetal corpus callosum agenesis by ultrasonography and magnetic resonance imaging. *Prenat Diagn* 1998;18:247.

130. Parrish M, Roessmann U, Lehvinsohn MW. Agenesis of the corpus callosum. A study on the frequency of associated malformations. *Ann Neurol* 1979;6:349.

131. Serur D, Jeret JS, Wisniewski K. Agenesis of the corpus callosum. Clinical, neuroradiological and cytogenetic studies. *Neuropediatr* 1986;19:87.

132. Donnenfeld AE, Packer RJ, Zackai EH, Chee CM, Sellinger B, et al. Clinical, cytogenetic and pedigree findings in

18 cases of Aicardi syndrome. *Am J Med Genet* 1989;32:461.

133. Byrd SE, Radkowski MA, Flannery A. The clinical and radiological evaluation of absence of the corpus callosum. *Eur J Radiol* 1990;10:65.

134. Bertino RE, Nyberg DA, Cyr DR, Mack LA. Diagnosis of agenesis of the corpus callosum. *J Ultrasound Med* 1988;7:251.

135. Blum A, André M, Droullé P, Husson S, Leheup B. Prenatal echographic diagnosis of corpus callosum agenesis. *Genet Counsel* 1990;38:115.

136. Vergani P, Ghidini A, Strobelt N, et al. Prognostic indicators in the prenatal diagnosis of agenesis of the corpus callosum. *Am J Obstet Gynecol* 1994;170:753.

137. Gupta JK, Lilford RJ. Assessment and management of fetal agenesis of the corpus callosum. *Prenat Diagn* 1995;15:301.

138. Fischer M, Ryan SB, Dobyns WB. Mechanisms of inter-hemispheric transfer and patterns of cognitive functions in acallosal patients of normal intelligence. *Arch Neurol* 1992;49:271.

139. Karnath HO, Schumacher M, Wallesch CW. Limitations of interhemispheric extracallosal transfer of visual information in callosal agenesis. *Cortex* 1991;27:345.

140. Jeeves MA. Stereoperception in callosal agenesis and partial callosotomy. *Neuropsychologia* 1991;29:19.

141. Temple CM, Jeeves MA, Villaroya OO. Reading in callosal agenesis. *Brain Lang* 1990;39:235.

142. Temple CM, Jeeves MA, Villaroya O. Ten pen men: rhyming skills in two children with callosal agenesis. *Brain Lang* 1989;37:548.

143. Swayze VM, Andreasen NC, Ehrardt JC, Yuh WT, Alliger RJ, et al. Developmental abnormalities of the corpus callosum in schizophrenia. *Arch Neurol* 1990;47:805.

144. Dattani MT, Martinez-Barbera JP, Thomas P, et al. Mutations in the homeobox gene HESX1/Hesx1 associated with septo-optic dysplasia in human and mouse. *Nature Genet* 1998;19:125.

145. de Morsier G. Etudes sur le dysraphies cranioencephaliques. III. Agenesie du septum pellucidum avec malformations du traits optique: la dysplasie septo-optique. *Schweiz Arch Neurochir Psychiatry* 1956;77:267.

146. Hoyt WF, Kaplan SL, Grumbach MMM, Glaser JS. Septo-optic dysplasia and pituitary dwarfism. *Lancet* 1970;11:894.

147. Masera N, Grant DB, Stanhope R, Preece MA. Diabetes insipidus with impaired osmotic regulation in septo-optic dysplasia and agenesis of the corpus callosum. *Arch Dis Child* 1994;70:51.

148. Margalith D, Jan JE, McCormick AQ, Tze WJ, Lapointe J. Clinical spectrum of congenital optic nerve hypoplasia: review of 51 patients. *Dev Med Child Neurol* 1984;26:311.

149. Pilu G, Sandri F, Cerisoli M, Alvisi C, Salvioli GP, et al. Sonographic findings in septo-optic dysplasia in the fetus and newborn infant. *Am J Perinatol* 1990;7:337.

150. Menelfe C, Rocchioli P. CT of septo-optique dysplasia. *AJR Am J Roentgenol* 1979;133:1157.

151. Sarwar M. The septum pellucidum: normal and abnormal. *AJNR Am J Neuroradiol* 1989;10:989.

152. Wales JKH, Quarrell OWJ. Evidence for possible Mendelian inheritance of septo-optic dysplasia. *Acta Paedr* 1996; 85:391.

153. Williams J, Brodsky MC, Griebel M, Glasier CM, Caldwell D, et al. Septo-optic dysplasia: the clinical insignificance of an absent septum pellucidum. *Dev Med Child Neurol* 1993;35:490.

154. Wales JKH, Quarrell OWJ. Evidence for possible Mendelian inheritance of septo-optic dysplasia. *Acta Paedr* 1996;85:391.

155. Jones KL. Septo-optic dysplasia sequence. In: *Smith's recognizable patterns of human malformation*, 5th ed. Philadelphia: WB Saunders, 1997:612.

156. Barkovich AJ, Chuang SH, Norman D. MR of neuronal migration anomalies. *AJR Am J Roentgenol* 1988;150:179.

157. Barkovich AJ, Koch TT, Carrol CL. The spectrum of lissencephaly: report of ten patients analyzed by magnetic resonance imaging. *Ann Neurol* 1991;30:139.

158. Dobyns WB, Kirkpatrick JB, Hittner HM, et al. Syndromes with lissencephaly II: Walker-Warburg and cerebro-oculo-muscular syndromes and a new type I lissencephaly. *Am J Med Genet* 1985;22:157.

159. Blaas HG, Eok-Nes SH, Kiserud T, van der Hagen CB, Smedvig E. Lissencephaly type I. *The Fetus* [online journal] 1992;2:1.

160. McGahan JP, Grix A, Gerscovich EO. Prenatal diagnosis of lissencephaly—Miller-Dieker syndrome. *Clin Ultrasound* 22:560–563.

161. Saltzman DH, Krauss CM, Goldman JM, Benaceraff BR. Prenatal diagnosis of lissencephaly. *Prenat Diagn* 1991;11:139.

162. Muller LM, de Jong G, Mouton SCE, et al. A case of the Neu-Laxova syndrome: prenatal ultrasonographic monitoring in the third trimester and the histopathological findings. *Am J Med Genet* 1987;26:421.

163. Monteagudo A, Timor-Tritsch IE. Development of fetal gyri, sulci and fissures: a transvaginal sonographic study. *Ultrasound Obstet Gynecol* 1997;9:222.

164. Dobyns WB, Stratton RF, Greenberg F. Syndromes with lissencephaly I: Miller-Dieker and Norman Roberts syndrome and isolated lissencephaly. *Am J Med Genet* 1984;18:509.

165. Jones K, Gilbert EF, Kaveggia EG, Opitz JM. The Miller-Dieker syndrome. *Pediatrics* 1980;66:277.

166. Barkovich AJ, Chuang SH. Unilateral megalencephaly: correlation of MR imaging and pathologic characteristics. *AJNR Am J Neuroradiol* 1990;11:523.

167. Sandri F, Pilu G, Dallacasa P, Foschi F, Salvioli GP, et al. Sonography of unilateral megalencephaly in the fetus and newborn infant. *Am J Perinatol* 1991;8:18.

168. Ramirez M, Wilkins I, Kramer L, Slopis J, Taylor SR. Prenatal diagnosis of unilateral megalencephaly by real-time ultrasonography. *Am J Obstet Gynecol* 1994;170:1384.

169. Hafner E, Bock W, Zoder G, Schuchter K, Rosen A, Plattner M. Prenatal diagnosis of unilateral megalencephaly by 2D and 3D ultrasound: a case report. *Prenat Diagn* 1999;19:159.

170. Cavenagh EC, Hart BL, Rose D. Association of linear sebaceous nevus syndrome and unilateral megalencephaly. *AJNR Am J Neuroradiol* 1993;14:405.

171. Parikh JR, Mak K, Shalay KM. Unilateral megalencephaly in association with Dandy-Walker complex. *Can Assoc Radiol J* 1994;45:394.

172. Maloof J, Sledz K, Hogg JF, Bodensteiner JB, Schwartz T, et al. Unilateral megalencephaly and tuberous sclerosis: related disorders? *Child Neurol* 1994;9:443.

173. Walters BC, Burrows PE, Musewe N, Chuang SH, Armstrong D. Unilateral megalencephaly associated with neonatal high output cardiac failure. *Childs Nerv Syst* 1990;6:123.

174. King M, Stephenson JBP, Ziervogel M, Doyle D, Galbraith S. Hemimegalencephaly—a case for hemispherectomy? *Neuropediatrics* 1985;16:46.

175. Yakovlev PI, Wadsworth RC. Schizencephalies: a study of the congenital clefts in the cerebral mantle. I: Clefts with fused lips. *J Neuropatol Exp Neurol* 1946;5:116.

176. Yakovlev PI, Wadsworth RC. Schizencephalies: a study of the congenital clefts in the cerebral mantle. II: Clefts with hydrocephalus and lips separated. *J Neuropathol Exp Neurol* 1946;5:169.

177. Barkovich AJ, Norman D. MR imaging of schizencephaly. *AJR Am J Roentgenol* 1988;50:1391.

178. McGahan JP, Ellis W, Lindfors K, et al. Congenital cerebrospinal fluid containing intracranial abnormalities: a sonographic classification. *J Clin Ultrasound* 1988;16:531.

179. Lituana M, Passamonti U, Cordone MS, et al. Schizencephaly: prenatal diagnosis by computed tomography and magnetic resonance imaging. *Prenat Diagn* 1989;9:649.

180. Klingensmith WC, Coiffi-Ragan DT. Schizencephaly: diagnosis and progression in utero. *Radiology* 1986;159:617.

181. Komarnski CA, Cyr DR, Mack LA, Weinberger E. Prenatal diagnosis of schizencephaly. *J Ultrasound Med* 1990;9:305.

182. Pilu G, Falco P, Perolo A, et al. Differential diagnosis and outcome of fetal intracranial hypoechoic lesions: report of 21 cases. *Ultrasound Obstet Gynecol* 1997;9:229.

183. Barkovich AJ, Norman D. Absence of the septum pellucidum: a useful sign in the diagnosis of congenital brain malformations. *AJR Am J Roentgenol* 1989;152:353.

184. Osborne RE. Schizencephaly and septo-optic dysplasia: separate entities. *Pediatr Radiol* 1989;20:137.

185. Robinson RG. Congenital cysts of the brain: arachnoid malformations. *Prog Neurol Surg* 1971;4:133.

186. Langer B, Haddad J, Favre R, Frigne V, Schlaeder G. Fetal arachnoid cysts: report of two cases. *Ultrasound Obstet Gynecol* 1994;4:68.

187. Oliver LC. Primary arachnoid cysts: report of two cases. *BMJ* 1958;1:1147.

188. Shaw CM, Alvord EC. Congenital arachnoid cysts and their differential diagnosis. In: Vinken PJ, Bruyn GW, eds. *Handbook of clinical neurology*, vol 31. Amsterdam: Elsevier/North Holland Biomedical Press, 1977:75.

189. Lewis AJ. Infantile hydrocephalus caused by arachnoid cyst: case report. *J Neurosurg* 1962;19:431.

190. Wester K. Peculiarities of intracranial arachnoid cysts: location, sidedness, and sex distribution in 126 consecutive patients. *Neurosurgery* 1999;45:775.

191. Williams B, Guthkelch AN. Why do central arachnoid pouches expand? *J Neurol Neurosurg Psychiatry* 1974;37:1085.

192. Blaicher W, Prayer D, Kuhle S, Deutinger J, Bernaschek. Combined prenatal ultrasound and magnetic resonance imaging in two fetuses with suspected arachnoid cysts. *Ultrasound Obstet Gynecol* 2001;18:166–168.

193. D'Addario V, Pinto V, Meo F, Resta MJ. The specificity of ultrasound in the detection of fetal intracranial tumors. *Perinat Med* 1998;26:480.

194. Weinberg P, Flom R. Intracranial subarachnoid cysts. *Radiology* 1973;106:329.

195. Marinov M, Undjian S, Wetzka P. An evaluation of the surgical treatment of intracranial arachnoid cysts in children. *Childs Nerv Syst* 1989;5:177.

196. Richard KE, Dahl K, Sanker P. Long-term follow-up of children and juveniles with arachnoid cysts. *Childs Nerv Syst* 1989;5:184.

197. Kwon TH, Jeanty P. Supratentorial arachnoid cyst. *The Fetus* [online journal] 1991;1:1.

198. Raman S, Rachagan SP, Lim CT. Prenatal diagnosis of a posterior fossa cyst. *J Clin Ultrasound* 1991;19:434.

199. Chervenak FA, Berkowitz RL, Tortora M, Hobbins JC. The management of fetal hydrocephalus. *Am J Obstet Gynecol* 1985;151:933.

200. Friede RL, Yasargil MG. Supratentorial intracerebral epithelial (ependymal) cysts: review, case reports and fine structure. *J Neurol Neurosurg Psychiatr* 1977;40:127.

201. Hassan J, Sepulveda W, Teixeira J, Cox PM. Glioependymal and arachnoid cysts: unusual causes of early ventriculomegaly in utero. *Prenat Diagn* 1996;16:729.

202. Pelkey TJ, Ferguson JE II, Veille JC, Alston SR. Giant glioependymal cyst resembling holoprosencephaly on prenatal ultrasound: case report and review of the literature. *Ultrasound Obstet Gynecol* 1997;9:200.

203. Karstaedt P, Jeanty P. Interhemispheric cyst. *The Fetus* [online journal] 1994;4:11.

204. Barkovich AJ, Simon EM, Walsh CA. Callosal agenesis with cyst: a better understanding and new classification. *Neurology* 2001;56:220.

205. Gupta JK, Cave M, Lilford RJ, Farrell TA, Irving HC, et al. Clinical significance of fetal choroid plexus cysts. *Lancet* 1995;346:724.

206. Chinn DH, Miller EI, Worthy LM, Towers CV. Sonographically detected fetal choroid plexus cysts. Frequency and association with aneuploidy. *J Ultrasound Med* 1991;10:255.

207. Neblett CR, Robertson JW. Symptomatic cysts of the telencephalic choroid plexus. *J Neurol Neurosurg Psychiatr* 1971;34:324.

208. Sullivan A, Giudice T, Vavelidis F, Thiagarajah S. Choroid plexus cysts: is biochemical testing a valuable adjunct to targeted ultrasonography? *Am J Obstet Gynecol* 1999;181:260.

209. Levene MI, Wigglesworth JS, Dubowitz V. Hemorrhage periventricular leukomalacia in the neonate: a real-time ultrasound study. *Pediatrics* 1983;71:794.

210. Papile L-A, Burstein J, Burstein R, Koffler H. Incidence and evaluation of subependymal and intraventricular hemorrhage: a study of infants with birth weights less than 1,500 gm. *J Pediatr* 1978;92:529.

211. Vergani P, Stroblet N, Locatelli A, Praterlini G, Tagliabue P, et al. Clinical significance of fetal intracranial hemorrhage. *Am J Obstet Gynecol* 1996;3:536.

212. Frank DA, McCarten KM, Robson CD, et al. Level of in utero cocaine exposure and neonatal ultrasound findings. *Pediatrics* 1999;104:1101.

213. Robinson R, Iida H, O'Brien TP, Pane MA, Traystman RJ, et al. Comparison of cerebrovascular effects of intravenous cocaine injection in fetal, newborn, and adult sheep. *Am J Physiol Heart Circ Physiol* 2000;279:H1.

214. Malinger G, Katz R, Amsel S, Gewurtz G, Zakut H. Brain hemorrhage, germinal matrix. *The Fetus* 1992;2:1.

215. Bose C. Hydrops fetalis and in utero intracranial hemorrhage. *J Pediatr* 1978;93:1023.

216. Portman M, Brouillette RT. Fatal intracranial hemorrhage complicating amniocentesis. *Am J Obstet Gynecol* 1982; 144:731.

217. Zalneraitis EL, Young RSK, Krishnamoorthy KS. Intracranial hemorrhage in utero as a complication of isoimmune thrombocytopenia. *J Pediatr* 1979;95:611.

218. Khouzami AN, Kickler TS, Callan NA, Shumway JB, Perlman EJ, et al. Devastating sequelae of alloimmune thrombocytopenia: an entity that deserves more attention. *J Matern Fetal Med* 1996;5:137.

219. Sherer DM, Anyaegbunam A, Onyeije C. Antepartum fetal intracranial hemorrhage, predisposing factors and prenatal sonography: a review. *Am J Perinatol* 1998;15:431–441.

220. Johnson JA, Ryan G, al-Musa A, Farkas S, Blanchette VS. Prenatal diagnosis and management of neonatal alloimmune thrombocytopenia. *Sem Perinatol* 1997;21:45.

221. Dickinson JE, Marshall LR, Phillips JM, Barr AL. Antenatal diagnosis and management of fetomaternal alloimmune thrombocytopenia. *Am J Perinatol* 1995;12:333.

222. Bussel JB, Zabusky MR, Berkowitz RL, McFarland JG. Fetal alloimmune thrombocytopenia. *N Engl J Med* 1997;337:22.

223. Fujimori K, Ohto H, Honda S, Sato A. Antepartum diagnosis of fetal intracranial hemorrhage due to maternal Bernard-Soulier syndrome. *Obstet Gynecol* 1999 Nov; 94:817–819.

224. Tchernia G, Morel-Kopp MC, Yvart J, Kaplan C. Neonatal thrombocytopenia and hidden maternal autoimmunity. *Br J Haematol* 1993;84:457.

225. De Spirlet M, Goffinet F, Philippe HJ, Bailly M, Couderc S, et al. Prenatal diagnosis of a subdural hematoma associated with reverse flow in the middle cerebral artery: case report and literature review. *Ultrasound Obstet Gynecol* 2000;16:72.

226. Volpe JJ. Intracranial hemorrhage: periventricular-intraventricular hemorrhage of the premature infant. In: Volpe JJ, ed. *Neurology of the newborn*, 2nd ed. Philadelphia: WB Saunders, 1987:311.

227. Rypens F, Avni EF, Dussaussois L, et al. Hyperechoic thickened ependyma: sonographic demonstration and significance in neonates. *Pediatr Radiol* 1994;24:550.

228. McGahan JP, Haesslein HC, Meyers M, Ford KB. Sonographic recognition of in utero intraventricular hemorrhage. *AJR Am J Roentgenol* 1984;142:171.

229. Achiron R, Pinchas OH, Reichmann B, Heymal Z, Schimel M, et al. Fetal intracranial hemorrhage: clinical significance of in utero ultrasonographic diagnosis. *Br J Obstet Gynecol* 1992;100:995.

230. Guerriero S, Ajossa S, Mais V, et al. Color Doppler energy imaging in the diagnosis of fetal intracranial hemorrhage in the second trimester. *Ultrasound Obstet Gynecol* 1997;10:205.

231. Tampakoudis P, Bili H, Lazaridis E, Anastasiadou E, Andreou A, et al. Prenatal diagnosis of intracranial hemorrhage secondary to maternal idiopathic thrombocytopenic purpura: a case report. *Am J Perinatol* 1995;12:268–270.

232. Mullaart RA, Van Dongen P, Gabreels FJ, van Oostrom C. Fetal periventricular hemorrhage in von Willebrand's disease: short review and first case presentation. *Am J Perinatol* 1991;8:190–192.

233. Smulian JC, Sigman RK. In utero intraventricular hemorrhage and growth discordancy in a quadruplet pregnancy. *Eur J Ultrasound* 1998;7:115–119.

234. Fusch C, Ozdoba C, Kuhn P, Durig P, Remonda L, et al. Perinatal ultrasonography and magnetic resonance imaging findings in congenital hydrocephalus associated with fetal intraventricular hemorrhage. *Am J Obstet Gynecol* 1997; 177:512–518.

235. Groothuis AM, de Kleine MJ, Oei SG. Intraventricular haemorrhage in utero. A case-report and review of the literature. *Eur J Obstet Gynecol Reprod Biol* 2000;89:207–211.

236. Felderhoff-Muser U, Brauer M, Buhrer C, Wagner M, Hierholzer J, et al. Familial recurrence of spontaneous fetal intracranial hemorrhage: ultrasonographic diagnosis and postnatal magnetic resonance imaging (MRI). *Ultrasound Obstet Gynecol* 2001;17:248–251.

237. McGahan JP. Fetal head and brain. In: McGahan JP, Goldberg BB, eds. *Diagnostic ultrasound: a logical approach*. Philadelphia: Lippincott–Raven, 1998:255.

238. Fuku K, Morioka T, Nishio S, Mihara F, Nakayama H, et al. Fetal germinal matrix and intraventricular haemorrhage diagnosed by MRI. *Neuroradiology* 2001;43:68–72.

239. Edmondson SR, Hallak M, Carpenter RJ Jr, Cotton DB. Evolution of hydranencephaly following intracerebral hemorrhage. *Obstet Gynecol* 1992;79:870–871.

240. Solak MM, Katz M, Lell ME. Neonatal survival after traumatic fetal subdural hematoma. *J Reprod Med* 1980;24:131.

241. Akman CI, Cracco J. Intrauterine subdural hemorrhage. *Dev Med Child Neurol* 2000;42:843–846.

242. Kawabata I, Imai A, Tamaya T. Antenatal subdural hemorrhage causing fetal death before labor. *Int J Gynaecol Obstet* 1993;43:57–60.

243. Rotmensch S, Grannum PA, Nores JA, Hall C, Keller MS, et al. In utero diagnosis and management of fetal subdural hematoma. *Am J Obstet Gynecol* 1991;164:1246–1248.

244. Sonigo PC, Rypens FF, Carteret M, Delezoide AL, Brunelle FO. MR imaging of fetal cerebral anomalies. *Pediatr Radiol* 1998;28:212–222.

245. Barozzino T, Sgro M, Toi A, Akouri H, Wilson S, et al. Fetal bilateral subdural haemorrhages. Prenatal diagnosis and spontaneous resolution by time of delivery. *Prenat Diagn* 1998;18:496–503.

246. Akman CI, Cracco J. Intrauterine subdural hemorrhage. *Dev Med Child Neurol* 2000;42:843–846.

247. Kirkinen P, Partanen K, Ryynanen M, Orden MR. Fetal intracranial hemorrhage. Imaging by ultrasound and magnetic resonance imaging. *J Reprod Med* 1997;42:467–472.

248. Hashimoto I, Tada K, Nakatsuka M, Nakata T, Inoue N, et al. Fetal hydrocephalus secondary to intraventricular hemorrhage diagnosed by ultrasonography and in utero fast magnetic resonance imaging. A case report. *Fetal Diagn Ther* 1999;14:248–253.

249. Shinnar S, Molteni RA, Gammon K, D'Souza BJ, Altman J, et al. Intraventricular hemorrhage in the premature infant. A changing outlook. *N Engl J Med* 1982;306:1464.

250. Cook RL, Miller RC, Katz VL, Cefalo RC. Immune thrombocytopenic purpura in pregnancy: a reappraisal of management. *Obstet Gynecol* 1991;78:578.

251. Thrombocytopenia in pregnancy. *ACOG practice bulletin*, 6, September 1999.

252. Nicolini U, Rodeck CH, Kochenour NK, et al. In utero platelet transfusions for alloimmune thrombocytopenia. *Lancet* 1988;2:506.

253. Bussel JB, Berkowitz RL, McFarland JG, Lynch L, Chitkara U. Antenatal treatment of maternal alloimmune thrombocytopenia. *N Engl J Med* 1988;319:1374.

254. Johnson JA, Ryan G, al-Musa A, Farkas S, Blanchette VS. Prenatal diagnosis and management of neonatal alloimmune thrombocytopenia. *Sem Perinatol* 1997;21:45.

255. Barkovich AJ. Metabolic and destructive brain disorders. In: Barkovich AJ, ed. *Pediatric neuroimaging*. New York: Raven Press, 1990:35.

256. Vintzileos AM, Hovick TX, Escoto DT, et al. Congenital midline porencephaly—prenatal sonographic findings and review of the literature. *Am J Perinatol* 1987;4:125.

257. Fleischer AC, Hutchison AA, Bundy AL, et al. Serial sonography of posthemorrhagic ventricular dilatation and porencephaly after intracranial hemorrhage in the preterm neonate. *AJR Am J Roentgenol* 1983;141:451.

258. Jung JH, Graham JM, Schultz N, Smith DW. Congenital hydranencephaly/porencephaly due to vascular disruption in monozygotic twins. *Pediatrics* 1984;73:467.

259. Eller KM, Kuller JA. Fetal porencephaly: a review of etiology, diagnosis, and prognosis. *Obstet Gynecol Surv* 1995; 50:684.

260. Viljoen DL. Porencephaly and transverse limb defects following severe maternal trauma in early pregnancy. *Clin Dysmorphol* 1995;4:75.

261. Youraoukos S, Papdelis F, Matsaniotis N. Porencephalic cysts after amniocentesis. *Arch Dis Child* 1980;55:814.

262. Eller KM, Kuller JA. Porencephaly secondary to fetal trauma during amniocentesis. *Obstet Gynecol* 1995;85:865.

263. Berg R, Aleck K, Kaplan A. Familial porencephaly. *Arch Neurol* 1983;40:567.

264. Bonnemann CG, Meinecke P. Bilateral porencephaly, cerebellar hypoplasia, and internal malformations: two siblings representing a probably new autosomal recessive entity. *Am J Med Genet* 1996;63:428.

265. Muir CS. Hydranencephaly and allied disorders. *Am J Dis Child* 1959;34:231.

266. Ho SS, Kuzniecky RI, Gilliam F, Faught E, Bebin M, et al. Congenital porencephaly: MR features and relationship to hippocampal sclerosis. *AJNR Am J Neuroradiol* 1998; 19:135.

267. Halsey JH, Allen N, Chamberlin HR. *Hydranencephaly. Handbook of clinical neurology*, vol. 30. Amsterdam: Elsevier/North Holland Biomedical Press, 1977:661.

268. Myers R. Brain pathology following fetal vascular occlusion: an experimental study. *Invest Ophthalmol* 1969;8:41.

269. Dixon A. Hydranencephaly. *Radiography* 1988;54:12.

270. Sutton L, Bruce D, Schut L. Hydranencephaly vs. maximal hydrocephalus: an important clinical distinction. *Neurosurgery* 1980;63:35.

271. Warkany J. *Congenital malformation*. Chicago: Year Book Medical Publishers, 1981.

272. Fernandez F, Perez-Higueras A, Hernandez R, et al. Hydranencephaly after maternal butane gas intoxication during pregnancy. *Develop Med Child Neurol* 1986;28:361.

273. Hutto C, Arvin A, Jacobs R, et al. Intrauterine herpes simplex infections. *J Pediatrics* 1987;110:97.

274. Christie J, Rakusan T, Martinez M, et al. Hydranencephaly caused by congenital infection with herpes simplex virus. *Pediatric Inf Disease* 1986;5:473.

275. Nahmias AJ, Keyserling HL, Kerrick GM. Herpes simplex. In: Remington JS, Klein JO, eds. *Infectious diseases of the fetus and newborn infant*, 2nd ed. Philadelphia: WB Saunders, 1983:636.

276. Hanigan W, Aldrich W. MRI and evoked potentials in a child with hydranencephaly. *Pediatric Neurol* 1988;4:185.

277. Fusi L, Mc Parland P, Fisk N, Nicolini U, Wigglesworth J. Acute twin-twin transfusion: a possible mechanism for brain-damaged survivors after intrauterine death of monochorionic twin. *Obstet Gynecol* 1991;78:517.

278. Greene M, Benacerraf B, Crawford J. Hydranencephaly: ultrasound appearance during in utero evolution. *Radiology* 1985;156:779.

279. Carrasco CR, Stierman ED, Harnsberger HR, Lee TG. An algorithm for prenatal ultrasound diagnosis of congenital central nervous system abnormalities. *J Ultrasound Med* 1985;4:163.

280. Aguirre Villa Coro A, Dominquey R. Intrauterine diagnosis of hydranencephaly by magnetic resonance. *Magn Reson Imaging* 1989;7:105.

281. Bendon R, Siddiqi J, de Courten-Myers G, Dignan P. Recurrent developmental anomalies: 1. Syndrome of hydranencephaly with renal aplastic dysplasia: 2. Polyvalvular developmental heart defect. *Am J Genet Suppl* 1987;3:357.

282. Bordarier C, Robain D. Familial occurrence of prenatal encephaloclastic damage: anatomoclinical report of 2 cases. *Neuropediatrics* 1989;20:103.

283. Pooh RK, Aono T. Transvaginal power Doppler angiography of the fetal brain. *Ultrasound Obstet Gynecol* 1996;8:417.

284. Pooh RK, Pooh KH, Nakagawa Y, Maeda K, Fukui R, et al. Transvaginal Doppler assessment of fetal intracranial venous flow. *Obstet Gynecol* 1999;93:697.

285. Laurichesse-Delmas H, Grimaud O, Moscoso G, Ville Y. Color Doppler study of the venous circulation in the fetal brain and hemodynamic study of the cerebral transverse sinus. *Ultrasound Obstet Gynecol* 1999;13:34.

286. Mari G, Moise KJ Jr, Deter RL, Kirshon B, Carpenter RJ Jr, et al. Doppler assessment of the pulsatility index in the cerebral circulation of the human fetus. *Am J Obstet Gynecol* 1989;160:698.

287. Bahado-Singh RO, Kovanci E, Jeffres A, Oz U, Deren O, et al. The Doppler cerebroplacental ratio and perinatal outcome in intrauterine growth restriction. *Am J Obstet Gynecol* 1999;180:750.

288. Ruchox MM, Renjard L, Monegier du Sorbier C, et al. Histopathologie de la veine de Galen. *Neurochirurgie* 1987; 33:272.

289. Padget DH. The cranial venous system in man in reference to development, adult configuration and relation to the arteries. *Am J Anat* 1956;98:307.

290. Lasjaunias P, Manelfe C, Terbrugge K, et al. Endovascular treatment of cerebral arteriovenous malformations. *Neurosurgery* 1986;9:265.

291. Lasjaunias P, Terbrugge K, Piske R, et al. Dilatation de la veine de Galien. Formes anatomo-cliniques et traitement endovasculaire a propos de 14 cas explores et/ou traites entre 1983 et 1986. *Neurochirurgie* 1986;33:315.

292. Rayboud CA, Hold JK, Strother CM. Aneurysm of the vein of Galen. Angiographic study and morphogenetic considerations. *Neurochirurgie* 1987;33:302.

293. Sepulveda W, Platt CC, Fisk NM. Prenatal diagnosis of cerebral arteriovenous malformation using color Doppler ultrasonography: case report and review of the literature. *Ultrasound Obstet Gynecol* 1995;6:282.

294. Heling KS, Chaoui R, Bollmann R. Prenatal diagnosis of an aneurysm of the vein of Galen with three-dimensional color power angiography. *Ultrasound Obstet Gynecol* 2000;15:333–336.

295. Lee TH, Shih JC, Peng SS, Lee CN, Shyu MK, et al. Prenatal depiction of angioarchitecture of an aneurysm of the vein of Galen with three-dimensional color power angiography. *Ultrasound Obstet Gynecol* 2000;15:337–340.

296. Kurihara N, Tokieda K, Ikeda K, Mori K, Hokuto I, et al. Prenatal MR findings in a case of aneurysm of the vein of Galen. *Pediatr Radiol* 2001;31:160–162.

297. Doren M, Tercanli S, Holzgreve W. Prenatal sonographic diagnosis of a vein of Galen aneurysm: relevance of associated malformations for timing and mode of delivery. *Ultrasound Obstet Gynecol* 1995;6:287.

298. Johnston IH, Whittle IR, Besser M, et al. Vein of Galen malformation: diagnosis and management. *Neurosurgery* 1987;20:747.

299. Stanbridge R de L, Westaby S, Smallhorn J, et al. Intracranial arteriovenous malformation with aneurysm of the vein of Galen as cause of heart failure in infancy. Echocardiographic diagnosis and results of treatment. *Br Heart J* 1983;49:157.

300. Pun KK, Yu YL, Huang CY, et al. Ventriculo peritoneal shunting of acute hydrocephalus in vein of Galen malformation. *Clin Exp Neurol* 1987;23:209.

301. Wilkins RH. Natural history of intracranial vascular malformations: a review. *Neurosurgery* 1985;16:421.

302. Phillips SJ, Dooley JM, Camfield PR. Vein of Galen malformation with cerebral calcification: a reversible cause of neurodegenerative disease. *Can J Neurol Sci* 1986;13:103.

303. Remington G, Jeffries JJ. The role of cerebral arteriovenous malformations in psychiatric disturbances: case report. *J Clin Psychiatry* 1984;45:226.

304. Aleem A, Knesevich MA. Schizophrenia like psychosis associated with vein of Galen malformation: a case report. *Can J Psychiatry* 1987;32:226.

305. Rosenfeld JV, Fabinyi GC. Acute hydrocephalus in an elderly woman with an aneurysm of the vein of Galen. *Neurosurgery* 1984;15:852.

306. Rodesch G, Hui F, Alvarez H, Tanaka A, Lasjaunias P. Prognosis of antenatally diagnosed vein of Galen malformations. *Child Nerv Syst* 1994;10:79.

307. Mitchell PJ, Rosenfeld JV, Dargaville P, Loughnan P, Ditchfield MR, et al. Endovascular management of vein of Galen aneurysmal malformations presenting in the neonatal period. *AJNR Am J Neuroradiol* 2001;22:1403–409.

308. Visentin A, Falco P, Pilu G, et al. Prenatal diagnosis of thrombosis of the dural sinuses with real-time and color Doppler ultrasound. *Ultrasound Obstet Gynecol* 2001;17:322.

309. Konishi Y, Kuriyama M, Sudo M, Konishi K, Hayakawa K, et al. Superior sagittal sinus thrombosis in neonates. *Pediatr Neurol* 1987;3:222.

310. Shevell MI, Silver K, O'Gorman AM, Watters GV, Montes JL. Neonatal dural sinus thrombosis. *Pediatr Neurol* 1989;5:161.

311. Marciniak E, Wilson HD, Mariar RA. Neonatal purpura fulminates: a genetic disorder related to the absence of protein C in the blood. *Blood* 1985;65:15.

312. Vielhaber H, Ehrenforth S, Koch HG, Scharrer I, Van der Werf N, et al. Cerebral venous sinus thrombosis in infancy and childhood: role of genetic and acquired risk factors of thrombophilia. *Eur J Pediatr* 1998;157:555.

313. Wong VK, Le Mesurier J, Francescini R, Heikali M, Hanson R. Cerebral venous thrombosis as a cause of neonatal seizures. *Pediatr Neurol* 1987;3:235.

314. Meldock M, Olivero WC, Hanigan W, Wright R, Winek S. Children with cerebral venous thrombosis diagnosed with magnetic resonance imaging and magnetic resonance angiography. *Neurosurgery* 1992;31:870.

315. Barron TF, Gusnard DA, Zimmerman RA, Clancy RR. Cerebral venous thrombosis in neonates and children. *Pediatric Neurol* 1992;8:112.

316. Hanigan WC, Tracy PT, Tadros WS, Wright RM. Neonatal cerebral venous thrombosis. *Pediatr Neurosci* 1988;14:177.

317. Pryor HB, Thelander H. Abnormally small head size and intellect in children. *J Pediatr* 1968;73:593.

318. Book JA, Schut JW, Reed SC. A clinical and genetical study of microcephaly. *Am J Ment Defic* 1953;57:637.

319. Brandon MWG, Kirman BH, Williams CE. Microcephaly. *J Ment Sci* 1959;105:721.

320. Daniel WL. A genetic and biochemical investigation of primary microcephaly. *Am J Ment Defic* 1971;75:653.

321. Van Den Bosch J. Microcephaly in the Netherlands: a clinical and genetic study. *Ann Hum Genet* 1959;23:91.

322. Myrianthopoulos NC, Chung CS. Congenital malformations in singletons: epidemiologic survey. *Birth Defects* 1974;10:1.

323. Davies H, Kirman BH. Microcephaly. *Arch Dis Child* 1962;37:623.

324. Chervenak FA, Jeanty P, Cantraine F. The diagnosis of fetal microcephaly. *Am J Obstet Gynecol* 1984;149:512.

325. Goldstein I, Reece EA, Pilu G, O'Connor TZ, Lockwood CJ, et al. Sonographic assessment of the fetal frontal lobe: a potential tool for prenatal diagnosis of microcephaly. *Am J Obstet Gynecol* 1988;158:1057.

326. Pilu G, Falco P, Milano V, Perolo A, Bovicelli L. Prenatal diagnosis of microcephaly assisted by vaginal sonography and power Doppler. *Ultrasound Obstet Gynecol* 1998;11:357.

327. Kurtz AB, Wapner RJ, Rubin CS. Ultrasound criteria for in utero diagnosis of microcephaly. *J Clin Ultrasound* 1980;8:11.

328. Jaworsky M, Hersh JH, Donat J, Shearer B, Weisskopf B. Computed tomography of the head in the evaluation of fetal microcephaly. *Pediatrics* 1986;79:1064.

329. Steinlin M, Zurrer M, Martin E, Boesch Ch, Largo RH, et al. Contribution of magnetic resonance imaging in the evaluation of microcephaly. *Neuropediatrics* 1991;22:184.

330. Libicher M, Troger J. US measurements of the subarachnoid space in infants: normal values. *Radiology* 1992;184:749.

331. Govaert P, De Vries L. Microcephaly. In: *Atlas of neonatal brain sonography*. Cambridge: Mac Keith Press, 1997:64.

332. Chervenak FA, Rosenberg J, Brightman RC, Chitkara U, Jeanty P. A prospective study of the accuracy of ultrasound in predicting fetal microcephaly. *Obstet Gynecol* 1987; 69:908.

333. Jaffe M, Tirosh E, Oren S. The dilemma in prenatal diagnosis of idiopathic microcephaly. *Dev Med Child Neurol* 1987;29:187.

334. Bromley B, Benacerraf BR. Difficulties in the prenatal diagnosis of microcephaly. *J Ultrasound Med* 1995;14:303.

335. Avery GB, Meneses L, Lodge A. The clinical significance of "measurement microcephaly." *Am J Dis Child* 1972; 123:214.

336. De Myer W. Megalencephaly in children. Clinical syndromes, genetic patterns and differential diagnosis from other causes of megalencephaly. *Neurology* 1972;22:634.

337. Schlembach D, Bornemann A, Rupprecht T, Beinder E. Fetal intracranial tumors detected by ultrasound: a report of two cases and review of the literature. *Ultrasound Obstet Gynecol* 1999;14:407.

338. DiGiovanni LM, Sheikh Z. Prenatal diagnosis, clinical significance and management of fetal intracranial teratoma: a case report and literature review. *Am J Perinatol* 1994; 11:420.

339. Doren M, Tercanli S, Gullotta F, Holzgreve W. Prenatal diagnosis of a highly undifferentiated brain tumour—a case report and review of the literature. *Prenat Diagn* 1997; 17:967.

340. Sherer DM, Onyeije CI. Prenatal ultrasonographic diagnosis of fetal intracranial tumors: a review. *Am J Perinatol* 1998;15:319.

341. Winter TC 3rd, Laing FC, Mack LA, Born DE. Prenatal sonographic diagnosis of a pontine lipoma. *J Ultrasound Med* 1992;11:559–561.

342. Sosa-Olavarria A, Diaz-Guerrero L, Reigoza A, Bermudez A, Murillo M. Fetal craniopharyngioma: early prenatal diagnosis. *J Ultrasound Med* 2001;20:803–806.

343. Wakai S, Aarai T, Nagai M. Congenital brain tumors. *Surg Neurol* 1984;21:597.

NEURAL TUBE DEFECTS AND THE SPINE

Neural tube defects (NTDs) are a heterogeneous group of malformations resulting from failure of normal neural tube closure between the third and fourth week of embryologic development. Anencephaly, encephalocele, and spina bifida are the three most common forms of NTDs. Less common types of NTDs include iniencephaly, amniotic bands, and other types of spinal abnormalities. For the purposes of this chapter, NTDs and spinal malformations are considered by their primary location as either primary cranial malformations or primary spinal abnormalities. These topics are preceded by a general discussion of NTDs.

EPIDEMIOLOGY

NTDs are the second most common fetal malformation in the United States, surpassed only by congenital heart defects. The incidence of NTDs varies with race, geographic location, and various other predisposition factors[1,2] (Table 1). In the United States, the incidence is approximately 1 to 2 per 1,000. Anencephaly and spina bifida are most common with nearly equal prevalence of 1 per 1,000.[3] The prevalence is much higher during early pregnancy, especially among pregnancy losses. Approximately 3% of all spontaneous abortions show evidence of an NTD.[4] It is estimated that of all embryos with NTDs at 8 weeks' gestation, approximately one-fourth will be live born, one-fourth stillborn, and one-half spontaneously aborted.

The vast majority of NTDs is sporadic and is believed to be multifactorial in origin. Geographic variation in the prevalence of open NTDs has been noted, with the highest rates reported in the United Kingdom and the lowest rates in Japan.[5] In the United States, considerable variation exists in the prevalence of NTDs by race or ethnicity and by type of NTD, with Hispanic women exhibiting the highest overall NTD rate.[6]

It has long been observed that lower socioeconomic classes have a predisposition for NTDs, leading to the theory that nutritional deficiency may be a causative factor. In 1976, Smithells et al.[7] implicated vitamin deficiencies among pregnancies with NTDs, observing decreased levels of folate, ascorbate, and riboflavin in lower socioeconomic groups.

This was confirmed by others.[8] In 1991, a landmark prospective, randomized, double blind study was published that showed women who had previous pregnancies with isolated NTDs had a 72% reduction of a recurrence of the NTD when supplemented with 4 mg per day of folate at least four weeks before conception through the twelfth week of gestation.[9] Questions still remain regarding the lowest effective dosage of folate supplementation, the optimal duration of pre- and post-conception supplementation, and the possible protective effect of folate supplementation in patients without a previous history of NTDs. In September 1992, the U.S. Public Health Service recommended that all women attempting pregnancy take the recommended daily allowance (0.4 mg) of folate for 1 month before conception and for at least 3 months after conception.[10]

Several teratogens have been implicated in the etiology of NTDs. Two anticonvulsant medications, carbamazepine and valproic acid, have been demonstrated to cause these defects, which some believe is secondary to lower levels of serum folate when on these medications.[11] This risk has been estimated as approximately 1%. Other agents that have been implicated include zinc deficiency, hyperthermia, aminopterin, clomiphene citrate, and insulin-dependent diabetes mellitus.[12] Other patients considered to be at increased risk for carrying a fetus with an NTD include women with a history of other types of vertebral defects including scoliosis and sacrococcygeal teratoma. It is important, however, to remember that 90% to 95% of NTDs occur in families without a prior family history of an NTD.

The link between environmental and genetic factors has been the object of many studies, and different genes involved in the folate metabolism pathway have been investigated, including the most commonly studied thermolabile mutation (C677T) in the MTHFR gene.[13] Rarely, NTDs occur as part of a mendelian syndrome or chromosomal anomalies, or result from teratogenic exposure. Table 2 lists the recognized causes of NTDs.

Table 3 describes the recurrence risk for NTDs according to different risk factors. Families who have had a child with NTD have a tenfold increase in recurrence risk in the range of 1% to 2%. However, Stevenson et al.[14] reported no recurrence of NTDs in 113 subsequent pregnancies to

TABLE 1. INCIDENCE OF NEURAL TUBE DEFECTS (1 PER 1,000 BIRTHS) IN VARIOUS GEOGRAPHIC AREAS

	Spina bifida	Anencephaly
South Wales, U.K.	4.1	3.5
Southampton, U.K.	3.2	1.9
Birmingham, U.K.	2.8	2.0
Charleston, U.S., whites	1.5	1.2
Charleston, U.S., blacks	0.6	0.2
Alexandria, U.S.	2.0	3.6
Japan	0.3	0.6

Modified from Brocklehurst. In: Vinken GW, Bruyn PW, eds. *Handbook of clinical neurology*, vol. 32. Amsterdam: Elsevier/North Holland Biomedical Press, 1978:519–578.

TABLE 2. RECOGNIZED CAUSES OF NEURAL TUBE DEFECTS

Multifactorial inheritance
Single mutant genes
  Meckel syndrome, autosomal recessive (phenotype includes occipital encephalocele and, rarely, anencephaly)
  Median-cleft face syndrome, possibly autosomal dominant (phenotype includes anterior encephalocele)
  Roberts syndrome, autosomal recessive (phenotype includes anterior encephalocele)
  Syndrome of anterior sacral meningomyelocele and anal stenosis dominant, either autosomal or X-linked
  Jarcho-Levin syndrome, autosomal recessive (phenotype includes meningomyelocele)
  HARD syndrome autosomal recessive (phenotype includes encephalocele)
Chromosome abnormalities
  Trisomy 13 syndrome
  Trisomy 18 syndrome
  Triploidy
  Other abnormalities, such as unbalanced translocation and ring chromosome
Probably hereditary, but mode of transmission not established
  Syndrome of occipital encephalocele, myopia, and retinal dysplasia
  Anterior encephalocele among Bantu and Thai
Teratogens
  Valproic acid (phenotype includes spina bifida)
  Aminopterin/amethopterin (phenotype includes anencephaly and encephalocele)
  Thalidomide (phenotype includes, rarely, anencephaly and meningomyelocele)
Maternal predisposing factors
  Diabetes mellitus (anencephaly more frequent than spina bifida)
  Specific phenotypes, but without known cause
  Syndrome of craniofacial and limb defects secondary to aberrant tissue bands (phenotype includes multiple encephaloceles)
  Cloacal exstrophy (phenotype includes myelocystocele)
  Sacrococcygeal teratoma (phenotype includes meningomyelocele)

HARD, hydrocephalus, agyria, retinal dysplasia.
Modified from Main DM, Mennuti MT. Neural tube defects: issues in prenatal diagnosis and counseling. *Obstet Gynecol* 1986;67:1–16.

TABLE 3. ESTIMATED INCIDENCE OF NEURAL TUBE DEFECTS BASED ON SPECIFIC RISK FACTORS IN THE UNITED STATES (INCIDENCE PER 1,000 LIVE BIRTHS)

Mother as reference	
General incidence	1.4–1.6
Women with diabetes mellitus	20
Women on valproic acid in first trimester	10–20
Fetus as reference	
One sibling with neural tube defect	15–30
Two siblings with neural tube defect[a]	57
Parent with neural tube defect	11
Half sibling with neural tube defect	8
First cousin (mother's sister's child)	10
Other first cousins	3
Sibling with severe scoliosis secondary to multiple vertebral defects	15–30
Sibling with occult spina dysraphism	15–30
Sibling with sacrococcygeal teratoma or hamartoma	Approximately 15–30

[a]Risk is higher in British studies. Risk increases further for three or more siblings or combinations of other close relatives.
Modified from Main DM, Mennuti MT. Neural tube defects: issues in prenatal diagnosis and counseling. *Obstet Gynecol* 1986;67:1–16.

mothers of infants with isolated NTDs who took periconceptional folic acid.

There has been a trend toward decreasing prevalence of NTDs. Some attribute this improvement to the use of folic acid,[14] whereas others believe that other factors must also be contributory.[3] Certainly, screening protocols with maternal serum alpha-fetoprotein (MS-AFP) and obstetric ultrasound have contributed to a dramatically decreased prevalence of liveborn infants with NTDs in some countries.[15]

SCREENING PROTOCOLS

The association of NTDs and elevated levels of amniotic fluid AFP, first reported in 1972 by Brock and Sutcliffe, represented a major technological advance in prenatal detection of NTDs.[16] The United Kingdom Collaborative Study subsequently reported that testing amniotic fluid AFP could detect 98% of anencephaly and 98% of open spina bifida.[17] This encouraging experience quickly led investigators to test for AFP in the maternal serum. Using a cutoff of 2.5 multiples of the median, screening programs have shown that elevated MS-AFP can detect 90% of anencephaly and approximately 80% of open spina bifida. Different strategies for alpha-fetoprotein screening in pregnancy exist, and the interested reader is referred to specific publications on this subject.[18,19]

During the same time period, ultrasound significantly improved so that expert sonography (also referred to in the United States as a level 2 ultrasound examination) has nearly a 100% diagnostic accuracy for malformations associated with increased MS-AFP.[20] As a consequence of these considerations, some centers have elected to limit examination of the patients with positive screen tests to ultrasound. Others prefer to continue to perform amniocentesis on positive patients to select patients for level 2 examinations, because of various considerations, the most important ones being probably represented by the decrease in the need for expert sonographic examinations. Where expert sonography is available, however, targeted ultrasound has been shown to be superior to AFP serum screening for detection of open spina bifida and is also superior to amniocentesis. This experience is not uniformly shared by all centers. Detection of virtually all NTDs remains an achievable goal that is not yet fulfilled. It is believed that continued improvements in wide-scale application of obstetric ultrasound by experienced sonographers and sonologists will eventually lead to fulfillment of this goal.

EMBRYOLOGY

The neural tube is the early embryonic structure that gives rise to the central nervous system. The neural tube forms early from an infolding of the neural plate, the embryonic ectoderm. This infolding of the ectoderm or neurulation forms the neural tube (Fig. 1). The neural tube begins as a neural groove, which fuses posteriorly to form the neural tube. The fusion of the neural groove starts in the mid-dorsal aspect of the embryo and proceeds anteriorly as the anterior neuropore and posteriorly as the posterior neuropore. The anterior neuropore closes in or about day 23 of embryotic life (42 menstrual days).[21] If this process is interrupted, it can result in a defect in either end of the neural tube. On occasion, this process can be interrupted on both ends, explaining the association of anterior neuropore defects such as cephaloceles or anencephaly with spina bifida.

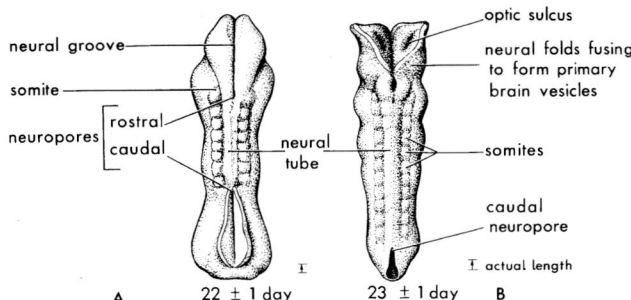

FIGURE 1. Normal development of the neural tube. **A:** Dorsal view at 37 menstrual days (23 fetal days) shows closure of the neural fold developing rostrally and caudally. **B:** Dorsal view at 38 menstrual days (24 fetal days) shows normal prominence of the forebrain and closing of the rostral neuropore. (Reproduced with permission from Moore KL. *The developing human*, 4th ed. Philadelphia: WB Saunders, 1988.)

HEAD AND CALVARIA

The head is scanned with several basic planes (see Chapter 6; Fig. 1). This scan includes the transventricular, transthalamic, and transcerebellar views. These views should detect all cases of acrania, anencephaly, and nearly all cephaloceles.

Acrania/Anencephaly

Synonyms

A synonym for acrania/anencephaly is exencephaly/anencephaly sequence.

Description

Acrania is absence of the cranial vault above the bony orbits. This may be considered as two subtypes: exencephaly and anencephaly. Exencephaly shows relatively normal amounts of cerebral tissue, although abnormally developed.[22,23] Anencephaly is associated with absence of the cerebral hemispheres with residual covering variable amounts of angiomatous stroma (area cerebrovasculosa).[24]

Incidence

The incidence for acrania/anencephaly is approximately 1 per 1,000 births, although live birth rates are decreasing. As noted in the previous Epidemiology section, geographic and ethnic differences are well known. Females are usually more commonly affected than males with a 4 to 1 ratio. Other data, however, indicate that when all NTDs are considered together, there is probably an equal female to male incidence.[25] While maternal obesity has been associated with an increased incidence of NTDs, it has not been specifically associated with an increased risk of anencephaly.[26]

Pathogenesis and Pathology

Acrania is part of the spectrum of NTDs—multifactorial disorders resulting from a combination of genetic, nutritional, and environmental factors. Isolated reports exist of reciprocal translocations[27] or genetic polymorphism associated with anencephaly.

Acrania is characterized pathologically by absence of the cranial vault. This absence affects the membranous flat bones above the orbits, while the base of the cranium is usually intact. With exencephaly, exposed brain is visualized, whereas anencephaly shows little disorganized tissue (angiomatous stroma) protruding from the defect. Good reason exists to believe that anencephaly develops from exencephaly as the exposed brain tissue is disrupted by relatively minor trauma produced by fetal movement.[28] This hypothesis is well supported by prenatal

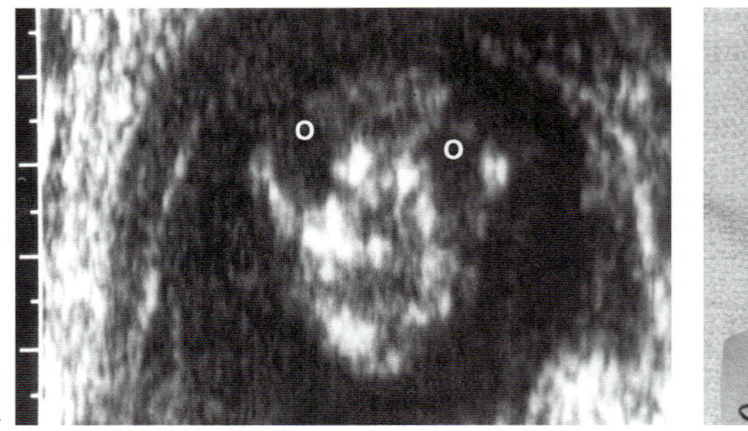
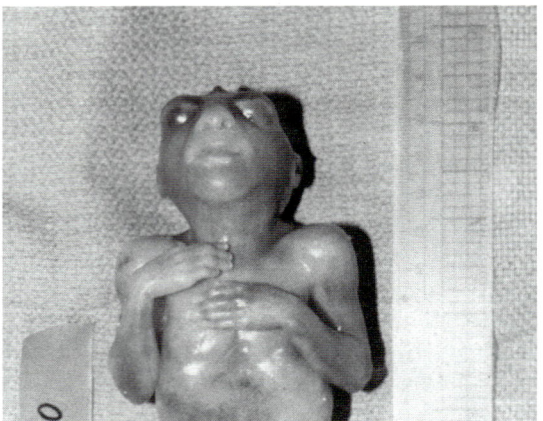

FIGURE 2. Anencephaly. **A:** Coronal scan at 16 weeks shows anencephaly with absence of brain and calvaria cephalad to the orbits (*O*). **B:** Corresponding pathologic photograph.

imaging studies,[29–31] although it lacks clear histologic confirmation.[31]

Diagnosis

The sonographic appearance of acrania in the second and third trimester is well documented. The most striking feature is absence of the calvaria above the bony orbits (Figs. 2 and 3). This is best appreciated in a coronal image of the face. The base of the skull is present, and the orbits appear prominent. The ventricles and thalami are not visualized. With anencephaly, little to no cerebral tissue is recognized, although small amounts of tissue may be seen protruding from the defect (Figs. 2 and 3). Exencephaly also shows absence of the calvaria cephalad to the orbits but with relatively normal amount of brain tissue. Exencephaly observed during the first trimester typically evolves into anencephaly (Fig. 4).

Ultrasound is highly accurate for detection of acrania during the midtrimester, with detection rates of 100%.[33,34] Vaginal sonography may be necessary when the fetal head is low in the maternal pelvis (Fig. 5). Reliable detection of acrania is also possible early in gestation, by 11 weeks if the head is carefully evaluated, and has been made as early as 9 to 10 weeks.[35] Care must be taken, however, as acrania appears as exencephaly during the first trimester and the lack of calvaria can be overlooked. In one first-trimester (10 to 14 weeks) study, sonograms were divided into two time periods. In the earliest portion of the study, acrania was diagnosed in 23 of 31 cases.[36] In the chronologically later portion of the study, after the first-trimester appearance of acrania was recognized, it was diagnosed in all 16 cases. During the first trimester, acrania may give the appearance of a Mickey Mouse face on coronal scans.[37,38] Certainly, this appearance may be confusing and could potentially be

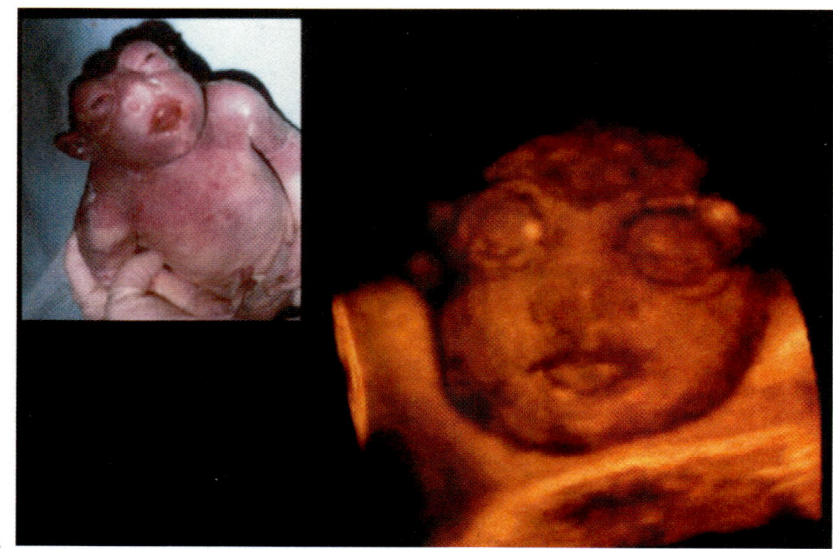

FIGURE 3. Anencephaly. **A:** Three-dimensional ultrasound shows anencephaly. **B:** Pathologic correlation. (Courtesy of Dr. R. Ximenes, San Paulo, Brazil.)

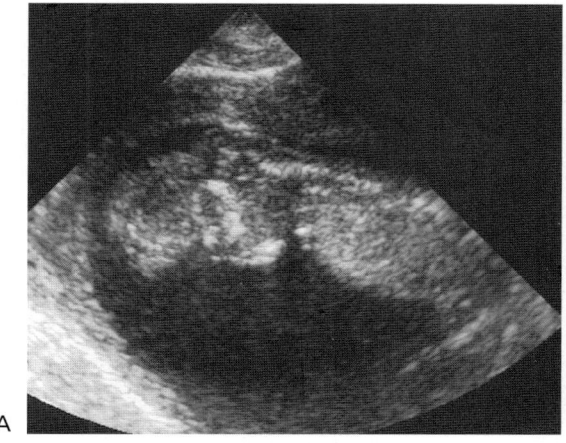
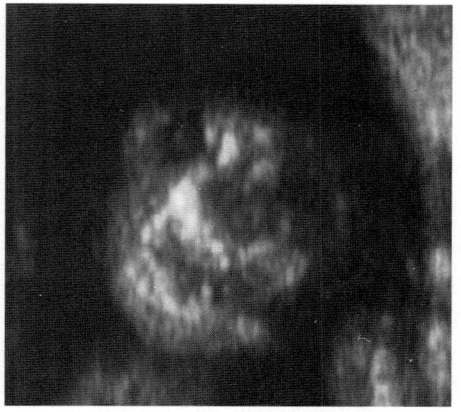

FIGURE 4. Acrania progressing to anencephaly. **A:** Scan at 12 weeks shows acrania with protruding brain lacking a calvaria. **B:** Follow-up scan at 17 weeks shows anencephaly without visible brain.

overlooked without focusing on detailed visualization of the brain and the absent calvaria.

Other associated anomalies may be detected by ultrasound, including spina bifida with or without a meningomyelocele. Recognition of these associated abnormalities, however, is of secondary importance as anencephaly in itself is a lethal condition. Polyhydramnios is common among affected fetuses with acrania after 25 weeks.

Differential Diagnosis

The correct diagnosis of acrania is not difficult, at least after the first trimester. The primary differential is distinguishing exencephaly from a large cephalocele (Table 4). Amniotic band syndrome (Fig. 6) may cause destruction of the brain

and cranial vault. The primary clues are unusual amputation defects of the calvaria and evidence of other defects elsewhere. Lack of mineralization of the skull in certain skeletal dysplasias, such as hypophosphatasias and lethal forms of osteogenesis imperfecta, show normal intracranial anatomy, and the brain is surrounded by a thick layer of tissue representing soft tissues and unossified bone. Bowing, fractures, or shortening of long bones is also evident.

Associated Anomalies

As anencephaly is rapidly lethal, most infants die early before anomalies are detected. Associated anomalies, however, were well documented in one series. These anomalies included spina bifida (27%), urinary tract anomalies

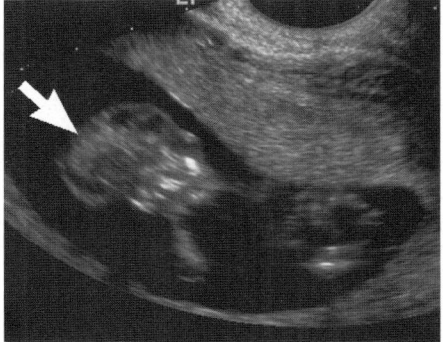

FIGURE 5. Acrania/anencephaly. Transvaginal scan in coronal plane shows protruding brain (*arrow*) with absent calvaria. This has a "Mickey Mouse" shape on coronal scans.

TABLE 4. DISTINGUISHING FEATURES OF CRANIAL DEFECTS

Anencephaly	Absent bony calvaria above orbits
	Orbits well visualized
	Absence of supratentorial brain
	Residual brain (angiomatous stroma)
	With or without spina bifida
	Polyhydramnios
Exencephaly/acrania	Calvaria absent
	Supratentorial brain tissue present but disorganized
Amniotic band syndrome	Asymmetric cephalocele
	Fixed fetal parts
	Other deformities, including limb amputation
Limb-body wall complex	Asymmetric encephaloceles
	Similar to amniotic band syndrome except fetal body to placenta
	Usually more severe than amniotic band syndrome, associated bizarre defects of fetal body, scoliosis, omphaloceles
Cephalocele	Midline defect
	Extracranial cyst or brain tissue
	With or without ventriculomegaly
	Lemon sign possible

Reproduced with permission from McGahan JP, Goldberg BG, eds. *Fetal head and brain, diagnostic ultrasound—a logical approach.* Philadelphia: Lippincott–Raven, 1998:231–270.

(16%), cleft lip and palate (10%), gastrointestinal abnormalities (6%), and cardiac abnormalities (4%).[39]

Prognosis and Management

Anencephaly is uniformly fatal, although not all infants die immediately. In a review of 181 liveborn infants with anencephaly, 40% were alive at 24 hours of age and 5% lived to 1 week of age.[40] Another study of 205 anencephalic infants weighing more than 2,500 g showed that 9% survived a week. Management is as with other lethal conditions.

Recurrence Risk

If a woman has one pregnancy with anencephaly, her risk is increased to approximately tenfold the background population risk. If she has a second pregnancy affected by anencephaly, the risk is increased to 20-fold the background population risk. Increased risk also exists for those who have relatives affected by anencephaly, with the highest risk in first-degree relatives.[41] A detailed list of risk factors is reported in Table 3. However, the risk is lower with periconceptual ingestion of folic acid.

Prevention

In 1991, the Medical Research Council Vitamin Study Group reported that the daily intake of 4 mg of folic acid periconceptually prevented 71% of recurrent NTDs in women with one affected offspring.[9] In September 1992, the U.S. Public Health Service recommended that all women attempting pregnancy take the recommended daily allowance (0.4 mg) of folate during pregnancy for 1 month before conception and for at least 3 months after conception.[10]

Amniotic Band Syndrome

Synonyms

Synonyms for amniotic band syndrome (see also Amniotic Band Syndrome in Chapter 5) include amniotic band sequence; amniotic deformities, adhesions, mutilation complex; amniotic disruption complex; amniotic bands; annular grooves; constricting bands; and Streeter bands.

Description

Amniotic band syndrome is a destructive fetal complex that is caused by disruption of the amnion. The fetus becomes entangled in these bands resulting in bizarre and asymmetrical defects that can involve the cranium base or spine.[42,43]

Incidence

The incidence for amniotic band syndrome is 1 in 1,200 live births.[44] Figures as high as 178 in 10,000 have been described in spontaneous abortions.[45]

Pathogenesis and Pathology

The precise etiology is unknown although the generally accepted theory is disruption of the amnion with fetal entanglement in the amnion. The fetus may also pass through a defect in the amnion and stick to the chorion. As the fetus grows, there is resultant asymmetrical amputation of fetal parts. If the defect occurs early in pregnancy, cranial or spinal defects may exist.[46] Others suggest a focal developmental error of connective tissue as the etiology of amniotic band syndrome to better explain the range of defects that may occur.[47–49]

Diagnosis

Amniotic band syndrome should be considered whenever unusual types of clefts are identified (Fig. 6). The presence of clefts involving more than one area should further suggest amniotic band syndrome. Asymmetrical spina defects, cephaloceles, or amputation defects of extremities should also suggest amniotic band syndrome. Facial defects can occur if the fetus swallows the amniotic band.[50,51]

Differential Diagnosis

The differential diagnosis is lengthy. This includes differential by each body part. For instance, for cranial defects caused by amniotic band syndrome, open NTDs, including

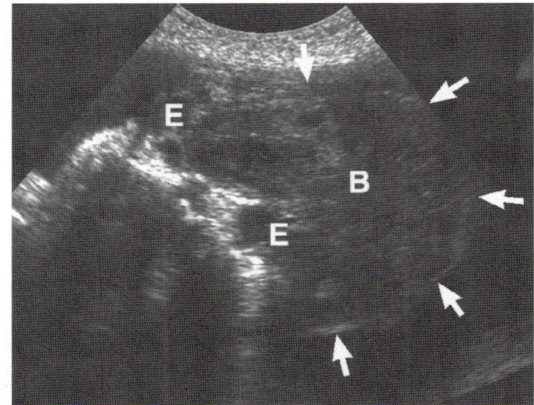

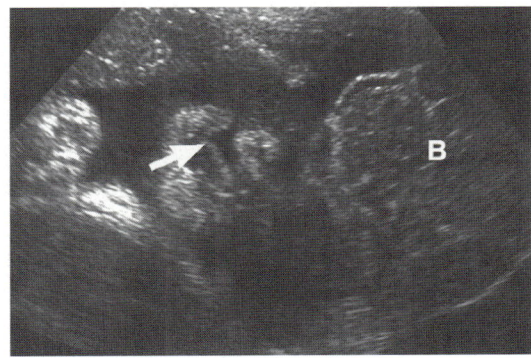

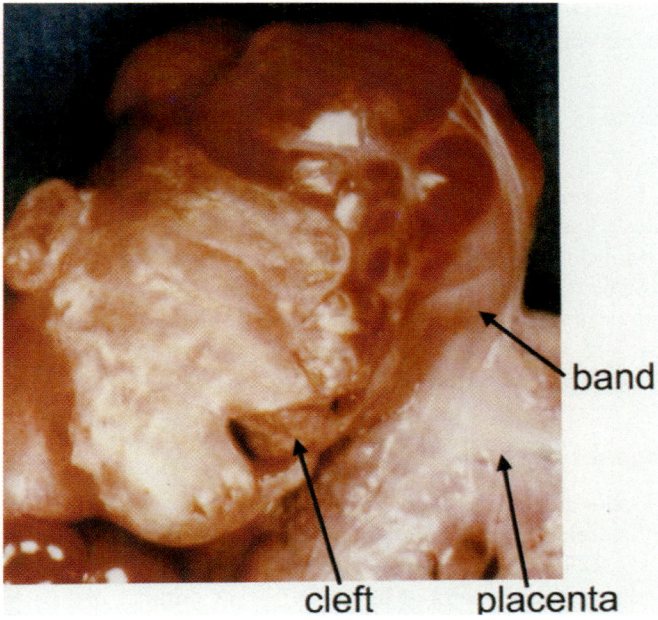

FIGURE 6. Amniotic band syndrome. **A:** Large amount of exposed brain (*B, arrows*) is identified. The eyes (*E*) are also involved and separated laterally. **B:** Coronal image shows facial cleft (*arrow*), indicating that this is not typical anencephaly alone. **C:** Pathologic photograph of similar case shows protruding brain adherent to the placenta and facial cleft secondary to amniotic bands.

anencephaly or encephaloceles, should be considered. Multisystem abnormalities favor the diagnosis of amniotic band syndrome. Limb body wall complex, also called *body stalk anomaly*, may show very similar findings. Some consider this a distinct entity from amniotic band syndrome, whereas others consider this to be a spectrum of the amniotic band syndrome.[52,53]

Associated Anomalies

Anomalies can be variable and multiple. They may vary from a single digit abnormality to major abnormalities of the cranium, face, thorax, or abdomen. Defects can include encephalocele; intra-abdominal wall defects; limb defects including asymmetrical constriction of limbs or digits; other defects including asymmetrical amputations, club feet, or amputated hands; facial clefting, which is asymmetrical; and scoliosis or thoracic deformities. No association exists with chromosome abnormalities.

Prognosis and Management

The prognosis varies considerably depending on the size and location of the defects. Defects involving the cranium,

face, spine, or thorax usually have an unfavorable outcome. More isolated defects such as limb defects have a very favorable prognosis, although they result in specific deformities such as constriction of limb digits or amputational defect. Obstetric management depends on the severity of the defect.

Recurrence Risk

The recurrence risk for amniotic band syndrome is not known to increase.

Cephalocele

Synonyms

Synonyms for cephalocele include encephalocele, cranial or occipital meningocele, cranium bifidum, encephalomeningocele, and encephalomeningocystocele.

Description

Encephaloceles are protrusions of intracranial structures through a defect in the skull. Most commonly, this herniated sac contains meninges of brain tissue (i.e., encephalocele) or less commonly only meninges (i.e., meningocele).

Incidence

Differences in type and frequency among various ethnic groups have been described. In the Western hemisphere, the incidence is between 1 to 3 per 10,000 births.[54] In Southeast Asia, the incidence is slightly higher, in the range of 1 in 5,000 live births. Occipital cephaloceles are most common in populations of European extraction, whereas frontal cephaloceles are 5 to 12 times more common than other cephaloceles in populations of Southeast Asian descent.

Pathogenesis and Pathology

Cephaloceles are a heterogenous group of disorders. Occipital cephaloceles are generally considered part of the spectrum of NTDs (i.e., anencephaly, iniencephaly, spina bifida) that are multifactorial in nature.[55,56] A number of genetic and nongenetic syndromes, however, may also occur with occipital cephaloceles (Table 5). In contrast, frontal cephaloceles are not associated with an increased risk of NTDs in first-degree relatives and, in fact, have shown some geographic predilection in some areas of Southeast Asia across diverse racial groups. This predilection suggests a possible environmental cause. Cephaloceles can be produced experimentally in animals by the administration of several teratogens, such as x-ray radiation, trypan blue, and hypervitaminosis A. Maternal obesity has been suggested to be a risk factor for cephaloceles.

Around 44 days, cranial ossification begins, proceeding dorsally and posteriorly. It is likely that the insulting event, which will result in a cephalocele, must occur at least by day 45 to 50. Etiologic theories include neural ectodermal maldevelopment (i.e., failure of anterior fusion of the neural folds with resulting failure of skull formation) as well as mesodermal maldevelopment (i.e., herniation of brain through bony malformation). Rapport et al. concluded that the presence of normal skin over a cephalocele suggests that the defect is probably more than just failure of anterior neurulation.[57] Monteagudo suggested that because cephaloceles are always smooth and rounded rather than cleft-shaped, the protrusion of brain or meninges occurs before the bony defect.[58]

Cephaloceles are commonly distinguished according to the content of the lesion and the location of the bony defect. Cephaloceles containing meninges only; brain tissue only; meninges and brain tissue; and meninges, brain tissue, and lateral ventricles are referred to as *meningocele*, *encephalocele*, *encephalomeningocele*, and *encephalomeningocystocele*, respectively. According to the site of the lesion, cephaloceles can be classified as follows: *occipital* cephaloceles occur when the defect lies between the lambdoid suture and foramen magnum; *parietal* cephaloceles occur

TABLE 5. CONDITIONS ASSOCIATED WITH CEPHALOCELES

Amniotic band syndrome (sporadic)
Multiple cephaloceles, predominantly anterior
Amputations of digits or limbs
Bizarre oral clefts
Chemke syndrome (autosomal recessive)
Hydrocephaly
Agyria
Cerebellar dysgenesis
Cryptophthalmos syndrome (autosomal recessive)
Forehead skin covers one or both eyes
Ear abnormalities
Soft tissue syndactyly
Dyssegmental dysplasia (autosomal recessive)
Short-limb dysplasia
Metaphyseal widening
Small thorax
Micrognathia
Frontonasal dysplasia (sporadic, some cases are familial)
Frontal cephalocele
Ocular hypertelorism
Meckel syndrome (autosomal recessive)
Polycystic kidneys
Polydactyly
Microphthalmia
Orofacial clefting
Ambiguous genitalia
DK-phocomelia syndrome
Agenesis of the corpus callosum
Phocomelia
Urogenital anomalies
Thrombocytopenia
Warfarin syndrome
Nasal hypoplasia
Bone stippling
Limb shortening
Hydrocephaly
Associations
   Absence of corpus callosum
   Cleft lip or palate
   Cleft lip–palate
   Craniostenosis
   Dandy-Walker syndrome
   Ectrodactyly
   Hemifacial microsomia
   Iniencephaly
   Meningomyelocele

Modified from Cohen MM Jr, Lemire RJ. Syndromes with cephaloceles. *Teratology* 1982;25:161.

between the bregma and the lambda; and *anterior* cephaloceles lie between the bregma and the anterior aspect of the ethmoid bone and are further classified into *frontal* and *basal* varieties. The *frontal* cephaloceles are always external lesions that occur near the root of the nose (glabella) and are subdivided into *nasofrontal* (i.e., a lesion protruding through the junction of the frontal and nasal bones); *nasoethmoidal* (i.e., a lesion protruding between the ethmoids, the nasal and the frontal process of the maxillary bones); and *nasoorbital* types (i.e., a lesion

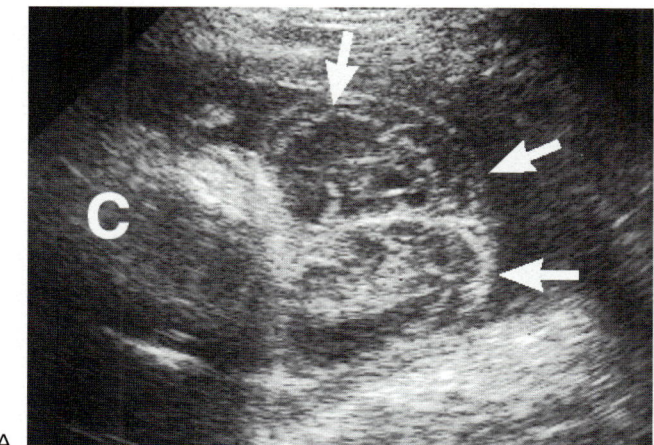

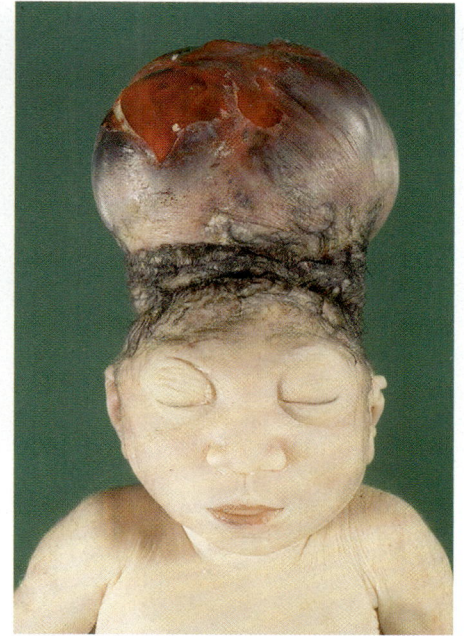

FIGURE 7. Large encephalocele. **A:** Scan of cranium (*C*) shows large amount of brain protruding posteriorly (*arrows*). **B:** Pathologic correlation.

emerging through a defect between the frontal and the lacrimal bones).

Basal cephaloceles are internal lesions that occur within the nose, the pharynx, or the orbit.

Diagnosis

Cephaloceles are highly variable in size and appearance.[59,60] Most cases are easily diagnosed on standard cranial views with brain protruding through a midline occipital defect (Figs. 7 and 8). Other cephaloceles are small and could be overlooked (Figs. 9 and 10). Some cases of cephaloceles

have been detected as early as the first trimester, especially those associated with Meckel-Gruber syndrome.[61–63]

Although, in general, ultrasound can predict the presence of brain tissue within the defect, individual cases suggest that the pathology cannot always be accurately predicted (Figs. 8 and 9). It is expected that magnetic resonance imaging (MRI) is helpful in this evaluation.

Serial examination of fetuses with cephaloceles has demonstrated that the sonographic appearance of the lesion may change throughout gestation. Transition from a solid to a fluid pattern[64] and transient disappearance have been described.[65]

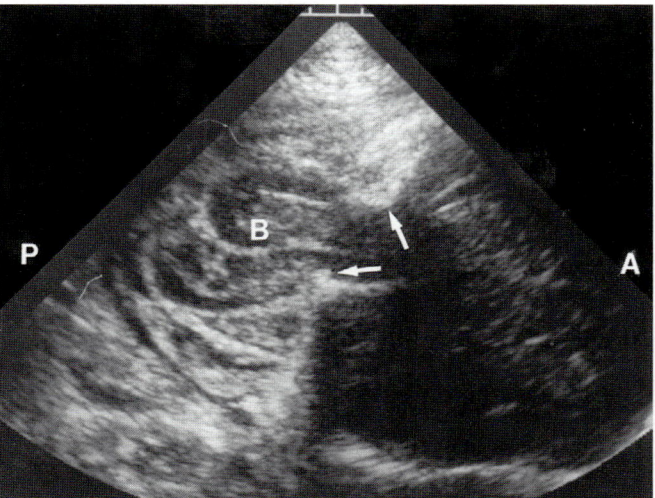

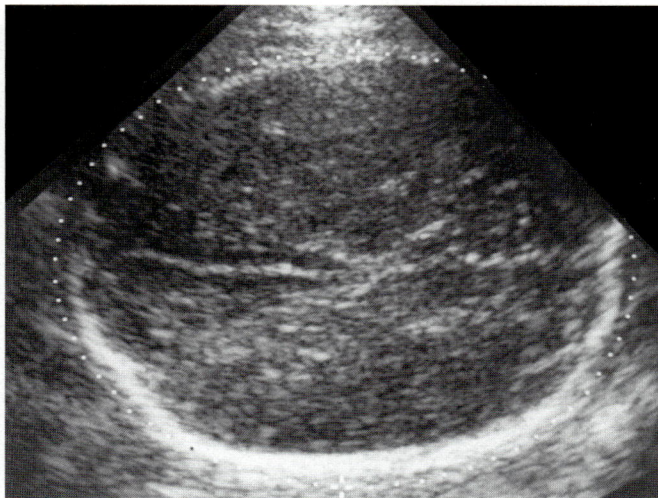

FIGURE 8. Large encephalocele. **A:** Transverse view shows defect of posterior calvaria (*arrows*) with protrusion of brain (*B*). A, anterior; P, posterior. **B:** View through mid-head shows distortion of normal brain landmarks secondary to traction by the cephalocele.

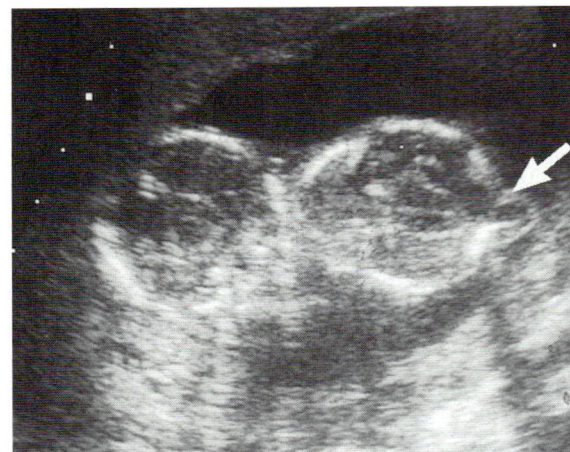

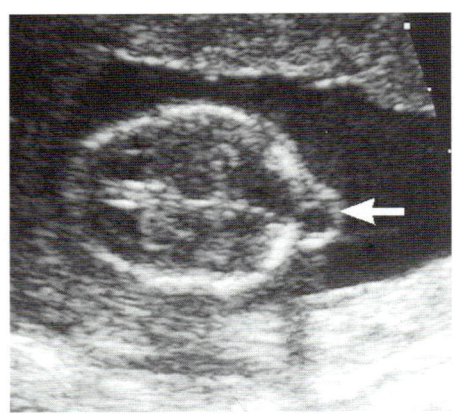

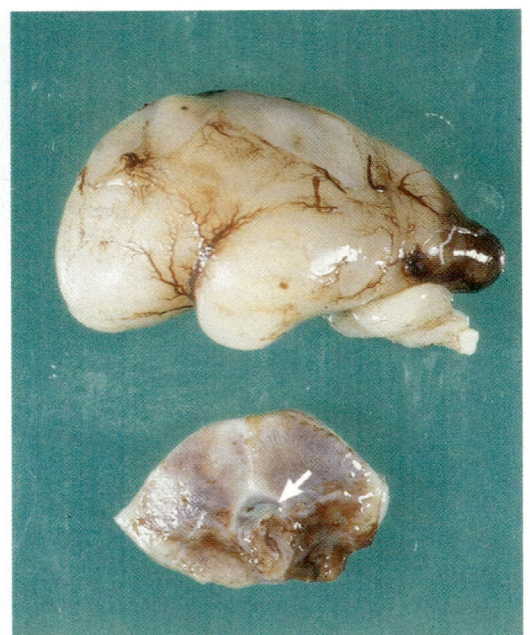

FIGURE 9. Small encephalocele. **A:** Scan at 14 weeks shows a monoamniotic twin gestation. The right twin appeared normal, whereas the left twin shows a small calvarial defect (*arrow*). **B:** Magnified view of affected twin shows posterior cephalocele (*arrow*). It appears to contain fluid, only suggesting a meningocele. **C:** Pathologic photograph shows the defect contains brain tissue and, therefore, represents an encephalocele. The tiny defect (*arrow*) of the calvaria is shown from the resected posterior skull. (Part **C** courtesy of Dr. Raj Kapur, Pathology Department, Children's Medical Center, Seattle, WA.)

Cephaloceles are often associated with other abnormal findings, similar to those encountered with open spina bifida, such as ventriculomegaly, frontal bossing, obliteration of the cisterna magna, and distortion of normal landmarks.

Anterior cephaloceles are difficult to detect, especially those protruding through the base of skull inside the pharynx. Occasional antenatal diagnoses of these lesions have been reported.[66] One clue to the diagnosis is hypertelorism because the eyes may be displaced laterally. Derangement of intracranial morphology may also suggest the correct diagnosis. MRI is expected to be useful for diagnosing anterior cephaloceles.

The use of biochemical markers such as alpha-fetoprotein has not added to diagnostic accuracy because the lesions are covered with intact meninges. One study was unable to detect even a single case of abnormally elevated alpha-fetoprotein in a series of 74 cephaloceles.[67]

Differential Diagnosis

Occipital meningocele should be easily distinguished from cystic hygromas. Demonstration of the bony defect in the skull allows a proper diagnosis but cranial meningoceles are often associated with extremely small defects that are not amenable to antenatal sonographic recognition. A more difficult, and more serious, error is to confuse a scalp hemangioma or cyst for a cephalocele (Fig. 11). A number of case reports suggest that this is possible unless care is taken to distinguish these possibilities (see also Hemangioma in Chapter 8).[68–73]

The differential diagnosis of frontal cephaloceles includes dermoid cyst of the anterior fontanelle, which may have fluid present in the mass with the presence of a bony defect,[74] and dacryocystocele. Basal cephaloceles protruding through the mouth must be differentiated from rare oral tumors such as epignathus.

Associated Anomalies

Cephaloceles are often part of specific syndromes (Table 5).[75] The Meckel-Gruber syndrome (Fig. 12) is important to recognize for counseling subsequent pregnancies because this condition carries a 25% chance of recurrence.[76] Cephaloceles are also associated with other malformations, most frequently involving the central nervous system. Overt ventriculomegaly has been reported in 80% of occipital meningoceles, 65% of occipital cephaloceles, and 15% of frontal cephaloceles.[77] Spina bifida is found in 7% to 15% of all cephaloceles.[78]

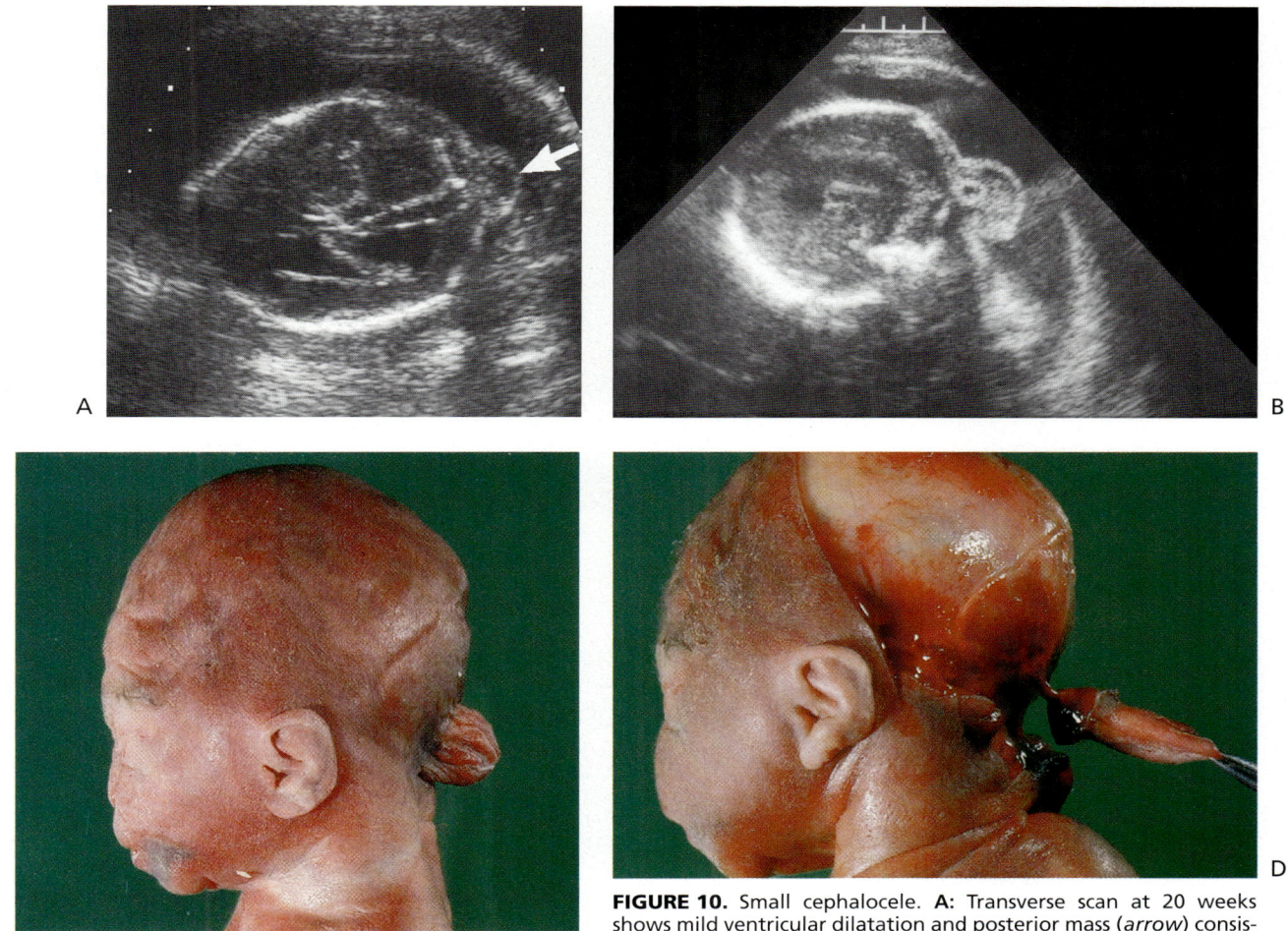

FIGURE 10. Small cephalocele. **A:** Transverse scan at 20 weeks shows mild ventricular dilatation and posterior mass (*arrow*) consistent with cephalocele. **B:** Transvaginal scan shows solid-appearing tissue, suggesting an encephalocele. **C:** Pathologic photograph shows posterior soft tissue. **D:** Further dissection shows only a small string of tissue protruding through the defect into the cephalocele.

Microcephaly was observed in 20% of cases in postnatal studies. Displacement of the cerebellum inside the cephalocele is occasionally observed, and it is referred to as *Chiari's deformity type III*. This deformity, combined with aqueductal stenosis, is the major cause of hydrocephalus in these infants. Frontal cephaloceles are often associated with median cleft face syndrome, characterized by hypertelorism and median cleft lip or palate.[79] Chromosomal aberrations have been described as well, mostly in prenatal studies.[80]

Prognosis

Ultrasound can help distinguish those with a more favorable prognosis from those with a worse prognosis.[81] The prognosis depends on the site and extent of the lesion, as well as the presence or absence of additional major abnormalities.

In two postnatal series, the overall mortality was 29% to 36%.[82,83] Mortality is usually the result of the impact of other abnormalities or the inability to repair a defect safely. Infants with posterior defects have poorer prognoses than those with anterior defects, largely because of the association with other anomalies, including other brain anomalies. Brown et al.[82] found the mortality was confined entirely to infants with posterior defects. Seizures and hydrocephalus were often secondary problems in those infants who did worse. Martinez-Lage et al.[83] reported that a favorable outcome correlated with an average head size at birth, a normal initial neurologic condition, operability of the condition, and an absence of disorders of neuronal migration.

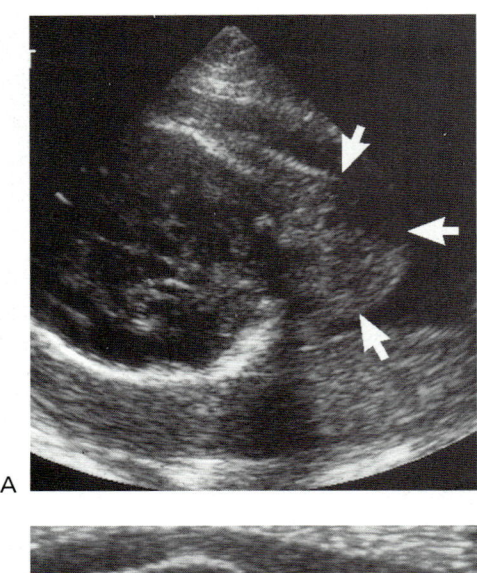

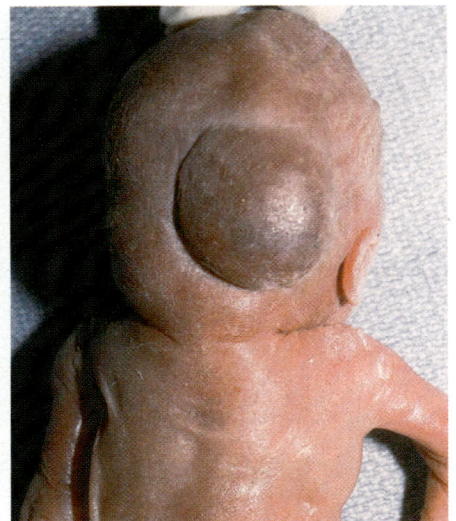

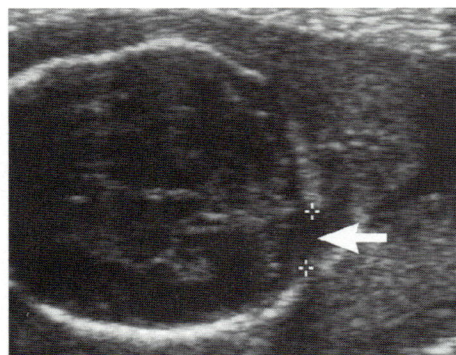

FIGURE 11. False-positive diagnosis of cephalocele. **A:** Transverse view shows soft tissue mass in occipital region (*arrows*). Note that the soft tissue mass is not midline. **B:** Artifact suggests a posterior calvarial defect (*arrow*). **C:** Pathologic correlation shows hemangioma just to right of midline. (Part **C** courtesy of Dr. Raj Kapur, Pathology Department, Children's Medical Center, Seattle, WA.)

Cephaloceles detected prenatally have a poor outcome compared to postnatal reports. This is undoubtedly related to the occipital location of most defects identified prenatally as well as the presence of brain tissue and other anomalies. On the other hand, those with a simple meningocele containing fluid or only a *nubbin* of brain tissue can survive with little or no disabilities.[81]

The influence of hydrocephalus on intellectual development is controversial. Lorber observed no significant difference in the groups of infants with and without ventriculomegaly.[55] In another series reported by Guthkelch, 86% of patients with meningocele without hydrocephalus had an IQ higher than 70, whereas only 50% of those with hydrocephalus had IQs above this level.[84]

Management

A thorough targeted ultrasound and chromosomal analysis is indicated to search for additional anomalies. MRI should also be considered to evaluate the defect and disorders of neuronal migration. In continuing pregnancies, obstetric management depends on the size of the defect, the amount of herniated brain tissue, and associated anomalies. Theoretically, a cesarean section could improve prognosis by avoiding birth trauma and contamination of brain tissue with vaginal flora.

Recurrence Risk

Recurrence risk varies with underlying etiology. Meckel-Gruber syndrome, an autosomal recessive disorder, is the most common single gene defect associated with NTDs. A number of other syndromes may be associated with cephaloceles (Table 5).

THE SPINE

The spine itself is a series of separate bony structures surrounded by muscles, ligaments, and covered by subcutaneous tissue and skin. The bony skeleton protects the spinal cord and nerve rootlets. To begin an approach to spinal anomalies requires a basic understanding of some of the embryologic events leading to formation of these structures.

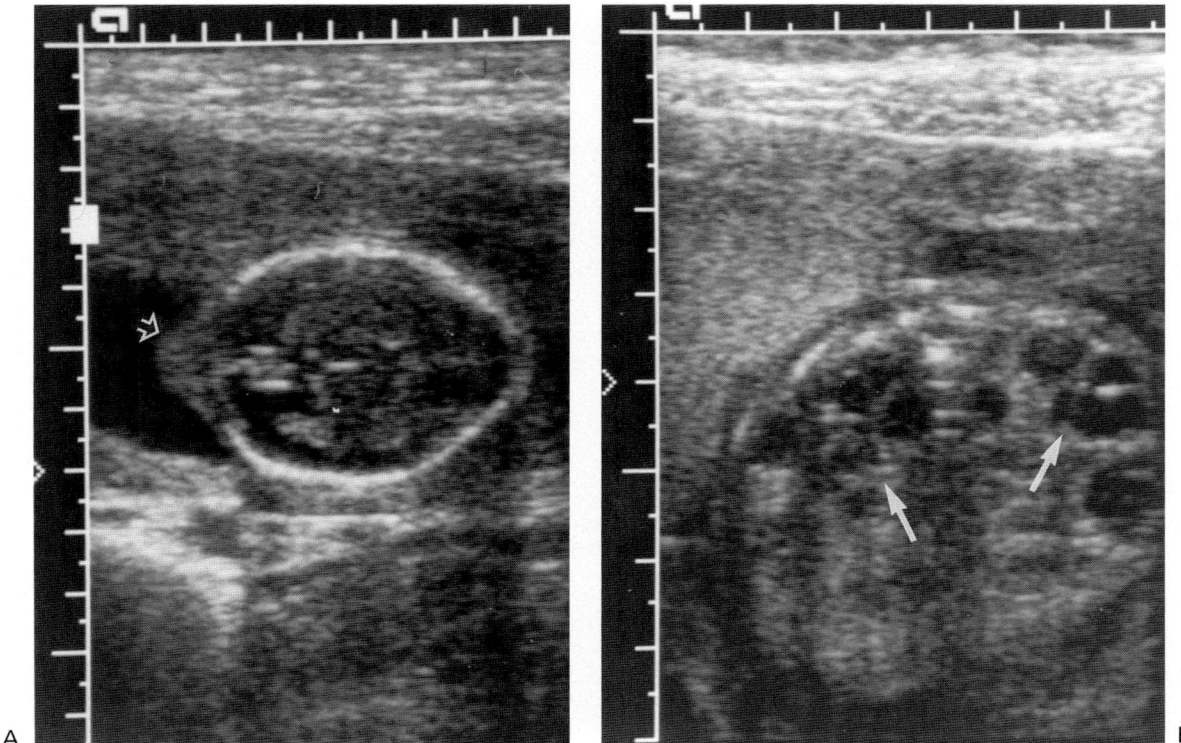

FIGURE 12. Meckel-Gruber syndrome. **A:** Small echogenic encephalocele noted in this midline occipital region (*open arrow*). **B:** Scans of the kidneys demonstrate multiple cysts of varying sizes within both kidneys (*arrows*), consistent with multicystic dysplastic kidneys. Associated polydactyly was also present in this case of Meckel-Gruber syndrome. (Reproduced with permission from McGahan JP, Coates TL, Lescale KB, et al. The fetal neck and spine. In: McGahan JP, Goldberg BB. *Diagnostic ultrasound: a logical approach.* Philadelphia: Lippincott–Raven, 1997:271–308.)

Mineralization of the spine begins in or about the sixth embryotic week (eighth menstrual week). Three ossification centers occur for each vertebra and include the vertebral body (centrum) and the lateral masses (dorsum centers or neural processes).[85] The centrum forms the vertebral body while each neural process begins ossification at the junction of the lamina and the pedicle and proceeds to form the transverse process, the spinous process, and the articular process.[86] By understanding this embryology, it is easy to understand even minor defects such as spina bifida occulta, in which there is absence of the spinous process owing to nonfusion of the two neural processes posteriorly. By approximately 13 menstrual weeks, not only is there ossification of the centrum (vertebral body), but ossification of the individual neural processes from the spine to the sacrum has begun.[87] By 16 weeks, these ossification centers can be seen sonographically, but the ossification of the lamina in the lower lumbar region is not observed until approximately 19 weeks (Fig. 13).[3,88] During the third trimester, the vertebral body, pedicles, laminae, transverse process, and spinous process may be identified sonographically (Fig. 14). Detailed scans of the spinal cord as well as the spine can be obtained in some cases (see Chapter 1).

Three basic scanning planes are used when evaluating the fetal spine. This includes the transverse (axial), sagittal, and rarely coronal views of the spine. Remembering that real-time imaging is used, the spine can be examined in a rapid and systematic approach. Many authors prefer the use of the transverse plane, as all three ossification centers can be observed in one scanning view.[89] A great deal of attention has been placed on the diagnosis of spinal defects, especially in patients with high MS-AFP levels. Previous publications, however, have shown some of these defects were difficult to recognize.[90] It has only been with the recognition of secondary cranial signs such as the *banana sign* or the *lemon head shape* that we can be more assured regarding the presence, or more commonly absence, of spinal defects.[91] However, a number of spinal abnormalities, even spinal defects, can occur without the presence of intracranial abnormalities.[92] Thus careful scanning technique is indicated. Furthermore, sagittal or coronal imaging may be helpful with vertebral anomalies such as scoliosis or hemivertebra.[93] These scan planes are helpful to localize the caudal extent of spinal cord and can be used to recognize the extent of spinal defects.

Three-dimensional ultrasound may also be used to evaluate the spine in multiple planes (Figs. 15 and 16). Unique display of the spine can be obtained with this method. Two-dimensional ultrasound, however, remains the primary means for assessing the spine.

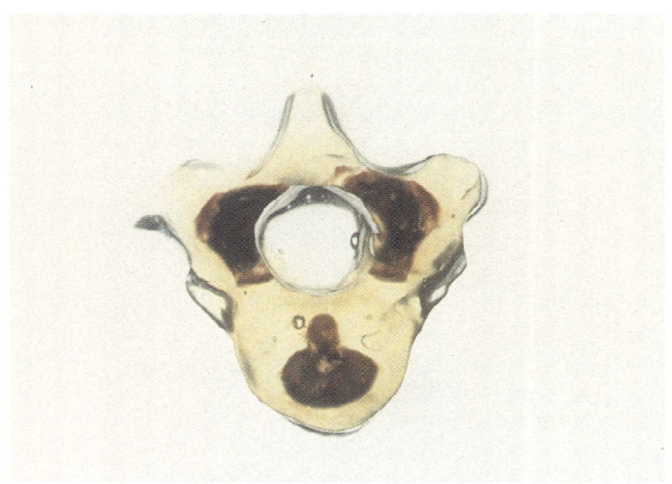
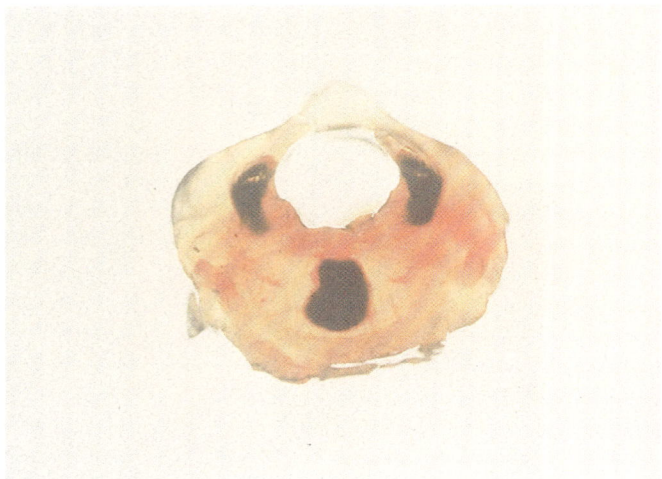

A   B

FIGURE 13. Normal spine. Histologic specimens at 18 menstrual weeks of **(A)** mid-thoracic spine (T 8) and **(B)** lower lumbar spine (L 5). Note ossification of the dorsal arch is incomplete for the lumbar spine. (Courtesy of Eric Sauerbrei, BSc, MSc, MD, FRCPC, Kingston, Ontario, Canada.)

Spina Bifida

Synonyms

Synonyms for spina bifida are spinal dysraphism, rachischisis, meningocele, and myelomeningocele.

Description

Spina bifida is a defect of the vertebrae resulting in exposure of the contents of the neural canal. In the vast majority of cases, the defect is localized to the posterior arch (dorsal) of the vertebrae. In rare cases, the defect consists of a splitting of the vertebral body. A classification of cranial and spinal dysraphism is presented in Table 6.

Incidence

The incidence for spina bifida is approximately 1 per 1,000. The epidemiologic factors of NTDs are discussed in Epidemiology. Spinal defects are more frequent in whites than in Asians or blacks and are most prevalent

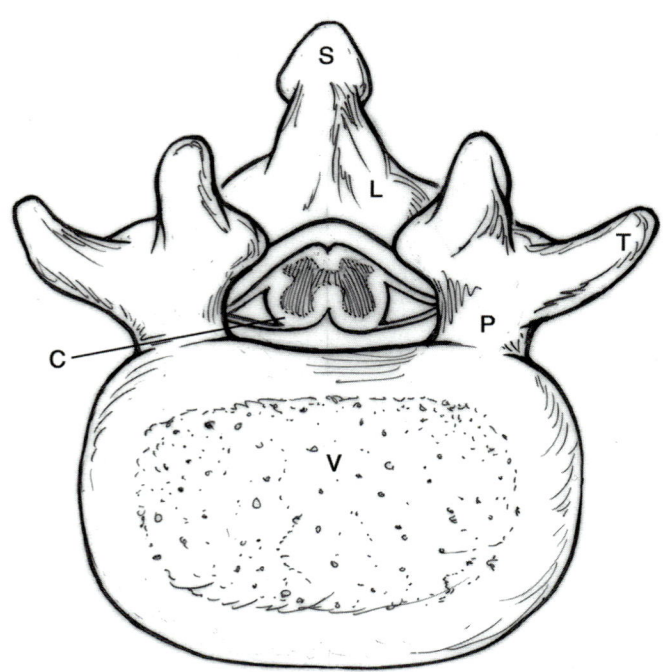

A

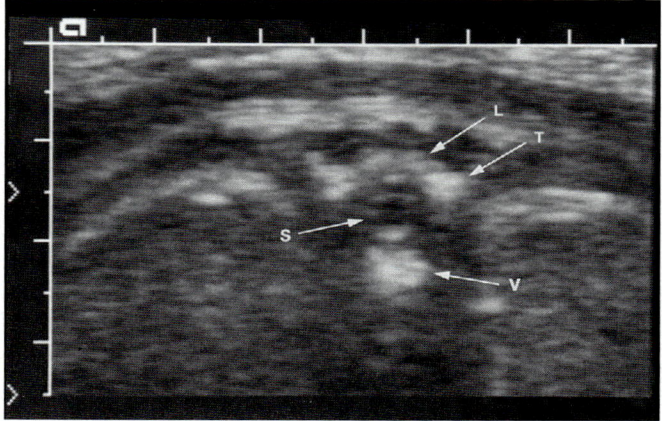

B

FIGURE 14. Normal transverse view of fetal spine. **A:** Depiction of fetal vertebra. C, spinal cord; L, lamina; P, pedicle; S, spinous process. **B:** Transverse ultrasound of the lumbar spine at 30 weeks demonstrating posterior ossification centers from which the laminae (*L*) are converging toward the midline. Note the hypoechoic spinal cord (*S*). T, transverse process; V, vertebral body. (Reproduced with permission from McGahan JP, Coates T, LeScale K, et al. In: McGahan JP, Goldberg BB, eds. *Diagnostic ultrasound: a logical approach.* Philadelphia: Lippincott–Raven, 1998.)

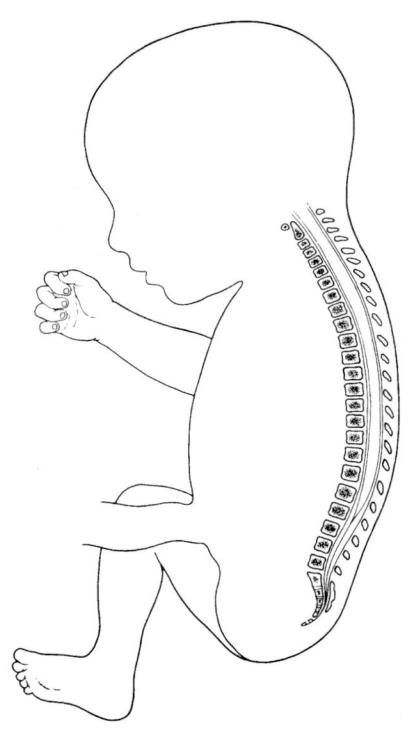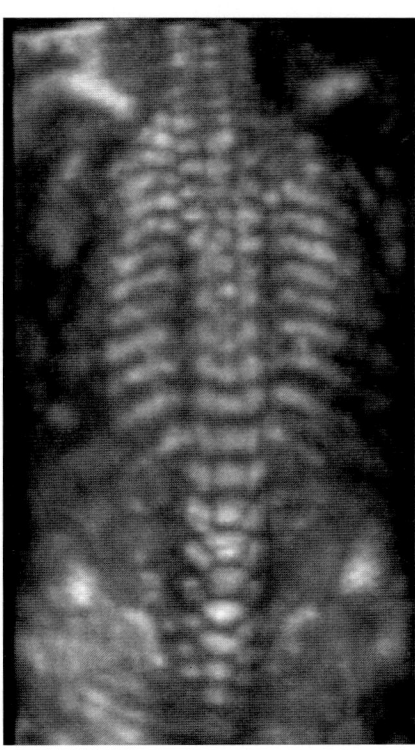

A,B

FIGURE 15. Normal sagittal spine. **A:** Sagittal view of the fetal spine demonstrating vertebral bodies and spinous processes. **B:** Three-dimensional ultrasound during third trimester shows cervical, thoracic, and lumbar spine. (Part **B** courtesy of Dr. Benoit, Nice, France.)

among Hispanics. These differences seem to persist even after migration, suggesting a genetic rather than an environmental effect.

Pathogenesis and Pathology

According to the classic arrhaphia theory, NTDs are the consequence of a primary failure of closure of the neuropores.[94] According to a more recent hydromyelic theory, dysraphism is caused by an imbalance between the production and reabsorption rate of cerebrospinal fluid in the embryonic period. Excessive accumulation of fluid in the normally closed neural tube (hydromyelia) leads to secondary separation of the dorsal wall.[95] The absence of skin and muscle directly above the defect results from failure of induction of the ectodermal and mesodermal tissues.

Spina bifida encompasses a broad spectrum of abnormalities. Lesions are commonly subdivided into ventral and dorsal defects. Ventral defects are extremely rare and are characterized by the splitting of the vertebral body and the occurrence of a cyst that is neuroenteric in origin. The lesion is generally seen in the lower cervical or upper thoracic vertebrae. Dorsal defects are by far the most common. They are subdivided into two types: spina bifida occulta and spina bifida aperta. Spina bifida occulta represents approximately 15% of the cases and is characterized by a small defect completely covered by skin. In many cases, this condition is completely asymptomatic and is diagnosed only incidentally at radiographic examination of the spine. In other instances, there is an area of hypertrichosis, pigmented or dimpled skin, or the presence of subcutaneous lipomas.[96] A dermal sinus connecting the skin to the verte-

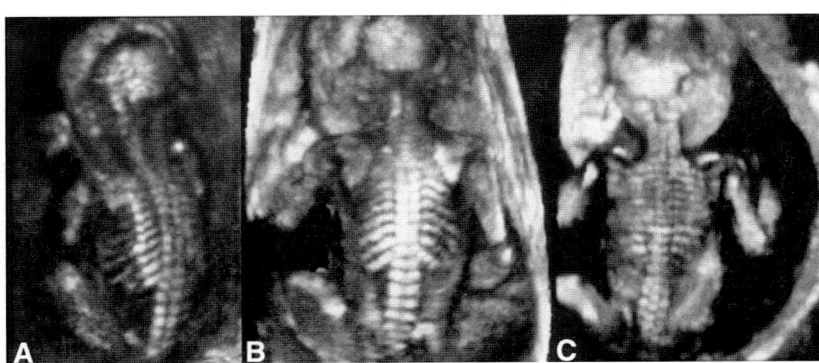

FIGURE 16. **A–C:** Views of spine from three different fetuses. (Reproduced with permission from Bega G, Lev-Toaff A, Kuhlman K, Kurtz A, Goldberg B, et al. Three-dimensional ultrasonographic imaging in obstetrics: present and future applications. *J Ultrasound Med* 2001;20:391–408.)

TABLE 6.   CLASSIFICATION OF CRANIAL AND SPINAL DYSRAPHISM

Spina bifida aperta
  Myeloschisis
  Myelomeningocele
  Hemimyelomeningocele
  Syringomyelomeningocele
  Spinal meningocele
Arnold-Chiari malformation
Dandy-Walker malformation
Cranium bifidum
  Cranial meningocele
  Encephalomeningocele
Occult cranial dysraphism
  Cranial dermal sinus
Occult spinal dysraphism
  Spinal dermal sinus
  Tethered cord syndrome
  Lumbosacral lipoma
  Diastematomyelia
  Neurenteric cyst
  Combined anterior and posterior spina bifida
  Anterior sacral meningocele
  Occult intrasacral meningocele
Nondysraphic malformations
  Perineurial (Tarlov's) cyst
  Spinal extradural cyst
  Nondysraphic spinal meningocele
  Caudal regression syndrome
  Sacrococcygeal teratoma

Reproduced with permission from Youmans JR. *Neurological surgery.* Philadelphia: WB Saunders, 1982:1082.

brae and to the dura mater can occasionally be seen. The clinical importance of this lesion is its frequent association with infection of the neural contents.

Spina bifida aperta is the most frequent lesion, resulting in 85% of dorsal defects. The neural canal may be exposed, or a thin meningeal membrane may cover the defect. More often, the lesion appears as a cystic tumor (spina bifida cystica). If the tumor contains purely meninges, the lesion is referred to as a *meningocele*. More frequently, neural tissue is part of the mass, and the name *myelomeningocele* is used (Fig. 17). The term *myeloschisis* is sometimes used to refer to a condition in which the spinal cord is widely opened dorsally and is part of the wall of the myelomeningocele. The vertebrae are lacking the dorsal arches, and the pedicles are typically spread apart.[97] Rarely, a meningocele may be covered by intact skin.

Diagnosis

The diagnosis of spina bifida has been greatly enhanced by the recognition of associated abnormalities in the skull and brain. These are among the most powerful prenatal screening *markers* available to every sonographer who performs obstetric ultrasounds. These abnormalities include frontal bone scalloping (lemon sign) and obliteration of the cisterna magna with either an *absent* cerebellum or abnormal anterior curvature of the cerebellar hemispheres (banana sign) (Fig. 18).[98–106] These easily recognizable alterations in skull and brain morphology are often more readily attainable than detailed spinal views. Ventricular dilatation is a less reliable finding during the second trimester.

The sensitivity of cranial signs in identifying spina bifida exceeds 99%.[107] Obliteration of the cisterna magna is the most consistent of the cranial findings due to compression of the posterior fossa as part of the Arnold-

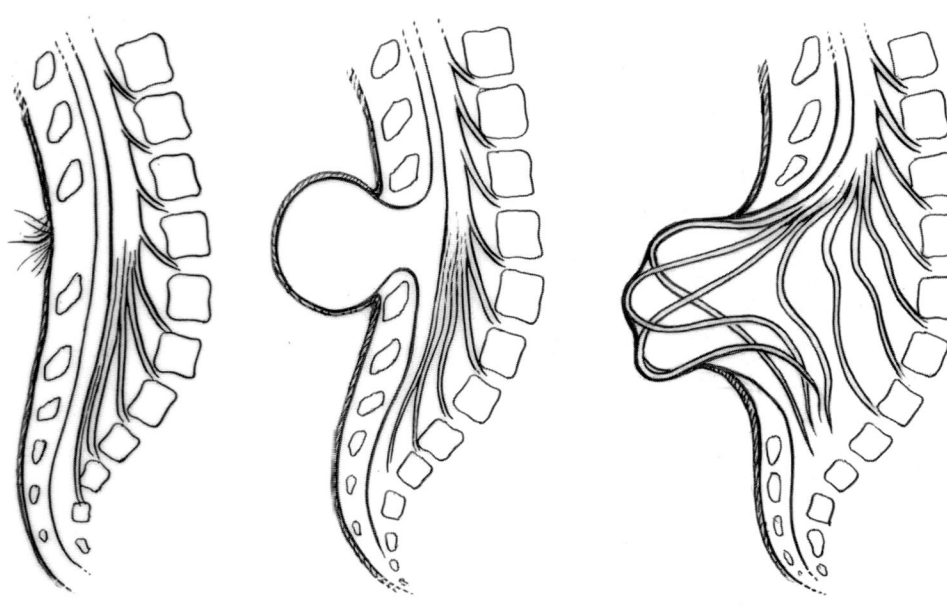

A–C

FIGURE 17. Classification of spina bifida. **A:** Spina bifida occulta is characterized by a defect in one or more vertebrae, but intact skin and no alternation in the spinal cord. **B:** Meningocele is characterized by protrusion of meninges and cerebrospinal fluid through the spinal defect. **C:** Myelomeningocele is characterized by protrusion of neural elements as well as meninges through the spinal defect.

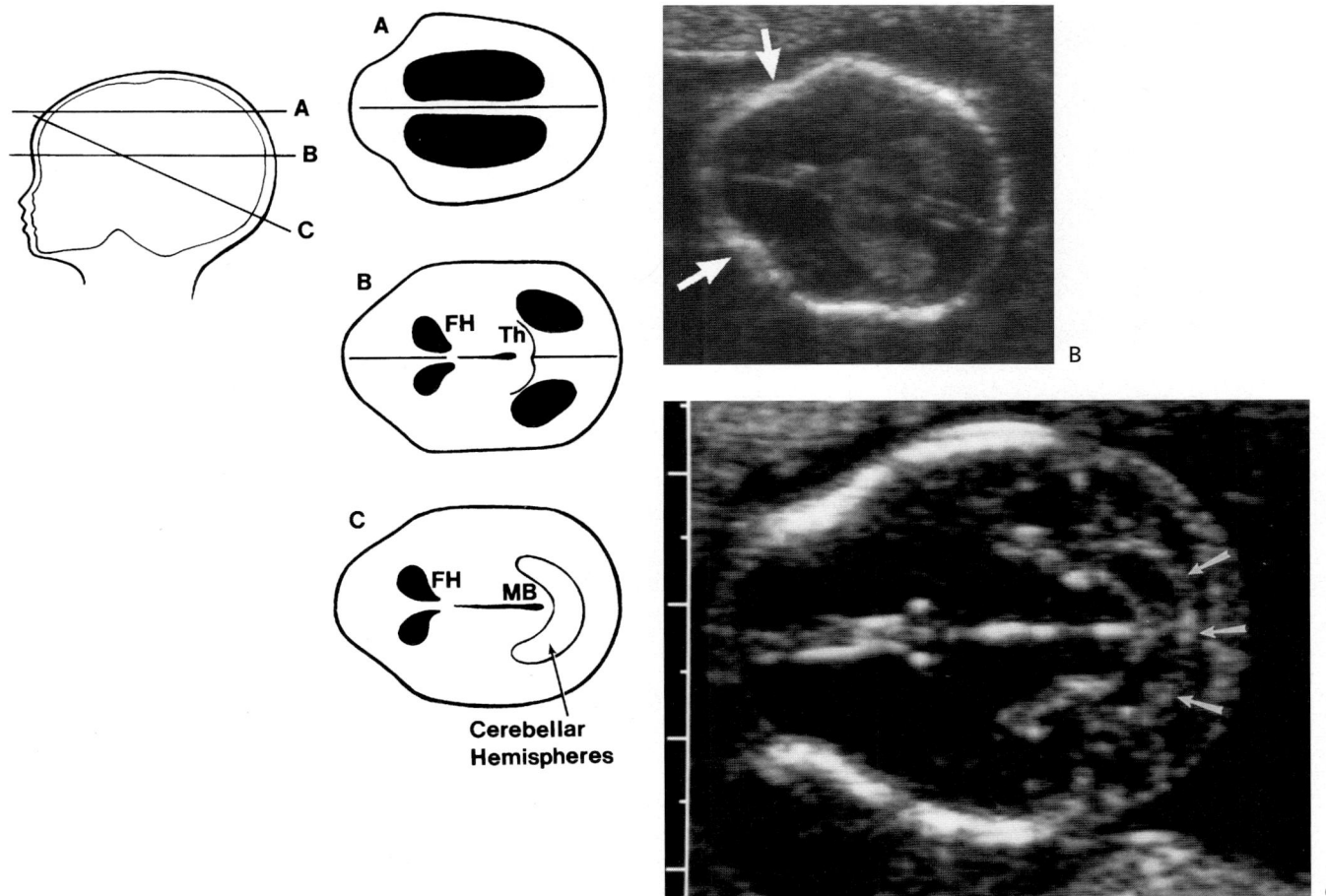

FIGURE 18. Cranial findings associated with spina bifida. **A:** Diagram demonstrating the typical cranial findings associated with spina bifida during the second trimester—the lemon-shaped calvaria, dilatation of the lateral cerebral ventricles (typically borderline or mild), and obliteration of the normal cisterna magna with distortion of the cerebellum to form the banana sign. FH, frontal horn; MB, midbrain; Th, thalamus. **B:** Axial ultrasound in the fetal head demonstrates bifrontal deformity of the calvaria (*arrows*) or so-called lemon sign. Note the absence of ventricular dilatation in this case. **C:** Scan of the posterior fossa demonstrates compression of the cerebellar hemispheres, or so-called banana sign (*arrows*). Complete obliteration of the cisterna magna exists.

Chiari malformation. This also can be visualized on MRI (Fig. 19). The cisterna magna should be sought and visualized in virtually all normal fetuses during the second and early third trimesters. Demonstration of a normal cisterna magna is reassuring in high-risk pregnancies and nearly eliminates the possibility of the Arnold-Chiari malformation, whereas obliteration of the cisterna magna should suggest a spinal defect. Available evidence suggests that false-negatives are probably limited only to cases with lipomeningoceles, meningoceles, or very low myelomeningoceles associated with an excellent prognosis. False-positives are virtually nonexisting for the cerebellar signs. The lemon sign is found however in 1% of normal fetuses.

A variable degree of ventricular enlargement is present in approximately 90% of cases of open spina bifida at birth, but in only approximately 70% of cases in the midtrimester. Even when present, only a minority of cases shows moderate to severe ventricular dilatation during the second trimester (Fig. 20), and in most cases it is borderline or mild.

The diagnosis of spina bifida obviously requires detection of the spinal defect itself, although this, perhaps surprisingly, is less helpful than the cranial findings for screening of spina bifida during the second trimester. With spina bifida, the lateral processes are separated, and the neural canal is exposed posteriorly. The skin and muscles above the defect are absent. With open spina bifida, the posterior line and over-

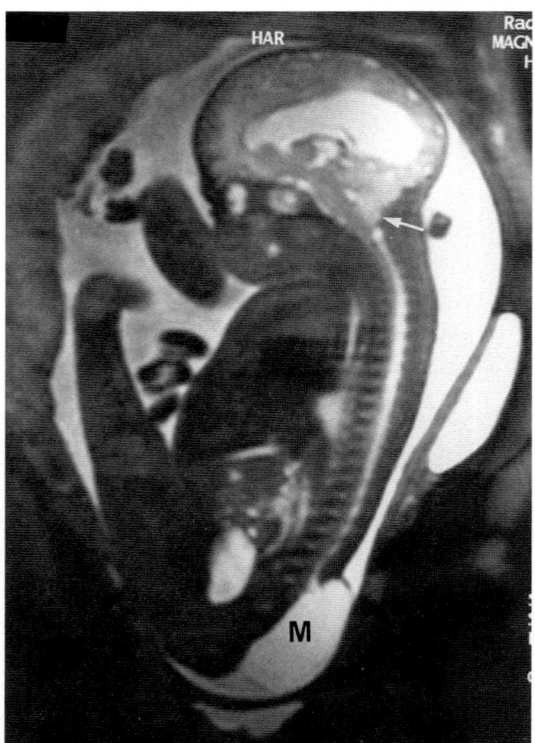

FIGURE 19. Sagittal magnetic resonance imaging scan (half-Fourier acquisition single-shot turbo spin-echo sequence) at 37 weeks shows myelomeningocele (*M*) of lumbar spine and Arnold-Chiari malformation with inferior herniation of cerebellar vermis (*arrow*). Hydrocephalus is also evident. (Reproduced with permission from Poutamo J, Vanninen R, Partanen K, et al. Magnetic resonance imaging supplements ultrasonographic imaging of the posterior fossa, pharynx and neck in malformed fetuses. *Ultrasound Obstet Gynecol* 1999;13:327–334.)

lying soft tissues are absent at the level of the lesion (Figs. 21 and 22). The appearance of the spinal defect is variable, however (Fig. 23). The spinal defect may be difficult to detect in some cases, in which case endovaginal ultra-

sound may be helpful (Fig. 24). It is uncertain whether three-dimensional ultrasound (Fig. 25) may add diagnostic information.

A surrounding myelomeningocele sac may or may not be present. The presence of a sac certainly aids the diagnosis of the spinal defect (Figs. 24 and 25) whereas the absence of a sac can make detection difficult (Fig. 23A). This myelomeningocele sac should not be confused for a skin-covered defect, however.

Ultrasound can predict the location and extent of the spinal defect with a high degree of accuracy. Sagittal and coronal views are most useful in this evaluation.[108] Closed spinal defects are extremely difficult to diagnose, with the possible exception of lipomeningoceles (Figs. 26 and 27).

The accuracy in the diagnosis of spina bifida depends heavily on the experience of the operator, the quality of the equipment, and the amount of time dedicated to the scan. We believe the accuracy of referral centers should be close to 100%, in large part due to recognition of associated cranial findings. The fact that not all centers have reached this rate means further improvements in overall screening for fetal anomalies can be expected.

The accuracy of routine nontargeted examinations is uncertain. In the RADIUS (routine antenatal diagnostic imaging with ultrasound) trial, in which routine ultrasound was performed in conjunction with maternal AFP screening, the sensitivity was 80%.[109] In a survey of European centers, Boyd et al.[110] reported overall sensitivity of 75%, but large variation between centers from 33% to 100%. In one retrospective study conducted in Great Britain, the estimated sensitivity was marginally higher for serum AFP screening, 84% to 92%, than for ultrasound screening, 70% to 84%.[111] In all of these studies, it is unclear whether the cranial signs of fetal spina bifida were systematically researched. In a more recent retrospective multicentric study using the cranial signs, the sensitivity of ultrasound was 85%.[112]

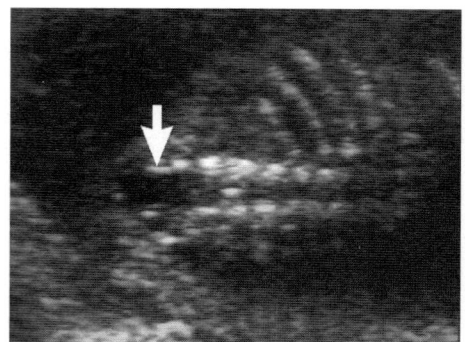

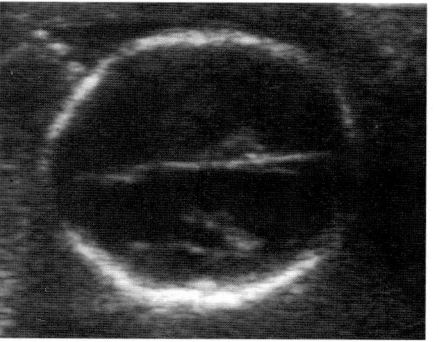

FIGURE 20. Ventricular dilatation and spina bifida. **A:** Longitudinal scan of lumbothoracic spine shows large lumbar defect (*arrow*). **B:** Moderate dilatation of the lateral ventricles (16 mm) is present on this transverse view of head.

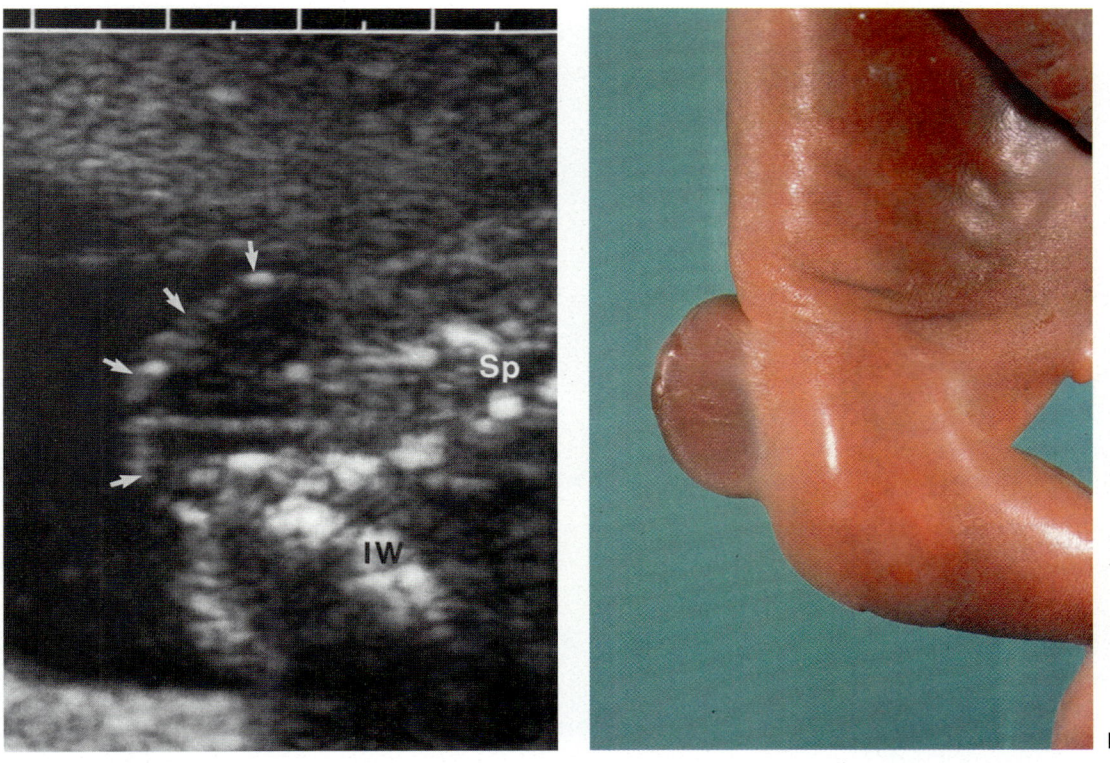

FIGURE 21. Cystic myelomeningocele. **A:** Longitudinal view of lumbar spine (*Sp*) shows cystic myelomeningocele (*arrows*). IW, iliac wing. **B:** Pathologic correlation, lateral view, confirms prenatal findings.

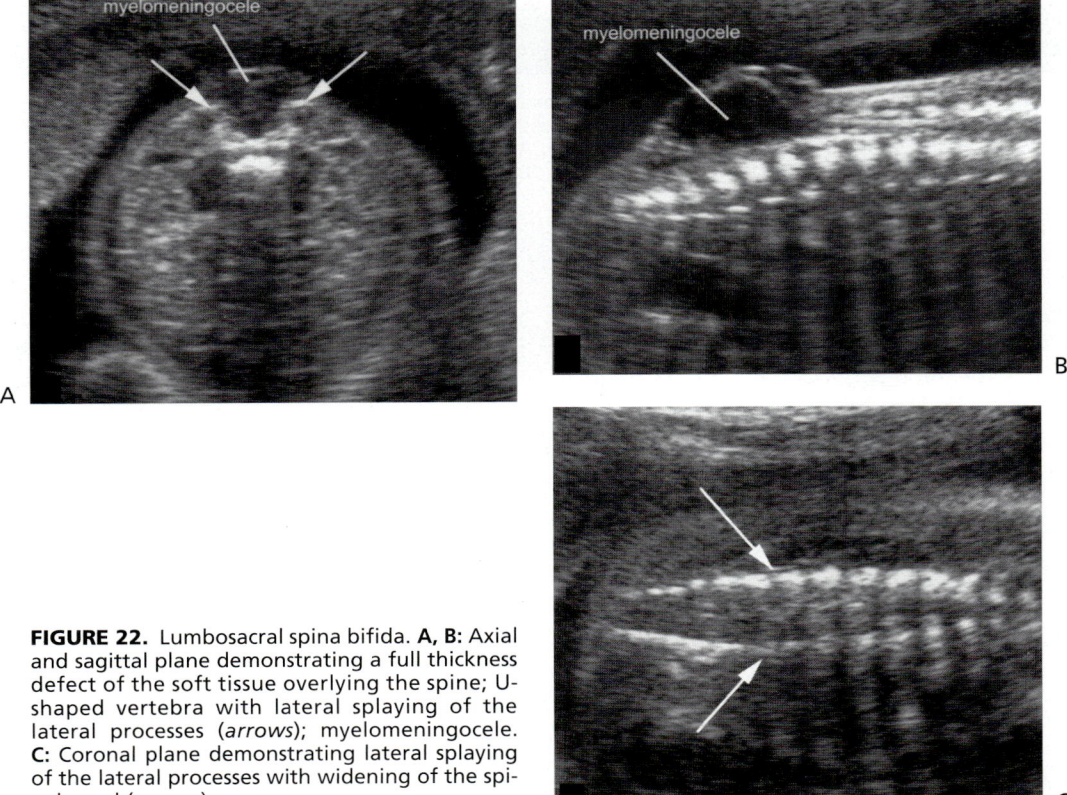

FIGURE 22. Lumbosacral spina bifida. **A, B:** Axial and sagittal plane demonstrating a full thickness defect of the soft tissue overlying the spine; U-shaped vertebra with lateral splaying of the lateral processes (*arrows*); myelomeningocele. **C:** Coronal plane demonstrating lateral splaying of the lateral processes with widening of the spinal canal (*arrows*).

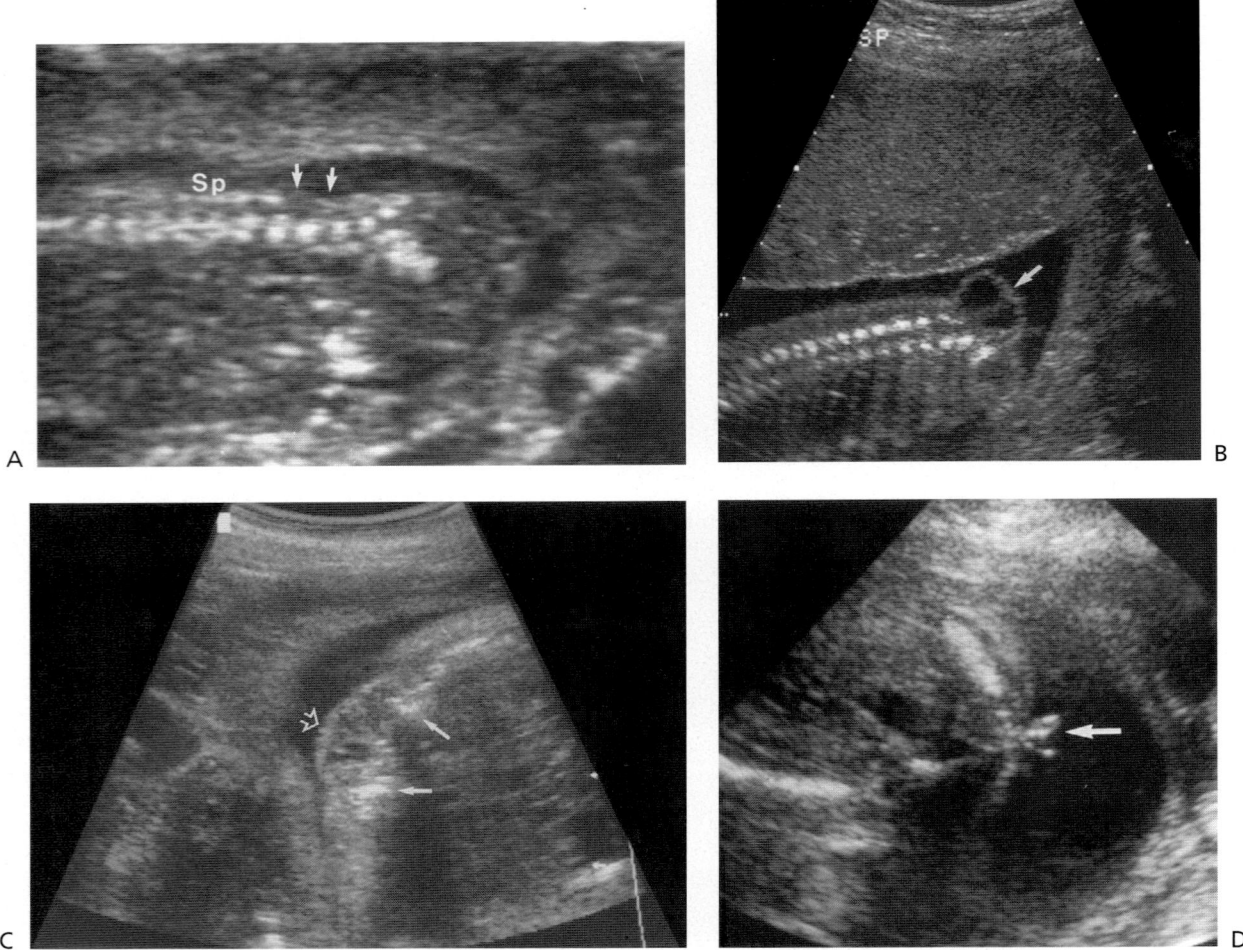

FIGURE 23. Variable appearance of neural tube defects. **A:** Sagittal scan showing a flat nonprotruding defect (*arrows*). Sp, spine. **B:** Cystic-appearing dorsal sac (*arrow*). **C:** Transverse scan shows solid-appearing dorsal sac (*open arrow*). Also note splaying of the posterior elements of the spine (*solid arrows*). **D:** Unusual appearing "tag" (*arrow*) was the only evidence for a closed lipomeningocele.

Lipomeningoceles are a variation of spinal dysraphism. They may be associated with tethered spinal cord and an echogenic lipoma within the spinal canal. This lipoma may protrude through the spinal dysraphism and be detected as an echogenic mass (lipoma) posterior to the lumbosacral spine. This midline mass almost has the appearance of the fetal tail (Figs. 26B and 27C). Careful scanning of the rest of the fetus should be performed to exclude associated abnormalities.

Differential Diagnosis

Cystic sacrococcygeal teratomas should be considered when cystic myelomeningocele is diagnosed (Table 7). The presence of cranial findings should help distinguish these possibilities in most cases. Incorrect angling can artifactually create the appearance of spinal defects. A mild degree of a *lemon* sign may be seen in 1% of normal fetuses during the second trimester, whereas false-positive diagnoses of cerebellar findings are virtually nonexistent when adequate views of the posterior fossa are obtained.

Associated Anomalies

The two main categories of anomalies associated with spina bifida are other central nervous system defects and foot deformities. In almost all cases of spina bifida aperta, Chiari's malformation type II is present. This malformation is characterized by a herniation of the cerebellar vermis through the foramen magnum and downward displacement of the fourth ventricle inside the neural canal. The posterior fossa is shallow, and the tentorium is displaced

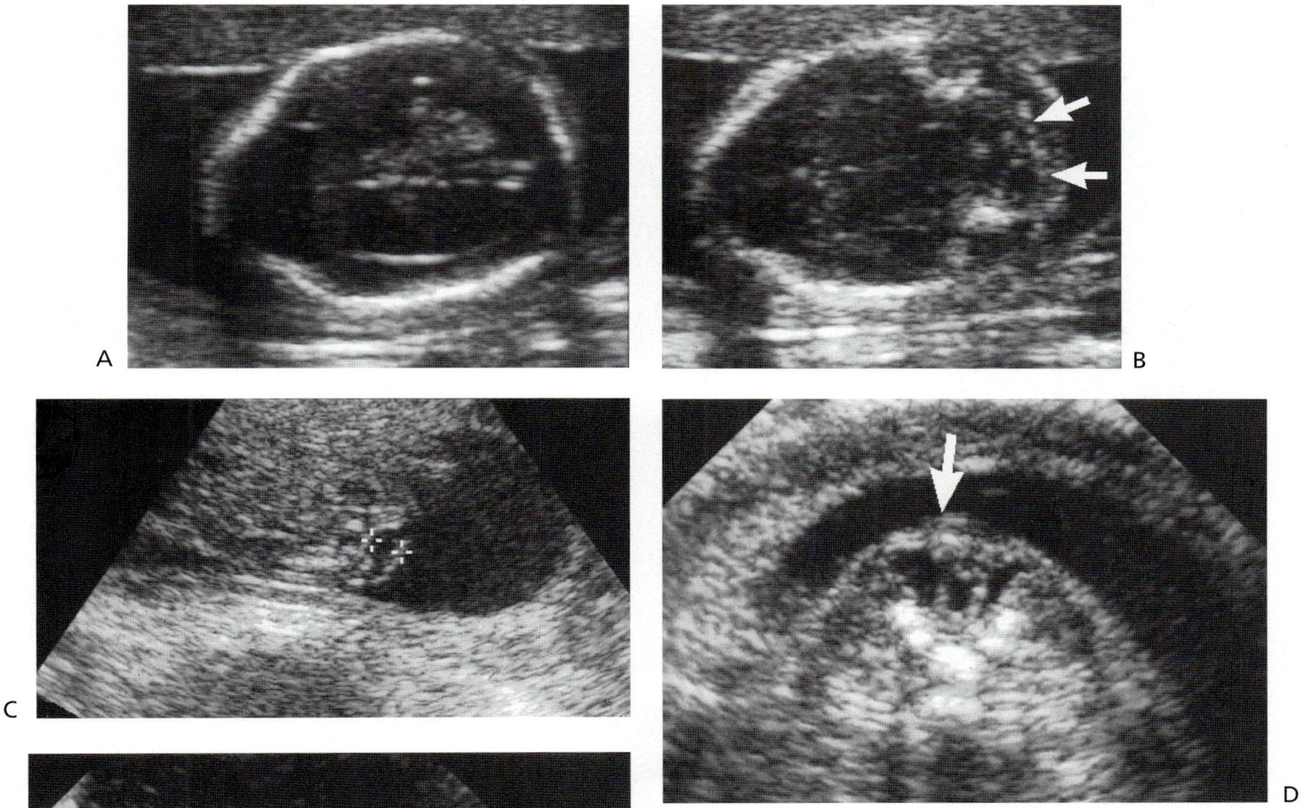

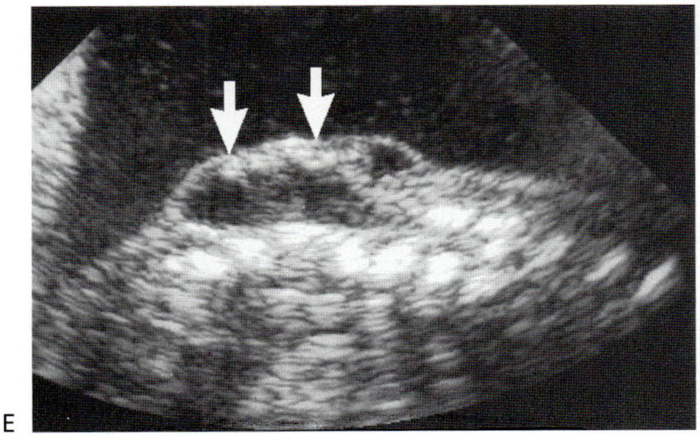

FIGURE 24. Transvaginal scan of cystic myelomeningocele. **A:** View at ventricular level at 17 weeks shows lemon-shaped calvaria and mild dilatation of the lateral cerebral ventricles. **B:** View through posterior fossa shows obliteration of cisterna magna (*arrows*). **C:** Transabdominal view shows small cystic defect of lower spine. **D:** Transverse and longitudinal **(E)** views, with transvaginal scanning, better show the extent of the spinal defect (*arrows*).

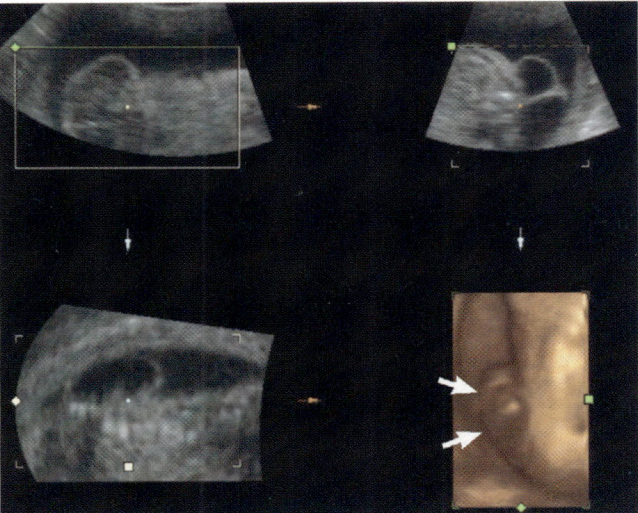

FIGURE 25. Three-dimensional ultrasound of cystic myelomeningocele (*arrows*). Three-dimensional ultrasound at 22 weeks shows cystic myelomeningocele in three orthogonal planes plus surface-rendered view **(bottom right)**.

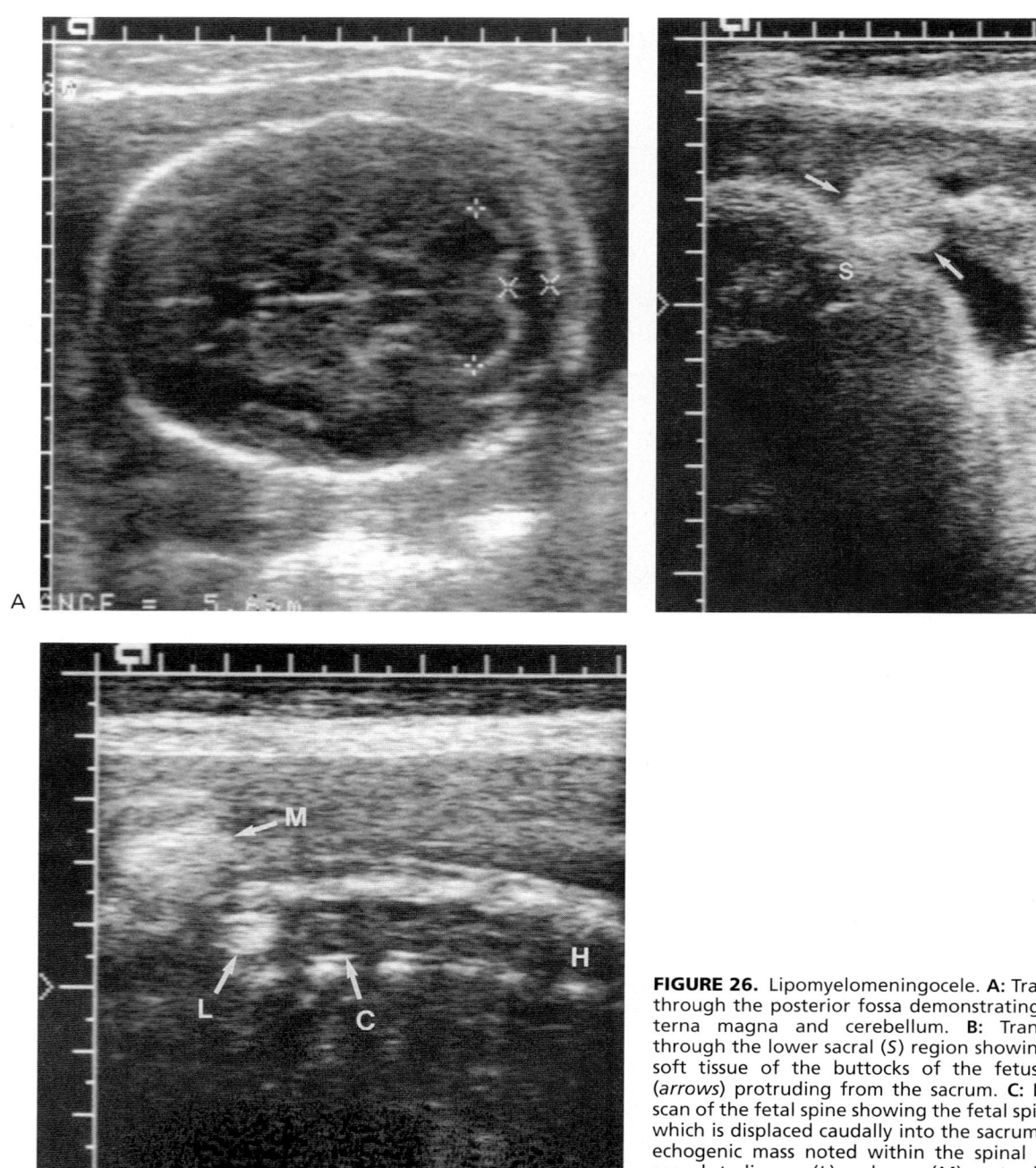

FIGURE 26. Lipomyelomeningocele. **A:** Transverse scan through the posterior fossa demonstrating normal cisterna magna and cerebellum. **B:** Transverse scan through the lower sacral (*S*) region showing symmetric soft tissue of the buttocks of the fetus with mass (*arrows*) protruding from the sacrum. **C:** Longitudinal scan of the fetal spine showing the fetal spinal cord (*C*), which is displaced caudally into the sacrum. Associated echogenic mass noted within the spinal canal corresponds to lipoma (*L*) and mass (*M*) protruding through the spinal canal external to the fetus. H, toward the head of the fetus. (Reproduced with permission from Kim S, McGahan JP, Boggan J, et al. Prenatal diagnosis of lipomyelomeningocele. *J Ultrasound Med* 2000;19:801.)

downward. Displacement and kinking of the medulla are also observed.

Arnold-Chiari malformation is almost invariably associated with obstructive hydrocephalus. The genesis of hydrocephalus seems to be related to the low position of the exit foramen of the fourth ventricle, which drains the cerebrospinal fluid inside the spinal canal. The cerebellum that obstructs the foramen magnum then blocks reentry of the fluid to the intracranial cavity. In many cases, deformities of the aqueduct are found, and these are believed to be secondary to ventricular enlargement and brain stem compression.[113]

Dislocations of the hip and foot deformities (e.g., clubfoot, rockerbottom foot) are frequently seen in association with spina bifida (Fig. 28). The pathogenesis of the malformation is related to the unopposed action of muscle groups

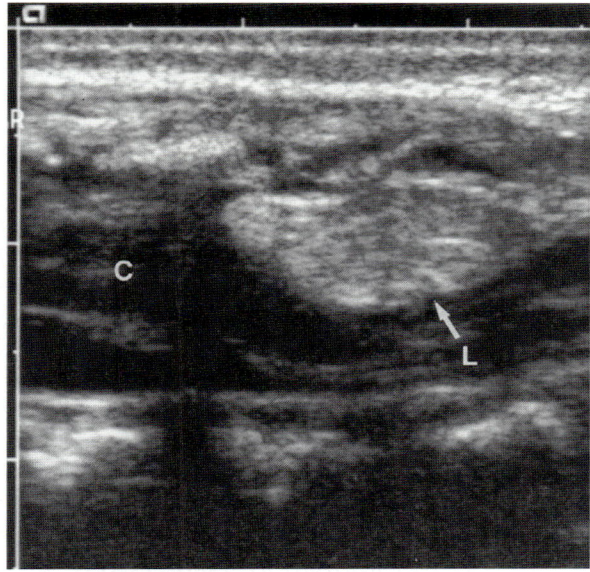

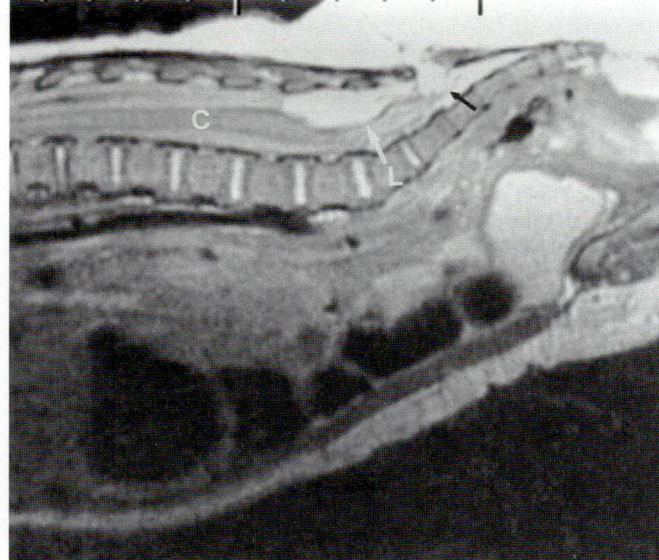

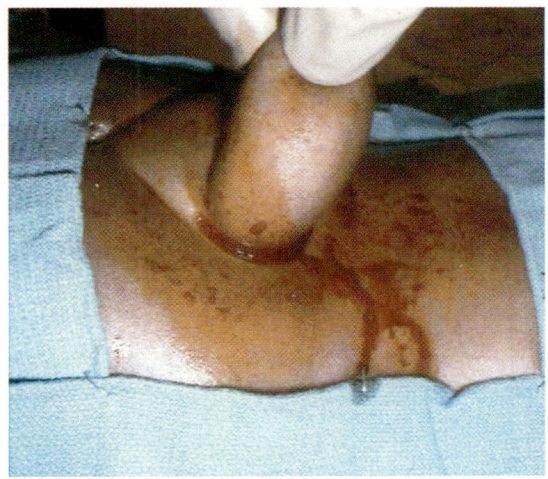

FIGURE 27. Postnatal imaging of lipomyelomeningocele. **A:** Sagittal ultrasound obtained posteriorly through the sacrum showing the spinal cord (*C*), which extends into the lower sacral region and is displaced dorsally by echogenic mass corresponding to lipoma (*L*). **B:** Postnatal magnetic resonance imaging fast spin-echo proton density–weighted sequence (TR, 3750 MS; TE, 33.3 MS) shows spinal cord (*C*), which extends into the lower sacral region and is displaced by high-intensity mass corresponding to the lipoma (*L*). Also note extension of the high-intensity signal (*black arrow*) posterior to the sacrum. **C:** Gross specimen obtained at the time of surgery showing the subcutaneous lipoma being held by the surgeon's fingers. (Reproduced with permission from Kim S, McGahan JP, Boggan J, et al. Prenatal diagnosis of lipomyelomeningocele. *J Ultrasound Med* 2000;19:801.)

because of a defect of the peripheral nerve corresponding to the involved myotomes.[114]

Prognosis

Spina bifida is associated with a high stillbirth rate. Approximately 20% of liveborn infants that undergo surgery die in the first year of life, and approximately 35% die within the first 5 years.[115] Approximately 50% of individuals reach an intellectual quotient greater than 80. Twenty-five percent of patients are totally paralyzed, 25% are almost totally paralyzed, 25% require intense rehabilitation, and only 25% have no significant lower limb dysfunction. Only 17% of infants at late follow-up have normal continence.[1] It is impossible to predict precisely *in utero* the outcome of affected fetuses. Prognostic factors include the level and extent of the lesion (Table 8).

All infants with spina bifida have some degree of Arnold-Chiari malformation. However, only in a relative minority of cases this condition is symptomatic (e.g., dyspnea, swallowing difficulties, opisthotonus) and represents a potentially fatal complication. Death is usually related to respiratory failure. In a series of 45 infants with symptomatic Arnold-Chiari malformation treated with laminectomy, the mortality rate was 38%.[116]

The prognosis for lipomeningocele is excellent, although meticulous surgery is needed to separate the lipoma from the nerve rootlets.

Management

In continuing pregnancies, delivery can occur at term. An indication for preterm delivery could be the rapid development of severe ventriculomegaly and macrocrania. The opti-

TABLE 7. TYPICAL LUMBOSACRAL MASSES AND ASSOCIATED ULTRASOUND FEATURES

	Type of mass	Ultrasound features
Common	Open neural tube defects	Symmetric cystic, complex, or solid mass in the lumbosacral region Associated with cranial defect, lemon or banana sign
Uncommon	Amniotic band syndrome	Asymmetric defect with scoliosis Cystic to complex mass Associated amputational defects
	Limb-body wall complex	Limb-body wall complex Similar to amniotic band syndrome Plus fetus in continuity with placental surface and umbilical cord
	Sacrococcygeal teratoma	Usually solid mass from buttocks Often intrapelvic components Rarely a cystic mass
Rare	Tumors	Rare tumors such as lipomas that are echogenic or other neural or cutaneous tumors Ultrasound appearance depending on tumor type

Reproduced with permission from LeScale KB, Eddleman KA, Chervenak FA. The fetal neck and spine. In: McGahan JP, Porto M, eds. *Diagnostic obstetrical ultrasound*, 1st ed. Philadelphia: JB Lippincott 1994:172.

mal mode of delivery is controversial. Theoretically, the vaginal route could traumatize the defect and increase the risk of infection to the exposed neural tissues. It has been therefore recommended that all fetuses with spina bifida should be electively delivered by cesarean section.[117] This view is supported by one large retrospective case-control study that demonstrated that infants with spina bifida delivered by cesarean section before the onset of labor were significantly less likely to have severe paralysis than those exposed to labor.[118] No difference in the frequency of neonatal complications or later intellectual performance, however, was found.

Some experimental evidence exists that *in utero* closure of spina bifida may reduce the risk of handicap because the amniotic fluid in the third trimester is thought to be neurotoxic. Intrauterine repair of myelomeningocele has been performed in several fetuses. The available experience suggests that prenatal surgery decreases the incidence of hindbrain herniation and shunt-dependent hydrocephalus.[119] The degree of paralysis and bladder dysfunction does not seem to be influenced, while the rate of premature delivery is increased.[120–122] At present, the role of intrauterine treatment is debated.[123] In the words of Olutoye and Adzick, "until the benefits of fetal [meningomyelocele] repair are carefully elucidated, weighed against maternal and fetal risks, and compared to conventional postnatal therapy, this procedure should be restricted to a few centers that are committed (clinically and experimentally) to investigating these issues."[120]

Recurrence Risk

In 1991, the Medical Research Council Vitamin Study Group reported that the daily intake of 4 mg of folic acid periconceptually prevented 71% of recurrent NTDs in women with one affected offspring.[9]

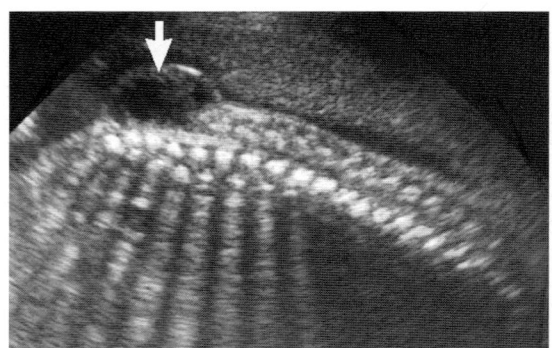

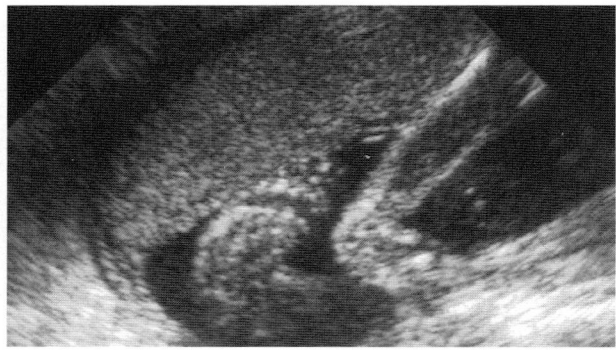

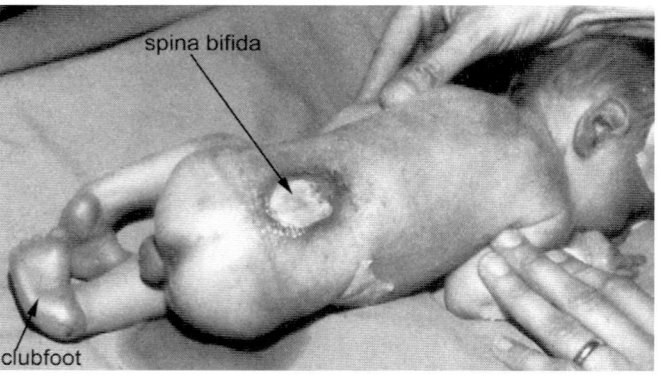

FIGURE 28. Myelomeningocele with clubfeet. **A:** Longitudinal scan of spine at 20 weeks shows cystic myelomeningocele (*arrow*). **B:** Views of feet show marked bilateral clubbed feet. **C:** Newborn with similar findings shows spina bifida and clubfeet.

TABLE 8. OUTCOME OF 171 INFANTS WITH MYELOMENINGOCELE

Level of lesion	Thoracolumbar	Lumbosacral	Sacral
Affected infants (%)	37	59	4
Mortality (%)	35	11	0
IQ >80 (%)	44	65	100
Able to walk (%)	71	81	100
Able to walk without appliances (%)	0	16	83

Modified from Main DM, Mennuti MT. Neural tube defects: issues in prenatal diagnosis and counseling. *Obstet Gynecol* 1986;67:1–16.

Iniencephaly

Synonyms

No synonyms are associated with iniencephaly.

Incidence

The incidence for iniencephaly is 0.1 to 10 per 10,000.

Description

Iniencephaly is an NTD involving the occiput and inion combined with rachischisis of the cervical and thoracic spine with retroflexion of the head.[124,125]

Etiology

The etiology for iniencephaly is probably the same as for the other NTDs. Seasonal and yearly variations exist.

Pathogenesis and Pathology

Iniencephaly is an NTD involving the occiput and inion combined with rachischisis of the cervical and thoracic spine with retroflexion of the head.[124,125] The time of onset is probably only a few days later than anencephaly.[126] Two main groups were classified by Lewis: iniencephaly apertus, which has an encephalocele, and iniencephaly clausus, which has a spinal defect but no cephalocele.[124]

The main features of iniencephaly are

1. A variable deficit of the occipital bones resulting in an enlarged foramen magnum
2. Partial or total absence of cervical and thoracic vertebrae with an irregular fusion of those present, accompanied by incomplete closure of the vertebral arches and bodies
3. Significant shortening of the spinal column due to marked lordosis and hyperextension of the malformed cervical-thoracic spine
4. Upward-turned face and mandibular skin directly continuous with that of the chest owing to the lack of neck

On microscopic examination of the brain, several anomalies have been detected including microencephaly, polymicrogyria, heterotopic glial tissue in the leptomeninges, atresia of the ventricular system, marked disorganization of the brain stem, vermian agenesis, large cerebellar cyst, and disorganization of the spinal cord tissue.[127]

Diagnosis

Iniencephaly is associated with gross alterations of intracranial anatomy, spine and fetal position, that should be easily detected in a standard sonographic examination (Fig. 29).[13,128–132] The sonographic diagnosis is made on the extreme dorsal flexion of the head, the abnormally short and deformed cervical and thoracic spine, and the overall shortening of the fetus. The retroflexion of the head and the spinal disorganization is visible on medial-sagittal scans of the spinal column. Anencephaly or cephaloceles are present in the open forms.

Most cases of iniencephaly diagnosed prenatally have presented with high AFP and polyhydramnios.

Differential Diagnosis

The differential diagnosis includes Klippel-Feil syndrome (shortness of the neck associated with fusion of cervical vertebrae), anencephaly, and a cervical myelomeningocele.[133] The differentiation between iniencephaly clausus and Klippel-Feil syndrome is difficult and controversial. Some authors believe that Klippel-Feil syndrome may be the mildest form of iniencephaly.[134,135]

Associated Anomalies

Associated anomalies are frequently found and include cephalocele, holoprosencephaly, spina bifida, omphalocele, gastroschisis, diaphragmatic hernia or agenesis, pulmonary hypoplasia or hyperplasia, cardiac malformations, renal anomalies, overgrowth of the arms compared to the legs, genu recurvatum, arthrogryposis, clubfoot, and gastrointestinal atresia.[125,136]

Prognosis

Iniencephaly apertus is always fatal in the neonatal period. A few cases of long-term survival of very mild iniencephalus clausus have been reported.[137]

Management

Management is as for any lethal diseases, with the exception of very mild and closed cases. Such cases, however, may not be amenable to antenatal diagnosis. Iniencephaly is frequently associated with polyhydramnios and is a well-established cause of dystocia.[138] Early induction of

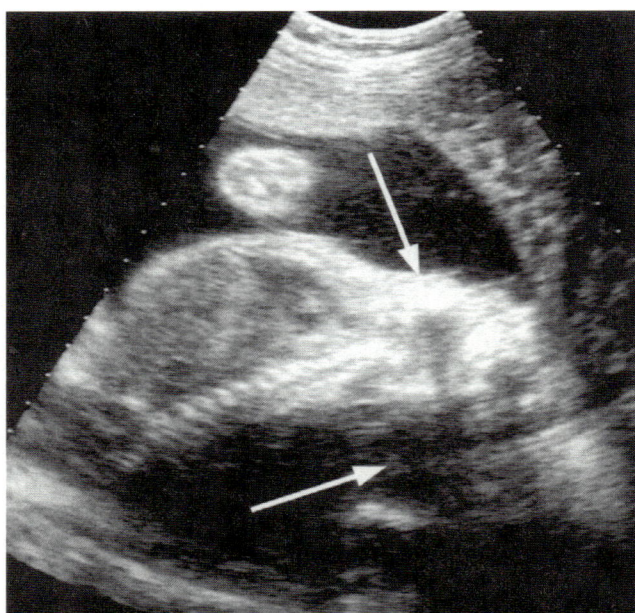
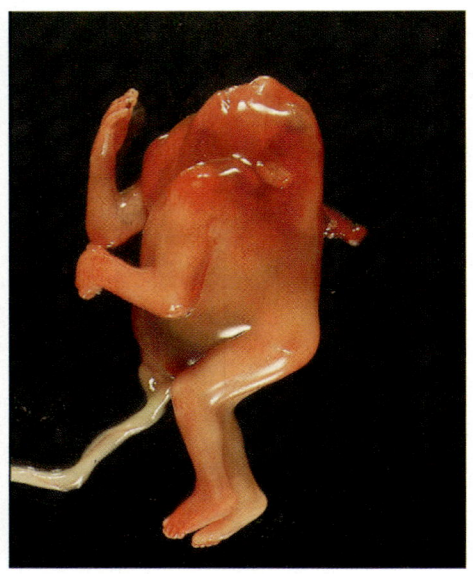

FIGURE 29. Iniencephaly. **A:** Sonogram shows the anterior neck (*top arrow*) is contiguous with the chest and the chin, without normal protrusion of the mandible. Also note retroflexion of the neck (*bottom arrow*). Anencephaly is also present. **B:** Postnatal photograph of similar case shows typical features of iniencephaly with anencephaly and marked retroflexion of neck.

labor should be considered to avoid the need of a cesarean section at term.[51]

Scoliosis/Kyphosis

Because scoliosis or kyphosis may be specific to a number of specific entities, abnormal curvature of the spine is discussed in general with more specific information given throughout the chapter on specific etiologies of scoliosis or kyphosis. Scoliosis is an abnormal lateral curvature of the spinal column of any cause. Kyphosis is abnormal anterior angulation of the spine and may occur in conjunction with scoliosis or so-called *kyphoscoliosis*. In 1992, Harrison et al. published their series of 20 fetuses detected by ultrasound with an abnormal spinal curvature[139] (Table 9). Most commonly, the etiology of the abnormal spinal curvature is a fetus with an associated open NTD (Fig. 30). These NTDs were most commonly myelomeningoceles. Other etiologies of scoliosis may include vertebral abnormalities, such as fused vertebrae (Fig. 31); hemivertebra (Fig. 32) or arthrogryposis; skeletal dysplasias; vertebral, anal, cardiac, tracheal, esophageal, renal, and limb (VACTERL) association; amniotic band syndrome; and limb body wall complex.[140,141] Rarely, diffuse spinal abnormalities may be observed from other causes (Fig. 33).

Curvature of the spinal canal *in utero* may be minor or as great as 90 degrees. As the fetal skeleton is flexible, it conforms to the *in utero* position and surrounding forces. As such, in a fetus with an associated decreased amniotic fluid, there may be an appearance of scoliosis. This diagno-

sis should be made with caution. Minor degrees of scoliosis may be secondary to isolated hemivertebra, whereas larger degrees of scoliosis may be secondary to such abnormalities as amniotic band syndrome or limb body wall complex.[142]

The prognosis of fetuses with abnormal spinal curvature is dependent on the underlying etiology of the scoliosis. For instance, prognosis of the fetus with an isolated hemivertebra should be excellent. However, a fetus with a more com-

TABLE 9. DIAGNOSES IN FETUSES WITH ABNORMAL SPINAL CURVATURE

Diagnosis	Number (n = 20)
Neural tube defect	12
Myelomeningocele	6
Frontal encephalocele with ectrodactyly	1
Exencephaly	1
Anencephaly	1
Anencephaly with trisomy 18	1
Iniencephaly	1
Craniorachischisis	1
Limb-body wall complex	2
Amniotic band syndrome	1
Multiple congenital anomalies, likely limb-body wall complex or amniotic band syndrome	2
Caudal regression syndrome	1
Thoracic dysplasia with multiple anomalies	1
Hemivertebra, no other anomalies	1

Reproduced with permission from Harrison LA, Pretorius DH, Budorick NE. Abnormal spinal curvature in the fetus. *J Ultrasound Med* 1992;11:473.

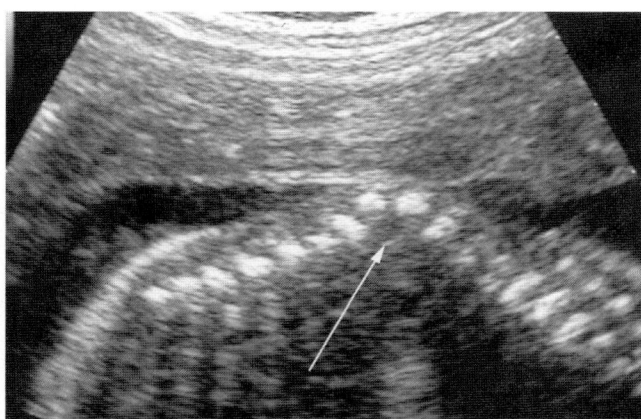

FIGURE 30. Kyphoscoliosis (*arrow*) in this fetus was secondary to a thoracolumbar spina bifida.

plex abnormality such as an open NTD or amniotic band syndrome has a more guarded prognosis.

Scoliosis/Hemivertebra

Synonyms

Synonyms for hemivertebra include congenital scoliosis (one of the causes of hemivertebra), unilateral aplasia of the vertebral body, and complete unilateral failure of formation of the vertebral body.

Description

Hemivertebra is a congenital anomaly of the spine in which only one-half of the vertebral body develops.

Incidence

The incidence of hemivertebra is estimated at 5 to 10 per 10,000 births with a male to female ratio of 0.31 for multiple vertebral anomalies and 0.68 for solitary vertebral anomalies.[143]

Pathogenesis and Pathology

At 6 weeks' gestational age, two lateral chondrification centers arise in the developing vertebral bodies. These chondrification centers then unite by 7 to 8 weeks' gestational age to form the primary ossification center of the vertebral body. A hemivertebra results from the failure of one of the lateral chondrification centers to develop. The defective vertebra acts as a wedge in the spine leading to excessive lateral curvature (i.e., scoliosis). Only one-half of the vertebral body is present, causing a deformation in the shape of the spine.

Diagnosis

The sonographic findings associated with fetal hemivertebra include a distortion in the shape of the spine that can be assessed by sagittal and coronal scans. A specific diagnosis requires meticulous scanning, but it is usually possible by demonstrating, usually in coronal scans, that at the level of the spinal distortion there is triangular bony structure, smaller than a vertebra, that acts as a wedge against the normal vertebral bodies (Fig. 32). It is expected that three-dimensional ultrasound may be useful for illustrating the affected vertebrae (Fig. 32B).

Differential Diagnosis

Hemivertebra may have a similar ultrasonic appearance to the other vertebral abnormalities (wedge vertebra, butter-

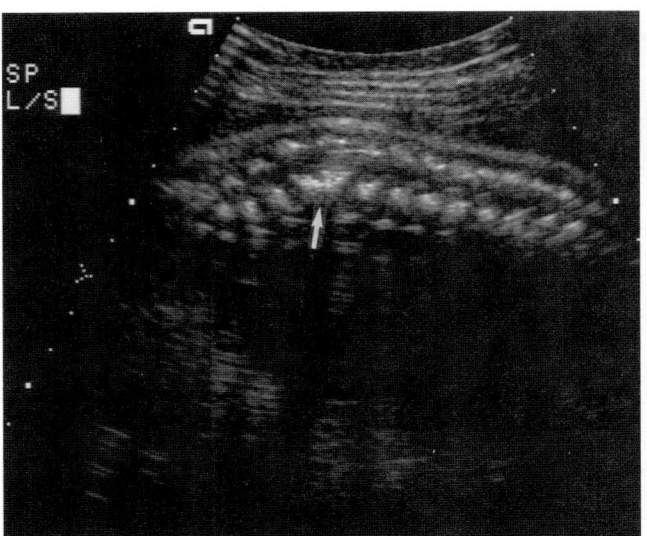

A

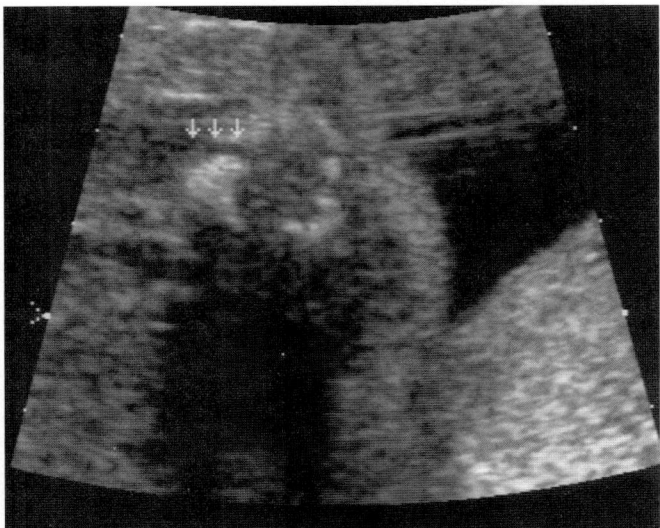

B

FIGURE 31. Scoliosis owing to block vertebra. Sagittal **(A)** and transverse **(B)** scan in the lumbar spine showing fused vertebral bodies (*arrows*). This was an isolated fetal malformation.

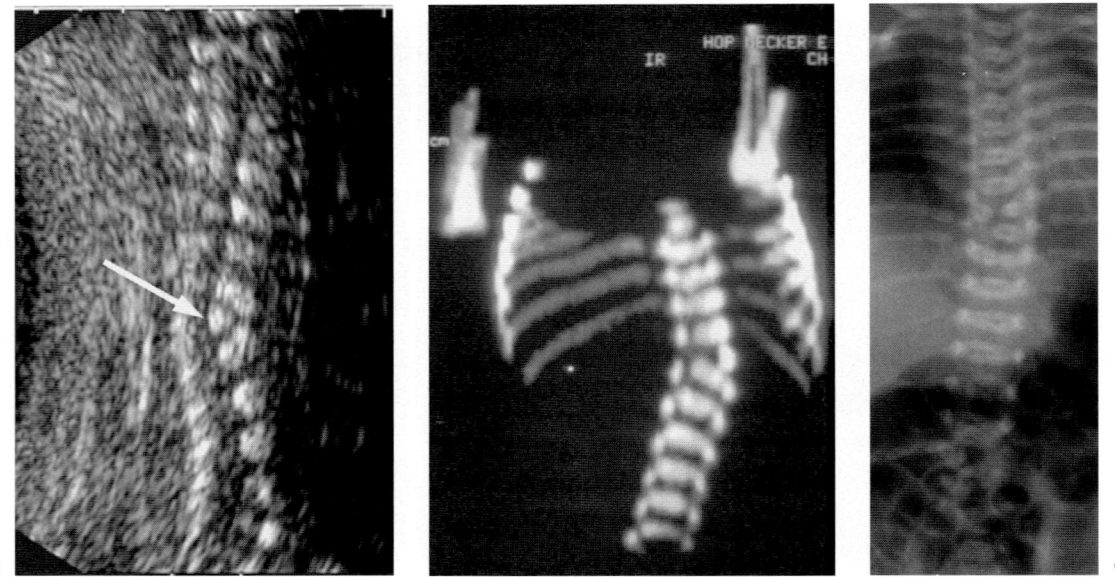

FIGURE 32. Hemivertebra. **A:** Coronal sonogram of the spine demonstrating small triangular vertebra (hemivertebra) ossification center (*arrow*), with resultant mild scoliosis. **B:** Three-dimensional ultrasound of another case showing hemivertebra with scoliosis. **C:** Postnatal radiograph showing hemivertebra. (Part **B** reproduced with permission from Brunelle F. Fetal imaging in a new era. *Ultrasound Obstet Gynecol* 2001;18:91–94.)

fly vertebra, bloc vertebra, bar vertebra, or any combination) that cause congenital scoliosis and in some cases may only be differentiated after careful neonatal radiologic evaluation. Open NTDs may also be associated with abnormal curvature of the spine but should have other findings differentiating it from hemivertebra. These include the intracranial changes associated with open NTDs as well as disruption of the skin over the defect and possibly the presence of a meningocele/myelomeningocele sac.

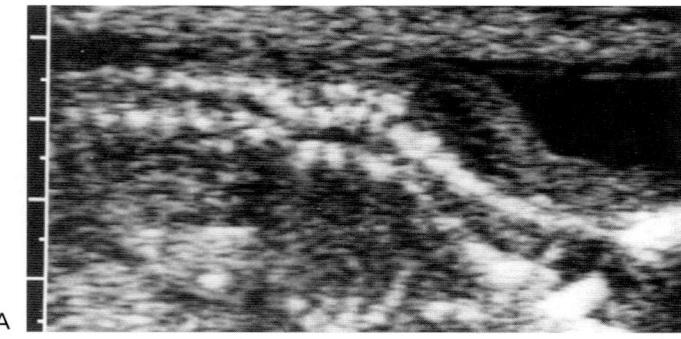

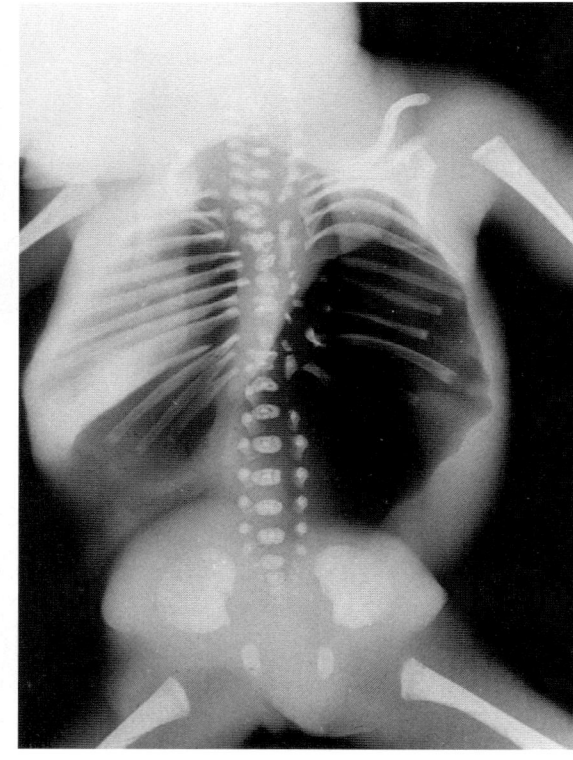

FIGURE 33. Multiple vertebral anomalies. **A:** Longitudinal view of thoracic spine at 19 weeks shows marked disorganization of spinal elements. **B:** Radiograph of pathologic specimen confirms multiple anomalies of the thoracic spine and ribs. Other anomalies included agenesis of the corpus callosum. This possibly represents spondylothoracic dysostosis (Jarcho-Levin syndrome). (Reproduced with permission from Nyberg DA, Mack LA. The spine and neural tube defects. In: Nyberg DA, Mahony BS, Pretorius DH, eds. *Diagnostic ultrasound of fetal anomalies: text and atlas.* Chicago: Yearbook Medical Publishers, 1990.)

Diastematomyelia may be associated with sonographic findings very similar to hemivertebra. A specific diagnosis can be difficult at times, but it is usually possible because in a transverse view diastematomyelia results in a typical image: a vertebra with three posterior ossification centers, the central one protruding toward the skin and the neural canal.

Associated Anomalies

Hemivertebra is commonly associated with other musculoskeletal anomalies, including those of the spine, ribs, and limbs. Cardiac and genitourinary tract anomalies are the more common extra-musculoskeletal anomalies seen with hemivertebra, with anomalies of the central nervous system and gastrointestinal tract also being reported. Hemivertebra may be part of a syndrome, including Jarcho-Levin, Klippel-Feil, and VACTERL.[144] The incidence of karyotypic abnormalities in fetuses with isolated vertebral anomalies is thought to be small. In the largest series, Zelop et al. performed amniocentesis on 18 fetuses with isolated vertebral anomalies and obtained a normal karyotype in all 18 cases.[145]

Prognosis

The prognosis is directly related to the presence or absence of associated anomalies. The prognosis of isolated hemivertebra is good. Left untreated, 25% of patients with congenital scoliosis show no progression, 50% progress slowly, and 25% progress rapidly during growth.[146] Spinal fusion is the treatment of choice for cases of congenital scoliosis that are progressive or are of the short, rigid type. The treatment of congenital scoliosis should occur before significant deformity occurs.

Management

When the prenatal diagnosis of hemivertebra is made, a meticulous search for associated anomalies should be performed. Chromosomal analysis can be offered, especially in the presence of associated anomalies. Amniotic fluid AFP concentration can be assessed if there is a question of an open NTD and the patient is of appropriate gestational age. Serial ultrasonic evaluation is recommended to follow fetal growth and evaluate for signs of an open NTD that may not be present at an initial early ultrasound.

If no other complicating factors exist, standard management of labor and delivery is recommended. A careful neonatal assessment for associated cardiac and genitourinary anomalies needs to be performed and the infant should receive long-term orthopedic follow-up so treatment can occur, if necessary, before the development of serious deformity.

Recurrence Risk

Recurrence risk for hemivertebra is uncertain. An increased risk of NTDs in siblings may exist.[147]

Diastematomyelia

Synonyms

Synonyms for diastematomyelia include split cord, occult spinal dysraphism, and diplomyelia with bony spur.

Description

Diastematomyelia involves longitudinal clefting of the spinal cord that is divided into two hemicords.[148]

Incidence

Incidence for diastematomyelia is unknown. Prenatal diagnosis has been infrequently reported.

Pathogenesis and Pathology

Diastematomyelia is characterized by a bony, fibrous or cartilaginous septum that subdivides partially or completely the vertebral canal. This produces a sagittal cleft in the spinal cord, conus medullaris, and filum terminale. The hemicords usually have a distinct arachnoid membrane, each with a common dura. Diastematomyelia may involve a single vertebra or extend to several vertebral segments. The cleft may be found at any level but in most cases is found at the lower thoracic or upper lumbar regions. It may be isolated or associated with other segmental anomalies of the vertebral bodies.

Several hypothesis have been formulated regarding the pathogenesis:

1. The neurenteric canal that transiently connects the yolk sac to the amnion via the primitive knot is retained. This knot migrates distally to the region of the coccyx, where it disappears. If an accessory canal develops, it splits the neural ectoderm with underlying endoderm and results in a midline fistula. The fistula eventually disappears, but not until abnormal vertebral and neural elements have been formed.[149]
2. A dorsal and ventral cleft exists that severs the neural plate near the midline, resulting in separate closure of the two hemicords. Mesenchymal tissue filling the gap results in mesodermal and bony abnormalities.[150]
3. Excessive dilatation of the neural tube exists, resulting in subdivision of the cord and internal penetration by mesodermal structures originating from the vertebral body.[151]

The vertebral column and the spinal cord have the same length up to the third month of embryonal life, after which growth proceeds with a different speed. The vertebral column elongates more rapidly, and at birth the conus medullaris is at the level of the lower margin of the second lumbar vertebra. This different growth continues up to the age of 5 years, when the conus medullaris reaches the upper margin of the body of the second lumbar vertebra.

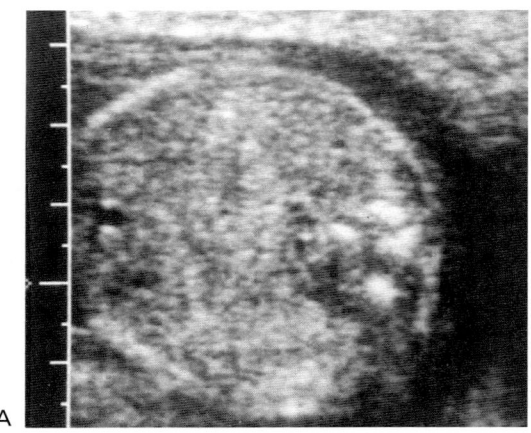 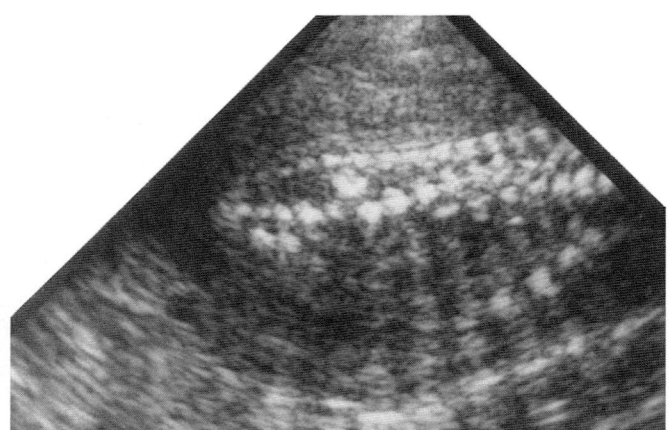

FIGURE 34. Diastematomyelia. Transverse **(A)** and longitudinal **(B)** views show bony spur projecting into the spinal canal.

Diastematomyelia acts as a restraint that slows the normal growth of the spinal cord by impeding the upward migration of the neural elements, with progressive neurologic deficits in the limbs.

Diagnosis

The experience with the antenatal diagnosis of diastematomyelia as a closed neural defect is limited to a few cases, most of which were associated with vertebral abnormalities (Figs. 34 and 35). Identification of an extra-echogenic posterior focus in the spinal canal is considered a highly specific prenatal sign of diastematomyelia.[152–155] This may be seen (a) in a coronal section with widening of the spinal canal or (b) in a transverse section of the affected vertebrae with three instead of two posterior ossification centers, with the central one protruding posteriorly toward the skin and anteriorly toward the spinal canal. The overlying soft tissues and skin are intact.

Cases without either spina bifida or bony alterations of the vertebrae are unlikely to be identified even by expert sonography.

Differential Diagnosis

Antenatally, the diagnostic problem is distinguishing diastematomyelia from open spina bifida and hemivertebra. The available experience suggests that the appearance of the spine in coronal and sagittal sections is aspecific, whereas the transverse section that demonstrates three ossification centers is strongly indicative of diastematomyelia.[71] Demonstrating the integrity of the soft tissues overlying the abnormal vertebrae and of the intracranial anatomy can be of further help in ruling out spina bifida. Amniotic fluid AFP concentration and acetylcholinesterase can be assessed if the doubt of an associated spina bifida cannot be ruled out by sonography alone.

Associated Anomalies

The anomalies that have been described in association with diastematomyelia[156,157] include

1. Open spina bifida.
2. Closed abnormalities of the vertebrae: scoliosis, kyphosis, hemivertebra, butterfly vertebra.
3. Cutaneous manifestations on the dorsal midline consisting of telangiectasias, atrophic skin, hemangiomas, subcutaneous lipomas, and cutaneous nevi. Among the cutaneous nevi, the most characteristic is the nevus pilosus, a large patch of long silky hairs that is situated over the site of the cleft in the cord in 50% to 70% of the cases. The location of the cutaneous abnormality, however, is not necessarily indicative of the level of the lesion.
4. Orthopedic deformities of the feet, especially clubfoot, are found in approximately one-half of the patients.

Prognosis

The presence of diastematomyelia has no influence on the prognosis when spina bifida is present. When diastematomyelia presents as a closed NTD, the prognosis for neurologic function may be enhanced by early surgical removal of the septum, dural reconstruction into a single tube, excision of associated developmental masses, and division of the tethering filum. Most of the cases identified antenatally thus far had a good outcome. Sepulveda reviewed 15 cases diagnosed antenatally.[154] Information on the postnatal outcome of diastematomyelia without additional abnormal findings was available from six cases. Of these cases, one had severe orthopedic problems, including a spinal deformity, shortening of one leg, and a small foot. The remaining cases were free from neurologic and orthopedic sequelae, although one underwent spinal surgery.

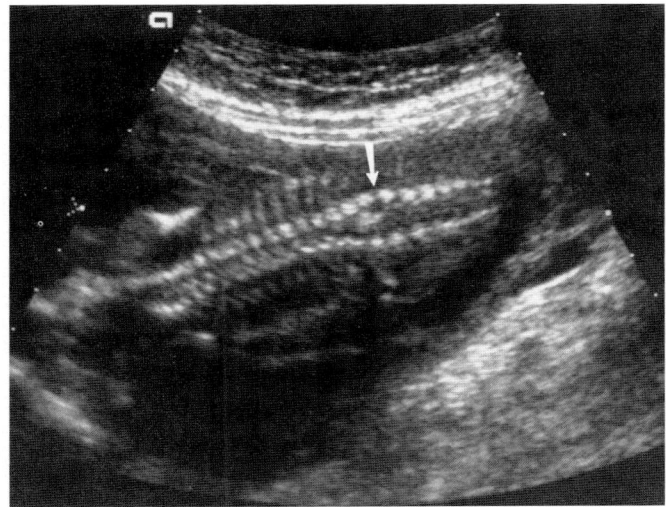

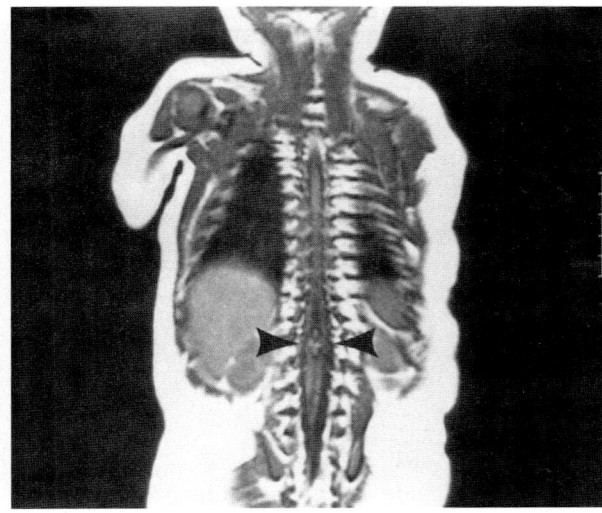

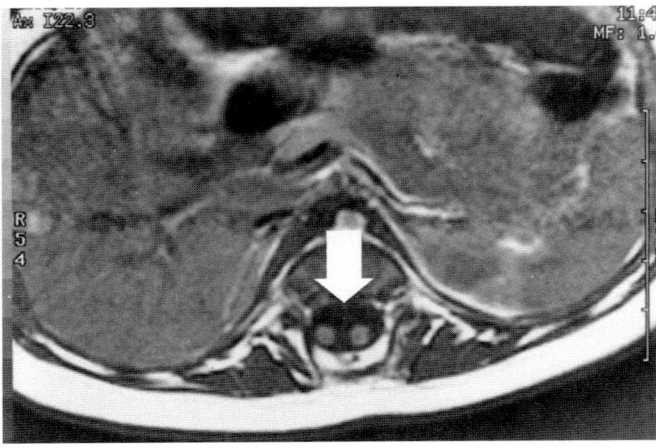

FIGURE 35. Diastematomyelia. **A:** Coronal sonogram shows diagnostic features of diastematomyelia with central bony spur (*arrow*) and associated widening of lumbar spine. **B:** Postnatal magnetic resonance image of spine in coronal plane shows central spur (*arrowheads*). **C:** Magnetic resonance image, transverse plane, shows division of spinal cord (*arrow*) by diastematomyelia. [Reproduced with permission from Allen LM, Silverman RK. Prenatal ultrasound evaluation of fetal diastematomyelia: two cases of type I split cord malformation. *Ultrasound Obstet Gynecol* 2000;15(1):78–82.]

Management

Counseling patients with a prenatal diagnosis of diastematomyelia without evidence of either spina bifida or other vertebral anomalies is difficult. Although the outcome is usually favorable, neurosurgical and orthopedic surgery may be necessary, and a chance of neurologic compromise exists.

Recurrence Risk

The risk of recurrence is unknown. Autosomal dominant transmission has been described in rare cases.[158]

Limb-Body Wall Complex

Limb-body wall complex produces severe scoliosis, body wall defects, and craniofacial defects. Limb-body wall complex is discussed in further detail in Chapter 5.

Sacral Agenesis

Agenesis of the sacrum is rarely identified in only a few abnormalities. The spectrum of sacral agenesis and dysgenesis is associated with caudal regression syndrome and sirenomelia. Considerable overlap between these abnormalities may exist, with some considering them spectrums of the same entity. A more recent theory, however, suggests that caudal regression syndrome and sirenomelia are pathologically distinct entities. A number of entities exist that are associated with abnormal sacrum and renal agenesis that are listed in Table 10.[159,160]

Sacral Agenesis/Caudal Regression

Synonyms

Synonyms for caudal regression include caudal dysplasia sequence, sacral agenesis, and caudal dysgenesis.

TABLE 10. LIST OF CONDITIONS OR SYNDROMES ASSOCIATED WITH SACRAL DYSGENESIS AND BILATERAL RENAL AGENESIS

VATER (VACTERL-H) association
Cloacal exstrophy sequence
Femoral hypoplasia—unusual facies syndrome
Fraser's syndrome
Muro's association
Renal agenesis (Potter's syndrome)

VACTERL, *v*ertebral, *a*nal, *c*ardiac, *t*racheal, *e*sophageal, *r*enal, and *l*imb; VATER, *v*ertebral defects, imperforate *a*nus, *t*racheoesoph*ageal fistula, and *r*enal dysplasia.

Description

This syndrome is associated with absence of the sacrum and absence of variable portions of the lumbar spine.

Incidence

Exact incidence is difficult to estimate because prior reports often combine cases of sirenomelia with caudal regression syndrome. Approximately 16% of cases are associated with infants of diabetic mothers.[161–163] Some have shown an increased frequency among siblings[164] and families.[165]

Pathogenesis and Pathology

The pathogenesis of caudal regression syndrome is probably related to disruption of formation of the more caudal portion of the neural tube, thus causing dysplasia or absence of the sacrum. Few reports indicate metabolic or teratogenic causes of caudal regression syndrome.[161,166]

Diagnosis

Ultrasound is used to establish the diagnosis of caudal regression syndrome. Diagnosis has been made as early as the first trimester by noting the short crown-rump length.[167] Such early diagnosis, however, is rare. Most commonly, diagnosis is made in the second trimester usually after there is ossification of the sacrum. The sonographic appearance may vary from abnormalities of the sacrum to complete absence of the sacrum and lower lumbar spine (Fig. 36). Agenesis of the thoracic spine may exist, and often there are abnormalities of the lower limb such as flexion deformities or clubbed feet.[168–170] Normal or increased amniotic fluid (polyhydramnios) is common.

Associated Anomalies

Other abnormalities of the genitourinary or gastrointestinal system have been reported with caudal regression syndrome.[168,170] These abnormalities have included renal agenesis, renal dysplasia, and gastrointestinal abnormalities such as duodenal atresia and tracheoesophageal atresia.

Differential Diagnosis

The main differential diagnosis includes sirenomelia and vertebral defects, imperforate anus, tracheoesophageal fistula, and radial and renal dysplasia association. (Also see Sirenomelia in Chapter 15.)

Prognosis

The prognosis is dependent on the severity of sacral agenesis and accompanying defects. If caudal regression is associ-

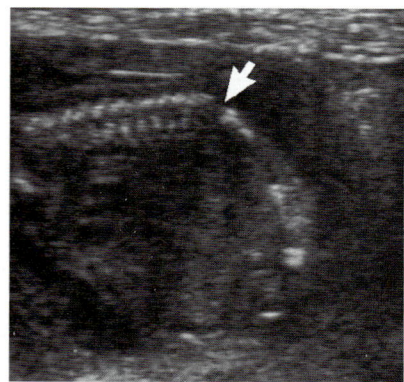

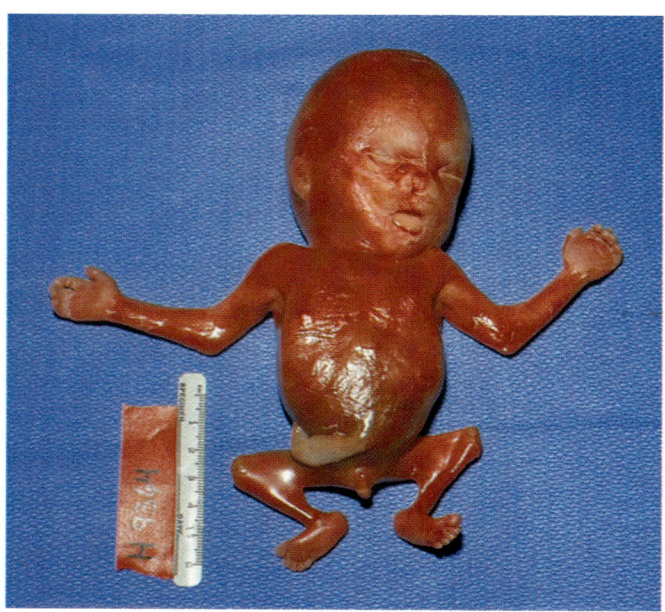

FIGURE 36. Caudal regression syndrome. **A:** Longitudinal sonogram in a woman with insulin-dependent diabetes at 18 weeks shows termination of spine below lower thoracic level (*arrow*). Only an ossified focus is demonstrated for the lumbar spine. The pelvis was also hypoplastic. **B:** Pathologic photograph shows marked shortening of lower extremities.

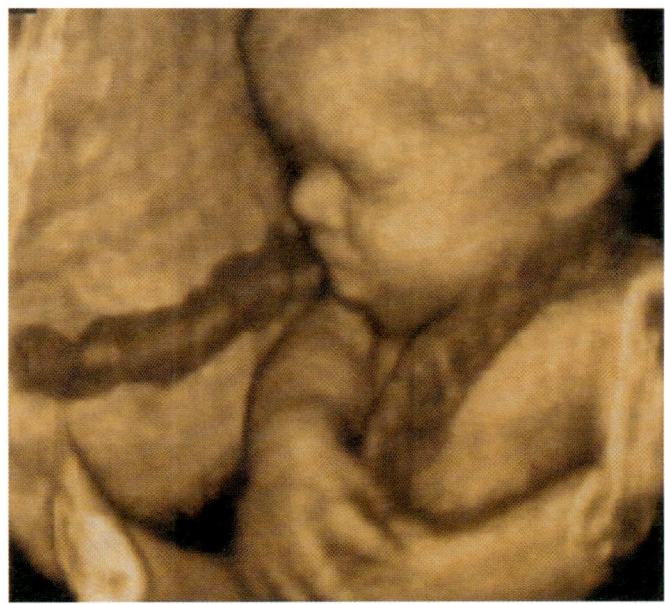
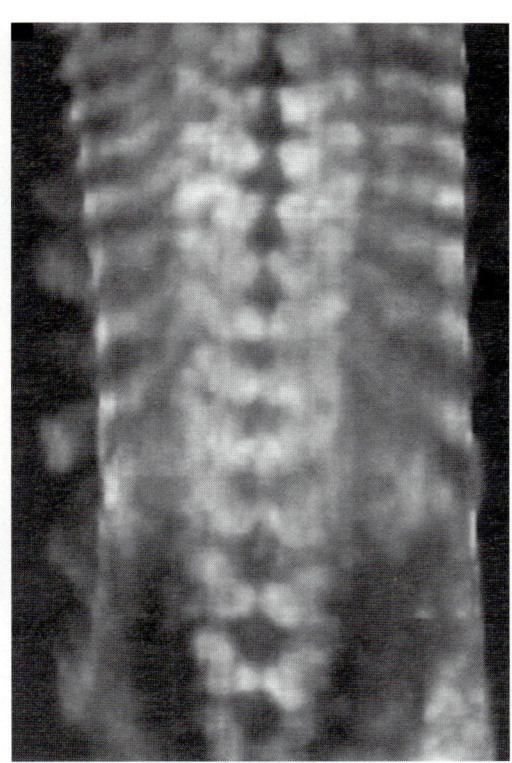

FIGURE 37. Achondroplasia. **A:** Three-dimensional ultrasound showing abnormal craniofacial appearance. **B:** Three-dimensional ultrasound of the spine shows caudal narrowing of intrapedicular distance, characteristic for achondroplasia. (Reproduced with permission from Moeglin D, Benoit B. Three-dimensional sonographic aspects in prenatal diagnosis of achondroplasia. *J Ultrasound Med* 2001;18:81–84.)

ated with bilateral renal agenesis, the defect is lethal. Severe sacral agenesis is associated with lower extremity neurologic compromise, and there may be severe bowel and bladder dysfunction.

Recurrence Risk

Most cases of caudal regression are sporadic. However, there is increased risk in familial cases of caudal regression syndrome or increased risk in diabetic mothers.

Skeletal Dysplasia

Skeletal dysplasias (see Chapter 15) commonly affect the spine. For example, achondroplasia is characterized by a narrower intrapedicular distance extending caudally (Fig. 37), in contrast to the normal situation when the intrapedicular distance widens. Focal hypomineralization of the spine indicates achondrogenesis. A number of conditions may be associated with flattened vertebrae, including thanatophoric dysplasia and spondyloepiphyseal dysplasia. Camptomelic dysplasia has narrow pelvic angles with wide pelvic outlet, and this is expected to be demonstrated by three-dimensional ultrasound.

Disorganized thoracic vertebrae and abnormal ribs are the primary manifestations of spondylothoracic dysostosis (Jarcho-Levin syndrome), also referred to as spondylocostal dysplasia, costovertebral dysplasia, and spondylothoracic

dysplasia, an autosomal recessive disorder characterized by multiple fused vertebrae and hemivertebrae in the cervical, thoracic, and lumbar regions that results in a crab-like thorax. The rest of the skeleton is unaffected, although other associated anomalies include a single umbilical artery and genitourinary, diaphragmatic, and anorectal malformations. Other considerations for multiple rib and vertebral anomalies include dyssegmental dysplasia, mesomelic dysplasia of the Robinow type, and VACTERL anomalies. Unlike Jarcho-Levin syndrome, dyssegmental dysplasia is characterized by severe micromelia (marked shortening of all extremities) and occipital encephalocele. Robinow mesomelic dysplasia is characterized by segmentation defects (hemivertebra, butterfly vertebrae, and vertebral fusion), facial abnormalities, and mesomelia, particularly of the upper extremities.[1]

LUMBOSACRAL MASSES

Lumbosacral masses are most commonly secondary to open NTDs. These can include simple meningoceles to more complex meningomyeloceles (myelomeningoceles). Meningoceles are usually cystic, as there is only herniation of dura; arachnoid; and they accompany cerebral spinal fluid. Meningomyeloceles may appear solid or complex due to the presence of neural elements within the herniated sac. These defects are typically midline and associated with the

Type 1

Type II

Type III

Type IV

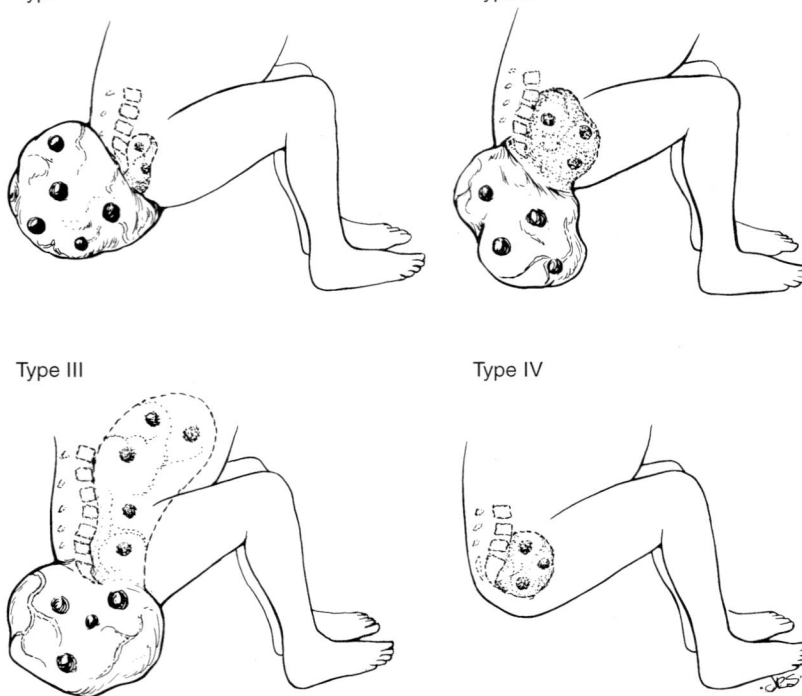

FIGURE 38. Types of sacrococcygeal teratomas. Sacrococcygeal teratomas may be almost entirely external or combined internal and external, or, as in type III, mainly internal. Those that are mainly external are less commonly malignant, whereas type IV tumors, which are mainly internal, usually have a delayed diagnosis and often are malignant. (Reproduced with permission from Altman RP, et al. *Sacrococcygeal teratoma.* American Academy of Pediatrics Surgical Section Survey, 1973.)

lemon-shaped head and the banana-shaped cerebellar hemispheres. Other spinal defects with accompanying masses may occur with either limb-body wall complex or amniotic band syndrome. These defects and masses are asymmetric and accompanied by other defects of the body or limbs.

Rare tumors may occur in the spine. These include sacrococcygeal teratoma and rare lipomas originating from the

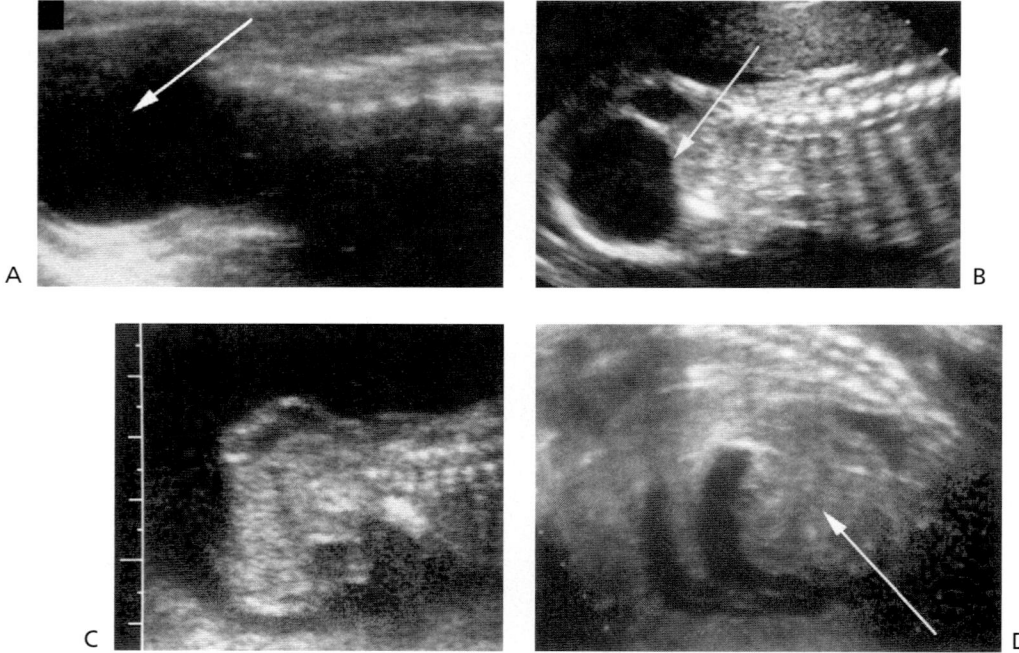

FIGURE 39. The spectrum of sacrococcygeal teratomas. **A:** Type 1 with predominately cystic teratoma (*arrow*). **B:** Type 2 teratoma with cystic and solid elements (*arrow*). **C:** Type 2 solid teratoma. **D:** Type 4 teratoma presenting as nonimmune fetal hydrops with a large intraabdominal mass (*arrow*).

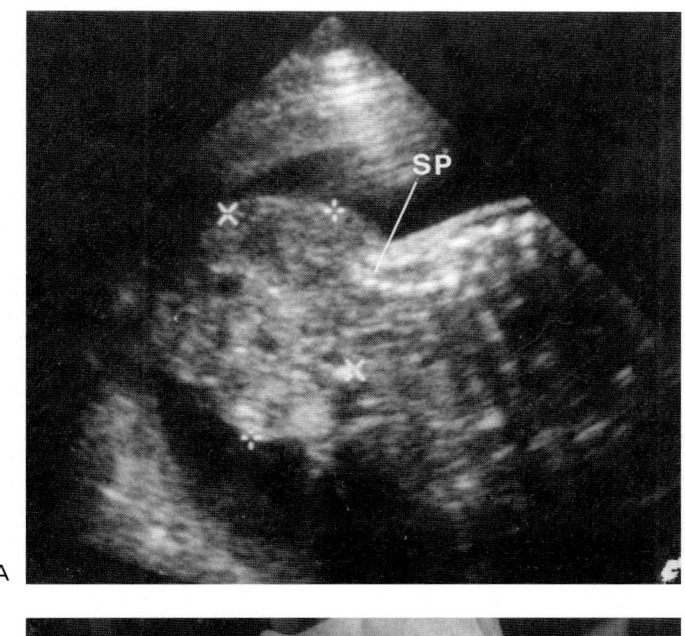

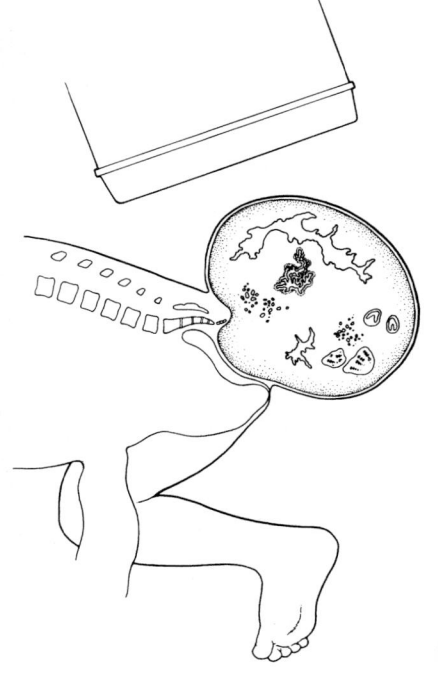

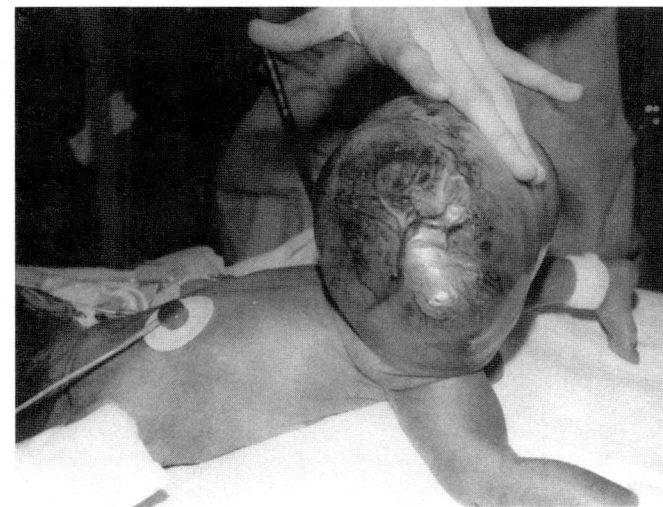

FIGURE 40. Solid sacrococcygeal teratomas. **A:** Sacrococcygeal teratomas outlined by calipers. SP, spine. **B:** Artist's conception of fetal sacrococcygeal teratoma. **C:** Neonate with sacrococcygeal teratomas. (Reproduced with permission from McGahan JP, Coates T, LeScale K, et al. In: McGahan JP, Goldberg BG, eds. *Diagnostic ultrasound: a logical approach.* Philadelphia: Lippincott–Raven, 1998.)

spinal canals. Some of these typical lumbosacral masses are outlined in Table 8.

Sacrococcygeal Teratoma

Description

Sacrococcygeal teratoma is a germ cell tumor arising from the presacral area.

Incidence

The incidence of sacrococcygeal teratoma is 1 per 40,000 births. The female to male ratio is 4 to 1, but malignant changes are seen more frequently in males.[171,172]

Pathogenesis and Pathology

Sacrococcygeal teratoma is believed to arise from the primitive knot or Hensen's node, an aggregation of totipotential cells that act as the primary organizers of embryonic development. Originally located in the lower dorsal area of the embryo, the Hensen's node migrates caudally inside the tail of the embryo during the first week post-conception, eventually resting anterior to the coccyx. This theory provides an explanation for the more frequent occurrence of teratomas in the sacral area rather than in other parts of the body.[173] An alternative theory of *twinning accident* with incomplete separation during embryogenesis has also been proposed.

The American Academy of Pediatric Surgery[102] distinguishes four types of sacrococcygeal teratomas (Fig. 38):

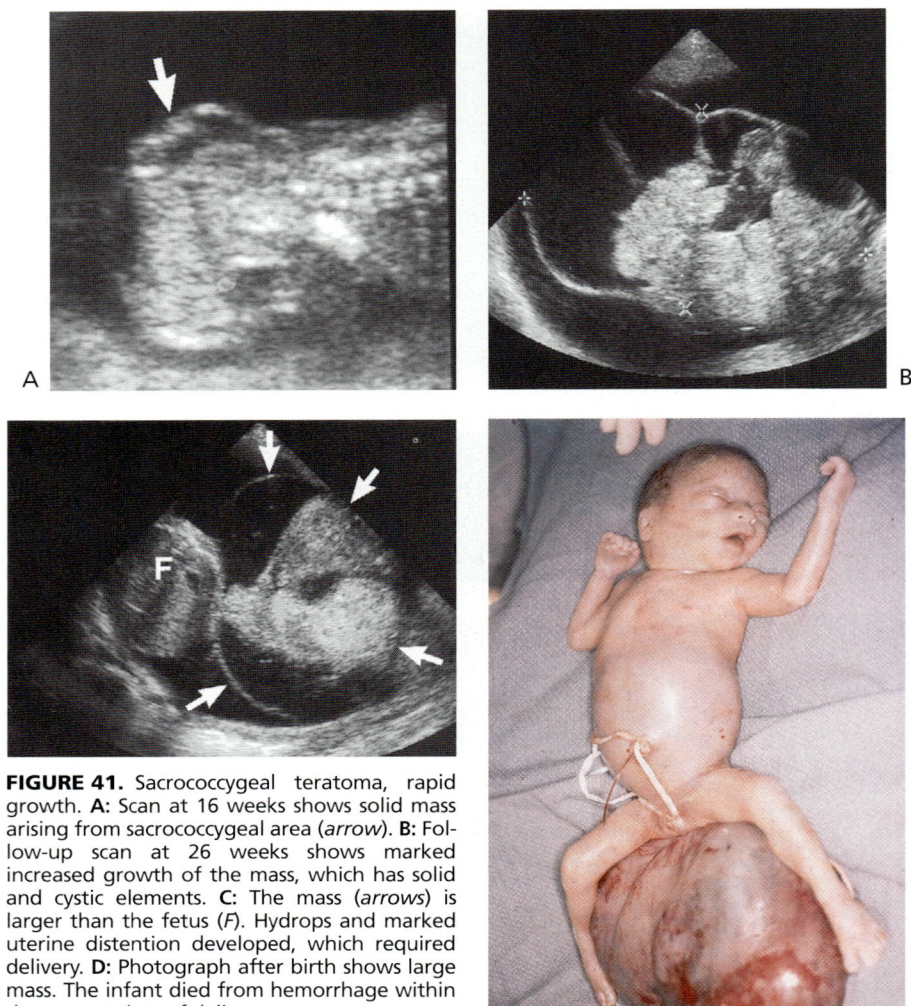

FIGURE 41. Sacrococcygeal teratoma, rapid growth. **A:** Scan at 16 weeks shows solid mass arising from sacrococcygeal area (*arrow*). **B:** Follow-up scan at 26 weeks shows marked increased growth of the mass, which has solid and cystic elements. **C:** The mass (*arrows*) is larger than the fetus (*F*). Hydrops and marked uterine distention developed, which required delivery. **D:** Photograph after birth shows large mass. The infant died from hemorrhage within the mass at time of delivery.

Type 1: Predominantly external, with minimal presacral component.

Type 2: Predominantly external, with significant intrapelvic component.

Type 3: Predominantly internal, with abdominal extension.

Type 4: Entirely internal with no external component.

Types 1 and 2 include 80% of the cases. Only 10% of the sacrococcygeal teratomas are of type 4.

In 15% of cases, the tumor is entirely cystic, with the remaining 85% of cases being either solid or mixed.

Histologically, sacrococcygeal teratomas are categorized in three main groups. Mature (or benign) teratomas consist of tissues similar to normal, well-developed structures (skin appendage, bone, glia, bowel, pancreas). Fully formed organs may be present, such as bowel loops, fingers, and teeth. Choroid plexus is frequently found and is responsible for the production of the fluid that forms cysts within the tumor. Immature teratomas contain different proportions of embryonal tissues, usually of neuroepithelial or renal origin. Malignant teratomas are yolk sac or endodermal sinus tumor and produce alpha-fetoprotein. Mature and immature teratomas are frequently cystic; malignant forms are predominantly solid. Solid tumors have usually an important vascular component and may be complicated by high-output cardiac failure, hydrops, and spontaneous hemorrhage. Mature, immature, and malignant forms account in different series for 55% to 75%, 11% to 28%, and 7% to 13%, respectively.[174]

Diagnosis

Sacrococcygeal teratoma has been reported by many authors,[175–190] including Kivilevich[191] who reviewed a total

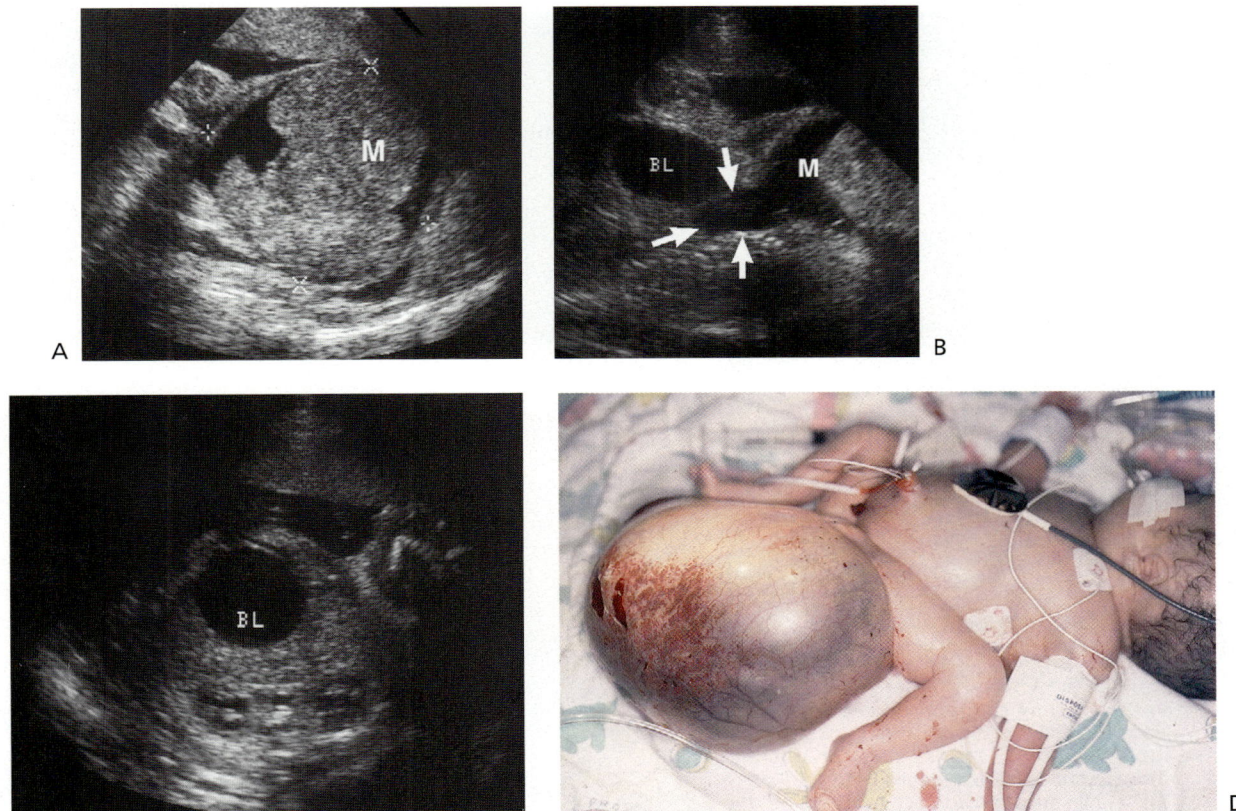

FIGURE 42. Sacrococcygeal teratoma with intrapelvic component. **A:** Scan at 34 weeks shows large mass (*M*) measuring 11 cm in diameter, which arose from sacrococcygeal region. **B:** Longitudinal scan of pelvis shows intrapelvic cystic component (*arrows*) posterior to urinary bladder (*BL*). **C:** Transverse view shows mild pyelectasis of both kidneys, reflecting distal obstruction. **D:** Photograph at delivery shows large size of tumor. This tumor was successfully resected surgically.

of 134 cases. These usually appear as cystic, solid, or mixed cystic and solid masses arising from the sacrococcygeal region (Figs. 39 and 40). Large, solid teratomas have an important vascular component, which is easily demonstrated using color Doppler technique. These tumors may rapidly increase in size (Fig. 41). Sometimes the intrapelvic component of type 3 may be detected (Fig. 42). However, type 4 masses that are entirely intra-abdominal may be difficult to detect.

Polyhydramnios and hydrops may develop as a consequence of hypervascularity and/or anemia following intratumoral hemorrhage, leading to high output cardiac failure. This appears to be much more likely for solid tumors or mixed solid/cystic tumors compared to cystic tumors (Fig. 43).

Three dimensional ultrasound[192,193] and MRI[194] have been used to assess sacrococcygeal teratomas. MRI is expected to be useful for demonstrating the size and extent of sacrococcygeal teratomas, particularly intrapelvic extension (Fig. 44).

Differential Diagnosis

The primary consideration is myelomeningocele. Characteristic cranial findings associated with myelomeningocele usually permit the correct diagnosis.

Associated Anomalies

Postnatal studies report an incidence ranging between 5% and 25%, involving various systems with no specific pattern. Prenatal series, in contrast, only rarely reported associated malformations, with the exception of hydrops.

Prognosis

The prognosis is related to three factors: the development of fetal hydrops, histology of the lesion, and size of the tumor. Hydrops occurs typically with large solid tumors with significant vascular component and is most frequently associated with perinatal death. Malignant tumors are

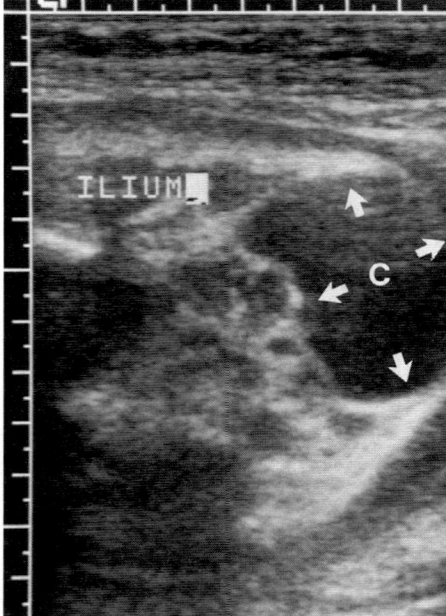

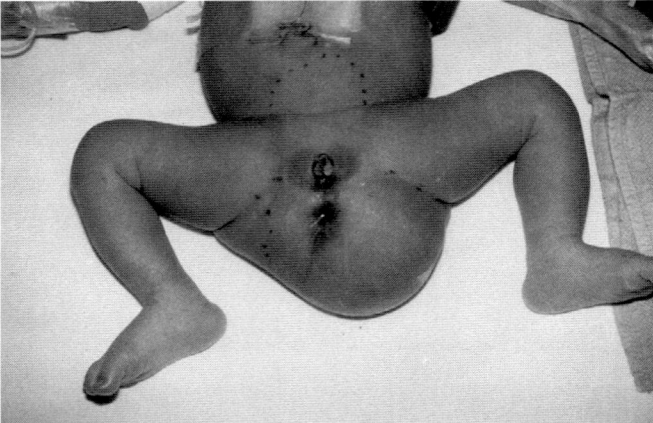

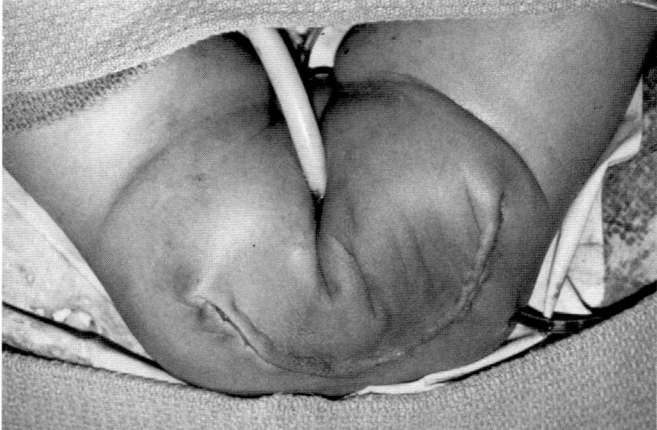

FIGURE 43. Cystic sacrococcygeal teratoma. **A:** Axial scan through the sacrum demonstrates splaying of the sacral elements and a large cystic (*C*) mass protruding posterior in the midline. **B:** Preoperative photograph shows cystic sacrococcygeal teratoma. Part of the cystic mass protruded from inside the fetal pelvis. **C:** Postoperative image with rectal tube demonstrating good cosmetic result after resection of the sacrococcygeal teratoma. (Reproduced with permission from McGahan JP, Coates T. LeScale K, et al. In: McGahan JP, Goldberg BG, eds. *Diagnostic ultrasound: a logical approach.* Philadelphia: Lippincott–Raven, 1998.)

almost invariably rapidly fatal. With this regard, the classification of the macroscopic type is relevant. In fact, type I is rarely if ever malignant, whereas with types II, III, and IV the probability of metastases is 6%, 20%, and 76%, respectively.[102] The size of the tumor does not seem to predict malignancies but is important as well, because very large lesions are associated to a greater surgical risk. In a review of 134 cases diagnosed in utero,[103] the perinatal mortality rate was 35%, excluding 17 cases of elective abortion. The available evidence suggests that a good outcome is expected from small lesions, predominantly external, cystic, and avascular. Conversely, the outcome is poor when a solid vascular lesion with significant internal component is seen.

Management

Termination of pregnancy can be offered to the parents before viability. In continuing pregnancies, serial sonograms and Doppler ultrasonography to follow up the growth and the vascularization of the tumor are indicated. Fetal intervention by open surgery and removal of the tumor has been performed[195] (see Chapter 26). Attempts at radiofrequency ablation of the tumor have resulted in a disproportionate number of fetal deaths and so is not considered necessary.[196,197]

With a large tumor, elective cesarean section is necessary because of soft tissue dystocia. With predominantly cystic lesions, aspiration may reduce the volume of the tumor, however, and allow a vaginal delivery.

Recurrence Risk

Although the majority of sacrococcygeal teratomas occurs sporadically, some cases typically associated with anorectal stenosis and sacrococcygeal defects (Currarino triad) are transmitted with autosomal dominant inheritance.[198–200]

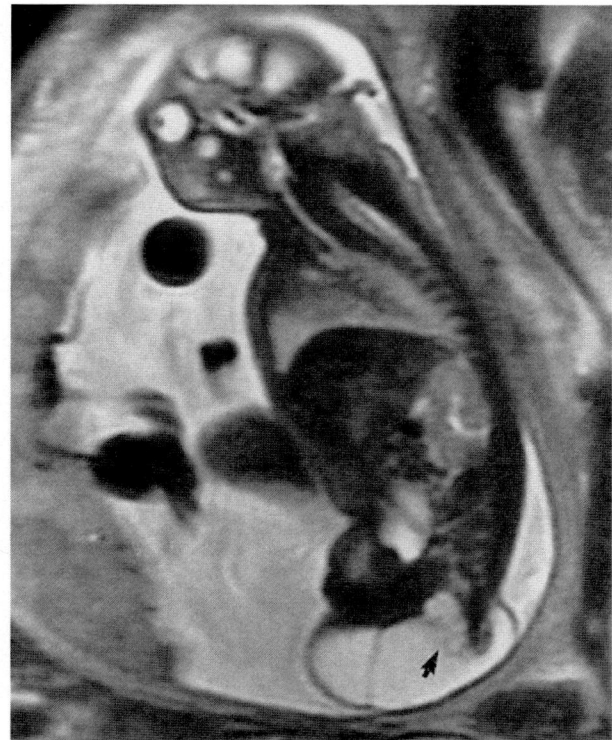

FIGURE 44. Sacrococcygeal teratoma. Sagittal single-shot fast spin-echo magnetic resonance image at 31 weeks shows a large multilocular cystic mass in the sacrococcygeal region. A solid nodular component is seen (*arrow*). Sacrococcygeal teratoma was confirmed after birth. [Reproduced with permission from Shinmoto H, Kashima K, Yuasa Y, et al. MR imaging of non-CNS fetal abnormalities: a pictorial essay. *Radiographics* 2000;20(5):1227–1243.]

REFERENCES

Epidemiology, Risk Factors, Screening

1. Main DM, Mennuti MT. Neural tube defects: issues in prenatal diagnosis and counseling. *Obstet Gynecol* 1986;67:1–15.
2. Leck I. Causation of neural tube defects: clues from epidemiology. *Br Med Bull* 1974;30:158.
3. Honein MA, Paulozzi LJ, Mathews TJ, et al. Impact of folic acid fortification of the US food supply on the occurrence of neural tube defects. *JAMA* 2001;285(23):2981–2986.
4. Creasy MR, Albeman ED. Congenital malformations of the central nervous system in spontaneous abortions. *J Med Genet* 1976;13:9.
5. Holmes LB, Driscoll SG, Atkins L. Etiologic heterogeneity of neural-tube defects. *N Engl J Med* 1976;294:365–369.
6. Feuchtbaum LB, Currier RJ, Riggle S, et al. Neural tube defect prevalence in California (1990–1994): eliciting patterns by type of defect and maternal race/ethnicity. *Genet Test* 1999;3(3):265–272.
7. Smithells RW, Sheppard S, Schorah CJ. Vitamin deficiencies and neural tube defects. *Arch Dis Child* 1976; 51(12):944–950.
8. Shaw GM, Velie EM, Schaffer DM. Is dietary intake of methionine associated with a reduction in risk for neural tube defect-affected pregnancies? *Teratology* 1997;56:295.
9. MRC Vitamin Study Research Group. Prevention of neural tube defects: results of the medical research council vitamin study. *Lancet* 1991;338:131.
10. Centers for Disease Control. Recommendations for the use of folic acid to reduce the number of cases of spina bifida and other neural tube defects. *MMWR Morb Mortal Wkly Rep* 1992;41(RR 14):1–7.
11. Lewis DP, Van Dyke DC, Stumbo PJ, et al. Drug and environmental factors associated with adverse pregnancy outcomes. Part I: antiepileptic drugs, contraceptives, smoking, and folate. *Ann Pharmacother* 1998;37:802.
12. Lemire RJ. Neural tube defects. *JAMA* 1988;259:558–562.
13. Northrup H, Volcik KA. Spina bifida and other neural tube defects. *Curr Probl Pediatr* 2000;30:313–332.
14. Stevenson RE, Allen WP, Pai GS, et al. Decline in prevalence of neural tube defects in a high-risk region of the United States. *Pediatrics* 2000;106(4):677–683.
15. Rankin J, Glinianaia S, Brown R, et al. The changing prevalence of neural tube defects: a population-based study in the north of England, 1984–96. Northern Congenital Abnormality Survey Steering Group. *Paediatr Perinat Epidemiol* 2000;14(2):104–110.
16. Brock DJH, Sutcliffe RG. Alpha-fetoprotein in the antenatal diagnosis of anencephaly and spina bifida. *Lancet* 1972;ii:197.
17. United Kingdom collaborative study on alphafetoprotein measurement in antenatal screening for anencephaly and spina bifida in early pregnancy. *Lancet* 1977;1:1323–1332.
18. Filly RA, Callen PW, Goldstein RB. Alpha-fetoprotein screening programs: what every obstetric sonologist should know. *Radiology* 1993;188:1–9.
19. Nadel AS, Green JK, Holmes LB, et al. Absence of need for amniocentesis in patients with elevated levels of maternal serum alphafetoprotein and normal ultrasonographic examinations. *N Engl J Med* 1990;323:557–561.
20. Nadel AS, Norton ME, Wilkins-Haug L. Cost-effectiveness of strategies used in the evaluation of pregnancies complicated by elevated maternal serum alpha-fetoprotein levels. *Obstet Gynecol* 1997;89:660–665.

Acrania/Anencephaly

21. Moore KL, Persaud TVN. *The developing human: clinically oriented embryology*, 5th ed. Philadelphia: WB Saunders, 1993.
22. Mannes EJ, Crelin ES, Hobbins JS, et al. Sonographic demonstration of fetal acrania. *AJR Am J Roentgenol* 1982; 139:181.
23. Kwon TH, King J, Jeanty P. Acrania: review of 13 cases. *The Fetus* [online journal] 1991;1:1.
24. Goldstein RB, Filly RA. Prenatal diagnosis of anencephaly: spectrum of sonographic appearances and distinction from the amniotic band syndrome. *AJR Am J Roentgenol* 1988; 151:547.
25. Seller MJ. Sex, neural tube defects, and multisite closure of the human neural tube. *Am J Med Genet* 1995;58:332.

26. Shaw GM, Velie EM, Schaffer D. Risk of neural tube defect–affected pregnancies among obese women. *JAMA* 1996;275:1093.

27. Winsor SH, McGrath MJ, Khalifa M, et al. A report of recurrent anencephaly with trisomy 2p23-2pter: additional evidence for the involvement of 2p24 in neural tube development and evaluation of the role for cytogenetic analysis. *Prenat Diagn* 1997;17:665.

28. Hendricks SK, Cyr DR, Nyberg DA, et al. Exencephaly—clinical and ultrasonic correlation to anencephaly. *Obstet Gynecol* 1988;72(6):898–901.

29. Wilkins-Haug L, Freedman W. Progression of exencephaly to anencephaly in the human fetus—an ultrasound perspective. *Prenat Diagn* 1991;11(4):227–233.

30. Beinder E, Gruner C, Erhardt I, et al. [The exencephaly-anencephaly sequence. Ultrasound diagnosis in early pregnancy]. [Article in German] *Ultraschall Med* 1995;16(4): 192–195.

31. Timor-Tritsch IE, Greenebaum E, Monteagudo A, et al. Exencephaly-anencephaly sequence: proof by ultrasound imaging and amniotic fluid cytology. *J Matern Fetal Med* 1996;5(4):182–185.

32. Reference deleted.

33. Chervenak FA, Isaacson G, Mahoney MJ. Advances in the diagnosis of fetal defects. *N Engl J Med* 1986; 315:305.

34. Williamson P, Alberman E, Rodeck C, et al. Antecedent circumstances surrounding neural tube defect births in 1990–1991. The Steering Committee of the National Confidential Enquiry into Counseling for Genetic Disorders. *Br J Obstet Gynaecol* 1997;104:51.

35. Becker R, Mende B, Stiemer B, et al. Sonographic markers of exencephaly at 9 + 3 weeks of gestation. *Ultrasound Obstet Gynecol* 2000;16(6):582–584.

36. Johnson SP, Sebire NJ, Snijders RJ, et al. Ultrasound screening for anencephaly at 10–14 postmenstrual weeks. *Ultrasound Obstet Gynecol* 1997;9:14–16.

37. Nishi T, Nakano R. First trimester diagnosis of exencephaly by transvaginal ultrasound. *J Ultrasound Med* 1994; 13:149.

38. Chatzipapas IK, Whitlow BJ, Economides DL. The 'Mickey Mouse' sign and the diagnosis of anencephaly in early pregnancy. *Ultrasound Obstet Gynecol* 1999; 13:196.

39. David TJ, Nixon A. Congenital malformations associated with anencephaly and iniencephaly. *J Med Genet* 1976; 13:263.

40. Baird PA, Sadovnick AD. Survival in liveborn infants with anencephaly. *Am J Med Genet* 1987;28(4):1019–1020.

41. Toriello HV, Higgins JV. Occurrence of neural tube defects among first-, second-, and third-degree relatives of probands: results of a United States study. *Am J Hum Genet* 1983;15:601.

Amniotic Band Syndrome

42. Higgenbottom MC, Jones KL, Hall BD. The amniotic band disruption complex: timing of amniotic rupture and variable spectra of consequent defects. *J Pediatr* 1979; 95:544.

43. Torpin R. Amniochorionic mesoblastic fibrosis strings and amniotic bands. *Am J Obstet Gynecol* 1965;91:65.

44. Burton DJ, Filly RA. Sonographic diagnosis of the amniotic band syndrome. *AJR Am J Roentgenol* 1991;156:555.

45. Buyse ML. *Birth defects encyclopedia.* Cambridge, England: Blackwell Science, 1990.

46. Moessinger AC, Blanc WA, Byrne J. Amniotic band syndrome associated with amniocentesis. *Am J Obstet Gynecol* 1981;141:588.

47. Herva R, Karinen-Jaaskelainen M. Amniotic adhesion malformation syndrome: fetal and placental pathology. *Teratology* 1984;29:11.

48. Lockwood C, Ghidini ARR, Romero R, et al. Amniotic band syndrome: reevaluation of its pathogenesis. *Am J Obstet Gynecol* 1989;160:1030.

49. Kino Y. Clinical and experimental studies of the congenital constriction band syndrome, with an emphasis on its etiology. *J Bone Joint Surg Am* 1987;57:636.

50. Fiske CE, Filly RA, Golbus MS. Prenatal ultrasound diagnosis of amniotic band syndrome. *J Ultrasound Med* 1982;1:45.

51. Mahony BS, Filly RA, Gallen PW, et al. The amniotic band syndrome: antenatal sonographic diagnosis and potential pitfalls. *Am J Obstet Gynecol* 1985;152:63.

52. Goldstein I, Winn HN, Hobbins JC. Prenatal diagnosis criteria for body stalk anomaly. *Am J Perinatol* 1989;6:84.

53. Gorczyca DP, Lindfors KK, McGahan JP, et al. Limb-body-wall complex: another cause for elevated maternal serum alpha-fetoprotein. *J Clin Ultrasound* 1990;18:198.

Cephaloceles

54. David D, Proudman T. Cephaloceles: classification, pathology and management. *World J Surg* 1989;13:349.

55. Lorber J. The prognosis of occipital encephalocele. *Dev Med Child Neurol* 1966;13[Suppl]:75.

56. McLaurin RL. Cranium bifidum and cranial cephaloceles. In: Vinken GW, Bruyn PW, eds. *Handbook of clinical neurology*, vol. 30. Amsterdam: Elsevier/North Holland Biomedical Press, 1977:209.

57. Rapport R, Dunn R, Elhady F. Anterior encephalocele. *J Neurosurg* 1981;54:213.

58. Monteagudo A, Timor-Tritsch IE. Cephalocele, anterior. *The Fetus* [online journal] 1992;2:1.

59. Nicolini U, Ferrazzi E, Minonzio M, et al. Prenatal diagnosis of cranial masses by ultrasound: report of five cases. *J Clin Ultrasound* 1983;11:170.

60. Jeanty P, Dinesh S, Ulm J, et al. Fetal cephalocele: a sonographic spectrum. *Am J Perinatol* 1991;8:144.

61. Weinstein BJ, Benacerraf BR. Meckel syndrome, first trimester diagnosis. *The Fetus* [online journal] 1994;4:7598.

62. Sepulveda W, Sebire NJ, Souka A, et al. Diagnosis of the Meckel-Gruber syndrome at eleven to fourteen weeks' gestation. *Am J Obstet Gynecol* 1997;176:316.

63. Braithwaite JM, Economides DL. First-trimester diagnosis of Meckel-Gruber syndrome by transabdominal sonography in a low-risk case. *Prenat Diagn* 1995;15(12):1168–1170.

64. Budorick NE, Pretorius DH, McGahan MC, et al. Cephalocele detection in utero: sonographic and clinical features. *Ultrasound Obstet Gynecol* 1995;5:77.

65. Bronshtein M, Zimmer EZ. Transvaginal sonographic follow-up on the formation of fetal cephalocele at 13–19 weeks' gestation. *Obstet Gynecol* 1991;78:528.

66. Carlan SJ, Angel JL, Leo J, et al. Cephalocele involving the oral cavity. *Obstet Gynecol* 1990;75:494.

67. Simpson D, David D, White J. Cephaloceles: treatment, outcome and antenatal diagnosis. *Neurosurgery* 1984;15:14.

68. Winter TC 3rd, Mack LA, Cyr DR. Prenatal sonographic diagnosis of scalp edema/cephalohematoma mimicking an encephalocele. *AJR Am J Roentgenol* 1993;161(6):1247–1248.

69. Sherer DM, Perillo AM, Abramowicz JS. Fetal hemangioma overlying the temporal occipital suture, initially diagnosed by ultrasonography as an encephalocele. *J Ultrasound Med* 1993;12(11):691–693.

70. Bronshtein M, Bar-Hava I, Blumenfeld Z. Early second-trimester sonographic appearance of occipital haemangioma simulating encephalocele. *Prenat Diagn* 1992;12:695.

71. Shahabi S, Busine A. Prenatal diagnosis of an epidermal scalp cyst simulating an encephalocele. *Prenat Diagn* 1998;18(4):373–377.

72. Mitchell CS. Vertex hemangioma mimicking an encephalocele. *J Am Osteopath Assoc* 1999;99(12):626–627.

73. Noriega CA, Fleming AD, Bonebrake RG. A false-positive diagnosis of a prenatal encephalocele on transvaginal ultrasonography. *J Ultrasound Med* 2001;20(8):925–927.

74. Kang AH, Bruner JP. Cephalocele, anterior fontanelle. *The Fetus* [online journal] 1994;4:5.

75. Wininger SJ, Donnenfeld AE. Syndromes identified in fetuses with prenatally diagnosed cephaloceles. *Prenat Diagn* 1994;14(9):839–843.

76. Nyberg DA, Hallesy D, Mahony BS, et al. Meckel-Gruber syndrome. Importance of prenatal diagnosis. *J Ultrasound Med* 1990;9(12):691–696.

77. Fitz CR. Midline anomalies of the brain and spine. *Radiol Clin North Am* 1982;20:95.

78. Chervenak FA, Isaacson G, Mahoney MJ, et al. Diagnosis and management of fetal cephalocele. *Obstet Gynecol* 1984;64:86.

79. DeMyer W. The median cleft face syndrome: differential diagnosis of cranium bifidum occultum, hypertelorism, and median cleft nose, lip, and palate. *Neurology* 1967;17:961.

80. Goldstein RB, LaPidus AS, Filly RA. Fetal cephaloceles: diagnosis with ultrasound. *Radiology* 1991;180:803.

81. Bannister CM, Russell SA, Rimmer S, et al. Can prognostic indicators be identified in a fetus with an encephalocele? *Eur J Pediatr Surg* 2000;10[Suppl 1]:20–23.

82. Brown M, Sheridan-Pereira M. Outlook for a child with a cephalocele. *Pediatrics* 1992;90:914.

83. Martinez-Lage JF, Poza M, Sola J, et al. The child with a cephalocele: etiology, neuroimaging, and outcome. *Childs Nerv Syst* 1996;12(9):540–550.

84. Guthkelch AN. Occipital cranium bifidum. *Arch Dis Child* 1970;45:104.

Spine: Normal Development

85. O'Rahilly R, Muller F, Meyer DB. The human vertebral column at the end of the embryonic period proper: the column as a while. *J Anat* 1980;131:565–575.

86. Flecker H. Time of appearance and fusion of ossification centers as observed by roentgenographic methods. *AJR Am J Roentgenol* 1942;47:97–159.

87. Cochlin DL. Ultrasound of the fetal spine. *Clin Radiol* 1982;33:641–650.

88. Filly RA, Simpson GF, Linkowski G. Fetal spine morphology and maturation during the second trimester. *J Ultrasound Med* 1987;6:631–636.

89. Gray DL, Crane JP, Rudloff MA. Prenatal diagnosis of neural tube defects: origin of midtrimester vertebral ossification centers as determined by sonographic water-bath studies. *J Ultrasound Med* 1988;7:421–427.

Spina Bifida

90. Lindfors KK, McGahan JP, Tennant F, et al. Midtrimester screening for open neural tube defects: correlation of sonography with amniocentesis results. *AJR Am J Roentgenol* 1987;149(1):141–145.

91. Nicolaides KH, Campbell S, Gabbe SG. Ultrasound screening for spina bifida: cranial and cerebellar signs. *Lancet* 1986;2:72–74.

92. Kim SY, McGahan JP, Boggan JE, et al. Prenatal diagnosis of lipomyelomeningocele. *J Ultrasound Med* 2000;19(11):801–805.

93. McGahan JP, Leeba JM, Lindfors KK. Prenatal sonographic diagnosis of VATER association. *J Clin Ultrasound* 1988;16:588–591.

94. Patten DM. Embryological stages in the establishing of myeloschisis with spina bifida. *Am J Anat* 1953;93:365.

95. Gardner WI. Myelomeningocele, the result of rupture of the embryonic neural tube. *Cleve Clin Q* 1960;27:88.

96. Emery JL, Lendon RG. Lipomas of the cauda equina and other fatty tumours related to neurospinal dysraphism. *Dev Med Child Neurol* 1969;20[Suppl]:62.

97. Brocklehurst G. Spina bifida. In: Vinken PL, Bruyn GW, eds. *Handbook of clinical neurology*, vol. 30. Amsterdam: Elsevier/North Holland Biomedical Press, 1977:519–578.

98. Furness ME, Barbary JE, Verco PW. A pointer to spina bifida: fetal head shape in the second trimester. In: Gill RW, Dadd MJ, eds. *WFUMB* [World Federation of Ultrasound in Medicine and Biology] *1985 Proceedings*. Sydney: Pergamon Press, 1985:296.

99. Nicolaides KH, Campbell S, Gabbe SG. Ultrasound screening for spina bifida: cranial and cerebellar signs. *Lancet* 1986;2:72–74.

100. Pilu G, Romero R, Reece A, et al. Subnormal cerebellum in fetuses with spina bifida. *Am J Obstet Gynecol* 1988;158:1052–1056.

101. Furness ME, Barbary JE, Verco PW. Fetal head shape in spina bifida in the second trimester. *J Clin Ultrasound* 1987;15:451–453.

102. Goldstein RB, Podrasky AE, Filly RA, et al. Effacement of the fetal cisterna magna in association with myelomeningocele. *Radiology* 1989;172:409–413.

103. Benacerraf BR, Stryher J, Figoletto JD Jr, et al. Abnormal US appearance of the cerebellum (banana sign). Indirect sign of spina bifida. *Radiology* 1989;171:151–153.

104. Nyberg DA, Mack LA, Hirsch J, et al. Abnormalities of fetal cranial contour in sonographic detection of spina bifida: evaluation of the "lemon" sign. *Radiology* 1988;167(2):387–392.

105. Van den Hof MC, Nicolaides KH, Campbell J, et al. Evaluation of the lemon and banana signs in one hundred thirty fetuses with open spina bifida. *Am J Obstet Gynecol* 1990;162(2):322–327.

106. Thiagarajah S, Henke J, Hogge WA, et al. Early diagnosis of spina bifida: the value of cranial ultrasound markers. *Obstet Gynecol* 1990;76(1):54–57.

107. Watson WJ, Cheschier NC, Katz VL, et al. The role of ultrasound in the evaluation of patients with elevated maternal serum alpha-fetoprotein: a review. *Obstet Gynecol* 1991;78:123–128.

108. Kollias SS, Goldstein RB, Cogen PH, et al. Prenatally detected myelomeningoceles: sonographic accuracy in estimation of the spinal level. *Radiology* 1992;185:109–112.

109. Crane JP, LeFevre ML, Winborn RC, et al. A randomized trial of prenatal ultrasonographic screening: impact on the detection, management, and outcome of anomalous fetuses. The RADIUS Study Group. *Am J Obstet Gynecol* 1994; 171:392–399.

110. Boyd PA, Wellesley DG, De Walle HE, et al. Evaluation of the prenatal diagnosis of neural tube defects by fetal ultrasonographic examination in different centres across Europe. *J Med Screen* 2000;7(4):169–174.

111. Williamson P, Alberman E, Rodeck C, et al. Antecedent circumstances surrounding neural tube defect births in 1990–91. The Steering Committee of the National Confidential Enquiry into Counseling for Genetic Disorders. *Br J Obstet Gynaecol* 1997;104:51–55.

112. Sebire NJ, Noble PL, Thorpe-Beeston JG, et al. Presence of the "lemon" sign in fetuses with spina bifida at the 10–14-week scan. *Ultrasound Obstet Gynecol* 1997;10:403–407.

113. Williams B. Is aqueduct stenosis a result of hydrocephalus? *Brain* 1973;96:399.

114. Sharrard W. The mechanism of paralytic deformity in spina bifida. *Dev Med Child Neurol* 1962;4:310.

115. Hunt GM, Poulton A. Open spina bifida: a complete cohort reviewed 25 years after closure. *Dev Med Child Neurol* 1995;37:19–29.

116. Park TS, Hoffman HJ, Hendrick EB, et al. Experience with surgical decompression of the Arnold-Chiari malformation in young infants with myelomeningocele. *Neurosurgery* 1983;13:147.

117. Chervenak FA, Duncan C, Ment L, et al. Perinatal management of myelomeningocele. *Obstet Gynecol* 1984;63:376.

118. Luthy DA, Wardinsky T, Shurtleff DB, et al. Cesarean section before the onset of labor and subsequent motor function in infants with meningomyelocele diagnosed antenatally. *N Engl J Med* 1991;324:662–666.

119. Sutton LN, Adzick NS, Bilaniuk LT, et al. Improvement in hindbrain herniation demonstrated by serial fetal magnetic resonance imaging following fetal surgery for myelomeningocele. *JAMA* 1999;282(19):1826–1831.

120. Olutoye OO, Adzick NS. Fetal surgery for myelomeningocele. *Semin Perinatol* 1999;23:462–473.

121. Bruner JP, Tulipan N, Paschall RL, et al. Fetal surgery for myelomeningocele and the incidence of shunt-dependent hydrocephalus. *JAMA* 1999;282:1819–1825.

122. Holzbeierlein J, Pope JC IV, Adams MC, et al. The urodynamic profile of myelodysplasia in childhood with spinal closure during gestation. *J Urol* 2000;164:1336–1339.

123. Bannister CM. The case for and against intrauterine surgery for myelomeningoceles. *Eur J Obstet Gynecol Reprod Biol* 2000;92:109–113.

Iniencephaly

124. Lewis HL. Iniencephalus. *Am J Obstet* 1897;35:11–53.

125. Nishimura H, Okamoto N. Iniencephaly. In: Vinken PJ, Bruyn GW, eds. *Handbook of clinical neurology*, vol. 30. New York: North-Holland Biochemical Press, 1977:257–268.

126. Gardner WJ. Klippel-Feil syndrome, iniencephalus, anencephalus, hindbrain hernia and minor movements: overdistension of the neural tube. *Child Brain* 1979;5:361–369.

127. Aleksic S, Budzilovich G, Greco MA, et al. Iniencephaly: a neuropathologic study. *Clin Neuropathol* 1983;2:55–61.

128. Morocz I, Szeifert T, Molnar P, et al. Prenatal diagnosis and pathoanatomy of iniencephaly. *Clin Genet* 1986;30:81–86.

129. Meizner I, Bar-Ziv J. Prenatal ultrasonic diagnosis of a rare case of iniencephaly apertus. *J Clin Ultrasound* 1987;15:200–203.

130. Romero R, Pilu G, Jeanty P, et al. *Prenatal diagnosis of congenital anomalies.* Norwalk, CT: Appleton & Lange, 1988:64–67.

131. Sahid S, Sepulveda W, Dezerega V, et al. Iniencephaly: prenatal diagnosis and management. *Prenat Diagn* 2000;20:202–205.

132. Shoham Z, Caspi B, Chemke J, et al. Iniencephaly: prenatal ultrasonographic diagnosis—a case report. *J Perinat Med* 1988;16:139–143.

133. Gunderson CH, Greenspan RH, Glaser G, et al. The Klippel-Feil syndrome: genetic and clinical reevaluation of cervical fusion. *Medicine* 1967;46:491–512.

134. Gilmour JR. The essential identity of Klippel-Feil syndrome and iniencephaly. *J Pathol* 1941;53:117–131.

135. Sherk HH, Shut L, Chung S. Iniencephalic deformity of the cervical spine with Klippel-Feil anomalies and congenital evaluation of the scapula. *J Bone Joint Surg* 1974;56-A:1254.

136. Lemire, RJ, Beckwith, B, Shepard TH. Iniencephaly and anencephaly with spinal retroflexion: a comparative study of eight human specimens. *Teratology* 1972;6:27–36.

137. Katz VL, Aylsworth AS, Albright SG. Iniencephaly is not uniformly fatal. *Prenat Diagn* 1989;9:595–599.

138. Cunningham I. Iniencephalus: a case of dystocia. *Br J Obstet Gynaecol* 1965;72:299–301.

Hemivertebra

139. Harrison LA, Pretorius DH, Budorick NE. Abnormal spinal curvature in the fetus. *J Ultrasound Med* 1992;11(9):473–479.

140. Benacerraf BR, Greene MF, Barss VA. Prenatal sonographic diagnosis of congenital hemivertebrae. *J Ultrasound Med* 1986;5:257.

141. Nyberg DA, Mack LA. The spine defects. In: Nyberg DA, Mahoney BS, Pretorius DH, eds. *Diagnostic ultrasound of fetal anomalies.* Chicago: Year Book Medical Publishers, 1990:146–192.

142. Patten DM, Van Allen M, Mack LA, et al. Limb-body wall complex: in utero sonographic diagnosis of a complicated fetal malformation. *AJR Am J Roentgenol* 1986;146:1019–1024.

143. Wynne-Davies R. Congenital vertebral anomalies: aetiology and relationship to spina bifida cystica. *J Med Genet* 1975;12:280–288.

144. McMaster MJ, David CV. Hemivertebra as a cause of scoliosis. *J Bone Joint Surg* 1986;68:588–595.

145. Zelop CM, Pretorius DH, Benacerraf BR. Fetal hemivertebrae: associated anomalies, significance, and outcome. *Obstet Gynecol* 1993;81:412–416.

Diastematomyelia

146. Winter RB. Congenital scoliosis. *Orthop Clin North Am* 1988;19:395–408.

147. Connor JM, Conner AN, Connor RAC, et al. Genetic aspects of early childhood scoliosis. *Am J Med Genet* 1987;27:419–424.

148. Guth Kelch AN, Jones RA, Zierski J. Diastematomyelia. *Dev Med Child Neurol* 1971;13[Suppl]:137–138.

149. Bremer JL. Dorsal intestinal fistula. Accessory neuroenteric canal: diastematomyelia. *Arch Pathol* 1952;54:132–138.

150. Padget DH. Neuroschisis and human embryonic maldevelopment. *J Neuropathol Exp Neurol* 1970;29:192.

151. Gardner WS. Diastematomyelia and the Klippel-Feil syndrome: relationship to hydrocephalus, syringomyelia, meningocele, meningomyelocele and miencephalus. *Clev Clin A* 1964;31:19–44.

152. Winter RK, McKnight L, Byrne RA, et al. Diastematomyelia: prenatal ultrasonic appearances. *Clin Radiol* 1989;40:291–294.

153. Anderson NG, Jordan S, McFarlane MR, et al. Diastematomyelia: diagnosis by prenatal sonography. *AJR Am J Roentgenol* 1994;163:911–914.

154. Sepulveda W, Kyle PM, Hassan J, et al. Prenatal diagnosis of diastematomyelia: case reports and review of the literature. *Prenat Diagn* 1997;17:2,161–165.

155. Allen LM, Silverman RK. Prenatal ultrasound evaluation of fetal diastematomyelia: two cases of type I split cord malformation. *Ultrasound Obstet Gynecol* 2000;15(1):78–82.

156. Schut L, Sutton NL, Duhaine AC. Congenital neurological disorders of the lumbar spine presenting in the adult. In: Frymover WJ, ed. *The adult spine: principles and practice.* New York: Raven Press, 1991.

157. Rothman RH, Simeone FA. Anomalie congenite del rachide. In: *Il Rachide.* Bologna: Gaggi, 1978.

Caudal Regression

158. Carter CO. Spinal dysraphism: genetic relation to neural tube malformations. *J Med Genet* 1976;13:343–350.

159. Mok PM. Sirenomelia: a morphological study of 33 cases and review of the literature. *Perspect Pediatr Pathol* 1987;10:7.

160. Onyeije CI, Sherer DM, Handwerker S, et al. Prenatal diagnosis of sirenomelia with bilateral hydrocephalus: report of a previously undocumented form of VACTERL-H association. *Am J Perinatol* 1998;15(3):193–197.

161. Mills JL. Malformations in infants of diabetic mothers. *Teratology* 1982;25:385.

162. Passarge E, Lenze W. Syndrome of caudal regression in infants of diabetic mothers: observations of further cases. *Pediatrics* 1965;37:672.

163. Rusnak SL, Driscoll SG. Congenital spinal anomalies in infants of diabetic mothers. *Pediatrics* 1965;35:989.

164. Finer NN, Bowen P, Dunbar LG. Caudal regression anomalad (sacral agenesis) in siblings. *Clin Genet* 1978;13:353.

165. Stewart JM, Stoll S. Familial caudal regression anomalad and maternal diabetes. *J Med Genet* 1979;16:17.

166. Hotston S, Carty H. Lumbosacral agenesis: a report of three new cases and a review of the literature. *Br J Radiol* 1982;55:629.

167. Baxi L, Warren W, Collins MH, et al. Early detection of caudal regression syndrome with transvaginal scanning. *Obstet Gynecol* 1990;75:486.

168. Lowey JA, Richards DG, Toi A. In utero diagnosis of the caudal regression syndrome: report of three cases. *J Clin Ultrasound* 1987;15:469.

169. Meizner I, Press F, Jaffe A, et al. Prenatal ultrasound diagnosis of complete absence of the lumbar spine and sacrum. *J Clin Ultrasound* 1992;20:77.

170. Sonek JD, Gabbe SG, Landon MB, et al. Antenatal diagnosis of sacral agenesis syndrome in a pregnancy complicated by diabetes mellitus. *Am J Obstet Gynecol* 1990;162:806.

Sacrococcygeal Teratoma

171. Altman RP, Randolph JG, Lilley JR. Sacrococcygeal teratoma: American Academy of Pediatrics Surgical Section Survey. *J Pediatr Surg* 1974;9:389–398.

172. Donnellan WA, Swenson O. Benign and malignant sacrococcygeal teratomas. *Surgery* 1968;64:834.

173. Gross RE, Clatworthy HW Jr, Meeker IA. Sacrococcygeal teratomas in infants and children. A report of 40 cases. *Surg Gynecol Obstet* 1951;92:341.

174. Valdiserri RO, Yunis EJ. Sacrococcygeal teratoma: a review of 68 cases. *Cancer* 1981;48:217–221.

175. Gross SJ, Benzie RJ, Sermer M, et al. Sacrococcygeal teratoma: prenatal diagnosis and management. *Am J Obstet Gynecol* 1987;156:393–396.

176. Hogge WA, Thiagarajah S, Barber VG, et al. Cystic sacrococcygeal teratoma: ultrasound diagnosis and perinatal management. *J Ultrasound Med* 1987;6:707–710.

177. Sheth S, Nussbaum AR, Sanders RC, et al. Prenatal diagnosis of sacrococcygeal teratoma: sonographic-pathologic correlation. *Radiology* 1988;169:131–136.

178. Teal LN, Angtuaco TL, Jimenez JF, et al. Fetal teratomas: antenatal diagnosis and clinical management. *J Clin Ultrasound* 1988;16:329–336.

179. Bond SJ, Harrison MR, Schmidt KG, et al. Death due to high output cardiac failure in fetal sacrococcygeal teratoma. *J Pediatr Surg* 1990;25:1287–1291.

180. Evans MJ, Danielian PJ, Gray ES. Sacrococcygeal teratoma: a case of mistaken identity. *Pediatr Radiol* 1994:24:52–53.

181. Shipp TD, Shamberger RC, Benacerraf BR. Prenatal diagnosis of a grade 4 sacrococcygeal teratoma. *J Ultrasound Med* 1996;15:175–177.

182. Winderl LM, Silverman RK. Prenatal identification of completely cystic internal sacrococcygeal teratoma (type 4). *Ultrasound Obstet Gynecol* 1997;9:425–428.

183. Sherer DM, Fromberg RA, Rindfusz DW, et al. Color Doppler–aided prenatal diagnosis of a type 1 cystic sacrococcy-

geal teratoma simulating a meningomyelocele. *Am J Perinatol* 1997;14:13–15.

184. Kirkinen P, Heinonen S, Vanamo K, et al. Maternal serum alpha-fetoprotein and epithelial tumor marker concentration are not increased by fetal sacrococcygeal teratoma. *Prenat Diagn* 1997;17:47–50.

185. Montgomery ML, Lillehei C, Acker D, et al. Intra-abdominal sacrococcygeal mature teratoma or fetus in fetus in a third-trimester fetus. *Ultrasound Obstet Gynecol* 1998;11:219–221.

186. Burgess I, Hines B, Stevenson P. Cystic type 4 sacrococcygeal teratoma detected at 18 week prenatal diagnosis. *Ultrasound Obstet Gynecol* 1998;11:305.

187. Holterman AX, Filiatrault D, Lallier M, et al. The natural history of sacrococcygeal teratoma diagnosed through routine obstetric sonogram: a single institute experience. *J Pediatr Surg* 1998;33:899–903.

188. Chisholm CA, Heider AL, Kuller JA, et al. Prenatal diagnosis and perinatal management of fetal sacrococcygeal teratoma. *Am J Perinatol* 1999;16:89–92.

189. Westerburg B, Feldstein VA, Sandberg PL, et al. Sonographic prognostic factors in fetuses with sacrococcygeal teratoma. *J Pediatr Surg* 2000;35:322–325.

190. Brace V, Grant SR, Brackley KJ, et al. Prenatal diagnosis and outcome in sacrococcygeal teratomas: a review of cases between 1992 and 1998. *Prenat Diagn* 2000;20(1):51–55.

191. Kivilevich Z. Sacrococcygeal teratoma. *The Fetus* [online journal] 2000.

192. Presti F, Sanusi FA, Hamid R. Three-dimensional prenatal ultrasound study of a large sacrococcygeal teratoma. *Int J Gynaecol Obstet* 2001;73(1):61–63.

193. Bonilia-Musoles F, Machado LE, Raga F, et al. Prenatal diagnosis of sacrococcygeal teratomas by two- and three-dimensional ultrasound. *Ultrasound Obstet Gynecol* 2002;19(2):200–205.

194. Avni FE, Guibaud L, Robert Y, et al. MR imaging of fetal sacrococcygeal teratoma: diagnosis and assessment. *AJR Am J Roentgenol* 2002;178(1):179–183.

195. Graf JL, Albanese CT, Jennings RW, et al. Successful fetal sacrococcygeal teratoma resection in a hydropic fetus. *J Pediatr Surg* 2000;35(10):1489–1491.

196. Paek BW, Jennings RW, Harrison MR, et al. Radiofrequency ablation of human fetal sacrococcygeal teratoma. *Am J Obstet Gynecol* 2001;184(3):503–507.

197. Lam YH, Tang MH, Shek TW. Thermocoagulation of fetal sacrococcygeal teratoma. *Prenat Diagn* 2002;22(2):99–101.

198. Sonnino RE, Chou S, Guttman FM. Hereditary sacrococcygeal teratoma. *J Pediatr Surg* 1989;24:1074–1075.

199. Hunt PT, et al. Radiography of hereditary presacral teratoma. *Radiology* 1977;122:187–191.

200. Kochling J, Pistor G, Marzhauser Brands S, et al. The Currarino syndrome—hereditary syndrome of anorectal, sacral and presacral anomalies. Case report and review of the literature. *Eur J Pediatr Surg* 1996;6:114.

8

THE FACE AND NECK

This chapter discusses a wide range of abnormalities that may affect the face. Three-dimensional (3-D) ultrasound is discussed in detail elsewhere (see Chapter 24). However, due to its increasing importance in prenatal detection and display of facial abnormalities, 3-D ultrasound is also incorporated throughout this chapter. A related chapter is Chapter 5, because the face is often involved in multiple anomalies.

INTRODUCTION

The fetal face is an important part of the sonographic structural survey and should be examined whenever feasible. In human fetuses, the facial abnormalities are among the more common malformations that have many different etiologies. Craniofacial abnormalities occur as isolated malformations of the face or as a result of syndromes such as chromosomal anomalies, genetic and nongenetic syndromes with multiple congenital anomalies of other systems, or environmental insults. When associated with a syndrome and other anomalies, facial defects are sometimes easier to identify sonographically than many of the more subtle anomalies of other organs (such as cardiac defects). It is important to evaluate the fetal face during all structural sonographic surveys of the fetus, as facial defects may indicate the presence of other, more subtle anomalies involving other organs.

Prenatal evaluation of the face and detection of facial anomalies dates back to the early 1980s, when several authors first reported the sonographic detection of fetal cleft lip and palate, anophthalmia, micrognathia, and so forth.[1-4] One of the largest early studies evaluating the detection of fetal facial defects showed a sensitivity of 89% for the detection of craniofacial malformations.[3] Another study suggests that the detection rate of craniofacial malformations remains essentially unchanged, at 72%.[5] It is of interest that in the presence of anomalies involving other organs the detection rate of craniofacial malformations was 100%, whereas, for *isolated* facial malformations, the detection rate was no more than 50%. These data suggest that, even today, the fetal face is not always evaluated completely during routine prenatal sonograms—particularly in the absence of any other major malformations.

The American Institute of Ultrasound and Medicine has yet to include the examination of the fetal face in its guidelines for second- and third-trimester fetal sonography. Evaluation of the fetal face, however, is an extremely important part of the structural survey and is necessary to demonstrate that the fetus is normal or to characterize the abnormality in an anomalous fetus. The fetal face lends itself beautifully to evaluation by sonography because of its surrounding fluid. Imaging of the fetal face in three planes (if possible) should not add more than a minute or two to the general screening sonographic fetal examination.

EMBRYOLOGY

The first step in learning about craniofacial malformations is to understand the embryology leading to the formation of the face; the following section, Technique for the Sonographic Examination of the Face, is a very brief overview of this important subject.[6-8] The branchial arches appear in the fourth and fifth weeks of development, and the four branchial arches represent bars of mesenchymal tissue that are separated by clefts. At the end of the fourth week, the stomodeum (rudimentary mouth) is formed at the center of the face and is surrounded by the first pair of branchial arches. Each branchial arch has a core of mesenchyme covered on the outside by ectoderm and on the inside by epithelium (endodermal in origin). Each arch contains neural crest cells, which contribute to the skeletal development of the face. The mesoderm of the arches results in the musculature of the face and neck. The first branchial arch gives rise to the maxilla and the mandible, including the premaxilla, zygoma, and part of the temporal bone.

The fetal face develops around the fifth week of embryonic life (Fig. 1). The nasal placodes evaginate to form the nasal pits. The ridges that result are called the *frontal nasal prominences*, and these form the upper boundary of the stomodeum. Coming from the first branchial arch, the paired maxillary prominences form the lateral boundaries of the stomodeum. The paired mandibular prominences (also from

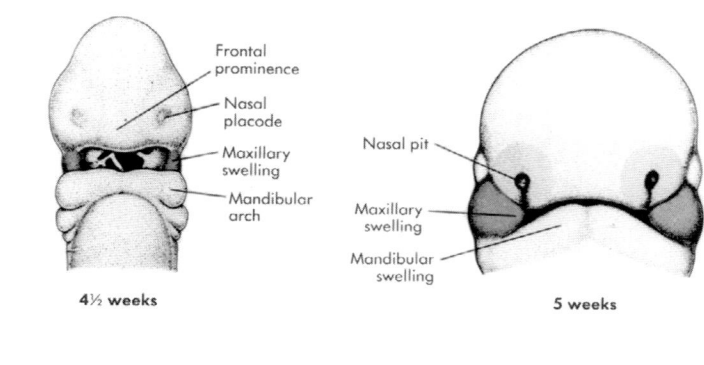

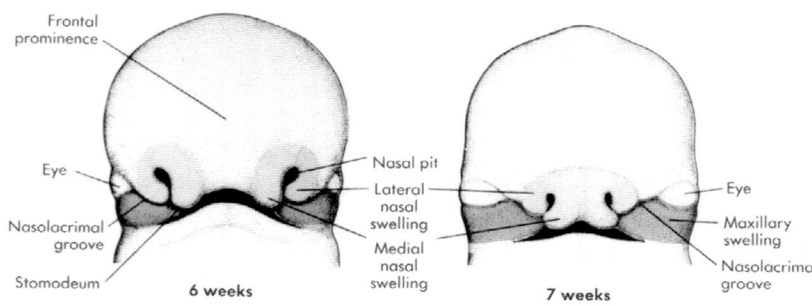

FIGURE 1. Embryologic development of the face from 4.5 to 7.0 weeks. (Reproduced with permission from Sadler TW. *Langman's medical embryology*, 5th ed. Baltimore: Williams & Wilkins, 1985.)

the first branchial arch) form the caudal boundary. Between weeks 5 and 8, the maxillary prominences grow medially, thus obliterating the grooves between the nasal prominences and the maxillary prominences. Hence, the upper lip is formed by the fusion of the maxillary prominences with the medial nasal prominences (otherwise known as the *intermaxillary segment*). The mandibular prominences merge to form the lower lip, chin, and mandible.

The nose is formed by five prominences: the frontal prominence forms the bridge of the nose; the two medial nasal prominences form the crest, tip, and central portion of the lip, or the intermaxillary segment; and the lateral nasal prominences form the sides, or the alae. The two medial nasal prominences, which fuse together to form the intermaxillary segment, not only form the philtrum component of the upper lip, but also the incisor teeth and the front portion of the palate, or *primary* palate. It is the partial or complete lack of fusion of one or both of the maxillary prominences with the medial nasal prominences (or the intermaxillary segment) that results in a unilateral or bilateral cleft lip and palate. The split occurs between the lateral incisors and canine teeth and along the side of the upper lip in the paramedian position. The median cleft lip is caused by incomplete merging of the two medial nasal prominences and results in a midline cleft. This is more likely to be associated with severe multiple congenital anomalies such as holoprosencephaly.

Abnormalities that originate from the first branchial arch are the result of insufficient migration of the cranial neural crest cells into the first branchial arch, and syndromes resulting from this defect include Treacher Collins syndrome (mandibulofacial dysostosis) and Pierre Robin

syndrome. Neural crest cells also contribute to the formation of the aortic and pulmonary arteries; therefore, some first arch syndromes can be accompanied by congenital heart defects.

TECHNIQUE FOR THE SONOGRAPHIC EXAMINATION OF THE FACE

In general, most practitioners evaluate the fetal face qualitatively, using three views: the coronal view, looking at bone and soft tissue from the surface well into the palate and orbits; the transverse view, looking at the mandible, maxilla, tooth buds, and orbits; and, last, the sagittal view, evaluating the nasal bridge, the frontal bone, the mandible, and the symmetry of the face. Ultrasound can optimally demonstrate external contour of the face when it is outlined by fluid (Figs. 2 through 4). Magnetic resonance imaging (MRI) has the potential to better visualize the palate and internal anatomy (Fig. 4B) although it is infrequently used to evaluate the fetal face. Color Doppler can also be used to evaluate the integrity of the alveolar ridge and palate. During respiratory activity, one can visualize flow of amniotic fluid, usually coming through the nostrils. Facial features can also be seen from a unique perspective using 3-D sonography (Figs. 5 and 6) as well as MRI (Fig. 4B).

The technique for the evaluation of the face—particularly when looking for a facial cleft—includes the coronal scan of the anterior mid-face, extending from the bony aspects of the maxilla and mandible out to the soft tissue components of the coronal view (Fig. 2). Rocking the

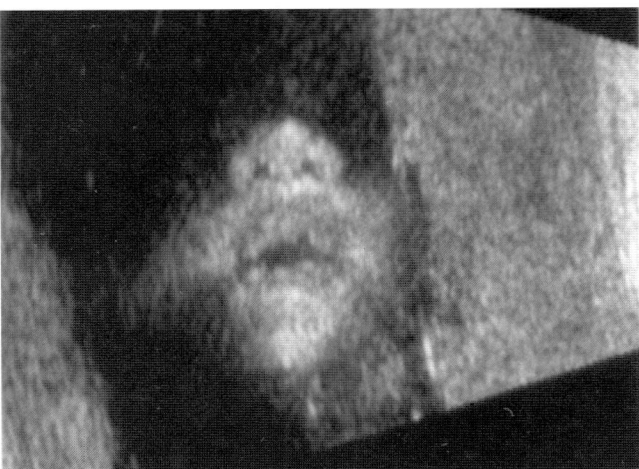

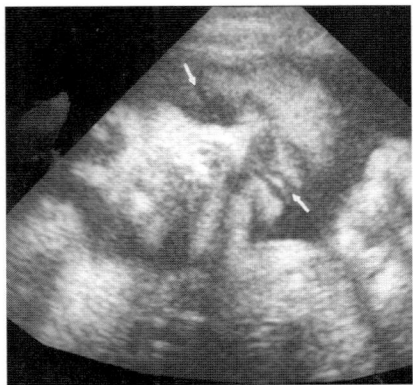

FIGURE 3. Coronal view of the face in the third trimester, showing the soft tissues, including the eyelids (*arrows*).

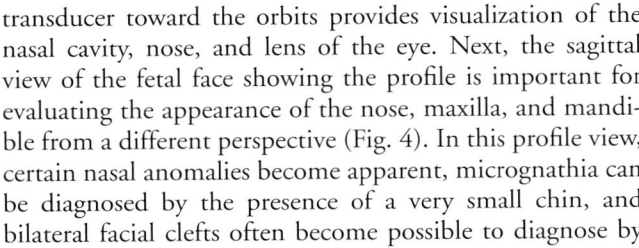

FIGURE 2. Coronal view of face. Ultrasound image in semicoronal plane aligned along the anterior contour shows lips, nose, and nostrils.

transducer toward the orbits provides visualization of the nasal cavity, nose, and lens of the eye. Next, the sagittal view of the fetal face showing the profile is important for evaluating the appearance of the nose, maxilla, and mandible from a different perspective (Fig. 4). In this profile view, certain nasal anomalies become apparent, micrognathia can be diagnosed by the presence of a very small chin, and bilateral facial clefts often become possible to diagnose by

the visualization of an anterior projection of the inner maxillary segment in combination with the nose, which forms a mass projecting forward from the midface.[9]

Measurements of various aspects of the abnormal facial development have been studied, in an attempt to quantify facial anomalies.[10–15] These measurements are helpful in evaluating a fetus with either a significant family history or a questionable abnormality. Such measurements as the

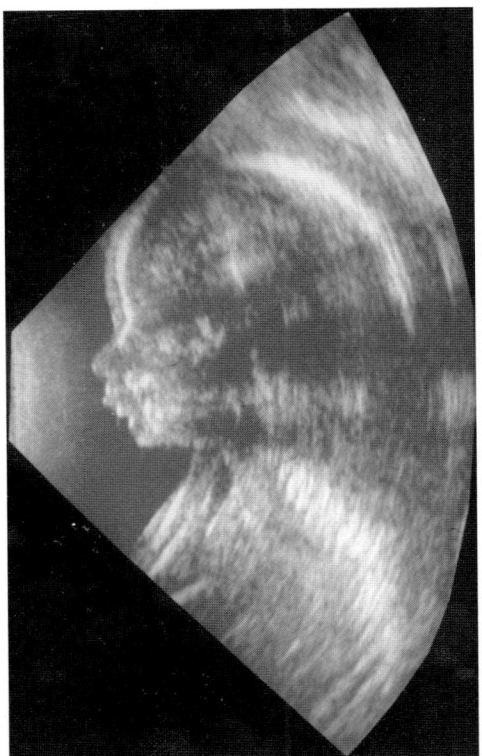

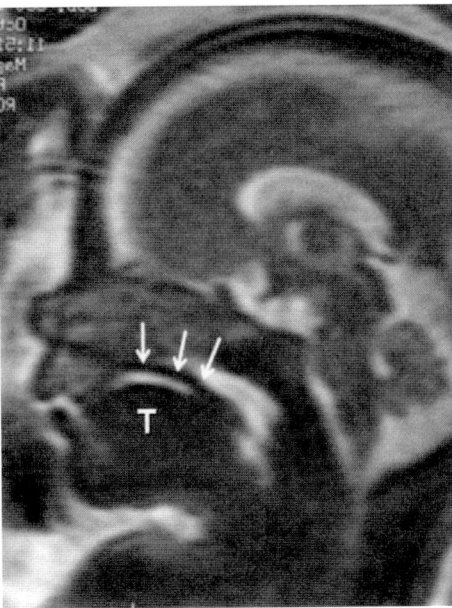

FIGURE 4. Facial profile. **A:** Ultrasound from late second trimester. Note the differentiation between the echogenic bony structures and the soft tissues. **B:** Magnetic resonance image at 25 weeks. Note that the palate (*arrows*) separates the high-intensity fluid in the oral cavity and hypopharynx. T, tongue.

A,B

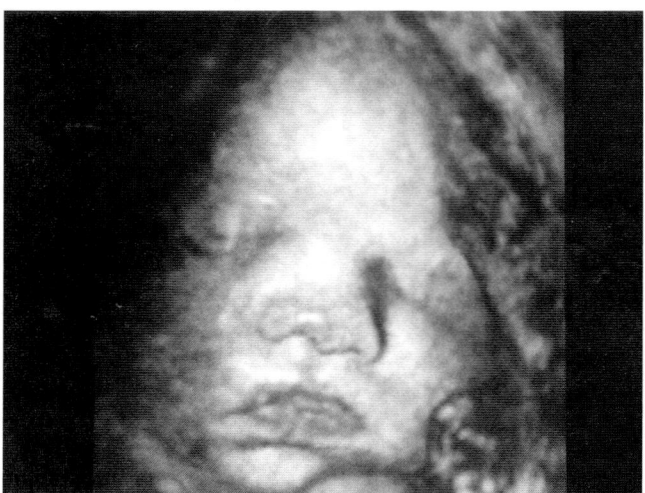

FIGURE 5. Three-dimensional surface rendering views of a third-trimester fetal face. The ability to change orientation permits recognition of subtle structures.

upper lip width, chin length, and others are available for normal second- and third-trimester fetuses.

Evaluating tooth buds is helpful for detecting different types of cleft palate or syndromes that have associated oligodontia or partial anodontia. In a study of 124 obstetric patients, at least four tooth buds were found in the jaws of each fetus between 19 and 34 weeks.[16] Before 19 weeks, the exact number and location of tooth buds could not be determined.

Evaluation of the fetal nose is usually done subjectively. However, the width and length of nasal bones have been characterized quantitatively, and these normal biometric measurements are available.[17–19] For normal fetuses between 14 and 40 weeks, nasal widths and internostral distances

have been established, showing a linear growth relationship between those measurements and gestational age.

Evaluation of the jaw is also usually subjective. However, mandibular measurements may be obtained in several different ways. Chitty advocates measuring the length of the mandibular rami and provides normative data between 12 and 28 weeks. Another approach[15] involves assessing the mandible on an axial plane at the base of the cranium and measuring the lateral and anteroposterior diameters. A line joining the bases of the two rami describes the lateral diameter. The anteroposterior diameter extends from the symphysis menti to the middle of the lateral diameter. One can also calculate the *jaw index* as follows:

$$\left(\frac{\text{Anteroposterior mandibular diameter}}{\text{biparietal diameter}}\right) \times 100$$

Measurements of the fetal tongue while inside the mouth have been correlated with gestational age. The tongue circumference as a function of gestational age is expressed as follows: tongue circumference in millimeters = –23.9 + 2.75 × gestational age in weeks.[20] Abnormal tongue measurements can be seen in fetuses with macroglossia (as in Beckwith-Wiedemann syndrome) or microglossia (as in certain chromosomal abnormalities).

Brief evaluation of the orbits can be routinely obtained on a transverse sweep of the face. Two orbits equal in size should be present (Fig. 7). As an estimate, the distance between the orbits (interorbital distance) should be slightly greater than the diameter of the globe (see Appendix 1, Table 23). If these relationships do not appear to be true, or the fetus is considered at high risk for facial abnormalities, measurements of the eyes may be obtained including orbital diameters, interorbital distance, and intraorbital distance (binocular distance).[21–23] The normal outer orbital dis-

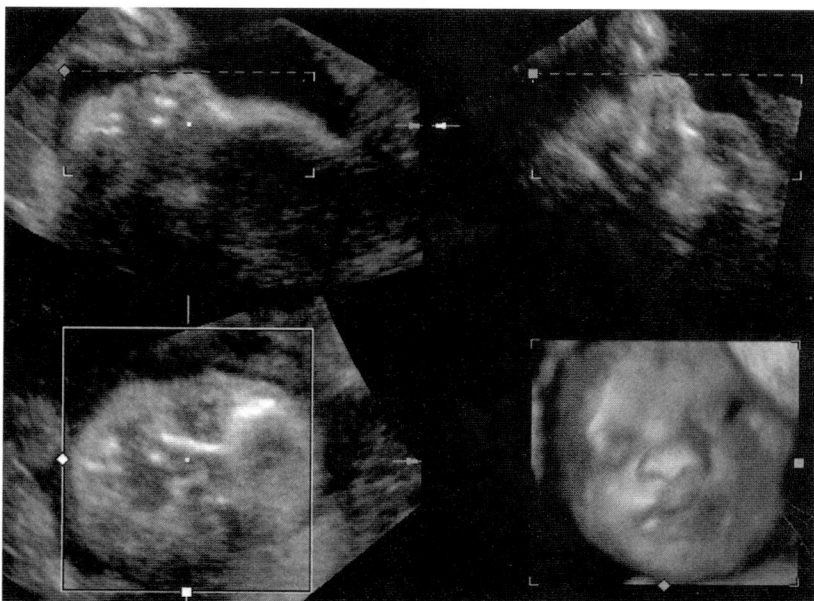

FIGURE 6. Three-dimensional ultrasound in multiplanar mode permits precise imaging in three orthogonal planes simultaneously (**upper left**, sagittal view; **upper right**, axial view; **lower left**, coronal view). This is very helpful for deeper structures. Surface-rendered mode **(lower right)** best delineates outer contour.

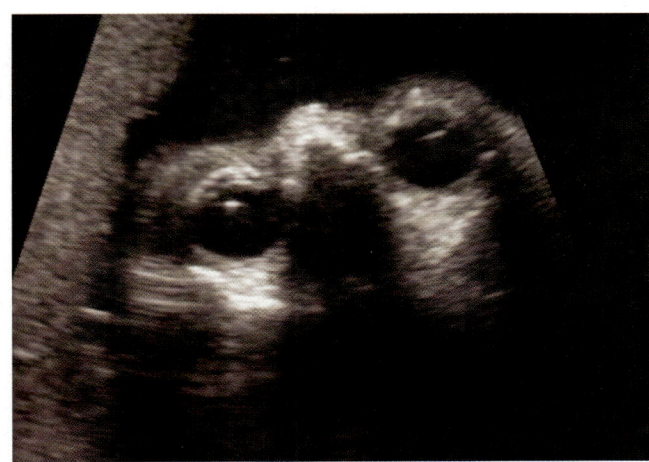

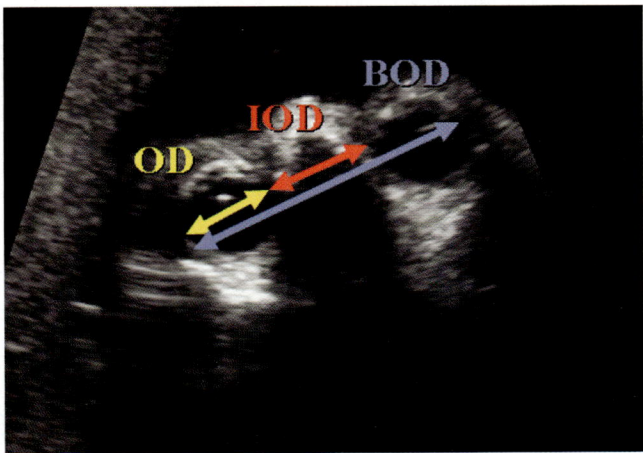

FIGURE 7. Normal orbits. **A:** Transverse view shows normal orbits. **B:** Normal orbital measurements of ocular diameter (*OD*), interocular diameter (*IOD*), and binocular diameter (*BOD*). Note that the interocular distance is only slightly greater than the ocular diameter.

range of 87 to 90 degrees, an abnormal downward slant was identified in a fetus with Seckel syndrome and an abnormal upward slant in a fetus with Down syndrome.

THREE-DIMENSIONAL ULTRASOUND

A number of studies have shown the benefits of using 3-D ultrasound for evaluating fetal facial malformations, including cleft lip with or without cleft lip/palate (CL/P).[25–28] Using not only surface display but also multiplanar reconstruction in three planes, Merz et al.[27] used transvaginal and abdominal 3-D scanning to better define malformations of the fetal face. A total of 25 fetuses with facial anomalies were detected by two-dimensional (2-D) abdominal sonography, and, although 20 cases were clearly seen using 3-D and 2-D sonography, in five cases 3-D sonography provided additional information not detectable by 2-D sonography. This included unilateral orbital hypoplasia, cranial ossification defects, and a flat profile.

Hata et al.[25] studied 94 healthy fetuses between 15 and 40 weeks, using 2-D and 3-D images.[25] The investigators showed that no significant difference in image quality of the face could be detected between 2-D and 3-D imaging. However, they suggested that 3-D sonography was found to be quite helpful in the evaluation of sutures, such as in fetuses suspected of having craniosynostosis, and in the depiction of fetal ear anomalies often overlooked using 2-D sonography.

Because of its unique display, 3-D ultrasound aids parents and referring physicians to understanding the extent of the defects.[29,30] Patient decisions may be affected in evaluation of CL/P, because they can view the abnormality on a recognizable 3-D–rendered image.[31] 3-D ultrasonographic imaging of fetal tooth buds can accurately classify clefts.[32]

FACIAL ABNORMALITIES

Facial abnormalities are important themselves but may also indicate an underlying problem, particularly a chromosome abnormality or syndromic condition (see Chapter 5). Therefore, it is important to evaluate the face when other anomalies are demonstrated and, conversely, search for additional anomalies when facial abnormalities are evident.

The frequency of chromosome abnormalities varies with reasons for referral, patient population, and the sensitivity of detecting isolated facial abnormalities. In one referred population, Nicolaides et al. reported 146 fetuses with facial defects who underwent chromosome analysis and, therefore, were considered to be at high risk. Chromosomal anomalies were present in 37 of 56 fetuses (66%) with micrognathia; 10 of 13 fetuses (77%) with macroglossia; 31 of 64 fetuses (48%) with cleft lip and palate; 5 of 11 fetuses (45%) with hypotelorism or cyclopia; and 6 of 19 fetuses (32%) with nasal hypoplasia or proboscis.[33]

tance (in millimeters) = −22.17 + 3.36 × gestational age − 0.03 × (gestational age)^2. The normal intraorbital distance (in millimeters) is −4.14 + 0.94 × gestational age − 0.007 × (gestational age)^2.[21] Mayden et al. also developed normative data for inner orbital and outer orbital distances as early as 1982,[22] and Jeanty et al. reported the normal ocular measurements in 1982.[23] These normative data are still in use today. Measurements of the normal orbit and lens are also available.[11] There is a linear growth function between gestational age and orbital width as well as between gestational age and diameter of the fetal lens. Other investigators have produced tables showing measurements of the vitreous circumference and lens circumference for fetuses between 12 and 37 weeks.[12]

Practitioners have tried to identify abnormal palpebral fissure slants, in attempts to diagnosis certain syndromes. Mielke et al.[24] developed a technique for the measurement of the palpebral fissure slant, using a frontal view of the face and the interior angle between the palpebral fissure and the midline of the skull. Assuming a normal interior angle

In 1986, Benacerraf et al. reviewed abnormal facial features in association with trisomies 18 and 13 and found that all the fetuses with trisomy 13 had associated intracranial anomalies (mostly holoprosencephaly), whereas the fetuses with trisomy 18 tended to have abnormal extremities, intrauterine growth retardation, and congenital heart disease.[34,35]

In the following sections, various facial anomalies are discussed. Because facial abnormalities associated with holoprosencephaly are more severe and distinctive, they are summarized separately. Holoprosencephaly is discussed in depth elsewhere (see Chapter 6).

Holoprosencephaly

A wide spectrum of facial features associated with holoprosencephaly has been described (Fig. 8). All show abnormalities of the palate, with the most severe form showing absence of the primary palate (premaxillary agenesis).[36]

De Meyer et al. pointed out that the "face predicts the brain," indicating that affected fetuses with the most severe facial abnormalities are associated with holoprosencephaly, usually alobar type.[37] The converse is not true, however, because fetuses with holoprosencephaly may not have one of these defects. Detection of facial abnormalities in holoprosencephaly helps predict the outcome as well as the likelihood of concomitant extracraniofacial malformations.

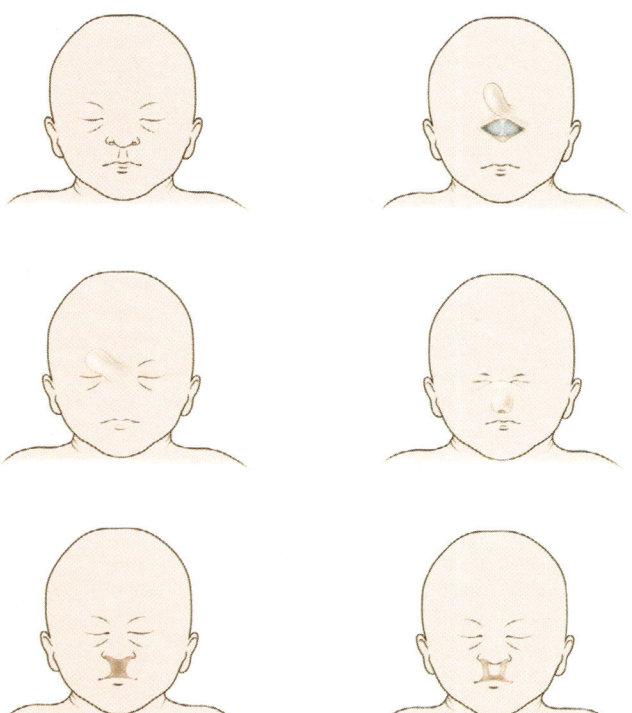

FIGURE 8. The many faces of holoprosencephaly. From top, left to right: normal, cyclopia, ethmocephaly, cebocephaly, median cleft lip and palate, and bilateral cleft lip and palate.

The facial defects associated with holoprosencephaly can be categorized as follows:

1. *Cyclopia* (Fig. 9) *with a proboscis*: A single eye globe with varying degrees of doubling of intrinsic ocular structures, arrhinia, and a blind-ending proboscis located above the median eye are found.
2. *Ethmocephaly*: Extreme orbital hypotelorism, arrhinia, and a blind-ended proboscis located between the eyes.
3. *Cebocephaly*: Orbital hypotelorism that is associated with a single-nostril nose (see Fig. 18).
4. *Cleft lip with palate*: Usually representing a median facial cleft. Premaxillary agenesis is characterized by a median agenesis of nasal bones and primary palate, and ocular hypotelorism (Fig. 10).
5. *Other rare defects*: Defects such as astomia agnathia[38] (mandibular atresia, absence of the mouth, and rotation of the ears underneath the eyes).[39–47]

The whole range of facial abnormalities associated with holoprosencephaly can be detected prenatally.[48–55] McGahan et al.[50] found facial abnormalities in 24 of 27 fetuses with holoprosencephaly. These included the range of abnormalities associated with holoprosencephaly, including cyclopia, ethmocephaly, cebocephaly, midline CL/P, unilateral CL/P, and mild hypotelorism.

Fetuses with cyclopia have a high incidence of trisomy 13 and alobar holoprosencephaly. These findings are usually detectable sonographically, as early as the first trimester.

Orbital Abnormalities

A multitude of orbital abnormalities may be detected prenatally. These include hypo- and hypertelorism, anophthalmia, and microphthalmia, cataracts, and masses (Tables 1 through 4).

Hypertelorism

Hypertelorism is associated with a variety of different syndromes and conditions (Table 1). Disorders include craniosynostosis syndromes such as Apert syndrome, Crouzon disease, and Pfeiffer syndrome; chromosomal anomalies; syndromes featuring other facial defects, such as encephaloceles (Fig. 11) and median clefts; some skeletal dysplasias; and other syndromes of multiple congenital abnormalities, including Pena Shokeir and Noonan syndrome.[56] Trout et al. derived normative data on 422 normal fetuses, to evaluate 11 fetuses with abnormal orbital diameters.[21] Of these 11 fetuses, eight had holoprosencephaly with hypotelorism and three had hypertelorism.

Hypotelorism

Hypotelorism is usually associated with many other abnormalities (Table 2), most of which are severe (e.g., holoprosencephaly) (Fig. 10).

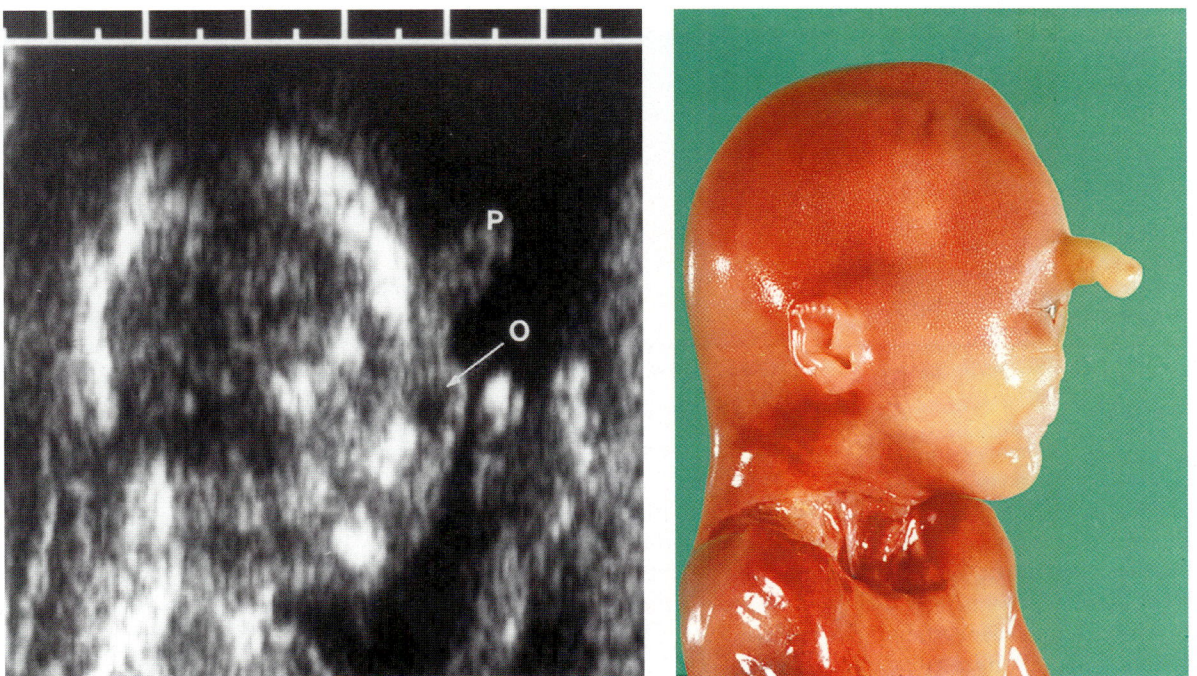

FIGURE 9. Cyclopia. **A:** Sagittal view at 16 weeks show proboscis (*P*) overlying midline orbit (*O*). Microcephaly is also apparent, and alobar holoprosencephaly was identified. The karyotype was trisomy 13. **B:** Pathologic photograph of similar case shows proboscis and cyclopia.

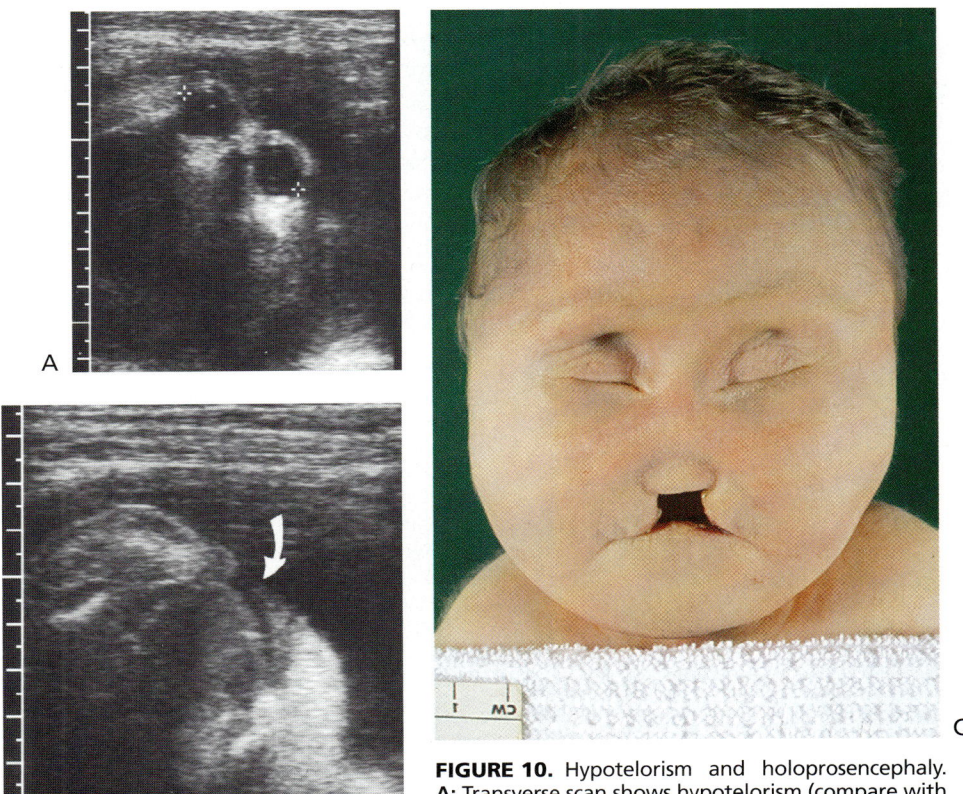

FIGURE 10. Hypotelorism and holoprosencephaly. **A:** Transverse scan shows hypotelorism (compare with Fig. 8). Also note absence of bony nose. **B:** Axial view lower, through the upper lip, shows midline cleft lip and palate (premaxillary agenesis) (*arrow*). **C:** Postnatal photograph confirms sonographic findings.

TABLE 1. ASSOCIATIONS WITH HYPOTELORISM

Holoanencephaly
Chromosomal abnormality
Microcephaly
Maternal phenylketonuria
Meckel-Gruber syndrome
Myotonic dystrophy
Severe hypotelorism/cyclopia
Cleft lip and palate
Crouzon disease
Trisomy 13 (Patau syndrome)
Holoprosencephaly

Adapted from Benacerraf BR. *Ultrasound of fetal syndromes.* New York: Churchill Livingstone, 1997:1–8.

Anophthalmia

Anophthalmia results from failure of the optic vesicle to form. Anophthalmia demonstrates striking absence of the globe and often the orbit on the axial view through the expected level of the orbits (Fig. 12). It occurs more rarely than microphthalmia, but its manifestations are more obvious. The most common cause of unilateral anophthalmia detected prenatally is the Goldenhar-Gorlin syndrome (hemifacial microsomia). Other association with anophthalmia includes trisomy 13, Lenz syndrome (X-linked microphthalmia), and microphthalmia with digital anomalies.

Microphthalmia

Microphthalmia (Fig. 13) is seen as a small globe and can be confirmed by objective measurements.[57,58] Microph-

TABLE 2. ASSOCIATIONS WITH HYPERTELORISM

Noonan syndrome
Encephalocele (anterior)
Gorlin syndrome
Median cleft face
Neu-Laxova
Camptomelic dysplasia
Chondrodysplasia punctata
Larsen syndrome
Multiple pterygium
Roberts syndrome
Apert syndrome
Crouzon disease
Pfeiffer syndrome
Deletion 4p (Wolf-Hirschhorn syndrome)
Deletion 11p
Tetrasomy 12p (Pallister Killian syndrome)
Triploidy
Trisomy 10
Trisomy 18 (Edwards syndrome)
CHARGE association
Pena Shokeir

CHARGE, coloboma, *heart anomaly, choanal atresia, retardation,* and genital and ear anomalies.
Adapted from Benacerraf BR. *Ultrasound of fetal syndromes.* New York: Churchill Livingstone, 1997:1–8.

TABLE 3. ASSOCIATIONS WITH MICRO- OR ANOPHTHALMIA (UNILATERAL OR BILATERAL)

CHARGE association
Fanconi anemia
Fraser syndrome
Fryns syndrome
Goldenhar syndrome
Meckel-Gruber syndrome
Median cleft face
Neu-Laxova
Proteus syndrome
Roberts syndrome
TORCH infection (rubella)
Triploidy
Trisomy 13 (Patau syndrome)
Trisomy 18 (Edwards syndrome)
Trisomy 9
Walker-Warburg syndrome

CHARGE, coloboma, heart anomaly, choanal atresia retardation, and genital and ear anomalies.
Adapted from Benacerraf BR. *Ultrasound of fetal syndromes.* New York: Churchill Livingstone, 1997:1–8.

thalmia may be familial. Cryptophthalmia indicates that the eyes are hidden, with absence of the palpebral fissures. Often, this is associated with microphthalmia and is a feature of Fraser syndrome[59–63] (Table 3). Although the prenatal diagnosis of cryptophthalmia is difficult, affected fetuses are identified by their associated microphthalmia, which has been detected early in the second trimester—particularly among patients at genetic risk.[64] The prognosis for microphthalmia and anophthalmia varies with the underlying etiology and severity of associated malformations. In general, however, it is frequently associated with mental retardation. Suspicion of anophthalmia or microphthalmia should prompt chromosomal analysis as

TABLE 4. ASSOCIATIONS WITH CONGENITAL CATARACTS

Arthrogryposis
Chondrodysplasia punctata
Coloboma
Congenital aniridia
G6PD deficiency
Hallermann-Streiff syndrome
Homocystinuria
Hypochondroplasia
Kniest
Marfan syndrome
Microphthalmia
Neu-Laxova
Roberts syndrome
Rubella
Smith-Lemli-Opitz syndrome
Toxoplasmosis
Walker-Warburg syndrome

G6PD, glucose-6-phosphate dehydrogenase.
Adapted from Benacerraf BR. *Ultrasound of fetal syndromes.* New York: Churchill Livingstone, 1997:1–8.

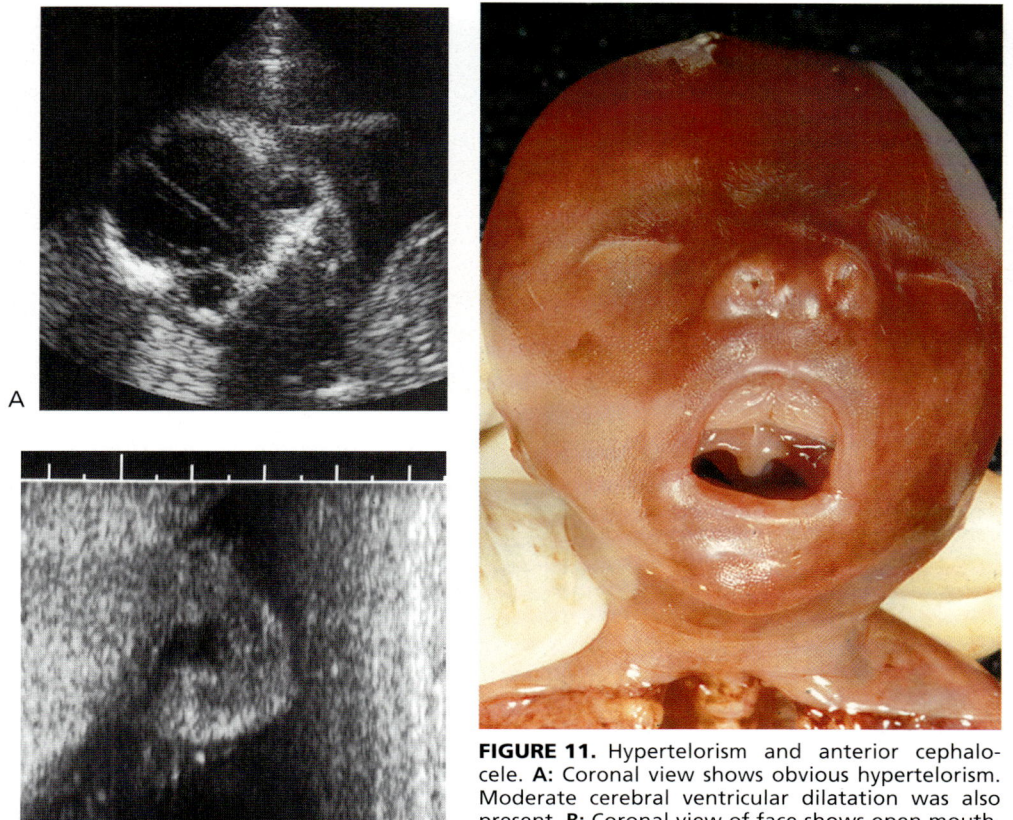

FIGURE 11. Hypertelorism and anterior cephalocele. **A:** Coronal view shows obvious hypertelorism. Moderate cerebral ventricular dilatation was also present. **B:** Coronal view of face shows open mouth. **C:** Pathologic photograph shows anterior cephalocele projecting from roof of mouth.

well as careful search of the fetus, especially for other potentially subtle facial or extremity malformations.

Cataracts

Cataracts are small round echogenic masses in the anterior aspect of the eye, in which the usually thin-walled, rounded, cystic lens appears solid and completely echo-genic. The diagnosis of cataracts (Fig. 14) can be made *in utero* and has been suspected as early as 14 weeks—particularly among fetuses at increased risk due to genetic disorders.[65–68] Cataracts can develop later in fetuses infected with cytomegalovirus, rubella, toxoplasmosis, or varicella and can be associated with other ocular abnormalities such as microphthalmia as well as a number of syndromes (Table 4). The diagnosis of cataracts *in utero* has been made largely

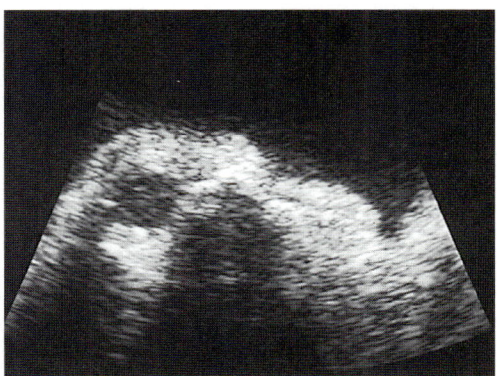

FIGURE 12. Anophthalmia and Goldenhar syndrome. Transverse view of face shows unilateral absence of orbit. Other facial anomalies were also consistent with Goldenhar syndrome.

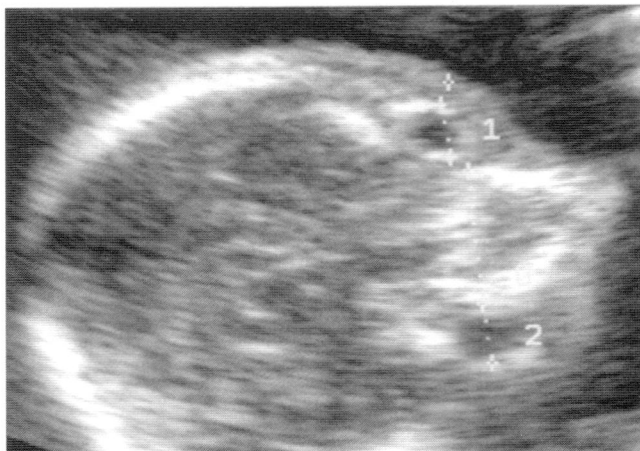

FIGURE 13. Microphthalmia. Transverse view shows small eyes (*1, 2*). The transverse orbital diameter should normally be approximately one-half the distance between the orbits. (Courtesy of Gianluigi Pilu, MD, Bologna, Italy.)

among patients at increased risk for cataracts in their offspring. The sensitivity for the prenatal identification of cataracts in the general population is unclear, as reports thus far are confined to patients who present with increased risks for this disorder.

Dacrocystocele

Dacrocystoceles are dilatations of the lacrimal drainage system, secondary to obstruction of proximal and distal ducts, resulting in a pooling of mucous or amniotic fluid in an enclosed space. Approximately 30% of newborns have nonpatent nasal lacrimal ducts, yet only 2% are symptomatic and develop a mass (dacrocystocele). Dacrocystoceles or lacrimal duct cysts have been frequently diagnosed by prenatal

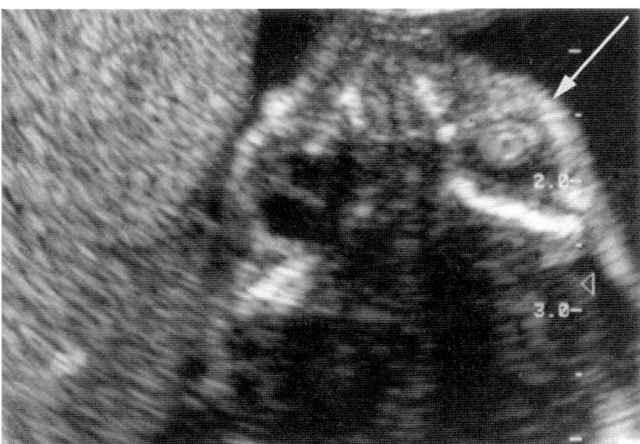

FIGURE 14. Cataract. Tangential anterior coronal section at 16 weeks shows a hyperechogenic ring containing another hyperechogenic ring (*arrow*), representing a cataract. (Courtesy of Ana Montegudo, MD, New York, NY.)

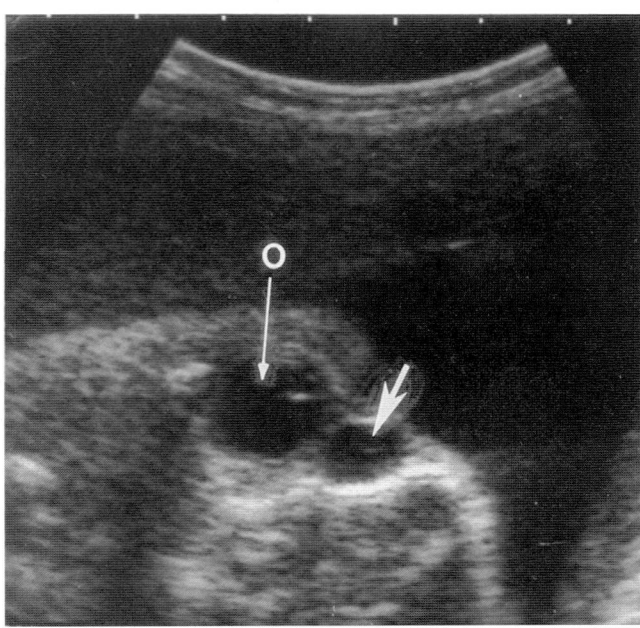

FIGURE 15. Dacrocystocele. Axial scan shows cyst (*arrow*) just medial to orbit (*O*).

ultrasound (Figs. 15 and 16).[69–73] The typical cystic appearance of dacrocystocele should be distinguished from other periorbital masses, including anterior encephalocele, hemangioma, dermoid cyst, and glioma. Dacrocystocele may be associated with other anomalies[74] although it is typically isolated. These cysts often spontaneously resolve *in utero*.[75]

Nose

The nose can be well visualized with 2-D or 3-D ultrasound (Fig. 17). Abnormalities of the nose may include a flattened, small, broad, beaked, large, or bulbous nose in addition to the abnormalities associated with holoprosencephaly (Fig. 18). Detection of nose abnormalities prenatally is particu-

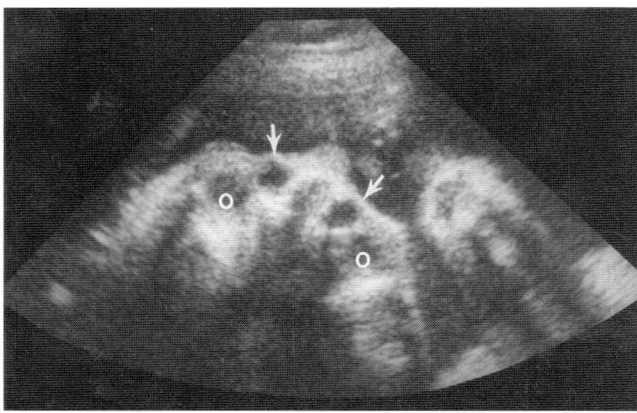

FIGURE 16. Bilateral dacrocystoceles. Axial scan shows bilateral cysts (*arrows*) just medial to orbits (*O*).

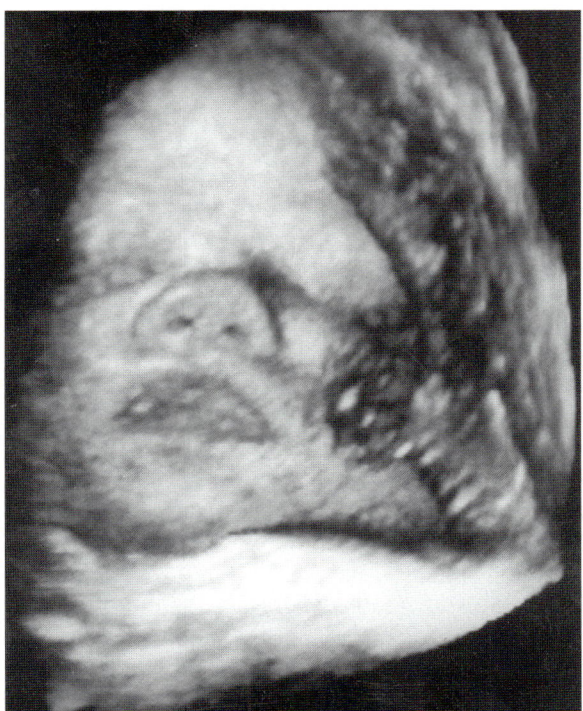

FIGURE 17. Normal nose. Three-dimensional ultrasound shows normal nose and nares.

larly likely to be associated with chromosome abnormalities or syndromes. In a series of 15 cases of nasal anomalies, Bronshtein et al.[76] reported three cases of trisomy 18 and one case each of trisomy 21, triploidy, and tetrasomy 12p.

A flattened or small nose may be seen with a variety of conditions, including Binder syndrome[77]; Aarskog syndrome[39]; Raine syndrome[40]; Brachmann-de Lange syndrome[41]; Roberts syndrome; or exposure to valproic acid,[42] warfarin,[43] or thalidomide, among other associations. Complete or total arhinia, in which there is absence of the soft tissue of the nose, is extremely rare. The embryologic origin of the defect is thought to be maldevelopment of the paired nasal placodes.[44]

Mouth and Lip

Cleft Lip and Palate

Definition and Incidence

CL/P is etiologically distinct from cleft palate alone. Together, these are among the more common congenital abnormalities, present in 0.15% of births (representing 7.5% of all anomalies). Of these, approximately 50% are combined cleft lip and palate, 20% are cleft lip alone, and 30% are cleft palate alone. Cleft lip with or without cleft palate (CL/P) may be considered separately from cleft palate alone. Among whites, the incidence of CL/P is approximately 1 per 1,000—although in the fetal population, it is much more common.[45] Marked ethnic variation is also noted, with a higher incidence among American Indians (1 per 300) and Asians (1 per 600) but lower incidence in blacks (1 per 2,500) compared to whites. Conversely, the rate of isolated cleft palate alone is constant among ethnic groups. Males are affected more commonly than females for CL/P, but females are more likely to have cleft palate alone. For unknown reasons, unilateral CL/P is more commonly on the left side than the right.[46]

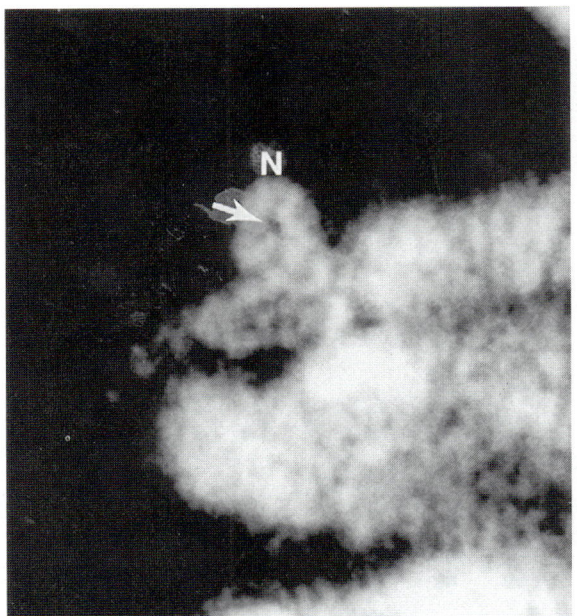

A

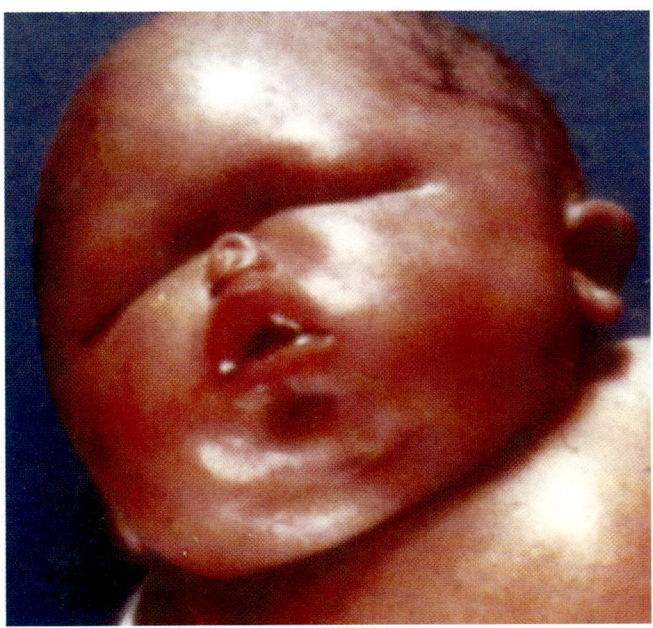

B

FIGURE 18. Cebocephaly. **A:** Coronal view shows abnormal nose (*N*) with single nares (*arrow*). **B:** Pathologic correlation. Holoprosencephaly was also present. (Courtesy of Gianluigi Pilu, MD, Bologna, Italy.)

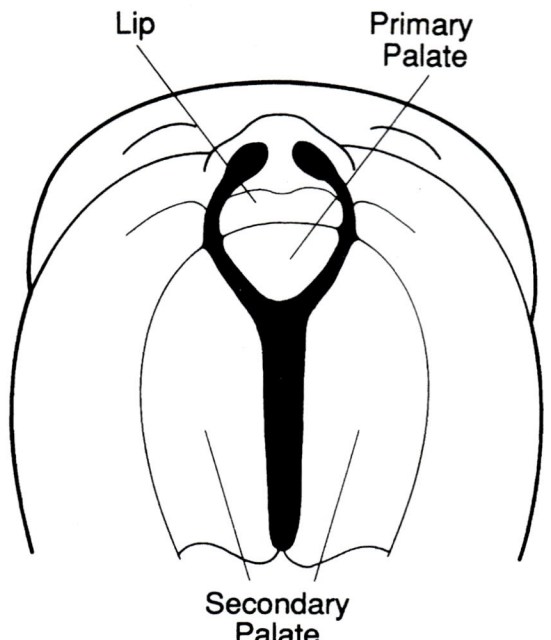

FIGURE 19. Embryologic basis of cleft lip and palate. The normal face results from fusion of lips, primary palate, and secondary palates. Clefts result from incomplete or lack of fusion of one or more of these structures. (Reproduced with permission from Nyberg DA, Sickler GK, Hegge FN, Kramer DJ, Kropp RJ. Fetal cleft lip with and without cleft palate: US classification and correlation with outcome. *Radiology* 1995;195:677–683.)

The prevalence of fetal facial clefting changes with different stages of pregnancy, due to the high incidence of associated fatal trisomies and other fatal multiple congenital anomalies. Clefts are present in 0.15% of births (representing 7.5% of all anomalies), whereas 12% of fetuses aborted at 8 weeks have cleft lip and palate.[35,47] This enormous difference in incidences underscores the common associated abnormalities that are most often lethal to affected fetuses.[78] Attrition of severely abnormal fetuses results in the shift in incidence of associated malformations between fetuses and newborns.

Embryology and Pathology

A review of normal embryologic development of the face is important for understanding formation of cleft lip and palate (Fig. 19). The lip usually closes by 7 to 8 weeks', and the palate closes by 12 weeks' gestation. Nonfusion parts of these structures produce CL/P.

A sonographic classification of CL/P has been proposed by Nyberg et al. (Table 4). Figure 20 illustrates normal anatomy and the first four types of clefts and their relationship with the primary and secondary palates. Type 5 cleft does not follow embryologic patterns but rather shows random types of defects, often large and devastating.

Factors associated with CL/P include exposure to rubella, some medications (thalidomide isotretinoin or retinoic acid, valproic acid, phenytoin or hydantoin, aminop-

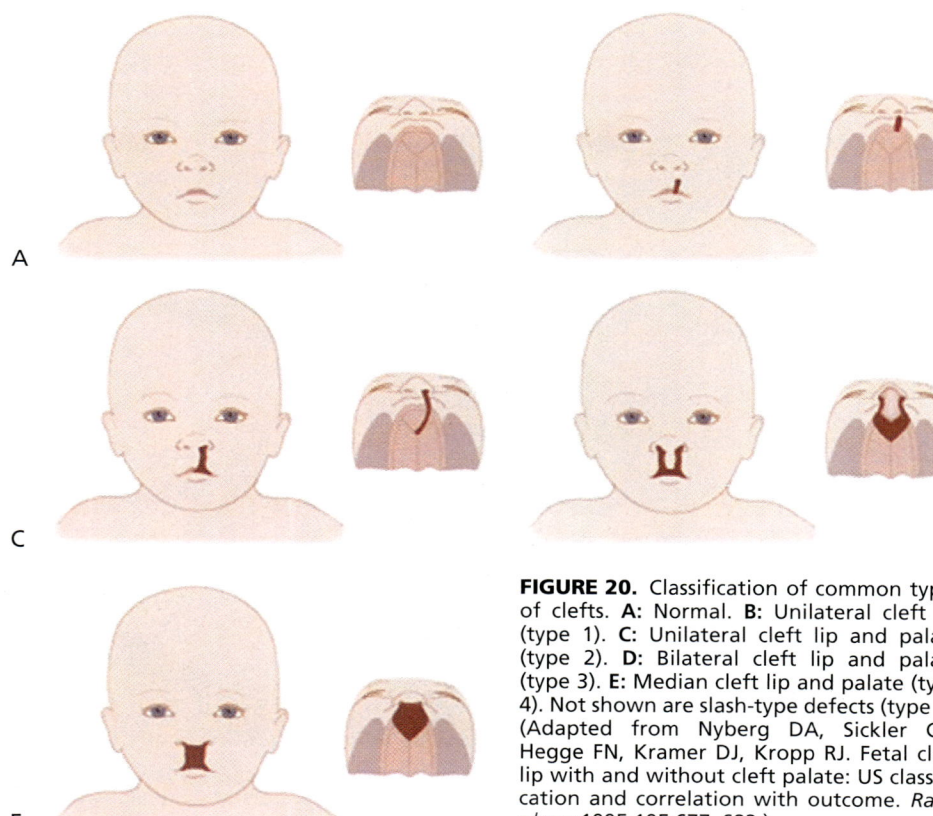

FIGURE 20. Classification of common types of clefts. **A:** Normal. **B:** Unilateral cleft lip (type 1). **C:** Unilateral cleft lip and palate (type 2). **D:** Bilateral cleft lip and palate (type 3). **E:** Median cleft lip and palate (type 4). Not shown are slash-type defects (type 5). (Adapted from Nyberg DA, Sickler GK, Hegge FN, Kramer DJ, Kropp RJ. Fetal cleft lip with and without cleft palate: US classification and correlation with outcome. *Radiology* 1995;195:677–683.)

TABLE 5. CLEFT LIP AND PALATE TYPES

Type 1: Cleft lip
Type 2: Unilateral cleft lip and palate
Type 3: Bilateral cleft lip and palate
    Usually with premaxillary protrusion
Type 4: Midline cleft lip and palate
    Gaping midline with hypoplastic midface, absence primary
    palate
Type 5: Amniotic bands and slash-type defects

Reproduced with permission from Nyberg DA, Sickler GK, Hegge FN, Kramer DJ, Kropp RJ. Fetal cleft lip with and without cleft palate: US classification and correlation with outcome. *Radiology* 1995;195:677–683.

terin), alcohol and drug use, and cigarette smoking. Folic acid deficiency has also been implicated.

Diagnosis

In 1981, Christ et al.[80] first reported the ultrasound diagnosis of cleft lip and palate in two third-trimester fetuses. Since then, prenatal detection has been reported by many others.[81,82] Coronal and axial images are most useful for evaluation of CL/P.[83] Prenatal sonographic evaluation of the axial view of the tooth-bearing alveolar ridge of the maxilla allows accurate determination of whether a cleft is confined to the lip or involves the lip and the palate.

Most centers now routinely include views of the face and lips, partly because parents so commonly request the views. As a result, prenatal detection of CL/P has markedly improved, especially for moderate-to-severe clefts. However, the sensitivity of CL/P remains low for milder forms of cleft or for nonsyndromic conditions.[84] A European registry reported detection of just 18% (65 of 366) of isolated clefts compared to 58% (21 of 36) for syndromic conditions and 52% (32 of 62) of those associated with a chromosome abnormality. Stoll et al.[85] reported that detection of isolated CL/P was low but improved during a 10-year survey. Overall, detection was 17.8%; however, this detection rate increased from 5.3% during the period of 1979–1988 to 26.5% during the period of 1989–1998.

The sonographic appearance of clefts depends on the type of cleft (Table 5), severity, gestational age at diagnosis, and associated anomalies. The least severe type is incomplete cleft lip without cleft palate (Fig. 21). Benacerraf and Mulliken reported that all seven cases of incomplete cleft

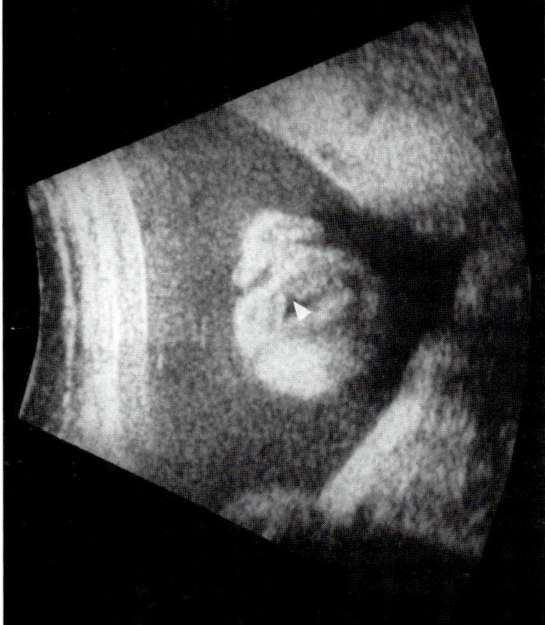

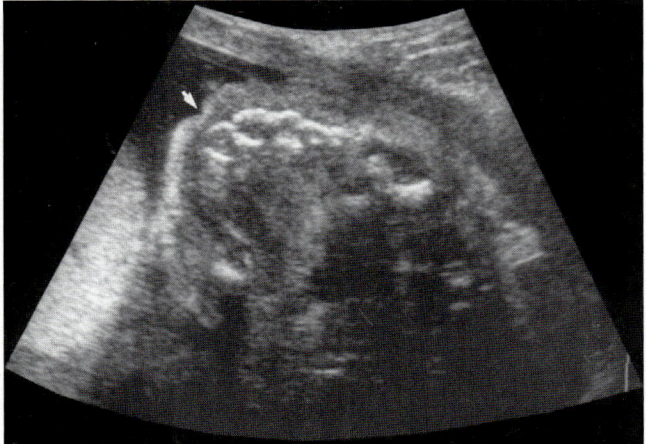

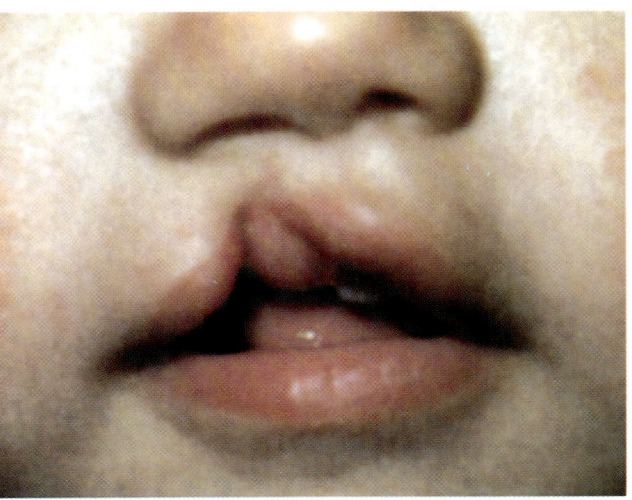

FIGURE 21. Unilateral incomplete cleft lip, 28 weeks. **A:** Coronal view shows partial defect of upper lip (*arrowhead*). **B:** Transverse view through the maxilla at the level of the teeth buds shows that the cleft (*arrow*) involves the lip only and does not extend into the palate. **C:** Photograph after birth from similar case as fetus in **(A)** and **(B)**.

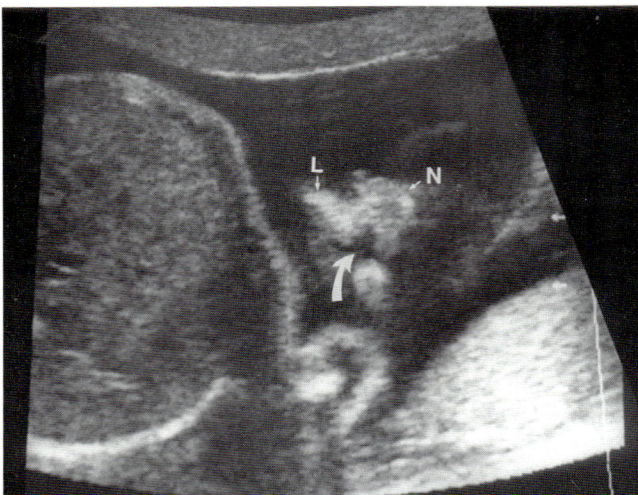

FIGURE 22. Unilateral cleft lip (type 1), 20 weeks. Coronal scan shows unilateral cleft lip extending to nares (*arrow*). This did not involve the palate. L, lip; N, nose.

lips were detected after 27 weeks' gestation even though three patients were scanned in the second trimester.[78] Many cases of isolated cleft lip (Fig. 22) without cleft palate are also difficult to diagnose before 20 weeks.

The various forms of cleft lip with cleft palate are much more likely to be detected by prenatal sonography than cleft lip alone and can usually be seen before 20 weeks. Unilateral cleft lip and palate (Figs. 23 through 25) is most common but varies widely in severity. Some clefts are large and produce marked distortion and depression of the nose (Figs. 24 and 25). Some cases produce marked distortion of

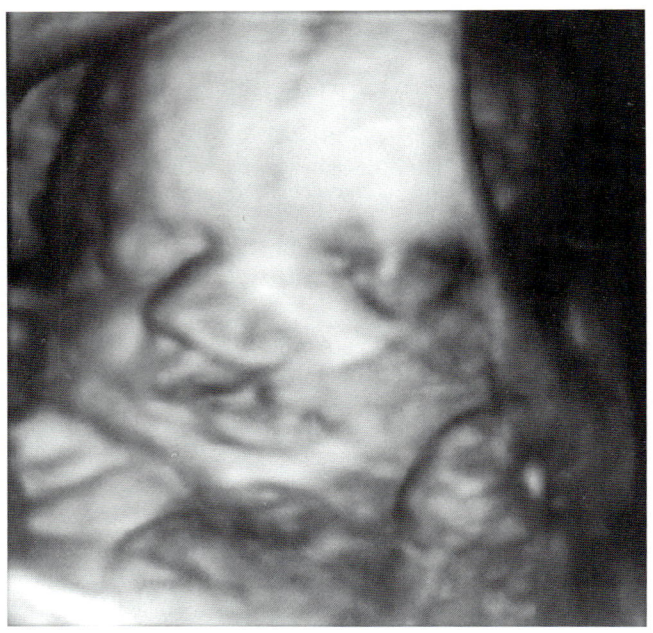

A

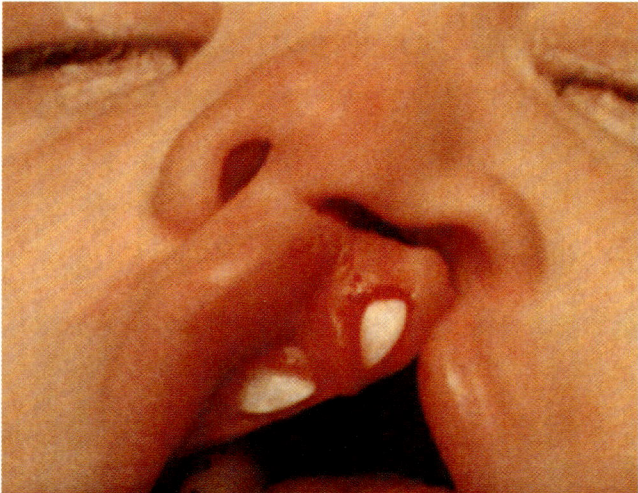

B

FIGURE 24. Unilateral cleft lip and palate (type 2). **A:** Three-dimensional ultrasound shows unilateral cleft lip and palate with associated nasal deformity. This type of information is extremely useful for the plastic surgeons. **B:** Similar case at time of surgical repair showing unilateral cleft lip and palate with depression of nose on side of cleft.

soft tissues that project anteriorly, and this can be confused for the premaxillary protrusion of bilateral clefts (Fig. 26).

Babcook and McGahan also evaluated the accuracy of characterizing facial clefts antenatally.[86] They found that prenatal characterization of unilateral versus bilateral clefts was correct in all cases, and the prenatal sonographic evaluation of the axial view of the tooth-bearing alveolar ridge made it possible to determine whether the cleft involved the palate.

Bilateral cleft lip and palate (type 3) is a more severe cleft than unilateral clefts. It can be subcategorized as those that

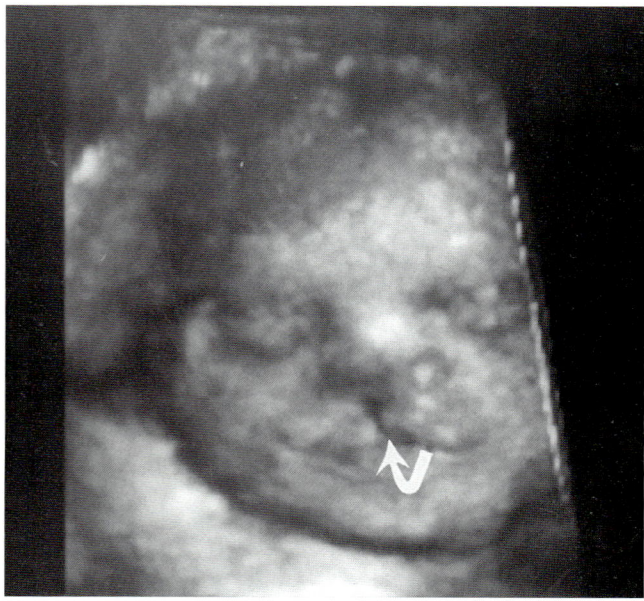

FIGURE 23. Three-dimensional surface rendering of a fetus with a unilateral cleft lip and palate (*arrow*).

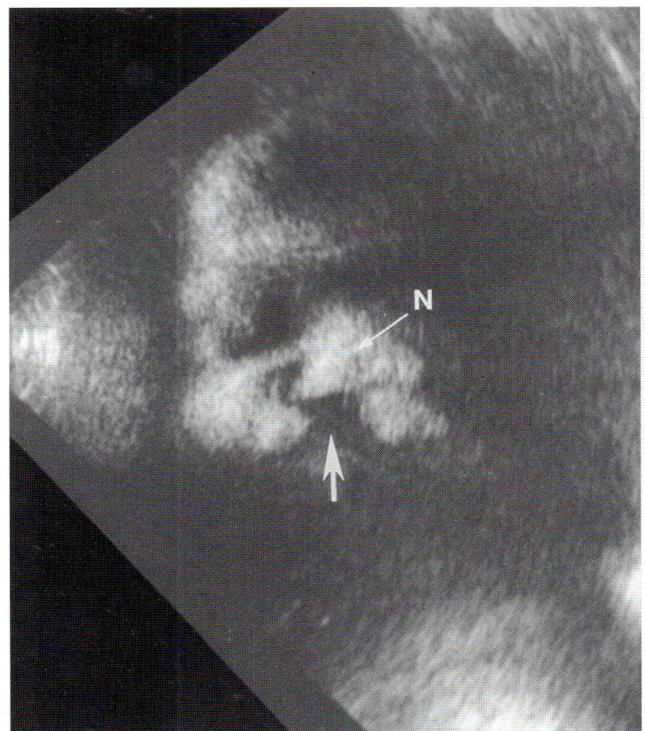

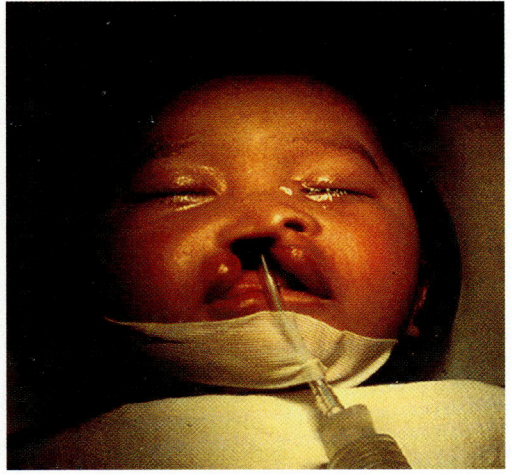

FIGURE 25. Unilateral cleft lip and palate. **A:** Coronal scan shows large unilateral cleft lip and palate (*arrow*). Polyhydramnios was also present at 26 weeks. N, nose. **B:** Photograph at surgical repair shows large cleft with unilateral nasal depression.

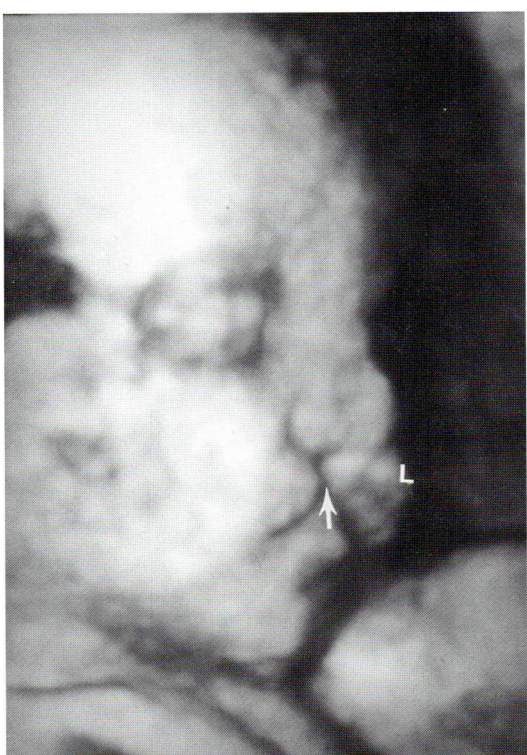

FIGURE 26. Unilateral cleft lip and palate. Three-dimensional ultrasound in early third trimester shows unilateral cleft lip and palate (*arrow*) seen in partial profile. Distorted soft tissues of upper lip (*L*) project anteriorly and could be confused for the premaxillary segment of bilateral cleft lip and palate.

have a protuberant premaxillary segment (Figs. 27 through 30) and those without (Fig. 31). The premaxillary segment may appear as a prominent soft tissue and echogenic mass just below the nose. This may be prominent during the second trimester and give the appearance of a *beak* (Fig. 30). It may be much more apparent than the cleft itself and helps to confirm the correct diagnosis of bilateral cleft lip and palate. Prenatal identification of this premaxillary protru-

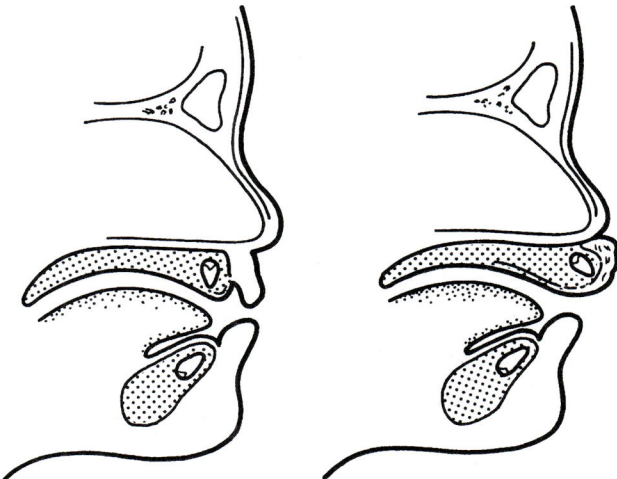

FIGURE 27. Development of premaxillary protrusion with bilateral cleft lip and palate. **A:** Normal sagittal view. **B:** Bilateral cleft lip and palate permits forward migration of the premaxillary segment.

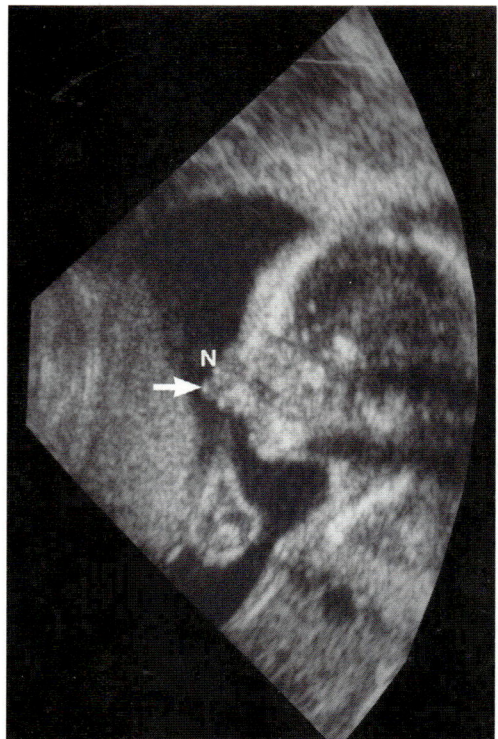
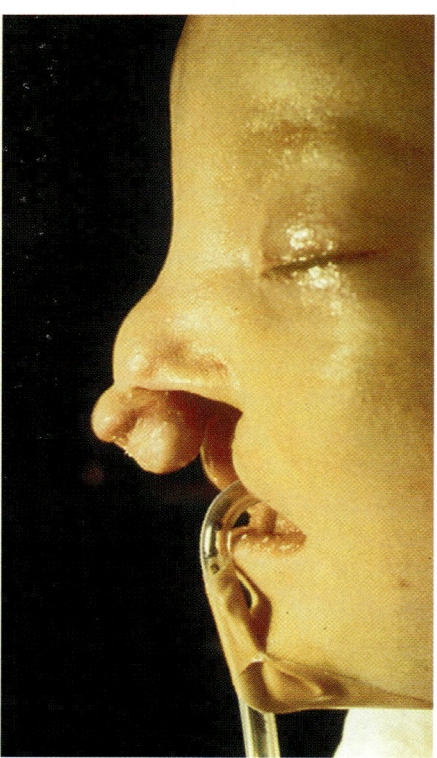

A,B

FIGURE 28. Premaxillary protrusion. **A:** Sagittal sonogram in a fetus with bilateral cleft lip and palate showing prominent premaxillary protrusion (*arrow*). N, nose. **B:** Photograph of similar case as **A** at time of surgical repair.

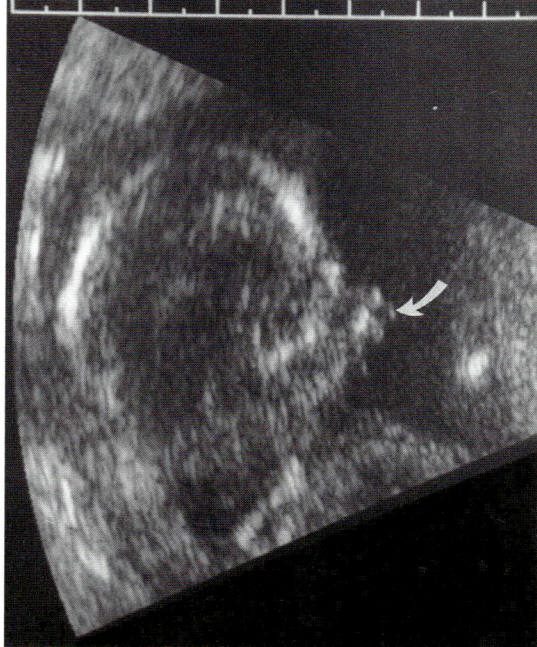
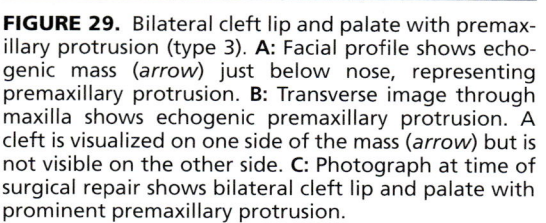

A

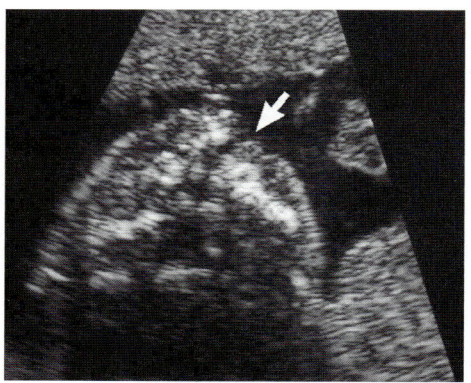

B

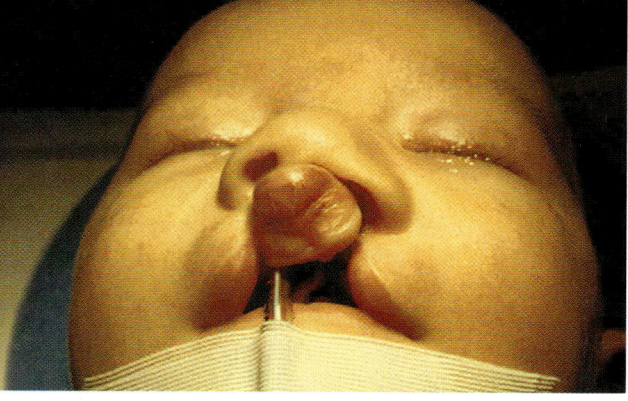

C

FIGURE 29. Bilateral cleft lip and palate with premaxillary protrusion (type 3). **A:** Facial profile shows echogenic mass (*arrow*) just below nose, representing premaxillary protrusion. **B:** Transverse image through maxilla shows echogenic premaxillary protrusion. A cleft is visualized on one side of the mass (*arrow*) but is not visible on the other side. **C:** Photograph at time of surgical repair shows bilateral cleft lip and palate with prominent premaxillary protrusion.

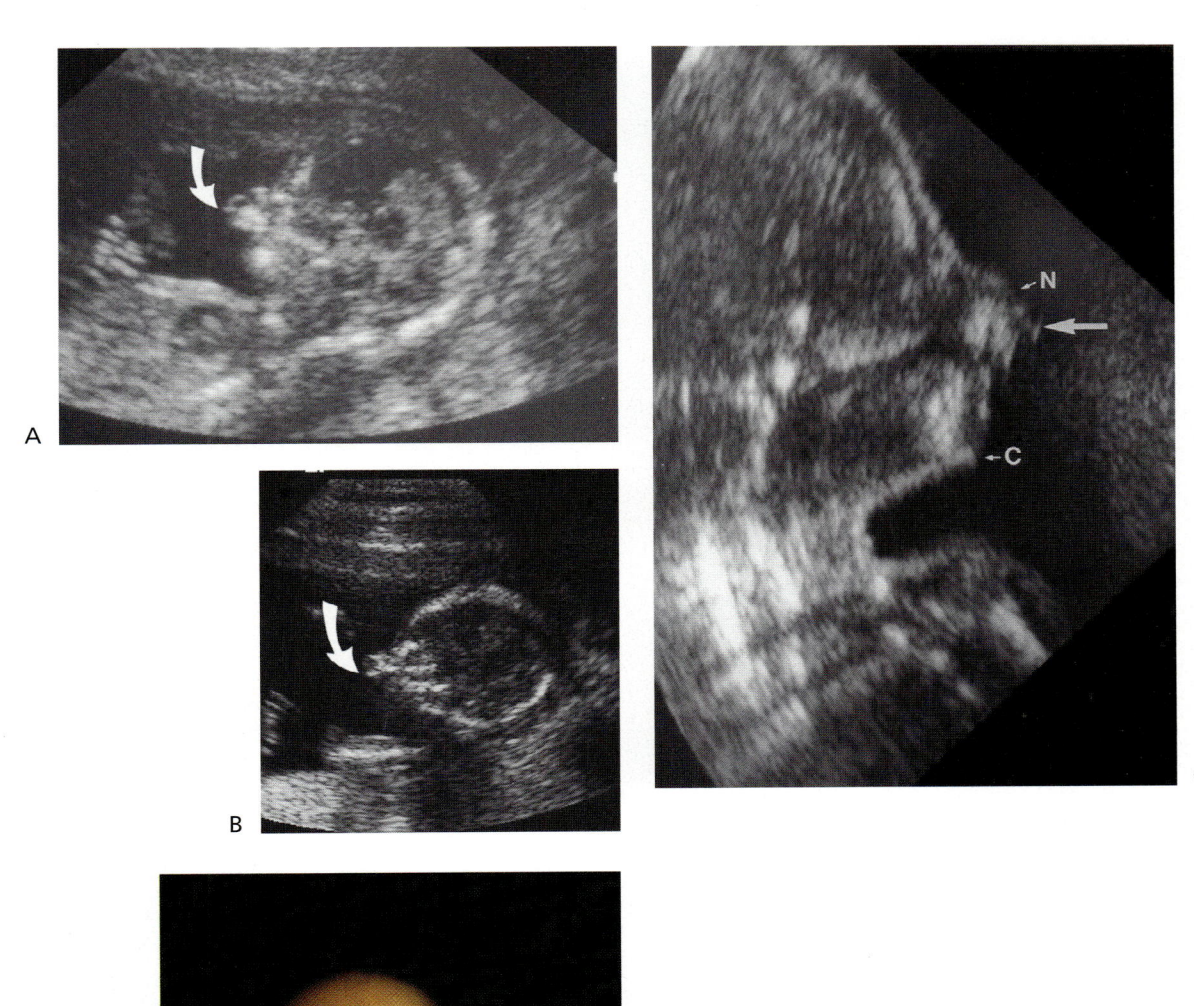

FIGURE 30. Bilateral cleft lip and palate with premaxillary protrusion. Facial profile **(A)** and transverse **(B)** scans at 15 weeks show prominent echogenic mass below nose (*arrows*). **C:** Follow-up scan, facial profile view, at 24 weeks again shows prominent premaxillary protrusion (*arrow*). C, chin; N, nose. **D:** Photograph at time of surgical repair shows bilateral cleft lip and palate with prominent premaxillary protrusion.

sion is also helpful to plastic surgeons in planning the type of surgery necessary for repair after birth.

Some cases of bilateral CL/P do not show a protuberant premaxillary segment but instead show a hypoplastic midface with depressed nose (Fig. 31). Nyberg et al. have referred to these as type 3B clefts. These cases are very similar to type 4 clefts—characterized as midline cleft lip and palate with absence of the primary palate, the only difference being a ridge of intact skin and lip in the midline.

Midline cleft lip and palate (type 4) is the most severe of the common types of clefts (Fig. 32). These probably represent absence of the primary palate, leaving a gaping midline cleft. These types of clefts are particularly likely to be associated with other anomalies, chromosome abnormalities, and poor outcome.

Slash types of defects (type 5) do not follow embryologic patterns but rather are random defects caused by amniotic bands. They are usually severe and fatal (Fig. 33).

Cleft palate without an associated cleft lip is very difficult to detect. Most cases of cleft palate alone involve the soft palate but not the hard palate. In these cases, color Doppler may be helpful in identifying the simultaneous flow of fluid in the nasal and oral cavities, although the only cases to date in which this phenomenon has been

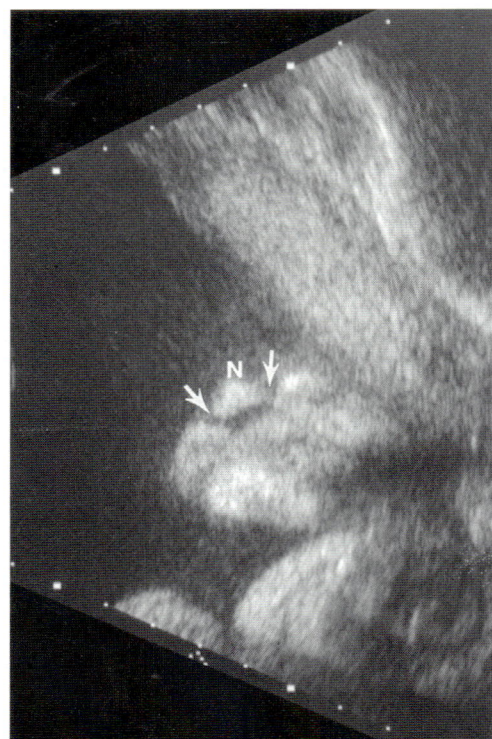

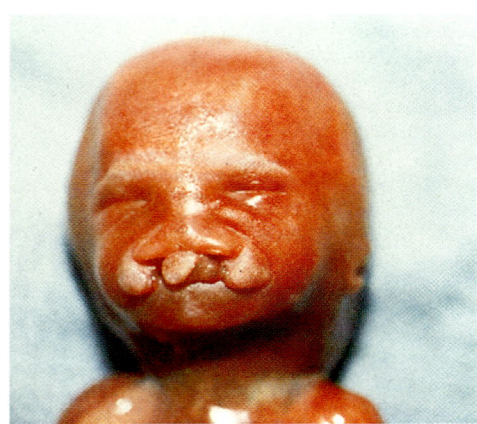

FIGURE 31. Bilateral cleft lip and palate without premaxillary protrusion. **A:** Coronal sonogram shows bilateral clefts (*arrows*). There is no premaxillary protuberance; rather, the nose (*N*) and midface is flat. **B:** Corresponding pathologic photograph in a fetus with trisomy 13 shows bilateral cleft lip and palate with depressed nose.

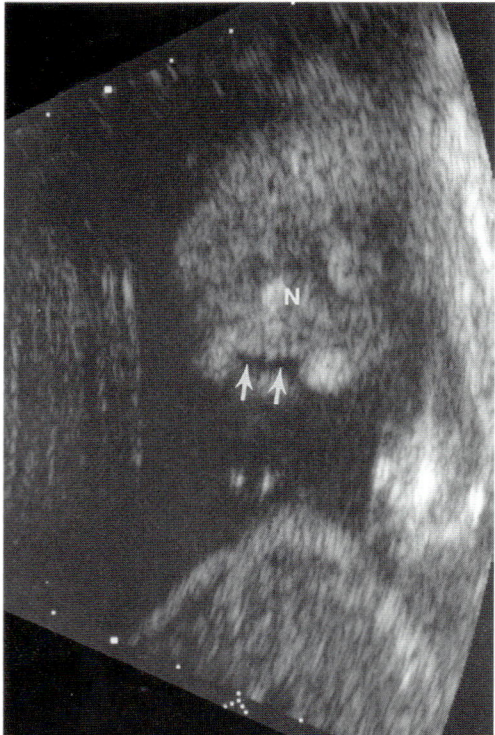

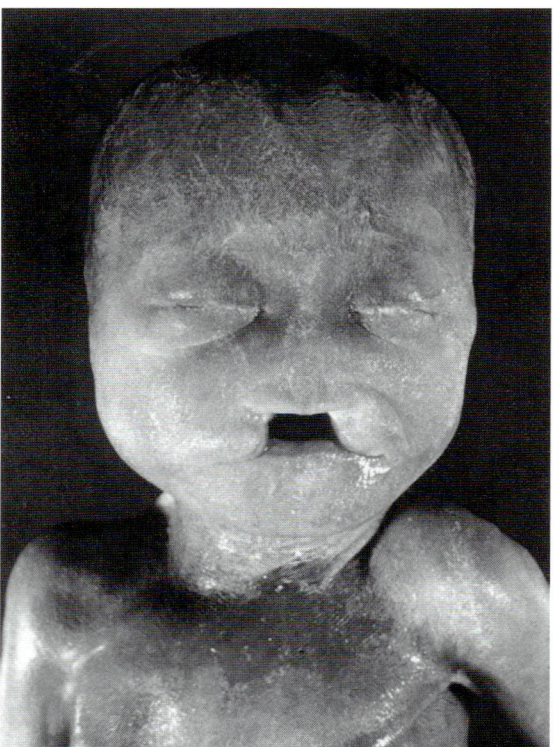

FIGURE 32. Midline cleft lip and palate (type 4). **A:** Coronal scan at 17 weeks shows large midline cleft lip and palate (*arrows*). Also note hypoplastic midface with depressed nose (*N*). **B:** Pathologic photograph confirms ultrasound findings. The karyotype was trisomy 13. (Reproduced with permission from Nyberg DA, Sickler GK, Hegge FN, Kramer DJ, Kropp RJ. Fetal cleft lip with and without cleft palate: US classification and correlation with outcome. *Radiology* 1995;195:677–683.)

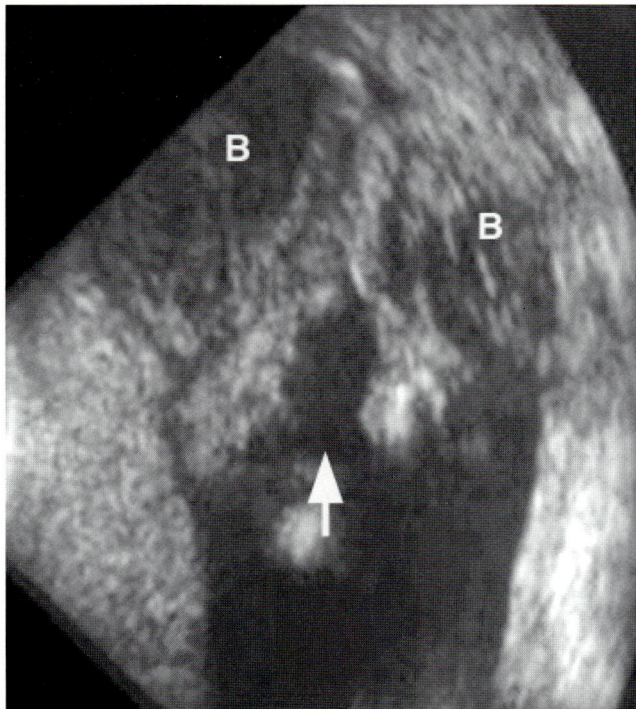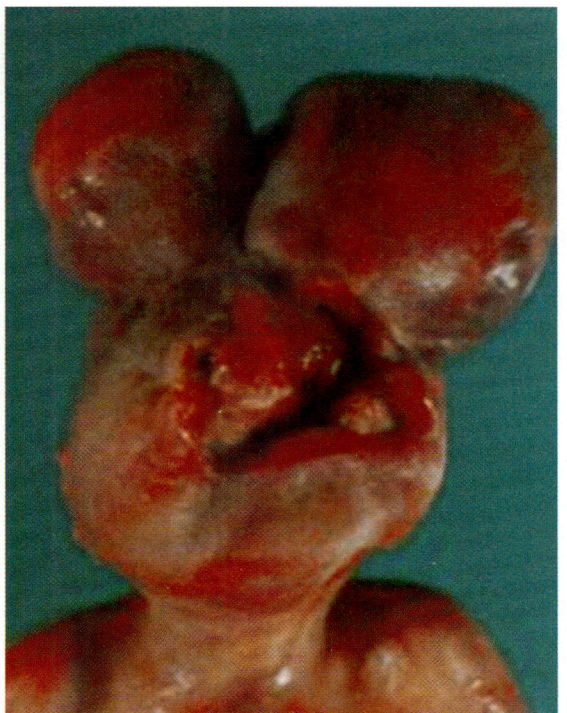

FIGURE 33. Slash type of facial cleft. **A:** Coronal view shows large defect through the face and head (*arrow*), making it difficult to identify normal landmarks. Exencephaly is also present. B, brain. **B:** Pathologic correlation confirms severity of defect.

demonstrated also included a cleft lip (Fig. 34).[87–89] Indirect sonographic features of cleft palate may include a small or nonvisualized fetal stomach and polyhydramnios, due to the fetus's difficulty in swallowing normally.[90] MRI can image the palate and face, although this has not yet been used for detection of clefts.

Abnormal levels of some enzymes (lactate dehydrogenase and creatine phosphokinase) in the amniotic fluid of affected pregnancies have been reported in association with CL/P.[91]

Differential Diagnosis

It is important to distinguish the normal philtrum from a midline cleft lip. Premaxillary protrusion associated with bilateral cleft lip and palate could be confused for other facial masses.

Associated Anomalies

Chromosome abnormalities are common with CL/P, although these fetuses usually have other anomalies that can be detected prenatally. In the multicenter study by Clementi et al., 10% of clefts had a chromosome abnormality and 27% had associated anomalies.

Chromosome abnormalities also vary with the type of defect, are especially common with median CL/P, and are least likely for unilateral cleft lip without cleft palate.[92]

Nyberg et al. found chromosome abnormalities varied with the type of cleft: (a) 0%, (b) 20%, (c) 30%, and (d) 52%. Trisomy 13 is particularly common among these types of clefts detected prenatally. Conversely, Snijders et al. reported that, among 54 fetuses with trisomy 13 and among 102 fetuses with trisomy 18, cleft palate was present in 40.7% and 6.9%, respectively.[93]

Facial clefting is associated with 100 different syndromes,[94] many of which are recognizable antenatally by ultrasound (Table 6).[56] Twenty-five percent of newborns with cleft lip and palate have reported associated anomalies versus as many as 80% in the fetal population.[9] Syndromes with CL/P include ectrodactyly, ectodermal dysplasia, clefting syndrome; Opitz syndrome; Meckel's syndrome; oral-facial-digital syndrome type I; short rib polydactyly; Majewski type; and Van der Woude's syndrome. Syndromes associated with cleft palate alone include Apert syndrome (see Chapter 5), diastrophic dysplasia, Fryns syndrome (see Chapter 5), Larsen syndrome, Treacher Collins syndrome (see Chapter 5), ot(o)-palat(o)-digital syndrome types I and II, Stickler's syndrome, and velocardiofacial syndrome (see Chapter 5).

A rare syndrome associated with an unusual pattern of clefting is median cleft face syndrome or frontonasal dysplasia sequence[95] (Fig. 12). This syndrome consists of a range of midline facial defects involving hypertelorism, a bifid nose, a midline cleft of the frontal bone and of the

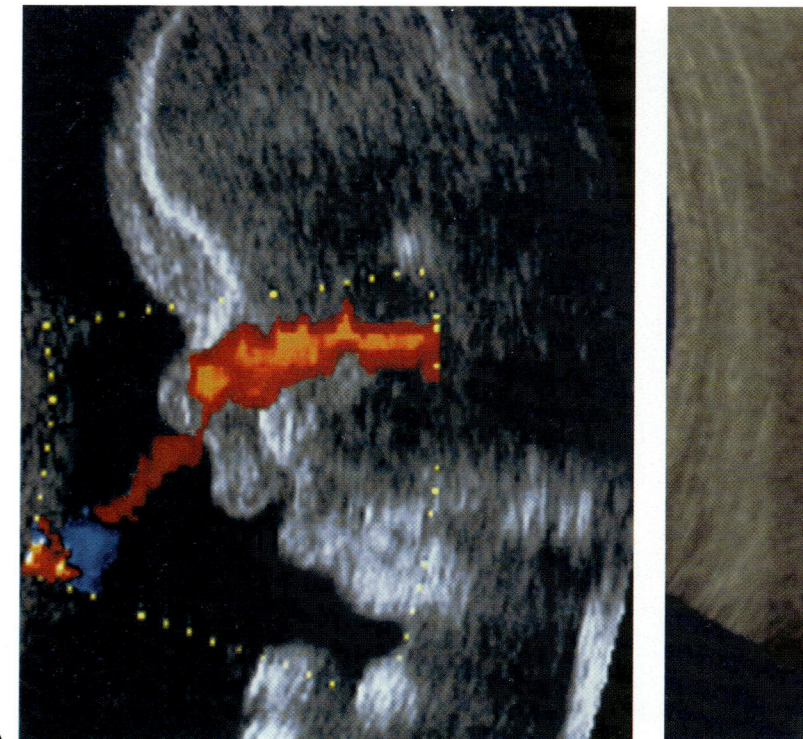
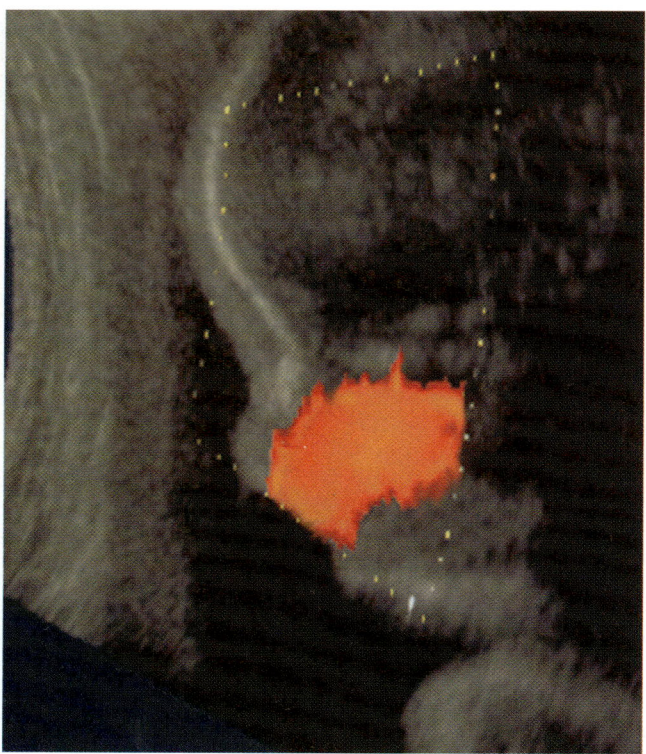

A   B

FIGURE 34. Normal and cleft palate. **A:** Color-flow imaging of normal fetus with respiratory activity shows amniotic fluid in the nasopharynx, separated from the oral pharynx inferiorly by the intact palate. **B:** Similar view in a fetus with cleft palate shows the nasopharynx and oral pharynx communicating in a single cavity. (Courtesy of Gianluigi Pilu, MD, Bologna, Italy.)

maxilla, with a completely flat profile. This is an extremely rare syndrome in which the findings are limited to the fetal face and frontal region of the brain, with the possibility of an associated frontal encephalocele. Other causes of facial clefting include trauma such as that resulting from amniotic band syndrome (a fetus can swallow an amniotic band, which can disrupt the fetal face).

Associated anomalies may be present, even after excluding aneuploidies or syndromic conditions. Associated malformations are more frequent in infants with cleft palate (46.7%) compared to those with cleft lip and palate (36.8%) or infants with isolated cleft lip (13.6%).[96] Malformations in the central nervous system and skeletal system are the most common, followed by malformations in the urogenital and cardiovascular systems. Although the absence of other anomalies is reassuring, subtle anomalies can be missed. We encountered one case diagnosed with isolated cleft but after birth was found to have critical pulmonary stenosis, which was fatal.

Prognosis and Management

The prognosis is directly related to associated anomalies and any underlying condition or chromosome abnormality. Lopoo et al. showed that patients and referring physicians highly depend on prenatal ultrasound to predict the severity of clefting and to exclude associated anomalies, so

that appropriate postnatal therapy can be planned.[97] These investigators studied a group of 40 fetuses with prenatally diagnosed clefts and found that severe associated anomalies were seen in 30 of the 40 cases. Life-threatening anomalies, such as central nervous system and cardiac defects, were the most common. As a result, many of the fetuses diagnosed with facial clefting were aborted therapeutically or died before obtaining plastic surgery. Only 12 of 40 fetuses survived, and only six had isolated facial clefts. This information is important for counseling patients whose fetuses are potential candidates for facial cleft repair. Certainly, the fetuses with median cleft face have the worst prognosis and usually have associated, fatal central nervous system anomalies.

Prenatal counseling is also beneficial when CL/P is isolated. Of those who had an antenatal diagnosis, 85% believed that the diagnosis prepared them psychologically for the birth of the cleft child.[98] Only one parent had actually terminated her pregnancy due solely to the antenatal diagnosis of a bilateral cleft lip and palate. Results suggest that parents of affected children have a strong desire for information and involvement in prenatal testing and counseling decisions. Parents appear to value preparation in spite of acknowledging anxiety associated with prenatal information.[99] All who had prenatal contact with the cleft team believed it was valuable.[100]

TABLE 6. ASSOCIATIONS WITH FACIAL CLEFTS

Amniotic band syndrome
Arthrogryposis
Camptomelic dysplasia
Caudal regression syndrome/sirenomelia
CHARGE association
Crouzon disease
Deletion 4p (Wolf-Hirschhorn syndrome)
Diastrophic dysplasia
Ectrodactyly, ectodermal dysplasia, clefting
Femoral hypoplasia, unusual facies
Fryns syndrome
Goldenhar syndrome
Gorlin syndrome
Holoprosencephaly
Hydrolethalus
Klippel-Feil syndrome
Larsen syndrome
Majewski (short rib–polydactyly syndrome, type II)
Marfan syndrome
Meckel-Gruber syndrome
Median cleft face (frontonasal dysplasia)
Multiple pterygiums
MURCS association
Nager syndrome
Neu-Laxova
Oral-facial-digital syndrome (Mohr syndrome)
Pena Shokeir
Pentalogy of Cantrell [diaphragm and diaphragmatic pericardium (occasional)]
Pierre Robin syndrome
Roberts syndrome
Shprintzen syndrome
Smith-Lemli-Opitz syndrome
Treacher Collins syndrome
Trisomy 10
Trisomy 13 (Patau syndrome)
Trisomy 18 (Edwards syndrome) (occasional)
Trisomy 22
Trisomy 9
Van der Woude syndrome
Walker-Warburg syndrome

CHARGE, *c*oloboma, *h*eart anomaly, choanal *a*tresia, *r*etardation, and *g*enital and *e*ar anomalies; MURCS, *m*üllerian, *r*enal, *c*ervicothoracic, *s*omite abnormalities.
Adapted from Benacerraf BR. *Ultrasound of fetal syndromes.* New York: Churchill Livingstone, 1997:1–8.

Postnatal management of CL/P requires a multidisciplinarian approach. A *cleft team* might include a plastic surgeon, a pediatrician, a dentist, a speech and language specialist, a social worker, a hearing specialist, an ear-nose-throat specialist, a psychologist, a nurse, and a genetic counselor. Surgical correction of clefts depends on the type. Some advocate early closure of the lip and palate, and others recommend delayed closure of the hard palate, thereby affording a high priority to the growth of the maxilla.[101] Primary repair of the lip is usually performed at a few months of age. It is important that parents be taught how to feed the baby during this period. For more severe clefts, breast-feeding may not be possible. Repair of the palate involves more extensive surgery and is usually done at 9 to 18 months of age. However, every case is individual and some patients require multiple surgeries.

Recurrence Risk

CL/P and isolated cleft palate carry an increased recurrence risk for their disorder, but not of the other. That is, patients with affected infants of CL/P are at increased risk for recurrent CL/P but not of cleft palate alone. If one parent has a facial cleft, there is a 3% to 5% risk to the offspring. If both a parent and child are affected, there is a 14% to 17% risk to other children in the family. If a family has Van der Woude's syndrome, an autosomal dominant syndrome of isolated facial clefting, the risk to subsequent children may be as high as 50%.[102] Folic acid supplementation may add some protective effect for CL/P.[103]

Macroglossia

Macroglossia appears as an unusually protuberant tongue (Fig. 35). Protrusion of the tongue can be a sign of several syndromes such as Beckwith-Wiedemann syndrome and Down syndrome.[104] In Beckwith-Wiedemann syndrome, the tongue is too large to fit in the fetal mouth. This is in contrast to fetuses with Down syndrome and other forms of mental deficiency, whose tongues may protrude forward due to hypotonia. Occasionally, an anterior encephalocele or intraoral tumor may extend through the ethmoid sinuses into the mouth and resemble an enlarged tongue.

Jaw and Mandible

Evaluation of the mandible and its relationship to the rest of the face is part of the sonographic examination of the fetal face. Biometric nomograms exist, although visual inspection of the mandible—particularly in the sagittal view—is the best way to determine the size of the mandible with respect to the rest of the face.[105] The transverse view along the mandibular rami is also helpful in obtaining biometric measurements and evaluating the symmetry of the rami.

Micrognathia

Syndromes associated with micrognathia include Treacher Collins syndrome,[106–110] Goldenhar syndrome, Roberts syndrome, Pierre Robin syndrome,[111,112] Nager acrofacial dysostoses, and many chromosomal abnormalities such as trisomies 13 and 18 (Table 7) (Fig. 36).[51,78–90,113] Other syndromes associated with micrognathia include oral-facial-digital syndromes in which micrognathia is seen together with polydactyly, double hallux, and other anomalies.

Syndromes with micrognathia are often associated with limb defects such as oral-mandibular-limb hypogenesis syndrome; Nager syndrome; ectrodactyly, ectodermal dysplasia, clefting syndrome; Roberts syndrome; and others (Table 7).[114]

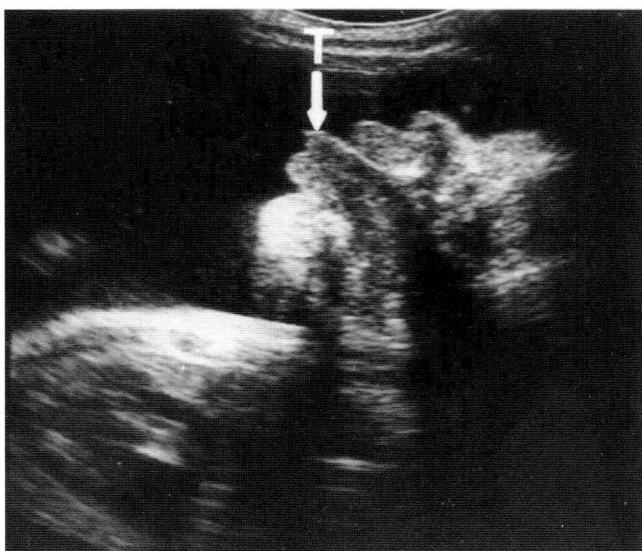

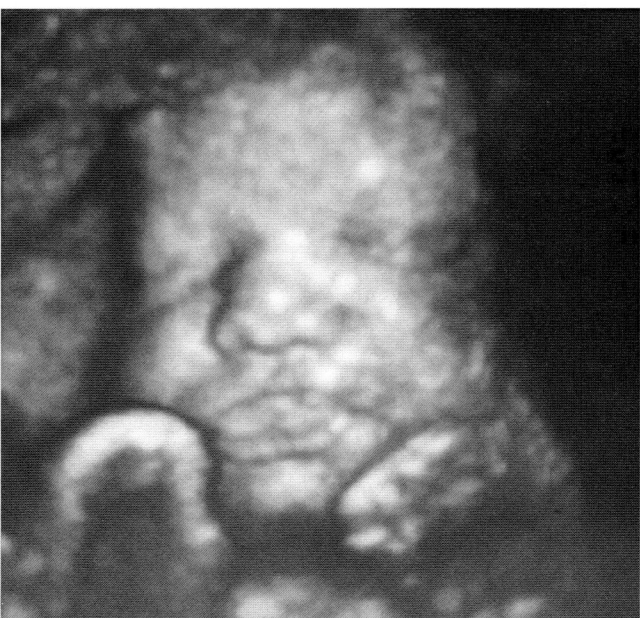

FIGURE 35. Macroglossia. **A:** Sagittal view in third trimester shows macroglossia with protruding tongue (*T*) in a fetus who proved to have Beckwith-Wiedemann syndrome. (Courtesy of L. Hill, MD, Pittsburgh, PA.) **B:** Three-dimensional ultrasound of another fetus shows enlarged tongue protruding through mouth.

The prognosis depends entirely on associated anomalies. In a retrospective study from Harvard Medical School's database, 20 fetuses with prenatally diagnosed micrognathia were identified—only four of whom (20%) survived.[115] Twenty-five percent had abnormal karyotypes, including three fetuses with trisomy 18, one with trisomy 13, and one with trisomy 9. There were two fetuses with Pena Shokeir syndrome, two with Treacher Collins syndrome, and two with multiple pterygium syndrome. One fetus each had Beckwith-Wiede-

TABLE 7. ASSOCIATIONS WITH MICROGNATHIA

Achondrogenesis
Amniotic band syndrome
Atelosteogenesis
Camptomelic dysplasia
Carpenter syndrome
Cerebrocostomandibular syndrome
CHARGE association
Cornelia de Lange syndrome
Crouzon disease
Deletion 11q (Jacobsen syndrome)
Deletion 4p (Wolf-Hirschhorn syndrome)
Diastrophic dysplasia
Ectrodactyly, ectodermal dysplasia, clefting
Femoral hypoplasia, unusual facies
Fryns
Goldenhar syndrome
Hydrolethalus
Infantile polycystic kidney disease
Joubert syndrome
Meckel-Gruber syndrome
Multiple pterygiums
MURCS association
Nager syndrome
Neu-Laxova
Oral-facial-digital syndrome (Mohr syndrome)
Pena Shokeir
Pierre Robin syndrome
Roberts syndrome
Seckel syndrome
Shprintzen syndrome
Smith-Lemli-Opitz syndrome
Thrombocytopenia
Treacher Collins syndrome
Triploidy
Trisomy 10
Trisomy 18 (Edwards syndrome)
Trisomy 9

CHARGE, coloboma, *h*eart anomaly, choanal *a*tresia, *r*etardation, and *g*enital and *e*ar anomalies; MURCS, *m*üllerian, *r*enal, *c*ervicothor-acic, *s*omite abnormalities.
Adapted from Benacerraf BR. *Ultrasound of fetal syndromes.* New York: Churchill Livingstone, 1997:1–8.

mann syndrome, arthrogryposis, Pierre Robin syndrome, harlequin syndrome, and osteochondrodysplasia with hydrocephalus. Other fetuses had multiple congenital abnormalities, which did not fit into a specific syndrome. Only three fetuses (15%) had micrognathia as the only sonographic finding, two of which survived: one with intrauterine growth restriction and one with mild Pierre Robin syndrome. These results demonstrate that the *in utero* diagnosis of micrognathia is associated with a poor prognosis and a high incidence of other serious congenital defects.

Robin Syndrome

Synonyms for Robin syndrome are cleft palate-micrognathia-glossoptosis, Pierre Robin syndrome, and Robin

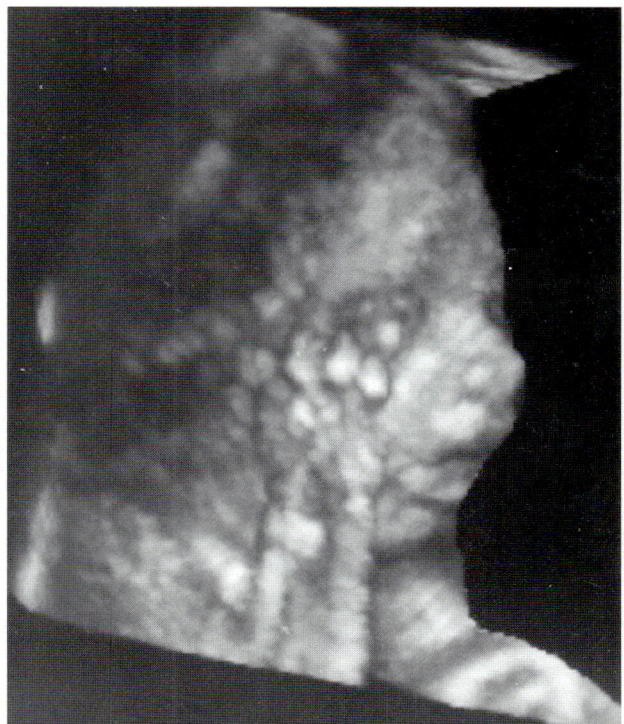
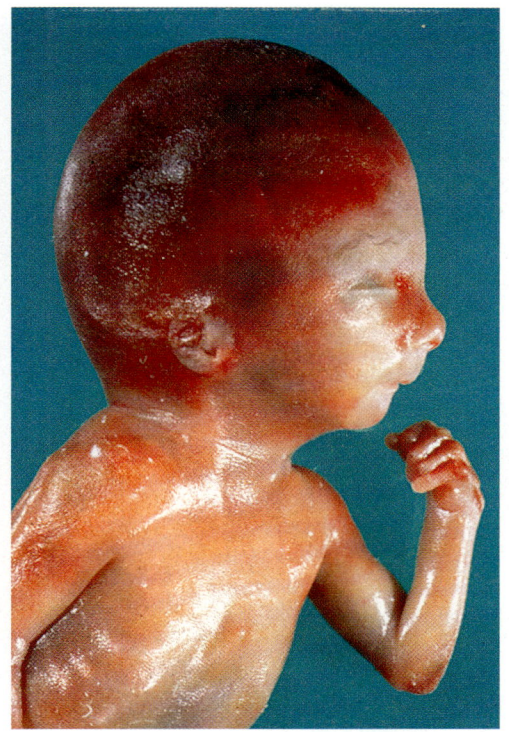

A   B

FIGURE 36. Micrognathia with trisomy 18. **A:** Three-dimensional surface rendering shows micrognathia. **B:** Pathologic photograph of another case of trisomy 18 shows micrognathia and clenched hand.

anomalad. Robin syndrome consists of triad of micrognathia, glossoptosis, and cleft palate.

Incidence
Robin syndrome is uncommon.

Embryology and Pathology
Pierre Robin syndrome is characterized by micrognathia, cleft palate with high arch palate, and glossoptosis. The primary abnormality is thought to be a small mouth. This produces glossoptosis (tongue falls back) and inhibits fusion of the palate to form a cleft palate.

Diagnosis
The main prenatal sonographic findings of Pierre Robin syndrome are micrognathia and polyhydramnios.[116] Cleft palate with high arch palate is not usually detected sonographically although it may occasionally be seen (Fig. 34). In 20 fetuses with Pierre Robin syndrome studied at the China Medical College Hospital, 12 fetuses (60%) had polyhydramnios and nine fetuses (45%) had cleft palate.[111]

Differential Diagnosis
The agnathia-microstomia-synotia syndrome (otocephaly) resembles a severe form of Pierre Robin syndrome. Other causes of micrognathia include trisomy 13 and trisomy 18.

Associated Anomalies
In approximately 80% of newborns with Pierre Robin syndrome, the triad of anomalies is part of an underlying genetic condition.[117] These may include trisomy 18, Stickler syndrome, velocardiofacial syndrome, or other syndromes.[118] Cardiac anomalies are also associated with Pierre Robin syndrome.

Prognosis and Management
Prognosis for Pierre Robin syndrome includes upper airway obstruction, neonatal respiratory distress, and feeding problems. Standard prenatal care is not altered when continuation of the pregnancy is opted. Among 20 cases reported by Hseih et al., there were two neonatal deaths and three children with mental retardation. Confirmation of diagnosis after birth is important for genetic counseling.

Recurrence Risk
Pierre Robin syndrome is autosomal recessive with a few X-linked cases.

Otocephaly

Synonyms for otocephaly are agnathia-microstomia-synotia and synotia. Otocephaly is defined as a failure of the assent of the developing auricles. The ears may be low set to mark-

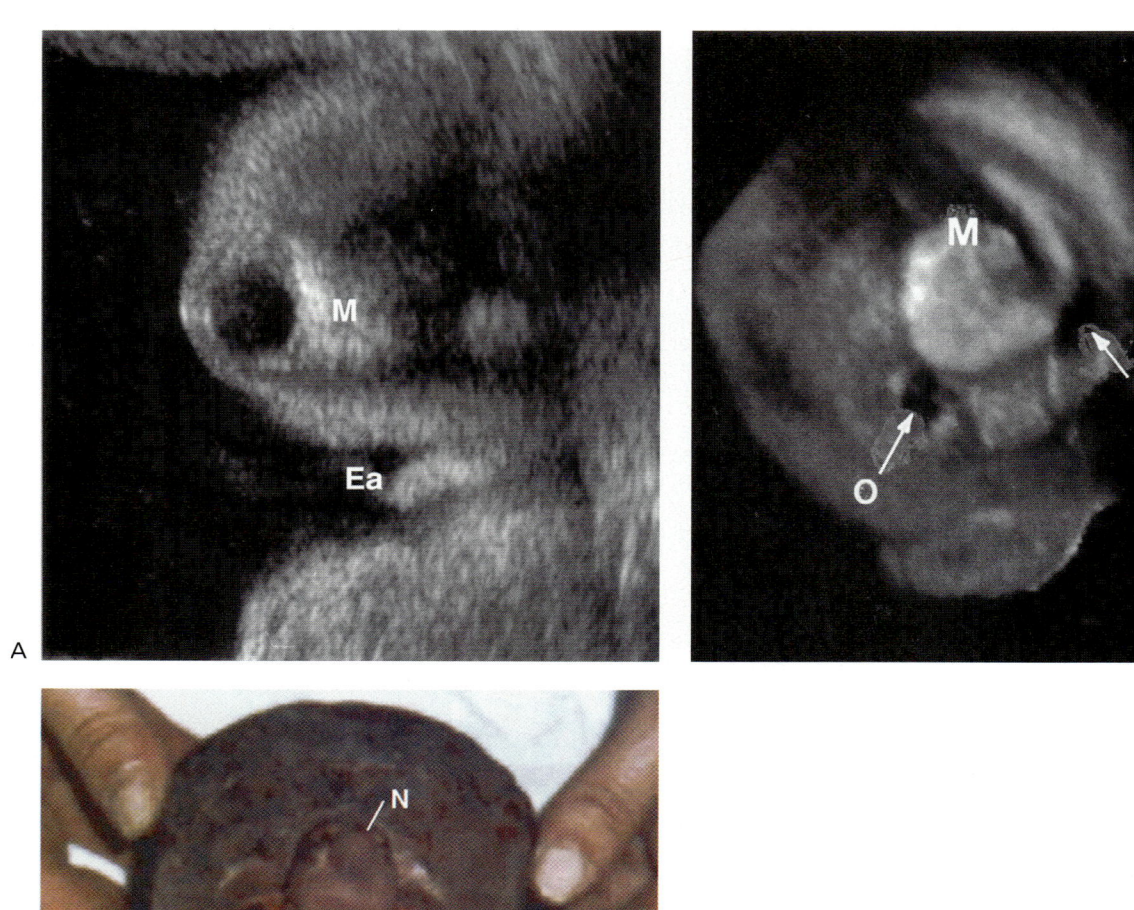

FIGURE 37. Otocephaly. **A:** Coronal view shows unusual face with ears (*Ea*) under jaw and mass-like area of midface (*M*). **B:** Three-dimensional ultrasound better shows unusual mass (*M*) of the midface and downward displacement of the orbits (*O*). **C:** Postnatal photograph shows striking features of otocephaly, which correlates well with ultrasound findings. Ea, ears; N, nose. (Courtesy of Dr. Adrian Clavelli, Diagnóstico Maipú, Buenos Aires, Argentina; republished in part from http://www.TheFetus.net.)

edly displaced along the anterior lower neck. It is always associated with agnathia or micrognathia.

Incidence

Otocephaly is rare and sporadic.

Embryology and Pathology

Otocephaly represents deficient development of the first branchial arch. Failure in assent of the developing auricles may be secondary to a defect in the neural crest's migration to the distal end of the mandibular arch.[119,120] Characteris-

tically, affected patients have ventrally displaced ears, small (microstomia) or absent mouth, and an absent (agnathia) or hypoplastic (micrognathia) mandible. In severe cases, failure of neural crest development and migration results in absence of the eyes and forebrain.[121]

Diagnosis

Several reports have described prenatal diagnosis of otocephaly.[120–122] This condition should be suspected when it is impossible to visualize the jaw, and the ears are not visible or in a very low position (Fig. 37). Other findings include hypo- or hypertelorism, prominent eyes, and proboscis, absence of visible stomach, and polyhydramnios. 3-D ultrasound or computed tomography scanning can provide additional information by better illustrating the striking facial features (Fig. 37).[123]

Differential Diagnosis

Agnathia may occur in isolation or with holoprosencephaly (agnathia-holoprosencephaly syndrome), situs inversus, or visceral anomalies.

Associated Anomalies

Associated anomalies may include holoprosencephaly, cephalocele, tracheoesophageal fistula, choanal atresia, cardiac defects, adrenal hypoplasia, situs inversus totalis, renal defects, vertebral and rib abnormalities, and single umbilical artery.[124]

Prognosis and Management

The prognosis is uniformly dismal. Ventilatory difficulties typically lead to the death of these infants shortly after birth. Occasional reports of survival beyond the perinatal period have been reported.[125]

Recurrence Risk

No recurrence risk is known.

The Ears

The ears can be seen by prenatal ultrasound and may be particularly well seen with 3-D ultrasound (Fig. 38). A number of papers have addressed normal ear size and length.[126–128] All have found that ear length is linearly correlated with gestational age and other fetal biometric measurements. Shimizu et al.[126] found that ear length is approximately one-third the biparietal diameter, independent of gestational age.

Small ears may be useful in detection of abnormalities. Awwad et al.[128] found that measured-to-expected ear length ratio of less than 0.8 was 75.0% sensitive and 98.8% specific in detecting Down syndrome fetuses. Lettieri et al.[129] reported that 10 of 14 fetuses with aneuploidy had ear lengths at or below the tenth percentile for a sensitivity of 71%, with a false-positive rate of 8%. On the other hand, Gill et al. suggests that the wide range of normal variation seen at each gestational age means that the fetal ear measurements are unlikely to be useful as a screening test.[130]

Other abnormalities of the ears may include dysplastic, absent (anotia), large, low-set, or otherwise malpositioned ears (Figs. 39 and 40). Preauricular tags may also provide useful clues on postnatal evaluation. Although low-set ears are a common feature of many syndromes, accurate prenatal diagnosis has been difficult. It is expected that 3-D ultrasound should better demonstrate many of these ear abnormalities.[131]

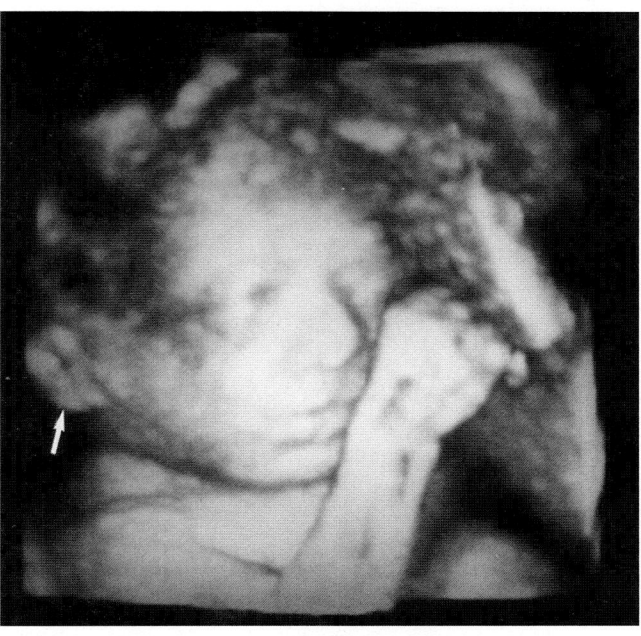

FIGURE 38. Normal ear. Three-dimensional surface sonogram shows normal ear (*arrow*).

OTHER FACIAL ABNORMALITIES

Maxillary hypoplasia with a depressed nasal bridge is associated with many syndromes, including several of the skeletal dysplasias (Table 8). Chromosomal anomalies such as Down syndrome are also associated with maxillary hypoplasia. Teratogens such as alcohol, hydantoin, valproic acid, and carbamazepine (Tegretol) have been associated with the development of maxillary hypoplasia.[56]

Prenatal ultrasound can detect facial abnormalities of the craniosynostosis syndromes. These include Apert syndrome,[132–134] Carpenter syndrome,[135,136] Pfeiffer syndrome,[137–139] and Crouzon disease.[140–142] Similar facial abnormalities for all of these disorders include high cranial vault (acrocephaly), prominent forehead (frontal bossing), hypertelorism and proptosis, depressed nasal bridge with parrot-beaked nose, and hypoplastic maxilla.

Apert syndrome [see also Craniosynostosis Syndromes (Fibroblast Growth Factor Receptor–Related) in Chapter 5] is characterized by craniosynostosis and midfacial hypoplasia together with bilateral syndactyly ("mitten hands"). The sutures of fetuses with craniosynostosis can be best evaluated using 3-D ultrasound, with which open and closed sutures are easily distinguishable.[143] Prenatal computed tomography scan has also been used.[144] Crouzon disease, one of the best known of many craniofacial syndromes, is an autosomal dominant disorder characterized by craniosynostosis, prominent eyes, and midfacial hypoplasia due to abnormal development and premature fusion of the skull.

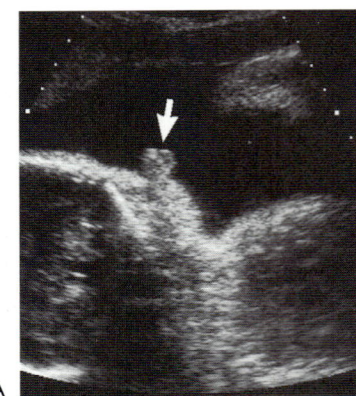

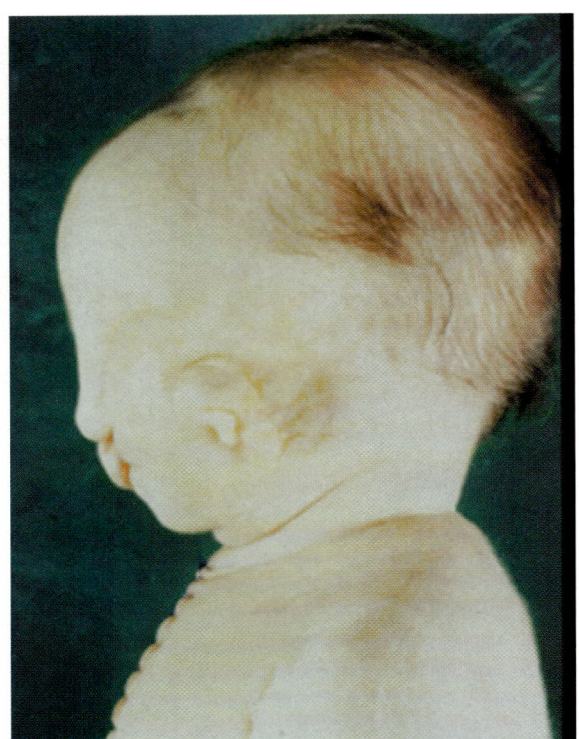

FIGURE 39. Dysmorphic, low-lying ear. **A:** Coronal scan shows abnormally low and malformed ear (*arrow*) in a fetus with Goldenhar syndrome. **B:** Pathologic photograph shows dysmorphic ear.

The twinning process can affect the fetal face, and incomplete duplication of the embryo can result in a duplicated face or diprosopus.[145–147] Diprosopus represents partial duplication of the face and intracranial contents, with a central double orbit similar to what is seen in cyclopia. However, there are two noses with another orbit on the outer side of each nose. If the intracranial malformations and facial defects are not recognized properly *in utero*, these fetuses can be mistaken for having holoprosencephaly with cyclopia.

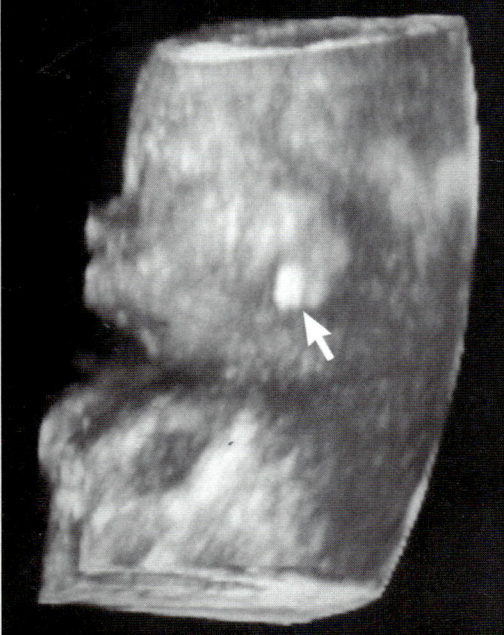

FIGURE 40. Dysmorphic ear (*arrow*). Three-dimensional surface rendering in a sagittal view of a fetus with multiple congenital abnormalities, which include severe micrognathia and abnormal ears.

TABLE 8. ASSOCIATIONS WITH MAXILLARY HYPOPLASIA/DEPRESSED NASAL BRIDGE

Achondroplasia
Apert syndrome
Atelosteogenesis
Camptomelic dysplasia
Carpenter syndrome
CHARGE association
Chondrodysplasia punctata
Cleft lip and palate (all types)
Cleidocranial dysostosis
Deletion 11q (Jacobsen syndrome)
Freeman-Sheldon syndrome (whistling face)
Holoprosencephaly
Larsen syndrome
Pena Shokeir
Pfeiffer syndrome
Thanatophoric dysplasia
Trisomy 13 (Patau syndrome)
Trisomy 21 (Down syndrome)

CHARGE, coloboma, *heart anomaly*, choanal atresia, retardation, and genital and ear anomalies.
Adapted from Benacerraf BR. *Ultrasound of fetal syndromes.* New York: Churchill Livingstone, 1997:1–8.

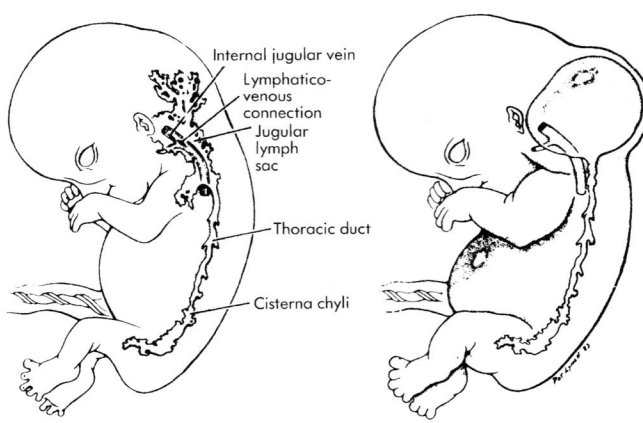

,B

FIGURE 41. Diagram of normal lymphatic system **(A)** and cystic hygroma **(B)**. (Reproduced with permission from Chervenak FA, Isaacson G, Blakemore KJ, Breg WR, Hobbins JC, et al. Fetal cystic hygroma. Cause and natural history. *N Engl J Med* 1983; 309:822–825.)

The Neck

Most neck abnormalities produce a mass effect. The most common are cystic hygroma, goiter, and tumors.

Cystic Hygroma

Synonyms for cystic hygroma are jugular lymphatic obstructive sequence and hygroma colli cysticum. The term *hygroma* means *moist tumor*. Cystic hygromas are anomalies of the lymphatic system characterized by single or multiple cysts within the soft tissue, usually involving the neck (Fig. 41). Cystic hygromas contain a clear or cloudy fluid.

Incidence
The incidence of cystic hygroma varies with gestational age and patient group. Cystic hygromas are certainly the most common cause for a neck *mass* detected prenatally. Cystic hygromas are observed in 1 per 200 spontaneously aborted fetuses with crown-rump length greater than 30 mm[148] compared to 1 per 1,000 live births. Trauffer et al.[149] reported 39 cases of cystic hygroma among 7,189 patients referred for chorionic villus sampling between 9 to 14 postmenstrual weeks for an incidence of 0.54% of cystic hygroma.

Embryology and Pathology
The fetal lymphatic system begins to develop at around the fifth week of gestation. Six lymphatic sacs form. Two are located lateral to the jugular veins, two are iliac, one is retroperitoneal, and the last one is the cisterna chyli. These sacs eventually develop communications with the venous system. The right and left thoracic duct joins the jugular sacs with the cisterna chyli.[150] Failure of establishing these lymphatic connections results in accumulation of lymphatic fluid in the jugular lymphatic sacs and tissues, eventually giving the appearance of the typical cystic hygroma (Fig. 41).[151,152]

A communication between this primitive structure and the jugular vein is formed at 40 days of gestation (conceptional age). Failure of development of this communication results in lymphatic stasis. Dilatation of the jugular lymphatic sac leads to the formation of a cystic structure in the cervical region. Overdistention of the jugular lymphatic sacs, which are located in both sides of the neck, results in the formation of a cystic structure that is usually partitioned by a thick fibrous band corresponding to the nuchal ligament. Within the cystic structure, thinner septa are seen and are thought to derive from either fibrous structure of the neck or deposits of fibrin. Resolution of the cystic hygroma may result in redundant skin and clinical appearance of *webbed neck* (pterygium colli). This is a common feature of Turner syndrome and other genetic and nongenetic conditions.

Diagnosis
Cystic hygroma is one of the easiest and earliest anomalies that can be detected by prenatal sonography. It may be seen as early as 12 weeks' gestation. However, cystic hygromas vary considerably in size and appearance. The typical appearance of cystic hygroma is a symmetric or bilateral cystic structure of the posterior neck, typically one or more characteristic septations (Figs. 42 and 43).[153–159] A midline septum frequently divides the cyst along the anteroposterior axis and corresponds to the nuchal ligament. Large cystic hygromas may fill the amniotic cavity whereas small cystic hygromas are localized to the posterior-inferior neck and may be missed.

Although typically considered separately, there is wide overlap between cystic hygroma, nuchal translucency, and nuchal thickening (Figs. 43 through 45). *Nuchal thickening* (see Chapter 21) does not show discrete fluid although cystic hygroma may resolve to nuchal thickening alone, and this is associated with aneuploidy.[160,161] Also, some cases of cystic hygroma show features of nuchal translucency (Fig. 44), and some cases of nuchal thickening appear *edematous* or may show subtle septations (Fig. 45).

Nuchal translucency refers to the sonolucent space optimally seen in all fetuses during specific times during the first trimester (10 to 14 weeks). It is described in greater detail in Chapter 20. Increased nuchal translucency is also associated with fetal aneuploidy and hydropic changes. When nuchal translucency is increased, fine internal trabeculae may occasionally be seen, especially with high-resolution probes (Fig. 44),[162] and this also shows overlap with cystic hygroma. However, cystic hygroma is distinguished by thick septations and loculated fluid.[163] Unilateral fluid collections of the neck, typically lateral or anterior in location, are referred to as a lymphangioma. Similar masses may be seen in the axilla.

Differential Diagnosis
The differential diagnosis of cystic hygroma includes cervical meningocele, cephaloceles, neck tumors, subcutaneous edema, goiter, cystic teratoma, and hemangioma. However, an experienced sonographer should have no difficulty in making the correct diagnosis.

sarcomas, or melanomas.[197] This risk increases with children who have received radiation therapy and is most common in the field of radiation. The cumulative risk is approximately 26% in nonirradiated and 58% in irradiated patients by 50 years of age.[198]

Patients with retinoblastoma need close follow-up after treatment. Children with germline retinoblastoma should be screened using magnetic resonance neuroimaging every 3 months for the first year after diagnosis and at least two times a year for the next 3 years.[199]

Recurrence Risk

Retinoblastoma has hereditary and sporadic forms. The familial form is inherited as an autosomal dominant with high penetrance. If a parent has been treated for bilateral retinoblastoma, almost one-half (45%) of their children develop retinoblastoma. If a parent had unilateral retinoblastoma, 7% to 15% of his or her offspring has retinoblastoma. The most common situation is when neither parent has been affected but has a child born with retinoblastoma. If the parents are genetically normal, the chance of another child having retinoblastoma is 1 in 15,000 to 1 in 20,000.

Epignathus

Synonyms for epignathus include oral teratoma, nasopharyngeal teratoma, extragonadal teratoma, and facial teratoma. Epignathus is a teratoma that arises from the oral cavity and the pharynx.

Incidence

The incidence for epignathus is approximately 1 per 35,000 live births. Approximately 2% of all pediatric teratomas occur in the nasopharyngeal area.[95]

Embryology and Pathology

Teratomas are tumors that usually have at least one tissue type from each of the three embryonic layers. They tend to be midline in location, supporting the hypothesis that primordial germ cells migrate along the dorsal midline from the hindgut into the embryonic genital ridge. Some cells continue their cephalad migration to eventually settle in the mediastinum, neck, nasopharynx, and brain.

Epignathus is a teratoma that arises from the palate or pharynx in the region of the basisphenoid (Rathke's pouch). These tumors can completely replace brain as they grow intracranially or fill the oral pharynx.

Diagnosis

Epignathus is seen as a complex mass, predominantly solid, emanating from the fetal mouth and nose (Fig. 49). Hyperextension of the head has been reported for large tumors. Large tumors are invariably associated with polyhydramnios, most likely due to the tumor itself or obstruction of fetal swallowing. The earliest reported case has been 15

weeks.[200–202] MRI has been used in combination with ultrasound and should be better able to show the intracranial extension of large tumors.[203,204]

Differential Diagnosis

The differential diagnosis for a mass in the region of the mouth includes macroglossia, cysts such as salivary gland cyst (ranula), hemangioma, lymphangioma, neurofibroma, anterior cephalocele (Fig. 50),[205] cervical teratoma, and gingival cell tumors (Fig. 51).[206–210] Lymphangiomas and ranula are predominantly cystic, whereas fibromas, granulosa cell tumors, and teratomas are solid.

Granulosa cell tumor (epulis) is a benign, pedunculated tumor, arising anteriorly from the maxillary alveolar ridge. Granulosa cell tumor has been rarely reported prenatally.[211,212] Meizner et al. demonstrated that a granulosa cell tumor may develop late in gestation; they described a fetus who had normal structural surveys at 15 and 22 weeks and yet developed such a tumor at 29 weeks.[212] Although fetal facial tumors are not usually associated with chromosomal anomalies, there is one report of a female XXX fetus with a congenital epulis.[207]

Associated Anomalies

Associated anomalies are seen in approximately 6% of these cases and include facial clefts, bronchial cysts, hypertelorism, and congenital heart defects. One case was reported in association with trisomy 13 and multiple other anomalies.[214] Nasopharyngeal teratomas are often associated with polyhydramnios, nonimmune fetal hydrops, and exophthalmos.

Prognosis

Although the majority of these tumors are benign, numerous reports of such tumors describe an extremely poor prognosis[215–220] with few exceptions.[221] The prognosis depends on the size of the tumor and destruction or compression of adjacent structures.

Management

Management usually involves planned cesarean section to avoid dystocia and fetal trauma with immediate establishment of an airway followed by surgical excision. A pediatric surgeon and neonatologist should be present at the time of delivery to provide immediate resuscitation, endotracheal intubation, and even a tracheotomy if an airway cannot be secured.

Recurrence

No recurrence of epignathus is known.

Cervical Teratoma

Cervical teratomas are tumors that arise in the neck, typically the anterior neck.

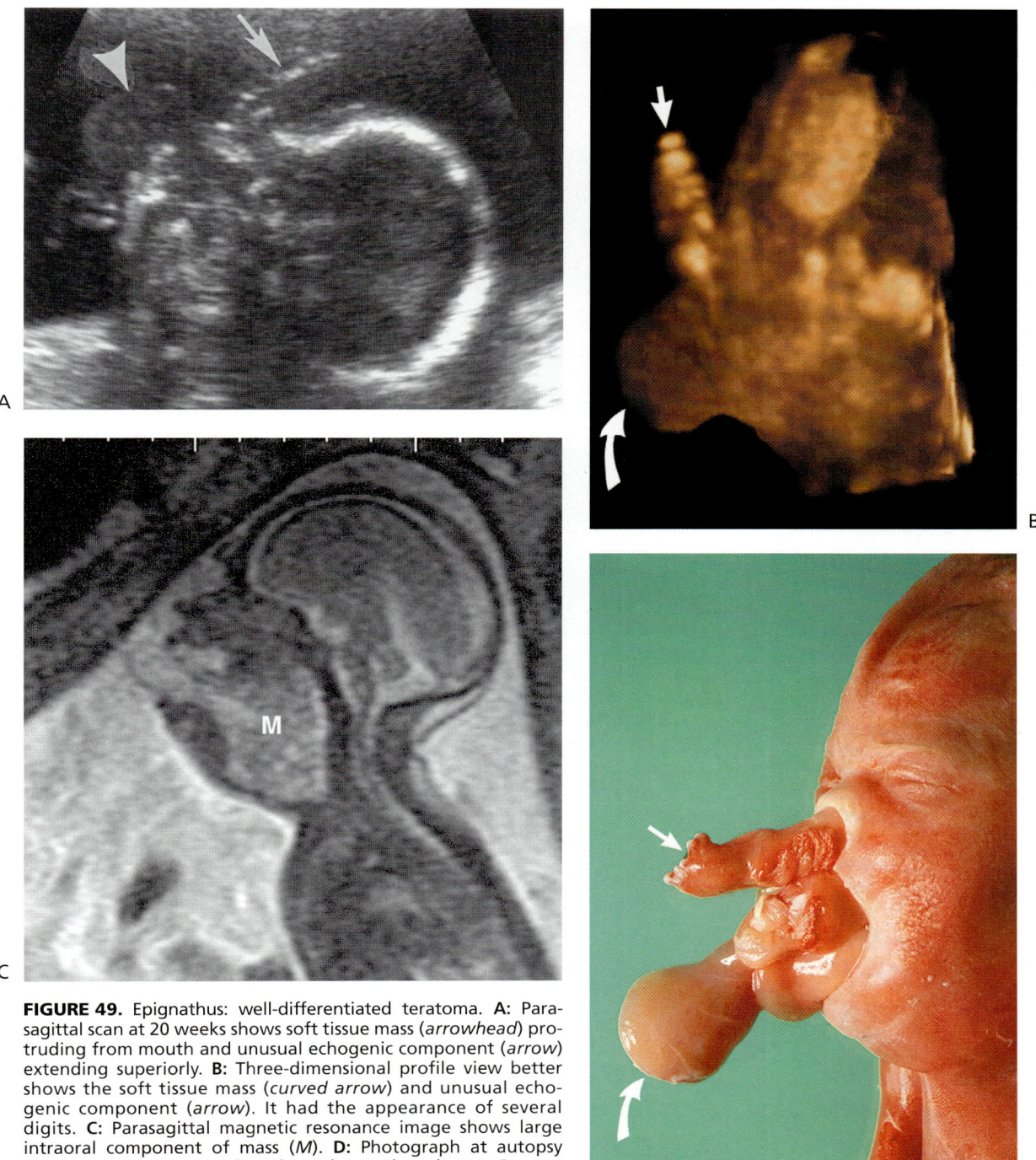

FIGURE 49. Epignathus: well-differentiated teratoma. **A:** Parasagittal scan at 20 weeks shows soft tissue mass (*arrowhead*) protruding from mouth and unusual echogenic component (*arrow*) extending superiorly. **B:** Three-dimensional profile view better shows the soft tissue mass (*curved arrow*) and unusual echogenic component (*arrow*). It had the appearance of several digits. **C:** Parasagittal magnetic resonance image shows large intraoral component of mass (*M*). **D:** Photograph at autopsy shows large mass protruding through mouth and nose. Component extending superiorly through nose (*arrow*) had features of a foot, whereas the soft tissue component (*curved arrow*) protruded through the mouth. (Part **D** courtesy of Joseph R. Siebert, PhD, Department of Pathology, Children's Hospital, Seattle, WA.)

Incidence

Cervical teratoma is rare. In a large series of 4,257 childhood neoplasms, only four teratomas of the neck were recorded, representing an incidence of less than 0.1%. The incidence of congenital teratoma is reported as 1 per 20,000 to 1 per 40,000 live births.[3,222] They are most frequently found in the sacrococcygeal area, although other sites include cranial, orbital, nasopharyngeal, thyroidal, cervical, mediastinal, retroperitoneal, and gonadal sites.

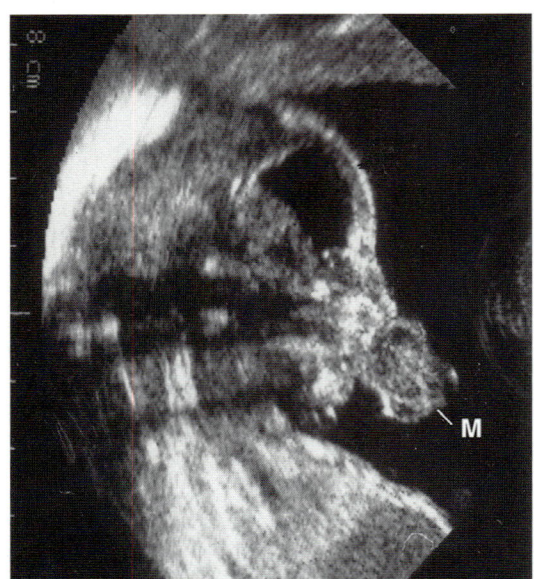

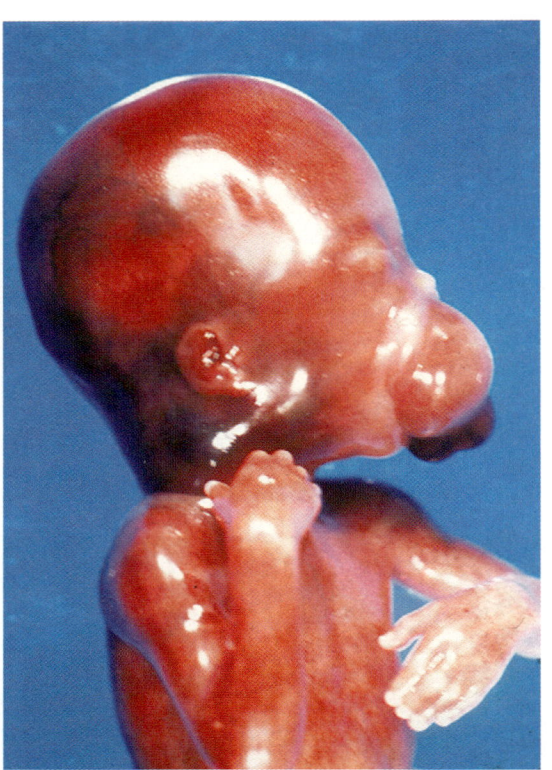

FIGURE 50. Anterior cephalocele. **A:** Sagittal scan shows large mass (*M*) protruding through mouth. Cerebral ventricular dilatation was also present. **B:** Postmortem photograph shows large mass, which represented anterior cephalocele. (Courtesy of Philippe Jeanty, MD, PhD, Nashville, TN.)

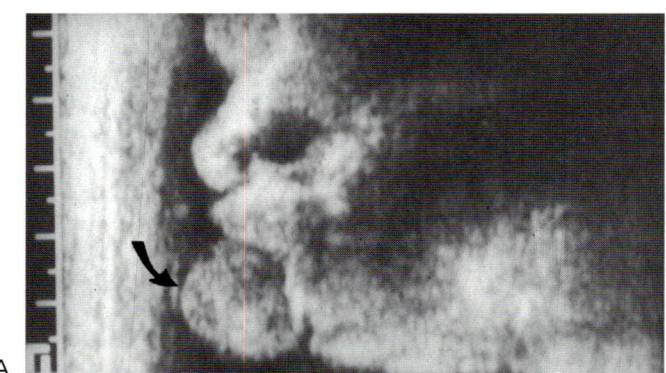

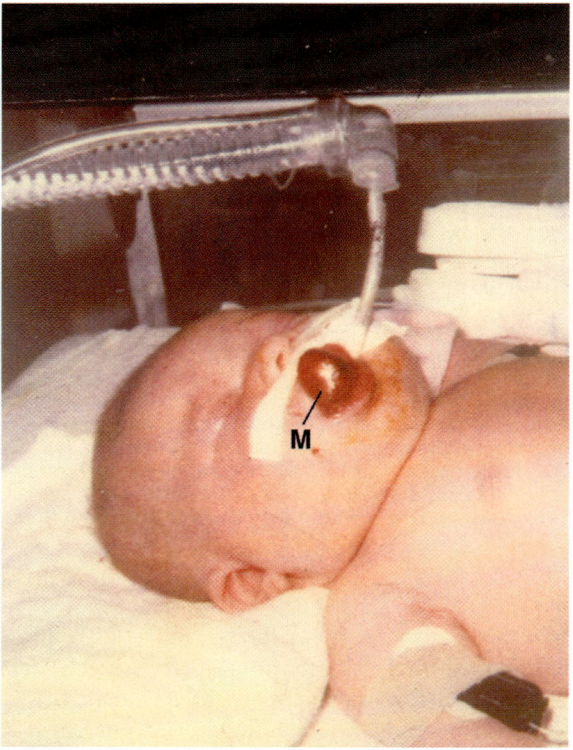

FIGURE 51. Gingival cell tumor of tongue. **A:** Sagittal view shows mass (*arrow*) protruding through mouth. **B:** Postnatal photograph shows mass (*M*), which proved to be gingival cell tumor of tongue. (Courtesy of Richard Bowerman, MD, Ann Arbor, MI.)

Embryology and Pathology

Teratomas are tumors comprised of all three germ layers. Cervical teratomas are usually detected at birth, but can occasionally present in adulthood. Although termed a *teratoma*, in fact many of the tumors detected prenatally are malignant.[223] Even when histologically benign, the tumors compress critical structures of the neck.

Diagnosis

Cervical teratomas have been frequently detected prenatally.[224–226] They appear as solid or mixed solid-cystic tumors, sometimes with internal calcifications located in the anterior or anterolateral neck (Fig. 52).[227,228] Large tumors produce hyperextension of the neck. Like teratomas in other areas, they are aggressive and may grow rapidly. They can be detected as early as 16 weeks.

MRI has also been used in evaluation of cervical teratomas.[229]

Differential Diagnosis

Differentiation from other cervical masses is usually not difficult. Primary possibilities include lymphangioma and hemangioma, or goiter.

Associated Anomalies

Cervical teratomas can contribute to pulmonary insufficiency and chondromalacia because of a mass effect *in utero* and underdevelopment of the fetal lungs.[230]

Prognosis

Polyhydramnios, preterm delivery, and perinatal death have, respectively, been reported as 25%, 17%, and 43%. Large tumors may produce dystocia. If the airway is stabilized and resection of the tumor can be performed, the prognosis is good.[231,232]

Management

Obstruction of the airway is the major challenge in the neonatal period. In one multicenter study of 14 cases of cervical teratoma, two of six infants with a prenatal diagnosis survived only because tracheostomies were performed by pediatric surgeons in the delivery.[233]

The *ex utero* intrapartum treatment has been proposed in cases of potential airway obstruction.[234] The infant is delivered but maintained on placental support until an airway can be established.[235]

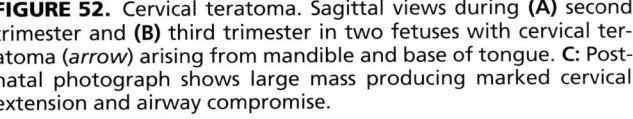

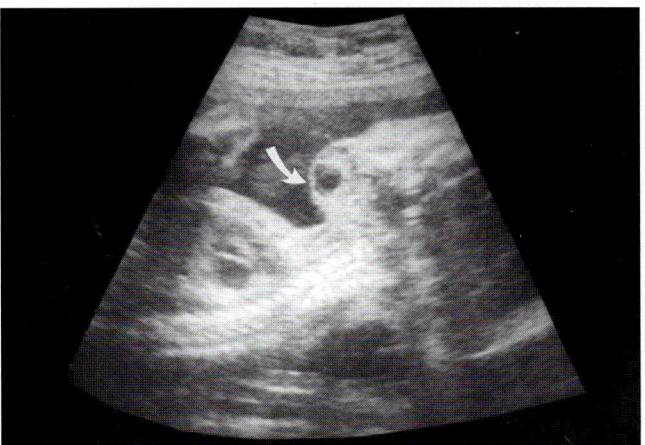

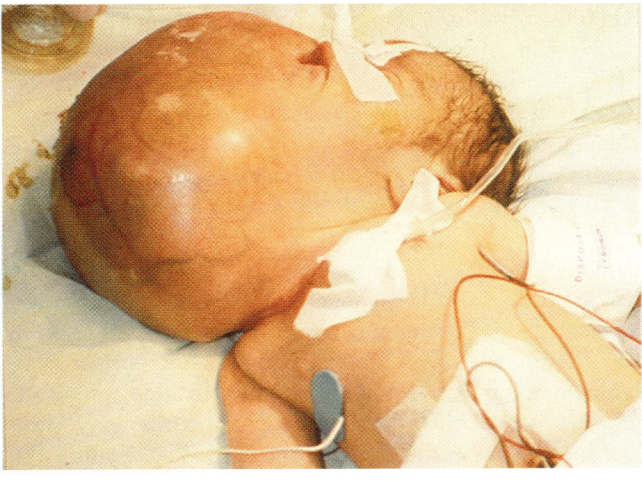

FIGURE 52. Cervical teratoma. Sagittal views during **(A)** second trimester and **(B)** third trimester in two fetuses with cervical teratoma (*arrow*) arising from mandible and base of tongue. **C:** Postnatal photograph shows large mass producing marked cervical extension and airway compromise.

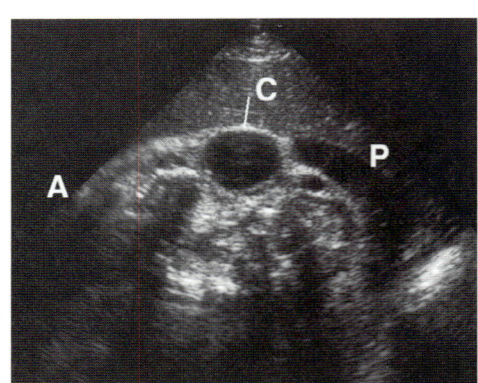
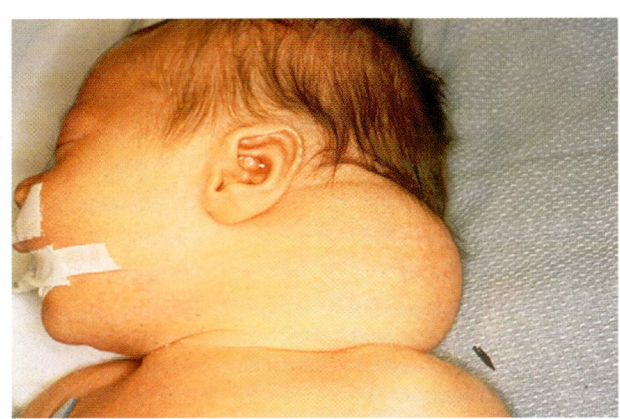

FIGURE 53. Lymphangioma. **A:** Axial view at base of neck shows unilateral cyst (*C*). A, anterior; P, posterior. **B:** Preoperative postnatal photograph shows unilateral mass. (Part **B** courtesy of Ian Nielsen, MD, Swedish Medical Center, Seattle, WA.)

Recurrence Risk

There is no known recurrence risk for cervical teratomas.

Hemangioma and Lymphangioma

Hemangiomas and lymphangiomas are the most common tumors of infancy. Most of these lesions are present at birth, and 90% are recognized before 3 years of age.[236]

Incidence

Hemangioma and lymphangioma are rare. Lymphangiomas are most frequently lesions of vascular origin during the first year of life, most commonly arising on the head, neck, and axilla.

Embryology and Pathology

Hemangioma and lymphangioma show overlapping pathologic and sonographic features. Hemangiolymphangioma is a malformation of lymphatic and blood vessels. Strawberry hemangiomas affect 1% to 3% of infants, with girls affected three times more commonly than boys. They may be solitary or multiple.

Cavernous hemangiomas are masses of dilated vessels deep in the skin. They appear as pale, skin-colored, red, or blue masses that are not as sharply defined as the strawberry hemangiomas.

Lymphangiomas are congenital malformations of lymphatic vessels. They are common in the neck and axillary region.[237]

Diagnosis

Hemangioma and lymphangioma have been frequently reported.[238] Lymphangiomas appear as cystic structures, often multilocular (Fig. 53). Hemangiomas appear as *solid* or mixed solid and cystic. Color-flow imaging or power Doppler may be helpful.[239] Some lesions are large and spread to the chest wall or extremity. MRI has occasionally been performed to differentiate from a cephalocele, but the

ultrasound appearance is usually characteristic.[240–242] The earliest reported case has been 14 weeks.[239]

Differential Diagnosis

Some cases of hemangioma have been mistaken for cephalocele (see Fig. 11, Chapter 7).[243–247]

Associated Findings

Unilateral lymphangiomas or hemangiomas are usually isolated. The Klippel-Trenaunay-Weber syndrome is characterized by vascular abnormalities with associated limb hypertrophy.

Prognosis and Management

Large hemangiomas may be associated with hydrops.[248] Spontaneous regression is common (60%) with hemangiomas, with many of these lesions involuting within the first 5 years of life.[249] Treatment for persistent hemangiomas includes administration of corticosteroids or interferon, and, in some instances, embolization or surgical resection.[250] Because these lesions may infiltrate adjacent tissue, surgical resection may be difficult. The local recurrence rate is 6% for incomplete excision in cases of complicated surgery. Surgery involving the operation on placental support procedure has been proposed when the airway is compromised.[213]

Recurrence Risk

There is no known recurrence risk for hemangioma and lymphangioma.

REFERENCES

1. Hegge FN, Prescott GH, Watson PT. Fetal facial abnormalities identified during obstetric sonography. *J Ultrasound Med* 1986;5:679–684.
2. Benacerraf BR, Frigoletto FD, Bieber FR. The fetal face: ultrasound examination. *Radiology* 1984;153:495–497.

3. Pilu G, Reece EA, Romero R, et al. Prenatal diagnosis of craniofacial malformations with ultrasonography. *Am J Obstet Gynecol* 1986;155:45–50.

4. Seeds JW, Defalo RC. Technique of early sonographic diagnosis of bilateral cleft lip and palate. *Obstet Gynecol* 1983;62:23–75.

5. Hafner E, Sterniste W, Scholler J, Schuchter K, Philip K. Prenatal diagnosis of facial malformations. *Prenat Diagn* 1997;17:51–58.

6. Sadler TW. *Langman's embryology*, 6th ed. Baltimore: Williams & Wilkins, 1990:297–305.

7. Moore KL. *The developing fetus*, 4th ed. Philadelphia: WB Saunders, 1988:189–206.

8. O'Rahilly R, Muller F. *Human embryology and teratology*, 2nd ed. New York: Wiley-Liss, 1996:207–213.

9. Nyberg DA, Mahoney BS, Kramer D. Paranasal echogenic mass: sonographic sign of bilateral complete cleft lip and palate before 20 menstrual weeks. *Radiology* 1992;184:757–759.

10. Sivan E, Chan L, Mallozzi-Eberte A, Reece EA. Sonographic imaging of the fetal face and the establishment of normative dimensions for chin length and upper lip width. *Am J Perinatol* 1997;14:191–194.

11. Goldstein I, Tamir A, Zimmer EZ, Itskovitz-Eldor J. Growth of the fetal orbit and lens in normal pregnancies. *Ultrasound Obstet Gynecol* 1998;12:175–179.

12. Achiron R, Gottlieb Z, Yaron Y, Gabbay M, Gabbay U, et al. The development of the fetal eye: in utero ultrasonographic measurements of the vitreous and lens. *Prenat Diagn* 1995;15:155–160.

13. Ben Ami M, Weiner E, Perlitz V, Shalev E. Ultrasound evaluation of the width of the fetal nose. *Prenat Diagn* 1998;18:1010–1013.

14. Chitty LS, Campbell S, Altman DG. Measurement of the fetal mandible—feasibility and construction of a centile chart. *Prenat Diagn* 1993;13:749–756.

15. Paladini D, Morra T, Teodoro A, Lamberti A, Tremolaterra F, et al. Objective diagnosis of micrognathia in the fetus: the jaw index. *Obstet Gynecol* 1999;93:382–386.

16. Ulm MR, Chalubinski K, Ulm C, Plockinger B, Deretinger J, et al. Sonographic depictions of fetal tooth germs. *Prenat Diagn* 1995;15:368–372.

17. Guis F, Ville Y, Vincent Y, Doumerc S, Pons JC, et al. Ultrasound evaluation of the length of the fetal nasal bones throughout gestation. *Ultrasound Obstet Gynecol* 1995;5:304–307.

18. Goldstein I, Tamir A, Itskovitz-Eldor J, Zimmer EZ. Growth of the fetal nose width and nostril distance in normal pregnancies. *Ultrasound Obstet Gynecol* 1997;9:35–38.

19. Pinette MG, Blackstone J, Pan Y, Pinette SG. Measurement of fetal nasal width by ultrasonography. *Am J Obstet Gynecol* 1997;177:842–845.

20. Achiron R, Ben Arie A, Gabbay U, Mashiach S, Rotstein Z, et al. Development of the fetal tongue between 14 and 26 weeks of gestation: in utero ultrasonographic measurements. *Ultrasound Obstet Gynecol* 1997;9:39–41.

21. Trout T, Budorict NE, Pretorius DH, McGahan JP. Significance of orbital measurements in the fetus. *J Ultrasound Med* 1994;13:937–943.

22. Mayden KL, Tortora M, Berkowitz RL, Bracken M, Hobbins JC. Orbital diameters: a new parameter for prenatal diagnosis and dating. *Am J Obstet Gynecol* 1982;144:289–297.

23. Jeanty P, Dramaix-Wilmet M, Van Gansbeke D, Van Regemorter N, Rodesch F. Fetal ocular biometry by ultrasound. *Radiology* 1982;143:513–516.

24. Mielke G, Dietz K, Franz H, Reiss I, Gembruch U. Sonographic assessment of the fetal palpebral fissure stant—an additional tool in the prenatal diagnosis of syndromes. *Prenat Diagn* 1997;17:323–326.

25. Hata T, Yonehara T, Aoki S, Manabe A, Hata K, et al. Three-dimensional sonographic visualization of the fetal face. *AJR Am J Roentgenol* 1998;170:481–483.

26. Lai TH, Chang CH, Yu CH, Kuo PL, Chang FM. Prenatal diagnosis of alobar holoprosencephaly by two-dimensional and three-dimensional ultrasound. *Prenat Diagn* 2000;20:400–403.

27. Merz E, Weber G, Bahlmann F, Miric-Fesanic D. Application of transvaginal and abdominal three-dimensional ultrasound for the detection or exclusion of malformations of the fetal face. *Ultrasound Obstet Gynecol* 1997;9:237–243.

28. Bonilla-Musoles F, Machado LE, Osborne NG, Raga F, Chamusca L, et al. Ultrasound diagnosis of facial and cephalic pole malformations: comparative study of different three-dimensional modalities and two-dimensional ultrasound. *Ultrasound Quarterly* 2000;16:97–105.

29. Pretorius DH, House M, Nelson TR, Hollenback KA. Evaluation of normal and abnormal lips in fetuses: comparison between three- and two-dimensional sonography. *AJR Am J Roentgenol* 1995;165:1233–1237.

30. Pretorius DH, Nelson TR. Fetal face visualization using three-dimensional ultrasound. *J Ultrasound Med* 1995;14:349–356.

31. Johnson DD, Pretorius DH, Budorick NE, Jones MC, Lou KV, et al. Fetal lip and primary palate: three-dimensional versus two-dimensional US. *Radiology* 2000;217:236–239.

32. Ulm MR, Kratochwil A, Ulm B, Lee A, Bettelheim D, et al. Three-dimensional ultrasonographic imaging of fetal tooth buds for characterization of facial clefts. *Early Hum Dev* 1999;55:67–75.

33. Nicolaides KH, Salvesen DR, Snijders RJM, Gosden CM. Fetal facial defects: associated malformations and chromosomal abnormalities. *Fetal Diagn Ther* 1993;8:1–9.

34. Benacerraf BR, Frigoletto FD, Greene MF. Abnormal facial features and extremities in human trisomy syndromes: prenatal ultrasound appearance. *Radiology* 1986;159:243–246.

35. Benacerraf BR, Miller WA, Frigoletto FD. Sonographic detection of fetuses with trisomies 13 and 18: accuracy and limitations. *Am J Obstet Gynecol* 1988;158:404–409.

36. Kjaer I, Keeling J, Russell B, Daugaard-Jensen J, Fischer Hansen B. Palate structure in human holoprosencephaly correlates with the facial malformation and demonstrates a new palatal developmental field. *Am J Med Genet* 1997;73:387–392.

37. De Meyer W, Zeman W, Palmer CG. The face predicts the brain: diagnostic significance of median facial anomalies for holoprosencephaly (arrhinencephaly). *Pediatrics* 1964;34:256–263.

38. Rolland M, Sarramon MF, Bloom MC. Astomia-agnathia-holoprosencephaly association. Prenatal diagnosis of a new case. *Prenat Diagn* 1991;11:199–203.

39. Lev-Gur M, Maklad NF, Patel S. Ultrasonic findings in fetal cyclopia. *J Reprod Med* 1983;28:554–557.

40. Rolland M, Sarramon MF, Bloom MC. Astomia agnathia-holoprosencephaly association. Prenatal diagnosis of a new case. *Prenat Diagn* 1991;11:199–203.

41. McGahan JP, Nyberg DA, Mack LA. Sonography of facial features of alobar and semilobar holoprosencephaly. *AJR Am J Roentgenol* 1990;154:143–148.

42. Toth Z, Csecsei K, Szeifert G, Torok O, Papp Z. Early prenatal diagnosis of cyclopia associated with holoprosencephaly. *J Clin Ultrasound* 1986;14:550–553.

43. Greene MF, Benacerraf BR, Frigoletto FD. Reliable criteria for the prenatal sonographic diagnosis of alobar holoprosencephaly. *Am J Obstet Gynecol* 1987;156:687–689.

44. Van Zalen-Sprock R, van Vugt JMG, van der Harten HJ, Nieuwint AWM, van Geijn HP. First trimester diagnosis of cyclopia and holoprosencephaly. *J Ultrasound Med* 1995; 14:631–633.

45. Bundy AL, Lidov H, Soliman M, Doubilet PM. Antenatal sonographic diagnosis of cebocephaly. *J Ultrasound Med* 1988;7:345–398.

46. Mehta L, Petrikovsky B, Tydings L, Lundberg J. Lateral nasal proboscis: antenatal diagnosis and counseling. *Obstet Gynecol* 1999;94:815–816.

47. Benacerraf BR. *Ultrasound of fetal syndromes*. New York: Churchill Livingstone, 1997:1–14, 97–117, 200–206.

48. Shulman LP, Gordon PL, Emerson DS, Wilroy RS, Elias S. Prenatal diagnosis of isolated bilateral microphthalmia with confirmation by evaluation of products of conception obtained by dilation and evacuation. *Prenat Diagn* 1993;13:403–409.

49. Feldman E, Shalev E, Weiner E, Cohen H, Zuckerman H. Microphthalmia—prenatal ultrasonic diagnosis: a case report. *Prenat Diag* 1985;5:205–207.

50. Boyd PA, Keeling JW, Lindenbaum RH. Fraser syndrome (cryptophthalmos-syndactyly syndrome): a review of eleven cases with postmortem findings. *Am J Med Genet* 1988;31: 159–168.

51. Levine RS, Powers T, Rosenberg HK, et al. The cryptophthalmos syndrome. *AJR Am J Roentgenol* 1984;143:375–376.

52. Gattuso J, Patton MA, Baraitser M. The clinical spectrum of the Fraser syndrome: report of three new cases and review. *J Med Genet* 1987;24:549–555.

53. Ramsing M, Rehder H, Holzgreve W, Meinecke P, Lenz W. Fraser syndrome (cryptophthalmos with syndactyly) in the fetus and newborn. *Clin Genet* 1990;37:84–96.

54. Schauer GM, Dunn LK, Godmilow L, Eagle RC Jr, Knisely AS. Prenatal diagnosis of Fraser syndrome at 18.5 weeks gestation, with autopsy findings at 19 weeks. *Am J Med Genet* 1990;37:583–591.

55. Feldman E, Shalev E, Weiner E, et al. Microphthalmia: prenatal sonographic diagnosis, a case report. *Prenat Diagn* 1985;5:205–207.

56. Monteagudo A, Timor-Tritsch IE, Friedman AH, Santos R. Autosomal dominant cataracts of the fetus: early detection by transvaginal ultrasound. *Ultrasound Obstet Gynecol* 1996;8:104–108.

57. Zimmer EZ, Bronshtein M, Ophir E, Meizner I, Auslender R, et al. Sonographic diagnosis of fetal congenital cataracts. *Prenat Diagn* 1993;13:503–511.

58. Gaary EA, Rawnsley E, Marin-Padilla JM, Morse CL, Crow HC. In utero detection of fetal cataracts. *J Ultrasound Med* 1993;4:234–236.

59. Drysdale K, Kyle PM, Sepulveda W. Prenatal detection of congenital inherited cataracts. *Ultrasound Obstet Gynecol* 1997;9:62–63.

60. Davis WK, Mahony BS, Carroll BA, Bowie JD. Antenatal sonographic detection of benign dacrocystoceles (lacrimal duct cysts). *J Ultrasound Med* 1987;6:461–465.

61. Battaglia C, Artini PG, DíAmbrogio G, Genazzani AR. Prenatal ultrasonographic evidence of transient dacryocystoceles. *J Ultrasound Med* 1994;13:897–900.

62. Kivikoski AI, Amin N, Cornell C. Antenatal sonographic diagnosis of dacrocystocele. *J Maternal-Fetal Med* 1997;6: 273–275.

63. Walsh G, Dubbins PA. Antenatal sonographic diagnosis of a dacryocystocele. *J Clin Ultrasound* 1994;22:457–460.

64. Alper CM, Chan KH, Hill LM, Chenevey P. Antenatal diagnosis of a congenital nasolacrimal duct cyst by ultrasonography: a case report. *Prenat Diagn* 1994;14:623–626.

65. Sharony R, Raz J, Aviram R, Cohen I, Beyth Y, et al. Prenatal diagnosis of dacryocystocele: a possible marker for syndromes. *Ultrasound Obstet Gynecol* 1999;14:71–73.

66. Bronshtein M, Zimmer EZ, Gershoni-Baruch R, Yoffe N, Meyer H, et al. First and second trimester diagnosis of fetal ocular defects and associated anomalies: report of eight cases. *Obstet Gynecol* 1991;77:443–449.

67. Bronshtein M, Blumenfeld I, Zimmer EZ, Ben-Ami M, Blumenfeld Z. Prenatal sonographic diagnosis of nasal malformations. *Prenat Diagn* 1998;18:447–454.

68. Cook K, Prefumo F, Presti F, Homfray T, Campbell S. The prenatal diagnosis of Binder syndrome before 24 weeks of gestation: case report. *Ultrasound Obstet Gynecol* 2000; 16:578–581.

69. Sepulveda W, Dezerega V, Horvath E, Aracena M. Prenatal sonographic diagnosis of Aarskog syndrome. *J Ultrasound Med* 1999;18:707–710.

70. Shalev SA, Shalev E, Reich D, Borochowitz ZU. Osteosclerosis, hypoplastic nose, and proptosis (Raine syndrome): further delineation. *Am J Med Genet* 1999;86:274–277.

71. Boog G, Sagot F, Winer N, David A, Nomballais MF. Brachmann-de Lange syndrome: a cause of early symmetric fetal growth delay. *Eur J Obstet Gynecol Reprod Biol* 1999;85:173–177.

72. Kozma C. Valproic acid embryopathy: report of two siblings with further expansion of the phenotypic abnormalities and a review of the literature. *Am J Med Genet* 2001;98:168–175.

73. Tongsong T, Wanapirak C, Piyamongkol W. Prenatal ultrasonographic findings consistent with fetal warfarin syndrome. *J Ultrasound Med* 1999;18:577–580.

74. Cusick W, Sullivan CA, Rojas B, Poole AE, Poole DA. Prenatal diagnosis of total arhinia. *Ultrasound Obstet Gynecol* 2000;15:259–261.

75. Melnick M. Cleft lip and cleft palate: etiology and pathogenesis. In: Kernahan DA, Rosenstein SW, Dado D, eds. *Cleft lip and palate: a system of management.* Baltimore: Williams & Wilkins, 1990:3–12.

76. Tolarova M. Orofacial clefts in Czechoslovakia. Incidence, genetics and prevention of cleft lip and palate over a 19-year period. *Scand J Plast Reconstr Surg* 1987;21:19–25.

77. Kraus BS, Kitamura H, Ooe T. Malformations associated

with cleft lip and palate in human embryos and fetuses. *Am J Obstet Gynecol* 1963;86:321–328.

78. Benacerraf BR, Mulliken JB. Fetal cleft lip/palate: sonographic diagnosis and postnatal outcome. *Plast Reconstr Surg* 1993;92:1045–1051.

79. Nyberg DA, Sickler GK, Hegge FN, Kramer DJ, Kropp RJ. Fetal cleft lip with and without cleft palate: US classification and correlation with outcome. *Radiology* 1995;195:677–683.

80. Christ JE, Meininger MG. Ultrasound diagnosis of cleft lip and cleft palate before birth. *Plast Reconstr Surg* 1981;8:854–859.

81. Savoldelli G, Schmid W, Schinzel A. Prenatal diagnosis of cleft lip and palate by ultrasound. *Prenat Diag* 1982;2:313–317.

82. Saltzman DH, Benacerraf BR, Frigoletto FD. Diagnosis and management of fetal facial clefts. *Am J Obstet Gynecol* 1986;155:377–379.

83. Babcook CJ, McGahan JP, Chong BW, Nemzek WR, Salamat MS. Evaluation of fetal midface anatomy related to facial clefts: use of US. *Radiology* 1996;201:113–118.

84. Clementi M, Tenconi R, Bianchi F, Stoll C. Evaluation of prenatal diagnosis of cleft lip with or without cleft palate and cleft palate by ultrasound: experience from 20 European registries. *Prenat Diagn* 2000;20:870–875.

85. Stoll C, Dott B, Alembik Y, Roth M. Evaluation of prenatal diagnosis of cleft lip/palate by fetal ultrasonographic examination. *Ann Genet* 2000;43:11–14.

86. Babcook CJ, McGahan JP. Axial ultrasonographic imaging of the fetal maxilla for accurate characterization of facial clefts. *J Ultrasound Med* 1997;16:619–625.

87. Monni G, Ibba RM, Olla G, Cao A, Crisponi G. Color Doppler ultrasound and prenatal diagnosis of cleft palate. *J Clin Ultrasound* 1995;23:189–191.

88. Sherer DM, Abramowicz JS, Jaffe R, Woods JR. Cleft palate: confirmation of prenatal diagnosis by colour Doppler ultrasound. *Prenat Diag* 1993;13:953–956.

89. Aubry MC, Aubry JP. Prenatal diagnosis of cleft palate: contribution of color Doppler ultrasound. *Ultrasound Obstet Gynecol* 1992;2:221–224.

90. Bundy AL, Saltzman DH, Emerson D, Fine C, Doubilet P, et al. Sonographic features associated with cleft palate. *J Clin Ultrasound* 1986;14:486–489.

91. Raposio E, Panarese P, Santi P. Fetal unilateral cleft lip and palate: detection of enzymic anomalies in the amniotic fluid. *Plast Reconstr Surg* 1999;103:391–394.

92. Chervenak FA, Tortora M, Mayden K, et al. Antenatal diagnosis of median cleft face syndrome: sonographic demonstration of cleft lip and hypertelorism. *Am J Obstet Gynecol* 1984;149:94–97.

93. Snijders RJM, Sebire NJ, Psara N, Souka A, Nicolaides KH. Prevalence of fetal facial cleft at different stages of pregnancy. *Ultrasound Obstet Gynecol* 1995;6:327–329.

94. Smith DW. *Recognizable patterns of human malformations*, 3rd ed. Philadelphia: WB Saunders, 1982.

95. Frattarelli JL, Boley TJ, Miller RA. Prenatal diagnosis of frontonasal dysplasia (median cleft syndrome). *J Ultrasound Med* 1996;15:81–83.

96. Stoll C, Alembik Y, Dott B, Roth MP. Associated malformations in cases with oral clefts. *Cleft Palate Craniofac J* 2000;37:41–47.

97. Lopoo JB, Hedrick MH, Chaser S, Montgomer L, Cherve-

nak FA, et al. Natural history of fetuses with cleft lip. *Plast Reconstr Surg* 1999;103:34–38.

98. Davalbhakta A, Hall PN. The impact of antenatal diagnosis on the effectiveness and timing of counseling for cleft lip and palate. *Br J Plast Surg* 2000;53:298–301.

99. Berk NW, Marazita ML, Cooper ME. Medical genetics on the cleft palate-craniofacial team: understanding parental preference. *Cleft Palate Craniofac J* 1999;36:30–35.

100. Matthews MS, Cohen M, Viglione M, Brown AS. Prenatal counseling for cleft lip and palate. *Plast Reconstr Surg* 1998;101:1–5.

101. Molsted K. Treatment outcome in cleft lip and palate: issues and perspectives. *Crit Rev Oral Biol Med* 1999;10:225–239.

102. Jones KL. *Smith's recognizable patterns of human malformations*, 5th ed. Philadelphia: WB Saunders, 1997:236.

103. Loffredo LC, Souza JM, Freitas JA, Mossey PA. Oral clefts and vitamin supplementation. *Cleft Palate Craniofac J* 2001;38:76–83.

104. Weissman A, Mashiach S, Achiron R. Macroglossia: prenatal ultrasonographic diagnosis and proposed management. *Prenat Diagn* 1995;15:66–69.

105. Paladini D, Morra T, Teodoro A, Lamberti A, Tremolaterra F, et al. Objective diagnosis of micrognathia in the fetus: the jaw index. *Obstet Gynecol* 1999;93:382–386.

106. Meizner I, Carmi R, Katz M. Prenatal ultrasonic diagnosis of mandibulofacial dysostosis (Treacher Collins syndrome). *J Clin Ultrasound* 1991;19:124–127.

107. Crane JP, Beaver HA. Midtrimester sonographic diagnosis of mandibulofacial dysostosis. *Am J Med Genet* 1986;25:251–255.

108. Behrents RG, McNamara JA, Avery JK. Prenatal mandibulofacial dysostosis (Treacher Collins syndrome). *Cleft Palate J* 1977;14:13–34.

109. Nicolaides KH, Johansson D, Donnai D, Rodeck CH. Prenatal diagnosis of mandibulofacial dysostosis. *Prenat Diagn* 1984;4:201–205.

110. Cohen J, Ghezi F, Goncalves L, Fuentes JD, Paulyson KJ, et al. Prenatal sonographic diagnosis of Treacher Collins syndrome: a case and review of the literature. *Am J Perinatol* 1995;12:416–419.

111. Hsieh YY, Chang CC, Tsai HD, Yank TC, Lee CC, et al. The prenatal diagnosis of Pierre-Robin sequence. *Prenat Diagn* 1999;19:567–569.

112. Pilu G, Romero R, Reece A, Jeanty P, Hobbins JC. The prenatal diagnosis of Robin anomalad. *Am J Obstet Gynecol* 1986;154:630–632.

113. Suresh S, Rajesh K, Suresh I, Raja V, Gopish D, et al. Prenatal diagnosis of orofaciodigital syndrome: Mohr type. *J Ultrasound Med* 1995;14:863–866.

114. Benson CB, Pober BR, Hirsh MP, Doubilet PM. Sonography of Nager acrofacial dysostosis syndrome in utero. *J Ultrasound Med* 1988;7:163–167.

115. Bromley B, Benacerraf BR. Fetal micrognathia: associated anomalies and outcome. *J Ultrasound Med* 1994;13:529–533.

116. Pilu G, Romero R, Reece EA, Jeanty P, Hobbins JC. The prenatal diagnosis of Robin anomalad. *Am J Obstet Gynecol* 1986;154:630–632.

117. Prows CA, Bender PL. Beyond Pierre Robin sequence. *Neonatal Netw* 1999;18:13–19.

118. van den Elzen AP, Semmekrot BA, Bongers EM, Huygen PL, Marres HA. Diagnosis and treatment of the Pierre

Robin sequence: results of a retrospective clinical study and review of the literature. *Eur J Pediatr* 2001;160:47–53.

119. Lawrence DL, Bersu ET. An anatomical study of human otocephaly. *Teratology* 1984;30:155–165.

120. Persutte WH, Lenke RR, DeRosa RT. Prenatal ultrasonographic appearance of the agnathia malformation complex. *J Ultrasound Med* 1990;9:725–728.

121. Cayea PD, Bieber FR, Ross MJ, Davidoff A, Osathanond HR, et al. Sonographic findings in otocephaly (synotia). *J Ultrasound Med* 1985;4:377–379.

122. Rahmani R, Dixon M, Chitayat D, Korb E, Silver M, et al. Otocephaly: prenatal sonographic diagnosis. *J Ultrasound Med* 1998;17:595–598.

123. Lin HH, Liang RI, Chang FM, Chang CH, Yu CH, et al. Prenatal diagnosis of otocephaly using two-dimensional and three-dimensional ultrasonography. *Ultrasound Obstet Gynecol* 1998;11:361–363.

124. Hersh JH, McChane RH, Rosenberg EM, Powers WH Jr, Corrigan C, et al. Otocephaly-midline malformation association. *Am J Med Genet* 1989;34:246–249.

125. Shermak MA, Dufresne CR. Nonlethal case of otocephaly and its implications for treatment. *J Craniofac Surg* 1996;7:372–375.

126. Shimizu T, Salvador L, Allanson J, Hughes-Benzie R, Nimrod C. Ultrasonographic measurements of fetal ear. *Obstet Gynecol* 1992;80:381–384.

127. Chitkara U, Lee L, El-Sayed YY, Holbrook RH Jr, Bloch DA, et al. Ultrasonographic ear length measurement in normal second- and third-trimester fetuses. *Am J Obstet Gynecol* 2000;183:230–234.

128. Awwad JT, Azar GB, Karam KS, Nicolaides KH. Ear length: a potential sonographic marker for Down syndrome. *Int J Gynaecol Obstet* 1994;44:233–238.

129. Lettieri L, Rodis JF, Vintzileos AM, Feeney L, Ciarleglio L, et al. Ear length in second-trimester aneuploid fetuses. *Obstet Gynecol* 1993;81:57–60.

130. Gill P, Vanhook J, Fitzsimmons J, Pascoe-Mason J, Fantel A. Fetal ear measurements in the prenatal detection of trisomy 21. *Prenat Diagn* 1994;14:739–743.

131. Shih JC, Shyu MK, Lee CN, Wu CH, Lin GJ, et al. Antenatal depiction of the fetal ear with three-dimensional ultrasonography. *Obstet Gynecol* 1998;91:500–505.

132. Chenoweth-Mitchell C, Cohen GR. Prenatal sonographic findings of Apert syndrome. *J Clin Ultrasound* 1994;22:510–514.

133. Kaufmann K, Baldinger S, Pratt L. Ultrasound detection of Apert syndrome: a case report and literature review. *Am J Perinatol* 1997;14:427–430.

134. Hill LM, Thomas ML, Peterson CS. The ultrasonic detection of Apert syndrome. *J Ultrasound Med* 1987;6:601–604.

135. Balci S, Onol B, Eryilmaz M, Haytoglu T. A case of Carpenter syndrome diagnosed in a 20-week-old fetus with postmortem examination. *Clin Genet* 1997;51:412–416.

136. Ashby T, Rouse GA, De Lange M. Prenatal sonographic diagnosis of Carpenter syndrome. *J Ultrasound Med* 1994;13:905–909.

137. Bernstain PS, Gross SJ, Cohen DJ, Tiller GR, Shanske AL, et al. Prenatal diagnosis of type 2 Pfeiffer syndrome. *Ultrasound Obstet Gynecol* 1996;8:425–428.

138. Martinelli P, Paladini D, D'Armiento M, Scarano G. Prena-

tal diagnosis of cloverleaf skull in the subtype 2 Pfeiffer syndrome. *Clin Dysmorphol* 1997;6:89–90.

139. Hill LM, Grzybek PC. Sonographic findings with Pfeiffer syndrome. *Prenat Diagn* 1994;14:47–49.

140. Gollin YG, Abuhamad AZ, Inati MN, Shaffer WK, Copel JA, et al. Sonographic appearance of craniofacial dysostosis (Crouzon syndrome) in the second trimester. *J Ultrasound Med* 1993;12:625–628.

141. Leo MV, Suslak L, Ganesh VL, Adhate A, Apuzzio JJ. Crouzon syndrome: prenatal ultrasound diagnosis by binocular diameters. *Obstet Gynecol* 1991;78:906–908.

142. Menashe Y, Ben Baruch G, Rabinovitch O, Shalev Y, Katzenlson MB, et al. Exophthalmus—prenatal ultrasonic features for diagnosis of Crouzon syndrome. *Prenat Diagn* 1989;9:805–808.

143. Benacerrraf BR, Spiro R, Mitchell A. Using 3-D ultrasound to detect craniosynostosis in a fetus with Pfeiffer syndrome. *Ultrasound Obstet Gynecol* 2000;16:391–394.

144. Mahieu-Caputo D, Sonigo P, Amiel J, Simon I, Aubry MC, et al. Prenatal diagnosis of sporadic Apert syndrome: a sequential diagnostic approach combining three-dimensional computed tomography and molecular biology. *Fetal Diagn Ther* 2001;16:10–12.

145. Strauss S, Tamarkin M, Engelberg S, Ben Ami T, Goodman RM. Prenatal sonographic appearance of diprosopus. *J Ultrasound Med* 1987;6:93–95.

146. Okazaki JR, Wilson JL, Holmes SM, Vandermark LL. Diprosopus: diagnosis in utero. *AJR Am J Roentgenol* 1987;149:147–148.

147. Chervenak FA, Pinto MM, Heller CI, Norooz H. Obstetric significance of fetal craniofacial duplication: a case report. *J Reprod Med* 1985;30:74–76.

148. Byrne J, Blanc WA, Warburton D, et al. The significance of cystic hygroma in fetuses. *Hum Pathol* 1984;15:61–67.

149. Trauffer PM, Anderson CE, Johnson A, Heeger S, Morgan P, et al. The natural history of euploid pregnancies with first-trimester cystic hygromas. *Am J Obstet Gynecol* 1994;170:1279–1284.

150. Sadler T. *Lymphatic system. Langman's medical embryology.* Baltimore: Williams & Wilkins, 1990:225–227.

151. Chervenak FA, Isaacson G, Blakemore KJ, Breg WR, Hobbins JC, et al. Fetal cystic hygroma. Cause and natural history. *N Engl J Med* 1983;309:822–825.

152. Pijpers L, Reuss A, Stewart PA, Wladimiroff JW, Sachs ES. Fetal cystic hygroma: prenatal diagnosis and management. *Obstet Gynecol* 1988;72:223–224.

153. Phillips HE, McGahan JP. Intrauterine fetal cystic hygromas: sonographic detection. *AJR Am J Roentgenol* 1981;136:799–802.

154. Toftager-Larsen K, Benzie RJ, Doran TA, Miskin M, Allen LC, et al. Alpha-fetoprotein and ultrasound scanning in the prenatal diagnosis of Turner's syndrome. *Prenat Diagn* 1983;3:35–40.

155. Newman DE, Cooperberg PL. Genetics of sonographically detected intrauterine fetal cystic hygromas. *J Can Assoc Radiol* 1984;35:77–79.

156. Brown BS, Thompson DL. Ultrasonographic features of the fetal Turner syndrome. *J Can Assoc Radiol* 1984;35:40–46.

157. Redford DH, McNay MB, Ferguson-Smith ME, Jamieson ME. Aneuploidy and cystic hygroma detectable by ultrasound. *Prenat Diagn* 1984;4:377–382.

158. Marchese C, Savin E, Dragone E, Carozzi F, De Marchi M, et al. Cystic hygroma: prenatal diagnosis and genetic counseling. *Prenat Diagn* 1985;5:221–227.

159. Garden AS, Benzie RJ, Miskin M, Gardner HA. Fetal cystic hygroma colli: antenatal diagnosis, significance, and management. *Am J Obstet Gynecol* 1986;154:221–225.

160. Benacerraf BR, Barss V, Laboda LA. A sonographic sign for detection in the second trimester of the fetus with Down's syndrome. *Am J Obstet Gynecol* 1985;151:1078–1079.

161. Benacerraf BR, Gelman R, Frigoletto FD. Sonographic identification of second trimester fetuses with Down's syndrome. *N Engl J Med* 1987;317:1371–1376.

162. Ville Y, Lalondrelle C, Doumerc S, Daffos F, Frydman R, et al. First-trimester diagnosis of nuchal anomalies: significance and outcome. *Ultrasound Obstet Gynecol* 1992;2:314–316.

163. Bronshtein M, Rottem S, Yoffe N, Blumenfeld Z. First-trimester and early second-trimester diagnosis of nuchal cystic hygroma by transvaginal sonography: diverse prognosis of the septated from the nonseptated lesion. *Am J Obstet Gynecol* 1988;161:78–82.

164. Bronshtein M, Bar-Hava I, Blumenfeld I, Bejar J, Toder V, et al. The difference between septated and nonseptated nuchal cystic hygroma in the early second trimester. *Obstet Gynecol* 1993;81:683–687.

165. Ville Y, Lalondrelle C, Doumerc S, Daffos F, Frydman R, et al. First-trimester diagnosis of nuchal anomalies: significance and outcome. *Ultrasound Obstet Gynecol* 1992;2:314–316.

166. Malone FD, Ball BH, Nyberg DA, Gross SJ, Comstock CH, et al. First trimester cystic hygroma—a population based screening study (the FASTER trial). *Am J Obstet Gynecol* 2001;185:S99.

167. Brumfield CG, Wenstrom K, Davis RO, Owen J, Cosper PP. Second-trimester cystic hygroma: prognosis of septated and nonseptated lesions. *Obstet Gynecol* 1996;88:979–982.

168. Azar GB, Snijders RJM, Gosden C, Nicolaides KH. Fetal nuchal cystic hygroma: associated malformations and chromosomal defects. *Fetal Diagn Ther* 1991;6:46–57.

169. Rosati P, Guariglia L. Prognostic value of ultrasound findings of fetal cystic hygroma detected in early pregnancy by transvaginal sonography. *Ultrasound Obstet Gynecol* 2000;16:245–250.

170. Yang YH, Cho JS, Min HW, Lee CH, Song CH. Rapid chromosome analysis and prenatal diagnosis using fluid from the cystic hygroma, hydrothorax and isolated ascites: new source for chromosome analysis. *J Obstet Gynaecol* 1995;21:443–450.

171. Donnenfeld AE, Lockwood D, Lamb AN. Prenatal diagnosis from cystic hygroma fluid: the value of fluorescence in situ hybridization. *Am J Obstet Gynecol* 2001;185:1004–1008.

172. Mehta PS, Mehta SJ, Vorherr H. Congenital iodide goiter and hypothyroidism: a review. *Obstet Gynecol Surv* 1983;38: 237–247.

173. Friedland DR, Rothschild MA. Rapid resolution of fetal goiter associated with maternal Grave's disease: a case report. *J Pediatr Otorhinolaryngol* 2000;54:59–62.

174. Momotani N, Noh JY, Ishikawa N, Ito K. Effects of propylthiouracil and methimazole on fetal thyroid status in mothers with Graves' hyperthyroidism. *J Clin Endocrinol Metab* 1997;82:3633–3636.

175. De Catte L, De Wolf D, Smitz J, Bougatef A, De Schepper J, et al. Fetal hypothyroidism as a complication of amiodarone treatment for persistent fetal supraventricular tachycardia. *Prenat Diagn* 1994;14:762–765.

176. Thorpe-Beeston JG, Nicolaides KH. *Maternal and fetal thyroid function in pregnancy. Frontiers in fetal medicine series.* Parthenon Publishing, 1996.

177. Bromley B, Frigoletto FD Jr, Cramer D, Osathanondh R, Benacerraf BR. The fetal thyroid: normal and abnormal sonographic measurements. *J Ultrasound Med* 1992;11:25–28.

178. Ho SS, Metreweli C. Normal fetal thyroid volume. *Ultrasound Obstet Gynecol* 1998;11:118–122.

179. Wenstrom KD, Weiner CP, Williamson RA, Grant SS. Prenatal diagnosis of fetal hyperthyroidism using funipuncture. *Obstet Gynecol* 1990;76:513–517.

180. Rakover Y, Weiner E, Mosh N, Shalev E. Fetal pituitary negative feedback at early gestational age. *Endocrinol (Oxf)* 1999;50:809–814.

181. Polak M, Leger J, Luton D, Oury JF, Vuillard E, et al. Fetal cord blood sampling in the diagnosis and the treatment of fetal hyperthyroidism in the offsprings of a euthyroid mother, producing thyroid stimulating immunoglobulins. *Ann Endocrinol (Paris)* 1997;58:338–342.

182. Insoft RM, Hurvitz J, Estrella E, Krishnamoorthy KS. Prader-Willi syndrome associated with fetal goiter: a case report. *Am J Perinatol* 1999;16:29–31.

183. Mitsuda N, Tamaki H, Amino N, Hosono T, Miyai K, et al. Risk factors for developmental disorders in infants born to women with Graves disease. *Obstet Gynecol* 1992;80:359–364.

184. Watson WJ, Fiegen MM. Fetal thyrotoxicosis associated with nonimmune hydrops. *Am J Obstet Gynecol* 1995;172: 1039–1040.

185. Ochoa-Maya MR, Frates MC, Lee-Parritz A, Seely EW. Resolution of fetal goiter after discontinuation of propylthiouracil in a pregnant woman with Graves' hyperthyroidism. *Thyroid* 1999;9:1111–1114.

186. Davidson KM, Richards DS, Schatz DA, Fisher DA. Successful in utero treatment of fetal goiter and hypothyroidism. *N Engl J Med* 1991;324:543–546.

187. Johnson RL, Finberg HJ, Perelman AH, Clewell WH. Fetal goitrous hypothyroidism. A new diagnostic and therapeutic approach. *Fetal Ther* 1989;4:141–145.

188. Volumenie JL, Polak M, Guibourdenche J, Oury JF, Vuillard E, et al. Management of fetal thyroid goitres: a report of 11 cases in a single perinatal unit. *Prenat Diagn* 2000;20:799–806.

189. Luton D, Fried D, Sibony O, Vuillard E, Tebeka B, et al. Assessment of fetal thyroid function by colored Doppler echography. *Fetal Diagn Ther* 1997;12:24–27.

190. Zajaczek S, Jakubowska A, Kurzawski G, et al. Age at diagnosis to discriminate those patients for whom constitutional DNA sequencing is appropriate in sporadic unilateral retinoblastoma. *Eur J Can* 1998;34:1919–1921.

191. Maat-Kievit JA, Oepkes D, Hartwig NG, Vermeij-Keers C, Van Kamp IL, et al. A large retinoblastoma detected in a fetus at 21 weeks of gestation. *Prenat Diagn* 1993;13:377–384.

192. Salim A, Wiknjosastro GH, Danukusumo D, Barnas B, Zalud I. Fetal retinoblastoma. *J Ultrasound Med* 1998;17:717–720.

193. Wiggs J, Nordenskjold M, Yandell D, et al. Prediction of the risk of hereditary retinoblastoma, using DNA polymor-

phisms within the retinoblastoma gene. *N Engl J Med* 1988;318:151–157.

194. Paulino AC. Trilateral retinoblastoma: is the location of the intracranial tumor important? *Cancer* 1999;86:135–141.

195. Beck MN, Balmer A, Dessing C, Pica A, Munier F. First-line chemotherapy with local treatment can prevent external-beam irradiation and enucleation in low-stage intraocular retinoblastoma. *J Clin Oncol* 2000;18:2881–2887.

196. Friedman DL, Himelstein B, Shields CL, Shields JA, Needle M, et al. Chemoreduction and local ophthalmic therapy for intraocular retinoblastoma. *J Clin Oncol* 2000;18:12–17.

197. Gallie BL, Dunn JM, Chan HS, et al. The genetics of retinoblastoma: relevance to the patient. *Pediatr Clin North Am* 1991;38:299–315.

198. Wong FL, Boice JD, Abramson DH, et al. Cancer incidence after retinoblastoma: radiation dose and sarcoma risk. *JAMA* 1997;278:1262–1267.

199. Kivela T. Trilateral retinoblastoma: a meta-analysis of hereditary retinoblastoma associated with primary ectopic intracranial retinoblastoma. *J Clin Oncol* 1999;17:1829–1837.

200. Papageorgiou C, Papathanasiou K, Panidis D, Vlassis G. Prenatal diagnosis of epignathus in the first half of pregnancy: a case report and review of the literature. *Clin Exp Obstet Gynecol* 2000;27:67–68.

201. Bruhwiler H, Mueller MD, Rabner M. [Ultrasound diagnosis of epignathus in the 17th week of pregnancy. Case report and review of the literature]. *Ultraschall Med* 1995;16:238–240.

202. Gull I, Wolman I, Har-Toov J, Amster R, Schreiber L, et al. Antenatal sonographic diagnosis of epignathus at 15 weeks of pregnancy. *Ultrasound Obstet Gynecol* 1999;13:271–273.

203. Abendstein B, Auer A, Pumpel R, Mark E, Desch B, et al. [Epignathus: prenatal diagnosis by sonography and magnetic resonance imaging]. *Ultraschall Med* 1999;20:207–211.

204. Levine AB, Alvarez M, Wedgwood J, Berkowitz RL, Holzman I. Contemporary management of a potentially lethal fetal anomaly: a successful perinatal approach to epignathus. *Obstet Gynecol* 1990;76:962–966.

205. Carlan SJ, Angel JL, Leo J, Feeney J. Cephalocele involving the oral cavity. *Obstet Gynecol* 1990;75:494–496.

206. McMahon MJ, Clescheir NC, Kuller JA, Wells SR, Wright LN, et al. Perinatal management of a lingual teratoma. *Obstet Gynecol* 1996;87:848–850.

207. Pellicano M, Zullo F, Catizone C, Guida F, Catizone F, et al. Prenatal diagnosis of congenital granular cell epulis. *Ultrasound Obstet Gynecol* 1998;11:144–146.

208. Kim ES, Gross TL. Prenatal ultrasound detection of a congenital epulis in a triple X female fetus: a case report. *Prenat Diagn* 1999;19:774–776.

209. Moya JMF, Sulzberger SC, Recasens JD, Ramos C, Sang R, et al. Antenatal diagnosis and management of a ranula. *Ultrasound Obstet Gynecol* 1998;11:147–148.

210. Paladini D, Morra T, Guida F, Lamberti A, Martinelli P. Prenatal diagnosis and perinatal management of a lingual lymphangioma. *Ultrasound Obstet Gynecol* 1998;11:141–143.

211. Hulett RL, Bowerman RA, Marks T, Silverstein A. Prenatal ultrasound detection of congenital gingival granular cell tumor. *J Ultrasound Med* 1991;10:185–187.

212. Meizner I, Shalev J, Mashiach R, Vardimon D, Ben-Rafael Z. Prenatal ultrasonographic diagnosis of congenital oral granular cell myoblastoma. *J Ultrasound Med* 2000;19:337–339.

213. Skarsgard ED, Chitkara U, Krane EJ, Riley ET, Halamek LP, et al. The OOPS procedure (operation on placental support): in utero airway management of the fetus with prenatally diagnosed tracheal obstruction. *J Pediatr Surg* 1996;31:826–828.

214. Yapar EG, Ekici E, Gokmen O. Sonographic diagnosis of epignathus (oral teratoma), prosencephaly, meromelia and oligohydramnios in a fetus with trisomy 13. *Clin Dysmorphol* 1995;4:266–271.

215. Smith NM, Chambers SE, Bileson VR, Laing I, West CP, et al. Oral teratoma (epignathus) with intracranial extension: a report of two cases. *Prenat Diagn* 1993;13:945–952.

216. Chervenak FA, Tortora M, Moya FR, Hobbins JC. Antenatal sonographic diagnosis of epignathus. *J Ultrasound Med* 1984;3:235–237.

217. Gaucherand P, Rudigoz RC, Chappuis JP. Epignathus: clinical and sonographic observations of two cases. *Ultrasound Obstet Gynecol* 1994;4:241–244.

218. Smith NM, Chambers SE, Bileson VR, Laing I, West CP, et al. Oral teratoma (epignathus) with intracranial extension: a report of two cases. *Prenat Diagn* 1993;13:945–952.

219. Sherer DM, Woods JR, Abramowicz JS, Diprete JA, Metlay LA, et al. Prenatal sonographic assessment of early, rapidly growing fetal cervical teratoma. *Prenat Diagn* 1993;13:1079–1084.

220. Gaucherand P, Rudigoz RC, Chappuis JP. Epignathus: clinical and sonographic observations of two cases. *Ultrasound Obstet Gynecol* 1994;4:241–244.

221. Todd DW, Votava HJ, Telander RL, Shoemaker CT. Giant epignathus. A case report. *Minn Med* 1991;74:27–28.

222. Teal LN, Antuaco TL, Jimenez JF, et al. Fetal teratomas: antenatal diagnosis and clinical management. *J Clin Ultrasound* 1988;16:329–336.

223. Schoenfeld A, Ovadia J, Edelstein T, et al. Malignant cervical teratoma of the fetus. *Acta Obstet Gynecol Scand* 1982;61:7–12.

224. Trecet JC, Claramunt V, Larraz J, et al. Prenatal ultrasound diagnosis of fetal teratoma of the neck. *J Clin Ultrasound* 1984;12:509–511.

225. Kerner B, Flaum E, Mathews H, Carlson DE, Pepkowitz SH, et al. Cervical teratoma: prenatal diagnosis and long-term follow-up. *Prenat Diagn* 1998;18:51–59.

226. Catte LD, De Backer A, Goosens A, Bougatef A, Volckaert M, et al. Teratoma, neck. Jeanty P, ed. Available at: http://www.TheFetus.net. Accessed September 3, 2002.

227. Shipp TD, Bromley B, Benacerraf B. The ultrasonographic appearance and outcome for fetuses with masses distorting the fetal face. *J Ultrasound Med* 1995;14:673–678.

228. Filston HC. Hemangiomas, cystic hygromas, and teratomas of the head and neck. *Semin Pediatr Surg* 1994;3:147–159.

229. Rothschild MA, Catalano P, Urken M, Brandwein M, Som P, et al. Evaluation and management of congenital cervical teratoma. Case report and review. *Arch Otolaryngol Head Neck Surg* 1994;120:444–448.

230. Larsen ME, Larsen JW, Hamersley SL, McBride TP, Bahadori RS. Successful management of fetal cervical teratoma using the EXIT procedure. *J Matern Fetal Med* 1999;8:295–297.

231. Kerner B, Flaum E, Mathews H, Carlson DE, Pepkowitz

SH, et al. Cervical teratoma: prenatal diagnosis and long-term follow-up. *Prenat Diagn* 1998;18:51–59.

232. Elmasalme F, Giacomantonio M, Clarke KD, Othman E, Matbouli S. Congenital cervical teratoma in neonates. Case report and review. *Eur J Pediatr Surg* 2000;10:252–257.

233. Azizkhan RG, Haase GM, Applebaum H, Dillon PW, Coran AG, et al. Diagnosis, management, and outcome of cervicofacial teratomas in neonates: a Childrens Cancer Group study. *J Pediatr Surg* 1995;30:312–316.

234. Ward VM, Langford K, Morrison G. Prenatal diagnosis of airway compromise: EXIT (ex utero intra-partum treatment) and fetal airway surgery. *Int J Pediatr Otorhinolaryngol* 2000;53:137–141.

235. Liechty KW, Crombleholme TM, Weiner S, Bernick B, Flake AW, Adzick NS. The ex utero intrapartum treatment procedure for a large fetal neck mass in a twin gestation. *Obstet Gynecol* 1999;93:824–825.

236. Clavelli A. Lymphangioma, case of day. Jeanty P, ed. Available at: http://www.thefetus.net. Accessed August 1999.

237. Reichler A, Bronshtein M. Early prenatal diagnosis of axillary cystic hygroma. *J Ultrasound Med* 1995;14:581–584.

238. Yang WT, Ahuja A, Metreweli C. Sonographic features of head and neck hemangiomas and vascular malformations: review of 23 patients. *J Ultrasound Med* 1997;16:39–44.

239. Viora E, Grassi Pirrone P, Comoglio F, Bastonero S, Campogrande M. Ultrasonographic detection of fetal craniofacial hemangioma: case report and review of the literature. *Ultrasound Obstet Gynecol* 2000;15:431–434.

240. Kramer LA, Crino JP, Slopis J, Hankins L, Yeakley J. Capillary hemangioma of the neck: prenatal MR findings. *AJNR Am J Neuroradiol* 1997;18:1432–1434.

241. Shiraishi H, Nakamura M, Ichihashi K, Uchida A, Izumi A, et al. Prenatal MRI in a fetus with a giant neck hemangioma: a case report. *Prenat Diagn* 2000;20:1004–1007.

242. Kaminopetros P, Jauniaux E, Kane P, Weston M, Nicolaides KH, et al. Prenatal diagnosis of an extensive fetal lymphangioma using ultrasonography, magnetic resonance imaging and cytology. *Br J Radiol* 1997;70:750–753.

243. Winter TC III, Mack LA, Cyr DR. Prenatal sonographic diagnosis of scalp edema/cephalohematoma mimicking an encephalocele. *AJR Am J Roentgenol* 1993;161:1247–1248.

244. Sherer DM, Perillo AM, Abramowicz JS. Fetal hemangioma overlying the temporal occipital suture, initially diagnosed by ultrasonography as an encephalocele. *J Ultrasound Med* 1993;12:691–693.

245. Bronshtein M, Bar-Hava I, Blumenfeld Z. Early second-trimester sonographic appearance of occipital haemangioma simulating encephalocele. *Prenat Diagn* 1992;12:695.

246. Shahabi S, Busine A. Prenatal diagnosis of an epidermal scalp cyst simulating an encephalocele. *Prenat Diagn* 1998;18:373–377.

247. Mitchell CS. Vertex hemangioma mimicking an encephalocele. *J Am Osteopath Assoc* 1999;99:626–627.

248. Sharara FI, Khoury AN. Prenatal diagnosis of a giant cavernous hemangioma in association with nonimmune hydrops. A case report. *J Reprod Med* 1994;39:547–549.

249. Boon LM, MacDonald DM, Mulliken JB. Complications of systemic corticosteroid therapy for problematic hemangioma. *Plast Reconstr Surg* 1999;104:1616–1623.

250. Mueller BU, Mulliken JB. The infant with a vascular tumor. *Semin Perinatol* 1999;23:332–340.

9

THE THORAX

Abnormalities of the thorax represent an important and diverse group of fetal anomalies. Sonography plays a central role in the diagnosis and management of these often complicated pregnancies. The role of sonography is not limited to an accurate fetal diagnosis. Sonography is also used in discriminating between the fetuses who are critically ill and may require urgent *in utero* therapy from those who are stable and can be safely treated and evaluated after birth. In some, though *in utero* therapy is not required, the site of delivery may be altered due to anticipated need for urgent postpartum neonatal therapy. These are all important decisions that are made with the help of prenatal ultrasound.

Sonographic observations include diagnosing the severity of the anomaly and presence of associated malformations. Sonographic findings when used with the natural history of the abnormality are central in making the many important management decisions in these pregnancies and for parental counseling. This chapter focuses on the most common fetal thoracic abnormalities.

FETAL LUNG DEVELOPMENT: EMBRYOLOGIC CONSIDERATIONS

Human lung development is generally divided into five stages: embryonic (conception to sixth week); pseudoglandular (sixth to sixteenth week); canalicular (sixth to twenty-eighth week); saccular (twenty-eighth to thirty-sixth week); and alveolar (thirty-sixth week to term).[1-3] Many thoracic anomalies observed sonographically can be linked to interruption in the normal embryologic sequences.

The human fetal lung arises as a ventral diverticulum from the caudal end of the laryngotracheal groove of the foregut at the end of the fourth week. These embryologic origins probably explain why some lung lesions communicate through a primitive connection to the gastrointestinal tract (also derived from the foregut). This diverticulum from the foregut grows caudally as the primitive trachea and the end divides into two sacs, the lung buds.

A series of dichotomous divisions occur resulting in the bronchial tree, up to and including the terminal bronchioles (Fig. 1). While they may increase in size, new bronchial branches are not formed after 16 weeks. It is impressive that the bronchial tree is already complete by the time of the usual mid-trimester sonogram.

Between the sixteenth and twenty-eighth weeks, the basic architecture of the gas-exchanging portion of the lung is roughly established and vascularized.[4] Flattening and changes of the acinar epithelium at approximately 22 to 24 weeks mark the initial differentiation of type II pneumocytes from which type I pneumocytes are derived later. Type II pneumocytes produce surfactant. Structural maturation of the lung is influenced by physical factors; biochemical maturation appears to be controlled by endocrine factors. Between 28 and 36 weeks, saccular stage airways, which terminate in large smooth-walled cylindrical structures, evolve into subsaccules that become alveoli.

Between the thirty-second and thirty-sixth weeks, type II pneumocytes mature. By the thirty-sixth week alveolar structures are uniformly present in the fetal lung.[4] Alveoli continue to increase in number after birth and are not complete until the eighth year of life. The greatest increase in the number of alveoli occurs during the first 2 years of life. For a more detailed discussion of the complexities of lung development, readers are referred to an excellent summary by Laudy and Wladimiroff.[4]

The lungs can be well visualized by ultrasound as well as with magnetic resonance imaging (MRI) throughout the second and third trimester (Fig. 2). The lungs appear as homogenously echogenic, glandular-appearing tissue surrounding the heart. On longitudinal scans the diaphragm can also be visualized; this is more apparent during the third trimester.

ALTERATIONS IN LUNG DEVELOPMENT AND FETAL PHYSIOLOGY CAUSED BY LUNG MASSES: GENERAL CONSIDERATIONS

The influence of the physical factors required for normal lung development helps to understand how thoracic masses may adversely influence lung development and growth.

For example, it has been shown that lung fluid, which is produced by the lung and functions to distend the developing airways, is critical for normal lung growth. Pulmonary hypopla-

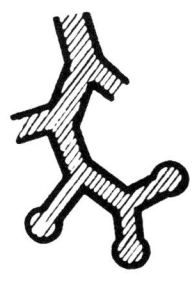 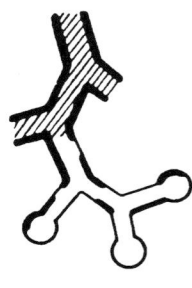 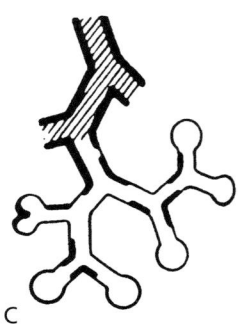

FIGURE 1. Development of the bronchial tree. **A:** At 16 weeks, at the end of the pseudoglandular period, airways have developed to the level of the terminal bronchioles. They are lined by thick columnar or cuboidal cells. **B:** At 24 weeks, the canalicular phase, the respiratory airways branch and differentiate. **C:** At 32 weeks, the alveolar phase, progressive branching and differentiation of the respiratory airways occur. (Reproduced with permission from Bucher U, Reid L. Development of the intrasegmental bronchial tree: the pattern of branching and development of cartilage at various stages of intrauterine life. *Thorax* 1961;16:207–218.)

sia can be produced experimentally after tracheal drainage in the fetal lamb, presumably due to the loss of the intrapulmonary fluid required for normal development.[5,6] In a similar way, a lung mass compressing the developing lung or a small, maldeveloped bony thorax may impair lung growth and maturation by diminishing the room for lung expansion and thereby lung distension by fluid within the tiny developing airways. As a corollary to the fetus with a lung mass, pulmonary hypoplasia has been produced in a fetal lamb by surgically placing an inflatable balloon in the thorax of the fetal lamb.[7,8]

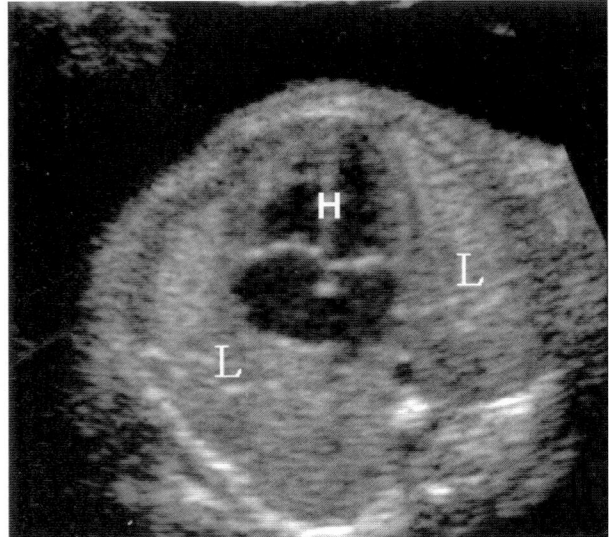 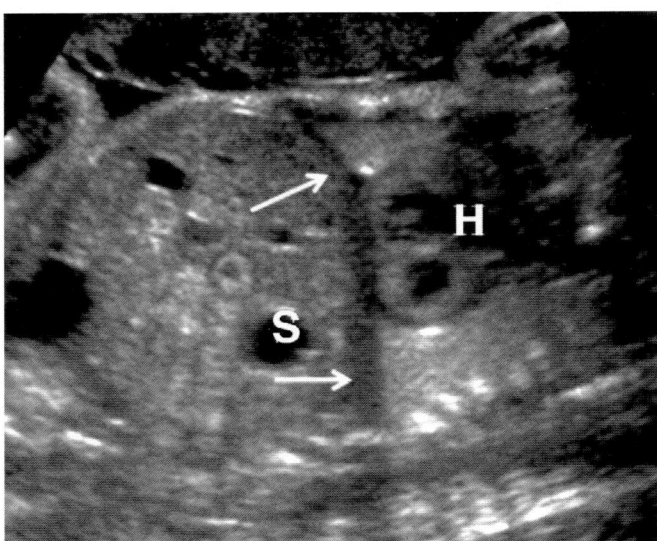 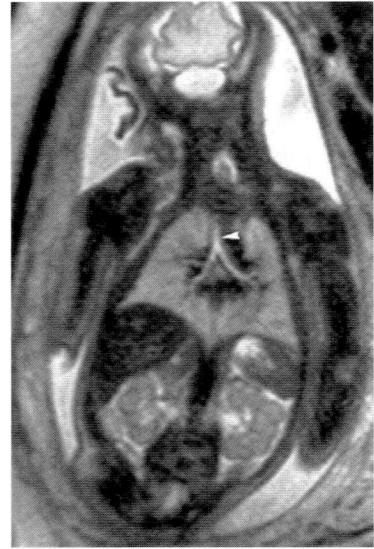

FIGURE 2. Normal lungs. **A:** Transverse view of thorax shows homogenously echogenic lungs (*L*) surrounding the heart (*H*). **B:** Coronal ultrasound at 30 weeks shows lungs and diaphragm (*arrows*). S, stomach. **C:** Magnetic resonance image, coronal plane shows normal lungs and trachea (*arrowhead*). (**C:** Reproduced with permission from Rypens F, Metens T, Rocourt N, Sonigo P, Brunelle F, et al. Fetal lung volume: estimation at MR imaging—initial results. *Radiology* 2001;219:236–41.)

More important, removal of such a mass in the fetal lamb has been shown to interrupt this adverse effect and allow continued lung growth.

Fetal chest masses, unlike those found in adults, are rarely malignant. In the fetus, the chest mass is threatening due to the secondary physiologic and anatomic alterations which result. Lung hypoplasia is one of the most important sequelae, but polyhydramnios, cardiac/mediastinal shift, and hydrops fetalis are also evidence of important physiologic derangements, which may be observed on the sonogram. Hydrops fetalis represents an especially significant finding, heralding fetal decompensation, and associated with a mortality rate greater than 90%.[9]

Compression of the mass on the heart and great vessels is thought to be the cause of hydrops. Central venous pressure, measured in experimental animals, has been shown to correlate with the occurrence and disappearance of hydrops, and this, in turn, has been associated with the placement (appearance of hydrops) and removal (disappearance of hydrops) of an artificial chest mass.[10] It makes sense that small lesions in the chest, with little mass effect on the heart and vessels, are very unlikely to result in hydrops.

Normal lung development and fetal physiology can be interrupted by a variety of thoracic lesions in the fetus, but the effect is sometimes unpredictable. Some lung masses rarely produce life-threatening lung hypoplasia and some defects, such as congenital diaphragmatic hernia (CDH), commonly result in pulmonary hypoplasia. In the following discussion of some of the more common fetal chest lesions, rates of associated anomalies, prognosis, and management strategies are emphasized.

PULMONARY HYPOPLASIA

Description

Pulmonary hypoplasia is caused by a decrease in the number of lung cells, airways, and alveoli, with a resulting decrease in organ size and weight. A decreased ratio of lung weight to body weight is the most consistent method of diagnosing pulmonary hypoplasia,[11] although alternative pathologic criteria have been suggested.[12]

Incidence

Pulmonary hypoplasia is relatively common, occurring in 1.4% of all live births[13] and 6.7% of all stillborns.[14] Pulmonary hypoplasia is the final common pathway for poor outcomes associated with a wide range of pathologic processes affecting the lung.

Pathology

Pathologic changes vary in degree from a mild reduction in acinar number to complete absence of acini.[15] The severity of pulmonary hypoplasia depends on the gestational age at onset, duration of the inciting conditions, and severity of the insult. Other factors such as pulmonary fluid dynamics, fetal breathing movements, and hormonal influences, may contribute to the resultant pulmonary hypoplasia.[16] Among these factors, the timing of the pathologic process affecting the lung is critical[17]; early impairment of pulmonary development causes reduced bronchiolar branching, cartilage development, and acinar vascularization and maturation.[18]

Most common, pulmonary hypoplasia results from either an intrathoracic or extrathoracic condition that restricts growth of the lung.[19,20]

Early onset oligohydramnios restricts normal growth and expansion of the lungs, resulting in histologically immature lungs with severe pulmonary hypoplasia. The histologic appearance may be indistinguishable when oligohydramnios is due to ruptured membranes before 20 weeks or renal agenesis.[21] Even a period of oligohydramnios as short as 6 days may interfere with fetal lung development and cause some degree of pulmonary hypoplasia.[20,22]

Intrathoracic masses result in pulmonary hypoplasia secondary to the mass effect. The degree of pulmonary hypoplasia correlates with the time of onset, duration, and severity of the underlying condition. Severe pulmonary hypoplasia may occur with early onset diaphragmatic hernia with large mass effect, whereas late-onset diaphragmatic hernia may produce histologically normal and mature acini but small lungs.

In addition to oligohydramnios and intrathoracic masses, less common etiologies for pulmonary hypoplasia include cardiovascular abnormalities, which restrict pulmonary blood flow (right-sided obstructive lesions); skeletal abnormalities producing a small or deformed thoracic cage; and neural abnormalities leading to reduced or absent fetal breathing.

Diagnosis

An accurate prenatal test for detecting pulmonary hypoplasia is highly desirable, especially for prediction of lethal pulmonary hypoplasia. Methods that have been proposed include thoracic measurements, various lung measurements, estimation of lung volume, Doppler studies of the pulmonary arteries, and assessment of fetal breathing activity. The existence of so many methods suggests that no one method has been found to be uniformly acceptable.[23] Visible comparison of the thoracic circumference to the abdominal circumference can also identify those fetuses with severe pulmonary hypoplasia, without intrathoracic mass (Fig. 3).

A good correlation exists between thoracic size and gestational age. However, discrepancies in thoracic circumference are noted between reported studies. Table 1 shows normal thoracic circumference values reported by Chitkara et al.[24] This varies from the more recent data of Laudy et al.[25] (Fig.

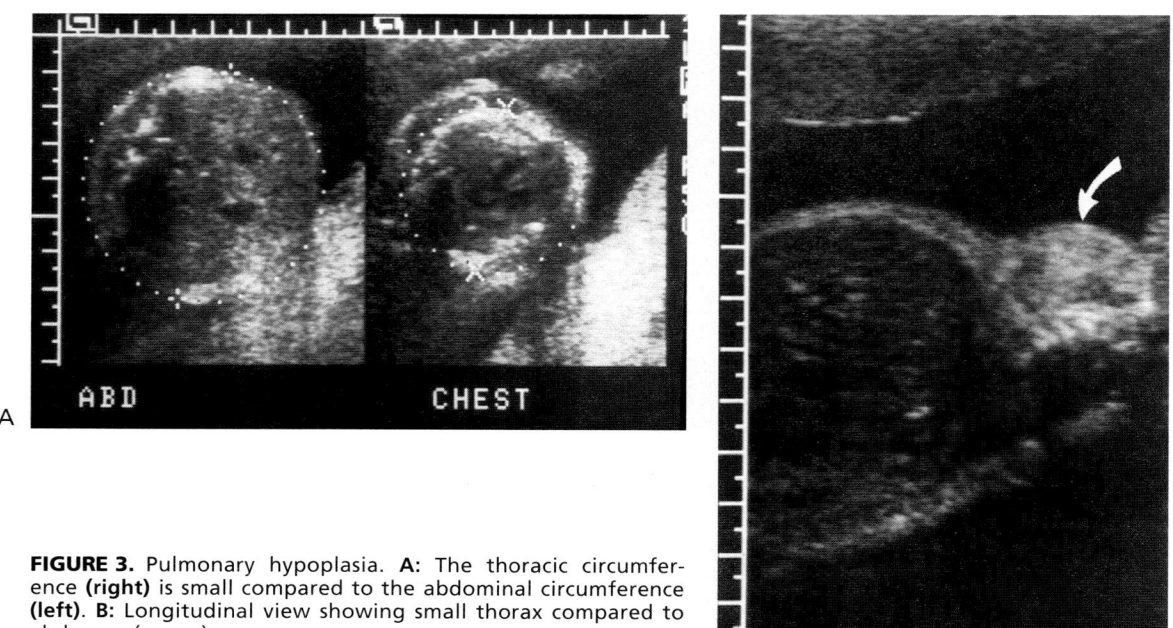

FIGURE 3. Pulmonary hypoplasia. **A:** The thoracic circumference **(right)** is small compared to the abdominal circumference **(left)**. **B:** Longitudinal view showing small thorax compared to abdomen (*arrow*).

4), especially during the late third trimester. However, Laudy et al. did not provide numerical data for the fifth and ninety-fifth percentiles. Ratios between thoracic size and other biometric indices (biparietal, head circumference diameter, abdominal circumference, and femur length) have also been used with a high correlation with gestational age in normal pregnancies.[26–28] Thoracic measurements can help predict pulmonary hypoplasia when the thoracic size is reduced, for

TABLE 1. FETAL THORACIC CIRCUMFERENCE MEASUREMENTS: PREDICTIVE PERCENTILES

Gestational age (wk)	No.	2.5	5	10	25	50	75
16	6	5.9	6.4	7.0	8.0	9.1	10.3
17	22	6.8	7.3	7.9	8.9	10.0	11.2
18	31	7.7	8.2	8.8	9.8	11.0	12.1
19	21	8.6	9.1	9.7	10.7	11.9	13.0
20	20	9.5	10.0	10.6	11.7	12.9	13.9
21	30	10.4	11.0	11.6	12.6	13.7	14.8
22	18	11.3	11.9	12.5	13.5	14.6	15.7
23	21	12.2	12.8	13.4	14.4	15.5	16.6
24	27	13.2	13.7	14.3	15.3	16.4	17.5
25	20	14.1	14.6	15.2	16.2	17.3	18.4
26	25	15.0	15.5	16.1	17.1	18.2	19.3
27	24	15.9	16.4	17.0	18.0	19.1	20.2
28	24	16.8	17.3	17.9	18.9	20.0	21.2
29	24	17.7	18.2	18.8	19.8	21.0	22.1
30	27	18.6	19.1	19.7	20.7	21.9	23.0
31	24	19.5	20.0	20.6	21.6	22.8	23.9
32	28	20.4	20.9	21.5	22.6	23.7	24.8
33	27	21.3	21.8	22.5	23.5	24.6	25.7
34	25	22.2	22.8	23.4	24.4	25.5	26.6
35	20	23.1	23.7	24.3	25.3	26.4	27.5
36	23	24.0	24.6	25.2	26.2	27.3	28.4
37	22	24.9	25.5	26.1	27.1	28.2	29.3
38	21	25.9	26.4	27.0	28.0	29.1	30.2
39	7	26.8	27.3	27.9	28.9	30.0	31.1
40	6	27.7	28.2	28.8	29.8	30.9	32.1

Note: Measurements in centimeters.
Reproduced with permission from Chitkara U, Rosenberg J, Chervenak FA, et al. Prenatal sonographic assessment of the fetal thorax: normal values. *Am J Obstet Gynecol* 1987;156:1069–1074.

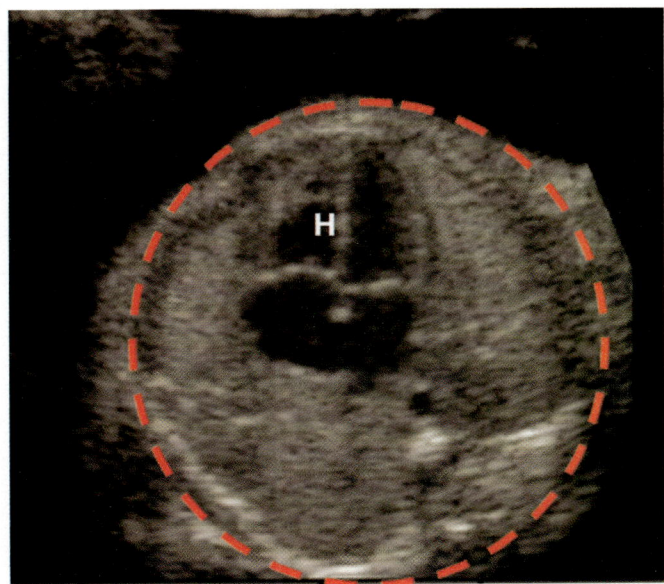

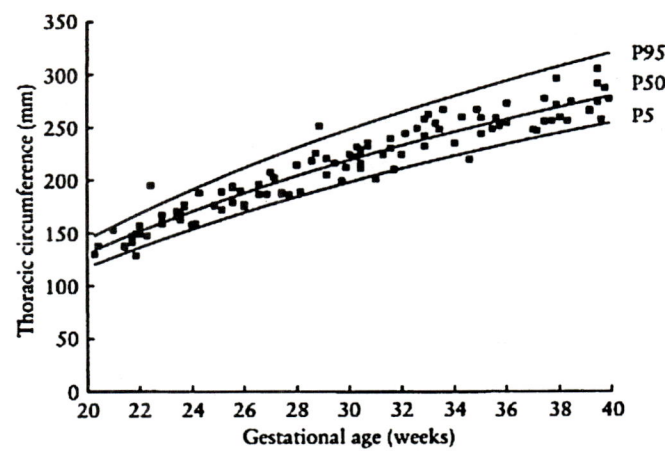

FIGURE 4. Normal thoracic circumference. **A:** Transverse view shows normal thoracic circumference measurement. H, heart. **B:** Thoracic circumference compared with gestational age in 111 normal pregnancies. (Reproduced with permission from Laudy JA, Wladimiroff JW. The fetal lung. 2. Pulmonary hypoplasia. *Ultrasound Obstet Gynecol* 2000;16:482–494.)

example, from oligohydramnios or skeletal dysplasia. However, measurements of thoracic size have a relatively low sensitivity and accuracy for prediction of other causes of lung hypoplasia.[27,28] Direct measurements of the lung appear to be more sensitive than thoracic measurements in these conditions. Methods proposed for measuring the lung include lung length, lung area, and lung diameter.[28,29]

Lung volumes have also been determined using MRI and three-dimensional ultrasonography (Fig. 5).[30–36] These studies have shown a good correlation between lung volume and gestational age. As expected, the right lung volume is slightly greater than the left. The potential role of fetal lung volume in predicting pulmonary hypoplasia is intriguing but remains uncertain at this time. Technical limitations of three-dimensional ultrasound may include poor visualization secondary to oligohydramnios, maternal size, and the lack of clear tissue borderlines. MRI and three-dimensional ultrasound may also experience motion artifacts.

Doppler studies have been proposed for prediction of pulmonary hypoplasia.[37–40] Most Doppler studies of the human fetal pulmonary circulation have been performed in the proximal pulmonary arteries. Whereas some studies appear promising, discrepancies have been reported in the appearance of the normal waveform, especially the end diastolic component, and the values of peak systolic velocities. For these reasons, the usefulness of Doppler velocimetry in prediction of pulmonary hypoplasia remains questionable.[41,42] Most evidence suggests that the presence or absence of fetal breathing movements does not prevent or confirm pulmonary hypoplasia. Many factors affect fetal respiratory activity, including time of day, maternal smoking, drugs, and glucose load.[43]

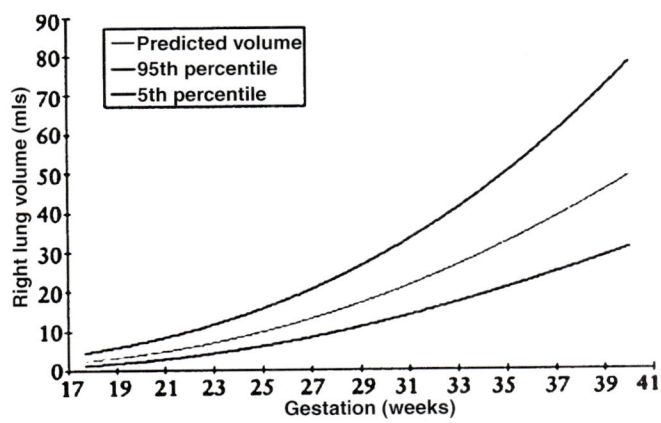

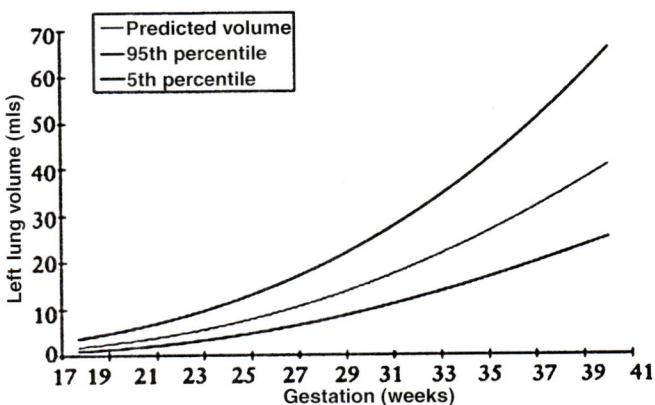

FIGURE 5. Right lung **(A)** and left lung **(B)** volumes calculated by three-dimensional ultrasound from 54 pregnancies. (Reproduced with permission from Bahmaie A, Hughes SW, Clark T, Milner A, Saunders J, et al. Serial fetal lung volume measurement using three-dimensional ultrasound. *Ultrasound Obstet Gynecol* 2000;16:154–158.)

Associated Abnormalities

A large number of conditions may be associated with pulmonary hypoplasia[44,45] (Table 2). The majority of cases with pulmonary hypoplasia result from associated major structural or chromosomal abnormalities, and one-half of all cases of pulmonary hypoplasia are attributed to a space-occupying lesion in the thorax that compresses or replaces normal lung parenchyma. Diaphragmatic hernia is the most common of these processes. Large pleural effusions or rare intrathoracic tumors (neuroblastoma, foregut abnormalities, teratomas) may act in a similar fashion. Primary parenchymal abnormalities of the lungs, such as cystic adenomatoid malformation of the lung, sequestration, and bronchial atresia, may also lead to pulmonary hypoplasia by replacing normal pulmonary parenchyma.

Prognosis and Management

The prognosis varies with the severity of pulmonary hypoplasia, with a high mortality rate observed for those with a clinical diagnosis of pulmonary hypoplasia. Infants with severe respiratory distress at delivery usually die as a result of respiratory difficulties or associated anomalies. Management of pulmonary hypoplasia also varies with the underlying condition. Removal of the intrathoracic mass effect is usually performed soon after birth to permit reexpansion of the lung.

TABLE 2. ANOMALIES ASSOCIATED WITH PULMONARY HYPOPLASIA

Intrathoracic masses	Congenital diaphragmatic hernia
	Congenital cystic adenomatoid malformation
	Bronchopulmonary sequestration
	Bronchogenic cyst and so forth
	Pleural effusions from any cause
	Thoracic neuroblastoma (rare)
Oligohydramnios based on renal or urinary tract anomalies	Bilateral renal agenesis or dysplasia
	Bladder outlet obstruction
	Bilateral multicystic dysplastic kidney disease
	Unilateral renal agenesis with contralateral multicystic dysplastic kidney
	Unilateral renal agenesis or multicystic dysplasia with contralateral severe obstruction
	Autosomal recessive (infantile) polycystic kidney disease
Nonrenal oligohydramnios	Prolonged preterm rupture of membranes
	Idiopathic
Skeletal malformations	Thanatophoric osteogenesis imperfecta, dwarfism
	Other skeletal dysplasias
	Chest wall hamartoma (rare)
Neuromuscular and central nervous system anomalies	Fetal akinesia, anencephaly, and so forth
	Intrauterine anoxic or ischemic damage
	Congenital myopathy
	Pena-Shokeir syndrome
	Phrenic nerve abnormalities
Cardiac lesions	Hypoplastic right or left heart, pulmonary stenosis, and so forth
	Cardiomyopathy
	Ebstein's anomaly
Abdominal wall defects	Omphalocele
Syndromes associated with pulmonary hypoplasia	Trisomies 13, 18, 21, Roberts syndrome, and so forth

CONGENITAL DIAPHRAGMATIC HERNIA

Description

CDH is a herniation of abdominal viscera into the fetal chest, which results from a congenital defect in the fetal diaphragm.

Incidence

CDH is the most common developmental abnormality of the diaphragm, occurring in 1 to 4.5 per 10,000 live births.[46] The incidence may be higher due to the fact that some deaths owing to CDH occur before or shortly after birth, and, in these cases, the CDH may not be clinically recognized. Males and females are affected roughly equally.

Embryology and Pathology

CDHs are most common on the left (75% to 90%), but diaphragmatic defects also occur on the right (approximately 10%) and bilaterally (less than 5%).

Most authorities believe that CDH results from failure of the pleuroperitoneal canals to close at the end of organogenesis. The muscular diaphragm forms between the sixth and fourteenth menstrual week as a result of a chain of events involving the fusion of four structures: the septum transversum (future central tendon), pleuroperitoneal membranes, dorsal mesentery of the esophagus (future crura), and body wall. Normally, the primitive diaphragm is intact by the end of the eighth menstrual week. The most posterior aspect of the diaphragm, derived from the body wall, is the part of the diaphragm that forms last and is most commonly defective.[47]

Reduction of the physiologic umbilical hernia (completed around 12 menstrual weeks) is thought to produce sufficient intraabdominal pressure so that if fusion of the primitive diaphragmatic structures is incomplete, abdominal viscera can herniate into the thorax.

In left-sided hernias, the stomach, some portion of the small and large intestines, and the left lobe of the liver and spleen are most commonly found in the chest. The content of the hernia does not change much during gestation, although, in theory, the visceral herniation may be intermittent. Serial sonograms rarely demonstrate intermittent herniation.

The size of the diaphragmatic defects can be quite variable. Some are small, others large, and, in some, there is complete absence of one or both diaphragms. In most cases, the stomach and bowel are found in the chest as well as a part of the left lobe of the liver. A portion of the left

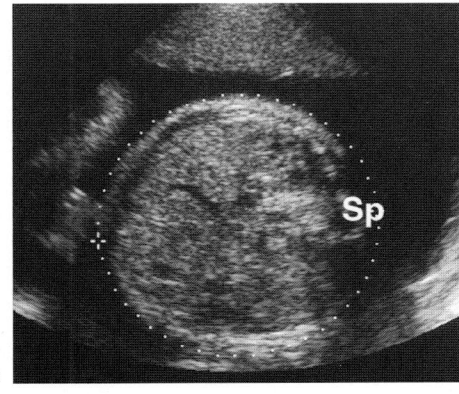

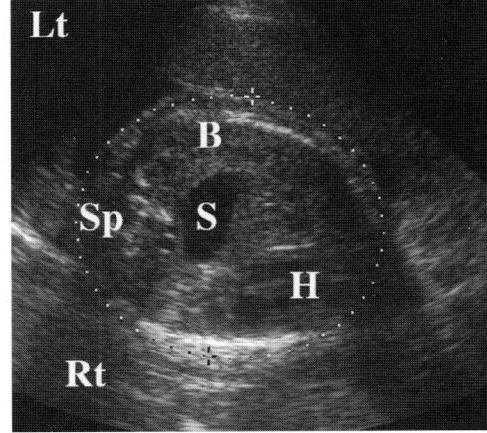

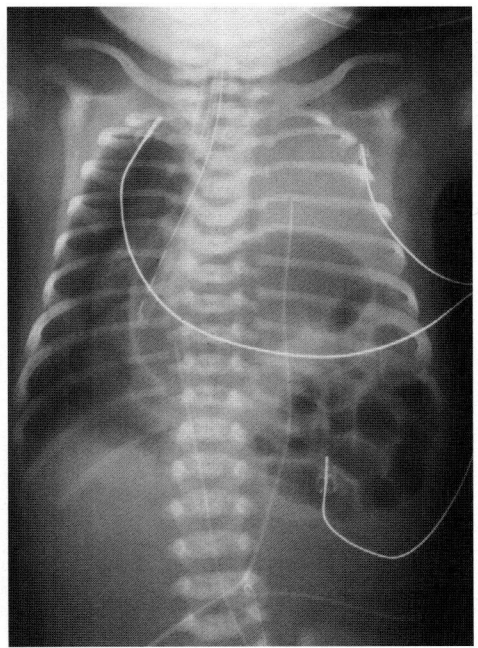

FIGURE 6. Diaphragmatic hernia. **A:** Transverse view of abdomen shows absent fetal stomach. **B:** View of chest shows heart (*H*) displaced to the right. The fluid-filled stomach (*S*) and more echogenic bowel (*B*) fill the left hemithorax. Lt, left; Rt, right; Sp, spine. **C:** Postnatal radiograph.

lobe of the liver, usually the lateral segment, is found in the chest in at least two-thirds of left-sided CDHs.[48,49]

The herniated gut produces mass effect on the heart and developing lungs. While small defects result in smaller hernias, these are often not diagnosed prenatally with sonography. More commonly, the diaphragmatic defects detected are large, with a large volume of bowel and liver herniated into the chest. The most common and important sequela of a CDH is lung hypoplasia and pulmonary hypertension. Hydrops is more commonly associated with lung masses and is rarely associated with left-sided CDH unless there are associated fetal malformations. This low rate of hydrops, despite the presence of fairly marked mass effect and cardiomediastinal shift, is not explained.

The diaphragmatic defect is of lesser importance to fetal prognosis than the derangements in normal development of the lung that the hernia causes—mainly life-threatening pulmonary hypoplasia and hypertension. These pulmonary alterations are most severe in the ipsilateral lung and are nearly always also present in the contralateral lung.

Pulmonary hypoplasia of varying degrees is found in nearly all fetuses with CDH. The lungs are volumetrically smaller than expected for age and histologically demonstrate arrested development. There is also a commonly associated alteration of the pulmonary arteries associated with CDH,

characterized by thickening of the walls of the small pulmonary arteries (medial wall muscular hypertrophy.) This wall thickening of the arteries can and often does extend as far peripherally as the small preacinar vessels. This is the cause of pulmonary hypertension in affected neonates, clinically recognized as persistent fetal circulation.

CDH remains an especially vexing clinical problem because, although the diaphragmatic defect can be repaired after birth, the pulmonary hypoplasia and vascular physiology cannot. Pulmonary and vascular changes, similar to those found in fetuses with CDH, have been produced in an experimental model of CDH in fetal lambs. In the animal model these abnormalities have been shown to be somewhat reversible after *in utero* repair of the CDH.[50] This provides the hope and incentive for correcting the defect during fetal life.

Diagnosis

Left-Sided Congenital Diaphragmatic Hernia

Left CDH is usually detected as a result of two sonographic observations: the displaced heart (to the right) and an ectopic stomach in the chest (present in 90% of cases) (Figs. 6 and 7).[49]

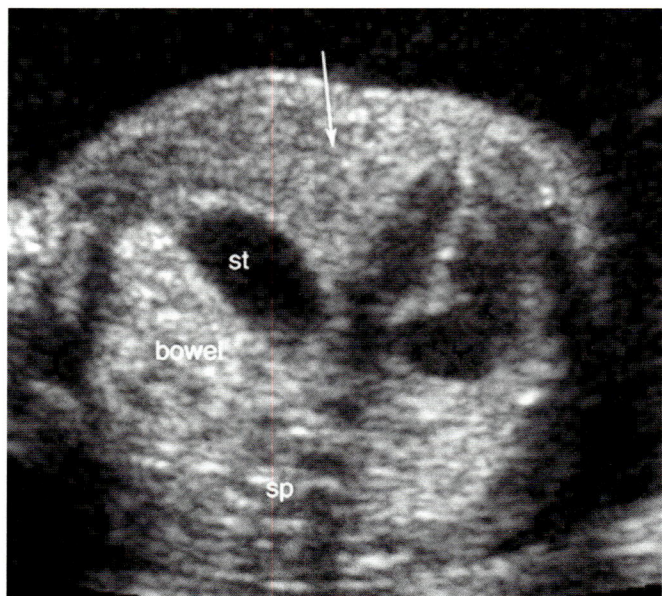
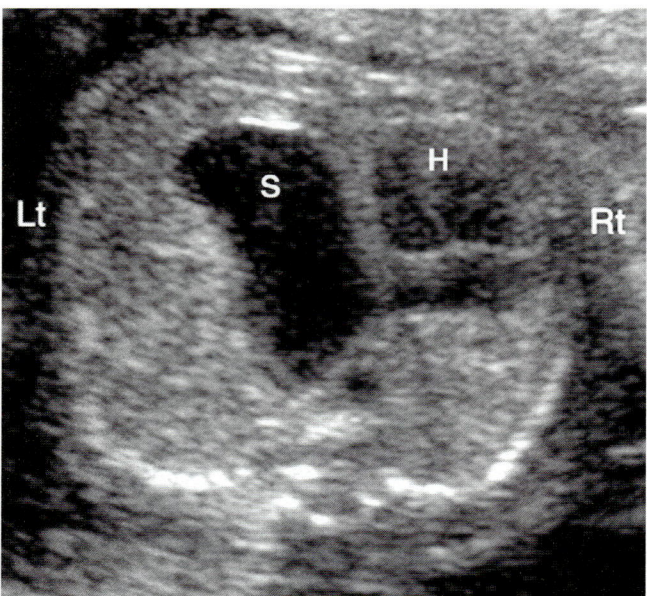

FIGURE 7. A: Left-sided (*liver up*) congenital diaphragmatic hernia, 20 weeks. The heart is shifted to the right by the intrathoracic viscera. The stomach (*st*) is displaced posteriorly by the liver (*arrow*). sp, spine. **B:** A different fetus with a left-sided (*liver down*) congenital diaphragmatic hernia shows displacement of the heart (*H*) to the right, but the fetal stomach (*S*) is not displaced posteriorly because the liver was not herniated into the chest. Lt, left; Rt, right.

The intrathoracic stomach is often the most conspicuous finding. Attention to the position of the heart on the *four-chamber* image of the fetal heart, as recommended by the American Institute of Ultrasound in Medicine and American College of Radiology,[51] greatly facilitates antenatal detection of CDH. For large diaphragmatic hernias, the abdomen may also be *scaphoid* (Fig. 8).

Unless a systematic survey is performed, diaphragmatic hernia can be easily missed. Among 136 newborns diagnosed with CDH over a 10-year period (1985–1995), Lewis et al.[52] reported that the false-negative rate remained approximately 55%. Multicenter experience suggests that approximately 60% of CDHs are detected before birth with sonographic screening,[53,54] and single centers report a much higher detection rate.[49] As expected, the largest CDHs are most easily detected. Smaller hernias with little or no visceral herniation or those in which the stomach remains intraabdominal may be missed on *dating* sonograms (Fig. 9). These seem to be associated with better outcomes, perhaps because they are the smaller of the hernias. Recognizing the cardiomediastinal shift is critical to making the diagnosis if the stomach is not in the chest.

The contents of the hernia should be characterized as fully as possible on the sonogram, because this influences prognosis and management. Small bowel and colon are commonly intrathoracic but are often collapsed and difficult to identify specifically. The fetal stomach in the chest is the *signpost* of fetal CDH. The presence of an intrathoracic

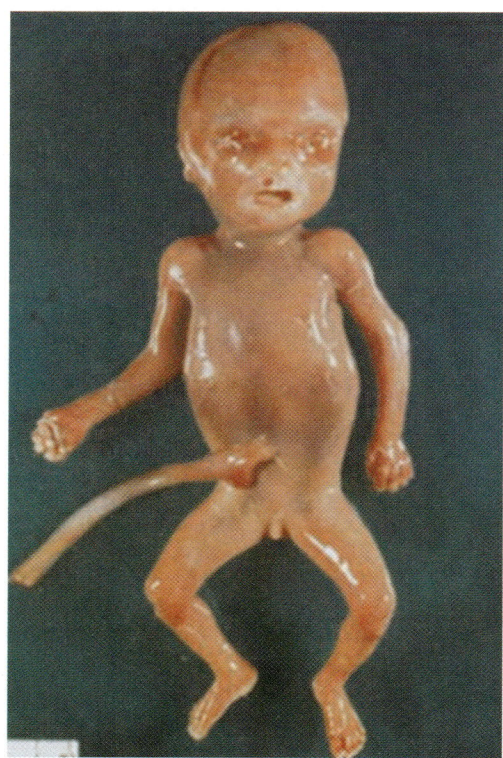

FIGURE 8. Pathologic photograph of fetus diagnosed with left-sided diaphragmatic hernia. Note the scaphoid appearance of the abdomen.

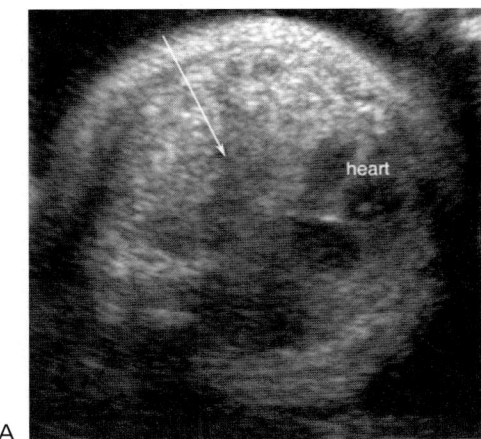 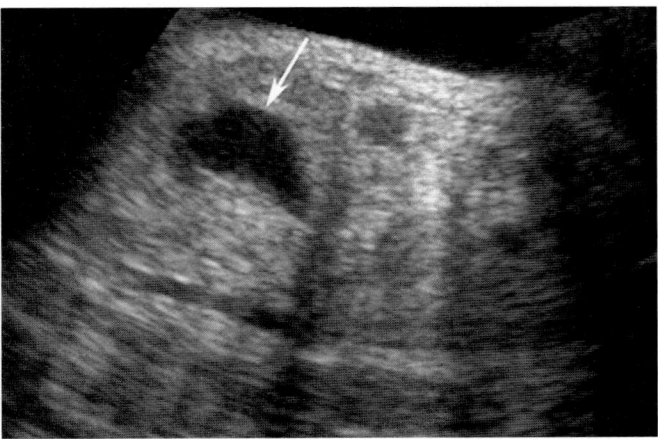

FIGURE 9. A: Unusual left-sided congenital diaphragmatic hernia. The stomach is not herniated into the chest, the expected location of the stomach for most left-sided congenital hernias, as indicated by the arrow. **B:** Same fetus as (**A**). Coronal image shows the stomach (*arrow*) in the abdomen.

cystic structure in the absence of an identifiable stomach in the abdomen is pathognomonic of a CDH.

The ipsilateral fetal lung (left lung) is very small and camouflaged by the hernia and, thus, is usually not visible on the sonogram.

A portion of the liver herniates into the chest in approximately two-thirds of cases, and the presence or absence of intrathoracic liver is an important observation because intrathoracic liver is associated with poorer outcomes (Tables 3 and 4). The sonographic diagnosis of intrathoracic liver in a left-sided CDH can be difficult.

The way in which the liver herniates in a left CDH is fairly predictable. Familiarity with the expected anatomy can be extremely helpful to the examiner. In most cases, the left lobe (or lateral segment) *flips up* adjacent to the heart, perpendicular to the horizontal axis of the normal liver. In addition, there is a fairly predictable displacement of the stomach, posteriorly, by the herniated liver. This can be appreciated on an axial image, even when the diagnosis of intrathoracic liver is uncertain (Fig. 8).

Sonographically, herniated livers appear as homogeneous soft tissue adjacent to the right cardiac ventricle, anteriorly in the chest. Because liver and collapsed bowel have a similar grey-scale appearance, additional effort is required to be certain that the tissue displacing the stomach

posteriorly is the liver. Color (and duplex) Doppler imaging can be extremely helpful by allowing identification of portal veins within this tissue. A posterior stomach in the chest is highly suggestive, but visualization of branches of the left portal vein is definitive (Fig. 10). Using higher frequency transducers (6 to 8 MHz), the intrathoracic liver and tiny portal triads can sometimes be recognized on greyscale images (Fig. 11).[55] Finally, if the location of the liver cannot be made confidently with sonography, fetal MRI can be safely performed and exquisitely demonstrates liver herniated into the chest (Fig. 12).[56]

A variety of methods have been proposed to estimate the degree of functional lung in the right thorax.[29] These methods include lung length, lung diameter,[28] lung area, lung area to head circumference ratio (LHR), and estimation of volume with three-dimensional ultrasound. These methods are important for predicting the prognosis (see Prognosis section).

Right-Sided Congenital Diaphragmatic Hernia

Right-sided CDHs account for less than 10% of congenital diaphragmatic defects and are more difficult to detect than

TABLE 3. IMPACT OF LIVER LOCATION ON SURVIVAL AND EXTRACORPOREAL MEMBRANE OXYGENATION REQUIREMENT

	Liver up	Liver down
Survival	43%	93%
Extracorporeal membrane oxygenation	53%	19%

TABLE 4. PROGNOSTIC FEATURES OF LEFT CONGENITAL DIAPHRAGMATIC HERNIA

Chromosomal abnormality
Other anomalies
Early diagnosis (less than 24 wk gestation) and early delivery
Large hernia
Intrathoracic stomach
Intrathoracic liver
Small right lung
Small left ventricle (cardiac)

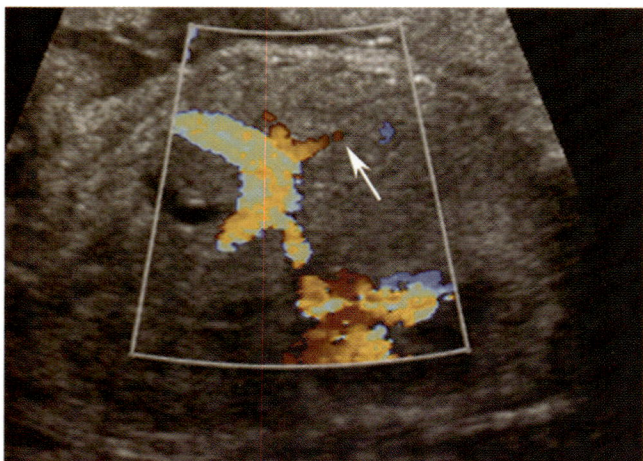

FIGURE 10. Color Doppler image of fetus with left-sided congenital diaphragmatic hernia demonstrating the lateral segment branch of the portal vein (*arrow*) in the chest above the level of the expected diaphragm.

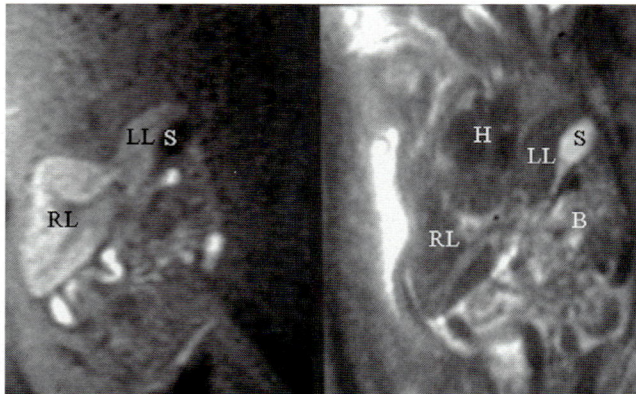

FIGURE 12. *Liver up* left-sided congenital diaphragmatic hernia. Fetal magnetic resonance image showing T1-weighted **(A)** and T2-weighted **(B)** coronal images. The lateral segment of the left lobe (*LL*) of the liver is in the fetal chest between the heart (*H*) and the stomach (*S*). B, bowel; RL, right lobe.

left-sided CDHs. The fetal stomach, conspicuously intrathoracic in left-sided CDH, is below the diaphragm in right-sided CDHs. The herniated viscera of a right CDH consist predominantly of liver and collapsed bowel, and, in these cases, mediastinal shift (heart to left) is the signpost of a right CDH (Fig. 13A). At first glance, a right CDH appears like a right-sided lung mass. If care is not taken to identify portal veins within the mass, this lesion can easily be misinterpreted as a mass, such as a microcystic adenomatoid malformation.

There are a few sonographic clues that a right-sided fetal chest mass is a CDH. First, portal veins should be sought

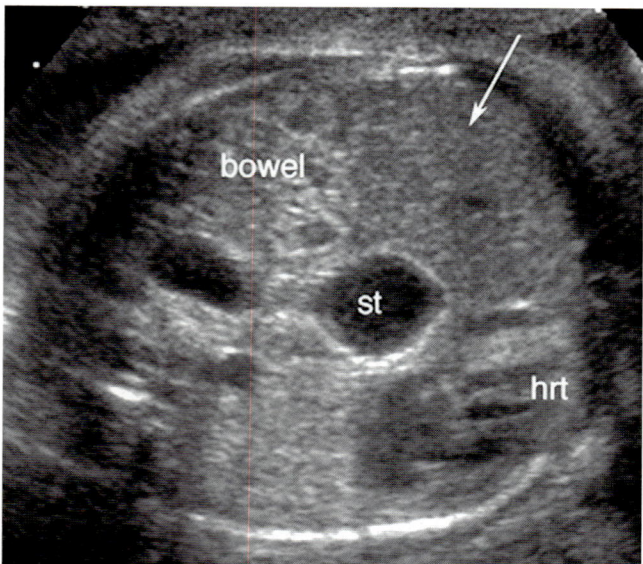

FIGURE 11. *Liver up* left-sided congenital diaphragmatic hernia. The liver (*arrow*) can be distinguished from the bowel and stomach (*st*) on this 8-MHz grey-scale image. hrt, heart.

and can be usually recognized within the *mass* (Fig. 13B), either with grey-scale or color Doppler imaging (Fig. 13C). Second, the gallbladder often herniates into the chest with the liver. The gallbladder should always be considered in the differential diagnosis when a single *cyst* is identified in a solid right-sided *mass* (Fig. 13D). Third, as an ancillary finding, there is often a small amount of ascitic fluid seen in the chest adjacent to the right lobe of the liver in association with right-sided CDH (Fig. 14). Pleural fluid is unusual in association with other chest masses (except for a large hydrothorax sometimes seen with sequestrations), so the examiner should suspect a right CDH if fluid is associated with a mass in the right hemithorax. Finally, absence of the hypoechoic diaphragmatic muscle on the right may help in further confirming the presence of diaphragmatic defect and the correct diagnosis.

Bilateral Diaphragmatic Hernias

Bilateral diaphragmatic hernias are rare and also tricky to detect because there may be little or no cardiomediastinal shift (Fig. 15). In these fetuses, the heart may appear to be displaced anteriorly and superiorly. In some bilateral hernias, the stomach is found within the left chest, but the degree of cardiomediastinal shift is much less than expected with a unilateral CDH.[57] Bilateral CDH may be associated with an autosomal recessive pattern of inheritance.[58]

Differential Diagnosis

The differential diagnosis of a mass in the left side of the fetal chest includes CDH, congenital cystic adenomatoid malformation (CCAM), sequestration, bronchogenic cyst, teratoma, or neuroenteric cyst (Table 5). In considering this

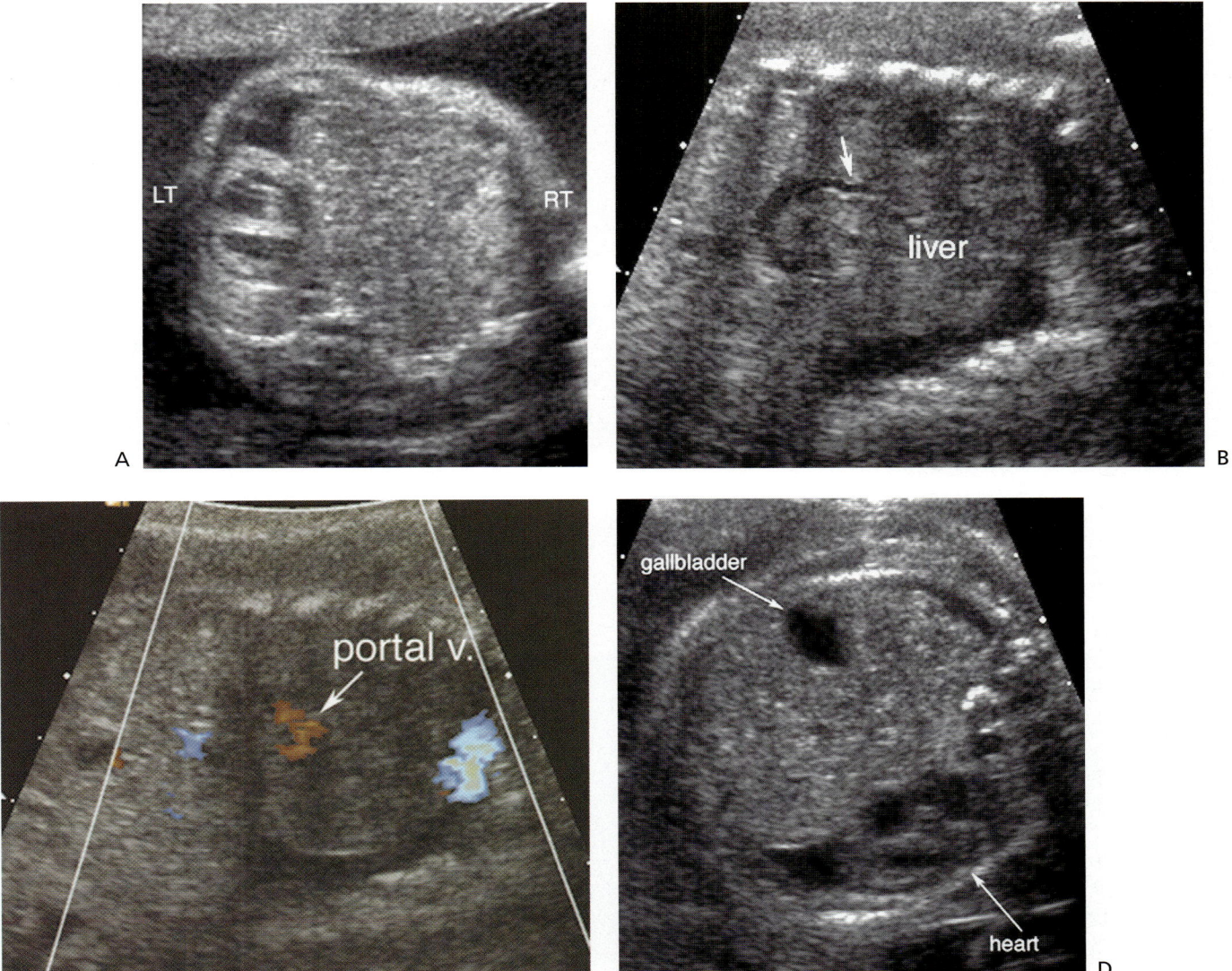

FIGURE 13. Right-sided congenital diaphragmatic hernia. **A:** Grey-scale image shows mass and small amount of fluid in right chest. LT, left; RT, right. **B:** Same fetus as **(A)**, sagittal images. Arrow indicates a portal vein within the mass. **C:** Same fetus as **(A)**. Color Doppler indicates flow within the portal vein (*v.*) confirming that the mass is liver. **D:** Transaxial image shows the gallbladder herniated into the chest.

differential diagnosis, the position of the stomach is critical. If the stomach cannot be found below the diaphragm, left-sided CDH is likely. Left-sided solid-appearing lesions include CCAM; sequestration; bronchial atresia (*obstructed* lung); and CDH (*stomach down*). In the latter case, the collapsed bowel appears as a solid mass, but peristalsis of the bowel may help to establish the correct diagnosis of CDH.

Diagnostic considerations of a right-sided chest mass include CCAM, CDH, sequestration, bronchial atresia, teratoma, and neuroenteric cyst. Multiple cysts are suggestive of a CCAM; portal veins and gallbladder in the chest suggest a right-sided CDH, and vertebral anomalies suggest neuroenteric cyst (see Neuroenteric Cyst).

If the diagnosis remains uncertain, fetal MRI can be performed without sedation of the fetus. MRI can very nicely demonstrate bowel and liver within the chest. MRI can also very sensitively and accurately distinguish *liver up* from *liver down* left-sided CDHs (Fig. 12).[56]

First Trimester

Sebire et al.[59] reported an interesting association between nuchal translucency and diaphragmatic hernia. Among 78,639 pregnancies presumed to have normal karyotype, 19 proved to have diaphragmatic hernia. In four cases, the parents opted for termination of the pregnancy; the

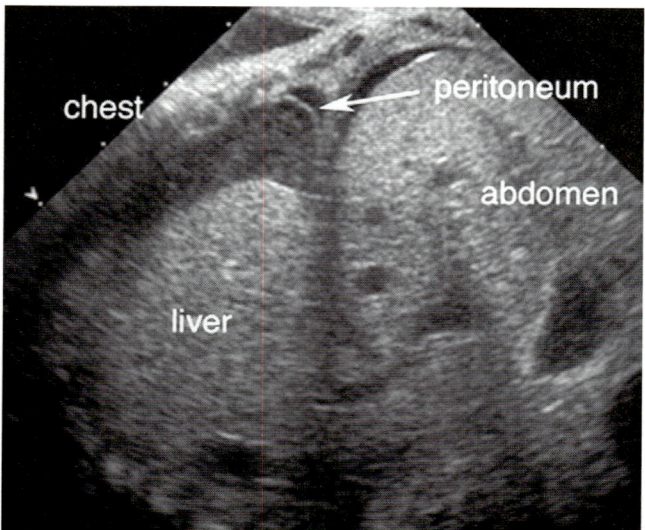

FIGURE 14. Intraoperative image of right-sided diaphragmatic hernia. The peritoneal membrane can be seen surrounding the intrathoracic liver and a small amount of ascitic fluid. In addition, a tiny pleural effusion can be seen adjacent to the peritoneum.

remaining 15 resulted in live births. Nuchal translucency was increased in 7 of 19 (37%) cases of diaphragmatic hernia, including five of six cases that resulted in neonatal death caused by pulmonary hypoplasia. This limited information suggests that, although nuchal translucency is nonspecific, nearly 40% of fetuses with diaphragmatic hernia may have increased nuchal translucency at 10 to 14 weeks, and it may be a marker of intrathoracic compression–related pulmonary hypoplasia.

Associated Anomalies

Associated anomalies and syndromes are found in 15% to 45% of fetuses with CDH. A variety of multiple anomaly syndromes and conditions have been associated with CDH (Table 6). Chromosomal abnormalities occur in 5% to 15%, with the most common being trisomy 18.[60–63]

The presence of associated anomalies greatly influences perinatal outcomes.[63] The presence of other anomalies, especially cardiac, is associated with poor outcomes. Survival is poor when associated anomalies are present (less

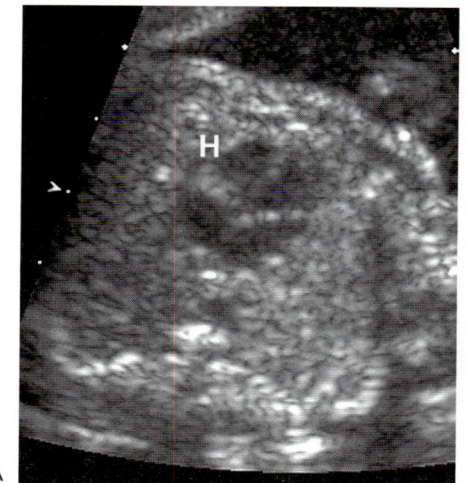

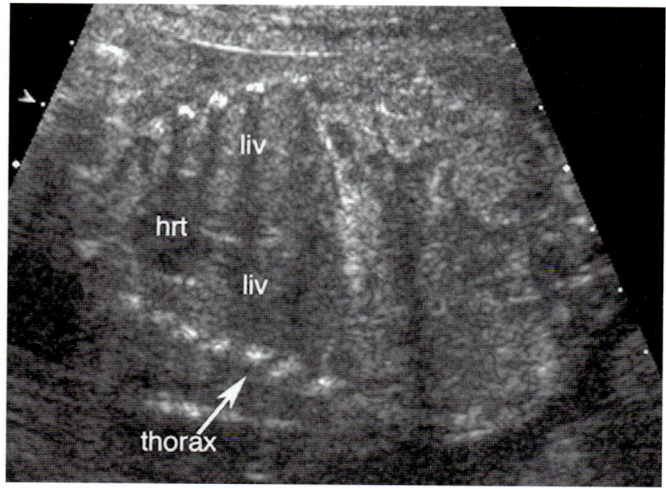

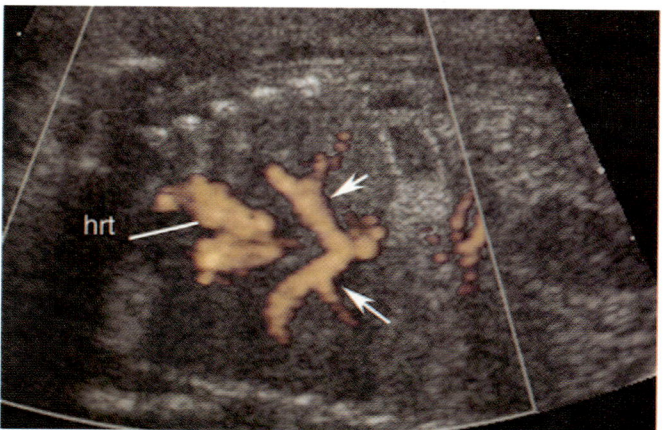

FIGURE 15. Bilateral diaphragmatic hernia. **A:** Prenatal diagnosis of bilateral congenital diaphragmatic hernia can be very difficult, owing to the subtle influence on cardiac position. In this transaxial image of the chest, note the midline position of the heart (*H*). The axis is somewhat more vertical than normal, but the findings are subtle. **B:** Coronal image of same fetus as in **(A)**. There is a bilateral herniation of liver (*liv*) into the chest. **C:** Coronal color Doppler image of same fetus as **(A)** shows portal veins (*arrows*) within the intrathoracic stomach. The heart (*hrt*) is displaced somewhat superiorly but remains in the midline.

TABLE 5. MAJOR ETIOLOGIES FOR AN INTRATHORACIC MASS

Diaphragmatic hernia or eventration
Cystic adenomatoid malformation
Bronchopulmonary sequestration
Bronchial, laryngeal, tracheal atresia
Tracheal, bronchial obstruction
Neurenteric or duplication cyst
Bronchogenic cyst
Tumor

than 20%) compared to the group with isolated CDH (greater than 60%). Some of the commoner syndromes associated with CDH include Fryns syndrome (autosomal recessive inheritance, craniofacial abnormalities, cystic hygroma, microcystic kidneys, digital hypoplasia, Dandy-Walker malformation, agenesis of corpus callosum)[64]; Pallister Killian syndrome (tetrasomy 12p, coarse face, skin pigmentary anomalies, profound mental retardation); as well as lethal pterygium, Beckwith-Wiedemann, Simpson-Golabi-Behmel, Brachmann-de Lange, and Perlman syndromes.[65]

As a general rule, malformations that are most frequently associated with CDH include heart and brain malformations. These are usually accurately detected with sonography, but subtle abnormalities (e.g., low-set ears, broad nasal bridge, micrognathia, digital anomalies, and even some heart defects) may elude even very experienced examiners' detection in as many as one-third of affected fetuses.[65]

Prognosis

In unselected groups of fetuses with CDH, the survival rate may be as low as 20%. Poor prognostic factors of left-sided CDH include associated morphologic anomalies, chromosomal abnormalities, early gestational age at diagnosis, premature delivery, large hernia, presence of intrathoracic stomach and liver, small size of the contralateral lung, and

TABLE 6. SYNDROMES ASSOCIATED WITH DIAPHRAGMATIC HERNIA

Asplenia/polysplenia
Beckwith-Wiedemann syndrome
Caudal regression syndrome
Chromosome abnormalities
de Lange syndrome
Fryns syndrome
Goldenhar syndrome
Klippel-Feil syndrome
Myelodysplasia complex
Pentalogy of Cantrell
Pallister-Killian syndrome
Rubinstein-Taybi syndrome
Stickler syndrome

cardiac ventricular disproportion (small left ventricle) (Table 4).[48,49,60,63] Bilateral CDH is the worst end of the spectrum, and no survivors have been reported.

Survival rates may be as high as 60% when CDH is isolated, without additional anomalies and chromosomal abnormalities.[48,49,66] However, the prognosis in this group of patients remains dependent on the volume of functional lung. In particular, three factors associated with a worse prognosis are (a) earlier diagnosis before 25 weeks, (b) intrathoracic liver, and (c) small size of the contralateral, right lung.

As prenatal detection of intrathoracic liver became more reliable, the correlation with worsened survival rate became evident[49] (Table 3). When the liver remains intraabdominal (*liver down*), postnatal survival rates are impressively optimistic (93%) compared to much poorer survival rates (43%) among those in whom the liver is intrathoracic (*liver up*).

As previously noted, a variety of methods have been used to help estimate the quantity of right lung in cases of left diaphragmatic hernia. This has included lung length, lung diameter, lung area, and LHR.[67,68]

This ratio is calculated by measuring the area of the right lung, in square millimeters, on a four-chamber image of the chest between 23 and 28 weeks (Fig. 16). Two diameters of the lung are multiplied and divided by the head circumference, in millimeters, yielding a gestational age–independent index.

In a study of 40 affected fetuses, Guibaud et al.[49] reported that the only significant predictor of survival was the quantification of the contralateral lung area at the level of an axial four-chamber view; the survival rate was 86% when the con-

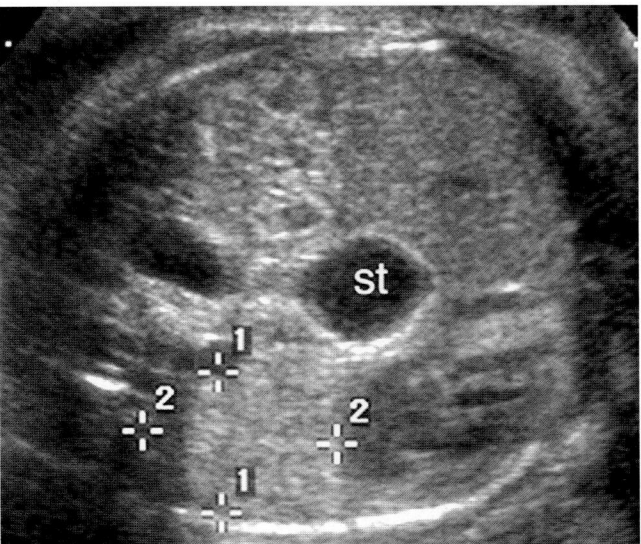

FIGURE 16. Fetal lung measurement for the calculation of the lung to head ratio in left-sided congenital diaphragmatic hernia. The measurement of the right lung is performed on a transaxial image demonstrating four cardiac chambers. The two diameters of the right lung, in millimeters, are multiplied and divided by the head circumference, also in millimeters. A lung to head ratio greater than or equal to 1.4 is considered favorable, and less than or equal to 0.8 is considered unfavorable. st, stomach.

tralateral lung area was equal to or greater than one-half the area of the hemithorax compared to only 25% survival if the right lung occupied less than 50%. Similarly, Metkus et al.[69] evaluated sonographic prognostic factors in 55 fetuses with diaphragmatic hernia. The overall survival rate was 65%. If the diagnosis was made after 25 weeks' gestation, the survival rate was 100% (12 of 12); the rate was 56% if the diagnosis was made at or before 25 weeks ($p <.005$). All five neonates with an LHR of less than 0.6 died; the survival rate was 100% for those whose LHR was greater than 1.35, and those with an LHR between 0.6 and 1.35 had a 61% survival rate ($p <.001$). Stomach position, polyhydramnios, and abdominal circumference were not found to be useful survival predictors. No prenatal sonographic parameter was absolutely predictive of postnatal death except very small right lung size, which was present in only 5 of the 55 patients. At University of California San Francisco there have been no survivors without fetal intervention when the LHR was less than 0.8, and there has been 100% survival among those with an LHR greater than 1.4.[70] Study on the efficacy (ROC curves, inter- and intraobserver variability) of the LHR is ongoing.

For survivors of surgical repair of the diaphragmatic hernia, morbidity may still be considerable and should be factored into parental counseling. Common complications include feeding dysfunction, gastroesophageal reflux, chronic lung disease, and delays in motor development.[71] Among fetuses with large CDHs, many require extracorporeal membrane oxygenation (ECMO) therapy. Survivors who require ECMO have a greater incidence of neurologic delay than those who do not, but this may reflect the severity of the presenting illness rather than the effects of ECMO.[72]

Management

Identification of CDH requires a detailed morphologic survey (including cardiac evaluation) and karyotype testing followed by parental counseling. Management options include (a) termination of the pregnancy, (b) repair of the defect after birth, or (c) fetal surgery.

Postnatal surgical options are immediate repair or delayed repair.[73] Repair of the diaphragmatic defect after birth does not reverse the pulmonary hypoplasia and pulmonary hypertension caused by the CDH.

ECMO may provide adequate oxygenation to permit nonemergent surgical repair later in the neonatal period. ECMO support is required more often in those with intrathoracic liver (53%) compared to those without (19%). High-frequency oscillatory ventilation with delayed surgical repair also appears encouraging. Use of surfactant and nitric oxide also appears beneficial.

Fetal Surgery

Because it is likely that the effects of the hernia are ongoing during gestation, the purpose of fetal intervention is to arrest the ongoing damage to the developing lung and vascular bed. While there is evidence that some fetuses may benefit from fetal therapy, the benefits (survival and morbidity) have not yet been proven. A multicenter, randomized controlled trial is under way. To determine the potential benefit of the surgery, not only the *local* benefit to the fetal lungs but also the risk of preterm delivery, ruptured membranes, and the risk of the procedure must be considered. Clearly the fetuses on the bad end of the spectrum of CDH are the ones who have the greatest potential to benefit from *in utero* surgery. Thus, the fetal treatment group at University of California San Francisco (and those at other fetal therapy centers) has tried to refine the sonographic prognostic indicators. The goal is to offer fetal intervention to only those who are expected to have the poorest prognosis—those who would potentially benefit the most.

In the 1980s, attempts to surgically repair the CDH *in utero* failed due to the intra-operative fetal deaths. These were attributed to the kinking of the umbilical vein and ductus venosus while attempting to reduce the liver, resulting in circulatory collapse. As a result of this experience and the known dependence of the fetus on the umbilical venous flow, it was concluded that the presence of liver in the chest should preclude primary fetal repair of the diaphragmatic defect.

Another approach to prenatal surgery of CDH is occlusion of the trachea, resulting in lung distension and accelerated lung growth. This approach was based on a natural *experiment* occurring with tracheal atresia in which the lungs were found, by some measures, to be more *mature* than expected for age and even *hyperplastic* in some cases. Further, experimentally produced, high airway obstruction in fetal animals demonstrated a similar benefit to the developing lamb lung as that observed with naturally occurring high airway obstruction.[74,75]

It was reasoned that tracheal occlusion might be a *stimulant* for lung development for fetuses with CDH. At University of California San Francisco, methods of tracheal occlusion have used first an expandable plug, then a tracheal clip, and finally a floatable balloon occlusion. This latter approach, using a temporary method of tracheal occlusion, is now the favored mode of surgical therapy in human fetuses and this is being investigated at University of California San Francisco. This can be accomplished endoscopically in the fetus using a video-fetoscopic technique [fetal endoscopic (FETENDO)]. Placement of the occluding balloon without hysterotomy (Fig. 17A) reduces the complications of prematurely ruptured membranes and uterine irritability. Within 1 or 2 weeks, the lungs appear increased in size and echogenic in most fetuses (Fig. 17B). Once a fetal tracheal balloon has been placed, however, the fetus must be delivered by cesarean section, maintained on placental circulation while the tracheal balloon is deflated, and the fetus can be incubated. This is known as the *ex utero intrapartum treatment* procedure.[76]

In 1998, Harrison and coworkers reported their experience with eight fetuses that had undergone fetoscopic tra-

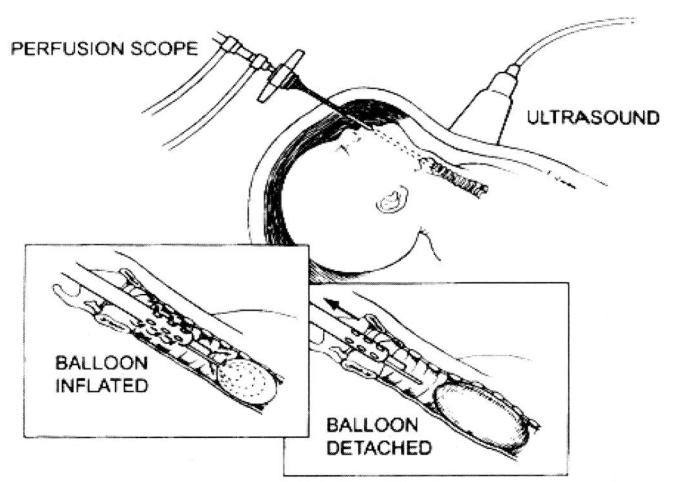

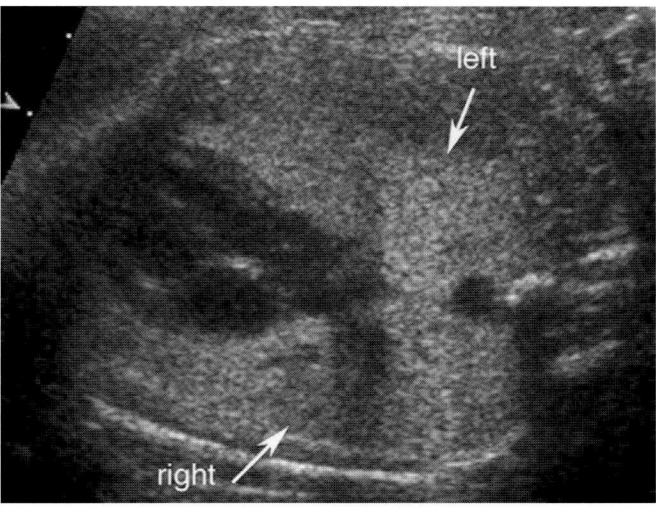

FIGURE 17. A: Fetal endoscopic procedure. In fetuses with congenital diaphragmatic hernia, the fetal trachea is occluded by a balloon to prevent efflux of lung fluid and to distend the tiny airways of the lung. A small endoscope is placed in the fetal mouth while the fetus remains in the uterus. Sonographic guidance aids in the correct placement of the balloon in the midtrachea before detachment of the balloon. **B:** Posttracheal balloon placement. Both lungs are echogenic and can now be identified (*arrows*).

cheal occlusion.[77] Survival rate was 75% in the FETENDO group compared to 38% in the group treated with standard postnatal therapy. While this procedure does not reduce the hernia, these authors reported striking enlargement of the lungs of *clipped* fetuses on imaging studies after birth and at the time of postnatal surgical repair. This intervention resulted in better than expected clinical respiratory function despite factors of CDH and premature delivery. In 1996 a National Institutes of Health randomized trial began to test this technique in fetuses with CDH in the poor prognosis group (*liver up* and low LHR).

Fetuses who may most benefit from this procedure include those identified as *poor prognosis* on the basis of associated anomalies, liver herniation, early diagnosis (before 25 weeks' gestation), and a low LHR. Harrison et al.[68] reported their results in 34 of 86 fetuses with an isolated left CDH who met criteria for the poor prognosis group. Thirteen families chose postnatal treatment at an ECMO center, 13 underwent open fetal tracheal occlusion, and eight underwent fetoscopic tracheal occlusion. The survival rate was 38% in the group treated by standard postnatal therapy, 15% in the open tracheal occlusion group, and 75% in those who underwent fetoscopic tracheal occlusion. Those treated with fetoscopic tracheal occlusion showed dramatic lung expansion. These results are encouraging for use of fetoscopic tracheal occlusion among fetuses identified in the poor prognosis group.

Recurrence Risk

CDH is usually a sporadic disorder with low recurrence risk. Teratogenic and genetic factors may play a role in the embryogenesis of some affected individuals.[58,65] Familial cases of CDH account for the minority of cases, representing less than 2% of recognized cases.[78] In some families, however, particularly those with bilateral CDH, the lesion may be inherited with an autosomal recessive mode of inheritance.

CONGENITAL CYSTIC ADENOMATOID MALFORMATION OF THE LUNG

Description

CCAM is a multicystic mass within the lung consisting of primitive lung tissue and abnormal bronchial and bronchiolar-like structures. CCAM is one of the bronchopulmonary foregut malformations.

Incidence

The precise incidence of CCAM is unknown. When detection is made after birth, reports on this lesion probably underestimate its incidence because more than two-thirds of neonates with CCAMs have no symptoms at birth.[79] Once considered a rare abnormality, detection of CCAM before birth has increased rather dramatically since the early 1990s. This may be due to improved resolution of sonographic equipment and increased popularity of antepartum screening. In a single health maintenance facility in Northern California, approximately three CCAMs were detected among 11,500 fetuses in *nonreferred* (screening) antepartum sonograms. This translates to a prevalence of approximately 1 per 4,000 (M. Caponigro; Kaiser Permanente; Oakland, CA; *personal communication*, 2001) and approaches the incidence of CDH.

CCAMs are reported to account for 25% of all congenital lung lesions in pathologic series,[80] but CCAMs account for more than 75% of lung lesions detected in fetuses.[81]

Embryology and Pathology

CCAM is thought to result from an embryogenetic alteration in the developing lung during the first 8 to 9 gestational weeks.[82] The arterial supply to a CCAM is due to a branch of the pulmonary artery reflecting its origin as an aberration of the normal lung anlage. The cause is not known.

Whereas CCAM is usually restricted to one lobe of the lung, the lesion may involve more than one lobe, an entire lung, or, rarely, may be bilateral. CCAMs often communicate with the bronchial tree through poorly supported primitive bronchi or bronchioles. The cysts within the mass can be large or small, and the mass can be predominantly solid, mixed, or cystic.

The vast majority of CCAMs are unilateral. Bilateral lesions are rare and account for approximately 3% of lung masses prenatally detected.[83,84] The right lung is involved approximately equally to the left, and CCAM occurs slightly more commonly in males.

Histologically, the lesion demonstrates abnormal proliferation of the terminal respiratory bronchioles and poorly organized primitive tissue. Because skeletal muscle may be present in the cyst walls,[85] some consider CCAM to be similar to focal dysplasia,[86] with features of dysplasia, hamartoma, and neoplasm being described in CCAMs.[87] While the pathogenesis is not understood, decreased apoptosis and increased cell proliferation has been noted in some fetal CCAM specimens.[88] These factors may play a role in the medical treatment of affected fetuses in the future.

The mass may be mainly cysts, mainly solid, or cystic and solid. Based on microscopic and gross features, Stocker suggested three forms of CCAM: type I (macrocystic) with cysts 2 to 10 cm; type II (macrocystic with a microcystic component) with cysts less than 2 cm; and type III (microcystic) with cysts less than 0.5 cm. Sonographically, macrocysts are seen in types I and II, but type III lesions appear solid and echogenic. Histologically, the solid tissue is composed of multiple, curved, branched structures that resemble immature or dysplastic bronchioles.

There is growing enthusiasm for a unifying theory of embryogenesis of CCAM, sequestration, lobar emphysema, and bronchial atresia,[89,90] because a combination of these lesions may be found in one fetus.[79,91,92] In some cases, CCAM has been associated with bronchial atresia, and some have even suggested that bronchial atresia may be the primary abnormality and the dysplastic lung tissue, distal to the atresia, a secondary phenomenon.[93–96] In many cases, elements of sequestration are found in CCAMs and

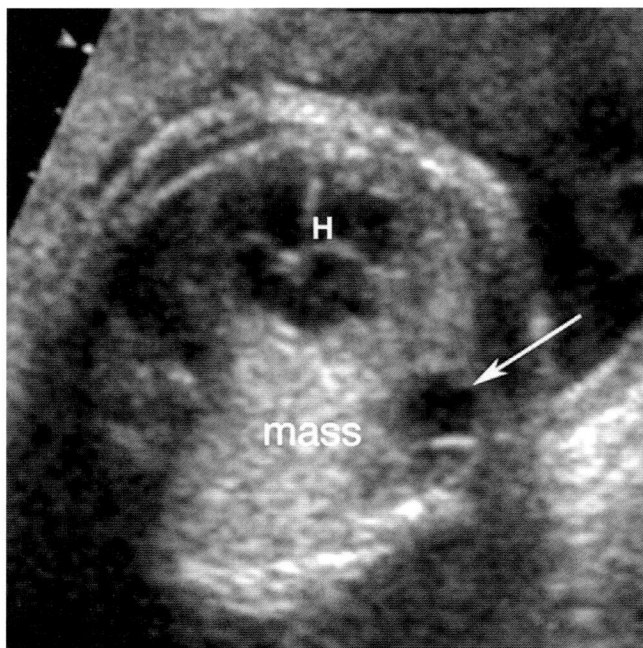

FIGURE 18. Cystic adenomatoid malformation of the lung. Medium-sized right-sided congenital adenomatoid malformation with mild-to-moderate shift of the mediastinum. The borders of the mass are ill defined. A single cyst is seen within the mass (*arrow*). H, heart.

vice versa. These have been called *hybrid* lesions. The mixed histology is not known to influence prognosis.

Diagnosis

A CCAM appears as a cystic and solid mass in the lung (Figs. 18 and 19). Among 122 cases detected prenatally in one study, 60% appeared macrocystic and 40% microcystic.[97] Sonographically, most lesions have cystic and solid components, although, in some, the size of the cyst may be only 1 or 2 mm (Fig. 19). In others, the mass consists almost entirely of cysts, and, occasionally, a single large (4 or 5 cm) cyst occupies nearly the entire volume of the mass (Fig. 20).

The size and appearance of a CCAM are variable, although large ones are more easily detected with antenatal sonography. CCAMs are often first detected because of the mass effect in the chest. Large lesions are associated with marked cardiomediastinal shift and flattening or inversion of the diaphragm. Although CCAMs *develop* in the first trimester, the abnormality is usually not detected until mid-gestation.[98] Presumably these lesions and cysts grow and become more conspicuous as the fetus reaches mid-gestation. The side of the CCAM is usually a straightforward assessment (right = left) but it may be difficult to determine which lobe of the lung is involved. Neither the side of the lesion or the lobe involved is known to have any influence on outcome.

As previously mentioned in Embryology and Pathology, the pulmonary artery supplies the CCAM, and color Dop-

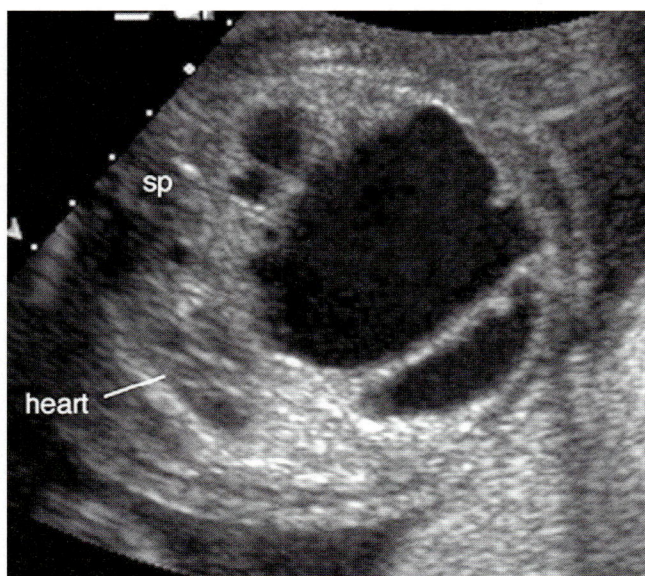

FIGURE 19. Cystic adenomatoid malformation of the lung. Large left-sided congenital cystic adenomatoid malformations. Mediastinal shift is severe, and the lesion is mainly large cysts. sp, spine.

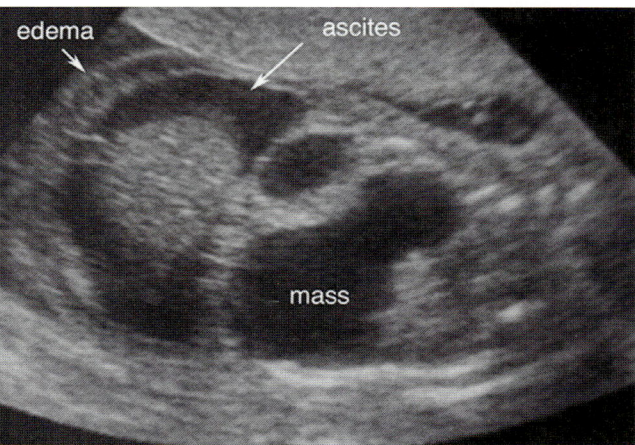

FIGURE 21. Cystic adenomatoid malformation of the lung with hydrops. Hydrops fetalis (integumentary *edema*, *ascites*) associated with congenital cystic adenomatoid malformation (*mass*).

pler imaging may be used to demonstrate this (Fig. 21). Demonstrating the pulmonary arterial supply to the mass helps to distinguish it from an extralobar sequestration (ELS), which is fed by a systemic artery.

Pleural effusion is almost never associated with CCAM unless hydrops is present. Even then, the mass usually occupies so much volume in the chest that pleural effusions are either absent or relatively small compared to the other serous effusions. Hydrops fetalis (Fig. 21) occurs in the

minority of fetuses with CCAMs but is extremely important evidence of fetal decompensation. As a rule, hydrops is only associated with large lesions.

The size of the mass—not the size of the cysts within the mass—is the feature that most greatly influences prognosis. There is no standard categorical description of the size of a CCAM. The lesion is usually described as large if it occupies greater than two-thirds of the hemithorax, medium sized if it occupies greater than one-third and less than two-thirds, and small if it occupies less than one-third of the hemithorax (Fig. 22). Mediastinal shift is considered severe if the heart is displaced to the contralateral rib cage (Fig. 23).

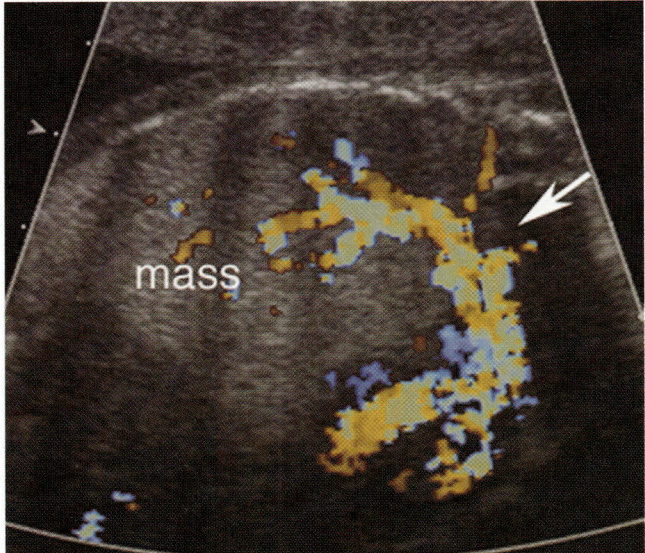

FIGURE 20. Cystic adenomatoid malformation of the lung. Large solid lung mass is fed by the pulmonary artery (*arrow*), suggesting a cystic adenomatoid malformation.

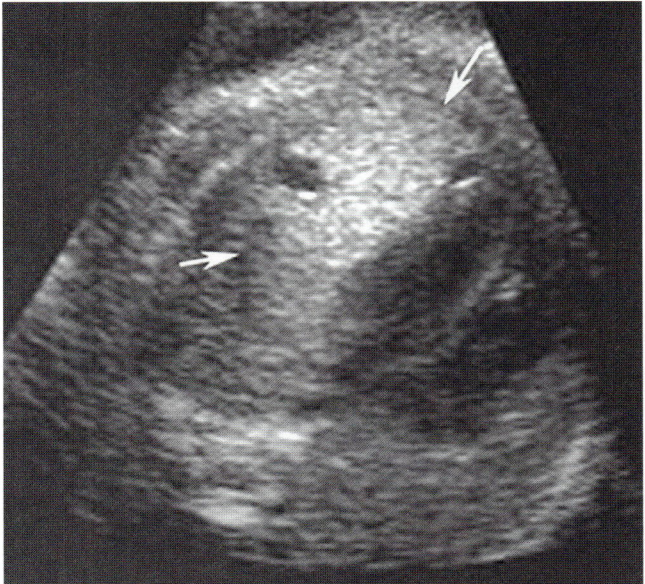

FIGURE 22. Left-sided cystic adenomatoid malformation (*arrows*). The mass is largely echogenic in nature and also contains a small cyst. The heart is shifted mildly to the right.

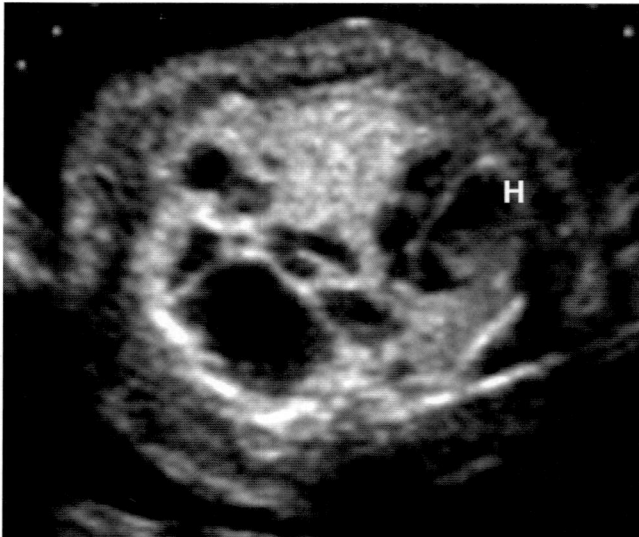

FIGURE 23. Large cystic adenomatoid malformation with heart (*H*) shifted to contralateral rib cage. The mass is mixed echogenic and multicystic. Skin thickening and ascites (not shown) indicate hydrops.

The presence of cysts within a lung mass makes the diagnosis of CCAM most likely (once CDH has been excluded). The size of the cysts, while not as important for prognosis, may be important in planning management of the pregnancy because percutaneous aspiration and drainage of a large, dominant cyst can decrease the size of the mass sufficiently to be a life-saving intervention in some.

Differential Diagnosis

If the mass is cystic, diagnostic considerations include CCAM; hybrid CCAM and sequestration; CDH; teratoma; neuroenteric cyst; esophageal duplication; or, less likely, pulmonary sequestration. CCAMs may appear cystic or solid, and sequestrations usually appear solid. However, *hybrid* masses contain elements of CCAM and sequestration but are sonographically interpreted to be a CCAM owing to the presence of cysts.[81,99] Currently we are not able to accurately identify hybrid lesions, but this is not known to influence outcome.

If the mass appears predominantly solid, the two most likely diagnoses are microcystic CCAM or sequestration. Less likely considerations include congenital lobar emphysema (CLE)[100] (Fig. 24) or an obstructed lung or lung lobe due to bronchial atresia or bronchogenic cyst. A small, rather inconspicuous bronchogenic cyst strategically positioned can cause the entire lung or lobe to distend into a solid-appearing mass (see Bronchogenic Cyst), and this may be misinterpreted as a CCAM. Thus the mediastinum should be scrutinized for a possible small obstructing bronchogenic cyst.

Associated Anomalies

CCAMs are not commonly associated with extrapulmonary anomalies or chromosomal defects, but renal and chromosomal anomalies have been associated with CCAM, mostly with Stocker's type II lesions. However, the rate of associated anomalies reported varies widely—from a high of 26% in postmortem studies by Stocker,[80] to 8% to 12% in prenatal

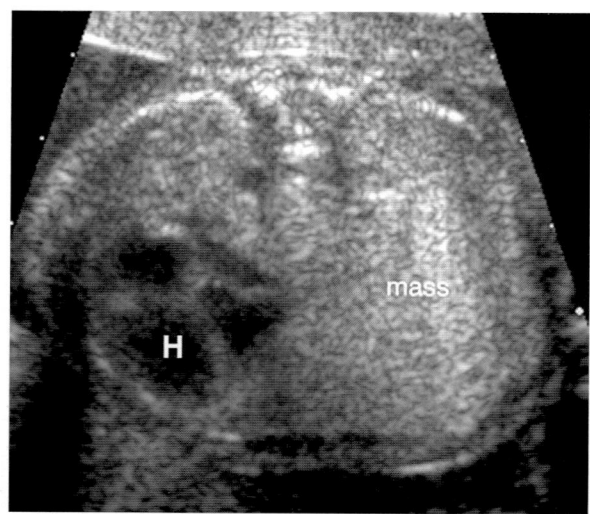

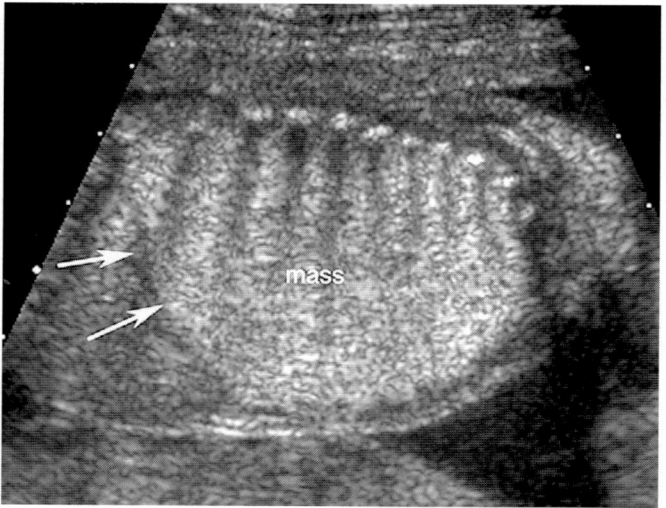

FIGURE 24. Left-sided solid lesion pathologically proven to be congenital lobar emphysema. **A:** Transaxial image demonstrates solid left-sided lesions, which were misinterpreted as a cystic adenomatoid malformation. H, heart. **B:** The mass is large with mass effect on the diaphragm (*arrows*).

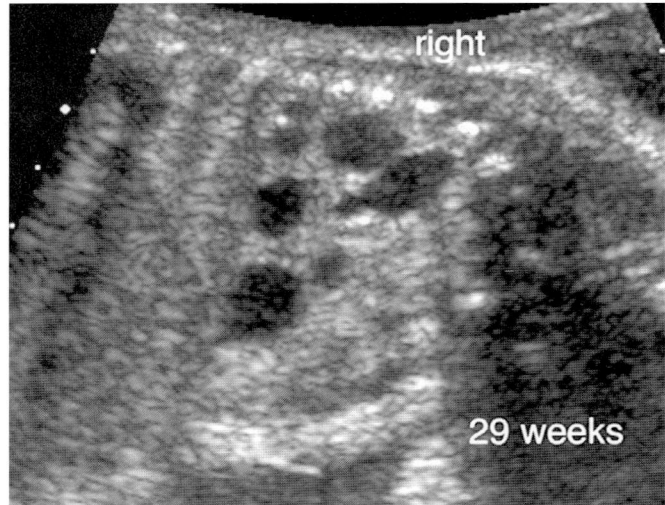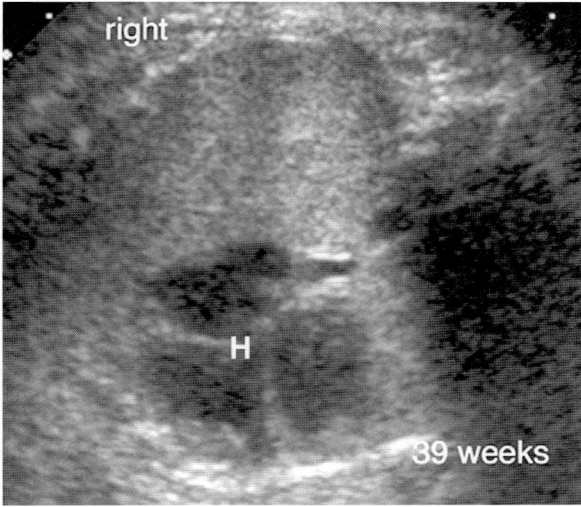

FIGURE 25. Regression of cystic adenomatoid malformation. **A:** Sagittal image at 29 weeks shows a moderate-sized right-sided lesion with many cysts. **B:** Axial image of same fetus as **(A)** at 39 weeks. The mass is imperceptible, and the cardiac shift has resolved. H, heart.

series,[81,97] to 3% in infants diagnosed postnatally and reported by pediatric surgeons.[101–103] The association of CCAM with other abnormalities has not been confirmed by all investigators.[104,105] Associated nonpulmonary malformations may be more common in fetuses with bilateral CCAMs.[97] As mentioned in Embryology and Pathology, some CCAMs are *hybrid* with other developmental abnormalities of the lung (such as sequestration, bronchogenic cyst, or bronchial atresia), but this diagnosis is usually not made until after birth.

The risk of chromosomal anomalies in association with CCAM may be slightly increased over the average patient, but the precise risk is not known. Among 25 cases reported by Bromley et al., two (8%) had chromosomal abnormalities (trisomy 21 and 18), and both fetuses had additional sonographic abnormalities.[81] In another series, only one (0.8%) fetus among 132 fetuses with CCAMs had an abnormal karyotype (trisomy 18).[97] Until there is convincing evidence that the rate of chromosomal abnormalities is not increased significantly in these fetuses, consideration for chromosomal analysis (as well as careful fetal anatomic survey) is probably warranted after diagnosis of CCAM in the fetus.

Prognosis and Management

Survival rate of fetuses with CCAMs is generally good, and most large series report 70% to 85% survival rates.[106,107] Among nonhydropic fetuses, survival approaches 100%. This is contrary to what was known about this fetal lesion before the early 1990s when most reports described the sickest fetuses. In the majority of fetuses with CCAMs detected today, no prenatal therapy is required or indicated.

After associated anomalies are excluded, the most important prognostic factor in a fetus with a CCAM is the presence or absence of hydrops. It was once thought that solid-appearing lesions were associated with the worst outcomes. The size of the mass might also be important, although even large masses have been seen to resolve spontaneously with a normal outcome.[9]

Despite an often-worrisome appearance during the second trimester, CCAMs rarely enlarge after the beginning of the third trimester. In fact, most lesions appear to get smaller, either absolutely or relatively, with advancing gestational age[81,108,109] (Figs. 25 through 27). The first signs of regression can occur as early as the second trimester but may not be evident until the third trimester. In the majority of cases, the mass gets smaller relative to the size of the growing fetal chest.[110] In some, the mass regresses so much that it is completely imperceptible on the sonogram by term, and the lesion may be *invisible* on plain chest x-ray at birth (Fig. 27B). However, in our experience, the lesions don't really disappear,[79] as they can always be detected on computed tomography scans after birth (Fig. 27C).[111,112]

Fetal outcome is poor in the presence of hydrops, with a rate of fetal or neonatal death more than 90%.[113] In one series,[9] in 1998, there were no survivors among hydropic fetuses with CCAMs who were treated expectantly. Thus the "don't touch" approach must be seriously reconsidered once hydrops develops. If fetal salvage is desired, fetal treatment or preterm delivery is considered. If the mass is predominantly cystic and there is a large cyst, percutaneous aspiration and catheter drainage may be attempted. If the fetus is already hydropic, however, there may not be enough time to determine whether the fetus will respond to aspiration, and fetal surgery must be considered. Because the fetus is so sick, the decision to deliver or perform fetal surgery must be made expeditiously.

Hydrops is much less common than once thought. Despite the tertiary referral pattern of the practice at Uni-

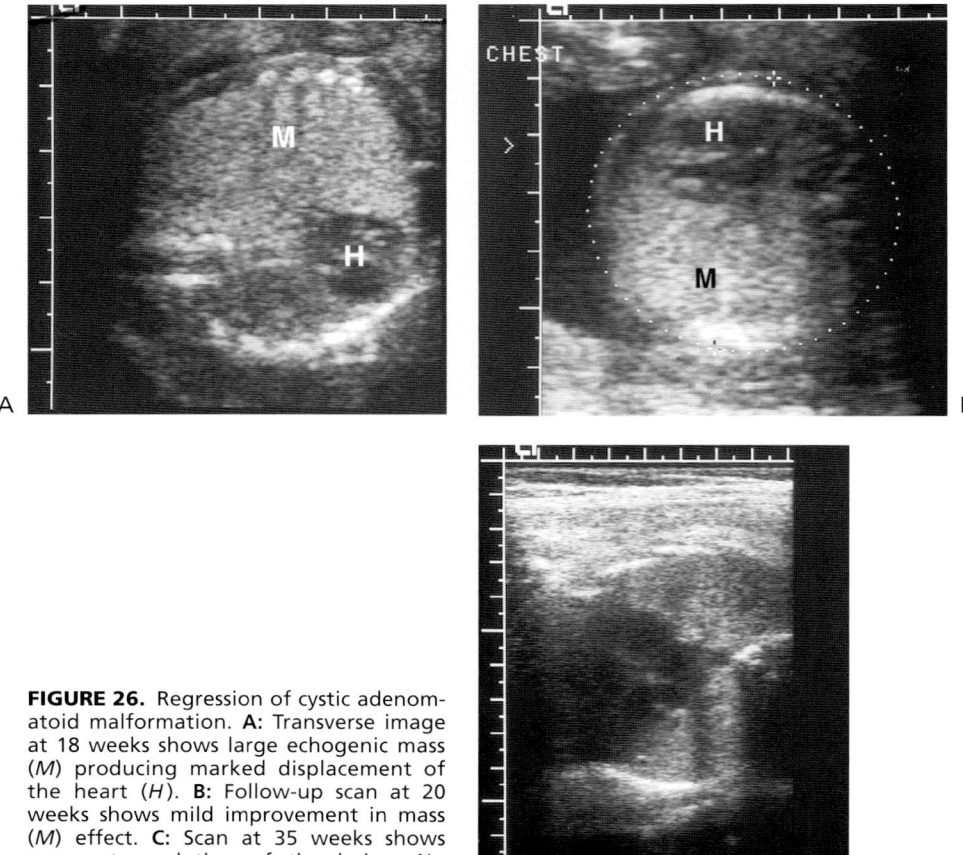

FIGURE 26. Regression of cystic adenomatoid malformation. **A:** Transverse image at 18 weeks shows large echogenic mass (*M*) producing marked displacement of the heart (*H*). **B:** Follow-up scan at 20 weeks shows mild improvement in mass (*M*) effect. **C:** Scan at 35 weeks shows apparent resolution of the lesion. No mass effect is appreciated.

versity of California San Francisco, hydrops is seen in fewer than 10% of fetuses with CCAMs. This is similar to the 8% rate of hydrops reported by Monni et al. in 2000.[114] While development of hydrops appears somewhat related to the size of the mass, because small lesions never become hydropic, development of hydrops is not predictable. Also, even large lesions typically are associated with a normal outcome and do not develop hydrops.

Resection of all masses is the preferred treatment at University of California San Francisco. This is usually delayed a variable amount of time after birth but performed during the first year of life. While expectant surveillance is an attractive treatment option, especially because 70% of neonates with CCAMs are asymptomatic at birth, many feel that CCAMs should be resected. Reasons for resection are the high rate of infection and air trapping and an increased risk (albeit small) of developing a carcinoma, particularly pleuropulmonary blastoma (i.e., rhabdosarcoma).[115–119] It is uncertain, however, whether prior resection is protective against development of such tumors.[120] Postnatal embolization of the mass has also been successfully performed.[121]

At University of California San Francisco, the following plan for management of a fetal CCAM has evolved since the late 1980s. No antenatal treatment is offered if the fetus does not show signs of hydrops. Frequent surveillance is performed (serial sonograms) until the third trimester or good evidence that the mass is stable in size or regressing (very few get bigger in the third trimester). If hydrops is detected before 24 weeks' gestational age, termination is offered. If hydrops is detected after 32 weeks, early delivery is offered in most cases. If the gestational age is 25 to 32 weeks, *in utero* resection or drainage of the fetal chest mass is offered. In our experience, following fetal surgery on hydropic fetuses, survival rates can be improved to greater than 50%.[118]

Recurrence Risk

There is no known recurrence risk for CCAM of the lung.

PULMONARY SEQUESTRATION

Description

Pulmonary sequestration is a supernumerary lobe of the lung, separated from the normal tracheobronchial tree

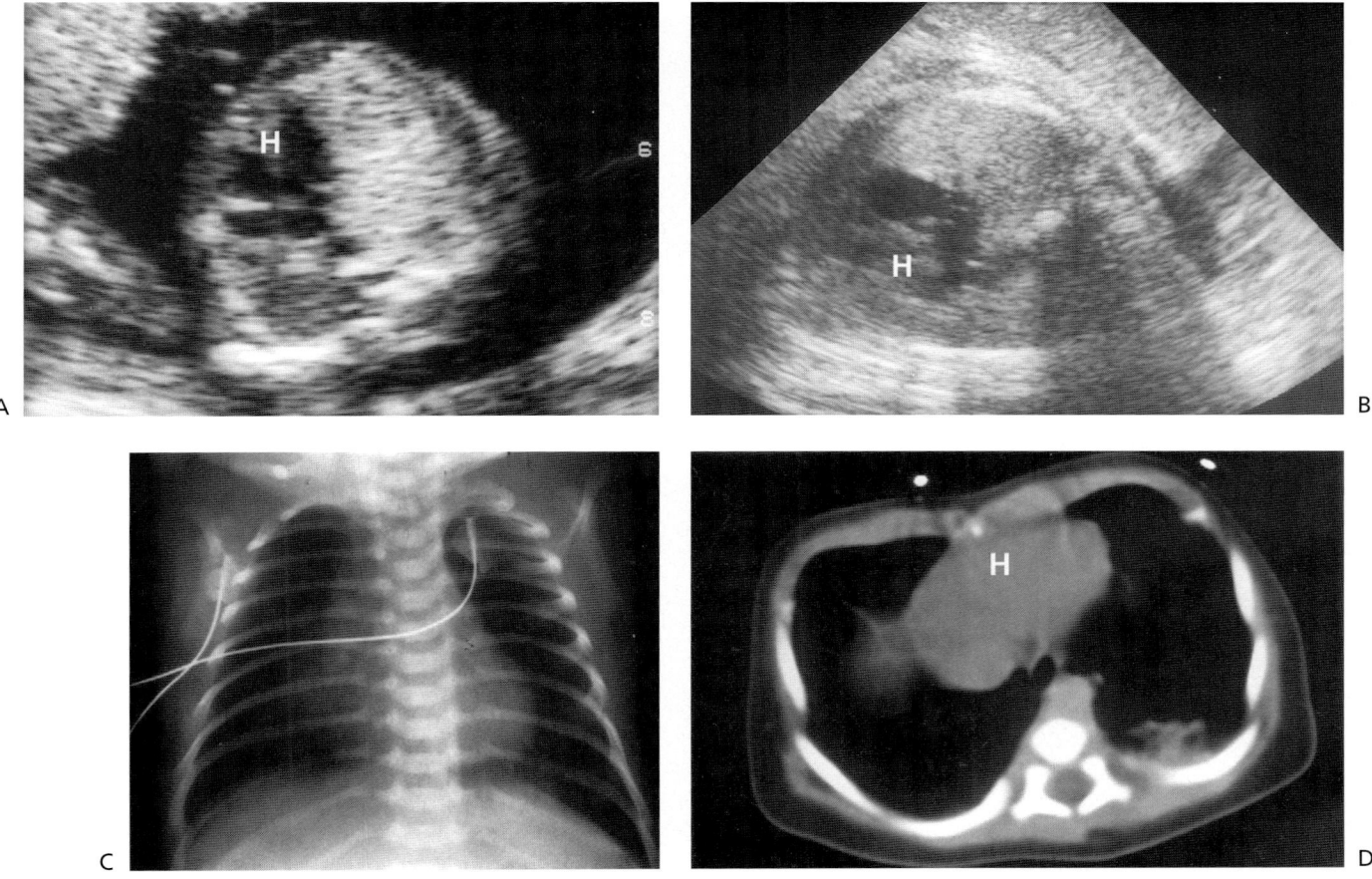

FIGURE 27. Resolution of cystic adenomatoid malformation. **A:** Transverse scan at 17 weeks shows echogenic mass in left thorax. Some displacement of the heart (*H*) to the right is shown. **B:** Follow-up scan at 32 weeks shows apparent resolution of mass. **C:** Postnatal radiograph appears normal, and the infant was asymptomatic. **D:** Computed tomography scan shows density in left lower lobe. Cystic adenomatoid malformation was resected at 9 months of age.

(from Latin *sequestrate*, which means to separate).[122,123] These lesions are also considered bronchopulmonary foregut malformations.

Prevalence

Pulmonary sequestration is divided into intralobar and extralobar types. Intralobar sequestrations account for 75% to 85% of all sequestrations diagnosed in adults and are only rarely detected in fetuses. Conversely, ELS accounts for nearly all of the sequestrations diagnosed prenatally. ELS is an uncommon anomaly with an estimated incidence of 0.15% to 1.7% in the general population,[124] but the precise incidence is not known. While ELSs are reported to account for approximately 0.5% to 6.0% of all congenital lesions of the thorax,[125] ELSs are known to account for a greater proportion of lung masses detected before birth. In one series, pulmonary sequestrations accounted for at least 12% to 16% of fetal chest masses misdiagnosed as CCAMs,[109] and ELSs accounted for 23% of the 175 fetal chest masses reported by Adzick et al.[9]

ELS had originally been reported to be more common in males (4 to 1)[126] but have been more recently reported to occur roughly as equal in males and females.[91]

Pathology

ELS is invested by its own pleura (*Rokitansky's lobe*), and the intralobar form resides within the pleural investment of a pulmonary lobe.[127] The two forms also differ in their blood supply and drainage. Intralobar sequestrations are nearly always drained by pulmonary veins, whereas extralobar forms most commonly drain into systemic veins (80%). Systemic arteries feed both forms, but the extralobar form characteristically receives its arterial supply from a large single vessel off the descending aorta. ELS is considered to represent a true congenital malformation, whereas many intralobar sequestrations are thought to be acquired during postnatal life. Microscopic chronic inflammation and fibrosis are typical of intralobar sequestrations.

ELS most likely results from the growth of an anomalous or supernumerary lung bud that receives its blood supply from the primitive splanchnic vessels of the foregut. These splanchnic vessels are connected to the primitive dorsal aorta and persist as the systemic feeding artery, present in nearly all ELSs.[128] The artery to the ELS from the thoracic or abdominal aorta is usually a single vessel (80%), but it may be supplied by multiple systemic arteries.[129] The venous drainage is usually systemic through the azygous system, the hemiazygous system, or the vena cava. Approximately 25% the ELS is partly drained through the pulmonary veins. The embryologic connection with the foregut typically involutes but may persist as a fibrous pedicle that accompanies the feeding and draining vessels.[130] In some cases, the foregut connection persists, accounting for a communication with the gastrointestinal tract that is occasionally found.[131]

Grossly, the lesion is *lobar* in shape, well circumscribed, and grossly appears *spongy*. Microscopically, the ELS resembles normal lung except that there is diffuse dilatation of the bronchioles, alveolar ducts, alveoli, and lymphatics. Dilated subpleural lymph vessels are seen in more than 85%. This may account for the hydrothorax that occurs in approximately 5% to 10% of fetuses with ELS.

The majority (80% to 90%) of ELSs occurs at the base of the left hemithorax,[129] between the left lung and diaphragm. In approximately 10%, the sequestration is located in the abdomen in the retroperitoneum hemithorax.[129,132]

Intraabdominal sequestrations are thought to develop just before closure of the diaphragm so that the sequestered lung tissue is *trapped* in the abdomen. Rarely, an ELS may even be found in the mediastinum or within the pericardium.[133]

In many cases, the lung mass pathologically demonstrates elements of sequestration and CCAM (*hybrid lesion*). Histologically, CCAM type II has been described in as many as 50% of ELSs.[91,134] The cysts of a CCAM in a hybrid lesion may increase the conspicuity of the mass and improve antenatal detection of ELS. Hybrid lesions seem to be more common among sequestrations, which are diagnosed before birth. Conran and Stocker[91] noted that 11 out of 12 prenatally detected ELSs had elements of CCAM in contrast to 50% of the whole series of ELSs they evaluated.[91] Intrathoracic and intraabdominal sequestrations may demonstrate elements of sequestration and CCAM.[135,136]

Diagnosis

ELSs are detected sonographically as well-circumscribed echogenic masses, lobar or triangular in shape, in the base of the left fetal chest (Figs. 28 and 29A). Like CCAMs, sequestrations come in all sizes—small, medium, or large—but, on average, they tend to be small- or moderate-sized lesions. Large sequestrations, however, may occur and can cause mediastinal shift and hydrops.

The majority of ELSs is homogeneous in echotexture although cysts (dilated bronchioles or hybrid lesions containing CCAM) are occasionally observed. A well-formed bronchus is located at one edge of the lesion in approxi-

mately one-half of the pathologically assessed lesions.[129] In my experience, this is much less commonly appreciated in the antenatal evaluation.

The fetal diagnosis of ELS has been made on sonograms as early as 16 weeks.[137] Visualization of a systemic artery arising from the thoracic or abdominal aorta feeding the mass strongly favors the diagnosis of ELS (Fig. 29B), because the arterial supply to most other masses considered in the differential diagnosis (i.e., CCAM, lobar emphysema, bronchial atresia) is from the pulmonary artery. Color and spectral Doppler can be extremely helpful in visualizing the large, commonly single, feeding systemic artery but may be inconsistently detected prenatally.[138] Whereas the venous drainage of most ELSs is to systemic veins, the nature of the venous drainage is difficult to visualize sonographically. Many of these lesions are of mixed histology and the precise pathologic diagnosis is less important for prognosis than the size, mediastinal shift, and the absence or presence of hydrops.

A hydrothorax ipsilateral to the mass may occur in approximately 5% to 10% of cases of ELS (Fig. 30).[9,96,97,138,139] Because hydrothorax is almost never seen in association with a CCAM, this observation lends support for the diagnosis of ELS. While not common, hydrothorax is an important complication of ELS since a large *tension* hydrothorax, causing cardiomediastinal shift and hydrops, can convert a rather modestly sized mass into a life-threatening situation. In these cases, the hydrothorax is much more conspicuous on the sonogram than the sequestered lobe (Fig. 31).

The precise pathophysiologic mechanism for the development of hydrothorax is not known, but torsion on the vascular pedicle of the mass or lymph secretion from the dilated lymphatic channels in the mass are believed to be the most likely explanation.[140,141] It is not known how to predict which fetuses with sequestrations are prone to this complication.

Approximately 10% to 15% of ELSs are found within or below the diaphragm (usually on the left) (Fig. 32).[129,132] Subdiaphragmatic sequestrations do not seem to influence fetal health, have not been associated with hydrops, and tend to be asymptomatic after birth.

Differential Diagnosis

Pulmonary sequestration should be considered in any fetus with a solid chest mass, especially if the mass has a lobar shape and is found in the left lower thorax. Other masses to consider are CCAM, lobar emphysema, and bronchial atresia resulting in an obstructed and distended lobe.[142] Cysts are not typical in a pulmonary sequestration but can be observed. If cysts are seen in a chest mass in the fetus, the lesion is likely to be misinterpreted as a CCAM. This probably does not alter the prognosis or management, especially if there is no evidence of hydrops. A systemic feeding artery in association with cysts in the mass is suggestive of a hybrid CCAM/ELS. Distinguishing bronchial atresia or lobar overinflation from an ELS is based mainly on location

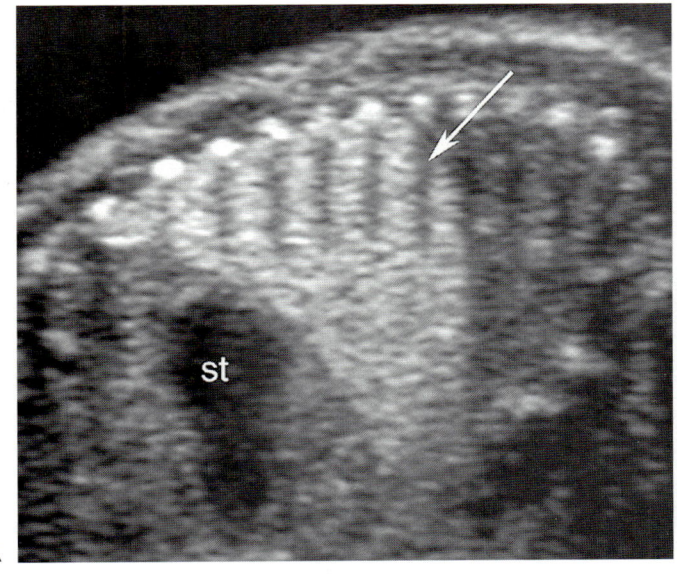

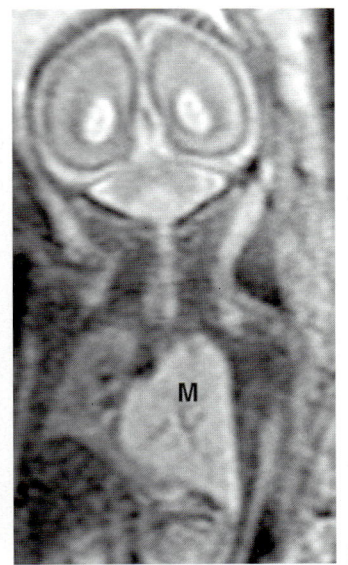

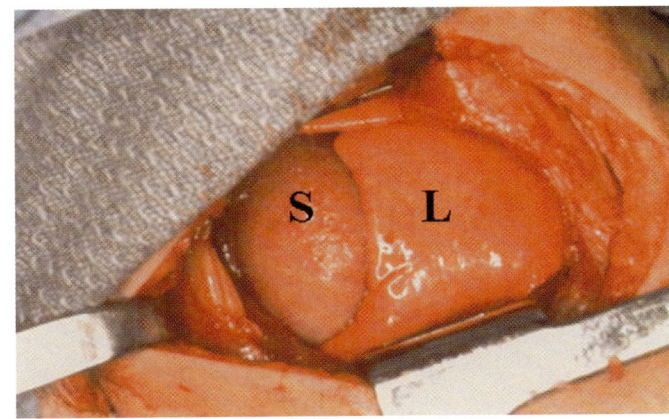

FIGURE 28. Small extralobar sequestration. **A:** Small, solid, lobar-shaped mass (*arrow*) at the left lung base. The stomach (*st*) is in normal position below the diaphragm. **B:** Magnetic resonance imaging scan, T2 weighted, in similar patient shows triangular-shaped mass (*M*) of high signal intensity in left lower lobe. **C:** Photograph at time of surgical resections shows sequestered lobe (*S*) separate from the lung (*L*).

(ELS tends to be left and lower lobe, the others upper lobe) and the systemic arterial supply of the ELS.

Other considerations for an intrathoracic mass include diaphragmatic hernia, duplication cyst, or tumor. An angioma mimicked pulmonary sequestration in one case.[143] This mass resolved completely after treatment by partial embolization.

A suprarenal echogenic mass in the left abdomen usually represents ELS but can also suggest neuroblastoma or adrenal hemorrhage. As distinguishing features, an ELS is typically echogenic, solid, left-sided, and can be identified in the second trimester, whereas neuroblastoma is most often cystic, right-sided, and most often detected in the third trimester (Table 7).[144] This is discussed further in Chapter 13.

Associated Anomalies

The likelihood of other anomalies is increased slightly in association with ELS. Some authors report an associated anomaly rate as high as 50% to 65% in individuals with ELS,[123,131] but the prevalence of associated anomalies seems to be lower in fetal studies. The cause of this discrepancy is not completely understood but may be due to selection bias (anomalous fetuses not referred to fetal therapy centers) or, perhaps, due to more complete reporting of smaller, potentially asymptomatic and isolated lesions that have been increasingly detected antenatally in recent years. Adzick et al. described 41 fetuses with ELSs in the largest series of fetal lung masses published to date.[9] In contrast to other reports, these authors found no significant anatomic or karyotypic anomalies in these fetuses. However, one-half of the reported 10 cases detected prenatally (all pathologically proven) by Becmeur et al.[138] had associated anomalies although some of the anomalies were minor (including contralateral lung segmental anomalies, *prune belly* due to fetal ascites, accessory diaphragm, aortic coarctation, and CCAM within the sequestration). It is conceivable that minor abnormalities may be missed on prenatal sonograms. In a review of subdiaphragmatic ELSs reported by Curtis et al., only 2 of the 18 (11%) cases described were associated with significant congenital anomalies.[144]

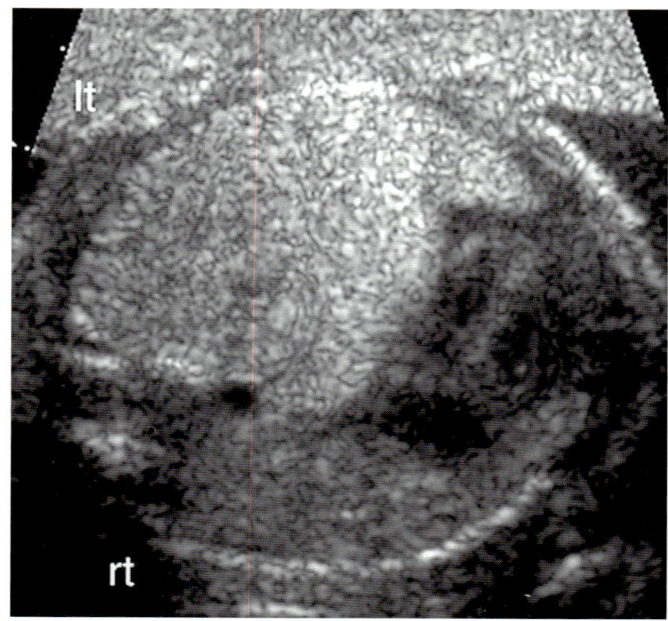
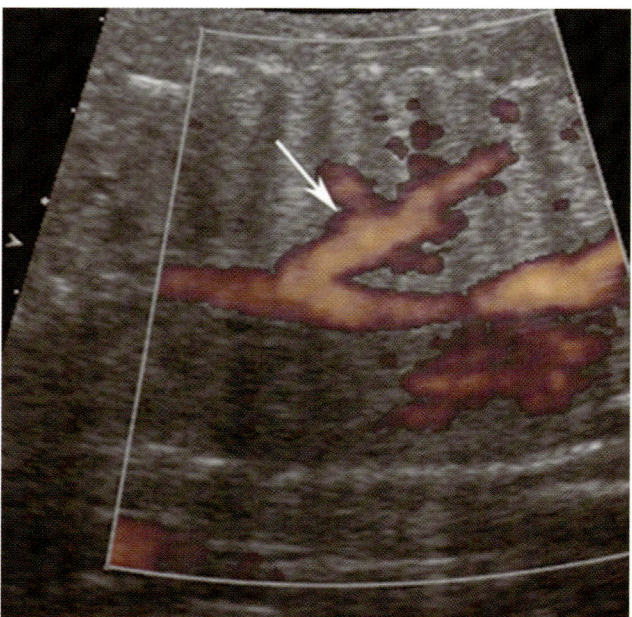

A   B

FIGURE 29. Medium-sized extralobar sequestration. **A:** Axial image shows solid, echogenic mass at the left lung base. lt, left; rt, right. **B:** Coronal image demonstrates a large feeding artery (*arrow*) directly from the descending aorta.

The anomalies most commonly associated with ELS are CDH[129] and diaphragmatic eventration or paralysis.[58] It is speculated that failure of the developing diaphragm too close around the embryologic connection to the foregut may explain the association with CDH. Other reported anomalies have included communication of the ELS with the esophagus or stomach, bronchogenic cyst, pericardial defect, CCAM, foregut duplication or diverticulum, ectopic pancreas, vertebral anomalies, and pectus excavatum. Of 15 ELSs reported by Stocker, three also had bronchogenic cysts.[129] Some favor a common embryologic origin of bronchopulmonary foregut malformations, and many of the fetal lung lesions detected prenatally ultimately have more than one pathologic diagnosis.

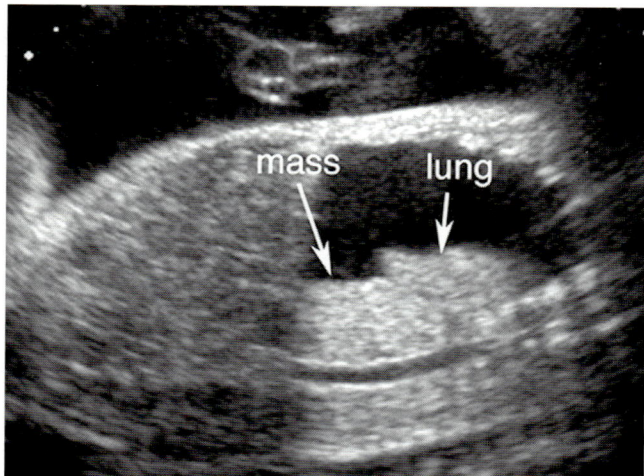

FIGURE 30. Left-sided hydrothorax associated with an extralobar sequestration (*mass*). Mass effect on the flattened diaphragm (*arrow*) is due to the large hydrothorax, not the sequestration. st, stomach.

FIGURE 31. Hydrothorax associated with a right-sided extralobar sequestration. Coronal image shows large hydrothorax and relatively inconspicuous mass inferior to right lung.

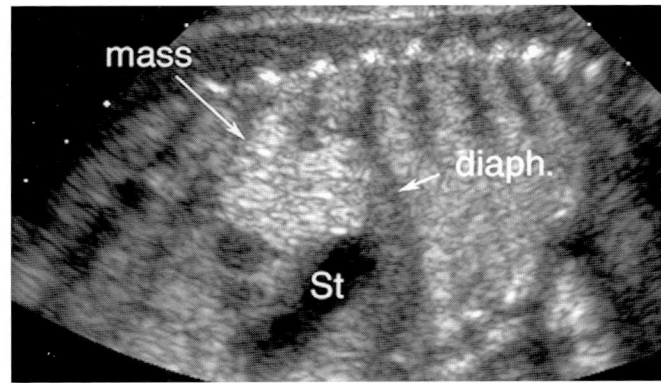

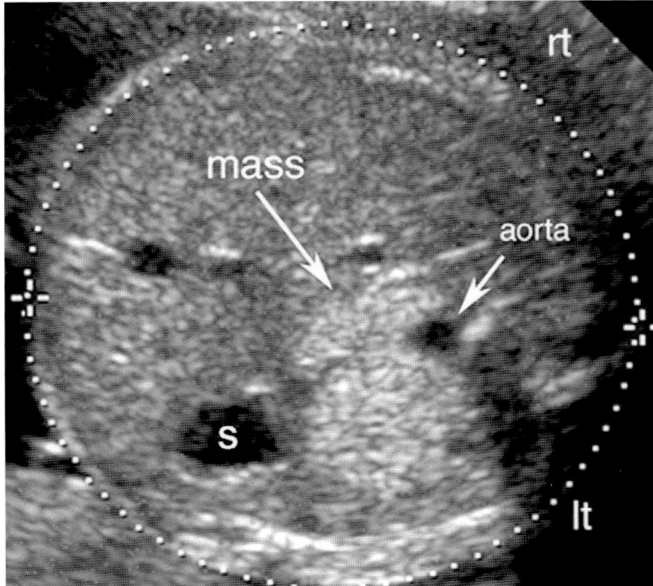

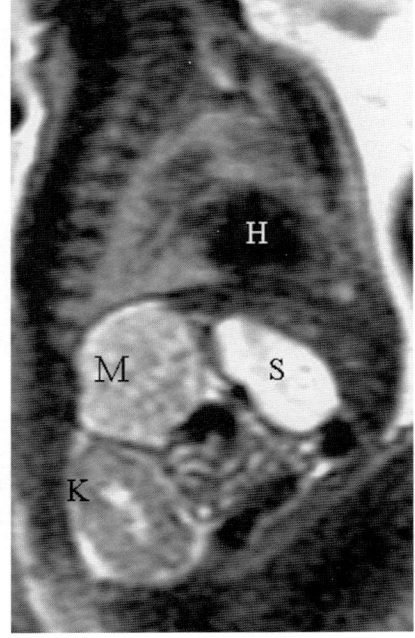

FIGURE 32. Subdiaphragmatic extralobar pulmonary sequestration. **A:** Sagittal image shows a solid mass below the diaphragm, posterior to the stomach (*St*) and superior to the left kidney. One or two small cysts are seen within the mass. diaph., diaphragm. **B:** Axial image of the same fetus as in (**A**) shows an echogenic mass posterior to the stomach (*S*) on the left (*lt*) and adjacent to the aorta. rt, right. **C:** Magnetic resonance imaging shows mass (*M*) of high signal below diaphragm and posterior to stomach (*S*). H, heart; K, kidney.

Prognosis and Management

The prognosis of fetuses with sequestrations is usually excellent. Lopoo et al. reported 100% survival among 13 fetuses with 15 pulmonary sequestrations.[139] Only one patient required prenatal intervention. In this fetus, a large hydrothorax resulted in hydrops, which was successfully treated with a thoracoamniotic shunt.

The prognosis is mainly related to the frequency of serious secondary physiologic derangements seen with any chest mass—pulmonary hypoplasia and hydrops. The true incidence of hydrops is not known and varies considerably among centers. Earlier reports suggested a relatively high (35%) rate of hydrops,[145] but more recent series suggest a rate no higher than 7% to 18%.[9,139] The one case reported by Lopoo et al.[139] was presumably caused by the large tension hydrothorax that was present.

Because sequestrations tend to be small- or medium-sized lesions, it is likely that many small sequestrations are not detected before birth. These small lesions are thought to have a benign clinical course and usually are not associated with any respiratory symptoms at birth.[91,139]

What is known about the natural history of fetal sequestrations also allows us to remain optimistic in most cases. Similar to CCAMs, sequestrations may regress during gestation and may have an even greater propensity to do so than CCAMs. It is estimated that 50% to 75% of prenatally detected sequestrations demonstrate partial or complete regression on serial sonograms.[138,146] Especially impressive is the description of one fetus initially diagnosed at 24 weeks

TABLE 7. INFRADIAPHRAGMATIC EXTRALOBAR SEQUESTRATION VERSUS NEUROBLASTOMA

	Distinguishing features	
	Extralobar sequestration	**Neuroblastoma**
Echotexture	Echogenic, solid	Cystic
Laterality	Left	Right
Time of diagnosis	Second trimester	Third trimester

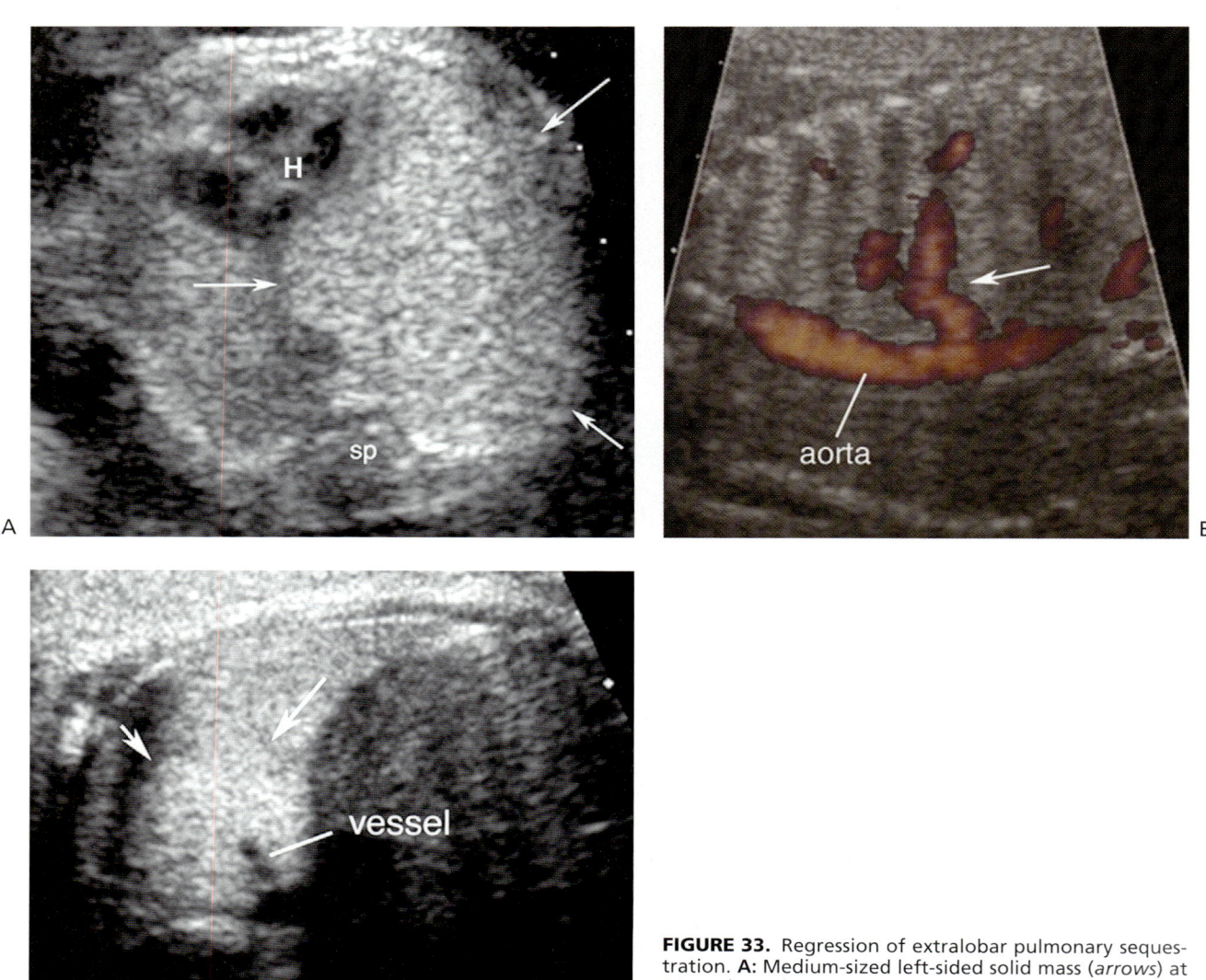

FIGURE 33. Regression of extralobar pulmonary sequestration. **A:** Medium-sized left-sided solid mass (*arrows*) at 21 weeks. H, heart; sp, spine. **B:** Same fetus as in **(A)** at 21 weeks. Large feeding artery (*arrow*) from the descending aorta. **C:** Same fetus as in **(A)** at 32 weeks. The sequestration (*arrows*) and feeding artery are both considerably smaller.

with signs of hydrops, which disappeared as the lesion regressed during the third trimester, underscoring the potential for even ominous cases to improve.[9] Further, all of the babies with regressed sequestrations in Adzick's series were asymptomatic at birth and have been followed without resection.[9] We have observed at least one very large ELS with a large feeding artery regress dramatically during gestation, which resulted in an asymptomatic neonate (Fig. 33).

Before birth, if hydrothorax and hydrops are present, treatment is directed at draining the fluid because, in most cases, the tension hydrothorax, not the lung mass, is the cause of the hydrops. A thoracentesis alone is usually insufficient treatment of the hydrothorax owing to the rapid reaccumulation of fluid, but the fluid can be safely drained with a percutaneously placed thoracoamniotic shunt (Fig. 34).[138,147] The potential occurrence of this complication

mandates that all fetuses with suspected sequestrations, even small- or medium-sized lesions, are followed closely during gestation.

After birth, management is usually surgical resection. However, treatment with arterial embolization has also been used. Curros et al.[148] treated 16 children with sequestrations by vascular embolization. Of these, ten were considered successful from embolization alone with complete resolution, three showed partial resolution, one was unsuccessful and underwent resection, and two were still being followed at the time of the report.

Recurrence Risk

There is no known recurrent risk with pulmonary sequestration.

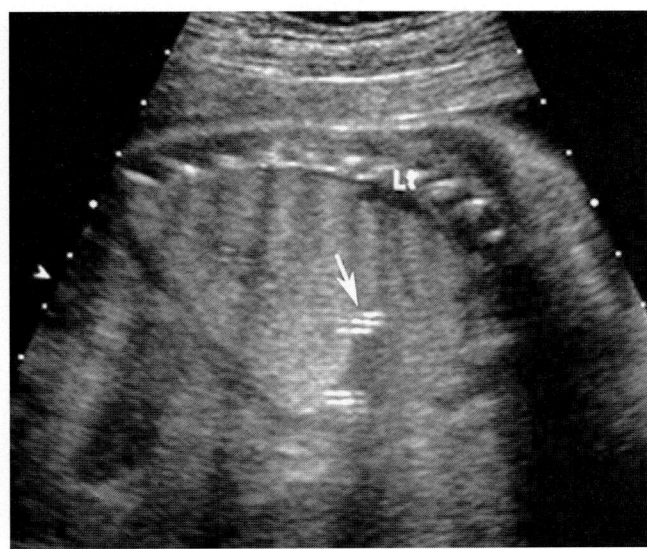

FIGURE 34. Catheter drainage of large hydrothorax of fetus in Figure 29 was successfully accomplished. Arrow indicates catheter. Lt, left.

BRONCHOGENIC CYST

Description

Bronchogenic cysts are cystic lesions lined by bronchial epithelium that may occur in the mediastinum or lung.

Prevalence

Prevalence for bronchogenic cyst is rare. Bronchogenic cysts account for approximately 8% of mediastinal masses detected in children.[149]

Embryology and Pathology

Bronchogenic cysts are considered bronchopulmonary foregut abnormalities. They arise due to abnormal budding of the tracheobronchial tree and foregut, in many cases as accessory lung buds of the ventral diverticulum of the foregut.[149] The cysts probably form between the twenty-sixth and fortieth day of fetal life, when the most active tracheobronchial development is occurring.[149] The cysts are lined by mucus-secreting respiratory epithelium and, as a result, may be filled with mucinous secretions.

Most bronchogenic cysts occur in the middle mediastinum, usually near the tracheal carina, but more than 15% can occur in the lung, pleura, and diaphragm. Rarely may the cysts also occur in unusual locations including the neck and abdomen.[150] Mediastinal cysts usually do not communicate with the bronchial tree but are often attached to the airway through a common wall or pedicle.[151] Intrapulmonary bronchogenic cysts, which may be more common than once

thought, may result from a later insult in embryogenesis, and, unlike the mediastinal cysts, intrapulmonary cysts usually communicate with the bronchial tree.

Because bronchogenic cysts are rarely detected antenatally, most information about the appearance and natural history of these cysts is derived from the postnatal imaging, surgical, and pathologic reports.

Bronchogenic cysts can be tiny or large—a few millimeters to more than 5 cm. They may appear as uni- or multilocular and may contain layering echogenic material.[152,153] Approximately two-thirds of intrapulmonary cysts occur in the lower lobes.[152–154]

Diagnosis

Very few cases of bronchogenic cysts have been detected before birth. The cyst may be fluid filled or contain layering debris. While they may be small and difficult to detect antenatally, the *effects* of the cyst on the fetal lung can be much more conspicuous and serious. An enlarged obstructed fetal lung may be detected despite the fact that the obstructing cyst is not detected[154] or incorrectly diagnosed, as another lesion such as a CCAM. Most bronchogenic cysts are small and located in the mediastinum. Because the thoracic cavity is small in the fetus, it may be difficult to detect a small mediastinal cyst, particularly if it contains echogenic fluid. If unilateral fetal lung hyperinflation is observed, however, the mediastinum should be carefully scrutinized for an obstructing mass. Fetal MRI has been helpful in further evaluation of the anatomy.[155]

Differential Diagnosis

Differential diagnosis of a cystic mass in the mediastinum or lung includes CCAM, bronchogenic cyst, neuroenteric cyst, or duplication cyst (usually esophagus). If the cyst causes obstruction of the lung, the lung appears enlarged and echogenic, and the differential diagnosis includes causes of bronchial obstruction, such as bronchogenic cyst, bronchial atresia, and CLE.

Associated Anomalies

Other congenital pulmonary malformations such as sequestration, lobar emphysema, and even CDH are occasionally associated with bronchogenic cysts. The coexistence of three anomalies, bronchogenic cyst, ELS, and CCAM, has led some to suggest a common embryologic link.[92]

Prognosis and Management

In the fetus, if a mediastinal cyst, thought to be a bronchogenic cyst, is detected, frequent surveillance is recommended. Too few bronchogenic cysts have been observed before birth to accurately predict their natural history during gestation.

Most bronchogenic cysts are detected in the first few decades of life. After birth, bronchogenic cysts may be detected incidentally or in symptomatic individuals (usually pain or infection). Intrapulmonary cysts tend to be more symptomatic than mediastinal cysts, presumably due to the connection with the bronchial tree. There is a small risk of a future cancer developing within a bronchogenic cyst.[156,157] Thus, once detected, most cysts are surgically removed.

BRONCHIAL ATRESIA

Description

Congenital bronchial atresia is a rare anomaly in which a segmental bronchus does not communicate with the central airways.

PREVALENCE

Although bronchial atresia has been reported to be the second most common congenital tracheobronchial malformation, this lesion has only rarely been diagnosed prenatally.[142,158]

Embryology and Pathology

The cause of bronchial atresia is unknown, but a vascular insult has been postulated. Others have suggested that this occurs because of separation of the bronchial bud, which may explain why bronchial atresia may coexist with sequestrations and bronchogenic cysts. Bronchial atresia is characterized by a focal obliteration of a segment of the bronchial lumen, which presumably occurred during the fifth fetal week when segmental airways develop. In some cases the lung distal to the bronchial atresia has been noted to be dysplastic compatible with a CCAM.[93]

The most common site of bronchial atresia is the left upper lobe (two-thirds), followed by the right upper and middle lobes. This lesion rarely occurs in the lower lobe.[97]

Diagnosis

In normal fetuses, the bronchi are not visualized. If a fetal main stem or segmental bronchus can be visualized on the sonogram, it is probably because it is fluid-filled and abnormal. The obstructed lung segment or lobe distally appears enlarged and echogenic.[142] In fact, the diagnosis of fetal bronchial atresia is really only considered if an enlarged echogenic lung, presumably obstructed by a stenotic or atretic bronchus, is observed. After birth, a mucous plug is often found distal to the area of atresia.[87]

Differential Diagnosis

The differential diagnosis of an enlarged echogenic lobe or lung suggests the presence of a *mass* obstructing the bronchus, an atresia/stenosis of the airway, or a lung mass such as a sequestration or microcystic CCAM. If the lung is enlarged due to obstruction, considerations include bronchogenic cyst, bronchial atresia, or other mass. It may be difficult to be more specific if the offending obstructing mass is not identified.

Associated Anomalies

Bronchial atresia may be associated with bronchogenic cyst, sequestrations, or CCAMs.

Prognosis and Management

Prognosis is related to the secondary effects, how distended the lung is postnatally and postoperative course. Bronchial atresia is not known to be associated with an increased risk of chromosomal abnormality.

CONGENITAL LOBAR EMPHYSEMA

Description

CLE, also known as *congenital lobar overinflation*, is lobar overinflation of the lung without destruction of alveolar septa. It usually occurs in the upper (left more than right) or middle lobe[159] and is located within the normal pleural envelope.

Prevalence

Few cases of CLE have been detected prenatally, and, therefore, this lesion is under-represented in fetal studies compared with pediatric series.[160] Children with this abnormality usually present in the first year of life,[161,162] often in the first few days, with respiratory symptoms.

Embryology and Pathology

CLE may occur secondary to anomalous development of a lobar or segmental bronchus[163] or intrinsic/extrinsic bronchial compression. It is postulated that the cause may also include an intrinsic cartilage deficiency or dysplasia of the bronchus. In more than 50% of cases, the cause is not found at surgery. The abnormality usually involves the upper lobes or right middle lobe. The lower lobes account for only 5% of cases.

Diagnosis

Sonographically, fetal CLE can appear identical to a microcystic CCAM, presenting as a large *solid* mass[100,142] (Fig.

24). In a single case reported by Richards et al.,[100] the large mass regressed (after treatment with indomethacin for preterm labor) at 34 weeks and was undetectable on the sonogram by 37 weeks.

Differential Diagnosis

There is nothing specific about the appearance of this mass in the fetus. Because CLE appears similar to a microcystic CCAM, the differential diagnosis includes CCAM, sequestration, bronchial atresia/stenosis, and overinflated lung, or other obstructing bronchial abnormality.

Associated Anomalies

Associated abnormalities have been reported in 14% to 50% of children with this diagnosis, and congenital heart disease tops the list of associated abnormalities (70%).[122] The most common cardiac defects associated include patent ductus arteriosus, ventricular septal defect, and tetralogy of Fallot.[164]

Prognosis and Management

Treatment is usually lobectomy due to childhood studies suggesting that most children with CLE become symptomatic during the neonatal period.

NEUROENTERIC CYST

Description

Neuroenteric cysts are posterior enteric remnants that result in a cystic mass in the posterior aspect of the thorax.

Prevalence

The incidence is not known but neuroenteric cysts are rare.

Embryology and Pathology

Neuroenteric cysts are thought to result from incomplete separation of the notochord from the foregut in the third week of embryogenesis. It is speculated that the cause is a persistent communication or adhesion between the ectoderm of the spinal cord and endoderm of the foregut before neural tube closure. The cysts are lined with epithelium of endodermal origin.

Neuroenteric cysts may occur in the chest or spinal canal. In the chest, they are most commonly located in the mediastinum, 90% posteriorly and 66% on the right side.[165] The cysts can penetrate the diaphragm and communicate with the small bowel.[166] Vertebral anomalies are always associated and are usually found more cephalad than the cystic chest mass owing to the differential rates of longitudinal growth of the spine and thorax.[167] When a neuroenteric cyst occurs in the spinal canal, it is usually in the lower cervical or upper thoracic spine.

Diagnosis

Few prenatally detected thoracic neuroenteric cysts have been reported,[168,169] but the abnormality has been detected as early as 22 weeks.[166] The typical sonographic appearance is that of a septated or bilobed cystic mass in the posterior chest (Fig. 35A). The mediastinal origin is difficult to appreciate sonographically. Thoracic or cervical spinal anomalies are always present (often hemi-vertebra), so any bony abnormality associated with a fetal thoracic cyst should suggest the diagnosis of neuroenteric cyst (Fig. 35B).

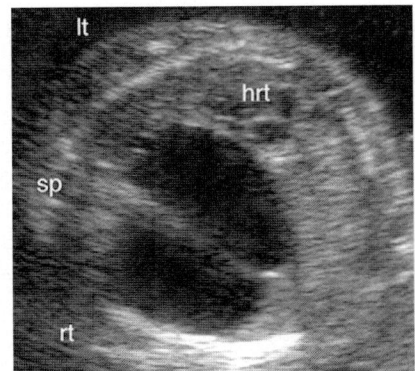 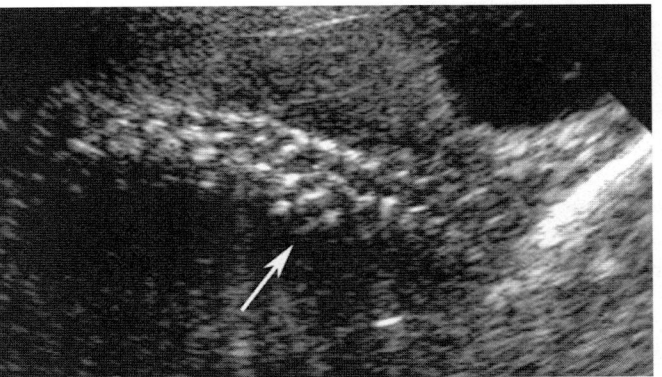

FIGURE 35. Neuroenteric cyst. **A:** Transaxial image demonstrates a large bilobed right (*rt*)-sided cystic mass in the posterior chest. hrt, heart; lt, left; sp, spine. **B:** Same fetus as in **(A)**. Abnormality of the cervicothoracic spine (*arrow*) suggests hemi- or butterfly vertebrae. A skeletal abnormality in association with a cystic chest mass in the fetus favors neuroenteric cyst.

Differential Diagnosis

Differential diagnosis includes macrocystic CCAM, CDH, gut duplication, and bronchogenic or neuroenteric cyst. The presence of vertebral anomalies implicates a neuroenteric cyst.

Associated Anomalies

The associated vertebral anomalies (Fig. 35B) include hemivertebrae, cleft vertebral body, posterior spina bifida, absent and fused vertebrae, and diastematomyelia. Less commonly occurring anomalies include elements of split notochord syndrome (cloacal/bladder exstrophy, renal agenesis) and intestinal anomalies such as imperforate anus, duplication, and malrotation. A stalk may connect the intraspinal and extraspinal spaces, although this connection is usually not appreciated sonographically.

Prognosis and Management

If large enough, fetal neuroenteric cysts may lead to hydrops,[169] a poor prognostic indicator. Fetal hydrops have accompanied fetal neuroenteric cysts in only two of the seven prenatally diagnosed cases reported. Once diagnosed, the mass is resected after birth. *In utero*, if the fetus develops hydrops, the cyst can be drained with a thoracoamniotic shunt. After birth, respiratory distress, often on the first day of life, is typical.

CONGENITAL HIGH AIRWAY OBSTRUCTION OR LARYNGEAL AND TRACHEAL ATRESIA

Description

Laryngeal and tracheal atresia, along with tracheal cysts or webs, are included in the category of congenital high airway obstructions (CHAOS). These entities are discussed under one heading because the sonographic findings of affected fetuses are similar—enlarged, bilateral, symmetric distended echogenic fetal lungs.

Three types of laryngeal atresia are recognized: type I, in which supraglottic and infraglottic parts of the larynx are atretic; type II, infraglottic atresia; and type III, glottic atresia. Tracheal atresia occurs when the mid-portion of the foregut develops into esophagus only and no endoderm is left to form trachea. The distinction between laryngeal and tracheal atresia is not possible with sonography.

Prevalence

The incidence of high airway obstruction in the fetus is not known. Once thought to be extremely rare, more than 22 cases have been reported since 1989.[170–173] High airway obstruction of one form or another is probably more common than appreciated because many fetuses die *in utero* or are stillborn before clinical recognition.

Embryology and Pathology

The precise cause is not known, although abnormal persistent fusion of the sixth bronchial arches may be involved. Sporadic, genetic, and vascular causes have been proposed.[174,175] In most cases, the subglottic portion of the airway (laryngeal) or proximal trachea is atretic, stenotic, or there may be a thick web obstructing the proximal airway. It is even more rare for the obstruction to occur distally in the trachea, although this has been described.[176]

Tracheal atresia is often associated with an abnormality of the esophagus, usually a fistula. A fistula may decompress the obstructed lungs, thus making the prenatal diagnosis more difficult.

Pathologically the high airway obstruction results in lungs that are distended, filled with fluid, and often demonstrating rib impressions on the surface, corroborating the enormously increased intrathoracic pressure generated by this abnormality. Obstruction of the airways leads to overdistension of the developing air spaces, which promotes alveolar development.[177] Paradoxically, the lungs demonstrate more advanced development than expected for gestational age when examined pathologically. Lung weights and radial alveolar count correspond to an older gestational age and, in some cases, to what might be expected for 2 or 3 months postnatal age.[178]

Diagnosis

This abnormality has been detected in the fetus as early as 16 weeks.[179,180] The sonographic findings are very characteristic (an *Aunt Minnie*). The lungs are symmetrically enlarged, echogenic, and homogeneous. This appearance is due to the fluid distension of the tiny air spaces, which are too small to be perceived as cysts on the sonogram. The distended lungs have mass effect on the diaphragm, which appears flattened or inverted, and the heart is displaced anteriorly in the midline (Fig. 36). The heart often appears *dwarfed* by the surrounding enlarged lungs. In many fetuses, the two fluid-filled main bronchi and trachea, distended by lung fluid, can be visualized (Fig. 36A). Neither the precise level of obstruction nor etiology (web vs. stenosis vs. atresia) can be determined accurately with sonography. One can safely assume, however, that the high airway obstruction is severe if the lungs are enlarged and diaphragm is flattened.

Fetal ascites is nearly universal at the time of diagnosis but may not be associated with other findings of hydrops. Poly- and oligohydramnios are reported. Presumably, polyhydramnios is caused by esophageal compression. Oligohydramnios is not fully understood but may be due to cardiac compromise or diminished lung fluid efflux into the amni-

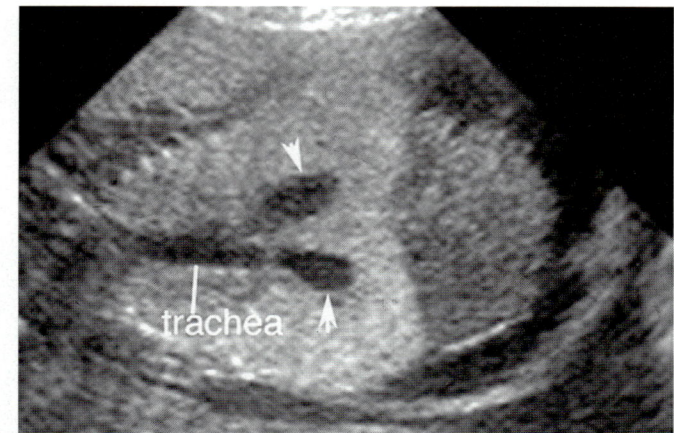

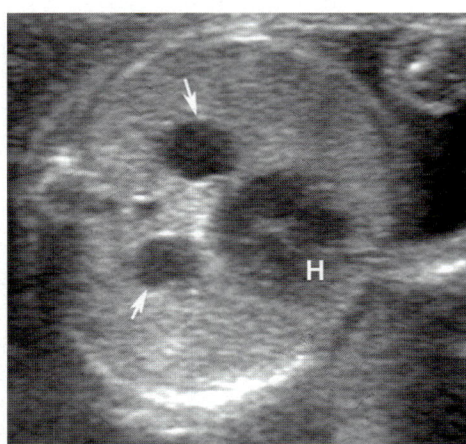

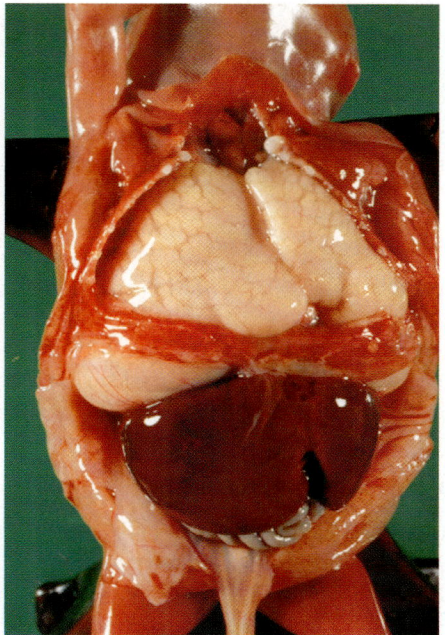

FIGURE 36. Congenital high airway obstruction. **A:** Coronal image shows a fluid-filled trachea and bilateral bronchi (*arrowheads*). Ascites is also present in the abdomen, typical of this abnormality. **B:** Axial image of the same fetus as in (**A**). The two fluid-filled bronchi (*arrows*) flank the heart (*H*), which is midline. **C:** Pathologic photograph of similar case shows markedly hyperexpanded lungs secondary to laryngeal atresia.

otic space. Integumentary edema is not always associated but, when present, is evidence of hydrops.

Differential Diagnosis

There are few entities that should be considered seriously in a fetus with bilateral, symmetrically enlarged, homogeneous lungs. These entities include an obstruction of the central airway, either tracheal or laryngeal atresia, or severe stenosis and bilateral lung masses such as microcystic CCAMs or sequestrations. The observation of bilateral fluid-filled main stem bronchi mitigates against CCAM and favors high airway obstruction. In addition, the symmetry of the lungs expected with CHAOS is usually not present with bilateral lung masses such as CCAM or sequestration.

Associated Anomalies

More than 50% of fetuses with laryngeal obstruction have additional abnormalities, most commonly renal, central nervous system malformations, and tracheoesophageal atresia.[181,182] Laryngeal atresia may occur as part of Fraser's syndrome (tracheal or laryngeal atresia, renal agenesis,

microphthalmia, cryptophthalmos, and syn- or polydactyly) with autosomal recessive inheritance.[175] It may be associated with the vertebral defects imperforate anus, tracheoesophageal fistula, and radial and renal dysplasia association and rhizomelic chondrodysplasia punctata, maternal pertussis infection.[183] Most CHAOS cases are sporadic malformations, however, without risk of recurrence.

Prognosis and Management

Little is known about the natural history of fetal CHAOS. If CHAOS is recognized prenatally, it is because the fetal high airway obstruction is severe and nearly complete, and therefore it is uniformly fatal without intervention before or during delivery. What is not known is how many and which fetuses may develop hydrops and die before birth. In some, the *ex utero* intrapartum treatment procedure may be helpful as a means of establishing a functional airway before the fetus is completely removed from placental support. This strategy, which allows bronchoscopy, laryngoscopy, and tracheostomy to be performed during operative (cesarean) delivery, has now been used to accomplish successful delivery of at least three infants prenatally diagnosed with CHAOS.[184,185]

FETAL HYDROTHORAX

Description

Fetal hydrothorax is an accumulation of fluid in the pleural space. Pleural fluid in the fetus is always abnormal.

Incidence

The incidence is unknown but has been estimated to be 1 per 15,000 pregnancies in tertiary care centers.[186] Slightly more males are affected than females.[187,188] Primary chylothorax is the most frequent cause of an isolated pleural effusion leading to respiratory distress in the newborn.

Embryology and Pathology

Pleural fluid may accumulate in the chest as a primary abnormality (primary chylothorax) or as one of the manifestations of the generalized conditions that causes hydrops fetalis (see Chapter 16). There are many causes of immune and nonimmune hydrops (see Chapter 16), and pleural effusion may be one of the earliest signs.[189]

Primary hydrothorax is chylous in origin. In most fetuses, the cause is not known although atresia, fistula, or absence of the thoracic duct has been diagnosed pathologically in some fetuses.[190,191] Intrathoracic masses should be considered, including subtle diaphragmatic hernia or ELS (Figs. 29 and 31). Rarely, a cause such as congenital pulmonary lymphangiectasia may be linked with hydrothorax.[192] Down and Turner's syndromes are also associated, presumably due to a related lymphatic abnormality.

Fetal hydrothorax can be unilateral or bilateral. When the hydrothorax is unilateral, it occurs roughly equally on the right and left sides.[188,193] The thoracic duct crosses from right to left in the posterior mediastinum at the fifth thoracic level. Thus an abnormality of the thoracic duct above or below this level could theoretically lead to a left- or right-sided chylothorax.

Diagnosis

Sonographically, pleural effusions appear as anechoic fluid collections in the pleural space that conform to the normal chest and diaphragmatic contour (Fig. 37). The lung appears to *float* in the fluid. The echogenicity of the fluid is the same regardless of its origin. Fetal hydrothorax is usually detected in the second or third trimesters. It is rarely detected before 15 weeks except in association with Down or Turner's syndromes.[194]

From a diagnostic perspective, the most important determination is whether the hydrothorax is likely to be the primary abnormality or a manifestation of a more global derangement resulting in generalized hydrops. Treatment of the hydropic fetus with hydrothorax focuses on the cause of

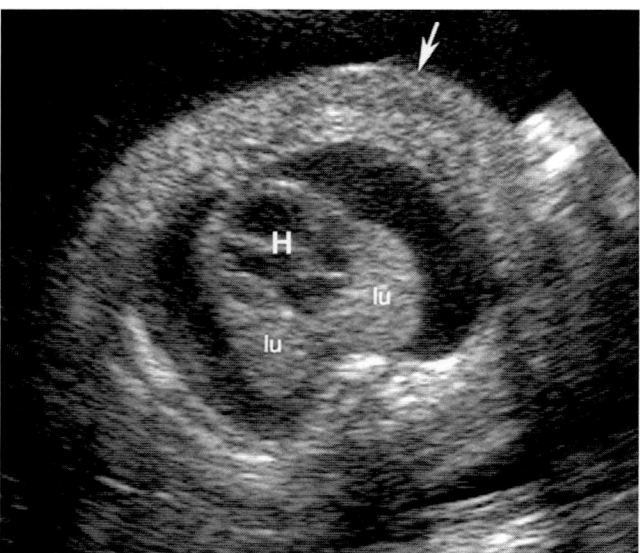

FIGURE 37. Bilateral hydrothorax with generalized hydrops fetalis. The pleural effusions are symmetric, the heart (*H*) is not displaced, and there is fetal integumentary edema (*arrow*). lu, lung.

the hydrops. Treatment of the fetus with a primary hydrothorax focuses on ameliorating the potential effects of the effusion on the fetus (i.e., pulmonary hypoplasia and hydrops).

Distinguishing between primary and secondary hydrothorax relies on a number of sonographic observations. If the pleural effusion is unilateral, shifts the mediastinum, and flattens the diaphragm, it is likely to be a primary chylothorax (Fig. 38).[188] If the effusions are bilateral, roughly symmetric, do not shift the heart dramatically, and are associated with other serous effusions and integumentary edema, the hydrothoraces are much more likely to be sec-

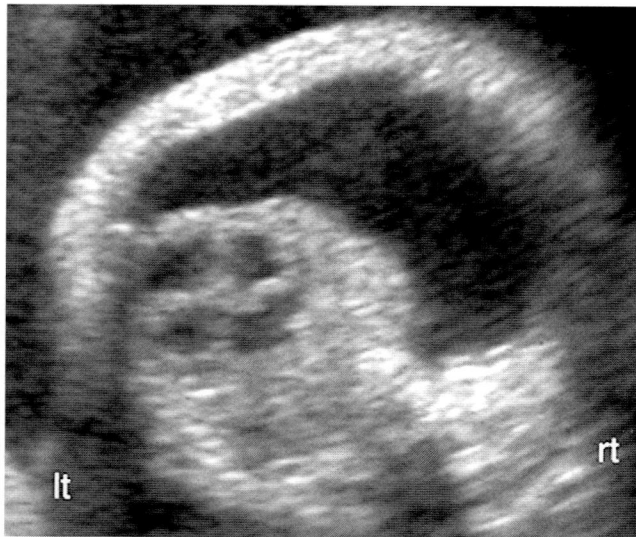

FIGURE 38. Primary chylothorax. Large unilateral right (*rt*)-sided hydrothorax shifts the mediastinum to the left (*lt*).

ondary to an underlying cause of the hydrops fetalis (anemia, infection, heart defect, arrhythmia, chromosomal anomaly, and so forth). Examiners should keep in mind that a primary chylothorax could be the cause of hydrops as well. This is one of the most treatable causes of hydrops and a diagnosis well worth the effort to make. Hydrops caused by a hydrothorax is suggested if there is obvious mass effect of one of the effusions and they are asymmetric in size. In this case, therapy is directed at draining the larger of the two hydrothoraces.

After birth, the diagnosis of chylothorax relies on the characteristic *milky* appearance resulting from the chylomicrons in the lymph fluid. In the *fasting* fetus, the aspirated fluid is clear and *straw-colored*.[195–199] Cellular analysis of chylous effusion in the fetus typically shows a large number of lymphocytes. Some have suggested that less than 80% lymphocytes in the fluid is diagnostic of chylothorax,[199] but others have found this analysis to be less consistent.[200]

Differential Diagnosis

The diagnosis of fluid in the fetal chest is straightforward. Any fluid is abnormal. The crux of the differential diagnostic considerations is the determination of whether the effusion(s) is (are) the primary abnormality or a secondary phenomenon. Secondary causes included chromosomal abnormality, infection, tumor, cardiovascular abnormalities, and syndromes.

Associated Anomalies

Pleural effusion may be associated with a number of underlying conditions (Table 8). Other major congenital anomalies are found in 25% to 40% of fetuses with nonimmune hydrops fetalis, most commonly cardiac.[201,202] If there are generalized findings of hydrops, detection of any associated anomaly is a poor prognostic feature and is associated with a perinatal mortality rate of greater than 90%.[202]

Primary chylothorax is often an isolated anomaly, but a chromosomal abnormality should be considered because

TABLE 8. MAJOR ETIOLOGIES FOR PLEURAL EFFUSIONS

Hydrops fetalis
Chylothorax
Intrathoracic mass
Cystic adenomatoid malformation of the lungs
Bronchopulmonary sequestration
Diaphragmatic hernia
Chromosome (trisomy 21, monosomy X)
Infection
Syndromic condition (Noonan)
Tumor
Vascular (pulmonary vein atresia)
Idiopathic

fetuses with Down, Turner's, and Noonan's syndromes may manifest with hydrothorax, unilateral or bilateral.[203,204] Further, hydrothorax may be the only abnormality observed sonographically. The rate of aneuploidy in association with primary chylothorax has been estimated to be 1.8% to 5.8%.[205–207]

A specific lesion in the chest may be associated with a fetal hydrothorax, and these include ELS and pulmonary lymphangiectasia.[191] Transient pleural effusion has also been reported as the only prenatal sonographic finding of diaphragmatic hernia. The potential for associated generalized abnormalities underscores the recommendation that any fetus with a hydrothorax should undergo a careful anatomic survey, viral screening, and karyotype testing.

Prognosis and Management

Prognosis associated with fetal hydrothorax is variable and generally considered to be guarded. Perinatal mortality rate of fetuses with hydrothorax is 35% to 50%.[187,188,208] The best outcomes are reported for fetuses with unilateral effusions and no other obvious anomalies.[188] Those who do most poorly have evidence of generalized hydrops, are delivered before 32 weeks, and have no fetal intervention.[152] If all of these *risk factors* were present, Weber and Philipson reported a 97% fetal/neonatal death rate.[187] Aubard and coworkers added *bilaterally* and *absence of spontaneous regression* to the list of poor prognostic indicators.[153]

Of all the poor prognostic indicators, however, hydrops is the most important.[188] The perinatal mortality rate of untreated hydropic fetuses was 76% in one series compared to only 25% among those without hydrops.[188] This is similar to observations of other investigators.[209–211]

The natural history of primary chylothorax is highly variable and difficult to predict. Spontaneous resolution occurs in approximately 9% to 22% of primary chylothoraces.[187,193] This has been associated with nearly 100% survival.[188] It is difficult to predict which effusions will spontaneously resolve, but early diagnosis (early in the second trimester), unilaterally, and absence of polyhydramnios or hydrops favor spontaneous resolution.[188]

The two most feared complications of fetal hydrothorax are pulmonary hypoplasia and hydrops caused by the effusion. The former is extremely difficult to predict, and predictions based on sonographic observations are imperfect. Management is usually based on the overall impression of fetal health. When the hydrothorax is small, isolated, and seemingly well tolerated by the fetus, frequent surveillance may be the most prudent management. In these cases, significant pulmonary hypoplasia is unlikely. If the hydrothorax spontaneously resolves, no invasive therapy is necessary. If the hydrothorax is very large or increases over time accompanied by signs of clinical deterioration (i.e., hydrops), a fetal thoracentesis and/or thoracoamniotic shunt should be considered (Fig. 39).[188]

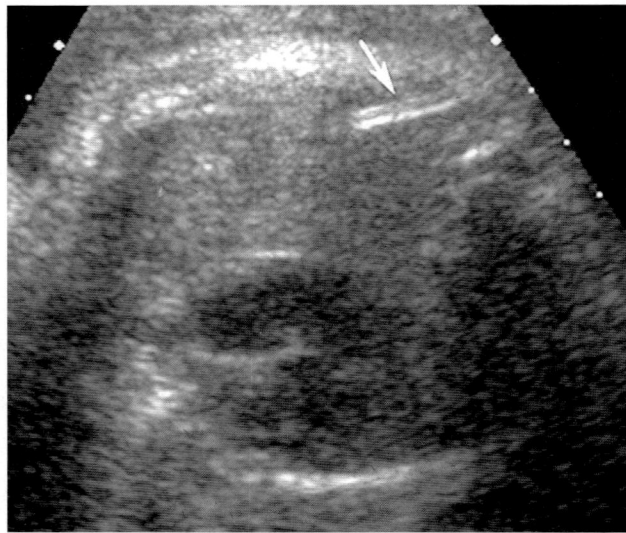
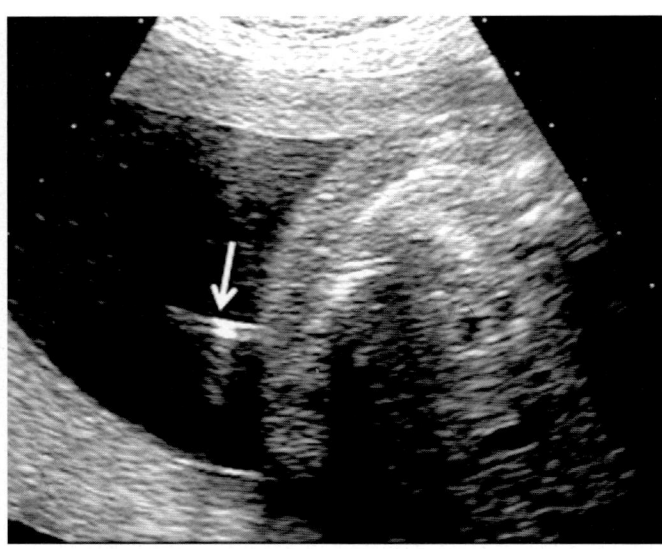

A   B

FIGURE 39. Primary chylothorax drained by the thoracoamniotic catheter. Two different fetuses **(A, B)** show catheter (*arrows*) placed within the chest.

Fetal thoracentesis can accomplish short-term drainage of the hydrothorax and aspiration just before delivery and may improve ventilation in the newborn. Fetal thoracentesis, however, is often not effective as a *cure* remote from delivery because the fluid re-accumulates rapidly in most cases.[188] An aspiration can be performed to see if it is effective. If the fetus does not improve after the aspiration or the fluid re-accumulates, a thoracoamniotic shunt can be placed relatively safely using sonographic guidance (Fig. 39). Allowing the pleural fluid to drain into the amniotic space may be especially useful in mid-gestation, because the risk of delivery before 32 weeks is associated with increased morbidity and mortality.

To accomplish thoracoamniotic shunting, a metal trocar with cannula is introduced through the maternal abdominal wall and uterus into the fetal thorax as close as possible to the mid-axillary line of the fetus. Once the trochar has been introduced into the thorax, a double pigtail catheter is passed through the trochar, and the *internal* loop is deployed into the thorax with an introducer rod. As the trochar and introducer rods are removed, the *external* end of the catheter is left in the amniotic space. Aubard et al.[188] summarized 80 reports of thoracoamniotic shunting in fetuses with bilateral or unilateral pleural effusions. This series suggests that shunting has the most dramatic effect on survival among fetuses already showing signs of hydrops. In this series, only 10% of hydropic fetuses survived after thoracentesis alone, whereas 67% of hydropic fetuses survived following thoracoamniotic shunting. Shunting is not always successful. Shunt failures have been reported in 26%,[188] and complications, including shunt migration (usually into the amniotic space) and clogging of the catheter, can be serious, resulting in fetal death in some cases.

REFERENCES

1. Snyder JM, Mendelson CR, Johnston JM. The morphology of lung development in the human fetus. In: Nelson GH, ed. *Pulmonary development.* New York: Marcel Dekker 1985;19–46.
2. Wigglesworth JS. Pathology of the lung in the fetus and neonate, with particular reference to problems to growth and maturation. *Histopathology* 1987;11:671–690.
3. Burri PH. Fetal and postnatal development of the lung. *Ann Rev Physiol* 1984;46:617–628.
4. Laudy JA, Wladimiroff JW. The fetal lung. I. Developmental aspects. *Obstet Gynecol* 2000;16:284–290.
5. Alcorn D, Adamson TM, Lambert TF, Maloney JE, Ritchie RC, et al. Morphological effects of chronic tracheal ligation and drainage in the fetal lamb lung. *J Anat* 1977;123:649–660.
6. Fewell JE, Hislop AA, Kitterman JA, Johnson P. Effect of tracheostomy on lung development in fetal lambs. *J Appl Physiol* 1983;55:1103–1108.
7. Fewell JE, Lee CC, Kittennan JA. Effects of phrenic nerve section on the respiratory system of fetal lambs. *J Appl Physiol* 1981;51:293–297.
8. Harrison MR, Bressack MA, Churg AM, deLorimier AA. Correction of congenital diaphragmatic hernia in utero. II. Simulated correction permits fetal lung growth with survival at birth. *Surgery* 1980;88:260–268.
9. Adzick NS, Harrison MR, Crombleholme TM, Flake AW, Howell LJ. Fetal lung lesions: management and outcome. *Am J Obstet Gynecol* 1998;179:884–889.
10. Rice HE, Estes JM, Hedrick MH, Bealer JF, Harrison MR, et al. Congenital cystic adenomatoid malformation: a sheep model of fetal hydrops. *Pediatr Surg* 1994;29:692–696.
11. Lauria MR, Gonik B, Romero R. Pulmonary hypoplasia: pathogenesis, diagnosis and antenatal prediction. *Obstet Gynecol* 1995;86:466–475.

12. Askenazi SS, Perlman M. Pulmonary hypoplasia: lung weight and radial alveolar count as criteria of diagnosis. *Arch Dis Child* 1979;54:614–618.

13. Knox WF, Barson AJ. Pulmonary hypoplasia in a regional perinatal unit. *Early Hum Dev* 1986;14:33–42.

14. Wigglesworth JS, Desai R. Use of DNA estimation for growth assessment in normal and hypoplastic fetal lungs. *Arch Dis Child* 1981;56:601–605.

15. Thurlbeck WM. Prematurity and the developing lung. *Clin Perinatol* 1992;19:497–519.

16. Hislop A, Hey E, Reid L. The lungs in congenital bilateral renal agenesis and aplasia. *Arch Dis Child* 1979;54:32–38.

17. Rotschild A, Ling EW, Puterman ML, Farquharson D. Neonatal outcome after prolonged preterm rupture of the membranes. *Am J Obstet Gynecol* 1990;162:46–52.

18. Nakamura Y, Harada K, Yamamoto I, Uemura Y, Okamoto K, et al. Human pulmonary hypoplasia: statistical, morphological, morphometric and biochemical study. *Arch Pathol Lab Med* 1992;116:635–642.

19. Lawrence S, Rosenfeld CR. Fetal pulmonary development and abnormalities of amniotic fluid volume. *Semin Perinatol* 1986;10:142–153.

20. Swischuk LE, Richardson CJ, Nichols MM, Ingman MJ. Primary pulmonary hypoplasia in the neonate. *J Pediatr* 1979;95:573–577.

21. Wigglesworth JS, Desai R, Gueffini P. Fetal lung hypoplasia: biochemical and structural variations and their possible significance. *Arch Dis Child* 1981;56:606–615.

22. Moessinger AC, Collins MH, Blanc WA, Rey HR, James LS. Oligohydramnios-induced lung hypoplasia: the influence of timing and duration in gestation. *Pediatr Res* 1986;20:951–954.

23. Harstad TW, Twickler DM, Leveno KJ, Brown CEL. Antepartum prediction of pulmonary hypoplasia: an elusive goal? *Am J Perinatol* 1993;10:8–11.

24. Chitkara U, Rosenberg J, Chervenak FA, et al. Prenatal sonographic assessment of the fetal thorax: normal values. *Am J Obstet Gynecol* 1987;156:1069–1074.

25. Laudy JA, Wladimiroff JW. The fetal lung. 2. Pulmonary hypoplasia. *Ultrasound Obstet Gynecol* 2000 Oct;16:482–494.

26. Hilpert PL, Pretorius DH. The thorax. In: Nyberg DA, Mahony BS, Pretorius DH, eds. *Diagnostic ultrasound of fetal anomalies text and atlas*. Chicago: Year Book Medical Publishers, Inc., 1990:262–299.

27. Vintzileos AM, Campbell WA, Rodis JF, Nochimson DJ, Pinette MG, et al. Comparison of six different ultrasonographic methods for predicting lethal fetal pulmonary hypoplasia. *Am J Obstet Gynecol* 1989;161:606–612.

28. Merz E, Miric-Tesanic D, Bahlmann F, Weber G, Hallermann C. Prenatal sonographic chest and lung measurements for predicting severe pulmonary hypoplasia. *Prenat Diagn* 1999;19:614–619.

29. Yoshimura S, Masuzaki H, Gotoh H, Fukuda H, Ishimaru T. Ultrasonographic prediction of lethal pulmonary hypoplasia: comparison of eight different ultrasonographic parameters. *Am J Obstet Gynecol* 1996;175:477–483.

30. D'Arcy TJ, Hughes SW, Chiu WSC, Clark R, Milner AD, et al. Estimation of fetal lung volume using enhanced 3-dimensional ultrasound: a new method and first result. *Br J Obstet Gynaecol* 1996;103:1015–1020.

31. Lee A, Kratochwil A, Stiimpflen L, Deutinger J, Bernaschek G. Fetal lung volume determination by three dimensional ultrasonography. *Am J Obstet Gynecol* 1996;175:588–592.

32. Pohls UG, Rempen A. Fetal lung volumetry by three-dimensional ultrasound. *Obstet Gynecol* 1998;11:6–12.

33. Walsh DS, Hubbard AM, Olutoye OO, Howell LJ, Crombleholme TM, et al. Assessment of fetal lung volumes and liver herniation with magnetic resonance imaging in congenital diaphragmatic hernia. *Am J Obstet Gynecol* 2000; 183:1067–1069.

34. Rypens F, Metens T, Rocourt N, Sonigo P, Brunelle F, et al. Fetal lung volume: estimation at MR imaging—initial results. *Radiology* 2001;219:236–241.

35. Laudy JA, Janssen MM, Struyk PC, Stijnen T, Wladimiroff JW. Three-dimensional ultrasonography of normal fetal lung volume: a preliminary study. *Ultrasound Obstet Gynecol* 1998;11:13–16.

36. Bahmaie A, Hughes SW, Clark T, Milner A, Saunders J, et al. Serial fetal lung volume measurement using three-dimensional ultrasound. *Ultrasound Obstet Gynecol* 2000; 16:154–158.

37. Van Eyck J, van der Mooren K, Wladimiroff JW. Ductus arteriosus flow velocity modulation by fetal breathing movements as a measure of fetal lung development. *Am J Obstet Gynecol* 1990;163:558–566.

38. Stanley JR, Veille JC, Zaccaro D. Description of right pulmonary artery blood flow by Doppler echocardiography in the normal human fetus 17–40 weeks gestation. *J Matern Fetal Invest* 1994;4:S14.

39. Twining P. The value of fetal pulmonary artery flow as a predictor of pulmonary hypoplasia in congenital diaphragmatic hernia. *Ultrasound Med Biol* 1997;23:S106.

40. Assali NS, Morris JA, Beck R. Cardiovascular hemodynamics in the fetal lamb before and after lung expansion. *Am J Physiol* 1965;208:122–29.

41. Yoshimura S, Masuzaki H, Miura K, Gotoh H, Ishimaru T. Diagnosis of fetal pulmonary hypoplasia by measurement of blood flow velocity waveforms of pulmonary arteries with Doppler ultrasonography. *Am J Obstet Gynecol* 1999;180:441–446.

42. Chaoui R, Kalache K, Tennstedt C, Lenz F, Vogel M. Pulmonary arterial Doppler velocimetry in fetuses with hypoplasia. *Eur J Obstet Gynecol Repr Biol* 1999;84:179–185.

43. Blott N, Greenough A, Nicolaides KH, Moscoso G, Gibb D, et al. Fetal breathing movements as a predictor of favorable pregnancy outcome after oligohydramnios due to membrane rupture in second trimester. *Lancet* 1987;1:129–131.

44. Sherer DM, Davis JM, Woods JR. Pulmonary hypoplasia: a review. *Obstet Gynecol Surg* 1990;45:792–803.

45. Page DV, Stocker JT. Anomalies associated with pulmonary hypoplasia. *Am Rev Respir Dis* 1982;125:216–221.

46. Katz AL, Wiswell TE, Baumgart S. Contemporary controversies in the management of congenital diaphragmatic hernia. *Clin Perinatol* 1998;25:219–248.

47. Moore KL. *The developing human: clinically oriented embryology*, 4th ed. Philadelphia: WB Saunders, 1988.

48. Albanese CT, Lopoo J, Goldstein RB, Filly RA, Feldstein VA, et al. Fetal liver position and perinatal outcome for congenital diaphragmatic hernia. *Prenat Diagn* 1998;18:1138–1142.

49. Guibaud L, Filiatrault D, Garel L, Grignon A, Dubois J, et al. Fetal congenital diaphragmatic hernia: accuracy of sonography in the diagnosis and prediction of the outcome after birth. *AJR Am J Roentgenol* 1996;166:1195–1202.

50. Adzick NS, Outwater KM, Harrison MR, Davies P, Glick PL, et al. Correction of congenital diaphragmatic hernia in utero. IV. An early gestational fetal lamb model for pulmonary vascular morphometric analysis. *J Pediatr Surg* 1985;20:673–680.

51. American Institute of Ultrasound in Medicine. Guidelines for the performance of the antepartum obstetrical ultrasound examination. *J Ultrasound Med* 1996;15:185–187.

52. Lewis DA, Reickert C, Bowerman R, Hirschl RB. Prenatal ultrasonography frequently fails to diagnose congenital diaphragmatic hernia. *J Pediatr Surg* 1997;32:352–356.

53. Grandjean H, Larroque D, Levi S. The performance of routine ultrasonographic screening of pregnancies in the Euro Fetus Study. *Am J Obstet Gynecol* 1999;181:446–454.

54. Chitty LS. Ultrasound screening for fetal abnormalities. *Prenat Diagn* 1995;15:1241–1257.

55. Bootstaylor BS, Filly RA, Harrison MR, Adzick NS. Prenatal sonographic predictors of liver herniation in congenital diaphragmatic hernia. *Ultrasound Med* 1995;14:515–520.

56. Hubbard AM, Adzik NS, Cromblehome TM, Haselgrove JC. Left-sided congenital diaphragmatic hernia: value of prenatal MR imaging in preparation for fetal surgery. *Radiology* 1997;203:636–640.

57. Paek BW, Danzer E, Machin GA, Coakley F, Albanese CT, et al. Prenatal diagnosis of bilateral diaphragmatic hernia: diagnostic pitfalls. *Ultrasound Med* 2000;19:495–500.

58. Gibbs DL, Rice HE, Farrell JA, Adzick NS, Harrison MR. Familial diaphragmatic agenesis: an autosomal-recessive syndrome with a poor prognosis. *Pediatr Surg* 1997;32:366–368.

59. Sebire NJ, Snijders RJ, Davenport M, Greenough A, Nicolaides KH. Fetal nuchal translucency thickness at 10–14 weeks gestation and congenital diaphragmatic hernia. *Obstet Gynecol* 1997;90:943–946.

60. Geary MP, Chitty LS, Morrison JJ, Wright V, Pierro A, et al. Perinatal outcome and prognostic factors in prenatally diagnosed congenital diaphragmatic hernia. *Ultrasound Obstet Gynecol* 1998;12:107–111.

61. Chitty LS. The thorax. In: Dewbury K, Meir H, Cosgrave D, eds. *Ultrasound obstetrics and gynecology.* Edinburgh: Churchill Livingstone, 1993:405–416.

62. Losty PD, Vanamo K, Rintala RJ, Donahoe PK, Schnitzer JJ, et al. Congenital diaphragmatic hernia—does the side of the defect influence the incidence of associated malformations? *Pediatr Surg* 1998;33:507–510.

63. Cannon C, Dildy GA, Ward R, Varner MW, Dudley DJ. A population-based study of congenital diaphragmatic hernia in Utah: 1988–1994. *Obst Gynecol* 1996;87:959–963.

64. Sheffield JS, Twickler DM, Timmons C, Land K, Harrod MJ, et al. Fryns syndrome: prenatal diagnosis and pathologic correlation. *Ultrasound Med* 1998;17:585–589.

65. Enns G, Cox VA, Goldstein RB, Gibbs DL, Harrison MR, et al. Congenital diaphragmatic defects and associated syndromes, malformations, and chromosome anomalies: a retrospective study of 60 patients and literature review. *Am J Med Genet* 1998;79:215–225.

66. Dommergues M, Louis-Sylvestre C, Mandelbrot L, Oury JF, Herlicovierz M, et al. Congenital diaphragmatic hernia: can prenatal ultrasonography predict outcome. *Am J Obstet Gynecol* 1996;174:1377–1381.

67. Geary M. Management of congenital diaphragmatic hernia diagnosed prenatally: an update. *Prenat Diagn* 1998;18:1155–1158.

68. Harrison MR, Adzik S, Estes JM, Howell LJ. A prospective study of the outcome for fetuses with diaphragmatic hernia. *JAMA* 1994;271:382–388.

69. Metkus AP, Filly RA, Stringer MD, Harrison MR, Adzick NS. Sonographic predictors of survival in fetal diaphragmatic hernia. *J Pediatr Surg* 1996;31:148–151.

70. Lipshutz GS, Albanese CT, Feldstein VA, Jennings RW, Housley HT, et al. Prospective analysis of lung-to-head ratio predicts survival for patients with prenatally diagnosed congenital diaphragmatic hernia. *J Pediatr Surg* 1997;32:1634–1636.

71. Bembaum J, Schwartz IP, Gerdes M, D'Agostino JA, Coburn CE, et al. Survivors of extracorporeal membrane oxygenation at 1 year of age: the relationship of primary diagnosis with health and neurodevelopmental sequelae. *Pediatrics* 1995;96:907–913.

72. McGahren ED, Mallik K, Rodgers BM. Neurological outcome is diminished in survivors of congenital diaphragmatic hernia requiring extracorporeal membrane oxygenation. *J Pediatr Surg* 1997;32:1216–1220.

73. Reyes C, Chang LK, Waffam F, Mir H, Warden MJ, et al. Delayed repair of congenital diaphragmatic hernia with early high-frequency oscillatory ventilation during preoperative stabilization. *J Pediatr Surg* 1998;33:1010–1016.

74. Kanai M, Kitano Y, von Allmen D, Davies P, Adzick NS, et al. Fetal tracheal occlusion in the rat model of nitrofen-induced congenital diaphragmatic hernia: tracheal occlusion reverses the arterial structural abnormality. *J Pediatr Surg* 2001;36:839–845.

75. Bratu L, Flageole H, Laberge M, Chen MF, Piedboeuf B. Pulmonary structural maturation and pulmonary artery remodeling after reversible fetal ovine tracheal occlusion in diaphragmatic hernia. *J Pediatr Surg* 2001;36:739–744.

76. Mychaliska GB, Bealer JF, Graf JL, Rosen MA, Adzick NS, et al. Operating on placental support: the ex utero intrapartum treatment procedure. *J Pediatr Surg* 1997;32:227–230.

77. Harrison MR, Mychalska GB, Albanese CT, Jennings RW, Farrell JA, et al. Correction of congenital diaphragmatic hernia in utero IX: fetuses with poor prognosis (liver herniation and low lung-to-head ratio) can be saved by fetoscopic temporary tracheal occlusion. *J Pediatr Surg* 1998;33:1017–1022.

78. Tibboel D, Gaag AV. Etiologic and genetic factors in congenital diaphragmatic hernia. *Clin Perinatol* 1996;23:689–699.

79. Waszak P, Claris O, Lapillone A, Picaud JC, Basson E, et al. Cystic adenomatoid malformation of the lung: neonatal management of 21 cases. *Pediatr Surg Int* 1999;15:326–31.

80. Stocker JT, Drake RM, Madewell JE. Cystic and congenital lung disease in the newborn. *Perspec Pediatr Pathol* 1978;4:93–154.

81. Bromley B, Parad R, Estroff JA, Benacerraf BR. Fetal lung masses: prenatal course and outcome. *Ultrasound Med* 1995;14:927–936.

82. Stocker JT, Madewell JE, Drake RM. Congenital cystic adenomatoid malformation of the lung. Classification and morphologic spectrum. *Hum Pathol* 1977;8:155–171.

83. Lipshutz GS, Lopoo JB, Jennings RW, Farrell J, Harrison MR, et al. Are bilateral fetal lung masses double trouble? *Fetal Diagn Ther* 1999;14:348–350.

84. Maas KL, Feldstein VA, Goldstein RB, Filly RA. Sonographic detection of bilateral fetal chest masses: report of three cases. *Ultrasound Med* 1997;16:647–652.

85. Samuel M, Burge DM. Management of antenatally diagnosed pulmonary sequestration associated with congenital cystic adenomatoid malformation. *Thorax* 1999;54:701–706.

86. Buntain WL, Issacs H Jr, Payne VC Jr, Lindesmith GG, Rosenkrantz JG. Lobar emphysema, cystic adenomatoid malformation, pulmonary sequestration, and bronchogenic cyst in infancy and childhood: a clinical group. *J Pediatr Surg* 1974;9:85–93.

87. Askin F. Respiratory tract disorders in the fetus and neonate. In: Wigglesworth JS, Singer DB, eds. *Textbook of fetal and perinatal pathology.* Boston: Blackwell Science, 1991:643–688.

88. Cass DL, Yang EY, Liechty KW, Quinn TM, Crombleholme TM, et al. Increased cell proliferation and decreased apoptosis in congenital cystic adenomatoid malformation: insights into pathogenesis. *Surg Forum* 1997;48:659–661.

89. Kwittken J, Reiner L. Congenital cystic adenomatoid malformation of the lung. *Pediatrics* 1962;30:759–768.

90. Clements BS, Warner JO. Pulmonary sequestration and related congenital bronchopulmonary-vascular malformations: nomenclature and classification based on anatomical and embryological considerations. *Thorax* 1987;42:401–408.

91. Conran RM, Stocker JT. Extralobar sequestration with frequently associated congenital cystic adenomatoid malformation, type 2: report of 50 cases. *Pediatr Dev Pathol* 1999;2:454–463.

92. MacKenzie TC, Guttenberg ME, Nisenbaum HL, Johnson MP, Adzick NS. A fetal lung lesion consisting of bronchogenic cyst, bronchopulmonary sequestration, and congenital cystic adenomatoid malformation: the missing link? *Fetal Diagn Ther* 2001;16:193–195.

93. Moerman P, Fryns J-P, Vandenberghe K, Devlieger H, Lauweryns JM. Pathogenesis of congenital cystic adenomatoid malformation of the lung. *Histopathology* 1992;21:315–321.

94. van Dijk C, Wagenvoort CA. The various types of congenital adenomatoid malformation of the lung. *J Pathol* 1973;110:131–134.

95. Wolf SA, Hertzler JR, Philippart Al. Cystic adenomatoid dysplasia of the lung. *J Pediatr Surg* 1980;15:925–930.

96. Fraser RG, Pard JAP. *Diagnosis of diseases of the chest*, 2nd ed. Philadelphia: WB Saunders, 1977.

97. Thorpe-Beeston JG, Nicolaides KH. Cystic adenomatoid malformation of the lung: prenatal diagnosis and outcome. *Pren Diagn* 1994;14:677–688.

98. Catanzarite V, Mendoza A, Chapman T, Muller W, Maida C. Early prenatal diagnosis of type II cystic adenomatoid malformation of the lung: sonographic and histological findings. *Ultrasound Obstet Gynecol* 1992;2:129–132.

99. Cass DL, Crombleholme TM, Howell LJ, Stafford PW, Ruchelli ED, et al. Cystic lung lesions with systemic arterial blood supply: a hybrid of congenital cystic adenomatoid malformation and bronchopulmonary sequestration. *J Pediatr Surg* 1997;32:986–990.

100. Richards DS, Langham MR Jr, Mahaffey SM. The prenatal ultrasonographic diagnosis of cloacal exstrophy. *J Ultrasound Med* 1992;11:507–510.

101. Heij HA, Ekkelkamp S, Vos A. Diagnosis of congenital cystic adenomatoid malformation of the lung in newborn infants and children. *Thorax* 1990;45:122–125.

102. Neilson IR, Russ P, Laberge JM, Filiatrault D, Ngujen LT, et al. Congenital adenomatoid malformation of the lung: current management and prognosis. *J Pediatr Surg* 1991; 26:975–80; discussion 980–981.

103. Bunduki V, Ruano R, da Silva MM, Miguelez J, Miyadahilra S, et al. Prognostic factors associated with congenital cystic adenomatoid malformation of the lung. *Prenat Diagn* 2000;20:459–464.

104. Bale PM. Congenital cystic malformation of the lung. A form of congenital bronchiolar ("adenomatoid") malformation. *Am J Clin Pathol* 1979;71:411–420.

105. Ostor AG, Fortune DW. Congenital cystic adenomatoid malformation of the lung. *Am J Clin Pathol* 1978;70:59–56.

106. Miller JA, Corteville JE, Langer JC. Congenital cystic adenomatoid malformation in the fetus: natural history and predictors of outcome. *J Pediatr Surg* 1996;31:805–808.

107. Dumez Y, Mandelbrot L, Radunovic N, Revillon Y, Dommergues M, et al. Prenatal management of congenital cystic adenomatoid malformation of the lung. *J Pediatr Surg* 1993;28:36–41.

108. van Leeuwen K, Teitelbaum DH, Hirschl RB, Austin E, Adelman SH, et al. Prenatal diagnosis of congenital cystic adenomatoid malformation and its postnatal presentation, surgical indications, and natural history. *J Pediatr Surg* 1999;34:794–798.

109. Dommergues M, Louis-Sylvestre C, Mandeolbrot L, Aubry MC, Revillon Y, et al. Congenital adenomatoid malformation of the lung: when is active fetal therapy indicated? *Am J Obstet Gynecol* 1997;177:953–958.

110. Winters WD, Effmann EL, Nghiem HV, Nyberg DA. Congenital masses of the lung: changes in cross-sectional area during gestation. *J Clin Ultrasound* 1997;25:372–377.

111. Winters WD, Effmann EL, Nghiem HV, Nyberg DA. Disappearing fetal lung masses: importance of postnatal imaging studies. *Pediatr Radiol* 1997;27:535–539.

112. van Leeuwen K, Teitelbaum DH, Hirschl RB, Austin E, Adelman SH, et al. Prenatal diagnosis of congenital cystic adenomatoid malformation and its postnatal presentation, surgical indications, and natural history. *J Pediatr Surg* 1999;34:794–798.

113. De Santis M, Masini L, Noia G, Cavaliere AF, Oliva N, et al. Congenital cystic adenomatoid malformation of the lung: antenatal ultrasound findings and fetal-neonatal outcome. Fifteen years of experience. *Fetal Diagn Ther* 2000;15:246–250.

114. Monni G, Paladini D, Ibba RM, Teodoro A, Zoppi MA, et al. Prenatal ultrasound diagnosis of congenital cystic adenomatoid malformation of the lung: a report of 26 cases and review of the literature. *Ultrasound Obstet Gynecol* 2000;16:159–162.

115. Prichard MG, Brown PJ, Sterrett GF. Bronchoalveolar carcinoma arising in long-standing lung cysts. *Thorax* 1984; 39:545–549.

116. Sheffield EA, Addis BJ, Corrin B, McCabe MM. Epithelial hyperplasia and malignant change in congenital lung cysts. *Clin Pathol* 1987;40:612–664.

117. Weinblatt ME, Siegel SE, Isaacs H. Pulmonary blastoma associated with cystic lung disease. *Cancer* 1982;49:669–671.

118. Adzick NS. The fetus with a lung mass. In: Harrison MR, Evans MI, Adzick NS, Holzgreve W, eds. *The unborn patient: the art and science of fetal therapy.* Philadelphia: WB Saunders 2001:287–296.

119. Ozcan C, Celik A, Ural Z, Veral A, Kandiloglu G, et al. Primary pulmonary rhabdomyosarcoma arising within cystic adenomatoid malformation: a case report and review of the literature. *J Pediatr Surg* 2001;36:1062–1065.

120. Papagiannopoulos KA, Sheppard M, Bush AP, Goldstraw P. Pleuropulmonary blastoma: is prophylactic resection of congenital lung cysts effective? *Ann Thorac Surg* 2001; 72:604–605.

121. Revillon Y, Jan D, Plattner V, Sonigo P, Dommergues M, et al. Congenital cystic adenomatoid malformation of the lung: prenatal management and prognosis. *J Pediatr Surg* 1993;28:1008–1011.

122. Pryce DM. Lower accessory pulmonary artery with intralobar sequestration of lung: a report of seven cases. *J Pathol Bact* 1946;58:457–467.

123. Piccione W Jr, Burt ME. Pulmonary sequestration in the neonate. *Chest* 1990;97:244–246.

124. Weinbaum PJ, Bors-Koefoed R, Green KW, Prenatt L. Antenatal sonographic findings in a case of intra-abdominal pulmonary sequestration. *Obstet Gynecol* 1989;73:860–862.

125. Levi A, Findler MI, Dolfin T, Di Segni E, Vidne BA. Intrapericardial extralobar pulmonary sequestration in a neonate. *Chest* 1990;98:1014–1015.

126. Carter R. Pulmonary sequestration. *Ann Thorac Surg* 1969; 7:68–88.

127. Rokitansky K. *Lehrbuch der pathologischen anatomie.* 3d revised. Vienna: Wilhelm Braumuller, 1855–1861.

128. Sade RM, Clouse M, Ellis FH Jr. The spectrum of pulmonary sequestration. *Ann Thorac Surg* 1974;18:644–658.

129. Stocker JT. Sequestrations of the lung. *Semin Diagn Pathol* 1986;3:106–121.

130. Flye MW, Izant RJ. Extralobar pulmonary sequestration with esophageal communication and complete duplication of the colon. *Surgery* 1972;71:744–752.

131. Gerle RD, Jaretzki A 3rd, Ashley CA, Berne AS. Congenital bronchopulmonary-foregut malformation. Pulmonary sequestration communicating with the gastrointestinal tract. *N Engl J Med* 1968;278:1413–1419.

132. Lager DJ, Kuper KA, Haake CK. Subdiaphragmatic extralobar pulmonary sequestration. *Arch Pathol Lab Med* 1991;115:536–538.

133. Case Records of the Massachusetts General Hospital. Weekly clinicopathological exercises. Case 14-1991. A 17 year old boy with a left posterior intrathoracic mass. *N Engl J Med* 1991;324:980–986.

134. Zangwill BC, Stocker JT. Congenital cystic adenomatoid malformation within an extralobar pulmonary sequestration. *Pediatr Pathol* 1993;13:309–315.

135. Aulicino MR, Reis ED, Dolgin SE, Unger PD, Shah KD. Intra-abdominal pulmonary sequestration exhibiting congenital cystic adenomatoid malformation. Report of a case and review of the literature. *Arch Pathol Lab Med* 1994; 118:1034–1037.

136. Rosado-de-Christenson ML, Frazier AA, Stocker JT, Templeton PA. From the archives of the AFIP. Extralobar sequestration: radiologic-pathologic correlation. *Radiographics* 1993;13:425–441.

137. Langer B, Donato L, Riethmuller C, Becmeur F, Dreyfus M, et al. Spontaneous regression of fetal pulmonary sequestration. *Obstet Gynecol* 1995;6:33–39.

138. Becmeur F, Horta-Geraud P, Donato L, Sauvage P. Pulmonary sequestrations: prenatal ultrasound diagnosis, treatment, and outcome. *J Pediatr Surg* 1998;33:492–499.

139. Lopoo JB, Goldstein RB, Lipshutz GS, Goldberg JD, Harrison MR, et al. Fetal pulmonary sequestration: a favorable congenital lung lesion. *Obstet Gynecol* 1999;94:567–571.

140. Thomas CS, Leopold GR, Hilton S, Key T, Coen R, et al. Fetal hydrops associated with extralobar pulmonary sequestration. *Ultrasound Med* 1986;5:668–671.

141. Hernanz-Schulman M, Stein SM, Neblett WW, Atkinson JB, Kirchner SG, et al. Pulmonary sequestration: diagnosis with color Doppler sonography and a new theory of associated hydrothorax. *Radiology* 1991;180:817–821.

142. Lacy DE, Shaw NJ, Pilling DW, Walkinshaw S. Outcome of congenital lung abnormalities detected antenatally. *Acta Paediatr* 1999;88:454–458.

143. Curros F, Brunelle F. Prenatal thoracoabdominal tumor mimicking pulmonary sequestration: a diagnosis dilemma. *Eur Radiol* 2001;11:167–170.

144. Curtis MR, Mooney DP, Vaccaro TJ, Williams JC, Cendron M, et al. Prenatal ultrasound characterization of the suprarenal mass: distinction between neuroblastoma and subdiaphragmatic extralobar pulmonary sequestration. *J Ultrasound Med* 1997;16:75–83.

145. Dolkart LA, Reimers FR, Helmuth WV, Porte MA, Eisinger G. Antenatal diagnosis of pulmonary sequestration: a review. *Obstet Gynecol Surv* 1992;47:515–520.

146. Morin L, Crombleholme TM, Louis F, D'Alton ME. Bronchopulmonary sequestration: prenatal diagnosis with clinicopathologic correlation. *Curr Opin Obstet Gynecol* 1994;6: 479–481.

147. Slotnick RN, McGahan JP, Milo L, Schwartz M, Ablin D. Antenatal diagnosis and treatment of fetal bronchopulmonary sequestration. *Fetal Therapy* 1990;5:33–39.

148. Curros F, Chigot V, Edmond S, Sayegh N, Revillon Y, et al. Role of embolization in the treatment of bronchopulmonary sequestration. *Pediatr Radiol* 2000;11:769–773.

149. Pare JAP, Fraser RG. *Synopsis of diseases of the chest.* Philadelphia: WB Saunders, 1983:863.

150. Bagolan P, Bilancioni E, Nahom A, Trucchi A, Inserra A, et al. Prenatal diagnosis of a bronchogenic cyst in an unusual site. *Obstet Gynecol* 2000;15:66–68.

151. Condon VR. The heart and great vessels. In: Silverman FN, Kuhn JP, eds. *Essentials of Caffey's pediatric x-ray diagnosis.* Chicago: Year Book, 1990;383–492.

152. Mayden KL, Tortora M, Chervenak FA, Hobbins JC. The antenatal sonographic detection of lung masses. *Am J Obstet Gynecol* 1984;148:349–351.

153. McAdams HP, Kirejczyk WM, Rosado-de-Christenson ML, Matsumoto S. Bronchogenic cyst: imaging features with clinical and histopathologic correlation. *Radiology* 2000; 217:441–446.

154. Young G, L'Heureux PR, Krueckeberg ST, Swanson DA. Mediastinal bronchogenic cyst: prenatal sonographic diagnosis. *AJR Am J Roentgenol* 1989;152:125–127.

155. Levine D, Jennings R, Barnewolt C, Mehta T, Wilson J, et al. Progressive fetal bronchial obstruction caused by a bronchogenic cyst diagnose of using prenatal MR imaging. *AJR Am J Roentgenol* 2001;176:49–52.

156. dePerrot M, Pache JC, Spiliopoulos A. Carcinoma arising in congenital lung cysts. *Thorac Cardiovasc Surg* 2001;49: 184–185.

157. Sullivan SM, Okada S, Kudo M, Ebihara Y. A retroperitoneal bronchogenic cyst with malignant change. *Pathol Int* 1999;49:338–341.

158. Beigelman C, Howarth NR, Chartrand-Lefebvre C, Grenier P. Congenital anomalies of tracheobronchial branching patterns: spiral CT aspects in adults. *Eur Radiol* 1998;8:79–85.

159. Hendren WH, McKee DM. Lobar emphysema of infancy. *J Pediatr Surg* 1966;1:24–39.

160. Schwartz MZ, Ramachandan P. Congenital malformations of the lung and mediastinum—a quarter century of experience from a single institution. *J Pediatr Surg* 1997;32: 44–47.

161. Bailey PV, Tracy T Sr, Connors RH, Demello D, Lewis JE, et al. Congenital bronchopulmonary malformations. Diagnostic and therapeutic considerations. *J Thorac Cardiovasc Surg* 1990;99:597–602.

162. Takeda S, Miyoshi S, Inoue M, Omori K, Okumura M, et al. Clinical spectrum of congenital cystic disease of the lung in children. *Eur J Cardiothorac Surg* 1999;15:11–17.

163. Haller JA Jr, Golladay ES, Pickard LR, Tepas JJ 3rd, Shorter NA, et al. Surgical management of lung bud anomalies: lobar emphysema, bronchogenic cyst, cystic adenomatoid. *Ann Thorac Surg* 1979;28:33–43.

164. Hedlund GL, Griscom NT, Cleveland RH, Kirks DR. Respiratory system. In: Kirks DR, ed. *Practical pediatric imaging: diagnostic radiology of infants and children.* Philadelphia: Lippincott–Raven 1998:619–910.

165. Reed JC, Sobonya RE. Morphologic analysis of foregut cysts in the thorax. *Am J Roentgenol Radium Ther Nucl Med* 1974;120:851–860.

166. Fernandes ET, Custer MD, Burton EM, Boulden TF, Wrenn EL Jr, et al. Neuroenteric cyst: surgery and diagnostic imaging. *J Pediatr Surg* 1991;26:108–110.

167. Haddon MJ, Bowen A. Bronchopulmonary and neuroenteric forms of foregut anomalies. Imaging for diagnosis and management. *Radiol Clin North Am* 1991;29:241–254.

168. Macaulay KE, Winter TC 3rd, Shields LE. Neuroenteric cyst shown by prenatal sonography. *AJR Am J Roentgenol* 1997;169:563–565.

169. Wilkinson CC, Albanese CT, Jennings RW, Feldstein VA, Goldberg JD, et al. Fetal neuroenteric cyst causing hydrops: case report and review of the literature. *Prenat Diagn* 1999;19:118–121.

170. Hedrick MH, Ferro MM, Filly RA, Flake AW, Harrison MR, et al. Congenital high airway obstruction syndrome (CHAOS): a potential for perinatal intervention. *J Pediatr Surg* 1994;29:271–274.

171. Schauer GM, Dun LK, Godmilow L, Eagle RC Jr, Knisely AS. Prenatal diagnosis of Fraser syndrome at 18.5 weeks gestation, with autopsy findings at 19 weeks. *Am J Med Gen* 1990;37:583–591.

172. Fang SH, Ocejo R, Sin M, Finer NN, Wood BP. Radiological cases of the month. Congenital laryngeal atresia. *Am J Dis Child* 1989;143:625–627.

173. DeCou JM, Jones DC, Jacobs HD, Touloukian RJ. Successful ex utero intrapartum treatment (EXIT) procedure for congenital high airway obstruction syndrome (CHAOS) owing to laryngeal atresia. *J Pediatr Surg* 1998;33:1563–1565.

174. McAlister WH, Wright JR Jr, Crane JP. Main-stem bronchial atresia: intrauterine sonographic diagnosis. *AJR Am J Roentgenol* 1987;148:364–366.

175. King SJ, Pilling DW, Walkinshaw S. Fetal echogenic lung lesions: prenatal ultrasound diagnosis and outcome. *Pediatr Radiol* 1995;25:208–210.

176. Scott JN, Trevenen CL, Wiseman DA, Elliott PD. Tracheal atresia: ultrasonographic and pathologic correlation. *Ultrasound Med* 1999;18:357.

177. Wigglesworth JS, Desai R, Hislop AA. Fetal lung growth in congenital laryngeal atresia. *Pediatr Pathol* 1987;7:515–25.

178. Silver MM, Thurston WA, Patrick JE. Perinatal pulmonary hyperplasia due to laryngeal atresia. *Hum Pathol* 1988;19: 110–113.

179. Morrison PJ, Macphail S, Williams D, McCusker G, McKeever P, et al. Laryngeal atresia or stenosis presenting as second-trimester fetal ascites—diagnosis and pathology in three independent cases. *Prenat Diagn* 1998;18:963–967.

180. Choong KKL, Trudinger B, Chow C, Osborn RA. Fetal laryngeal obstruction: sonographic detection. *Obstet Gynecol* 1992;2:357–359.

181. Myer CM 3rd. Larynx, atresia. In: Buyse ML. *Birth defects encyclopedia.* Dover, MA: Center for Birth Defects Information Services, 1990:1034–1035.

182. Witters IP, Moerman D, Fryns JP. Prenatal echographic diagnosis of laryngeal atresia as part of a multiple congenital anomalies (MCA) syndrome. *Genet Couns* 2000;11:215–219.

183. Haugen G, Jenum PA, Scheie D, Sund S, Stray-Pedersen B. Prenatal diagnosis of tracheal obstruction: possible association with maternal pertussis infection. *Ultrasound Obstet Gynecol* 2000;15:69–73.

184. Bui TH, Grunewald C, Frenckner B, Frenckner B, Kuylenstierng R, et al. Successful EXIT (ex utero intrapartum treatment) procedure in a fetus diagnosed prenatally with congenital high-airway obstruction syndrome due to laryngeal atresia. *Eur Pediatr Surg* 2000;10:328–333.

185. Crombleholme TM, Sylvester K, Flake AW, Adzick NS. Salvage of a fetus with congenital high airway obstruction syndrome by ex utero intrapartum treatment (EXIT) procedure. *Fetal Diagn Ther* 2000;15:280–282.

186. Longaker MT, Laberge JM, Dansereau J, Langer JC, Crombleholme TM, et al. Primary fetal hydrothorax: natural history and management. *Pediatr Surg* 1989;24:573–576.

187. Weber AM, Philipson EH. Fetal pleural effusion: a review and meta-analysis for prognostic indicators. *Obstet Gynecol* 1992;79:281–286.

188. Aubard Y, Derouineau I, Aubard V, Chalifor V, Preux PM. Primary fetal hydrothorax: a literature review and proposed antenatal clinical strategy. *Fetal Diagn Ther* 1998;3:325–333.

189. DeVore GR, Acherman RJ, Cabal LA, Siassi B, Platt LD. Hypoalbuminemia: the etiology of antenatally diagnosed pericardial effusion in rhesus-hemolytic anemia. *Am J Obstet Gynecol* 1982;142:1056–1057.

190. Van Arede J, Campbell AN, Smyth JA, Lloyd D, Bryan MH. Spontaneous chylothorax in newborns. *Am J Dis Child* 1984;138:961–964.

191. Sardet A. Chylothorax in children and newborn infants. *Arch Fr Pediatr* 1981;38:455.

192. Hunter WS, Becroft DM. Congenital pulmonary lymphangiectasis associated with pleural effusions. *Arch Dis Child* 1984;59:278–279.

193. Hagay Z, Reece A, Roberts A, Hobbins JC. Isolated fetal pleural effusion: a prenatal management dilemma. *Obstet Gynecol* 1993;81:147–152.

194. Cadkin A, Pergament E. Bilateral pleural effusion at 8.5 weeks gestation with Down syndrome and Turner syndrome. *Prenat Diagn* 1993;13:659–660.

195. Benacerraf BR, Frigoleto FD Jr. Mid-trimester fetal thoracentesis. *J Clin Ultrasound* 1985;13:202–204.

196. Vain NE, Swamer OW, Cha CC. Neonatal chylothorax: a report and discussion of nine consecutive cases. *J Pediatr Surg* 1980;15:261–265.

197. Chernick V, Reed MH. Pneumothorax and chylothorax in the neonatal in the neonatal period. *J Pediatr* 1970;76:624–632.

198. Petres RE, Redwine FO, Cruikshank DP. Congenital bilateral chylothorax. Antepartum diagnosis and successful intrauterine surgical management. *JAMA* 1982;248:1360–1361.

199. Lange IR, Manning FA. Antenatal diagnosis of congenital pleural effusions. *Am J Obstet Gynecol* 1981;140:839–840.

200. Eddleman KA, Levine AB, Chitkara U, Berkowitz RL. Non-immune hydrops fetalis: clinical experience and factors related to a poor outcome. *Am J Obstet Gynecol* 1986;155:530–532.

201. Hutchison AA, Drew JH, Yu VY, Williams ML, Gortune DW, et al. Nonimmunologic hydrops fetalis: review of 61 cases. *Obstet Gynecol* 1982;59:347–352.

202. Castillo RA, Devoe LD, Hadi HA, Martin S, Geist D. Non-immune hydrops fetalis: clinical experience and factors related to a poor outcome. *Am J Obstet Gynecol* 1986;155:812–816.

203. Petrikovsky BM, Shmoys SM, Baker DA, Monheit AG. Pleural effusion in aneuploidy. *Am J Perinatol* 1991;8:214–216.

204. Sherer DM, Abramowicz JS, Sanko SR, Woods JR Jr. Trisomy 21 presented as a transient unilateral pleural effusion at 18 weeks gestation. *Am J Perinatol* 1993;10:12–13.

205. Achiron R, Weissman A, Lipitz S, Mashiach S, Goldman B. Fetal pleural effusion: the risk of fetal trisomy. *Gynecol Obstet Invest* 1995;39:153–156.

206. Shimizu T, Hashimoto K, Shimizu M, Ozaki M, Murata Y. Bilateral pleural effusion in the first trimester: a predictor of chromosomal abnormality and embryonic death? *Am J Obstet Gynecol* 1997;177:470–471.

207. Nicolaides K, Rodeck CH, Gosden CM. Rapid karyotyping in non-lethal fetal malformations. *Lancet* 1985–1989;1:283–287.

208. Wilkins-Haug LE, Doubilet P. Successful thoracoamniotic shunting and review of the literature in unilateral pleural effusion with hydrops. *Ultrasound Med* 1997;16:153–160.

209. Holzgreve W. Management of the fetus with nonimmune hydrops. In: Harrison MR, Golbus MS, Filly RA, eds. *The unborn patient.* Orlando: Grune & Stratton 1984;193–216.

210. Mahony BS, Filly RA, Callen PW, Chinn DH. Severe non-immune hydrops fetalis: sonographic evaluation. *Radiology* 1984;151:757–761.

211. Estroff JA, Parad RB, Frigoletto FD Jr, Benacerraf BR. The natural history of isolated fetal hydrothorax. *Ultrasound Obstet Gynecol* 1992;162–165.

CARDIAC ANATOMY AND SONOGRAPHIC APPROACH

Congenital heart disease is one of the more common and often devastating congenital anomalies, with an estimated incidence just less than 1% of all live births.[1,2] *In utero* diagnosis of cardiac malformations is important, as it is often associated with a high rate of morbidity or mortality in the fetus and the neonate. Although sonography has been used for more than 30 years in diagnosis of congenital abnormalities, only more recently have we become more proficient in diagnosing a number of congenital heart abnormalities by ultrasound. In many instances, only a four-chamber view of the heart and an M-mode ultrasound through the heart are obtained as the portion of the screening examination of the fetal heart.[3,4] However, it is estimated that the screening four-chamber view of the heart may detect only 50% to 60% of cardiac malformations.[5,6] Others have shown that visualization of the right and the left ventricular outflow tracts, when performed by trained personnel, increases the sensitivity of the ultrasound examination to approximately 75% in detecting congenital cardiac defects.[5,6] However, this limited screening examination does not constitute a thorough examination of the fetal heart. Thus, other real-time views combined with color-flow mapping, pulsed Doppler, and M-mode echocardiography are needed to obtain a complete study for understanding more complex cardiac malformations.

The purpose of this chapter is to discuss the ultrasound approach used to examine the fetal heart. In preparing this material, the first inclination is to systematically list the views and the imaging modalities that are available to accomplish this task without considering the purpose of the examination, the skill of the examiner, and the type of ultrasound equipment available. However, the material is presented using a logical, stepwise progression that begins with the *screening* examination, offered by the radiologist, obstetrician, or sonographer, and evolves to the *diagnostic* examination performed by the specialist in fetal cardiovascular imaging.

FOUR-CHAMBER SCREENING EXAMINATION OF THE FETAL HEART

Technique

High-resolution real-time equipment using linear array, curved array, or sector scanners may be used for fetal echocardiography. It is important to use transducer frequencies as high as possible, in the range of 5 to 8 MHz. Image magnification and cine loops for instantaneous playback of information are recommended. Digital storage of information in real time, either with software available within the ultrasound equipment or a separate attached video recorder, is helpful for review of the study and to further analyze data frame by frame to elucidate some of the more subtle findings. This type of examination involves the most common imaging modality available to practitioners of fetal ultrasound—grey-scale real-time ultrasound. Using this approach, basic cardiovascular anatomy can be identified. Although useful, there may be limitations, especially during the second trimester, when grey-scale imaging can be limited by fetal position, maternal adipose tissue, or abdominal wall scar from previous abdominal or pelvic surgery.[7]

Position of the Heart within the Chest

In the normal fetus, the stomach and the four-chamber view of the heart are positioned within the left side of the body (Figs. 1 and 2). If the stomach and heart are in opposite positions, then there is an abnormality of situs in which either the stomach or the heart is on the incorrect side of the body.[8] Rarely, the stomach and heart are located on the right side of the body. When this occurs, complete situs inversus may be present. To identify normal situs of the heart, the preferred method is the following:

1. Identify the position of the fetus *in utero*.
2. Determine if the left side is up or down.
3. Identify the stomach and heart to be on the left side. Some examiners have found that having a *doll* to position on the maternal abdomen after the fetal

verse plane used in obtaining the four chambers of the fetal heart. **B:** Artist's conception of the four-chamber view of the heart, with the blood entering the right atrium from the inferior vena cava, being directed primarily across the foramen ovale. Two of the four pulmonary veins that enter into the left atrium are illustrated. Other structures are labeled. *Continued.*

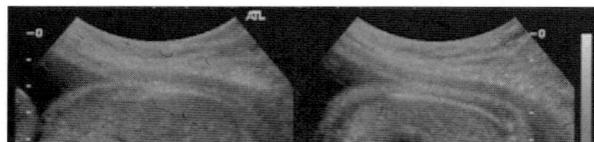

sidedness and usually presents with less severe cardiac malformations.

In either situs solitus or situs inversus, the cardiac apex may point to the left, as with levocardia, or to the right, as

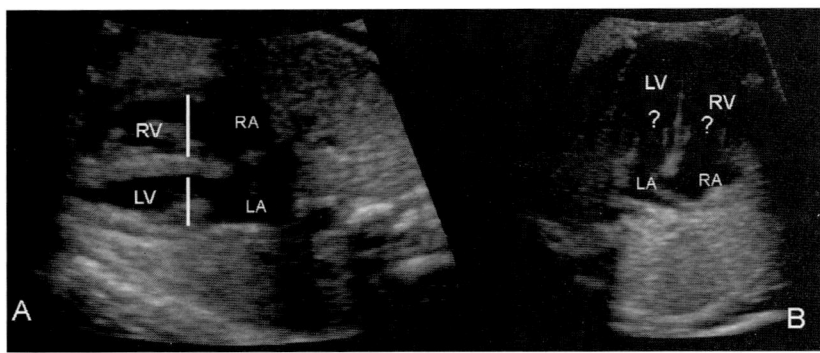

FIGURE 6. Ventricular size. The left ventricle (*LV*) and the right ventricle (*RV*) are nearly equal in size, most accurately identified when the ultrasound beam is oriented perpendicular **(A)** rather than parallel **(B)** to the ultrasound beam. Note the lines depicting the ventricular size as measured at the valve openings are approximately equal. LA, left atrium; RA, right atrium.

TRANSITION BETWEEN THE SCREENING AND DIAGNOSTIC EXAMINATION

Real-Time Grey-Scale Outflow Tracts Examination

Although the outflow tracts examination is considered by some to be part of the screening examination of the fetal heart, it has not been endorsed at this time by the American College of Obstetricians and Gynecologists, the American College of Radiology, or the American Institute of Ultrasound in Medicine. However, in a recent American Institute of Ultrasound in Medicine Technical Bulletin the outflow tracts examination is listed as part of the *extended* cardiovascular examination.[16] Three approaches to the examination of the outflow tracts exist, all of which use the four-chamber view as the reference point. When the outflow tracts are imaged, the following should be identified:

1. The aortic outflow tract originates from the left ventricle.
2. The pulmonary outflow tract originates from the right ventricle.
3. These two outflow tracts are of similar size.

4. The ascending aorta and the main pulmonary artery are perpendicular to each other as they exit their respective ventricles.
5. The ascending aorta becomes the aortic arch, with the corresponding arch vessels branching from the cephalad portion of the vessel.
6. The main pulmonary artery bifurcates into the right and left pulmonary arteries, with the ductus arteriosus branching from the point of bifurcation.

Four-Chamber View Cephalad Sweep

The four-chamber view cephalad sweep is best used when the fetus is supine or when the left side of the fetus is nearest the transducer. Using the four-chamber view as the reference point, the transducer beam is directed cephalad in a transverse plane until the neck is imaged. Using this imaging technique, all the criteria previously listed are met except identification of the vessels originating from the aortic arch. There are five imaging planes that the examiner must be familiar with as one directs the transducer beam cephalad from the four-chamber view.[17]

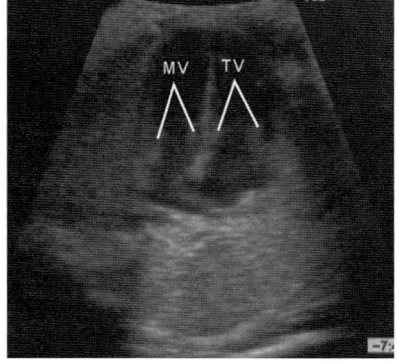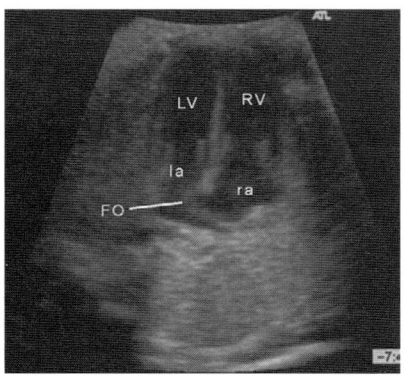

FIGURE 7. Four-chamber view of the heart. **A:** The openings for the mitral (*MV*) and tricuspid valves (*TV*) are similar in size, best appreciated with the ultrasound beam oriented parallel to the interventricular septum, during this scan, in which the valve leaflets are open. **B:** The foramen ovale (*FO*) is located in the middle third of the atrial septum and opens into the left atrium (*la*) from the right atrium (*ra*). LV, left ventricle; RV, right ventricle.

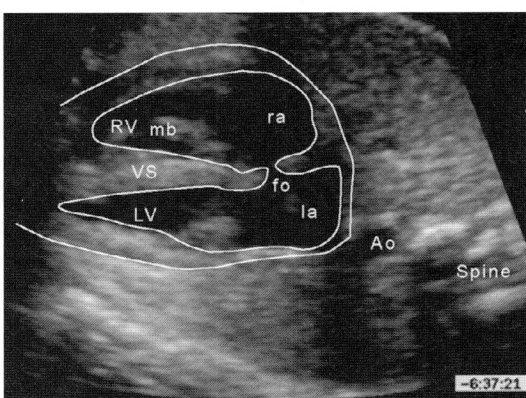

FIGURE 8. Four-chamber view of the heart with the interventricular septum perpendicular to the ultrasound beam. This view illustrates an intact ventricular septum (*VS*), foramen ovale (*fo*), and the thickened muscle of the moderator band (*mb*) in the right ventricle. Ao, descending aorta; la, left atrium; LV, left ventricle; ra, right atrium; RV, right ventricle.

1. *Level I: Four-chamber view.* From this image the examiner identifies the right and left sides of the heart (Fig. 8).

2. *Level II: Ascending aorta.* This is identified as it exits the left ventricle. The posterior wall of the aorta is contiguous with the anterior leaflet of the mitral valve, and the superior wall of the ascending aorta is contiguous with the interventricular septum (Fig. 9).

3. *Level III: Main pulmonary artery.* This level demonstrates the main pulmonary artery originating from the right ventricle and running perpendicular to the ascending aorta. At this level, the bifurcation of the right and left pulmonary arteries can be observed (Fig. 10).

4. *Level IV: Ductus arteriosus.* Further sweeping the beam cephalad demonstrates the ductus arteriosus originating from the bifurcation of the main pulmonary artery. The

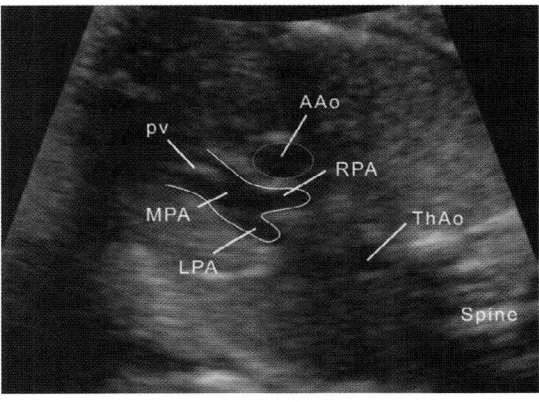

FIGURE 10. Pulmonary artery. By angling the transducer further cephalad, the main pulmonary artery (*MPA*) can be identified exiting the right ventricle. In this view, the pulmonary artery should be perpendicular rather than parallel to the aorta that was identified in Figure 9. AAo, ascending aorta; LPA, left pulmonary artery; pv, pulmonary valve; RPA, right pulmonary artery; ThAo, thoracic aorta.

ductus arteriosus runs directly posterior and to the left of the spine when it empties into the thoracic aorta (Fig. 11).

5. *Level V: Transverse aortic arch.* The highest level of the sweep identifies the transverse aortic arch going from the right side of the chest into the descending thoracic aorta (Fig. 12).

The full aortic and ductal arches can be identified using the previous technique through a simple modification of this technique. The aortic arch can be identified when the ultrasound beam is oriented perpendicular to the interventricular septum. By directing the ultrasound beam cephalad, the transverse arch is identified parallel to the beam (Fig. 12). Once the transverse

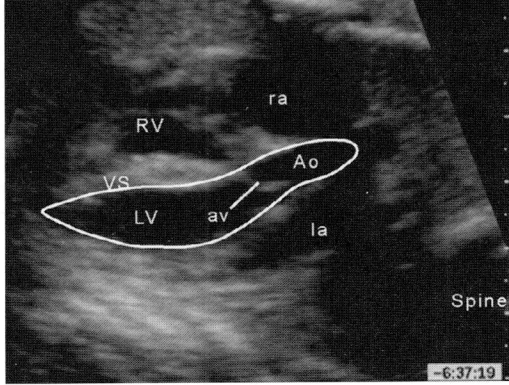

FIGURE 9. Ascending aorta. As the ultrasound probe is angled and directed more cephalad from four-chamber view, the ascending aorta (*Ao*) is identified exiting from the left ventricle (*LV*). This view may be useful to identify a defect in the ventricular septum (*VS*), which is contiguous with the superior wall of the ascending aorta. av, aortic valve; la, left atrium; ra, right atrium; RV, right ventricle.

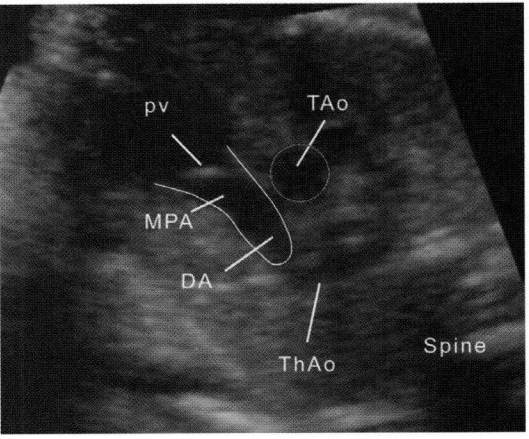

FIGURE 11. Ductus arteriosus. Directing the ultrasound beam further cephalad, the ductus arteriosus (*DA*) can be identified originating from the main pulmonary artery (*MPA*) that runs posterior and to the left of the spine to empty into the thoracic aorta (*ThAo*). pv, pulmonary valve; TAo, transverse aorta.

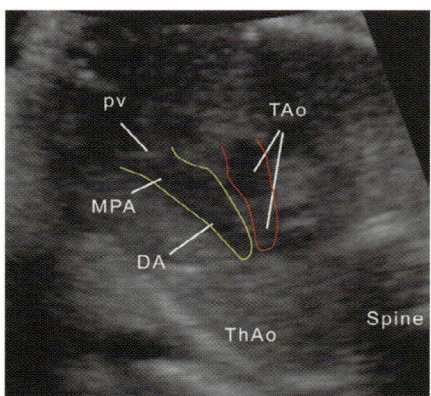

FIGURE 12. Transverse aortic arch (*TAo*). At the highest level of the sweep, the main pulmonary artery (*MPA*) emptying into the ductus arteriosus (*DA*) can be identified, with the transverse aortic arch identified to the right side of the chest emptying into the thoracic aorta (*ThAo*). pv, pulmonary valve.

arch is identified, the transducer is rotated 90 degrees (Fig. 13A). The full aortic arch then comes into view. It is important to identify that the head and neck vessels originate from the aortic arch (Fig. 14). These vessels may be more readily identified using color or power Doppler ultrasound (Fig. 13B and C). In abnormalities of the aortic arch, such as hypoplastic left heart syndrome, the more proximal portion of the arch may be atretic compared to the descending aorta. In this view, the arch of the aorta appears like a *cane*. The ascending aorta rises more centrally within the thorax and connects through the arch to the descending aorta that lies against the spine. The ductal arch can be identified when the ultrasound beam is oriented tangential to the interventricular septum, with the fetus in the supine position. By directing the ultrasound beam cephalad, the ductus arteriosus is identified parallel to the beam. Once the ductus is identified, the transducer is rotated 90 degrees until the full ductal arch comes into view (see Fig. 16A). This view has been thought to appear like a *hockey stick* and may be more readily identified with color Doppler ultrasound (Figs. 15 and 16B and C).

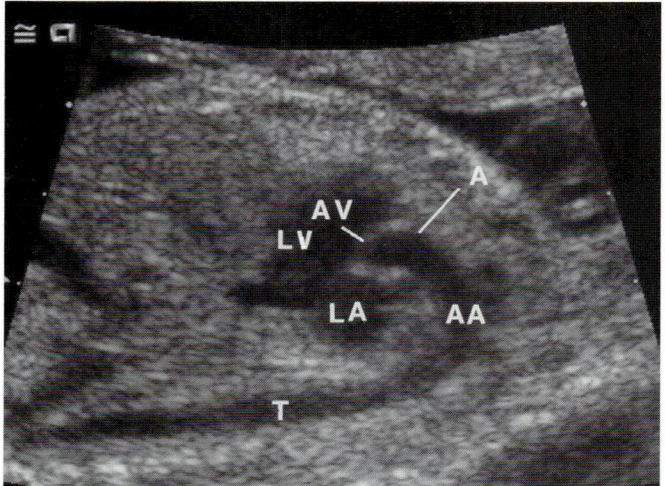

A

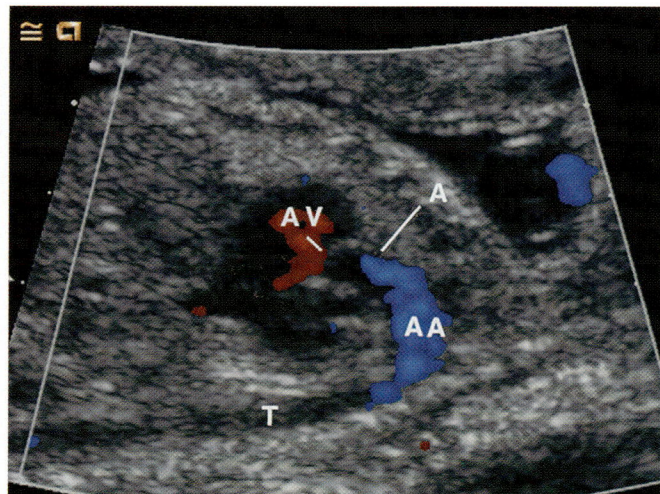

B

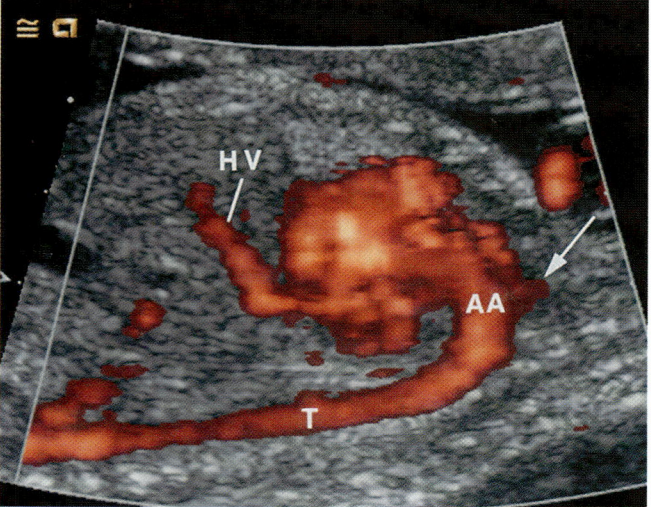

C

FIGURE 13. Aortic arch (*AA*) view. **A:** In the real-time image, after identifying the transverse aortic arch, the ultrasound probe is rotated 90 degrees to identify the entire aortic arch, which appears as a *cane*. The entire arch from the aortic valve (*AV*), including the ascending aorta (*A*), the aortic arch, and the thoracic aorta (*T*), are identified in this fetus, in the supine position. LA, left atrium; LV, left ventricle. **B, C:** Aortic arch view. Similar findings are identified with color (**B**) and power (**C**) Doppler ultrasound showing the aortic arch. In the power Doppler image, a hepatic vein (*HV*) and a head and neck vessel (*arrow*) are identified.

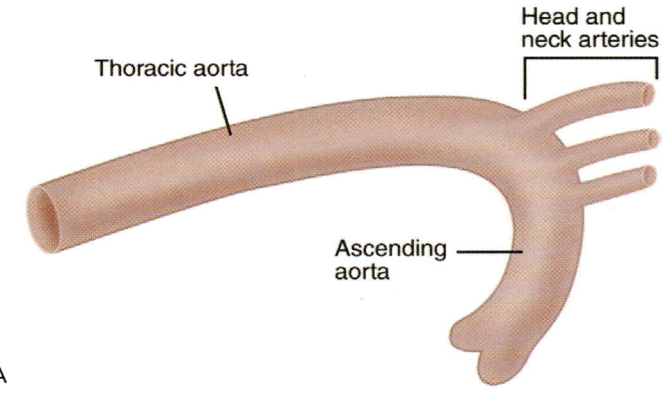

A

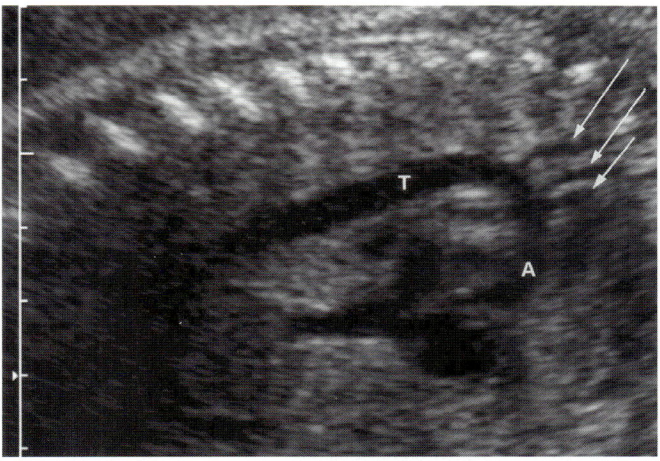

B

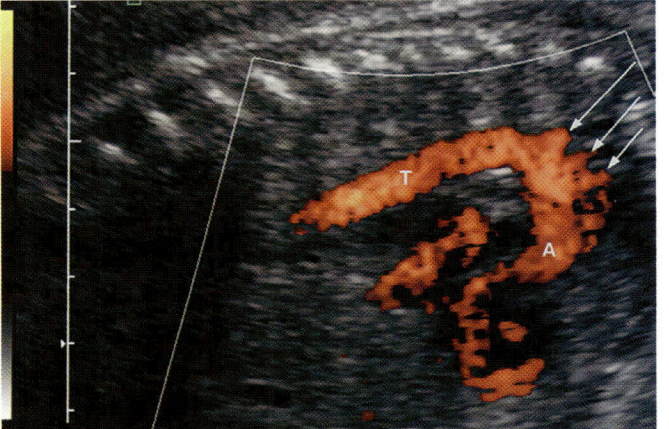

C

FIGURE 14. Aortic arch-head and neck vessels. **A:** Artist's conception demonstrating the head and neck arteries arising from the aortic arch, with the ascending aorta and the thoracic aorta illustrated. **B, C:** In this fetus, in the prone position, the ascending aorta (*A*) and the thoracic aorta (*T*) are noted appearing as a cane. It is important to identify the head and neck vessels (*arrows*) originating from the aortic arch. This is seen with the real-time image in **(B)** and in the power Doppler image in **(C)** of this figure.

Yagel et al. proposed an examination of the fetal heart by five short axis views (Fig. 17) as a proposed screening method for a comprehensive cardiac evaluation. This is similar to the four-chamber view cephalad sweep. This simplified, comprehensive fetal heart examination is based on five transverse planes. These include the following[18]:

1. The most caudal view is the transverse view of the upper abdomen, demonstrating the fetal stomach as well as the abdominal aorta, spine, and liver. This is helpful to determine the fetal situs.

2. The traditional four-chamber view, which remains the key to the fetal cardiographic examination.

3. The third plane is the five-chamber view of the heart. In this view, the aortic route is identified most centrally, as well as the two ventricles and two atria.

4. A transverse view above this level revealing the bifurcation of the pulmonary arteries. This cross-sectional view of the major vessels is a quick and accurate method to identify the great vessels, including the bifurcation of the left and right pulmonary arteries and cross sections of the ascending and descending aortas.

5. The fifth short axis view complements the traditional planes and includes the three vessels and the trachea. In this

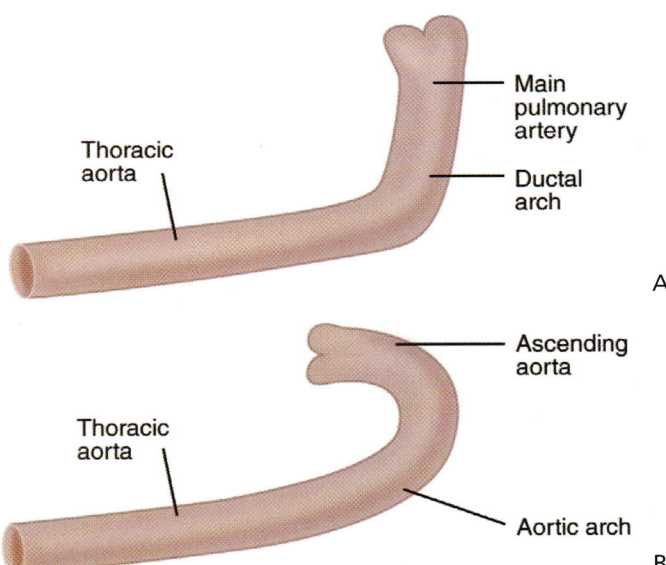

A

B

FIGURE 15. Artist's conception demonstrating the ductal arch **(A)** appearing as a hockey stick. The main pulmonary artery gives rise to the ductal arch and connects to the thoracic aorta. **B:** The aortic arch appears more like a candy cane, with the ascending aorta giving rise to the aortic arch and connecting to the thoracic arch. This is the artist's illustration for the corresponding figures of the ductal and aortic arch.

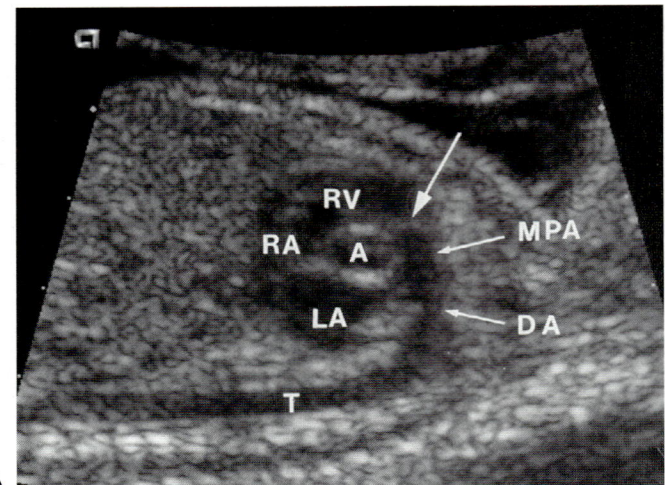

A

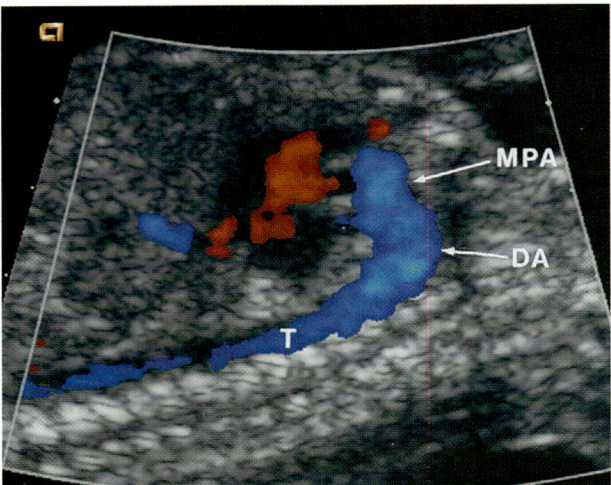

B

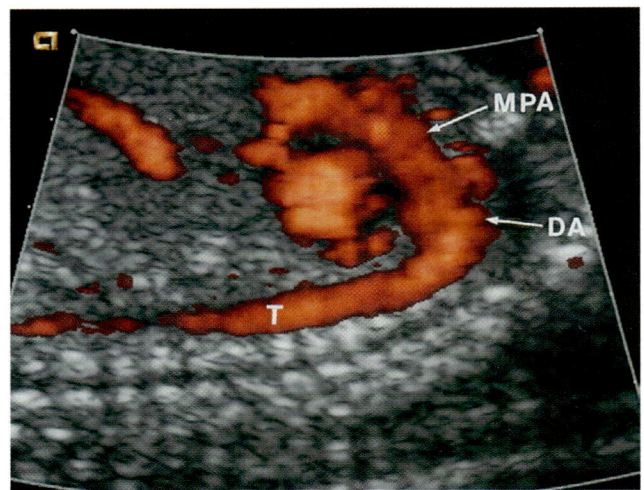

C

FIGURE 16. The ductal arch. **A:** The ductal arch is observed in this fetus in the supine position. The right ventricle (*RV*) lies anterior to the aorta (*A*) and gives rise to the main pulmonary artery (*MPA*). The pulmonary artery then connects through the ductus arteriosis (*DA*) into the thoracic aorta. The arrow in this figure points to the pulmonary valve. LA, left atrium; RA, right atrium; T, thoracic arch. **B, C:** The ductal arch. The ductal arch is identified in color (**B**) and power (**C**) Doppler ultrasound. The main pulmonary artery (*MPA*), the ductus arteriosis (*DA*), and the thoracic arch (*T*) are identified.

view, the pulmonary trunk, proximal aorta, and ductus arteriosus are identified. The distal aorta, superior vena cava, and trachea are also visualized.

Four-Chamber Rotational Sweep: Interventricular Septum Perpendicular to the Ultrasound Beam

The four-chamber rotational sweep is most useful when the interventricular septum is perpendicular to the ultrasound beam.[19] There are three movements of the transducer required to evaluate the outflow tracts when using this technique.

1. The four-chamber view is identified with the interventricular septum perpendicular to the ultrasound beam (Fig. 18).

2. The transducer is then rotated approximately 45 degrees so that the beam bisects a plane between the left hip and right shoulder of the fetus. This identifies the ascending aorta as it exits the left ventricle (Fig. 19A and B). In this view, a portion of the transverse arch is also identified.

3. Once the ascending aorta and transverse arch are identified, the transducer, remaining in the same position, is rocked cephalad (Fig. 19D). This movement results in the display of the main pulmonary artery exiting the right ventricle and coursing perpendicular to the ascending aorta.

In a study reported in 1992, DeVore et al. reported that 80% of fetuses imaged during the second trimester were in a position such that this approach could be used. In the third trimester, more than 90% of fetuses were in a position that allowed the outflow tracts to be imaged using this maneuver.[19]

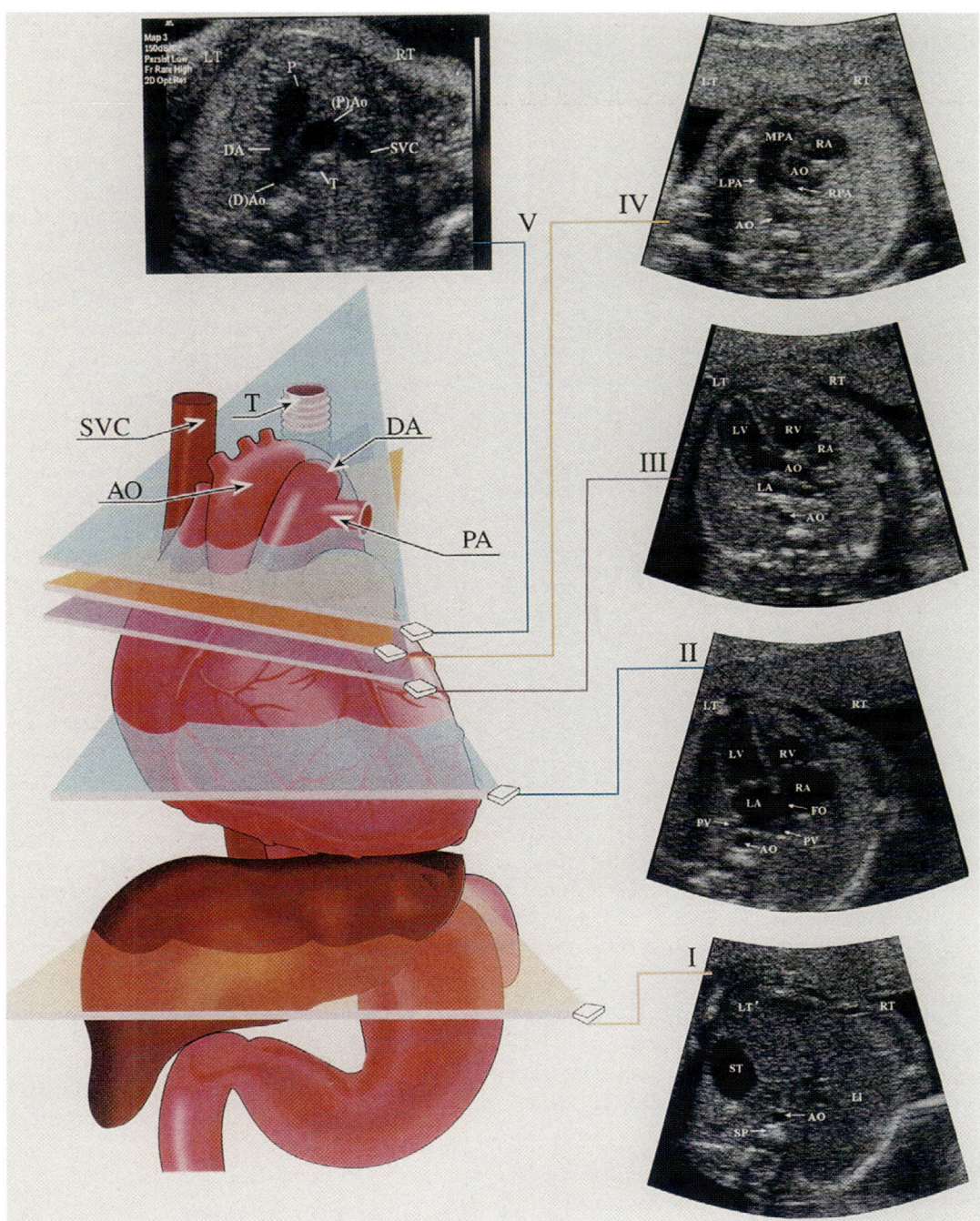

FIGURE 17. The five short axis views for optimal fetal heart screening. The color image shows the trachea (*T*), heart and great vessels, liver, and stomach with the five planes of insonation superimposed. AO, aorta; DA, ductus arteriosus; PA, pulmonary artery; SVC, superior vena cava. Polygons show the angle of the transducer and are assigned to the relevant grey-scale images. **I:** The most caudal plane, showing the fetal stomach (*ST*), cross section of the abdominal aorta (*AO*), spine (*SP*), and liver (*Li*). LT, left; RT, right. **II:** The four-chamber view of the heart, showing the right and left ventricles (*RV* and *LV*) and atria (*RA* and *LA*), foramen ovale (*FO*), and pulmonary veins (*PV*) to the right (*RT*) and left (*LT*) of the aorta (*AO*). **III:** The five-chamber view, showing the aortic root (*AO*), left and right ventricles (*LV* and *RV*) and left and right atria (*LA* and *RA*), and a cross section of the descending aorta (*AO* with *arrow*). **IV:** The slightly more cephalad view, showing the main pulmonary artery (*MPA*), the bifurcation of left and right pulmonary arteries (*LPA* and *RPA*), and cross sections of the ascending and descending aorta (*AO* and *AO* with *arrow*, respectively). **V:** The 3VT plane of insonation, showing the pulmonary trunk (*P*), proximal aorta [(*P*)*Ao*], ductus arteriosus (*DA*), distal aorta [(*D*)*Ao*], superior vena cava (*SVC*), and the trachea (*T*). (Reproduced with permission from Yagel S, Cohen SM, Achiron R. Examination of the fetal heart by five short-axis views: a proposed screening method for comprehensive cardiac evaluation. *Ultrasound Obstet Gynecol* 2001;17:367–369.)

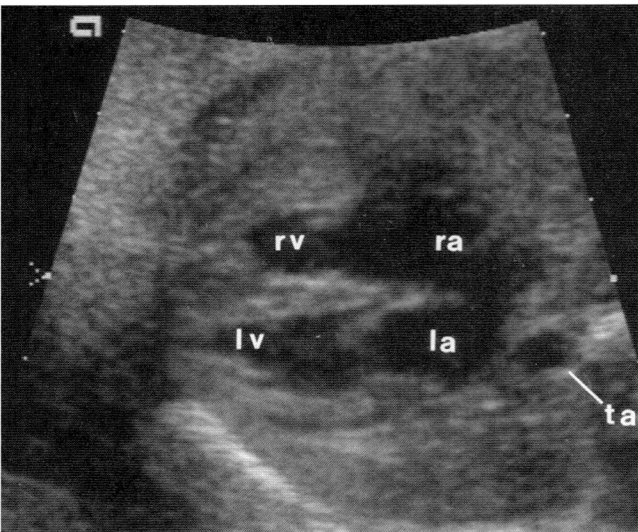

FIGURE 18. Four-chamber view of the heart. This is the orientation of the four-chamber view of the heart with the ultrasound beam oriented perpendicular to the interventricular septum. Note that the right ventricle (*rv*) is retrosternal. The left ventricle (*lv*) forms the majority of the left heart border. The corresponding right atrium (*ra*) and the left atrium (*la*) are noted. The thoracic aorta (*ta*) is labeled.

Four-Chamber Rotational Sweep: Interventricular Septum Tangential to the Ultrasound Beam

The four-chamber rotational sweep is most useful when the fetus is supine and the interventricular septum tangential to the ultrasound beam. There are two movements of the transducer to evaluate the outflow tracts using this technique.

1. The four-chamber view is identified with the interventricular septum tangential to the ultrasound beam.
2. The transducer is then rotated more parallel to the long axis of the spine and is angled cephalad (Fig. 20A and B).

In this view the aorta is central, with the similar-sized pulmonary artery and its bifurcation anterior and perpendicular to the aorta (Fig. 20B). The right atrium is seen emptying into the right ventricle. The valves of the pulmonary artery are noted at the root of the aorta. In general, the aorta and pulmonary outflow tract have a one-to-one relationship in early pregnancy. Later in pregnancy, the pulmonary artery becomes slightly enlarged as compared to the aorta. However, if the aorta is increased in size compared to the pulmonary artery, this may indicate such an abnormality as tetralogy of Fallot, whereas if the aorta is smaller as compared to the pulmonary artery, it may indicate certain abnormalities such as hypoplastic left heart syndrome.[20]

Color Doppler of the Four-Chamber View and the Outflow Tracts

Background

Real-time grey-scale ultrasound identifies anatomic relationships but does not provide information regarding blood flow. Because the fetal heart consists of two components, anatomy and blood flow, color Doppler ultrasound is useful during the screening examination of the heart. Color Doppler uses the principle of velocity change to display the color pixels on the screen. Using color Doppler, the direction and velocity of moving objects such as blood can be detected. The color spectrum is usually displayed on the side of the real-time image (Fig. 21). The color Doppler scale can be displayed in any color combination. Usually the scale is displayed in such a way that if the Doppler shift is toward the transducer, the color is displayed as red. If blood flow is away from the transducer, the color display is in blue. This color display is arbitrary, and any color or color combination may be used. This color bar is usually not displayed in red and blue but is often shaded in different color combinations, such as red shaded to orange or even yellow, that may reflect changes in velocity or disturbed flow. If the velocity of blood flow recording the Doppler shift of the red blood cell movement is above that at which the scale is set, then *aliasing* occurs. In this situation, within the vessel or ventricular chamber there may be a mixture of different colors. Typically, the velocity of blood is less along the edges of the vessel and appears as red, while centrally in the vessel with increased velocity there is increased color shift, maybe to yellow or even blue. This occurs when the maximum velocity or *Nyquist* limit is too low or when there is increased velocity of blood resulting in aliasing (Fig. 22). To overcome this problem, the Doppler scale is changed to a higher frequency shift so that aliasing is avoided. However, in some situations, aliasing may be important to note, as this can be a clue to increased velocity of blood in an area of stenosis. Regurgitant flow may be observed with color Doppler ultrasound. If, however, the scale is set too high, minimal amounts of regurgitant flow are not detected.

Optimizing the Image

To display color Doppler in the fetal heart, the examiner must adjust the settings to optimize the image. We have found, for example, that the fetal heart is best imaged when the persistence is 0, the wall filter is at its highest setting, and the velocity is adjusted to demonstrate flow within the entire cardiac chambers. However, if the velocity settings are too high, the color Doppler is not observed to fill all of the chambers. This can be corrected by decreasing the velocity setting but results in aliasing (Fig. 23). Aliasing should not be a problem if the only purpose is to identify where blood flow is present.

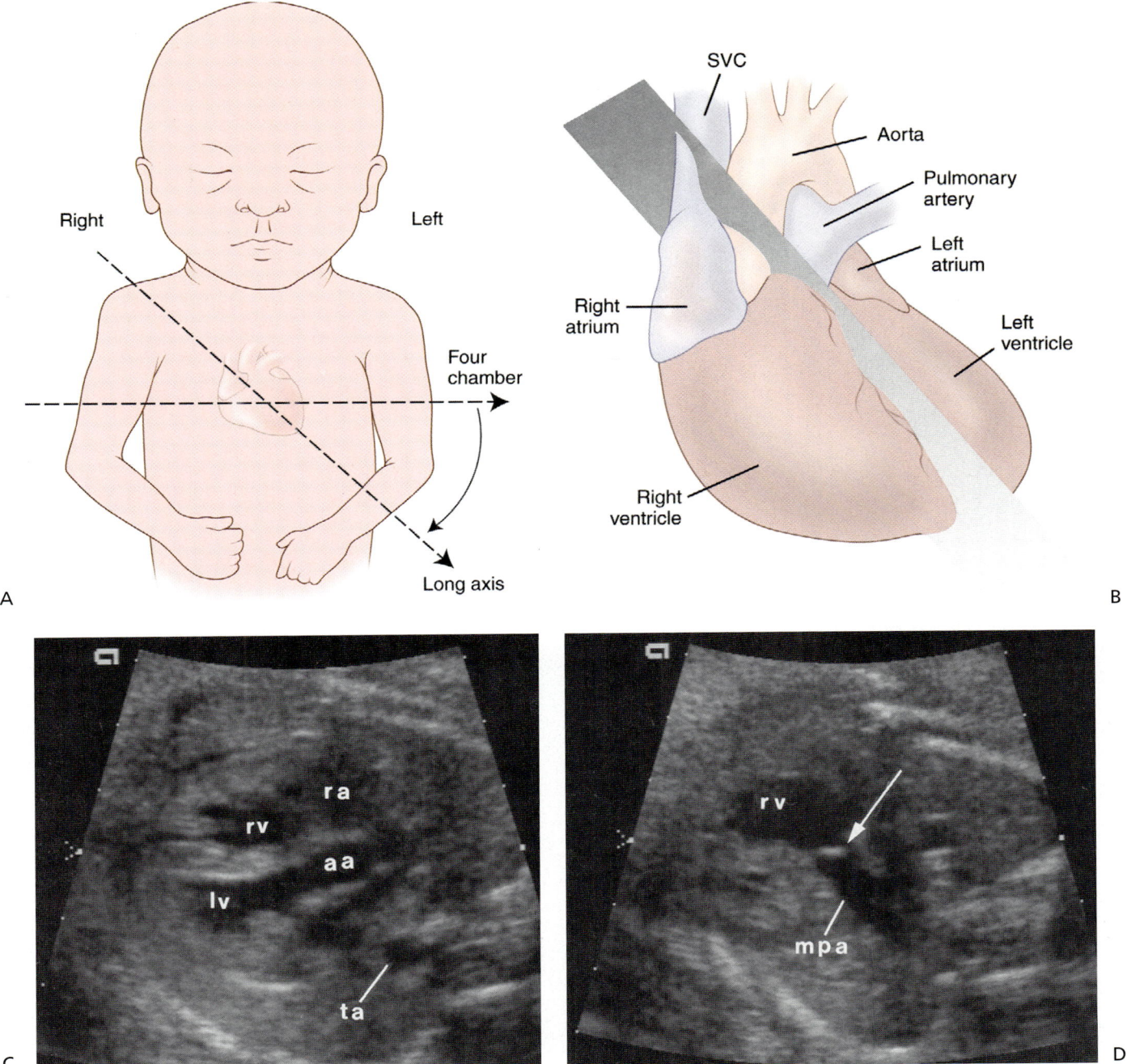

A

B

C

D

FIGURE 19. Outflow tracts of the heart. **A:** From the four-chamber view of the heart, the transducer is angled in a plane that bisects the left upper quadrant of the abdomen and the right shoulder to obtain a long axis view of the heart. **B:** The artist's conception of the plane used to obtain a long axis view of the heart, which intercepts part of the right atrium and right ventricle but, most important, demonstrates the aorta originating from the left ventricle. SVC, superior vena cava. **C:** In the same fetus as in Figure 18, the transducer is rotated in the proper plane; the ascending aorta (*aa*) is identified originating from the left ventricle (*lv*). This view may also be helpful to check for a ventricular septal defect between the left ventricle and the right ventricle (*rv*). ra, right atrium; ta, thoracic aorta. **D:** With the transducer approximately in the same position as it is in **C**, but rocked cephalad, the main pulmonary artery (*mpa*) is identified exiting the right ventricle (*rv*). A long arrow points to the pulmonic valve. Again, the pulmonary artery should course perpendicular to the ascending aorta as compared to the previous view in **C**.

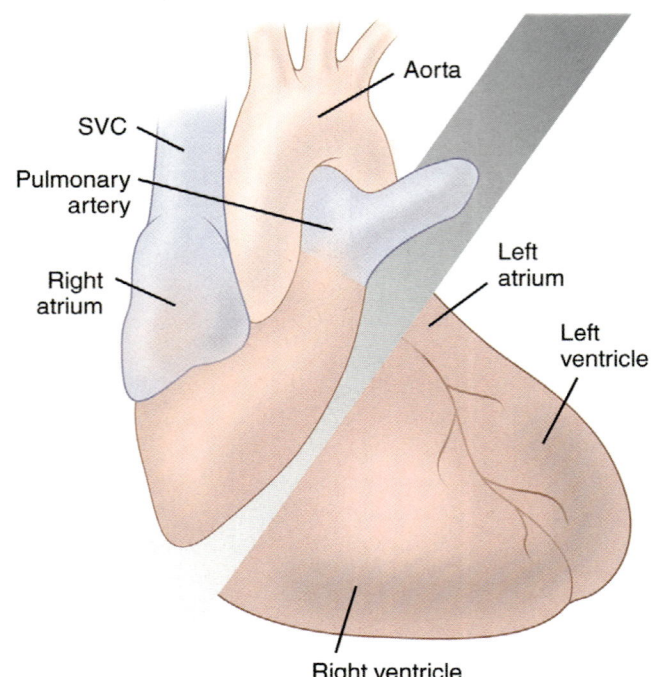

A

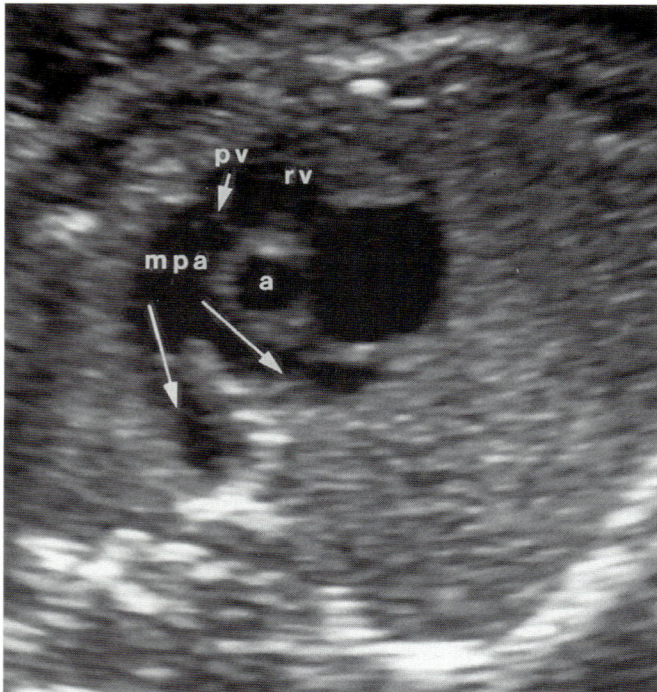

B

FIGURE 20. Short axis view of the heart. **A:** The ultrasound transducer is placed in a plane that identifies the pulmonary artery arising from the right ventricle. **B:** Axis view of the heart with the fetus supine. The beam is directed so the circular aorta (*a*) is noted centrally. The right ventricle (*rv*) gives rise to the main pulmonary artery (*mpa*), which then bifurcates to the corresponding arteries (*arrows*). The pulmonary valve is identified (*pv*).

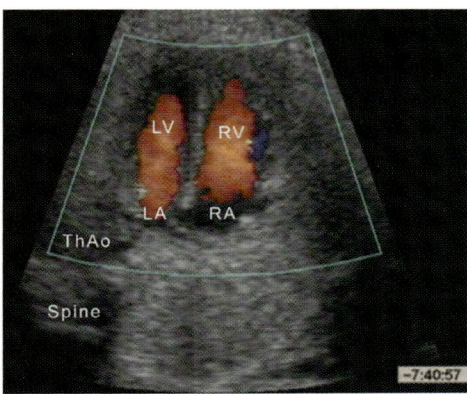

FIGURE 21. Color Doppler of the four-chamber view of the heart. Four-chamber view of the heart with the color Doppler scale adjusted to produce fairly uniform color within the heart and demonstrating blood flow toward the transducer from the left and the right atria (*LA* and *RA*) into the left and right ventricles (*LV* and *RV*), respectively. ThAo, thoracic aorta.

Examination of the Fetal Heart

Color Doppler ultrasound has been proposed as a method of investigating the normal and abnormal fetal heart.[21–27] Color Doppler has been useful in the difficult-to-image patient in whom grey-scale ultrasound does allow the examiner to identify the characteristic features of the four-chamber view and the outflow tracts. Using color Doppler is extremely important in the first-trimester fetus or in the obese patient (Fig. 24). In addition to identifying the presence or absence of blood flow, it also allows the examiner to screen for abnormal flow patterns such as valvular stenosis or regurgitation. In fact, on some occasions the structural defect may be difficult to detect without the use of color Doppler (Fig. 25).[21–27]

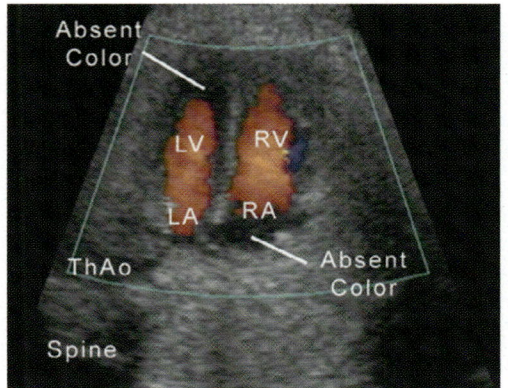

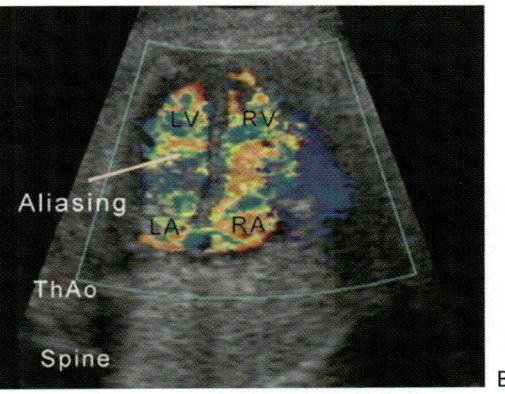

FIGURE 23. Flow detection versus aliasing. **A:** Color scale is adjusted to produce a similar red hue throughout the cardiac chambers. However, note there is absence of color flow within the apex of the left ventricle (*LV*) and within the right atrium (*RA*). **B:** To identify flow within these regions, the color scale is decreased, which produces aliasing within the cardiac chamber but demonstrates flow within all regions of the heart. LA, left atrium; RV, right ventricle; ThAo, thoracic aorta.

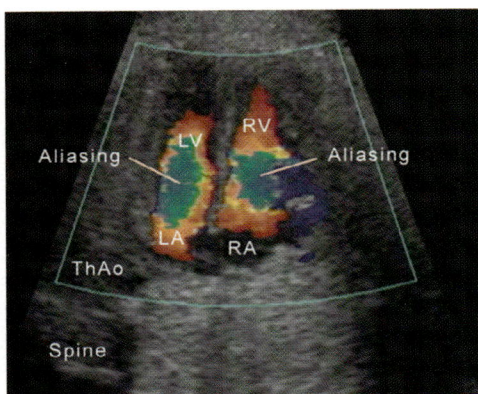

FIGURE 22. Four-chamber view—color aliasing. Note in this figure that the color scale is altered from Figure 21. In this example, the highest velocity exceeds the (Nyquist) limit and appears as aliasing with a different color hue (in this case, blue rather than red), toward the center of the ventricle. LA, left atrium; LV, left ventricle; RA, right atrium; RV, right ventricle; ThAo, thoracic aorta.

Color Doppler evaluation can be helpful to assess flow across the tricuspid and mitral valves, can visualize normal flow in the intra-atrial septum, or can be helpful to observe abnormal flow in the tricuspid or mitral valves or in the interatrial or the interventricular septum. Without color Doppler, the interventricular and interatrial septa may not always be clearly identified (Fig. 26). When color Doppler is used, the ventricular chambers fill with a single color or a color hue. If the maximum velocity of the scale is set too low, as previously described in Background, aliasing occurs. When aliasing occurs, adjusting the color baseline to the bottom or top of the range results in a *color ventriculogram* (Fig. 27). In normal systole, color flow is observed to exit through the outflow tracts of the heart. The atrioventricular valve should have no evidence of regurgitant flow. However, tricuspid regurgitation is more common than mitral valve regurgitation in the fetus (Fig. 28). It may be secondary to a number of different etiologies. In this situation, color flow may be observed during

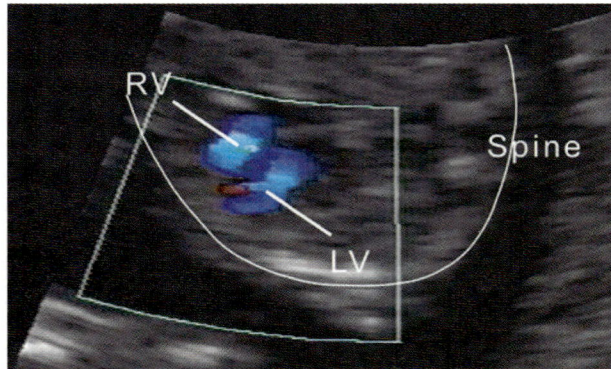

FIGURE 24. Color flow in a difficult-to-image patient. In technically difficult examinations, color flow may be useful to identify the presence of the normal four chambers of the heart, as observed in this 13-week-old fetus. LV, left ventricle; RV, right ventricle.

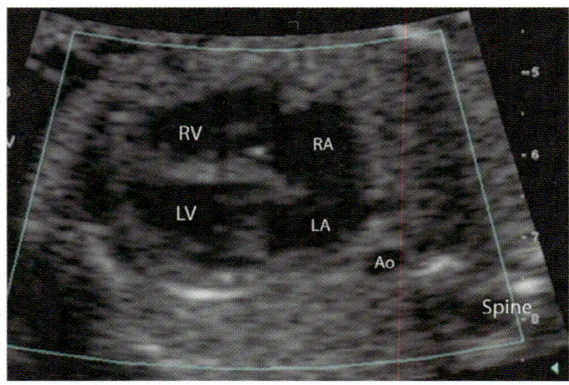

FIGURE 26. Four-chamber view of the heart in which the borders of the interventricular septum and atrial septum are not clearly identified. Ao, aorta; LA, left atrium; LV, left ventricle; RA, right atrium; RV, right ventricle.

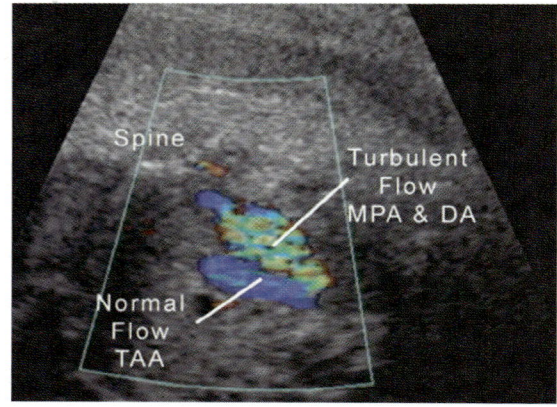

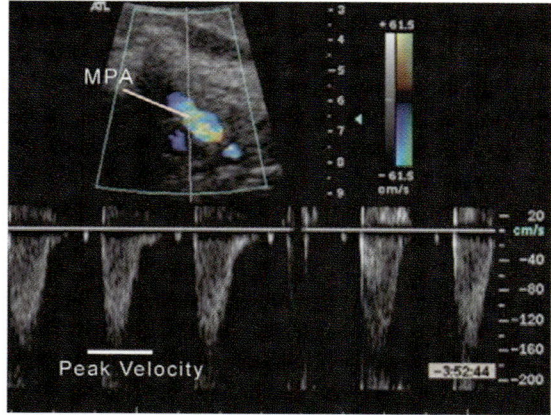

FIGURE 25. Pulmonic stenosis—turbulent flow. **A:** Color settings are adjusted in such a fashion that there is normal flow within the transverse aortic arch (*TAA*), as identified by blue hue. However, note there is color aliasing caused by increased velocity within the main pulmonary artery (*MPA*) and ductus arteriosus (*DA*), indicating possible pulmonary stenosis. **B:** Pulsed Doppler examination with appropriate angle correction demonstrates increased velocity in the main pulmonary artery (*MPA*) in the range of 160 cm per second, indicating pulmonic stenosis.

ventricular systole as it exits from the right ventricle and regurgitates into the right atrium.

Color Doppler imaging may also be helpful to evaluate the ventricular septum for defects. Whereas the septum is first identified when it is tangential to the ultrasound beam, a ventricular septal defect may be difficult to detect with such an orientation. By angling the transducer so the septum is more perpendicular to the ultrasound beam, color may be noted to cross the septum during either systole or diastole, or during systole and diastole (Fig. 29).

Furthermore, color flow may be very useful to identify the outflow tracts. In cases in which it is difficult to identify the outflow tracts, use of color flow may be helpful to identify the normal *criss-cross* relationship of the outflow tracts (Fig. 30A, B, and C). Thus, it may make the examiner more confident that he or she has adequately examined and

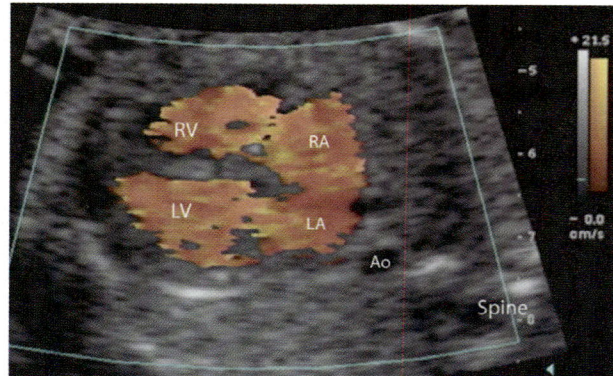

FIGURE 27. Same image as Figure 26, with low-velocity color Doppler activated. In this image, the baseline has been adjusted downward to give the effect of a ventriculogram. This clearly demonstrates the boundary between the interatrial and interventricular septa in the cardiac chambers. Ao, aorta; LA, left atrium; LV, left ventricle; RA, right atrium; RV, right ventricle.

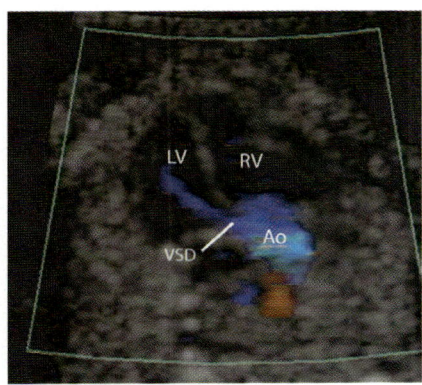

FIGURE 28. Color Doppler demonstrating a ventricular septal defect. Blood flow can be observed exiting the left ventricle (*LV*), crossing the ventricular septal defect (*VSD*), and emptying into the misaligned aortic outflow tract (*Ao*). This fetus had a double-outlet right ventricle (*RV*).

identified the outflow tracts of the heart. Also, color Doppler imaging may be helpful to identify abnormalities of the great vessels. For instance, if there is hypoplastic left heart, there may be retrograde flow from the pulmonary artery through the ductus to fill the more proximal aorta. Also, when there is a region of valvular stenosis, this may be identified with color flow.

Power Color Doppler of the Four-Chamber and Outflow Tracts

Power Doppler uses the amplitude change in the Doppler waveform to display the presence or absence of blood flow. This technique is different from color Doppler in that it does not display direction of blood flow, only its presence or absence. The advantage of power color Doppler is that it is not dependent on the angle of the ultrasound beam to display the flow of blood and has better edge discrimination. For this reason, it is extremely useful when the interventricular septum is oriented perpendicular to the ultrasound beam (Fig. 31). We have found this imaging modality useful for identifying the presence or absence of blood flow within the atrial and ventricular chambers, as well as the relationships of the outflow tracts in difficult-to-image patients. By using power color Doppler, the examiner can change an inadequate examination of the fetal heart into one in which much of the information described in the screening examination of the four-chamber view can be obtained (i.e., size, location, and disproportion of the chambers). It also enables the examiner to identify the presence or absence of the outflow tracts in difficult-to-image fetuses.

DIAGNOSTIC EXAMINATION

The purpose of the screening examination of the fetal heart is to identify fetuses at risk for congenital heart defects. Whereas the screening examination may identify disproportion between the atria and ventricles, it is not designed to determine the specific diagnosis or cause of the disproportion. To accomplish this task, the examiner must have all of the information available from the four-chamber and outflow tracts examination using real-time, color, or power Doppler ultrasound but must consider quantitative evaluation of cardiac structures and hemodynamic flow patterns. This section describes the use of quantitative evaluation of the heart and focuses on M-mode, real-time, and pulsed Doppler measurements.

M-Mode Echocardiography

In the late 1970s and early 1980s, M-mode ultrasound was used to elucidate fetal arrhythmias and to measure ventricular chamber size, ventricular wall thickness, ventricular contractility, atrioventricular valve size, and the dimensions of the aortic and pulmonary outflow tracts.[28–32] M-mode is still a useful adjunct to the fetal cardiovascular examination because it enables the physician or sonographer to obtain exact measurements of the structures. This section describes how to obtain the M-mode recording and an approach to making the necessary measurements. In addition, M-mode echocardiography is a useful method to evaluate abnormal cardiac rhythm.

Placement of the M-Mode Cursor

Unlike the postnatal period, in which an echocardiogram can be obtained to identify systole and diastole, an echocardiogram of the fetus cannot be obtained for this purpose. Therefore, it is important to place the M-mode cursor

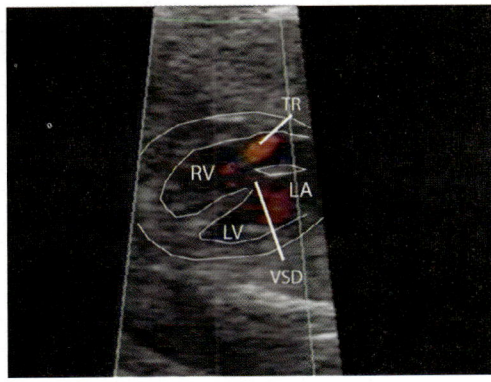

FIGURE 29. Tricuspid regurgitation (*TR*) is observed with color Doppler in a 17-week-old fetus with trisomy 21. In addition, there is a ventricular septal defect (*VSD*). LA, left atrium; LV, left ventricle; RV, right ventricle.

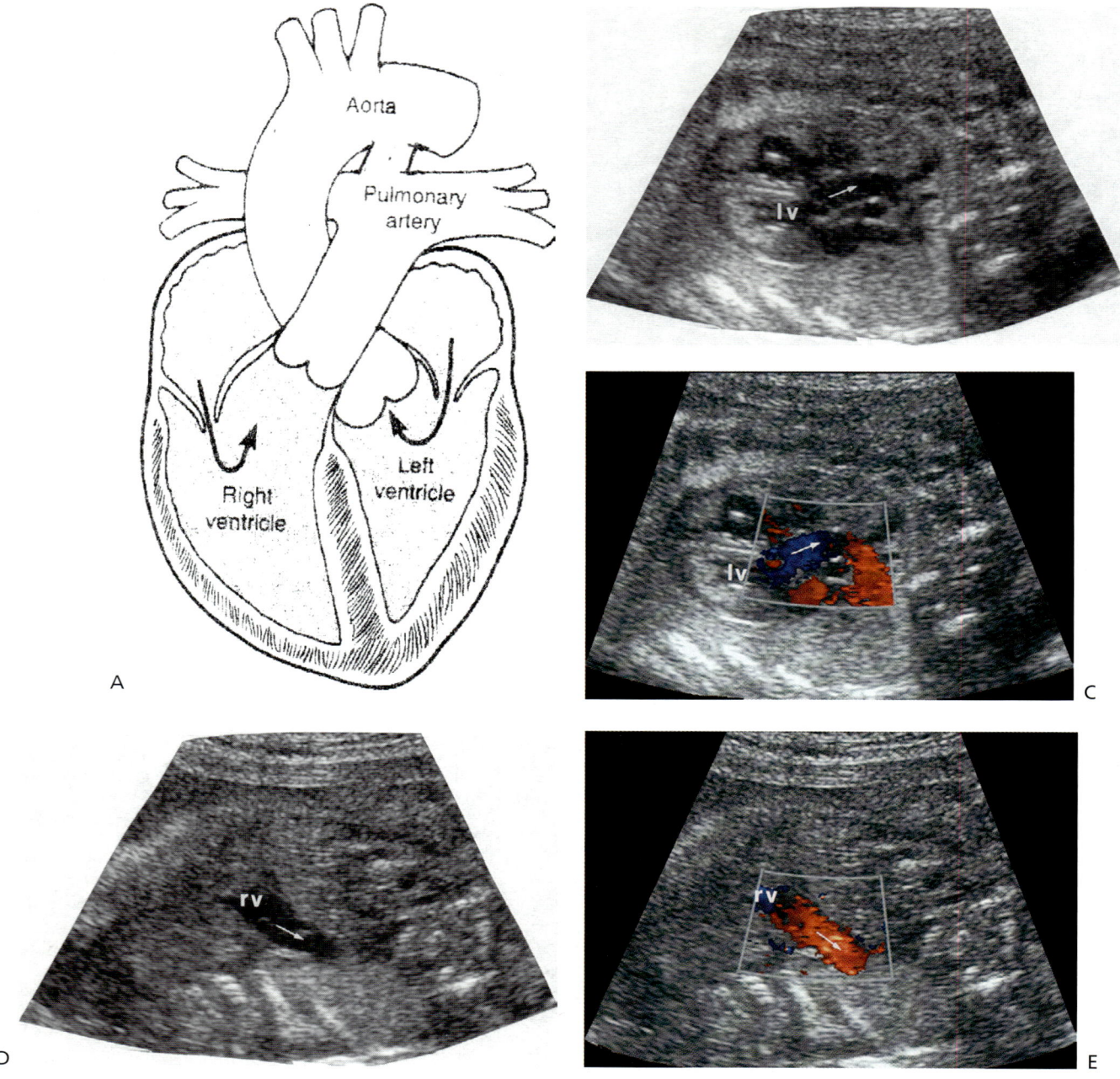

FIGURE 30. Criss-cross of the outflow tracts. **A:** Diagram showing the pulmonary artery lying anterior and crossing the aorta. **B, C:** Real-time and color-flow image showing the direction of the flow in the ascending aorta (*arrow*) as it exits from the left ventricle (*lv*). **D, E:** Without the fetus moving—and the transducer approximately in the same position—it is rocked approximately 30 degrees toward the left side of the fetus. This shows the direction of flow in the pulmonary artery (*arrow*) arising from the right ventricle (*rv*) to be in a different direction to the aortic flow. Thus, the aorta and the pulmonary outflow tracts criss-cross each other.

through the heart so that the mechanical equivalent of ventricular systole and diastole can be identified. To accomplish this, the M-mode cursor is placed perpendicular to the interventricular septum at the level of the mitral and tricuspid valves and the M-mode recorded (Fig. 32). This allows the examiner to identify end-systole (maximal inward excursion of the ventricular walls) and maximal end-diastole (closure of the atrioventricular valves).

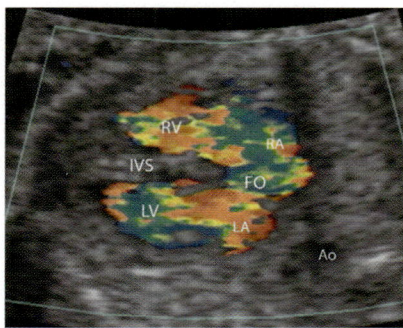

FIGURE 31. Color ventriculogram using power Doppler. This illustrates blood filling the atrial and ventricular chambers when the septum is perpendicular to the ultrasound beam. Ao, aorta; FO, foramen ovale; IVS, interventricular septum; LA, left atrium; LV, left ventricle; RA, right atrium; RV, right ventricle.

Adjusting for Gestational Age

Several studies have been published in which the M-mode measurements have been compared to gestational age that was determined from ultrasound measurements of noncardiovascular structures.[29,30] From these data, confidence intervals were constructed. The problem with this approach is that gestational age is a derived value from regression analysis of measurements of the fetal head, abdomen, and femur that introduces an additional error. In the postnatal period, cardiac measurements are compared to the size of the individual and not his or her age. For these reasons, we prefer to compare M-mode measurements with the fetal biparietal diameter, femur length, or abdominal circumference.[28,31,32] This allows for the comparison of heart size with the size of the fetus, independent of age.

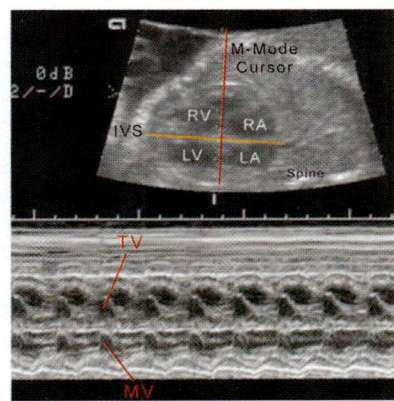

FIGURE 32. M-mode examination of the heart. After identifying the four-chamber view of the heart, the M-mode cursor is placed perpendicular to the interventricular septum (*IVS*) at the level of the mitral and tricuspid valves. The opening and closing of the tricuspid valve (*TV*) and the mitral valve (*MV*) is identified on the M-mode tracing. LA, left atrium; LV, left ventricle; RA, right atrium; RV, right ventricle.

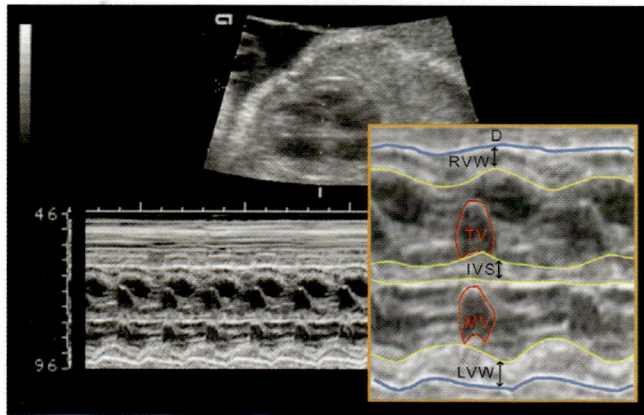

FIGURE 33. Ventricular dimensions. The right ventricular inner dimension and the left ventricular inner dimension may be obtained from the M-mode tracing. Note the motion of the tricuspid valve (*TV*) and the mitral valve (*MV*) and the change in the ventricular size between systole (*S*) and diastole (*D*). LVW, left ventricular wall; RVW, right ventricular wall.

Measurements of Ventricular Chamber Size

There are three measurements that are used to determine ventricular size, all of which are obtained at end-diastole.

Biventricular outer dimension is measured from the epicardium of the left ventricle to the epicardium of the right ventricle. This measurement includes the thickness of the right and left ventricular walls and interventricular septum and the dimensions of the ventricular chambers (Fig. 33).

Right ventricular inner dimension is measured from the endocardium of the right ventricular wall to the endocardium of the right side of the interventricular septum. This is the widest dimension of the right ventricle (Fig. 34).

Left ventricular inner dimension is measured from the endocardium of the left ventricular wall to the endocardium of the left side of the ventricular septum. This is the widest dimension of the left ventricle (Fig. 31).

Measurements of Ventricular Wall Thickness

There are two methods to evaluate the thickness of the ventricular walls and interventricular septum. The first method is to evaluate the total wall thickness that includes the right and left ventricular wall and the interventricular septum. This is computed by measuring the biventricular outer dimension and subtracting the right and left inner dimensions. The second method is to measure the right and left walls and interventricular septum separately (Fig. 35). For screening purposes, we have found the first method to be easiest to use.

Measurements of Ventricular Function

Evaluation of cardiac contractility is easily accomplished using M-mode echocardiography. In addition to the ven-

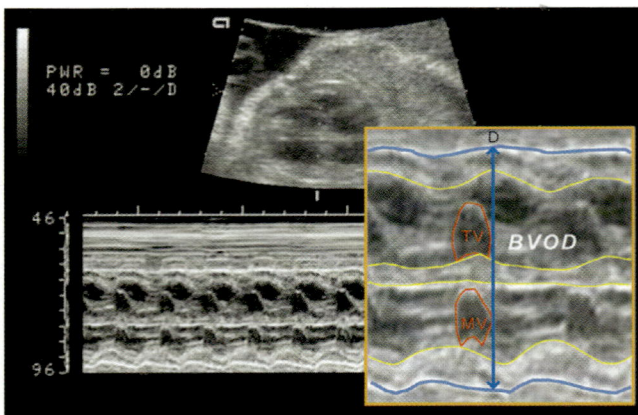

FIGURE 34. Ventricular wall thickness. Separate measurements can be made from the M-mode cursor of the right ventricular wall, the interventricular septum, and the left ventricular wall. BVOD, biventricular outer dimension; D, diastole; MV, mitral valve; TV, tricuspid valve.

tricular diastolic dimensions, measurements at end-systole of the right and left ventricular chambers are required. To accomplish this, the examiner measures the dimension of each chamber at the point of maximal inward excursion of the walls (systole). Ventricular function is computed by subtracting the systolic dimension from the diastolic dimension and dividing it by the diastolic dimension.

Evaluation of Cardiac Rhythm

Rhythm disturbances in the fetus are not uncommon. The clinician often auscultates an irregular rhythm. The

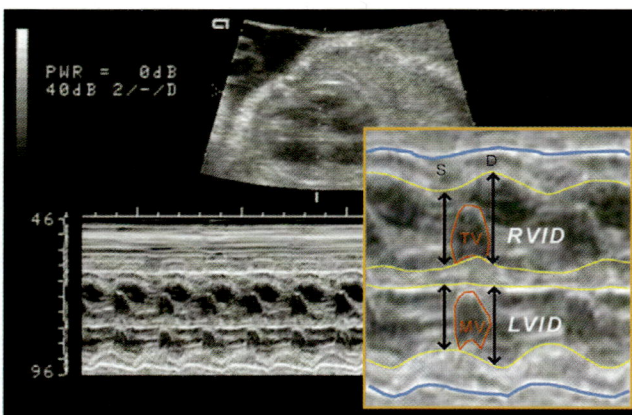

FIGURE 35. Biventricular outer dimension. The biventricular outer dimension can be obtained from the M-mode tracing. This includes the thickness of the right ventricular wall (between *blue* and *yellow lines*), the right ventricular inner dimension (*RVID*), the interventricular septum (between *yellow lines*), the left ventricular inner dimension (*LVID*), and the left ventricular wall (between *yellow* and *blue lines*). Combined ventricular and septal wall thickness may be obtained by measuring the biventricular outer dimension and subtracting the right ventricular inner dimension and the left ventricular inner dimension, as illustrated in Figure 33. D, diastole; S, systole.

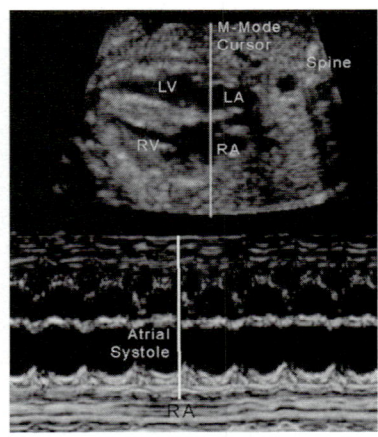

FIGURE 36. M-mode for atrial rhythm. M-mode cursor is placed perpendicular to the atrial septum, showing the wall motion within the left atrium (*LA*) and the right atrium (*RA*) pertaining to the atrial rate and rhythm. LV, left ventricle; RV, right ventricle.

most common cause of this type of rhythm disturbance is premature atrial contractions, with or without block. To elucidate an abnormal rhythm, the M-mode cursor is first placed perpendicular to the atrial septum to record the wall motion of the right and left atrial walls (Fig. 36). From this recording, premature atrial beats, bradycardia, or tachycardia can be readily identified.[33] Once the atrial rate is identified, the next question that the examiner must address is whether the atrial contraction is conducted to the ventricles. To accomplish this, the M-mode cursor is placed at a 30-degree angle such that it records atrial wall motion as well as ventricular wall motion (Fig. 37). Another method is to record atrial wall motion and opening and closing of the aortic valve using M-mode color Doppler (Fig. 38).

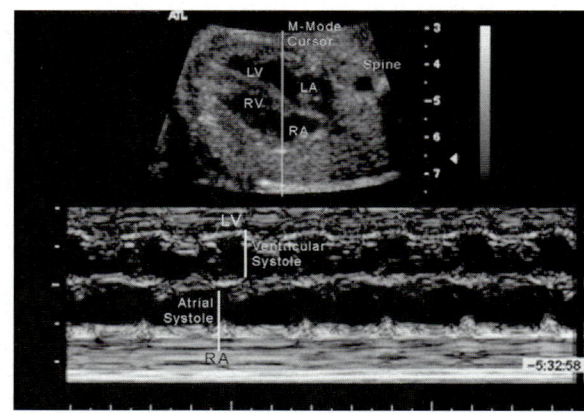

FIGURE 37. M-mode—atrial-ventricular rate. The M-mode cursor is angled in such a way to identify ventricular wall motion and atrial wall motion to identify if each atrial beat is conducted into the ventricle. LA, left atrium; LV, left ventricle; RA, right atrium; RV, right ventricle.

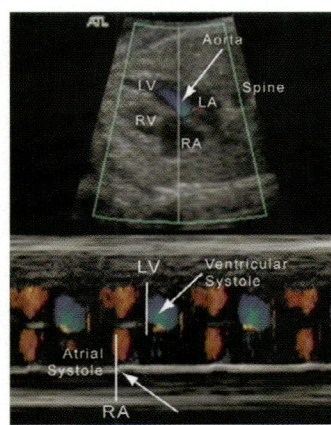

FIGURE 38. M-mode color Doppler—atrial-ventricular rate. The M-mode color Doppler cursor is placed through the ventricular and atrial wall to identify the ventricular and the atrial rate by combining wall motion changes and the flow of blood. Ventricular systole is identified by the blue from the color Doppler and the atrial rate by the change in the atrial wall motion identified by M-mode ultrasound. LA, left atrium; LV, left ventricle; RA, right atrium; RV, right ventricle.

Real-Time Measurements

In the early 1980s, the real-time image was not clear enough to identify fetal cardiac anatomy from which to obtain adequate measurements of the chambers or other cardiovascular dimensions. However, as the frequency of transducers increased and the ability to record and evaluate the real-time image with computerized, digitized images evolved, accurate measurements could be made. Although there are several papers in which real-time measurements have been reported, the most comprehensive study was reported by Tan et al.[34,35] Although the paper included numerous measurements, we have included those that are the most useful during the screening examination:

1. Width of the ventricular and atrial chambers (Fig. 39)
2. Length of the ventricular and atrial chambers (Fig. 40)
3. Measurements of the aortic arch and ductus arteriosus (Fig. 41)
4. Measurements of the aorta and main pulmonary artery (Fig. 42)

Pulsed Doppler Examination

Background

Pulsed Doppler examination provides important information and demonstrates the direction and the characteristics of blood flow within the heart. Pulsed Doppler devices use one crystal that transmits and receives the ultrasound signal. This is performed by placing a small *box* that is a sample volume on the cursor that can be steered through any sector line or depth of the image. Doppler signals that are received from moving red blood cells are then displayed either above or below a baseline. They are displayed above the baseline if the red blood cells are traveling toward the transducer and displayed below the baseline if the red blood cells are flowing away from the transducer. It is ideal to obtain the Doppler signal parallel to the main direction of the blood flow, as the more perpendicular the Doppler is to the flowing blood the less is the frequency shift. The Doppler frequency, which returns to the transducer, is the frequency shift that can be displayed as a signal on the output of the ultrasound monitor. Older ultrasound equipment measured and displayed the frequency shift, whereas most current equipment using state-of-the-art pulsed wave Doppler technology automatically uses fast Fourier analysis to convert the frequency shift into a velocity display (Table 2). Velocity display is obtained with the formula in which

$$v = (f_d \times c)/(2f_o \times \cos \varnothing)$$

Using this formula, the velocity (v) is recorded in meters per second and recorded on the video output of the ultrasound monitor. c is the velocity of sound in water, which is a constant at 1,560 m per second, and f_o is the transmitted frequency (i.e., the frequency used within the transducer, such as 3 MHz). f_d is the frequency shift in hertz, which is the returning frequency that is recorded in the ultrasound equipment. $\varnothing$ is the angle of insonation of the ultrasound beam as it interrogates the red blood cells. Thus, if the ultrasound beam is parallel to the flow of the red blood cells, the angle is 0 and cos $\varnothing$ is 1. If the ultrasound beam is perpendicular to the flow of the red blood cells, the angle is 90 degrees, and cos $\varnothing$ is 0. The angle $\varnothing$ should always be less than 60 degrees and ideally less than 30 degrees for most accurate measurements. Thus, using this formula, velocity is then recorded in meters per second.

Velocities can be measured using continuous wave instrumentation. With continuous wave instrumentation, two transducers are used—one to transmit and the other to receive the Doppler signal. Use of continuous wave Doppler is nonselective in that all signals along the ultrasound beam are recorded. Therefore, most individuals use pulsed wave Doppler for examining the fetal heart.

Doppler ultrasound also exposes the fetus to higher levels of ultrasound energy than real-time imaging or M-mode ultrasound. As such, the amount of time one uses in performing pulsed Doppler ultrasound of the fetus should be limited. It is known that the Doppler ultrasound energy should be kept below 100 mW/cm² spatial peak-temporal average.[36]

Measurement of blood flow volume (Q) requires measurement of the cross-sectional area (A) through which blood is flowing, which is then multiplied by an average velocity (V).

$$Q = V \times A$$

To obtain an average velocity, one needs to integrate the entire Doppler signal, which can usually be done by mov-

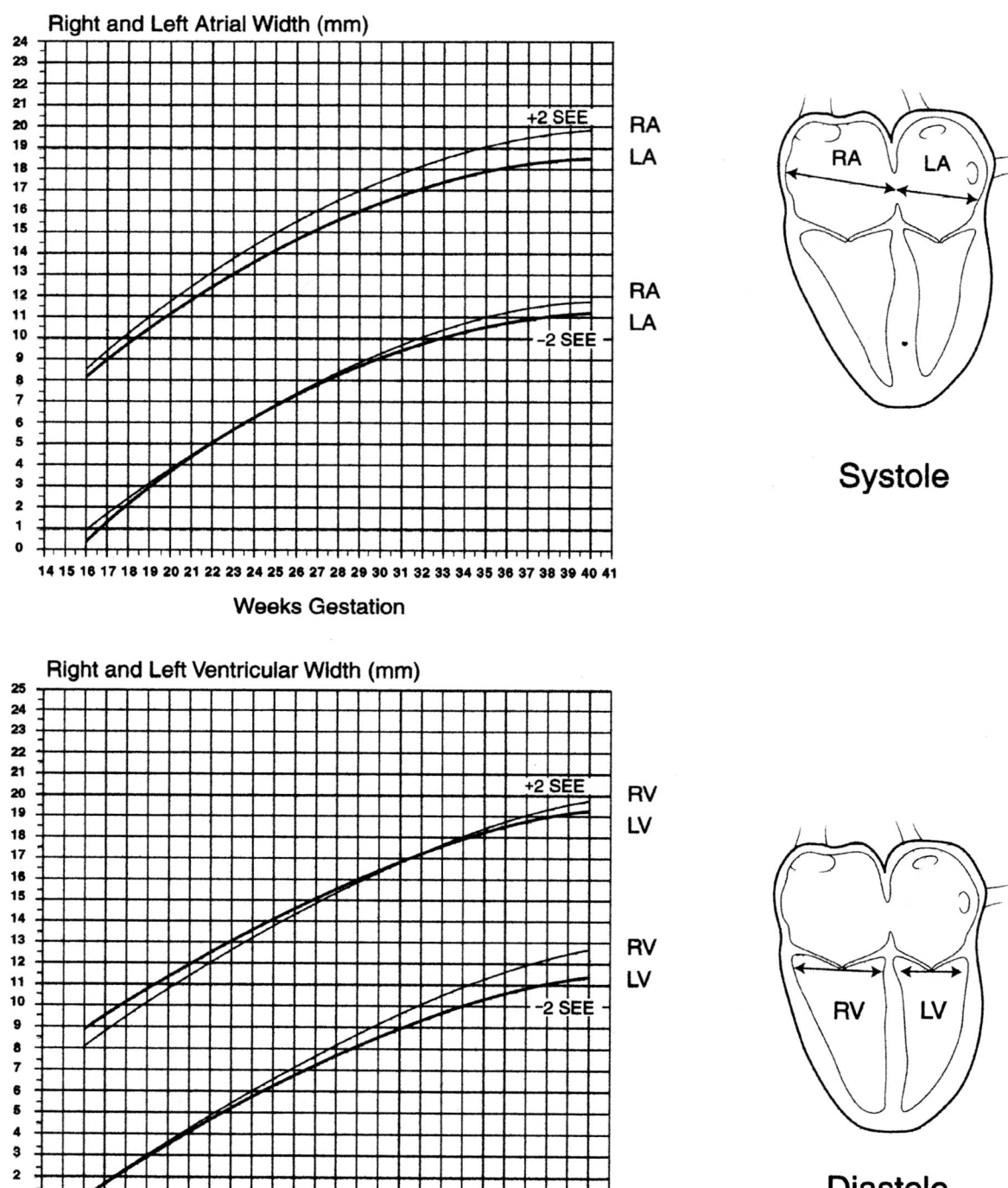

FIGURE 39. Real-time measurements of atrial and ventricular width. The graphs illustrate the upper and lower boundaries for the right and left atria (*RA* and *LA*) and ventricular chambers. LV, left ventricle; RV, right ventricle; SEE, standard error of the estimate.

Right and Left Atrial Length (mm)

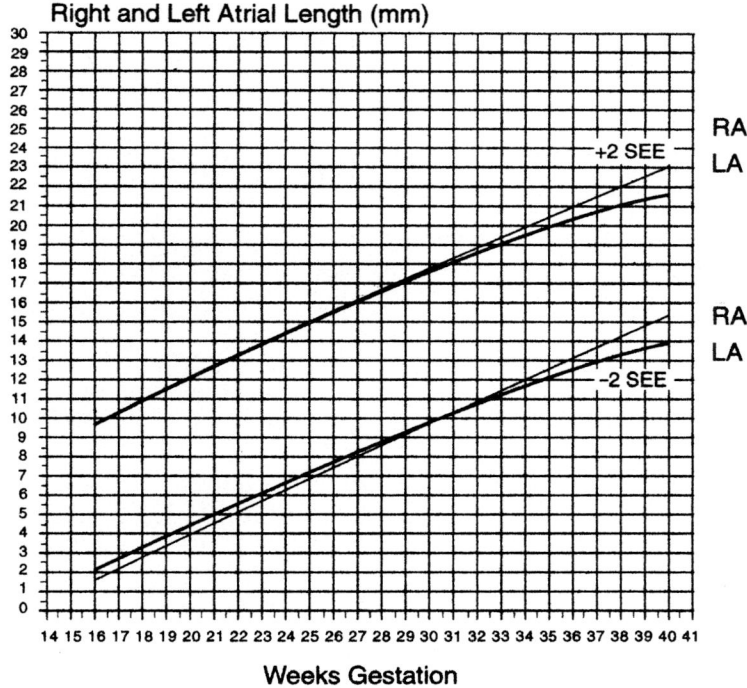

Weeks Gestation

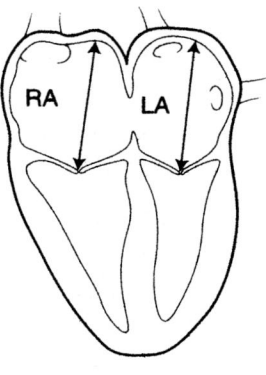

Systole

Right and Left Ventricular Length (mm)

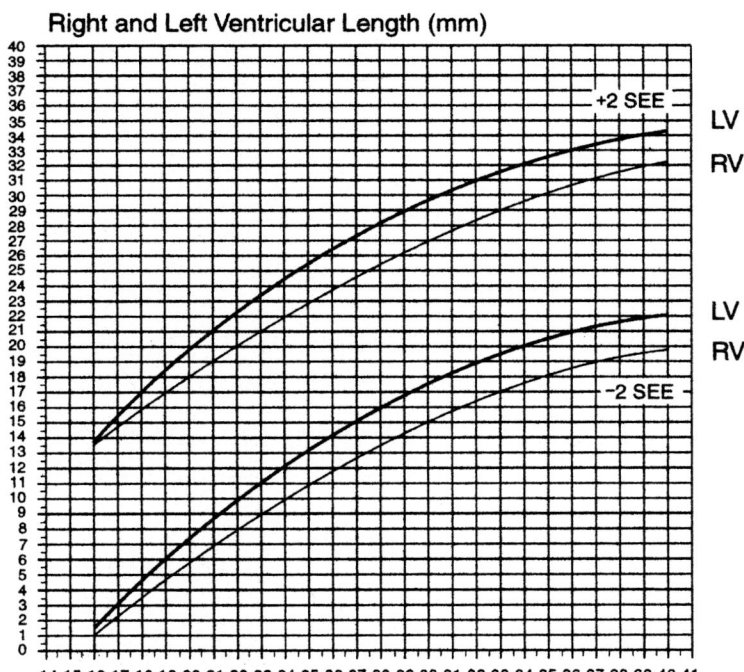

Weeks Gestation

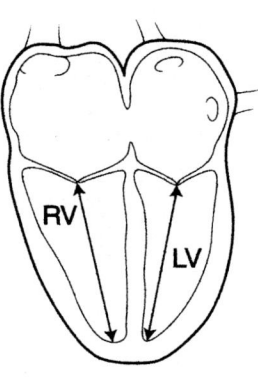

Diastole

FIGURE 40. Real-time measurements of atrial and ventricular length. The graphs illustrate the upper and lower boundaries for the right and left atria (*RA* and *LA*) and ventricular chambers. LV, left ventricle; RV, right ventricle; SEE, standard error of the estimate.

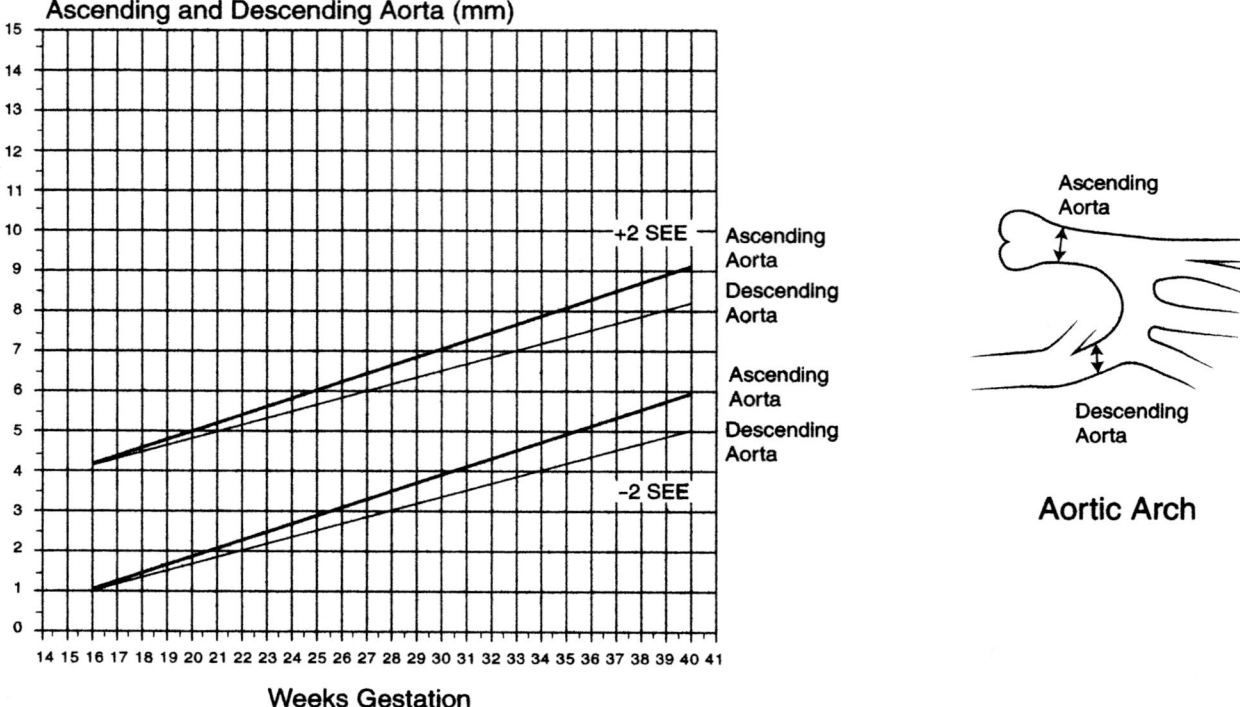

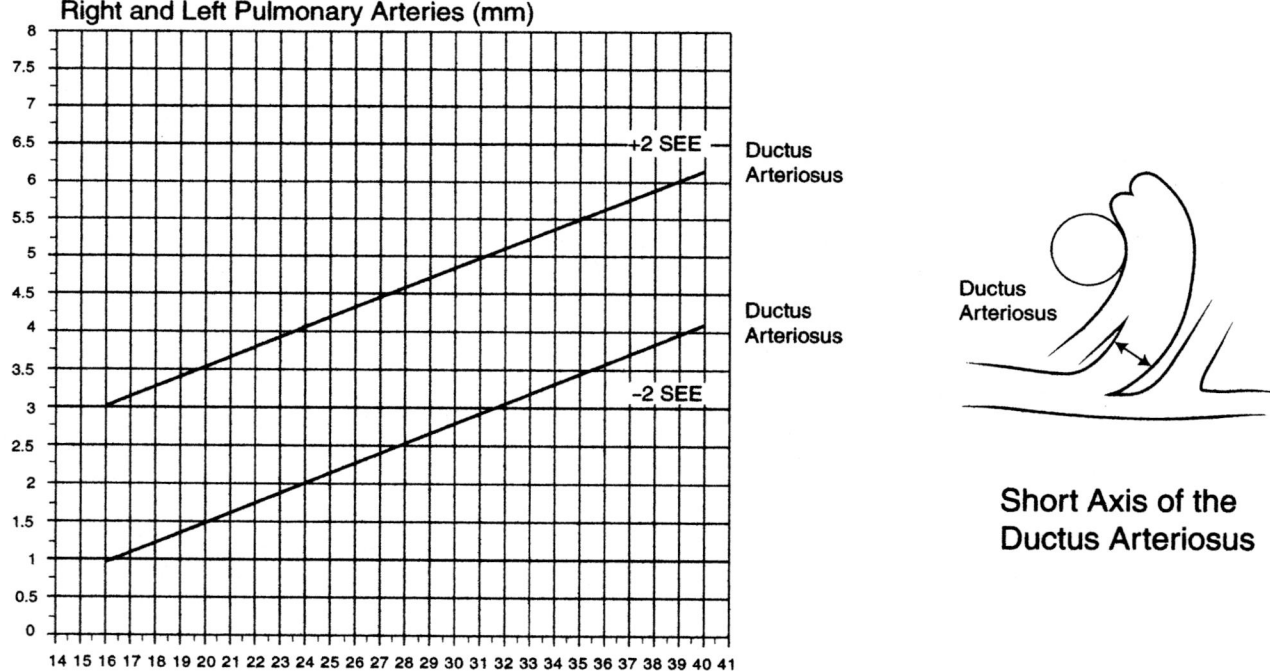

FIGURE 41. Real-time measurements of the ascending aorta, descending aorta, and ductus arteriosus. The graphs illustrate the upper and lower boundaries for these structures. SEE, standard error of the estimate.

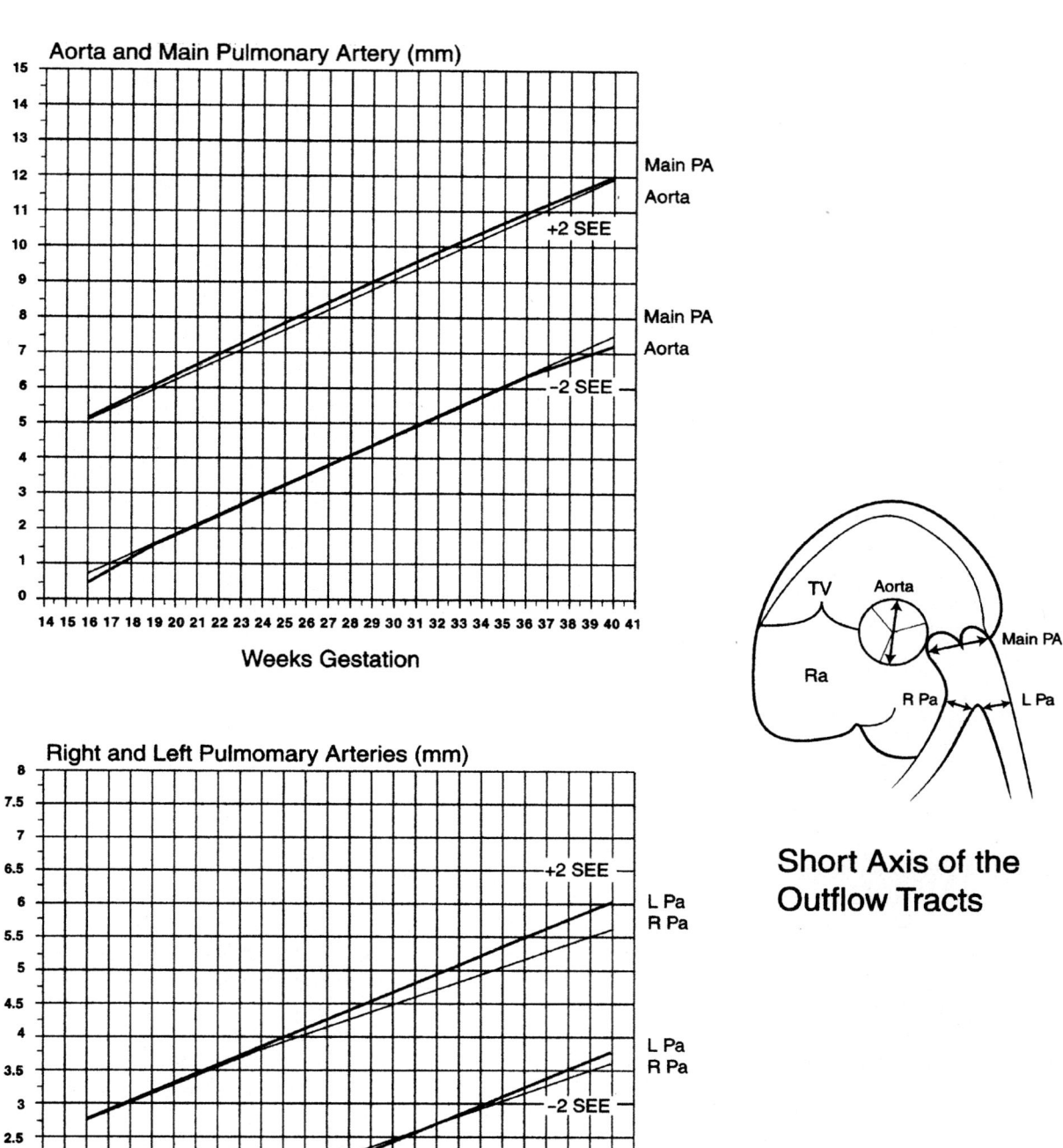

FIGURE 42. Real-time measurements of the main pulmonary artery (*PA*), aorta, and right and left pulmonary arteries (*R Pa* and *L Pa*). The graphs illustrate the upper and lower boundaries for these structures. SEE, standard error of the estimate; TV, tricuspid valve.

TABLE 2. NORMAL DOPPLER ECHOCARDIOGRAPHY IN THE FETUS

Valve	Tricuspid	Mitral	Pulmonary	Aorta
Maximal velocity (cm/sec)	51 ± 4	47 ± 4	60 ± 4	70 ± 3
Mean velocity (cm/sec)	12 ± 1	11 ± 1	16 ± 2	18 ± 2
Valve diameter (mm)[a]	8 ± 0.5	6.6 ± 0.4	7.6 ± 0.3	6.7 ± 0.2
Cardiac output (ml/kg/min)[a]	307 ± 30	232 ± 25	312 ± 11	250 ± 9
Atrial contraction/early diastole ratio[a]	1.29 ± 0.04	1.35 ± 0.01	—	—
Deceleration time (msec)[a]	97 ± 29	110 ± 31	—	—
Acceleration time (msec)[a]	—	—	50.6 ± 12.0	46.7 ± 9.1

[a]Varies with gestational age.
Reproduced with permission from Reed KL. Fetal Doppler echocardiography. *Clin Obstet Gynecol* 1989;32:728–737.

ing electronic calipers from the beginning of the Doppler pulse to the end of the Doppler pulse. This is then multiplied by the heart rate (HR) of the fetus. Integration of the entire Doppler signal is the velocity time integral (VTI). When this is multiplied by the heart rate, it gives the average velocity. The area of the valve is then obtained by multiplying pi by radius^2, or one-half of the diameter^2. This volume flow (Q) can be estimated at the valve levels using the following formula:

$$Q = \pi \times (D/2)^2 \times VTI \times HR$$

Again, Q is the flow per minute where D is the diameter of the valve. The VTI is the velocity time integral and HR is the heart rate (Table 3).

Intracardiac Doppler

Intracardiac Doppler examination can be performed for either the tricuspid or mitral valve or the aortic or pulmonary artery. Evaluation of the ductus arteriosus can be performed using pulsed Doppler ultrasound. In most instances it is best to have the pulsed Doppler cursor placed in such a way that it is parallel to the moving red blood cells. As such, in the fetus it is best to have the four-chamber view of the heart oriented in such a way that the interventricular septum is parallel to the ultrasound beam. Velocities can be angle corrected, but small errors in estimation of the angle may result in unacceptably large errors of velocity measure-

ments. Ideally, angle measurement between the ultrasound beam and the direction of the flowing blood should be less than 30 degrees and must always be less than 60 degrees.

When examining either the tricuspid or the mitral valve, the Doppler sample is placed immediately distal to the valve leaflets in the right or the left ventricle, respectively (Fig. 43). If valvular insufficiency is suspected, the Doppler sample may be placed through the mitral or tricuspid valve into the respective atrium for detection of valvular insufficiency. When flow velocity is detected across the tricuspid or mitral valve with the cursor placed within either the right or the left ventricle, there is usually a biphasic portion to the Doppler signal (Fig. 44). The flow velocity curve across the valve is normally characterized by an "e" component followed by a higher "a" component. The "e" component is a result of venous filling, and the "a" component is the result of atrial contraction. The maximum velocities in the tricuspid and mitral valves have been established in or approximately 50 cm per second (Table 2). Thus, increased velocities through the valve may indicate valvular stenosis.[37]

Aortic or pulmonary arterial Doppler waveforms may be obtained as either the aorta or the pulmonary artery leaves the respective ventricle (Fig. 45). The aortic blood flow velocities may be obtained using a long axis view of the heart, whereas pulmonary Doppler flow velocities are best obtained from a short axis view of the heart. In this fashion, the pulmonary artery or the aorta is most parallel to the ultrasound beam. Maximum velocities for the aorta

TABLE 3. DOPPLER MEASUREMENTS

Measurement[a]	Method	Units
Peak or maximal velocity	Zero line to peak	cm/sec
Mean velocity	Time velocity integral/time of cardiac cycle	cm/sec
Volume flow	Mean velocity × area[b] × 60	mL/min
Acceleration time	Time from onset to peak	msec
Deceleration time	Time from peak to zero line along slope of descent	msec
Atrial contraction/early diastole ratio	Peak velocity with atrial contraction/peak velocity during early diastole	—

[a]Velocities should be measured within 30 degrees of estimated direction of flow or be angle corrected.
[b]Area obtained from diameters measured with two-dimensional ultrasound.
Reproduced with permission from Reed KL. Fetal Doppler echocardiography. *Clin Obstet Gynecol* 1989;32:728–737.

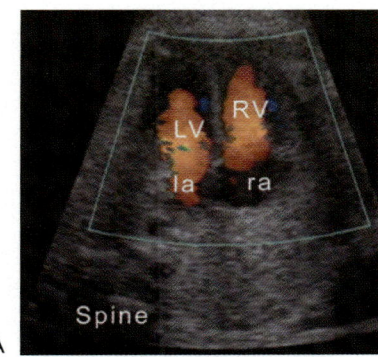

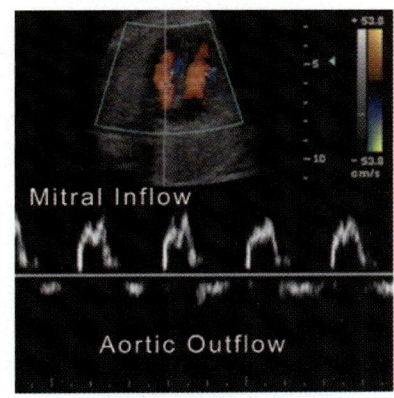

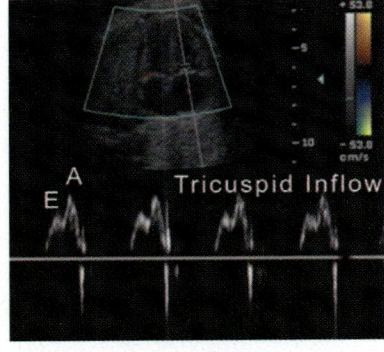

FIGURE 43. Mitral-tricuspid Doppler. **A:** Color Doppler four-chamber view of the heart with ultrasound beam oriented parallel to interventricular septum. la, left atrium; LV, left ventricle; ra, right atrium; RV, right ventricle. **B:** Doppler cursor is placed just distal to the leaflet of the mitral valve, demonstrating biphasic velocity peaks just beyond the mitral valve. Negative Doppler flow in this example is caused by aortic outflow. **C:** Doppler cursor is placed just beyond the leaflets of the tricuspid valve, demonstrating biphasic velocity peaks as seen within the mitral inflow. The first peak is during early diastole due to venous filling end (*E*) and the second peak is the result of atrial contraction (*A*). This is the typical flow pattern within the mitral and the tricuspid inflow.

and the pulmonary artery are 70 and 60 cm per second, respectively (Table 2). For the pulmonary artery and the aorta, there is usually only one peak noted on the Doppler waveform, rather than the two peaks, as noted for either the tricuspid or the mitral valve. Peak velocities are then

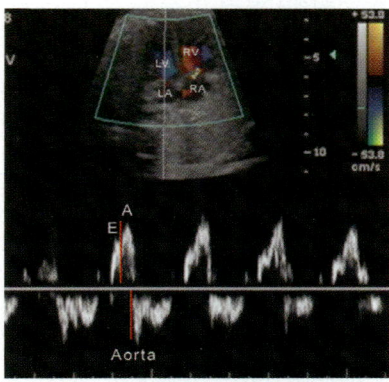

FIGURE 44. Simultaneous mitral valve and aorta pulsed Doppler tracing. Placement of the pulsed Doppler sample volume at the junction of the mitral inflow and the aortic outflow may identify the mitral inflow toward the transducer with early diastolic filling (*E*) and atrial contraction (*A*). Aortic velocities are noted away from the transducer, as is depicted below the baseline. LA, left atrium; LV, left ventricle; RA, right atrium; RV, right ventricle.

obtained by measuring the highest velocities of the time velocity Doppler signal that is angle corrected. The mean velocities are then computed by the time velocity integral divided by the time of the cardiac cycle. Normal Doppler measurements in the fetus are demonstrated in Table 2 with Doppler measurements and the explanation of these measurements in Table 3.

With the use of prostaglandin synthesis inhibitors for preterm labor tocolysis, it has been noted that there is increased constriction of the ductus arteriosus.[38] Systolic ductus velocities in normal fetuses range from approxi-

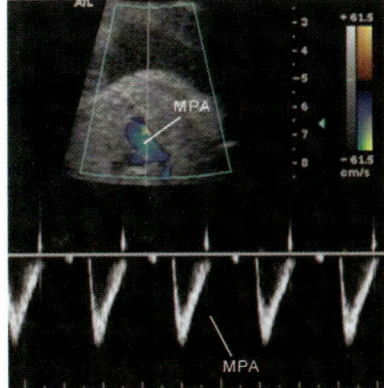

FIGURE 45. Pulsed Doppler—main pulmonary artery (*MPA*). Pulsed Doppler examination angle corrected the MPA demonstrate a single peak for the MPA. A single peak is also seen in the aorta. Velocity measurements, including maximum velocity and other velocity measurements for the pulmonary artery, aorta, or mitral tricuspid valve, can be calculated and compared to normal, as shown in Tables 2 and 3.

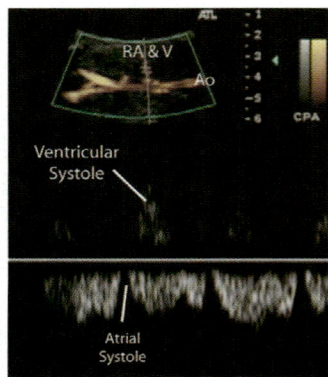

FIGURE 46. Pulsed Doppler of the renal artery and vein. This simultaneous recording is obtained at the level of the bifurcation of the renal artery and vein from the abdominal aorta (*Ao*). Atrial systole is identified by the notching in the venous waveform and ventricular systole by the peak of the arterial waveform. RA &V, right atrium and ventricle.

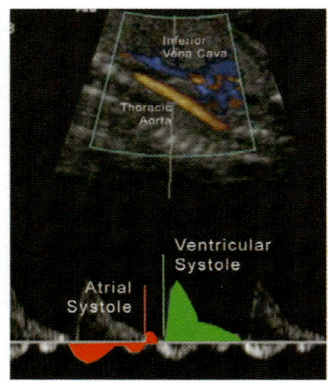

FIGURE 47. Pulsed Doppler of aorta and inferior vena cava. By widening the Doppler gate, the sample may be obtained across the aorta and the inferior vena cava. Typical aortic pulsations are depicted toward the transducer in green. Pulsations within the inferior vena cava are generally away from the transducer or toward the heart and are depicted in red. In atrial systole, flow in the inferior vena cava is away from the heart.

mately 90 to 135 cm per second, and diastolic velocities range from approximately 15 to 25 cm per second. Fetuses with ductal constrictions have elevated systolic velocities in the range of 140 to 235 cm per second and elevated diastolic velocities in the range of 35 to 170 cm per second.[39] Certain other drugs, such as indomethacin and other antiinflammatory medications, can constrict the fetal ductus arteriosus.[40]

Timing Relationships of the Cardiac Cycle

Like M-mode echocardiography, pulsed Doppler may be useful to identify normal and abnormal rhythm disturbances. There are four areas of the fetal cardiovascular system that may be sampled with pulsed Doppler to record the timing relationships.

Left Ventricle

Placement of the pulsed Doppler sample volume at the junction of mitral inflow and aortic outflow allows the examiner to simultaneously record atrial and ventricular systole (Fig. 44). Atrial systole is represented by the A wave of the mitral valve and ventricular systole by the peak velocity of the aortic valve.

Renal Artery and Vein

By placing the pulsed Doppler parallel to the renal artery and vein, atrial and ventricular systole can simultaneously be recorded (Fig. 46). Atrial systole is represented by an *indentation* in the venous waveform (equivalent to the A wave) and ventricular systole by the arterial waveform.

Abdominal Aorta and the Inferior Vena Cava

These two vessels converge as the inferior vena cava enters the heart.[41] By placing the pulsed Doppler sample volume

in this area, both waveforms may be recorded simultaneously (Fig. 47). However, because of the fetal position, obtaining the waveforms from blood flowing parallel to the ultrasound beam is difficult. From these waveforms atrial and ventricular systole can be identified.

Pulmonary Artery and Vein

The fetal lungs are highly vascular, with arteries and veins adjacent to each other (Fig. 48).[42] By placing the pulsed Doppler in the lung field, one can usually record simultaneous venous and arterial waveforms. Atrial systole is represented by the A wave or an indentation in the venous

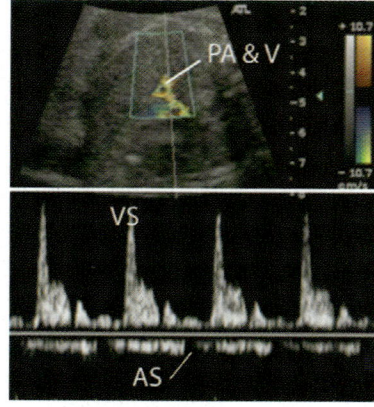

FIGURE 48. Pulsed Doppler of the pulmonary vein and artery from the lungs. During atrial systole (*AS*), a notch appears in the pulmonary vein, followed by a spike in the pulmonary artery, representing ventricular systole. These waveforms have the appearance of an echocardiogram. PA &V, pulmonary artery and vein; VS, ventricular septum.

waveform. Ventricular systole is represented by the peak of the waveform of the pulmonary artery.

REFERENCES

1. Allan LD, Crawford DC, Chita SK, Tynan MJ. Prenatal screening for congenital heart disease. *BMJ* 1986;292: 1717–1719.
2. Moller JH, Neal WA. Incidence of cardiac malformations. In: *Heart disease in infancy.* New York: Appleton-Century-Crofts, 1981:1–13.
3. American Institute of Ultrasound in Medicine. AIUM guidelines. *J Ultrasound Med* 1991;10:576.
4. McGahan JP. Sonography of the fetal heart: findings on the four-chamber view. *AJR Am J Roentgenol* 1991;156: 547–553.
5. Achiron R, Glaser J, Gelernter I, Hegesh J, Yagel S. Extended fetal echocardiographic examination for detecting cardiac malformations in low risk pregnancies. *BMJ* 1992; 304:671–674.
6. Bromley B, Estroff JA, Sanders SP, Parad R, Roberts D, et al. Fetal echocardiographic accuracy: accuracy and limitations in a population at high and low risk for heart defects. *Am J Obstet Gynecol* 1992;166:1473–1481.
7. DeVore GR, Medearis AL, Brar MB, Horenstein J, Platt LD. Fetal echocardiography: factors that influence imaging of the fetal heart during the second trimester of pregnancy. *J Ultrasound Med* 1993;11:659–663.
8. Van Praagh R, Weinberg PM, Smith SD, et al. Malpositions of the heart. In: Adams FH, Emmanouilides GC, Riemenschneider TA, eds. *Moss' heart disease in infants, children, and adolescents,* 4th ed. Baltimore: Williams & Wilkins, 1989:530.
9. McGahan JP, Benacerraf BR. Real-time examination of the fetal heart. In: McGahan JP, Goldberg BB, eds. *Diagnostic ultrasound: a logical approach.* Philadelphia: Lippincott–Raven Publishers, 1998:257–281.
10. Smith RS, Comstock CH, Kirk JS, Lee W. Ultrasonographic left axis deviation: a marker for fetal anomalies. *Obstet Gynecol* 1995;85:187–191.
11. Crane JM, Ash K, Fink N, Desjardins C. Abnormal fetal cardiac axis in the detection of intrathoracic anomalies and congenital heart disease. *Ultrasound Obstet Gynecol* 1997; 10:90–93.
12. Comstock CH. Normal heart axis and position. *Obstet Gynecol* 1987;70:255.
13. Shipp TD, Bromley B, Hornberger LK, Nadel A, Benacerraf BR. Levorotation of the fetal cardiac axis: a clue for the presence of congenital heart disease. *Obstet Gynecol* 1995;85:97–102.
14. McGahan JP, Choy M, Parrish MD, Brant WE. Sonographic spectrum of fetal cardiac hypoplasia. *J Ultrasound Med* 1991;10:539–546.
15. DeVore GR. The prenatal diagnosis of congenital heart disease: a practical approach for the fetal sonographer. *J Clin Ultrasound* 1985;13:229.
16. Lee W. Performance of the basic fetal cardiac ultrasound examination. *J Ultrasound Med* 1998;17:601–607.
17. Yoo SJ, Lee YH, Kim ES, Ryu HM, Kim MY, et al. Three-vessel view of the fetal upper mediastinum: an easy means of detecting abnormalities of the ventricular outflow tracts and great arteries during obstetric screening. *Ultrasound Obstet Gynecol* 1997;9:173–182.
18. Yagel S, Cohen SM, Achiron R. Examination of the fetal heart by five short-axis views: a proposed screening method for comprehensive cardiac evaluation. *Ultrasound Obstet Gynecol* 2001;17:367–369.
19. DeVore GR. The aortic and pulmonary outflow tract and screening examination in the human fetus. *J Ultrasound Med* 1992;11:345–348.
20. Lee W, Smith RS, Comstock CH, Kirk JS, Rigs T, et al. Tetralogy of Fallot: prenatal diagnosis and postnatal survival. *Obstet Gynecol* 1995;86:583–588.
21. DeVore GR, Horenstein J, Siassi B, Platt LD. Fetal echocardiography. VII Doppler color flow mapping: a new technique for the diagnosis of congenital heart disease. *Am J Obstet Gynecol* 1987;156:1054–1064.
22. DeVore GR. The role of color Doppler in the screening examination of the fetal heart. In: McGahan JP, Goldberg BB, eds. *Diagnostic ultrasound: a logical approach.* Philadelphia: Lippincott–Raven Publishers, 1998:282–296.
23. Chiba Y, Kanzaki T, Kobayashi H, et al. Evaluation of fetal structural heart disease using color flow mapping. *Ultrasound Med Biol* 1990;16:221–229.
24. DeVore GR, Brar HS, Platt LD. Doppler ultrasound in the fetus: a review of current applications. *J Clin Ultrasound* 1987;15:687–703.
25. Gembruch U, Chatterjee MS, Bald R, et al. Color Doppler flow mapping of fetal heart. *J Perinat Med* 1991;19:27–32.
26. Sharland GK, Chita SK, Allan LD. The use of colour Doppler in fetal echocardiography. *Int J Cardiol* 1990;28:229–236.
27. Matsuura T. Study on intracardiac blood flow with color flow mapping in human fetus: the reverse flow at tricuspid valve in human fetus during labor. *Nippon Sanka Fujinka Gakkai Zasshi* 1989;41:1373–1379.
28. DeVore GR, Siassi B, Platt LD. Fetal echocardiography. IV. M-mode assessment of ventricular size and contractility during the second and third trimesters of pregnancy in the normal fetus. *Am J Obstet Gynecol* 1984;150:981–988.
29. Allan LD, Joseph MC, Boyd EG, Campbell S, Tynan M. M-mode echocardiography in the developing human fetus. *Br Heart J* 1982;47:573–583.
30. St. John Sutton MG, Gewitz MH, Shah B, Cohen A, Reichek N, et al. Quantitative assessment of growth and function of the cardiac chambers in the normal human fetus: a prospective longitudinal echocardiographic study. *Circulation* 1984;69:645–654.
31. DeVore GR, Siassi B, Platt LD. The use of the abdominal circumference as a means of assessing M-mode ventricular dimensions during the second and third trimesters of pregnancy in the normal human fetus. *J Ultrasound Med* 1985;4:175–182.
32. DeVore GR, Siassi B, Platt LD. Use of femur length as a means of assessing M-mode ventricular dimensions during second and third trimesters of pregnancy in normal fetus. *J Clin Ultrasound* 1985;13:619–625.
33. DeVore GR, Siassi B, Platt LD. Fetal echocardiography. III. The diagnosis of cardiac arrhythmias using real-time-directed M-mode ultrasound. *Am J Obstet Gynecol* 1983; 146:792–799.

34. Tan J, Silverman NH, Hoffman JI, Villegas M, Schmidt KG. Cardiac dimensions determined by cross-sectional echocardiography in the normal human fetus from 18 weeks to term. *Am J Cardiol* 1992;70:1459–467.

35. Shapiro I, Degani S, Leibovitz Z, Ohel G, Tal Y, et al. Fetal cardiac measurements derived by transvaginal and transabdominal cross-sectional echocardiography from 14 weeks of gestation to term. *Ultrasound Obstet Gynecol* 1998;12:404–418.

36. Schulman H. Doppler ultrasound. In: Eden RD, Boehm FH, eds. *Assessment and care of the fetus.* Norwalk, CT: Appleton & Lange, 1990:397–407.

37. Reed KL. Fetal Doppler echocardiography. *Clin Obstet Gynecol* 1989;32:728–737.

38. Moise KJ, Huhta JG, Sharif DS. Indomethacin in the treatment of premature labor. *N Engl J Med* 1988;319:327–330.

39. Reed KL, Sahn DJ, Marx GR. Cardiac Doppler flow during fetal arrhythmias: physiologic consequences. *Obstet Gynecol* 1987;70:1–5.

40. Momma K, Konishi T, Hagiwara H. Characteristic morphology of the constricted fetal ductus arteriosus following maternal administration of indomethacin. *Pediatr Res* 1985;19:493–500.

41. Chan FY, Woo SK, Ghosh A, Tang M, Lam C. Prenatal diagnosis of congenital fetal arrhythmias by simultaneous pulsed Doppler velocimetry of the fetal abdominal aorta and inferior vena cava. *Obstet Gynecol* 1990;76:200–205.

42. DeVore GR, Horensstein J. Simultaneous Doppler recording of the pulmonary artery and vein: a new technique for the evaluation of a fetal arrhythmia. *J Ultrasound Med* 1993;12:669–671.

CARDIAC MALFORMATIONS

Congenital heart defects are the most common congenital abnormalities found at birth, with a prevalence of 5 per 1,000 live births[1] (Table 1). In 25% to 30% of cases, extra-cardiac anomalies are present. Of isolated cardiac defects, approximately 50% (approximately 2 per 1,000 births) continue to be life threatening despite current treatment and are commonly referred therefore as major cardiac defects.[2] During antenatal life, the prevalence of cardiac anomalies is higher because of a high selection rate of affected fetuses.[3]

This chapter concentrates on congenital heart defects and their appearance on ultrasound. Pioneer studies on the ultrasound investigation of the fetal heart were reported in the early 1970s. Fetal echocardiography is now a well-established technique for prenatal diagnosis of cardiac heart defects. However, it requires specific skills and expertise, and therefore continues to have a limited diffusion. The standard of practice in the United States as well as in most European countries is to refer pregnant patients with risk factors for fetal cardiac anomalies in specialized settings for a complete fetal echocardiographic examination. Such risk factors include mostly a family history of congenital heart disease, maternal disease, teratogens, chromosomal abnormalities, extracardiac anomalies, arrhythmias, and nonimmune hydrops, and are discussed in detail. The magnitude of the risks of a cardiac anomaly when one of these indications is present is listed in Table 2.

In the standard sonographic examination of low-risk patients, the general recommendation is to evaluate the heart rate and obtain a four-chamber view. The limitations of this approach are well appreciated. The first large multicentric studies reported low sensitivities, in the range of 5% to 15%.[4–6] More recent studies suggest better results, and one large study conducted in pediatric cardiology units in England reported a sensitivity in the antenatal detection in the range of 25%.[7] As cardiac defects are one of the most common types of congenital anomalies, we anticipate that in the future the standard sonographic examination of the fetus will include a basic echocardiographic examination. Several studies have now shown improved detection of congenital heart disease using views that demonstrate the outflow tracts and great arteries (sensitivity improved from 50% to greater than 80%).[8–11] It is clear that this will demand a significant improvement over the present level of expertise and training.

INDICATIONS FOR FETAL ECHOCARDIOGRAPHY

Family History

A positive family history of congenital heart disease is probably the most common reason for referral for fetal echocardiography. In the past, most congenital heart defects were considered sporadic or multifactorial but many defects have been found to have an underlying genetic basis.[12–14] There are inheritable syndromes that often follow autosomal recessive or dominant inheritance patterns. Some families with heterotaxy syndrome appear to have an X-linked recessive pattern of inheritance. Holt-Oram syndrome is autosomal dominant with family members most commonly having atrial septal defects and upper limb abnormalities. In most families, we do not know what the recurrence risks are but use estimates based on previous studies. The recurrence risk with one previous child with congenital heart defects is 2% to 5% and increases to 3% to 10% with two children. Mothers with congenital heart defects have a higher recurrence risk of 5% to 10%.[13] There is less information regarding the recurrence risk in fathers.

Certain types of defects have higher recurrence risks (Table 3). The highest risk is for left heart obstructive defects such as hypoplastic left heart syndrome, aortic stenosis, and coarctation of the aorta, with recurrence rates up to 10% to 15%. Septal defects and conotruncal anomalies have a moderate recurrence risk of 2% to 5%. Transposition of the great arteries and single ventricle anomalies have lower recurrences of less than 2%.

Maternal Disease

Diabetes Mellitus

The incidence of congenital heart defects in infants of diabetic mothers was approximately 5%, but with better diabetic con-

TABLE 1. FREQUENCY OF CONGENITAL HEART DISEASE IN THE BALTIMORE-WASHINGTON INFANT STUDY (4,390 INFANTS WITH CONGENITAL HEART DISEASE OF 906,626 BIRTHS IN 1981–1989)

Defect	N	%
Ventricular septal defect	1,411	32.1
Pulmonary stenosis	395	9.0
Atrial septal defect, secundum	340	7.7
Atrioventricular septal defect	326	7.4
Tetralogy of Fallot	297	6.8
Complete transposition	208	4.7
Coarctation of aorta	203	4.6
Hypoplastic left heart syndrome	167	3.8
Aortic stenosis	128	2.9
Patent arterial duct	104	2.4
Heterotaxy	99	2.3
Double-outlet right ventricle	86	2.0
Bicuspid aortic valve	84	1.9
Pulmonary atresia with intact ventricular septum	73	1.7
Total anomalous pulmonary venous return	60	1.4
Truncus arteriosus	51	1.2
Corrected transposition	47	1.1
Ebstein anomaly	43	1.0
Tricuspid atresia	32	0.7
Interrupted aortic arch	31	0.7
Double-inlet single ventricle	18	0.4
Divided left atrium (cor triatriatum)	5	0.1
Other miscellaneous problems	182	4.2

Adapted from Ferencz C, Rubin JD, Loffredo CA, Magree CA. *Perspectives in pediatric cardiology. Vol. 4. Congenital heart disease: The Baltimore-Washington Infant Study 1981–9.* New York: Futura Publishing, 1993.

TABLE 2. RISK FACTORS FOR CONGENITAL HEART DISEASE

Risk factor	%
Family history of congenital heart disease	
Inheritable syndrome	Variable
Parent	See Table 3
Maternal disease	
Diabetes	≤5
Collagen vascular disease	0.5–8.0[a]
Phenylketonuria	≤13
Teratogens	
Alcohol	≤25
Retinoic acid	≤40
Anticonvulsants: valproic acid, phenytoin, trimethadione	2–3
Thalidomide	5–10
Lithium	1
Infection: rubella	2–8
Chromosomal abnormalities	See Table 4
Extracardiac anomalies	See Table 5
Nonimmune fetal hydrops	10–23

[a]0.5% Risk for mother with positive antibodies only, 8% after first child with congenital heart block.

TABLE 3. RECURRENCE RISKS OF CONGENITAL HEART DISEASE

Defect	Recurrence risk (%)		
	One sibling affected[a]	Father affected[b]	Mother affected[b]
Aortic stenosis	2	3	13–18
Atrial septal defect	2.5	1.5	4.0–4.5
Atrioventricular septal defect	2	1	14
Coarctation	2	2	4
Patent ductus arteriosus	3	2.5	3.5–4.0
Pulmonary stenosis	2	2	4.0–6.5
Tetralogy of Fallot	2.5	1.5	2.5
Ventricular septal defect	3	2	6–10

[a]Data derived from Nora JJ, Nora AH. *Genetics and counseling in cardiovascular disease.* Springfield, MA: Charles C. Thomas, 1978.
[b]Data derived from Nora JJ, Nora AH. Maternal transmission of congenital heart disease: new recurrence risk figures and the questions of cytoplasmic inheritance and vulnerability to teratogens. *Am J Cardiol* 1987;59:459–465.

trol the incidence has fallen. Structural defects most commonly seen in infants of diabetic mothers are ventricular septal defects, transposition of the great arteries, coarctation of the aorta, and other conotruncal anomalies such as double-outlet right ventricle and truncus arteriosus. Hypertrophic cardiomyopathy is seen in insulin-dependent and gestational diabetics, usually in the last months of pregnancy. Its incidence and severity have also decreased with better diabetic control.[15–19]

Collagen Vascular Disease

Women with anti–Sjögren syndrome A antibodies or Sjögren syndrome B antibodies (anti-Ro or anti-La) are at risk for the fetus's developing congenital heart block and myocarditis. The women often do not have clinical collagen vascular disease. Congenital heart block in a fetus with no structural heart disease is almost always associated with one or both of these antibodies, and they should be looked for. The antibodies are usually gone by 3 months of age, but the damage to the conduction system has been done. Perinatal mortality for isolated congenital heart block is 10% to 15%.[20] Recurrence risk in subsequent pregnancies has been reported at 8%.[21]

Phenylketonuria

Like diabetes, phenylketonuria adversely affects the fetus when the mother is not adequately treated.[22] Treatment is with a low phenylalanine diet to prevent mental retardation in the mother and congenital heart disease, microcephaly, intrauterine growth retardation, and mental retardation in the infant. Good dietary control results in a decreased incidence of malformations but should be started before conception, keeping phenylalanine levels lower than 400 to 600 μmol per L. Structural defects seen most commonly with phenylketonuria are ventricular septal defects, coarctation of the aorta, hypoplastic left heart syndrome, and tetralogy of Fallot.

Teratogens

Numerous pharmacologic agents have been associated with congenital heart defects, but there is clearly an increased risk in only a few.[23–25] Exposure of the fetus to alcohol, especially if fetal alcohol syndrome develops, can be associated with congenital heart defects in up to 25%.[26–28] The most common defects are a patent ductus arteriosus and septal defects. Isotretinoin (retinoic acid) is also very teratogenic with many exposed fetuses developing congenital heart defects. The most common defects are conotruncal and great artery abnormalities, such as transposition of the great arteries, tetralogy of Fallot, double-outlet right ventricle, truncus arteriosus, and interrupted aortic arch. Historically, exposure to thalidomide had a 5% to 10% incidence of cardiac defects, especially tetralogy of Fallot, truncus arteriosus, and septal defects.[29]

Many of the anticonvulsants have been implicated as causes of congenital heart defects. Valproic acid has the strongest evidence for teratogenic effects, with phenytoin and trimethadione also implicated.[29–31] The cardiac defects most frequently seen are patent ductus arteriosus, aortic stenosis, ventricular septal defect, tetralogy of Fallot, coarctation of the aorta, and transposition of the great arteries.

The teratogenic effects of lithium have been questioned.[23,32–34] The overall incidence of congenital heart disease is probably not increased with lithium exposure, but when congenital heart disease is found it usually is Ebstein anomaly, an otherwise rare cardiac defect.

With the exception of daunorubicin, which appears to cause myocardial necrosis, the antineoplastic drugs have not been associated with congenital heart disease.[31,35] Other drugs, such as amphetamines, tranquilizers, and cocaine, remain controversial.

Of the infectious agents, rubella is the only one associated with structural defects, especially as part of the congenital rubella syndrome. The defects most commonly seen are patent ductus arteriosus, pulmonary stenosis, and septal defects. The effect of parvovirus on the heart has been mainly secondary to anemia and the fetal hydrops that develops, but parvovirus can also affect the myocardial cell itself.[36,37] Other viruses, such as coxsackievirus, may also affect the heart prenatally.

Chromosomal Anomalies

Fetuses with a chromosomal abnormality frequently have congenital heart defects (Table 4). Fetuses with congenital heart disease also have a significant risk of having a chromosomal abnormality. In liveborn infants with congenital heart disease, the incidence of chromosomal abnormalities was 11.8%.[1] In prenatal series, the incidence varies from 15% to 38% depending on gestational age.[29] The detection

TABLE 4. CONGENITAL HEART DISEASE AND CHROMOSOMAL ABNORMALITIES

Chromosomal anomaly[a]	Cardiac defects (%)	Types of cardiac defects
Trisomy 21	50	AVSD, VSD, ASD, TOF, COARC
Trisomy 18	100	VSD, DORV, TOF, PVND, HLHS
Trisomy 13	80	VSD, ASD, PDA, AS, PS
Trisomy 8	25	VSD
Trisomy 9	80	VSD
Partial trisomy 22q	60	ASD, VSD, PDA
Turner XO	35	COARC, AS, HLHS, MS
Klinefelter XXY	50	MVP
Triploidy	50	VSD, ASD, PDA
Deletion 22	95	IAA, TA, TOF
Deletion 4p	30	ASD, PS
Deletion 5p	40	VSD, ASD, PS
Deletion 4q21, 32+	60	VSD, PDA, ASD, COARC
Recombinant chromosome 8 syndrome	90	TOF, DORV, TA, VSD, PDA, ASD, HLHS
Cat-eye	40	TAPVC
Fragile X	70	MVP
Penta –X	<50	PDA, VSD

AS, aortic stenosis; ASD, atrial septal defect; AVSD, atrioventricular septal defect; COARC, coarctation of the aorta; DORV, double-outlet right ventricle; HLHS, hypoplastic left heart syndrome; IAA, interrupted aortic arch; MS, mitral stenosis; MVP, mitral valve prolapse; PDA, patent ductus arteriosus; PS, pulmonary stenosis; PVND, polyvalvular nodular dysplasia; TA, truncus arteriosus; TAPVC, total anomalous pulmonary venous connection; TOF, tetralogy of Fallot; VSD, ventricular septal defect.
[a]Other deletion syndromes include 9p, 13q, 18p, 18q, and 17p13, with 20% to 40% having congenital heart disease of variable type. Duplication syndromes, 3q2, 9p, and 11p15 (Beckwith-Wiedemann), are rare, with 15% to 35% having congenital heart disease of variable type.

of a cardiac defect alone is often enough to recommend genetic testing and if any other abnormality is present testing is strongly recommended.

Extracardiac Malformations

Extracardiac malformations are present in 25% to 45% of children with congenital heart disease.[29] Extracardiac malformations are more common in children with atrioventricular septal defects, other septal defects, heterotaxy syndromes, and conotruncal defects; less common in left heart defects; and uncommon in transposition of the great arteries. Table 5 reviews the extracardiac malformations most commonly associated with congenital heart disease. Increased nuchal translucency without chromosomal abnormalities is associated with cardiac defects, especially narrowing of the aorta.[38]

Twins are not a malformation, but monozygotic twins do have twice the incidence of congenital heart disease seen in dizygotic twins and the concordance rate is higher.[29,39] In conjoined twins, those with thoracopagus or thoracoomphalopagus have a 75% incidence of congenital heart

TABLE 5. CONGENITAL HEART DISEASE AND EXTRACARDIAC MALFORMATIONS

Extracardiac malformation	Risk of congenital heart defect (%)		Risk of cardiac malformation in cases with congenital heart defect (%)	Type of congenital heart defect
	Postnatal	Prenatal		
Central nervous system[a]	6–7	—	3–7	
Hydrocephalus	4.5	10–15	—	VSD, ASD
Agenesis of corpus callosum	15	14	—	DORV, TOF
Tracheoesophageal fistula and/or esophageal atresia	15–39	—	1	VSD, ASD, TOF, COARC
Gastrointestinal	5–22	—	2.2–7.0	
Duodenal atresia	17	27	—	VSD, AVSD
Jejunal/ileal atresia	5.2	—	—	Septal defects
Imperforate anus	12	—	—	TOF, VSD
Ventral wall defects				
Gastroschisis	0–12	—	—	TGA, AVSD, VSD
Omphalocele	19.5–32.0	26–35	—	TOF
Diaphragmatic hernia	9.6	14–18	0.3	TOF, DORV
Genitourinary[b]	8	—	—	VSD, COARC
Skeletal	—	—	4.6–16.1	
Short rib polydactyly	—	—	—	TGA
Thrombocytopenia-absent radius	33	—	—	TOF, ASD
Fanconi syndrome	14	—	—	—
Crouzon disease	Low	—	—	COARC, AS
Apert syndrome	10	—	—	VSD, TOF, COARC
Carpenter syndrome	3.2	—	—	—
Pierre Robin syndrome	9	—	—	—
Arthrogryposis	Up to 25%	—	—	—
de Lange syndrome	Occasional	—	—	—

AS, aortic stenosis; ASD, atrial septal defect; AVSD, atrioventricular septal defect; COARC, coarctation of the aorta; DORV, double-outlet right ventricle; TGA, transposition of the great arteries; TOF, tetralogy of Fallot; VSD, ventricular septal defect.
[a]Also abnormalities of the eyes and ears, meningomyelocele, holoprosencephaly, and Dandy-Walker malformation.
[b]Especially renal agenesis, hydronephrosis, and horseshoe kidney.

disease, usually involving shared structures between the two hearts. In most of the others the pericardium is shared. Even in omphalopagus, congenital heart disease is found in at least one twin in 25%.[29,39]

Arrhythmias

The most frequent types of fetal arrhythmia are premature atrial and ventricular contractions that have little clinical significance and are not associated with an increased risk of structural abnormalities. Tachycardias frequently cause *in utero* heart failure but are rarely associated with structural anomalies. Conversely, 50% of fetuses with complete atrioventricular block have cardiac malformations, mostly atrioventricular septal defects or corrected transposition of the great arteries.[40]

Nonimmune Fetal Hydrops

Nonimmune fetal hydrops is secondary to a cardiac abnormality in 25% of cases.[41] Two-thirds of the cardiac cases are due to arrhythmias, and one-third are due to structural heart disease. Occasionally both an arrhythmia and structural heart disease can be present, such as an atrioventricular septal defect with heart block or Ebstein anomaly with atrial flutter. The arrhythmias can be tachyarrhythmias, such as supraventricu-

lar tachycardia or atrial flutter, or bradyarrhythmias, such as heart block. The structural anomalies most commonly associated with fetal hydrops are (a) valve insufficiency, particularly Ebstein anomaly and other tricuspid valve abnormalities, but also absent pulmonary valve syndrome and atrioventricular septal defect and (b) outflow obstructions, particularly hypoplastic right or left heart syndromes, when associated with tricuspid valve insufficiency. The presence of fetal hydrops with either arrhythmia or structural heart disease worsens the prognosis. In particular, structural heart disease and complete heart block have an ominous prognosis when associated with hydrops, with exceedingly rare survivors. On the other hand, tachycardias can be treated effectively *in utero* and have a much more favorable outlook.

DIAGNOSIS OF FETAL CARDIAC DEFECTS

Almost all cardiac defects have been described *in utero* using echocardiography.[42–44] The ability to obtain accurate imaging depends on the ultrasound equipment used, the experience of the sonographer, and maternal and fetal factors such as maternal size, gestational age, fetal position, and amount of amniotic fluid. In general, a satisfying examination of the fetal heart can be obtained in virtually all cases by an experienced examiner at 18 to 23 weeks. Repeat examinations a few weeks after the initial examination can also improve accuracy if a complete examination could not be obtained initially. Diagnosis of some defects may be possible as early as 11 to 15 weeks.[45–48]

Certain defects are more readily detected because the four-chamber view is abnormal. These include atrioventricular septal defects, single ventricle, hypoplastic left and right heart, and tricuspid valve abnormalities. The diagnosis of conotruncal anomalies is more complex because the demonstration of the ventriculoarterial connections requires the use of specific sections that are usually more difficult to obtain. Eventually, the diagnosis of some defects may be impossible either because they are minor or because of the difference in fetal anatomy and physiology. These include atrial septal defects, anomalous pulmonary venous return, aortic coarctation, and minor valve abnormalities. A patent ductus arteriosus, of course, cannot be diagnosed *in utero*.

The sensitivity of a detailed fetal echocardiographic examination in the detection of cardiac abnormalities is widely reported to be approximately 85%.[8,10,49] False-negatives include mostly minor anomalies, such as septal defects. False-positives are exceedingly rare. In most studies they are limited only to two specific types of defects: ventricular septal defects and coarctation of the aorta.[8,50] Fetal echocardiography is accurate in the identification of the specific type of cardiac anomaly in greater than 90% of cases.[50]

The result of the examination will affect the prenatal care in several ways. When the examination is normal, the parents can be reassured. This is particularly valuable for couples at increased risk for fetal cardiac anomalies. When a severe anomaly is identified in early gestation, termination of pregnancy can be offered. Many believe that once a cardiac anomaly is diagnosed *in utero*, optimization of perinatal care, including delivery in a tertiary care center and early cardiologic treatment, may decrease mortality and morbidity. Studies focusing on selected ductal dependent anomalies that require rapid treatment after birth, such as transposition of the great arteries and hypoplastic left heart syndrome, suggest a decrease in operative mortality and morbidity.[51,52]

PROGNOSIS OF CARDIAC ANOMALIES DIAGNOSED *IN UTERO*

In countries where selective abortion is an option, the proportion of couples that request pregnancy termination after the early diagnosis of fetal cardiac defects is variable. Figures ranging from 30% to 50% are reported in most studies.[50,53] The severity of the cardiac anomaly, the association with extracardiac anomalies, and the availability of postnatal treatment probably represent the most important factors influencing the parents' decisions.

In continuing pregnancies, the earliest series of congenital heart disease detected prenatally demonstrated a higher mortal-

TABLE 6. INCIDENCE OF CONGENITAL HEART DISEASE

Congenital heart disease	Incidence (%)		Perinatal survival[a] (%)
	Postnatal	Prenatal	
Ventricular septal defect	20–30	8.2–9.7	42–63
Tetralogy of Fallot	9.7–11.0	6.5–8.3	21–33
Atrial septal defect	6–10	—	100
Pulmonary stenosis	8–10	2.4	67–100
Hypoplastic left heart syndrome	7–9	5.5–12.9	0–9
Coarctation of the aorta	6–8	2.9–6.8	17–100
Transposition of the great arteries	5–7	3.5–5.5	60–100
Aortic stenosis	3–6	2.7–6.5	0
Atrioventricular septal defect	4–5	13.8–21.7	28–53
Truncus arteriosus	1–4	1.3–1.8	0–50
Hypoplastic right heart syndrome	0.7–3.1	2.9	0–22
Tricuspid atresia	1.1–2.4	2.4	14
Double-outlet right ventricle	2	1.3–8.8	0
Single ventricle	1.5	4.1–10.9	33
Ebstein anomaly	0.5	4.1–5.6	13–20
Atrial isomerism	—	3.5	20

[a]Perinatal survival with prenatally diagnosed heart defect.

ity rate than studies of cardiac defects detected after birth. This discrepancy was most likely due to three factors: (a) the prenatal series include fetuses with defects that die *in utero*; (b) fetuses with more severe cardiac defects as well as other anomalies were more likely to be detected prenatally; and (c) an excess of fetuses with associated extracardiac anomalies was present. In these preliminary studies, the predominant anomalies were univentricular lesions, atrioventricular septal defect, and tricuspid valve abnormalities associated with hydrops. In more recent series, the spectrum of cardiac anomalies detected antenatally has widened to include a greater number of less severe conditions, which are more amenable to postnatal treatment. This was most likely the consequence of increased awareness of cardiac malformations in standard sonographic examinations. In one antenatal series,[50] the overall survival of fetal cardiac anomalies not associated with extracardiac anomalies at a mean postnatal follow-up of 3 years was 80%. In particular, survival exceeded 90% with conotruncal anomalies and was approximately 60% for univentricular lesions (Table 6).

CLASSIFICATION OF CONGENITAL HEART DEFECTS

Cardiac defects have traditionally been classified into groups with similar anatomy and physiology; however, there is a lot of variation within the groups and some overlap between groups. Tetralogy of Fallot, for example, can have very mild pulmonary stenosis with similar physiology to a large ventricular septal defect, or it can be accompanied by pulmonary atresia and depend on ductal patency. *Transposition* really refers to the relationship of the great arteries, but it is commonly used to describe a heart with situs solitus, atrioventricular concordance, ventriculoarterial discordance, and *d*-transposition of the great arteries. This latter description arises from a segmental approach to cardiac anatomy, which describes the anatomy in a specific heart rather than placing it in a category.[54,55] Both classifications are useful, but in complex disease, the segmental approach allows a more detailed anatomic description. The segmental approach also allows a systemic way of evaluating a heart defect and accounting for all of its structures and connections, whether they are present or not. Using the segmental approach, determination of the location of the heart and atrial situs is followed by determination of the atrioventricular and ventriculoarterial connections.

Concordance means that the right atrium is connected to the right ventricle, which is connected to the pulmonary artery, and the left atrium is connected to the left ventricle, which is connected to the aorta. Discordance occurs when other connections are found. Finally, associated anomalies of venous return, atrial anatomy, the atrioventricular junction, ventricular anatomy, infundibular (outflow) anatomy, aorta, aortic arch, and pulmonary arteries are described.

Septal Defects

Ventricular Septal Defects

A ventricular septal defect is an opening of the ventricular septum causing communication between the two ventricles.

Incidence

Ventricular septal defects are the most common cardiac defects seen postnatally, accounting for 30% of all structural defects.

Pathology and Hemodynamics

Four types of ventricular septal defects are identified, based on location in the ventricular septum: muscular, perimembranous, inlet, or subpulmonary. Muscular or trabecular defects occur in the muscular portion of the septum. Perimembranous defects involve the membranous septum below the aortic valve and extend to variable degrees into the adjacent portion of the muscular septum. Inlet defects occur in the inlet septum, close to the insertion of the atrioventricular valves. The subpulmonary defects are on the inflow tract of the right ventricle and thus affect the implantation of the septal chordae of the tricuspid valve. The most common are muscular and perimembranous. Ventricular septal defects can be isolated or associated with other cardiac defects. Ventricular septal defects associated with conotruncal defects are outlet in location and usually associated with malalignment of the ventricular and infundibular septa.

There is no evidence that ventricular septal defects are responsible for hemodynamic compromise *in utero*. Even a large interventricular communication probably gives rise only to small shunts in the fetus, because during intrauterine life the right and left ventricular pressures are very similar. The vast majority of infants are not symptomatic in the neonatal period. Rare exceptions are represented by very large defects causing massive left to right shunt, which can indeed be associated with congestive heart failure soon after birth.

Associated Anomalies

Most ventricular septal defects are isolated, but they are also found in association with almost every other kind of structural cardiac defect. Therefore when a ventricular septal defect is detected, a thorough echocardiographic examination is necessary. A specific diagnosis may be difficult at times. For example, in some cases of tetralogy of Fallot, a ventricular septal defect may be the only abnormal finding in early gestation.[56] The opposite is also true: A thorough search for a ventricular septal defect should be done when other structural heart defects are demonstrated. The available experience suggests that even seemingly isolated ventricular septal defects detected *in utero* are not infrequently associated with aneuploidies, particularly autosomal trisomies.[57]

Diagnosis

The echocardiographic diagnosis depends on the demonstration of a dropout of echoes in the ventricular septum (Fig. 1). Ventricular septal defects that are large are usually easily demonstrated on two-dimensional echocardiography, but small defects may not be easily seen. Defects smaller than 1 to 2 mm during intrauterine life, which represent the bulk of all ventricular septal defects, will fall beyond the resolution power of current two-dimensional ultrasound. Color Doppler may enhance the diagnosis of even small defects by demonstrating shunting across the septum. However, because ventricular pressures and compliance are similar prenatally, the color jets are usually not turbulent and flow can be either "left to right" or "right to left" at different times even in the same fetus, making detection of small defects challenging (Fig. 2).

Inlet or posterior defects are usually large and well seen on the four-chamber view. Many muscular defects can be seen on the four-chamber view as well, but some are more anteriorly located. Perimembranous and subpulmonary ventricular septal defects are best visualized from the long- and short-axis views of the heart, with the perimembranous ventricular septal defect located just below the aortic valve and the subpulmonary defect more anteriorly underneath the pulmonary valve. Ventricular septal defects associated with conotruncal defects are outlet in location and usually

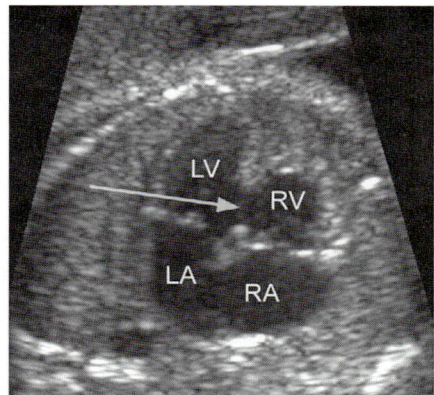
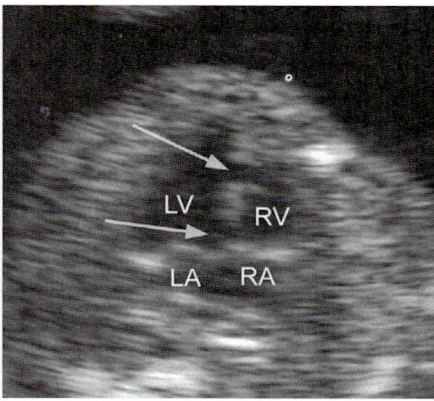
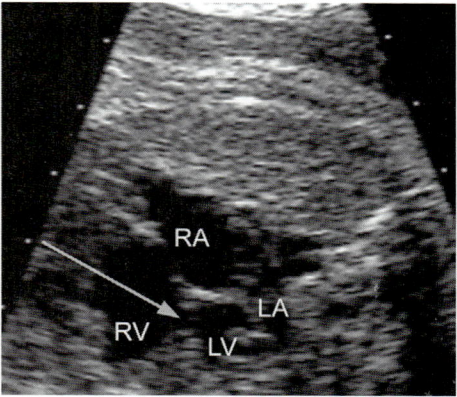

FIGURE 1. A: This four-chamber view of the fetal heart demonstrates a large posterior inlet ventricular septal defect (*arrow*). **B:** This four-chamber view demonstrates combined inlet and muscular ventricular septal defects (*arrows*). **C:** A large subaortic malalignment ventricular septal defect (*arrow*) in a fetus with a complex cardiac abnormality. LA, left atrium; LV, left ventricle; RA, right atrium; RV, right ventricle.

associated with malalignment of the ventricular and infundibular septa.

Ventricular septal defects used to be commonly missed. In a large series of pregnant patients screened at midgestation with the four-chamber view only, none of the 53 cases were identified.[6] Even in series of patients undergoing detailed fetal echocardiography, most of the ventricular septal defects that are detected are the ones associated with more complex cardiac malformations.[58,59] With better equipment, more experienced sonographers, and the use of color Doppler we expect an increase in the detection rate. The positive predictive value for the diagnosis of ventricular septal defects is similarly low. In one series, only 40% of isolated defects diagnosed *in utero* were confirmed after

birth.[50] This is probably due to a combination of false diagnosis and intrauterine closure of the defects.

Prognosis

Isolated ventricular septal defects should not cause hemodynamic compromise prenatally because ventricular pressures and compliance are not significantly different. Even in the neonatal period, the vast majority of infants are asymptomatic. Most (80% to 90%) small muscular and perimembranous ventricular septal defects that are detected at birth close in the first 2 years of life. Evidence suggests that prenatal closure is also possible.[60–62] In one large antenatal series, 46% of all defects closed *in utero*, 23% closed during the first year of life, and 31% remained patent. Spontaneous closure was more likely when

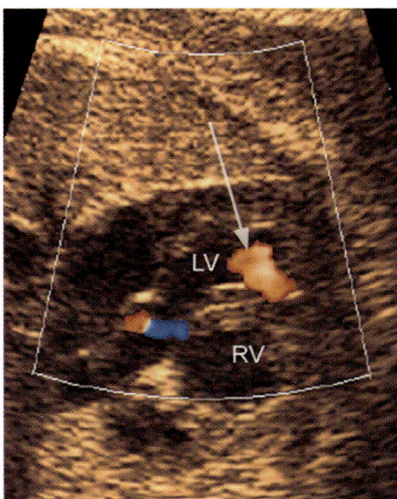
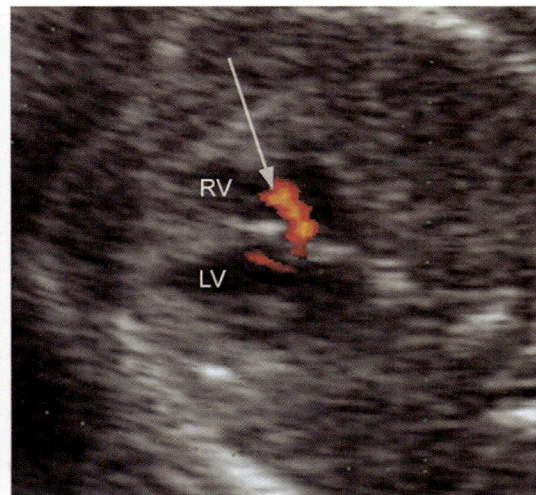
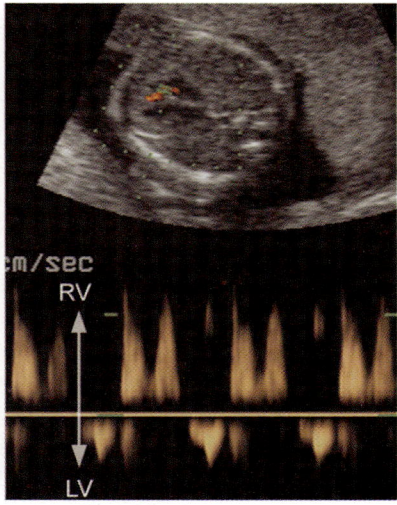

FIGURE 2. Doppler imaging facilitates the diagnosis of ventricular septal defects. **A:** Right to left shunt (*arrow*) across a muscular ventricular septal defect. **B:** Left to right shunt (*arrow*) across a perimembranous ventricular septal defect. **C:** Spectral Doppler imaging demonstrates a bidirectional shunt across the ventricular septum in the same case imaged in **B**. LV, left ventricle; RV, right ventricle.

the defect was smaller than 3 mm in diameter. None of the malalignment defects closed, in comparison to 69% of the perimembranous and 60% of the muscular defects.[57] Inlet and subpulmonary ventricular septal defects, as well as large muscular and perimembranous ventricular septal defects patent at birth, usually require surgical closure in the first year or two of life at low surgical risk with few long-term sequelae. The vast majority of patents will have a normal life span and a normal level of activity. Ventricular septal defects associated with other structural cardiac defects have a less favorable prognosis.

Obstetric Management
A careful search for associated anomalies, intracardiac and extracardiac as well, is indicated. Determination of fetal karyotype should be considered. Isolated ventricular septal defects, independent of their size and location, should not alter standard obstetric care. Prompt cardiologic evaluation after birth is recommended, however.

Atrial Septal Defect

Incidence
An opening of the atrial septum causing communication between the two atria, atrial septal defects account for 8% of structural heart defects.

Pathology and Hemodynamics
Three types of atrial septal defects are identified based on their location in the atrial septum: secundum, sinus venosus, and primum. By far the most common is the secundum type, which is characterized by a deficiency of tissue in this area of the atrial septum and often by a thickened appearance to the septal tissue around it. An atrial septal aneurysm may also be present. These aneurysms result from a redundancy of the valve of the fossa ovalis and usually completely close the atrial septum postnatally but occasionally remain patent postnatally. Prenatally, these aneurysms can be associated with atrial arrhythmias, usually benign premature atrial contractions, but occasionally more serious arrhythmias such as supraventricular tachycardia.[63,64] Sinus venosus atrial septal defects account for 5% to 10% of atrial septal defects. They are located posterior to the foramen ovale, usually inferior to the superior vena cava. Special views are often needed postnatally to visualize this defect, such as the right parasternal and subcostal short-axis views, making this defect difficult to visualize prenatally. A primum atrial septal defect is a type of atrioventricular septal defect and is discussed later [see Atrioventricular Septal Defect (Endocardial Cushion Defect)].

Atrial septal defects are not a cause of impairment of cardiac function *in utero*, as a large right-to-left shunt at the level of the atria is a physiologic condition in the fetus. Most affected infants are asymptomatic even in the neonatal period.

Associated Anomalies
Secundum atrial septal defects are most frequently isolated, but they may be related to other cardiac lesions associated with ventricular septal defects or pulmonary valve stenosis. Later in life, mitral valve prolapse can develop. Secundum atrial septal defects are also seen with complex defects causing interatrial shunts (e.g., mitral, pulmonary, tricuspid, or aortic atresia). Occasionally, they may be found as part of syndromes, including Holt-Oram syndrome (ostium secundum defect, hypoplasia of the thumb and radius, triphalangeal thumb, abrachia, and phocomelia).[65] The sinus venosus defect is commonly associated with anomalous connection of the right pulmonary veins to the right atrium or superior vena cava. These anomalous veins can be very difficult to detect prenatally.

Diagnosis
The prenatal diagnosis of an isolated atrial septal defect is very difficult or impossible. Secundum atrial septal defects are located at the fossa ovalis and most frequently cannot be distinguished from a normal foramen ovale. Sinus venosus defects are usually small. Furthermore, postnatally, special views are needed to visualize these defects, such as the right parasternal and subcostal short-axis views, that are difficult to replicate in the fetus. Only a few cases of secundum defects have been diagnosed *in utero*, and we expect that these were particularly large. We are not aware of any case of sinus venosus defect recognized *in utero*.

Prognosis
Isolated atrial septal defects should be asymptomatic prenatally, and the right heart enlargement seen postnatally is not present. Some defects become smaller or close, especially if they are initially small or associated with an atrial septal aneurysm. For moderate to large defects, closure is usually recommended either surgically or with catheterization closure devices. Both procedures are done at very low risk of morbidity or mortality with few long-term sequelae. Sinus venosus atrial septal defects are closed surgically because of their location and the frequently associated anomalous pulmonary veins.

Obstetric Management
When an atrial septal defect is either seen or suspected, a careful search for associated anomalies, intracardiac and extracardiac, is indicated. Determination of fetal karyotype may be considered. However, there are no clear-cut data suggesting an increased risk of associated aneuploidy when an isolated secundum atrial septal defect is present. Isolated atrial septal defects, independent of their size and location, should not alter standard obstetric care. However, prompt cardiologic evaluation after birth is recommended.

Atrioventricular Septal Defect (Endocardial Cushion Defect)

An atrioventricular septal defect is a defect in the central core of the heart, featuring the combination of a primum

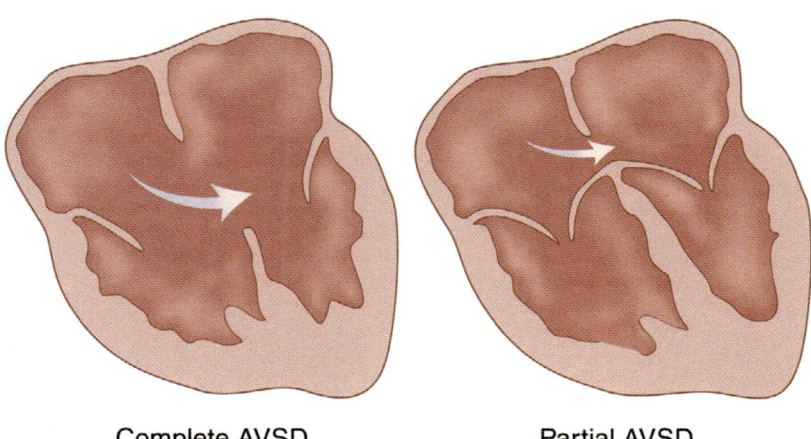

Complete AVSD   Partial AVSD

FIGURE 3. Schematic representations of partial and complete atrioventricular septal defects (AVSDs). (Courtesy of Philippe Jeanty, MD, Nashville, TN.)

atrial septal defect, a ventricular septal defect, and a variable degree of abnormality of the atrioventricular valves.

Incidence

Atrioventricular septal defects account for 7% of structural heart defects.

Pathology and Hemodynamics

Atrioventricular septal defects form because of incomplete fusion of the endocardial cushions, which form the crux of the heart. Two main varieties exist (Fig. 3). The complete defect, which is more common, includes an atrial septal defect located in the inferior part of the atrial septum, a large ventricular septal defect located posteriorly, and abnormal atrioventricular valves that are variable in their insufficiency (Fig. 4). The partial defect includes the atrial septal defect and a cleft mitral valve. There are also variants such as an intermediate atrioventricular septal defect with a small ventricular septal defect and a common atrium. Atrioventricular septal defects may be associated with marked asymmetry between the two ventricles (unbalanced defects). This variation has important prognostic implications because if one side of the heart is too hypoplastic, biventricular repair may not be possible postnatally.

Atrioventricular septal defects usually do not alter fetal hemodynamics, as the pressure in the left and right ventricles is similar and a mixture of blood occurs normally during intrauterine life. The exception is represented by cases with insufficiency of the atrioventricular valve that causes regurgitation and may result in heart failure and hydrops.

Associated Anomalies

Other cardiac defects commonly associated with atrioventricular canal defect include tetralogy of Fallot, double-outlet right ventricle, coarctation of the aorta, subaortic stenosis, ventricular hypoplasia, and pulmonary valve stenosis. Atrioventricular septal defects are usually encountered in fetuses either with chromosomal aberrations (50% of cases are associated with aneuploidy, 60% being trisomy 21, 25% trisomy 18)[66] or with heterotaxy syndromes. In the former cases, an atrioventricular septal defect is frequently found in association with extracardiac anomalies. In the latter cases, multiple cardiac anomalies are usually present (see Heterotaxy Syndromes). Abnormalities of the mitral valve, such as parachute deformity or a double orifice mitral valve, may also be present. Congenital heart block is also associated, especially in the heterotaxy syndromes. The association with aneuploidies is less likely if heterotaxy or a left ventricular hypoplasia is found. The risk of recurrence is 7% to 17% in families with normal karyotype.[67, 68]

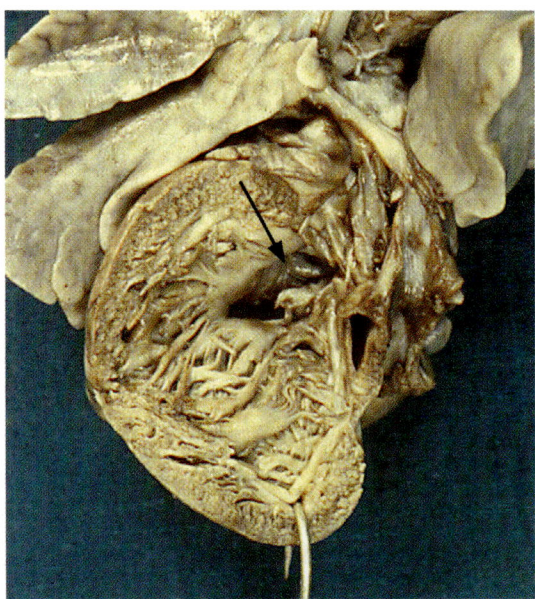

FIGURE 4. Pathologic specimen of complete atrioventricular septal defect. The arrow indicates the central deficiency of tissue at the core the heart involving both the inlet ventricular septum and the atrial septum primum.

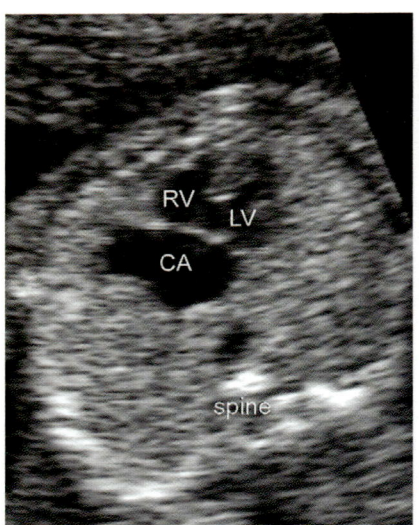
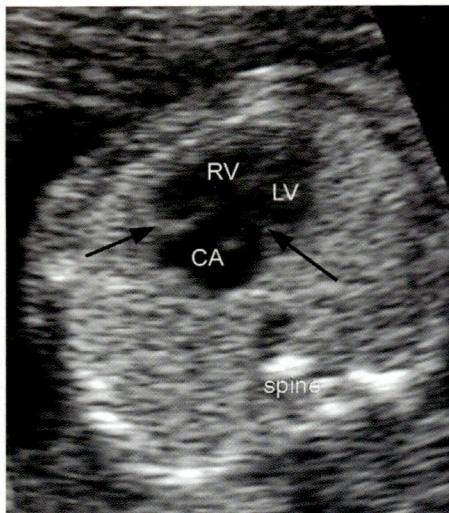
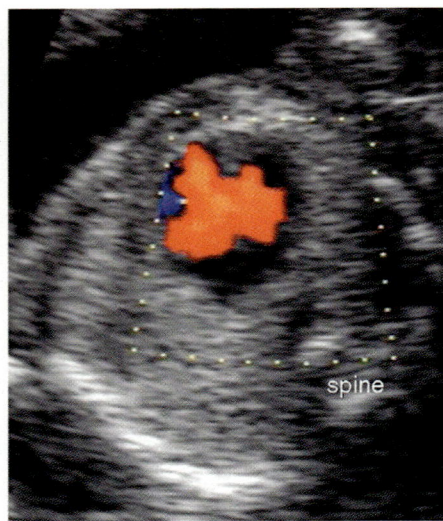

A–C

FIGURE 5. Four-chamber view demonstrates a complete atrioventricular septal defect in a fetus at 22 weeks. **A:** The systolic frame of the four-chamber view demonstrates a common atrium (*CA*) and a large atrioventricular septal defect. **B:** The diastolic frame demonstrates the central opening of the common atrioventricular valve (*arrow*). **C:** Color Doppler imaging in diastole demonstrates the mixture of blood at the level of the defect. LV, left ventricle; RV, right ventricle.

Diagnosis

Complete atrioventricular septal defects are well visualized in the four-chamber view since this view demonstrates the crux of the heart where the atrial and ventricular septal defects are located as well as visualizing the atrioventricular valves, often a "single" common valve. The defect is best detected during diastole when the common valve is patent and the defect becomes more evident. Color Doppler helps in visualizing mixture of flow between both ventricles during diastole (Fig. 5). Insufficiency of valves is very often found and can be demonstrated by color Doppler during systole.[69] It is still important, however, to visualize the other cardiac structures since there can be associated anomalies. The diagnosis can be performed in late first trimester by transabdominal or transvaginal ultrasound, especially in fetuses presenting with an increased nuchal translucency thickness.[48] However, missed diagnosis has been reported even in expert centers.[70] The reason for such erroneous diagnoses remains uncertain. We suspect that in early gestation an atrioventricular septal defect with a relatively small ventricular defect may be overlooked. Similarly, the partial form of atrioventricular septal defect involving only the septum primum may be difficult to demonstrate at times. A useful clue is the demonstration that both atrioventricular valves insert at the same level on the ventricular septum (Fig. 6).

While assessing the prognosis from a cardiologic point of view, the critical factors are the association with other cardiac malformations (e.g., heterotaxy syndromes), the presence of atrioventricular insufficiency, and hypoplasia of one of the ventricles and/or great artery (unbalanced atrioventricular septal defects) (Fig. 7).

Prognosis

Because of the high incidence of other structural and chromosomal abnormalities, prenatal mortality is high, ranging from 14% to 22%. These fetuses are also at risk for the development of hydrops particularly when there is insufficiency of the atrioventricular valve or complete heart block.[66,69] Post-

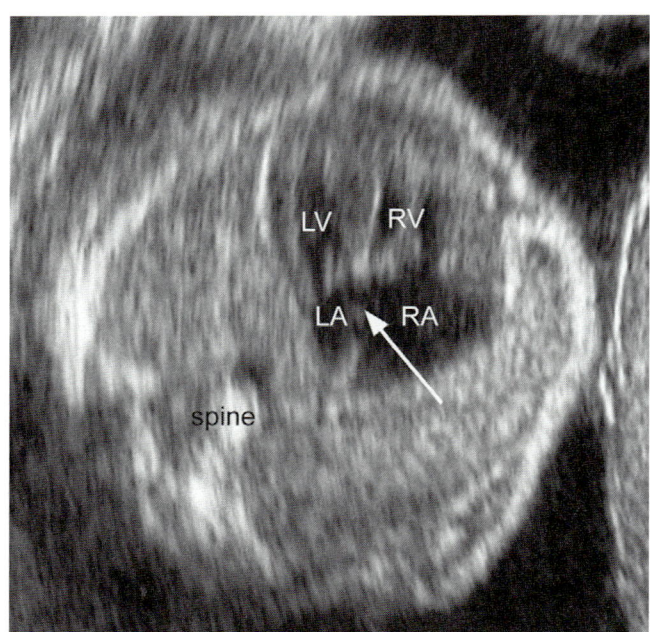

FIGURE 6. Partial atrioventricular septal defect. This four-chamber view demonstrates a primum atrial septal defect (*arrow*) and the insertion of the two atrioventricular valves at the same level on the septum. LA, left atrium; LV, left ventricle; RA, right atrium; RV, right ventricle.

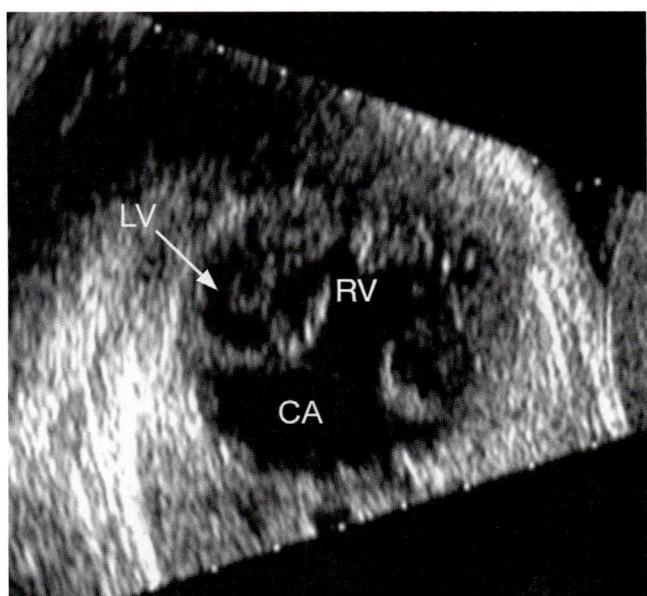

FIGURE 7. Unbalanced complete atrioventricular septal defect in a fetus with a complex cardiac malformation (right isomerism). Hypoplasia of the left ventricle (*LV*) is marked (*arrow*). The ascending aorta was severely hypoplastic as well, and, after birth, single ventricle repair with a Norwood-like operation was necessary. CA, common atrium; RV, right ventricle.

natally, most isolated atrioventricular canal defects can be repaired with an 85% to 90% survival rate. There is usually only mild residual mitral valve regurgitation, and the recent incidence of postoperative heart block is low. With other associated cardiac defects or extracardiac abnormalities, the mortality is higher. Marked hypoplasia of one ventricle/great artery may render biventricular repair impossible.

Obstetric Management

A careful search for associated anomalies, intracardiac and extracardiac, is indicated. Determination of fetal karyotype should be offered. Isolated atrioventricular septal defects, independent of their size and location, should not alter standard obstetric care. Serial sonography is recommended, however, particularly when atrioventricular valve insufficiency or heart block is seen, given the high risk of fetal hydrops. In these cases, anticipation of delivery should be considered when fetal maturity is achieved. Delivery in a tertiary care center is recommended.

Right Heart Abnormalities

Ebstein Anomaly and Other Tricuspid Valve Anomalies

Incidence
Tricuspid valve anomalies are rare, accounting for only 1% of cardiac anomalies.

Pathology and Hemodynamics
Ebstein anomaly is rare postnatally and is characterized by displacement of the septal and posterior leaflets of the tri-

cuspid valve into the right ventricle (Fig. 8). The degree of displacement is variable.[71] This creates an "atrialized" portion of the right ventricle, and the functional tricuspid valve orifice is displaced into the ventricle. Two other tricuspid valve abnormalities are (a) tricuspid valve dysplasia, in which the tricuspid valve is not displaced but its leaflets show nodular thickening and do not coapt, often with abnormal chordae and papillary muscles as well, and (b) unguarded tricuspid valve, in which little if any tricuspid valve tissue is present.[72,73] All three defects can be accompanied by right ventricular dysplasia and dysfunction. They usually have moderate to severe tricuspid valve regurgitation and a large right atrium. The heart is often very enlarged, which can lead to lung hypoplasia.[74,75] The association of Ebstein anomaly with lithium exposure is discussed earlier in this chapter, under Teratogens. Although Ebstein anomaly can remain undetected until adulthood (10%), 10% were detected *in utero* in a study by Celermajer et al.[76] Of the other 80%, one-half are diagnosed as neonates (less than 1 month of age) and the other half as infants and children. Tricuspid valve regurgitation with normal cardiac anatomy is usually secondary to abnormal physiology and not significant.[77]

Atrioventricular insufficiency is a well-established cause of fetal heart failure. Regurgitation of blood from the ventricles into the venous system causes a decrease in preload

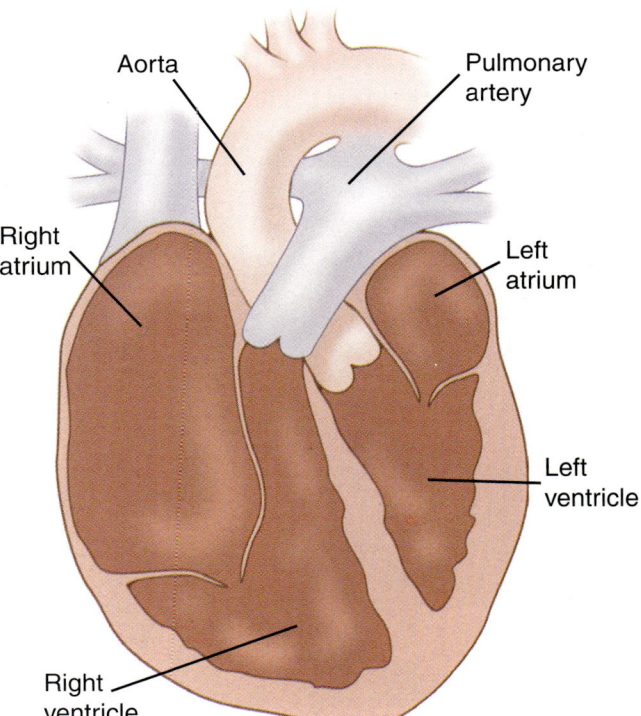

FIGURE 8. Schematic representation of Ebstein malformation of the tricuspid valve. The tricuspid valve is displaced into the right ventricle.

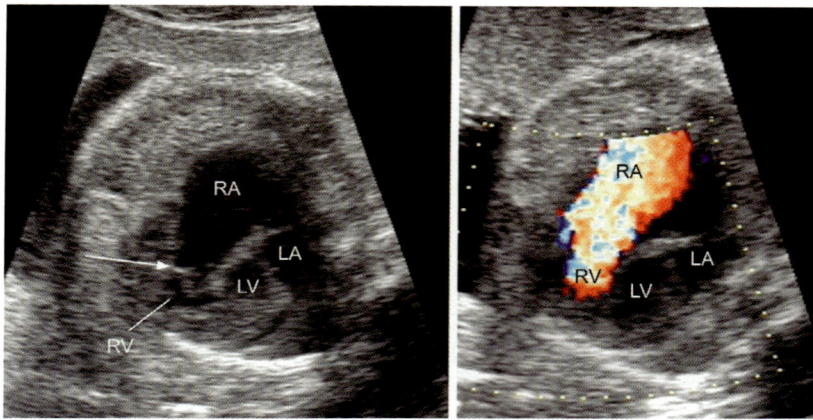

A,B

FIGURE 9. Basal four-chamber view of Ebstein anomaly associated with severe cardiomegaly. **A:** The tricuspid valve is displaced into the right ventricle (*RV, arrow*), and a large right atrium (*RA*) is demonstrated. **B:** Color Doppler imaging shows severe tricuspid valve regurgitation. LA, left atrium; LV, left ventricle.

and an increase in central venous pressure that may eventually lead to hydrops. In cases with massive tricuspid insufficiency, the output of the right ventricle may be greatly diminished and the pulmonary circulation supplied by the ductus arteriosus may be retrograde.

Associated Anomalies

The most common associated structural defect is a large foramen ovale or atrial septal defect. This atrial defect is often caused by a distended right atrium. A more serious defect often acquired during fetal life is pulmonary valve stenosis or atresia.[72,73,78] Lack of forward flow across the pulmonary valve secondary to severe tricuspid valve regurgitation and/or right ventricular dysfunction causes the pulmonary valve to not grow normally, eventually leading to pulmonary stenosis or atresia.[79] The presence of pulmonary atresia can make

Ebstein anomaly hard to distinguish from a hypoplastic right heart. Celermajer et al.[76] found pulmonary stenosis or atresia in 20% of their patients with Ebstein anomaly. They also found that associated cardiac defects were more common in those diagnosed prenatally (80%), with the majority of the defects being pulmonary stenosis or atresia. Other associated defects are ventricular septal defect, coarctation of the aorta, and patent ductus arteriosus.

Diagnosis

The severe forms of Ebstein anomaly and other tricuspid valve abnormalities are well visualized from the four-chamber view. There is overall enlargement of the heart, particularly affecting the right atrium, and color and spectral Doppler will reveal massive regurgitation across the tricuspid valve (Figs. 9 and 10). Mild forms can sometimes be hard to dis-

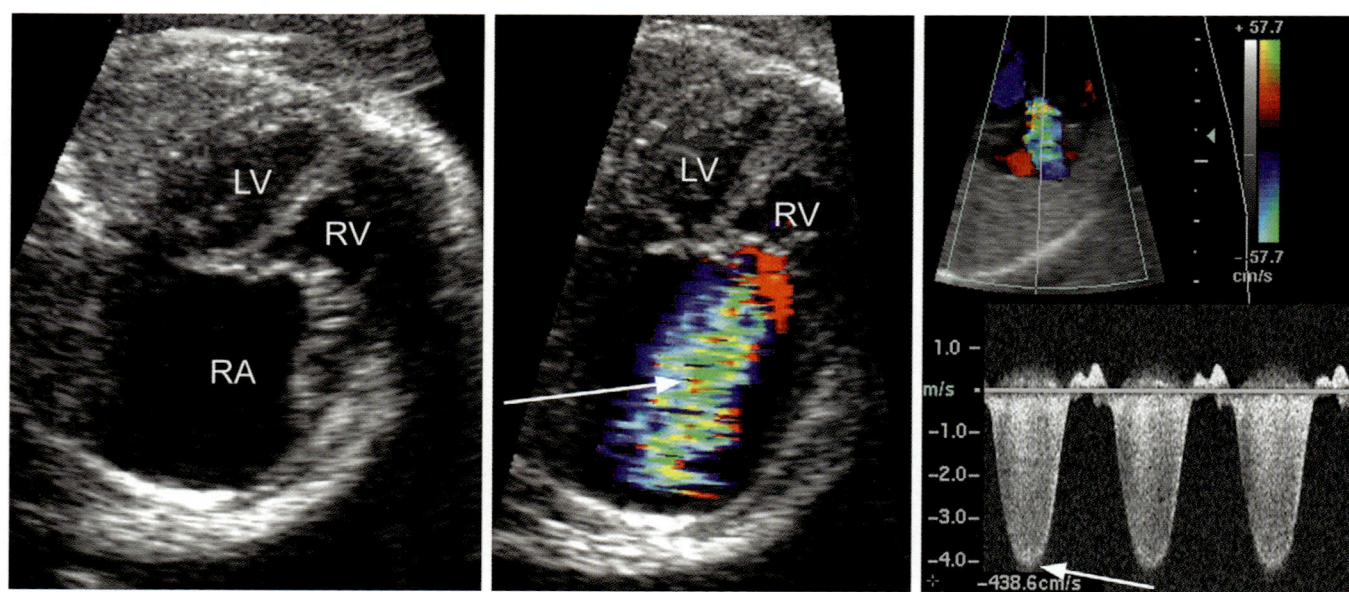

A–C

FIGURE 10. **A:** A four-chamber view shows a dysplastic tricuspid valve, which has thickened leaflets but is not displaced into the right ventricle (*RV*). The right atrium (*RA*) is enlarged. Severe tricuspid valve regurgitation (*arrow*) as seen by color Doppler **(B)** and continuous spectral Doppler **(C)**. The peak velocity of the regurgitant jet exceeds 4 m per second. LV, left ventricle.

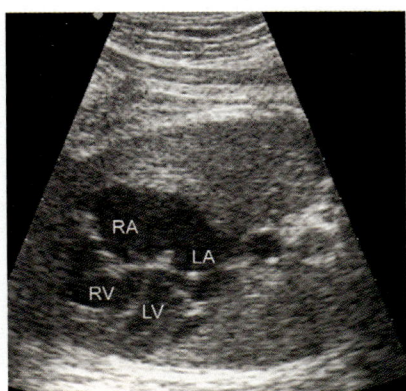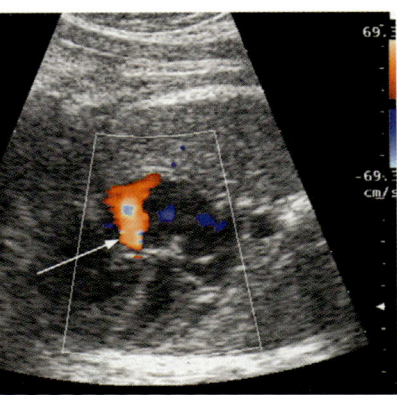

FIGURE 11. Mild tricuspid insufficiency (*arrow*) in a third-trimester fetus with normal cardiac structures. This was confirmed at birth. The infant was asymptomatic and required no treatment. LA, left atrium; LV, left ventricle; RA, right atrium; RV, right ventricle.

tinguish from normal anatomy, especially early in gestation, but color Doppler usually detects more than mild tricuspid valve regurgitation. Tricuspid valve abnormalities often progress during fetal life with increasing tricuspid valve regurgitation and right heart enlargement, primarily the right atrium. The pulmonary artery may be normal in size, but it is frequently small. When severe regurgitation from the tricuspid valve is present, there is usually no forward flow detectable with color Doppler within the pulmonary artery. In these cases, the differential diagnosis from pulmonary atresia with intact ventricular septum may be impossible. The left heart can appear small, but measurements are usually normal. The ascending aorta is of normal size. On the other hand, the occasional demonstration of mild tricuspid valve regurgitation with normal cardiac structures and a right atrium and ventricle of normal size is usually of no consequence and may be a transient phenomenon during fetal life[80] (Fig. 11).

Prognosis

Fetuses with Ebstein anomaly or other tricuspid valve abnormalities diagnosed *in utero* frequently develop hydrops from tricuspid valve regurgitation and/or right heart failure, which usually results in perinatal death. When severe regurgitation and cardiomegaly are present, newborns are often found to have hypoplastic lungs.[72–76,78,81] Therefore, the perinatal mortality can be as high as 85%. Once they survive infancy, the prognosis is much better. Patients are stratified according to clinical status and morphology, then treated with observation, valve repair, conversion to single ventricle, or transplantation. The mortality rate is 1% per year during childhood, increasing to 1.4% during adolescence and adulthood.[82,83] Some patients require closure of their atrial septal defects because of cyanosis, and some will require tricuspid valve repair or replacement, usually as adolescents or adults. The presence of severe right ventricular outflow obstruction usually makes the neonate ductus dependent and requires opening the pulmonary valve, either surgically or by interventional catheterization, or placement of a systemic to pulmonary artery shunt. Before opening the pulmonary valve, the degree of right ventricular dysfunction should be assessed. The force the right

ventricle can generate can be determined from the tricuspid valve regurgitation peak flow velocity, which is usually greater than 3.0 to 3.5 m per second in the presence of right ventricular outflow tract obstruction. If lower flow velocities are detected, the adequacy of the right ventricle to maintain forward flow once the pulmonary valve is opened should be questioned. Opening the pulmonary valve in the presence of inadequate right ventricular function can decrease flow to the lungs by creating wide open pulmonary valve insufficiency. Patients with Ebstein anomaly often have accessory connections that make them susceptible to atrial tachyarrhythmia, especially supraventricular tachycardia and atrial flutter. The development of a tachyarrhythmia during fetal life significantly worsens the prognosis, and most of these fetuses will die *in utero*.

Obstetric Management

A careful search for other cardiac anomalies is indicated. When severe tricuspid insufficiency and cardiomegaly are detected in early gestation, the prognosis is poor. Termination of pregnancy should be offered to the couples. In continuing pregnancies, serial sonograms are indicated. Whether the fetuses would benefit from early delivery is uncertain. It has been postulated that the drop in pulmonary resistances following the closure of the fetal circulatory pathways may improve hemodynamics. Certainly, the development of hydrops is an ominous sign, with no fetuses surviving the perinatal period in the authors' own experience. Experience with regard of the optimal mode of delivery is limited. There are no known contraindications to vaginal delivery.

Pulmonary Valve Atresia with Intact Ventricular Septum (Hypoplastic Right Heart)

Atresia of the pulmonary valve is usually associated with hypoplastic pulmonary artery and right ventricle (Fig. 12).

Incidence

Pulmonary valve atresia with intact ventricular septum is uncommon, accounting for only 1.7% of structural heart defects.

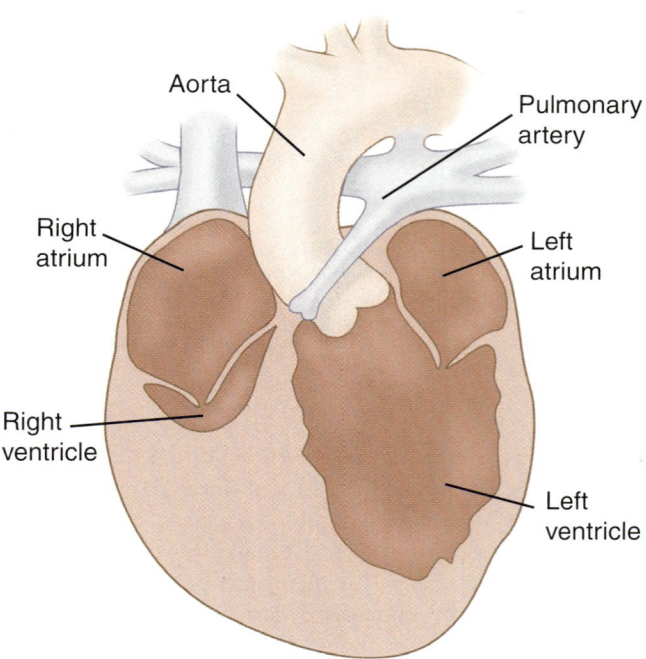

FIGURE 12. Schematic representation of pulmonary atresia with intact ventricular septum.

Pathology

The pulmonary valve is usually imperforate, though rarely a tiny opening is present. The pulmonary arteries are usually small, often measuring only 2 to 3 mm in diameter (Fig. 13). What is more variable is the degree of right ven-

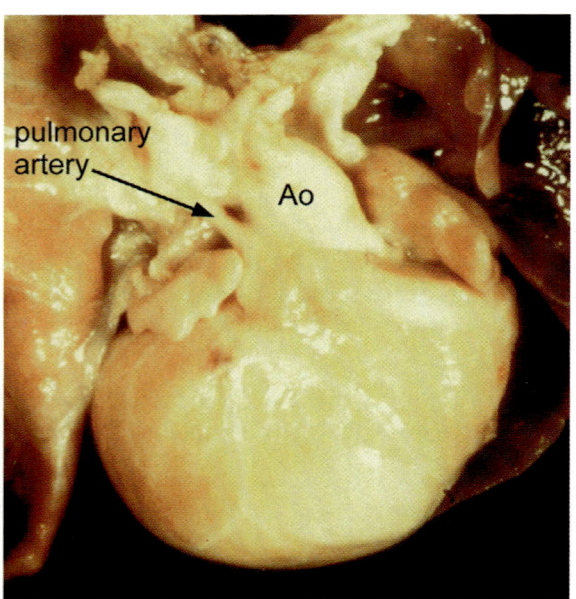

FIGURE 13. Anatomic specimen in one fetus with pulmonary atresia with intact ventricular septum. Ao, aorta.

tricular and tricuspid valve hypoplasia. The right ventricle has three parts: inflow, trabecular, and outflow. In some of the most severe cases the right ventricle is not hypoplastic but can be enlarged and dysfunctional, usually with dilation of a normal tricuspid valve that is severely incompetent. This form can be very hard to distinguish from Ebstein anomaly or other primarily tricuspid valve abnormalities. Even if the right ventricle and tricuspid valve are hypoplastic, significant tricuspid valve regurgitation may be causing severe right atrial enlargement. These hearts can be significantly enlarged, predisposing these fetuses to lung hypoplasia.[84,85] The coronary arteries can be stenotic and even occluded so that coronary flow is from the high-pressure right ventricle and not the aorta. In these cases, perfusion of the myocardium occurs by way of the right ventricle through dilated sinusoids.

Associated Anomalies

Most associated anomalies are secondary to the underlying right heart abnormalities as described above, and the presence of other unrelated defects is rare.

Diagnosis

It is important to distinguish a hypoplastic right heart from other "single" ventricle anomalies. In hypoplastic right heart there is always atrioventricular and ventriculoarterial concordance. In most cases, the entire right heart, with the exception of the right atrium, is small or hypoplastic from the tricuspid valve to the pulmonary arteries. The tricuspid valve may be small, but it is patent, thus distinguishing these defects from tricuspid atresia. Although rarely a problem, there must be a good-sized atrial septal defect. The left heart is usually normal. Color Doppler imaging is extremely important because it will usually demonstrate either minimal or no flow across the tricuspid valve (at times tricuspid valve regurgitation is present) and no forward flow across the pulmonary valve. A color Doppler cross section of the fetal chest conducted above the base of the heart and passing though the transverse aortic arch and ductus arteriosus/pulmonary artery is particularly valuable in these cases to demonstrate reversal of flow in the ductus arteriosus/pulmonary artery[86,87] (Fig. 14). The diagnosis of pulmonary atresia with intact ventricular septum may be difficult in early gestation because the right ventricle may be minimally underdeveloped. Indeed, a case with a normal cardiac ultrasound at 20 weeks' gestation and development of severe pulmonary stenosis at 34 weeks has been reported.[88] In the authors' experience, the most useful clues for a diagnosis in early gestation are the evaluation of right ventricular contractility in real-time, which is usually severely impaired in early gestation, and above all the use of color Doppler imaging to demonstrate reduced or absent flow across the tricuspid valve and reverse flow in the ductus arteriosus/pulmonary artery[89] (Fig. 15).

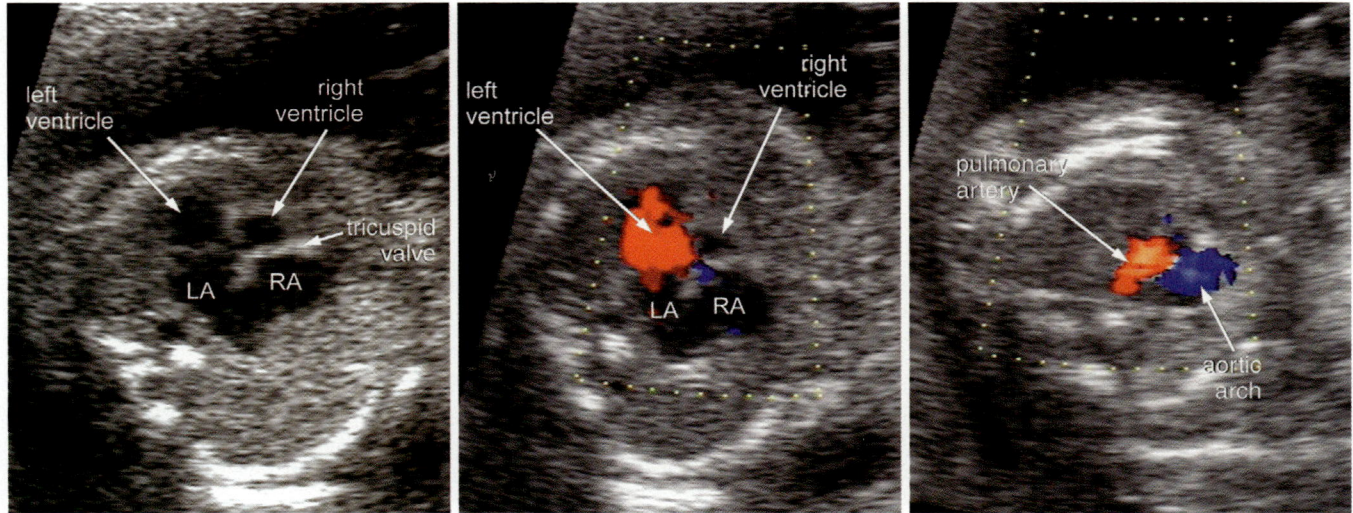

FIGURE 14. Pulmonary artery with intact ventricular septum at 21 weeks. **A:** A four-chamber view demonstrates a right ventricle of slightly smaller size than normal, with a bright endocardium, and minimal contractility on the real-time examination. **B:** Color Doppler imaging documents absence of blood flow across the tricuspid valve. **C:** A transverse scan in the upper chest demonstrates retrograde blood flow in the pulmonary artery/ductus arteriosus. LA, left atrium; RA, right atrium.

Prognosis

The prognosis is severe when severe tricuspid regurgitation and cardiomegaly are present, similar to that described for Ebstein anomaly. Infants who do not develop hydrops are ductus dependent, however, and undergo a pulmonary valvotomy or valvuloplasty and/or right ventricular outflow tract reconstruction. Rarely, a systemic to pulmonary artery shunt is also necessary for adequate pulmonary blood flow. In a few patients, the right ventricle and/or tricuspid valve is too hypoplastic, and these patients require a Fontan procedure typically used

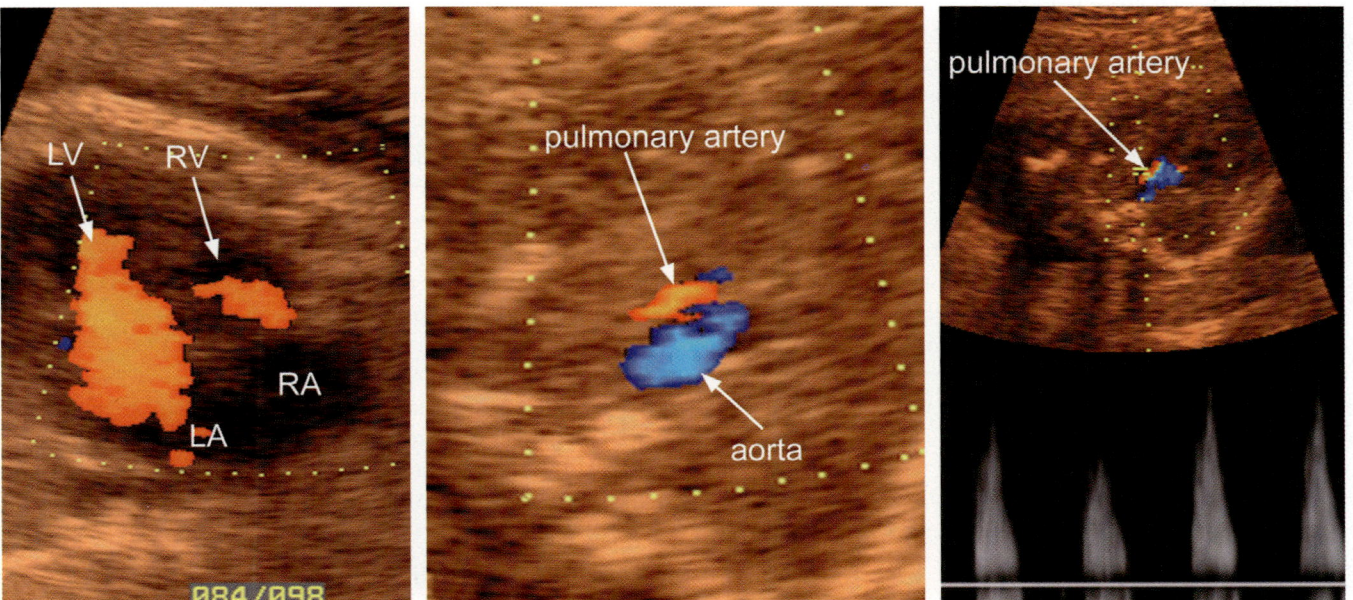

FIGURE 15. **A:** In this 22 weeks' gestational age fetus, the right ventricle (*RV*) is slightly diminished in size. Color Doppler imaging demonstrates decreased blood flow across the tricuspid valve when compared to the mitral valve. Color **(B)** and spectral **(C)** Doppler imaging reveals reverse blood flow in the pulmonary artery/ductus arteriosus. LA, left atrium; LV, left ventricle; RA, right atrium.

for single ventricle anatomy. Postnatally, approximately 65% survive their right ventricular outflow tract reconstruction surgeries and require few other interventions except for closure of atrial septal defects. Very few patients have survived beyond childhood after a Fontan operation for single ventricle anatomy, so the long-term prognosis is unknown.[90]

Obstetric Management

A search for associated anomalies is indicated. Fetal karyotyping should be considered, although the risk of aneuploidy with isolated pulmonary atresia with intact ventricular septum is low. Termination of pregnancy should be offered. In continuing pregnancy, serial sonography is recommended to identify signs of cardiac decompensation, such as severe tricuspid insufficiency, cardiomegaly, and hydrops. In the absence of these findings, delivery can occur at term and there is no contraindication to the vaginal route. The infants will be ductus dependent, and delivery in a tertiary care center is recommended.

Pulmonary Stenosis

Pulmonary stenosis is an anatomic lesion of the pulmonary valve, right ventricular infundibulum, or pulmonary arteries that leads to obstruction of right ventricular output.

Incidence

Pulmonary valve stenosis accounts for 8% to 10% of structural heart defects.

Pathology and Hemodynamics

Pulmonary stenosis encompasses a wide spectrum of severity, from mild to critical.[84] The most common form is the valval type due to the fusion of the pulmonary leaflets. The valve may be bicuspid or dysplastic. Dysplastic valves are often associated with Noonan's syndrome. As a consequence, the work of the right ventricle is increased, as well as the pressure, leading to hypertrophy of the ventricular walls. Apart from hypertrophy, the right ventricle is normal. The pulmonary arteries are usually normal in size. With more severe pulmonary stenosis, subpulmonary (infundibular) stenosis can develop. At the severe end of the spectrum, the right ventricular output may be so decreased that pulmonary circulation is supplied in a retrograde manner via the ductus arteriosus.

Associated Anomalies

The most common associated defects are atrial and ventricular septal defects. Other associated defects include anomalous pulmonary venous connection and valvular aortic stenosis. In addition to Noonan's syndrome, pulmonary valve stenosis can be seen in Williams syndrome, although more typically peripheral pulmonary stenosis and supravalvular aortic stenosis are associated with Williams syndrome. Chromosomal abnormalities are rare, but pulmonary valve stenosis has been associated with trisomy 13 and with dele-

tions of 4p and 5p. Prenatal exposure to the rubella virus has also been associated with valvular and peripheral pulmonary stenosis. Severe pulmonary stenosis has been described in the recipient twin in cases of twin-to-twin transfusion.[91] The pathophysiology in unclear, but it is thought to derive from chronic volume and pressure overload and, possibly, humoral factors.

Diagnosis

Sonographically, stenosis of the pulmonary valve is diagnosed by demonstrating with real-time ultrasound incomplete opening (doming) of the pulmonary valve. If the valve is dysplastic it may also appear thicker than normal. Stenosis may also be associated, independent from the degree of valval obstruction, with poststenotic dilation of the main pulmonary artery. Occasionally in severe or critical pulmonary stenosis, the pulmonary arteries are small, but they are usually normal in size The right ventricular hypertrophy is often hard to distinguish from the normal relative right ventricular hypertrophy and dominance seen during fetal life. Doppler imaging can be helpful. Doppler flow velocities in the pulmonary artery are often higher than those in the aorta, which is the opposite of normal. Color Doppler imaging demonstrates turbulence in the main pulmonary artery (Fig. 16) and occasionally tricuspid valve regurgitation or pulmonary valve insufficiency.[84,92] In practice, it is extremely difficult to identify mild to moderate stenosis antenatally, unless poststenotic enlargement of the main pulmonary trunk is present. In severe pulmonary stenosis, reverse of flow in the ductus arteriosus may be observed.[89]

Prognosis

The prognosis for pulmonary stenosis depends on the severity but is generally good. Mild forms rarely need any intervention. However, a progression in the severity of the stenosis has been described in some cases.[88,92] Critical pulmonary stenosis can be ductus dependent. Most patients with pulmonary stenosis undergo valvuloplasty, although a few patients with dysplastic valves or a small pulmonary annulus require surgery. Outcome for either procedure is excellent, and long-term problems are few.

Obstetric Management

A search for associated anomalies is warranted. Serial sonography is recommended. Unless tricuspid regurgitation and signs of heart failure develop, delivery can occur at term by the vaginal route.

Left Heart Abnormalities

Aortic Stenosis

Aortic stenosis is an anatomic lesion of the aortic valve, left outflow tract, or ascending aorta that obstructs the output of the left ventricle.

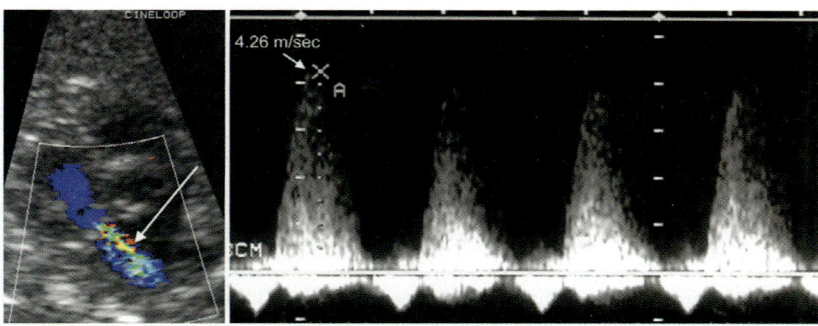

FIGURE 16. Severe pulmonary valve stenosis. **A:** Color Doppler imaging of the pulmonary outflow tract in a short-axis view demonstrates turbulent flow in the main pulmonary artery (*arrow*). **B:** Continuous spectral Doppler imaging of the pulmonary artery demonstrates increased flow velocities across the pulmonary valve. Mild pulmonary valve insufficiency is also present.

Incidence

Aortic stenosis accounts for 3% of structural heart defects and is more common in males.

Pathology and Hemodynamics

Stenosis can be valvular, subvalvular, or supravalvular. In valvular aortic stenosis the valve can be trileaflet with fused commissures, bicuspid, unicuspid, or noncommissural. The stenosis can vary from mild, never requiring intervention, to critical, causing left ventricular dysfunction and death. When aortic stenosis occurs in females, Turner syndrome should be considered. Subvalvular stenosis includes a fixed type, representing the consequence of a fibrous or fibromuscular obstruction, and a dynamic type, which is due to a thickened ventricular septum obstructing the outflow tract of the left ventricle. The latter is also known as *asymmetric septal hypertrophy* or *idiopathic hypertrophic subaortic stenosis.* Shone syndrome is a syndrome of multiple left heart obstructive lesions with valvular and/or subvalvular aortic stenosis. Supravalvular aortic stenosis is rare and is usually either associated with Williams syndrome or familial. Aortic stenosis can be associated with trisomy 13. A transient form of dynamic obstruction of the left outflow tract is seen in infants of diabetic mothers and is probably the consequence of fetal hyperglycemia and hyperinsulinemia.

Associated Anomalies

Valvular aortic stenosis is most commonly associated with other left heart defects, particularly coarctation of the aorta but also mitral valve abnormalities, especially a parachute mitral valve. Other associated defects include patent ductus arteriosus, ventricular septal defects, and pulmonary stenosis. Supravalvular aortic stenosis is often associated with peripheral pulmonary stenosis in Williams syndrome. Aortic stenosis is one of the congenital cardiac defects most frequently found in association with intrauterine growth restriction.

Diagnosis

Mild forms of aortic stenosis can be undetectable prenatally because it is usually impossible to obtain sonographic images with enough resolution to demonstrate incomplete opening (doming) of the aortic valve, particularly in early gestation. In severe aortic stenosis the valve is thickened and more obviously doming, limited in its motion, or both. The left ventricle can be hypertrophied. In critical aortic stenosis, the left ventricle is usually dilated with decreased systolic function and endocardial fibroelastosis and mitral valve regurgitation are often present. Pulsed Doppler imaging can detect increased flow velocities across the aortic valve (Fig. 17). Flow velocities that decrease during gestation are usually an ominous sign of decreased cardiac output from worsening left ventricular failure.[93] Color

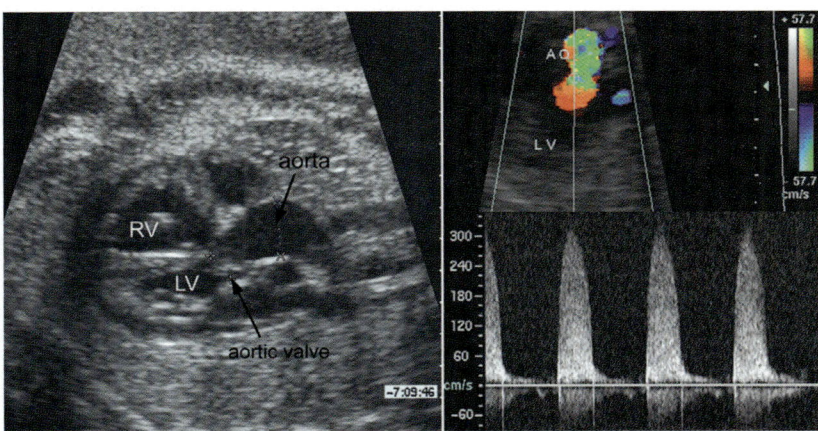

FIGURE 17. Severe aortic stenosis. **A:** A long-axis view of the left ventricle (*LV*) demonstrates a thickened aortic valve and enlarged ascending aorta. **B:** Color Doppler imaging demonstrates a turbulent jet in the ascending aorta (*AO*), and continuous Doppler demonstrates high flow velocity (3.2 m per second). RV, right ventricle.

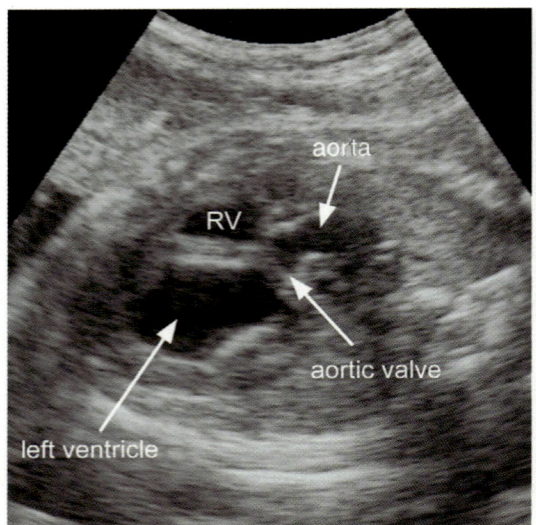
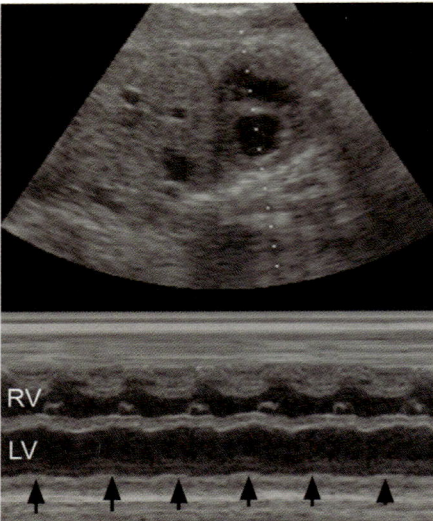
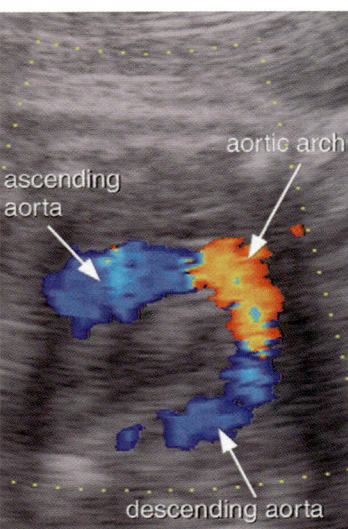

A–C

FIGURE 18. Critical aortic stenosis with ductus dependence. **A:** A long-axis view of the left ventricle demonstrates a thickened aortic valve and enlarged ascending aorta. The left ventricle is also enlarged, with a bright and thick endocardial lining suggestive of endocardial fibroelastosis. **B:** M-mode tracing demonstrates severely decreased contractility of the left ventricle (*LV*). **C:** Color Doppler imaging of the aorta demonstrates reversed flow across the arch and ascending portions. RV, right ventricle.

Doppler imaging demonstrates turbulence in the ascending aorta and, in critical cases, reversal of blood flow across the aortic arch[89] (Fig. 18). Mitral valve regurgitation and aortic valve insufficiency can also be identified when present.

Asymmetric septal hypertrophy has been identified *in utero*.[94] The only reported case is likely to be an exception, however, as this anomaly usually evolves over time and is not apparent in the neonatal period. Hypertrophic cardiomyopathy in fetuses of diabetic mothers has been reported on several occasions.[16,95,96] We are not aware of cases of supravalvular aortic stenosis detected *in utero*.

Progression of aortic stenosis *in utero* has been documented. In an antenatal series, the left ventricle and aortic root were of normal size until early in the third trimester. In some cases, failure of growth occurred, and at birth several infants had critical aortic stenosis requiring a Norwood operation.[97]

Prognosis

The prognosis for aortic stenosis depends on its severity, but it is a lifelong disease often requiring multiple procedures. The subvalvular and supravalvular types of stenoses are not generally manifest in the neonatal period. Conversely, the valvular type can be a cause of congestive heart failure in the newborn as well as the fetus.[98] Significant endocardial fibroelastosis is usually present in these cases.[99] Attempts have been made to balloon dilate these valves prenatally[100] but thus far without significant success.[97] However, the prognosis for this defect could be significantly altered by fetal intervention if the valve could be safely opened, allowing the left ventricle to recover func-

tion. Most valves that require intervention in infancy and childhood undergo valvuloplasty, but surgical commissurotomy can also be done. Most of these valves eventually require replacement surgically with either the pulmonary valve (Ross procedure), homograft valves, or prosthetic valves. Aortic stenosis has a low but significant risk of sudden death throughout life and has one of the highest recurrence risks, especially for women with the defect.

Obstetric Management

In the absence of signs of cardiac compromise, delivery can occur at term vaginally. The optimal management of cases with signs of cardiac decompensations, severe growth restriction, or both is unknown. It has been suggested that anticipation of delivery and early treatment may improve the outcome of critical cases.[101]

Coarctation of the Aorta

Coarctation of the aorta is a constriction of the aortic arch that ranges from a discrete shelf-like lesion within the lumen to a segmental narrowing of a portion of the arch.

Incidence

Coarctation of the aorta accounts for 4.6% of structural heart defects.

Pathology and Hemodynamics

Coarctation is a localized narrowing of the juxtaductal arch, most commonly between the left subclavian artery and the ductus. A discrete shelf between the isthmus and the

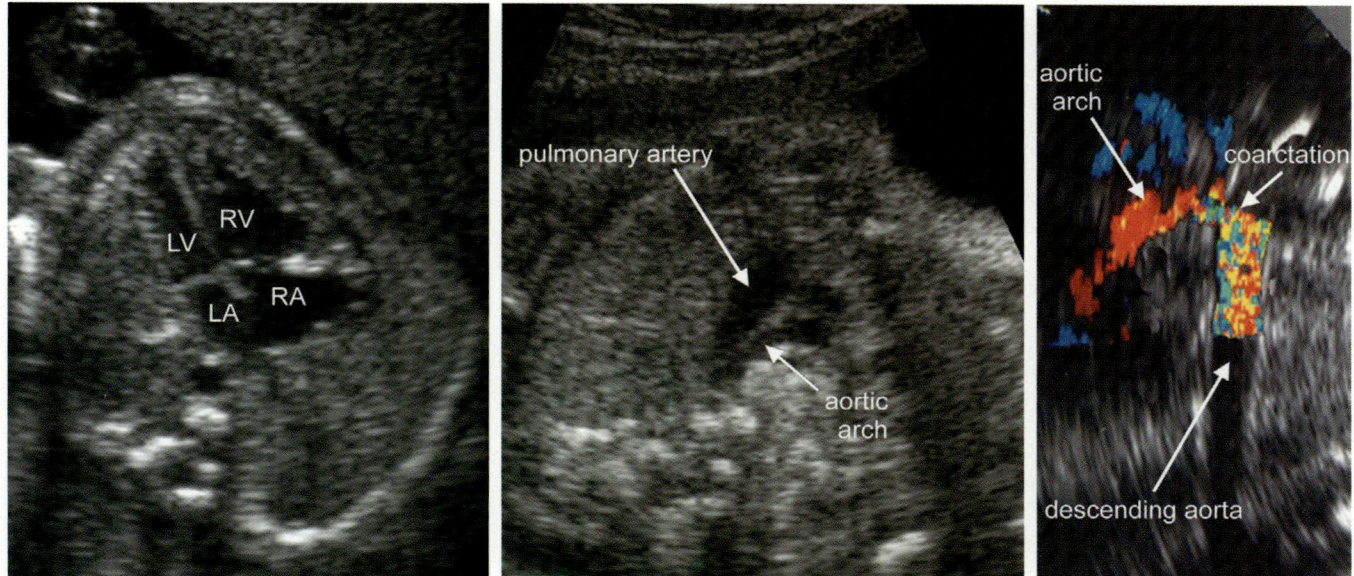

A–C

FIGURE 19. Fetal coarctation of the aorta. **A:** In the four-chamber view, a discrepancy in the sizes of the ventricles is demonstrated. The left ventricle (*LV*) is narrower than the right ventricle (*RV*). LA, left atrium; RA, right atrium. **B:** In the three-vessel view, the aortic arch is shown to be tinier than usual compared with the pulmonary artery. **C:** Color Doppler imaging of the aortic arch demonstrates turbulence in the descending aorta.

descending aorta is the most common finding at anatomic dissection. In infants, however, many coarctations involve tubular hypoplasia of the aortic isthmus and even the transverse arch. Tubular hypoplasia is a generalized narrowing of the aorta that affects the proximal arch, most commonly the segment between the left common carotid and the left subclavian artery or the isthmus, and may extend in the brachiocephalic vessels. Interrupted aortic arch, type A, is a severe type of coarctation in which the arch is interrupted distal to the left subclavian artery. The pathogenesis of coarctation of the aorta is heterogeneous. Coarctation may be a true malformation, due to an embryogenetic abnormality, the consequence of aberrant ductal tissue in the aortic wall, resulting in narrowing of the isthmus at the time of closure of the ductus or, finally, the anatomic result of an intrauterine hemodynamic perturbation, due to an intracardiac anomaly diverting blood flow from the aorta into the pulmonary artery and ductus arteriosus.

As the blood flow through the isthmus is minimal during intrauterine life, the descending aorta being mainly supplied via the ductus arteriosus, isolated coarctation does not significantly alter fetal hemodynamics.

Associated Anomaly

A bicuspid aortic valve occurs in up to 85% of patients with coarctation. Other defects commonly associated with coarctation are patent ductus arteriosus and ventricular septal defects. Less commonly associated defects are subaortic stenosis, atrioventricular septal defect, transposition of the great arteries, and double-outlet right ventricle. Like other left heart defects, coarctation can be familial. Extracardiac anomalies include chromosomal aberrations, mostly Turner syndrome (approximately 35% of infants with Turner syndrome have a coarctation). Coarctations are also associated with trisomy 21 and found in infants of diabetic mothers.

Diagnosis

Although visualization of the fetal aortic arch is usually possible, good images can sometimes be difficult to obtain.[102,103] Even with good visualization, a discrete coarctation may not be detectable. Therefore indirect findings that suggest the presence of a coarctation are most commonly used for diagnosis. Right ventricular and pulmonary artery enlargement relative to the left ventricle and aorta without right heart disease or ductal constriction can indicate the presence of a coarctation.[102,103] Hornberger et al.[104,105] found that the transverse arch and aortic isthmus measurements were significantly smaller and the ratio of the left common carotid to transverse aorta was significantly greater in fetuses with coarctation when compared to normal subjects. Color Doppler imaging can be helpful in better delineating the aortic arch, the area of coarctation, or demonstrating turbulence through this area (Fig. 19). The main difficulty in the diagnosis depends on the fact that aortic coarctation is suspected in many cases because of indirect findings (predominance of the right cardiac sections, small aortic isthmus) that may be present in normal fetuses. In the authors' experience, the positive predictive values of fetal echocardiography in the antenatal diagnosis of isolated aortic coarctation was 80%.[50]

Prognosis

The prognosis for coarctation of the aorta depends on its severity and when it is repaired.[106–108] These two factors are often related, in that more severe or extensive coarctations usually require repair in infancy. The mortality for unrepaired symptomatic coarctation in infancy is as high as 84%. When repaired in infancy, the surgical mortality can be 5% to 15% especially if other cardiac defects are present but drops to 0% by 2 to 3 years of age. The long-term prognosis is good but problems can occur. Recurrence of coarctation is highest when surgical repair is in infancy, often 15% to 30%, whereas the recurrence rate is only 5% when coarctation is repaired beyond infancy. The risk for systemic hypertension and its complications is greater when coarctations are repaired after 5 years of age. Aortic aneurysms at the coarctation site can also occur, especially with patch aortoplasty repair or angioplasty. In a subgroup of fetuses in whom aortic coarctation is diagnosed early in gestation, progression of the disease leads to severe hypoplasia of the left heart structures. Parents of fetuses diagnosed early in gestation with severe coarctation of the aorta need to be advised that if growth of the left heart is poor as pregnancy advances, a biventricular repair may be impossible at birth and the postnatal management will follow that for hypoplastic left heart syndrome.[97]

Obstetric Management

Termination of pregnancy can be offered, particularly if a severe lesion is detected early in gestation. A search for associated anomalies and fetal karyotyping are indicated. The diagnosis of isolated coarctation does not alter obstetric management.

Interrupted Aortic Arch

Incidence

Discontinuity in the aortic arch is rare.

Pathology and Hemodynamics

The interruption can be complete or there may be an atretic fibrous segment between the arch and the descending aorta. The lesion has been considered an extreme form of coarctation.[109] Indeed, the occurrence of coarctation of the aorta, interrupted aortic arch, and hypoplastic left heart syndrome in the same families suggests that the three lesions are etiologically related.[110] The interruptions are categorized according to their level compared to the brachiocephalic vessels (Fig. 20). In type A (42%), the aorta supplies the three brachiocephalic vessels and the pulmonary artery supplies the descending aorta via the ductus. In type B (53%), the interruption is proximal to the left subclavian artery. In type C (4%), the interruption is between the right innominate and left common carotid arteries. Type C is the most lethal form. Ventricular septal

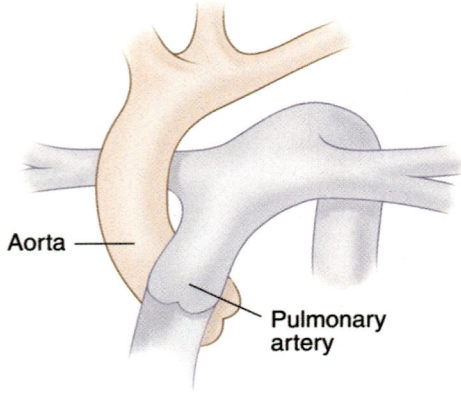

Type A

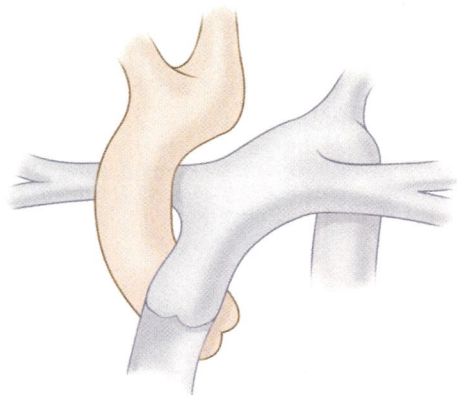

Type B

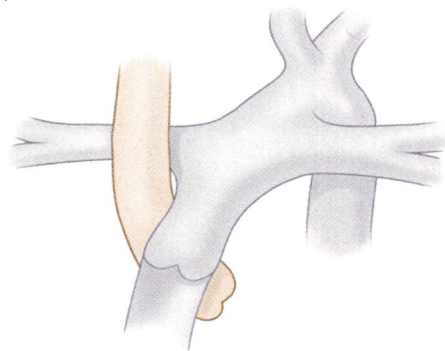

Type C

FIGURE 20. Schematic representation of the three types of interrupted aortic arch.

defects are almost always present in type B and occur in 50% of type A cases. The ventricular septal defect is of the malalignment type and is usually associated with obstruction of the aortic outflow. The same hemodynamic considerations discussed for aortic coarctation

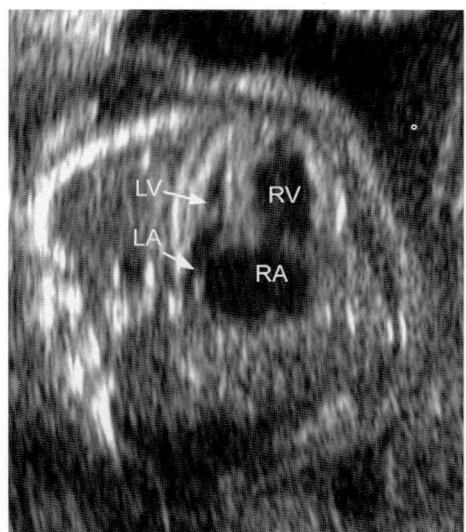 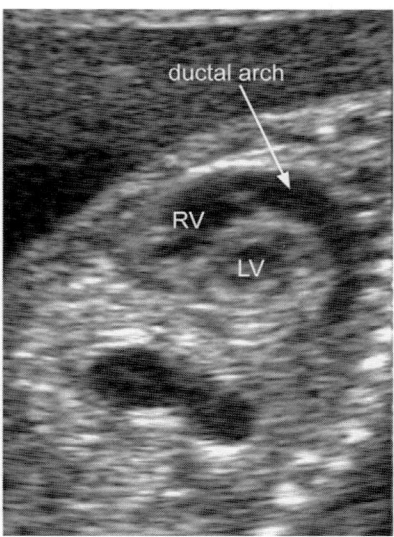 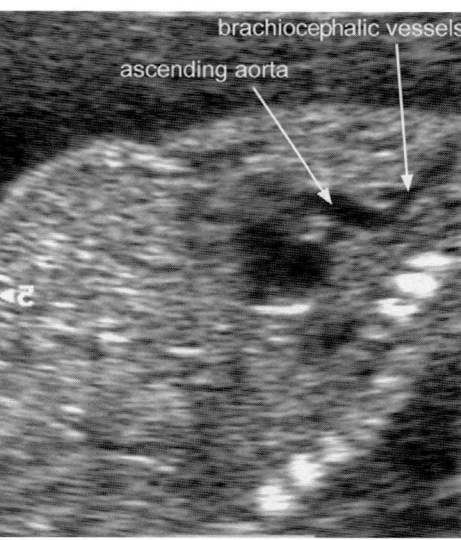

FIGURE 21. Interrupted aortic arch in a second-trimester fetus. **A:** The four-chamber view reveals a discrepancy in the sizes of the ventricles. The left ventricle (*LV*) is narrower than the right ventricle (*RV*). **B:** The ductal arch is increased in size and gives rise to some brachiocephalic vessels. **C:** The ascending arch has a steep vertical course, gives rise to only one brachiocephalic vessel, and is not connected to the descending aorta. LA, left atrium; RA, right atrium.

apply to interrupted aortic arch. The lesion does not cause cardiac compromise during intrauterine life. In types B and C, brachiocephalic vessels are supplied by the ductus arteriosus.

Associated Anomalies

Major associated cardiac abnormalities are commonly seen: In one postnatal series approximately one-third of infants had ventricular septal defect with patent ductus arteriosus, one-third had complex ventricular septal defect with left ventricular outflow obstruction, and one-third had complex intracardiac lesions.[111] Extracardiac anomalies include holoprosencephaly, cleft lip/palate, esophageal atresia, duplicated stomach, diaphragmatic hernia, horseshoe kidneys, bilateral renal agenesis, oligodactyly, claw hand, and sirenomelia. Interruption of the aortic arch may be associated with microdeletion 22q11,[112] which is discussed later, under Conotruncal Defects.

Diagnosis

The characteristic findings of an arch that cannot be traced into the descending aorta should suggest the diagnosis. Another finding is the discrepancy in the size of the ventricles, with a predominance of the right ventricle (Fig. 21). Differentiation from a severe aortic coarctation is always difficult. A useful clue is the straight vertical appearance of the ascending aorta (Fig. 22). Complex cardiac anomalies diverting blood flow from the aorta may be present.

Prognosis

In a large series of patients seen between 1987 and 1992, preoperatory death occurred in 5% and survival at 4 years after repair with different techniques was 63%.[113] One-stage primary repair including the associated cardiac defects is currently considered the method of choice and can be accomplished with low operative risk, although the long-term prognosis is strongly influenced by the presence of subaortic obstruction. Elective repair is performed at 2 to 3 months or earlier if signs of cardiac failure are present.

Obstetric Management

A search for associated anomalies including fetal karyotype and diagnosis of microdeletion 22q11 is indicated.[114,115] Termination of pregnancy can be offered. In continuing pregnancies, the lesion is usually well tolerated by the fetus and does not alter standard obstetric management.

Hypoplastic Left Heart Syndrome

Hypoplastic left heart syndrome is a spectrum of conditions associated with severe hypoplasia of the left ventricle and left ventricular outflow tract (Fig. 23).

Incidence

Hypoplastic left heart syndrome accounts for 7% to 9% of structural heart defects. It is one of the anomalies most frequently identified with prenatal ultrasound and is the leading cause of cardiac death in the neonatal period.

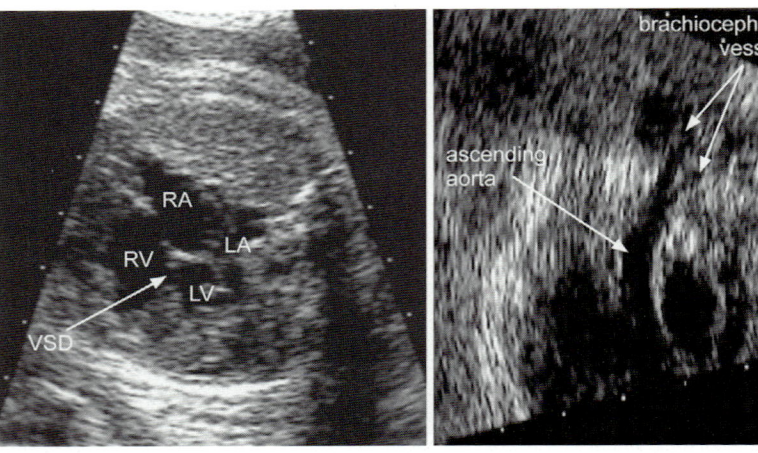

A,B

FIGURE 22. Interrupted aortic arch with complex intracardiac malformations. **A:** The four-chamber view demonstrates a large malalignment ventricular septal defect (*VSD*). LA, left atrium; LV, left ventricle; RA, right atrium; RV, right ventricle. **B:** A longitudinal view of the fetus demonstrates a steep vertical ascending aorta.

Pathology and Hemodynamics

A wide spectrum of left heart hypoplasia is seen with hypoplastic left heart syndrome. The common denominator is that the left ventricle is unable to support the systemic circulation, which is ductal dependent. Three main varieties can be recognized: (a) With combined mitral and aortic atresia, there is no communication between the left atrium and left ventricle. The ventricle is either slitlike or a virtual cavity that is not demonstrable with ultrasound. (b) With aortic atresia the left ventricle is hypoplastic but globular and has a very echogenic lining. In each of the first two types, the ascending aorta is very small (1 to 3 mm), and a

coarctation is often present as well (Fig. 24). (c) With critical aortic stenosis, the left ventricle is more prominent than with the other two varieties, but it is also hypertrophic and echogenic and it demonstrates poor contractility. The mitral and aortic valves are usually patent, at least in early gestation. Eventually, severe coarctation of the aorta and hypoplastic left heart and unbalanced atrioventricular septal defects with hypoplastic left heart may need to be managed after birth as classic forms of hypoplastic left heart.[116]

With obstruction to left ventricular output, the aortic arch is supplied in a retrograde manner via the ductus arteriosus. Unless other complications develop (e.g., tricuspid insufficiency), the condition does not compromise fetal hemodynamics. Neonates have normal birth weight and do not seem to have an increased rate of intrapartum distress.

Associated Anomalies

Aortic atresia in association with other heart defects mimics hypoplastic left heart physiology. Other defects that can be associated with aortic atresia are atrioventricular canal, transposition of the great arteries with a hypoplastic right ventricle, single ventricle, and corrected transposition. Hypoplastic left heart is twice as common in boys; when present in a girl, Turner syndrome should be considered. Incidence of trisomy 18 is also increased, and 10% have extracardiac malformations. Deletion 22q11 may be present.[112]

Diagnosis

A hypoplastic left heart is usually easily seen on a four-chamber view as either complete absence of the left ventricle (mitral and aortic atresia) or as a small globular left ventricle with poor contractility and an internal echogenic lining, probably representing endocardial fibroelastosis[116,117] (Fig. 25). In these cases it is important to distinguish it from other "single" ventricle anomalies. The size of the aorta and where it arises will determine the prognosis postnatally, so a complete evaluation of this defect always includes determination of the size of the aorta from the aortic valve to the ductus arteriosus.[118] The left atrium is small to normal in size. Some

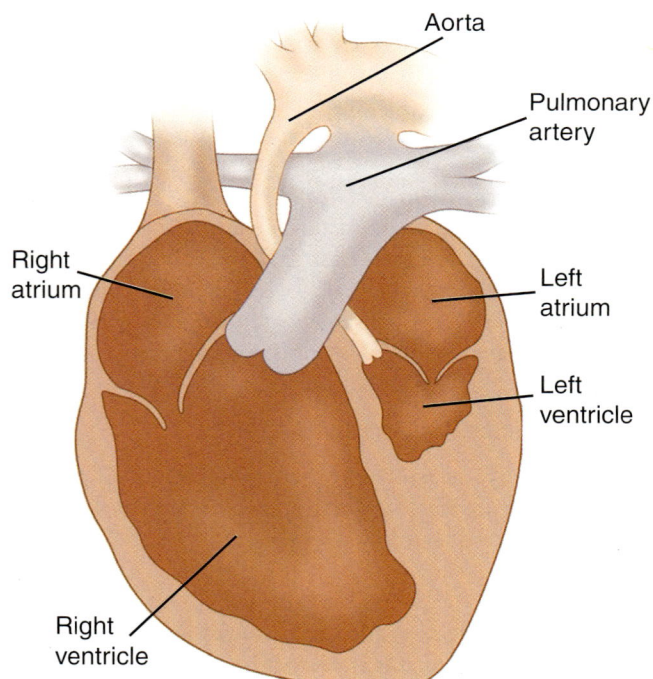

FIGURE 23. Schematic representation of hypoplastic left heart syndrome.

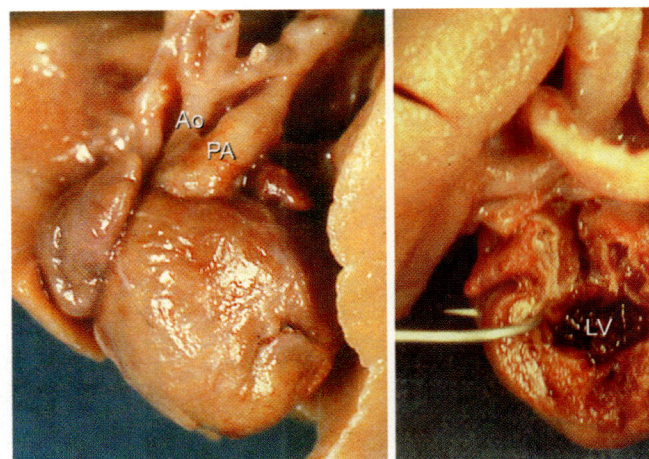

\,B

FIGURE 24. Pathologic specimen obtained from a midtrimester fetus with hypoplastic left heart. The ascending aorta (*Ao*) is small **(A)**, and the cavity of the left ventricle (*LV*) is extremely hypoplastic **(B)**. PA, pulmonary artery.

authors think a restrictive foramen ovale causes pulmonary vascular disease to develop, worsening the prognosis.[119] With aortic atresia there is retrograde flow in the aortic arch and ascending aorta. The differential diagnosis between critical aortic stenosis and severe coarctation and hypoplastic left heart syndrome may be difficult at times. Failure to demonstrate forward blood flow across the mitral or aortic valve (and particularly the demonstration of retrograde blood flow in the ascending aorta) favors the diagnosis of hypoplastic left heart syndrome (Fig. 26).

The presence of tricuspid regurgitation is not frequently seen in fetuses, but when present worsens the prognosis.

Hypoplastic left heart, like other left and right heart obstructive defects, can progress *in utero*. Some fetal hearts have appeared normal at 16 to 18 weeks' gestation and found to have a hypoplastic left heart later in gestation or at birth.[119] This can occur either when relatively minor structural abnormalities in the left heart redirect flow away from the left heart or when obstruction subsequently occurs at the foramen ovale.

Prognosis

Hypoplastic left heart syndrome is associated with a 5% intrauterine death rate.[120] Without surgical intervention,

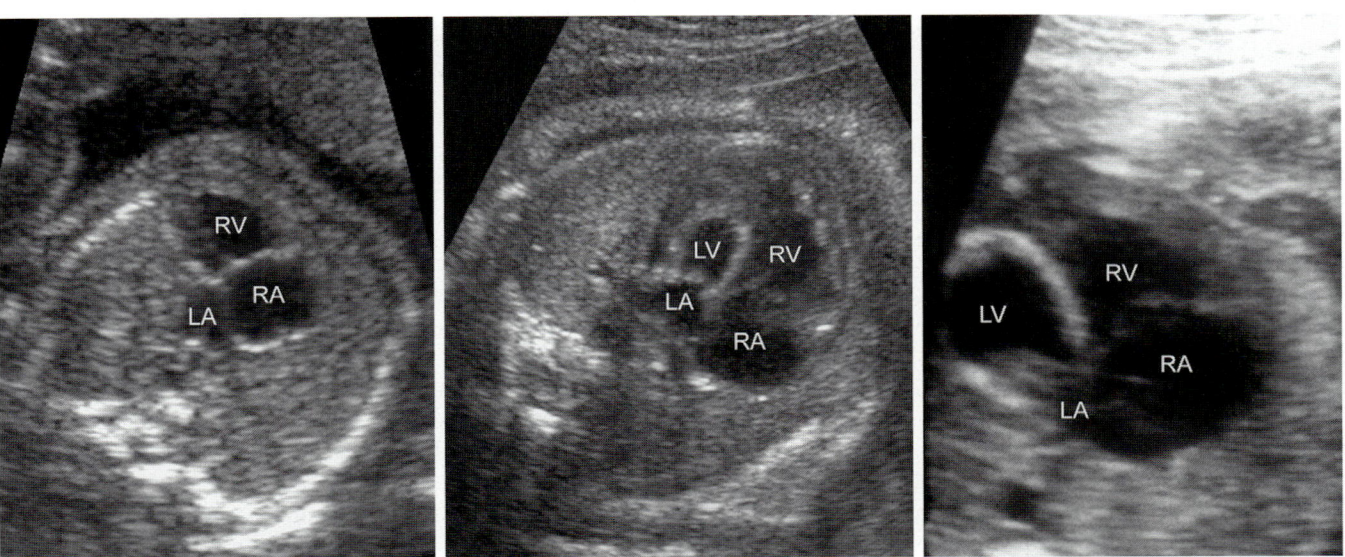

A–C

FIGURE 25. The spectrum of hypoplastic left heart syndrome in the fetus, as seen in the four-chamber view. **A:** The left ventricle is not demonstrated with ultrasound and was found to be only a virtual cavity at pathology. **B:** The left ventricle (*LV*) is small and globular with an internal echogenic lining suggesting endocardial fibroelastosis. On real-time examination, there was no obvious contractility. **C:** A slightly underdeveloped left ventricle (*LV*) is demonstrated with a bright endocardium. This fetus was diagnosed to have aortic stenosis in early gestation. The stenosis progressed *in utero*, and, at birth, univentricular repair was necessary. LA, left atrium; RA, right atrium; RV, right ventricle.

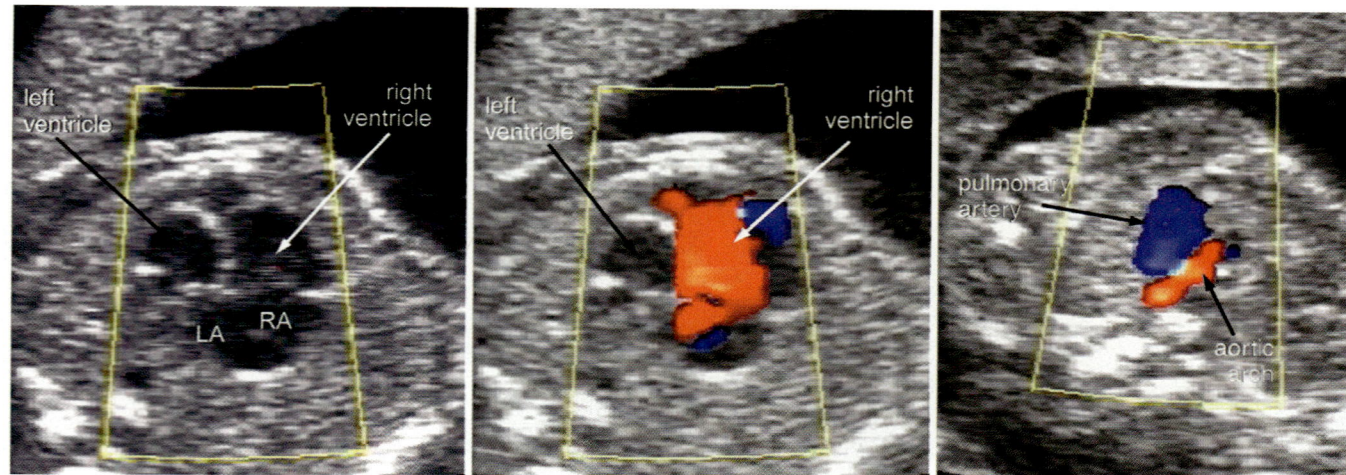

A–C

FIGURE 26. Hypoplastic left heart syndrome in the midtrimester. **A:** The four-chamber view demonstrates an underdeveloped left ventricle with bright endocardium. LA, left atrium; RA, right atrium. **B:** Color Doppler imaging fails to demonstrate blood flow across the mitral valve. **C:** A transverse section of the upper chest demonstrates retrograde blood flow into the transverse aortic arch.

95% of liveborn infants will die in the first month of life. Surgical choices are heart transplantation or the Norwood procedure followed by a least two other surgeries or a heart transplant. Heart transplant itself confers relatively low risk, but there are problems with donor availability and long-term complications.[121] Some cardiac surgeons now have survival rates of 60% to 75% for the Norwood procedure, but there are further surgeries and complications. The long-term prognosis is essentially unknown. Abnormal neurodevelopment has also been documented in survivors, and it remains uncertain whether this is the consequence of preoperative circulatory compromise or is somehow related to the surgical procedure that requires prolonged circulatory arrest.[122] It is controversial whether the prenatal diagnosis of hypoplastic left heart syndrome is beneficial to the affected infants by allowing *in utero* transfer to a tertiary care center and thus optimizing neonatal care. Some studies have demonstrated a decreased mortality rate for stage 1 surgery.[51] Four large antenatal series suggest that after the diagnosis of fetal isolated left heart syndrome the midterm survival rate is only in the range of 25% to 40%.[50,120,123,124]

Obstetric Management

A careful search for associated anomalies, including fetal karyotype, is indicated. Diagnosis of microdeletion 22q11 has also been suggested. Termination of pregnancy should be offered before viability. In continuing pregnancy, hypoplastic left syndrome is usually well tolerated by the fetus, with the exception of the rare cases associated with tricuspid regurgitation. There is no contraindication to vaginal delivery at term. A slight increase in premature delivery has been noted in one series.[120] Delivery should occur within a tertiary care center.

Mitral Valve Disease

Isolated mitral valve disease is rare. It is usually associated with other left heart disease of greater or equal hemodynamic significance. Mitral stenosis is usually produced by tethering or shortening of the mitral valve support apparatus with the most severe being a parachute mitral valve with a single papillary muscle. Other mitral valve abnormalities producing mitral stenosis are double-orifice mitral valve and supravalvular membrane. Mitral regurgitation is seen in atrioventricular canal defects but also commonly seen secondary to left ventricular dilation, ventricular dysfunction, or both.

Conotruncal Defects

Conotruncal malformations are a heterogeneous group of defects that involve two different segments of the heart: the conotruncus and the ventricles.

Conotruncal anomalies occur relatively frequently. They account for 20% to 30% of all cardiac anomalies and are the leading cause of symptomatic cyanotic heart disease in the first year of life. Prenatal diagnosis is of interest for several reasons. Given the parallel model of fetal circulation, conotruncal anomalies are well tolerated *in utero*. The clinical presentation occurs frequently hours to days after delivery and is often severe, representing a true emergency and leading to considerable morbidity and mortality. Yet, these malformations have a good prognosis when promptly treated. Two ventricles of adequate size and two great vessels are commonly present, giving the premise for biventricular surgical correction. The outcome is indeed much more favorable than with most other cardiac defects detected antenatally.

The first reports on prenatal echocardiography of conotruncal malformations date from the beginning of the 1980s.[125–128] Nevertheless, despite improvement in the technology of diagnostic ultrasound, the recognition of these anomalies remains difficult today. The four-chamber view, which many recommend be included in the standard sonographic examination of fetal anatomy, is frequently unremarkable in these cases. A specific diagnosis requires meticulous scanning and at times may represent a challenge even for experienced sonologists. Indeed, referral centers with special expertise in fetal echocardiography have reported both false-positive and false-negative diagnoses.

Conotruncal anomalies may be associated with deletion of chromosome 22q11.2 (the DiGeorge syndrome chromosome region), which may be associated with a variety of phenotypes: DiGeorge syndrome (hypocalcemia arising from parathyroid hypoplasia, thymic hypoplasia, and outflow tract defects of the heart); Shprintzen, or velocardiofacial, syndrome (abnormal facies, cardiac defects, and cleft palate); conotruncal anomaly face (or Takao syndrome); and isolated outflow tract defects of the heart, including tetralogy of Fallot, truncus arteriosus, and interrupted aortic arch. Because these syndromes clinically overlap, the general term *chromosome 22 deletion syndrome* is frequently used. The acronyms *CATCH22* (cardiac *a*bnormality/abnormal facies, *T*-cell deficit due to thymic hypoplasia, *c*left palate, and *h*ypocalcemia due to hypoparathyroidism resulting from *22*q11 deletion)[112] and *CATCH* phenotype (cardiac *a*bnormality, *T*-cell deficit, *c*lefting, and *h*ypocalcemia)[129] have also been proposed. DiGeorge syndrome is, however, etiologically heterogeneous with a small number of cases presenting defects in other chromosomes, notably 10p13.

Specific diagnosis of microdeletion 22q11 is possible by fluorescence *in situ* hybridization (FISH) analysis and should be considered when evaluating a fetus with a conotruncal anomaly, particularly tetralogy of Fallot and truncus arteriosus. It is indicated as well with the spectrum of aortic coarctation, interrupted aortic arch, and hypoplastic left heart that has already been discussed. Apart from the cardiac malformation, short stature and mild to moderate learning difficulties are common. A variety of psychiatric disorders have been described in a small proportion of adult cases, including paranoid schizophrenia and major depressive illness.[112,129]

Tetralogy of Fallot

Tetralogy of Fallot is the association of a subaortic ventricular septal defect, aortic valve overriding the defect, infundibular pulmonic stenosis, and hypertrophy of the right ventricle; hypertrophy of the right ventricle only develops after birth.

Incidence

Tetralogy of Fallot is the most common cyanotic heart defect, accounting for 7% of structural heart defects.

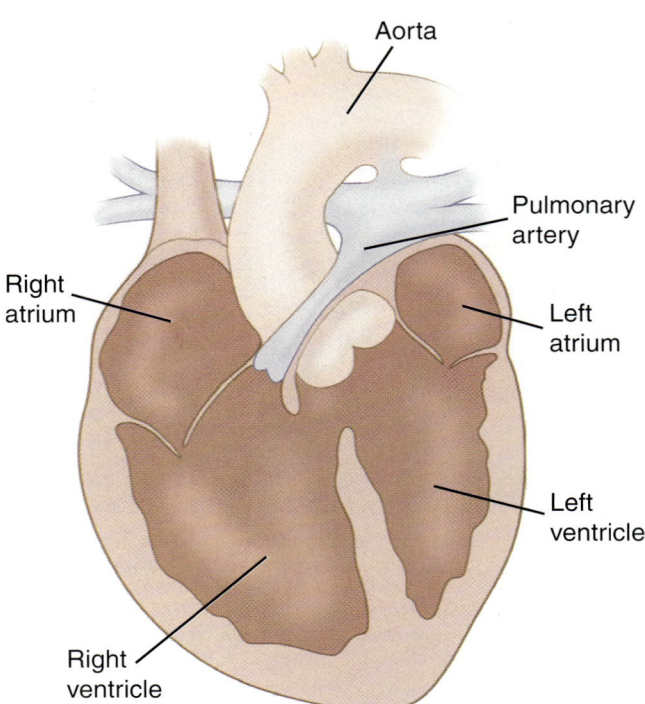

FIGURE 27. Schematic representation of tetralogy of Fallot. A large aorta overrides a ventricular septal defect, and the pulmonary outflow tract is restricted. Cardiac hypertrophy is usually not seen during fetal life.

Pathology and Hemodynamics

The essential features of this malformation are (a) malalignment ventricular septal defect with anterior displacement of the infundibular septum associated with subpulmonary narrowing and overriding aortic root and (b) demonstrable continuity between the right outflow tract and the pulmonary trunk (Fig. 27). In approximately 20% of cases this continuity is lacking, leading to atresia of the pulmonary valve, a condition commonly known as *pulmonary atresia with ventricular septal defect*. Hypertrophy of the right ventricle, one of the classic elements of the tetrad, is always absent in the fetus and only develops after birth. Stenosis of the outflow tract of the right ventricle diverts the blood flow from the pulmonary artery to the ascending aorta, which is usually enlarged. With tight pulmonic stenosis or atresia, pulmonary circulation is supplied via reverse flow in the ductus arteriosus. Tetralogy of Fallot does not cause cardiocirculatory compromise during fetal life, with the exception of cases with absent pulmonary valve, in which regurgitation from the massively dilated pulmonary artery into the right ventricle is seen.

Associated Anomalies

Pulmonary atresia, rather than pulmonary stenosis, can be present in tetralogy of Fallot. With pulmonary atresia, the infant is ductal dependent, has systemic to pulmonary artery

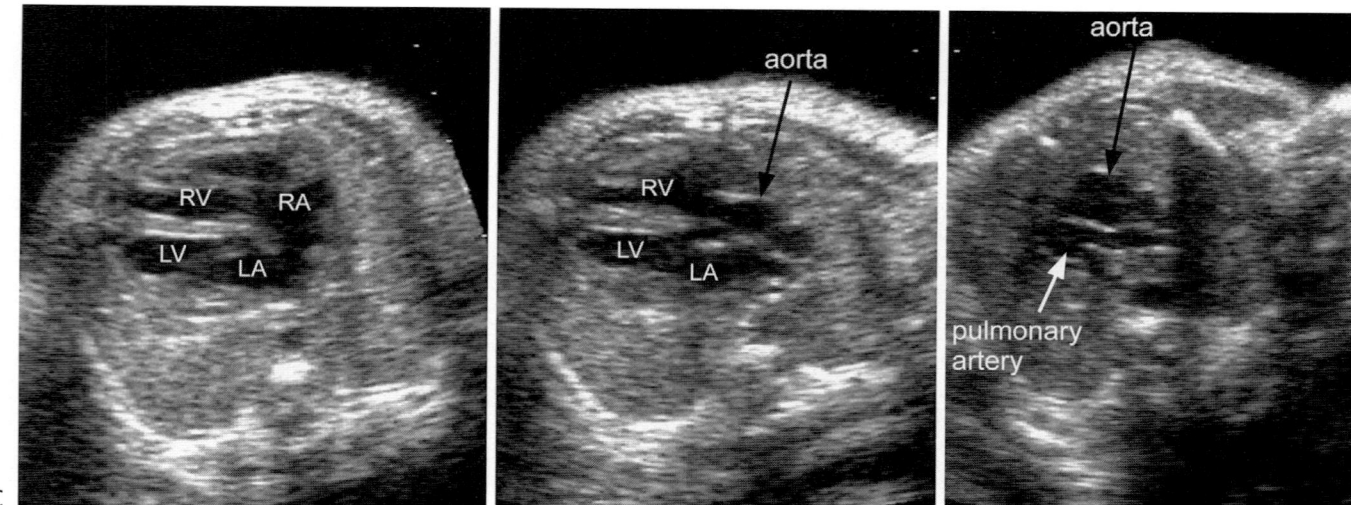

FIGURE 28. Tetralogy of Fallot in a third-trimester fetus. **A:** The four-chamber view is unremarkable except for a marked deviation in the cardiac axis, a frequent finding with this condition. **B:** A long-axis view of the left ventricle (*LV*) demonstrates a large aorta overriding the ventricular septum by approximately 50%. **C:** A short-axis view demonstrates a striking disproportion in the relative size of the great vessels; the aorta is larger than normal, and the pulmonary artery is smaller. LA, left atrium; RA, right atrium; RV, right ventricle.

collaterals, or both. An even more serious associated anomaly is absent pulmonary valve, found in 3% to 4%. Not only is the fetus at risk for fetal hydrops but postnatally there is usually tracheobronchial malacia from *in utero* compression by large pulmonary arteries.[130,131] Other associated anomalies are atrial septal defects, atrioventricular septal defect, and a right aortic arch. Tetralogy of Fallot may be associated with trisomy 18, trisomy 21, extracardiac malformations including the VATER (*v*ertebral defects, *a*nal atresia, *t*racheoesophageal fistula, *e*sophageal atresia, *r*adial and renal anomalies)/VACTERL (*v*ertebral anomalies, *a*norectal atresia, *c*ardiac anomalies, *t*racheoesophageal fistula, *r*enal anomalies, and *l*imb abnormalities) syndromes, gastrointestinal abnormalities such as omphalocele and diaphragmatic hernia, central nervous system abnormalities, and skeletal syndromes. In one prenatal series, other abnormalities, chromosomal and extracardiac, were found in 60% of fetuses with tetralogy of Fallot.[132] In a clinical study, seven of 33 infants with tetralogy of Fallot were found to have 22q11 microdeletion, but only four had other clinical features associated with 22q11 deletion syndrome.[133]

Diagnosis

Tetralogy of Fallot is frequently not detected on prenatal ultrasound if only the four-chamber view of the heart is obtained.[9] The ventricular septal defect in tetralogy of Fallot is not usually visualized in the four-chamber view but rather in the long-axis view of the left ventricular outflow tract. A useful sign that alerts the physician to the presence of this condition is an increased rotation of the cardiac axis, which tends to be significantly increased (Fig. 28). Echocardiographic diagnosis of tetralogy of Fallot relies on the demonstration of a ventricular septal defect in the outlet portion of the septum and an overriding aorta.[56,132,134] There is an inverse relationship between the size of the ascending aorta and pulmonary artery, with a disproportion that is often striking (Fig. 28). A large aortic root is indeed an important diagnostic clue.[135] Doppler studies provide valuable information. The finding of increased peak velocities in the pulmonary artery corroborates the diagnosis of tetralogy of Fallot by suggesting obstruction of blood flow in the right outflow tract. Conversely, demonstration with color and/or pulsed Doppler imaging that in the pulmonary artery there is either no forward flow or reverse flow allows a diagnosis of pulmonary atresia.[89] Diagnostic problems arise at the extremes of the spectrum of tetralogy of Fallot. In cases with minor forms of right outflow obstruction and aortic overriding, differentiation from a simple ventricular septal defect can be difficult. Indeed, in one of the largest antenatal series of tetralogy of Fallot, ventricular septal defect could be demonstrated at first in only a handful of cases and aortic overriding and pulmonary stenosis only appeared late in gestation. Conversely, in those cases in which the pulmonary artery is not imaged, a differential diagnosis between pulmonary atresia with ventricular septal defect and truncus arteriosus communis is similarly difficult.

The sonographer should also be alerted to a frequent artifact that resembles overriding of the aorta. Incorrect orientation of the transducer may demonstrate apparent septo-aortic discontinuity in a normal fetus. The mechanism of the artifact is probably related to the angle of incidence of the sound beam. Such an artifact caused the only false-positive in the authors' preliminary series, and our further experience suggests that careful visualization of the left outflow tract with

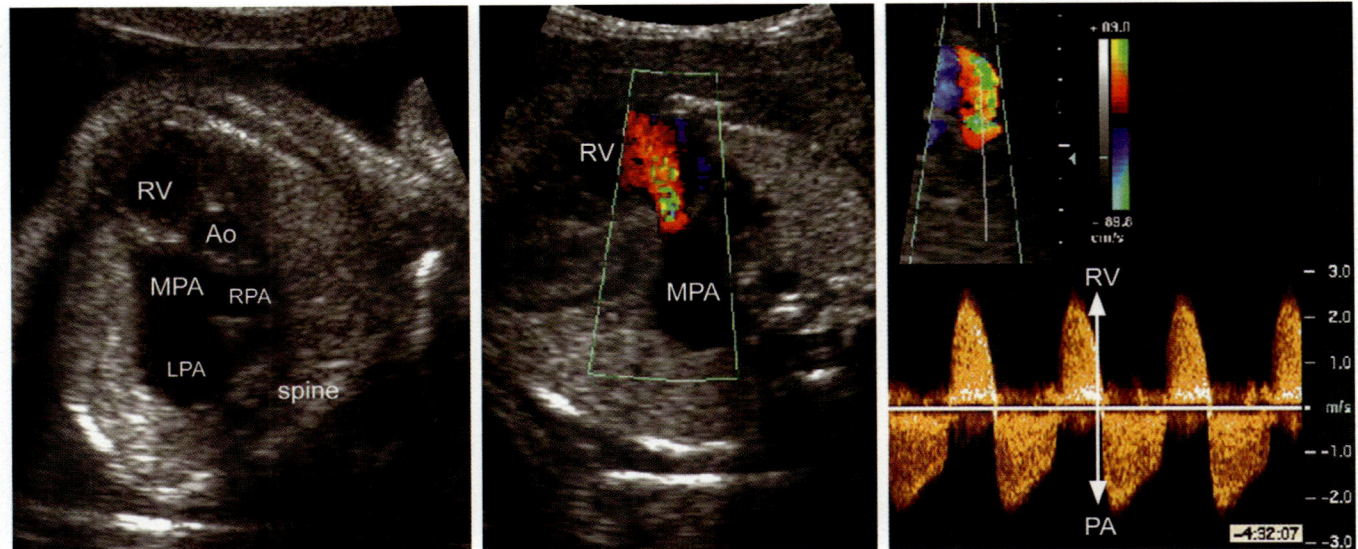

FIGURE 29. A: The most striking finding with tetralogy of Fallot and absent pulmonary valve is the massive dilatation of the pulmonary artery that can be seen on real-time imaging as a large fluid-filled space occupying most of the upper mediastinum. In these cases, color Doppler **(B)** and spectral Doppler **(C)** imaging demonstrate high-velocity holodiastolic regurgitation of blood flow from the pulmonary artery (*PA*) into the right ventricle (*RV*). Ao, aorta; LPA, left pulmonary artery; MPA, main pulmonary artery; RPA, right pulmonary artery; RV, right ventricle.

different insonation angles, as well as the use of color Doppler imaging and the research of the other elements of the tetralogy, should virtually eliminate this problem.[126]

Atrioventricular connections need to be carefully assessed to rule out the possible association with atrioventricular septal defects. Such combination is associated with an increased risk of concomitant autosomal trisomies, Down syndrome in particular, and results per se in a worse prognosis. Abnormal enlargement of the right ventricle, main pulmonary trunk and artery, suggests absence of the pulmonary valve (Fig. 29).

Evaluation of other variables, such as multiple ventricular septal defects and coronary anomalies, would be valuable for a better prediction of surgical timing and operative prognosis. Unfortunately, these findings cannot be recognized for sure by prenatal echocardiography at present.

Right ventricular hypertrophy is not evident prenatally. Pulmonary stenosis can progress *in utero* so that repeat studies throughout the rest of the pregnancy are indicated.

Prognosis

Surgical series of tetralogy of Fallot have very low operative mortality rates, approximately 2%. Total repair is the surgery of choice, and palliative shunts initially are needed only occasionally. Tetralogy of Fallot with pulmonary atresia or absent pulmonary valve usually requires placement of a right ventricle to pulmonary artery conduit. Long-term prognosis is generally good during childhood and adolescence, but long-term problems include residual defects, pulmonary insufficiency with right ventricular dysfunction, and arrhythmias. Conduits usually require replacement because they become obstructed. Surgical series report a 20-year survival rate of 98% with tetralogy of Fallot and 88% with pulmonary atresia with ventricular septal defect. Virtually all survivors are in New York Heart Association class I.[136,137] Antenatal series document a poor outcome with fetal conotruncal anomalies, but this is mainly due to the frequent association with extracardiac malformations and chromosomal aberrations.[134,138] The outcome of isolated tetralogy of Fallot diagnosed *in utero* is good, similar to postnatal studies.[50,134] An exception is represented by cases with absence of the pulmonary valve, which may develop intrauterine heart failure, polyhydramnios, hydrops, and postnatal respiratory complications.[130,131]

Obstetric Management

A search for associated anomalies including fetal karyotype and FISH study for chromosome 22q11 deletion is indicated. Isolated tetralogy of Fallot does not alter standard obstetric management. Absence of the pulmonary valve may, however, cause hydrops and polyhydramnios, either as a manifestation of heart failure or as the consequence of obstruction to fetal swallowing by the very enlarged pulmonary arteries. Anticipation of delivery when fetal maturity is achieved may be an option in these cases.

Double-Outlet Right Ventricle

Double-outlet right ventricle is a cardiac abnormality with most of the great arteries connected to the right ventricle.

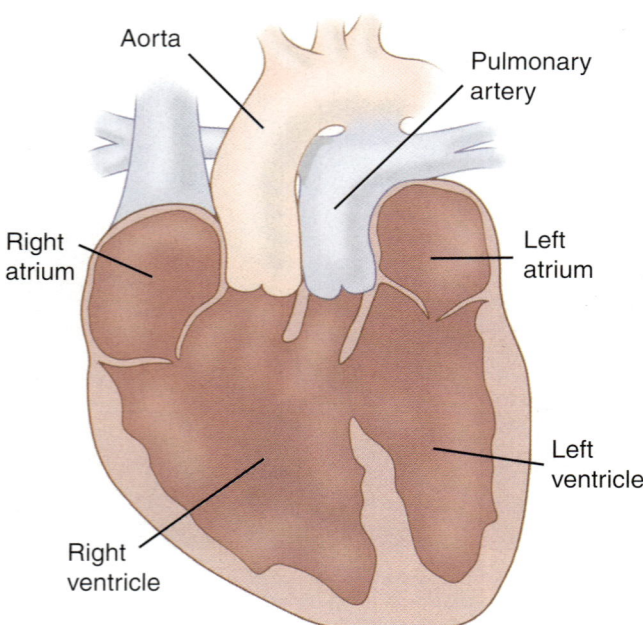

FIGURE 30. Schematic representation of double-outlet right ventricle, in this instance, illustrates a side-to-side relationship between the two great vessels, with the aorta anterior to the pulmonary artery, but this may vary.

Incidence

Double-outlet right ventricle is a rare cardiac defect accounting for 2% of structural heart defects.

Pathology and Hemodynamics

In double-outlet right ventricle, both great arteries arise from the right ventricle, but because the great artery relationship and degree of stenosis can vary, the defect can clinically mimic a ventricular septal defect, transposition of the great arteries, or tetralogy of Fallot (Fig. 30). *Taussig-Bing syndrome* refers to a frequent variety: double-outlet right ventricle with the two arteries arising side by side. The ventricular septal defect is usually large and subaortic or sub-

pulmonary but may be doubly committed or remote. Rarely the ventricular septal defect is small or absent. The hemodynamics may vary greatly depending on the anatomy of the defect, but usually this condition does not cause cardiac compromise during fetal life.

Associated Anomalies

Double-outlet right ventricle is commonly associated with other cardiac defects. It can be seen with single ventricle anatomy with both great arteries arising from a small right ventricle or outlet chamber. A hypoplastic left ventricle can also be associated with double-outlet right ventricle. Atrioventricular valve abnormalities are also frequently seen. Double-outlet right ventricle can be associated with aneuploidies (trisomy 18 in particular) and chromosome 22q11 deletion.[112,129]

Diagnosis

In double-outlet right ventricle, the four-chamber view is usually normal because the ventricular septal defect is usually anterior under the great arteries. However, deviation of the cardiac axis is frequently present. Both great arteries arise from the right ventricle, but their relationship to each other and the ventricular septal defect varies (Fig. 31). It is sometimes difficult to distinguish double-outlet right ventricle from a large ventricular septal defect, tetralogy of Fallot, and transposition of the great arteries with a large ventricular septal defect. In one study, seven of 17 fetuses with double-outlet right ventricle anatomy had incorrect prenatal assessment of the great artery relationships.[134]

Prognosis

The prognosis for double-outlet right ventricle is not clearcut. The outcome varies depending on the associated defects. Double-outlet right ventricle with pulmonary stenosis has a similar outcome to tetralogy of Fallot. The Taussig-Bing anomaly has a hospital mortality rate of approximately 14% and a 10-year survival rate of approximately 80%.[139] The prognosis is more guarded if there is a remote ventricular septal defect or hypoplasia of one of the

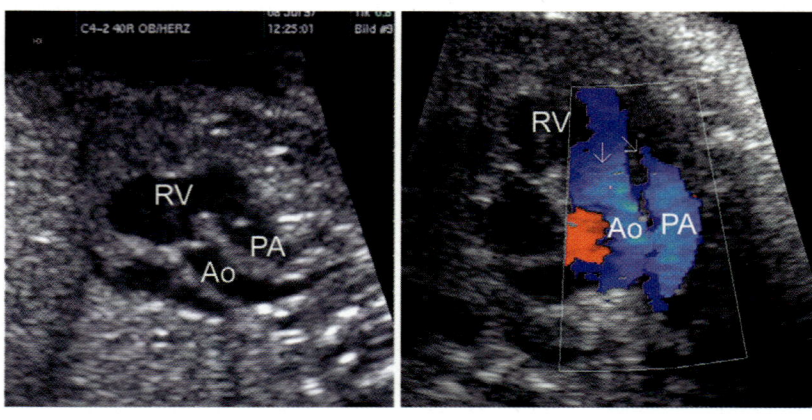

A,B

FIGURE 31. Double-outlet right ventricle. **A:** Anterior angulation from the four-chamber view demonstrates double-outlet right ventricle with malposition and parallel course of the great arteries (Taussig-Bing heart). **B:** Color Doppler imaging further demonstrates the parallel course of the great arteries both arising from the right ventricle (*arrows, RV*). Ao aorta; PA, pulmonary artery.

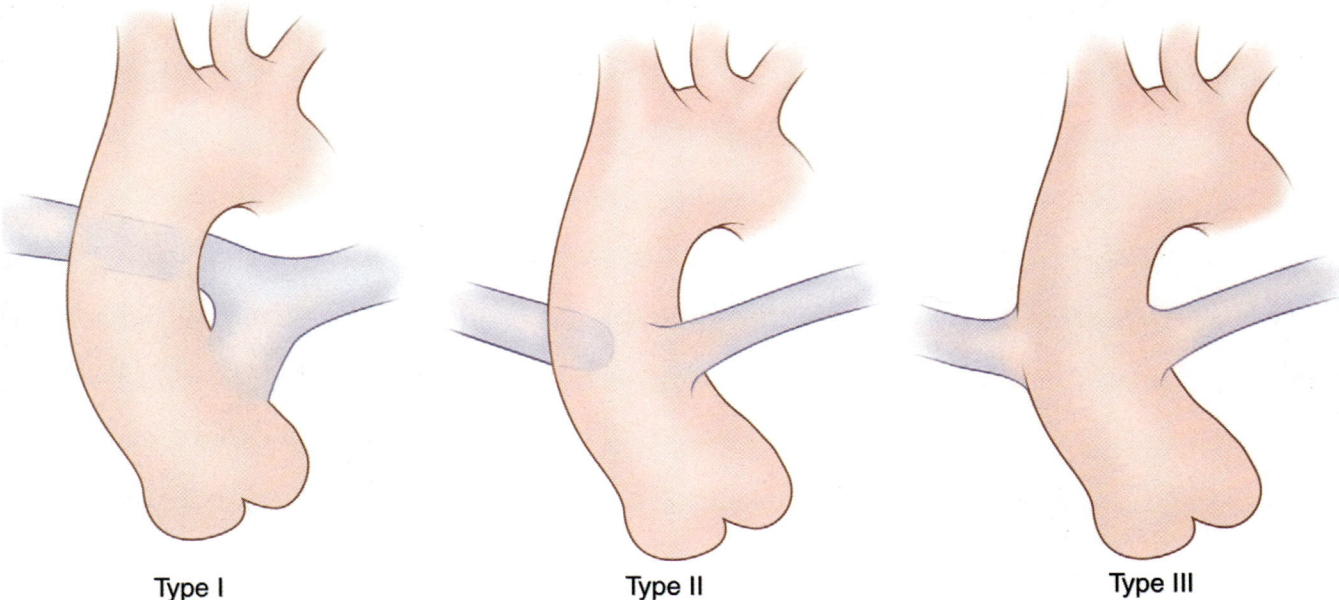

| Type I | Type II | Type III |

FIGURE 32. Schematic representation of the three main types of truncus arteriosus.

ventricles. Postoperatively, obstruction to left ventricular outflow at the ventricular septal defect and heart block can occur.

Obstetric Management

A search for associated anomalies, including fetal karyotype and FISH study for chromosome 22q11 microdeletion, is indicated. Isolated double-outlet right ventricle does not alter standard obstetric management. Serial sonography is recommended, however.

Truncus Arteriosus

In truncus arteriosus, a single arterial vessel arises from the base of the heart and gives rise to both systemic and pulmonary circulation.

Incidence

Truncus arteriosus is a rare cardiac defect accounting for 1% of structural heart defects.

Pathology and Hemodynamics

In truncus arteriosus, a large ventricular septal defect is almost always present. The pulmonary arteries arise from the truncal root either as a common trunk that bifurcates (type I), separately but close together (type II), or separately at some distance from each other (type III) (Fig. 32). The truncal valve is usually tricuspid (69%), occasionally quadricuspid (22%) or bicuspid (9%), and rarely pentacuspid or unicommissural. The truncal valve is often insufficient and rarely stenotic. Truncus arteriosus is well tolerated during

fetal life and does not cause hemodynamic compromise unless the truncal valve is insufficient or stenotic.

Associated Anomalies

Moderate or severe truncal valve regurgitation occurs in 23% of patients, interrupted aortic arch in 12%, and coronary artery abnormalities in 18%. One pulmonary artery is absent in 16%.[140] The ductus arteriosus is absent in 50% but when present remains patent in two-thirds. Other less frequently associated defects include secundum atrial septal defect, aberrant left subclavian artery, and persistent left superior vena cava. Truncus arteriosus is one of the cardiac anomalies most frequently seen with chromosome 22q11 deletion.[112,129]

Diagnosis

In truncus arteriosus, the four-chamber view is usually normal, although a deviation of the cardiac axis is frequent. The ventricular septal defect in the outlet is large and malalignment in type. The truncal root usually overrides the ventricular septum, but in 20% it arises from the right ventricle. Visualization of the pulmonary arteries is essential to distinguish this defect from tetralogy of Fallot with pulmonary atresia where the pulmonary arteries are supplied by the ductus arteriosus and/or systemic to pulmonary artery collateral vessels. In truncus type I the main pulmonary trunk arises from the posterolateral aspect of the common trunk and then bifurcates into the two pulmonary arteries (Fig. 33). In types II and III, the pulmonary arteries arise separately and usually on both sides of the common trunk (Fig. 34). At times, however, differentiation of truncus arteriosus from pulmonary

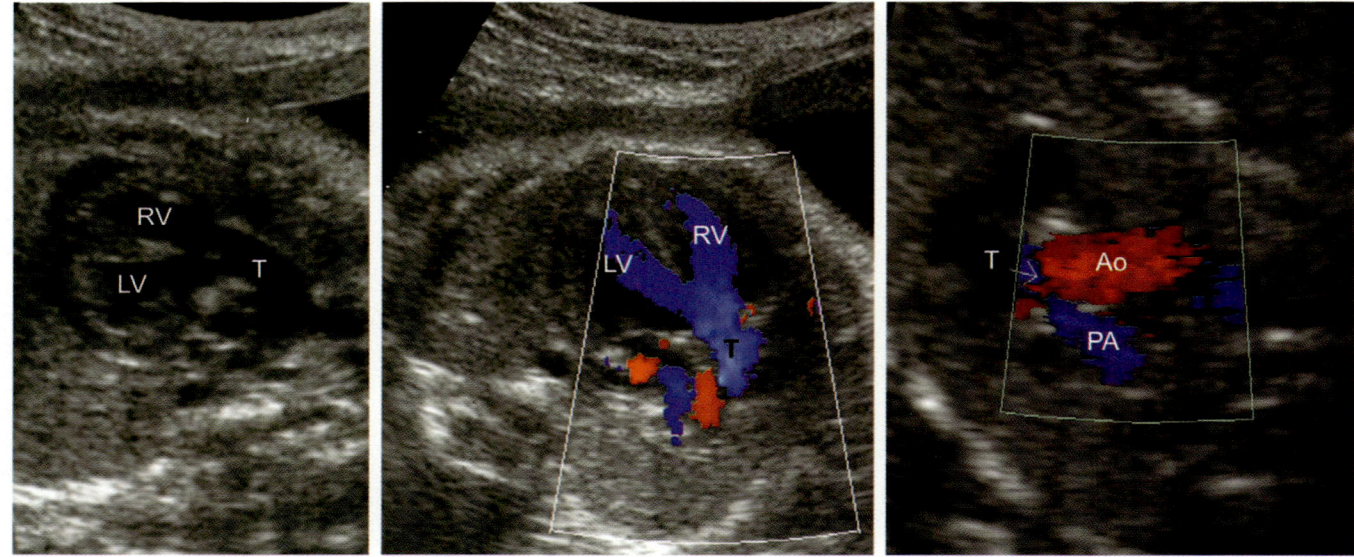

A–C

FIGURE 33. Truncus arteriosus type I. **A:** A single large vessel [common arterial trunk (*T*)] arises from the base of the heart, overriding the ventricular septum by approximately 50%. **B:** Overriding is further demonstrated by the use of color Doppler imaging. **C:** A definitive diagnosis of truncus arteriosus type I is made by demonstrating the bifurcation of the common arterial trunk into the aortic arch and main pulmonary artery. Ao, aorta; LV, left ventricle; PA, pulmonary artery; RV, right ventricle.

atresia with ventricular septal defect may be difficult.[50,134] A useful sign favoring the diagnosis of truncus arteriosus in an uncertain situation is the demonstration of abnormal truncal valve because of an abnormal number of cusps, thickening, stenosis, or insufficiency. Color Doppler imaging may aid in the identification of the pulmonary arteries. Color and spectral Doppler imaging can also help assess the degree of truncal valve dysfunction[134,138,141] (Fig. 35).

Prognosis

Unless truncal valve dysfunction is severe, the anomaly is usually well tolerated during intrauterine life. After birth, surgery consists of complete repair with closure of the ventricular septal defect, detachment of the pulmonary arteries from the truncal root, and attachment to the right ventricle

with a conduit. This is usually done within the first 3 months of life. These children require further surgeries mainly for replacement of their right ventricular to pulmonary artery conduits. In one large series, the overall 80-month survival rate was 80%.[142] The mortality can be as low as 5% to 10% when there is no significant truncal valve abnormality. The presence of truncal valve insufficiency and interrupted aortic arch is commonly regarded as a risk factor, although some series report a favorable outcome in most cases.[143] These figures are derived from pediatric tertiary care centers. Such good results may not apply entirely to cases diagnosed *in utero*, as they probably do not take into account those cases that develop congestive heart failure early in postnatal life and die before reaching a tertiary care center.[50]

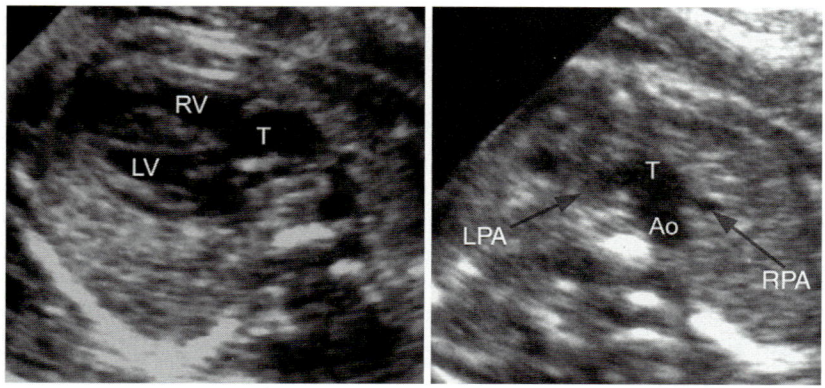

A,B

FIGURE 34. Truncus arteriosus type II. **A:** A single large vessel [common arterial trunk (*T*)] arises from the base of the heart, overriding the ventricular septum by more than 50%. **B:** The common arterial trunk gives origin to the aortic arch and left and right pulmonary arteries (*LPA* and *RPA*). Ao, aorta; LV, left ventricle; RV, right ventricle.

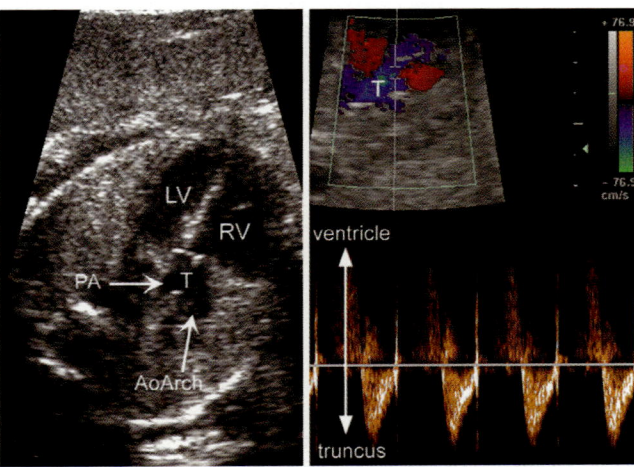

FIGURE 35. In a fetus with truncus arteriosus, spectral Doppler imaging demonstrates a holodiastolic regurgitation of the dysplastic truncus valve. AoArch, aortic arch; LV, left ventricle; PA, pulmonary artery; RV, right ventricle; T, common arterial trunk.

Obstetric Management

A search for associated anomalies, including fetal karyotype and FISH analysis for chromosome 22q11 deletion, is indicated. Isolated truncus arteriosus does not alter standard obstetric management. Stenosis or insufficiency of the truncal valve may be present, however, and cause cardiac compromise and heart failure *in utero*. Serial sonography is recommended.

Complete Transposition of the Great Arteries

In the presence of a normal atrioventricular connection, the aorta arises from the right ventricle and the pulmonary artery from the left ventricle (atrioventricular concordance, ventriculoarterial discordance).

Incidence

Complete transposition of the great arteries accounts for approximately 5% of congenital heart defects.

Pathology and Hemodynamics

The two great arteries arise side-by-side from the base of the heart. The aorta arises from the right ventricle and lies anterior and to the left of the pulmonary artery, which is connected to the left ventricle and lies posteriorly and medially (Figs. 36 and 37). As anticipated from the parallel model of fetal circulation, complete transposition of the great arteries is uneventful *in utero*. The lack of hemodynamic compromise is indirectly attested to by the frequency of a normal birth weight in these infants.

Associated Anomalies

Other than a patent ductus arteriosus and a patent foramen ovale, the most common associated defect is a ventricular septal defect seen in 40% to 45%, though varying from small to large. Left ventricular outflow tract obstruction is seen in

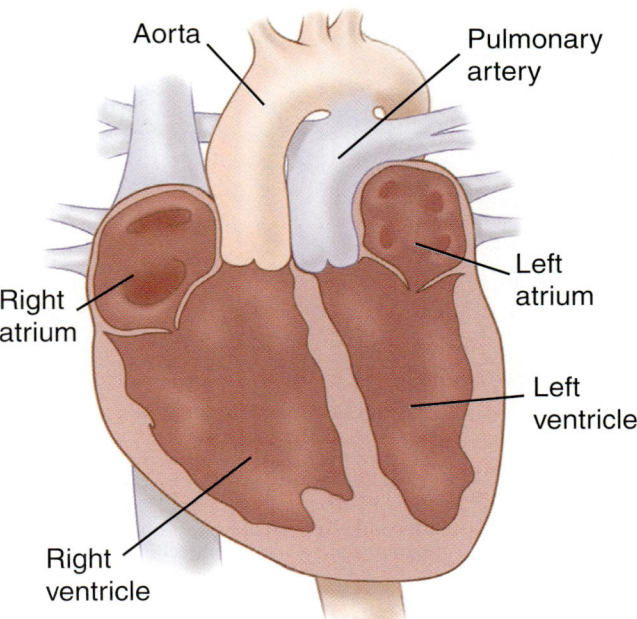

FIGURE 36. Schematic representation of complete transposition of the great arteries. (Courtesy of Philippe Jeanty, MD, Nashville, TN.)

25% and can be subpulmonary or valvular. Tricuspid and mitral valve abnormalities are each seen in 4%, and coarctation of the aorta occurs in 5%. These anomalies are often accompanied by hypoplasia of the respective ventricle. Complete transposition is rarely associated with chromosomal

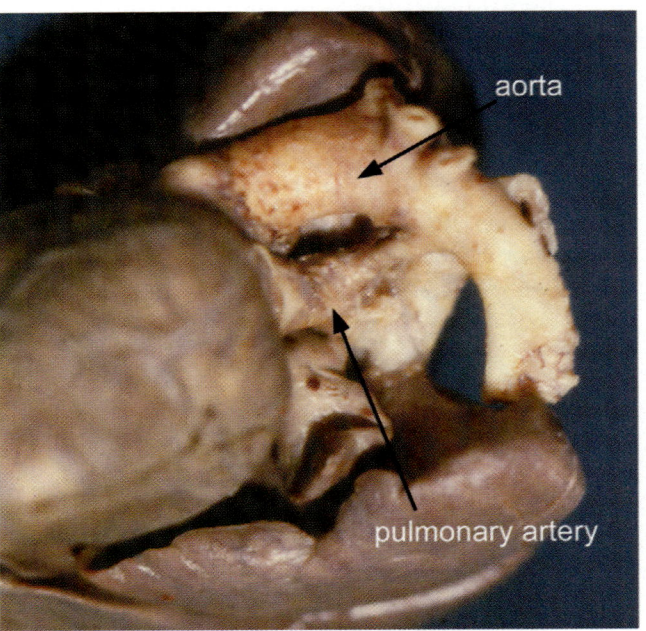

FIGURE 37. This pathologic specimen from a fetus with complete transposition of the great arteries demonstrates the parallel course of the great arteries. Note the characteristic steep posterior course of the pulmonary artery.

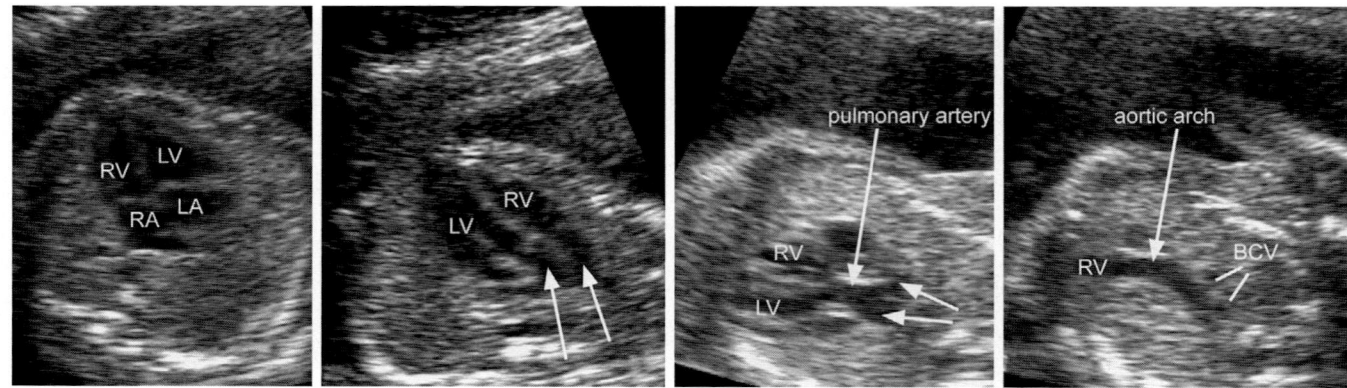

FIGURE 38. Complete transposition of the great vessels with intact ventricular septum in a 22-week-old fetus. **A:** The four-chamber view is unremarkable. **B:** The outflow view demonstrates the parallel course of the great arteries (*arrows*); the artery arising from the left ventricle (*LV*) has a steep posterior course that identifies it as the pulmonary artery. **C:** This vessel is further identified as the pulmonary artery by demonstrating its bifurcation into the two pulmonary arteries (*two shorter arrows*). **D:** The artery arising from the right ventricle (*RV*) is identified as the aorta by demonstrating that is has a long upward course and is connected to brachiocephalic vessels (*BCV*). LA, left atrium; RA, right atrium.

abnormalities or extracardiac malformations (less than 10%) especially when compared to other conotruncal defects (30% to 50%).[134,138] Transpositions are among the cardiac defects most frequently seen in infants of diabetic mothers.

Diagnosis

Complete transposition is probably one of the most difficult cardiac lesions to recognize *in utero*. The four-chamber view is usually unremarkable, and the cardiac cavities and vessels are normal in size.[134,138] One important clue to the diagnosis is the demonstration that the two great vessels do not cross but arise parallel from the base of the heart. The most useful echocardiographic view *in utero* is the equivalent of the subcostal oblique in postnatal life, demonstrating that the vessel connected to the left ventricle has a posterior course and bifurcates into the two pulmonary arteries. Conversely, the vessel connected to the right ventricle has a long upward course and gives rise to the brachiocephalic vessels (Fig. 38). Difficulties may arise in case of huge malalignment ventricular septal defect with overriding of the posterior semilunar root. This combination makes the differentiation with double-outlet right ventricle very difficult.[134]

Prognosis

Complete transposition is well tolerated *in utero*. After birth, survival depends on the amount and size of the mixing of the two otherwise independent circulations. Patients with transposition and an intact ventricular septum present shortly after birth with cyanosis and tend to deteriorate rapidly. When a large ventricular septal defect is present, cyanosis can be mild. Clinical presentation may be delayed up to 2 to 4 weeks and usually occurs with signs of congestive heart failure. When severe stenosis of the pulmonary artery is associated with a ventricular septal defect, symptoms are similar to those in patients with tetralogy of Fallot. Balloon septostomy to create mixing at the atrial level and prostaglandins to keep the ductus

arteriosus are used to stabilize infants until definitive surgery can be performed. The technique of choice is the arterial switch operation, which is performed in the first 2 weeks of life, currently with mortality rates less than 5%. An atrial switch (Mustard or Senning operation) is now infrequently performed, avoiding all the long-term consequences of the atrial baffle. The presence of a ventricular septal defect or other cardiac anomalies complicates the repair and increases the risk. In some series, hospital mortality is in the range of 3% to 5% for simple transposition, 10% with an associated ventricular septal defect, and 14% for the Taussig-Bing syndrome (double-outlet right ventricle with side-by-side arteries).[139] Cumulative survival at 10 years is approximately 90%, with more than 96% of patients unlimited in physical activity.[144] One large study suggests that prenatal diagnosis is likely to be beneficial by reducing hospital mortality as much as 15%.[52]

Obstetric Management

A search for associated anomalies, including fetal karyotyping and FISH analysis for chromosome 22q11 deletion, is indicated. Complete transposition is well tolerated *in utero*, and there is no contraindication to standard obstetric care. However, cardiologic treatment may be necessary in the very first hours of life, and delivery in a tertiary care center is therefore mandatory.

Corrected Transposition of the Great Arteries

In corrected transposition of the great arteries, a discordance in the atrioventricular connection is associated with a discordance in the ventriculoarterial connection.

Incidence

Corrected transposition of the great arteries is rare, accounting for approximately 1% of all congenital cardiac defects.

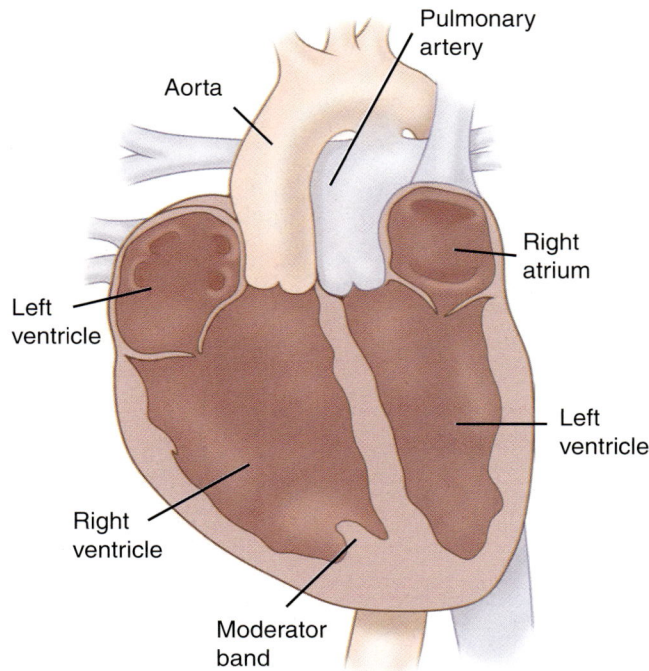

FIGURE 39. Schematic representation of corrected transposition of the great vessels. This anomaly can be considered as an inversion of the ventricles. The morphologic right ventricle, indicated by the moderator band, is interposed between the left atrium and aorta. The morphologic left ventricle is interposed between the right atrium and pulmonary artery.

Pathology and Hemodynamics

Corrected transposition of the great vessels is characterized by a double discordance at the atrioventricular and ventriculoarterial levels. The left atrium is connected to the right ventricle, which is in turn connected to the ascending aorta. Conversely, the right atrium is connected with the right ventricle, which is in turn connected to the ascending aorta (Fig. 39).

Associated Anomalies

A ventricular septal defect, usually of the perimembranous type, is present in approximately one-half of the cases. Overriding of the pulmonary artery over the ventricular septal defects and pulmonic stenosis is common. Dextrocardia and abnormal visceral situs are frequently seen. Malalignment of the atrial and ventricular septa may result in derangement of the conduction tissue and dysrhythmias, namely complete atrioventricular block. Indeed, corrected transposition is the single most common cardiac anomaly associated with complete heart block.[40] As anticipated from the parallel model of fetal circulation, complete transposition of the great arteries is uneventful *in utero*, with the exception of cases associated with complete heart block and bradycardia.

Diagnosis

Unlike complete transposition, the four-chamber view carries important diagnostic information for suspecting and even diagnosing corrected transposition. The cardiac axis is frequently deviated, dextrocardia may be present, and ventricular inversion can be recognized by the identification of anatomic markers of ventricular morphology: moderator band, papillary muscles, and insertion of the atrioventricular valves. Demonstration that the pulmonary veins are connected to an atrium that is in turn connected to a ventricle with the moderator band at the apex is an important clue. A definitive diagnosis, however, requires meticulous scanning to carefully assess all cardiac connections. As in the complete form, the great arteries arise parallel from the base of the heart without crossing[134,138] (Fig. 40). The presence of atrioventricular block increases the index of suspicion.[40]

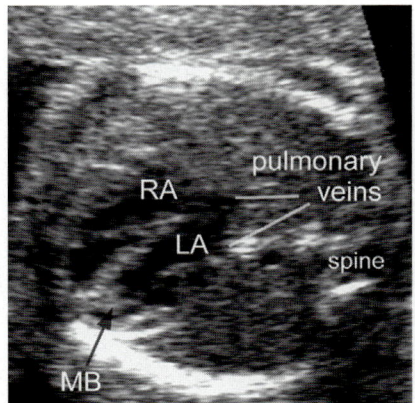
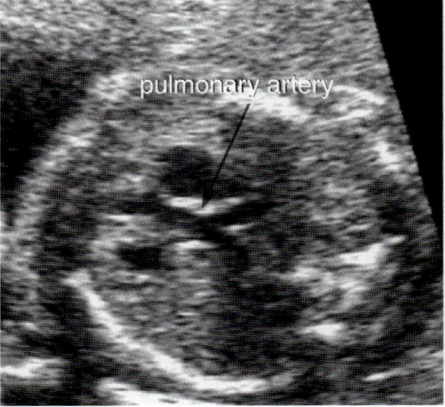
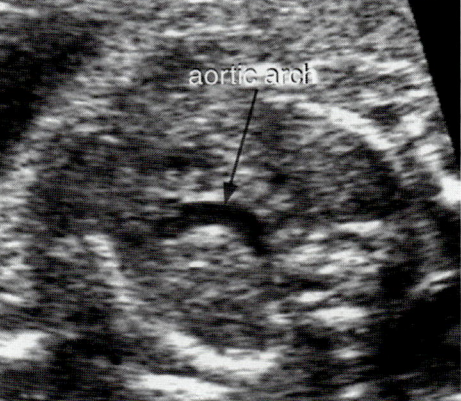

FIGURE 40. Corrected transposition of the great vessels in a 21-week-old fetus. **A:** The diagnosis can be made with the four-chamber view. The moderator band (*MB*) is in the posterior ventricle, the one connected to the left atrium (*LA*, identified by the presence of the pulmonary veins). A marked deviation of the cardiac axis is also noted. RA, right atrium. **B, C:** The diagnosis is further confirmed by demonstrating that the two vessels arise parallel from the base of the heart without crossing: the pulmonary artery from the anterior ventricle and the aorta from the posterior ventricle.

Prognosis

It is difficult to state clear-cut prognostic figures for corrected transpositions. The time and mode of clinical presentation depend on the concomitant cardiac defects (ventricular septal defects, pulmonary stenosis, bradycardia, etc.), which are extremely variable. When necessary, surgery aims at the correction of the associated defects. These patients have the anatomic right ventricle as their systemic pumping chamber, with ventricular dysfunction and heart failure being relatively common in older adults. In a large multicentric study,[145] by age 45, 67% of patients with associated lesions had chronic heart failure and 25% of patients without associated lesions had this complication. The rates of systemic ventricular dysfunction and chronic heart failure were higher with increasing age, significant associated anomalies, arrhythmias, pacemaker implantation, prior surgery of any type, and particularly with tricuspid valvuloplasty or replacement.

Obstetric Management

A search for associated anomalies, including fetal karyotyping and diagnosis of microdeletion 22q11, is indicated. Termination of pregnancy can be offered. Corrected transposition is well tolerated *in utero*, and there is no contraindication to standard obstetric care, with the exception of cases with concomitant heart block. In these cases, if severe bradycardia develops, heart failure may ensue.

Single Ventricle Defects

Tricuspid Atresia

Incidence

Tricuspid atresia is rare, accounting for less than 1% of all congenital cardiac defects.

Pathology and Hemodynamics

Tricuspid atresia occurs when the tricuspid valve does not form, leaving no communication between the right atrium and right ventricle, which is usually markedly hypoplastic. There is an obligatory atrial septal defect and usually a ventricular septal defect. In three-fourths of cases the great arteries are normally related, with 85% having pulmonary outflow obstruction at the ventricular septal defect, pulmonary valve, or both.[146] In one-fourth of cases transposition of the great arteries is present and either pulmonary or aortic outflow obstruction may be present.[147] In a minority of cases, there is no recognizable right ventricular cavity, usually in association with pulmonary atresia (Fig. 41). As with the other forms of univentricular heart, the condition is usually well tolerated during fetal life without signs of cardiac compromise.

Associated Anomalies

Besides the septal defects and outflow obstruction already discussed, coarctation of the aorta is seen in 8%, persistent

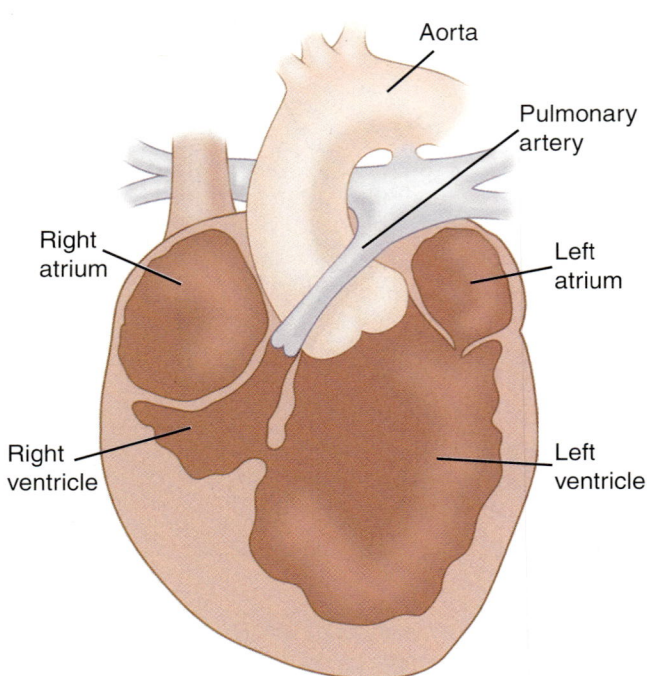

FIGURE 41. Schematic representation of tricuspid atresia. There is a rudimentary right ventricle, a ventricular septal defect, and outflow obstruction to the pulmonary artery.

left superior vena cava in 16%, and a patent ductus arteriosus and right aortic arch in 3% each. Chromosomal defects are rare. Extracardiac malformations are seen in 20%, mainly gastrointestinal and musculoskeletal.

Diagnosis

In tricuspid atresia, no tricuspid valve tissue is present and there is only one patent atrioventricular valve, the mitral valve. The atretic tricuspid valve is typically fixed, thick, and echogenic. The right ventricle is hypoplastic, but the right atrium is normal in size unless there is a restrictive atrial septal defect (rare), in which case it is enlarged. A large ventricular septal defect is well visualized. Less frequently, usually in association with pulmonary atresia, the right ventricle may not be demonstrable[146–148] (Fig. 42). The great artery anatomy should be defined as well as the location and degree of outflow obstruction. The degree of outflow obstruction can progress *in utero*.

Prognosis

Palliation in tricuspid atresia is aimed at optimizing the anatomy and physiology for eventual total cavopulmonary artery connection, the Fontan procedure. Palliation can include increasing or decreasing pulmonary blood flow or increasing aortic outflow. The Fontan procedure is often done in two stages, first a bidirectional Glenn operation

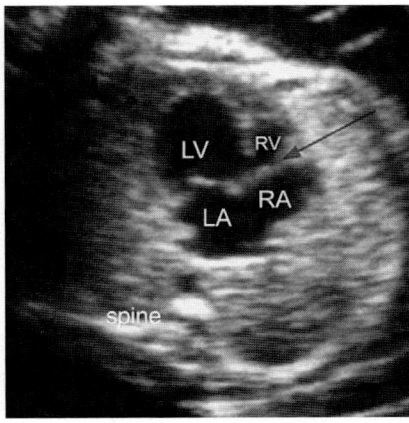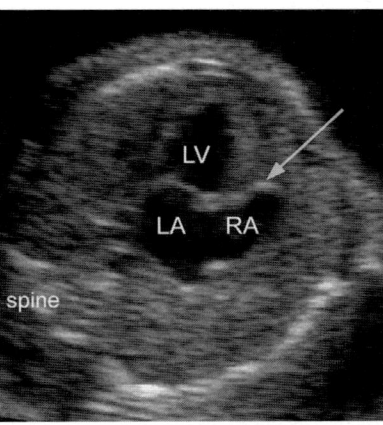

,B

FIGURE 42. Tricuspid atresia. Four-chamber views demonstrating the following. **A:** A very small right ventricle (*RV*) communicating with the dominant left ventricular (*LV*) cavity through a defect in the ventricular septum. The atretic tricuspid valve (*arrow*) is thickened and echogenic and did not move on the real-time examination. **B:** Atresia of the tricuspid valve (*arrow*) with no demonstrable right ventricular cavity. LA, left atrium; RA, right atrium.

(superior vena cava to right pulmonary artery connection) followed by a baffle between the inferior vena cava and pulmonary artery, but it can be done as a single procedure. Patents with tricuspid atresia have a better prognosis than other forms of single ventricle, and currently the mortality for the Fontan operation is 5% to 10%. However, the long-term prognosis for Fontan patients is guarded and many develop long-term sequelae from residual shunts, systemic venous hypertension, and arrhythmias and may eventually require cardiac transplantation.[90]

Single Ventricle

Single ventricle is a group of anomalies in which the entire atrioventricular junction is connected to only one chamber in the ventricular mass.

Incidence
Single ventricle is rare, accounting for less than 0.5% of all congenital cardiac anomalies.

Pathology
Single ventricle is a broad category encompassing a wide variety of complex cardiac defects but can be analyzed using the segmental approach to cardiac anatomy.[149] There are three types of atrioventricular valve anatomy: (a) double inlet, in which each atrium has a separate atrioventricular valve, both emptying into a single ventricle; (b) single inlet, in which only one atrioventricular valve is connected to only one of the atria, with the other atrium communicating with the rest of the heart only via the foramen ovale; (c) common inlet, in which only one atrioventricular valve is present, but it communicates with both atria, and a primum atrial septal defect is present. There are at least four types of single ventricle anatomy, but the most common is a left ventricular type with an anterior outlet chamber giving rise to one or, rarely, both great arteries. There is usually transposition of the great arteries, but they can be normally related. Outflow obstruction, either pulmonary or aortic, is also commonly seen.

Associated Anomalies
Other than coarctation of the aorta and the associated defects described earlier, other defects associated with single ventricle are those of the systemic and pulmonary venous systems, which are discussed in the next section, Heterotaxy Syndromes.

Diagnosis
Although the anatomy can be variable and complex, there is always one main ventricle to which all atrioventricular valves connect[149] (Fig. 43). Although the type of ventricular anatomy is important in determining outcome from the Fontan procedure, it is the great vessel anatomy and outflow obstruction that will determine newborn need for palliation. Therefore it is important to define this anatomy as well. As in less complex forms of cardiac disease, the outflow obstruction can progress *in utero* so serial fetal echocardiograms are indicated.

Prognosis
As with tricuspid atresia, palliative procedures are done so that eventually a Fontan physiology can be obtained. However, because the anatomy is more complex, the mortality before and with the Fontan procedure is greater than seen with tricuspid atresia. The mortality with the Fontan procedure varies depending on the associated defects but on average is 15%. These patients also have the guarded long-term prognosis and long-term sequelae seen in Fontan patients.[90]

Heterotaxy Syndromes

Heterotaxy syndromes (also called *cardiosplenic syndromes*) are disorders characterized by a tendency toward symmetric development of normally asymmetric organs or organ systems (see also heterotaxy section in Chapter 5).

Incidence
Heterotaxy syndromes account for 2% of all congenital cardiac defects.

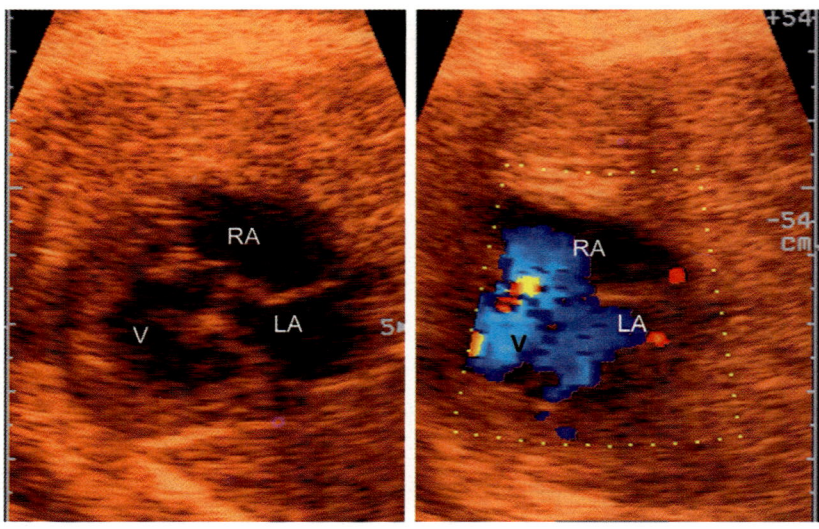

FIGURE 43. Double-inlet single ventricle. **A:** A four-chamber view demonstrates two atria with two atrioventricular valves connected with a single ventricular cavity (*V*). **B:** Color Doppler imaging further confirms the absence of the ventricular septum demonstrating the mixture of blood from the two atrioventricular valves during diastole. LA, left atrium; RA, right atrium.

Pathology and Hemodynamics

Heterotaxy syndromes are characterized by situs ambiguous, in which the chest and abdominal structures are often a mixture of bilateral, inversus, or midline structures. Isolated dextrocardia with situs inversus totalis is a different abnormality and is usually not associated with the complex heart defects seen with situs ambiguous. In heterotaxy syndromes, there can be bilateral right-sidedness, also called *asplenia syndrome*,[150–152] or bilateral left-sidedness, also called *polysplenia syndrome*.[151–153] Both syndromes usually have complex heart defects often with a single ventricle, common atrioventricular valve, and common atrium; however, there can be two ventricles and two atria although they are usually both right or both left atria.[154] There are also often abnormal venous connections, systemic venous abnormalities such as an interrupted inferior vena cava or bilateral superior vena cava, or anomalous pulmonary venous connections. In asplenia syndrome, there is no spleen; in polysplenia syndrome, there are usually several smaller spleens with overall normal splenic function. The bilateral sidedness can also be seen in the bronchi and pulmonary arteries. The abdominal organs can be inverted, absent, or malrotated.[154]

The anatomic derangement in heterotaxy is variable and so are the hemodynamics. Heart failure and hydrops are not infrequent, however, mostly as a consequence of atrioventricular valve insufficiency, bradycardia secondary to complete heart block, or both.

Associated Anomalies

Since the heterotaxy syndromes are usually complex, any cardiac abnormality can be seen. The less complex the cardiac defect, the less likely there is to be a heterotaxy syndrome. Almost all have systemic or pulmonary venous abnormalities but the actual abnormality can vary considerably. Interestingly, despite the cardiac anatomy often resembling that of an atrioventricular septal defect, Down syndrome as well as other trisomies are not associated. Heterotaxy syndromes can be associated with congenital heart block.[40,152,155] When fetal congenital heart block is detected and structural heart disease is present, it is most commonly one of the heterotaxy syndromes.[155]

Diagnosis

Heterotaxy syndromes should be suspected if a cardiac anomaly is seen in association with an abnormal disposition of the thoracic and/or abdominal organs[55,151,152,154] (Fig. 44). For example, the stomach may be contralateral to the heart or the liver ipsilateral to the heart or midline. Evaluation of the abdominal aorta and inferior vena cava is valuable in particular. In a transverse view of the upper abdomen, the descending aorta is normally to the left and close to the spine and the inferior vena cava is to the right and more anterior. Any variation can suggest a heterotaxy syndrome but particularly so if both vessels are ipsilateral and close to the spine.[55] Interruption of the inferior vena cava is characteristic of left isomerism or polysplenia. In these cases, the cava is interrupted and continues into the hemiazygos, which is ipsilateral and posterior to the aorta (Fig. 45). The azygos vein may drain to either superior vena cava. In asplenia, the aorta and cava are on the same side (either left or right) of the spine.

In general, any abnormality of the disposition of the visceral organs should always prompt a careful evaluation of fetal anatomy.

In addition, heterotaxy syndromes are suggested when complex congenital heart disease is present, usually with a single ventricle without an outlet chamber, a common atrioventricular valve, and a primum atrial septal defect or common atrium. The most common systemic venous anomalies have been mentioned. The anomalous pulmonary venous connections can be partial, total, or mixed and connect to any of the systemic veins or atria. The great

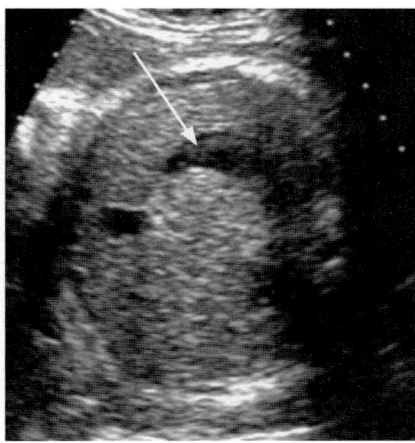 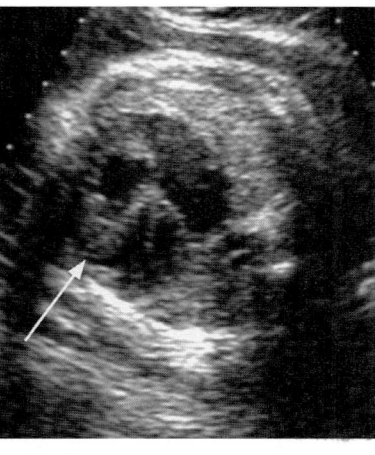

FIGURE 44. Fetal heterotaxy. A transverse cross section of the upper fetal abdomen and chest demonstrates that the stomach and cardiac apex (*arrows*) are on different sides of the abdomen. A complete atrioventricular septal defect can also be noted.

arteries can be normally related or transposed, and outflow obstruction is frequently seen. The anatomy in the heterotaxy syndromes can be so complex that, even postnatally, further imaging studies such as angiography and magnetic resonance imaging are needed to delineate the anatomy.

In one large study, the most frequent echocardiographic markers of heterotaxy syndromes included a large azygos continuation of an interrupted inferior vena cava, atrioventricular block with structural heart disease, and viscerocardiac heterotaxy. At least one of these markers was usually present.[154]

Prognosis

In the heterotaxy syndromes, fetal hydrops can develop. If either fetal hydrops or congenital heart block is present along with complex structural heart defects, the mortality *in utero* is almost 100%. If they survive to postnatal life, the

often primitive ventricles and venous anomalies complicate initial palliation, surgical survival following Fontan procedures, as well as long-term survival and complications. In some centers that routinely perform complex Fontan procedures, survival rates approach those of other single ventricles. However, the mortality rates for these patient remains higher than any other type of single ventricle anatomy.[90,149] In severe cases, cardiac transplantation is an option.[156]

Obstetric Management

A search for associated anomalies is indicated. Fetal karyotype may be offered, but the risk of aneuploidy is exceedingly low. Termination of pregnancy should be offered prior to viability. Serial sonography is recommended. In the absence of hydrops or severe bradycardia there is no contraindication to standard obstetric management.

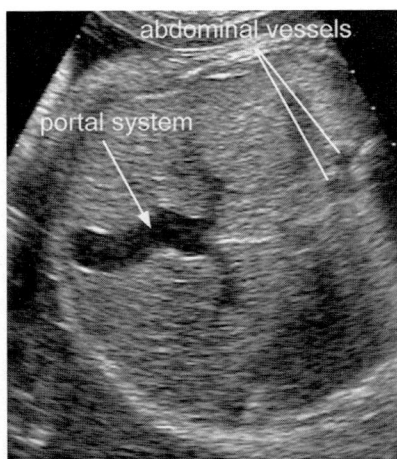 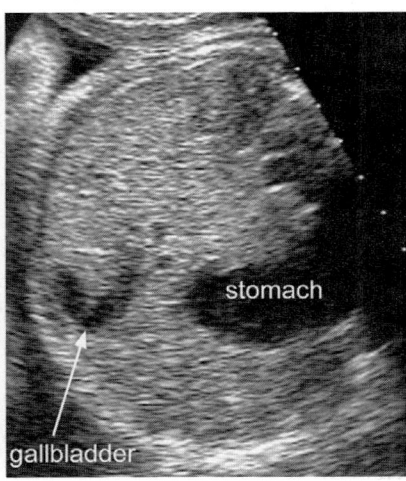 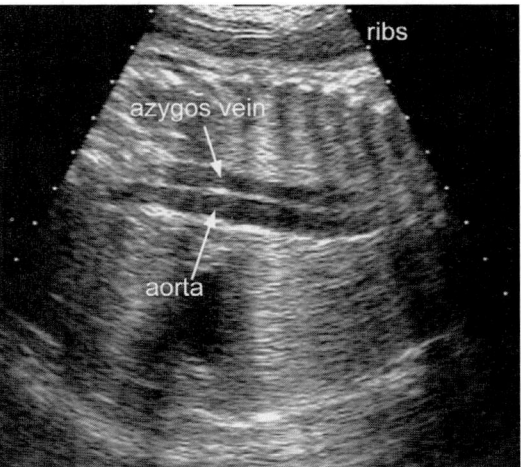

A–C

FIGURE 45. Fetal heterotaxy: left atrial isomerism with interruption of the inferior vena cava and azygos continuation. **A, B:** Transverse views of the upper abdomen demonstrate a number of findings typically associated with fetal heterotaxy. The abdominal vessels are seen on the same side of the spine; the liver circulation has an abnormal pattern, suggesting hepatic symmetry; the gallbladder is seen on the left side of the portal vein; and, in this case, the stomach is on the left side. **C:** The inferior vena cava could not be demonstrated; the great vein posterior to the abdominal aorta was identified as an enlarged azygos vein by following its course into the chest.

Other Cardiac Defects

Anomalous Pulmonary Venous Connection

Anomalous pulmonary venous connection is an abnormal connection between one or more of the pulmonary veins and the atria.

Incidence

Anomalous pulmonary venous connection accounts for approximately 1.5% of congenital cardiac defects.

Pathology and Hemodynamics

Anomalous pulmonary venous connection can involve from one to all four pulmonary veins. Instead of connecting to the left atrium, the anomalous veins connect to the right atrium or one of the systemic veins. In partial anomalous pulmonary venous connection, there is often an atrial septal defect, usually of the sinus venosus type. Partial anomalous pulmonary venous connection, is usually supradiaphragmatic, but when it is infradiaphragmatic the veins enter the inferior vena cava, forming the scimitar syndrome.[157] In total anomalous pulmonary venous connection, 20% to 25% are infradiaphragmatic, connect with the portal-hepatic veins, and are obstructed. In one-third of cases, the connection is to the innominate vein via a vertical vein. The rest are to the superior vena cava, right atrium, coronary sinus, or mixed. There is an obligatory "right to left" atrial shunt with total anomalous pulmonary venous connection. Because of the presence of the foramen ovale mixing atrial blood, abnormal connection of the pulmonary vein does not cause any compromise during fetal life.

Associated Anomalies

Besides atrial septal defects, partial and total anomalous pulmonary venous connections are associated with other major cardiac defects in one-third of cases. Other than the heterotaxy syndromes, it is also seen with a hypoplastic left ventricle, coarctations, truncus arteriosus, transposition of the great arteries, and pulmonary atresia.

Diagnosis

The antenatal diagnosis of anomalous pulmonary venous return is a challenge and very few cases have been reported thus far, most frequently associated with complex cardiac anomalies and heterotaxy in particular.[158–161] The condition is suspected when a pulmonary venous confluence or vein is seen posterior to the atria and shown to drain anomalously (Fig. 46). With total anomalous pulmonary venous connection, the right heart is usually enlarged and the left heart small. Indeed, when a significant disproportion is seen between the ventricles, the possibility of total anomalous pulmonary vein connection should be considered even if the anomaly cannot be directly demonstrated.[158] However, in the presence of an atrial septal defect or with infradiaphragmatic drainage, right heart

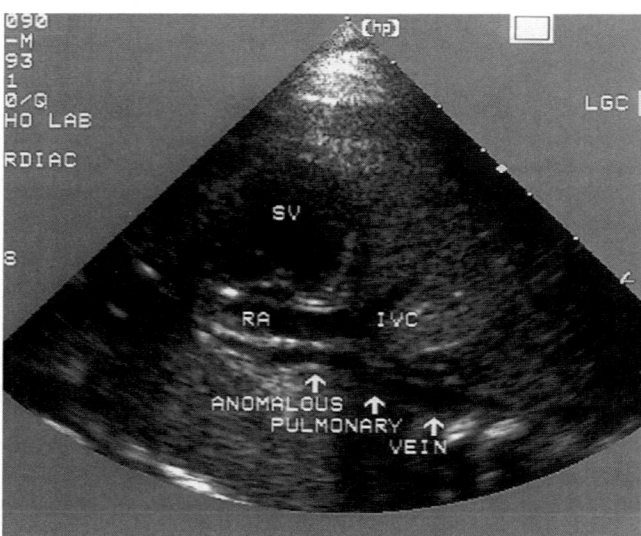

FIGURE 46. An infradiaphragmatic anomalous pulmonary vein courses below the diaphragm, posterior to the inferior vena cava (*IVC*). This fetus has a single ventricle (*SV*) and asplenia syndrome. RA, right atrium.

dilatation may not occur until late in pregnancy. Color Doppler imaging may aid in the demonstration of the normal confluence of the pulmonary veins, although it has been reported that a normal appearance does not rule out with complete certainty abnormal pulmonary venous return. Spectral Doppler imaging may be useful, as atypical waveforms in the venous circulation have been described.[159] As the diagnosis of anomalous venous drainage is difficult, particularly in the absence of other cardiac malformations, it is not surprising that both false-negatives[162] and false-positives[163] have been reported.

Prognosis

The prognosis in total anomalous pulmonary venous connection is adversely influenced by the presence of pulmonary venous obstruction, inadequate interatrial communication, the degree of pulmonary vascular disease, and the presence of other major cardiac defects. The surgical mortality is 10% to 15%. Reobstruction of the pulmonary veins is most commonly seen in those patients with a small pulmonary venous confluence or small pulmonary veins, most often seen in heterotaxy syndromes. One major factor influencing the prognosis is the rapid deterioration soon after clinical presentation. Thus, prenatal diagnosis is of great benefit. Unfortunately, this proves difficult in most cases.

Obstetric Management

A search for associated anomalies is indicated. Fetal karyotyping should be offered. The diagnosis of anomalous pulmonary venous return does not alter obstetric management. In practice this diagnosis is rarely made, but it could be suspected in cases with significant disproportion between the ventricular cavities.[158] In these cases (that are at risk for aortic coarctation as well), cardiologic evaluation is recommended soon after birth.

Ectopia Cordis

There are two types of ectopia cordis: the thoracic type, in which the heart protrudes from the chest cavity with a cephalic orientation of the cardiac apex, and the thoracoabdominal type, in which defects in the diaphragm and pericardium allow pericardial to peritoneal communication and the cardiac ventricles are displaced through the diaphragmatic defect and into the abdomen. There is usually structural heart disease as well, most commonly conotruncal defects. The prognosis is usually severe. The small thoracic cavity and the presence of structural cardiac defects make surgical repair difficult.

Cardiomyopathies and Endocardial Fibroelastosis

Cardiomyopathies are a heterogeneous group of disorders rarely seen *in utero* that can be caused by structural defects, infectious agents, metabolic disease, or myocardial ischemia or be familial. There are two major types, hypertrophic and dilated. Hypertrophic cardiomyopathy is usually familial or metabolic and characterized by ventricular hypertrophy, which can cause outflow obstruction and myofibril disarray.[94] The cause of dilated cardiomyopathy is much more variable and is characterized by dilated ventricles with decrease systolic function and cardiac failure.[164]

Endocardial fibroelastosis is characterized by thickening of the ventricular endocardium usually leading to both systolic and diastolic dysfunction. There are two types, primary and secondary. The cause is unknown in the primary type, although a few are familial. The secondary type is caused by left ventricular outflow obstruction, primarily aortic valve stenosis or atresia.

Cardiomyopathies more commonly involve the left ventricle but can involve the right ventricle particularly in infants and children. In hypertrophic cardiomyopathy the ventricular septum and walls are thickened with good, even hyperdynamic, systolic function[16,17,165] (Fig. 47). Ventricular outflow obstruction can be detected by Doppler imaging. In dilated cardiomyopathy the ventricles are enlarged with thin walls and decreased systolic function. Often, there is significant atrioventricular valve regurgitation, and cardiac output can be inadequate. Cardiac failure can be present, leading to fetal hydrops.[164]

In endocardial fibroelastosis the ventricular endocardium and papillary muscles appear bright and echogenic (Fig. 48). It usually resembles a dilated cardiomyopathy of the primary type, but the ventricles can be hypertrophied when secondary to structural cardiac defects. In all cases,

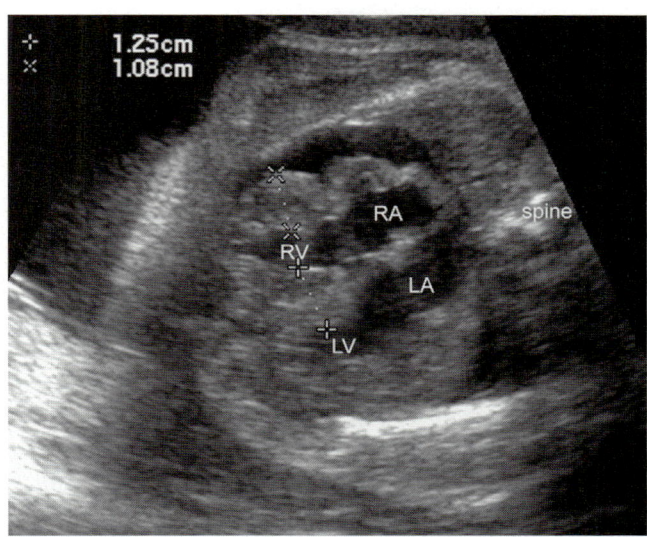

FIGURE 47. Hypertrophic cardiomyopathy in a 32-week-old fetus. Notice the thickened myocardium and the pericardial effusion. LA, left atrium; LV, left ventricle; RA, right atrium; RV, right ventricle.

ventricular systolic function is decreased and there is usually atrioventricular valve dysfunction as well.[82,166,167] When not caused by structural cardiac defects, associated cardiac defects are uncommon. The hypertrophic cardiomyopathy seen in infants of diabetic mothers is becoming uncommon with better control of the diabetes during pregnancy. Many of the cardiomyopathies seen in infants and children are found to be associated with metabolic or genetic disease. Endocardial fibroelastosis can be associated with fetal hydrops.[166,168]

The prognosis varies with the type and underlying etiology. However, cardiomyopathy detected *in utero* carries a worse prognosis and almost all cases of endocardial

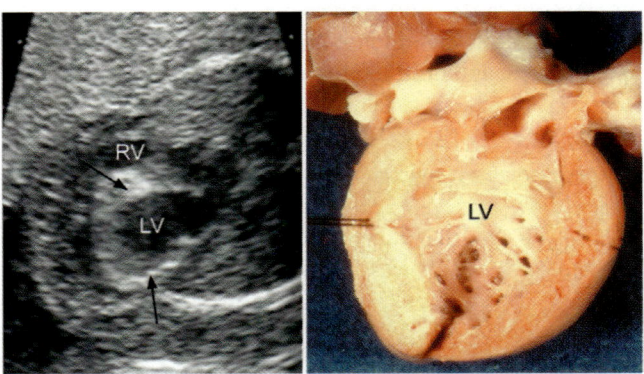

A,B

FIGURE 48. Endocardial fibroelastosis with enlargement of the left ventricle in a hydropic fetus. **A:** On ultrasound, the left ventricle (*LV*) is dilated, with markedly decreased contractility and a bright internal lining (*arrows*). **B:** The pathologic specimen reveals diffuse thickening of the endocardium of the walls and papillary muscles of the left ventricle (*LV*). RV, right ventricle.

fibroelastosis die *in utero*. Postnatally many require cardiac transplantation if medical and surgical therapy fail.

Obstructed Foramen Ovale

The foramen ovale is a normal and necessary structure in the fetal heart. During fetal life there is a predominately right to left shunt through the foramen ovale and this shunt provides the majority of flow through the left heart since pulmonary venous flow is small. Obstruction or closure of the foramen ovale can be associated with increased flow to the right heart and pulmonary arteries with increased muscularity of pulmonary arteries, supraventricular tachycardia, fetal hydrops, right ventricular failure, tricuspid regurgitation, and fetal and neonatal death.[169] Left heart abnormalities are commonly associated with an obstructed foramen ovale, but it can also be an isolated structural defect. This has led to two theories regarding the pathogenesis of the obstructed foramen ovale. The first is that it is the primary defect causing decreased flow to the left heart with development of left heart abnormalities and hypoplasia. The second is that left heart abnormalities or tachycardia is causing elevated left atrial pressure and obstruction or premature closure of the foramen ovale.[170,171] Probably both mechanisms can occur or even a combination of the two.

Obstructed foramen ovale is most commonly associated with left heart obstructive defects such as hypoplastic left heart, mitral stenosis, and aortic stenosis. It can also be associated with severe mitral valve regurgitation, supraventricular tachycardia, or fetal hydrops.

The foramen ovale is usually a flap-like structure with low velocity, phasic flow, and a predominately right to left shunt. Its diameter is usually 75% to 100% of the aortic root diameter, and peak flow velocity is less than 45 cm per second. Color Doppler imaging is usually helpful in assessing foramen ovale size and flow. Reversal of flow with a left to right shunt is associated with severe left heart abnormalities, usually hypoplastic left heart.

Obstruction or closure of the foramen ovale is an ominous finding prenatally, whether isolated or associated with other cardiac abnormalities. Prenatally, it can lead to right heart failure, hydrops, and death. When it is an isolated finding, delivery when possible is usually the best option. When associated with left heart abnormalities, their severity often predicts postnatal morbidity and mortality. Even when isolated the postnatal course can be complicated by persistent fetal circulation and right heart failure. Prenatal treatment of arrhythmias is of course indicated, and some have treated the heart failure and hydrops with digitalis and diuretics. Many of these fetuses die, and before recognition by ultrasound these cases were primarily in autopsy series of spontaneous miscarriage or fetal hydrops.

Cardiac Tumors

Cardiac tumors are rare both prenatally and postnatally. The most common cardiac tumor in children is the rhabdomyoma,[172,173] which accounts for 50% of childhood cardiac tumors and up to 90% of prenatally diagnosed cardiac tumors.[173,174] Other cardiac tumors seen in children are fibromas, teratomas (usually intrapericardial), myxomas, and hemangiomas. Myxomas have not been seen prenatally.

Rhabdomyomas are associated with tuberous sclerosis in at least 50% when diagnosed prenatally.[175] In patients with tuberous sclerosis, at least 50% have rhabdomyomas.[176] Multiple rhabdomyomas are more commonly associated with tuberous sclerosis. Tuberous sclerosis is an autosomal dominant disorder linked to chromosome 9; 50% of cases are due to a spontaneous mutation. Whereas fetal hydrops and pericardial effusions are rarely seen with rhabdomyomas, these associated findings are often seen with fibromas, teratomas, and hemangiomas. Arrhythmias, ventricular or atrial, and brady- or tachycardia can be seen in up to 15% of cases of rhabdomyomas and fibromas.[177,178] Occasionally, cardiac tumors are associated with structural heart disease. If the cardiac tumors are large or strategically located they can cause cardiac obstruction, heart failure, and, rarely, development of hypoplastic left heart.[179] Emboli occur most commonly with myxomas and have not been reported to occur prenatally.

Cardiac tumors have been seen as early as 20 weeks' gestation. One-half of rhabdomyomas are multiple and one-half single tumors. They are homogeneous and usually found originating from the ventricular septum but can originate from the ventricular free walls and the atria. They often extend into the cardiac chambers (Fig. 49). Fibromas

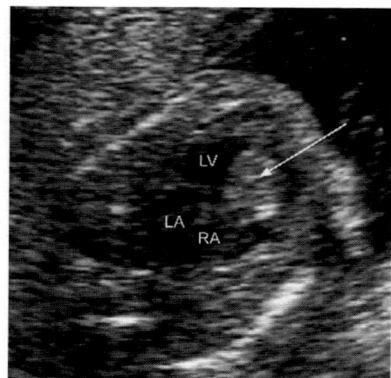
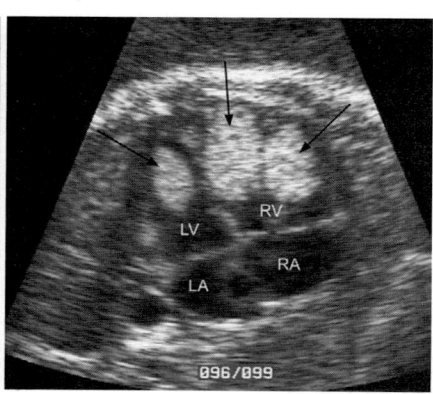

A,B

FIGURE 49. Fetal cardiac rhabdomyomas. **A:** A single echogenic mass (*arrow*) impinges on the cavity of the left ventricle (*LV*). **B:** Multiple tumors (*arrows*) involve both ventricles. LA, left atrium; RA, right atrium; RV, right ventricle.

are usually solitary and originate from the left ventricular apex. Although most are homogeneous, they can have areas of calcification and cysts. Teratomas are usually extracardiac with attachment to the aortic root or pulmonary artery. They have a mixed echogenicity due to cysts and calcifications. Hemangiomas are rare and usually located at the base of the heart adjacent to the atria. They are usually of mixed echogenicity due to cysts and calcifications.[173]

Although cardiac tumors were initially thought to lead to cardiac compromise and require surgical removal, studies have shown most are benign.[174,180] Most rhabdomyomas regress postnatally, either partially or completely.[181–183] Therefore unless rhabdomyomas cause problems prenatally or in the first 6 months of life, they are very unlikely to cause problems later. The other cardiac tumors usually do not regress, often enlarge, and usually require surgical removal. There is a small incidence of sudden death in the first 6 months of life with cardiac tumors, presumably secondary to a fatal arrhythmia.

Ventricular Echogenic Focus

The ventricular echogenic focus has been reported to occur in 0.17% to 20% of fetuses and seems more prevalent later in gestation (Fig. 50). An echogenic focus should have the echogenicity of bone, which usually distinguishes it from cardiac tumors. The echogenic focus is usually smaller than cardiac tumors and does not change in size with gestation. They are usually due to calcification of the papillary muscles or less commonly the chordal attachment of the atrioventricular valves. Most are in the left ventricle (90%), but a few are in the right ventricle or are bilateral. Usually, there is just one but occasionally two. Initially there was concern

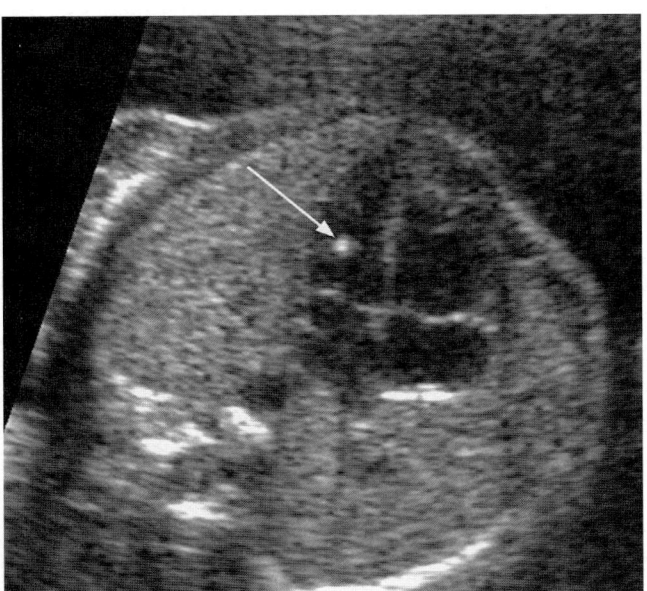

FIGURE 50. Echogenic focus (*arrow*) of the left ventricle.

that these echogenic foci were associated with structural heart disease or myocardial ischemia as seen in children and adults but no association has been found prenatally. More recently, the echogenic focus has been associated with Down syndrome. This issue is considered elsewhere (see Chapter 21).

Premature Constriction of the Ductus Arteriosus

The ductus arteriosus is a normal and necessary structure in the fetal heart providing one of two shunts that make fetal cardiac physiology possible. Although its patency postnatally can cause hemodynamic compromise, especially in premature infants, its constriction prenatally can lead to cardiac compromise and possibly persistent pulmonary hypertension postnatally. Spontaneous ductal constriction is rare. Ductal constriction is more likely to be seen with maternal administration of prostaglandin syntheses inhibitors, usually indomethacin. Indomethacin is used as a second-line tocolytic agent but has also been used to decrease polyhydramnios. The prenatal effects of indomethacin have been documented by several authors,[184] but the consequences of ductal constriction in the fetus and the newborn are controversial.

Diagnosis

It is important to document the ductal arch and patency of the ductus arteriosus in all fetuses. With ductal constriction the ductus may be very small and only detected using color Doppler or continuous wave Doppler imaging.[185] Normal ductal flow velocities are less than 150 cm per second in systole and less than 40 cm per second in diastole so that flow velocities higher than these may indicate ductal constriction.[186] Systolic flow velocities greater than 150 cm per second can be seen in the last 4 to 6 weeks of pregnancy or with conditions that increase cardiac output, such as treatment with terbutaline, but an increased diastolic flow velocity is pathognomonic for ductal constriction (Fig. 51). With ductal constriction, right ventricular enlargement and hypertrophy, right atrial enlargement, and tricuspid regurgitation can develop.[187] Pericardial and pleural effusions and pulmonary insufficiency have also been reported.[188] All these findings suggest an increase in stress on the right ventricle and even right heart failure.

Prognosis

The incidence of ductal constriction with indomethacin depends on gestational age: It is rare under 24 weeks but occurs in more than 50% of fetuses treated with indomethacin between 28 and 34 weeks.[189,190] Length of treatment can also be significant in that the ductal constriction seen with indomethacin appears to be reversible if the constriction occurs for 48 to 72 hours but may not be reversible if constriction is present longer.[191–193] Therefore the use of indomethacin beyond 28 weeks gestation should

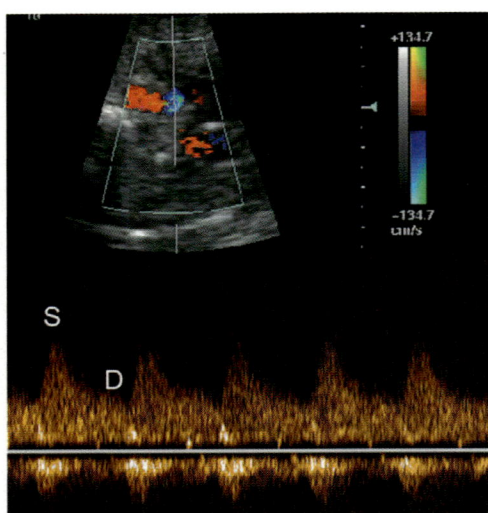

FIGURE 51. Fetus with moderate ductal constriction. Continuous wave Doppler imaging reveals flow velocities of 160 cm per second in systole (*S*) and 60 to 80 cm per second in diastole (*D*).

be very limited. Initial assessment for ductal constriction can be done between 48 to 72 hours after starting indomethacin, thereby allowing some tocolysis but avoiding irreversible ductal constriction.[194–196] To avoid ductal constriction in ductal dependent structural heart disease, normal cardiac anatomy should be determined before starting indomethacin.[197,198] The increase in muscularization of the pulmonary arteries and the increase in pulmonary artery pressure and resistance demonstrated in fetal lambs has not been demonstrated convincingly in newborns by persistence of pulmonary hypertension.[197–201] Prenatal exposure to indomethacin does not appear to affect spontaneous or indomethacin-induced closure of the ductus arteriosus postnatally, but an increased incidence of ductal reopening with prenatal exposure to indomethacin has been reported.[202] Ductal closure is usually associated with fetal demise and reported in autopsy series.

Absence of the Ductus Venosus

Incidence
Absence of the ductus venosus is rare.

Pathology
Absence of the ductus venosus is most commonly due to an abnormal connection of the intraabdominal umbilical vein. In a review of the antenatal literature,[203] three types were identified: (a) umbilical vein bypassing the liver and connecting directly to the right atrium (50% of cases); (b) umbilical vein bypassing the liver and connecting to the inferior vena cava by one iliac or renal vein (30% of cases); (c) umbilical vein connecting to the portal circulation without giving rise to the ductus venosus (20% of cases).

Associated Anomalies
Fetal malformations and/or chromosomal aberrations (trisomy 21, trisomy 18, Turner 45,X) and fetal hydrops were present in 25% and 33% of cases, respectively.[203]

Diagnosis
Absence of the ductus venosus is usually discovered due to an abnormal course and connection of the umbilical vein.[203] With connection to the inferior vena cava, iliac vein, or renal vein, the umbilical vein courses inferiorly. Furthermore, the inferior vena cava is always significantly enlarged since midgestation. With connection to the right atrium, a long aberrant vessel is seen coursing between the liver and the right abdominal wall and crossing the diaphragm. In these cases, cardiomegaly and cardiac hypertrophy are frequent. Polyhydramnios, hydrops, or both frequently develop. Eventually, in a handful of cases, the condition was suspected due to failure to visualize the ductus venosus with color Doppler imaging, with the umbilical vein normally connecting to the portal vein. In these cases, although there may be some distension of the hepatic veins, usually there are no signs of cardiac compromise (Fig. 52).

Prognosis
The available data do indicate a high proportion of associated malformations, including chromosomal aberrations, and a marked tendency towards the development of *in utero* heart failure.[203] The mechanism is unknown. Signs of fetal cardiac compromise are frequent with the umbilical circulation connecting directly to the heart or inferior vena cava. Conversely, they are rare in cases with direct connection of the umbilical vein to the portal circulation. It has been speculated that the umbilical vein bypassing the liver may result in increased cardiac preload, increased cardiac work, and progressive cardiac decompensation. In these cases, cardiomegaly and polyhydramnios may appear as early as midgestation and usually become very severe by the onset of the third trimester. Absence of the ductus venosus may also lead to significant long-term complications. Approximately one-half of the infants are found to have absence of the portal veins. Experience with this anomaly is limited, but the existing reports document a long list of severe complications including congestive heart failure, pulmonary edema, abnormal liver development with focal nodular hyperplasia and hepatic tumors, and portosystemic encephalopathy.[204,205]

Obstetric Management
A search for associated malformations and fetal karyotyping are indicated. If signs of cardiac compromise (cardiomegaly, tricuspid insufficiency, polyhydramnios) develop, anticipation of delivery should be considered.

Fetal Arrhythmia

Fetal arrhythmias have been observed in up to 2% of pregnancies.[206–210] Fortunately, 90% are benign and only

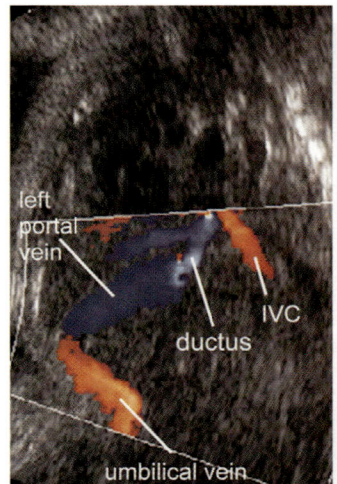 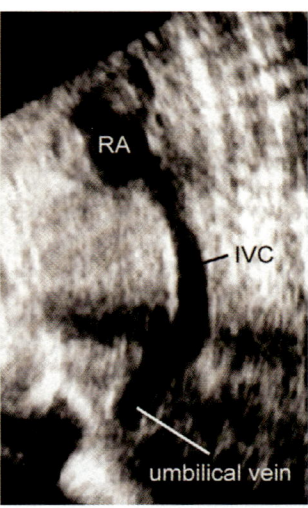 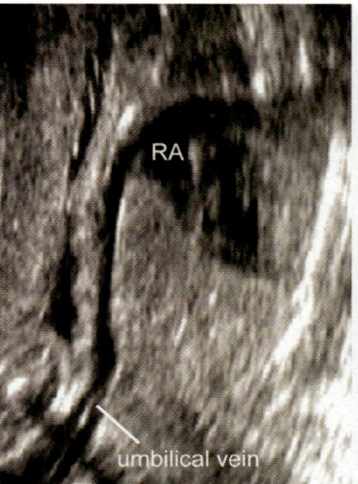 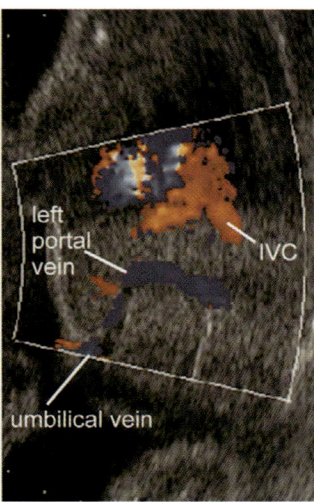

-D

FIGURE 52. **A:** Color Doppler imaging of a normal fetus demonstrates the ductus venosus connecting the left portal vein to the subdiaphragmatic venous vestibulum. **B:** Absence of the ductus venosus with connection between the umbilical vein and a dilated inferior vena cava (*IVC*) through the right iliac vein. **C:** Absence of the ductus venosus with a direct connection between the umbilical vein and the right atrium (*RA*) through a long aberrant vessel coursing between the liver and the right abdominal wall. **D:** Absence of the ductus venosus with a connection between the umbilical vein and the portal vein; despite meticulous scanning, it was impossible to demonstrate any connection between the portal system and the IVC. RA, right atrium. (Reproduced with permission from Contratti G, Banzi C, Ghi T, Perolo A, Pilu G, Visentin A. Absence of the ductus venosus: report of 10 new cases and review of the literature. *Ultrasound Obstet Gynecol* 2001;18:605–609.)

10% are significant, causing fetal morbidity and mortality.[207] Fetal arrhythmias can be evaluated by M-mode and/or Doppler ultrasound.[207,208] The effects of fetal arrhythmias should also be evaluated and include the presence of fetal hydrops, ventricular dysfunction, and atrioventricular valve insufficiency. The presence of structural heart defects can also be determined by cardiac ultrasound. Fetal arrhythmias can be categorized into three groups: those with an irregular rhythm, those with a tachyarrhythmia, and those with a bradyarrhythmia. The fetal heart rate typically demonstrates rapid variations. Tachycardia from possible cardiologic origin is generally considered to be a rate of greater than 200 beats per minute, whereas bradycardia is a rate of less than 100 beats per minute.[208]

Irregular Rhythm

An irregular rhythm is usually caused by premature atrial contractions (either conducted or nonconducted), sinus pauses, or premature ventricular beats. The rhythm is usually irregularly irregular but can be regularly irregular. Two studies have implicated caffeine as a cause of fetal ectopy.[210–212] Maternal antihypertensives, hydrazine and nifedipine, have also been associated with fetal ectopy, which resolves after discontinuing the drug.[212] The common consensus is that there is an increased chance for fetuses with irregular heart rhythm to develop supraventric-

ular tachycardia, but the risk is probably much less than the 1% originally suggested.

Associated Anomalies

Associated anomalies are rare. The only one consistently reported is an atrial septal aneurysm.[63,64,121,122] The incidence of structural cardiac defects is not increased compared to the general population.

Diagnosis

Fetal arrhythmias can be evaluated by both M-mode and Doppler ultrasound. With M-mode ultrasound, the cursor is placed through the atrial wall or foramen ovale to demonstrate atrial activity and rate and either the ventricular/septal wall or aortic valve to demonstrate ventricular activity and rate.[208,213] With Doppler ultrasound there are several methods to obtain simultaneous atrial and ventricular activity. The most commonly used is placing the sample volume between the inflow and outflow of the left ventricle.[214] Other methods include using the descending aorta and inferior vena cava[215,216] or pulmonary artery and vein, since these two sets of structures lie close to each other and flow can be obtained in both simultaneously. Repeated premature contractions can give rise to complex rhythm patterns. Premature atrial contractions may be either conducted to the ventricles or blocked, depending on the time of the cardiac cycle in which they occur, thus resulting in either an increased or decreased ventricular rate. Blocked

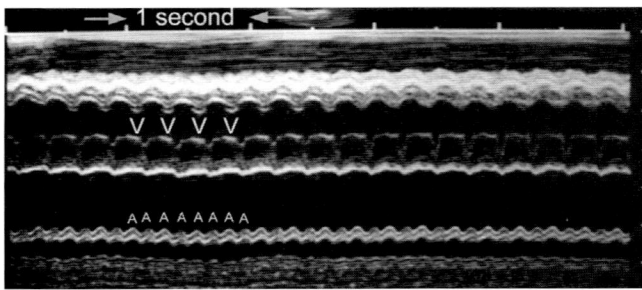

FIGURE 58. M-mode sonography demonstrates an atrial (*A*) rate of approximately 480 beats per minute and a ventricular (*V*) rate of approximately 240 beats per minute. This is atrial flutter.

tachycardias it is also important to assess ventricular function and the presence and degree of atrioventricular valve insufficiency since the presence of these abnormalities can affect treatment and outcome.

Treatment

Close to term, delivery of the infant is often the easiest and most effective treatment. If the fetal heart rate is less than 200 beats per minute or if there is no fetal hydrops, close observation without pharmacologic treatment may be considered. However, most fetuses with tachycardia require treatment. The most commonly used drugs are listed in Table 7. For supraventricular tachycardia and atrial flutter, the most commonly used drug is digoxin, especially in the nonhydropic fetus, where fetal levels are often 80% of maternal levels.[233–235] Fetal levels are considerably lower in the hydropic fetus, and other drugs are often needed in addition or used as first-line treatment. Flecainide by itself

or in combination with digoxin is the second most widely used drug.[236–238] The proarrhythmic effects seen in adults have not been seen in children or the fetus though there has been one report of fetal demise on flecainide.[235,239] There is also a potential risk to the mother so that electrocardiographic monitoring (telemetry) of the mother is probably appropriate. Amiodarone has also been used but may take longer to convert the tachycardia. There are several side effects, fortunately most with long-term use, but neonatal hypothyroidism has been reported.[240–246] Sotalol has been used with few side effects.[244,247,248]

Intraumbilical vein administration of antiarrhythmic drugs has been used in terminating tachycardia. Adenosine[249–252] and digoxin[253,254] have been used most commonly, but amiodarone has also been given via the umbilical vein.[241,242]

Procainamide is occasionally used, but its long-term use is complicated by accumulation of its active metabolite in the fetus.[218,255,256] Verapamil is no longer recommended because of its effects on myocardial function in infants and the fetus.[257] Propranolol is no longer used because much more effective drugs are now available. Both verapamil and propranolol also have low fetal levels (20% and 30% to 40%, respectively) when compared to maternal levels.[233–235]

In fetuses with atrial flutter, decreasing the ventricular rate without converting the atrial flutter is inadequate. Fetal hydrops and ventricular dysfunction will not resolve unless sinus rhythm is restored.

Cryoablation of the atrioventricular node for malignant supraventricular tachycardia has been successfully attempted in fetal lambs.[258] There have also been attempts to use vagal maneuvers to convert fetal tachycardia.[259]

TABLE 7. MEDICATIONS FOR FETAL ARRHYTHMIA

Drug	Loading dose	Maintenance dose	Plasma therapeutic level	Plasma toxic level	Maternal side effects	Other
Digoxin	0.5 mg + 0.25 mg q6–8h to 1.25–1.50 mg i.v.; or 1.5–2.0 mg in 1st 24 hr i.v. or p.o.	0.5–0.7 mg/d p.o.	1–2 ng/mL	>2.5 ng/mL	Bradycardia, atrioventricular block	Levels may increase with the addition of flecainide or amiodarone
Flecainide	100–150 mg b.i.d.	0.2–1.0 µg/mL p.o.	>1 µg/mL	—	Proarrhythmia, increased PR or QRS intervals, blurred vision, dizziness	Levels may increase with addition of amiodarone
Amiodarone	1,200 mg/d i.v. × 5; 2.5 mg/kg UV	600–800 mg/d p.o.	—	—	Hypothyroidism, increased liver function tests, pulmonary fibrosis, anorexia, nausea, vomiting, dizziness, paresthesias	Fetal hypothyroidism
Procainamide	15 mg/kg i.v., up to 1 g	0.5–1.0 g q4h p.o.	3–6 µg/mL	>8 µg/mL	Lupus-like syndrome, thrombocytopenia, gastrointestinal complaints, confusion	Active metabolite, N-acetyl procainamide, can accumulate in fetus
Adenosine	0.2 mg/kg UV	—	—	—	Bradycardia, asystole	—

UV, via umbilical vein.

Ventricular tachycardia usually does not need treatment since rates are usually less than 200 beats per minute. If fetal hydrops develops, type I antiarrhythmics (e.g., procainamide) or amiodarone have been used.[206]

A common problem is how and when to deliver a fetus whose tachycardia has been successfully controlled with medication. As antiarrhythmic medications do have potential side effects both for the fetus and the mother, a prudent approach would be to deliver the fetus as soon as adequate maturity has been achieved. There is, however, no contraindication to a vaginal delivery.

Prognosis

In 85% to 90% of supraventricular tachycardias, there will be *in utero* control of the tachycardia. With the current drugs available, even 80% of those with fetal hydrops will be controlled. *In utero* death is rare and exclusively in those with associated fetal hydrops or structural cardiac defects. In atrial flutter, only two-thirds are controlled *in utero* with medications and mortality can be as high as one-third. Those who die *in utero* have associated fetal hydrops, structural cardiac defects, or both. Postnatally 50% of tachycardias persist or recur, more commonly with atrial flutter (64%) than with supraventricular tachycardia (44%). Many that are present neonatally do not recur after 1 year of life.[206,238] One important problem that has emerged recently is that although treatment may restore a normal heart rate and function, fetuses—particularly if hydropic—may have already developed ischemic cerebral complications,[251] and these cerebral lesions may be difficult if not impossible to ascertain prenatally.

Bradycardia

Sinus bradycardia is often secondary to extracardiac causes such as cord or head compression, hypoxia, or maternal drugs. It has been associated in a few cases with heterotaxy syndromes. If the cardiac structure is normal and the heart rate is 80 to 100 beats per minute, the bradycardia is usually well tolerated.

Blocked or nonconducted premature atrial contractions usually are not frequent enough to cause significant bradycardia. Occasionally they are frequent enough, such as in atrial bigeminy, to produce an effective heart rate of less than 80 beats per minute, mimicking heart block.

In second-degree atrioventricular block, sinus beats are not regularly conducted through the atrioventricular node to the ventricles. Therefore the ventricular rate is slower than the atrial rate. The block may be regular, such as 2:1, or variable. Most fetuses with second-degree atrioventricular block progress to complete heart block *in utero* or postnatally. Structural cardiac defects have not been associated with second-degree atrioventricular block.

In complete heart block the atria and ventricles are completely dissociated, and the ventricular rate is almost always lower than the atrial rate. These fetuses fall into two groups. One-half have associated structural cardiac defects, primarily heterotaxy syndromes, ventricular inversion, or atrioventricular septal defect. Most of the other fetuses have mothers with autoantibodies, anti–SS-A, –SS-B, or both, but the mother is often clinically asymptomatic.[40,260–262] Not all infants with positive titers will develop complete heart block, and the antibodies are usually gone by 3 months of life. The maternal autoantibodies damage the fetal conduction system and appear to cause a congestive cardiomyopathy in some fetuses as well. The recurrence risk for subsequent pregnancies has been reported as high as 25% but is probably approximately 8%.[21]

Associated Anomalies

The associated structural cardiac defects and maternal autoantibodies have been discussed above. Fetal hydrops develops in one-third. Fetal hydrops is unlikely to develop with ventricular rates greater than 70 beats per minute but frequently develops with ventricular rates less than 55 beats per minute or when there is a rapid decrease in heart rate.[40,263]

Diagnosis

The same methods used to evaluate tachycardias are used to evaluate bradycardias. However, the atrial rate is normal and the ventricular rate is decreased, usually between 40 and 80 beats per minute (Fig. 59). An exception is represented by complete atrioventricular block associated with atrial isomerism in which the atrial rate can be reduced as well.[40] Intermittent atrioventricular conduction is present in second-degree atrioventricular block, but there is compete atrioventricular dissociation in complete heart block. As with tachycardias, it is important to evaluate ventricular function and the presence and degree of atrioventricular valve regurgitation. With autoimmune congenital heart block, bradycardia tends to worsen with gestation. We have seen a handful of these cases in which the heart rate was in the range of 70 to 90 beats per minute at midgestation and dropped to 40 to 60 beats per minute in the late third trimester.

Treatment

Beta agonists, such as terbutaline, have been used and fetal heart rates can be increased by as much as 50%, but the fetuses do not improve clinically because 1:1 atrioventricular conduction has not been restored. Salbutamol was used to increase fetal heart rate with improvement in ventricular function and resolution of fetal hydrops.[256,264] There have been attempts to pace the fetus either directly or through the maternal abdomen with limited success.[265–267] In two studies, fetal lambs have been paced after induced heart block. These studies show that combined cardiac output is 43% to 45% of normal and that with atrioventricular sequential pacing, the cardiac output increases to 77% to 80% of normal, with no further improvement with heart rate greater than 100 beats per

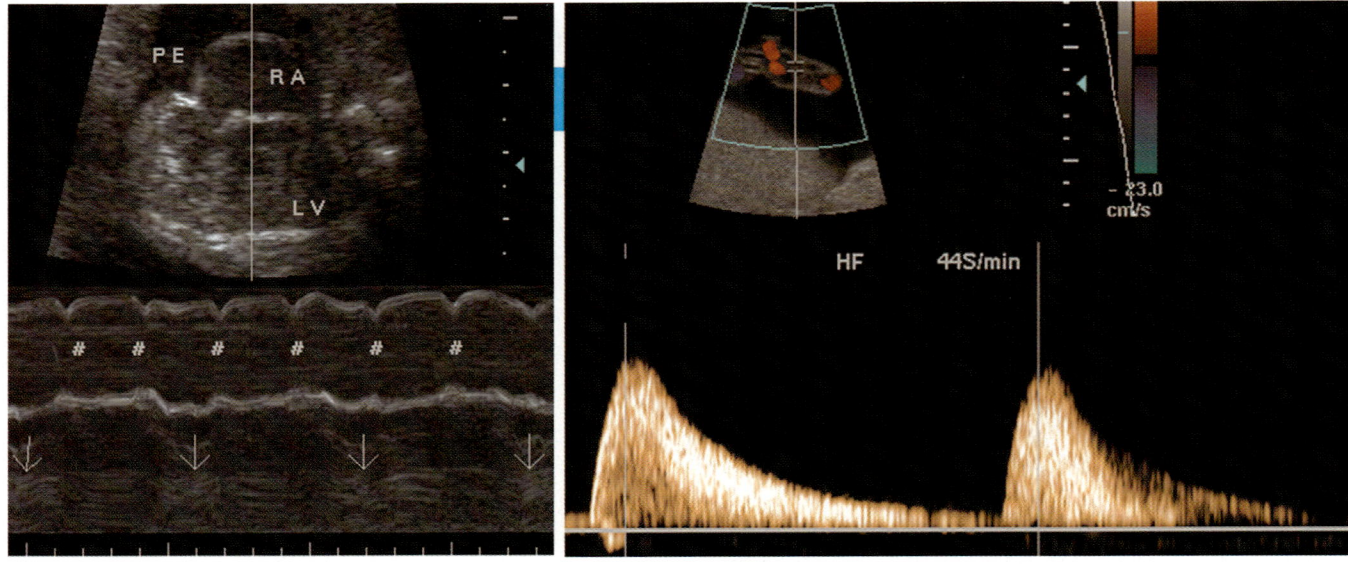

FIGURE 59. Complete atrioventricular block. Atria and ventricles activate independently, with a rate of 120 and 44 beats per minute, respectively. The fetus is hydropic. Velocimetry of the umbilical artery confirms the presence of severe bradycardia. LV, left ventricle; PE, pericardial effusion; RA, right atrium.

minute. Ventricular pacing improved combined cardiac output to only 62% of normal.[268,269]

More recently, steroids have been used. Dexamethasone, which crosses the placenta, has been used in fetuses with heart block and there have been reports of reversal of heart block to lesser degrees or return to sinus rhythm.[262,263] The dosage used is 4 mg per day. Prednisone and gamma globulin have been used prophylactically in women who have autoantibodies and have had a previous child with heart block.[264] There is no evidence that this treatment decreases the risk of heart block in subsequent pregnancies. Steroids have also been used to treat the myocarditis and fetal hydrops that are often associated with congenital heart block.[270–276] The side effects of high-dosage maternal steroid administration are well known, and include diabetes, hypertension, and premature rupture of the membranes. Digitalis and furosemide have also been used, presumably to treat the associated myocardial dysfunction and fetal hydrops. Plasmapheresis has also been used to decrease the maternal antibody levels with limited success.[20,271,272,277]

Prognosis

The prognosis for heart block is determined by the presence of structural cardiac defects or fetal hydrops.[40,262,278] If either is present, *in utero* demise is nearly 100%. Postnatally, most fetuses require pacemakers either as newborns or children. It has been demonstrated that infants with congenital complete heart block are at risk for developing dilated cardiomyopathy. In one study with long-term follow-up, this complication occurred in 6%, at a mean age of 6 years.[279] The affected infants either received heart transplantation or died. Most of the affected infants had intra-uterine diagnosis in the midtrimester and were born from mothers with anti–SS-A/SS-B antibodies.

REFERENCES

1. Ferencz C, Rubin JD, Loffredo CA, Magree CA. *Perspectives in pediatric cardiology. Vol. 4. Congenital heart disease: The Baltimore-Washington Infant Study 1981–9.* New York: Futura Publishing, 1993.
2. Allan LD, Benacerraf B, Copel JA, Carvalho AC, Chaoui R, et al. Isolated major congenital heart disease. *Ultrasound Obstet Gynecol* 2001;17:370–379.
3. Gertis LM. Cardiac malformations in spontaneous abortions. *Int J Cardiol* 1985;7:29–35.
4. Buskens E, Grobbee DE, Frohn-Mulder IM, Stewart PA, Juttmann RE, et al. Efficacy of routine fetal ultrasound screening for congenital heart disease in normal pregnancy. *Circulation* 1996;94(1):67–72.
5. Todros T, Faggiano F, Chiappa E, Gaglioti P, Mitola B, Sciarrone A. Accuracy of routine ultrasonography in screening heart disease prenatally. Gruppo Piemontese for Prenatal Screening of Congenital Heart Disease. *Prenat Diagn* 1997;17(10):901–906.
6. Tegnander E, Eik-Nes SH, Johansen OJ, Linker DT. Prenatal detection of heart defects at the routine fetal examination at 18 weeks in a non-selected population. *Ultrasound Obstet Gynecol* 1995;5(6):372–380.
7. Bull C. Current and potential impact of fetal diagnosis on prevalence and spectrum of serious congenital heart disease at term in the UK. British Paediatric Cardiac Association. *Lancet* 1999;354(9186):1242–1247.

8. Achiron R, Glaser J, Gelernter I, Hegesh J, Yagel S. Extended fetal echocardiographic examination for detecting cardiac malformations in low risk pregnancies. *BMJ* 1992;304(6828):671–674.

9. Benacerraf BR. Sonographic detection of fetal anomalies of the aortic and pulmonary arteries: value of four-chamber view vs direct images. *AJR Am J Roentgenol* 1994;163(6):1483–1489.

10. Bromley B, Estroff JA, Sanders SP, Parad R, Roberts D, et al. Fetal echocardiography: accuracy and limitations in a population at high and low risk for heart defects. *Am J Obstet Gynecol* 1992;166(5):1473–1481.

11. Kirk JS, Riggs TW, Comstock CH, Lee W, Yang SS, Weinhouse E. Prenatal screening for cardiac anomalies: the value of routine addition of the aortic root to the four-chamber view. *Obstet Gynecol* 1994;84(3):427–431.

12. Murphy EA, Pyeritz RE. Assessment of genetic risk in congenital heart disease. *J Am Coll Cardiol* 1991;18(2):311–342.

13. Nora JJ, Nora AH. Maternal transmission of congenital heart diseases: new recurrence risk figures and the questions of cytoplasmic inheritance and vulnerability to teratogens. *Am J Cardiol* 1987;59:459–463.

14. Nora JJ. Causes of congenital heart disease: old and new modes, mechanisms, and models. *Am Heart J* 1993;125(5 Pt 1):1409–1419.

15. Cooper MJ, Enderlein MA, Tarnoff H, Roge CL. Asymmetric septal hypertrophy in infants of diabetic mothers. Fetal echocardiography and the impact of maternal diabetic control. *Am J Dis Child* 1992;146(2):226–229.

16. Rizzo G, Arduini D, Romanini C. Accelerated cardiac growth and abnormal cardiac flow in fetuses of type I diabetic mothers. *Obstet Gynecol* 1992;80(3 Pt 1):369–376.

17. Rizzo G, Arduini D, Romanini C. Cardiac function in fetuses of type I diabetic mothers. *Am J Obstet Gynecol* 1991;164(3):837–843.

18. Veille JC, Sivakoff M, Hanson R, Fanaroff AA. Interventricular septal thickness in fetuses of diabetic mothers. *Obstet Gynecol* 1992;79(1):51–54.

19. Weber HS, Copel JA, Reece EA, Green J, Kleinman CS. Cardiac growth in fetuses of diabetic mothers with good metabolic control. *J Pediatr* 1991;118(1):103–107.

20. Olah KS, Gee H. Antibody mediated complete congenital heart block in the fetus. *Pacing Clin Electrophysiol* 1993;16(9):1872–1879.

21. Julkunen H, Kaaja R, Wallgren E, Teramo K. Isolated congenital heart block: fetal and infant outcome and familial incidence of heart block. *Obstet Gynecol* 1993;82:11–16.

22. Platt LD, Koch R, Azen C. Maternal phenylketonuria collaborative study, obstetric aspects and outcome: the first 6 years. *Am J Obstet Gynecol* 1992;166:1150–1162.

23. Zierler S. Maternal drugs and congenital heart disease. *Obstet Gynecol* 1985;65(2):155–165.

24. Hill LM. Effects of drugs and chemicals on the fetus and newborn (first of two parts). *Mayo Clin Proc* 1984;59:707–716.

25. Hill LM. Effects of drugs and chemicals on the fetus and newborn (second of two parts). *Mayo Clin Proc* 1984;59:755–765.

26. Loser H, Pfefferkorn JR, Themann H. [Alcohol in pregnancy and fetal heart damage]. *Klin Padiatr* 1992;204(5):335–339.

27. Clarren SK. Recognition of fetal alcohol syndrome. *JAMA* 1981;245:2436–2439.

28. Sandor GC, Smith DF, MacLeod PM. Cardiac malformations in the fetal alcohol syndrome. *J Pediatr* 1981;98:771–773.

29. Copel JA, Pilu G, Kleinman CS. Congenital heart disease and extracardiac anomalies: associations and indications for fetal echocardiography. *Am J Obstet Gynecol* 1986;154(5):1121–1132.

30. Briggs GG, Freeman RK, Yaffe SJ. *Drugs in pregnancy and lactation*, 4th ed. Baltimore: Williams & Wilkins, 1994.

31. Friedman JM, Polifka JE. *Teratogenic effects of drugs: a resource for clinicians.* Baltimore & London: The Johns Hopkins University Press, 1994.

32. Cohen LS, Friedman JM, Jefferson JW, Johnson EM, Weiner ML. A reevaluation of risk of in utero exposure to lithium. *JAMA* 1994;271(2):146–150.

33. Jacobson SJ, Jones K, Johnson K, Ceolin L, Kaur P, et al. Prospective multicentre study of pregnancy outcome after lithium exposure during first trimester. *Lancet* 1992;339(8792):530–533.

34. Schou M, Goldfield MD, Weinstein MR, Villeneuve A. Lithium and pregnancy-1, report from the register of lithium babies. *BMJ* 1973;2:135–136.

35. Takatsuki H, Abe Y, Goto T. Two cases of acute promyelocytic leukemia in pregnancy and the effect on anthracyclines of fetal development. *Jap J Clin Hematol* 1992;33(11):1736–1740.

36. Jordan EK, Sever JL. Fetal damage caused by parvoviral infections. *Reprod Toxicol* 1994;8(2):161–189.

37. Morey AL, Keeling JW, Porter HJ, Fleming KA. Clinical and histopathological features of parvovirus B19 infection in the human fetus. *Br J Obstet Gynaecol* 1992;99:566–574.

38. Hyett JA, Moscoso G, Papapanagiotou G, Perdu M, Nicolaides KH. Abnormalities of the heart and great arteries in chromosomally normal fetuses with increased nuchal translucency thickness at 11–13 weeks of gestation. *Ultrasound Obstet Gynecol* 1996;7(4):245–250.

39. Little J, Bryan E. Congenital anomalies in twins. *Semin Perinatol* 1986;10(1):50–64.

40. Schmidt KG, Ulmer HE, Silverman NH, Kleinman CS, Copel JA. Perinatal outcome of fetal complete atrioventricular block: a multicenter experience. *J Am Coll Cardiol* 1991;17(6):1360–1366.

41. Poeschmann RP, Verheijen HM, Van Dongen PWJ. Differential diagnosis and causes of nonimmunological hydrops fetalis: a review. *Obstet Gynecol Survey* 1991;46(4):223–231.

42. Allan LD. Antenatal diagnosis of heart disease. *Heart* 2000;83(3):367.

43. Todros T. Prenatal diagnosis and management of fetal cardiovascular malformations. *Curr Opin Obstet Gynecol* 2000;12(2):105–109.

44. Chaoui R. Fetal echocardiography: state of the art of the state of the heart. *Ultrasound Obstet Gynecol* 2001;17(4):277–284.

45. Bronshtein M, Zimmer EZ, Gerlis LM, Lorber A, Drugan A. Early ultrasound diagnosis of fetal congenital heart defects in high-risk and low-risk pregnancies. *Obstet Gynecol* 1993;82(2):225–229.

46. Achiron R, Weissman A, Rotstein Z, Lipitz S, Mashiach S, Hegesh J. Transvaginal echocardiographic examination of

the fetal heart between 13 and 15 weeks' gestation in a low-risk population. *J Ultrasound Med* 1994;13(10):783–789.

47. Achiron R, Rotstein Z, Lipitz S, Mashiach S, Hegesh J. First-trimester diagnosis of fetal congenital heart disease by transvaginal ultrasonography. *Obstet Gynecol* 1994;84(1):69–72.

48. Gembruch U, Knopfle G, Chatterjee M, Bald R, Hansmann M. First-trimester diagnosis of fetal congenital heart disease by transvaginal two-dimensional and Doppler echocardiography. *Obstet Gynecol* 1990;75(3 Pt 2):496–498.

49. Stumpflen I, Stumpflen A, Wimmer M, Bernaschek G. Effect of detailed fetal echocardiography as part of routine prenatal ultrasonographic screening on detection of congenital heart disease. *Lancet* 1996;348(9031):854–857.

50. Perolo A, Prandstraller D, Ghi T, Gargiulo G, Leone O, et al. Diagnosis and management of fetal cardiac anomalies: 10 years of experience at a single institution. *Ultrasound Obstet Gynecol* 2001;18:615–618.

51. Tworetzky W, McElhinney DB, Reddy VM, Brook MM, Hanley FL, Silverman NH. Improved surgical outcome after fetal diagnosis of hypoplastic left heart syndrome. *Circulation* 2001;103(9):1269–1273.

52. Bonnet D, Coltri A, Butera G, Fermont L, Le Bidois J, et al. Detection of transposition of the great arteries in fetuses reduces neonatal morbidity and mortality. *Circulation* 1999;99(7):916–918.

53. Jaeggi ET, Sholler GF, Jones OD, Cooper SG. Comparative analysis of pattern, management and outcome of pre- versus postnatally diagnosed major congenital heart disease: a population-based study. *Ultrasound Obstet Gynecol* 2001;17(5):380–385.

54. Becker AE, Anderson RH. *Pathology of congenital heart disease.* London: Butterworths, 1981.

55. Huhta JC, Hagler DJ, Seward JB, Tajik AJ, Julsrud PR, Ritter DG. Two-dimensional echocardiographic assessment of dextrocardia: a segmental approach. *Am J Cardiol* 1982;50(6):1351–1360.

56. Lee W, Smith RS, Comstock CH, Kirk JS, Riggs T, Weinhouse E. Tetralogy of Fallot: prenatal diagnosis and postnatal survival. *Obstet Gynecol* 1995;86:583–585.

57. Paladini D, Palmieri S, Lamberti A, Teodoro A, Martinelli P, Nappi C. Characterization and natural history of ventricular septal defects in the fetus. *Ultrasound Obstet Gynecol* 2000;16(2):118–122.

58. Crawford DC, Chita SK, Allan LD. Prenatal detection of congenital heart disease: factors affecting obstetric management and survival. *Am J Obstet Gynecol* 1988;159(2):352–356.

59. Benacerraf BR, Pober BR, Sanders SP. Accuracy of fetal echocardiography. *Radiology* 1987;165(3):847–849.

60. Orie J, Flotta D, Sherman FS. To be or not to be a VSD. *Am J Cardiol* 1994;74(12):1284–1285.

61. Nir A, Driscoll DJ, Edwards WD. Intrauterine closure of membranous ventricular septal defects: mechanism of closure in two autopsy specimens. *Pediatr Cardiol* 1994;15(1):33–37.

62. Nir A, Weintraub Z, Oliven A, Kelener J, Lurie M. Anatomic evidence of spontaneous intrauterine closure of a ventricular septal defect. *Pediatr Cardiol* 1990;11(4):208–210.

63. Stewart PA, Wladimiroff JW. Fetal atrial arrhythmias associated with redundancy/aneurysm of the foramen ovale. *J Clin Ultrasound* 1988;16(9):643–650.

64. Rice MJ, McDonald RW, Reller MD. Fetal atrial septal aneurysm: a cause of fetal atrial arrhythmias. *J Am Coll Cardiol* 1988;12(5):1292–1297.

65. Brons JT, van Geijn HP, Wladimiroff JW, van der Harten JJ, Kwee ML, et al. Prenatal ultrasound diagnosis of the Holt-Oram syndrome. *Prenat Diagn* 1988;8(3):175–181.

66. Machado MV, Crawford DC, Anderson RH, Allan LD. Atrioventricular septal defect in prenatal life. *Br Heart J* 1988;59(3):352–355.

67. Disegni E, Pierpont ME, Bass JL, Kaplinsky E. Two-dimensional echocardiography in detection of endocardial cushion defect in families. *Am J Cardiol* 1985;55(13 Pt 1):1649–1652.

68. Digilio MC, Marino B, Cicini MP, Giannotti A, Formigari R, Dallapiccola B. Risk of congenital heart defects in relatives of patients with atrioventricular canal. *Am J Dis Child* 1993;147(12):1295–1297.

69. Gembruch U, Knopfle G, Chatterjee M, Bald R, Redel DA, et al. Prenatal diagnosis of atrioventricular canal malformations with up-to-date echocardiographic technology: report of 14 cases. *Am Heart J* 1991;121(5):1489–1497.

70. Bronshtein M, Egenburg S, Auslander R, Zimmer EZ. Atrioventricular septal defect in a fetus: a false negative diagnosis in early pregnancy. *Ultrasound Obstet Gynecol* 2000;16(1):98–99.

71. Roberson DA, Silverman NH. Ebstein's anomaly: echocardiographic and clinical features in the fetus and neonate. *J Am Coll Cardiol* 1989;14(5):1300–1307.

72. Lang D, Oberhoffer R, Cook A, Sharland G, Allan L, et al. Pathologic spectrum of malformations of the tricuspid valve in prenatal and neonatal life. *J Am Coll Cardiol* 1991;17(5):1161–1167.

73. Hornberger LK, Sahn DJ, Kleinman CS, Copel JA, Reed KL. Tricuspid valve disease with significant tricuspid insufficiency in the fetus: diagnosis and outcome. *J Am Coll Cardiol* 1991;17(1):167–173.

74. Satomi G, Momoi N, Kikuchi N, Nakazawa M, Momma K. Prenatal diagnosis and outcome of Ebstein's anomaly and tricuspid valve dysplasia in relation to lung hypoplasia. *Echocardiography* 1994;11(3):215–220.

75. Oberhoffer R, Cook AC, Lang D, Sharland G, Allan LD, et al. Correlation between echocardiographic and morphological investigations of lesions of the tricuspid valve diagnosed during fetal life. *Br Heart J* 1992;68(6):580–585.

76. Celermajer DS, Bull C, Till JA, Cullen S, Vassillikos VP, et al. Ebstein's anomaly: presentation and outcome from fetus to adult. *J Am Coll Cardiol* 1994;23(1):170–176.

77. Respondek ML, Kammermeier M, Ludomirsky A, Weil SR, Huhta JC. The prevalence and clinical significance of fetal tricuspid valve regurgitation with normal heart anatomy. *Am J Obstet Gynecol* 1994;171(5):1265–1270.

78. Sharland GK, Chita SK, Allan LD. Tricuspid valve dysplasia or displacement in intrauterine life. *J Am Coll Cardiol* 1991;17(4):944–949.

79. Yeager SB, Parness IA, Sanders SP. Severe tricuspid regurgitation simulating pulmonary atresia in the fetus. *Am Heart J* 1988;115(4):906–908.

80. Smrcek JM, Gembruch U. Longitudinal observations in normally grown fetuses with tricuspid valve regurgitation: report of 22 cases. *Prenat Diagn* 1999;19(3):197–204.

81. Chaoui R, Bollmann R, Goldner B, Heling KS, Tennstedt C. Fetal cardiomegaly: echocardiographic findings and outcome in 19 cases. *Fetal Diagn Ther* 1994;9(2):92–104.

82. Di Russo GB, Gaynor JW. Ebstein's anomaly: indications for repair and surgical technique. *Semin Thorac Cardiovasc Surg Pediatr Card Surg Annu* 1999;2:35–50.

83. Gentles TL, Calder AL, Clarkson PM, Neutze JM. Predictors of long-term survival with Ebstein's anomaly of the tricuspid valve. *Am J Cardiol* 1992;69(4):377–381.

84. Hornberger LK, Benacerraf BR, Bromley BS, Spevak PJ, Sanders SP. Prenatal detection of severe right ventricular outflow tract obstruction: pulmonary stenosis and pulmonary atresia. *J Ultrasound Med* 1994;13(10):743–750.

85. Allan LD, Crawford DC, Tynan MJ. Pulmonary atresia in prenatal life. *J Am Coll Cardiol* 1986;8(5):1131–1136.

86. Yagel S, Arbel R, Auteby EY, Raveh D, Achiron R. The threee vessels and tracheo view (3VT) in fetal cardiac scanning. *Ultrasound Obstet Gynecol* 2002;20:360–365.

87. Vinals F, Tapia J, Giuliano A. Prenatal detection of ductal-dependent congenital heart disease: how can things be made easier? *Ultrasound Obstet Gynecol* 2002;19(3):246–249.

88. Todros T, Presbitero P, Gaglioti P, Demarie D. Pulmonary stenosis with intact ventricular septum: documentation of development of the lesion echocardiographically during fetal life. *Int J Cardiol* 1988;19(3):355–362.

89. Berning RA, Silverman NH, Villegas M, Sahn DJ, Martin GR, Rice MJ. Reversed shunting across the ductus arteriosus or atrial septum in utero heralds severe congenital heart disease. *J Am Coll Cardiol* 1996;27(2):481–486.

90. Driscoll DJ, Offord KP, Feldt RH, Schaff HV, Puga FJ, Danielson GK. Five- to fifteen-year follow-up after Fontan operation. *Circulation* 1992;85:469–496.

91. Murakoshi T, Yamamori K, Tojo Y, Naruse H, Seguchi M, et al. Pulmonary stenosis in recipient twins in twin-to-twin transfusion syndrome: report on 3 cases and review of literature. *Croat Med J* 2000;41(3):252–256.

92. Rice MJ, McDonald RW, Reller MD. Progressive pulmonary stenosis in the fetus: two case reports. *Am J Perinatol* 1993;10(6):424–427.

93. Jouk PS, Rambaud P. Prediction of outcome by prenatal Doppler analysis in a patient with aortic stenosis. *Br Heart J* 1991;65(1):53–54.

94. Stewart PA, Buis-Liem T, Verwey RA, Wladimiroff JW. Prenatal ultrasonic diagnosis of familial asymmetric septal hypertrophy. *Prenat Diagn* 1986;6(4):249–256.

95. Zielinsky P. Role of prenatal echocardiography in the study of hypertrophic cardiomyopathy in the fetus. *Echocardiography* 1991;8(6):661–668.

96. Sheehan PQ, Rowland TW, Shah BL, McGravey VJ, Reiter EO. Maternal diabetic control and hypertrophic cardiomyopathy in infants of diabetic mothers. *Clin Pediatr (Phila)* 1986;25(5):266–271.

97. Simpson JM, Sharland GK. Natural history and outcome of aortic stenosis diagnosed prenatally. *Heart* 1997;77(3):205–210.

98. Hornberger LK, Sanders SP, Rein AJ, Spevak PJ, Parness IA, Colan SD. Left heart obstructive lesions and left ventricular growth in the midtrimester fetus. A longitudinal study. *Circulation* 1995;92(6):1531–1538.

99. Sharland GK, Chita SK, Fagg NL, Anderson RH, Tynan M, et al. Left ventricular dysfunction in the fetus: relation to aortic valve anomalies and endocardial fibroelastosis. *Br Heart J* 1991;66(6):419–424.

100. Allan LD, Maxwell DJ, Carminati M, Tynan MJ. Survival after fetal aortic balloon valvoplasty. *Ultrasound Obstet Gynecol* 1995;5(2):90–91.

101. Huhta JC, Carpenter RJ Jr, Moise KJ Jr, Deter RL, Ott DA, McNamara DG. Prenatal diagnosis and postnatal management of critical aortic stenosis. *Circulation* 1987;75(3):573–576.

102. Sharland GK, Chan KY, Allan LD. Coarctation of the aorta: difficulties in prenatal diagnosis. *Br Heart J* 1994;71(1):70–75.

103. Allan LD, Chita SK, Anderson RH, Fagg N, Crawford DC, Tynan MJ. Coarctation of the aorta in prenatal life: an echocardiographic, anatomical, and functional study. *Br Heart J* 1988;59(3):356–360.

104. Hornberger LK, Sahn DJ, Kleinman CS, Copel J, Silverman NH. Antenatal diagnosis of coarctation of the aorta: a multicenter experience. *J Am Coll Cardiol* 1994;23(2):417–423.

105. Hornberger LK, Weintraub RG, Pesonen E, Murillo-Olivas A, Simpson IA, et al. Echocardiographic study of the morphology and growth of the aortic arch in the human fetus. Observations related to the prenatal diagnosis of coarctation. *Circulation* 1992;86(3):741–747.

106. Aeba R, Katogi T, Ueda T, Takeuchi S, Kawada S. Complications following reparative surgery for aortic coarctation or interrupted aortic arch. *Surg Today* 1998;28(9):889–894.

107. Hougen TJ, Sell JE. Recent advances in the diagnosis and treatment of coarctation of the aorta. *Curr Opin Cardiol* 1995;10(5):524–529.

108. Siblini G, Rao PS, Nouri S, Ferdman B, Jureidini SB, Wilson AD. Long-term follow-up results of balloon angioplasty of postoperative aortic recoarctation. *Am J Cardiol* 1998;81(1):61–67.

109. Van Praagh R, Bernhard WF, Rosenthal A, Parisi LF, Fyler DC. Interrupted aortic arch: surgical treatment. *Am J Cardiol* 1971;27(2):200–211.

110. Gerboni S, Sabatino G, Mingarelli R, Dallapiccola B. Coarctation of the aorta, interrupted aortic arch, and hypoplastic left heart syndrome in three generations. *J Med Genet* 1993;30(4):328–329.

111. Collins-Nakai RL, Dick M, Parisi-Buckley L, Fyler DC, Castaneda AR. Interrupted aortic arch in infancy. *J Pediatr* 1976;88(6):959–962.

112. Wilson DI, Burn J, Scambler P, Goodship J. DiGeorge syndrome: part of CATCH 22. *J Med Genet* 1993;30(10):852–856.

113. Jonas RA, Quaegebeur JM, Kirklin JW, Blackstone EH, Daicoff G. Outcomes in patients with interrupted aortic arch and ventricular septal defect. A multiinstitutional study. Congenital Heart Surgeons Society. *J Thorac Cardiovasc Surg* 1994;107(4):1099–1109; discussion 1109–1113.

114. Volpe P, Gentile M, Marasini M. Interrupted aortic arch type A with 22q11 deletion: prenatal detection of an unusual association. *Prenat Diagn* 2002;22(5):317–314.

115. Davidson A, Khandelwal M, Punnett HH. Prenatal diagnosis of the 22q11 deletion syndrome. *Prenat Diagn* 1997;17(4):380–383.

116. Simpson JM. Hypoplastic left heart syndrome. *Ultrasound Obstet Gynecol* 2000;15(4):271–278.

117. Cartier MS, Emerson D, Plappert T, St. John Sutton M. Hypoplastic left heart with absence of the aortic valve: prenatal diagnosis using two-dimensional and pulsed Doppler echocardiography. *J Clin Ultrasound* 1987;15:463–468.

118. Cartier MS, Davidoff A, Warneke LA, Hirsh MP, Bannon S, et al. The normal diameter of the fetal aorta and pulmonary artery: echocardiographic evaluation in utero. *AJR Am J Roentgenol* 1987;149(5):1003–1007.

119. Allan LD, Sharland G, Tynan MJ. The natural history of the hypoplastic left heart syndrome. *Int J Cardiol* 1989;25(3):341–343.

120. Brackley KJ, Kilby MD, Wright JG, Brawn WJ, Sethia B, et al. Outcome after prenatal diagnosis of hypoplastic left-heart syndrome: a case series. *Lancet* 2000;356(9236):1143–1147.

121. Razzouk AJ, Chinnock RE, Gundry SR, Johnston JK, Larsen RL, et al. Transplantation as a primary treatment for hypoplastic left heart syndrome: intermediate-term results. *Ann Thorac Surg* 1996;62(1):1–7; discussion 8.

122. Kern JH, Hinton VJ, Nereo NE, Hayes CJ, Gersony WM. Early developmental outcome after the Norwood procedure for hypoplastic left heart syndrome. *Pediatrics* 1998;102:1148–1152.

123. Munn MB, Brumfield CG, Lau Y, Colvin EV. Prenatally diagnosed hypoplastic left heart syndrome—outcomes after postnatal surgery. *J Matern Fetal Med* 1999;8(4):147–150.

124. Allan LD, Apfel HD, Printz BF. Outcome after prenatal diagnosis of the hypoplastic left heart syndrome. *Heart* 1998;79(4):371–373.

125. Allan LD, Tynan M, Campbell S, Anderson RH. Identification of congenital cardiac malformations by echocardiography in midtrimester fetus. *Br Heart J* 1981;46(4):358–362.

126. Pilu G, Baccarani G. Prenatal diagnosis of cardiac structural abnormalities. *Fetal Ther* 1986;1(2–3):86–88.

127. Kleinman CS, Hobbins JC, Jaffe CC, Lynch DC, Talner NS. Echocardiographic studies of the human fetus: prenatal diagnosis of congenital heart disease and cardiac dysrhythmias. *Pediatrics* 1980;65(6):1059–1067.

128. Kleinman CS, Donnerstein RL, DeVore GR, Jaffe CC, Lynch DC, et al. Fetal echocardiography for evaluation of in utero congestive heart failure. *N Engl J Med* 1982;306(10):568–575.

129. Burn J. Closing time for CATCH22. *J Med Genet* 1999;36:737–738.

130. Callan NA, Kan JS. Prenatal diagnosis of tetralogy of Fallot with absent pulmonary valve. *Am J Perinatol* 1991;8(1):15–17.

131. Fouron JC, Sahn DJ, Bender R, et al. Prenatal diagnosis and circulatory characteristics in tetralogy of Fallot with absent pulmonary valve. *Am J Cardiol* 1989;64:547–549.

132. Allan LD, Sharland GK. Prognosis in fetal tetralogy of Fallot. *Pediatr Cardiol* 1992;13:1–4.

133. Trainer AH, Morrison N, Dunlop A, Wilson N, Tolmie J. Chromosome 22q11 microdeletions in tetralogy of Fallot. *Arch Dis Child* 1996;74(1):62–63.

134. Tometzki AJ, Suda K, Kohl T, Kovalchin JP, Silverman NH. Accuracy of prenatal echocardiographic diagnosis and prognosis of fetuses with conotruncal anomalies. *J Am Coll Cardiol* 1999;33(6):1696–1701.

135. DeVore GR, Siassi B, Platt LD. Fetal echocardiography. VIII. Aortic root dilatation—a marker for tetralogy of Fallot. *Am J Obstet Gynecol* 1988;159(1):129–136.

136. Knott-Craig CJ, Elkins RC, Lane MM, Holz J, McCue C, Ward KE. A 26-year experience with surgical management of tetralogy of Fallot: risk analysis for mortality or late reintervention. *Ann Thorac Surg* 1998;66:506–511.

137. Alexiou C, Mahmoud H, Al-Khaddour A, Gnanapragasam J, Salmon AP, et al. Outcome after repair of tetralogy of Fallot in the first year of life. *Ann Thorac Surg* 2001;71:494–500.

138. Paladini D, Rustico M, Todros T, Palmieri S, Gaglioti P, et al. Conotruncal anomalies in prenatal life. *Ultrasound Obstet Gynecol* 1996;8(4):241–246.

139. Haas F, Wottke M, Poppert H, Meisner H. Long-term survival and functional follow-up in patients after the arterial switch operation. *Ann Thorac Surg* 1999;68:1692–1697.

140. Thompson LD, McElhinney DB, Reddy M, Petrossian E, Silverman NH, Hanley FL. Neonatal repair of truncus arteriosus: continuing improvement in outcomes. *Ann Thorac Surg* 2001;72(2):391–395.

141. deAraujo LML, Schmidt KG, Silverman NH, Finbeiner WE. Prenatal detection of truncus arteriosus by ultrasound. *Pediatr Cardiol* 1987;8:261–263.

142. Brizard CP, Cochrane A, Austin C, Nomura F, Karl TR. Management strategy and outcome for truncus arteriosus. *Eur J Cardiothorac Surg* 1997;11(4):687–695; discussion 695–696.

143. Jahangiri M, Zurakowski D, Mayer JE, del Nido PJ, Jonas RA. Repair of the truncal valve and associated interrupted arch in neonates with truncus arteriosus. *J Thorac Cardiovasc Surg* 2000;119(3):508–514.

144. von Bernuth G. 25 years after the first arterial switch procedure: mid-term results. *Thorac Cardiovasc Surg* 2000;48:228–232.

145. Graham TP, Bernard YD, Mellen GB, Celarmajer D, Baumgartner H, et al. Long-term outcome in congenitally corrected transposition of the great arteries: a multi-institutional study. *J Am Coll Cardiol* 2000;36(1):255–261.

146. DeVore GR, Siassi B, Platt LD. Fetal echocardiography: the prenatal diagnosis of tricuspid atresia (type Ic) during the second trimester of pregnancy. *J Clin Ultrasound* 1987;15(5):317–324.

147. Johnson BL, Fyfe DA, Gillette PC, Kline CH, Sade R. In utero diagnosis of interrupted aortic arch with transposition of the great arteries and tricuspid atresia. *Am Heart J* 1989;117(3):690–692.

148. McGahan JP, Choy M, Parrish MD, Brant WE. Sonographic spectrum of fetal cardiac hypoplasia. *J Ultrasound Med* 1991;10(10):539–546.

149. Williams RG. Echocardiography in the management of single ventricle: fetal through adult life. *Echocardiography* 1993;10(3):331–342.

150. Cesko I, Hajdu J, Toth T, Marton T, Papp C, Papp Z. Ivemark syndrome with asplenia in siblings. *J Pediatr* 1997;130(5):822–824.

151. Atkinson DE, Drant S. Diagnosis of heterotaxy syndrome by fetal echocardiography. *Am J Cardiol* 1998;82(9):1147–1149, A10.

152. Chitayat D, Lao A, Wilson RD, Fagerstrom C, Hayden M. Prenatal diagnosis of asplenia/polysplenia syndrome. *Am J Obstet Gynecol* 1988;158(5):1085–1087.

153. Cesko I, Hajdu J, Marton T, Tarnai L, Papp Z. Polysplenia and situs inversus in siblings. Case reports. *Fetal Diagn Ther* 2001;16(1):1–3.

154. Phoon CK, Villegas MD, Ursell PC, Silverman NH. Left atrial isomerism detected in fetal life. *Am J Cardiol* 1996;77(12):1083–1088.

155. Baschat AA, Gembruch U, Knopfle G, Hansmann M. First-trimester fetal heart block: a marker for cardiac anomaly. *Ultrasound Obstet Gynecol* 1999;14(5):311–314.

156. Larsen RL, Eguchi JH, Mulle NF, Johnston JK, Fitts J, et al. Usefulness of cardiac transplantation in children with visceral heterotaxy (asplenic and polysplenic syndromes and single right-sided spleen with levocardia) and comparison of results with cardiac transplantation in children with dilated cardiomyopathy. *Am J Cardiol* 2002;89(11):1275–1279.

157. Abdullah MM, Lacro RV, Smallhorn J, Chitayat D, van der Velde ME, et al. Fetal cardiac dextroposition in the absence of an intrathoracic mass: sign of significant right lung hypoplasia. *J Ultrasound Med* 2000;19(10):669–676.

158. Allan LD, Sharland GK. The echocardiographic diagnosis of totally anomalous pulmonary venous connection in the fetus. *Heart* 2001;85(4):433–437.

159. Feller Printz B, Allan LD. Abnormal pulmonary venous return diagnosed prenatally by pulsed Doppler flow imaging. *Ultrasound Obstet Gynecol* 1997;9(5):347–349.

160. Patel CR, Lane JR, Muise KL. In utero diagnosis of obstructed supracardiac total anomalous pulmonary venous connection in a patient with right atrial isomerism and asplenia. *Ultrasound Obstet Gynecol* 2001;17(3):268–271.

161. Yasukochi S, Satomi G, Iwasaki Y. Prenatal diagnosis of total anomalous pulmonary venous connection with asplenia. *Fetal Diagn Ther* 1997;12(5):266–269.

162. Allan LD, Chita SK, Sharland GK, Fagg NL, Anderson RH, Crawford DC. The accuracy of fetal echocardiography in the diagnosis of congenital heart disease. *Int J Cardiol* 1989;25(3):279–288.

163. Papa M, Camesasca C, Santoro F, Zoia E, Fragasso G, et al. Fetal echocardiography in detecting anomalous pulmonary venous connection: four false positive cases. *Br Heart J* 1995;73(4):355–358.

164. Schmidt KG, Birk E, Silverman NH, Scagnelli SA. Echocardiographic evaluation of dilated cardiomyopathy in the human fetus. *Am J Cardiol* 1989;63(9):599–605.

165. Rizzo G, Pietropolli A, Capponi A, Cacciatore C, Arduini D, Romanini C. Analysis of factors influencing ventricular filling patterns in fetuses of type I diabetic mothers. *J Perinat Med* 1994;22(2):149–157.

166. Bovicelli L, Picchio FM, Pilu G, Baccarani G, Orsini LF, et al. Prenatal diagnosis of endocardial fibroelastosis. *Prenat Diagn* 1984;4(1):67–72.

167. Veille JC, Sivakoff M. Fetal echocardiographic signs of congenital endocardial fibroelastosis. *Obstet Gynecol* 1988;72(2):219–222.

168. Newbould MJ, Armstrong GR, Barson AJ. Endocardial fibroelastosis in infants with hydrops fetalis. *J Clin Pathol* 1991;44:576–579.

169. Buis-Liem TN, Broekhuizen M, Ottenkam J, Gittenberger-deGroot AC, Meerman RJ. Obstructive foramen ovale: an underestimated cause of intrauterine and perinatal distress or death (abstract). *Pediatr Cardiol* 1988;9(3):186.

170. Chobot V, Hornberger LK, Hagen-Ansert S, Sahn DJ. Prenatal detection of restrictive foramen ovale. *J Am Soc Echocardiogr* 1990;3(1):15–19.

171. Bharati S, Patel AG, Varga P, Husain AN, Lev M. In utero echocardiographic diagnosis of premature closure of the foramen ovale with mitral regurgitation and large left atrium. *Am Heart J* 1991;122(2):597–600.

172. Crawford DC, Garrett C, Tynan M, Neville BG, Allan LD. Cardiac rhabdomyomata as a marker for the antenatal detection of tuberous sclerosis. *J Med Genet* 1983;20:303–304.

173. Holley DG, Martin GR, Brenner JI, Fyfe DA, Huhta JC, et al. Diagnosis and management of fetal cardiac tumors: a multicenter experience and review of published reports. *J Am Coll Cardiol* 1995;26(2):516–520.

174. Groves AM, Fagg NL, Cook AC, Allan LD. Cardiac tumours in intrauterine life. *Arch Dis Child* 1992;67(10 Spec No):1189–1192.

175. Harding CO, Pagon RA. Incidence of tuberous sclerosis in patients with cardiac rhabdomyoma. *Am J Med Genet* 1990;37:443–446.

176. Smith HC, Watson GH, Patel RG, Super M. Cardiac rhabdomyomata in tuberous sclerosis: their course and diagnostic value. *Arch Dis Child* 1989;64:196–200.

177. Mehta AV. Rhabdomyoma and ventricular preexitation syndrome. A report of two cases and review of literature. *Am J Dis Child* 1993;147(6):669–671.

178. Jan CJ, Wu FF, Sue WC, Chang CH, Lin YH. Tuberous sclerosis with cardiac rhabdomyoma manifested by fetal bradycardia: report of a case. *Zhonghua Min Guo Xiao Er Ke Yi Xue Hui Za Zhi* 1991;32(3):183–190.

179. Watanabe T, Hojo Y, Kozaki T, Nagashima M, Ando M. Hypoplastic left heart syndrome with rhabdomyoma of the left ventricle. *Pediatr Cardiol* 1991;12:121–122.

180. Leithiser RE, Fyfe D, Weatherby E, Sade R, Garvin AJ. Prenatal sonographic diagnosis of atrial hemangioma. *AJR Am J Roentgenol* 1986;147:1207–1208.

181. Alkalay AL, Ferry DA, Lin B, Fink BW, Pomerance JJ. Spontaneous regression of cardiac rhabdomyoma in tuberous sclerosis. *Clin Pediatr (Phila)* 1987;26(10):532–535.

182. Guereta LG, Burgueros M, Elorza MD, Alix AG, Benito F, Gamallo C. Cardiac rhabdomyoma presenting as fetal hydrops. *Pediatr Cardiol* 1986;7(3):171–174.

183. Brand JM, Friedberg DZ. Spontaneous regression of a primary cardiac tumor presenting as fetal tachyarrhythmias. *J Perinatol* 1992;12(1):48–50.

184. Bivins NIA, Newman RB, Fyfe DA, Campbell BA, Stramm SL. Randomized trial of oral indomethacin and terbutaline sulfate for the long-term suppression of preterm labor. *Am J Obstet Gynecol* 1993;169(4):1065–1070.

185. Brezinka C, Gittenberger-de Groot AC, Wladimiroff JW. The fetal ductus arteriosus: a review. *Zentralblatt Gynakol* 1993;115(10):423–432.

186. Huhta JC, Moise KJ, Fisher DJ, Sharif DS, Wasserstrum N, Martin C. Detection and quantitation of constriction of the

fetal ductus arteriosus by Doppler echocardiography. *Circulation* 1987;75(2):406–412.

187. Hofstadler G, Tulzer G, Altmann R, Schmitt K, Danford D, Huhta JC. Spontaneous closure of the human fetal ductus arteriosus—a cause of fetal congestive heart failure. *Am J Obstet Gynecol* 1996;174(3):879–883.

188. Takahashi Y, Harada K, Ishida A, Tanaka T, Tsuda A, Takada G. Doppler echocardiographic findings of indomethacin-induced occlusion of the fetal ductus arteriosus. *Am J Perinatol* 1996;13(1):15–18.

189. Van den Veyver IB, Moise KJ, Ou CN, Carpenter RJ. The effect of gestational age and fetal indomethacin levels on the incidence of constriction of the fetal ductus arteriosus. *Obstet Gynecol* 1993;82(4 Pt 1):500–503.

190. Moise KJ Jr. Effect of advancing gestational age on the frequency of fetal ductal constriction in association with maternal indomethacin use. *Am J Obstet Gynecol* 1993;168(5):1350–1353.

191. Respondek M, Weil SR, Huhta JC. Fetal echocardiography during indomethacin treatment. *Ultrasound Obstet Gynecol* 1995;5(2):86–89.

192. Mohen D, Newnham JP, D'Orsogna L. Indomethacin for the treatment of polyhydramnios: a case of constriction of the ductus arteriosus. *Aust N Z J Obstet Gynaecol* 1992;32(3):243–246.

193. Dudley DKL, Hardie MJ. Fetal and neonatal effects of indomethacin used as a tocolytic agent. *Am J Obstet Gynecol* 1985;151(2):181–184.

194. Sibony O, de Gayffier A, Carbillon L, et al. Has the use of indomethacin during pregnancy consequences in newborn infants? Prospective study of 83 pregnant women and 115 newborn infants. *Arch Pediatr* 1994;1(8):709–715.

195. Frejgin MD, Delpino NIL, Bidiwala KS. Isolated small bowel perforation following intrauterine treatment with indomethacin. *Am J Perinatol* 1994;11(4):295–296.

196. Marpeau L, Bouillie J, Barrat J, Milliez J. Obstetrical advantages and perinatal risks of indomethacin: a report of 818 cases. *Fetal Diagn Ther* 1994;9(2):110–115.

197. Saenger JS, Mayer DC, D'Angelo LJ, Manci EA. Ductus-dependent fetal cardiac defects contraindicate indomethacin tocolysis. *J Perinatol* 1992;12(1):41–47.

198. Menahem S. Administration of prostaglandin inhibitors to the mother; the potential risk to the fetus and neonate with duct-dependent circulation. *Reprod Fertil Dev* 1991;3(4): 489–494.

199. Belik J, Halayko AJ, Rao K, Stephens NL. Fetal ductus arteriosus ligation: pulmonary vascular smooth muscle biochemical and mechanical changes. *Circ Res* 1993;72(3):588–596.

200. Manchester D, Margolis HS, Sheldon RE. Possible association between maternal indomethacin therapy and primary pulmonary hypertension of the newborn. *Am J Obstet Gynecol* 1976;126(4):467–469.

201. Arcilla RA, Thilenius OG, Ranniger K. Congestive heart failure from suspected ductal closure in utero. *J Pediatr* 1969;75(1):74–78.

202. Eronen M, Pesonen E, Kurki T, Ylikorkala O, Hallman M. The effects of indomethacin and a beta-sympathomimetic agent on the fetal ductus arteriosus during treatment of premature labor: a randomized double-blind study. *Am J Obstet Gynecol* 1991;164(1 Pt 1):141–146.

203. Contratti G, Banzi C, Ghi T, Perolo A, Pilu G, Visentin A. Absence of the ductus venosus: report of 10 new cases and review of the literature. *Ultrasound Obstet Gynecol* 2001;18:605–609.

204. Grazioli L, Alberti D, Olivetti L, Rigamonti W, Codazzi F, et al. Congenital absence of portal vein with nodular regenerative hyperplasia of the liver. *Eur Radiol* 2000;10(5):820–825.

205. Howard ER, Davenport M. Congenital extrahepatic portocaval shunts—the Abernethy malformation. *J Pediatr Surg* 1997;32(3):494–497.

206. Kleinman CS. Prenatal diagnosis and management of intrauterine arrhythmias. *Fetal Ther* 1986;1(2–3):92–95.

207. Kleinman CS, Copel JA, Weinstein EM, Santulli TV Jr, Hobbins JC. In utero diagnosis and treatment of fetal supraventricular tachycardia. *Semin Perinatol* 1985;9(2):113–129.

208. Allan LD, Anderson RH, Sullivan ID, Campbell S, Holt DW, Tynan M. Evaluation of fetal arrhythmias by echocardiography. *Br Heart J* 1983;50(3):240–245.

209. Stewart PA, Tonge HM, Wladimiroff JW. Arrhythmia and structural abnormalities of the fetal heart. *Br Heart J* 1983;50(6):550–554.

210. Moser JC, Hatjis C. Transient fetal atrial flutter related to maternal caffeine intake: a case study. *J Diag Med Sonogr* 1991;9(6):331–333.

211. Oei SG, Vosters RPL, van der Hagen NLJ. Fetal arrhythmia caused by excessive intake of caffeine by pregnant women. *BMJ* 1989;298:568.

212. Lodeiro JG, Feinstein SJ, Lodeiro SB. Fetal premature atrial contractions associated with hydralazine. *Am J Obstet Gynecol* 1989;160(1):105–107.

213. Kleinman CS, Donnerstein RL, Jaffe CC, DeVore GR, Weinstein EM, et al. Fetal echocardiography. A tool for evaluation of in utero cardiac arrhythmias and monitoring of in utero therapy: analysis of 71 patients. *Am J Cardiol* 1983;51(2):237–243.

214. Strasburger JF, Huhta JC, Carpenter RJ Jr, Garson A Jr, McNamara DG. Doppler echocardiography in the diagnosis and management of persistent fetal arrhythmias. *J Am Coll Cardiol* 1986;7(6):1386–1391.

215. Chan FY, Woo SK, Ghosh A, Tang M, Lam C. Prenatal diagnosis of congenital fetal arrhythmias by simultaneous pulsed Doppler velocimetry of the fetal abdominal aorta and inferior vena cava. *Obstet Gynecol* 1990;76(2):200–205.

216. Lingman G, Marsal K. Fetal cardiac arrhythmias: Doppler assessment. *Semin Perinatol* 1987;11(4):357–361.

217. Copel JA, Liang RI, Demasio K, Ozeren S, Kleinman CS. The clinical significance of the irregular fetal heart rhythm. *Am J Obstet Gynecol* 2000;182(4):813–817; discussion 817–819.

218. Kleinman CS, Copel JA, Weinstein EM, Santulli TV Jr, Hobbins JC. Treatment of fetal supraventricular tachyarrhythmias. *J Clin Ultrasound* 1985;13(4):265–273.

219. Guntheroth WG, Cyr DR, Shields LE, Nghiem HV. Rate-based management of fetal supraventricular tachycardia. *J Ultrasound Med* 1996;15(6):453–458.

220. Gest AL, Hansen TN, Moise AA, Hartley CJ. Atrial tachycardia causes hydrops in fetal lambs. *Am J Physiol* 1990;258:H1159–H1163.

221. Nimrod C, Davies D, Harder J, et al. Ultrasound evaluation of tachycardia-induced hydrops in the fetal lamb. *Am J Obstet Gynecol* 1987;157(3):655–659.

222. Boxer RA, Seidman S, Singh S, LaCorte MA, Pek H, et al. Congenital intracardiac rhabdomyoma: prenatal detection by echocardiography, perinatal management, and surgical treatment. *Am J Perinatol* 1986;3(4):303–305.

223. Hoadley SD, Wallace RL, Miller JF, Murgo JP. Prenatal diagnosis of multiple cardiac tumors presenting as an arrhythmia. *J Clin Ultrasound* 1986;14(8):639–643.

224. Wiggins JW Jr, Bowes W, Clewell W, Manco-Johnson M, Manchester D, et al. Echocardiographic diagnosis and intravenous digoxin management of fetal tachyarrhythmias and congestive heart failure. *Am J Dis Child* 1986;140(3):202–204.

225. Birnbaum SE, McGahan JP, Janos GG, Meyers M. Fetal tachycardia and intramyocardial tumors. *J Am Coll Cardiol* 1985;6(6):1358–1361.

226. Buis-Liem TN, Ottenkamp J, Meerman RH, Verwey R. The concurrence of fetal supraventricular tachycardia and obstruction of the foramen ovale. *Prenat Diagn* 1987;7(6):425–431.

227. Haddad S, Degani S, Rahav D, Ohel G. The antenatal diagnosis of fetal atrial septal aneurysm. *Gynecol Obstet Invest* 1996;41(1):27–29.

228. Reed KL. Fetal arrhythmias: etiology, diagnosis, pathophysiology, and treatment. *Semin Perinatol* 1989;13(4):294–304.

229. Belhassen B, Pauzner D, Blieden L, Sherez J, Zinger A, et al. Intrauterine and postnatal atrial fibrillation in the Wolff-Parkinson-White syndrome. *Circulation* 1982;66(5):1124–1128.

230. Shah K, Walsh K. Giant right atrial diverticulum: an unusual cause of Wolff-Parkinson-White syndrome. *Br Heart J* 1992;68(1):58–59.

231. Simpson JM, Milburn A, Yates RW, Maxwell DJ, Sharland GK. Outcome of intermittent tachyarrhythmias in the fetus. *Pediatr Cardiol* 1997;18(2):78–82.

232. Spinnato JA, Shaver DC, Flinn GS, Sibai BM, Watson DL, Marin-Garcia J. Fetal supraventricular tachycardia: in utero therapy with digoxin and quinidine. *Obstet Gynecol* 1984;64(5):730–735.

233. Maxwell D, Chapman MG, Allan LD. The use of fetal blood sampling in the management of fetal tachycardias (abstract). *Pediatr Cardiol* 1988;9(3):190.

234. Scurry J, Watkins A, Acton C, Drew J. Tachyarrhythmia, cardiac rhabdomyomata and fetal hydrops in a premature infant with tuberous sclerosis. *J Paediatr Child Health* 1992;28(3):260–262.

235. Azancot-Benisty A, Jacqz-Aigrain E, Guirgis NM, Decrepy A, Oury JF, Blot P. Clinical and pharmacologic study of fetal supraventricular tachyarrhythmias. *J Pediatr* 1992;121(4):608–613.

236. Wren C, Hunter S. Maternal administration of flecainide to terminate and suppress fetal tachycardia. *Br Heart J* 1988;296:249.

237. Vautier-Rit S, Dufour P, Vaksmann G, Subtil D, Vaast P, et al. [Fetal arrhythmias: diagnosis, prognosis, treatment; apropos of 33 cases]. *Gynecol Obstet Fertil* 2000;28(10):729–737.

238. van Engelen AD, Weijtens O, Brenner JI, Kleinman CS, Copel JA, et al. Management outcome and follow-up of fetal tachycardia. *J Am Coll Cardiol* 1994;24(5):1371–1375.

239. Allan LD, Chita SK, Sharland GK, Maxwell D, Priestley K. Flecainide in the treatment of fetal tachycardias. *Br Heart J* 1991;65:46–48.

240. Darwiche A, Vanlieferinghen P, Lemery D, Paire M, Lusson JR. [Amiodarone and fetal supraventricular tachycardia. Apropos of a case with neonatal hypothyroidism]. *Arch Fr Pediatr* 1992;49(8):729–731.

241. Flack NJ, Zosmer N, Bennett PR, Vaughan J, Fish NM. Amiodarone given by three routes to terminate fetal atrial flutter associated with severe hydrops. *Obstet Gynecol* 1993;82(4 Pt 2 Suppl):714–716.

242. Gembruch U, Manz M, Bald R, et al. Repeated intravascular treatment with amiodarone in a fetus with refractory supraventricular tachycardia and hydrops fetalis. *Am Heart J* 1989;118:1335–1338.

243. Laurent M, Betremieux P, Biron Y, et al. Neonatal hypothyroidism after treatment by amiodarone during pregnancy. *Am J Cardiol* 1987;60:942.

244. Meijboom EJ, van Engelen AD, van de Beek EW, Weijtens O, Lautenschutz JM, Benatar AA. Fetal arrhythmias. *Curr Opin Cardiol* 1994;9(1):97–102.

245. Magee LA, Downar E, Sermer M, et al. Pregnancy outcome after gestational exposure to amiodarone in Canada. *Am J Obstet Gynecol* 1995;172(4 Pt 1):1307–1311.

246. Wladimiroff JW, Stewart PA. Treatment of fetal cardiac arrhythmias. *Br J Hosp Med* 1985;34(3):134–140.

247. Lisowski LA, Verheijen PM, Benatar AA, Soyeur DJ, Stoutenbeek P, et al. Atrial flutter in the perinatal age group: diagnosis, management and outcome. *J Am Coll Cardiol* 2000;35(3):771–777.

248. Meden H, Neeb U. Transplacental cardioversion of fetal supraventricular tachycardia using sotalol. *Zeitschrift Geburtshilfe Perinatol* 1990;194(4):182–184.

249. Leiria TL, Lima GG, Dillenburg RF, Zielinsky P. Fetal tachyarrhythmia with 1:1 atrioventricular conduction. Adenosine infusion in the umbilical vein as a diagnostic test. *Arq Bras Cardiol* 2000;75(1):65–68.

250. Kohl T, Tercanli S, Kececioglu D, Holzgreve W. Direct fetal administration of adenosine for the termination of incessant supraventricular tachycardia. *Obstet Gynecol* 1995;85(5 Pt 2):873–874.

251. Dangel JH, Roszkowski T, Bieganowska K, Kubicka K, Ganowicz J. Adenosine triphosphate for cardioversion of supraventricular tachycardia in two hydropic fetuses. *Fetal Diagn Ther* 2000;15(6):326–330.

252. Holmgren S, Ansved P, Selbing A, Larsson H. [A case report: fetal tachycardia—umbilical vein injection of adenosine restored the sinus rhythm]. *Lakartidningen* 1998;95(44):4857–4859.

253. Maeda FL, Shimokawa H, Nakano H. Effects of intrauterine treatment on nonimmunologic hydrops fetalis. *Fetal Ther* 1988;3(4):198–209.

254. Weiner CP, Thompson MB. Direct treatment of fetal supraventricular tachycardia after failed transplacental therapy. *Am J Obstet Gynecol* 1988;158:570–573.

255. Given BD, Phillippe M, Sanders SP, Dzau VJ. Procainamide cardioversion of fetal supraventricular tachyarrhythmia. *Am J Cardiol* 1984;53(10):1460–1461.

256. Dumesic DA, Silverman NH, Tobias S, Golbus MS. Transplacental cardioversion of fetal supraventricular tachycardia with procainamide. *N Engl J Med* 1982;307(18):1128–1131.

257. Owen J, Colvin EV, Davis RO. Fetal death after successful cardioversion of fetal supraventricular tachycardia with digoxin and verapamil. *Am J Obstet Gynecol* 1988;158:1169–1170.

258. Assad RS, Aiello VD, Jatene MB, et al. Cryosurgical ablation of fetal atrioventricular node: new model to treat fetal malignant tachyarrhythmias. *Ann Thorac Surg* 1995;60(6 Suppl):S629–S632.

259. Fernandez C, De Rosa GE, Guevara E, Velazquez H, Pueyrredon HR, et al. Reversion by vagal reflex of a fetal paroxysmal atrial tachycardia detected by echocardiography. *Am J Obstet Gynecol* 1988;159(4):860–861.

260. McCue CM, Mantakes ME, Tingelstad JB, et al. Congenital heart block in newborns of mothers with connective tissue disease. *Circulation* 1977;56:82.

261. Hull D, Binns BAO, Joyce D. Congenital heart block and widespread fibrosis due to maternal lupus erythematosus. *Arch Dis Child* 1966;41:688.

262. Machado MV, Tynan MJ, Curry PV, Allan LD. Fetal complete heart block. *Br Heart J* 1988;60(6):512–515.

263. Groves AM, Allan LD, Rosenthal E. Outcome of isolated congenital complete heart block diagnosed in utero. *Heart* 1996;75(2):190–194.

264. Groves AM, Allan LD, Rosenthal E. Therapeutic trial of sympathomimetics in three cases of complete heart block in the fetus. *Circulation* 1995;92(12):3394–3396.

265. Carpenter RJ Jr, Strasburger JF, Garson A Jr, Smith RT, Deter RL, Engelhardt HT Jr. Fetal ventricular pacing for hydrops secondary to complete atrioventricular block. *J Am Coll Cardiol* 1986;8(6):1434–1436.

266. Scagliotti D, Shimokochi DD, Pringle KC. Permanent cardiac pacemaker implant in the fetal lamb. *PACE* 1987;10:1253–1261.

267. Walkinshaw SA, Welch CR, McCormack J, Walsh K. In utero pacing for fetal congenital heart block. *Fetal Diag Ther* 1994;9(3):183–185.

268. Crombleholme TM, Harrison MR, Longaker MT, et al. Complete heart block in fetal lambs, 1. Technique and acute physiological response. *J Pediatr Surg* 1990;25(6):587–593.

269. Murotsuki J, Okamura K, Watanabe T, Kimura Y, Yajima A. Production of complete heart block and utero cardiac pacing in fetal lambs. *J Obstet Gynaecol* 1995;21(3):233–239.

270. Chua S, Ostman-Smith I, Sellars S, Redman CWG. Congenital heart block with hydrops fetalis treated with high-dose dexamethasone. *Eur J Obstet Gynecol Reprod Biol* 1991;42:155–158.

271. Buyon JP, Swersky SH, Fox HE, Bierman FZ, Winchester RJ. Intrauterine therapy for presumptive fetal myocarditis with acquired heart block due to systemic lupus erythematosus. Experience in a mother with a predominance of SS-B (La) antibodies. *Arthritis Rheum* 1987;30(1):44–49.

272. Carreira PE, Gutierrez-Larraya F, Gomez-Reino JJ. Successful intrauterine therapy with dexamethasone for fetal myocarditis and heart block in a woman with systemic lupus erythematosus. *J Rheumatol* 1993;20(7):1204–1207.

273. Buyon JP, Waltuck J, Kleinman C, Copel J. In utero identification and therapy of congenital heart block. *Lupus* 1995;4(2):116–121.

274. Copel JA, Buyon JP, Kleinman CS. Successful in utero therapy of fetal heart block. *Am J Obstet Gynecol* 1995;173(5):1384–1390.

275. Rosenthal D, Druzin M, Chin C, Dubin A. A new therapeutic approach to the fetus with congenital complete heart block: preemptive, targeted therapy with dexamethasone. *Obstet Gynecol* 1998;92(4 Pt 2):689–691.

276. Yamada H, Kato EH, Ebina Y, Moriwaki M, Yamamoto R, et al. Fetal treatment of congenital heart block ascribed to anti-SSA antibody: case reports with observation of cardiohemodynamics and review of the literature. *Am J Reprod Immunol* 1999;42(4):226–232.

277. Arroyave CM, Puente Ledezma F, Montiel Amoroso G, Martinez Garcia AC. [Myocardiopathy diagnosed in utero in a mother with SS-A antibodies treated with plasmapheresis]. *Ginecol Obstet Mex* 1995;63:134–137.

278. Eronen M. Outcome of fetuses with heart disease diagnosed in utero. *Arch Dis Child Fetal Neonatal Ed* 1997;77(1):F41–F46.

279. Udink ten Cate FE, Breur JM, Cohen MI, Boramanand N, Kapusta L, et al. Dilated cardiomyopathy in isolated congenital complete atrioventricular block: early and long-term risk in children. *J Am Coll Cardiol* 2001;37(4):1129–1134.

VENTRAL WALL DEFECTS

Ventral wall defects represent a common group of fetal anomalies, occurring in 1 in 2,000 live births. In conjunction with widespread maternal alpha-fetoprotein (AFP) screening, prenatal sonographic detection of ventral wall defects is now routine.[1–3] When detected before fetal viability (approximately 24 menstrual weeks), knowledge of a ventral wall defect gives the prospective parents the opportunity to make important decisions regarding the pregnancy.

Because excellent results can be expected following surgical correction of an isolated ventral wall defect, parents may choose to continue the pregnancy when the defect represents gastroschisis or an omphalocele that is not associated with concurrent anomalies or chromosome abnormalities. On the other hand, pregnancy termination may be elected when the defect is a complex malformation or when additional anomalies are present. These diverse options emphasize the importance of establishing the correct diagnosis and identifying major concurrent anomalies when a ventral wall defect is detected prenatally. Detection of ventral wall defects is also important in preparation for a planned delivery, so that pediatricians and surgeons can be notified and prompt treatment can be accomplished after birth.

The pathogenesis, typical pathologic and sonographic findings, associated anomalies, and prognosis for both common and less common types of ventral wall defects are discussed in this chapter. Sonographic findings that are considered to be of diagnostic or prognostic importance are emphasized. A discussion of embryogenesis and a general sonographic approach to ventral wall defects precedes the discussion of individual malformations.

EMBRYOGENESIS

Development of the anterior ventral wall occurs as the embryo folds in both cranial-caudal and lateral directions, changing the flat trilaminar embryonic disc into its curvilinear embryonic shape. With development of the cranial fold at the end of the third fetal week (menstrual week 5), the heart and pericardial cavity come to lie on the ventral surface of the embryo[4] (Fig. 1). The heart is later incorporated into the central chest, with development of the lateral folds in the thoracic region. The heart is intimately connected with the septum transversum, which will form the central tendon of the diaphragm.[4] As the primitive heart elongates and bends, it gradually invaginates into the pericardial cavity.

Lateral body walls (somatopleures) fold the sides of the embryo medially, changing the previously flattened embryonic disc to a roughly cylindrical form.[4] As the lateral and ventral wall forms, part of the yolk sac is incorporated into the embryo as the midgut. Concurrently, the connection of the midgut with the yolk sac is reduced to a narrow yolk stalk, and there is relative constriction at the umbilicus. Coalescence of the body stalk with the yolk stalk forms the umbilical cord at 5 to 6 fetal weeks (7 to 8 menstrual weeks). As the umbilical cord forms, ventral fusion of the lateral folds reduces the region of communication between the intraembryonic and extraembryonic coeloms to a narrow communication that persists until approximately the tenth fetal week (twelfth menstrual week). Rapid expansion of the amniotic cavity obliterates the extraembryonic coelom and forms the epithelial covering for the umbilical cord.

At approximately 6 fetal weeks (8 menstrual weeks), rapid elongation of the midgut forms a midgut loop that herniates into the base of the umbilical cord[4] (Fig. 2). This physiologic bowel migration occurs because of the lack of intraabdominal space, which is filled primarily by the relatively large liver and kidneys. Within the umbilical cord, the midgut loop rotates 90 degrees counterclockwise around the axis of the superior mesenteric artery. During the tenth fetal week (twelfth menstrual week), the intestines return rapidly to the abdomen. As the large intestines return, they undergo a further 180-degree counterclockwise rotation.

A false-positive diagnosis of ventral wall defect is possible between 6 and 12 weeks when the rapidly elongating midgut normally herniates into the base of the body stalk (umbilical cord) as part of normal gut migration[5–7] (Figs. 3 and 4). Because this embryologic process can be readily observed sonographically, in many fetuses a reliable diagnosis of certain types of ventral wall defects (gastroschisis and bowel-containing omphaloceles) may not be possible before 12 menstrual weeks.

However, a number of findings can aid in distinguishing between the normal midgut migration of the first trimester

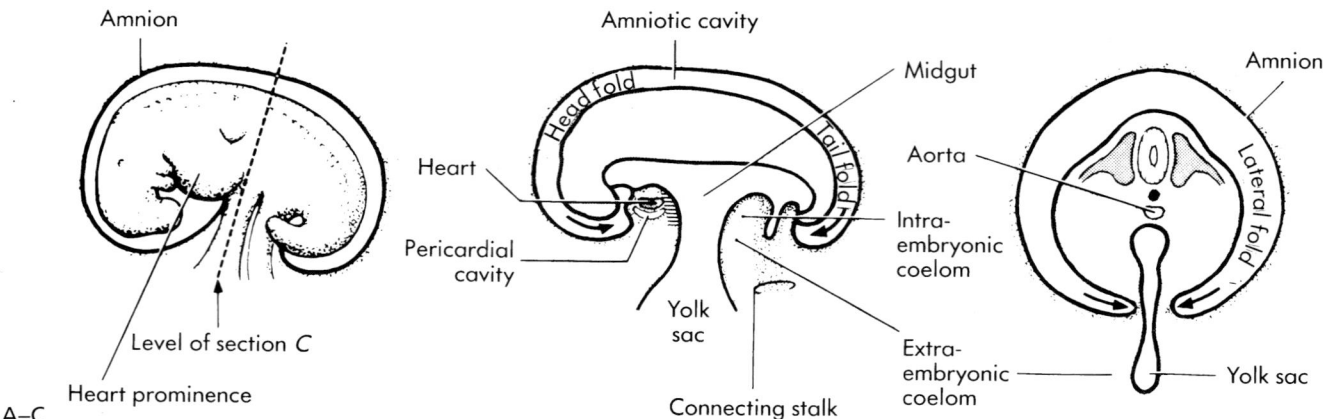

FIGURE 1. Normal embryologic development at 40 menstrual days (26 postconceptual days) demonstrates normal folding of the embryo. **A:** Lateral view of the embryo. **B:** A longitudinal section shows head and tail folds. The heart and pericardium lie on the ventral surface of the embryo. Further folding incorporates the heart into the central chest. **C:** A transverse section at the level shown in **A** illustrates the lateral folds. (Reproduced with permission from Moore KL. *The developing human*, 4th ed. Philadelphia: WB Saunders, 1988.)

and a pathologic ventral wall defect. The size of the herniated area can serve as an important sign, particularly when compared with the fetus' crown-rump length (CRL).[8–10] In the normal fetus, the maximum diameter of the midgut hernia-

tion increases in an approximately linear fashion from a diameter of 4 mm at a CRL of 19 mm to a diameter of 7 mm at a CRL of 41 mm.[8] Moreover, an anterior ventral wall mass that is equal in size or larger than the fetal abdomen, or

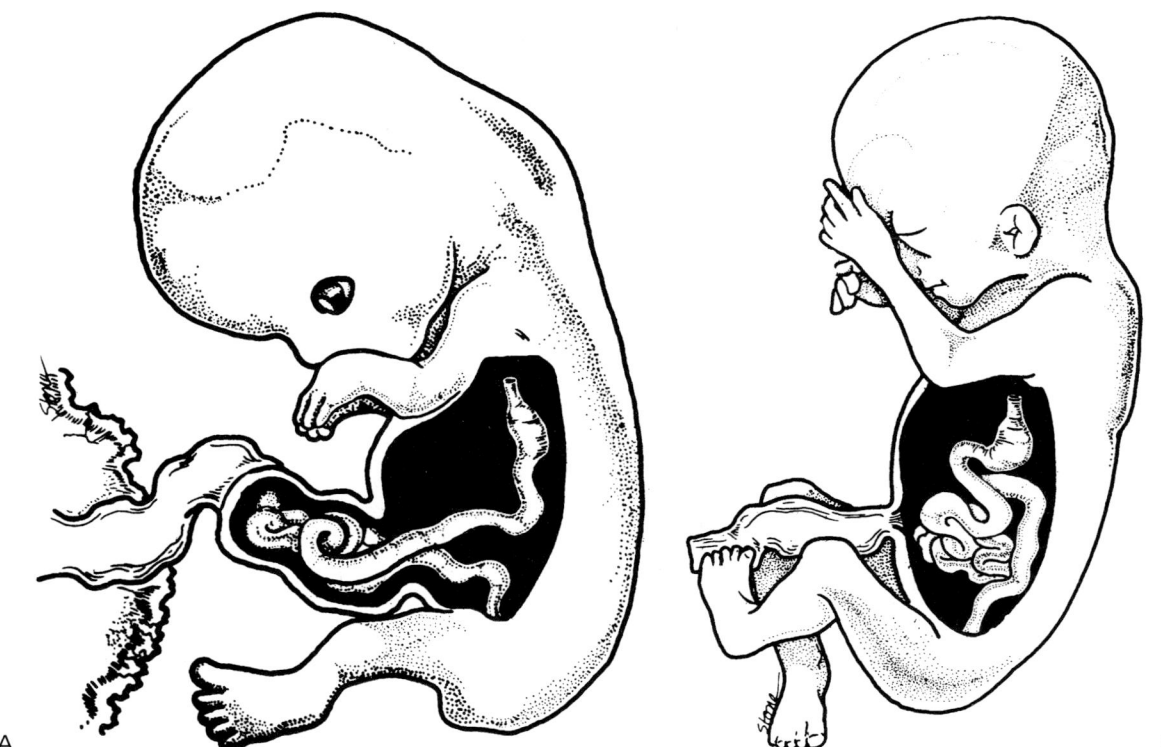

FIGURE 2. Normal gut migration. **A:** The midgut is positioned at the base of the umbilical cord during normal gut migration from 8 to 12 weeks (6 to 10 weeks postconception). **B:** The gut returns to the abdominal cavity by 12 menstrual weeks. (Reproduced with permission from Cyr DR, Mack LA, Schoenecker SA, Patten RM, Shepard TH, et al. Bowel migration in the normal fetus: US detection. *Radiology* 1986;161:119–121.)

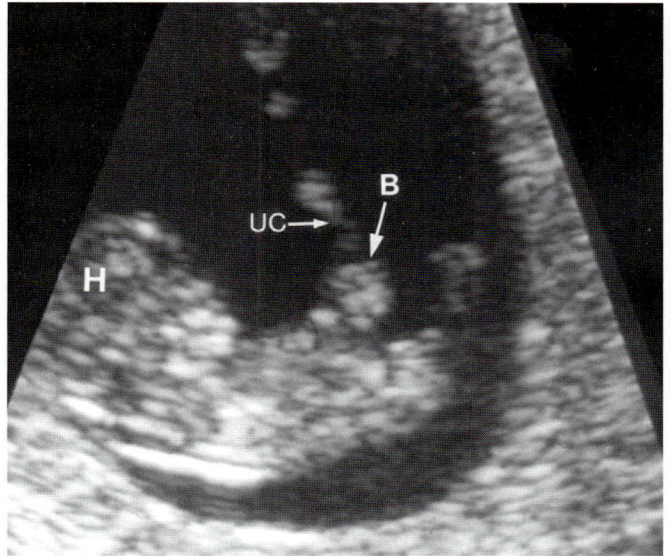

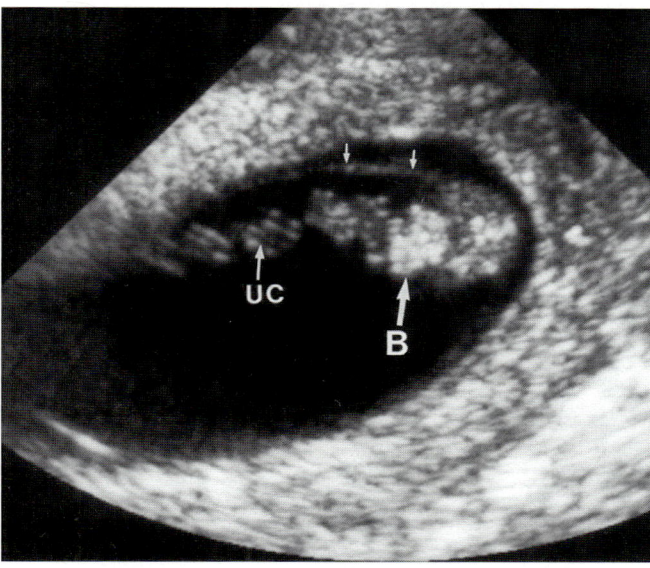

FIGURE 3. Normal gut migration. Longitudinal **(A)** and transverse **(B)** sonograms show echogenic bowel (*B*) herniated into the base of the umbilical cord (*UC*) at 9.5 menstrual weeks. The small arrows indicate amnion. H, head. (Reproduced with permission from Nyberg DA, Hill LM, Bohm-Velez M, Mendelson EB, eds. *Transvaginal ultrasound*. St. Louis: Mosby–Year Book, 1992:136.)

that measures more than 7 mm at any CRL, suggests a pathologic process.[8] Likewise, an early diagnosis may be possible in some fetuses with gastroschisis if a normal umbilical cord insertion can be depicted distinct from the exteriorized bowel loops.[11,12] Even so, definitive distinction between physiologic and pathologic gut herniation is not always possible, and when the herniated contents approach or exceed the maximum size limits a follow-up sonogram should be performed in the early second trimester.[13]

Delayed return of bowel to the abdomen can also serve as a sign of potential fetal abnormality, even when the bowel eventually completes its migration back to the abdomen and the anterior ventral wall is intact at follow-up sonography. For example, one report described a fetus who had persistent bowel herniation at 13 menstrual weeks but a normal-appearing, intact anterior ventral wall at 15 weeks, and who subsequently developed volvulus, bowel obstruction, and small bowel gangrene.[14]

SONOGRAPHIC APPROACH TO VENTRAL WALL DEFECTS

Because ventral wall defects occur early in embryologic development, it is theoretically possible to detect all major defects before the age of viability. In actual practice, small ventral wall defects may be missed during routine obstetric scanning. This emphasizes the importance of routine views of the anterior ventral wall and umbilical cord insertion site (Fig. 5), as recommended by the guidelines adopted by the American Institute of Ultrasound in Medicine (see Chapter 1). Routine views of the urinary bladder and pelvis should also permit improved prenatal diagnosis of bladder and cloacal exstrophy.

Once a ventral wall defect is identified, it is important to categorize correctly the type of malformation (Tables 1 and 2). Accurate prenatal diagnosis of ventral wall defects affects patient management and prognosis.[15] Gastroschisis and omphalocele are the two most common types of ventral wall defects, reported with nearly equal frequency in 1

FIGURE 4. Three-dimensional ultrasound, rendered mode, at 10 menstrual weeks, shows a bulge at the base of the umbilical cord (*UC*) that represents normal physiologic bowel herniation.

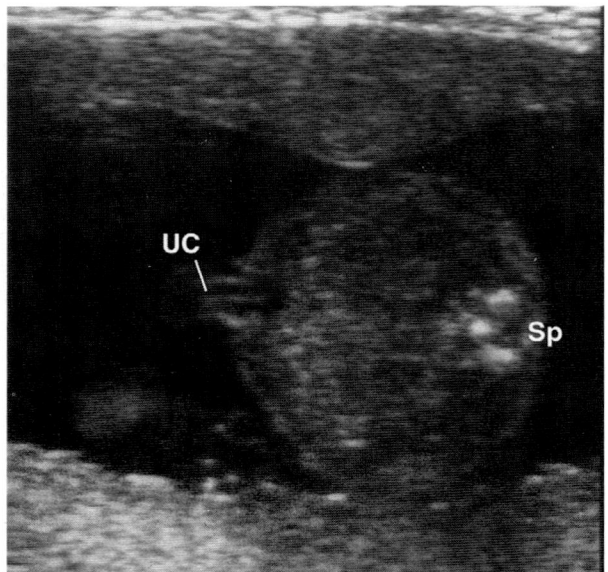

FIGURE 5. Normal cord insertion at 17 weeks; normal anterior abdominal wall. A transverse view of the abdomen shows normal insertion of the umbilical cord (*UC*) into the anterior abdominal wall. This normal appearance excludes the vast majority of anterior abdominal wall defects. Sp, spine.

TABLE 1. TYPES OF VENTRAL WALL DEFECTS

Gastroschisis
Omphalocele
    With extracorporeal liver
    With intracorporeal liver
Pentalogy of Cantrell
Cleft or absent sternum
Ectopia cordis
Bladder exstrophy
Cloacal exstrophy
Limb-body wall complex or amniotic band syndrome

in 4,000 live births. Antenatal distinction between omphalocele and gastroschisis is important because these two disorders differ markedly in their typical pathologic findings, frequency of associated malformations, and prognosis. The sonographic findings are also distinctive enough that a reliable diagnosis is possible in most cases.[16,17]

As an aid in distinguishing gastroschisis from omphalocele, we suggest answering a series of questions whenever a ventral wall defect is suspected. This approach should also permit recognition of less common, but more complex, types of ventral wall defects including ectopia cordis, blad-

TABLE 2. TYPICAL FEATURES OF VENTRAL WALL DEFECTS AND ASSOCIATED CONDITIONS

Type of defect	Description	Sonographic features	Other anomalies
Gastroschisis	Paraumbilical defect	Typically, only bowel is eviscerated; occasionally other organs but almost never the liver	Associated anomalies are uncommon; little to no risk of aneuploidy; high rate of bowel-related complications
Omphalocele	Midline defect, contained by membrane	Variable in appearance	High risk of other anomalies and/or aneuploidy
Extracorporeal liver	—	Typically large	When isolated without other detectable anomalies, risk of aneuploidy is very low; however, high rate of cardiac anomalies
Intracorporeal liver	—	Typically small	>50% risk of aneuploidy when detected prenatally
Beckwith-Wiedemann syndrome	Syndromic condition (see Chapter 5)	Macroglossia; omphalocele; visceromegaly	Omphalocele is typically intracorporeal liver type
Pentalogy of Cantrell	(1) Omphalocele, (2) anterior diaphragmatic hernia, (3) distal partial sternal defect, (4) pericardial defect, and (5) cardiac defect	May appear only as high omphalocele; pleural effusion, even transient, is highly suggestive of diaphragmatic hernia in this situation	—
Absent sternum	Absent sternum	Dynamic heart covered by skin	Rare; usually isolated
Ectopic cordis	Thoracic defect of sternum and skin	Dynamic heart not covered by skin	Rare; high rate of cardiac and other defects; may be associated with high omphalocele
Bladder exstrophy	Eviscerated urinary bladder	Nonvisualization of urinary bladder; soft-tissue mass of anterior abdominal wall may be subtle	Increased risk of fetal aneuploidy
Cloacal exstrophy	Eviscerated cloaca with two hemibladders	Nonvisualization of urinary bladder; in one variation, ileal prolapse produces "elephant trunk" appearance	Severe, complex anomaly
Limb-body wall complex	Multiple anomaly condition (see Chapter 5)	Bizarre, complex defect with ventral wall defect, close attachment to placenta, cranial defects, scoliosis	100% lethal, but no risk of aneuploidy

der and cloacal exstrophy, amniotic band syndrome, and the limb-body wall complex (LBWC). Although occasional exceptions invariably occur, this approach should permit correct categorization of nearly all ventral wall defects.

1. Is a limiting membrane present? Omphalocele is always covered by a "membrane" comprising the peritoneum and the outer layer of the umbilical cord (amnion). In contrast, gastroschisis is characterized by a through-and-through defect not limited by a membrane.[18,19] Sonographic identification of the membrane may actually be easier than clinical evaluation because the membrane may rupture during delivery but only rarely ruptures *in utero*.[20,21] Rupture of an omphalocele during delivery may explain why instances of chromosome abnormalities (trisomy 13 or 18) or externalized liver occasionally have been reported in neonatal series of "gastroschisis" but not in prenatal series.[22,23] Umbilical hernia can be distinguished from omphalocele because it is covered by skin and subcutaneous fat.

2. What is the relation of the umbilical cord to the defect? The ventral wall defect of omphalocele is located at the umbilical cord insertion site, whereas the defect of gastroschisis is paraumbilical in location. Bladder and cloacal exstrophy defects are infraumbilical, and the defect of ectopia cordis is located cephalad to the umbilical cord insertion. The defect and membranes of LBWC are intimately connected with the umbilical cord.

3. Which organs are eviscerated? Eviscerated liver usually represents an omphalocele, although other complex defects (LBWC, pentalogy of Cantrell, and cloacal exstrophy) should also be considered. Eviscerated bowel alone usually represents gastroschisis but may also be seen with an omphalocele that contains only bowel (intracorporeal liver). Eviscerated bowel may also be seen with LBWC and cloacal exstrophy.

4. Is the bowel normal in appearance? Near term, fetuses with gastroschisis commonly demonstrate mild bowel dilatation and bowel wall thickening, reflecting a chemical peritonitis caused by prolonged exposure of bowel to urine in the amniotic fluid.[24] In contrast, the bowel in an omphalocele sac does not become directly exposed to amniotic fluid and therefore demonstrates a more normal appearance. Marked bowel dilatation indicates an increased likelihood of intestinal complications such as atresia or bowel infarction, which frequently complicate gastroschisis but rarely are associated with omphalocele.

5. Are additional malformations present? Omphalocele is commonly associated with concurrent malformations (50% to 70%) and chromosome abnormalities (30% to 40%), whereas other anomalies are rarely demonstrated with gastroschisis.[25] An omphalocele seen in conjunction with severe scoliosis should suggest the diagnosis of LBWC, and an omphalocele associated with a nondetectable urinary bladder should suggest the possibility of cloacal exstrophy. Demonstration of other random defects (e.g., facial cleft, encephalocele) in combination with "gastroschisis" should suggest the amniotic band syndrome.

VENTRAL WALL MALFORMATIONS

Gastroschisis

Gastroschisis is a periumbilical defect nearly always located to the right of the umbilicus.

Incidence

The incidence of gastroschisis is approximately 1 in 3,000 births. However, this varies considerably with maternal age, with a strong association reported among younger women.[26,27] The reported incidence of gastroschisis has also increased.[28] This trend is thought to reflect both a greater recognition of gastroschisis and a real increase in affected fetuses.[23,29–31]

Embryology and Pathology

Gastroschisis is a relatively small (2- to 4-cm) defect involving all layers of the ventral wall (Fig. 6). The defect is nearly always located just to the right of the umbilicus, although left-sided defects have been rarely described.[32,33] The most widely accepted etiology of gastroschisis, proposed by DeVries,[34] suggests that the defect results from abnormal involution of the right umbilical vein, which normally occurs 28 to 33 days postconception (42 to 47 menstrual days). Other authors[35] suggest that the defect is caused by disruption of the omphalomesenteric artery.

Gastroschisis has been associated with substance abuse, especially when more than one type of recreational drug was used.[36,37] Various medications have also been associated with gastroschisis, including cyclooxygenase inhibitors (aspirin, salicylates, and ibuprofen) and decongestants (pseudoephedrine and phenylpropanolamine).[38,39] These agents are known to be vasoactive, supporting a vascular origin for the pathogenesis of gastroschisis.

Diagnosis

The majority of fetuses with gastroschisis are now detected before 24 weeks with serum AFP screening and a targeted sonogram (Figs. 7 and 8). Because eviscerated organs of gastroschisis come into direct contact with the amniotic fluid, AFP levels of gastroschisis tend to be higher than those associated with omphalocele.[2] Gastroschisis, and to a lesser extent omphalocele, occurs with increased incidence when the amniotic fluid acetylcholinesterase band is positive.[40,41]

The sonographic diagnosis of gastroschisis is highly reliable when the following characteristic findings are demonstrated: (a) the full-thickness ventral wall defect is located

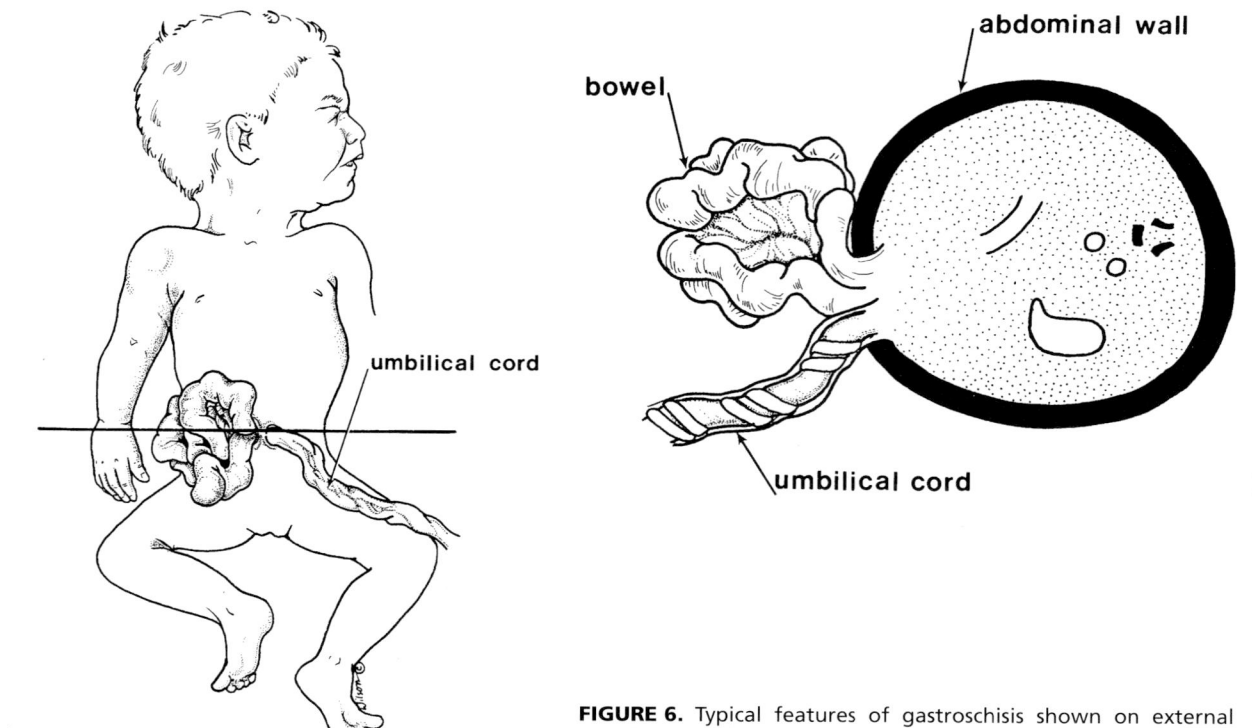

FIGURE 6. Typical features of gastroschisis shown on external examination **(A)** and on cross-sectional view **(B)**.

just to the right of a normal umbilical cord insertion site, and (b) a variable amount of bowel protrudes through the defect and floats in the surrounding amniotic fluid. The eviscerated bowel may appear disproportionately large relative to the abdominal cavity; yet the defect itself is often small, usually measuring less than 2 cm.[18] The abdominal cavity may be reduced in size, depending on the amount of eviscerated bowel.

Evaluation of eviscerated structures alone can usually suggest the correct diagnosis of gastroschisis.[20,42] Small bowel is always eviscerated, often accompanied by large bowel and, occasionally, the stomach or portions of the genitourinary system (Fig. 9). Rare reports have suggested that portions of the liver can also be eviscerated with gastroschisis.[24,43] although this should suggest an alternative diagnosis. In one clinical series,[44] liver was exposed in 3 of

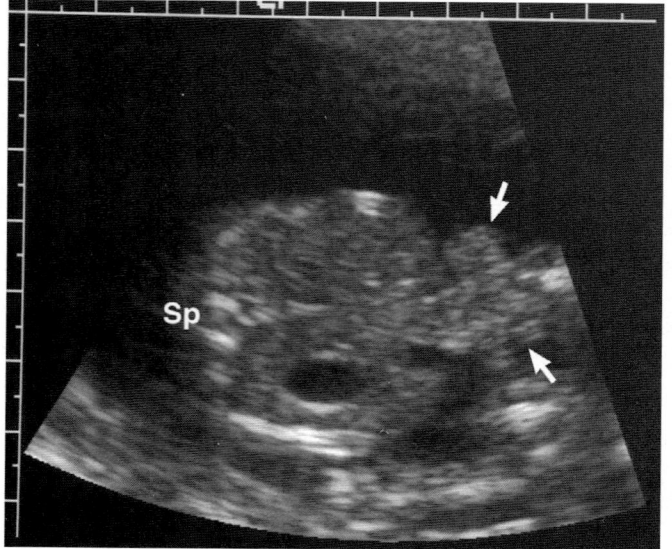

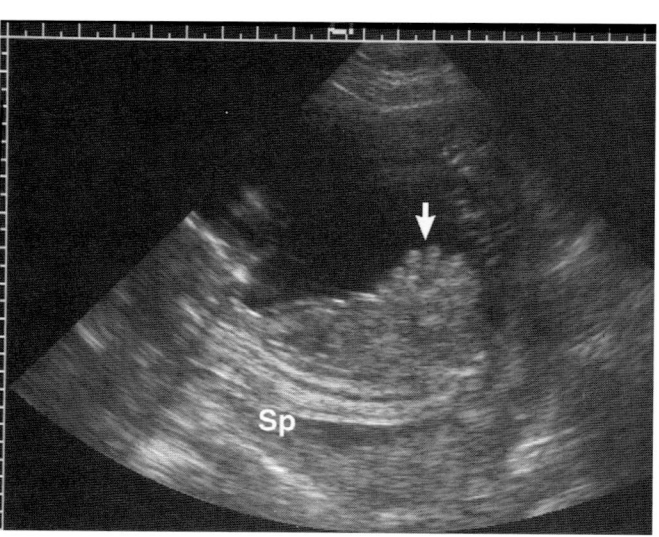

FIGURE 7. Gastroschisis at 16 menstrual weeks. Transverse **(A)** and longitudinal **(B)** scans of the abdomen show eviscerated bowel (*arrows*). The bowel herniates through a small paraumbilical defect, which is nearly always located just to the right of the umbilicus. Sp, spine.

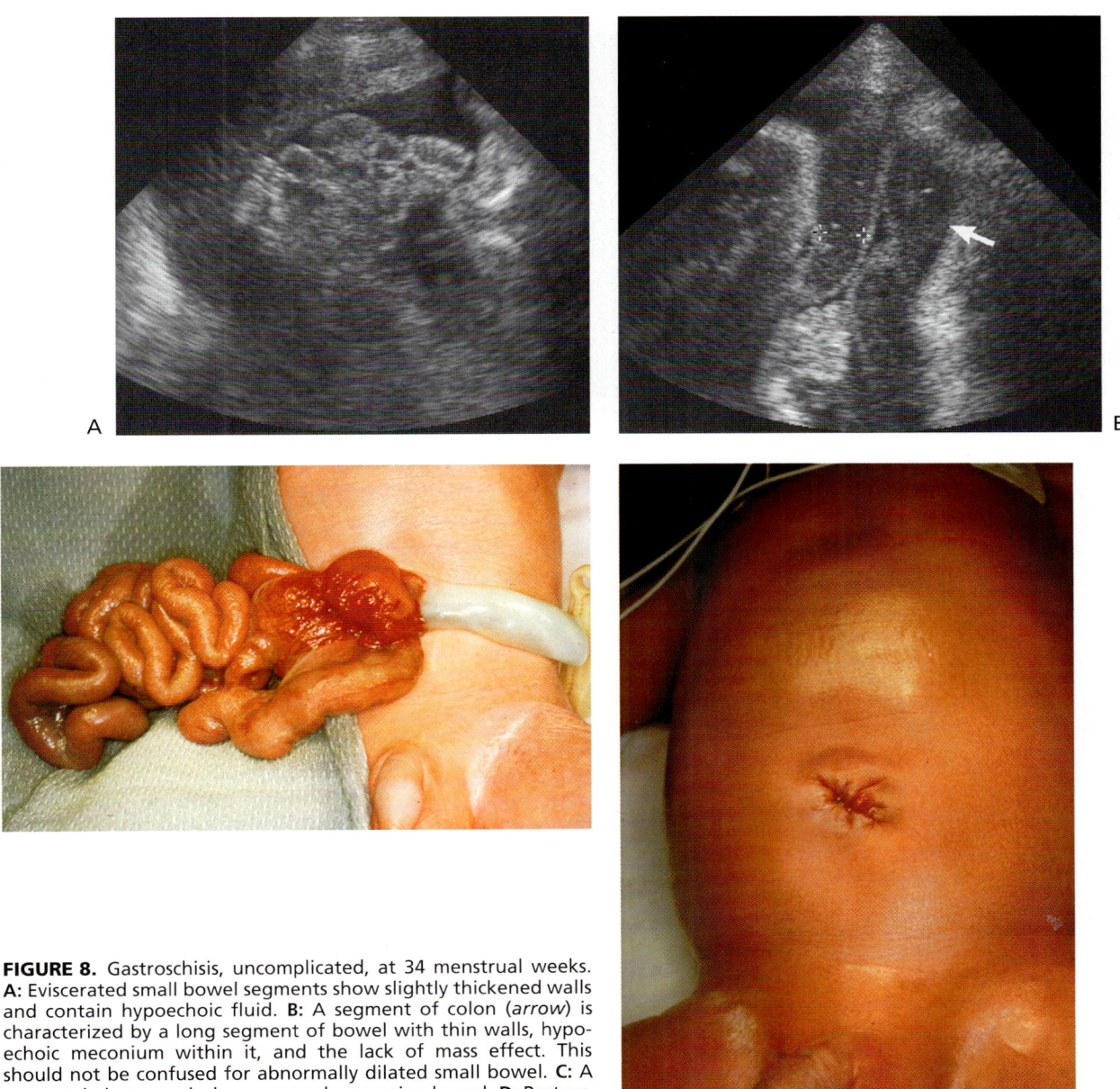

FIGURE 8. Gastroschisis, uncomplicated, at 34 menstrual weeks. **A:** Eviscerated small bowel segments show slightly thickened walls and contain hypoechoic fluid. **B:** A segment of colon (*arrow*) is characterized by a long segment of bowel with thin walls, hypoechoic meconium within it, and the lack of mass effect. This should not be confused for abnormally dilated small bowel. **C:** A postnatal photograph shows normal-appearing bowel. **D:** Postsurgical result.

64 (5%) infants with gastroschisis, whereas most prenatal studies and our own experience suggest that extracorporeal liver is never observed with true gastroschisis.[20]

Near term, eviscerated bowel exposed to amniotic fluid often appears slightly thickened and matted with gastroschisis[24] (Figs. 8 and 10), which corresponds to its appearance at birth, when the bowel is covered by a fibrinous "peel" on its serosal surface and may look edematous and foreshortened. This appearance is thought to result from a chemical peritonitis induced by prolonged exposure of bowel to fetal urine in the amniotic fluid.[45] The peel is the probable cause of the prolonged postoperative ileus experienced by many infants

with gastroschisis, but not by infants with omphalocele. This fibrinous peel usually resolves by 4 weeks after birth.[46]

Complications of bowel atresia, perforation, and meconium peritonitis can be identified by ultrasound[47,48] (Fig. 11). In some cases, eviscerated bowel segments may become matted near the umbilicus and hyperechoic. This may accompany progressive intraabdominal bowel dilation and associated polyhydramnios. These cases indicate high bowel obstruction, atresia, and poor neonatal outcome. Occasionally, abnormal bowel segments can be identified during the second trimester, suggesting that the atresia occurs early and may not be avoidable.

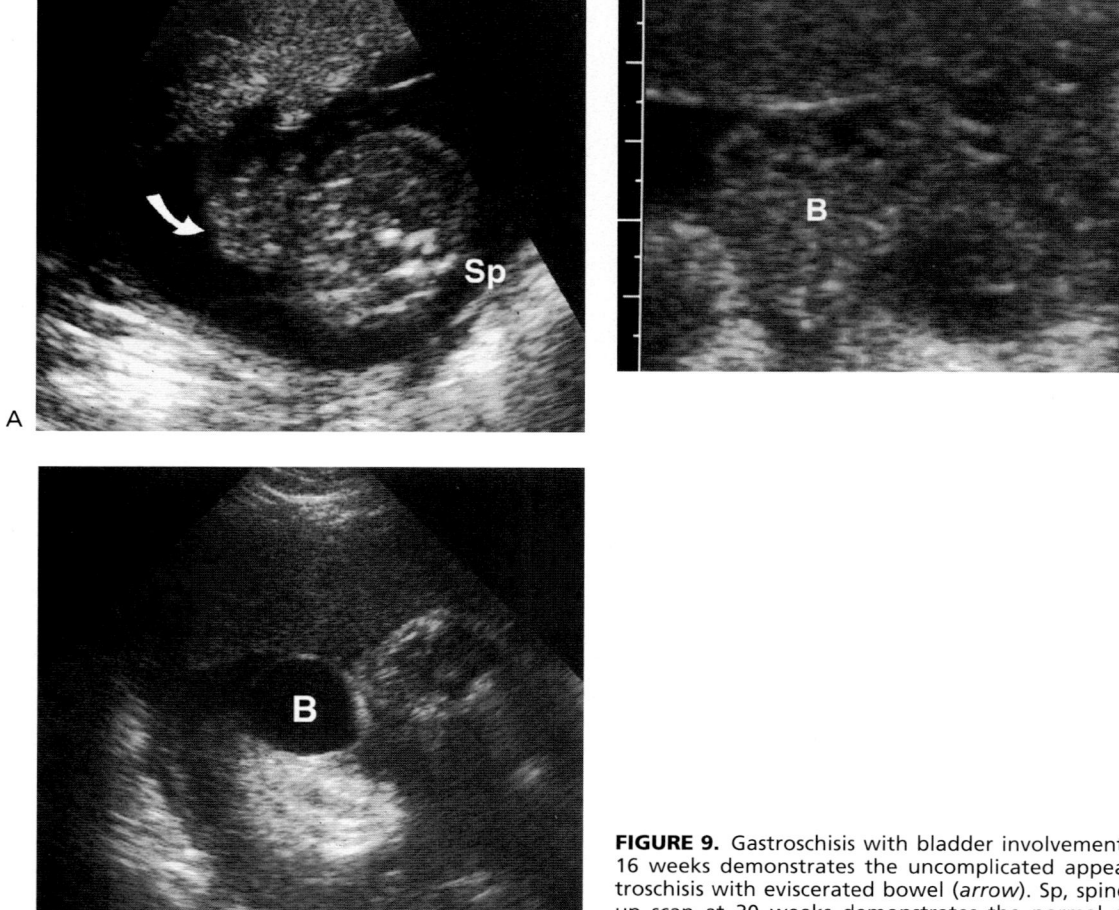

FIGURE 9. Gastroschisis with bladder involvement. **A:** A scan at 16 weeks demonstrates the uncomplicated appearance of gastroschisis with eviscerated bowel (*arrow*). Sp, spine. **B:** A follow-up scan at 30 weeks demonstrates the normal appearance of bowel (*B*). **C:** A scan of the pelvis shows a cystic structure on the anterior abdominal wall that represents the urinary bladder (*B*).

In severe cases, eviscerated bowel segments of gastroschisis may resorb entirely ("vanishing gut") secondary to bowel necrosis, resulting in bowel atresia and short bowel syndrome.[49–53] Reported cases have had a very tight defect with secondary vascular ischemia.[52,53] In some cases, the defect may even close entirely, so that at birth an infant with bowel atresia or the short-bowel syndrome has no obvious defect.

Mild dilatation of both the small and large bowel is commonly seen when eviscerated bowel is exposed to amniotic fluid and is unlikely to be of prognostic importance. In contrast, abnormally dilated bowel segments show long segments of dilated small bowel, thickened and sometimes irregular walls, and overall greater mass effect. A number of studies suggest that this appearance correlates with the bowel complications at birth.[54–63] For example, Bond et al.[54] reported that 4 of 11 fetuses with gastroschisis demonstrated bowel dilatation and wall nodularity, and all four infants showed complications of necrosis, atresias, or matted bowel after birth. Langer et al.[59] noted that fetuses with bowel dilatation of 18 mm or more took a significantly longer time to reach oral feeding and were more likely to require bowel resection. Adra et al.[63] observed that dilated bowel was significantly more likely to show bowel edema at birth, require a longer operative time, and have a higher rate of postoperative complications. Another study by Abuhamad et al.[64] found that bowel dilatation was also associated with adverse outcome, but this study suggests that bowel diameter of more than 10 mm between 28 and 32 weeks may be the best predictor of poor neonatal outcome.

Not all authors have found that intestinal dilatation predicts neonatal outcome in fetuses with gastroschisis.[65] However, in assessing eviscerated bowel segments, it is important to distinguish the colon from small bowel because it is significantly more dilated than small bowel as a normal finding.

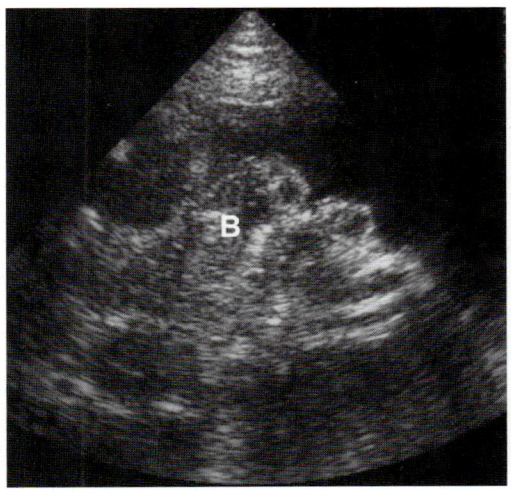
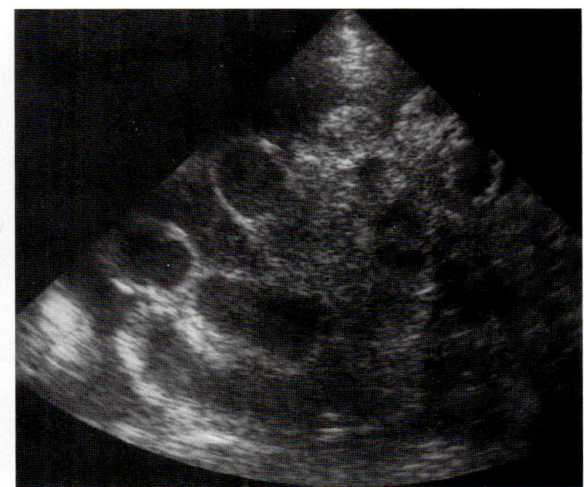

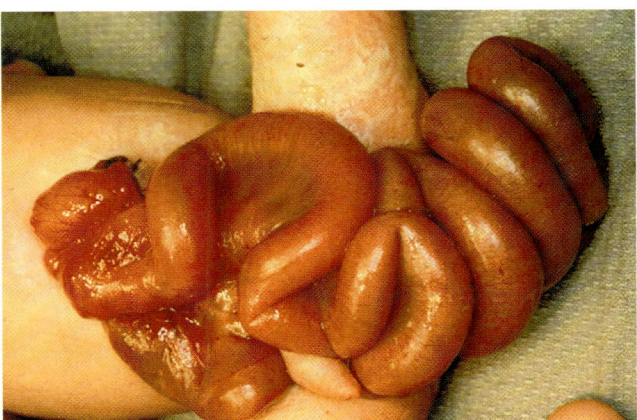

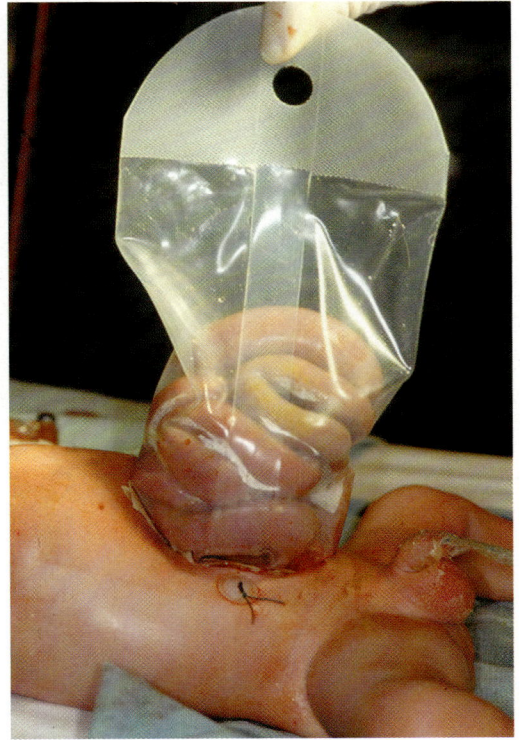

FIGURE 10. Gastroschisis with bowel peel. **A:** A scan at 28 weeks demonstrates the uncomplicated appearance of bowel (*B*). **B:** In a follow-up scan 1 month later, small bowel segments are dilated (2 cm), and the bowel wall appears thicker. **C:** A photograph at delivery shows mildly dilated bowel segments with thickened serosal layer, or "peel." This required secondary closure. **D:** A silo chimney keeps the bowel sterile and protected while gradually pushing bowel segments into the abdominal cavity. The defect was successfully closed by 2 weeks of age.

Eviscerated colon can be identified as a bowel segment that contains meconium and shows a thin outer wall, no peristalsis, and no significant mass effect (Fig. 8B).

Doppler velocimetry of the superior mesenteric artery and its branches has not been found to be predictive of outcome in fetuses with gastroschisis.[64]

Amniotic fluid is usually normal with gastroschisis but may be decreased. Oligohydramnios was observed in 36% of cases in one study.[66] Oligohydramnios probably correlates with fetal distress and may be associated with a higher rate of bowel complications. Polyhydramnios has been reported in the minority of cases of gastroschisis. When present, polyhydramnios should suggest the possibility of bowel obstruction or atresia. Fetuses with gastroschisis are prone to intrauterine growth restriction (IUGR).[22,66–70] The mean birth weight is 2,400 to 2,500 g with a mean age of 36 to 37 weeks at birth.[71–73] Term babies born with gastroschisis are more likely to be growth retarded compared with premature babies, suggesting that normal growth depends on a normally functioning gastrointestinal tract.[74] Ultrasound may underestimate fetal size because of small abdominal circumference related to the gastroschisis. In one series, IUGR was predicted in 43% of infants but was present in only 23%.[70]

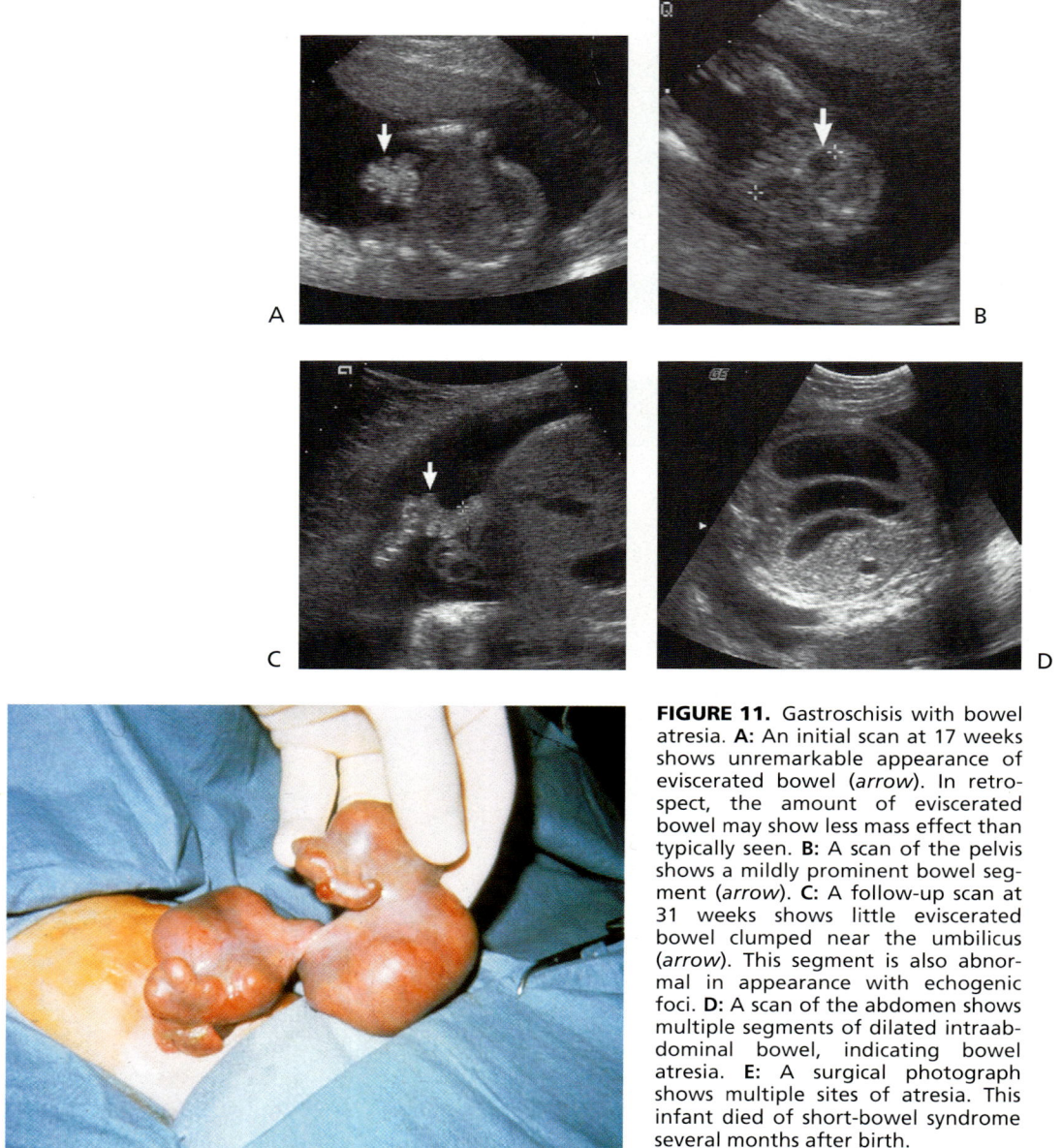

FIGURE 11. Gastroschisis with bowel atresia. **A:** An initial scan at 17 weeks shows unremarkable appearance of eviscerated bowel (*arrow*). In retrospect, the amount of eviscerated bowel may show less mass effect than typically seen. **B:** A scan of the pelvis shows a mildly prominent bowel segment (*arrow*). **C:** A follow-up scan at 31 weeks shows little eviscerated bowel clumped near the umbilicus (*arrow*). This segment is also abnormal in appearance with echogenic foci. **D:** A scan of the abdomen shows multiple segments of dilated intraabdominal bowel, indicating bowel atresia. **E:** A surgical photograph shows multiple sites of atresia. This infant died of short-bowel syndrome several months after birth.

Magnetic resonance imaging can provide an overall perspective of fetuses with ventral wall defects, including gastroschisis[75] (Fig. 12), and may be useful in cases that are difficult to image with ultrasound.

Differential Diagnosis

When only bowel is eviscerated, other types of ventral wall defects should be considered including a bowel-containing omphalocele, LBWC, and cloacal exstrophy. Omphalocele can be distinguished by its characteristic location at the base of the umbilical cord and the presence of a limiting membrane. LBWC usually demonstrates eviscerated liver, cranial and extremity defects, and scoliosis. Cloacal exstrophy is an infraumbilical defect associated with nonvisualization of the urinary bladder.

Associated Anomalies

Bowel-related abnormalities are the most common and the most clinically important complications related to gastroschisis.[18,44,48,54,55,76] By definition, the small bowel in gastroschisis is nonrotated and lacks secondary fixation to the dorsal ventral wall. Intestinal atresia or stenosis is found in 7% to 30% of fetuses secondary to intestinal and mesenteric ischemia that develops during embryologic develop-

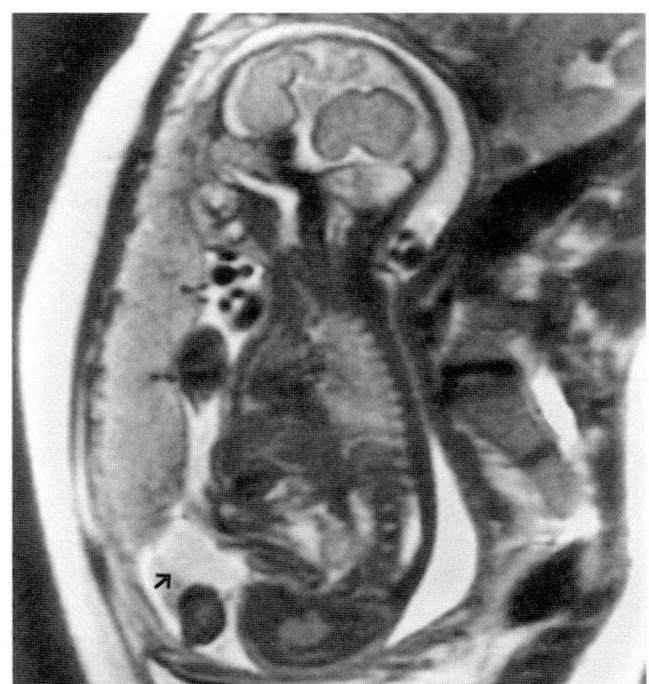 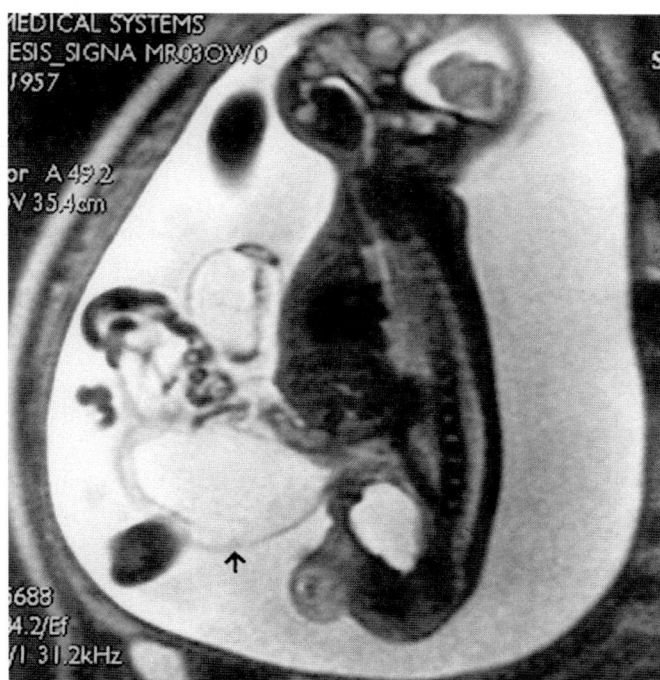

A

B

FIGURE 12. Gastroschisis in a 28-week-old fetus. **A:** A sagittal single-shot fast spin-echo magnetic resonance image shows a midline abdominal wall defect and prolapse of a bowel loop (*arrow*) into the amniotic fluid. **B:** A follow-up sagittal magnetic resonance image obtained 3 weeks later shows progressive change in the bowel prolapse; the markedly dilated small bowel loops are clearly identified (*arrow*). Polyhydramnios has increased in volume. [Reproduced with permission from Shinmoto H, Kashima K, Yuasa Y, Tanimoto A, Morikawa Y, et al. MR imaging of non-CNS fetal abnormalities: a pictorial essay. *Radiographics* 2000;20(5):1227–1243.]

ment. Ischemia may result either from compression of the mesenteric vessels by the relatively small ventral wall defect or from torsion of the eviscerated bowel around the mesenteric axis.[22,44] Ischemia may also cause bowel perforations and meconium peritonitis. The importance of bowel ischemia to the clinical outcome of gastroschisis is emphasized by two large neonatal series in which one-half of the 23 infants with gastroschisis who presented with ischemia or gangrene subsequently died.[22,44]

Most reports indicate that anomalies other than bowel abnormalities occur infrequently with gastroschisis. In a series of 41 cases of gastroschisis detected prenatally, Boyd et al.[77] reported other anomalies in two (5%). Cardiovascular malformations have been reported in up to 8% of fetuses with gastroschisis, but these tend to be minor and are not usually demonstrated on sonography.[23,46] An association between amyoplasia (a form of arthrogryposis) and gastroschisis has been noted, and this suggests vascular compromise as the etiology for this condition.[78] No association with gastroschisis and aneuploidy has been established.

Prognosis

The mortality rate for gastroschisis has significantly improved since the 1970s.[25,77,79–83] The mortality rate

for surgical series is now 10% or less, but for prenatally diagnosed cases, the mortality rate may be 15% or more.[66,76,77,82,83] Improved survival can be attributed to improved perinatal management, including fetal monitoring, use of total parenteral nutrition, and improved surgical technique. The major causes of neonatal death today are prematurity, sepsis, and intestinal complications related to bowel ischemia.[46] Risk factors for sepsis are low gestational age and development of necrotizing enterocolitis.[71]

Fetuses with gastroschisis are at significant risk of fetal distress, observed in 43% of cases in one study.[84] Oligohydramnios is probably related to development of fetal distress and may also be related to bowel complications. However, IUGR alone may not be a risk factor for adverse outcome.[85] Bowel dilatation may also be a nonspecific marker of fetal distress rather than bowel complications.[83]

Approximately 10% to 20% of infants with gastroschisis have bowel complications, including intestinal atresia, stenosis, necrosis, and perforation. Proximal atresias may be difficult to repair or exteriorize and may be repaired later, whereas distal atresias are often complicated by perforation or infarction and may benefit from early enterostomy.[86] Infants with bowel atresia are more likely to require prolonged parenteral nutrition and hospitalization.[87] Delayed complications, particularly obstruction, are more likely to develop in infants with bowel atresia and infants who require small bowel resection during the neonatal period.[77,78,88]

Fetuses with gastroschisis also appear to be at risk for developmental or neurologic abnormalities. Boyd et al.[77] observed that 12% of survivors had long-term developmental problems, and Burge and Ade-Ajayi[84] noted abnormal neurologic outcome in 10.5% (6 of 57), including two newborns who died of perinatal brain injury. Seizures and cerebral palsy were also observed. Fetal monitoring may lower the rate of these complications.

Management

The vast majority of fetuses with gastroschisis are now detected before 24 weeks with serum AFP screening and targeted sonograms. Chromosomal analysis is not necessary after sonographic identification of gastroschisis, but it can be performed if the diagnosis is in doubt or if amniocentesis is performed for other reasons. In-depth patient counseling should include discussions with a pediatric surgeon.

Assuming the pregnancy is continued, serial sonograms are performed to evaluate fetal growth and well-being and to detect possible bowel complications.[89] Close antenatal surveillance of fetal well-being is recommended in the third trimester.[66,83,84]

Both experimental and limited clinical evidence suggests that amnioinfusion may improve the outcome of gastroschisis.[90–93] In a series of ten fetuses with gastroschisis who underwent amnioinfusion, Luton et al.[93] showed a shorter delay before full oral feeding (49.7 ± 21.5 days vs. 72.3 ± 56.6 days) and a shorter overall length of hospitalization (59.5 ± 19.7 days vs. 88.5 ± 73.6 days), although these differences were not statistically significant. The potential beneficial effect of amnioinfusion is presumably related to dilution of the inflammatory exudate that characterizes the amniotic fluid of fetuses with gastroschisis.[94] This potential therapeutic option merits further study.

Patients carrying a fetus with gastroschisis are delivered at, or near, a referral center staffed by experienced pediatric surgeons to facilitate prompt surgical correction of the abdominal defect.[95] The optimal mode of delivery remains controversial, largely because of a lack of large prospective randomized trials comparing outcomes of vaginal and cesarean deliveries.[96] Some authorities recommend elective cesarean delivery to reduce the risk of bowel trauma, contamination, and the bowel "peel" before onset of labor.[87–100] Dunn et al.[101] found that infants born vaginally were more likely to require silo staged repair than those delivered by cesarean section and tended to have a longer hospital stay (53 days vs. 39 days, *p* = .19). Moore et al.[100] reported a 6.4-fold reduction in the occurrence of gastroschisis complications (3% vs. 19%) and complete elimination of the

disabling peel when cesarean delivery is performed before the onset of labor. Others, however, have questioned the value of cesarean delivery to the eventual outcome.[102,103]

Preterm delivery at 36 weeks (after confirmation of lung maturity) has been suggested to minimize the risk of intrauterine bowel ischemia and possibly to decrease the time of postoperative ileus caused by prolonged exposure of bowel to amniotic fluid. However, others suggest that early delivery be considered only in fetuses in whom fetal distress or bowel complications are suspected, and others suggest a near-term delivery may be beneficial.[104]

Prompt repair and closure of gastroschisis minimizes problems of bacterial contamination, sepsis, hypothermia, and metabolic acidosis. Primary closure of the abdominal wall defect is preferred when the bowel can be returned to the abdominal cavity without producing bowel compromise or excessive abdominal pressure. Primary closure has been associated with better survival rates, reduced risk of sepsis, and a shorter hospital stay.[105] In a series of 90 infants with gastroschisis (98% of whom were diagnosed prenatally), surgery was performed a mean of 5 hours (range, 0.5 to 17.0 hours) after delivery.[106] Primary closure of the abdominal defect was possible in 80% of cases, and a silo was required in the remaining 20%.

When primary repair is performed, it is important not to produce increased intraabdominal pressure or overdistention of the abdomen.[107] Increased intraabdominal pressure may cause intestinal and renal ischemia in addition to respiratory difficulty. Some authorities recommend monitoring of intraabdominal or bladder pressure during operative repair to determine whether staged repair is necessary.[107]

When primary repair is not performed, a silo placement helps protect eviscerated bowel from trauma and infection; definitive surgical repair of the ventral wall defect is performed later. Although a silo placement has been associated with longer time to oral feeding and longer hospital stays, these findings may be related to the underlying condition of the bowel itself. Minkes et al.[108] recommend a novel approach using an initial spring-loaded silo device followed by elective closure for all infants with gastroschisis. This device can be placed at the patient's bedside. Infants treated in this way required fewer days on a ventilator (4 days vs. 6 days, *p* = .03) and had lower peak airway pressures and a lower median hospital charge. The time to tolerate full feedings was 21 days compared with 27 days for those treated with the standard approach of emergent surgical closure.

Infants with gastroschisis universally experience some degree of bowel dysfunction, which requires delayed oral feeding, total parenteral nutrition, and prolonged hospitalization. The median time of parenteral nutrition is in the range of 20 to 23 days, time to full oral feeding is 24 to 30 days, and median hospitalization time is 40 to 42 days.[87,95,106] However, variation among patients is wide. Infants with intestinal atresia require significantly more time to achieve full oral feeding, longer time on parenteral

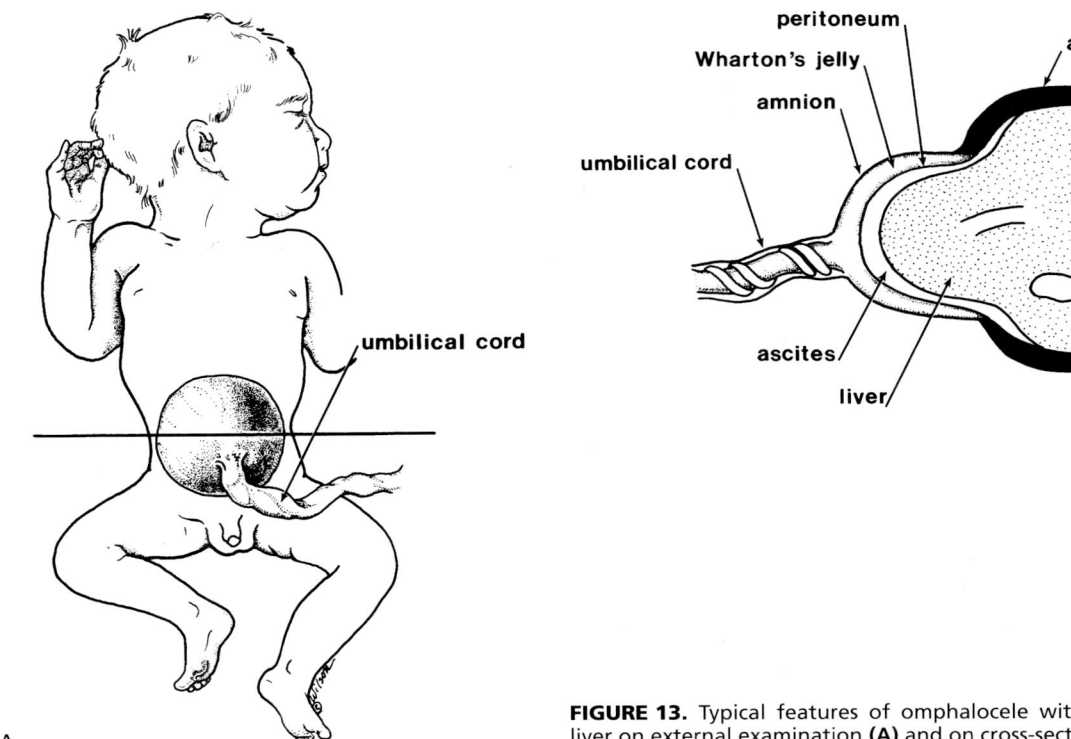

FIGURE 13. Typical features of omphalocele with extracorporeal liver on external examination **(A)** and on cross-sectional view **(B)**.

nutrition, and longer hospitalization stays. Some infants on prolonged parenteral nutrition develop liver abnormalities, and this is a poor prognostic finding.[87]

Recurrence Risk

Gastroschisis is typically sporadic, although occasional familial cases have been reported and there has been one report in a pair of monozygotic twins.[109,110] One study of 127 families suggested a sibling recurrence rate of 3.5%.[109]

Omphalocele

Omphalocele is a central defect involving the umbilicus that is contained in a covering membrane.

Incidence

Omphalocele occurs in 1 in 4,000 births. An increased incidence of omphalocele has been observed with advancing maternal age, and infants born to older mothers are more likely to have an underlying chromosome abnormality.[111]

Embryology and Pathology

Pathologically, omphalocele is characterized by a midline defect of the abdominal muscles, fascia, and skin that

results in herniation of intraabdominal structures into the base of the umbilical cord (Figs. 13 and 14). Eviscerated abdominal structures are limited by a "membrane" that is actually composed of two layers: the peritoneum and amnion. Although rupture of the membrane has been reported in 10% to 20% of omphaloceles in clinical series, this complication only rarely occurs *in utero*.[19–21] The limiting membrane presents a relative barrier to leakage of AFP into the amniotic fluid so that maternal serum AFP levels associated with omphalocele are generally lower and show a broader range than those observed with gastroschisis.[2]

Omphaloceles can be subcategorized pathologically as either (a) those that contain liver within the omphalocele sac, termed *omphaloceles with extracorporeal liver* (Fig. 13); or (b) those that contain a variable amount of bowel but no liver, termed *omphaloceles with intracorporeal liver* (Fig. 14). This categorization is useful because each type produces a distinctive sonographic appearance and has a different prognostic significance (see Prognosis and Chromosomal Abnormalities sections). Furthermore, the embryogenesis of each type is likely to differ.[112] Omphaloceles with intracorporeal liver may simply be considered a persistence of the primitive body stalk beyond 12 menstrual weeks.[4] However, given that the liver is never found outside the abdominal cavity during normal embryologic development, omphaloceles

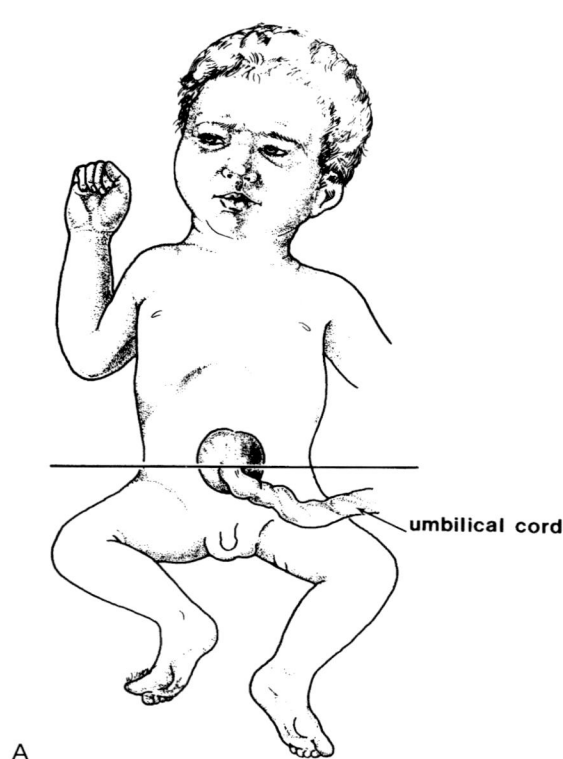

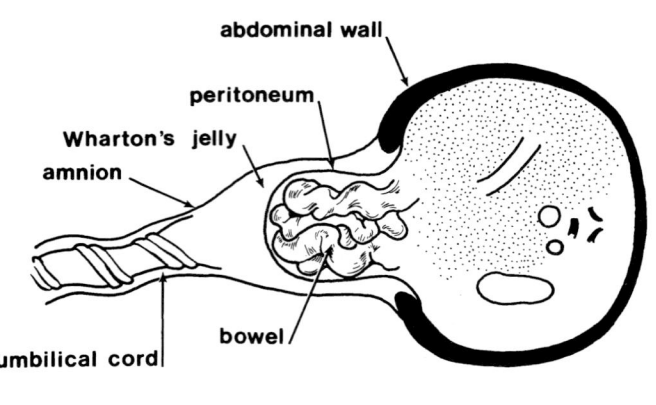

FIGURE 14. Typical features of omphalocele with intracorporeal liver on external examination **(A)** and on cross-sectional view **(B)**.

with extracorporeal liver may result from primary failure of body wall closure.[18,112]

Diagnosis

The ultrasound appearance of omphalocele is variable, depending on the size of the ventral wall defect, type of eviscerated organs, presence of ascites, and associated anomalies.[113,114] Therefore, it is important to keep in mind those features that permit a reliable diagnosis of omphalocele and distinction from gastroschisis. Failure to observe these differences can lead to errors in interpretation and inappropriate management of affected fetuses.[115]

The central location of the ventral wall defect at the base of the umbilical cord insertion site is a primary and diagnostic feature of omphalocele. However, because the umbilical cord inserts into the caudal-apical portion of the herniated sac, the relationship with the umbilical cord may be best visualized on sagittal or oblique scans rather than on transverse views alone. Demonstration of the intrahepatic umbilical vein coursing through the defect is also evidence of the central location of the ventral wall defect.

The presence of a limiting membrane (amnion and peritoneum) is another essential feature of omphalocele. However, the membrane itself may be difficult to visualize as a discrete structure when not outlined by ascites. In this situation, the existence of a membrane is often confirmed by showing that extracorporeal structures appear contained

rather than floating freely in the amniotic fluid. Amorphous material representing Wharton's jelly may also be observed between the amnion and peritoneum.

Ascites is commonly observed with omphalocele, and its presence can provide evidence of a limiting membrane. A large amount of ascites, however, can be confused with amniotic fluid and may lead to an erroneous diagnosis of gastroschisis. As a distinguishing finding, the bowel contained within an omphalocele sac is not directly exposed to amniotic fluid and does not become thickened or dilated.

As noted, omphaloceles differ in appearance depending on the presence or absence of liver from the omphalocele sac. Because the liver is never found outside the abdominal cavity during normal embryologic development,[4] demonstration of extracorporeal liver should permit a reliable diagnosis of omphalocele at any age (Figs. 15 through 18). The liver can usually be identified by its homogeneous appearance and the presence of intrahepatic vessels. Omphaloceles that contain liver typically demonstrate a relatively large ventral wall defect; however, the size of extracorporeal liver and the size of the central defect are highly variable (Figs. 15 through 18).

Some omphaloceles are large enough to be described as "giant" (Fig. 19), although there are no definitive criteria for this term. Omphaloceles can also be assessed with magnetic resonance imaging, although ultrasound should be able to provide the necessary information in most cases.

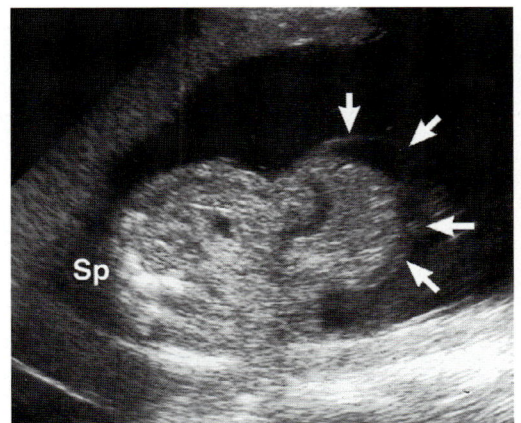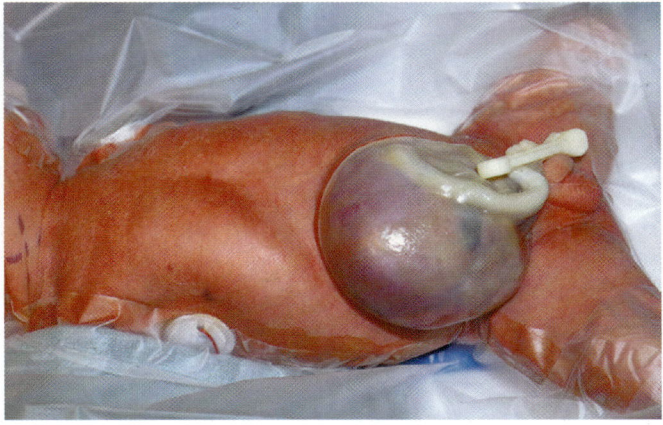

FIGURE 15. Omphalocele, extracorporeal liver. **A:** A transverse scan of the abdomen at 18 weeks shows a moderate-sized omphalocele sac containing liver (extracorporeal liver). The omphalocele sac is central and well contained by the surrounding membrane (*arrows*). Sp, spine. **B:** A photograph at surgery correlates well with prenatal findings. This moderate-sized defect was closed primarily without complications.

Omphaloceles with intracorporeal liver cannot be diagnosed with certainty until after 12 weeks when normal gut migration should be complete. Omphaloceles with intracorporeal liver demonstrate a variable appearance, depending on the amount of bowel present (Figs. 20 through 24). The bowel is characteristically more echogenic and irregular in appearance than the liver and does not contain intrahepatic vessels. This combination of a small midline defect with echogenic eviscerated tissue usually represents omphalocele with intracorporeal liver. However, exceptions occur when a small amount of liver is eviscerated and has the appearance of bowel (Figs. 25 and 26).

Omphaloceles with intracorporeal liver accounted for 50% to 70% of omphaloceles in several large neonatal studies,[19,44] but the minority of omphaloceles in prenatal series (10% to 25%).[20,116] Indeed, this discrepancy is a consistent finding in comparing prenatal and postnatal diagnoses. St-Vil et al.[117] observed that intracorporeal liver accounted for 30% of 50 cases diagnosed prenatally compared with 91% of 33 cases diagnosed only after birth. An

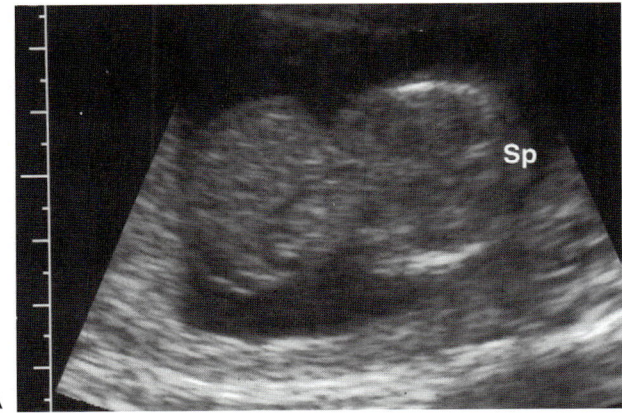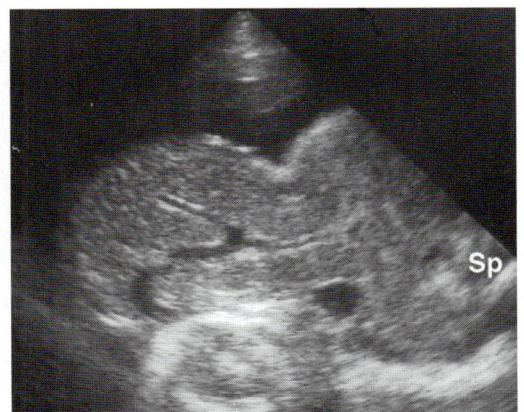

FIGURE 16. Omphalocele. **A:** A transverse scan of the abdomen at 16 weeks shows typical features of omphalocele with extracorporeal liver. The omphalocele sac is larger than the central defect. **B:** In a follow-up scan at 30 weeks, the relative size of the omphalocele sac and defect appears unchanged. Sp, spine.

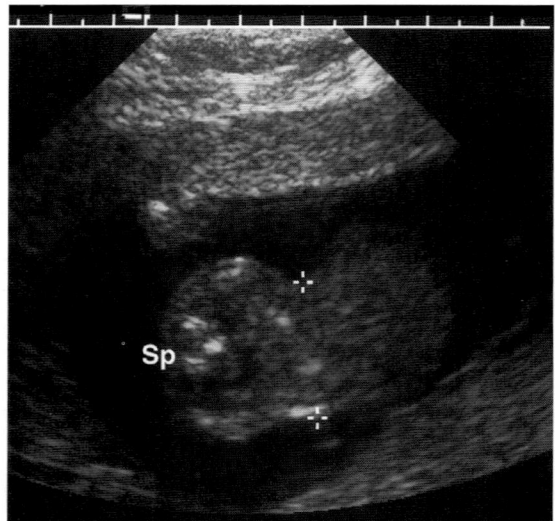
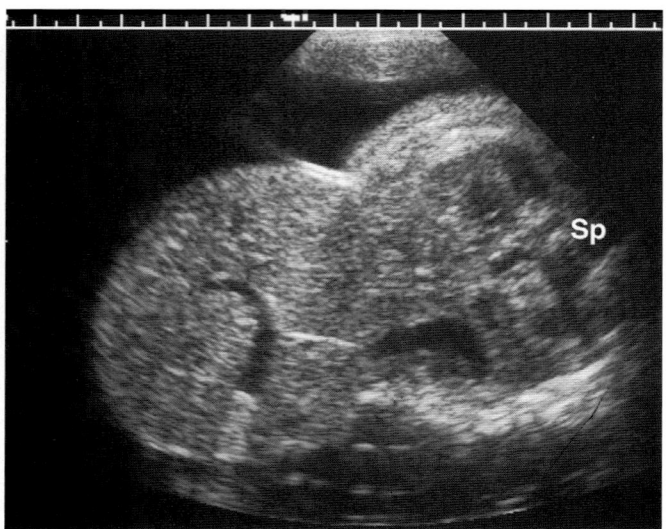

FIGURE 17. Omphalocele. **A:** A transverse scan of the abdomen at 15 weeks shows relatively large omphalocele with extracorporeal liver. The defect is also broad and nearly as large as the omphalocele. **B:** In a follow-up scan at 32 weeks, the relative size of the omphalocele and defect appears unchanged. This required secondary closure. Sp, spine.

obvious explanation is that small omphaloceles with intracorporeal liver are more likely to be missed by prenatal ultrasound or are less likely to present with clinical indications for an ultrasound. Mann et al.[118] reported missing six of seven small omphaloceles that presumably contained only bowel on prenatal sonography.

Just as ventral wall defects can be overdiagnosed, they are also occasionally missed.[119] Careful attention to demonstrating the intactness of the ventral wall and of the umbilical cord insertion into the abdomen is an important part of the routine obstetric ultrasound examination. It is likewise important to accurately identify any freely floating structures in the amniotic fluid.[120] Even large ventral wall defects can be missed when herniated loops of bowel are erroneously thought to represent the umbilical cord.[121]

Polyhydramnios has been noted in approximately one-third of fetuses with an omphalocele.[122] The etiology of polyhydramnios in this setting is not always clear. Nelson et al.[123] suggest that polyhydramnios may indicate the presence of a high gastrointestinal obstruction such as midgut volvulus. However, polyhydramnios might also result from a central nervous system anomaly, such as holoprosencephaly or a major chromosome disorder on the basis of decreased fetal swallowing. Whatever the mechanism, the presence of polyhydramnios may be associated with a worse fetal outcome. In considering 22 fetuses with omphalocele who were not terminated, Hughes et al.[122] observed deaths in seven of eight fetuses (88%) with abnormal amniotic fluid volume (polyhydramnios or oligohydramnios) compared with 3 of 12 fetuses (25%) with normal amniotic fluid volume.

Rarely, a transient omphalocele may be observed in fetuses with intracorporeal liver. In these cases, the bowel does not herniate through the defect until late in gestation or it returns into the abdomen before delivery. Bromley and Benacerraf[124] describe one such case in a fetus with trisomy 18 who showed an omphalocele with intracorporeal liver and other anomalies at 15.5 and 33.0 weeks, but no omphalocele was apparent at autopsy. A second fetus had an umbilical cord cyst and an apparently normal ventral wall umbilical cord insertion at 25 weeks but an omphalocele and multiple anomalies at birth. The latter fetus was subsequently shown to have trisomy 13.

Differential Diagnosis

Because of their variable appearance, omphaloceles can be confused with other types of ventral wall defects. When extracorporeal liver is demonstrated, it is important to distinguish omphalocele from LBWC, a disorder that has been uniformly associated with a fatal outcome. LBWC should be considered whenever marked scoliosis is demonstrated in association with omphalocele. Other typical findings of LBWC include scoliosis, cranial defects, limb defects, abnormal cord attachment to the placental membranes, and ventral wall defect.

Omphaloceles with intracorporeal liver should be distinguished from gastroschisis or umbilical hernia.[38] Gastroschisis can be readily distinguished by the absence of a limiting membrane, absent ascites, and its paraumbilical location.[20,124,125] Distinguishing a small omphalocele from umbilical hernia may be more difficult, however, because both defects are located at the umbilical cord insertion site. The defect of omphalocele is limited only by a membrane,

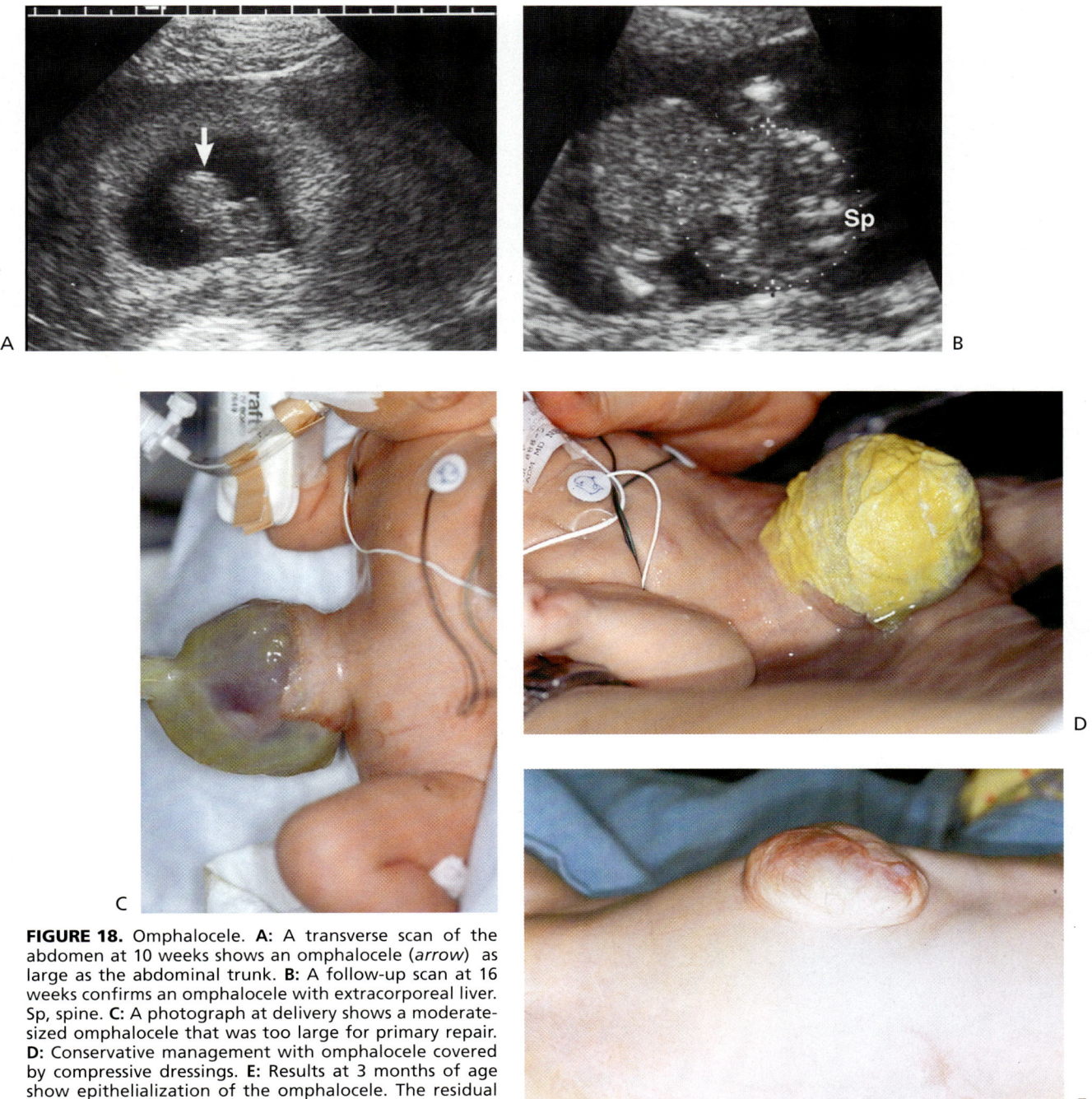

FIGURE 18. Omphalocele. **A:** A transverse scan of the abdomen at 10 weeks shows an omphalocele (*arrow*) as large as the abdominal trunk. **B:** A follow-up scan at 16 weeks confirms an omphalocele with extracorporeal liver. Sp, spine. **C:** A photograph at delivery shows a moderate-sized omphalocele that was too large for primary repair. **D:** Conservative management with omphalocele covered by compressive dressings. **E:** Results at 3 months of age show epithelialization of the omphalocele. The residual defect was then repaired surgically.

whereas the defect of umbilical hernia is covered by skin and subcutaneous fat.

Other complex syndromes that may include omphalocele as a prominent feature should be distinguished from omphalocele alone, if possible. Pentalogy of Cantrell (a cephalic fold defect)[126] is characterized by an omphalocele, anterior diaphragmatic defect, sternal cleft, pericardial defect, and a variety of cardiovascular malformations. Findings other than the omphalocele may be subtle (see Cleft Sternum, Ectopia Cordis, and Pentalogy of Cantrell, later in this chapter). Cloacal exstrophy (a caudal fold defect) consists of a low ventral wall defect associated with bladder or cloacal exstrophy.[18,126] The OEIS complex (*o*mphalocele, *e*xstrophy of the bladder, *i*mperforate anus, and *s*pinal

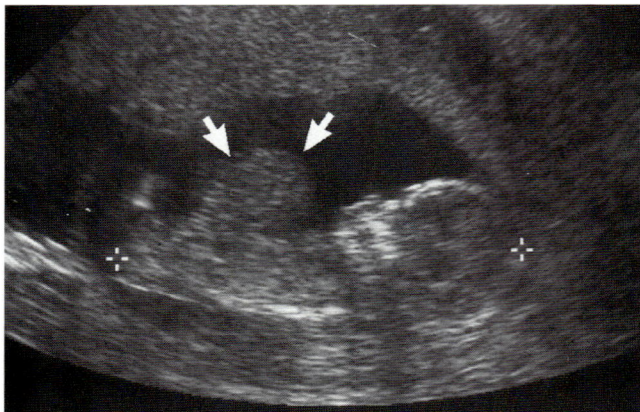

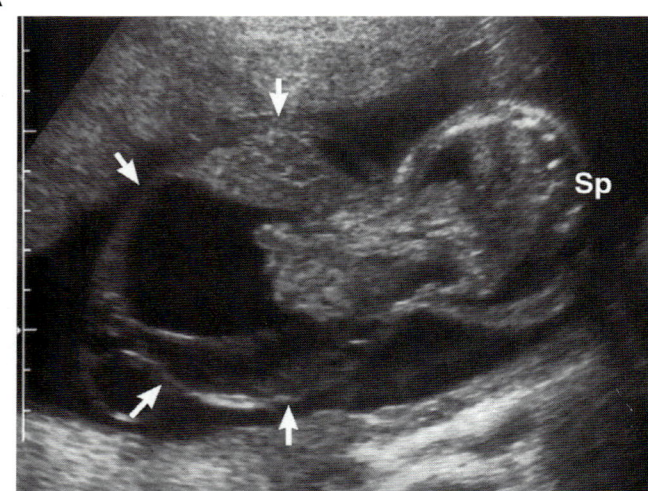

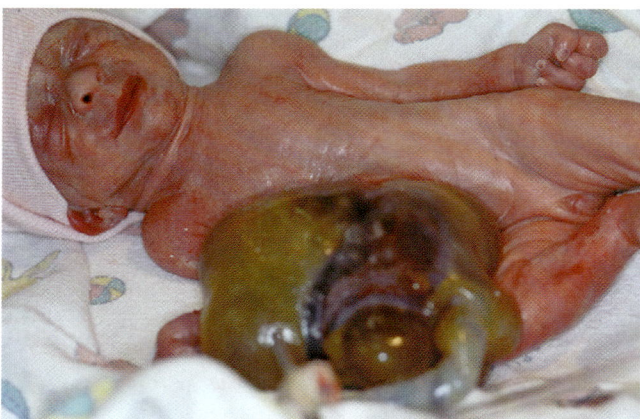

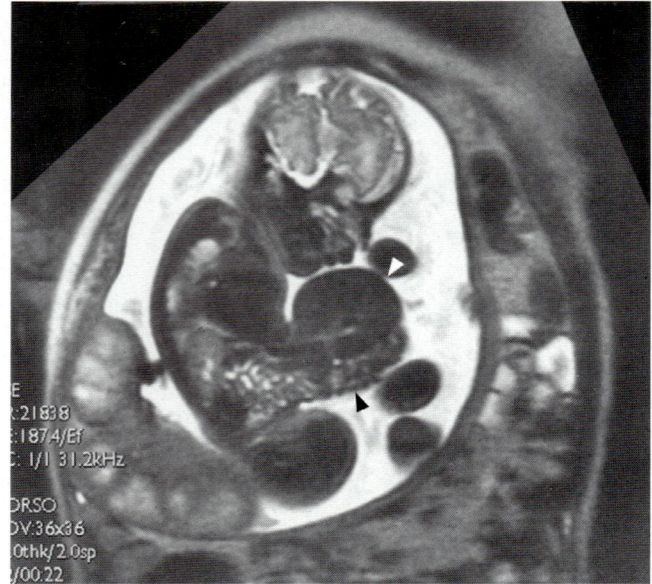

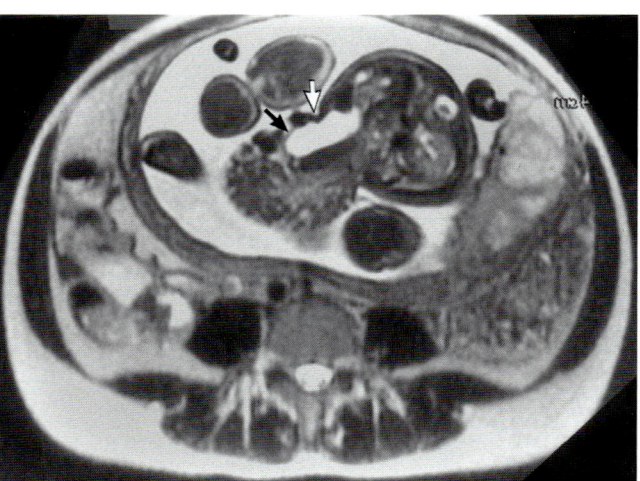

FIGURE 20. Omphalocele with extracorporeal liver at 35 weeks. **A:** A magnetic resonance image shows prolapse of the liver (*white arrowhead*) and small bowel loops (*black arrowhead*) into the omphalocele sac. **B:** An axial image shows prolapse of the stomach (*black arrow*) and colon (*white arrow*). [Reproduced with permission from Shinmoto H, Kashima K, Yuasa Y, Tanimoto A, Morikawa Y, et al. MR imaging of non-CNS fetal abnormalities: a pictorial essay. *Radiographics* 2000;20(5):1227–1243.]

FIGURE 19. Giant omphalocele. **A:** A longitudinal scan of the abdomen at 14 weeks shows an omphalocele containing liver (*arrows*). **B:** A follow-up scan at 22 weeks shows a huge, unusual omphalocele (*arrows*) containing nearly all of the abdominal contents. Sp, spine. **C:** A photograph at delivery shows a large omphalocele that required delayed closure and eventually resulted in demise.

abnormalities) demonstrates other characteristic defects (see Associated Anomalies below). The Miller-Dieker syndrome may show omphalocele with mild ventriculomegaly.

Fluorescent *in situ* hybridization analysis can detect a deletion in 17p13.3 in these cases.[127]

A false-positive diagnosis of omphalocele, or *pseudoomphalocele,* can be produced by scanning in an oblique plane or by compressing the fetal abdomen.[128] This mistake should be readily recognized by experienced sonographers. More often, false-positive diagnoses of omphalocele have been attributed to misidentification of the umbilical cord or of umbilical cord abnormalities such as a thickened umbilical cord, umbilical cord cyst, or urachal cyst.[121,129–131] Doppler evaluation may be helpful in distinguishing the

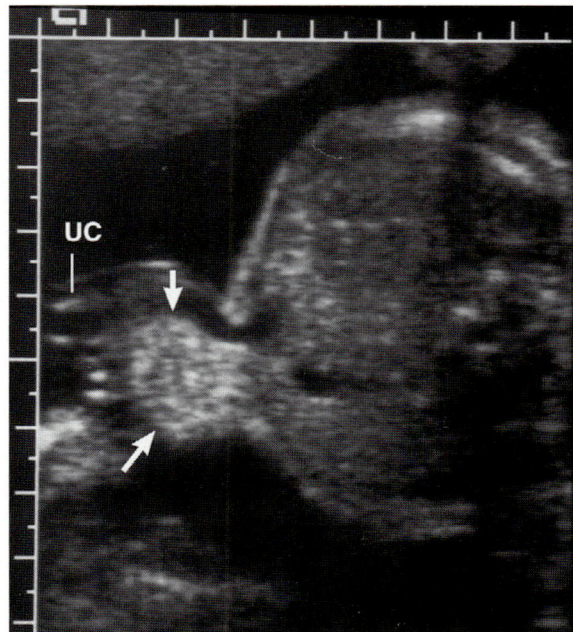

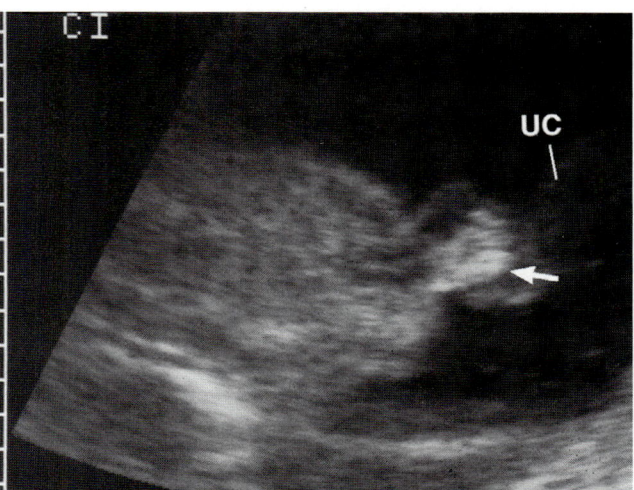

FIGURE 23. Omphalocele with intracorporeal liver, trisomy 21. A transverse scan at 18 weeks shows echogenic bowel (*arrow*) at the base of the umbilical cord (*UC*). No other abnormalities were noted. Fetal karyotype yielded trisomy 21.

FIGURE 21. Omphalocele with intracorporeal liver. A transverse scan shows an omphalocele containing echogenic bowel (*arrows*) at the base of the umbilical cord (*UC*). No other anomalies were present, and the karyotype was normal. This was easily repaired after delivery.

umbilical cord and umbilical cord lesions from an omphalocele. A skin lesion such as a hemangioma arising from the ventral wall can superficially resemble an omphalocele.[132] A skin lesion can be distinguished from a true ventral wall defect by demonstrating the integrity of the ventral wall.

Associated Anomalies

In a series of 732 neonates born with omphalocele, Calzolari et al.[3] reported additional anomalies in 54%. Similar

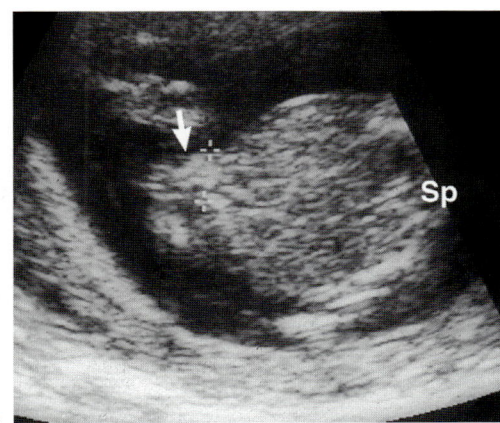

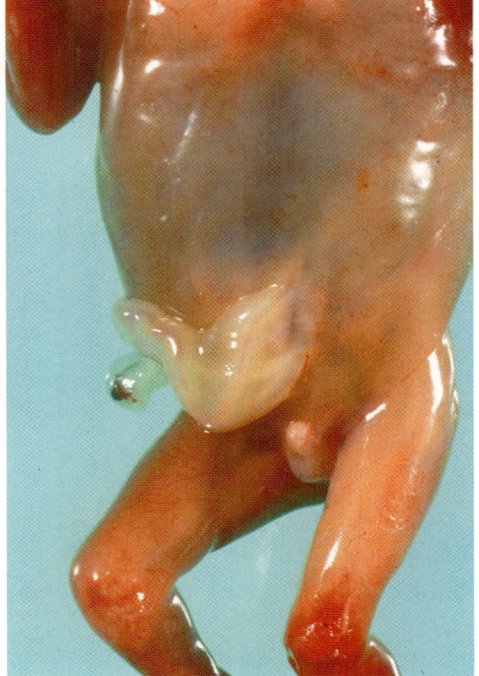

FIGURE 22. Omphalocele with intracorporeal liver, trisomy 18. **A:** A transverse scan at 16 weeks shows a tiny echogenic area that represents bowel (*arrow*) at the base of the umbilical cord. A strawberry-shaped head was also present. Sp, spine. **B:** A postmortem photograph shows a small omphalocele with bowel herniated through a central defect.

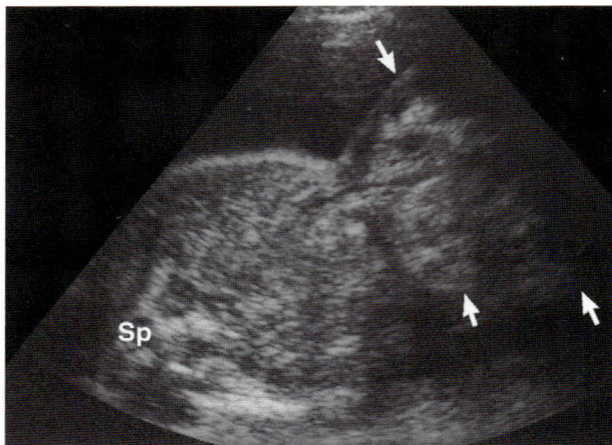

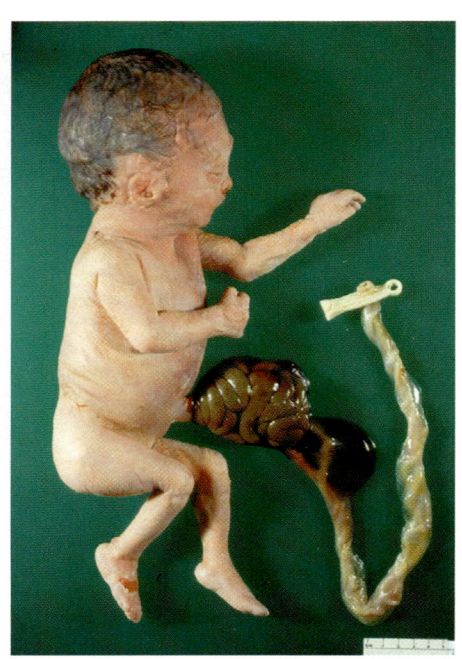

FIGURE 24. Omphalocele with intracorporeal liver, trisomy 18. **A:** A scan at 26 weeks shows an omphalocele containing a relatively large amount of bowel (*arrows*). Multiple other anomalies were identified. Sp, spine. **B:** A postmortem photograph shows an omphalocele containing only bowel. The size of the omphalocele is smaller than noted prenatally, suggesting that bowel could slide in and out of the omphalocele.

rates have been observed in other postnatal studies.[133] A higher frequency of other anomalies has been reported in prenatal studies.[24,66,67,111,121,122,134] Cardiac anomalies are present in 30% to 50% of affected fetuses and are often complex. Central nervous system anomalies occur less frequently, but are easier to detect on prenatal sonography.[122] An association with neural tube defects has been observed.[3] Genitourinary and gastrointestinal malformations are also relatively common.

Compared with gastroschisis, bowel complications are uncommon with omphalocele. This probably reflects both the protective effect of the covering membrane and the larger ventral wall defect, which is less likely to compromise mesenteric blood flow. Duodenal atresia secondary to midgut strangulation by an omphalocele has been reported.[135]

Detection of concurrent anomalies might suggest a diagnosis of another specific type of ventral wall defect (see the previous section, Differential Diagnosis). Beckwith-

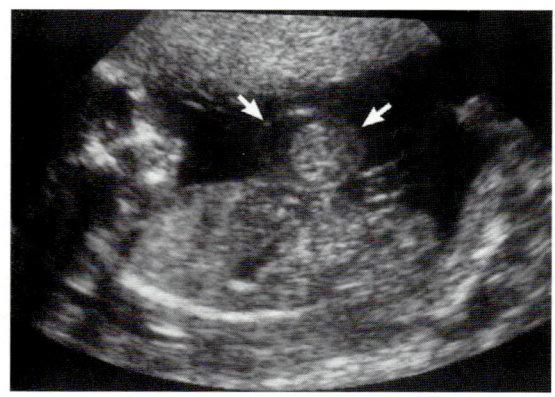

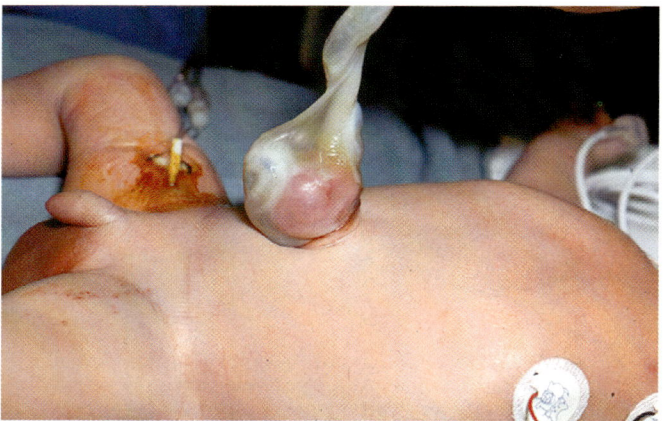

FIGURE 25. Omphalocele. **A:** A longitudinal scan at 16 weeks shows a small omphalocele with surrounding membrane (*arrows*). The appearance suggests that it represents only bowel within the omphalocele. **B:** A photograph at delivery. The omphalocele sac contained a small segment of liver (part of the quadratic lobe).

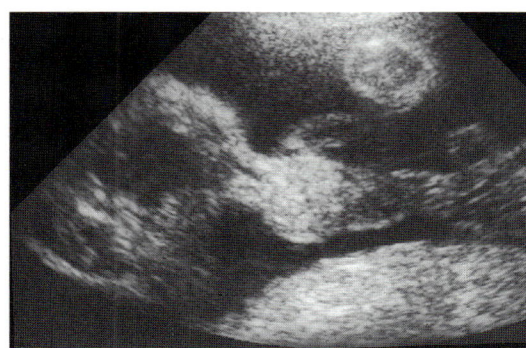

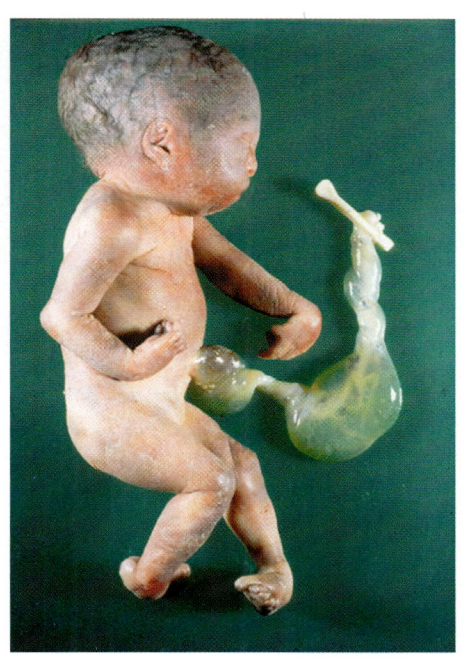

FIGURE 26. Omphalocele and trisomy 18. **A:** A transverse scan at 22 weeks shows a small omphalocele, echogenic in appearance, with surrounding membrane. The appearance suggested that the omphalocele sac contained only bowel. Other anomalies were detected, including umbilical cord pseudocyst. **B:** A photograph at delivery shows multiple anomalies. The omphalocele sac contained a small segment of liver (part of the quadratic lobe).

Wiedemann syndrome deserves mention here because it is relatively common, accounting for 5% to 10% of omphaloceles in postnatal series.[136] It is characterized by congenital overgrowth resulting in gigantism, macroglossia, and pancreatic hyperplasia (sometimes resulting in profound neonatal hypoglycemia).[137]

The diagnosis of Beckwith-Wiedemann syndrome can be suggested by characteristic findings on the ultrasound study, particularly in patients with a positive family history.[138–140] Beckwith-Wiedemann syndrome should be suspected if antenatal ultrasound demonstrates any combination of omphalocele, growth acceleration, macroglossia, and visceromegaly.[138–147] Omphaloceles associated with Beckwith-Wiedemann syndrome are nearly always of the type with intracorporeal liver. Therefore, Beckwith-Wiedemann syndrome should be considered whenever omphalocele with intracorporeal liver is associated with a normal karyotype. Polyhydramnios is common in fetuses with Beckwith-Wiedemann syndrome.

Chromosome Abnormalities

Omphalocele has been associated with trisomies 18 and 13 most often, followed by triploidy and 45,X (Turner syndrome). Conversely, omphalocele is found in approximately 22% of fetuses with trisomy 18, 9% of those with trisomy 13, and 12% of those with triploidy.[148] There are conflicting data whether trisomy 21 is associated with omphalocele,[149] but we have observed two such cases, suggesting to us that a weak association probably exists. Rarely,

Beckwith-Wiedemann syndrome may be associated with a cytogenetic abnormality involving chromosome 11p15 that is visible on standard cytogenetic studies.[150]

Omphalocele carries a high risk of aneuploidy.[149,151,152] This risk is substantially higher for omphaloceles diagnosed prenatally compared with neonatal data. Whereas neonatal studies suggest aneuploidy in 10% to 12%, prenatal series report aneuploidy in approximately 30%.[77,148,151–155] However, the actual risk of aneuploidy with omphalocele varies with a number of factors including maternal age, gestational age, associated anomalies, and the contents of the omphalocele. Boyd et al.[77] observed abnormal karyotype in 29% of cases detected prenatally, but this number increased to 54% when another anomaly was identified.

Nyberg et al.[155] were the first to suggest that omphaloceles with intracorporeal liver were associated with a greater risk for aneuploidy than omphaloceles with extracorporeal liver. This has been confirmed by a number of other studies and has been one of the most consistent observations of omphaloceles detected prenatally.[154–158] Combining data from several series, Getachew et al.[154] observed aneuploidy in approximately 87% of omphaloceles with intracorporeal liver compared with 9% of fetuses with extracorporeal liver. The absence of concurrent anomalies would further decrease the risk of aneuploidy so the "typical" appearance of omphalocele with extracorporeal liver and no other anomalies carries a very low risk of aneuploidy.

Umbilical cord cysts appear to further increase the risk of aneuploidy in fetuses with omphalocele, especially for trisomy 18.[159] The umbilical cord cysts most commonly associated with omphaloceles are pseudocysts and allantoic cysts.[160]

Prognosis

The prognosis for fetuses with omphalocele depends primarily on the presence and severity of concurrent anomalies.[122,137,146,161,162] One-year survival rates of 69% to 79% have been reported from postnatal studies.[158,163,164] Not surprisingly, the prognosis is not as favorable for cases detected antenatally. The presence of one or more concurrent malformations is associated with perinatal mortality of 80%, and the presence of a chromosome abnormality or a major cardiovascular malformation increases the mortality rate to nearly 100%.[23,122] On the other hand, fetuses with normal karyotype and no associated life-threatening anomalies have an excellent outcome, with a survival rate similar to that of gastroschisis.[46,122,165,166] Hughes et al.[122] found that a favorable outcome could be expected in fetuses with extracorporeal liver, no other detectable anomalies, and normal amounts of amniotic fluid.

When the karyotype is known to be normal, the size and content of the omphalocele sac are also important, but in this situation smaller omphaloceles with intracorporeal liver have the more favorable prognosis. St-Vil et al.[158] found that omphaloceles with intracorporeal liver have a higher survival rate than those with extracorporeal liver (88% vs. 48%) despite the significantly higher rate of karyotypic abnormalities (16% vs. 0%). The survival rate was also higher for omphaloceles detected postnatally compared with those detected prenatally (79% vs. 58%) because the latter group had a much higher percentage of extracorporeal liver (70% vs. 9%). Omphaloceles with extracorporeal liver also had a higher frequency of cardiac defects (33% vs. 18%), and the cardiac defects were more complex.

The worse prognosis observed for extracorporeal liver could also be explained by the higher rate of respiratory failure in these infants, particularly for large or "giant" (larger than 5 cm) omphaloceles.[18,23,158,167–170] Just as bowel complications are common with gastroschisis, respiratory insufficiency is an important cause of mortality and morbidity in infants with omphalocele. In a series of 30 infants with omphalocele, Tsakayannis et al.[170] reported that 12 (40%) experienced severe respiratory distress at birth including two who died within 48 hours. Cardiac or other major associated anomalies were present in nine infants (75%), and eight (67%) had a giant omphalocele. The average length of ventilatory support for the survivors was 57.7 days.

Affected patients with Beckwith-Wiedemann syndrome have an increased incidence of Wilms tumor, renal anomalies, nephromegaly, and hemihypertrophy. Less common complications include developmental delay, congenital heart defects, polydactyly, and cleft palate.[136]

Management

Chromosome analysis should be performed whenever omphalocele is diagnosed prenatally. However, this risk is considered to be very low when the omphalocele contains extracorporeal liver and no other anomalies are identified.[122] Because of the frequency of major cardiac defects, a careful fetal echocardiogram is also recommended whenever an omphalocele is identified prenatally.[171] After delivery, infants should undergo a thorough clinical examination and fetal echocardiography.

Beckwith-Wiedemann syndrome should be considered when the karyotype is normal, especially for those with intracorporeal liver. Although most cases are sporadic, approximately 15% are familial and a small number have cytogenetic abnormalities involving chromosome 11p15.[162–174] Uniparental disomy may be found in both familial and sporadic types; 17% to 28% of infants with nonfamilial Beckwith-Wiedemann syndrome and a normal karyotype have uniparental disomy.[150,173] Although this might suggest that uniparental disomy could be evaluated prenatally, several studies now indicate that patients with Beckwith-Wiedemann syndrome and omphalocele are unlikely to exhibit uniparental disomy.[150,173] Furthermore, these patients may not be at risk for development of embryonic tumors.[174]

Assuming the karyotype is normal and the pregnancy is continued,[175] most centers advise serial monitoring with ultrasound. However, compared with gastroschisis, the apparent risk of IUGR, fetal distress, or bowel complications with omphalocele is little to none, and close monitoring may not be required.

The appropriate mode of delivery for fetuses identified with an omphalocele is controversial.[96,126] Cesarean delivery has been suggested by some authorities to decrease the potential risk of infection and to avoid possible rupture of the sac during vaginal delivery. Others, however, have questioned the validity of this practice. There is no evidence that vaginal delivery is safer than cesarean for fetuses with isolated small omphalocele,[176] and there is not the same risk for bowel trauma that might occur with gastroschisis. On the other hand, cesarean section is generally recommended for large (larger than 5 cm) omphaloceles.[176]

Primary surgical closure has been the traditional approach to omphalocele. However, primary closure of large omphaloceles can produce abdominal compartment syndrome with bowel necrosis, sepsis, respiratory compromise, and dysfunction of the liver and kidneys.[165,177] Thus, various nonsurgical options have been proposed, including (a) use of a silo chimney with gradual reduction of the contents of the sac,[178] (b) delayed external compression reduction using elastic bandaging,[179–181] or (c) nonoperative management (epithelialization) of the omphalocele followed by delayed repair of the residual ventral hernia.[182]

Many infants with omphalocele, especially large ones, experience respiratory difficulty from low lung volumes.

This is temporarily worsened by closure of the defect.[166] Thus, nonsurgical management is recommended when respiratory distress is present. This is emphasized by Tsakayannis et al.[170] who reported that only one of six infants with omphalocele and respiratory distress survived when surgical repair was performed soon after birth, compared with three of four infants who were managed nonsurgically.

Cleft Sternum, Ectopia Cordis, and Pentalogy of Cantrell

Cleft sternum, ectopia cordis, and pentalogy of Cantrell each share a defect of the sternum. However, their sonographic and pathologic features are usually very different. These can be defined as three categories of sternal defects:

1. Pentalogy of Cantrell is an association of cleft distal sternum, diaphragmatic defect, midline anterior ventral wall defect, defect of the apical pericardium with communication into the peritoneum, and an internal cardiac defect.[183,184]
2. Cleft sternum, either partial or absent without ectopia cordis,[185] is typically a superior or total cleft.
3. In true ectopia cordis, the exposed heart presents outside the chest wall through a cleft sternum.[186]

Incidence

The incidence is unknown.

Embryology and Pathology

The embryologic basis of cleft sternum and ectopia cordis is uncertain. The most commonly ascribed theory suggests they result from failure of fusion of the lateral body folds in the thoracic region.[187] To help explain the association between cleft sternum and vascular malformations, Hersh et al.[188] suggest that an early disturbance affects midline mesodermal structures leading to both to lack of fusion of lateral sternal bands (or interference with a proposed medioventral unpaired structure, which may help form the sternum) and persistence/proliferation of midline angioblastic tissue. This mechanism is postulated to occur during the sixth to ninth gestational weeks. Other authors suggest that ectopia cordis is a manifestation of the amniotic band syndrome in some cases because rupture of the chorion or yolk sac (or both) at 5 menstrual weeks might interfere with normal cardiac descent.[189]

Ravitch[190] suggests that the pentalogy of Cantrell results from aplasia of both the transverse septum that forms the anterior diaphragm and the associated pericardium between 14 and 18 days of embryonic life.

True ectopia cordis has been classified into five categories: cervical, cervicothoracic, thoracic, thoracoabdominal, and abdominal.[190] Ninety-five percent of cases are of the thoracic or thoracoabdominal types.

Diagnosis

Each of the three types of sternal defects produces a very different sonographic appearance.

Pentalogy of Cantrell

An omphalocele is usually the primary finding of pentalogy of Cantrell (Fig. 27). Such omphaloceles are typically high or supraumbilical. One possible indication of the high position of an omphalocele is an omphalocele sac that may contain the stomach. If the diaphragmatic defect is large enough to produce a diaphragmatic hernia, displacement of the heart and mediastinum may be observed, whereas the sternal and pericardial defects are usually not detected. Cardiac defects may be subtle and are not universally present with pentalogy of Cantrell variants.

The presence of a pericardial or pleural effusion in association with an omphalocele may be an important clue to the pentalogy of Cantrell or its variants.[191,192] Siles et al.[191] report that pericardial effusion was noted on initial scan in two of three cases, and both of these had an anterior diaphragmatic hernia; the case without a pericardial effusion had an intact diaphragmatic pericardium. We have encountered similar cases in which the diaphragmatic hernia remained undetected, even after birth. We believe that in the setting of omphalocele, pleural effusion, even when transient, is a sign of a diaphragmatic hernia.

Cleft Sternum

In the absence of the protective sternum, the anterior chest wall is dynamic and moves with cardiac pulsations. The heart may appear to protrude through the chest, but the chest wall is intact (Fig. 28). An overlying hemangioma may dominate the sonographic appearance and hide the underlying sternal defect.[193,194]

Ectopia Cordis

Demonstration of an extrathoracic heart is a dramatic finding that is diagnostic of ectopia cordis[195–197] (Fig. 29). However, only a portion of the heart may herniate through the defect, in which case the diagnosis is more difficult.[194,195] Ectopia cordis and omphalocele may be missed in the presence of oligohydramnios.[198]

Differential Diagnosis

Demonstration of both ectopia cordis and omphalocele should suggest a more specific diagnosis of pentalogy of Cantrell[195]; however, this is uncommon.

Associated Anomalies

Cleft sternum is associated with vascular malformations, including cavernous hemangiomas, and omphalocele.[185,199] Rose et al.[193] describe prenatal detection of a chest wall hamartoma with underlying sternal cleft. Hebra et al.[194]

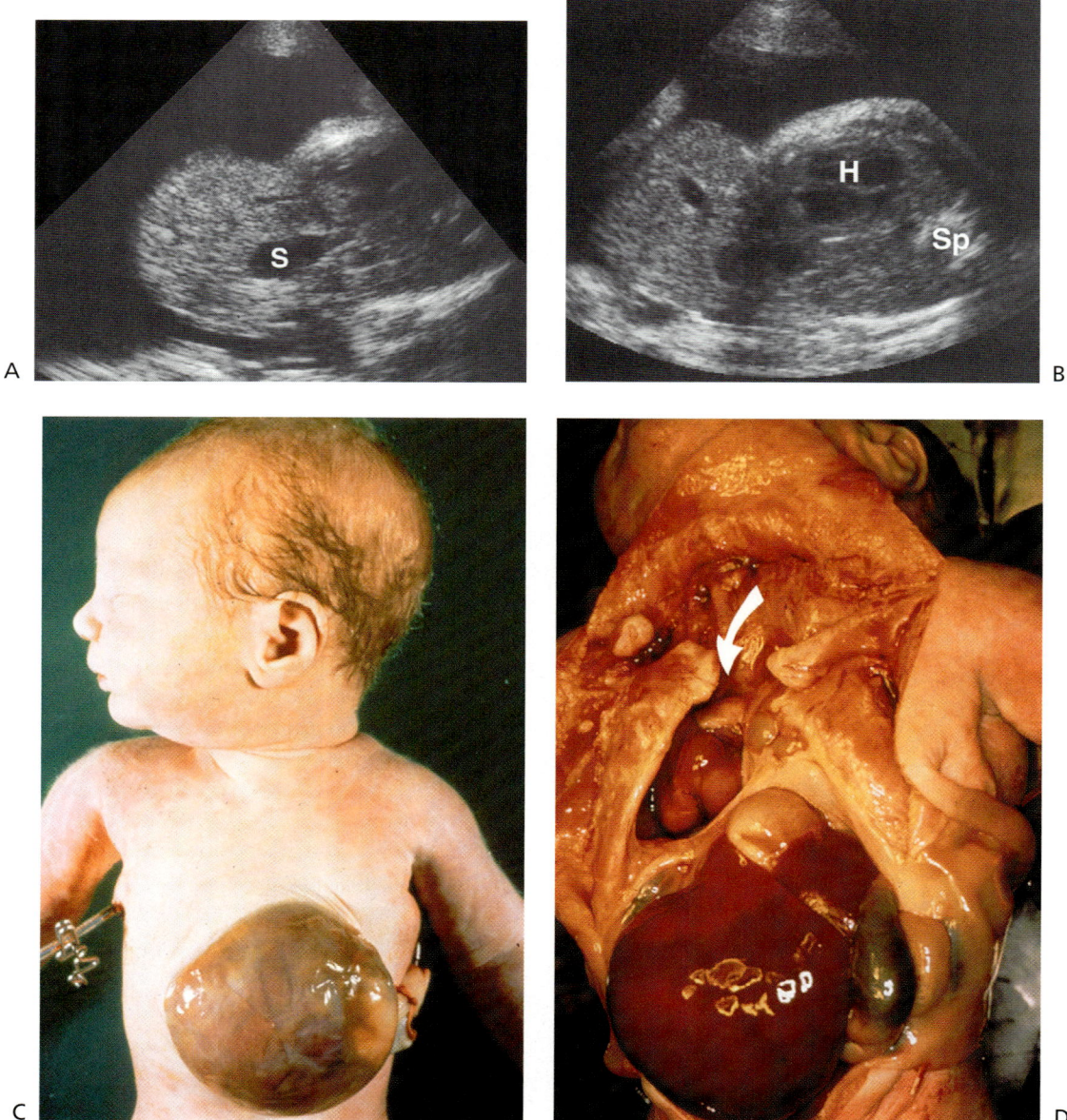

FIGURE 27. Pentalogy of Cantrell. **A:** A transverse scan shows an omphalocele containing liver as well as stomach (*S*). The presence of stomach suggests that this is a high omphalocele defect. **B:** A scan slightly higher shows the heart (*H*) displaced to the right. The infant died soon after birth from respiratory distress despite intervention. Sp, spine. **C:** A postmortem photograph. **D:** An internal examination shows a left-sided diaphragmatic defect and sternal defect (*arrow*).

describe a similar case in which an unusual exophytic cystic mass hid an underlying sternal defect.

Pentalogy of Cantrell may be associated with various cardiac defects, cleft lip with or without cleft palate, encephalocele, exencephaly, and sirenomelia.[200–202] Cystic hygroma may be present in the first trimester.[203] Pentalogy of Cantrell has also been associated with trisomies 13 and 18 and 45,X (Turner syndrome) in postnatal reports.[195,204]

Anomalies most frequently associated with ectopia cordis include omphalocele, cardiovascular malformations, and craniofacial defects.[195,205–207] In a series of eight fetuses with ectopia cordis reported by Klingensmith et al.,[207] five (63%) also had an omphalocele, and six (75%) fetuses also had structural cardiac defects. Cardiac defects usually include a ventricular septal defect with or without tetralogy of Fallot. Other cardiac defects that have been reported include tricuspid atresia, Ebstein anomaly, common atrium, atrioventricular canal defect, mitral atresia, total anomalous pulmonary venous return, single ventricle, pulmonary stenosis, pulmonary atresia, aortic stenosis, coarc-

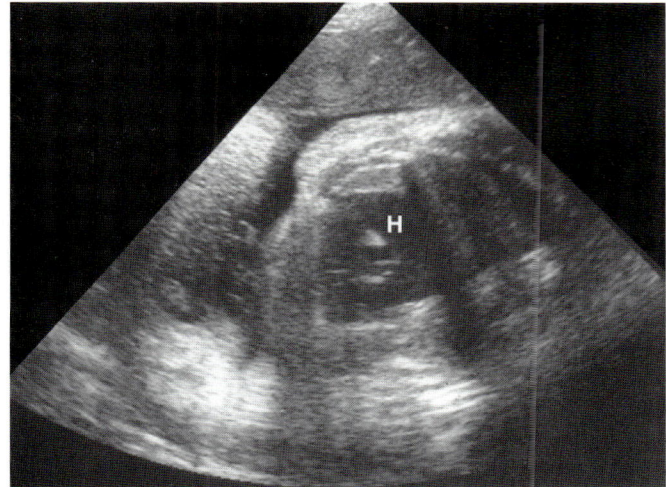

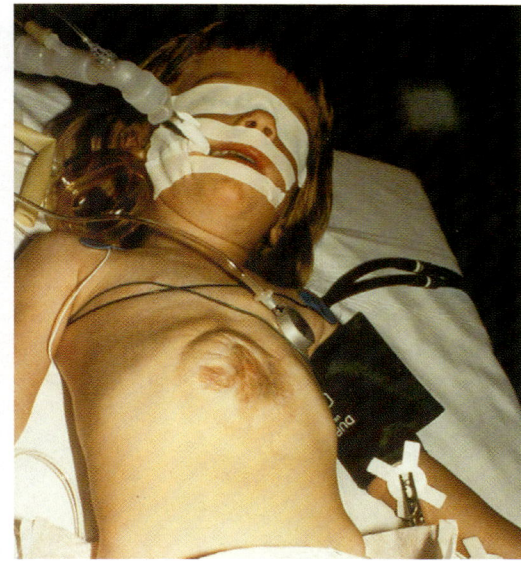

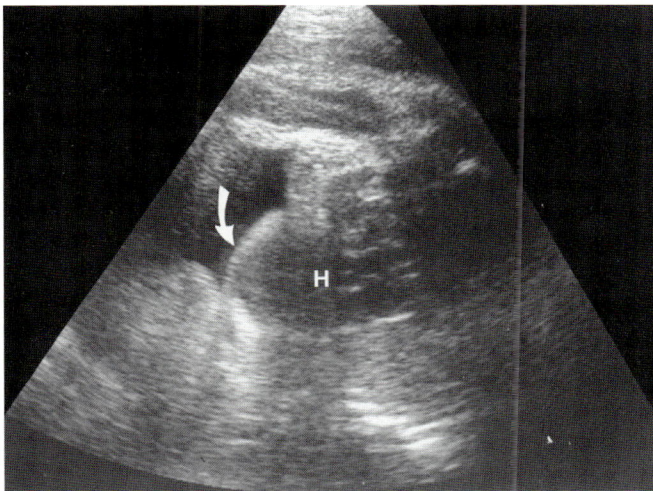

FIGURE 28. Absent sternum. **A:** A transverse view of the chest shows the normally positioned heart (*H*). **B:** A moment later the chest wall is displaced anteriorly (*arrow*) with systolic contraction. The dynamic movement of the heart (*H*) was striking on real-time examination. **C:** A photograph at surgical correction performed at 1 year of life shows protrusion from absent sternum.

tation of the aorta, transposition of the great arteries, and ventricular diverticulum. Other possible anomalies include pulmonary hypoplasia, cranial defects, facial cleft, clubfeet, and kyphoscoliosis.

Chromosome abnormalities have been associated with ectopia cordis including one case of trisomy 18 reported by Klingensmith et al.[207] and two cases of trisomy 18 among ten fetuses with the pentalogy of Cantrell reported by Ghidini et al.[195]

Prognosis and Management

Cleft sternum alone has an excellent prognosis following surgical repair. Primary surgical repair is best performed during the first weeks of life.[208] Partial clefts may be converted to a total cleft, with subsequent complete approximation of the two segments. Reinforcement with titanium plate has been recommended.[209]

True ectopia cordis carries a very high mortality rate, with most infants dying within a few days of birth and few patients living more than a few months.[184,210–212] The survival rate is no more than 5% to 10%, with the underlying cardiac defect being the primary determinant of survival. The surgical approach should be tailored to the severity of the defect and the presence of other complicating factors.[212,213] The omphalocele is covered to prevent infection and fluid losses. Use of a prosthetic covering can also protect a true ectopia cordis. Staging of cardiac repair may be necessary in true ectopic cordis because of severe abnormalities.

Cloacal and Bladder Exstrophy

Bladder and cloacal exstrophy share a common embryologic origin in abnormal cloacal development, but they differ in severity and extent of involvement.[214,215]

Incidence

Bladder exstrophy occurs in approximately 1 in 30,000 births and has a male to female ratio of 2:1. Cloacal exstro-

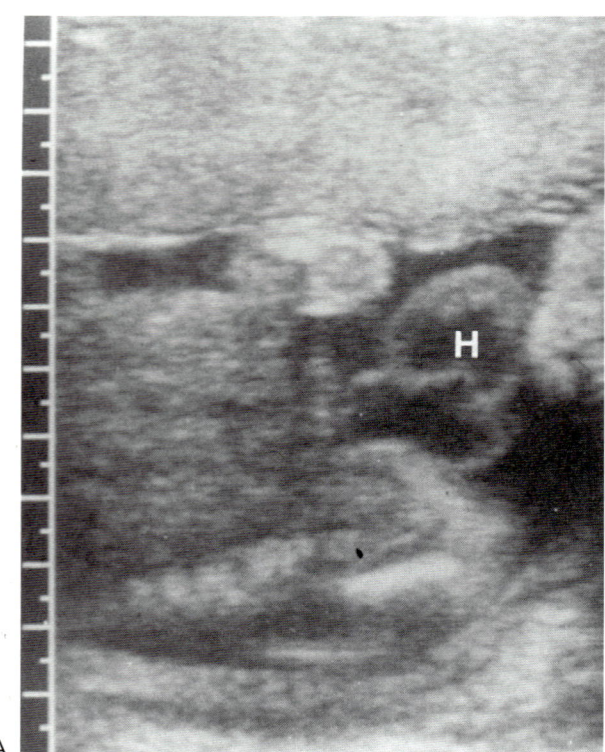

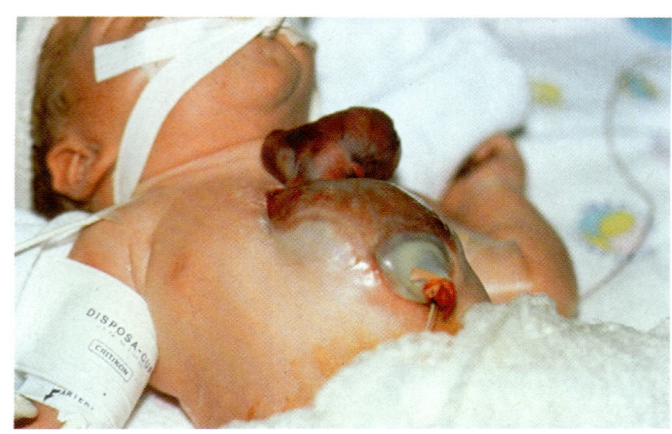

FIGURE 29. Ectopia cordis. **A, B:** The heart (*H*) is eviscerated into the amniotic fluid. An atrioventricular septal defect is also identified with a single atrioventricular valve separating a large atrial septal defect and ventricular septal defect. Other abnormalities found at necropsy included atrioventricular septal defect, double-outlet right ventricle, and pulmonic stenosis.

phy has an incidence of 1 in 50,000 births and may be more frequent in twins. It is estimated that 10% of all cases of cloacal exstrophy occur in like-sex twins.[216]

Embryology and Pathology

An understanding of bladder and cloacal exstrophy requires familiarity with normal embryologic development of the cloaca[217–219]: By the eighth menstrual week (sixth fetal week), downward growth of the urorectal septum normally reaches the cloacal membrane, separating the cloaca into the urogenital sinus anteriorly and the hindgut posteriorly. The urorectal septum also subdivides the cloacal membrane into the urogenital membrane anteriorly and the anal membrane posteriorly. These membranes normally rupture by 11 to 12 menstrual weeks to produce patent urogenital and rectal tracts. Closure of the lower ventral wall occurs at the same time the cloacal membrane retracts caudally.

As the urorectal septum develops, the mesonephric ducts fuse into the cloaca laterally. These ducts form the seminal vesicles in the male but atrophy in the female. Induced by the mesonephric ducts, the paired paramesonephric ducts (müllerian ducts) fuse in the midline to form the uterovaginal cord, which in turn fuses with the urogenital sinus posteriorly. The sinovaginal bulbs then join and extend distally to form the vagina.

In bladder exstrophy, the urorectal septum successfully divides the cloaca, but the cloacal membrane does not retract normally, and the cloacal membrane becomes the anterior wall of the bladder.[218] Regression of the cloacal membrane then results in direct exposure of the posterior bladder wall (Fig. 30). In cloacal exstrophy, the urorectal septum also fails to reach the cloacal membrane, so that when the cloacal membrane regresses, both the bladder and rectum are exposed (Fig. 31). The genitalia are also duplicated, because the genital tubercles did not fuse.

Bladder exstrophy results in an everted bladder that becomes exposed on the lower ventral wall. The severity of bladder exstrophy can be clinically graded from mild to severe. In the mild form, exstrophy of the urethra and external bladder sphincter is present but diastasis of the pubic symphysis and rectus abdominis muscles is minimal. In the typical form, bladder exstrophy is accompanied by wide diastasis of the symphysis pubis.[220] The most severe form may be accompanied by omphalocele, inguinal hernia, undescended testis, a ventrally located anal orifice, a relaxed anal sphincter, and intermittent rectal prolapse.[212,215]

Cloacal exstrophy is a more rare and more complex disorder than bladder exstrophy. It is embryologically related to persistent cloaca, but the latter condition does not have a ventral wall defect[221] (see Chapter 13). Cloacal exstrophy results in exstrophy of the bladder, in which two hemibladders (each with its ureteral orifice) are separated by intestinal mucosa[222] (Fig. 32). The intestinal mucosa probably corresponds to the cecum because the ileum enters it as an ileal-vesicle fistula. A zone of intestinal mucosal divides the bladder into two parts. The orifices of the terminal ileum, the rudimentary tailgut, and a single or paired appendix are

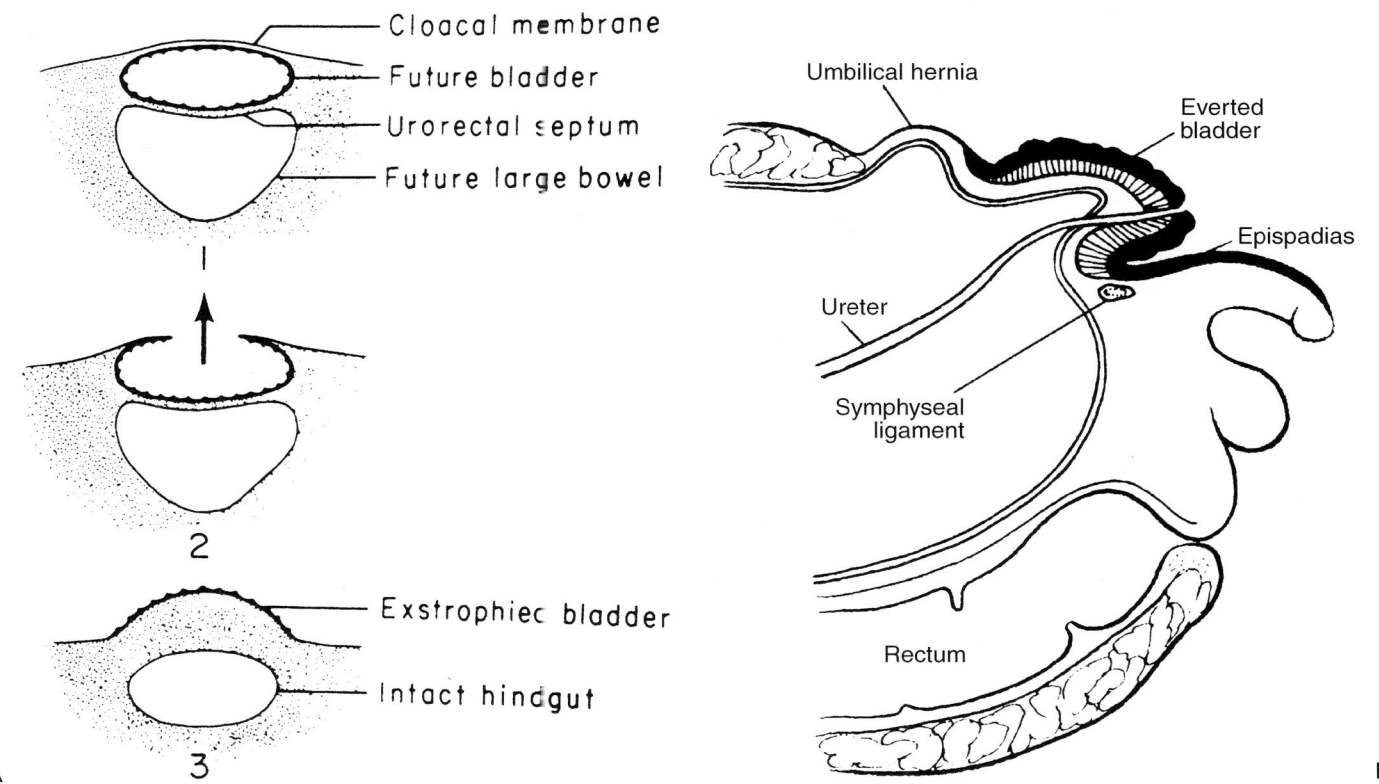

FIGURE 30. Bladder exstrophy. **A**: Events leading to bladder exstrophy. The anterior abdominal wall breaks down (*2*) and results in eversion of the urinary bladder (*3*). **B**: Typical findings of bladder exstrophy in a male. (Reproduced with permission from Muecke EC. In: Walsh PC, et al., eds. *Campbell's urology*, 5th ed. Philadelphia: WB Saunders, 1986:1856–1880.)

present on the surface of the everted intestine. The terminal ileum may be prolapsed outward at birth, creating an unusual appearance.

Diagnosis

Both bladder and cloacal exstrophy have been reported prenatally. More cases of cloacal exstrophy have been reported, suggesting that bladder exstrophy may be overlooked.[223–226] A primary finding in cases of bladder exstrophy has been failure to visualize a normal urinary bladder.[223–227] A soft-tissue mass, representing the exposed bladder mucosa, may also be demonstrated on the surface of the lower ventral wall with bladder exstrophy[228] (Fig. 33). Goldstein et al.[229] described a case in which a small cystic structure, thought to represent the normal urachus, initially simulated a small urinary bladder with bladder exstrophy.

Cloacal exstrophy is characterized by a ventral wall defect and a severe form of bladder exstrophy. Demonstration of the ventral wall defect may be the primary sonographic finding of cloacal exstrophy. Thus, cloacal exstrophy should be considered whenever an atypical low ventral wall defect is identified in association with failure to visualize a normal urinary bladder.[229–231] However, the ven-

tral wall defect may be difficult to visualize because of its small size, and visualization may be difficult in the presence of oligohydramnios caused by associated renal abnormalities.[224] Amnioinfusion may greatly improve the diagnostic image in this situation.[232]

Austin et al.[233] contributed nine cases (two prospective and seven retrospective) and reviewed a total of 22 prenatal cases of cloacal exstrophy. The typical sonographic features were nonvisualization of the bladder, a midline infraumbilical wall defect or cystic anterior wall structure (persistent cloacal membrane), and omphalocele. Other findings may include abnormalities of the spine, lower extremities, and kidneys; ascites; widened pubic arches; a narrow thorax; hydrocephalus; and a single umbilical artery. Meizner et al.[234] reported similar findings in six cases of cloacal exstrophy diagnosed prenatally. In all six cases, fetal bowel was observed floating in a large amount of ascites within the omphalocele sac. Polyhydramnios was present in four of the six cases.

A common feature of cloacal exstrophy at birth is a prolapsed distal ileum, which can be visualized by prenatal sonography. Hamada et al.[232] describe the unique appearance of a single thickened bowel segment protruding from the lower ventral wall and creating an appearance similar to

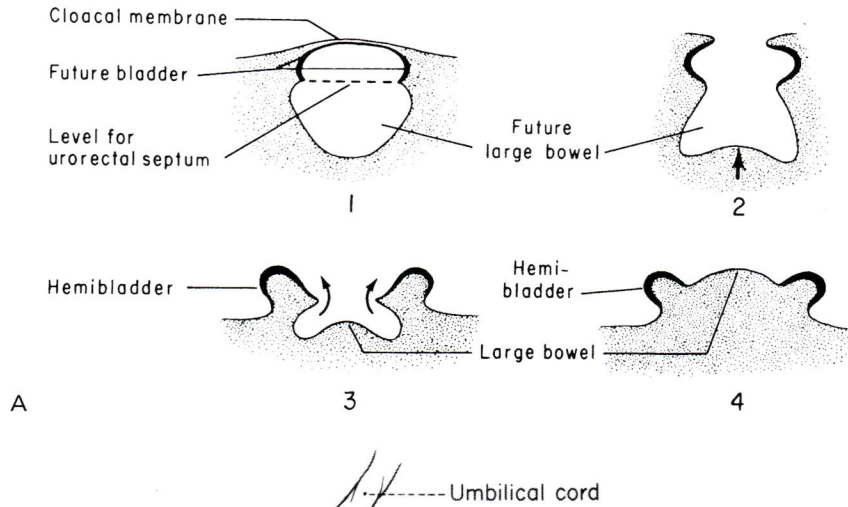

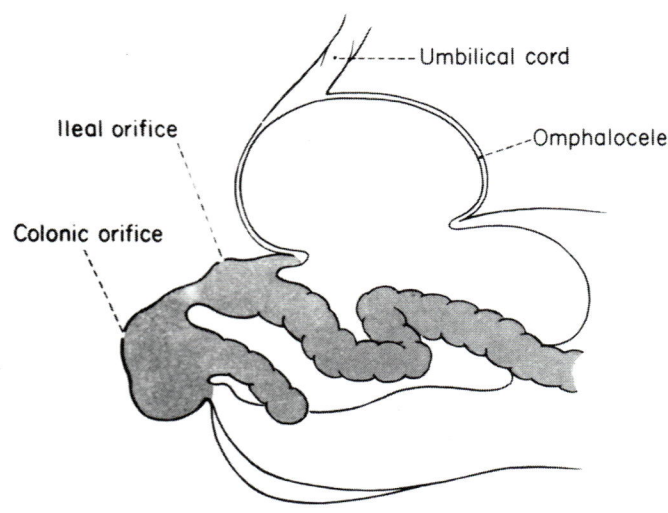

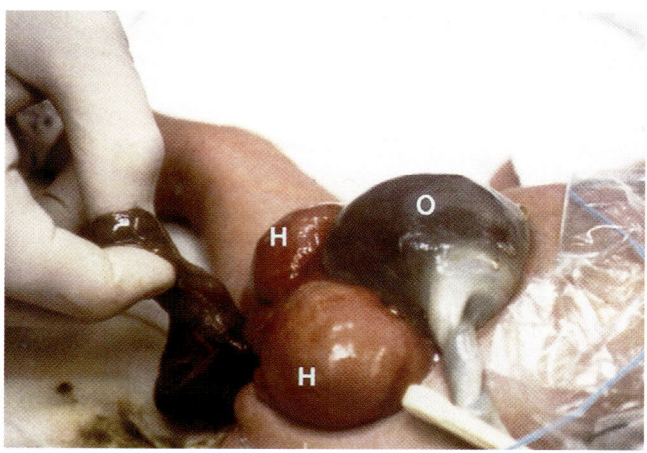

FIGURE 31. Cloacal exstrophy. **A:** Events leading to cloacal exstrophy. Both the anterior abdominal wall and urorectal septum break down. **B:** Anatomy of cloacal exstrophy on sagittal view. The distal ileum opens to the lower defect below the omphalocele. (Reproduced with permission from Muecke EC. In: Walsh PC, et al., eds. *Campbell's urology*, 5th ed. Philadelphia: WB Saunders, 1986:1856–1880.)

FIGURE 32. Pathologic features of cloacal exstrophy without prolapsed ileum. Meconium is passed between the two exstrophied hemibladders (*H*). O, omphalocele. (Reproduced with permission from Cullinan. In: Rumack CM, Wilson, Charboneau W, et al., eds. *Diagnostic ultrasound*, 2nd ed. Philadelphia: Mosby–Year Book, 1997.)

an "elephant trunk" (Fig. 34). This represents the prolapsed distal ileum. No other congenital anomaly creates an elephant trunk–like mass protruding from the ventral wall.

Several cases have now been reported of delayed rupture of the cloacal membrane between 18 and 24 weeks including two sets of twin pregnancies.[232,234–237] This is observed as a cystic mass that subsequently ruptures. For example, Bruch et al.[237] describe intact cloacal membrane at 18 weeks with a cystic mass associated with bilateral hydronephrosis and oligohydramnios. The cloacal membrane subsequently ruptured by 24 weeks, relieving the urinary tract outlet obstruction.

Differential Diagnosis

Persistent failure to demonstrate a normal urinary bladder may also reflect other genitourinary disorders such as a persistent cloaca.[237,238] This disorder typically shows a septated cystic mass in the pelvis and is not associated with a ventral wall defect[237] (see Chapter 13).

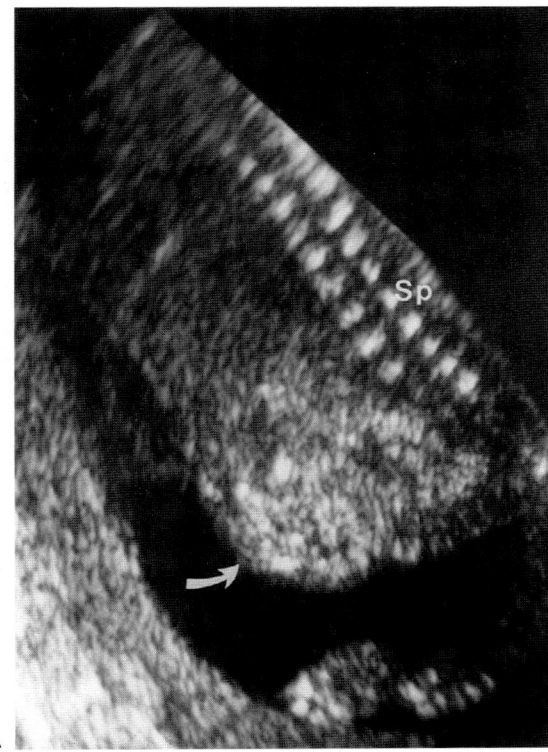

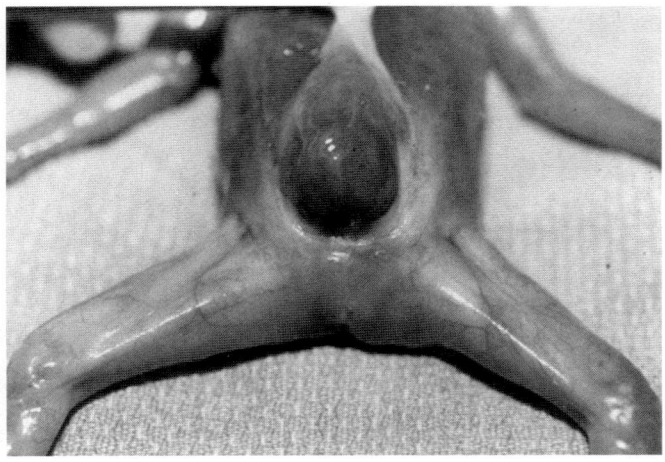

FIGURE 33. Bladder exstrophy. **A:** A transvaginal scan of the pelvis at 17 menstrual weeks shows absence of a normal urinary bladder and a soft-tissue mass on the anterior pelvic wall (*arrow*). The fetal karyotype was trisomy 13. Sp, spine. **B:** A postmortem photograph confirms ultrasound findings, with exstrophied bladder. (Reproduced with permission from Nyberg DA, Hill LM, Bohm-Velez M, Mendelson EB, eds. *Transvaginal ultrasound.* St. Louis: Mosby–Year Book, 1992.)

The bowel segment of bladder exstrophy should not be mistaken for gastroschisis. Also, the infraumbilical wall defect should not be mistaken for omphalocele alone.

Associated Anomalies

Abnormalities associated with bladder exstrophy relate principally to the primary malformation and associated genitourinary anomalies. The severity of abnormalities is variable, although common findings in males include epispadias, incomplete descent of the testes, and bilateral inguinal hernias.[220,239,240] Sex reassignment may be necessary in 1% to 2% of males if surgical correction does not result in an adequately functional penis. In females, cleft clitoris is common.

Cloacal exstrophy is associated with more severe anomalies than bladder exstrophy.[214] These include vertebral malformations (40% to 90%); myelomeningocele (30% to 70%); upper urinary tract anomalies, such as unilateral or bilateral renal agenesis (10% to 35%) or crossed-fused ectopia (10% to 60%); and lower extremity malformations, including clubfeet (20% to 45%), gastrointestinal malformations (50%), and single umbilical artery.[229] Other possible anomalies include didalphus (separation of the phallus); absence of the vagina; and malformations of the gastrointestinal tract, cardiovascular system, or central nervous system.

The combination of omphalocele, exstrophy of the bladder, imperforate anus, and spinal deformities has been called the *OEIS complex*.[241,242] This rare disorder, affecting 1 in 200,000 to 400,000 pregnancies,[243] is thought to arise from a single localized defect in the early development of the mesoderm that later contributes to infraumbilical mesenchyme, cloacal septum, and caudal vertebrae.[244] It may be considered the most severe end of a spectrum of birth defects that includes phallic separation with epispadias, pubic diastasis, exstrophy of the bladder, and cloacal exstrophy. Limb aplasia or hypoplasia may also be present.[244–246] It has been diagnosed during the first trimester.[247]

The frequency of chromosome abnormalities associated with bladder or cloacal exstrophy is unknown. However, we have observed fetuses with bladder exstrophy who had abnormal karyotypes, including trisomies 21 and 13 (Fig. 33).

Prognosis and Management

Bladder exstrophy can be surgically corrected with favorable results in most cases.[248,249] The major problems are the ventral wall defect itself, urinary incontinence, and associated genital abnormalities. Divergent levator ani and puborectal muscles may result in rectal incontinence and anal prolapse. Surgical correction of the defect is necessary, because untreated patients with exstrophy of the bladder usually die of ascending pyelonephritis. Infertility is common, particularly among males. Uterine prolapse is a common complication among females. There is an increased frequency of malignant tumors involving the exstrophic

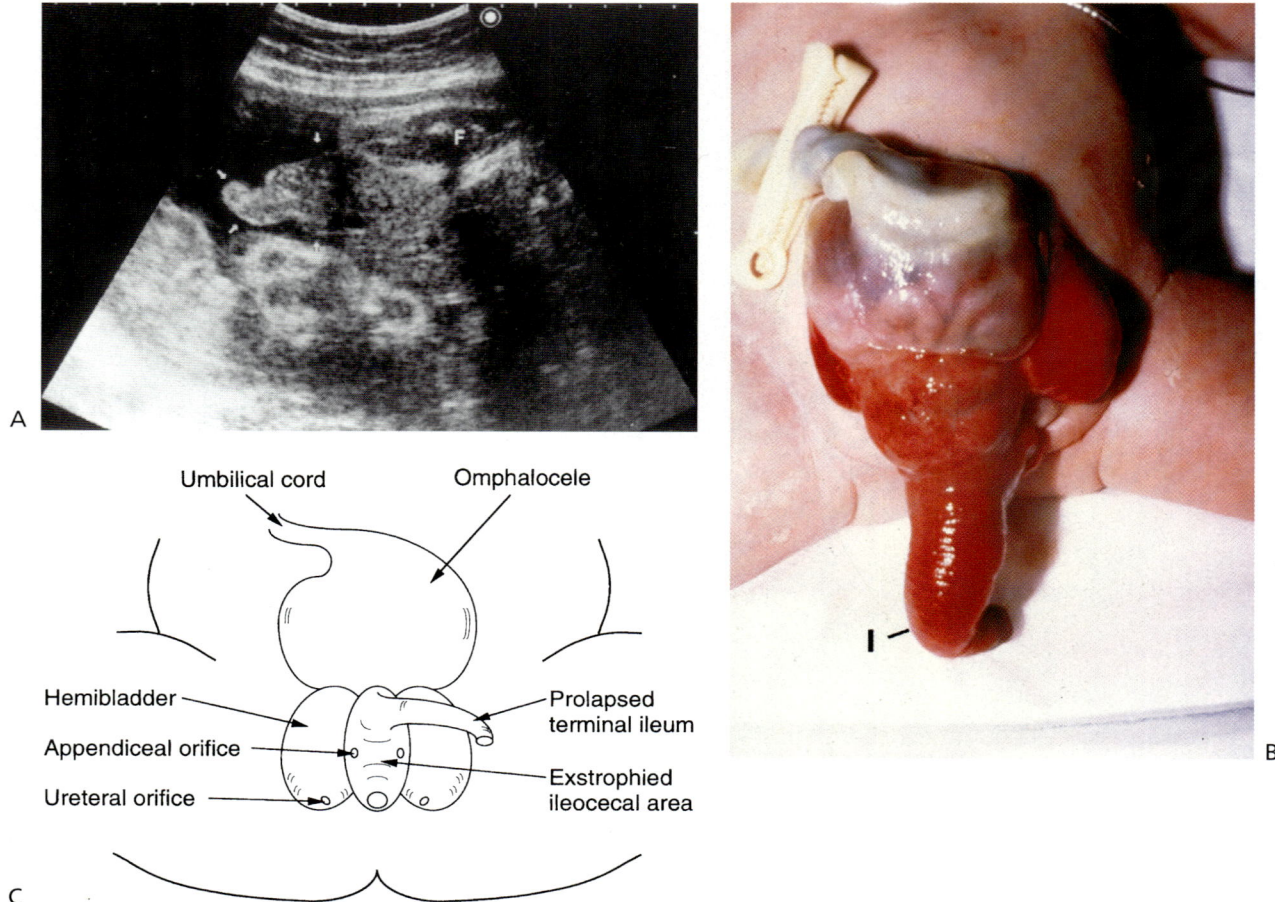

FIGURE 34. Cloacal exstrophy with prolapsed ileum. **A:** Ultrasound shows an elongated soft tissue mass of the lower pelvis similar in appearance to an elephant's trunk (*small arrows*). F, fetus. **B:** A postnatal photograph from a similar case shows a prolapsed ileum (*I*) and bladder exstrophy. **C:** Sonographic and pathologic findings. (Parts **A** and **C** reproduced with permission from Hamada H, Takano K, Shina H, Sakai T, Sohda S, Kubo T. New ultrasonographic criterion for the prenatal diagnosis of cloacal exstrophy: elephant-trunk like image. *J Urol* 1999;162:2123–2124.)

bladder; bladder carcinoma occurred in 7 (4%) of 170 cases observed at the Mayo Clinic.[250]

Cloacal exstrophy was uniformly fatal until 1960[251] due to the complexity of the malformation and the frequency of associated anomalies. Improvements in surgical technique have significantly improved mortality rates so that quality of life, rather than survival, has now become the primary issue facing most patients with cloacal exstrophy without other life-threatening anomalies.[252] Surgical correction requires a series of complex procedures beginning with separation of bowel from bladder, closure of the ventral wall defect, and functional bladder closure. The gastrointestinal tract is established first to make optimal use of available bowel, and then the genitourinary tract is reconstructed.[253] Later surgeries during childhood include anticontinence and antireflux procedures. Few achieve voluntary bowel or bladder control but depend on intermittent catheterization and enemas.[251,253,254] Surviving

females usually undergo vaginal reconstruction at 14 to 18 years of age. Typically, males are converted to females because of the poor results in attempting to create a functional penis.

Limb-Body Wall Complex and Amniotic Band Syndrome

LBWC and amniotic band syndrome may produce complex abdominal wall defects. Typically, the eviscerated organs of LBWC form a complex, bizarre-appearing mass (Figs. 35 and 36). Body defects are generally large, involving both the thorax and abdomen. The body wall defect or neural tube defect is often in direct continuity with the placenta (Fig. 35). Cranial defects (anencephaly and encephalocele), scoliosis, and abnormalities of the lower extremities are common. Because these defects affect multiple organs, they are discussed in greater detail in Chapter 5.

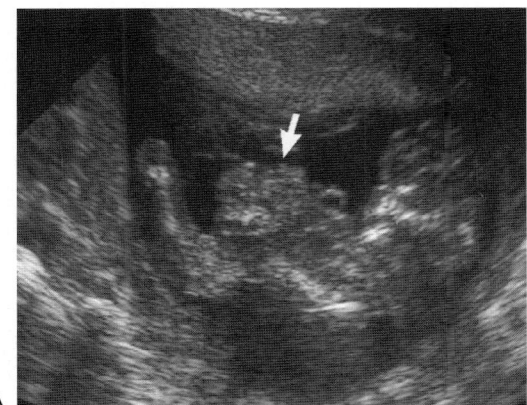 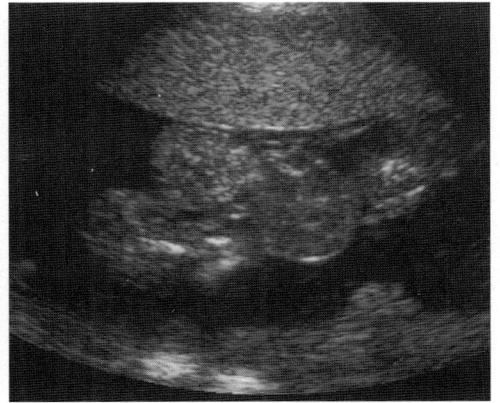

FIGURE 35. Limb-body wall complex. **A:** A scan at 16 weeks shows a complex ventral wall defect with eviscerated liver and bowel (*arrow*). Acrania and scoliosis were also noted. **B:** The ventral wall defect is in intimate contact with the anterior placenta.

Urachal and Allantoic Abnormalities

Urachal and allantoic abnormalities are the result of persistence of the embryologic urachus or allantois.

Incidence

Congenital patent urachus is a rare anomaly with an estimated incidence of 0.25 in 10,000 deliveries.[255] Males are affected twice as often as females.

Embryology and Pathology

The allantois develops as an outpouching or diverticulum from that part of the yolk sac that eventually forms the cloaca. In reptiles and birds, this diverticulum projects outside the umbilical cord and serves as the source of oxygen exchange through the porous eggshell. Because the placenta assumes the function of oxygen exchange in mammals, the allantois obliterates during the second month of gestation and has no apparent function except for possible early hematopoiesis. As the cloaca forms, the allantois remains connected to the urogenital sinus through the urachus. The urachus extends from the umbilical cord to the ventral aspect of the urogenital sinus (urinary bladder). It narrows to a small fibrous band at or about the time of birth to become the median umbilical ligament.

Occasionally, trace remnants of the allantois remain in the proximal umbilicus and may be seen between the umbilical arteries on pathologic examination of fetuses at this gestational age. Although not a true ventral wall defect, failure of the urachus to regress may result in complete or partial communication between the bladder and anterior ventral wall.

Failure of the urachal lumen to close can result in four primary anomalies (Fig. 37): (a) completely patent urachus,

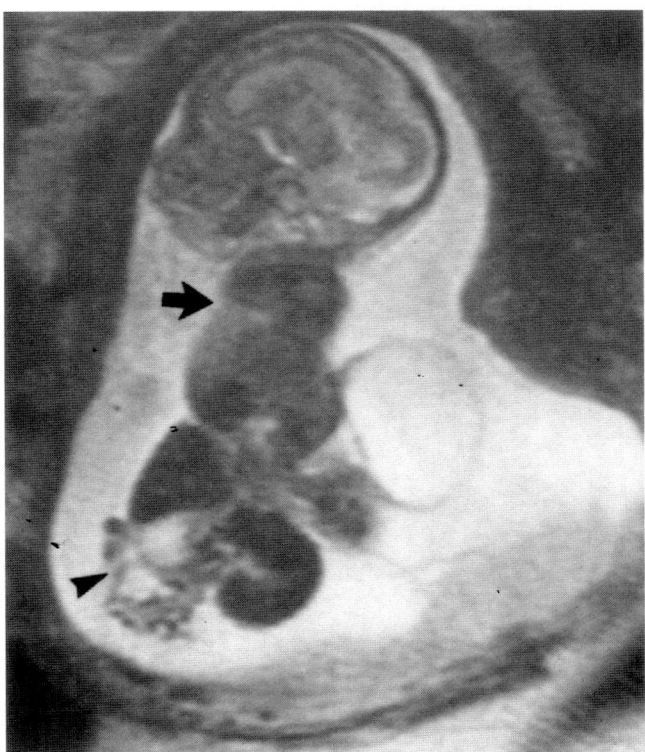

FIGURE 36. Limb-body wall defect in an 18-week-old fetus. A sagittal magnetic resonance image shows a large abdominal wall defect, with the liver, stomach, and bowel spilling into the amniotic fluid (*arrowhead*). The thorax and lungs appear hypoplastic and hypointense (*arrow*). A large myelomeningocele is seen protruding posteriorly. The normal pelvic girdle and the lower extremities are not visualized. (Reproduced with permission from Huppert BJ, Brandt KR, Ramin KD, King BF. Single-shot fast spin-echo MR imaging of the fetus: a pictorial essay. *Radiographics* 1999;19:S215–S227.)

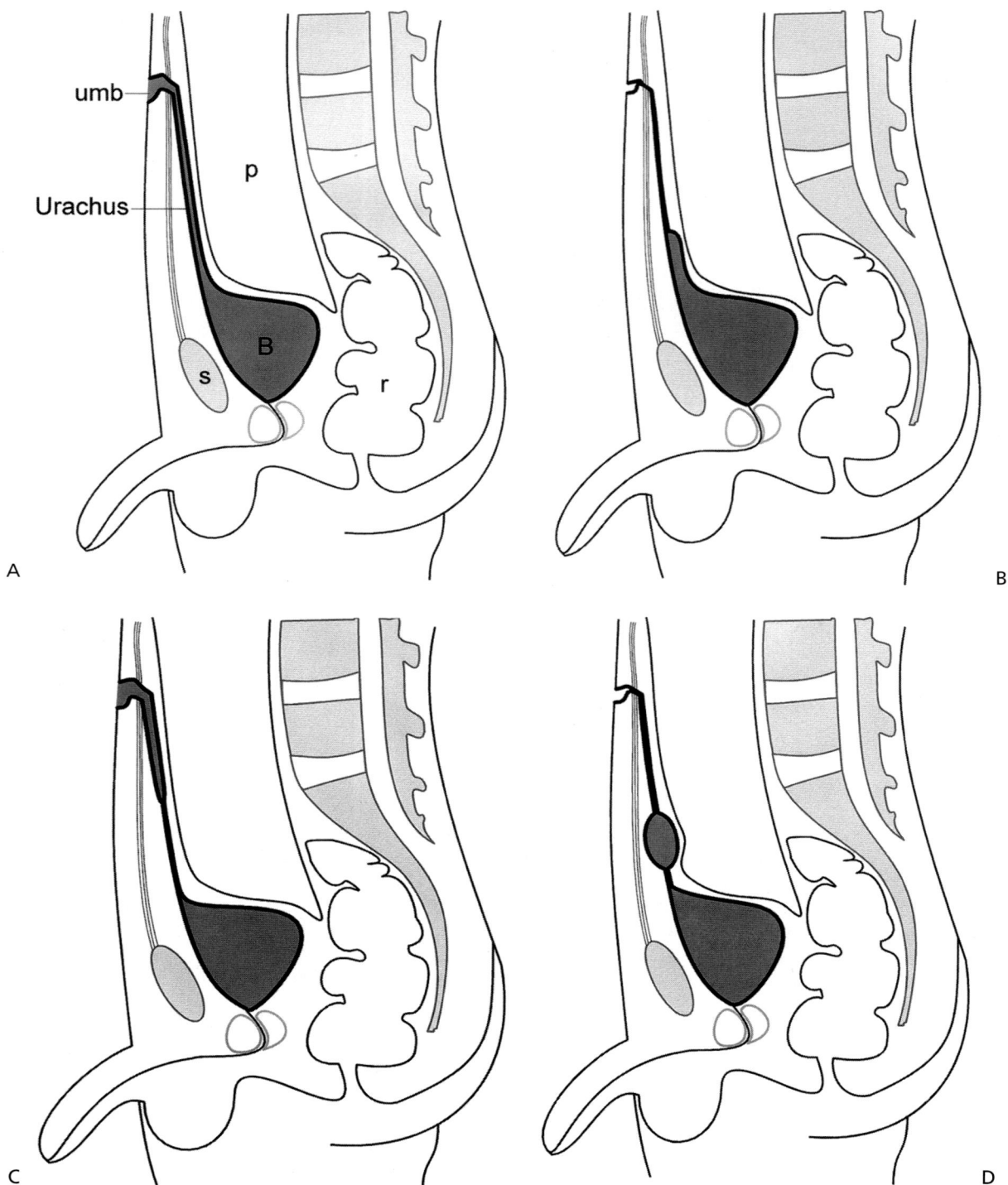

FIGURE 37. Four types of congenital urachal anomalies. **A:** Patent urachus. B, bladder; p, perito-neal cavity; r, rectum; s, symphysis pubis; umb, umbilicus. **B:** Urachal diverticulum. **C:** Urachal sinus. **D:** Urachal cyst. [Reproduced with permission from Yu JS, Kim KW, Lee HJ, Lee YJ, Yoon CS, Kim MJ. Urachal remnant diseases: spectrum of CT and US findings. *Radiographics* 2001;21(2): 451–461.]

(b) urachal diverticulum, (c) urachal sinus, and (d) urachal cyst.[256–258] In a review of 35 children with urachal abnormalities, Rich et al.[258] reported that 19 had patent urachus, 12 had urachal cyst, and four had urachal sinus.

Diagnosis

A urachal abnormality should be considered when a cystic mass is seen anterosuperior to the bladder, particularly if it extends toward the umbilical cord insertion into the ventral wall.[259] In Figure 38, the extraabdominal component of the patent urachus appears entirely cystic and communicates with the urinary bladder. The cystic mass subsequently resolved on serial sonograms, but a patent urachus was found after birth. Similar findings have been observed by others.[129,260–264] In these cases, a cystic mass is seen of the ventral wall, extending from the umbilical cord insertion to the anterior aspect of the bladder. Communication between the cyst and urinary bladder may be seen and helps to confirm the diagnosis of patent urachus. The umbilical cord may be dilated distal to the cystic mass and may be related to absorption of fetal urine by Wharton's jelly.[265]

Differential Diagnosis

The differential diagnosis includes ventral wall defects such as omphalocele or cloacal or bladder exstrophy.[129] An attempt should be made to distinguish the cystic appearance of a patent urachus or urachal cyst from a ven-tral wall defect, particularly from cloacal or bladder exstrophy. In the latter case, the urinary bladder is absent and bladder mucosa is demonstrated on the anterior ventral wall. Finally, the persistent urachus may demonstrate a solid appearance that may be difficult to distinguish from a small bowel-containing omphalocele or persistent omphalomesenteric duct.

Other considerations include vascular lesions of the umbilical cord (hemangioma, varix, true knot), umbilical cord cyst, and pseudocyst.

Associated Anomalies

Urachal cyst is usually isolated. However, Rich et al.[258] reported associated anomalies in 16 of 35 (46%) children with urachal abnormalities, including omphalocele, omphalomesenteric remnant, myelomeningocele, and various genitourinary anomalies (cryptorchidism, unilateral kidney, hydronephrosis, vaginal atresia). Umbilical cord cysts and pseudocysts have been associated with other abnormalities and aneuploidy.[266–269]

Prognosis and Management

The prognosis of urachal abnormalities depends on the presence of associated anomalies. In a neonatal series of 35 surgically corrected urachal abnormalities, Rich et al.[258] reported only one death. The clinical presentation of urachal abnormalities is variable in childhood. Although

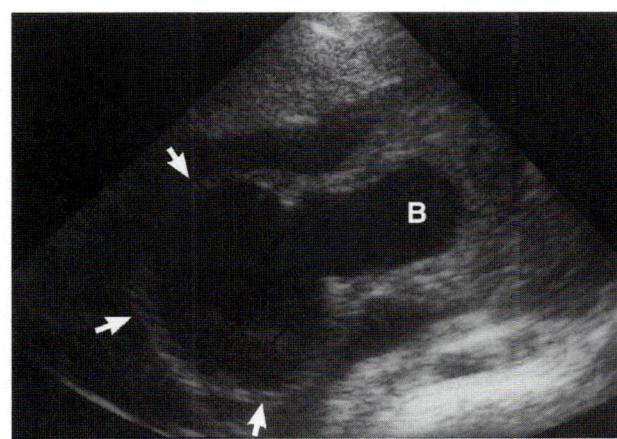

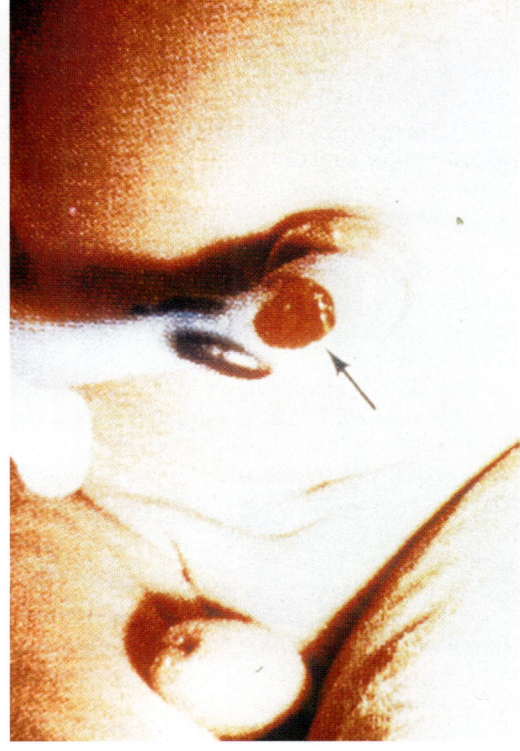

FIGURE 38. Urachal cyst. **A:** A scan of the pelvis shows a cystic mass (*arrows*) communicating with the urinary bladder (*B*). The cyst resolved on follow-up. **B:** A photograph at delivery shows a remnant of a urachal cyst (*arrow*).

usually asymptomatic, urachal cysts may present with infection or late malignancy.[270,271]

Urachal cysts are surgically resected. Infected cysts are first drained and excised later.[272] Neoplasms may develop in urachal remnants, including a variety of benign tumors and mucinous adenocarcinoma.

REFERENCES

1. Dibbins AW, Curci MR, McCrann DJ Jr. Prenatal diagnosis of congenital anomalies requiring surgical correction. *Am J Surg* 1985;149:528–533.
2. Palomaki GE, Hill LE, Knight GJ, Haddow JE, Carpenter M. Second-trimester maternal serum alpha-fetoprotein levels in pregnancies associated with gastroschisis and omphalocele. *Obstet Gynecol* 1988;71:906–909.
3. Calzolari E, Bianchi F, Dolk H, Milan M. Omphalocele and gastroschisis in Europe: a survey of 3 million births 1980–1990. EUROCAT Working Group. *Am J Med Genet* 1995;58(2):187–194.
4. Moore KL. *The developing human*, 4th ed. Philadelphia: WB Saunders, 1988:65–86.
5. Cyr DR, Mack LA, Schoenecker SA, Patten RM, Shepard TH, et al. Bowel migration in the normal fetus: US detection. *Radiology* 1986;161:119–121.
6. Timor-Tritsch IE, Warren WB, Peisner DB, Pirrone E. First-trimester midgut herniation: a high-frequency transvaginal sonographic study. *Am J Obstet Gynecol* 1989; 161:831–833.
7. Bronshtein M, Yoffe N, Zimmer EZ. Transvaginal sonography at 5 to 14 weeks' gestation: fetal stomach, abnormal cord insertion, and yolk sac. *Am J Perinatol* 1992;9:344–347.
8. Bowerman RA. Sonography of fetal midgut herniation: normal size criteria and correlation with crown-rump length. *J Ultrasound Med* 1993;5:251–254.
9. Brown DL, Emerson DS, Shulman LP, Carson SA. Sonographic diagnosis of omphalocele during 10th week of gestation. *AJR Am J Roentgenol* 1989;153:825–826.
10. Pagliano M, Mossetti M, Ragno P. Echographic diagnosis of omphalocele in the first trimester of pregnancy. *J Clin Ultrasound* 1990;18:658–660.
11. Guzman ER. Early prenatal diagnosis of gastroschisis with transvaginal ultrasonography. *Am J Obstet Gynecol* 1990; 162:1253–1254.
12. Kushnir O, Izquierdo L, Vigil D, Curet LB. Early transvaginal sonographic diagnosis of gastroschisis. *J Clin Ultrasound* 1990;18:194–197.
13. Gray DL, Martin CM, Crane JP. Differential diagnosis of first trimester ventral wall defect. *J Ultrasound Med* 1989; 8:255–258.
14. Finley BE, Burlbaw J, Bennett TL, Levitch L. Delayed return of the fetal midgut to the abdomen resulting in volvulus, bowel obstruction, and gangrene of the small intestine. *J Ultrasound Med* 1992;11:233–235.
15. Fogata ML, Collins HB 2nd, Wagner CW, Angtuaco TL. Prenatal diagnosis of complicated abdominal wall defects. *Curr Probl Diagn Radiol* 1999;28(4):101–128.
16. Walkinshaw SA, Renwick M, Hebisch G, et al. How good is ultrasound in the detection and evaluation of anterior abdominal wall defects? *Br J Radiol* 1992;65:298–301.
17. van de Geijn EJ, van Vugt JMG, Sollie JE, van Geijn HP. Ultrasonographic diagnosis and perinatal management of fetal abdominal wall defects. *Fetal Diagn Ther* 1991;6:2–10.
18. Hutchin P. Somatic anomalies of the umbilicus and anterior abdominal wall. *Surg Gynecol Obstet* 1965;120:1075–1090.
19. Martin LW, Torres AM. Omphalocele and gastroschisis. Symposium on pediatric surgery. *Surg Clin North Am* 1985;65:1235–1244.
20. Redford DH, McNay MB, Whittle MJ. Gastroschisis and exomphalos: precise diagnosis by midpregnancy ultrasound. *Br J Obstet Gynecol* 1985;92:54–59.
21. Hansen LK, Pedersen SA, Kristoffersen K. Prenatal rupture of omphalocele. *J Clin Ultrasound* 1987;15:191–193.
22. Luck SR, Sherman J, Raffensperger JG, Goldstein IR. Gastroschisis in 106 consecutive newborn infants. *Surgery* 1985;98:677–683.
23. Mayer T, Black R, Matlak ME, Johnson DG. Gastroschisis and omphalocele. An eight-year review. *Ann Surg* 1980; 192:783–787.
24. Bair JH, Russ PD, Pretorius DH, Manchester D, Manco-Johnson ML. Fetal omphalocele and gastroschisis: a review of 24 cases. *AJR Am J Roentgenol* 1986;147:1047–1051.
25. Eurenius K, Axelsson O. Outcome for fetuses with abdominal wall defects detected by routine second trimester ultrasound. *Acta Obstet Gynecol Scand* 1994;73:25–29.
26. Rankin J, Dillon E, Wright C. Congenital anterior abdominal wall defects in the north of England, 1986–1996: occurrence and outcome. *Prenat Diagn* 1999;19(7):662–668.
27. Nichols CR, Dickinson JE, Pemberton PJ. Rising incidence of gastroschisis in teenage pregnancies. *J Matern Fetal Med* 1997;6(4):225–229.
28. Tan KH, Kilby MD, Whittle MJ, Beattie BR, Booth IW, Botting BJ. Congenital anterior abdominal wall defects in England and Wales 1987–93: retrospective analysis of OPCS data. *BMJ* 1996;313(7062):903–906.
29. Grosfeld JL, Dawes L, Weber TR. Congenital abdominal wall defects: current management and survival. *Surg Clin North Am* 1981;61:1037–1049.
30. Schwaitzberg SD, Pokorny WJ, McGill CW, Harberg FJ. Gastroschisis and omphalocele. *Am J Surg* 1982;144:650–654.
31. Penman DG, Fisher RM, Noblett HR, Soothill PW. Increase in incidence of gastroschisis in the south west of England in 1995. *Br J Obstet Gynaecol* 1998;105:328–331.
32. Thepcharoennirund S. Left-sided gastroschisis: two case reports in Ratchaburi Hospital. *J Med Assoc Thai* 2000; 83(7):804–808.
33. Duhamel B. Embryology of exomphalos and allied malformations. *Arch Dis Child* 1968;38:142–147.
34. DeVries PA. The pathogenesis of gastroschisis and omphalocele. *J Pediatr Surg* 1980;15:245–251.
35. Hoyme HE, Higginbottom MC, Jones KL. The vascular pathogenesis of gastroschisis: intrauterine interruption of the omphalomesenteric artery. *J Pediatr* 1981;98:228–231.
36. Werler MM, Mitchell AA, Shapiro S. Demographic, reproductive, medical, and environmental factors in relation to gastroschisis. *Teratology* 1992;45:353–360.
37. Torfs CP, Velie EM, Oechsli FW, Bateson TF, Curry CJ. A

population-based study of gastroschisis: demographic, pregnancy, and lifestyle risk factor. *Teratology* 1994;50:44–53.

38. Martinez-Frias ML, Rodriguez-Pinilla E, Prieto L. Prenatal exposure to salicylates and gastroschisis: a case-control study. *Teratology* 1997;56(4):241–243.

39. Torfs CP, Katz EA, Bateson TF, Lam PK, Curry CJ. Maternal medications and environmental exposures as risk factors for gastroschisis. *Teratology* 1996;54(2):84–92.

40. Sadovsky Y, Robbin ML, Crandall BF, Filly RA, Golbus MS. The association between "faint-positive" amniotic fluid acetylcholinesterase and fetal malformations. *Prenat Diagn* 1993;13:1071–1074.

41. Tucker JM, Brumfield CG, Davis RO. Prenatal differentiation of ventral abdominal wall defects—are amniotic fluid markers useful adjuncts? *J Reprod Med* 1992;37:445–448.

42. Hasan S, Hermansen MC. The prenatal diagnosis of ventral abdominal wall defects. *Am J Obstet Gynecol* 1986;155:842–845.

43. Pinzon M, Barr RG. Extracorporeal liver and spleen in gastroschisis. *AJR Am J Roentgenol* 1995;164(4):1025.

44. Mabogunje OOA, Mahour GH. Omphalocele and gastroschisis: trends in survival across two decades. *Am J Surg* 1984;148:679–686.

45. Kluck P, Tibboel D, van der Kamp AW, Molenaar JC. The effect of fetal urine on the development of bowel in gastroschisis. *J Pediatr Surg* 1983;18:47–50.

46. Stringel G, Filler RM. Prognostic factors in omphalocele and gastroschisis. *J Pediatr Surg* 1979;14:515–519.

47. Tibboel D, Raine M, McNee M, Azmy A, Kluck P, et al. Developmental aspects of gastroschisis. *J Pediatr Surg* 1986;21:865–869.

48. Fitzsimmons J, Nyberg DA, Cyr DR, Hatch E. Perinatal management of gastroschisis. *Obstet Gynecol* 1988;71:910–913.

49. Pinette MG, Pan Y, Pinette SG, Jones M, Stubblefield PG, et al. Gastroschisis followed by absorption of the small bowel and closure of the abdominal wall defect. *J Ultrasound Med* 1994;13:719–721.

50. Johnson N, Lilford RJ, Irving H, Crabbe D, Cartmill R. The vanishing bowel: case report of bowel atresia following gastroschisis. *Br J Obstet Gynaecol* 1991;98:214–215.

51. Perrella RR, Ragavendra N, Tessler FN, Boechat I, Crandall B, Grant EG. Fetal abdominal wall mass detected on prenatal sonography: gastroschisis vs omphalocele. *AJR Am J Roentgenol* 1991;157:1065–1068.

52. Kimble RM, Blakelock R, Cass D. Vanishing gut in infants with gastroschisis. *Pediatr Surg Int* 1999;15(7):483–485.

53. Barsoom MJ, Prabulos A, Rodis JF, Turner GW. Vanishing gastroschisis and short-bowel syndrome. *Obstet Gynecol* 2000;95(5 Pt 2):818–819.

54. Bond SJ, Harrison MR, Filly RA, Callen PW, Anderson RA, Golbus MS. Severity of intestinal damage in gastroschisis: correlation with prenatal sonographic findings. *J Pediatr Surg* 1988;23:520–525.

55. Pokorny WJ, Harberg FJ, McGill CW. Gastroschisis complicated by intestinal atresia. *J Pediatr Surg* 1981;16:261–263.

56. Pryde PG, Bardicef M, Treadwell MC, Klein M, Isada NB, Evans MI. Gastroschisis: Can antenatal ultrasound predict infant outcomes? *Obstet Gynecol* 1994;84:505–510.

57. Babcook CJ, Hedrick MH, Goldstein RB, Callen PW, Harrison MR, et al. Gastroschisis: Can sonography of the fetal bowel accurately predict postnatal outcome? *J Ultrasound Med* 1994;13:701–706.

58. Lenke RR, Persutte WH, Nemes J. Ultrasonographic assessment of intestinal damage in fetuses with gastroschisis: is it of clinical value? *Am J Obstet Gynecol* 1990;163:995–998.

59. Langer JC, Khanna J, Caco C, Dykes EH, Nicolaides KH. Prenatal diagnosis of gastroschisis: development of objective sonographic criteria for predicting outcome. *Obstet Gynecol* 1993;81:53–56.

60. Nicholls EA, Ford WD, Barnes KH, Furness ME, Hayward C. A decade of gastroschisis in the era of antenatal ultrasound. *Aust N Z J Surg* 1996;66:366–368.

61. Sipes SL, Weiner CP, Williamson RA, Pringle KC, Kimura K. Fetal gastroschisis complicated by bowel dilatation: an indication for imminent delivery? *Fetal Diagn Ther* 1990;5:100–103.

62. Poulain P, Milon J, Fremont B, Proudhon JF, Odent S, et al. Remarks about the prognosis in case of antenatal diagnosis of gastroschisis. *Eur J Obstet Gynecol Reprod Biol* 1994;54: 185–190.

63. Adra AM, Landy HJ, Nahmias J, Gomez-Marin O. The fetus with gastroschisis: impact of route of delivery and prenatal ultrasonography. *Am J Obstet Gynecol* 1996;174(2):540–546.

64. Abuhamad AZ, Mari G, Cortina RM, Croitoru DP, Evans AT. Superior mesenteric artery Doppler velocimetry and ultrasonographic assessment of fetal bowel in gastroschisis: a prospective longitudinal study. *Am J Obstet Gynecol* 1997; 176(5):985–990.

65. Alsulyman OM, Monteiro H, Ouzounian JG, Barton L, Songster GS, Kovacs BW. Clinical significance of prenatal ultrasonographic intestinal dilatation in fetuses with gastroschisis. *Am J Obstet Gynecol* 1996;175(4 Pt 1):982–984.

66. Adair CD, Rosnes J, Frye AH, Burrus DR, Nelson LH, Veille JC. The role of antepartum surveillance in the management of gastroschisis. *Int J Gynaecol Obstet* 1996;52(2): 141–144.

67. Axt R, Quijano F, Boos R, Hendrik HJ, Jessberger HJ, et al. Omphalocele and gastroschisis: prenatal diagnosis and peripartal management. A case analysis of the years 1989–1997 at the Department of Obstetrics and Gynecology, University of Homburg/Saar. *Eur J Obstet Gynecol Reprod Biol* 1999;87(1):47–54.

68. Heydanus R, Raats MA, Tibboel D, Los FJ, Wladimiroff JW. Prenatal diagnosis of fetal abdominal wall defects: a retrospective analysis of 44 cases. *Prenat Diagn* 1996;16(5):411–417.

69. Blakelock RT, Upadhyay V, Pease PW, Harding JE. Are babies with gastroschisis small for gestational age? *Pediatr Surg Int* 1997;12(8):580–582.

70. Raynor BD, Richards D. Growth retardation in fetuses with gastroschisis. *J Ultrasound Med* 1997;16(1):13–16.

71. Snyder CL. Outcome analysis for gastroschisis. *J Pediatr Surg* 1999;34(8):1253–1256.

72. Ortiz VN, Villarreal DH, Gonzalez Olmo J, Ramos Perea C. Gastroschisis: a ten year review. *Bol Asoc Med P R* 1998;90(4–6):69–73.

73. Mercer S, Mercer B, D'Alton ME, Soucy P. Gastroschisis: ultrasonographic diagnosis, perinatal embryology, surgical and obstetric treatment and outcomes. *Can J Surg* 1988;31:25–26.

74. Blakelock R, Upadhyay V, Kimble R, Pease P, Kolbe A, Harding J. Is a normally functioning gastrointestinal tract nec-

essary for normal growth in late gestation? *Pediatr Surg Int* 1998;13(1):17–20.

75. Shinmoto H, Kashima K, Yuasa Y, Tanimoto A, Morikawa Y, et al. MR imaging of non-CNS fetal abnormalities: a pictorial essay. *Radiographics* 2000;20(5):1227–1243.

76. Kirk EP, Wah R. Obstetric management of the fetus with omphalocele or gastroschisis: a review and report of one hundred twelve cases. *Am J Obstet Gynecol* 1983;146:512–518.

77. Boyd PA, Bhattacharjee A, Gould S, Manning N, Chamberlain P. Outcome of prenatally diagnosed anterior abdominal wall defects. *Arch Dis Child Fetal Neonatal Ed* 1998; 78(3):F209–F213.

78. Reid CO, Hall JG, Anderson C, Bocian M, Carey J, et al. Association of amyoplasia with gastroschisis, bowel atresia, and defects of the muscular layer of the trunk. *Am J Med Genet* 1986;24(4):701–710.

79. Swartz KR, Harrison MW, Campbell JR, Campbell TJ. Long-term follow-up of patients with gastroschisis. *Am J Surg* 1986;151:546–549.

80. Novotny DA, Klein RL, Boeckman CR. Gastroschisis: an 18-year review. *J Pediatr Surg* 1993;28:650–652.

81. Gabriel R, Leroux B, Quéreux C, Daoud S, Wahl P. Gastroschisis: What part can the obstetrician play? *Eur J Obstet Gynecol Reprod Biol* 1992;45:101–105.

82. Fonkalsrud EW, Smith MD, Shaw KS, Borick JM, Shaw A. Selective management of gastroschisis according to the degree of visceroabdominal disproportion. *Ann Surg* 1993;218:742–747.

83. Crawford RA, Ryan G, Wright VM, Rodeck CH. The importance of serial biophysical assessment of fetal wellbeing in gastroschisis. *Br J Obstet Gynaecol* 1992;99(11):899–902.

84. Burge DM, Ade-Ajayi N. Adverse outcome after prenatal diagnosis of gastroschisis: the role of fetal monitoring. *J Pediatr Surg* 1997;32(3):441–444.

85. Fries MH, Filly RA, Callen PW, Goldstein RB, Goldberg JD, Golbus MS. Growth retardation in prenatally diagnosed cases of gastroschisis. *J Ultrasound Med* 1993;12:583–588.

86. Fleet MS, de la Hunt MN. Intestinal atresia with gastroschisis: a selective approach to management. *J Pediatr Surg* 2000;35(9):1323–1325.

87. Dimitriou G, Greenough A, Mantagos JS, Davenport M, Nicolaides KH. Morbidity in infants with antenatally-diagnosed anterior abdominal wall defects. *Pediatr Surg Int* 2000;16(5–6):404–407.

88. Davies BW, Stringer MD. The survivors of gastroschisis. *Arch Dis Child* 1997;77(2):158–160.

89. Dykes EH. Prenatal diagnosis and management of abdominal wall defects. *Semin Pediatr Surg* 1996;5(2):90–94.

90. Aktug T, Ucan B, Olguner M, Akgur FM, Ozer E, et al. Amnio-allantoic fluid exchange for the prevention of intestinal damage in gastroschisis. III: Determination of the waste products removed by exchange. *Eur J Pediatr Surg* 1998;8(6):326–328.

91. Luton D, de Lagausie P, Guibourdenche J, Peuchmaur M, Sibony O, et al. Influence of amnioinfusion in a model of *in utero* created gastroschisis in the pregnant ewe. *Fetal Diagn Ther* 2000;15(4):224–228.

92. Luton D, De Lagausie P, Guibourdenche J, Oury JF, Vuillard E, et al. Prognostic factors of prenatally diagnosed gastroschisis. *Fetal Diagn Ther* 1997;12(1):7–14.

93. Luton D, de Lagausie P, Guibourdenche J, Oury J, Sibony O, et al. Effect of amnioinfusion on the outcome of prenatally diagnosed gastroschisis. *Fetal Diagn Ther* 1999;14(3):152–155.

94. Morrison JJ, Klein N, Chitty LS, Kocjan G, Walshe D, et al. Intra-amniotic inflammation in human gastroschisis: possible aetiology of postnatal bowel dysfunction. *Br J Obstet Gynaecol* 1998;105(11):1200–1204.

95. Kitchanan S, Patole SK, Muller R, Whitehall JS. Neonatal outcome of gastroschisis and exomphalos: a 10-year review. *J Paediatr Child Health* 2000;36(5):428–430.

96. Sipes SL, Weiner CP, Sipes DR 2d, Grant SS, Williamson RA. Gastroschisis and omphalocele: does either antenatal diagnosis or route of delivery make a difference in perinatal outcome? *Obstet Gynecol* 1990;76:195–199.

97. Lenke RR, Hatch EI. Fetal gastroschisis: a preliminary report advocating the use of cesarean section. *Obstet Gynecol* 1986;67:395–398.

98. Sakala EP, Erhard LN, White JJ. Elective cesarean section improves outcomes of neonates with gastroschisis. *Am J Obstet Gynecol* 1993;169:1050–1053.

99. Swift RI, Singh MP, Ziderman DA, Silverman M, Elder MA, Elder MG. A new regime in the management of gastroschisis. *J Pediatr Surg* 1992;27:61–63.

100. Moore TC, Collins DL, Catanzarite V, Hatch EI Jr. Pre-term and particularly pre-labor cesarean section to avoid complications of gastroschisis. *Pediatr Surg Int* 1999;15(2):97–104.

101. Dunn JC, Fonkalsrud EW, Atkinson JB. The influence of gestational age and mode of delivery on infants with gastroschisis. *J Pediatr Surg* 1999;34(9):1393–1395.

102. How HY, Harris BJ, Pietrantoni M, Evans JC, Dutton S, et al. Is vaginal delivery preferable to elective cesarean delivery in fetuses with a known ventral wall defect? *Am J Obstet Gynecol* 2000;182(6):1527–1534.

103. Stringer MD, Brereton RJ, Wright VM. Controversies in the management of gastroschisis: a study of 40 patients. *Arch Dis Child* 1991;66:34–36.

104. Blakelock RT, Harding JE, Kolbe A, Pease PW. Gastroschisis: can the morbidity be avoided? *Pediatr Surg Int* 1997;12(4):276–282.

105. Puri A, Bajpai M. Gastroschisis and omphalocele. *Indian J Pediatr* 1999;66(5):773–789.

106. Driver CP, Bruce J, Bianchi A, Doig CM, Dickson AP, Bowen J. The contemporary outcome of gastroschisis. *J Pediatr Surg* 2000;35(12):1719–1723.

107. Lacey SR, Carris LA, Beyer AJ 3d, Azizkhan RG. Bladder pressure monitoring significantly enhances care of infants with abdominal wall defects: a prospective clinical study. *J Pediatr Surg* 1993;28(10):1370–1374.

108. Minkes RK, Langer JC, Mazziotti MV, Skinner MA, Foglia RP. Routine insertion of a Silastic spring-loaded silo for infants with gastroschisis. *J Pediatr Surg* 2000;35(6):843–846.

109. Torfs CP, Curry CJR. Familial cases of gastroschisis in a population-based registry. *Am J Med Genet* 1993;45:465–467.

110. Gorczyca DP, Lindfors KK, Giles KA, McGahan JP, Hanson FW, Tennant FP. Prenatally diagnosed gastroschisis in monozygotic twins. *J Clin Ultrasound* 1989;17:216–218.

111. Gilbert WM, Nicolaides KH. Fetal omphalocele: associated malformations and chromosomal defects. *Obstet Gynecol* 1987;70:633–635.

112. Seashore JH. Congenital abdominal wall defects. *Clin Perinatol* 1978;5:62–77.

113. Cameron GM, McQuown DS, Modanlou HD, Zenlyn S, Pillsbury SG Jr. Intrauterine diagnosis of an omphalocele by diagnostic ultrasonography. *Am J Obstet Gynecol* 1978;131:821–822.

114. Schaffer RM, Barone C, Friedman AP. The ultrasonographic spectrum of fetal omphalocele. *J Ultrasound Med* 1983;2:219–222.

115. Griffiths DM, Gough MH. Dilemmas after ultrasonic diagnosis of fetal abnormality. *Lancet* 1985;i:623–625.

116. Brown BSJ. The prenatal ultrasonographic features of omphalocele: a study of 10 patients. *J Can Assoc Radiol* 1985;36:312–316.

117. St-Vil D, Shaw KS, Lallier M, Yazbeck S, Di Lorenzo M, et al. Chromosomal anomalies in newborns with omphalocele. *J Pediatr Surg* 1996;31(6):831–834.

118. Mann L, Ferguson-Smith MA, Desai M, Gibson AAM, et al. Prenatal assessment of anterior abdominal wall defects and their prognosis. *Prenat Diagn* 1984;4:427–435.

119. Roberts JP, Burge DM. Antenatal diagnosis of abdominal wall defects: a missed opportunity? *Arch Dis Child* 1990;65:687–689.

120. Hertzberg BS. Sonography of the fetal gastrointestinal tract: anatomic variants, diagnostic pitfalls, and abnormalities. *AJR Am J Roentgenol* 1994;162:1175–1182.

121. Lindfors KK, McGahan JP, Walter JP. Fetal omphalocele and gastroschisis: pitfalls in sonographic diagnosis *AJR Am J Roentgenol* 1986;147:797–800.

122. Hughes MD, Nyberg DA, Mack LA, Pretorius DH. Fetal omphalocele: prenatal detection of concurrent anomalies and other predictors of outcome. *Radiology* 1989;173(2):371–376.

123. Nelson PA, Bowie JD, Filston HC, Crane LM. Sonographic diagnosis of omphalocele *in utero*. *AJR Am J Roentgenol* 1981;138:1178–1180.

124. Bromley B, Benacerraf BR. Transient omphalocele. *J Ultrasound Med* 1993;12:688–689.

125. Osborne J. Gastroschisis and omphalocele. Prenatal ultrasonic detection and its significance. *Australas Radiol* 1986;30:113–116.

126. Carpenter MW, Curci MR, Dibbins AW, Haddow JE. Perinatal management of ventral wall defects. *Obstet Gynecol* 1984;64:646–651.

127. Chitayat D, Toi A, Babul R, Blaser S, Moola S, et al. Omphalocele in Miller-Dieker syndrome: expanding the phenotype. *Am J Med Genet* 1997;69(3):293–298.

128. Salzman L, Kuligowska E, Semine A. Pseudoomphalocele: pitfall in fetal sonography. *AJR Am J Roentgenol* 1986;146:1283–1285.

129. Tolaymat LL, Maher JE, Kleinman GE, Stalnaker R, Kea K, Walker A. Persistent patent urachus with allantoic cyst: a case report. *Ultrasound Obstet Gynecol* 1997;10(5):366–368.

130. Colley N, Knott PD, Gould SJ. Misdiagnosis of omphalocele associated with Edwards syndrome and congenital heart disease. *Prenat Diagn* 1987;7:377–381.

131. Hughes HA, Feinstein SJ, Lodeiro JG, Byers JW, Srinivasan J, et al. Umbilical cord cyst presenting as an omphalocele at 15 weeks' gestation: a case report. *J Reprod Med* 1990;35:658–660.

132. Maynor CH, Hertzberg BS, Kliewer MA, Heyneman LE, Carroll BA. Antenatal ultrasonographic diagnosis of abdominal wall hemangioma: potential to simulate ventral abdominal wall defects. *J Ultrasound Med* 1995;14:317–319.

133. Calzolari E, Volpato S, Bianchi F, Cianciulli D, Tenconi R, et al. Omphalocele and gastroschisis: a collaborative study of five Italian congenital malformation registries. *Teratology* 1993;47(1):47–55.

134. Sermer M, Benzie RJ, Pitson L, Carr M, Skidmore M. Prenatal diagnosis and management of congenital defects of the anterior abdominal wall. *Am J Obstet Gynecol* 1987;156:308–312.

135. Shigemoto H, Horiya Y, Isomoto T, Yamamoto Y, Sano K, Saito M. Duodenal atresia secondary to intrauterine midgut strangulation by an omphalocele. *J Pediatr Surg* 1982;17:420–421.

136. Elliott M, Bayly R, Cole T, Temple IK, Maher ER. Clinical features and natural history of Beckwith-Wiedemann syndrome: presentation of 74 new cases. *Clin Genet* 1994;46:168–174.

137. Knight PJ, Sommer A, Clatworthy HW. Omphalocele: a prognostic classification. *J Pediatr Surg* 1981;16:599–604.

138. Weinstein L, Anderson C. *In utero* diagnosis of Beckwith-Wiedemann syndrome by ultrasound. *Radiology* 1980;134:474.

139. Winter SC, Curry CJR, Smith JC, Kassel S, Miller L, Andrea J. Prenatal diagnosis of the Beckwith-Wiedemann syndrome. *Am J Med Genet* 1986;24:137–141.

140. Viljoen DL, Jaquire Z, Woods DL. Prenatal diagnosis in autosomal dominant Beckwith-Wiedemann syndrome. *Prenat Diagn* 1991;11:167–175.

141. Wieacker P, Wilhelm C, Greiner P, Schillinger H. Prenatal diagnosis of Wiedemann-Beckwith syndrome. *J Perinat Med* 1989;17(5):351–355.

142. Whisson CC, Whyte A, Ziesing P. Beckwith-Wiedemann syndrome: antenatal diagnosis. *Australas Radiol* 1994;38:130–131.

143. Shal YG, Metlay L. Prenatal ultrasound diagnosis of Beckwith-Wiedemann syndrome. *J Clin Ultrasound* 1990;18:597–600.

144. Lodeiro JG, Byers JW 3rd, Chuipek S, Feinstein SJ. Prenatal diagnosis and perinatal management of the Beckwith-Wiedemann syndrome: a case and review. *Am J Perinatol* 1989;6:446–449.

145. Meizner I, Carmi R, Katz M, Insler V. *In utero* prenatal diagnosis of Beckwith-Wiedemann syndrome: a case report. *Eur J Obstet Gynecol Reprod Biol* 1989;32:259–264.

146. Cobellis G, Iannoto P, Stabile M, Lonardo F, Della Bruna M, et al. Prenatal ultrasound diagnosis of macroglossia in the Wiedemann-Beckwith syndrome. *Prenat Diagn* 1988;8:79–81.

147. Ranzini AC, Day-Salvatore D, Turner T, Smulian JC, Vintzileos AM. Intrauterine growth and ultrasound findings in fetuses with Beckwith-Wiedemann syndrome. *Obstet Gynecol* 1997;89(4):538–542.

148. Snijders RJ, Sebire NJ, Souka A, Santiago C, Nicolaides KH. Fetal exomphalos and chromosomal defects: relationship to maternal age and gestation. *Ultrasound Obstet Gynecol* 1995;6(4):250–255.

149. Torfs CP, Honore LH, Curry CJ. Is there an association of Down syndrome and omphalocele? *Am J Med Genet* 1997;73(4):400–403.

150. Catchpoole D, Lam WW, Valler D, Temple IK, Joyce JA, et al. Epigenetic modification and uniparental inheritance of H19 in Beckwith-Wiedemann syndrome. *J Med Genet* 1997;34(5):353–359.

151. Skupski DW. Prenatal diagnosis of gastrointestinal anoma-

lies with ultrasound. What have we learned? *Ann N Y Acad Sci* 1998;847:53–58.

152. Kilby MD, Lander A, Usher-Somers M. Exomphalos. *Prenat Diagn* 1998;18(12):1283–1288.

153. Nicolaides KH, Snijders RJ, Cheng HH, Gosden C. Fetal gastro-intestinal and abdominal wall defects: associated malformations and chromosomal abnormalities. *Fetal Diagn Ther* 1992;7(2):102–115.

154. Getachew MM, Goldstein RB, Edge V, Goldberg JD, Filly RA. Correlation between omphalocele contents and karyotypic abnormalities: sonographic study in 37 cases. *AJR Am J Roentgenol* 1992;158(1):133–136.

155. Nyberg DA, Fitzsimmons J, Mack LA, Hughes M, Pretorius DH, et al. Chromosomal abnormalities in fetuses with omphalocele: the significance of omphalocele contents. *J Ultrasound Med* 1989;8:299–308.

156. Benacerraf BR, Saltzman DH, Estroff JA, Frigoletto FD Jr. Abnormal karyotype of fetuses with omphalocele: prediction based on omphalocele contents. *Obstet Gynecol* 1990;75(3 Pt 1):317–319.

157. De Veciana M, Major CA, Porto M. Prediction of an abnormal karyotype in fetuses with omphalocele. *Prenat Diagn* 1994;14(6):487–492.

158. St-Vil D, Shaw KS, Lallier M, Yazbeck S, Di Lorenzo M, et al. Chromosomal anomalies in newborns with omphalocele. *J Pediatr Surg* 1996;31(6):831–834.

159. Chen CP, Liu FF, Jan SW, Sheu JC, Huang SH, Lan CC. Prenatal diagnosis and perinatal aspects of abdominal wall defects. *Am J Perinatol* 1996;13(6):355–361.

160. Chen CP, Jan SW, Liu FF, Chiang S, Huang SH, et al. Prenatal diagnosis of omphalocele associated with umbilical cord cyst. *Acta Obstet Gynecol Scand* 1995;74(10):832–835.

161. Tucci M, Bard H. The associated anomalies that determine prognosis in congenital omphaloceles. *Am J Obstet Gynecol* 1990;163:1646–1649.

162. Wakhlu A, Wakhlu AK. The management of exomphalos. *J Pediatr Surg* 2000;35(1):73–76.

163. Forrester MB, Merz RD. Epidemiology of abdominal wall defects, Hawaii, 1986–1997. *Teratology* 1999;60(3):117–123.

164. Martin RW. Screening for fetal abdominal wall defects. *Obstet Gynecol Clin North Am* 1998;25(3):517–526.

165. Fisher R, Attah A, Partington A, Dykes E. Impact of antenatal diagnosis on incidence and prognosis in abdominal wall defects. *J Pediatr Surg* 1996;31(4):538–541.

166. Langer JC. Gastroschisis and omphalocele. *Semin Pediatr Surg* 1996;5(2):124–128.

167. Towne BH, Peters G, Cheng JHT. The problem of "giant" omphalocele. *J Pediatr Surg* 1980;15:543–548.

168. Laubscher B, Greenough A, Dimitriou G, Davenport M, Nicolaides KH. Serial lung volume measurements during the perinatal period in infants with abdominal wall defects. *J Pediatr Surg* 1998;33(3):497–499.

169. Reynolds M. Abdominal wall defects in infants with very low birth weight. *Semin Pediatr Surg* 2000;9(2):88–90.

170. Tsakayannis DE, Zurakowski D, Lillehei CW. Respiratory insufficiency at birth: a predictor of mortality for infants with omphalocele. *J Pediatr Surg* 1996;31(8):1088–1090.

171. Crawford DC, Chapman MG, Allan LD. Echocardiography in the investigation of anterior abdominal wall defects in the fetus. *Br J Obstet Gynecol* 1985;92:1034–1036.

172. Pettenati MJ, Haines JL, Higgins RR, Wappner RS, Palmer CG, Weaver DD. Wiedemann-Beckwith syndrome: presentation of clinical and cytogenetic data on 22 new cases and review of the literature. *Hum Genet* 1986;74:143–154.

173. Slatter RE, Elliott M, Welham K, Carrera M, Schofield PN, et al. Mosaic uniparental disomy in Beckwith-Wiedemann syndrome. *J Med Genet* 1994;31(10):749–753.

174. Engel JR, Smallwood A, Harper A, Higgins MJ, Oshimura M, et al. Epigenotype-phenotype correlations in Beckwith-Wiedemann syndrome. *J Med Genet* 2000;37(12):921–926.

175. Chi LH, Stone DH, Gilmour WH. Impact of prenatal screening and diagnosis on the epidemiology of structural congenital anomalies. *J Med Screen* 1995;2(2):67–70.

176. Lurie S, Sherman D, Bukovsky I. Omphalocele delivery enigma: the best mode of delivery still remains dubious. *Eur J Obstet Gynecol Reprod Biol* 1999;82(1):19–22.

177. Rizzo A, Davis PC, Hamm CR, Powell RW. Intraoperative vesical pressure measurements as a guide in the closure of abdominal wall defects. *Am Surg* 1996;62(3):192–196.

178. Dunn JC, Fonkalsrud EW. Improved survival of infants with omphalocele. *Am J Surg* 1997;173(4):284–287.

179. DeLuca FG, Gilchrist BF, Paquette E, Wesselhoeft CW, Luks FI. External compression as initial management of giant omphaloceles. *J Pediatr Surg* 1996;31(7):965–967.

180. Belloli G, Battaglino F, Musi L. Management of giant omphalocele by progressive external compression: case report. *J Pediatr Surg* 1996;31(12):1719–1720.

181. Brown MF, Wright L. Delayed external compression reduction of an omphalocele (DECRO): an alternative method of treatment for moderate and large omphaloceles. *J Pediatr Surg* 1998;33(7):1113–1115.

182. Nuchtern JG, Baxter R, Hatch EI Jr. Nonoperative initial management versus silon chimney for treatment of giant omphalocele. *J Pediatr Surg* 1995;30(6):771–776.

183. Cantrell JR, Haller JA, Ravitch HH, et al. A syndrome of congenital defects involving the abdominal wall, sternum, diaphragm, and heart. *Surg Gynecol Obstet* 1958;107:602.

184. Toyama WM. Combined congenital defects of the anterior abdominal wall, sternum, diaphragm, pericardium, and heart: a case report and review of the syndrome. *Pediatrics* 1972;50:778–792.

185. Fokin AA. Cleft sternum and sternal foramen. *Chest Surg Clin N Am* 2000;10(2):261–276.

186. Firmin RK, Fragomeni LS, Lennox SC. Complete cleft sternum. *Thorax* 1980;35(4):303–306.

187. Heron D, Lyonnet S, Iserin L, Munnich A, Padovani JP. Sternal cleft: case report and review of a series of nine patients. *Am J Med Genet* 1995;59(2):154–156.

188. Hersh JH, Waterfill D, Rutledge J, Harrod MJ, O'Sheal SF, et al. Sternal malformation/vascular dysplasia association. *Am J Med Genet* 1985;21(1):177–186, 201–202.

189. Kaplan LC, Matsuoka R, Gilbert EF, Opitz JM, Kurnit DM. Ectopia cordis and cleft sternum: evidence of mechanical teratogenesis following rupture of the chorion or yolk sac. *Am J Med Genet* 1985;21:187–199.

190. Ravitch MM. Cantrell's pentalogy and notes on diverticulum of the left ventricle. In: *Congenital deformities of the chest wall and their operative corrections.* Philadelphia: WB Saunders, 1977:53–57.

191. Siles C, Boyd PA, Manning N, Tsang T, Chamberlain P.

Omphalocele and pericardial effusion: possible sonographic markers for the pentalogy of Cantrell or its variants. *Obstet Gynecol* 1996;87(5 Pt 2):840–842.

192. Lau TK, Fung HY, Fung TY. Fetal diaphragmatic hernia presented with transient unilateral pleural effusion. *Ultrasound Obstet Gynecol* 1997;9(2):125–127.

193. Rose NC, Coleman BG, Wallace D, Gaupman K, Fuchelli E. Prenatal diagnosis of a chest wall hamartoma and sternal cleft. *Ultrasound Obstet Gynecol* 1996;7(6):453–455.

194. Hebra A, Davidoff A, O'Neill JA Jr. Neonatal sternal cleft associated with an extrathoracic cystic mass. *J Pediatr Surg* 1997;32(4):627–630.

195. Ghidini A, Sirtori M, Romero R, Hobbins JC. Prenatal diagnosis of pentalogy of Cantrell. *J Ultrasound Med* 1988;7:567–472.

196. Seeds JW, Cefalo RC, Lies SC, Koontz WL. Early prenatal sonographic appearance of rare thoraco-abdominal eventration. *Prenat Diagn* 1984;4:437–441.

197. Fernandez MS, Lopez A, Vila JJ, Lluna J, Miranda J. Cantrell's pentalogy. Report of four cases and their management. *Pediatr Surg Int* 1997;12(5–6):428–431.

198. Baker ME, Rosenberg ER, Trofatter KF, Imber MJ, Bowie JD. The in utero findings in twin pentalogy of Cantrell. *J Ultrasound Med* 1984;3:525–527.

199. Pasic M, Carrel T, Tonz M, Niederhauser U, Von Segesser LK, Turina MI. Sternal cleft associated with vascular anomalies and micrognathia. *Ann Thorac Surg* 1993;56(1):165–168.

200. Carmi R, Boughman JA. Pentalogy of Cantrell and associated midline anomalies: a possible ventral midline developmental field. *Am J Med Genet* 1992;42:90–95.

201. Egan JFX, Petrikovsky BM, Vintzileos AM, Rodis JF, Campbell WM. Combined pentalogy of Cantrell and sirenomelia: a case report with speculation about a common etiology. *Am J Perinatol* 1993;10:327–329.

202. Denath FM, Romano W, Solcz M, Donnelly D. Ultrasonographic findings of exencephaly in pentalogy of Cantrell: case report and review of the literature. *J Clin Ultrasound* 1994;22:351–354.

203. Hsieh YY, Lee CC, Chang CC, Tsai HD, Hsu TY Tsai CH. Prenatal sonographic diagnosis of Cantrell's pentalogy with cystic hygroma in the first trimester. *J Clin Ultrasound* 1998;26(8):409–412.

204. Garson A, Hawkins EP, Mullins CE, Edwards SB, Sabiston DC Jr, Cooley DA. Thoracoabdominal ectopia cordis with mosaic Turner's syndrome: report of a case. *Pediatrics* 1978;62:218.

205. Abu-Yousel MM, Wray AB, Williamson RA, Bonsib SM. Antenatal ultrasound diagnosis of variant of pentalogy of Cantrell. *J Ultrasound Med* 1987;6:535–538.

206. Haynor DR, Shuman WP, Brewer DR, Mack LA. Imaging of fetal ectopia cordis: roles of sonography and computed tomography. *J Ultrasound Med* 1984;3:25–28.

207. Klingensmith WC III, Cioffi-Ragan DT, Harvey DE. Diagnosis of ectopia cordis in the second trimester. *J Clin Ultrasound* 1988;16:204–206.

208. Daum R, Zachariou Z. Total and superior sternal clefts in newborns: a simple technique for surgical correction. *J Pediatr Surg* 1999;34(3):408–411.

209. Hazari A, Mercer NS, Pawade A, Hayes AM. Superior sternal cleft: construction with a titanium plate. *Plast Reconstr Surg* 1998;101(1):167–170.

210. Greig DM. Cleft sternum and ectopia cordis. *Edinburgh Med J* 1926;33:480.

211. Dobell ARC, Williams HB, Long RW. Staged repair of ectopia cordis. *J Pediatr Surg* 1982;17:353.

212. Morales JM, Patel SG, Duff JA, Villareal RL, Simpson JW. Ectopia cordis and other midline defects. *Ann Thorac Surg* 2000;70(1):111–114.

213. Dillon E, Renwick M. The antenatal diagnosis and management of abdominal wall defects: the northern region experience. *Clin Radiol* 1995;50(12):855–859.

214. Bartholomew TH, Gonzales ET Jr. Urologic management in cloacal dysgenesis. *Urology* 1978;117:102.

215. Tank ES. Urologic complications of imperforate anus and cloacal dysgenesis. In: *Campbell's urology*, 5th ed. Philadelphia: WB Saunders, 1986:1889–2000.

216. Schinzel AAGL, Smith DW, Miller JR. Monozygotic twinning and structural defects. *J Pediatr* 1979;95:921–930.

217. Gray SW, Skandalakis JE. *Embryology for surgeons*. Philadelphia: WB Saunders, 1972.

218. Moore KL. *The developing human*, 4th ed. Philadelphia: WB Saunders, 1988:217–285.

219. Mildenberger H, Kluth D, Dziuba M. Embryology of bladder exstrophy. *J Pediatr Surg* 1988;23(2):166–170.

220. Engel RME. Exstrophy of the bladder and associated anomalies. *Birth Defects* 1974;10:146–149.

221. Kay R, Tank ES. Principles of management of the persistent cloaca in the female newborn. *J Urol* 1977;117:102–104.

222. Howell C, Caldamone A, Snyder H, Ziegler M, Duckett J. Optimal management of cloacal exstrophy. *J Pediatr Surg* 1983;18:365–369.

223. Mirk P, Calisti A, Fileni A. Prenatal sonographic diagnosis of bladder exstrophy. *J Ultrasound Med* 1986;5:291–293.

224. Haygood VP, Wahbeh CJ. Prospects for the prenatal diagnosis and obstetric management of cloacal exstrophy. *J Reprod Med* 1983;28:807–812.

225. Meizner I, Bar-Ziv J. *In utero* prenatal ultrasonic diagnosis of a rare case of cloacal exstrophy. *J Clin Ultrasound* 1985; 13:500–502.

226. Petrikovsky BM, Walzak MP Jr, D'Addario PF. Fetal cloacal anomalies: prenatal sonographic findings and differential diagnosis. *Obstet Gynecol* 1988;72:464–469.

227. Barth RA, Filly RA, Sondheimer FK. Prenatal sonographic findings in bladder exstrophy *J Ultrasound Med* 1990;9:359–361.

228. Jaffe R, Schoenfeld A, Ovadia J. Sonographic findings in the prenatal diagnosis of bladder exstrophy. *Am J Obstet Gynecol* 1990;162:675–678.

229. Goldstein I, Shalev E, Nisman D. The dilemma of prenatal diagnosis of bladder exstrophy: a case report and a review of the literature. *Ultrasound Obstet Gynecol* 2001;17(4):357–359.

230. Richards DS, Langham MR Jr, Mahaffey SM. The prenatal ultrasonographic diagnosis of cloacal exstrophy. *J Ultrasound Med* 1992;11:507–510.

231. Carr MC, Benacerraf BR, Mandell J. Prenatal diagnosis of an XY fetus with aphallia and cloacal exstrophy variant. *J Ultrasound Med* 1994;13:323–325.

232. Hamada H, Takano K, Shina H, Sakai T, Sohda S, Kubo T. New ultrasonographic criterion for the prenatal diagnosis of cloacal exstrophy: elephant-trunk like image. *J Urol* 1999; 162:2123–2124.

233. Austin PF, Homsy YL, Gearhart JP, Porter K, Guidi C, et al. The Langer prenatal diagnosis of cloacal exstrophy. *J Urol* 1998;160(3 Pt 2):1179–1181.

234. Meizner I, Levy A, Barnhard Y. Cloacal exstrophy sequence: an exceptional ultrasound diagnosis. *Obstet Gynecol* 1995;86(3):446–450.

235. Langer JC, Brennan B, Lappalainen RE, Caco CC, Winthrop AL, et al. Cloacal exstrophy: prenatal diagnosis before rupture of the cloacal membrane. *J Pediatr Surg* 1992;27:1352–1355.

236. Kaya H, Oral B, Dittrich R, Ozkaya O. Prenatal diagnosis of cloacal exstrophy before rupture of the cloacal membrane. *Arch Gynecol Obstet* 2000;263(3):142–144.

237. Bruch SW, Adzick NS, Goldstein RB, Harrison MR. Challenging the embryogenesis of cloacal exstrophy. *J Pediatr Surg* 1996;31(6):768–770.

238. Lande IM, Hamilton EF. The antenatal sonographic visualization of cloacal dysgenesis. *J Ultrasound Med* 1986;5:275–278.

239. Soper RT, Kilger K. Vesico-intestinal fissure. *J Urol* 1964; 92:490–501.

240. Tank ES, Lindenaner SM. Principles of management of exstrophy of the cloaca. *Am J Surg* 1970;119:95–100.

241. Carey JC, Greenbaum B, Hall BD. The OEIS complex (omphalocele, exstrophy, imperforate anus, spinal defects). *Birth Defects Orig Artic Ser* 1978;14(6B):253–263.

242. Gosden C, Brock DJH. Prenatal diagnosis of exstrophy of the cloaca. *Am J Med Genet* 1981;8:95–109.

243. Lee DH, Cottrell JR, Sanders RC, Meyers CM, Wulfsberg EA, Sun CC. OEIS complex (omphalocele-exstrophy-imperforate anus-spinal defects) in monozygotic twins. *Am J Med Genet* 1999;84(1):29–33.

244. Chen CP, Shih SL, Liu FF, Jan SW, Jeng CJ, Lan CC. Perinatal features of omphalocele-exstrophy-imperforate anus-spinal defects (OEIS complex) associated with large meningomyeloceles and severe limb defects. *Am J Perinatol* 1997;14(5):275–279.

245. Kallen K, Castilla EE, Robert E, Mastroiacovo P, Kallen B. OEIS complex—a population study. *Am J Med Genet* 2000;92(1):62–68.

246. Kutzner DK, Wilson WG, Hogge WA. OEIS complex (cloacal exstrophy): prenatal diagnosis in the second trimester. *Prenat Diagn* 1988;8:247–253.

247. Girz BA, Sherer DM, Atkin J, Venanzi M, Ahlborn L, Cestone L. First-trimester prenatal sonographic findings associated with OEIS (omphalocele-exstrophy-imperforate anus-spinal defects) complex: a case and review of the literature. *Am J Perinatol* 1998;15(1):15–17.

248. Hendren WH. Repair of cloacal anomalies: current techniques. *J Pediatr Surg* 1986;21:1159–1176.

249. Csontai A, Merksz M, Pirót L, Toth J. Results of surgical treatment in children with bladder exstrophy. *Br J Urol* 1992;70:683–685.

250. Wattenberg A, Beare JB, Tormey AR Jr. Exstrophy of the urinary bladder complicated by adenocarcinoma. *J Urol* 1956;76:583–594.

251. Hendren WH. Cloaca, the most severe degree of imperforate anus: experience with 195 cases. *Ann Surg* 1998;228(3):331–346.

252. Ricketts RR, Woodard JR, Zwiren GT. Modern treatment of cloacal exstrophy. *J Pediatr Surg* 1991;26:444–448.

253. Soffer SZ, Rosen NG, Hong AR, Alexianu M, Pena A. Cloacal exstrophy: a unified management plan. *J Pediatr Surg* 2000;35(6):932–937.

254. Davidoff AM, Hebra A, Balmer D, Templeton JM Jr, Schnaufer L. Management of the gastrointestinal tract and nutrition in patients with cloacal exstrophy. *J Pediatr Surg* 1996;31(6):771–773.

255. Reference deleted.

256. Hinman F. Surgical disorders of the bladder and umbilicus of urachal origin. *Surg Gynecol Obstet* 1961;113:605–614.

257. Perlmutter AD. Urachal disorders. In: *Campbell's urology*, 5th ed. Philadelphia: WB Saunders, 1986:1883–1888.

258. Rich RH, Hardy BE, Filler RM. Surgery for anomalies of the urachus. *J Pediatr Surg* 1983;18:370–372.

259. Persutte WH, Lenke RR, Kropp K, Ghareeb C. Antenatal diagnosis of fetal patent urachus. *J Ultrasound Med* 1988;7:399–403.

260. Donnenfeld AE, Mennuti MT, Templeton JM, Gabbe SG. Prenatal sonographic diagnosis of a vesico-allantoic abdominal wall defect. *J Ultrasound Med* 1989;8:43–45.

261. Frazier HA, Guerrieri JP, Thomas RL, Christenson PJ. The detection of a patent urachus and allantoic cyst of the umbilical cord on prenatal ultrasonography. *J Ultrasound Med* 1992;11:117–120.

262. Sachs L, Fourcroy JL, Wenzel DJ, Austin M, Nash JD. Prenatal detection of umbilical cord allantoic cyst. *Radiology* 1982;145:445–446.

263. Awwad J, Azar G, Soubra M. Sonographic diagnosis of a urachal cyst *in utero. Acta Obstet Gynecol Scand* 1994;73:156–157.

264. Hill LM, Kislak S, Belfar HL. The sonographic diagnosis of urachal cysts *in utero. J Clin Ultrasound* 1990;18:434–437.

265. Tsuchida Y, Ishida M. Osmolar relationship between enlarged umbilical cord and patent urachus. *J Pediatr Surg* 1969;4:465–467.

266. Ramirez P, Haberman S, Baxi L. Significance of prenatal diagnosis of umbilical cord cyst in a fetus with trisomy 18. *Am J Obstet Gynecol* 1995;173(3 Pt 1):955–957.

267. Sepulveda W, Gutierrez J, Sanchez J, Be C, Schnapp C. Pseudocyst of the umbilical cord: prenatal sonographic appearance and clinical significance. *Obstet Gynecol* 1999;93(3):377–381.

268. Smith GN, Walker M, Johnston S, Ash K. The sonographic finding of persistent umbilical cord cystic masses is associated with lethal aneuploidy and/or congenital anomalies. *Prenat Diagn* 1996;16(12):1141–1147.

269. Moore L, Russell S, Wilson L, Kiwanuka A. Re: allantoic cysts of the umbilical cord in trisomy 21. *Prenat Diagn* 1997;17(9):886–887.

270. Mesrobian HG, Zacharias A, Balcom AH, Cohen RD. Ten years of experience with isolated urachal anomalies in children. *J Urol* 1997;158(3 Pt 2):1316–1318.

271. Suita S, Nagasaki A. Urachal remnants. *Semin Pediatr Surg* 1996;5(2):107–115.

272. Pesce C, Costa L, Musi L, Campobasso P, Zimbardo L. Relevance of infection in children with urachal cysts. *Eur Urol* 2000;38(4):457–460.

13

ABDOMEN AND GASTROINTESTINAL TRACT

Intraabdominal anomalies present a particular challenge to the obstetric sonographer because they can arise from a variety of organs and anatomic sites. Potential sites of intraabdominal abnormalities include the urinary tract (kidneys, ureter, and bladder), adrenal glands, gastrointestinal tract (stomach, duodenum, jejunoileum, and colon). liver, spleen, gallbladder, pancreas, female reproductive tract (uterus and ovaries), and mesentery or peritoneal cavity.

Despite the diversity of causes of intraabdominal abnormalities, a likely diagnosis or a limited differential diagnosis can usually be suggested after carefully considering the location, distribution, and sonographic appearance of the abnormality in conjunction with gestational age at detection and associated findings (amniotic fluid, ascites. calcification, and other anomalies).[1,2] Familiarity with the underlying disease process, possible concurrent malformations, and the usual outcome is essential for determining the appropriate obstetric management of fetuses who have an intraabdominal abnormality.

As with other congenital malformations, correct interpretation of intraabdominal anomalies begins with a thorough understanding of normal embryologic development and normal sonographic appearances.

NORMAL EMBRYOLOGIC DEVELOPMENT AND FUNCTION

The primitive gut forms at the end of the fifth menstrual week (20 days postfertilization), when the dorsal part of the yolk sac invaginates into the growing embryonic disc.[3] It can be considered as three parts—foregut, midgut, and hindgut—that are supplied by the celiac artery, superior mesenteric artery, and inferior mesenteric artery, respectively. Derivatives of the foregut include the pharynx, respiratory tract, esophagus, stomach, proximal duodenum, liver, and pancreas; derivatives of the midgut include the small bowel and proximal large bowel; and derivatives of the hindgut include the distal colon, rectum, and portions of the vagina and urinary bladder (Fig. 1).

Intestinal peristalsis begins by 11 menstrual weeks, and fetal swallowing begins shortly thereafter.[4] Radioisotope dilution techniques have estimated that the fetus swallows 2 to 7 mL per day at 16 weeks, 16 mL per day by 20 weeks, and 450 mL per day by term.[5] Small bowel peristalsis propels the swallowed fluid to the large bowel where it is resorbed, leaving a residual of material called *meconium.*

Meconium begins to accumulate in the bowel by 4 to 5 months and completely fills the colon by term. In this regard, the large bowel may be considered a natural reservoir for the accumulating meconium until shortly after delivery, when it is normally evacuated. Meconium is composed of sloughed cells, lanugo hairs, mucoproteins, vernix caseosa, steroids, urea, and a sufficient amount of biliverdin to make it green.[4] It also contains a large portion of mucopolysaccharide that probably originates from the gastrointestinal tract by active secretion. Aristotle thought that meconium (mekonium = poppy) had a role in keeping the fetus asleep until delivery.

There is good evidence that normal bowel function is important for normal fetal growth in both human and animal studies.[6,7] At the same time, abolition of fluid ingestion early in gestation results in a profound restriction on growth of the gastrointestinal tract. Cytologic changes of abnormal or absent microvilli, inappropriate cell extrusion, glycogen accumulation, and altered lysosomal morphology resemble those seen in malnourished infants. This effect can be reversed in animal models.[8]

NORMAL SONOGRAPHIC APPEARANCE

The liver occupies most of the upper abdomen in the fetus (Fig. 2). Due to its greater supply of oxygenated blood *in utero,* the left lobe of the liver is larger than the right, a relationship that is reversed in the adult. The spleen is visualized on a transverse plane just posterior and to the left of the fetal stomach. Normal measurements of the liver, spleen, pancreas, stomach, gallbladder, and intestine have been reported[9] (see Appendix 1).

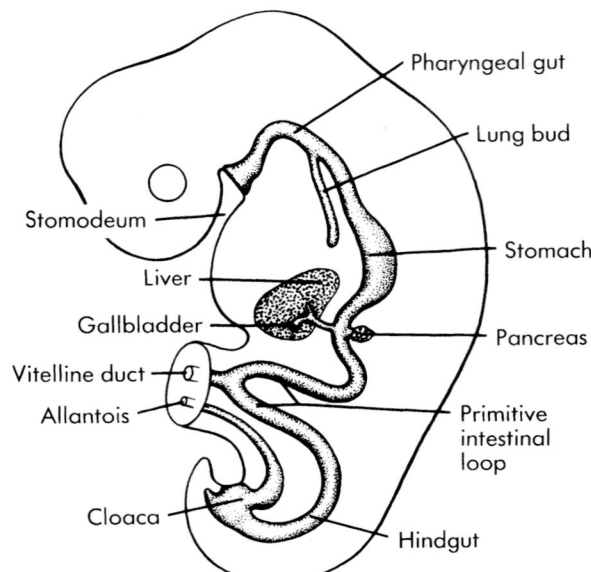

FIGURE 1. Derivatives of the foregut include the pharynx, respiratory tract, esophagus, stomach, proximal duodenum, liver, and pancreas; derivatives of the midgut include the small bowel and proximal large bowel; and derivatives of the hindgut include the distal colon, rectum, and portions of the vagina and urinary bladder. (Reproduced with permission from Sadler TW. *Langerman's medical embryology*, 5th ed. Williams & Wilkins, 1985.)

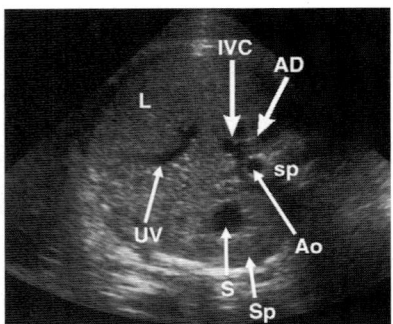

FIGURE 2. Normal abdominal anatomy. A transverse view at the level of abdominal circumference in a 38-week fetus shows normal landmarks of stomach (*S*), liver (*L*), spleen (*Sp*), umbilical vein (*UV*), aorta (*Ao*), inferior vena cava (*IVC*), right adrenal gland (*Ad*), and spine (*sp*).

The sonographic appearance of bowel varies with menstrual age (Fig. 3). By 11 menstrual weeks, the fetus is capable of swallowing sufficient amounts of amniotic fluid to permit sonographic visualization of the stomach. By 14 weeks, the stomach should be demonstrated in nearly all normal fetuses.

Because stomach size varies significantly among patients and even in the same fetus over time, nonvisualization of the stomach may require repeat scanning a few hours or even days later.

During the first and second trimesters, the bowel is normally visualized as an ill-defined area of increased echogenicity in the mid to lower abdomen (Fig. 3A). Distinguishing large bowel from small bowel is possible after 20 menstrual weeks, and this distinction becomes more obvious with advancing gestational age.[10] Characteristically, the large bowel appears as a continuous tubular structure located in the periphery of the abdomen that is filled with hypoechoic meconium (Fig. 3B). By comparison, the small bowel is located centrally and remains more echogenic in appearance until the late third trimester. Unlike the colon, the small bowel also undergoes active peristalsis that can be observed sonographically during the third trimester.

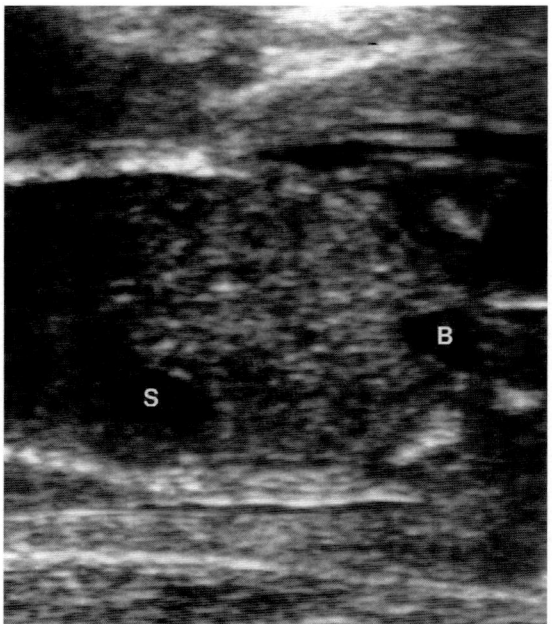

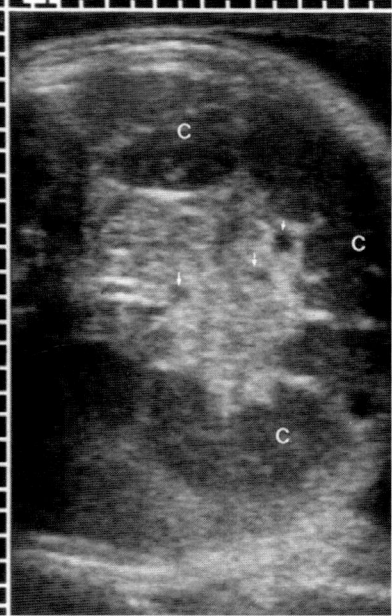

FIGURE 3. Variations in bowel with age. **A:** A longitudinal image at 16 weeks shows the bowel as an ill-defined area between the stomach (*S*) and urinary bladder (*B*). **B:** A transverse image at 40 weeks shows the prominent meconium-filled colon (*C*) at the periphery and the much smaller small bowel centrally (*small arrows*).

A,B

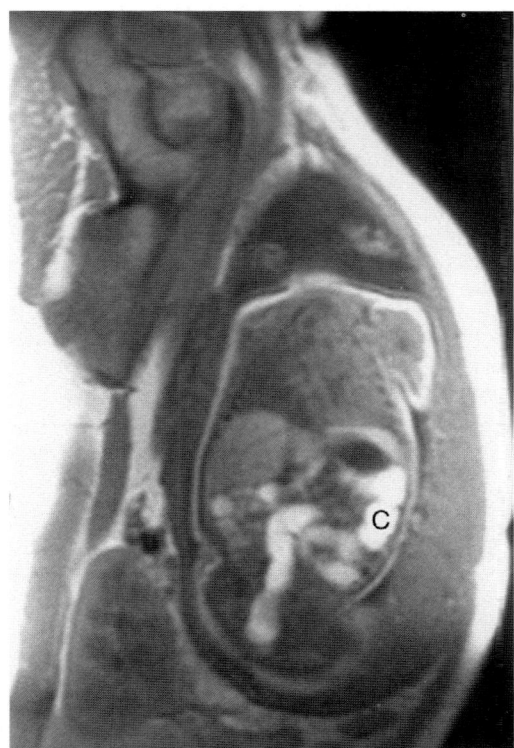

FIGURE 4. Normal abdominal magnetic resonance imaging: coronal view with T1-weighted fast spin-echo magnetic resonance images from fetus at 35 weeks. The colon (*C*) shows high-signal intensity on T1-weighted images but low signal on single-shot fast spin-echo images due to meconium. [Reproduced with permission from Shinmoto H, Kashima K, Yuasa Y, et al. MR imaging of non-CNS fetal abnormalities: a pictorial essay. *Radiographics* 2000;20(5):1227–1243.]

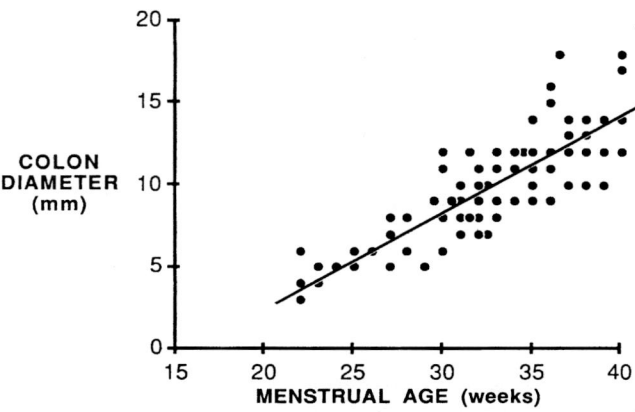

FIGURE 5. Growth in colon diameter with gestational age. Note the large variations in large bowel size by term. (Reproduced with permission from Nyberg DA, Mack LA, Patten RM, et al. Fetal bowel: normal sonographic findings. *J Ultrasound Med* 1987;6:3–6.)

Abdominal structures including the bowel can also be visualized by magnetic resonance imaging (MRI). The colon appears as high signal intensity on T1-weighted images but hypointense on single-shot fast spin-echo images due to the intraluminal meconium, at least during the third trimester (Fig. 4). In contrast, the proximal small bowel appears hypointense on T1-weighted images but hyperintense on T2-weighted images because of amniotic fluid within.[11,12]

The large bowel progressively enlarges with meconium throughout pregnancy, measuring 3 to 5 mm at 20 weeks and reaching 23 mm or occasionally even larger near term[13] (Fig. 5). Large variations in colon size and conspicuity may be seen near term. Although the small bowel also becomes more prominent with gestational age, individual segments do not normally exceed 5 mm in diameter or 15 mm in length even near term. The discrepancy between large and small bowel subsides soon after birth, when swallowed air distends the poorly muscularized small bowel at the same time the colon is evacuated.

Normal colon can be mistaken for abnormally dilated small bowel or other pathologic processes including renal cysts and pelvic masses.[14] This potential pitfall is especially likely when the meconium, which is usually hypoechoic compared to the bowel wall, has a more sonolucent appearance. Sonolucent meconium presumably reflects a greater content of water but has no known clinical significance. Conversely, unusually echogenic meconium, occasionally observed in the third trimester, might reflect decreased water content of meconium.

Normal stomach measurements have been described[15]; however, marked variation in stomach size can be seen, even in the same fetus. Echogenic debris can sometimes be seen laying in the dependent portion of the stomach.[16] These echoes could represent vernix, protein, or intraamniotic hemorrhage. It is important to ensure that the stomach is on the same side as the axis of the heart. Abdominal situs inversus is most frequently seen with polysplenia/asplenia syndromes [see Heterotaxy Syndromes (Cardiosplenic Syndrome; Polysplenia/Asplenia) in Chapter 5].

The normal esophagus can be visualized in the thorax during the second and third trimesters when carefully sought. Avni et al.[17] observed the esophagus as either two parallel echogenic lines or several parallel echogenic lines ("multilayered pattern"). The multilayered pattern was observed in 87% of cases after 26 weeks' gestation.

Detection of fetal anomalies requires a systematic approach. Guidelines proposed by the American Institute of Ultrasound in Medicine include five views of the abdominal structures: abdominal circumference, stomach, renal area, bladder, and cord insertion. Routine evaluation of just these views can identify the vast majority of fetuses with abdominal abnormalities.[18]

BOWEL DISORDERS

The fetal bowel can be altered by a number of pathologic processes. Typical sonographic findings and associated anomalies of common gastrointestinal abnormalities are shown in Table 1. Most commonly, a mechanical or functional bowel obstruction results in proximal bowel dilatation that is characteristically recognized as one or more tubular structures

TABLE 1. TYPICAL FEATURES OF COMMON GASTROINTESTINAL ABNORMALITIES

Abnormality	Typical ultrasound findings	Associated abnormalities
Esophageal atresia	Nonvisible stomach, polyhydramnios later	Increased risk of trisomies 18 and 21
Duodenal atresia	Double bubble sign	Trisomy 21 detected prenatally in >50%
Jejunoileal atresia	Dilated small bowel	Usually isolated
Meconium ileus	Hyperechoic bowel, dilated bowel	Cystic fibrosis
Anal atresia	Dilated colon occasionally	VATER syndrome

VATER, *v*ertebral defects, *a*nal atresia, *t*racheoesophageal fistula, *e*sophageal atresia, *r*adial and renal anomalies.

TABLE 2. CAUSES OF DILATED BOWEL

Small bowel
  Jejunoileal atresia
  Volvulus
  Meconium ileus
  Meconium peritonitis
  Hirschsprung disease
  Enteric duplications
  Congenital chloridorrhea
Large bowel (also consider causes of small bowel dilatation)
  Anorectal atresia
  Hirschsprung disease
Pitfall
  Normal bowel
  Hydroureter

TABLE 3. CAUSES AND ASSOCIATIONS OF INTRAABDOMINAL CYSTIC MASSES

Causes
  Renal cyst, hydronephrosis
  Urinary bladder
  Hydroureter
  Dilated bowel
  Persistent cloaca
  Ovarian cyst
  Meconium pseudocyst
  Hydrometrocolpos
  Mesenteric cyst
  Enteric duplication cyst
  Choledochal cyst
  Liver, splenic cysts
  Hemangioma, lymphangioma
  Cystic tumors

	Associations of some cystic lesions in abdomen				
Condition	Sonographic appearance	Amniotic fluid	Gestational age	Associated conditions	Fetal gender
Ovarian cyst	Usually sonolucent but may be complex, echogenic	Normal, occasionally increased	Third trimester	Usually none—may be associated with fetal hypothyroidism, Rh sensitization	Female
Hydrometrocolpos	Oval mass, may cause oval mass, mid lower abdomen	Normal	Third trimester	Genitourinary anomalies	Female
Megacystic-microcolon	Enlarged urinary bladder	Increased or normal	Third trimester	±Dilated bowel	Female
Persistent cloaca, urogenital sinus	Cystic mass, often septated	Decreased	Second, third trimester	Multiple anomalies	Usually female
Hydronephrosis, urinoma	Variable size, extends to retroperitoneum (near spine)	Variable	Any age	Variable	Either
Dilated bowel	Tubular in shape	Variable, increased with proximal obstruction	Third trimester > second	Usually isolated	Either
Choledochal cyst	Cyst right upper quadrant	Normal to increased	Second through third trimester	Usually isolated	Female > male in whites
Urachal cyst	Near umbilical cord insertion; may communicate with urinary bladder	Normal	Second, third trimesters?	Usually isolated	Either

Rh, rhesus.

within the fetal abdomen. Common causes of dilated bowel are summarized in Table 2.

Dilated bowel segments are usually sonolucent in appearance but may be normal or even increased in echogenicity. Before a bowel segment is diagnosed as abnormal, however, normal bowel should be specifically considered and excluded. It is important to recognize that a sonolucent appearance of bowel is not necessarily abnormal and that bowel diameter is a more reliable criterion for diagnosing bowel dilatation.

Other intraabdominal cystic masses should also be considered when dilated bowel is thought to be present (Table 3). Distinguishing hydroureter from dilated bowel may occasionally be difficult, particularly when cystic tubular structures are localized to the pelvis.

The vast majority of cases of bowel dilatation represent small bowel, although large bowel dilatation is occasionally observed. Many causes of bowel dilatation do not become apparent until after 20 weeks. An earlier age of diagnosis is occasionally possible for some proximal sites of obstruction, such as duodenal atresia, especially when combined with esophageal atresia (EA).

Polyhydramnios commonly accompanies obstruction of the gastrointestinal tract. Both the frequency and severity of polyhydramnios are related to proximal sites of obstruction (Fig. 6). Polyhydramnios rarely develops before 20 weeks from a gastrointestinal cause. These observations reflect the increasing contribution of fetal swallowing and bowel function to normal fluid dynamics during the third trimester.

In the remaining sections, major bowel disorders that can be identified sonographically are discussed as they arise along the course of the gastrointestinal tract, from proximal to distal.

PROXIMAL GASTROINTESTINAL DISORDERS

Esophageal Atresia

Incidence

Atresia of the esophagus, with or without tracheoesophageal fistula (TEF), occurs in 1 in 2,500 to 4,000 live births. In a survey of 1,546,889 births, the prevalence was 2.86 per

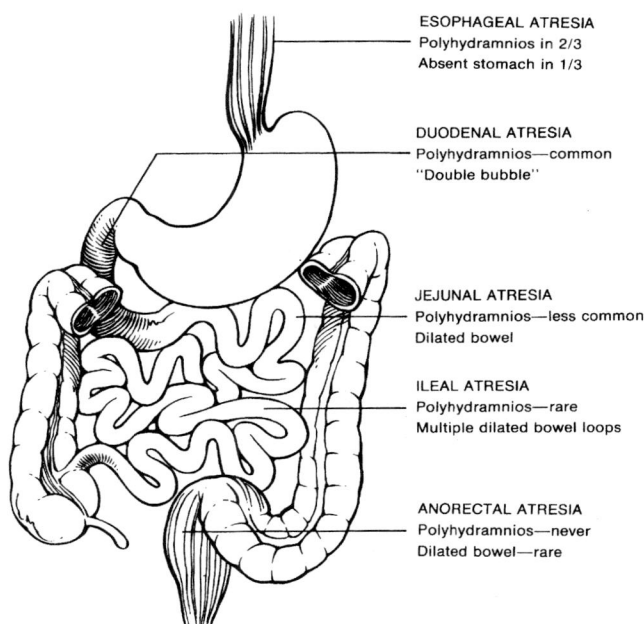

FIGURE 6. Sites of gastrointestinal obstruction and typical ultrasound findings. (Reproduced with permission from McGahan JP, Porto M, eds. *Diagnostic obstetrical ultrasound.* Philadelphia: JB Lippincott Co, 1994;343–385.)

10,000.[19] Males are affected slightly more than females. There is no known pattern of inheritance.

Embryology and Pathology

Esophageal malformations (EA and/or TEF) result from incomplete division of the foregut into the ventral respiratory portion and the dorsal digestive portion by the tracheoesophageal septum, a process that normally is complete by 8 weeks. EA is associated with TEF in greater than 90% of cases.[20,21] Fetuses with Down syndrome are more likely to have EA alone without TEF, perhaps in as many as 50% of cases.[22]

The pathologic classification of esophageal malformations as described by Gross[23] is as follows (Fig. 7):

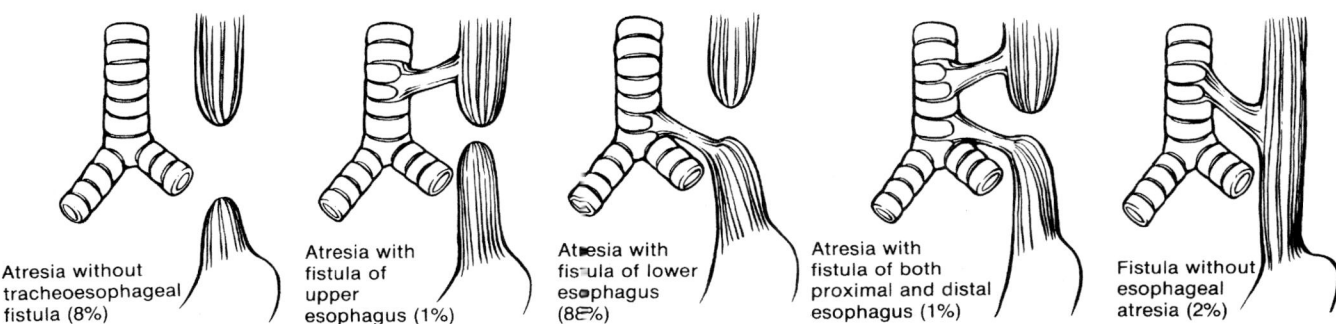

FIGURE 7. Types of esophageal malformations. Type C (esophageal atresia with fistula of lower esophageal segment) accounts for 88% of cases. (Reproduced with permission from McGahan JP, Porto M, eds. *Diagnostic obstetrical ultrasound.* Philadelphia: JB Lippincott Co, 1994;343–385.)

Type A: EA without TEF
Type B: EA with TEF of the upper esophageal segment
Type C: EA with TEF of the lower esophageal segment
Type D: EA with TEFs of both proximal and distal segments
Type E: TEF without EA

Type C is by far the most common, accounting for 88% of cases. EA alone (type A) accounts for 8% of cases, and the remaining types (B, D, and E) are each found in only 1% to 2% of cases. EA without TEF is much more difficult to surgically repair.

Diagnosis

Sonographic diagnosis of EA with or without TEF can be suspected based on either indirect or direct signs, which include the following:

1. Absent or small fetal stomach, usually associated with polyhydramnios after 20 weeks
2. Polyhydramnios combined with intrauterine growth restriction (IUGR)
3. A C loop representing a closed bowel segment from the combination of EA and duodenal atresia or stenosis
4. Proximal esophageal pouch

Absent or Small Stomach
Absence of a visible stomach is expected from EA alone (type A) but it may also occur with TEF since the fistula and distal esophageal segment are usually stenotic. An absent or small stomach (Figs. 8 and 9) reflects a relative obstruction to passage of amniotic fluid, even though it allows passage of air after birth.[24,25]

The constellation of a nonvisible stomach and polyhydramnios as a sign of EA was first suggested by Hobbins et al.[26] and first observed by Farrant in 1980.[27] Unfortunately, polyhydramnios does not usually occur until after 20 weeks since fetal swallowing contributes relatively little to amniotic fluid dynamics before this time. Also, although the combination of absent stomach and polyhydramnios is highly suggestive of EA, this combination proves to be EA in only approximately one-half of cases.[28–30]

The sensitivity of ultrasound for EA depends on gestational age, reasons for ultrasound, sonographic criteria, and the experience of the sonologist. Stringer et al.[30] reported a sensitivity of 42%. In 118,265 consecutive pregnancies, Stoll et al.[31] reported the sensitivity of detecting EA as 24.2% and none of these were isolated. In another series of 152 cases of EA from northern England, Sparey and colleagues[29] reported that 14 were suspected prenatally but an additional 28 cases should also have been suspected. These findings suggest that the sensitivity of ultrasound is low for EA unless a systematic survey is performed and the sonologist is familiar with the signs of EA.

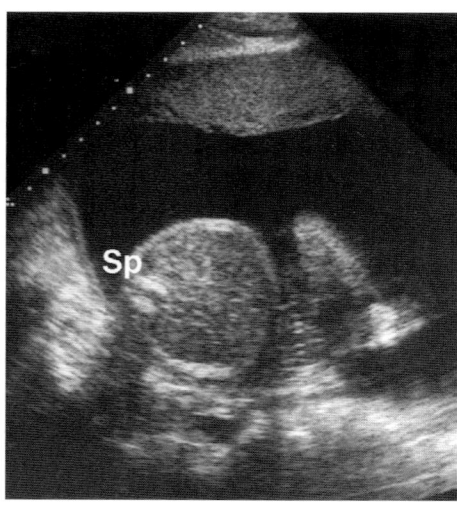

FIGURE 8. Esophageal atresia. The transverse view of an abdomen shows the classic finding of nonvisualization of the stomach and polyhydramnios. Approximately one-half of the fetuses showing these findings will prove to have esophageal atresia. Sp, spine.

Polyhydramnios and Intrauterine Growth Restriction
Gut atresia is a relatively common fetal cause of polyhydramnios,[32] reflecting the role of swallowing and fluid absorption by the fetal intestinal tract in the regulation of amniotic fluid. The risk of underlying fetal anomaly increases with the severity of polyhydramnios.[33,34]

IUGR is often found in association with EA[35] (Fig. 10). Approximately 40% of infants with EA are below tenth percentile for birth weight,[36] and greater than 20% are below the fifth percentile.[29] These findings support other clinical and experimental evidence suggesting that amniotic fluid ingestion and normal intestinal function is important for normal fetal growth, particularly late in gestation.[6]

"Idiopathic" polyhydramnios is most commonly associated with a large-for-gestational-age fetus, with or without maternal diabetes.[37–40] In contrast, the combination of polyhydramnios and IUGR is distinctly unusual and should suggest the presence of underlying anomalies, including EA[41–43] (Fig. 10). Among 39 fetuses with IUGR and polyhydramnios reported by Sickler et al.[41] major anomalies were present at birth in 92%. Among nine fetuses without other detectable anomalies, six (67%) proved to have anomalies at birth, including two with EA.

C Loop of Esophageal Atresia Plus Proximal Bowel Obstruction
A dilated distal esophageal segment has been reported both prenatally and postnatally, and in these cases a proximal bowel obstruction (duodenal or gastric atresia) was also present.[44,45] The combination of esophageal and duodenal atresia may show a characteristic C-shaped fluid collection

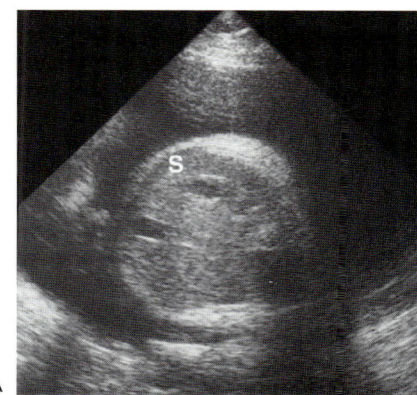

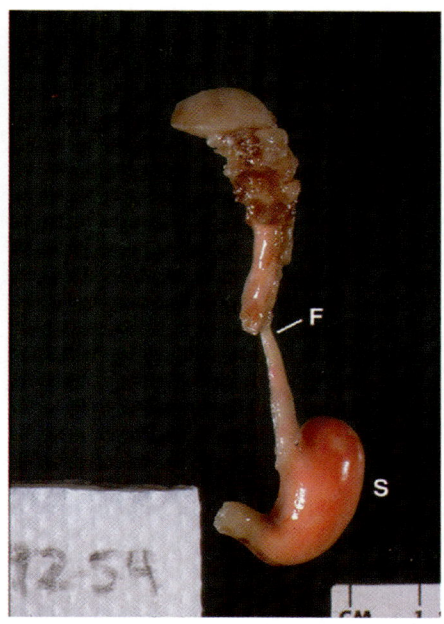

FIGURE 9. Esophageal atresia with tracheoesophageal fistula. **A:** A transverse scan at 34 weeks shows a small but visible stomach (*S*) and polyhydramnios. **B:** A pathologic photograph shows esophageal atresia with a tracheoesophageal fistula. F, fistula; S, stomach.

in the fetal abdomen.[46] This fluid represents a closed-loop bowel obstruction involving the distal esophagus, stomach, and duodenum. It can be diagnosed earlier in gestation and has been reported as early as 12 weeks of gestation.[47] Moreover, the presence of polyhydramnios at 20 weeks in a fetus with a suspected duodenal atresia should alert the physician to the possibility of combined esophageal and duodenal atresias. The combination of duodenal atresia and EA appears to carry a particularly high risk of fetal Down syndrome.

Proximal Esophageal Pouch

In some cases, more direct and specific evidence of EA is found by visualizing the proximal esophageal segment.[48–50] This evidence has been called the *pouch sign*.[48,49] Several reports emphasize that this is a transient finding, observed when the fetus swallows. Satoh and colleagues[49] reported eight such cases of esophageal pouch among ten fetuses that presented with polyhydramnios and a small stomach. EA was found in all eight of these cases but was not present in the two fetuses without a visible pouch (one had Nager syndrome and the other, a disorder of the central nervous system). Visualization of regurgitation after swallowing has also been observed with EA.[51]

Differential Diagnosis

The stomach may be small or not visible in up to 1% of normal fetuses on initial scan.[30] The likelihood that nonvisualization of the stomach represents a true malformation increases with its persistence over time, as well as with the presence of polyhydramnios.[52] Millener et al.[53] evaluated 31 fetuses (0.4% of all scans) who showed a nonvisible or very small stomach on one or more scans at 14 to 40 weeks. A normal fluid-filled stomach was observed on the next

FIGURE 10. Esophageal atresia with intrauterine growth restriction. A transverse view of the abdomen at 32 weeks shows a visible stomach (*S*). Polyhydramnios was unexplained, and the abdominal circumference was disproportionately small with an estimated weight less than the tenth percentile. Esophageal atresia with a tracheoesophageal fistula was found at birth.

TABLE 4. ABSENT VISUALIZATION OF STOMACH: DIFFERENTIAL DIAGNOSIS

Esophageal atresia/tracheoesophageal fistula
Diaphragmatic hernia
Hiatal hernia
Cleft lip/palate
Central nervous system disorders
Other swallowing disorders
Arthrogryposis
Twin-twin transfusion syndrome
Trisomy 18
Triploidy
Renal agenesis
Oligohydramnios from any cause
Pitfall: transient nonvisualization of stomach in normal fetuses

sonogram in 15 cases, but five of these had an abnormal outcome.

A nonvisible stomach may be seen in a number of other conditions (Table 4). Facial clefts probably cause ineffective fetal swallowing, and central nervous system disorders presumably result in depression of swallowing on a neurologic basis. Oligohydramnios from any cause also may result in failure to visualize the stomach because little amniotic fluid is available to swallow.

The dilated bowel segment of combined duodenal and esophageal atresia can be confused for other masses; a cystic mass in the chest was confused for a diaphragmatic hernia in a fetus with Down syndrome.[54]

Associated Findings

Concurrent malformations are present in 50% to 70% of infants with EA.[29] In a series of more than 1,000 cases reviewed by Holder et al.,[55] one-half had associated anomalies in the following sites: gastrointestinal 28%, cardiac 24%, genitourinary 13%, musculoskeletal 11%, central nervous system 7%, facial anomalies 6%, and other 12%. Common gastrointestinal anomalies associated with esophageal malformations include malrotation, anorectal atresia, duodenal atresia, Meckel diverticulum, and annular pancreas.[56] Combined esophageal and duodenal atresia may be seen with Down syndrome.[57]

A recognized group of malformations is identified as the VATER association: *v*ertebral defects, *a*nal atresia, *T*EF, *E*A, *r*adial and renal anomalies. This acronym has been modified to denote the VACTERL syndrome for *v*ertebral anomalies, *a*norectal atresia, *c*ardiac anomalies, *t*racheoesophageal fistula, *r*enal anomalies, and *l*imb abnormalities (see VATER/VACTERL Association in Chapter 5).

Ultrasound does not appear to be sensitive for detection of associated anomalies in many cases of EA. Sparey et al.[29] reported 63% of cases had associated anomalies, and 78% of these anomalies were missed prenatally.

Fetuses with EA and aneuploidy are probably more likely to be detected prenatally. Fetuses with trisomy 18 can be detected by a variety of abnormalities, including IUGR, limb abnormalities, and cardiac defects, and fetuses with trisomy 21 may show duodenal atresia and congenital heart disease.

The risk of fetal aneuploidy with EA varies between prenatal and postnatal studies.[58,59] A large postnatal study reported chromosomal abnormalities in 5.2% of 670 patients with EA.[22] Of the 35 affected cases, 16 had trisomy 18 and 12 had trisomy 21. Another postnatal series of EA cases reported that 10% had aneuploidy and one-half of the remaining cases had multiple anomalies.[19]

In a prenatal series, Pretorius[24] reported aneuploidy in 19% (two cases each of trisomy 21 and 18). Also, Stringer et al.[30] reported trisomy 18 in 44% (7 of 16) of fetuses with EA. Of the remaining nine, two had isolated EA and two had laryngeal atresia and EA.

Prognosis and Management

The prognosis for infants with EA depends primarily on the presence of other abnormalities, as well as the time of diagnosis and specific malformation. Among 152 cases reported by Sparey et al.,[29] the overall perinatal and infant mortality rate was 22%, including 12 pregnancy terminations, one spontaneous abortion, and 19 perinatal deaths (including nine stillbirths). Among survivors, 120 underwent surgical repair, including 102 (85%) who had a primary repair. One hundred and eight (90%) had EA with a distal TEF. The postoperative mortality rate was 9%.

The prognosis appears much worse for cases of EA diagnosed prenatally due to associated anomalies and aneuploidy. Among 16 cases of EA detected prenatally by Stringer et al.,[30] the mortality rate was 75% (12 of 16) through the neonatal period, including two late unexplained intrapartum deaths.

Kalache and colleagues[60] suggest that a proximal position of an esophageal pouch may identify a group with a worse prognosis. They described seven fetuses with EA who showed a proximal esophageal pouch in the neck (n = 3) or chest (n = 4). Only one of three fetuses with a neck pouch survived to surgery, and a staged repair was necessary because of a long atretic gap. Conversely, three of the four fetuses with a chest pouch survived after a successful corrective operation, and primary repair was possible in all cases.

For surviving infants, gastroesophageal reflux may produce repeated pneumonitis and recurrent stricture.[61] In the series of Sparey et al.,[29] 32.5% (n = 39) had postoperative gastroesophageal reflux, necessitating fundoplication in 21 cases. At 2-year follow-up, 23 of 89 infants had dysphagia, for which seven still required a gastrostomy or jejunostomy.

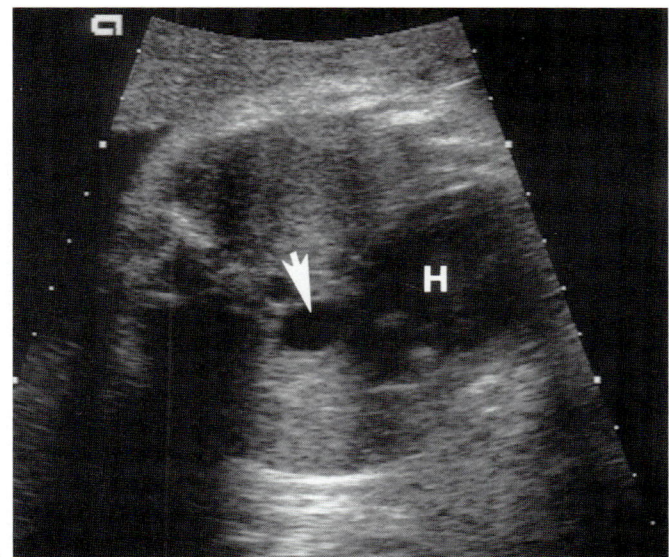

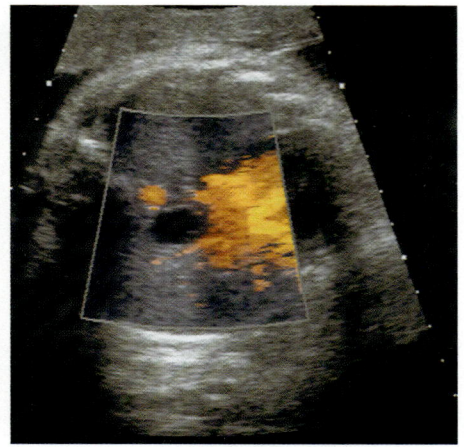

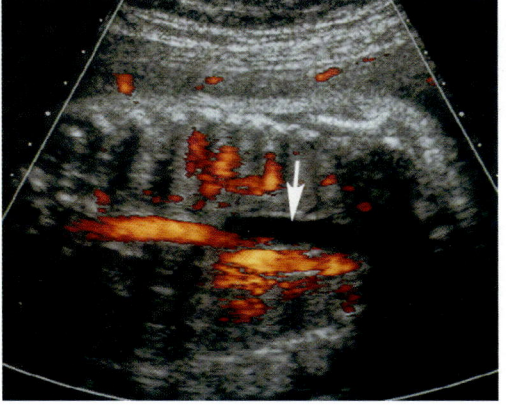

FIGURE 11. Hiatal hernia. **A:** A transverse view of the chest at 33 weeks shows a cystic structure (*arrowhead*) posterior to the heart (*H*). A previous scan at 25 weeks showed nonvisualization of the stomach but no mass. **B:** Power Doppler indicates that the mass is not vascular. **C:** The longitudinal scan shows that this is a tubular cystic structure (*arrow*) that was seen along the length of the thorax. Hiatal hernia was found after delivery. (Courtesy of Dotun Ogunyemi, MD, Los Angeles, CA.)

Infants in whom the condition was diagnosed prenatally were more likely to need prolonged mechanical ventilation, to have longer hospital stays, and to have long-term gastrointestinal problems.

Hiatal Hernia

Incidence

Hiatal hernia is rare in newborns.

Pathology and Embryology

Hiatal hernia is sliding of the stomach into the chest so that the gastroesophageal junction is above the diaphragm. Paraesophageal hernia is displacement through a defect in the diaphragm near the esophageal hiatus.

Diagnosis

A dilated esophagus may be seen with hiatal hernia during the third trimester[62–64] (Fig. 11). Ogunyemi[64] described a fetus on serial scans that showed absence of fetal stomach and polyhydramnios, suggestive of EA, during the second trimester (Fig. 11). Hiatal hernia has also been diagnosed by prenatal MRI (Fig. 12).

Differential Diagnosis

EA typically shows more proximal dilatation of the esophagus in a minority of fetuses with a proximal pouch.[65] Duplication cyst should also be considered. Hiatal hernia may also be mistaken for diaphragmatic hernia.[63]

Associated Anomalies

Hiatal hernia/paraesophageal hernia has been associated with Marfan syndrome[66] and asplenia/polysplenia syndrome.[67]

Prognosis and Management

The prognosis is good following surgical repair.[68] However, al-Arfaj et al.[69] reported deaths in two of ten (20%) newborns with giant hiatal hernia, probably as a result of delay in diagnosis and associated malformations.

Recurrence Risk

Familial cases have been rarely reported.[70]

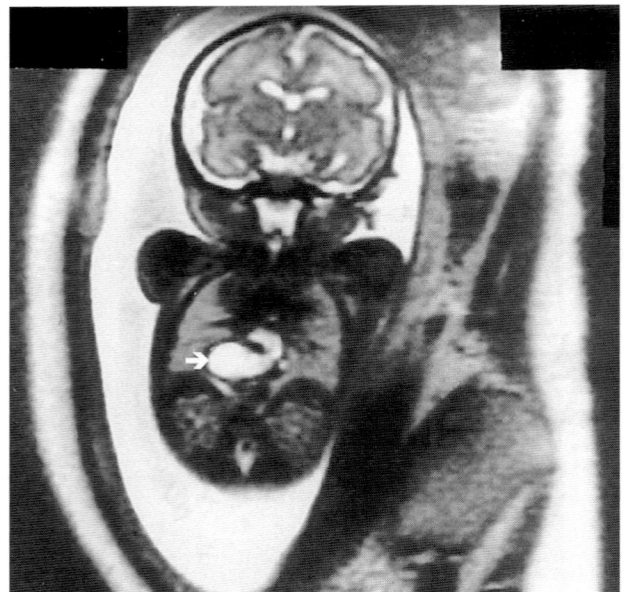

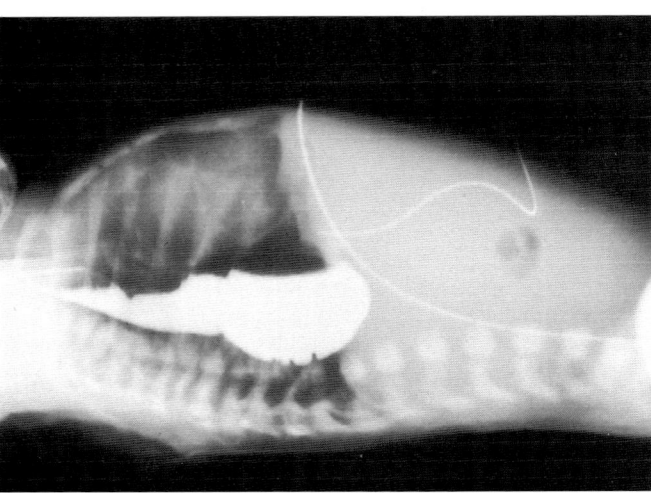

FIGURE 12. Hiatal hernia on magnetic resonance imaging. **A:** A coronal single-shot fast spin-echo magnetic resonance image at 31 weeks shows the stomach (*arrow*) protruding through the esophageal hiatus. **B:** Barium esophagography after delivery shows a sliding hiatal hernia. [Reproduced with permission from Shinmoto H, Kashima K, Yuasa Y, et al. MR imaging of non-CNS fetal abnormalities: a pictorial essay. *Radiographics* 2000;20(5):1227–1243.]

Duodenal Atresia/Obstruction

Incidence

Duodenal atresia affects 1 in 5,000 pregnancies.

Embryology and Pathology

The etiology of duodenal atresia is usually a blind-end atresia and less likely a diaphragm or membrane that interrupts the duodenal lumen.[71] The site of obstruction typically is near the ampulla of Vater, with 80% distal to the ampulla and 20% proximal to it.[71] Atresia of the common bile duct may be an associated abnormality. Annular pancreas is found in conjunction with duodenal atresia in many cases, although most authorities do not consider this the primary cause of obstruction.[71]

A previously cited explanation for development of duodenal atresia is failure to "recanalize" the duodenal lumen after a temporary solid state during early embryologic development. However, other authors[71] suggest that, similar to other small bowel atresias, duodenal atresia results from vascular impairment during gut development. Experimental studies also fail to support the idea of a "solid core" stage at any time during embryologic development.[72]

Diagnosis

Duodenal atresia is seen as the characteristic double bubble sign representing the fluid-filled stomach and duodenum (Fig. 13), an appearance initially reported by Loveday et al.[73] Because the obstruction is complete, all cases of duodenal atresia should ultimately show the double bubble finding. However, this appearance is usually not evident until after 20 weeks, reflecting the relative small volume of swallowed amniotic fluid before this time.[74,75] Duodenal stenosis may present late, and this may also be seen in association with Down syndrome.

Duodenal atresia can occasionally be diagnosed before 20 weeks (Fig. 14), and some cases have been diagnosed as early as the first trimester.[76] With duodenal atresia alone, this sonographic appearance may be a subtle finding with a small amount of fluid in the duodenum. A more prominent appearance with a C loop of dilated bowel may occur when duodenal atresia is associated with EA[54] (Fig. 15). As noted, this combination carries a particularly high risk of fetal Down syndrome.

Polyhydramnios occurs in all cases of typical duodenal atresia during the third trimester. Polyhydramnios develops when the amount of swallowed amniotic fluid exceeds the absorptive capacity of the stomach and proximal duodenum.

Differential Diagnosis

Continuity with the stomach should be demonstrated to distinguish a distended duodenum from other cystic masses in the right upper quadrant, such as choledochal cyst, hepatic cyst, and duplication cyst.[77] A mildly dilated duodenum may be seen from duodenal stenosis, and an

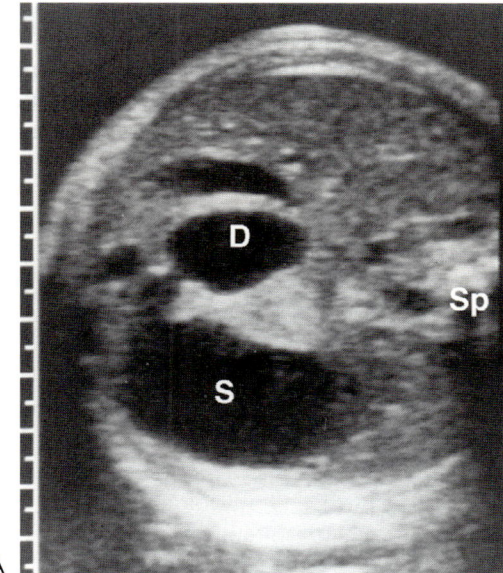

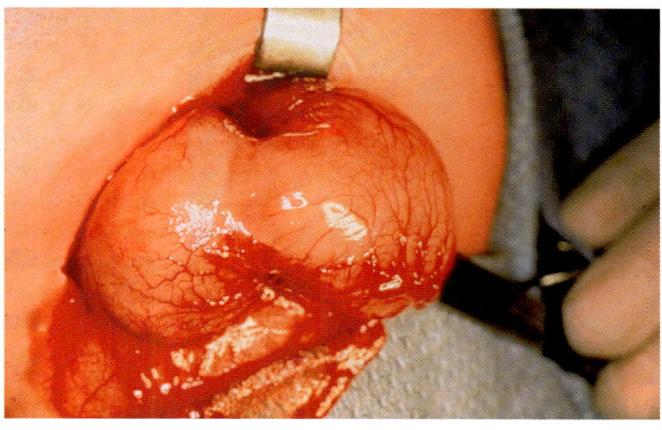

FIGURE 13. Duodenal atresia. **A:** A transverse sonogram at 30 weeks demonstrates a characteristic double bubble appearance representing the fluid-filled stomach (*S*) and duodenum (*D*). Polyhydramnios was also present. Sp, spine. **B:** A photograph taken at time of surgery shows the double bubble of dilated stomach and proximal duodenum.

enlarged stomach alone has been reported in association with an antral web.[78]

Associated Findings

Approximately one-half of the fetuses with duodenal atresia have concurrent malformations including skeletal, gastrointestinal, cardiovascular, genitourinary, and chromosomal abnormalities.[79] Associated skeletal abnormalities include vertebral and rib anomalies, sacral agenesis, radial abnormalities, and talipes equinovarus.[80] Concurrent gastrointestinal abnormalities include other sites of atresia: EA, intestinal jejunoileal atresia, biliary atresia, pancreatic ductal atresia, and anorectal atresia.[71] Trisomy 21 (Down syn-

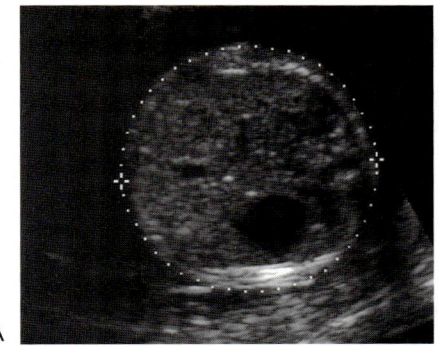

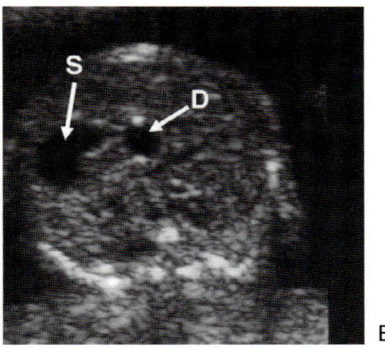

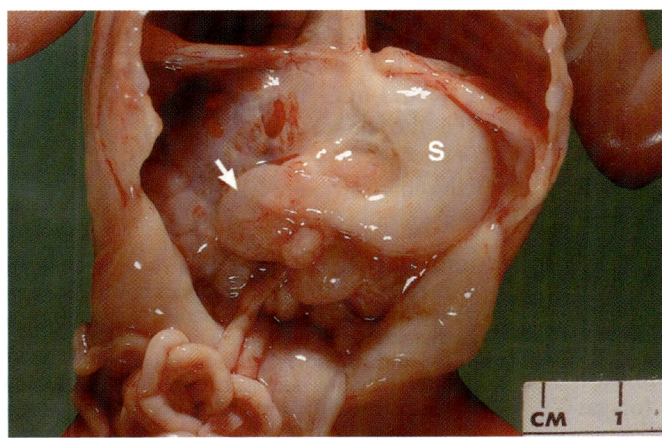

FIGURE 14. Duodenal atresia and trisomy 21 at 19 weeks. **A:** A transverse view of the upper abdomen, at the level of abdominal circumference, appears unremarkable. **B:** A slightly lower scan shows a mildly dilated duodenum (*D*). Trisomy 21 was found at genetic amniocentesis. **C:** A pathologic photograph confirms a mildly dilated duodenal bulb (*arrow*) and duodenal atresia. S, stomach.

trojejunostomy) as soon as possible. Delayed complications

Differential Diagnosis

When dilated small bowel is demonstrated, meconium ileus should be considered in addition to jejunoileal atresia and volvulus. Rare causes of small bowel dilatation and polyhydramnios include Hirschsprung disease and congenital chloridorrhea. The sonographic distinction between these possibilities is difficult, if not impossible. Unfortunately, measurement of amniotic fluid microvillar enzyme levels is also unlikely to be helpful in identification of meconium ileus, because low levels would be expected from any cause of bowel obstruction.

Care should be taken to distinguish dilated bowel from hydroureter, in which case oligohydramnios and/or hydronephrosis is often present. Occasionally small bowel atresia can present as a cystlike mass.[99] More common abdominal cystic masses include ovarian cysts, enteric duplication cysts, and mesenteric cysts.

Associated Anomalies

Unlike many other sites of intestinal atresia, extraintestinal anomalies are uncommon with small bowel atresias, although other bowel abnormalities are frequent. Associated bowel abnormalities that have been reported include the probable cause of atresia (malrotation, volvulus, intestinal duplications, meconium ileus, or gastroschisis) in 27%, complications of atresia (meconium peritonitis) in 6%, and concurrent bowel abnormalities (colon atresia, EA, anorectal atresia, enteric duplications) in 5%.[89]

Cystic fibrosis (CF) should also be considered in the setting of small bowel atresia. Surana and Puri[36] reported 59 fetuses with type I atresia (24 jejunal, 35 ileal). Ten (17%) had associated anomalies including CF (three), heart defects (two), malrotation (two), and one case each of vesicoureteric reflux, neural tube defect, and microcephaly.

Prognosis and Management

Fetuses with proximal obstructions more likely to be small and premature compared to distal obstructions. Surana and Puri[36] found that of 10 of 22 (45%) patients with jejunal atresia were born before 36 weeks, compared to only five of 35 (14%) patients with ileal atresia. Earlier delivery probably reflects the degree of polyhydramnios.[36,97] Small birth weights may also reflect the nutritive effect of amniotic fluid. Amniotic fluid contributes to the fetal growth in the last few weeks of gestation, and the higher the obstruction in the small intestine, the more pronounced the effect on the nutrition of the fetus.[36]

All patients with small bowel atresia present with symptoms of bowel obstruction, typically within a few days of life.[100] The prognosis depends primarily on the site and extent of bowel involvement and other anomalies or complications. The primary complication of bowel obstruction from small bowel atresia is ischemia and infarction. This leads to *in utero* bowel perforation and meconium peritonitis in approximately 6% of cases of jejunoileal atresia.

Jejunal atresia has a less favorable prognosis than distal obstructions, possibly due to the greater rate of premature delivery.[101] The mortality rate also increased with concurrent malformations, meconium peritonitis, and volvulus.[101] Multiple sites of atresia and apple-peel atresia have a poor prognosis. When an antenatal diagnosis is made, the atresia is more likely to be proximal, requiring intensive and prolonged postnatal treatment.[102]

Spinal radiographs and testing for CF have been recommended for infants with jejunoileal atresia.[103]

Cystic Fibrosis/Meconium Ileus

Meconium ileus is characterized by impaction of abnormally thick and sticky meconium in the distal ileum, producing a functional obstruction.[104] Nearly all newborns who develop meconium ileus prove to have CF. Conversely, meconium ileus affects 10% to 15% of patients with CF and is the earliest clinical manifestation of this disorder.

Incidence

CF is one of the most common autosomal recessive disorders in the United States today. One in 29 Americans is a carrier for this genetic abnormality, and approximately 1 in 3,000 newborns has the clinical disease. CF is rare among Black and Asian populations.

Embryology and Pathology

Meconium ileus is obstruction of the ileum with meconium but without an anatomic cause of obstruction. Characteristic pathologic findings of meconium ileus include a dilated ileum, relatively normal jejunum, and a collapsed empty colon. Analysis of meconium from fetuses with meconium ileus shows an abnormally high protein content including albumin, increased mucus, and decreased water content compared with normal meconium.[106] Abnormal meconium composition probably results from increased mucus secretion by the gastrointestinal tract and abnormalities of electrolytes that are characteristic of CF.

Inspissated meconium may also obstruct the colon, resulting in the mucus plug syndrome. In this disorder, transient colonic obstruction and failure to pass meconium in the first few days of life result from distal meconium impaction. Although not as strongly linked to CF as is meconium ileus, as many as 25% of infants with the mucus plug syndrome have been reported to have CF.[104]

Diagnosis

Definitive diagnosis of CF has traditionally rested on an abnormal sweat chloride test. In the last two decades, major advances have been made in the use of DNA probes to diagnose CF.[105–108] The gene disorder of CF has now been identified on the seventh chromosome. More than 900 gene mutations have been associated with CF. The most common probes (deltaF508, deltaI507, 1717-1G→A, G542X, G551D, R553X, W1282X, N1303K) can identify approximately 85% of cases.

Diagnosis of CF using gene mutations in large populations has been shown to be feasible.[109–113] Scotet et al.[113] reported that among 343,756 neonates screened, 118 cases of CF were identified, an incidence of 1 in 2,913. The cost of the screening program was $2.32 per screened child.

A National Institutes of Health panel now recommends testing for adults with a positive family history of CF, to partners of people with CF, to couples currently planning a pregnancy, and to couples seeking prenatal care but not to the general population or newborns.[114] The cost-benefit analysis of screening for CF has been favorable.[115,116] CF carrier screening is most cost-effective when the information is used for more than one pregnancy and when the intention of the couple is to identify and terminate affected pregnancies.[117]

In patients with a high risk (1 in 4) of CF, analysis of amniotic fluid during the second trimester may be highly accurate (98%) for diagnosis of CF.[118] Criteria for CF may include meconium ileus, significant increase of albumin content in the meconium, and periodic acid-Schiff–positive mucus-like material in some pancreatic acini.

Sonographic diagnosis of CF has been based on identification of meconium ileus or echogenic meconium [hyperechoic bowel (HB)]. Meconium ileus, seen as dilated bowel (Fig. 19), may be less common but may carry a higher risk for CF compared to HB.[119–122] Small bowel dilatation develops secondary to the impacted meconium that is characteristic of meconium ileus. Most cases of bowel dilatation have been diagnosed after 26 weeks, although bowel dilatation in the second trimester has also been observed.[120] Colon dilatation from the mucus plug syndrome has also been rarely noted in association with CF.[121]

Estroff et al.[123] reviewed the cases of 15 fetuses with dilated bowel distal to the duodenum and found that five (33%) had CF. A characteristic appearance, when present, is dilated bowel segments containing echogenic meconium (Fig. 19). A fluid-meconium interface may also be seen.

The association between HB and meconium ileus has been reported in both the second and third trimesters among fetuses with CF[124] (Fig. 20). Although initially observed in families with a 25% recurrence risk for CF, similar observations have been made in nonselected patients. In these cases, the echogenic "masses" probably represent the impacted meconium itself.

The risk of CF when HB is present is considered to be relatively low but is probably underestimated. A summary of cases suggests that 1% to 2% of fetuses with HB may be found to have CF (Table 5). In an ethnically diverse popu-

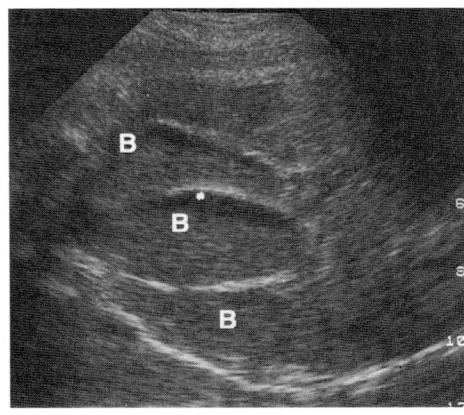

FIGURE 19. Dilated bowel and meconium ileus. A transverse sonogram at 33 weeks demonstrates several dilated loops of bowel (*B*) filled with meconium and with a fluid-meconium layer. Meconium ileus was found at birth.

lation of 159 fetuses with HB, Monaghan and Feldman[125] identified two (1.3%) with CF and eight with an identifiable CF mutation (5%). In another heterogeneous population of 244 fetuses with HB, Berlin et al.[126] found that two (0.8%) were positive for CF mutations, a third case was at high risk since both parents were carriers but the fetus was not tested, and nine (8%) of 113 fetuses tested had one CF mutation. In a study of 175 fetuses with HB after exclusion of fetuses with major anomalies or those referred for abnormal outside ultrasound, Al-Kouatly et al.[127] reported CF in five cases (2.9%). Seven of the ten parents were not previously aware that they carried a CF mutation. Of those tested, CF mutations were found in 7 of 138 (5%) mothers and 9 of 86 (10.5%) fathers.

Differential Diagnosis

Dilated bowel should suggest jejunoileal atresia and other bowel abnormalities. The differential diagnosis for HB is discussed further later in this chapter (see Hyperechoic Bowel).

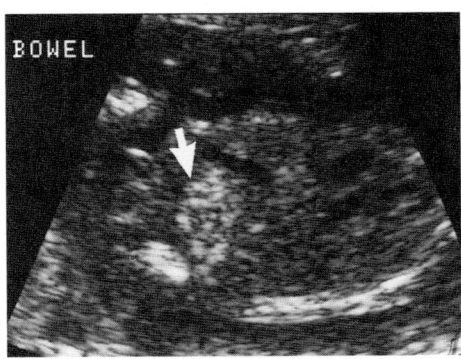

FIGURE 20. Cystic fibrosis and hyperechoic bowel. A scan at 17 weeks shows hyperechoic bowel (*arrow*). The fetus proved to have cystic fibrosis.

TABLE 5. SUMMARY OF LARGEST STUDIES OF HYPERECHOIC BOWEL AND OUTCOME

Study	n	Aneuploidy (N)	Cystic fibrosis (N)	Fetal demise or stillbirth (N)	Bowel complication (N)	Infection (N)	Other anomalies (N)	Other adverse outcome
Al-Kouatly[127]	171	5	5	—	a	1	a	—
Berlin[126]	244	3	2	—	—	—	—	—
Dicke[162]	30	1	4	5	—	—	—	6 IUGR
Ghose[163]	60	3	3	6	—	—	—	6 IUGR
Hill[138]	32	—	—	—	—	—	—	—
MacGregor[149]	45	—	2	3	—	4	1 fetal alcohol syndrome	5 IUGR
Muller[159]	182	1	—	24	9	3	23	1 sudden infant death
Nyberg[140]	95	—	—	—	—	—	—	—
Scioscia[147]	22	6	—	—	—	—	—	—
Sepulveda[153]	45	2	—	—	—	2	—	5 IUGR
Sipes[151]	7	1	—	—	—	—	—	—
Slotnick[139]	105b	8	7	—	—	—	—	—
Strocker[164]	131c	12	0	—	—	29	11	—
Yaron[156]	79	5	2	3	5	5	7	—
Total (%)	1,248	47 (3.8)	25 (2.0)	41 (3.3)	14 (1.1)	44 (3.5)	41 (3.3)	—

IUGR, intrauterine growth restriction.
[a]Nine cases with detectable major anomalies were excluded.
[b]Considering only grades 2 and 3 bowel echogenicity.
[c]Infection included recent influenza infection.

Associated Anomalies

Most, but not all, cases of meconium ileus are associated with CF. Up to 25% of those with meconium plug syndrome of the colon also have CF.[104] Cases of meconium ileus not related to CF have been reported,[128,129] and these include extreme prematurity (presumably related to intestinal dysmotility), swallowed blood, infection, or multiple-anomaly syndromes.[130]

Prognosis and Management

Up to 50% of infants with meconium ileus have other gastrointestinal complications including volvulus, atresia, bowel perforation, or meconium peritonitis. For patients with uncomplicated meconium ileus, the therapy of choice is nonoperative Gastrografin enema, with enterotomy and irrigation reserved for enema failures. Complicated cases require exploration and, in the absence of giant cystic meconium peritonitis, are usually amenable to bowel resection and primary anastomosis.[131]

The prognosis for patients with CF has been dramatically improved during the last few decades secondary to improved medical treatment. The average life span has now risen to 32 years. Approximately 80% of patients develop pancreatic insufficiency, and 95% develop recurrent respiratory infections and chronic lung disease. Affected males are invariably infertile.

Recurrence Risk

Because CF is an autosomal recessive disorder, the recurrence risk for those patients with a previously affected pregnancy is 25%.

Hyperechoic Bowel

HB is a subjective impression of unusually echogenic bowel, typically seen during the second trimester. Although not a pathologic entity, it is discussed in detail here because of its potential importance to prenatal diagnoses.

Incidence

HB is found in approximately 0.5% of second trimester pregnancies.

Embryology and Pathology

The pathologic equivalent of HB has been elusive. It could reflect one or more of the following[132]:

1. Alterations in meconium with decreased water content and/or increased protein content
2. Swallowed blood in some cases of intraamniotic hemorrhage
3. Bowel wall edema, for example, from thalassemia
4. Ischemia

Decreased water content, alterations of meconium, or both are the probable etiology in most fetuses with HB. Decreased water content could be secondary to hypoperistalsis given that fluid is normally resorbed by the small bowel. Hypoperistalsis, in turn, could be secondary to decreased bowel function or vascular compromise. Inspissated, altered meconium can even lead to calcification in some cases. We have observed some cases of HB that were correlated with calcified intraluminal meconium, seen only on low-power radiographs of postmortem specimens. Sickler et al.[133] reported the same observation in a fetus with trisomy 21.

Inspissated meconium is most likely during the second trimester because the bowel lumen is very small and the fetus swallows less fluid at this time. With advancing gestational age, an increase of swallowed fluid promotes passage of bowel contents down the gut.

Fluid microvillar enzymes are decreased in fetuses with trisomy syndromes as well as in fetuses with CF.[134] This finding supports the notion that these fetuses exhibit "constipation" *in utero.*

Diagnosis

The significance of HB probably varies with its location (small bowel vs. colon), menstrual age, and degree of echogenicity. The echogenicity of normal bowel also increases with transducer frequency,[135] although this effect is uniform whereas true HB tends to be focal. Despite its subjectivity, the prevalence of HB among normal fetuses (0.5%) has been remarkably consistent at our center in the last decade and is also similar to other reports, suggesting that different centers can agree on the presence of HB. Objective methods of determining HB have been proposed,[136,137] but clinical detection still requires subjective interpretation.

To minimize subjectivity, some authors consider only bowel that is markedly hyperechoic, whereas others[138,139] recognize both moderate and markedly hyperechoic bowel. We, and others, have used the following grading system for HB[140] (Fig. 21):

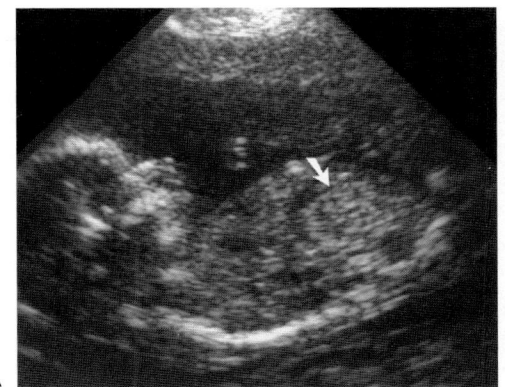

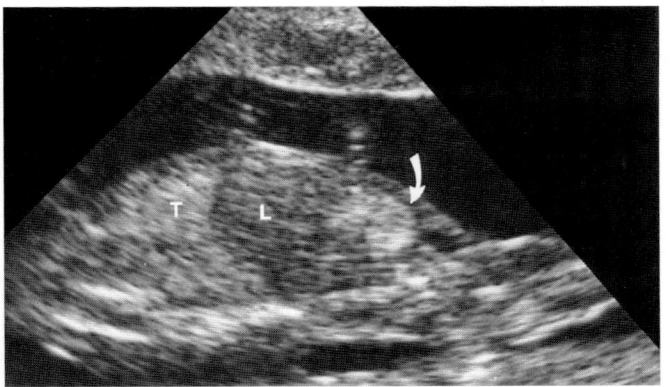

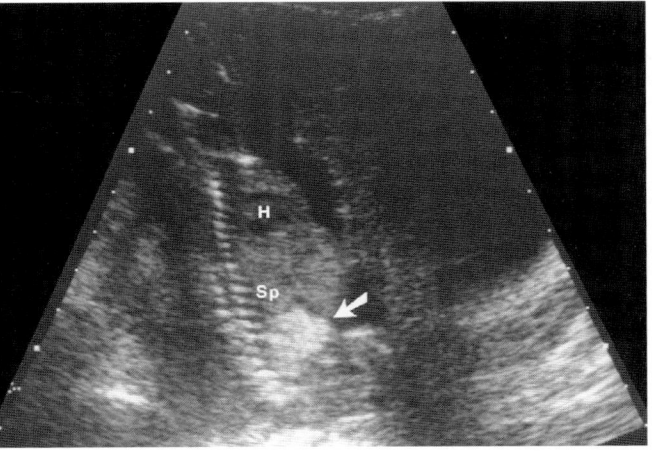

FIGURE 21. Gradation of hyperechoic bowel. **A:** Grade 1—bowel (*arrow*) is only mildly more echogenic than liver. **B:** Grade 2—bowel (*arrow*) is moderately echogenic compared to liver (*L*) but not as echogenic as bone (*T*). The fetus proved to have trisomy 21. **C:** Grade 3—bowel (*arrow*) is markedly hyperechoic with echogenicity approaching bone. H, heart; Sp, spine. (Reproduced with permission from Nyberg DA, Dubinsky T, Mahony BS, et al. Echogenic fetal bowel: clinical importance. *Radiology* 1993;188:527–531.)

Grade 1: mildly echogenic and typically diffuse
Grade 2: moderately echogenic and typically focal
Grade 3: very echogenic, similar to that of bone structures

Differential Diagnosis

HB should be distinguished from intraabdominal echogenic areas, especially meconium peritonitis, by both the location and appearance of the abnormality (Table 6). HB should also be distinguished from other echogenic intraabdominal masses including dysplastic kidneys, intraabdominal extrathoracic pulmonary sequestration, or duplication cyst based on the location. Other intraabdominal masses such as hemorrhagic ovarian cyst or neuroblastoma are not visualized until the third trimester.

Hyperechoic meconium during the third trimester can be normal[141] but this is usually confined to the colon.[142] Hyperechoic small bowel during the third trimester is uncommon and may also be associated with adverse outcome.[143]

Associated Anomalies and Conditions

HB is nonspecific and most commonly observed in normal fetuses. However, it is clearly associated with adverse outcomes including fetal aneuploidy (see Chapter 21), bowel obstruction or atresia, congenital infection (Fig. 22), IUGR, fetal demise, and CF.[144-167]

The risk of both aneuploidy and CF increases with the degree of echogenicity with HB. Slotnick and Abuhamad[139] identified 145 cases (1.9%) of HB from 7,400 second-trimester ultrasound examinations. CF was found in 0% (0 of 40) fetuses with mild increase in bowel (grade 1), 2.5% (2 of 81) fetuses with moderate increase (grade 2), and 20.8% (5 of 24) with markedly hyperechoic bowel (grade 3); trisomy 21 was found in 0%, 2.5%, and 25%, respectively. The authors conclude that both grades 2 and 3 HB carry an increased risk of CF and aneuploidy. Similar results were previously suggested by Nyberg et al.[140] and Hill et al.[138]

Prognosis and Management

The prognosis depends on the underlying condition as well as on the threshold for diagnosing HB and the degree of echogenicity. Nevertheless, some idea of the risk can be estimated from a summary of some of the larger series of HB (Table 5). These data indicate an increased risk of aneuploidy (approximately 3%), fetal or neonatal demise (3% to 4%), CF (1% to 2%), congenital infection (1% to 2%), bowel complication (1% to 2%), and other anomalies (3%). In addition there is a probable higher rate of fetal growth restriction among fetuses with HB. Among 79 fetuses with HB, Yaron et al.[156] reported two (2.5%) with CF; seven (8.9%) with multiple anomalies; and five (6.3%) each with aneuploidy, bowel obstruction or perforation,

TABLE 6. CAUSES OF ECHOGENIC AREAS IN THE FETAL ABDOMEN

Calcification
  Peritoneal calcification
    Meconium perititonitis
    Hydrometrocolpos
  Intraluminal meconium calcification
    Anorectal atresia
    Small bowel atresia
    Rarely isolated without bowel obstruction
  Parenchymal
    Liver
    Splenic
    Adrenal
    Complicated ovarian cyst (rare)
  Cholelithiasis—gallbladder
Noncalcified
  Echogenic meconium
  Intraabdominal, extrathoracic pulmonary sequestration
  Tumors
  Adrenal hemorrhage

and intrauterine infection [cytomegalovirus (CMV), herpes simplex virus, varicella-zoster virus, or parvovirus B19]. Three cases (3.8%) were associated with subsequent unexplained stillbirth. In another series of 182 fetuses with HB, Muller et al.[159] reported that 23 (13%) underwent termination of pregnancy for associated anomalies and another 24 (13%) experienced spontaneous demise. Of 135 newborns, 121 (90%) were normal, but nine (6.7%) had gastrointestinal obstruction requiring surgery, three (2.2%) had infection (CMV or parvovirus), one (0.7%) had a triple X chromosome, and one (0.7%) died from sudden infant death syndrome.

HB combined with maternal serum alpha-fetoprotein (AFP) levels is associated with poor fetal outcome, particularly fetal growth restriction with fetal and neonatal death. Among six patients with HB and elevated maternal serum AFP reported by Achiron et al.,[167] all showed IUGR and all died *in utero* (n = 4) or after birth (n = 2). In a series of 156 fetuses with HB, Al-Kouatly et al.[168] found that nine (5.8%) experienced fetal demise. Among five who had maternal serum AFP levels available, four (80%) had elevated levels. Among various factors evaluated, elevated maternal serum AFP was the strongest predictor of fetal demise. Fetuses with HB and abnormal Doppler studies probably also carry a much higher risk of IUGR and fetal demise.

When HB is demonstrated, other testing may be considered including fetal karyotype, maternal serologic studies for congenital infection, and DNA testing for CF. The prognosis is favorable once fetal aneuploidy, CF, structural abnormalities, infection, and IUGR have been excluded.

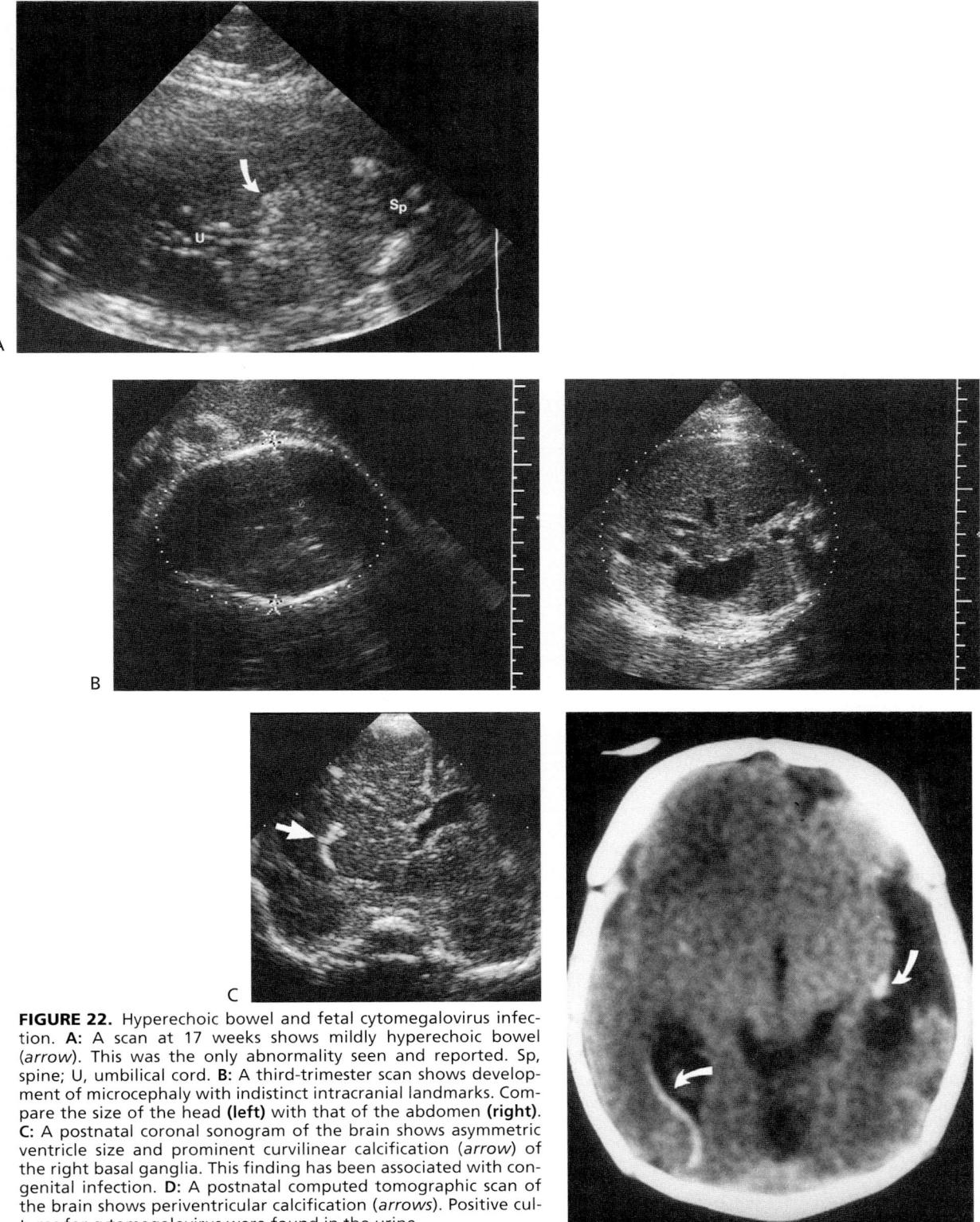

FIGURE 22. Hyperechoic bowel and fetal cytomegalovirus infection. **A:** A scan at 17 weeks shows mildly hyperechoic bowel (*arrow*). This was the only abnormality seen and reported. Sp, spine; U, umbilical cord. **B:** A third-trimester scan shows development of microcephaly with indistinct intracranial landmarks. Compare the size of the head **(left)** with that of the abdomen **(right)**. **C:** A postnatal coronal sonogram of the brain shows asymmetric ventricle size and prominent curvilinear calcification (*arrow*) of the right basal ganglia. This finding has been associated with congenital infection. **D:** A postnatal computed tomographic scan of the brain shows periventricular calcification (*arrows*). Positive cultures for cytomegalovirus were found in the urine.

Nonobstructive Small Bowel Dilatation

Rarely, bowel dilatation may be seen in the absence of obstruction from congenital chloridorrhea. This autosomal recessive disorder is characterized by absent or impaired cellular transport of chloride from the distal ileum and colon. It is thought to be secondary to deficiency of the chloride-bicarbonate ion-exchange pump. Postnatal clinical features of congenital chloridorrhea include profuse watery diarrhea, dehydration, and metabolic alkalosis. Congenital chloridorrhea has been observed as multiple loops of dilated bowel and polyhydramnios in several cases prenatally.[169–171] In a series of eight cases, Lundkvist et al.[172] reported that affected fetuses show dilated bowel segments with normal bowel peristalsis associated with marked polyhydramnios. This disorder can be fatal after birth if not correctly diagnosed and treated with volume replacement.

Megacystis-microcolon intestinal hypoperistalsis syndrome (MMIHS) is another rare case of functional bowel obstruction.[173] However, in all cases reported prenatally, an enlarged nonobstructed urinary bladder has dominated the sonographic findings.[165,174,175] Failure to empty the urinary bladder also results in hydronephrosis and a thickened urinary bladder wall. Prenatal diagnosis is difficult because of nonspecificity of ultrasound findings.[166] Greater than 90% of reported cases are females, unlike urethrovesical obstruction, which occurs predominantly in males. Also, unlike urethrovesical obstruction, amniotic fluid volume is normal to increased with MMIHS. Although the pathogenesis remains uncertain, some authors believe that MMIHS is secondary to a degenerative disease of smooth muscle resulting in absent peristalsis.[176] The prognosis is poor, with long-term survivors reported in only 11% of cases.

LARGE BOWEL ABNORMALITIES

Abnormalities of the large bowel are more rare, and less likely to be visualized with prenatal ultrasound than are abnormalities of the small bowel. Abnormalities of the large bowel include anorectal atresia, persistent common cloaca, and Hirschsprung disease. Of these, persistent common cloaca (a complicated form of anorectal atresia) is probably the most commonly encountered prenatally, even though it is rare postnatally.

Anorectal Atresia

Synonyms for anorectal atresia include *anal atresia* and *imperforate anus*.

Incidence

Anorectal malformations occur in as many as 1 in 2,000 births.[177]

Embryology and Pathology

A number of complex pathologic classifications have been derived for describing anal or rectal atresia. For simplification these are referred to here as *anorectal atresia*. Anorectal atresia can be categorized into two groups: high (supralevator) lesions that terminate above the levator sling and low (infralevator) lesions that terminate below the levator sling. High lesions are more common and are more frequently associated with fistulas and genitourinary malformations. Membranous atresia (imperforate anus), in its simplest form, is a rare condition that results from failure of the anal membrane to perforate. An especially complex type of atresia is a persistent cloaca (discussed below), in which the rectum, vagina, and urinary tract communicate with the perineum through a single opening.

Anorectal malformations result from abnormal partitioning of the cloaca by the urorectal septum. The cloaca represents the distal confluence of (a) the distal hindgut, (b) the allantois, and (c) the mesonephric ducts. During the ninth menstrual week, downgrowth of the urorectal septum separates the cloaca into the dorsal rectum and the ventral urogenital sinus. The urogenital sinus subsequently forms the urinary bladder and urethra, and the rectum remains a blind pouch until the anal membrane perforates by the tenth week.

Diagnosis

Anorectal atresia has rarely been recognized on prenatal sonography as dilated colon in the lower abdomen or pelvis.[178,179] Most cases have been reported during the third trimester. However, one case of anal atresia associated with the Johanson-Blizzard syndrome with dilated colon was reported at 21 weeks' gestation.[180]

Calcified intraluminal meconium is another possible manifestation of anorectal atresia[181–184] (Fig. 23). First observed by Berdon et al.,[181] this finding has now been confirmed by a number of other reports.[183,184] The calcified meconium pellets can be found either proximal or distal to the site of obstruction. The cause of the intraluminal calcification is unknown, although it is presumably related to prolonged stasis. Other authors[183] have proposed that alkaline urine from a colovesical fistula may predispose to intraluminal meconium calcification.

Amniotic fluid volume is either normal or, when associated with bilateral renal disorders, decreased in association with anorectal atresia. The presence of polyhydramnios should suggest either a diagnosis other than anorectal atresia or an additional anomaly such as EA. Fetuses with gastrointestinal obstruction, including anal atresia, also tend to be small.[31]

Decreased levels of microvillar enzymes have been associated with anal atresia in addition to other bowel abnormalities such as CF and nonobstructive anomalies, namely chromosomal abnormalities.[185,186] Decreased levels of

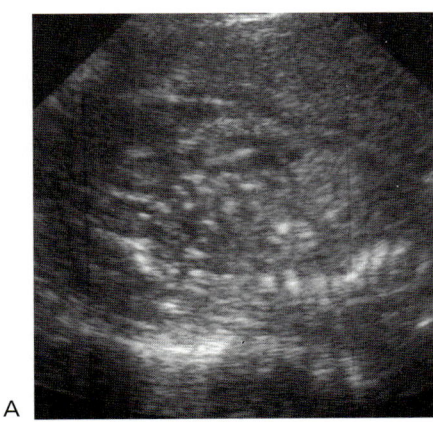
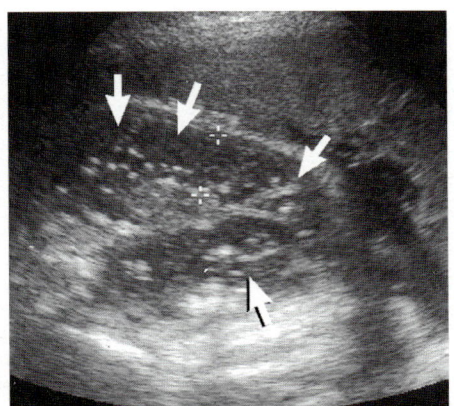
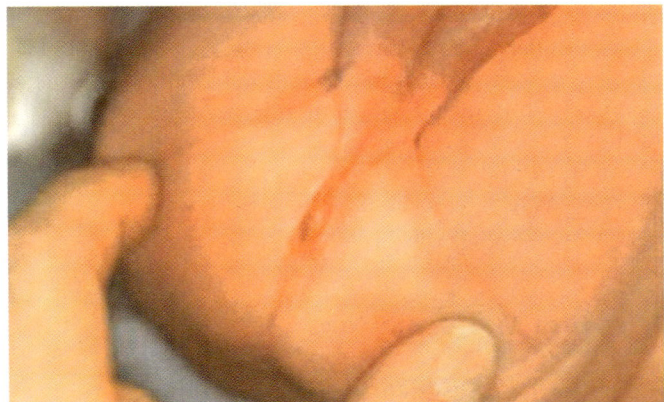

FIGURE 23. Anal atresia with enterolithiasis. **A:** A scan at 17 weeks shows scattered echogenic foci. The location of the foci was uncertain, and meconium peritonitis was considered. **B:** A follow-up scan at 35 weeks shows echogenic foci consistent with calcification within dilated bowel segments (*arrows*, calipers). **C:** A photograph taken at birth shows imperforate anus. Rectourinary fistulas were also present.

amniotic fluid and maternal serum AFP levels have also been observed with anal atresia.[187]

Differential Diagnosis

Because dilated small bowel can closely simulate large bowel, causes of small bowel dilatation should also be considered whenever large bowel dilatation is suspected (see Table 2). Persistent cloaca should always be considered when dilated large bowel is thought to be visualized, although this disorder should show a cystic structure in midpelvis. Other unusual causes of large bowel dilatation include colonic atresia,[188] meconium plug syndrome, and Hirschsprung disease.

Associated Anomalies

Additional malformations are present in up to 70% of neonates with anorectal atresia and in greater than 90% of fetuses in whom anorectal atresia is detected prenatally. The genitourinary system is the most frequently involved organ system, which is not surprising in view of the common embryogenesis of the cloaca and urogenital sinus. Esoph-

ageal malformations and spinal abnormalities are also commonly present. The frequent concurrence of anorectal atresia and genitourinary malformations is reflected by two major groups of disorders: the VACTERL syndrome and the caudal regression syndrome (renal agenesis or dysplasia, sacral agenesis, lower limb hypoplasia, and, in its severest form, sirenomelia). Many malformations associated with anorectal atresia are random and do not necessarily fit into one of these syndromes. Specific malformations that may be associated with anorectal atresia include the following:

1. Genitourinary
   A. Renal agenesis or dysplasia
   B. Horseshoe kidney
   C. Uterine duplication abnormalities
2. Skeletal, vertebral
   A. Vertebral anomalies
   B. Sacral agenesis
   C. Sirenomelia
3. Gastrointestinal: tracheoesophageal atresia
4. Cardiovascular malformations
5. Central nervous system anomalies
6. Chromosomal abnormalities (trisomies 21 and 18)

Prognosis and Management

The prognosis for fetuses with anorectal atresia is poor owing to the severity and high frequency of concurrent malformations. Bilateral renal agenesis or dysplasia is uniformly fatal, and cardiovascular or central nervous system malformations contribute to other deaths. Among survivors, bowel and bladder incontinence is common. Functional results appear to have improved with the development of a surgical technique (posterior sagittal anorectoplasty) described by Pena[189] and de Vries and Cox.[190] In this technique, careful dissection from the posterior approach permits the bowel to be pulled through the levator muscle complex and improves bowel continence. Using this technique, Chen[191] described his 10-year experience with 108 patients with imperforate anus. Of these, 66 were boys and 42 were girls. Thirty-five patients with a low lesion underwent a limited posterior sagittal anorectoplasty. Seventy-one patients had a high lesion and had three-stage operations including colostomy, posterior sagittal anorectoplasty, and takedown of colostomy. Most patients were continent and able to have voluntary bowel movements. Approximately one-half of the patients with high-type lesions complained of constipation.

Urorectal Septum Malformations

Persistent Cloaca/Urogenital Sinus

Persistent cloaca and urogenital sinus are complex abnormalities affecting the hindgut, urinary tract, and genital tract and are caused by abnormal formation of the urorectal septum. Persistent cloaca (Latin for "sewer") is persistence of the primitive common chamber formed by the urinary, gastrointestinal, and genital tracts. Persistent urogenital sinus is a common chamber of the urinary and genital tracts.

Incidence

Persistent cloaca is a rare disorder occurring in approximately 1 in 50,000 births.[192] It is much more common in females than in males. The prenatal literature also suggests that urorectal septum malformations (URSMs) may be more common in twin pregnancies.

Embryology and Pathology

The cloaca constitutes a functional definitive organ among premammals such as reptiles and birds, whereas in humans it represents a temporary embryonic structure where the genital, urinary and digestive systems join. Normally, downward growth of the urorectal septum divides the cloaca into the urogenital sinus, which will form the bladder, and the hindgut posteriorly (Fig. 24). It also divides the cloacal membrane into the urogenital membrane and anal membrane. A persistent cloaca results from failure of development of the urorectal septum. This forms a common chamber of the rectum, vagina, and urinary system, usually with a single common perineal opening. This disorder is more common in females because males usually produce a distal fistula by the developing urethral folds.[193]

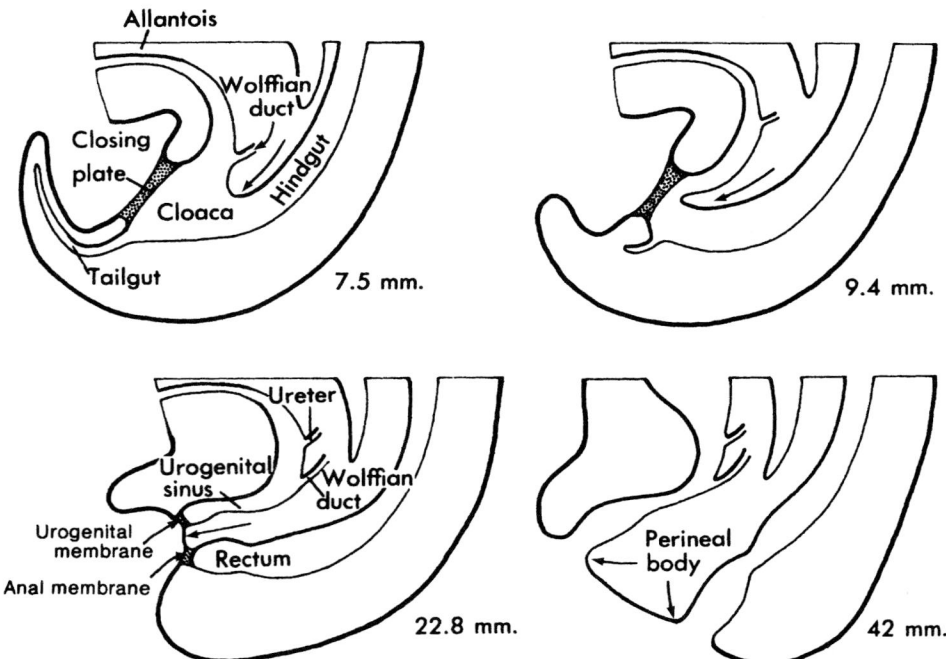

FIGURE 24. Normal development of the cloaca. The urorectal septum grows in a caudal direction to separate the cloaca into the hindgut posteriorly and the urogenital sinus anteriorly. The urorectal septum also divides the cloacal membrane into the urogenital and anal membranes. Abnormalities of the cloaca and urogenital sinus result from failure of normal development of these membranes. (Reproduced with permission from Gray SW, Skandalakis JE. *Embryology for surgeons.* Philadelphia: WB Saunders, 1972.)

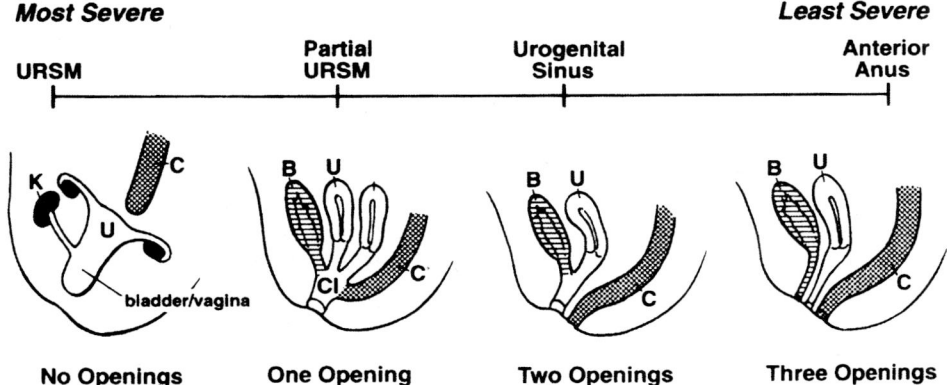

FIGURE 25. Spectrum of abnormalities related to the urorectal septum. Common cloaca is referred to as *partial urorectal septum malformation (URSM)* in this classification. Variations of these forms may also occur. B, bladder; C, colon; Cl, cloaca; K, kidney; U, uterus. (Reproduced with permission from Wheeler PG, Weaver DD. Partial urorectal septum malformation sequence: a report of 25 cases. *Am J Med Genet* 2001; 103:99–105.)

A urogenital sinus malformation occurs where there is a common channel for the urinary and genital tract. In this condition, two perineal orifices are present, one for the urogenital sinus and the other for the anus. Both common cloaca and urogenital sinus malformation show great internal and external anatomic variability among affected patients. The spectrum of defects involving the cloaca and urogenital sinus has been unified under the term *URSM sequence*.[194,195] In the classification of Wheeler and Weaver,[195] partial common cloaca is also termed *partial URSM* (Fig. 25).

Pathologic findings of persistent cloaca include confluence of the bladder, proximal urethra, upper two-thirds of the vagina, and rectum with connection to the perineum through a single common channel. Obstruction of the bladder, vagina, and intestine may result in dilated bowel, hydrocolpos, urethral obstruction, hydronephrosis, and oligohydramnios. Failure of the paired mullerian ducts to fuse also usually results in duplication of the uterus and vagina.

Hydrocolpos may also develop with urogenital sinus.[196] In some cases, a high position of the vaginal opening near the bladder neck is associated with reflux of urine from the bladder into the vagina without obstruction,[197] which may form a markedly dilated vagina and, to a lesser extent, a dilated uterus.

Diagnosis
Although rare, a number of cases of URSMs have been reported on prenatal sonography.[192,198–206] In fact, reports of persistent cloaca are more common than of anorectal atresia alone. The typical sonographic appearance is a cystic pelvic mass, often septated, in association with oligohydramnios and impaired fetal growth (Fig. 26).[207,208] Ascites, ambiguous genitalia, and nonvisualization of a normal urinary bladder are additional findings. Ascites, sometimes transient, may represent urine that has escaped from the cloaca into the peritoneal cavity via the fallopian tubes.

This mechanism could result in meconium peritonitis without bowel perforation.[209]

Urogenital sinus shows similar findings. A cystic mass may be demonstrated, usually representing the markedly dilated vagina (Fig. 27) or sometimes the uterus. With a urogenital sinus, the cyst may initially appear as a prominent urinary bladder because the bladder is not visualized as a separate structure. However, frequent variations occur in which a bladder may be identified and the mass may be suspected to be hydrocolpos (Fig. 28). A fluid-debris level has been reported to be highly suggestive.[210] The vagina may also become filled with echoes producing a solid mass-like appearance or complex cystic mass. The echoes are thought to be related to mucus, desquamated epithelium, and meconium.

Differential Diagnosis
The differential diagnosis for URSMs includes other anorectal atresia alone, other cystic masses, and a normal or prominent urinary bladder.

Associated Findings
Associated anomalies are common and tend to be more severe with the severity of the defect. Multiple associated anomalies are invariably present with persistent cloaca. Anomalies of the upper urinary tract are present in the majority of cases and may include renal agenesis, dysplasia, hydronephrosis, horseshoe kidney, and crossed renal ectopia. Other anomalies that have been associated with URSMs include vaginal and uterine duplication, urachal remnants, TEF, duodenal atresia, and myelomeningocele.

Prognosis and Management
The prognosis of URSMs is directly related to associated anomalies and the severity of the defect. Fetuses with the most severe type, with no external opening (Fig. 25), usually die from pulmonary hypoplasia secondary to renal

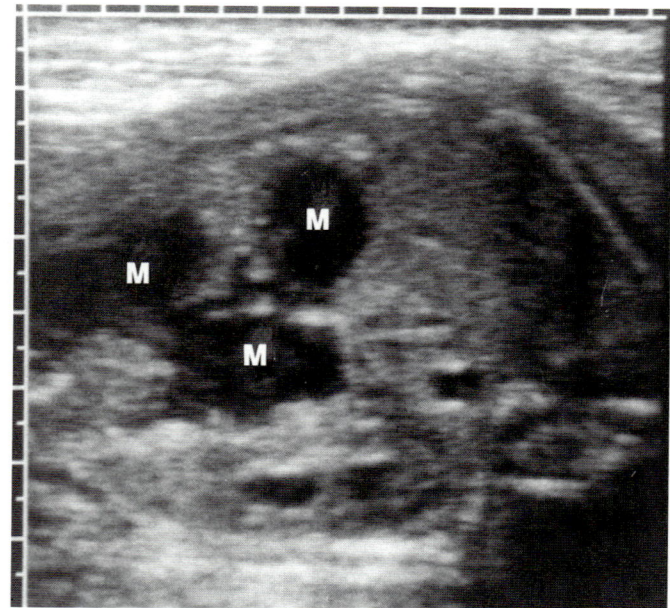
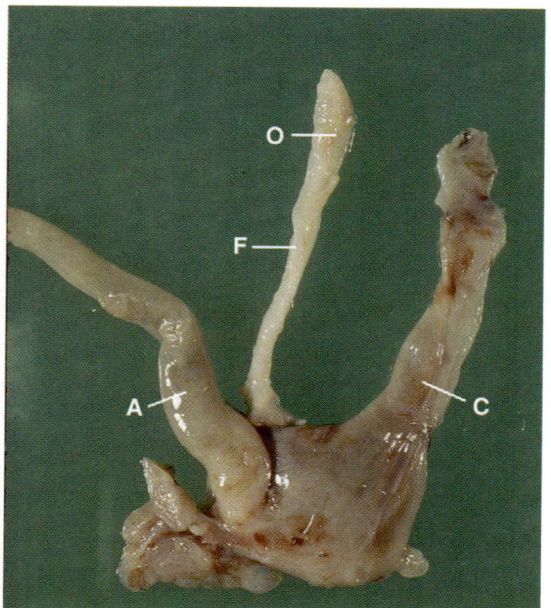

FIGURE 26. Persistent cloaca. **A:** This sonogram of a pelvis at 27 weeks shows a septated cystic mass (*M*). No urinary bladder was identified, and oligohydramnios was present. **B:** The postmortem examination shows single chamber of urinary, intestinal, and genital tracts. A, allantois and primitive bladder; C, colon; F, fallopian tube; O, ovary.

agenesis or dysplasia.[195] In survivors, repair of the defect is a surgical challenge.[211,212] Immediate colostomy is necessary after birth. Subsequent definitive surgical repair of all three systems (rectum, vagina, and urinary tract) can be accomplished simultaneously in most patients.[213] However, patients with life-threatening obstruction, reflux, or both require repair of the urinary tract first.[214]

Hendren[215] reviewed cases of 141 patients following surgical repair of a persistent cloaca. Of these, 82 had spontaneous bowel movements and continence and 83 voided spontaneously. Among 24 adults, seven had successful pregnancies, usually by cesarean delivery. The author concludes that, with comprehensive surgical planning, a rea-

sonable lifestyle can be achieved for most patients with persistent cloaca.

Hirschsprung Disease (Congenital Aganglionic Megacolon)

Hirschsprung disease is characterized by congenital absence of the intramural myenteric parasympathetic nerve ganglia and sympathetic nerve plexus in a bowel segment.

Incidence

Hirschsprung disease occurs in 1 in 10,000 to 20,000 births.[216] Males are affected three to four times more fre-

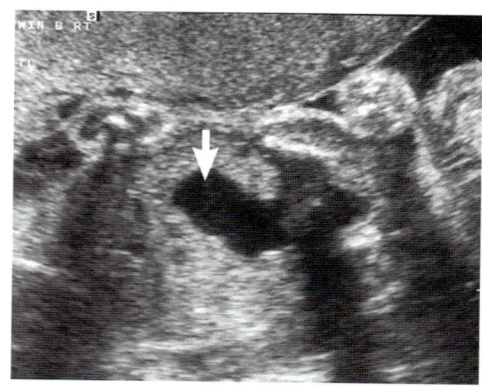
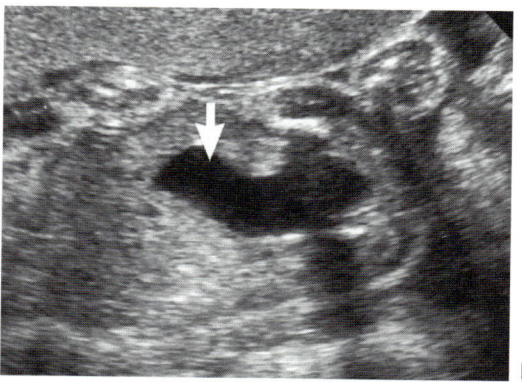

FIGURE 27. Urogenital sinus. **A, B:** Longitudinal views at 32 weeks from a twin pregnancy show an unusual cystic mass (*arrows*) arising from the pelvis. On earlier scans, only a prominent urinary bladder was visualized. Urogenital sinus was found after birth with the cystic structure representing the dilated vagina.

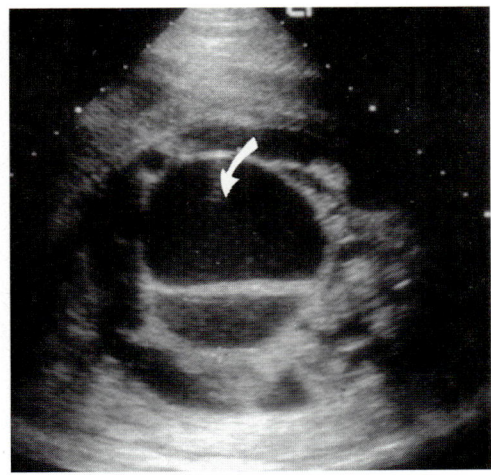

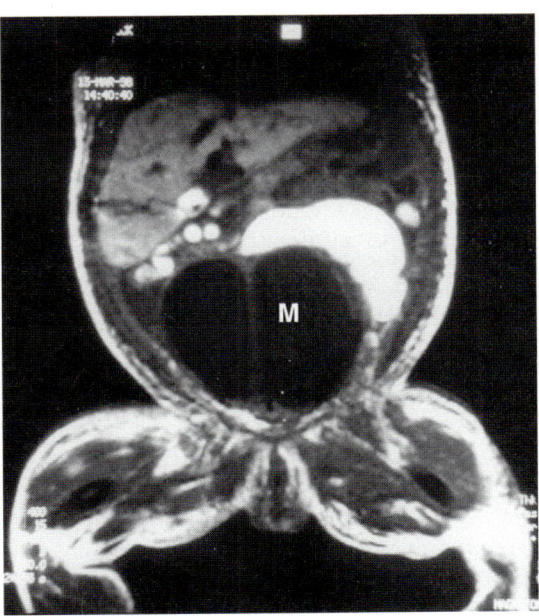
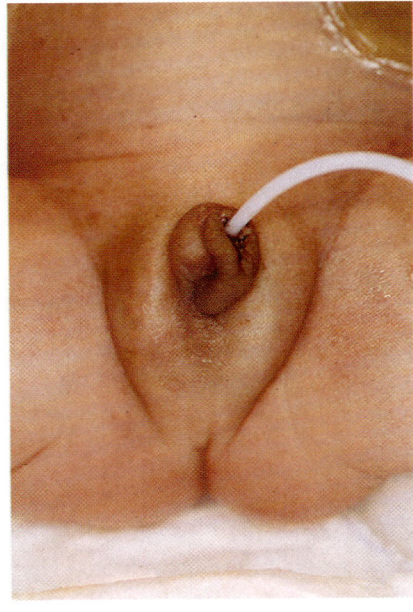

A

B,C

FIGURE 28. Dilated vagina and urogenital sinus malformation. **A:** Retrovesical septated cystic mass (*arrow*) with mild ascites at 35 weeks' gestation. **B:** Postnatal magnetic resonance image in coronal plane shows the septated cystic mass (*M*), which proved to be the dilated vagina. **C:** A postnatal photograph shows ambiguous genitalia. Anal atresia was also present. Other anomalies included horseshoe kidney with dilated renal pelvis and ureter, small muscular ventricular septal defect, vaginal atresia, and urethrovaginal and rectovaginal fistulas. The uterus was 0.8 cm long and appeared normal. This type of abnormality is closely related to persistent urogenital sinus, but in this case a separate bladder was present. [Parts **A** and **B** reproduced with permission from Geipel A, Berg C, Germer U, et al. Diagnostic and therapeutic problems in a case of prenatally detected fetal hydrocolpos. *Ultrasound Obstet Gynecol* 2001;18(2):169–172; and part **C** courtesy of Dr. Geipel.]

quently than are females, and whites are affected more frequently than blacks.

Embryology and Pathology

The rectum is invariably affected at the distal end, whereas the extent of proximal involvement is variable. Involvement is limited to the rectosigmoid in 74% of cases and distal to the splenic flexure in 90% of cases. The entire colon (total colonic aganglionosis) or distal ileum is involved in less than 10% of cases.[216]

Okamoto and Ueda[217] first suggested that the absence of ganglion cells in Hirschsprung disease was attributable to failure of migration of neural crest cells. In this theory, the earlier the arrest of migration, the longer the aganglionic segment. Another theory[218] favors the abnormal microenvironment hypothesis wherein the developing and migrating normal neural crest cells confront a segmentally abnormal and hostile microenvironment in the colon; nerve cells may

reach the correct position but then fail to develop or survive. An alternative hypothesis[219] has been proposed that the aganglionosis may be caused by failure of differentiation as a result of microenvironmental changes after migration.

Diagnosis

The clinical diagnosis of Hirschsprung disease can be made by demonstrating absent ganglion cells on (full-thickness) rectal biopsies. Accurate diagnoses have also been made with anorectal manometry and staining of mucosal biopsies for acetylcholinesterase. Hypertrophied nerve fibers are abundantly present in the bowel wall of patients with Hirschsprung disease, and these are rich in acetylcholinesterase.[220]

Hirschsprung disease rarely has been reported antenatally, even when specifically sought.[221–224] Eliyahu et al.[224] reported a case in the second trimester that showed dilated bowel segments and mild polyhydramnios. Similar to the case reported by Wrobleski and Wesselhoeft,[222] aganglionosis involved the entire colon up to the distal ileum. Based on this limited information, it appears that Hirschsprung disease may be detected prenatally when it affects the entire colon (total aganglionosis of the colon), resulting in small bowel dilatation and polyhydramnios during the third trimester.

Differential Diagnosis

Distinguishing Hirschsprung disease from other causes of small bowel dilatation may be impossible.

Associated Anomalies

Aneuploidy, usually trisomy 21, is present in approximately 2% of cases of Hirschsprung disease.[225,226] Associated anomalies include trisomy 21 in 10% of cases and neurologic abnormalities in 5%. Other reported associations include congenital heart defects (ventricular septal defects, transposition of the great arteries), imperforate anus in 3% of cases, and hypospadias.[218,220] Hirschsprung disease may be associated with a number of genetic conditions, including Bardet-Biedl syndrome, cartilage-hair hypoplasia, congenital central hypoventilation syndrome (Ondine's curse), Riley-Day syndrome, Mowat syndrome, and Waardenburg-Shah syndrome.[227] Mowat syndrome is associated with deletions or heterozygous mutations in the *ZFHX1B* (Zinc Finger Homeobox 1B) gene localized to 2q22, and Waardenburg-Shah may have mutations of the *SOX10* gene.[228]

Prognosis and Management

The major potential complication of Hirschsprung disease is bowel perforation proximal to the site of obstruction. Meconium peritonitis develops in 10% of cases by the time of birth.[218,220] After birth, clinical symptoms include failure to pass meconium, bile-stained vomiting, and abdominal distention. Delay in the correct diagnosis can lead to enterocolitis, bowel perforation, septicemia, and even death. The mortality rate during infancy is 20%[227] and 40% or more for total aganglionosis of the colon.[228,229] Major complications include sepsis and (a high-output) heavy fluid and electrolyte loss from the proximal stoma after enterostomy.

Patients with aganglionosis of the colon are generally treated with a two-stage surgery. The first stage creates a diverting stoma to relieve the obstruction. The definitive surgery consists of a pull-through procedure using one of several techniques. Surgery is performed in the first year of life.[230] Single-stage surgery without a colostomy can also be undertaken laparoscopically.

Recurrence Risk

Hirschsprung disease is usually sporadic. However, 4% to 6% of cases are familial. Mutations in the RET gene (del 10q11.2) are responsible for approximately one-half of familial cases and a smaller number of sporadic cases.[227]

MECONIUM PERITONITIS AND INTRAABDOMINAL CALCIFICATION

Intraabdominal calcification or echogenic areas arise from a variety of sites (Table 6), which can be categorized as follows:

1. Peritoneal
2. Intraluminal intestinal
3. Parenchymal (liver, splenic, adrenal, etc.)
4. Vascular
5. Biliary

It is important to distinguish calcification from HB alone (see Hyperechoic Bowel). Thus, acoustic shadowing should be demonstrated before calcification is reliably diagnosed. It is also important to precisely define the location of calcification and to search for other possible abnormalities.

Peritoneal calcification almost always results from meconium peritonitis. Retrograde secretion from vaginal obstruction and hydrocolpos can rarely result in peritoneal calcification.[231] Peritoneal and bladder wall calcification has also been described in association with obstruction of the urinary bladder related to posterior urethral valves.[183]

Meconium Peritonitis

Meconium peritonitis is a sterile chemical peritonitis resulting from *in utero* bowel perforation that nearly always involves the small bowel.

Incidence

Meconium peritonitis is estimated to occur in 1 in 2,000 pregnancies.[232]

Embryology and Pathology

Approximately one-half of meconium peritonitis cases are associated with an underlying bowel disorder, the most common being volvulus, atresia, intussusception, meconium ileus,[233] gastroschisis, or rarely cloaca.[209,231] The remaining cases are believed to result from idiopathic vascular impairment.[234] Occlusion and thrombosis of mesenteric arteries are frequently demonstrated on pathologic examination in these cases. The bowel is particularly prone to ischemia *in utero* because any cause of fetal or neonatal hypoxia leads to a selective decrease in mesenteric blood flow.[235] Cocaine exposure has been implicated in some cases.[236]

Whatever the underlying cause, the final common result of meconium peritonitis is bowel perforation. Extrusion of meconium and digestive enzymes into the peritoneal cavity incites an intense chemical peritonitis and secondary inflammatory response. Calcification may develop within days histologically, although radiographic evidence of calcification

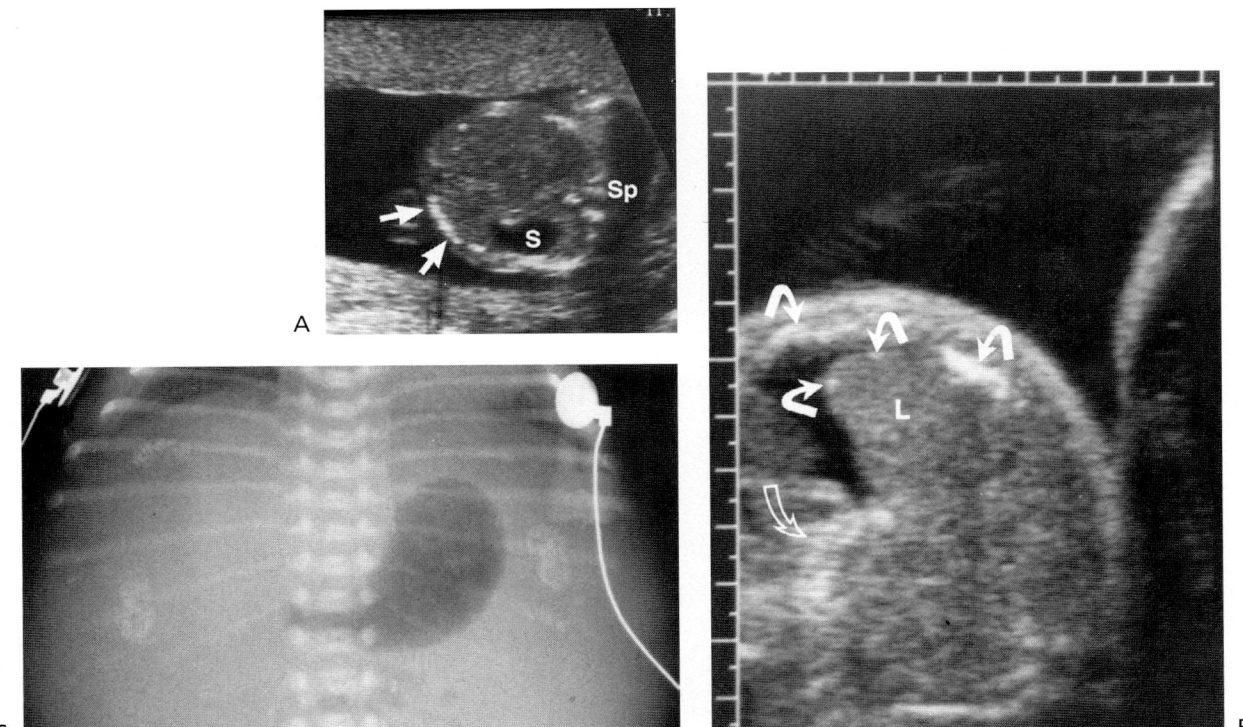

FIGURE 29. Meconium peritonitis. **A:** A scan at 28 weeks shows extensive calcification (*arrows*) along the peritoneum without ascites. S, stomach; Sp, spine. **B:** Another case shows peritoneal calcification (*solid arrows*) and mesenteric calcification (*open arrow*) with ascites. L, liver. **C:** A postnatal radiograph of the fetus in part **B** shows peritoneal calcifications. (Parts **B** and **C** reproduced with permission from Foster MA, Nyberg DA, Mahony BS, et al. Meconium peritonitis: prenatal sonographic findings and their clinical significance. *Radiology* 1987;165:661–665.)

usually requires 1 to 2 weeks.[237–239] Over time, the inflammatory response may seal the perforation spontaneously.

Diagnosis

Prenatal sonographic findings of meconium peritonitis are variable depending on the extent of meconium leakage, time elapsed since the bowel perforation, and the underlying bowel disorder[240] (Figs. 29 through 31). Peritoneal calcification is the most common and characteristic finding of meconium peritonitis on both prenatal sonography and postnatal radiography.[241] Other sonographic findings of meconium peritonitis include meconium pseudocyst, ascites, and bowel dilatation.[241] Polyhydramnios may also occur.

Peritoneal calcification may occur in any part of the peritoneal cavity including the parietal peritoneum overlying the liver, the visceral peritoneum in the mesentery, or through the process vaginalis into the scrotum. After resolution of the acute phase, these calcifications are usually the only visible signs of a previous meconium peritonitis.

Ascites is commonly demonstrated in association with meconium peritonitis, presumably reflecting the intense inflammatory response induced by the chemical peritonitis. The inflammatory response can also cause abdominal wall thickening and, in conjunction with

ascites, mimic fetal hydrops. Ascites may be the first manifestation of meconium peritonitis.[259] Because it may be the primary or only sonographic abnormality during the acute phase, meconium peritonitis should be considered whenever fetal ascites is demonstrated (Fig. 30). Serial sonograms may show development of characteristic peritoneal calcifications.

A meconium pseudocyst results from a contained bowel perforation.[242,243] It appears as a hypoechoic mass representing extraluminal meconium (Fig. 31). An echogenic wall forms around the mass, although calcification may not be obvious and acoustic shadowing may not be apparent.

The presence of bowel dilatation should suggest an associated bowel obstruction, most commonly from jejunoileal atresia, volvulus, or meconium ileus.

Differential Diagnosis

Meconium peritonitis should be distinguished from HB.

Peritoneal calcification of meconium peritonitis should be distinguished from intraluminal meconium calcification or inspissated meconium producing HB[244] (see Anorectal Atresia and Hyperechoic Bowel, earlier in this chapter). Calcification of meconium peritonitis is usually linear in appearance and should be localized to the peritoneum,

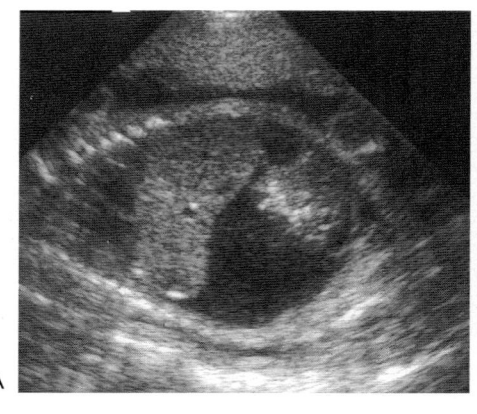
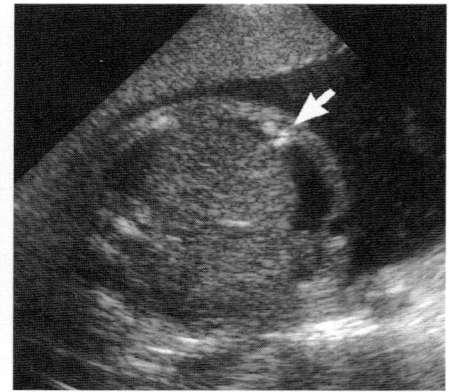
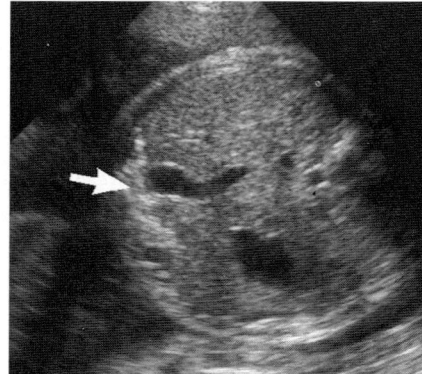

FIGURE 30. Meconium peritonitis presenting as ascites. **A:** A scan at 30 weeks shows a large amount of ascites. Echogenic mesentery was suggestive of meconium peritonitis. **B:** Small peritoneal calcifications are seen along the anterior peritoneal surface (*arrow*). **C:** A follow-up scan 4 weeks later shows complete resolution of ascites but persistent peritoneal calcification (*arrow*).

whereas intraluminal meconium calcification appears as punctate foci localized to the bowel lumen. Solitary echogenic foci near the stomach are not uncommon and should be diagnosed as meconium peritonitis (Fig. 32).

An evolving meconium pseudocyst may be difficult to distinguish from other intraabdominal masses, including hemorrhagic ovarian cysts. An unusual presentation of meconium pseudocyst has been described as simulating a sacrococcygeal teratoma.[245]

Ascites may be due to a large variety of abnormalities including hydrops, renal abnormalities, infection,[246] aneuploidy, hematologic conditions, cardiac abnormalities, and bowel disorders including volvulus,[247] meconium peritonitis, and laryngeal atresia.[248,249] Imperforate hymen[250] or hydrocolpos[251] may also rarely result in ascites. Infectious causes may include CMV, parvovirus, hepatitis, and syphilis.

Associated Anomalies

In infants diagnosed with meconium peritonitis in neonatal studies, CF has been reported in 15% to 40% of cases, although this association is distinctly unusual prenatally, probably reflecting the larger number of cases diagnosed by prenatal ultrasound.

Other bowel abnormalities leading to meconium peritonitis may include jejunoileal atresia, intussusception,[252] persistent cloaca, and gastroschisis.[253] Bowel atresia could be either the cause or consequence of ischemia and bowel perforation.

Evidence exists that meconium peritonitis may be associated with intrauterine infection. A number of infectious agents have been implicated, including parvovirus,[254,255] CMV,[256] rubella,[257] hepatitis B,[258] and hepatitis A.[259] In cases of true meconium peritonitis, infection presumably leads to vascular compromise and rupture of the bowel.

Prognosis and Management

In general, the prognosis for antenatally detected meconium peritonitis is excellent and much better than suggested by the neonatal literature.[129] Those fetuses showing only peritoneal calcification can be expected to have a favorable outcome without intervention,[260] whereas those with complex meconium peritonitis (i.e., with ascites, meconium cyst, or bowel dilatation) are more likely to require surgical resection of the perforated bowel segment.[261,262] Dirkes et al.[262] reported that only 22% of fetuses with a prenatal diagnosis of meconium peritonitis

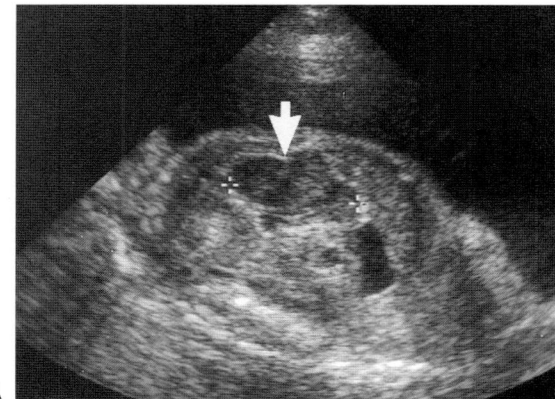

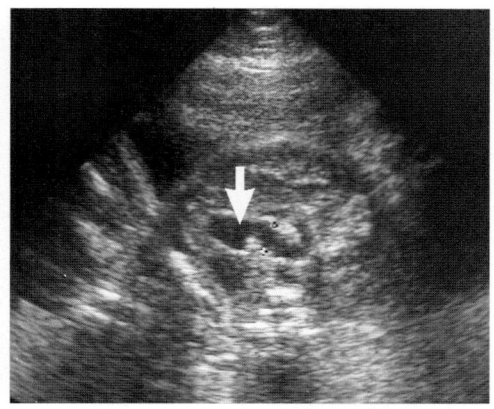

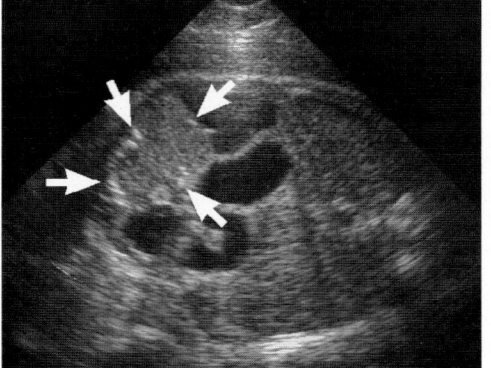

FIGURE 31. Meconium peritonitis and meconium pseudocyst. **A:** A scan at 30 weeks shows a hypoechoic mass (*arrow*) with a slightly echogenic rim, which is consistent with meconium pseudocyst. **B:** A mildly dilated bowel segment (*arrow*) is also present. **C:** A follow-up scan at 35 weeks shows a meconium pseudocyst (*arrows*) and dilated small bowel segment. Ileal atresia was found at surgery.

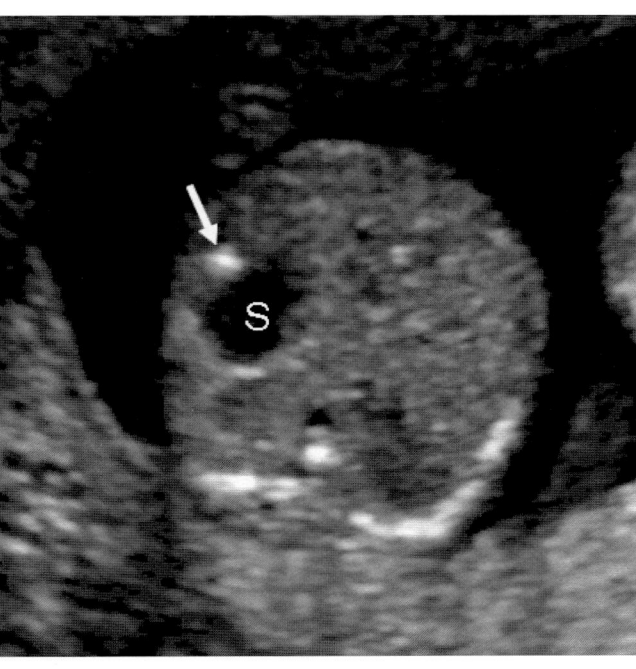

FIGURE 32. Echogenic focus near stomach. A transverse image at 18 weeks shows a solitary echogenic focus (*arrow*) near the stomach (*S*). This should not be diagnosed as meconium peritonitis.

require postnatal operation. Among nine fetuses with meconium peritonitis, two showing bowel dilatation and meconium pseudocyst required surgery (ileal resection and ileostomy) and two others showing bowel dilatation prenatally but not on postnatal radiographs required no intervention.

Infants with meconium ileus and CF as the underlying etiology have a poorer long-term prognosis (see the Cystic Fibrosis/Meconium Ileus section earlier in this chapter). Common complications include pancreatic insufficiency, multiple respiratory infections, chronic lung disease, and gastrointestinal disturbances.

Hepatic Calcification/Hyperechogenicities

Intrahepatic calcifications are punctate echogenic foci seen within the fetal liver by ultrasound.

Incidence

Intrahepatic calcifications (hyperechogenicities or echogenic foci) are not rare. Bronshtein and Blazer[263] estimated the incidence as 1 in 1,750 fetuses at 15 to 26 weeks, and Koopman and Wladimiroff[264] encountered intrahepatic echogenic foci in 1 in 1,037 pregnancies.

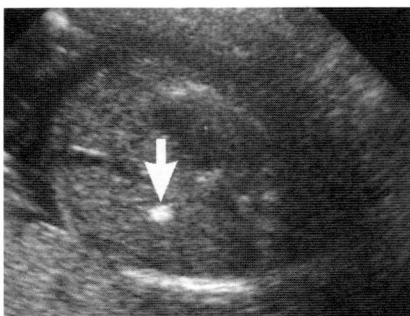

FIGURE 33. Hepatic calcification. An axial scan shows high-amplitude echogenic focus (*arrow*), consistent with calcification, in the liver. Acoustic shadowing was demonstrated on other images but may not be evident for smaller foci.

Pathology

The pathologic correlate of intrahepatic hyperechogenicities is uncertain. Avni et al.[265] suggest a vascular etiology: Localized infarct or ischemia could fibrose or calcify leading to segmental hyperechogenicities.

Diagnosis

Intrahepatic echogenic foci or calcifications are typically seen as one or two discrete echogenic foci within the liver[266,267] (Fig. 33). Occasionally, multiple calcifications may be seen, and these are more likely to be associated with underlying fetal infection or aneuploidy (see Associated Anomalies, below).

Differential Diagnosis

The most important differential diagnosis is meconium peritonitis, in which case calcified plaques are located on the peritoneal surface of the liver and not intraparenchymally. Small hemangiomas should also be distinguished from hepatic hyperechogenicities.

Associated Anomalies

Available evidence suggests that associated anomalies are unlikely when isolated, typical (one or two) foci are demonstrated. Among seven cases of intrahepatic echogenic foci, Koopman and Wladimiroff[264] reported two with major anomalies (one with trisomy 18) but both showed other major abnormalities on sonography. Among 14 cases of hepatic calcifications reported by Bronshtein and Blazer,[263] three (21%) had associated severe malformations: two with trisomy 18 and one with dwarfism and hydronephrosis. Similarly, Simchen et al.[268] evaluated 671 fetuses with liver calcification. Ten patients (1.5%) had abnormal karyotype including four with trisomy 13 and all of these showed additional anomalies. All 22 cases of isolated hepatic calcification had a normal outcome.

Widespread liver calcification can also represent fetal infection, especially from varicella or toxoplasmosis[269] (see Chapter 17).

Prognosis and Management

The prognosis is generally normal when one or two hepatic hyperechogenicities are demonstrated.[264] However, adverse outcome has been occasionally reported from widespread lesions.

Among 33 fetuses with intrahepatic calcifications evaluated by Stein et al.[270] at 16 to 38 weeks, four died including one with liver calcifications and no other findings. However, this fetus showed increasing numbers of calcifications on follow-up scans and proved to have CMV. Among 14 cases reported by Bronshtein and Blazer,[263] one fetus showed polyhydramnios and bowel calcifications and this fetus died *in utero*, whereas the ten fetuses with isolated calcifications were normal.

Fetal karyotyping is recommended when additional abnormalities are demonstrated, and a workup of infection is recommended when multiple intrahepatic echogenic foci are present.

Other Causes of Abdominal Calcification

Intraluminal intestinal calcification is nearly always associated with bowel obstruction, although exceptions have been reported.[271] Possible causes of bowel obstruction include anorectal atresia (see Anorectal Atresia, earlier in this chapter), multiple bowel atresia, small bowel stenosis, volvulus, persistent cloaca, and total colonic aganglionosis. The calcification may be located either proximal or distal to the site of obstruction.

Fetus *in fetu* can show as calcification and may be mistaken for meconium peritonitis or teratoma.[272,273]

Parenchymal calcifications are primarily confined to the liver, although adrenal calcification could result from infection or neuroblastoma.

ASCITES

Ascites may be secondary to a variety of etiologies (see Table 8 in Chapter 16), including hydrops of any cause, infection, chromosomal anomalies, urinary ascites, meconium peritonitis, laryngeal atresia, and primary lymphangiectasia.[274]

ABDOMINAL MASSES

A large variety of types of abdominal masses may be seen prenatally. Awareness of the location, gestational age, gender, and sonographic appearance of an abdominal mass should suggest the correct diagnosis or a limited differential diagnosis. In distinguishing abdominal masses, it is useful

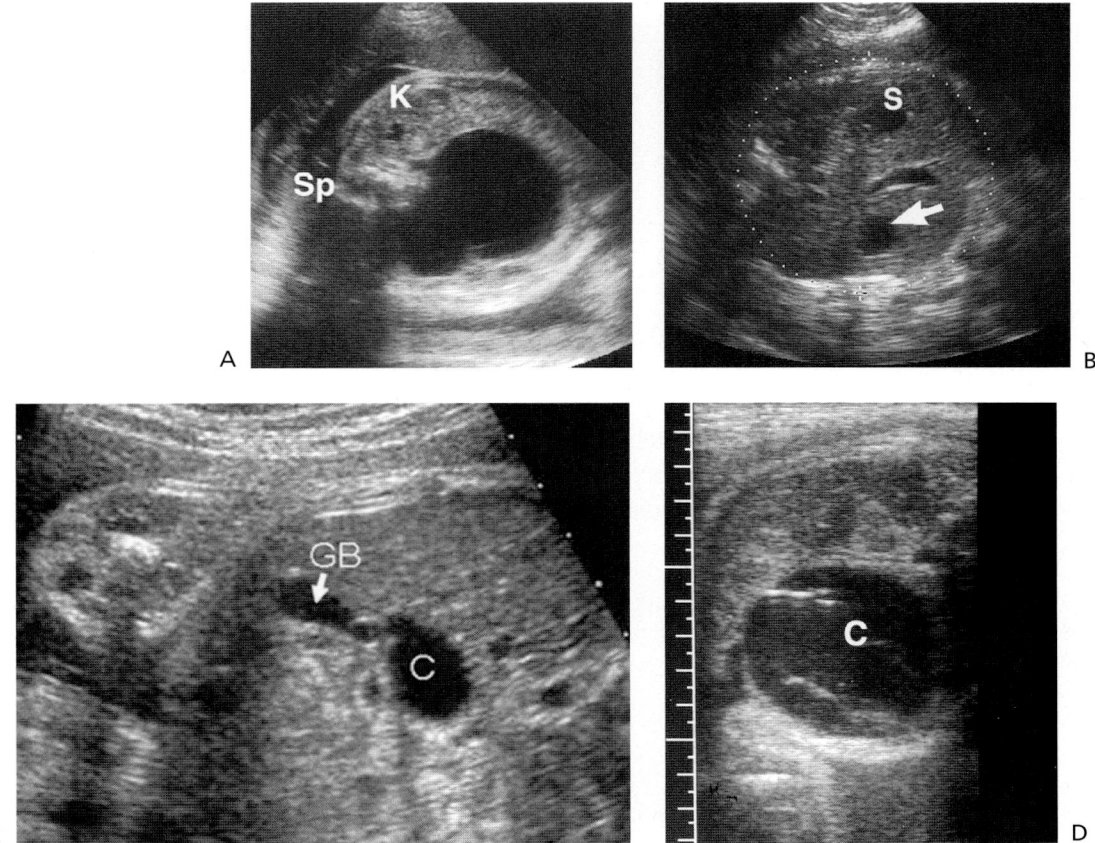

FIGURE 34. Various causes of intraabdominal cystic structures. **A:** Hydronephrosis. K, contralateral kidney; Sp, spine. **B:** Liver cyst (*arrow*). S, stomach. **C:** Choledochal cyst (*C*). GB, gallbladder. **D:** Ovarian cyst (*C*).

to distinguish echogenic from cystic masses, although certain types of cysts may appear either echogenic or cystic.

Echogenic or solid masses are less common than cystic masses in the abdomen. Echogenic masses may represent meconium pseudocyst, enteric duplication cyst,[275] adrenal hemorrhage or tumor, extrapulmonary intraabdominal pulmonary sequestration, hemorrhagic ovarian cyst, hydrocolpos, or various tumors.

Cystic masses of the abdomen may arise from many organ systems (Table 6, Fig. 34). Excluding cystic masses arising from the urinary system (hydronephrosis, multicystic dysplastic kidneys, paranephric pseudocysts, hydroureter, distended urinary bladder) or dilated bowel (discussed earlier), intraabdominal cystic masses may represent an ovarian cyst, enteric duplication cyst, mesenteric cyst (lymphangioma), choledochal cyst, liver or splenic cyst, hydrocolpos, urachal cyst, mesenchymal hamartoma, hemangioma, or varix of the umbilical vein.

Ovarian Cyst

Ovarian cysts are macroscopic cysts arising from the ovary.

Incidence

Fetal ovarian cysts are the most common cause of an intraabdominal cyst reported antenatally, excluding renal and bowel etiologies. The prevalence is uncertain, however.

Embryology and Pathology

Ovarian cysts are typically benign, functional cysts that result from enlargement of otherwise normal follicles known to be present during the third trimester and early neonatal period. Desa[276] found small follicular cysts in 34% (113 of 332) of newborns and infants who died within 28 days of life. However, these cysts are usually too small (less than 1 mm) to visualize sonographically.

Evidence suggests that ovarian cysts result from excessive stimulation of the fetal ovary by placental and maternal hormones. A higher prevalence of ovarian cysts has been noted in infants of mothers with diabetes, toxemia, or rhesus isoimmunization, presumably from excessive release of human chorionic gonadotropin by the enlarged placenta. An association between ovarian cysts and fetal hypothyroidism has also been suggested on the basis of

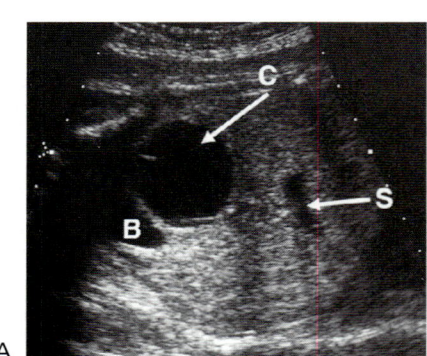
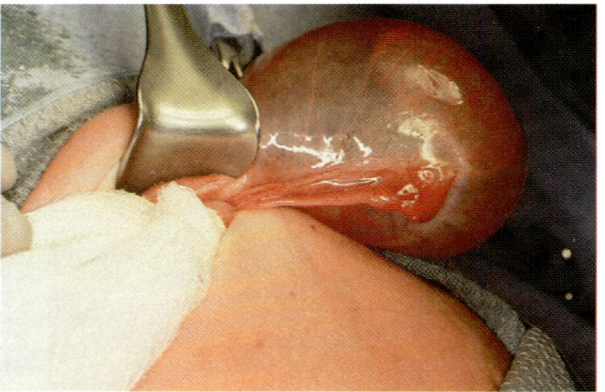

FIGURE 35. Ovarian cyst. **A:** This scan of a pelvis at 33 weeks shows a cystic mass (*C*) superior to the urinary bladder (*B*). S, stomach. **B:** Photograph of an ovarian cyst.

nonspecific stimulation of pituitary glycoprotein hormone synthesis.[277]

After birth, levels of human chorionic gonadotropin and estrogen plummet while levels of follicle-stimulating hormone and luteinizing hormone rise until approximately 3 months of age and then fall. These hormonal changes parallel typical resolution of ovarian cysts after birth.

Diagnosis

Ovarian cysts have been frequently diagnosed on prenatal sonography[278–285] (Figs. 35 and 36). In no case has a fetal ovarian cyst been reported before the third trimester, even when an earlier sonogram was performed.[286] This fact reflects insufficient hormonal stimulation until the third trimester of pregnancy.

Most ovarian cysts are unilateral, although several cases of bilateral ovarian cysts have also been reported.[278] The sonographic appearance of an ovarian cyst varies depending on its size and complications of torsion or hemorrhage. An uncomplicated ovarian cyst appears as a unilocular cystic mass, occasionally with internal septations. When complicated by torsion or hemorrhage, ovarian cysts may appear complex or even solid[287,288] (Fig. 36). Complicated ovarian cysts may also demonstrate a fluid-debris level, a retracting clot, and internal septa. The wall may be echogenic from dystrophic calcification associated with infarction.

Among 44 cases of ovarian cysts reported by Muller-Leisse et al.,[289] 39 were purely cystic and five were echogenic or had a mixed pattern. Meizner et al.[282] suggest that "intracystic flocculation," which typically was seen on the sloping part of the cyst, gave a characteristic liquid interface that was regarded as evidence of torsion. All six cases with this appearance were confirmed to have torsion at surgery.

The size of ovarian cysts is variable. Some ovarian cysts can become very large (8 to 10 cm) and extend to the upper abdomen. There is a general consensus that cysts larger than 5 cm in diameter may be at increased risk of torsion.[290,291] Meizner et al.[282] found that mean size of cysts with evidence of torsion was 5.41 ± 0.25 cm, and the mean

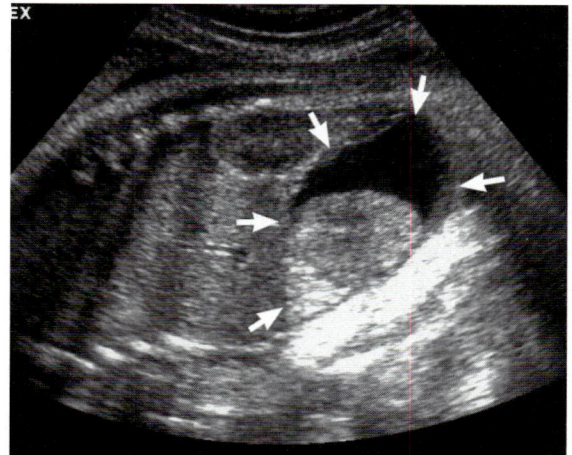
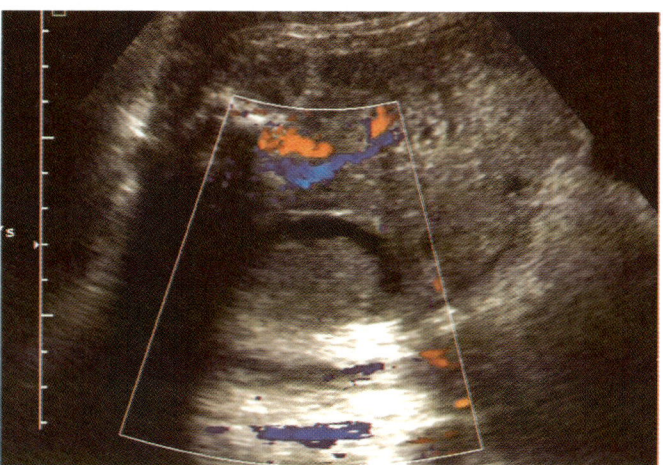

FIGURE 36. Hemorrhagic ovarian cyst. **A:** Oblique view of abdomen shows complex cystic mass (*arrows*) with an echogenic component. **B:** Color-flow imaging shows no vascularity to the echogenic component. Both the echogenic and the cystic components resolved on follow-up scans.

size of nine other cysts without torsion was 4.33 ± 0.3 cm (p <.01). On the other hand, Muller-Leisse et al.[289] found torsion in eight of 26 who underwent surgery and this was independent of the size of the cyst. The volume of these cysts varied from 5 to 71 mL (correlating to a diameter of up to 5.1 cm).

Polyhydramnios has been reported in at least 10% of cases, probably secondary to extrinsic small bowel obstruction.[292] Ascites may be present, presumably from ruptured ovarian cyst or torsion.[287,293]

Percutaneous aspiration can be diagnostic as well as potentially therapeutic by showing elevated estradiol levels and progesterone, in addition to hemosiderin-laden macrophages when the cyst is hemorrhagic.[290,294]

Differential Diagnosis

The differential diagnoses for a cystic mass in the fetal pelvis or lower abdomen is shown in Table 3. A mesenteric or enteric duplication cyst may appear indistinguishable from an ovarian cyst. Identification of male gender would exclude ovarian cyst or hydrocolpos and make persistent cloaca or MMIHS unlikely. Other considerations in both sexes include urachal cyst, mesenteric cyst, and enteric duplication cyst. If the urinary bladder is not identified separate from the mass, other considerations for a cystic pelvic mass should include obstructive uropathy, MMIHS, and persistent cloaca. A complex or solid mass similar in appearance to a complicated ovarian cyst can also be differentiated from a meconium pseudocyst.

Associated Findings

Few other anomalies have been associated with a fetal ovarian cyst. Fetal hypothyroidism has been observed.[277]

Prognosis and Management

Birth dystocia, respiratory distress, and gastrointestinal obstruction have been reported from very large cysts.[295,296] However, fetuses with cysts as large as 10 cm have been successfully delivered vaginally without complication. Fetal anemia has been reported secondary to hemorrhage into an ovarian cyst.[297]

Among 25 ovarian cysts reviewed by Bagolan and colleagues,[284] eight (32%) showed sonographic patterns of torsion and all were confirmed at surgery. In six additional cases the cysts increased or remained unchanged in size after 15 days of life, and three (50%) of these showed torsion at surgery. In the remaining six cases spontaneous resolution occurred within 1 to 4 months. One cyst was aspirated prenatally. Two of the affected infants reportedly had intestinal obstruction.

After delivery, therapeutic options are surgery (conventional or laparoscopic),[298] percutaneous aspiration, or observation alone. Intervention is often suggested for complex cysts,[299] cysts over 5 cm in diameter, as well as occasionally smaller cysts that do not decrease in size. However, others recommend expectant follow-up of ovarian cysts with surgery only for cysts with solid or complex components or cysts causing symptoms from large size or torsion.[300]

Given the large number of cases that end in oophorectomy in some surgical series, it is not apparent that surgery offers any advantages over expectant management. Muller-Leisse et al.[289] reported oophorectomy in 15 of the 26 who underwent surgery. Of the 23 cysts that were followed expectantly, 15 completely resolved within 14 months without correlation to the sonographic pattern.

In another series of 24 ovarian cysts, Suita and colleagues[301] reported surgical intervention in nine cases, each larger than 5 cm. Five of these neonates had clinical symptoms of abdominal distention or vomiting, and four showed hemorrhage with suspected torsion. Fifteen cysts, including two cysts larger than 5 cm, began to regress within 6 months after birth and ten of them disappeared between 2 weeks and 2 years.

Cystadenoma has rarely been reported in ovarian cysts during the first year of life[302] but has not been reported antenatally. Because ovarian cysts usually disappear spontaneously and rarely cause severe symptoms, Muller-Leisse et al.[289] suggest monitoring the cysts and reserve surgical intervention only if the cyst produces significant mass effect and percutaneous puncture cannot be performed.

Hydrocolpos

Hydrocolpos is dilatation of the vagina due to obstruction of the genital tract. Hydrometrocolpos is distention of the uterus and vagina. We use the term *hydrocolpos* here to refer to both conditions.

Incidence

Congenital hydrocolpos is rare, occurring in less than 1 in 16,000 female births.[303] In contrast, hematometrocolpos that develops at puberty is relatively common, with a prevalence of 1 in 1,000.

Embryology and Pathology

Development of hydrocolpos requires two conditions: vaginal obstruction and fluid secretion. The fluid can be secreted by glands or may accumulate from the urine in cases of urogenital sinus.

Diagnosis

Hydrocolpos has been reported as a cystic (Figs. 37 and 38) or solid mass in the mid-lower pelvis of a female fetus.[304–306]

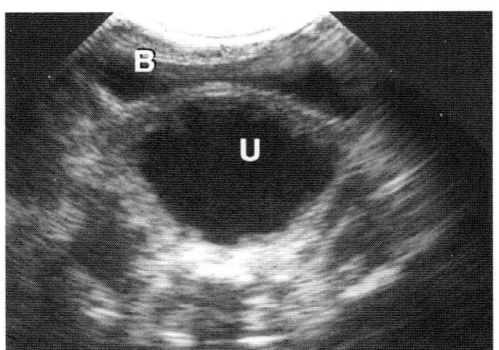

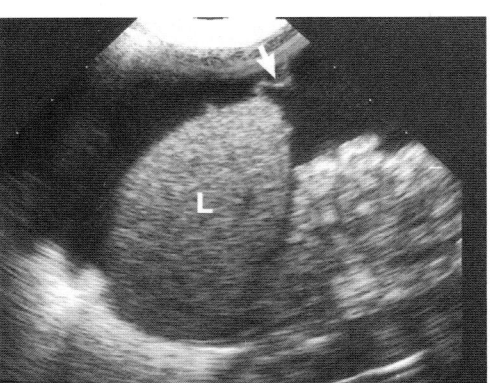

FIGURE 37. Hydrocolpos. **A:** A scan at 38 weeks shows a midline pelvic mass (*M*) posterior to the urinary bladder (*B*). A large amount of ascites (*A*) is also present. UA, umbilical artery. **B:** Postnatal scan of the pelvis confirms hydrocolpos with a dilated uterus (*U*) and vagina posterior to the urinary bladder (*B*). **C:** Large amount of ascites contains septations (*arrow*). The infant had bowel complications secondary to adhesions. Ascites was thought to arise from retrograde flow of fluid from hydrocolpos. L, liver.

A specific diagnosis may be suggested when the structure is duplicated[300] (Fig. 38), although this can also represent a septated vagina. In fact, it may be impossible to distinguish a dilated vagina from a dilated uterus,[307] and most suspected cases of hydrocolpos actually represent the dilated vagina.

Like ovarian cysts, no case has been reported before the third trimester, probably because maternal hormonal stimulation is insufficient for glandular secretion before this age. Hydronephrosis may result from ureteral obstruction by the enlarged uterus. Ascites may occur (Fig. 37). Peritoneal calcification has been observed with hydrocolpos, presumably because aseptic peritonitis resulted from retrograde flow of uterine secretions through the fallopian tube.[209,231]

Differential Diagnosis

The primary differential considerations for a cystic pelvic mass in a female fetus include a bladder or ureteral abnormality, dilated bowel, ovarian cyst, or mesenteric or enteric cyst. A specific diagnosis of hydrocolpos is suggested when the mass bulges through the perineum.

Associated Anomalies

Hydrocolpos is commonly associated with uterine duplication anomalies. Other malformations that may be associated with hydrocolpos include persistent urogenital sinus, anorectal atresia, renal agenesis, polycystic kidneys, EA, duodenal atresia, and caudal regression. Associated anomalies are more likely when the site of obstruction is high (cervical or high vaginal).[303] Combinations of associated anomalies may suggest the VACTERL syndrome. A triad of hydrocolpos, polydactyly, and congenital heart disease is

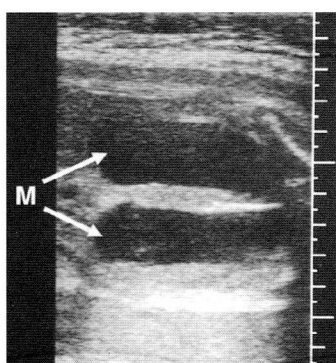

FIGURE 38. Hydrocolpos with duplicated uterus. A longitudinal scan shows a duplicated cystic mass (*M*) arising from the pelvis, characteristic for hydrocolpos with duplicated uterus. A septated vagina could also produce this appearance.

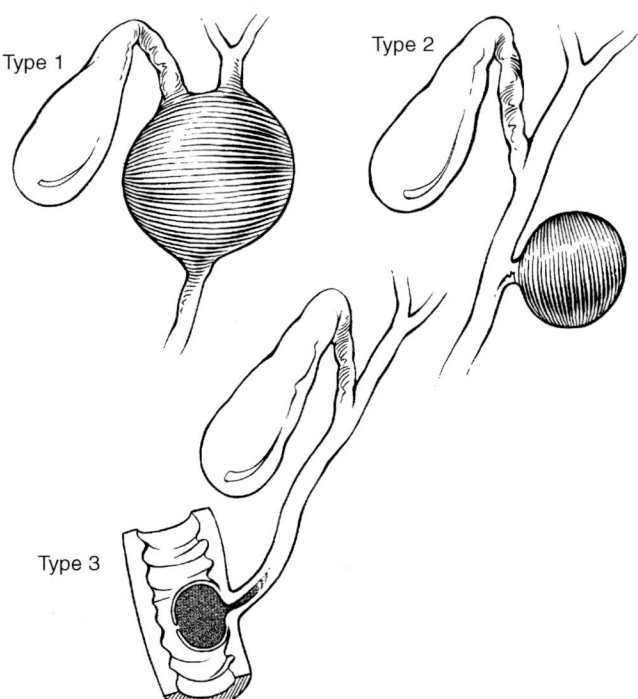

FIGURE 39. Different types of choledochal cysts. Type 1 is by far the most common and the type seen sonographically. Type 2 is focal diverticula of the common bile duct, and type 3 is a smaller diverticulum of the common bile duct as it enters the duodenum. (Reproduced with permission from McGahan JP, Porto M, eds. *Diagnostic obstetrical ultrasound.* Philadelphia: JB Lippincott Co, 1994;343–385.)

known as the *McKusick-Kaufman syndrome* and is inherited as an autosomal recessive trait.[308–310] MURCS (*mu*llerian duct, *r*enal agenesis/ectopia, and *c*ervical thoracic *s*omite dysplasia) association[311] should also be considered. There is overlap among these various syndromes.

Prognosis and Management

The prognosis depends primarily on the presence and severity of associated disorders. In a review of 44 infants with hydrocolpos, eight (18%) died.[312] An excellent outcome can be anticipated when abnormalities are confined to the uterus and vagina. Surgical intervention is necessary to relieve the obstruction.

Choledochal Cysts

Incidence

Choledochal cysts are rare.[313] Approximately one-third of reported cases have been in the Japanese population where the female to male ratio is nearly equal. By comparison, females are affected four to five times more frequently than males among whites.

Embryology and Pathology

Three types of choledochal cysts have been described[313] (Fig. 39):

Type 1 is a fusiform, sac-like dilatation of the common bile duct.
Type 2 is a diverticular dilatation of the common bile duct.
Type 3 is a dilatation of the distal, intramural portion of the common bile duct (choledochocele).

Other authors[330,331] add type 4 as cystic dilatation of intrahepatic biliary ducts (Caroli disease). Type 1 is by far the most common and the only type that has been reported on prenatal sonograms. Histologically, the cyst wall is thickened and fibrotic with dense connective tissue.

Diagnosis

A choledochal cyst can be identified as a simple, cystic mass in the upper abdomen or right upper quadrant[314–319] (Figs. 40 and 41). A definitive diagnosis of a choledochal cyst can be made by showing that biliary ducts lead to the cystic mass,[314] by evaluation of the fluid from aspiration,[320] or both.

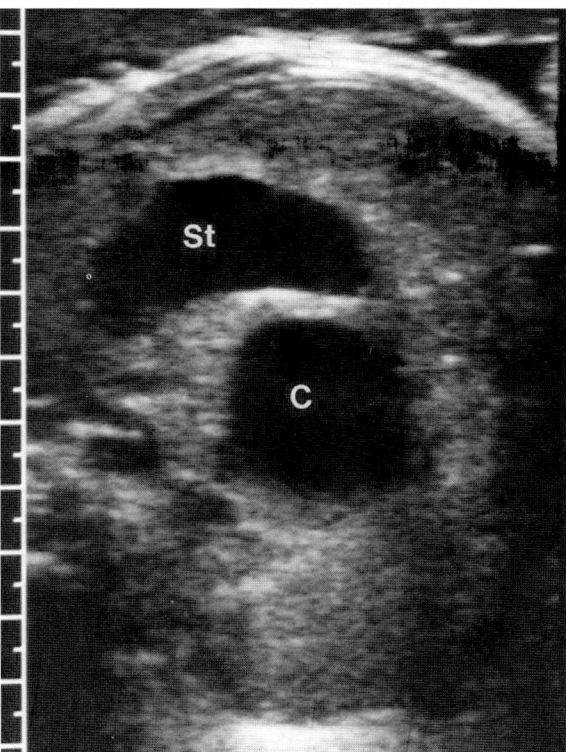

FIGURE 40. Choledochal cyst. A large cyst (*C*) is seen adjacent to the stomach (*St*) but not communicating with it.

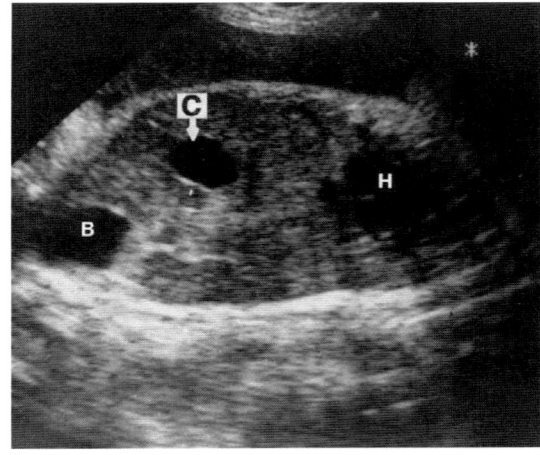

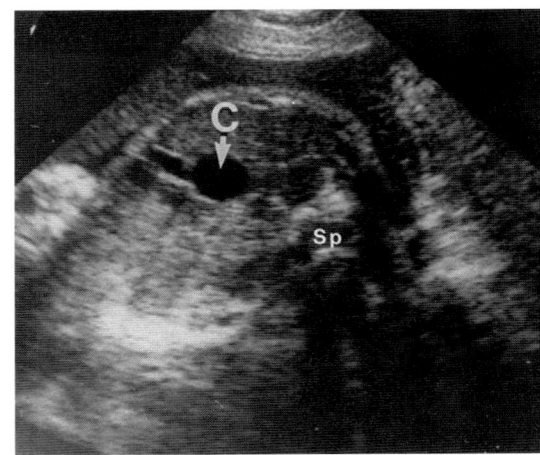

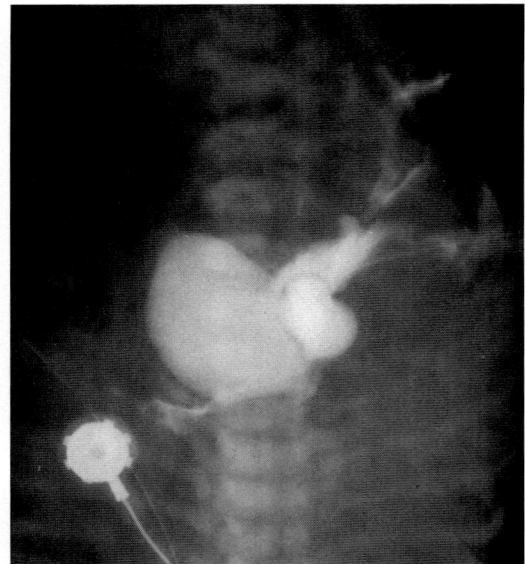

FIGURE 41. Choledochal cyst. **A:** A longitudinal view shows a cyst (C) in the upper abdomen. B, urinary bladder; H, heart. **B:** An oblique scan shows a cyst (C) is located at base of gallbladder. Sp, spine. **C:** A postnatal cholangiogram of another case shows a choledochal cyst communicating with the biliary system. (Courtesy of Lyndon M. Hill, MD, Pittsburgh, PA.)

Lugo-Vicente[321] reviewed 14 cases of choledochal cyst reported by prenatal sonography. The gestational age at time of detection was 26.9 weeks (range, 15 to 37 weeks). In a series by Redkar et al.[322] the median gestational age at antenatal detection was 20 weeks. Benhidjeb et al.[319] suggest that it is possible to make a presumptive prenatal diagnosis of choledochal cyst as early as 15 weeks.[323,324] However, another report showed a choledochal cyst at 31 weeks that was not apparent 4 to 5 weeks earlier.[314]

Differential Diagnosis

The differential diagnosis includes duodenal atresia, enteric duplication cyst, ovarian cyst, liver cyst, and gallbladder duplication.

Redkar et al.[322] reported that ultrasound was inaccurate for suggesting the correct diagnosis of choledochal cysts. Among 13 cases of biliary abnormalities (ten choledochal cysts, two type 1 cystic biliary atresia, and one with a noncommunicating segmental dilatation of the bile duct in a type 3 biliary atresia), the correct diagnosis of a biliary abnormality was made antenatally in only 15% (2 of 11)

cases. In the remaining cases, other types of cystic masses were suggested.

Associated Anomalies

Congenital biliary atresia may accompany choledochal cyst.[325] Tsuchida et al.[326] reviewed five cases of antenatally diagnosed biliary atresia. All were type 1 cysts, and antenatal diagnosis was made at 19 to 32 weeks. Matsubara et al.[325] suggest that a cyst that does not enlarge on serial examinations may represent biliary atresia.

Few extrabiliary anomalies have been associated with a choledochal cyst.[327] One case of trisomy 18 was reported among 19 cases of choledochal cyst reviewed by Cheng et al.[328]

Prognosis and Management

Unless correctly recognized and surgically removed following delivery, choledochal cysts can lead to complications of cholestasis, cholangitis, biliary cirrhosis, pancreatitis, portal hypertension, and liver failure. An increased incidence of bile duct cancer has also been noted. Clinical symptoms frequently are delayed until the second or third decade of life, at which time the mortality is high. Antenatal diagnosis offers the possibility of early definitive surgery for uncomplicated choledochal dilatation and the chance of improved outcome.[329,330]

Stringer et al.[331] reported that of 72 patients diagnosed postnatally (median age, 2.2 years), 50 (69%) presented with jaundice and only four (6%) showed the classic triad of jaundice, pain, and a right upper quadrant mass. Delayed referral was due to misdiagnosis as hepatitis (n = 12), incomplete investigation of abdominal pain (n = 6), or failure to note the significance of ultrasonographic findings (n = 10).

The preferred surgical treatment is total or subtotal resection of the cyst with Roux-en-Y hepaticojejunostomy (choledochojejunostomy).[332] Long-term results with this method are good, at least for those without biliary atresia. However, Cheng et al.[328] caution that biliary atresia can accompany choledochal cyst and these patients have a worse prognosis. In seven infants with biliary atresia, three are living and well. Of the remainder, two died due to delayed presentation, both with liver cirrhosis; another had recurrent cholangitis until 8 months and then was lost to follow-up; and one patient is living with liver cirrhosis. In the 12 without biliary atresia, nine patients are living and well.

Enteric Duplication Cyst

Incidence

Enteric duplication cysts—duplication cysts arising from the gastrointestinal tract—are not uncommon postnatally but are rarely detected prenatally. Males are affected twice as often as females.[71]

Embryology and Pathology

The two most accepted theories of embryogenesis regarding enteric duplication cysts involve (a) faulty recanalization of the gut lumen and (b) failure of separation of the notochord from the endoderm. The latter theory presupposes transient attachment of the endodermal roof with the notochord during the fifth week. This idea is supported by the association of enteric duplication cysts with vertebral anomalies.[71] Enteric duplication cysts may develop anywhere along the course of the digestive tract, although the stomach is the least frequent site of involvement. They are located on the mesenteric side of the intestine and do not usually communicate with the normal gut, unless tubular in type.

Diagnosis

Duplication cysts may be seen along the course of the gastrointestinal tract (Figs. 42 and 43). They are most common in the abdomen but have also been reported in the mouth[333] and thorax.[334] The stomach is a relatively com-

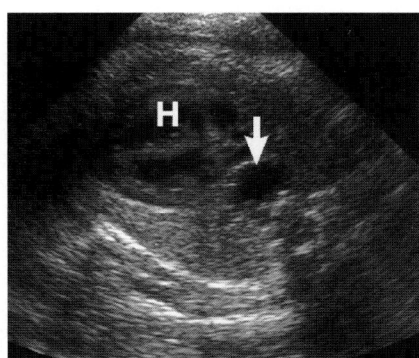

FIGURE 42. Esophageal duplication cyst. A well-defined cyst (*arrow*) is seen posterior to the heart (*H*) near the spine. This proved to be a duplication cyst.

mon site. The mass may appear cystic or even echogenic[77,335–337] (Fig. 43). Its location and mass effect on adjacent bowel can suggest the correct diagnosis. Demonstration of peristalsis in the cyst also allowed a specific diagnosis in one case.[338]

Differential Diagnosis

The differential diagnosis for an intraabdominal cyst includes ovarian cyst or mesenteric cyst. For subhepatic cysts in the right upper quadrant, the primary differential diagnosis is duodenal or antral duplication cyst vs. choledochal cyst.[337] The double bubble sign of duodenal atresia should also be considered. Other possibilities such as urachal cyst, renal cyst, and dilated bowel segments should be excluded based on their location and appearance.

Associated Anomalies

Enteric duplication cysts may be associated with other developmental defects including bronchopulmonary sequestration.[339] Vertebral defects may accompany esophageal duplication cysts.

Prognosis and Management

Approximately 85% of patients with enteric duplication cysts eventually become symptomatic from intussusception, pain, or bleeding.[71] Surgical resection is curative.

Mesenteric, Omental, and Retroperitoneal Cysts

Incidence

The precise prevalence of mesenteric, omental, and retroperitoneal cysts is unknown because they often are asymptomatic. The estimated incidence is 1 in 140,000 hospital admissions.[340]

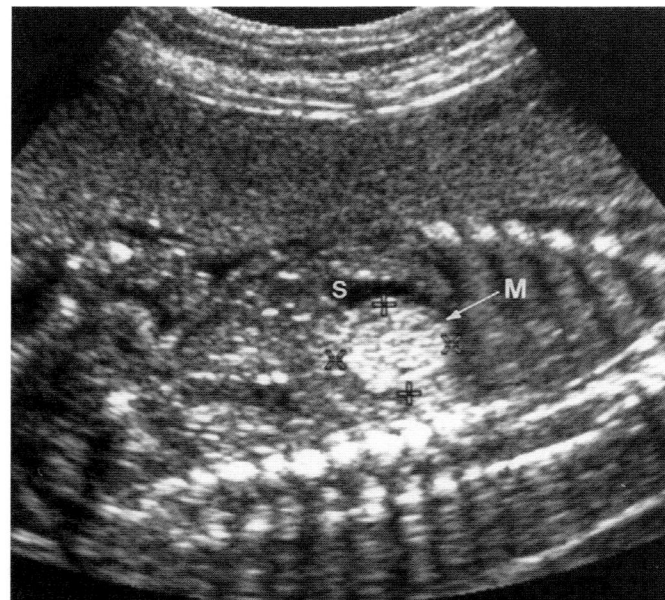

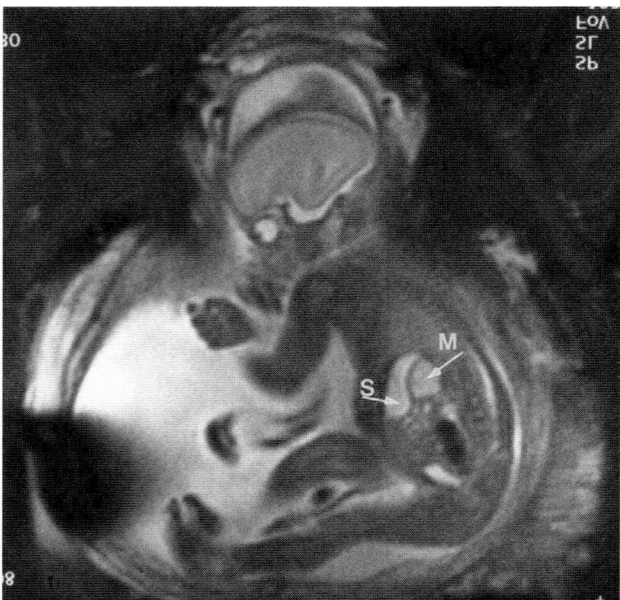

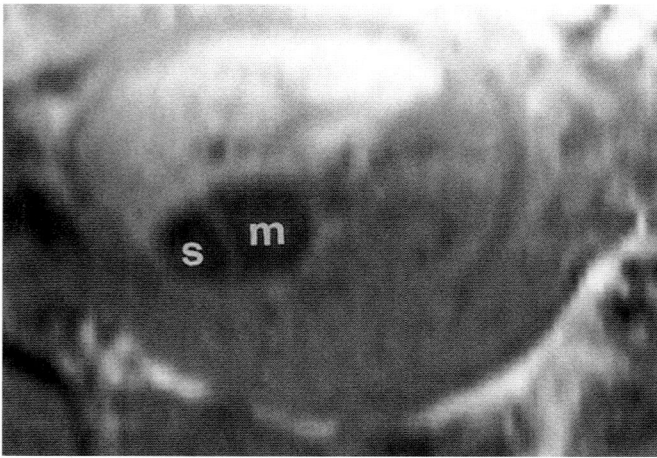

FIGURE 43. Gastric duplication cyst. **A:** An oblique coronal scan at 28 weeks shows an echogenic mass (*M*) posterior to the stomach (*S*) that suggested a meconium pseudocyst. **B:** A sagittal T2-weighted rapid acquisition with relaxation enhancement magnetic resonance image shows the mass (*M*) impressing on the stomach (*S*), suggesting the diagnosis of duplication cyst. **C:** An axial T1-weighted image shows that the mass (*m*) has similar signal intensity than that of adjacent stomach (*s*). The appearance of the mass suggested a duplication cyst, which was confirmed postnatally. (Reproduced with permission from Levine D, Barnes PD, Edelman RR. Obstetric MR imaging. *Radiology* 1999;211:609–617.)

Embryology and Pathology

These cysts usually represent abdominal lymphangiomas, although other etiologies have been identified.[341] The most common location is the small bowel mesentery, followed by the large bowel mesentery, omentum, and retroperitoneum.

They typically are solitary, unilocular, or multilocular cysts lined by a layer of endothelial cells. The fluid may be serous, chylous, or even bloody.

Diagnosis

The sonographic findings of mesenteric, omental, and retroperitoneal cysts are variable. They may be multiseptated or unilocular, small or large (Fig. 44). Although typically sonolucent,[342] they may appear solid or complex when hemorrhagic.[343] They are usually located in the mid-abdomen within the mesentery, omentum, or retroperitoneum,[344–349] but unusual sites of involvement include the kidneys,

spleen, liver, other abdominal organs. Mesenteric and omental cysts are characteristically mobile, so they may fluctuate in position.

Differential Diagnosis

An enteric duplication cyst or ovarian cyst may be indistinguishable from a mesenteric cyst. Less likely considerations include pancreatic cyst,[350] urachal cyst, renal cyst, or bowel dilatation.

Associated Anomalies

No significant anomalies are associated with mesenteric cysts.

Prognosis and Management

When symptomatic, these cysts should be surgically removed. Common presenting symptoms include abdominal distention,

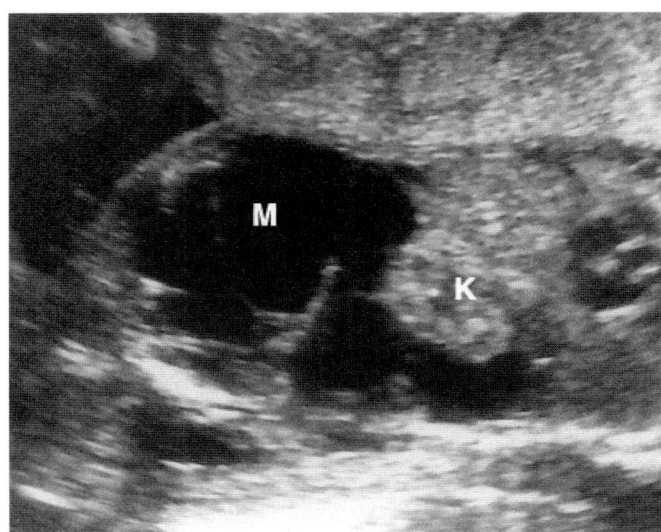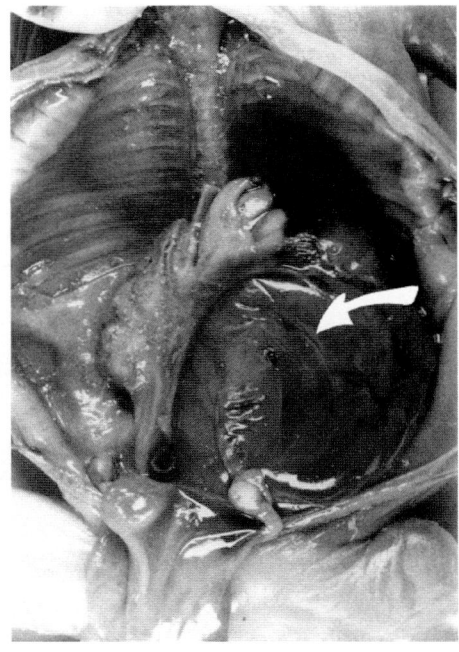

A   B

FIGURE 44. Lymphangioma. **A:** A scan at 20 weeks' gestation revealed a left-sided retroperitoneal abdominopelvic mass (*M*) associated with anterior displacement of the ipsilateral kidney (*K*). **B:** A postmortem photograph shows a large left-sided lymphangioma (*arrow*) displacing abdominal contents to the right. [Reproduced with permission from Deshpande P, Twining P, O'Neill D. Prenatal diagnosis of fetal abdominal lymphangioma by ultrasonography. *Ultrasound Obstet Gynecol* 2001;17(5):445–448.]

pain, and vomiting. Postsurgical recurrence is more likely for retroperitoneal cysts than for omental or mesenteric cysts.[351]

Liver/Spleen

Liver/Splenic Cyst

Incidence
Congenital liver cyst is a rare disorder. Females are affected four times more frequently than males are.

Embryology and Pathology
Congenital liver cyst possibly results from interruption of the intrahepatic biliary system.[352] The cysts are most frequently located at the inferior margin of the right lobe. Histologically, they are lined with an inner layer of cuboidal epithelial cells or a dense fibrous layer.

Diagnosis
Hepatic cysts have been reported prenatally, and these have been described as intrahepatic cystic masses[352] (Fig. 34B). These may develop following a normal second trimester ultrasound.[353] Splenic cysts have also been rarely detected *in utero*[354] (Fig. 45). Approximately 10% of hepatic cysts are multilocular.[327]

Differential Diagnosis
Less likely considerations for an intrahepatic cystic mass include cystic hepatoblastoma, mesenchymal hamar-

toma, hemangioendothelioma, or Caroli disease. Choledochal cyst should also be considered, although careful observation should reveal that hepatic cyst is confined to the liver whereas choledochal cyst is just inferior to the liver.

Associated Anomalies
There are no known associated anomalies with congenital solitary liver cysts.

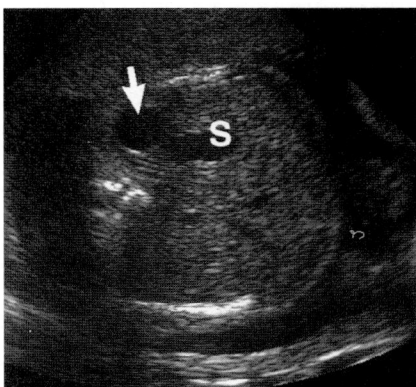

FIGURE 45. Splenic cyst. A cyst (*arrow*) is identified within the spleen, posterior to the stomach (*S*).

TABLE 7. CAUSES OF FETAL HEPATOMEGALY

Immune hydrops
Nonimmune hydrops
Congenital infection
Tumors
Hypothyroidism
Beckwith-Wiedemann syndrome
Zellweger (cerebrohepatorenal) syndrome
Myeloproliferative disorder (may be seen with trisomy 21)

Prognosis and Management

Many liver cysts remain asymptomatic throughout life and are noted only as an incidental finding at autopsy. Infection, hemorrhage, and torsion of the cysts are potential complications. Prenatal aspiration of a giant hepatic cyst has been described.[355]

Hepatosplenomegaly

Hepatosplenomegaly may result from a number of etiologies (Tables 7 and 8) including immune or nonimmune hydrops, hemolytic anemia, congenital infection (toxoplasmosis, CMV, syphilis, or rubella), and metabolic disorders (hypothyroidism). Splenomegaly has been correlated with severe anemia in rhesus disease.[356] Bahado-Singh et al.[356] found that splenic circumference was an excellent predictor of severe anemia (sensitivity, 100%, and specificity, 94.7%). Suspected hepatomegaly and splenomegaly can be compared with normal measurements, which have been reported.[357,358] Liver or splenic enlargement alone should be distinguished from tumor involvement or metastases.

Hepatomegaly is a constant feature of the Beckwith-Weidemann syndrome and cerebrohepatorenal syndrome (Zellweger syndrome).[359] It has been reported with metabolic abnormalities and glycogen storage disease.[360,361] Extramedullary hematopoiesis occasionally has been reported to produce an enlarged, heterogeneous appearance of the liver.[362] Hepatosplenomegaly, with or without hydrops, may be the only or primary sonographic finding among fetuses with Down syndrome and a myeloproliferative disorder. This situation has been reported in several cases[363–365] (Fig. 46). Smrcek and colleagues[365] found that 11 of 79 fetuses with Down syndrome had antenatal evidence of hydrops and at least three of these (a fourth fetus had unsuccessful karyotype) presented with hepatosplenomegaly and myeloproliferative disorder in the second and third trimesters. They conclude that transient myeloprolif-

TABLE 8. CAUSES OF FETAL SPLENOMEGALY

Immune hydrops
Nonimmune hydrops
Infection
Inborn errors of metabolism
   Gaucher disease
   Niemann-Pick disease
   Wolman disease
Leukemia

erative disorder with hepatomegaly may be more common among fetuses with Down syndrome than commonly realized.

Liver Masses

Incidence

Liver and splenic masses in the neonatal period are rare. Liver masses include hemangioma and various tumors, including hemangioendothelioma,[366–371] mesenchymal hamartoma, and liver metastases.[372,373]

Embryology and Pathology

Hemangioma of the liver is a congenital vascular malformation composed of innumerable capillary channels.[374]

Hepatoblastoma is the most common malignant tumor of the liver during the neonatal period. Hepatoblastomas are extremely vascular, and rupture of the tumor may occur. Mesenchymal hamartoma is a developmental abnormality characterized by edematous, acellular connective tissue and fluid-filled spaces lacking a cellular lining; it is histologically similar to lymphangioma.

Liver metastases are unusual prenatally but may occur with neuroblastoma.

Diagnosis

Hepatoblastoma has been rarely detected by prenatal ultrasound[372,375] (Fig. 47). They typically are solid and strongly echogenic on sonography. They may demonstrate a typical spoke-wheel appearance (Fig. 47). Calcifications may be demonstrated.[372] Hepatoblastomas are rarely cystic. They are typically highly vascular, which can be shown with Doppler studies.

Hemangioendothelioma has also been reported prenatally (Fig. 48). Meirowitz et al.[370] describe a case of hepatic hemangioendothelioma that was first suspected at 19 weeks' gestation. The patient presented at 16 weeks with a markedly elevated maternal serum AFP level.

Metastasis from neuroblastoma may be detected by ultrasound[376] (Fig. 49) or MRI.[377] They may show findings similar to hepatoblastoma.

Several cases of cavernous hemangioma have been detected antenatally[378–380] (Fig. 50). The sonographic appearance may be hyperechoic, hypoechoic, or mixed. Calcification occasionally may occur. Very small hemangiomas can also be detected prenatally.[381]

Mesenchymal hamartoma typically appears as a multilobulated cystic mass, with most tumors diagnosed before 2 years of age.

Differential Diagnosis

Other intraabdominal masses should be distinguished from liver masses by their location.

Prognosis and Management

Hepatomegaly, anemia, and congestive heart failure may complicate large liver hemangiomas.[382] Although histologi-

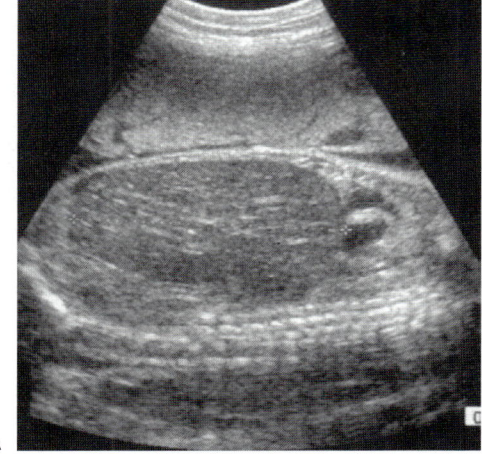

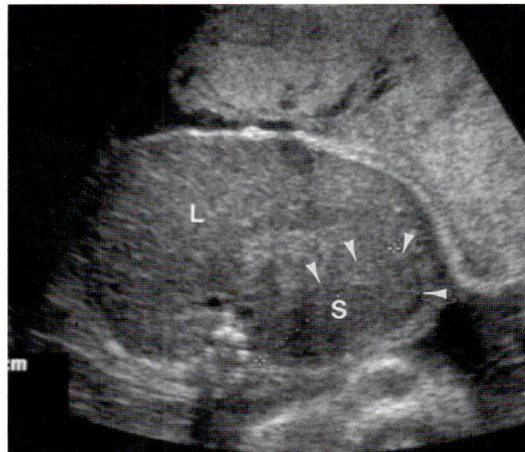

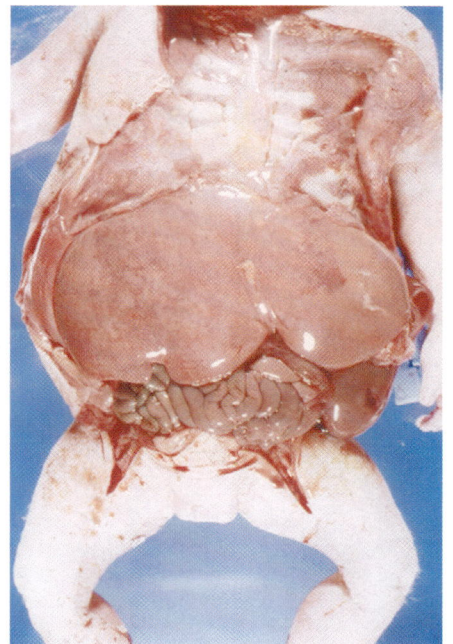

FIGURE 46. Hepatomegaly and myeloproliferative disease with Down syndrome. **A:** A longitudinal image at 28 weeks shows marked hepatomegaly. **B:** The transverse scan shows the markedly enlarged liver (*L*) and spleen (*S, arrowheads*). Hydropic, thickened placenta is also evident, and cardiomegaly was present. **C:** Postmortem examination confirms marked hepatomegaly and splenomegaly. [From Smrcek JM, Baschat AA, Germer U, et al. Fetal hydrops and hepatosplenomegaly in the second half of pregnancy: a sign of myeloproliferative disorder in fetuses with trisomy 21. *Ultrasound Obstet Gynecol* 2001;17(5):403–409.]

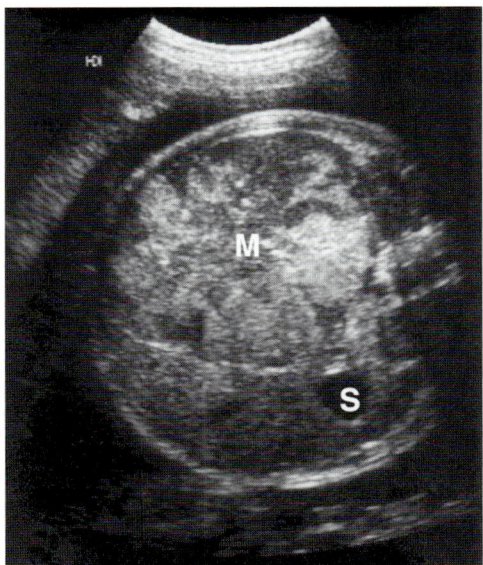

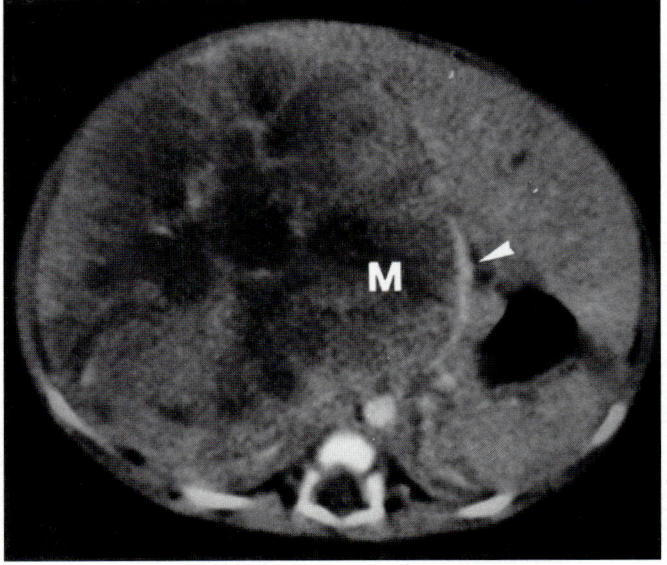

FIGURE 47. Hepatoblastoma. **A:** A transverse image of fetal abdomen at 36 weeks shows a large mass (*M*) arising from the liver. Note the typical spoke-wheel appearance. S, stomach. **B:** The postnatal computed tomographic scan confirms prenatal ultrasound findings. The mass (*M*) is necrotic and displaces hepatic vessels (*arrowhead*). [Reproduced with permission from Shih JC, Tsao PN, Huang SF, et al. Congenital hepatoblastoma. *Ultrasound Obstet Gynecol* 2000;16(1):103.]

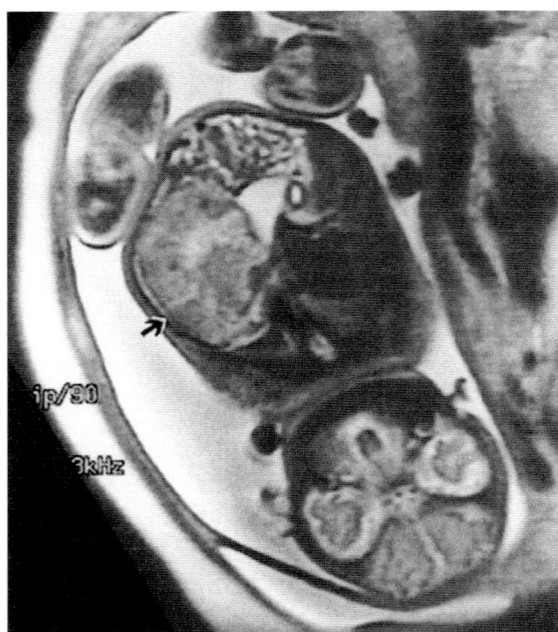

FIGURE 48. Liver tumor (infantile hemangioendothelioma). A coronal single-shot fast spin-echo magnetic resonance image at 40 weeks shows an inhomogeneous tumor (*arrow*) arising from the lower aspect of the left hepatic lobe. Infantile hemangioendothelioma was found at surgery. [Reproduced with permission from Shinmoto H, Kashima K, Yuasa Y, et al. MR imaging of non-CNS fetal abnormalities: a pictorial essay. *Radiographics* 2000;20(5):1227–1243.]

cally benign, the mortality rate is high (81%) when congestive heart failure develops from arteriovenous shunting. The mortality rate can be reduced to 29% with medical, radiation, and surgical therapy.[383] Hemangiomas can be successfully treated

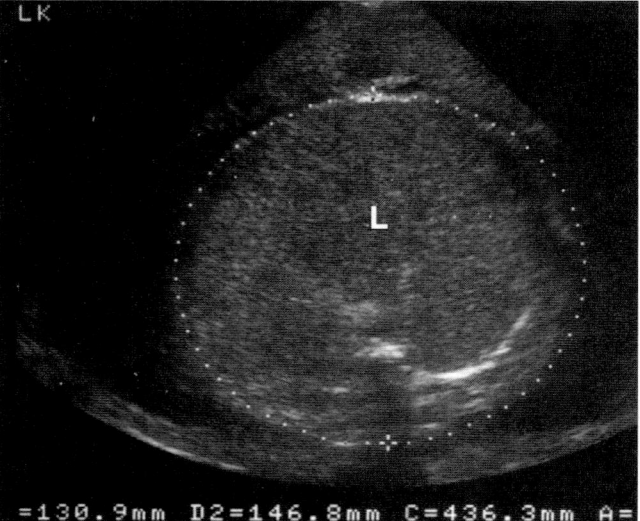

FIGURE 49. Metastatic neuroblastoma to the liver. A scan at 38 weeks shows the markedly enlarged liver (*L*) with a diffuse heterogeneous appearance. Neuroblastoma was found after birth. Despite treatment, the infant died after birth.

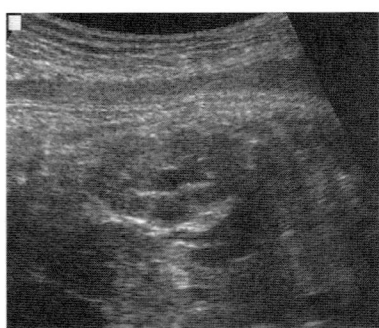

FIGURE 50. Hemangioma. A transverse view of an abdomen at term shows a small hypoechoic lesion with an echogenic outer rim, which proved to be a hemangioma.

with corticosteroids,[384] and maternal corticosteroid therapy has been successfully used to treat a fetal hemangioma.[385]

Mesenchymal hamartomas are benign and usually present in early infancy with symptoms that are related to the mass effect on adjacent organs.[386] Once the tumor is removed, the prognosis is generally good.

Adrenal Gland

Abnormalities that may affect the adrenal gland include hemorrhage,[387,388] adrenal cysts, hypertrophy, and tumor (neuroblastoma). Intraabdominal, extrapulmonary sequestration[389–391] may appear as an adrenal mass and is probably the most common mass that affects the adrenal area. It is nearly always left-sided and demonstrates a characteristic echogenic, homogenous appearance. The adrenal gland may be visibly displaced by the mass.

Neuroblastoma

A neuroblastoma is a specific type of tumor arising from the adrenal gland.

Incidence
Congenital neuroblastoma is the most frequent solid neoplasm in infancy, representing 25% of neonatal tumors. The incidence ranges from 1 in 7,100 to 10,000 live births.

Embryology and Pathology
Neuroblastoma originates in the autonomous nervous system. This tumor originates in the stem cells of the sympathetic nerve in at least 80% to 85% of all cases from the adrenal gland.

A relationship between progestational hormones given during pregnancy as a risk factor for neuroblastoma in infancy has been suggested by one paper.[392]

Diagnosis
Neuroblastoma has been frequently detected by prenatal sonography.[393–402] Neuroblastomas can have a solid, purely cystic or complex sonographic appearance. Nearly one-half

TABLE 9. DISTINGUISHING FEATURES OF INFRADIAPHRAGMATIC EXTRALOBAR SEQUESTRATION VERSUS NEUROBLASTOMA

	Extralobar sequestration	Neuroblastoma
Echotexture	Echogenic, solid	Cystic
Laterality	Left	Right
Time of diagnosis	Second trimester	Third trimester

are cystic. Approximately 93% of neuroblastomas identified prenatally are adrenal in origin.[396] Thoracic and rarely cervical neuroblastomas have also been reported.[399]

All cases of neuroblastoma have been detected in the third trimester, even when second trimester scans have also been performed.[390] For example, all four cases reported by Rubenstein et al.[390] were detected after 36 weeks and three of these had a normal ultrasound during the second trimester. The earliest case reported has been at 26 weeks.[399]

Liver metastases may appear as a mass with calcification. Metastasis may be detected prenatally by ultrasound or MRI.[377] Hydrops with placental metastases have also been reported. Tumor emboli to the placenta may appear as a bulky, hydropic placenta without macroscopic masses.[403]

Hydrops appears to be related to liver or placental metastasis. These fetuses also have a much worse prognosis.

Suprarenal masses may spontaneously resolve.[404] This may occur with neuroblastoma and is also expected from adrenal hemorrhage.

Differential Diagnosis

The primary differential diagnostic consideration is intraabdominal, extrapulmonary sequestration (Table 9).

Intraabdominal, extrapulmonary sequestration is typically echogenic, homogenous, and nearly always left-sided (Fig. 51). Unlike neuroblastoma, extrapulmonary sequestration may be seen during the second trimester. Neuroblastoma is more likely to be cystic, heterogeneous in appearance, right-sided, and identified in the third trimester. Adrenal hemorrhage is much less common and may have a variable echo pattern depending on the age of hemorrhage. Acute hemorrhage is echogenic, then becomes hypoechoic or mixed, and gradually becomes more cystic and sonolucent. Doppler should show no internal vascularity with hemorrhage, and MRI may show a typical appearance of hemorrhage.[405]

Prognosis and Management

Fetuses with neuroblastoma tend to have a favorable stage of disease, favorable biological features, and consequently an excellent prognosis compared to infants diagnosed after birth.[406] Among 55 cases of neuroblastoma reviewed by Acharya et al.,[396] 37 (67%) had stage I disease without metastasis. Twelve (22%) had stage IV-S disease, and only three (5%) had stage IV disease. Among 16 of these patients, the DNA index was favorable (greater than 1) in 14 and none had amplification of the N-*myc* oncogene. Of the 50 patients for whom follow-up was available, 45 (90%) were alive at a range of 2 to 120 months.

Maternal symptoms of headache, hypertension, and preeclampsia may result from excessive release of catecholamines. Catecholamines were elevated in 33% of patients reviewed by Acharya et al.[396] The presence of maternal symptoms appears to correlate with a more severe stage of disease. Preeclampsia increases the possibility of metastases

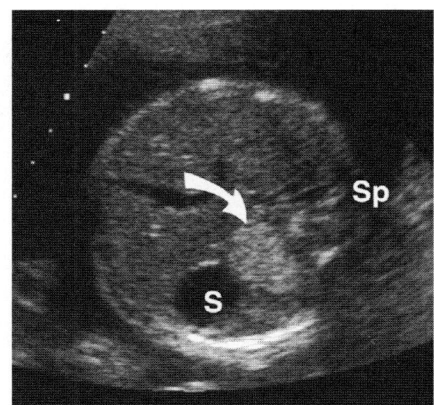
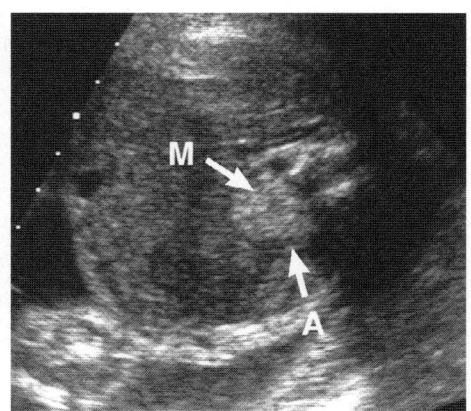

FIGURE 51. Intraabdominal extrapulmonary sequestration. **A:** A transverse scan of the upper abdomen at 28 weeks shows an echogenic mass (*arrow*) posterior to the stomach (*S*). Sp, spine. **B:** A scan slightly superiorly shows the left adrenal gland (*A*) is displaced laterally from the mass (*M*). Intraabdominal extrapulmonary sequestration was confirmed postnatally. The mass could have been mistaken for a neuroblastoma, but gestational age, location, and appearance are all diagnostic of the correct disorder.

and hydrops, whereas mothers without preeclampsia have a very low risk of widely disseminated metastasis.[399] Among 16 cases reviewed by Jennings et al.[399] four (25%) mothers had hypertension or preeclampsia. Three of these neonates had stage IV or IV-S disease with liver metastases, and all three had fetal hydrops.

Neuroblastomas may metastasize to the skeleton, skin and liver, the placenta, and even the umbilical cord. The liver is the most common site, observed in 25% of patients reviewed by Acharya et al.[396] Bone involvement was not observed in any patient in that series. Ultrasonography failed to detect liver metastasis in three patients. No cases of maternal metastases have been reported.

Surgery alone is curative for most patients. However, a period of observation may avoid surgery in some individuals whose tumors spontaneously regress.

Other Abdominal Masses

Other tumors may involve the abdomen. It may be difficult to distinguish a well-differentiated teratoma from fetus *in fetu* (Fig. 52).

The Gallbladder

The gallbladder is normally visualized as an ovoid, fluid-filled structure to the right and inferior to the intrahepatic portion

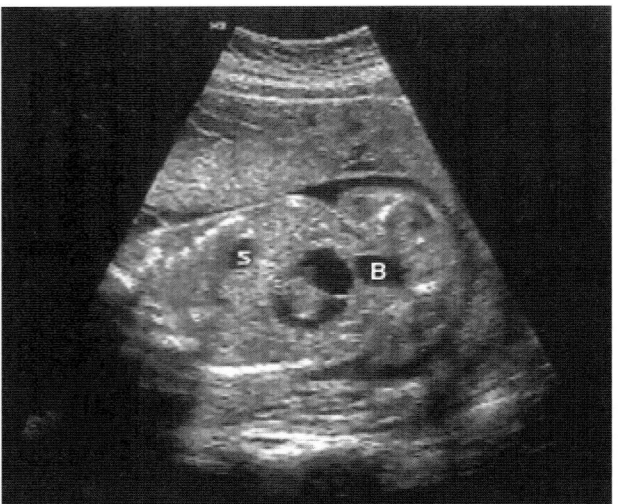

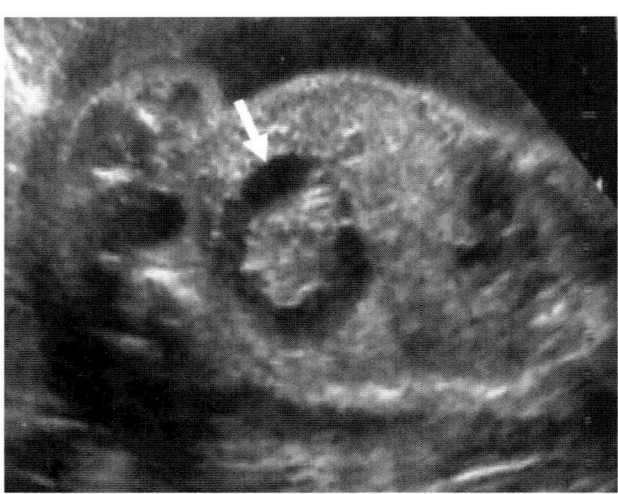

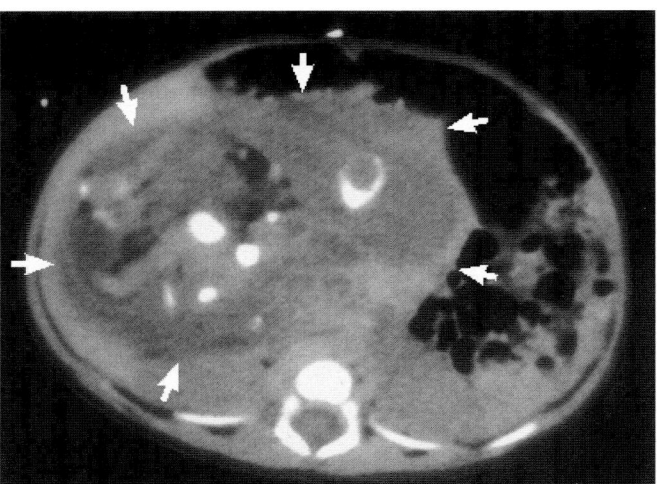

FIGURE 52. Fetus *in fetu* or well-differentiated teratoma. **A:** Longitudinal scan at 21 weeks shows a complex cystic and solid mass between the stomach (*S*) and urinary bladder (*B*). **B:** A follow-up scan at 27 weeks shows a persistent mass. The outer sac (*arrow*) suggested an amniotic cavity. **C:** A computed tomographic scan at 1 day of age shows a mass (*arrows*) in the right retroperitoneum that contains various calcified components. Pathologic examination showed a mass containing two well-formed appendages with paddle-shaped digits, rudimentary vertebrae, and a primitive notochord. There is overlap in findings between a well-differentiated teratoma and fetus *in fetu*. [Reproduced with permission from Nastanski F, Downey EC. Fetus in fetu: a rare cause of neonatal mass. *Ultrasound Obstet Gynecol* 2001;18(1):72–75.]

of the umbilical vein. It can be mistaken for the umbilical vein unless the characteristic course of the umbilical vein or its intrahepatic branches are visualized. The gallbladder increases linearly in size with gestational age between 15 and 30 weeks of gestation, after which a plateau is observed.[407–409] Muller et al.[408] showed that detection of the normal gallbladder increases from 28.5% before the sixteenth week up to 98% after the thirty-second week of gestation.

Cholecystomegaly
The gallbladder may occasionally appear quite prominent and should not be mistaken for an abnormal cystic mass. Enlargement of the fetal gallbladder has been implicated with fetal aneuploidy in one report[410] but not in another.[411] Hertzberg et al.[411] evaluated 43 fetuses with an enlarged gallbladder (area more than 2 SD above the mean for gestational age). All but one (isolated ventricular septal defect, which closed spontaneously) were normal without evidence of anatomic defects, biliary tract abnormality, or aneuploidy. Normal outcomes were reported in 94% (75 of 80) of fetuses with nonvisualized gallbladders who had follow-up.

Agenesis of the Gallbladder
Agenesis of the gallbladder occurs in approximately 20% of patients with biliary atresia. Absence of the gallbladder also can occur in association with polysplenia and rare multiple anomaly syndromes. Several reports suggest that failure to visualize the gallbladder may indicate gallbladder disease,[412] biliary atresia, or even CF.[413] Bronshtein et al.[412] reported absent visualization of the gallbladder in seven cases. Agenesis of the gallbladder was confirmed at autopsy or postpartum in all cases, and two of these had other anomalies. In another series of 80 fetuses with nonvisualization of the gallbladder, Hertzberg et al.[414] reported that one had trisomy 21 and four others had relatively minor, non–life-threatening problems that did not involve the gallbladder or biliary tract. However, these authors suggest that the rate of nonvisualization of the fetal gallbladder in normal fetuses is sufficiently high that nonvisualization of the gallbladder may not be clinically useful as a screening test. They reported that the likelihood of visualizing the gallbladder increases with gestational age, reaching a plateau of approximately 95% between 24 and 32 weeks.

Gallbladder Duplication
Gallbladder duplication is reported in 1 in 4,000 at autopsy examinations[415,416] and occasionally is seen on prenatal scans. Among 17 cases of gallbladder abnormalities reported by Bronshtein et al.,[412] two were septated or bilobed. The ultrasound appearance is distinctive (Fig. 53). The primary differential diagnosis is gallbladder folds.[417] Unlike gallbladder duplication, gallbladder folds are commonly transverse in orientation. Choledochal, hepatic, or mesenteric cyst should be readily excluded. An increased incidence of foregut malformations has been reported.[418]

Although several authors[419] report increased risk of acute and chronic cholecystitis, cholesterolosis, papilloma, carcinoma, biliary cirrhosis, and torsion, gallbladder duplication is typically an incidental finding with normal outcome.

Gallbladder Echogenic Foci (Gallstones, Sludge)
As it may be difficult to distinguish gallstones from sludge, we refer to both here as gallbladder echogenic foci.

Incidence. Detection of echogenic foci is unusual, but not rare. Although the exact incidence is unknown, Kiserud et al.[420] observed echogenic material in nearly 1% of referred patients after 28 weeks.

Embryology and Pathology. Possible causes of gallstone in neonates include hemolytic disorders (spherocytosis, sickle cell anemia, thalassemia, and erythroblastosis fetalis) and nonhemolytic disorders (pancreatitis, CF, and hyperalimentation).[421] Although the etiology of fetal gallstones/sludge is uncertain, it is likely related to increased cholesterol secretions and depressed bile acid synthesis caused by estrogens.[421] Breakdown of blood, possibly arising from placental hemorrhage, to bilirubin has also been suggested.[427]

Diagnosis. Gallbladder echogenic foci have been frequently reported in the third trimester but not before[421–427] (Fig. 54). In the series of Brown et al.[424] the mean gestational age at the time of diagnosis was 36.2 weeks, with a range of 28 to 32 weeks. In this series of 26 cases, 12% showed a single echogenic focus, 73% had multiple foci, and the remaining 15% had a diffuse filling of the lumen of the gallbladder.

Differential Diagnosis. Gallbladder echogenic foci could mimic intrahepatic calcification or HB.[428] Fetal gallstones in a contracted gallbladder can also simulate hepatic or peritoneal calcification.[429]

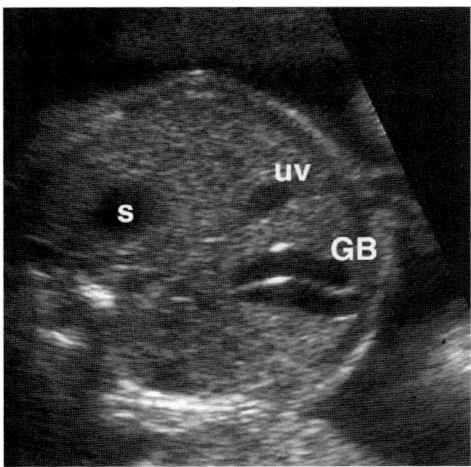

FIGURE 53. Duplicated gallbladder (*GB*). A transverse view of the abdomen shows a duplicated gallbladder. s, stomach; uv, umbilical vein.

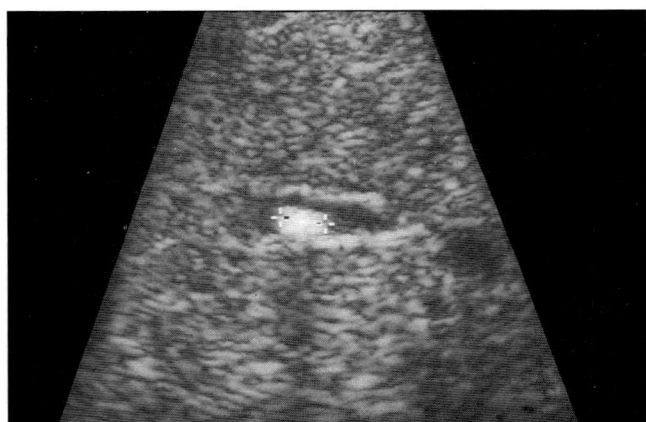

FIGURE 54. Gallstone. A scan at 36 weeks shows a well-defined echogenic focus within the gallbladder that is consistent with gallstone.

Associated Anomalies. Reports on possible associated anomalies with gallbladder echogenic foci are conflicting. Among a select group of six fetuses reported by Kiserud et al.,[420] five had other abnormalities: extraamniotic hematoma with IUGR and oligohydramnios, tetralogy of Fallot, trisomy 21 with atrioventricular septal defect and transient ascites, chromosomal aberration [t(10;11)] with bilateral clubfoot, and gastroschisis. In contrast, Brown et al.[424] reported no hemolytic anemias, predisposing risk factors, or clinical sequelae in any of 26 cases detected prenatally. Our own experience also suggests that gallbladder echogenic foci are generally benign without associated anomalies.

Prognosis and Management. Neonatal gallstones frequently resolve spontaneously,[430] and gallbladder echogenic foci seen prenatally also usually resolve. Brown et al.[424] reported postnatal sonographic or pathologic follow-up studies in 17 cases of gallbladder echogenic foci. In only three infants the foci persisted (longest follow-up, 4 to 12 years) and none of these became symptomatic. Among the six cases reported by Kiserud et al.,[420] five resolved by weeks of birth and one was still present at 8 months of age.

REFERENCES

1. Sohaey R, Woodward P, Zwiebel WJ. Fetal gastrointestinal anomalies. *Semin Ultrasound CT MR* 1996;17(1):51–65.
2. Skupski DW. Prenatal diagnosis of gastrointestinal anomalies with ultrasound. What have we learned? *Ann N Y Acad Sci* 1998;18(847):53–58.
3. Moore KL. *The developing human*, 4th ed. Philadelphia: WB Saunders, 1988:217–245.
4. Grelin ES. *Functional anatomy of the newborn*. New Haven: Yale University Press, 1973:54–60.
5. Pritchard JA. Fetal swallowing and amniotic fluid volume. *Obstet Gynecol* 1966;28:606–610.
6. Trahair JF, Harding R. Ultrastructural anomalies in the fetal small intestine indicate that fetal swallowing is important for normal development: an experimental study. *Virchows Arch A Pathol Anat Histopathol* 1992;420(4):305–312.
7. Blakelock R, Upadhyay V, Kimble R, et al. Is a normally functioning gastrointestinal tract necessary for normal growth in late gestation? *Pediatr Surg Int* 1998;13(1):17–20.
8. Trahair JF, Harding R. Restitution of fetal swallowing in the fetal sheep restores intestinal growth after midgestation on esophageal obstruction. *J Pediatr Gastroenterol Nutr* 1995;20:156–161.
9. Hata T, Deter RL. A review of fetal organ measurements obtained with ultrasound: normal growth. *J Clin Ultrasound* 1992;20(3):155–174.
10. Nyberg DA, Mack LA, Patten RM, et al. Fetal bowel: normal sonographic findings. *J Ultrasound Med* 1987;6:3–6.
11. Hubbard AM, Harty P. Prenatal magnetic resonance imaging of fetal anomalies. *Semin Roentgenol* 1999;34:41–47.
12. Shinmoto H, Kashima K, Yuasa Y, et al. MR imaging of non-CNS fetal abnormalities: a pictorial essay. *Radiographics* 2000;20:1227–1243.
13. Parulekar SG. Sonography of normal fetal bowel. *J Ultrasound Med* 1991;10:211–220.
14. Karcnik TJ, Rubenstein JB, Swayne LC. The fetal presacral pseudo-mass: a normal sonographic variant. *J Ultrasound Med* 1991;10:579–581.
15. Goldstein J, Reece AE, Yarkoni S, et al. Growth of the fetal stomach in normal pregnancies. *Obstet Gynecol* 1987;70:641–644.
16. Fakhry J, Shapiro LR, Schechter A, et al. Fetal gastric pseudomasses. *J Ultrasound Med* 1987;6:177–180.
17. Avni EF, Rypens F, Milaire J. Fetal esophagus: normal sonographic appearance. *J Ultrasound Med* 1994;13:175–180.
18. Levine D, Callen PW, Goldstein RB, et al. Imaging the fetal abdomen: how efficacious are the AIUM/ACR guidelines? *J Ultrasound Med* 1995;14:335–341.

Esophageal Atresia

19. Depaepe A, Dolk H, Lechat MF. The epidemiology of tracheo-oesophageal fistula and oesophageal atresia in Europe. EURO-CAT Working Group. *Arch Dis Child* 1993;68:743–748.
20. Gray SW, Skandalakis JE. The esophagus. In: *Embryology for surgeons*. Philadelphia: WB Saunders, 1972:63–100.
21. Waterson DJ, Bonham CRE, Aaberdeen E. Oesophageal atresia: tracheo-oesophageal fistula. *Lancet* 1962;21:819–822.
22. Beasley SW, Allen M, Myers N. The effects of Down syndrome and other chromosomal abnormalities on survival and management in oesophageal atresia. *Pediatr Surg Int* 1997;12(8):550–551.
23. Gross RE. *The surgery of infancy and childhood*. Philadelphia: WB Saunders, 1953.
24. Pretorius DH, Drose JA, Dennis MA, et al. Tracheoesophageal fistula in utero. *J Ultrasound Med* 1987;6:509–513.
25. Weinberg B, Diakoumakis EE. Three complex cases of foregut atresia: prenatal sonographic diagnosis with radiographic correlation. *J Clin Ultrasound* 1985;13:481–484.
26. Hobbins JC, Grannum PAT, Berkowitz RI, et al. Ultrasound in the diagnosis of congenital anomalies. *Am J Obstet Gynecol* 1979;134:331–344.
27. Farrant P. The antenatal diagnosis of oesophageal atresia by ultrasound. *Br J Radiol* 1980;53:1202–1203.

28. Pretorius DH, Meier PR, Johnson ML. Diagnosis of esophageal atresia *in utero. J Ultrasound Med* 1983;2:475.

29. Sparey C, Jawaheer G, Barrett AM, Robson SC. Esophageal atresia in the Northern Region Congenital Anomaly Survey, 1985–1997: prenatal diagnosis and outcome. *Am J Obstet Gynecol* 2000;182:427–431.

30. Stringer MD, McKenna KM, Goldstein RB, et al. Prenatal diagnosis of esophageal atresia. *J Pediatr Surg* 1995;30:1258–1263.

31. Stoll C, Alembik Y, Dott B, Roth MP. Evaluation of prenatal diagnosis of congenital gastro-intestinal atresias. *Eur J Epidemiol* 1996;12(6):611–616.

32. Kimble RM, Harding JE, Kolbe A. Does gut atresia cause polyhydramnios? *Pediatr Surg Int* 1998;13(2–3):115–117.

33. Barkin SZ, Pretorius DH, Beckett MK, et al. Severe polyhydramnios: incidence of anomalies. *AJR Am J Roentgenol* 1987;148:155–159.

34. Glantz JC, Abramowicz JS, Sherer DM. Significance of idiopathic midtrimester polyhydramnios. *Am J Perinatol* 1994;11:305–308.

35. Jolleys A. An examination of the birthweights of babies with some abnormalities of the alimentary tract. *J Pediatr Surg* 1981;16:160–163.

36. Surana R, Puri P. Small intestinal atresia: effect on fetal nutrition. *J Pediatr Surg* 1994;29:1250–1252.

37. Benson CB, Coughlin BF, Doubilet PM. Amniotic fluid volume in large-for-gestational-age fetuses of nondiabetic mothers. *J Ultrasound Med* 1991;10:149–151.

38. Panting-Kemp A, Nguyen T, Chang E, et al. Idiopathic polyhydramnios and perinatal outcome. *Am J Obstet Gynecol* 1999;181:1079–1082.

39. Maymon E, Ghezzi F, Shoham-Vardi I, et al. Isolated hydramnios at term gestation and the occurrence of peripartum complications. *Eur J Obstet Gynecol Repro Biol* 1998;77:157–161.

40. Sohaey R, Nyberg DA, Sickler GK, Williams MA. Idiopathic polyhydramnios: association with fetal macrosomia. *Radiology* 1994;190:393–396.

41. Sickler GK, Nyberg DA, Sohaey R, Luthy DA. Polyhydramnios and fetal intrauterine growth restriction: ominous combination. *J Ultrasound Med* 1997;16:609–614.

42. Furman B, Erez O, Senior L, et al. Hydramnios and small for gestational age: prevalence and clinical significance. *Acta Obstet Gynecol Scand* 2000;79:31–36.

43. Lazebnik N, Many A. The severity of polyhydramnios, estimated fetal weight and preterm delivery are independent risk factors for the presence of congenital malformations. *Gynecol Obstet Invest* 1999;48:28–32.

44. Hayden CK, Schwartz MZ, Davis M, Swischuk LE. Combined esophageal and duodenal atresia: sonographic findings. *AJR Am J Roentgenol* 1983;140:225–226.

45. Claiborne AK, Blocker SH, Martin CM, et al. Prenatal and postnatal sonographic delineation of gastrointestinal abnormalities in a case of the VATER syndrome. *J Ultrasound Med* 1986;5:45–47.

46. Estroff JA, Parad RB, Share JC, Benacerraf BR. Second trimester prenatal findings in duodenal and esophageal atresia without tracheoesophageal fistula. *J Ultrasound Med* 1994;13:375–379.

47. Tsukerman GL, Krapiva GA, Kirillova IA. First-trimester diagnosis of duodenal stenosis associated with oesophageal atresia. *Prenat Diagn* 1993;13:371–376.

48. Eyheremendy E, Pfister M. Antenatal real-time diagnosis of esophageal atresia. *J Clin Ultrasound* 1983;11:395–397.

49. Satoh S, Takashima T, Takeuchi H, et al. Antenatal sonographic detection of the proximal esophageal segment: specific evidence for congenital esophageal atresia. *J Clin Ultrasound* 1995;23:419–423.

50. Kalache KD, Chaoui R, Mau H, Bollmann R. The upper neck pouch sign: a prenatal sonographic marker for esophageal atresia. *Ultrasound Obstet Gynecol* 1998;11:138–140.

51. Bowie JD, Clair MR. Fetal swallowing and regurgitation: observation of normal and abnormal activity. *Radiology* 1982;144:877–878.

52. Pretorius DH, Gosink BB, Clautice-Engle T, et al. Sonographic evaluation of the fetal stomach: significance of nonvisualization. *AJR Am J Roentgenol* 1988;151:987–989.

53. Millener PB, Anderson NG, Chisholm RJ. Prognostic significance of nonvisualization of the fetal stomach by sonography. *AJR Am J Roentgenol* 1993;160(4):827–830.

54. Chitty LS, Goodman J, Seller MJ, Maxwell D. Esophageal and duodenal atresia in a fetus with Down's syndrome: prenatal sonographic features. *Ultrasound Obstet Gynecol* 1996;7:450–452.

55. Holder TM, Cloud DT, Lewis JE Jr, et al. Esophageal atresia and tracheoesophageal fistula. A survey of its members by the surgical section of the American Academy of Pediatrics. *Pediatrics* 1964;34:542–549.

56. Louhimo I, Lindahl H. Esophageal atresia: primary results of 500 consecutively treated patients. *J Pediat Surg* 1983;18:217–229.

57. Pameijer CR, Hubbard AM, Coleman B, Flake AW. Combined pure esophageal atresia, duodenal atresia, biliary atresia, and pancreatic ductal atresia: prenatal diagnostic features and review of the literature. *J Pediatr Surg* 2000;35:745–747.

58. German JC, Mahour GH, Wooley MM. Esophageal atresia and associated anomalies. *J Pediatr Surg* 1976;11:299–306.

59. Rabinowitz JG, Moseley JE, Mitty HA, et al. Trisomy 18, esophageal atresia, anomalies of the radius, and congenital hypoplastic thrombocytopenia. *Radiology* 1967;89:488–491.

60. Kalache KD, Wauer R, Mau H, et al. Prognostic significance of the pouch sign in fetuses with prenatally diagnosed esophageal atresia. *Am J Obstet Gynecol* 2000;182:978–981.

61. Ashcraft KW, Goodwin C, Amoury RA, et al. Early recognition and aggressive treatment of gastroesophageal reflux following repair of esophageal atresia. *J Pediatr Surg* 1977;12:317–321.

62. Bahado-Singh RO, Romero R, Vecchio M, Hobbins JC. Prenatal diagnosis of congenital hiatal hernia. *J Ultrasound Med* 1992;11:297–300.

63. Chacko J, Ford WD, Furness ME. Antenatal detection of hiatus hernia. *Pediatr Surg Int* 1998;13:163–164.

64. Ogunyemi D. Serial sonographic findings in a fetus with congenital hiatal hernia. *Ultrasound Obstet Gynecol* 2001;17:350–353.

65. Yadav K, Myers NA. Paraesophageal hernia in the neonatal period—another differential diagnosis of esophageal atresia. *Pediatr Surg Int* 1997;12:420–421.

66. Parida SK, Kriss VM, Hall BD. Hiatus/paraesophageal hernias in neonatal Marfan syndrome. *Am J Med Genet* 1997;72:156–158.

67. Nakada K, Kawaguchi F, Wakisaka M, et al. Digestive tract disorders associated with asplenia/polysplenia syndrome. *J Pediatr Surg* 1997;32:91.

68. Jawad AJ, al-Samarrai AI, al-Mofada S, et al. Congenital para-oesophageal hiatal hernia in infancy. *Pediatr Surg Int* 1998;13:91–94.

69. al-Arfaj AL, Khwaja MS, Upadhyaya P. Massive hiatal hernia in children. *Eur J Surg* 1991;157:465–468.

70. Baglaj SM, Noblett HR. Paraoesophageal hernia in children: familial occurrence and review of the literature. *Pediatr Surg Int* 1999;15:85–87.

Duodenal Atresia

71. Gray SW, Skandalakis JE. The small intestines. In: *Embryology for surgeons*. Philadelphia: WB Saunders, 1972:129–186.

72. Cheng W, Tam PK. Murine duodenum does not go through a "solid core" stage in its embryological development. *Eur J Pediatr Surg* 1998;8:212–215.

73. Loveday BJ, Barr JA, Aitken J. The intra-uterine demonstration of duodenal atresia by ultrasound. *Br J Radiol* 1975;48:1031–1032.

74. Lawrence MJ, Ford WD, Furness ME, et al. Congenital duodenal obstruction: early antenatal ultrasound diagnosis. *Pediatr Surg Int* 2000;16:342–345.

75. Rizzo N, Pittalis MC, Pilu G, et al. Distribution of abnormal karyotypes among malformed fetuses detected by ultrasound throughout gestation. *Prenat Diagn* 1996;16:159–163.

76. Petrikovsky BM. First-trimester diagnosis of duodenal atresia. *Am J Obstet Gynecol* 1994;171:569–570.

77. Malone FD, Crombleholme TM, Nores JA, et al. Pitfalls of the "double bubble" sign: a case of congenital duodenal duplication. *Fetal Diagn Ther* 1997;12:298–300.

78. Zimmerman HB. Prenatal demonstration of gastric and duodenal obstruction by ultrasound. *J Can Assoc Radiol* 1978;29:138–141.

79. Fonkalsrud EW, deLorimier AA, Hays DM. Congenital atresia and stenosis of the duodenum. A review compiled from the members of the Surgical Section of the American Academy of Pediatrics. *Pediatrics* 1969;43:79–83.

80. Atwell JD, Klidjian AM. Vertebral anomalies and duodenal atresia. *J Pediatr Surg* 1982;17:237–240.

81. Nyberg DA, Resta R, Luthy DA, et al. Prenatal sonographic findings of Down syndrome: review of 94 cases. *Obstet Gynecol* 1990;76:370–377.

82. Murshed R, Nicholls G, Spitz L. Intrinsic duodenal obstruction: trends in management and outcome over 45 years (1951–1995) with relevance to prenatal counselling. *Br J Obstet Gynaecol* 1999;106:1197–1199.

83. Grosfeld JL, Rescorla FJ. Duodenal atresia and stenosis: reassessment of treatment and outcome based on antenatal diagnosis, pathologic variance, and long-term follow-up. *World J Surg* 1993;17:301–309.

84. Romero R, Jeanty P, Gianluigi P, et al. The prenatal diagnosis of duodenal atresia. Does it make any difference? *Obstet Gynecol* 1988;71:739–741.

85. Nicolaides KH, Snijders RJ, Cheng HH, Gosden C. Fetal gastro-intestinal and abdominal wall defects: associated malformations and chromosomal abnormalities. *Fetal Diagn Ther* 1992;7:102–115.

86. Spigland N, Yazbeck S. Complications associated with surgical treatment of congenital intrinsic duodenal obstruction. *J Pediatr Surg* 1990;25:1127–1130.

Jejunoileal Atresia

87. Nixon HH, Tawes R. Etiology and treatment of small intestinal atresia: analysis of a series of 127 jejunoileal atresias and comparison with 62 duodenal atresia. *Surgery* 1971;69:41–51.

88. Grosfeld JL, Ballantine TVN, Shoemaker R. Operative management of intestinal atresia and stenosis based on pathologic findings. *J Pediatr Surg* 1979;14:368–375.

89. Touloukian RJ. Intestinal atresia. *Clin Perinatol* 1978;5:3–18.

90. De Lorimier AA, Fonkalsrud EW, Hays DM. Congenital atresia and stenosis of the jejunum and ileum. *Surgery* 1969;65:819–827.

91. Petrikovsky BM, Nochimson DJ, Campbell WA, et al. Fetal jejunoileal atresia with persistent omphalomesenteric duct. *Am J Obstet Gynecol* 1988;158:173–175.

92. Skoll AM, Marquette GP, Hamilton EF. Prenatal ultrasonic diagnosis of multiple bowel atresias. *Am J Obstet Gynecol* 1987;156:472–473.

93. Baxi LV, Yeh MN, Blanc WA, et al. Antepartum diagnosis and management of in utero intestinal volvulus with perforation. *N Engl J Med* 1983;308:1519–1521.

94. Samuel N, Dicker D, Feldberg D, et al. Ultrasound diagnosis and management of fetal intestinal obstruction and volvulus in utero. *J Perinat Med* 1984;12:333–337.

95. Morikawa N, Namba S, Fujii Y, et al. Intrauterine volvulus without malrotation associated with segmental absence of small intestinal musculature. *J Pediatr Surg* 1999;34:1549–1551.

96. Crisera CA, Ginsburg HB, Gittes GK. Fetal midgut volvulus presenting at term. *J Pediatr Surg* 1999;34:1280–1281.

97. Cheng W, Mya GH, Saing H. Does the amniotic fluid protein absorption contribute significantly to the fetal weight? *J Paediatr Child Health* 1996;32:39–41.

98. Benachi A, Sonigo P, Jouannic JM, et al. Determination of the anatomic location of an antenatal intestinal occlusion by magnetic resonance imaging. *Ultrasound Obstet Gynecol* 2001;18:163–165.

99. Kubota A, Nakayama T, Yonekura T, et al. Congenital ileal atresia presenting as a single cyst-like lesion on prenatal sonography. *J Clin Ultrasound* 2000;28:206–208.

100. Touloukian RJ. Diagnosis and treatment of jejunoileal atresia. *World J Surg* 1993;17:310–317.

101. Bergmans MGM, Merkus JWWM, Baars AM. Obstetrical and neonatological aspects of a child with atresia of the small bowel. *J Perinat Med* 1984;12:325–332.

102. Tam PK, Nicholls G. Implications of antenatal diagnosis of small-intestinal atresia in the 1990s. *Pediatr Surg Int* 1999;15:486–487.

103. Kimble RM, Harding J, Kolbe A. Additional congenital anomalies in babies with gut atresia or stenosis: when to investigate, and which investigation. *Pediatr Surg Int* 1997;12:565–570.

Cystic Fibrosis

104. Park RW, Grand RJ. Gastrointestinal manifestations of cystic fibrosis: a review. *Gastroenterology* 1981;81:1143–1161.

105. Buchanan DJ, Rapoport S. Chemical comparison of normal meconium and meconium from a patient with meconium ileus. *Pediatrics* 1952;9:304–310.

106. Wainwright BJ, Scambler PJ, Schmidtke J, et al. Localization of cystic fibrosis to human chromosome 7cen-q22. *Nature* 1985;318:384–385.

107. Beaudet AL, Spence JE, Montes M, et al. Experience with new DNA markers for the diagnosis of cystic fibrosis. *N Engl J Med* 1988;318:50–51.

108. Gilbert F, Kwei-Lan T, Mendoza A, et al. Prenatal diagnostic options in cystic fibrosis. *Am J Obstet Gynecol* 1988;158:947–952.

109. Witt DR, Schaefer C, Hallam P, et al. Cystic fibrosis heterozygote screening in 5,161 pregnant women. *Am J Hum Genet* 1996;58:823–835.

110. Brock DJ. Prenatal screening for cystic fibrosis: 5 years' experience reviewed. *Lancet* 1996;347:148–150.

111. Cuckle H, Quirke P, Sehmi I, et al. Antenatal screening for cystic fibrosis. *Br J Obstet Gynaecol* 1996;103:795–799.

112. Doherty RA, Bradley LA, Haddow JE. Prenatal screening for cystic fibrosis: an updated perspective. *Am J Obstet Gynecol* 1997;176:268–270.

113. Scotet V, de Braekeleer M, Roussey M, et al. Neonatal screening for cystic fibrosis in Brittany, France: assessment of 10 years' experience and impact on prenatal diagnosis. *Lancet* 2000;356:789–794.

114. National Institutes of Health Consensus Development Conference Statement on genetic testing for cystic fibrosis. Genetic testing for cystic fibrosis. *Arch Intern Med* 1999;159:1529–1539.

115. Rowley PT, Loader S, Kaplan RM. Prenatal screening for cystic fibrosis carriers: an economic evaluation. *Am J Hum Genet* 1998;63:1160–1174.

116. Vintzileos AM, Ananth CV, Smulian JC, et al. A cost-effectiveness analysis of prenatal carrier screening for cystic fibrosis. *Obstet Gynecol* 1998;91:529–534.

117. Asch DA, Hershey JC, Dekay ML, et al. Carrier screening for cystic fibrosis: costs and clinical outcomes. *Med Decis Making* 1998;18:202–212.

118. Boue A, Muller F, Nezelof C, et al. Prenatal diagnosis in 200 pregnancies with a 1-in-4 risk of cystic fibrosis. *Hum Genet* 1986;74:288–297.

119. Goldstein RB, Filly RA, Callen PW. Sonographic diagnosis of meconium ileus *in utero*. *J Ultrasound Med* 1987;6:663–666.

120. Caspi B, Elchalal U, Lancet U, et al. Prenatal diagnosis of cystic fibrosis: ultrasonographic appearance of meconium ileus in the fetus. *Prenat Diagn* 1988;8:379–382.

121. Nyberg DA, Hastrup W, Watts H, et al. Dilated bowel: a sonographic sign of cystic fibrosis. *J Ultrasound Med* 1987;6:257–260.

122. Konje JC, de Chazal R, MacFadyen U, Taylor DJ. Antenatal diagnosis and management of meconium peritonitis: a case report and review of the literature. *Ultrasound Obstet Gynecol* 1995;6:66–69.

123. Estroff JA, Parad RB, Benacerraf BR. Prevalence of cystic fibrosis in fetuses with dilated bowel. *Radiology* 1992;183:677–680.

124. Benacerraf BR, Chaudhury AK. Echogenic fetal bowel in the third trimester associated with meconium ileus secondary to cystic fibrosis. A case report. *J Reprod Med* 1989;34:299–300.

125. Monaghan KG, Feldman GL. The risk of cystic fibrosis with prenatally detected echogenic bowel in an ethnically and racially diverse North American population. *Prenat Diagn* 1999;19:604–669.

126. Berlin BM, Norton ME, Sugarman EA, et al. Cystic fibrosis and chromosome abnormalities associated with echogenic fetal bowel. *Obstet Gynecol* 1999;94:135–138.

127. Al-Kouatly HB, Chasen ST, Strelzoff J, Chervenak FA. The clinical significance of echogenic bowel. *Am J Obstet Gynecol* 2001;185:1035–1038.

128. Chang PY, Huang FY, Yeh ML, et al. Meconium ileus-like condition in Chinese neonates. *J Pediatr Surg* 1992;27:1217–1219.

129. Greenholz SK, Perez C, Wesley JR, Marr CC. Meconium obstruction in markedly premature infant. *J Pediatr Surg* 1996;31:117–120.

130. Gaillard D, Bouvier R, Scheiner C, et al. Meconium ileus and intestinal atresia in fetuses and neonates. *Pediatr Pathol Lab Med* 1996;16:25–40.

131. Rescorla FJ, Grosfeld JL. Contemporary management of meconium ileus. *World J Surg* 1993;17:318–325.

Hyperechoic Bowel

132. Ewer AK, McHugo JM, Chapman S, Newell SJ. Fetal echogenic gut: a marker of intrauterine gut ischaemia? *Arch Dis Child* 1993;69:510–513.

133. Sickler GK, Vang R, Maklad N. Echogenic fetal bowel and calcified meconium in a fetus with trisomy 21. *J Ultrasound Med* 1998;17:591–593.

134. Brock DJH. Prenatal diagnosis of cystic fibrosis. In: Rodeck CH, Nicolaides KH, eds. *Prenatal diagnosis.* New York: John Wiley and Sons, 1985:159–175.

135. Vincoff NS, Callen PW, Smith-Bindman R, Goldstein RB. Effect of ultrasound transducer frequency on the appearance of the fetal bowel. *J Ultrasound Med* 1999;18(12):799–803.

136. Caspi B, Blickstein I, Appelman Z. The accuracy of the assessment of normal fetal intestinal echogenicity—electro-optical densitometry versus the ultrasonographer's eye. *Gynecol Obstet Invest* 1992;33(1):26–30.

137. Khandelwal M, Silva J, Chan L, Reece EA. Three-dimensional ultrasonographic technology to assess and compare echodensity of fetal bowel, bone, and liver in the second trimester of pregnancy. *J Ultrasound Med* 1999;18(10):691–695.

138. Hill LM, Fries J, Hecker J, Grzybek P. Second-trimester echogenic small bowel: an increased risk for adverse perinatal outcome. *Prenat Diagn* 1994;14:845–850.

139. Slotnick RN, Abuhamad AZ. Prognostic implications of fetal echogenic bowel. *Lancet* 1996;347(8994):85–87.

140. Nyberg DA, Dubinsky T, Mahony BS, et al. Echogenic fetal bowel: clinical importance. *Radiology* 1993;188:527–531.

141. Paulson EK, Hertzberg BS. Hyperechoic meconium in the third trimester fetus: an uncommon normal variant. *J Ultrasound Med* 1991;10(12):677–680.

142. Fung AS, Wilson S, Toi A, Johnson JA. Echogenic colonic meconium in the third trimester: a normal sonographic finding. *J Ultrasound Med* 1992;11(12):676–678.

143. Sepulveda W, Bower S, Fisk NM. Third-trimester hyperchogenic bowel in Down syndrome. *Am J Obstet Gynecol* 1995;172(1 Pt 1):210–211.

144. Porter KB, Plattner MS. Fetal abdominal hyperechoic mass: diagnosis and management *Fetal Diagn Ther* 1992;7(2):116–122.

145. Nyberg DA, Resta RG, Luthy DA, et al. Echogenic bowel and Down's syndrome. *Ultrasound Obstet Gynecol* 1993;3:330–333.

146. Persutte WH, Lenke RR. Fetal intra-abdominal hyperchogenicity. *Fetal Diagn Ther* 1993;8(4):291–292.

147. Scioscia AL, Pretorius DH, Budorick NE, et al. Second-trimester echogenic bowel and chromosomal abnormalities. *Am J Obstet Gynecol* 1992;167:889–894.

148. Bromley B, Doubilet P, Frigoletto FD Jr, et al. Is fetal hyperechogenic bowel on second-trimester sonogram an indication for amniocentesis? *Obstet Gynecol* 1994;83:647–651.

149. MacGregor SN, Tamura R, Sabbagha R, et al. Isolated hyperechoic fetal bowel: significance and implications for management. *Am J Obstet Gynecol* 1995;173(4):1254–1258.

150. Sepulveda W, Nicolaidis P, Mai AM, et al. Ultrasound: Is isolated second-trimester hyperechogenic bowel a predictor of suboptimal fetal growth? *Obstet Gynecol* 1996;7(2):104–107.

151. Sipes SL, Weiner CP, Wenstrom KD, et al. Fetal echogenic bowel on ultrasound: Is there clinical significance? *Fetal Diagn Ther* 1994;9(1):38–43.

152. Forouzan I. Fetal abdominal echogenic mass: an early sign of intrauterine cytomegalovirus infection. *Obstet Gynecol* 1992;80(3 Pt 2):535–537.

153. Sepulveda W, Leung KY, Robertson ME, et al. Prevalence of cystic fibrosis mutations in pregnancies with fetal echogenic bowel. *Obstet Gynecol* 1996;87(1):103–106.

154. Bahado-Singh R, Morotti R, Copel JA, Mahoney MJ. Hyperechoic fetal bowel: the perinatal consequences. *Prenat Diagn* 1994;14(10):981–987.

155. Stipoljev F, Sertic J, Kos M, et al. Incidence of chromosomopathies and cystic fibrosis mutations in second trimester fetuses with isolated hyperechoic bowel. *J Matern Fetal Med* 1999;8(2):44–47.

156. Yaron Y, Hassan S, Geva E, et al. Evaluation of fetal echogenic bowel in the second trimester. *Fetal Diagn Ther* 1999;14(3):176–180.

157. Font GE, Solari M. Prenatal diagnosis of bowel obstruction initially manifested as isolated hyperechoic bowel. *J Ultrasound Med* 1998;17(11):721–723.

158. Muller F, Dommergues M, Simon-Bouy B, et al. Cystic fibrosis screening: a fetus with hyperechogenic bowel may be the index case. *J Med Genet* 1998;35(8):657–660.

159. Muller F, Dommergues M, Aubry MC, et al. Hyperechogenic fetal bowel: an ultrasonographic marker for adverse fetal and neonatal outcome. *Am J Obstet Gynecol* 1995;173(2):508–513.

160. Sepulveda W, Reid R, Nicolaidis P, et al. Second-trimester echogenic bowel and intraamniotic bleeding: association between fetal bowel echogenicity and amniotic fluid spectrophotometry at 410 nm. *Am J Obstet Gynecol* 1996;174(3):839–842.

161. Hogge WA, Hogge JS, Boehm CD, Sanders RC: Increased echogenicity in the fetal abdomen: use of DNA analysis to establish a diagnosis of cystic fibrosis. *J Ultrasound Med* 1993;12(8):451–454.

162. Dicke JM, Crane JP. Sonographically detected hyperechoic fetal bowel: significance and implications for pregnancy management. *Obstet Gynecol* 1992;80(5):778–782.

163. Ghose I, Mason GC, Martinez D, et al. Hyperechogenic fetal bowel: a prospective analysis of sixty consecutive cases. *Br J Obstet Gynaecol* 2000;107(3):426–429.

164. Strocker AM, Snijders RJ, Carlson DE, et al. Fetal echogenic bowel: parameters to be considered in differential diagnosis. *Ultrasound Obstet Gynecol* 2000;16(6):519–523.

Nonobstructive Small Bowel Dilatation

165. Chen CP, Wang TY, Chuang CY. Sonographic findings in a fetus with megacystis-microcolon-intestinal hypoperistalsis syndrome. *J Clin Ultrasound* 1998;26(4):217–220.

166. White SM, Chamberlain P, Hitchcock R, et al. Megacystis-microcolon-intestinal hypoperistalsis syndrome: the difficulties with antenatal diagnosis. Case report and review of the literature. *Prenat Diagn* 2000;20(9):697–700.

167. Achiron R, Seidman DS, Horowitz A, et al. Hyperechogenic fetal bowel and elevated serum alpha-fetoprotein: a poor fetal prognosis. *Obstet Gynecol* 1996;88(3):368–371.

168. Al-Kouatly HB, Chasen ST, Karam AK, et al. Factors associated with fetal demise in fetal echogenic bowel. *Am J Obstet Gynecol* 2001;185:1039–1043.

169. Groli C, Zucca S, Cesaretti A. Congenital chloridorrhea: antenatal ultrasonographic appearance. *J Clin Ultrasound* 1986;14:293–295.

170. Kirkinen P, Jouppila P. Prenatal ultrasonic findings in congenital chloride diarrhoea. *Prenat Diagn* 1984;4:457–461.

171. Langer JC, Winthrop AL, Burrows RF, et al. False diagnosis of intestinal obstruction in a fetus with congenital chloride diarrhea. *J Pediatr Surg* 1991;26(11):1282–1284.

172. Lundkvist K, Ewald U, Lindgren PG. Congenital chloride diarrhoea: a prenatal differential diagnosis of small bowel atresia. *Acta Paediatr* 1996;85(3):295–298.

173. Berdon WE, Baker DH, Blanc WA, et al. Megacystis-microcolon-intestinal hypoperistalsis syndrome: a new cause of intestinal obstruction in the newborn. Report of radiologic findings in five newborn girls. *AJR Am J Roentgenol* 1976;126:957–964.

174. Manco LG, Osterdahl P. The antenatal sonographic features of megacystis-microcolon-intestinal hypoperistalsis syndrome. *J Clin Ultrasound* 1984;12:595–598.

175. Ventzileos AM, Eisenfeld LI, Herson VC, et al. Megacystis-microcolon-intestinal hypoperistalsis syndrome: antenatal sonographic findings and review of the literature. *Am J Perinatol* 1986;3:297–302.

176. Puri P, Lake BD, Gorman F, et al. Megacystis-microcolon-intestinal hypoperistalsis syndrome: a visceral myopathy. *J Pediatr Surg* 1983;18:64–69.

Anorectal Atresia

177. Stoll C, Alembik Y, Roth MP, Dott B. Risk factors in congenital anal atresias. *Ann Genet* 1997;40(4):197–204.

178. Bean WJ, Calonge MA, Aprill CN, et al. Anal atresia: a prenatal ultrasound diagnosis. *J Clin Ultrasound* 1978;6:111–112.

179. Harris RD, Nyberg DA, Mack LA, et al. Anorectal atresia: prenatal sonographic diagnosis. *AJR Am J Roentgenol* 1987;149:395–400.

180. Auslander R, Nevo O, Diukman R, et al. Johanson-Blizzard syndrome: a prenatal ultrasonographic diagnosis. *Ultrasound Obstet Gynecol* 1999;13(6):450–452.

181. Berdon WE, Baker DH, Wigges HJ, et al. Calcified intraluminal meconium in newborn males with imperforate anus. *AJR Am J Roentgenol* 1975;125:449–455.

182. Mandell J, Lillehei CW, Greene M, Benacerraf BR. The prenatal diagnosis of imperforate anus with rectourinary fistula: dilated fetal colon with enterolithiasis. *J Pediatr Surg* 1992;27(1):82–84.

183. Hillcoat BL. Calcification of the meconium within the bowel of the newborn. *Arch Dis Child* 1962;37:86–89.

184. Shalev E, Weiner E, Zuzherman H. Prenatal ultrasound diagnosis of intestinal calcifications with imperforate anus. *Acta Obstet Gynecol Scand* 1983;62:95–96.

185. Szabo M, Veress L, Teichmann F, et al. Amniotic fluid

microvillar enzyme activity in fetal malformations. *Clin Genet* 1990;38(5):340–345.

186. Brock DJH. A comparative study of microvillar enzyme activities in the prenatal diagnosis of cystic fibrosis. *Prenat Diagn* 1985;5:129–134.

187. Van Rijn M, Christaens GC, Hagenaars AM, Visser GH. Maternal serum alpha-fetoprotein in fetal anal atresia and other gastrointestinal obstructions. *Prenat Diagn* 1998;18(9):914–921.

188. Anderson N, Malpas T, Robertson R. Prenatal diagnosis of colon atresia. *Pediatr Radiol* 1993;23(1):63–64.

189. Pena A. Surgical treatment of high imperforate anus. *World J Surg* 1985;9:236–243.

190. deVries PA, Cox KL. Surgery of anorectal anomalies. *Surg Clin North Am* 1985;65:1139–1169.

191. Chen CJ. The treatment of imperforate anus: experience with 108 patients. *J Pediatr Surg* 1999;34(11):1728–1732.

Urorectal Septum Malformations

192. Cilento BG Jr, Benacerraf BR, Mandell J. Prenatal diagnosis of cloacal malformation. *Urology* 1994;43(3):386–388.

193. Tank ES. The urologic complications of imperforate anus and cloacal dysgenesis. In: Harrison JH, Gittes RF, Perlmutter AD, et al., eds. *Campbell's urology,* 4th ed. Philadelphia: WB Saunders, 1979:1889–1900.

194. Escobar LF, Weaver DD, Bixler D, et al. Urorectal septum malformation sequence. *Am J Dis Child* 1987;141:1021–1024.

195. Wheeler PG, Weaver DD. Partial urorectal septum malformation sequence: a report of 25 cases. *Am J Med Genet* 2001;103:88–105.

196. Arena F, Romeo C, Cruccetti A, et al. The neonatal management and surgical correction of urinary hydrometrocolpos caused by a persistent urogenital sinus. *BJU Int* 1999;84(9):1063–1068.

197. Williams DI, Bloomberg S. Urogenital sinus in the female child. *J Pediatr Surg* 1976;11:51–56.

198. Ohno Y, Koyama N, Tsuda M, Arii Y. Antenatal ultrasonographic appearance of a cloacal anomaly. *Obstet Gynecol* 2000;95(6 Pt 2):1013–1015.

199. Carroll SG, Hyett J, Eustace D, et al. Evolution of sonographic findings in a fetus with agenesis of the urethra, vagina, and rectum. *Prenat Diagn* 1996;16(10):931–933.

200. Cacciaguerra S, Lo Presti L, Di Leo L, et al. Prenatal diagnosis of cloacal anomaly. *Scand J Urol Nephrol* 1998;32(1):77–80.

201. Odibo AO, Turner GW, Borgida AF, et al. Late prenatal ultrasound features of hydrometrocolpos secondary to cloacal anomaly: case reports and review of the literature. *Ultrasound Obstet Gynecol* 1997;9(6):419–421.

202. Zaccara A, Gatti C, Silveri M, et al. Persistent cloaca: are we ready for a correct prenatal diagnosis? *Urology* 1999;54(2):367.

203. Adams MC, Ludlow J, Brock JW III, Rink RC. Prenatal urinary ascites and persistent cloaca: risk factors for poor drainage of urine or meconium. *J Urol* 1998;160(6 Pt 1): 2179–2181.

204. Lande IM, Hamilton EF. The antenatal sonographic visualization of cloacal dysgenesis. *J Ultrasound Med* 1986;5:275–278.

205. Achiron R, Frydman M, Lipitz S, Zalel Y. Urorectal septum malformation sequence: prenatal sonographic diagnosis in two sets of discordant twins. *Ultrasound Obstet Gynecol* 2000;16(6):571–574.

206. Warne S, Chitty LS, Wilcox DT. Prenatal diagnosis of cloacal anomalies. *BJU Int* 2002;89(1):78–81.

207. Petrikovsky BM, Walzak MP Jr, D'Addaria PF. Fetal cloacal anomalies: prenatal sonographic findings and differential diagnosis. *Obstet Gynecol* 1988;72:464–469.

208. Shalev E, Feldman E, Weiner E, et al. Prenatal sonographic appearance of persistent cloaca. *Acta Obstet Gynecol Scand* 1986;65:517–518.

209. Stephenson CA, Ball TI Jr, Ricketts RR. An unusual case of meconium peritonitis associated with perforated hydrocolpos. *Pediatr Radiol* 1992;22(4):279–280.

210. Basl ARM, Sanders RC, Gearhart JP. Obstructed uterovaginal anomalies: demonstration with sonography. Part I. Neonates and infants. *Radiology* 1991;179:70–83.

211. Thomas DF. Cloacal malformations: embryology, anatomy and principles of management. *Prog Pediatr Surg* 1989;23:135–143.

212. Soffer SZ, Rosen NG, Hong AR, et al. Cloacal exstrophy: a unified management plan. *J Pediatr Surg* 2000;35(6):932–937.

213. Hendren WH. Repair of cloacal anomalies: current techniques. *J Pediatr Surg* 1986;21(12):1159–1176.

214. Hendren WH. Urological aspects of cloacal malformations. *J Urol* 1988;140(5 Pt 2):1207–1213.

215. Hendren WH. Cloaca, the most severe degree of imperforate anus: experience with 195 cases. *Ann Surg* 1998; 228(3):331–346.

216. Gray SW, Skandalakis JE. The colon and rectum. In: *Embryology for surgeons.* Philadelphia: WB Saunders, 1972:187–216.

Hirschsprung Disease

217. Okamoto E, Ueda T. Embryogenesis of intramural ganglia of the gut and its relation to Hirschsprung's disease. *J Pediatr Surg* 1967;2:437–443.

218. Sullivan PB. Hirschsprung's disease. *Arch Dis Child* 1996;74(1):5–7.

219. Puri P, Ohshiro K, Wester T. Hirschsprung's disease: a search for etiology. *Semin Pediatr Surg* 1998;7(3):140–147.

220. Ikeda K, Goto S. Diagnosis and treatment of Hirschsprung's disease in Japan: an analysis of 1628 patients. *Ann Surg* 1984;199:400–405.

221. Jarmas AL, Weaver DD, Padilla LM, et al. Hirschsprung disease: etiologic implications of unsuccessful prenatal diagnosis. *Am J Med Genet* 1983;16:163–167.

222. Wrobleski D, Wesselhoeft. Ultrasonic diagnosis of prenatal intestinal obstruction. *J Pediatr Surg* 1979;14:598–600.

223. Vermish M, Mayden KL, Confino E, et al. Prenatal sonographic diagnosis of Hirschsprung's disease. *J Ultrasound Med* 1986;5:37–39.

224. Eliyahu S, Yanai N, Blondheim O, et al. Sonographic presentation of Hrischsprung's disease. A case of an entirely aganglionic colon and ileum. *Prenat Diagn* 1994;14:1170–1172.

225. Blisard KS, Kleinman R. Hirschsprung's disease: a clinical and pathologic overview. *Hum Pathol* 1986;17:1189–1191.

226. Buyse ML. *Birth defects encyclopedia.* Cambridge: Blackwell Science, 1990:427–428.

227. Parisi MA, Kapur RP. Hirschsprung Disease Overview, in Gene Clinics (www.geneclinics.org), July, 2002.

228. Pingault V, Bondurand N, Kuhlbrodt K, et al. SOXIO mutations in patients with Waardenburg-Hirschsprung disease. *Nat Genet* 1998;18:171–173.

229. N-Fékété C, Ricour C, Martelli H, et al. Total colonic aganglionosis (with or without ileal involvement): a review of 27 cases. *J Pediatr Surg* 1986;21:251–254.

230. Dykes EH, Guiney EJ. Total colonic aganglionosis. *J Pediatr Gastr Nutr* 1989;8:129–132.

Meconium Peritonitis

231. Ceballos R, Hicks GM. Plastic peritonitis due to neonatal hydrometrocolpos: radiologic and pathologic observations. *J Pediatr Surg* 1970;5:63–70.

232. Soong JH, Hsieh CC, Chiu TH, et al. Meconium peritonitis—antenatal diagnosis by ultrasound. *Chang Keng I Hsueh Tsa Chih* 1992;15(3):155–160.

233. Forouhar F. Meconium peritonitis: pathology, evolution, and diagnosis. *Am J Clin Pathol* 1982;78:208–213.

234. Tibboel D, Gaillard JLJ, Molenaar JC. Importance of mesenteric vascular insufficiency in meconium peritonitis. *Hum Pathol* 1986;17:411–416.

235. Edelstone DI, Holzman IR. Regulation of perinatal intestinal oxygenation. *Semin Perinatol* 1984;8:226–233.

236. Hume RF Jr, Gingras JL, Martin LS, et al. Ultrasound diagnosis of fetal anomalies associated with *in utero* cocaine exposure: further support for cocaine-induced vascular disruption teratogenesis. *Fetal Diagn Ther* 1994;9(4):239–245.

237. Tucker AS, Izant RJ. Problems with meconium. *AJR Am J Roentgenol* 1971;112:135–142.

238. Finkel LI, Slovis TL. Meconium peritonitis, intraperitoneal calcifications, and cystic fibrosis. *Pediatr Radiol* 1982;12:92–93.

239. Neuhauser EB. The roentgen diagnosis of fetal meconium peritonitis. *AJR Am J Roentgenol* 1944;51:421–425.

240. Chalubinski K, Deutinger J, Bernaschek G II. Meconium peritonitis: extrusion of meconium and different sonographical appearances in relation to the stage of the disease. *Prenat Diagn* 1992;12(8):631–636.

241. Foster MA, Nyberg DA, Mahony BS, et al. Meconium peritonitis: prenatal sonographic findings and clinical significance. *Radiology* 1987;165:661–665.

242. Fleischer AC, Davis RJ, Campbell L. Sonographic detection of a meconium-containing mass in a fetus: a case report. *J Clin Ultrasound* 1983;11:103–105.

243. McGahan JP, Hanson F. Meconium peritonitis with accompanying pseudocyst: prenatal sonographic diagnosis. *Radiology* 1983;148:125–126.

244. Miller JP, Smith SD, Newman B, et al. Neonatal abdominal calcification: Is it always meconium peritonitis? *J Pediatr Surg* 1988;23:555–556.

245. Lockwood C, Ghidini A, Romero R, et al. Fetal bowel perforation simulating sacrococcygeal teratoma. *J Ultrasound Med* 1988;7:227–229.

246. Quinlivan JA, Newnham JP, Dickinson JE. Ultrasound features of congenital listeriosis—a case report. *Prenat Diagn* 1998;18(10):1075–1078.

247. Miyakoshi K, Tanaka M, Miyazaki T, Yoshimura Y. Prenatal ultrasound diagnosis of small-bowel torsion. *Obstet Gynecol* 1998;91(5 Pt 2):802–803.

248. Balci S, Altinok G, Ozaltin F, et al. Laryngeal atresia presenting as fetal ascites, olygohydramnios and lung appearance mimicking cystic adenomatoid malformation in a 25-week-old fetus with Fraser syndrome. *Prenat Diagn* 1999;19(9):856–858.

249. Morrison PJ, Macphail S, Williams D, et al. Laryngeal atresia or stenosis presenting as second-trimester fetal ascites—diagnosis and pathology in three independent cases. *Prenat Diagn* 1998;18(9):963–967.

250. Jacquemyn Y, De Catte L, Vaerenberg M. Fetal ascites associated with an imperforate hymen: sonographic observation. *Ultrasound Obstet Gynecol* 1998;12(1):67–69.

251. Manzella A, Filho PB. Hydrocolpos, uterus didelphys and septate vagina in association with ascites: antenatal sonographic detection. *J Ultrasound Med* 1998;17(7):465–468.

252. Shimotake T, Go S, Tsuda T, Iwai N. Ultrasonographic detection of intrauterine intussusception resulting in ileal atresia complicated by meconium peritonitis. *Pediatr Surg Int* 2000;16(1-2):43–44.

253. Brun M, Grignon A, Guibaud L, et al. Gastroschisis: are prenatal ultrasonographic findings useful for assessing the prognosis? *Pediatr Radiol* 1996;26(10):723–726.

254. Schild RL, Plath H, Thomas P, et al. Fetal parvovirus B19 infection and meconium peritonitis. *Fetal Diagn Ther* 1998;13(1):15–18.

255. Zerbini M, Gentilomi GA, Gallinella G, et al. Intra-uterine parvovirus B19 infection and meconium peritonitis. *Prenat Diagn* 1998;18(6):599–606.

256. Pletcher BA, Williams MK, Mulivor RA, et al. Intrauterine cytomegalovirus infection presenting as fetal meconium peritonitis. *Obstet Gynecol* 1991;78(5 Pt 2):903–905.

257. Radner M, Vergesslich KA, Weninger M, et al. Meconium peritonitis: a new finding in rubella syndrome. *J Clin Ultrasound* 1993;21(5):346–349.

258. Nigro G, La Torre R, Mazzocco M, et al. Multi-system cytomegalovirus fetopathy by recurrent infection in a pregnant woman with hepatitis B. *Prenat Diagn* 1999;19(11):1070–1072.

259. McDuffie RS Jr, Bader T. Fetal meconium peritonitis after maternal hepatitis A. *Am J Obstet Gynecol* 1999;180(4):1031–1032.

260. Estroff JA, Bromley B, Benacerraf BR. Fetal meconium peritonitis without sequelae. *Pediatr Radiol* 1992;22(4):277–278.

261. Moslinger D, Chalubinski K, Radner M, et al. [Meconium peritonitis: intrauterine follow-up—postnatal outcome]. [Article in German] *Wien Klin Wochenschr* 1995;107(4):141–145.

262. Dirkes K, Crombleholme TM, Craigo SD, et al. The natural history of meconium peritonitis diagnosed *in utero*. *J Pediatr Surg* 1995;30(7):979–982.

Hepatic Calcifications

263. Bronshtein M, Blazer S. Prenatal diagnosis of liver calcifications. *Obstet Gynecol* 1995;86(5):739–743.

264. Koopman E, Wladimiroff JW. Fetal intrahepatic hyperechogenic foci: prenatal ultrasound diagnosis and outcome. *Prenat Diagn* 1998;18(8):569–572.

265. Avni EF, Rypens F, Donner C, et al. Hepatic cysts and hyperechogenicities: perinatal assessment and unifying theory on their origin. *Pediatr Radiol* 1994;24(2):489–492.

266. Perez CG, Goldstein RB. Sonographic borderlands in the fetal abdomen. *Semin Ultrasound CT MR* 1998;19(4):336–346.

267. Achiron R, Seidman DS, Afek A, et al. Prenatal ultrasonographic diagnosis of fetal hepatic hyperechogenicities: clinical significance and implications for management. *Ultrasound Obstet Gynecol* 1996;7(4):251–255.

268. Simchen MJ, Bona M, Toi A, et al. Fetal hepatic calcifications: prenatal diagnosis and outcome. *Am J Obstet Gynecol* 2001;185(6):s238.

269. Schackelford GD, Kirks DR. Neonatal hepatic calcification secondary to transplacental infection. *Radiology* 1977;122:753–757.

270. Stein B, Bromley B, Michlewitz H, et al. Fetal liver calcifications: sonographic appearance and postnatal outcome. *Radiology* 1995;197(2):489–492.

271. Yousefzadeh DK, Jackson JH Jr, Smith WL, et al. Intraluminal meconium calcification without distal obstruction. *Pediatr Radiol* 1984;14:23–27.

272. Magnus KG, Millar AJ, Sinclair-Smith CC, Rode H. Intrahepatic fetus-in-fetu: a case report and review of the literature. *J Pediatr Surg* 1999;34(12):1861–1864.

273. Khadaroo RG, Evans MG, Honore LH, et al. Fetus-in-fetu presenting as cystic meconium peritonitis: diagnosis, pathology, and surgical management. *J Pediatr Surg* 2000;35(5):721–723.

274. Schmider A, Henrich W, Reles A, et al. Isolated fetal ascites caused by primary lymphangiectasia: a case report. *Am J Obstet Gynecol* 2001;184(2):227–228.

275. Levine D, Barnes PD, Edelman RR. Obstetric MR imaging. *Radiology* 1999;211(3):609–617.

Ovarian Cysts

276. Desa DJ. Follicular ovarian cysts in stillbirths and neonates. *Arch Dis Child* 1975;50:24–50.

277. Jafri SZH, Bree RL, Silver TM, et al. Fetal ovarian cysts: sonographic detection and association with hypothyroidism. *Radiology* 1984;150:809–812.

278. Jouppila P, Kirkinen P, Tuononen S. Ultrasonic detection of bilateral ovarian cysts in the fetus. *Eur J Obstet Gynecol Reprod Biol* 1982;13:87–92.

279. Lindeque BG, du Toit JP, Muller LMM, et al. Ultrasonographic criteria for the conservative management of antenatally diagnosed fetal ovarian cysts. *J Reprod Med* 1988;33:196–198.

280. Sakala EP, Leon ZA, Rouse GA. Management of antenatally diagnosed fetal ovarian cysts. *Obstet Gynecol Surv* 1991;46(7):407–414.

281. Garel L, Filiatrault D, Brandt M, et al. Antenatal diagnosis of ovarian cysts: natural history and therapeutic implications. *Pediatr Radiol* 1991;21(3):182–184.

282. Meizner I, Levy A, Katz M, et al. Fetal ovarian cysts: prenatal ultrasonographic detection and postnatal evaluation and treatment. *Am J Obstet Gynecol* 1991;164(3):874–878.

283. D'Addario V, Volpe G, Kurjak A, et al. Ultrasonic diagnosis and perinatal management of complicated and uncomplicated fetal ovarian cysts: a collaborative study. *J Perinat Med* 1990;18(5):375–381.

284. Bagolan P, Rivosecchi M, Giorlandino C, et al. Prenatal diagnosis and clinical outcome of ovarian cysts. *J Pediatr Surg* 1992;27(7):879–881.

285. Sapin E, Bargy F, Lewin F, et al. Management of ovarian cyst detected by prenatal ultrasounds. *Eur J Pediatr Surg* 1994;4(3):137–140.

286. O'Hagan DB, Pudifin J, Mickel RE, et al. Antenatal detection of a fetal ovarian cyst by real-time ultrasound. *S Afr Med J* 1985;67:471–473.

287. Nussbaum AR, Sanders RC, Hartman DS, et al. Neonatal ovarian cysts: sonographic-pathologic correlation. *Radiology* 1988;168:817–821.

288. Katz VL, McCoy MC, Kuller JA, et al. Fetal ovarian torsion appearing as a solid abdominal mass. *J Perinatol* 1996;16(4):302–304.

289. Muller-Leisse C, Bick U, Paulussen K, et al. Ovarian cysts in the fetus and neonate—changes in sonographic pattern in the follow-up and their management. *Pediatr Radiol* 1992;22(6):395–400.

290. Crombleholme TM, Craigo SD, Garmel S, D'Alton ME. Fetal ovarian cyst decompression to prevent torsion. *J Pediatr Surg* 1997;32(10):1447–1449.

291. Dolgin SE. Ovarian masses in the newborn. *Semin Pediatr Surg* 2000;9(3):121–127.

292. Ikeda K, Suita S, Nakano H. Management of ovarian cysts detected antenatally. *J Pediatr Surg* 1988;23:432–435.

293. Degani S, Lewinsky RM. Transient ascites associated with a fetal ovarian cyst. Case report. *Fetal Diagn Ther* 1995;10(3):200–203.

294. Meagher SE, Fisk NM, Boogert A, Russell P. Fetal ovarian cysts: diagnostic and therapeutic role for intrauterine aspiration. *Fetal Diagn Ther* 1993;8(3):195–199.

295. Carlson DH, Griscom NT. Ovarian cysts in the newborn. *AJR Am J Roentgenol* 1972;116:664–672.

296. Koc E, Turkyilmaz C, Atalay Y, et al. Neonatal ovarian cyst associated with intestinal obstruction. *Indian J Pediatr* 1997;64(4):555–557.

297. Abolmakarem H, Tharmaratnum S, Thilaganathan B. Fetal anemia as a consequence of hemorrhage into an ovarian cyst. *Ultrasound Obstet Gynecol* 2001;17(6):527–528.

298. Templeman CL, Reynolds AM, Hertweck SP, Nagaraj HS. Laparoscopic management of neonatal ovarian cysts. *J Am Assoc Gynecol Laparosc* 2000;7(3):401–404.

299. Brandt ML, Luks FI, Filiatrault D, et al. Surgical indications in antenatally diagnosed ovarian cysts. *J Pediatr Surg* 1991;26(3):276–282.

300. Campbell BA, Garg RS, Garg K, et al. Perinatal ovarian cyst: a nonsurgical approach. *J Pediatr Surg* 1992;27(12):1618–1619.

301. Suita S, Handa N, Nakano H. Antenatally detected ovarian cysts—a therapeutic dilemma. *Early Hum Dev* 1992;29:363–367.

302. Marshall JR. Ovarian enlargements in the first year of life. *Ann Surg* 1965;161:372–377.

Other Cystic Masses

303. Westerhout FC, Hodgman JE, Anderson GV, et al. Congenital hydrocolpos. *Am J Obstet Gynecol* 1964;89:957–961.

304. Russ PD, Zavitz WR, Pretorius DH, et al. Hydrometrocolpos, uterus didelphys and septate vagina: an antenatal sonographic diagnosis. *J Ultrasound Med* 1986;5:211–213.

305. Hill SJ, Hirsch JH. Sonographic detection of fetal hydrometrocolpos. *J Ultrasound Med* 1985;4:323–325.

306. Manzella A, Filho PB. Hydrocolpos, uterus didelphys and septate vagina in association with ascites: antenatal sonographic detection. *J Ultrasound Med* 1998;17(7):465–468.

307. Geipel A, Berg C, Germer U, et al. Diagnostic and therapeutic problems in a case of prenatally detected fetal hydrocolpos. *Ultrasound Obstet Gynecol* 2001;18:169–172.

308. McKusick VA, Bauer RL, Koop CE, et al. Hydrometrocolpos as a simply inherited malformation. *JAMA* 1964;189:813.

309. Robinow M, Shaw A. The McKusick-Kaufman syndrome: recessively inherited vaginal atresia, hydrometrocolpos, uterovaginal duplications, anorectal anomalies, postaxial polydactyly and congenital heart disease. *J Pediatr* 1979;94:776–778.

310. Hsu YR, Chuang JH, Huang CB, Changchien CC. The McKusick-Kaufman hydrometrocolpos-polydactyly syndrome—a case report. *Chang Keng I Hsueh Tsa Chih* 1994;17(2):173–177.

311. Lin HJ, Cornford ME, Hu B, et al. Occipital encephalocele and MURCS association: case report and review of central nervous system anomalies in MURCS patients. *Am J Med Genet* 1996;61:59–62.

312. Spencer R, Levy DM. Hydrometrocolpos: report of three cases and review of the literature. *Ann Surg* 1962;155:558–571.

313. Alonso-Lej F, Rever WB Jr, Pessagno DJ. Collective review. Congenital choledochal cyst, with a report of 2, and an analysis of 94 cases. *Int Abstract Surg* 1959;108:1–30.

314. Howel CG, Templeton JM, Weiner S, et al. Antenatal diagnosis and early surgery for choledochal cyst. *J Pediatr Surg* 1983;18:387–393.

315. Dewbury KC, Aluwihare M, Birch SJ, et al. Prenatal ultrasound demonstration of a choledochal cyst. *Br J Radiol* 1980;53:906–907.

316. Bancroft JD, Bucuvalas JC, Ryckman FC, et al. Antenatal diagnosis of choledochal cyst. *J Pediatr Gastroenterol Nutr* 1994;18(2):142–145.

317. Cramer B, Pushpanathan C, Kennedy R. Nonrenal cystic masses in neonates and children. *Can Assoc Radiol J* 1993;44(2):93–98.

318. Elrad H, Mayden KL, Ahart S, et al. Prenatal ultrasound diagnosis of choledochal cyst. *J Ultrasound Med* 1985; 4:553–555.

319. Benhidjeb T, Chaoui R, Kalache K, et al. Prenatal diagnosis of a choledochal cyst: a case report and review of the literature. *Am J Perinatol* 1996;13(4):207–210.

320. Chen CP. Ultrasound-guided needle aspiration of a fetal choledochal cyst. *Ultrasound Obstet Gynecol* 2001;17:175–176.

321. Lugo-Vicente HL. Prenatally diagnosed choledochal cysts: observation or early surgery? *J Pediatr Surg* 1995;30(9):1288–1290.

322. Redkar R, Davenport M, Howard ER. Antenatal diagnosis of congenital anomalies of the biliary tract. *J Pediatr Surg* 1998;33(5):700–704.

323. Greenholz SK. Antenatal diagnosis of choledochal cyst at 15 weeks' gestation: etiologic implications and management. *J Pediatr Surg* 1990;25(5):584.

324. Schroeder D, Smith L, Prain HC. Antenatal diagnosis of choledochal cyst at 15 weeks' gestation: etiologic implications and management. *J Pediatr Surg* 1989;24(9):936–938.

325. Matsubara H, Oya N, Suzuki Y, et al. Is it possible to differentiate between choledochal cyst and congenital biliary atresia (type I cyst) by antenatal ultrasonography? *Fetal Diagn Ther* 1997;12(5):306-308.

326. Tsuchida Y, Kawarasaki H, Iwanaka T, et al. Antenatal diagnosis of biliary atresia (type I cyst) at 19 weeks' gestation: differential diagnosis and etiologic implications. *J Pediatr Surg* 1995;30(5):697–699.

327. Gray SW, Skandalakis JE. Extrahepatic biliary ducts and the gallbladder. In: *Embryology for surgeons.* Philadelphia: WB Saunders, 1972:229–262.

328. Cheng MT, Chang MH, Hsu HY, et al. Choledochal cyst in infancy: a follow-up study. *Taiwan Erh Ko I Hsueh Hui Tsa Chih* 2000;41(1):13–17.

329. Gallivan EK, Crombleholme TM, D'Alton ME. Early prenatal diagnosis of choledochal cyst. *Prenat Diagn* 1996;16(10):934–937.

330. Rha SY, Stovroff MC, Glick PL, et al. Choledochal cysts: a ten year experience. *Am Surg* 1996;62(1):30–34.

331. Stringer MD, Dhawan A, Davenport M, et al. Choledochal cysts: lessons from a 20 year experience. *Arch Dis Child* 1995;73(6):528–531.

332. Yamaguchi M. Congenital choledochal cyst: analysis of 1,433 patients in the Japanese literature. *Am J Surg* 1980;140:653–657.

333. Chen MK, Gross E, Lobe TE. Perinatal management of enteric duplication cysts of the tongue. *Am J Perinatol* 1997;14(3):161–163.

334. Markert DJ, Grumbach K, Haney PJ. Thoracoabdominal duplication cyst: prenatal and postnatal imaging. *J Ultrasound Med* 1996;15(4):333–336.

335. Goyert GL, Blitz D, Gibson P, et al. Prenatal diagnosis of duplication cyst of the pylorus. *Prenat Diagn* 1991;11(7):483–486.

336. Bidwell JK, Nelson A. Prenatal ultrasonic diagnosis of congenital duplication of the stomach. *J Ultrasound Med* 1986;5:589–591.

337. Yamataka A, Pringle KC. A case with duodenal duplication cyst: prenatal diagnosis and surgical management. *Fetal Diagn Ther* 1998;13(1):39–41.

338. Richards DS, Langham MR, Anderson CD. The prenatal sonographic appearance of enteric duplication cysts. *Ultrasound Obstet Gynecol* 1996;7(1):17–20.

339. Fenton LZ, Williams JL. Bronchopulmonary foregut malformation mimicking neuroblastoma. *Pediatr Radiol* 1996;26(10):729–730.

340. Egozi EI, Ricketts RR. Mesenteric and omental cysts in children. *Am Surg* 1997;63(3):287–290.

341. Walker AR, Putnam TC. Omental, mesenteric, and retroperitoneal cysts: a clinical study of 33 new cases. *Ann Surg* 1973;178:13.

342. Benacerraf BR, Figoletto FD. Prenatal sonographic diagnosis of isolated congenital cystic hygroma, unassociated with lymphedema or other morphologic abnormality. *J Ultrasound Med* 1987;6:63–66.

343. Blumhagen JD, Wood BJ, Rosenbaum DM. Sonographic evaluation of abdominal lymphangiomas in children. *J Ultrasound Med* 1987;6:487–495.

344. Goyert GL, Blitz D, Gibson P, et al. Prenatal diagnosis of duplication cyst of the pylorus. *Prenat Diagn* 1991;11(7):483–486.

345. Ozmen MN, Onderoglu L, Ciftci AO, et al. Prenatal diagnosis of gastric duplication cyst. *J Ultrasound Med* 1997;16(3):219–222.

346. Duncan BW, Adzick NS, Eraklis A. Retroperitoneal alimentary tract duplications detected *in utero. J Pediatr Surg* 1992;27(9):1231–1233.

347. Degani S, Mogilner JG, Shapiro I. *In utero* sonographic appearance of intestinal duplication cysts. *Ultrasound Obstet Gynecol* 1995;5(6):415–418.

348. Steiner Z, Mogilner J. A rare case of completely isolated duplication cyst of the alimentary tract. *J Pediatr Surg* 1999;34(8):1284–1286.

349. May DA, Spottswood SE, Ridick-Young M, Nwomeh BC. Case report: prenatally detected dumbbell-shaped retroperitoneal duplication cyst. *Pediatr Radiol* 2000;30(10):671–673.

350. Daher P, Diab N, Melki I, et al. Congenital cyst of the pancreas. Antenatal diagnosis. *Eur J Pediatr Surg* 1996;6(3):180–182.

351. Kurtz RJ, Heimann Tomas M, Beck AR, et al. Mesenteric and retroperitoneal cysts. *Ann Surg* 1986;203:109–112.

352. Chung W-M. Antenatal detection of hepatic cyst. *J Clin Ultrasound* 1986;14:217–219.

353. Macken MB, Wright JR Jr, Lau H, et al. Prenatal sonographic detection of congenital hepatic cyst in third trimester after normal second-trimester sonographic examination. *J Clin Ultrasound* 2000;28(6):307–310.

354. Lichman JP, Miller EI. Prenatal ultrasonic diagnosis of splenic cyst. *J Ultrasound Med* 1988;7:637–638.

355. Ito M, Yoshimura K, Toyoda N, Tanaka H. Aspiration of giant hepatic cyst in the fetus *in utero*. *Fetal Diagn Ther* 1997;12(4):221–225.

Liver/Spleen

356. Bahado-Singh R, Oz U, Mari G, et al. Fetal splenic size in anemia due to Rh-alloimmunization. *Obstet Gynecol* 1998;92(5):828–832.

357. Vintzileos AM, Neckles S, Campbell WA, et al. Fetal liver ultrasound measurements during normal pregnancy. *Obstet Gynecol* 1985;66:477–480.

358. Schmidt W, Yarkoni S, Jeanty P, et al. Sonographic measurements of the fetal spleen: clinical implications. *J Ultrasound Med* 1985;4:667–672.

359. Weinstein L, Anderson C. In-utero diagnosis of Beckwith-Wiedemann syndrome by ultrasound. *Radiology* 1980;134:474.

360. Ghidini A, Sirtori M, Romero R, et al. Hepatosplenomegaly as the only prenatal finding in a fetus with pyruvate kinase deficiency anemia. *Am J Perinatol* 1991;8(1):44–46.

361. Rowlands S, Murray H. Prenatal ultrasound findings in a fetus diagnosed with Gaucher's disease (type 2) at birth. *Prenat Diagn* 1997;17(8):765–769.

362. Hill LH. Sonographic detection of fetal gastrointestinal anomalies. *Ultrasound Q* 1988;6:35–67.

363. Macones GA, Johnson A, Tilley D, et al. Fetal hepatosplenomegaly associated with transient myeloproliferative disorder in trisomy 21. *Fetal Diagn Ther* 1995;10(2):131–133.

364. Hartung J, Chaoui R, Wauer R, Bollmann R. Fetal hepatosplenomegaly: an isolated sonographic sign of trisomy 21 in a case of myeloproliferative disorder. *Ultrasound Obstet Gynecol* 1998;11(6):453–455.

365. Smrcek JM, Baschat AA, Germer U, et al. Fetal hydrops and hepatosplenomegaly in the second half of pregnancy: a sign of myeloproliferative disorder in fetuses with trisomy 21. *Ultrasound Obstet Gynecol* 2001;17(5):403–409.

366. Diakoumakis EE, Weinberg B, Seife B, et al. Infantile hemangioendothelioma of the liver. *J Clin Ultrasound* 1986;14:137–139.

367. de Bievre P, Dufour P, Lefebvre C, et al. [Prenatal diagnosis of hepatic hemangioendothelioma. Apropos of a case]. [Article in French] *J Gynecol Obstet Biol Reprod (Paris)* 1994;23(4):435–439.

368. Marton T, Silhavy M, Csapo Z, et al. Multifocal hemangioendothelioma of the fetus and placenta. *Hum Pathol* 1997;28(7):866–869.

369. Mhanni AA, Chodirker BN, Evans JA, et al. Fetal hepatic haemangioendothelioma: a new association with elevated maternal serum alpha-fetoprotein. *Prenat Diagn* 2000;20(5):432–435.

370. Meirowitz NB, Guzman ER, Underberg-Davis SJ, et al. Hepatic hemangioendothelioma: prenatal sonographic findings and evolution of the lesion. *J Clin Ultrasound* 2000;28(5):258–263.

371. Gonen R, Fong K, Chiasson DA. Prenatal sonographic diagnosis of hepatic hemangioendothelioma with secondary nonimmune hydrops fetalis. *Obstet Gynecol* 1989;73(3 Pt 2):485–487.

372. Brunnelle F, Chaumont P. Hepatic tumors in children: ultrasonic differentiation of malignant from benign lesions. *Radiology* 1984;150:695–699.

373. Stanley P, Hall TR, Woolley MM, et al. Mesenchymal hamartoma of the liver in childhood: sonographic and CT findings. *AJR Am J Roentgenol* 1986;147:1035–1039.

374. Berman B, Lim HW. Concurrent cutaneous and hepatic hemangioma in infancy: report of a case and review of the literature. *J Dermatol Surg Oncol* 1978;4:869–873.

375. Shih JC, Tsao PN, Huang SF, et al. Congenital hepatoblastoma. *Ultrasound Obstet Gynecol* 2000;16(1):103.

376. Liyanage IS, Katoch D. Ultrasonic prenatal diagnosis of liver metastases from adrenal neuroblastoma. *J Clin Ultrasound* 1992;20(6):401–403.

377. Toma P, Lucigrai G, Marzoli A, Lituania M. Prenatal diagnosis of metastatic adrenal neuroblastoma with sonography and MR imaging. *AJR Am J Roentgenol* 1994;162(5):1183–1184.

378. Platt LD, DeVore GR, Benner P, et al. Antenatal diagnosis of a fetal liver mass. *J Ultrasound Med* 1983;2:521–522.

379. Nakamoto SK, Dreilinger A, Dattel B, et al. The sonographic appearance of hepatic hemangioma in-utero. *J Ultrasound Med* 1983;2:239–241.

380. Chuileannain FN, Rowlands S, Sampson A. Ultrasonographic appearances of fetal hepatic hemangioma. *J Ultrasound Med* 1999;18(5):379–381.

381. Abuhamad AZ, Lewis D, Inati MN, et al. The use of color flow Doppler in the diagnosis of fetal hepatic hemangioma. *J Ultrasound Med* 1993;12(4):223–226.

382. Stone HH, Nielson IC. Haemangioma of the liver in the newborn. *Arch Surg* 1965;90:319–322.

383. Nguyen L, Shardling B, Ein S, et al. Hepatic hemangioma in childhood: medical management or surgical management? *J Pediatr Surg* 1982;17:576–579.

384. Padalkar JA, Bapat VS, Phadke MA, Ujjainwalla F. Successful treatment of hepatic hemangiomas with corticosteroids. *Indian Pediatr* 1992;29(6):769–770.

385. Morris J, Abbott J, Burrows P, Levine D. Antenatal diagnosis of fetal hepatic hemangioma treated with maternal corticosteroids. *Obstet Gynecol* 1999;94(5 Pt 2):813–815.

386. Hirata GI, Matsunaga ML, Medearis AL, et al. Ultrasonographic diagnosis of a fetal abdominal mass: a case of a mesenchymal liver hamartoma and a review of the literature. *Prenat Diagn* 1990;10(8):507–512.

Adrenal

387. Burbidge KA. Prenatal adrenal hemorrhage confirmed by postnatal surgery. *J Urol* 1993;150:1867–1869.

388. Vollersen E, Hof M, Gembruch U. Prenatal sonographic diagnosis of fetal adrenal gland hemorrhage. *Fetal Diagn Ther* 1996;11(4):286–291.

389. Gross E, Chen MK, Lobe TE, et al. Infradiaphragmatic extralobar pulmonary sequestration masquerading as an intra-abdominal, suprarenal mass. *Pediatr Surg Int* 1997;12(7):529–531.

390. Rubenstein SC, Benacerraf BR, Retik AB, Mandell J. Fetal

suprarenal masses: sonographic appearance and differential diagnosis. *Ultrasound Obstet Gynecol* 1995;5(3):164–167.

391. Curtis MR, Mooney DP, Vaccaro TJ, et al. Prenatal ultrasound characterization of the suprarenal mass: distinction between neuroblastoma and subdiaphragmatic extralobar pulmonary sequestration. *J Ultrasound Med* 1997;16(2):75–83.

392. Mandel M, Toren A, Rechavi G, et al. Hormonal treatment in pregnancy: a possible risk factor for neuroblastoma. *Med Pediatr Oncol* 1994;23(2):133–135.

393. Hamada Y, Ikebukuro K, Sato M, et al. Prenatally diagnosed cystic neuroblastoma. *Pediatr Surg Int* 1999;15(1):71–74.

394. Jaffa AJ, Many A, Hartoov J, et al. Prenatal sonographic diagnosis of metastatic neuroblastoma: report of a case and review of the literature. *Prenat Diagn* 1993;13(1):73–77.

395. Heling KS, Chaoui R, Hartung J, et al. Prenatal diagnosis of congenital neuroblastoma. Analysis of 4 cases and review of the literature. *Fetal Diagn Ther* 1999;14(1):47–52.

396. Acharya S, Jayabose S, Kogan SJ, et al. Prenatally diagnosed neuroblastoma. *Cancer* 1997;15;80(2):304–310.

397. Hosoda Y, Miyano T, Kimura K, et al. Characteristics and management of patients with fetal neuroblastoma. *J Pediatr Surg* 1992;27(5):623–625.

398. Saylors RL 3rd, Cohn SL, Morgan ER, Brodeur GM. Prenatal detection of neuroblastoma by fetal ultrasonography. *Am J Pediatr Hematol Oncol* 1994;16(4):356–360.

399. Jennings RW, LaQuaglia MP, Leong K, et al. Fetal neuroblastoma: prenatal diagnosis and natural history. *J Pediatr Surg* 1993;28(9):1168–1174.

400. Shen MR, Lin YS, Huang SC, Chou CY. Rapid growth of a fetal abdominal mass: a case report of congenital neuroblastoma. *J Clin Ultrasound* 1997;25(1):39–42.

401. Chen CP, Chen SH, Chuang CY, et al. Clinical and perinatal sonographic features of congenital adrenal cystic neuroblastoma: a case report with review of the literature. *Ultrasound Obstet Gynecol* 1997;10(1):68–73.

402. Grasso SN, Schwartz DS, Keller MS. Disappearing suprarenal masses in fetuses and infants. *Pediatr Radiol* 1998;28(9):732.

403. Smith CR, Chan HS, deSa DJ. Placental involvement in congenital neuroblastoma. *J Clin Pathol* 1981;34(7):785–789.

404. Holgersen LO, Subramanian S, Kirpekar M, et al. Spontaneous resolution of antenatally diagnosed adrenal masses. *J Pediatr Surg* 1996;31(1):153–155.

405. Schwarzler P, Bernard JP, Senat MV, Ville Y. Prenatal diagnosis of fetal adrenal masses: differentiation between hemorrhage and solid tumor by color Doppler sonography. *Ultrasound Obstet Gynecol* 1999;13(5):351–355.

406. Hayes F, et al. Neuroblastoma. In: Pizzo PA, Poplack DG, eds. *Principles and practice of pediatric oncology.* Philadelphia: JB Lippincott Co, 1989:608–622.

Gallbladder

407. Hata K, Aoki S, Hata T, et al. Ultrasonographic identification of the human fetal gallbladder *in utero. Gynecol Obstet Invest* 1987;23(2):79–83.

408. Muller R, Dohmann S, Kordts U. [Fetal gallbladder and gallstones]. [Article in German] *Ultraschall Med* 2000;21(3):142–144.

409. Chan L, Rao BK, Jiang Y, et al. Fetal gallbladder growth and development during gestation. *J Ultrasound Med* 1995;14(6):421–425.

410. Sepulveda W, Nicolaidis P, Hollingsworth J, Fisk NM. Fetal cholecystomegaly: a prenatal marker of aneuploidy. *Prenat Diagn* 1995;15(2):193–197.

411. Hertzberg BS, Kliewer MA, Bowie JD, McNally PJ. Enlarged fetal gallbladder: prognostic importance for aneuploidy or biliary abnormality at antenatal US. *Radiology* 1998;208(3):795–798.

412. Bronshtein M, Weiner Z, Abramovici H, et al. Prenatal diagnosis of gall bladder anomalies—report of 17 cases. *Prenat Diagn* 1993;13(9):851–861.

413. Duchatel F, Muller F, Oury JF, et al. Prenatal diagnosis of cystic fibrosis: ultrasonography of the gallbladder at 17–19 weeks of gestation. *Fetal Diagn Ther* 1993;8(1):28–36.

414. Hertzberg BS, Kliewer MA, Maynor C, et al. Nonvisualization of the fetal gallbladder: frequency and prognostic importance. *Radiology* 1996;199(3):679–682.

415. Boyden EA. The accessory gallbladder. *Am J Anat* 1926;38:177–231.

416. Gross RE. Congenital anomalies of the gallbladder: a review of 148 cases with a report of double gallbladder. *Arch Surg* 1936;32:131.

417. Goiney RC, Schoenecker SA, Cyr DR, et al. Sonography of gallbladder duplication and differential considerations. *AJR Am J Roentgenol* 1985;145:241–243.

418. Nichols DM. Superior mesenteric vein rotation: a CT sign of mid-gut malrotation. *AJR Am J Roentgenol* 1983;141:707–708.

419. Granot E. Duplication of gallbladder associated with childhood obstructive biliary disease and biliary cirrhosis. *Gastroenterology* 1983;85:946–950.

420. Kiserud T, Gjelland K, Bogno H, et al. Echogenic material in the fetal gallbladder and fetal disease. *Ultrasound Obstet Gynecol* 1997;10(2):103–106.

421. Beretsky I, Lanken DH. Diagnosis of fetal cholelithiasis using real-time high-resolution imaging employing digital detection. *J Ultrasound Med* 1983;2:381–383.

422. Penzias AS, Treisman O. Vitamin K–dependent clotting factor deficiency in pregnancy. *Obstet Gynecol* 1988;72:452–454.

423. Klingensmith WC 3d, Cioffi-Ragan DT. Fetal gallstones. *Radiology* 1988;167(1):143–144.

424. Brown DL, Teele RL, Doubilet PM, et al. Echogenic material in the fetal gallbladder: sonographic and clinical observations. *Radiology* 1992;182(1):73–76.

425. Suchet IB, Labatte MF, Dyck CS, Salgado LA. Fetal cholelithiasis: a case report and review of the literature. *J Clin Ultrasound* 1993;21(3):198–202.

426. Stringer MD, Lim P, Cave M, et al. Fetal gallstones. *J Pediatr Surg* 1996;31(11):1589–1591.

427. Suma V, Marini A, Bucci N, et al. Fetal gallstones: sonographic and clinical observations. *Ultrasound Obstet Gynecol* 1998;12(6):439–441.

428. Petrikovsky B, Klein V, Holsten N. Sludge in fetal gallbladder: natural history and neonatal outcome. *Br J Radiol* 1996;69(827):1017–1018.

429. Hertzberg BS, Kliewer MA. Fetal gallstones in a contracted gallbladder: potential to simulate hepatic or peritoneal calcification. *J Ultrasound Med* 1998;17(10):667–670.

430. Keller MS, Markle BM, Laffey PA, et al. Spontaneous resolution of cholelithiasis in infants. *Radiology* 1985;157:345–348.

GENITOURINARY MALFORMATIONS

It has been 30 years since Garrett et al.[1] reported the first prenatal diagnosis of a renal abnormality using ultrasound. Since that time, there have been enormous advances in ultrasound machine technology with dramatic improvements in image resolution. Despite these improvements, the diagnosis and management of fetal renal abnormalities remains controversial in a number of areas.[2]

It has been estimated that a significant fetal structural abnormality affects 1% of pregnancies and that 20% of these affect the genitourinary system.[2] In addition, severe bilateral renal abnormalities account for 10% of all terminations for lethal fetal abnormalities.[3] Genitourinary abnormalities are common and account for a significant proportion of lethal fetal anomalies.

The incidence of antenatally detected urinary tract abnormalities varies among centers and depends on the timing of the scan. Scanning later in pregnancy detects a higher proportion of urinary tract anomalies[4,5] (Table 1). In a retrospective study comparing routine scanning at 17 and 32 weeks' gestation, Fugelseth et al.[6] detected only 32% of urinary tract anomalies at the first scan but 62% at the second. The introduction of routine midtrimester scanning in the mid-1980s and improvements in ultrasound resolution have also increased the incidence of prenatally detected urinary tract abnormalities from approximately 1 in 1,000 in the late 1980s to 1 in 200 to 300 in the late 1990s[3–14] (Table 1).

Improvements in ultrasound technology and the appropriate timing of antenatal ultrasound has led to refined prenatal diagnosis and enhanced accuracy of diagnosis.[15,16] In most series, however, a high false-positive rate remains, in the range of 39% to 52%.[3,4,17,18] The primary cause for this high rate of false-positive diagnoses is the detection of mild hydronephrosis, which subsequently resolves later in pregnancy or in the neonatal period.[3,17,18] Another problem is the lack of a clear definition of prenatal hydronephrosis, as most series use different cutoff values for renal pelvic diameters, which makes comparison of different studies very difficult. Although the exact degree of renal pelvic dilatation that requires full postnatal investigation is still not entirely resolved, some fairly clear guidelines are gradually emerging.[14]

One further controversial area is the management of fetuses with bilateral obstruction, usually secondary to posterior urethral valves. This subject has prompted considerable debate within the literature,[10,19,20] and the exact role of intrauterine therapy has yet to be clearly defined.[21–23]

The assessment and management of fetal urinary tract abnormalities is still far from clear-cut; however, the vast body of work carried out since the 1980s has improved our understanding of the natural history of many conditions and their relation to uropathies developing in the postnatal period. The involvement of multidisciplinary groups of specialists can only improve the management protocols that have been developed for fetuses presenting with a urinary tract malformation.

EMBRYOLOGY

The kidneys arise from the intermediate mesoderm on either side of the dorsal body wall. The bladder is formed from the cloaca, a distal expansion of the hindgut, and the genital tracts develop from the genital ridges situated medial to the intermediate mesoderm and the paramesonephric ducts.[24]

At the beginning of the fourth week, the intermediate mesoderm on either side of the spine differentiates into the pronephros and mesonephros, which subsequently regress, and the metanephros or metanephric blastema situated in the sacral region, which ultimately develops into the definitive kidney (Fig. 1A).

The ureteric bud grows out of the distal mesonephric duct and induces formation of the kidney from the metanephric blastema. The ureteric bud penetrates the metanephric blastema and then divides to form the collecting systems and ureters. Similarly, the metanephric blastema differentiates to form the nephrons, and by the tenth week the kidney becomes functional[24] (Fig. 1B through D). If the ureteric buds fail to communicate with the metanephric blastema, the definitive kidney does not form and renal agenesis results. Similarly, if the nephrons fail to connect to the collecting ducts, cystic renal disease will result. During the sixth to ninth weeks, the kidneys move up from the sac-

TABLE 1. INCIDENCE OF PRENATALLY DETECTED UROPATHIES

Reference	Year	Center	Incidence
7	1984	Lund, Sweden	1:1,200
8	1986	Malmö, Sweden	1:330
9	1988	Nottingham, UK	1:935
10	1989	Leeds, UK	1:600
4[a]	1989	Stoke-on-Trent, UK	1:154
11	1990	Hameenlinna, Finland	1:208
3	1993	Northern Region, UK	1:333
12	1994	Westmead, Australia	1:200
5[a]	1995	Aukland, New Zealand	1:70
14	1998	Nottingham, UK	1:364
13	1998	Cleveland, UK	1:200

[a]Studies based on ultrasound scanning at 28 weeks' gestation. Reproduced with permission from Thomas DFM. Prenatally detected uropathies: epidemiological considerations. *Br J Urol* 1998;81(Suppl 2):8–12.

ral region to the lumbar position. Failure of ascent results in a pelvic kidney, and fusion of the lower poles of the kidneys produces a horseshoe kidney (Fig. 2).

During weeks 4 to 6, the urorectal septum separates the cloaca into an anterior primitive urogenital sinus and a posterior rectum.[24] The bladder is formed from the superior part of the primitive urogenital sinus, which is continuous with the allantois (Fig. 3). The part of the urogenital sinus just below the bladder forms the membranous urethra in females and the membranous and prostatic urethra in males. The definitive urogenital sinus develops into the vestibule of the vagina in females and the penile urethra in males[25] (Fig. 3). At the same time, the ureters (derived from the ureteric buds) implant into the posterior wall of the future bladder.

The genital tracts arise from the genital ridges just medial to the mesonephros. The genital ridges represent primordial germ cells that migrate from the yolk sac during the fourth week. The gonads arise from the genital ridges, and male-female differentiation occurs at approximately 8 weeks. In the female, the gonad forms the ovary and a paramesonephric duct forms, which develops into the fallopian tubes, uterus, and superior part of the vagina. In the male, the gonad forms the testis and the mesonephric duct forms the vas deferens. In the female, the mesonephric duct regresses[24] (Fig. 4).

The development of the external genitalia is remarkably similar for males and females up to 7 weeks. Early in the fifth week two swellings occur on either side of the cloacal membrane called the *cloacal folds*. These folds join anteriorly to form the genital tubercle and posteriorly develop into the urogenital folds on either side of the urogenital membrane. Two further labioscrotal swellings appear on either side of the urogenital folds. After 7 weeks in the male the genital tubercle becomes the penis and the urogenital folds become the penile urethra. In the female the

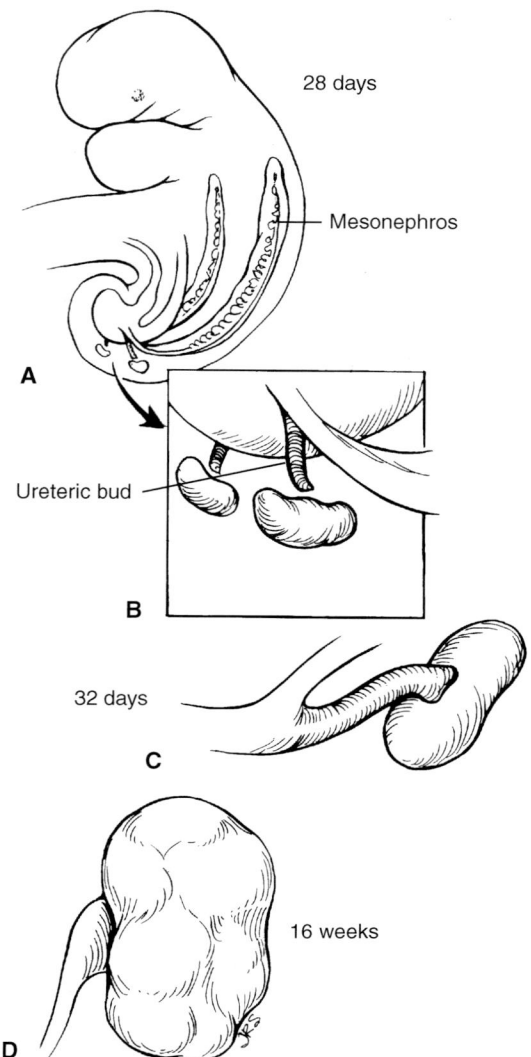

FIGURE 1. Formation of the definitive kidney. **A:** The metanephric blastema develops on each side of the body early in the fifth week. **B:** The ureteric bud grows out to the metanephric blastema. **C:** The ureteric bud bifurcates to produce superior and inferior lobes in the metanephros. **D:** Additional lobules form during the next 10 weeks in response to further bifurcation of the ureteric buds. (Reproduced with permission from Larson WJ. *Human embryology.* London: Churchill Livingstone, 1993.)

genital tubercle becomes the clitoris, the urogenital membrane breaks down to form the vagina, and the labioscrotal folds form the labia majora[24] (Fig. 5). In the male the labioscrotal folds develop into the scrotum, and later in fetal life the testes descend into the scrotum through the inguinal canals.

The end result of these complex series of events is that by approximately 10 weeks' gestation both kidneys have formed and are producing urine. By 20 weeks, when the collecting system is completely developed, approximately one-third of nephrons are present. Nephrogenesis continues at a nearly exponential rate and is complete by 36 weeks.[2]

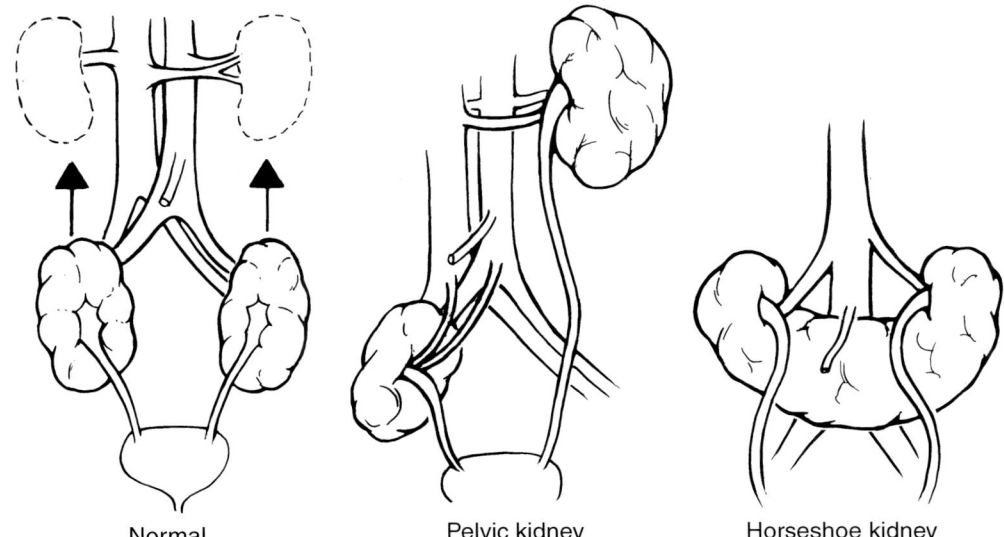

A–C   Normal   Pelvic kidney   Horseshoe kidney

FIGURE 2. Normal and abnormal ascent of the kidneys. **A:** The metanephros ascends from the sacral region to the definitive lumbar position between the sixth and ninth weeks. **B:** A kidney may fail to ascend, resulting in a pelvic kidney. **C:** If the inferior poles make contact and fuse, the result is a horseshoe kidney. (Reproduced with permission from Larson WJ. *Human embryology.* London: Churchill Livingstone, 1993.)

NORMAL APPEARANCES

Using transvaginal sonography the fetal kidneys can be demonstrated as early as 9 weeks' gestation.[26] However, at 12 weeks' gestation 86% to 99% of fetal kidneys can be demonstrated, whereas at 13 weeks 92% to 99% can be demonstrated.[27,28] At this stage of pregnancy the kidneys appear as bilateral hyperechoic structures in the paravertebral regions (Fig. 6). The renal pelves can often be seen as sonolucent areas medially. The bladder is identified as a rounded echo-free area situated centrally within the pelvis, and color-flow Doppler imaging is useful to localize it as both umbilical arteries split around the bladder (Fig. 7).

In scans at 18 to 20 weeks the kidneys are also slightly hyperechoic with regard to surrounding tissues such as bowel and paravertebral tissues. On coronal scans the kidneys are bounded medially by the psoas muscles and superiorly by the adrenal glands, which appear as crescentic hypoechoic structures embracing the upper poles of the kidneys (Fig. 8). The renal pyramids may be seen as hypo-

echoic structures within the renal parenchyma and should not be mistaken for renal cysts. The renal pelves may be seen as echo-free areas medially.

On transverse scanning the kidneys are demonstrated as circular structures and accurate measurements can be made of the renal pelves, particularly with the spine uppermost (Fig. 9). The upper limit of normal is 4 mm up to 33 weeks' gestation and 7 mm from 33 weeks to term.[29]

The ureters are not normally seen; however, with high-resolution scanners, ureters measuring 1 mm or less in diameter can occasionally be demonstrated during a midtrimester scan (Fig. 10). These appearances are likely to be physiologic; however, ureters measuring 2 to 3 mm or more in diameter should certainly raise the possibility of vesicoureteric reflux or obstruction.

As in the first trimester, the bladder is seen as a circular echo-poor area centrally positioned within the pelvis (Fig. 11). The rectum may be seen posteriorly on transverse scanning, and both umbilical arteries are seen to split around the bladder using color-flow Doppler imaging (Fig.

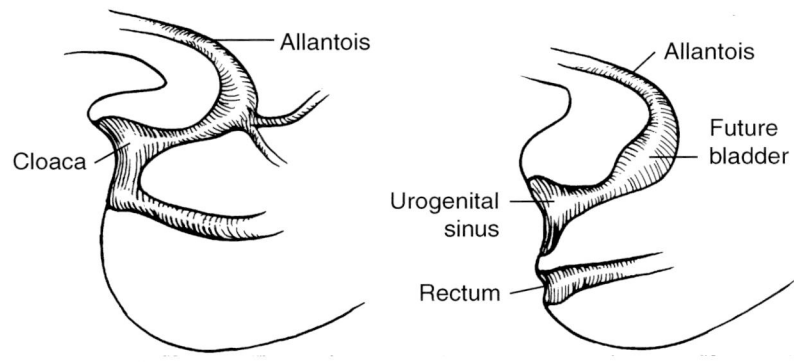

FIGURE 3. Formation of the bladder and rectum. The bladder and rectum form from the cloaca. The urorectal septum separates the bladder from the rectum. The urogenital sinus becomes the penile urethra in the male and the vestibule of the vagina in the female. (Reproduced with permission from Larson WJ. *Human embryology.* London: Churchill Livingstone, 1993.)

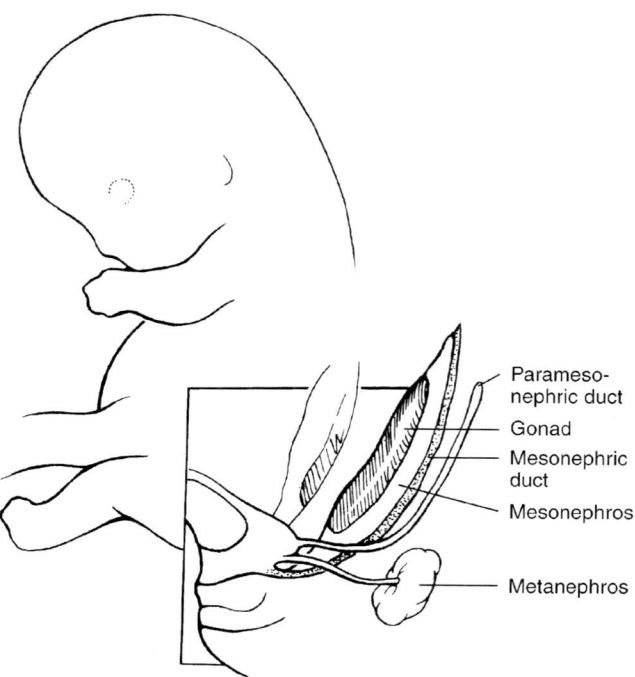

FIGURE 4. Formation of the genital ridges. The primitive gonads arise from the genital ridges, which are situated just medial to the developing mesonephros. (Reproduced with permission from Larson WJ. *Human embryology.* London: Churchill Livingstone, 1993.)

12). The normal bladder wall measures up to 2 mm in diameter and is best measured at the level of the umbilical artery (Fig. 13).

SONOGRAPHIC APPROACH

Assessment of the fetal urinary tract involves a logical approach with assessment of the fetal kidneys, bladder, and liquor volume.

Both kidneys should be present, as described in the previous section. The absence of a kidney should prompt a search for a kidney in an ectopic location, most commonly the fetal pelvis. If there is no pelvic kidney, then unilateral renal agenesis is the most likely diagnosis. Another possibility, however, is crossed renal ectopia, and in this condition the contralateral kidney is large and unusually shaped. If both kidneys are absent, severe oligohydramnios associated with absence of the bladder is usually seen.

The presence of macroscopic cysts affecting a kidney usually indicates a multicystic dysplastic kidney. In unilateral disease liquor volume is normal, but the presence of unilateral renal disease of whatever nature requires careful assessment of the contralateral kidney and a careful search for any associated abnormalities.

Although a multicystic kidney is usually a straightforward diagnosis to make, care should be taken not to con-

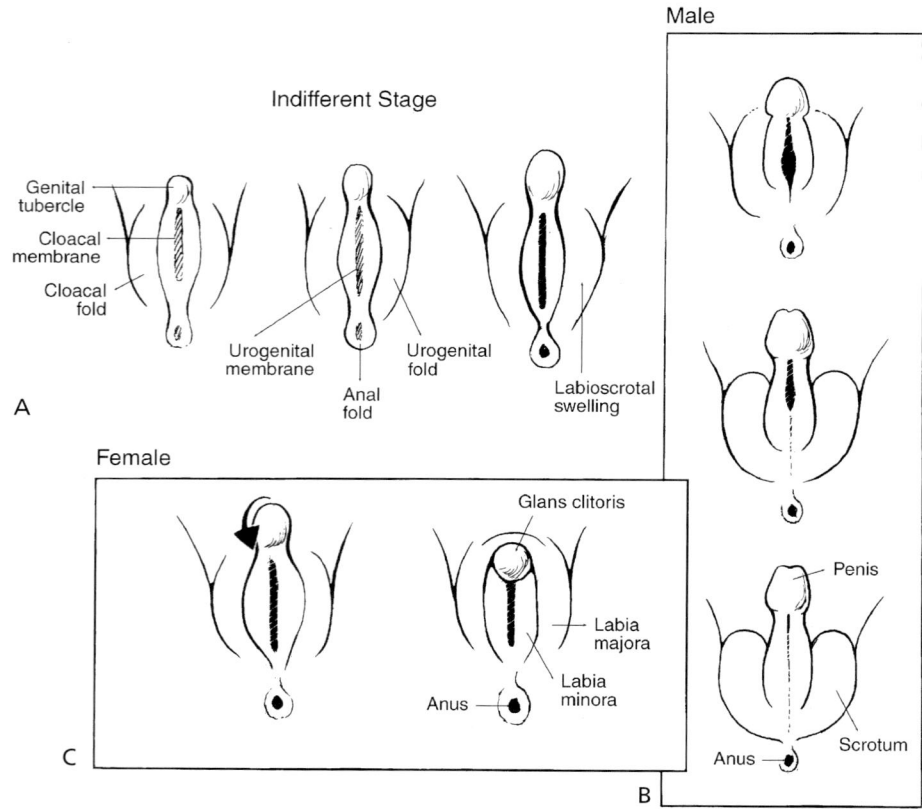

FIGURE 5. Formation of the external genitalia in males and females. **A:** The external genitalia form from a pair of labioscrotal folds, a pair of urogenital folds, and an anterior genital tubercle. Male and female genitalia are morphologically indistinguishable at this stage. **B:** In males, the urogenital folds fuse and the genital tubercle elongates to form the shaft and glans of the penis. Fusion of the urogenital folds encloses the definitive urogenital sinus to form most of the penile urethra. A small region of the distal urethra is formed by the invagination of ectoderm covering the glans. The labioscrotal folds give rise to the scrotum. **C:** In females, the genital tubercle bends inferiorly to form the clitoris, and the urogenital folds remain separated to form the labia minora. The labioscrotal folds form the labia majora.

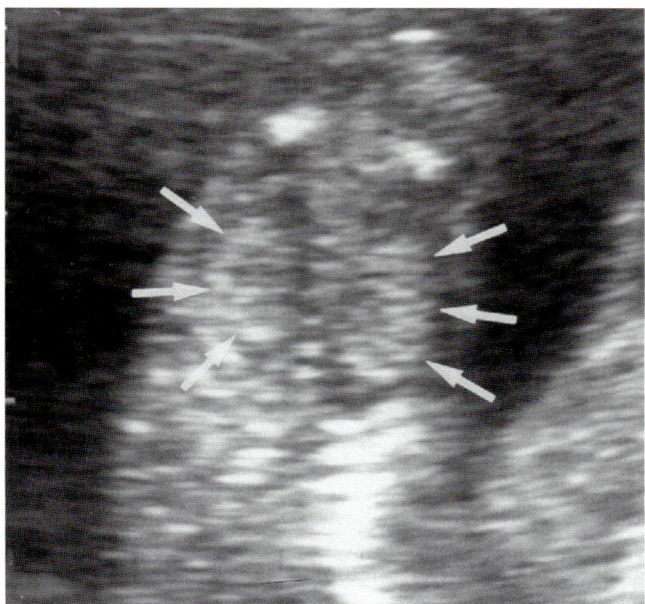

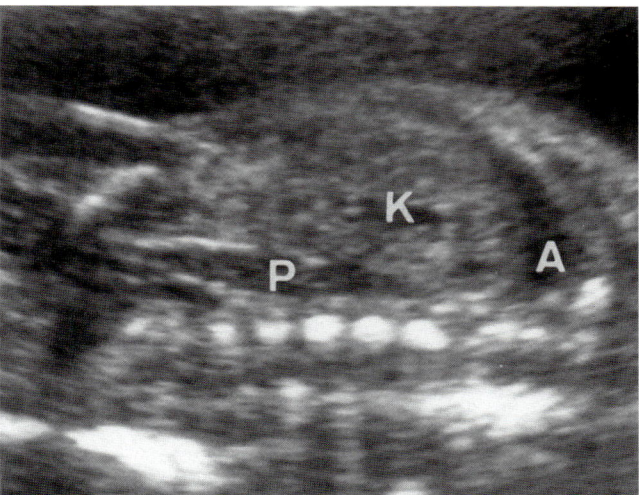

FIGURE 8. Coronal scan through the fetal kidneys. The fetal kidney (*K*) rests on the psoas muscle (*P*) and is outlined superiorly by the adrenal gland (*A*).

FIGURE 6. Normal fetal kidneys at 12 to 13 weeks. A transvaginal scan in the coronal plane shows both fetal kidneys (outlined by *arrows*). At this stage of gestation, the fetal kidneys have an increased echogenicity.

fuse this condition with hydronephrosis. On occasion, a multicystic kidney demonstrates a large central cyst with multiple small peripheral cysts, thus mimicking a pelviureteric junction obstruction. In this situation it is important to demonstrate that the cysts do not communicate, because this finding is more indicative of hydronephrosis.

In addition, the demonstration of a single macroscopic cyst usually indicates a simple renal cyst.

Large echogenic kidneys usually indicate either infantile polycystic renal disease or occasionally adult-type polycystic disease. Liquor volume is usually reduced in the former but normal in the latter. Large echogenic kidneys can also be part of a number of syndromes, such as trisomy 13 or Meckel-Gruber syndrome, so a careful search for associated anomalies is essential. Normal-sized echogenic kidneys may be a normal finding or can also be a sign of some form of renal dysplasia.

Dilatation of the renal collecting system suggests either hydronephrosis or reflux. Initially the affected kidney is scrutinized, and if the dilatation affects just the upper pole

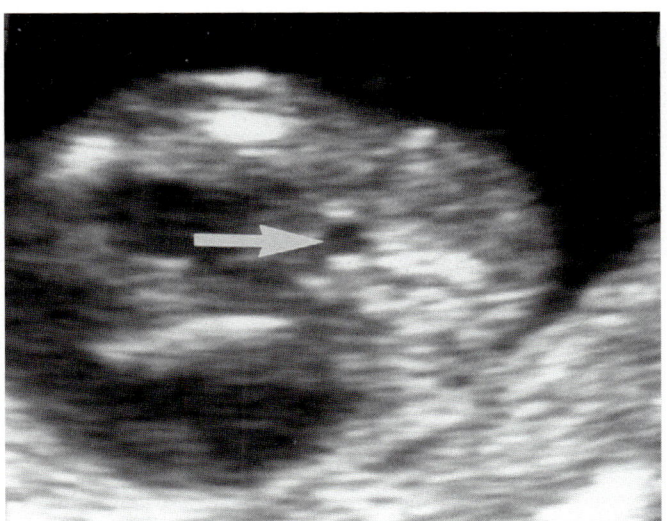

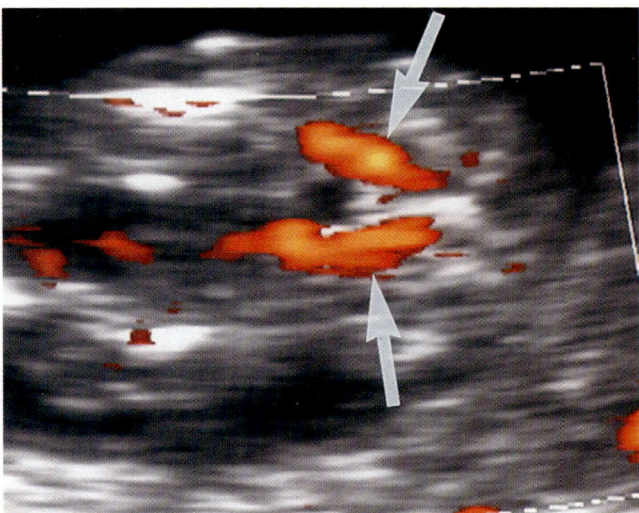

A

B

FIGURE 7. A: The fetal bladder: transvaginal scan in the transverse plane through the fetal pelvis. The bladder (*arrow*) is situated centrally within the pelvis. **B:** With color-flow Doppler imaging, both umbilical arteries (*arrows*) are shown separating around the bladder. This is a useful technique for demonstrating the position of the fetal bladder.

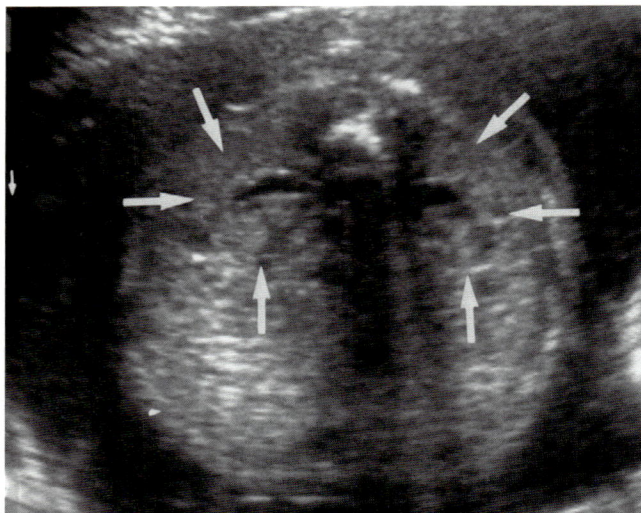

FIGURE 9. Transverse scan through the fetal kidneys. Both kidneys are seen in a paravertebral location and are outlined by arrows. Both renal pelvises are seen centrally.

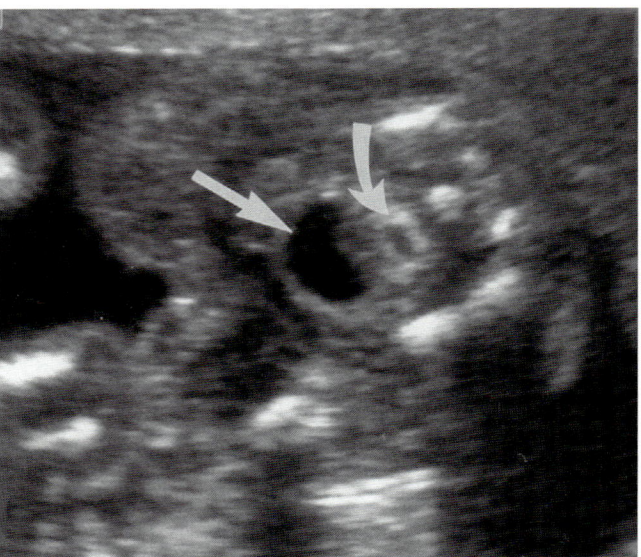

FIGURE 11. Normal bladder. A transverse scan through the fetal pelvis demonstrates the bladder (*straight arrow*) and rectum (*curved arrow*).

of the kidney then there may be a duplex system. In that setting the bladder is assessed with a view to demonstrate a ureterocele. When the whole collecting system is involved, a simple hydronephrosis may be the cause. The level of obstruction is determined by the degree of dilatation of the renal pelvis and ureter. Dilatation of the renal pelvis usually only indicates a pelviureteric junction obstruction, whereas ureteric dilatation suggests either a vesicoureteric junction obstruction or reflux.

In the presence of hydronephrosis the echogenicity of the renal parenchyma should be analyzed. The demonstration of echogenic cortex with subcapsular cysts indicates secondary renal dysplasia and poor function of the affected kidney.

As in all cases of unilateral disease the contralateral kidney must be assessed.

Bilateral hydronephrosis should always raise the possibility of bladder outlet obstruction, and ureteric dilatation should be present; the bladder wall may be thickened with dilatation of the posterior urethra. In the setting of bilateral hydronephrosis, assessment of liquor volume is extremely important. Although most experi-

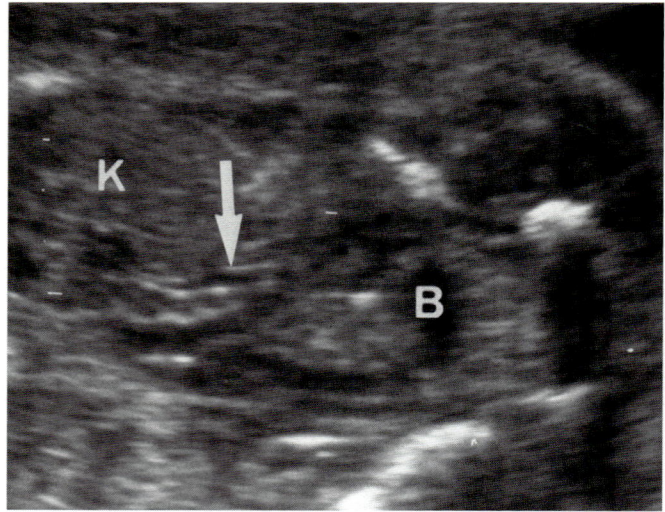

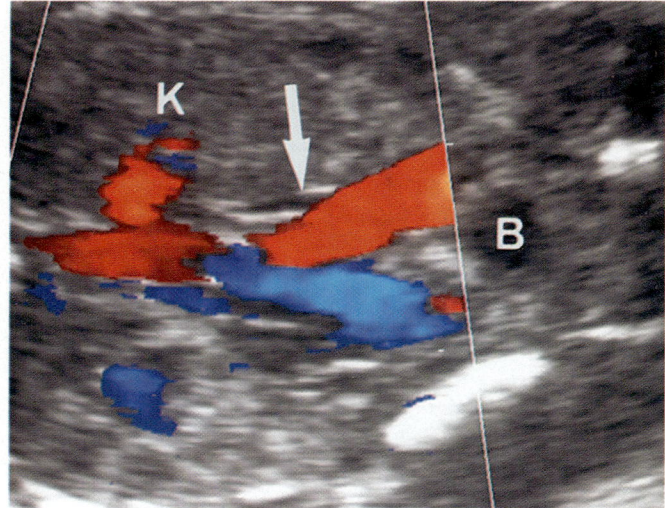

A   B

FIGURE 10. Ureter. **A:** A coronal scan through the paravertebral regions demonstrates the ureter (*arrow*). The normal fetal ureteric diameter is 1 to 2 mm. **B:** A color-flow scan in same plane shows the ureter (*arrow*) separate from the iliac artery (in red). B, bladder; K, kidney.

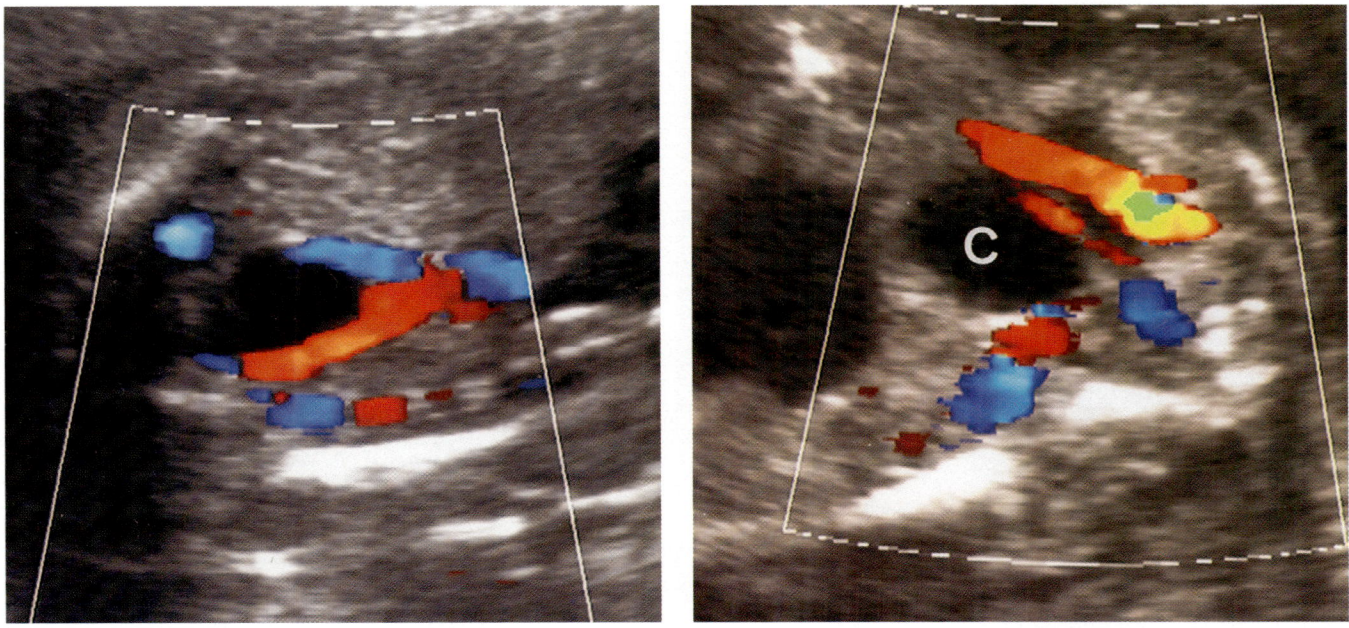

A

B

FIGURE 12. Bladder. **A:** Color-flow Doppler imaging demonstrates both umbilical arteries separating around the bladder. **B:** Large cyst (*C*) displacing the bladder. This color-flow Doppler image shows bladder position.

enced sonologists subjectively assess liquor, a more objective approach—particularly if serial measurements are to be made—is use of the amniotic fluid index.[30] Using this technique, amniotic fluid is measured in four quadrants, and the sum of the measurements is plotted on a normal range chart (Fig. 14). Bilateral hydronephrosis and hydroureters can be associated with vesicoureteric reflux; however, in this setting, even though the bladder

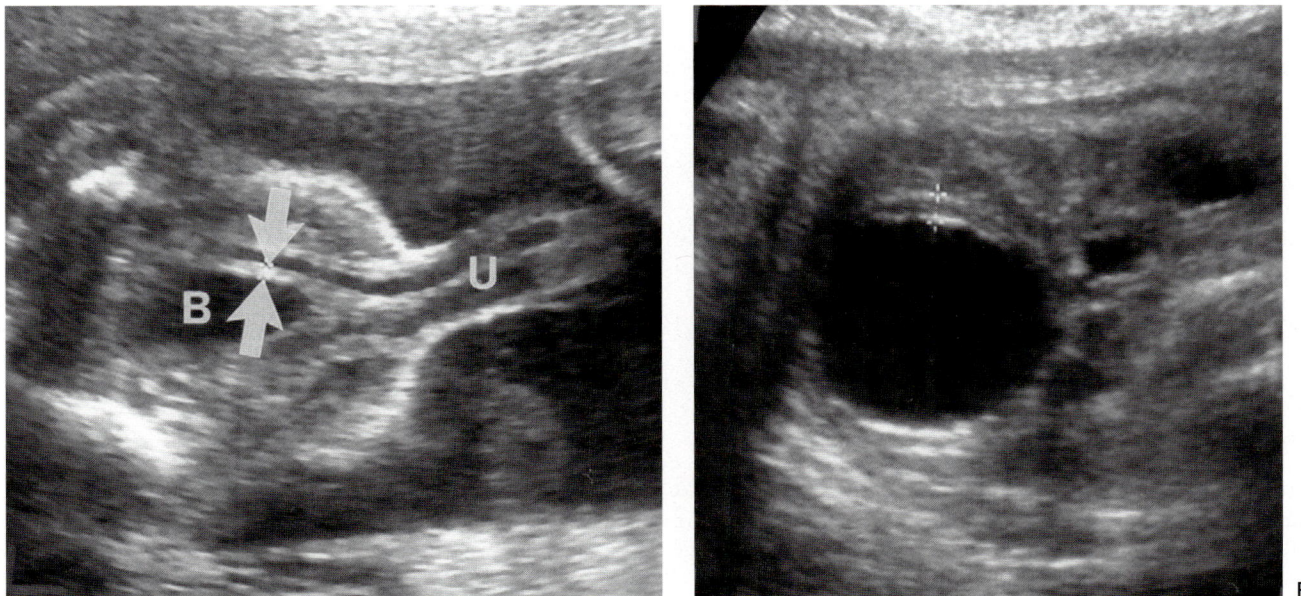

A

B

FIGURE 13. Measurement of bladder wall thickness. **A:** A transverse scan through the fetal pelvis shows the level at which the bladder wall is measured. The bladder wall is best measured at the point where the umbilical artery separates around the bladder (*B*). Arrows demonstrate the bladder wall thickness. U, umbilical cord. **B:** A thick-walled bladder. The measurement of the bladder wall thickness was 4.2 mm. The upper limit of normal is 2 mm. (Reproduced with permission from Twining P, McHugo J, Pilling D. *Textbook of fetal abnormalities*. London: Churchill Livingstone, 2000.)

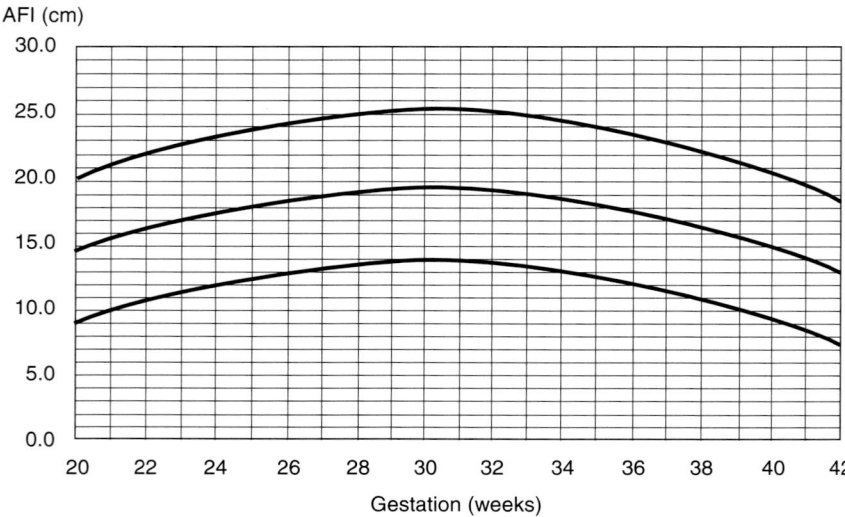

FIGURE 14. Graph of the normal range for amniotic fluid index (AFI). (Reproduced with permission from Ninosu EC, Welch CR, Manasse PR, Walkingshaw SA. Longitudinal assessment of amniotic fluid index. *Br J Obstet Gynaecol* 1993;100:816–819.)

may be distended, the wall is usually not thickened and liquor volume is normal.

The assessment of the urinary tract, therefore, requires a careful assessment of the location, size, and echogenicity of both kidneys and the presence or absence of cysts. In addition, when dilatation of the collecting system occurs, the level and degree of dilatation must be determined as well as whether it is unilateral or bilateral. The bladder should always be carefully evaluated, as should liquor volume (Fig. 15).

URINARY TRACT ABNORMALITIES

Renal Agenesis

Renal agenesis is the absence of one or both kidneys.

Incidence

The incidence of unilateral renal agenesis is 1 in 1,000 live births[31] and of bilateral renal agenesis is 1 in 4,000.[32] Unilateral renal agenesis occurs equally in males and females,[33] whereas bilateral renal agenesis occurs up to three times more frequently in boys.[34–36]

Etiology

The true etiology of renal agenesis is unknown; however, in the older child and adult it has been suggested that some cases could be caused by multicystic dysplastic kidneys that have involuted.[31,37]

Embryology

The definitive kidney arises from the metanephric blastema situated in the sacral region. The kidney appears to rely on an inductive signal from the ureteric bud that grows out from the distal mesonephric duct. If the ureteric bud fails to reach the metanephric blastema and induce formation of the kidney, renal agenesis results (Fig. 1).

Diagnosis

Bilateral renal agenesis is usually associated with severe oligohydramnios with absence of both kidneys and the bladder. However, liquor volume can be relatively normal up to 16 weeks' gestation in cases of bilateral renal agenesis.[32]

The diagnosis can be difficult to make because oligohydramnios is severe and the fetus is often curled up deep in the pelvis. In practice there are two approaches to this problem. When the fetus is cephalic, the fetal abdomen and pelvis can often be demonstrated using high-resolution transabdominal scanning. Absence of the kidneys is usually indicated by the adrenal glands' filling the renal fossae, producing the "lying down adrenal sign"[38] (Fig. 16). The diagnosis can be confirmed by demonstrating absence of both renal arteries using color-flow Doppler imaging[39] (Fig. 17). The bladder will be absent, and color-flow Doppler imaging can also be used to localize it, as both umbilical arteries split around the bladder before joining the iliac arteries (Fig. 18).

When the fetus is breech, transabdominal scanning is unable to demonstrate the fetal abdomen because it is usually deep within the maternal pelvis. Transvaginal scanning is very useful in this setting because the combination of a high-frequency transducer in close proximity to the fetus compensates for the lack of liquor and difficult fetal lie.[40,41]

Some workers have used other techniques to assess suspected renal agenesis, including intraamniotic and intraperitoneal infusion of fluid[42,43]; however, these measures are not indicated in most cases. Umbilical artery Doppler imaging, however, can be of value if intrauterine growth restriction is suspected, as the waveforms should be abnormal.[44]

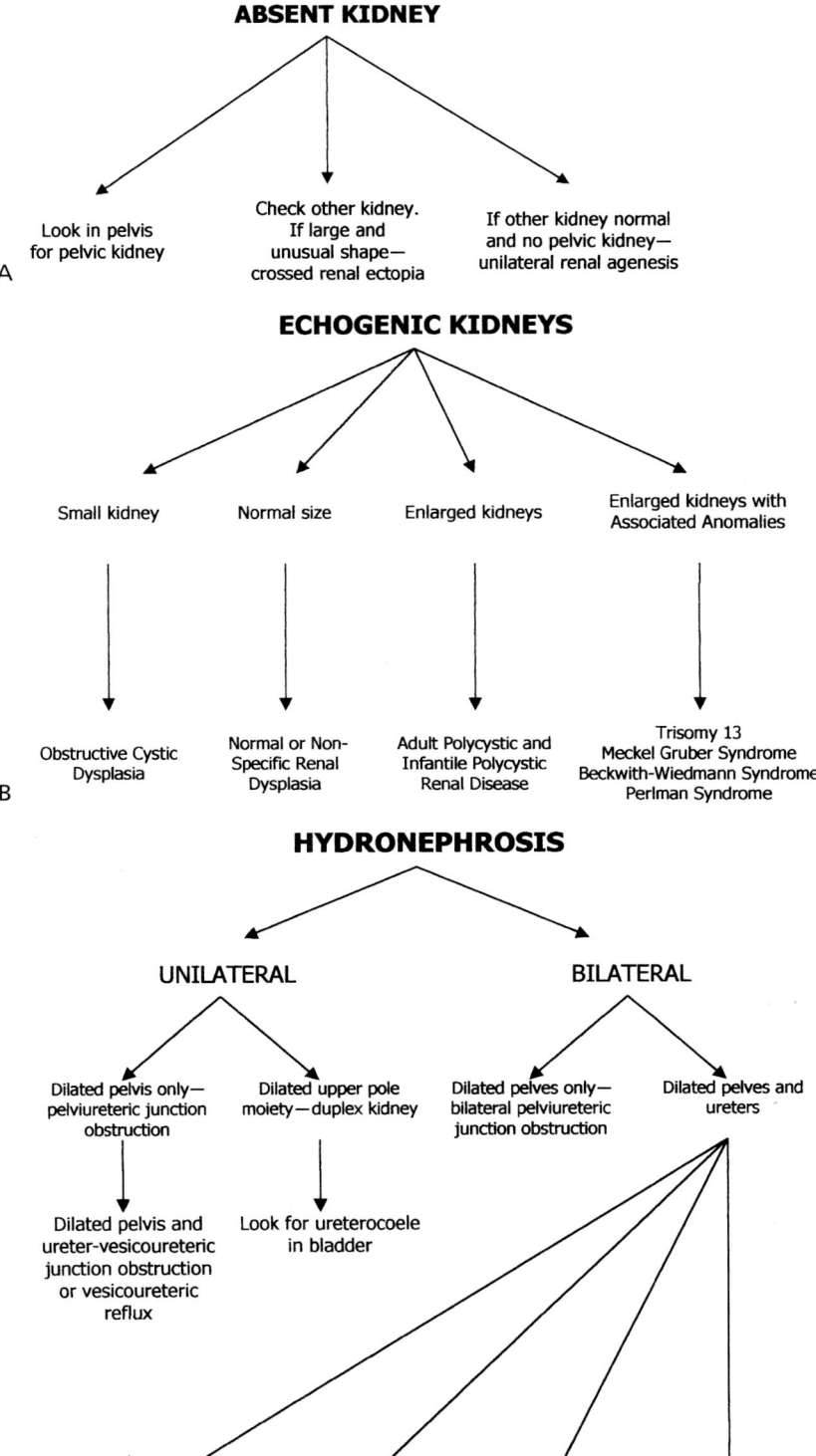

FIGURE 15. Algorithms for the assessment of absent kidney **(A)**, echogenic kidneys **(B)**, and hydronephrosis **(C)**.

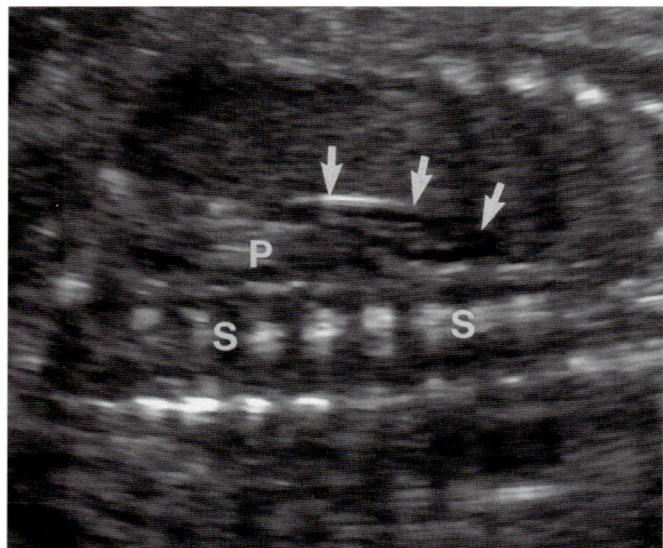

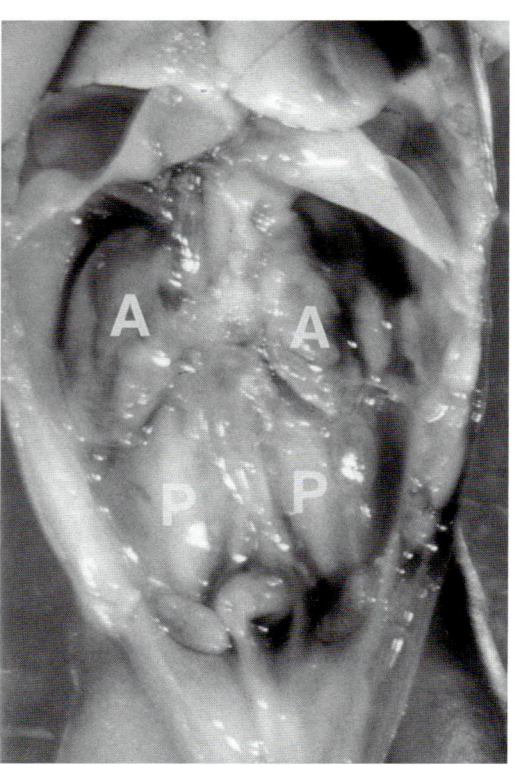

FIGURE 16. Renal agenesis. **A:** A coronal scan through a renal fossa shows absence of the kidney and the adrenal gland (*arrows*) flattened onto the psoas muscle (*P*). S, spine. **B:** A postmortem photograph of a fetus with renal agenesis. A, adrenal glands. (Reproduced with permission from Twining P, McHugo J, Pilling D. *Textbook of fetal abnormalities*. London: Churchill Livingstone, 2000.)

Unilateral renal agenesis is a diagnosis that can be very easy to miss unless a meticulous assessment is made of both renal fossae. In much the same way as in bilateral renal agenesis, the adrenal gland fills the renal fossa, producing a unilateral lying down adrenal sign, which can also be confirmed using color-flow Doppler imaging (Fig. 19). When absence of one kidney is demonstrated, a careful search should be made in the fetal pelvis for a pelvic kidney and the contralateral kidney should be evaluated to exclude crossed renal ectopia.[45]

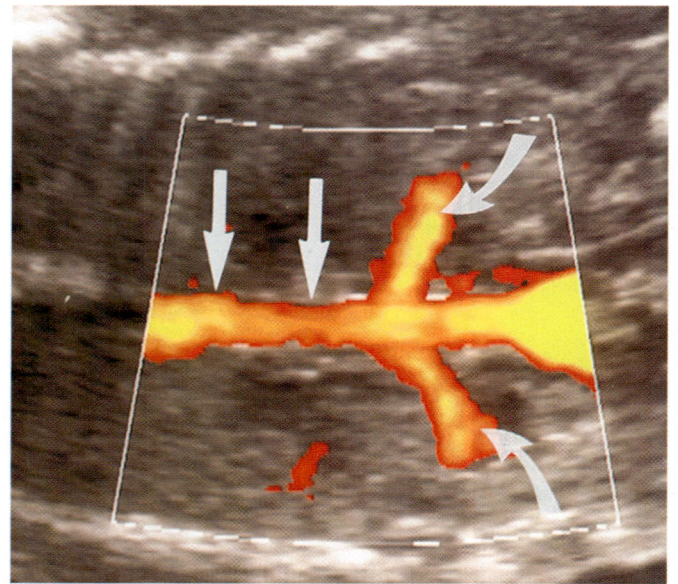

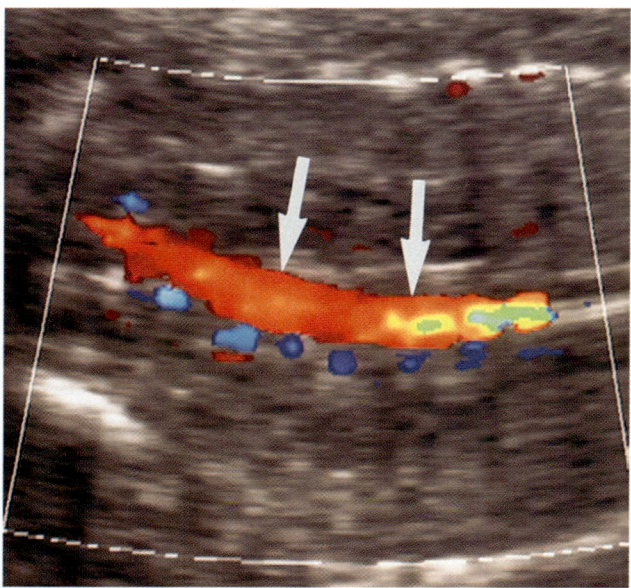

FIGURE 17. Color-flow Doppler assessment of renal agenesis. **A:** Normal appearance. Straight arrows outline the aorta, and curved arrows point to both renal arteries. **B:** Renal agenesis. Absence of the renal arteries is noted while the aorta is clearly shown (*arrows*).

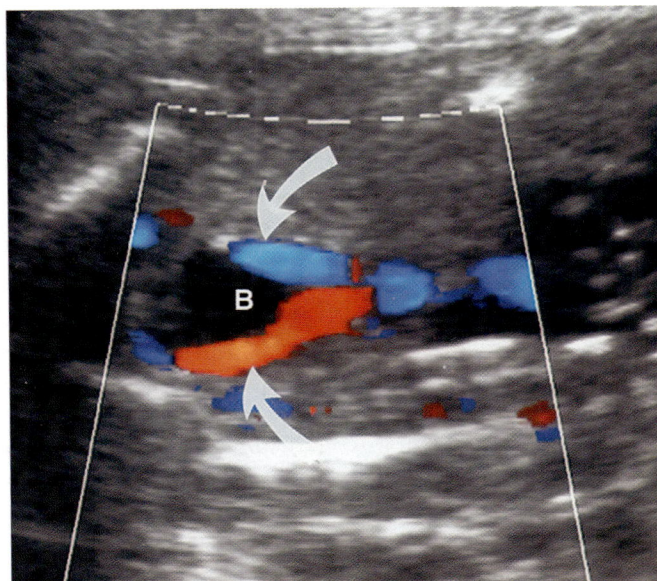 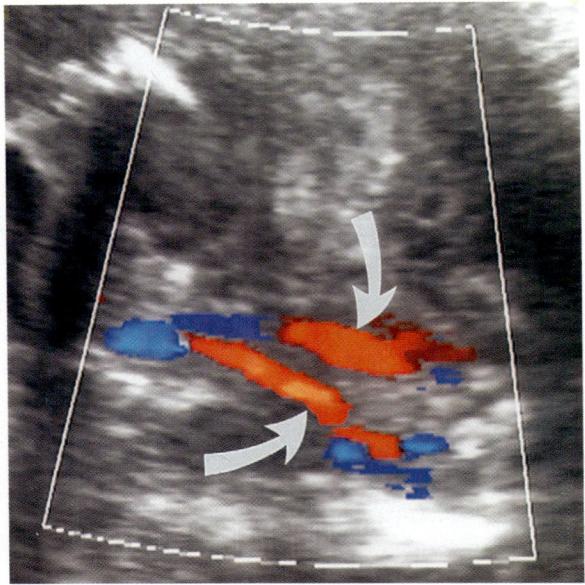

FIGURE 18. Color-flow Doppler assessment of bladder position. **A:** Normal appearance. Both umbilical arteries separate around the bladder (*B*). **B:** Renal agenesis. Both umbilical arteries (*curved arrows*) are seen to separate; however, there is absence of the bladder.

Differential Diagnosis

The differential diagnosis includes other causes of severe oligohydramnios in the second trimester, particularly severe bilateral renal disease. The most common include bilateral multicystic kidneys and infantile polycystic renal disease. Severe bladder outlet obstruction also pro-

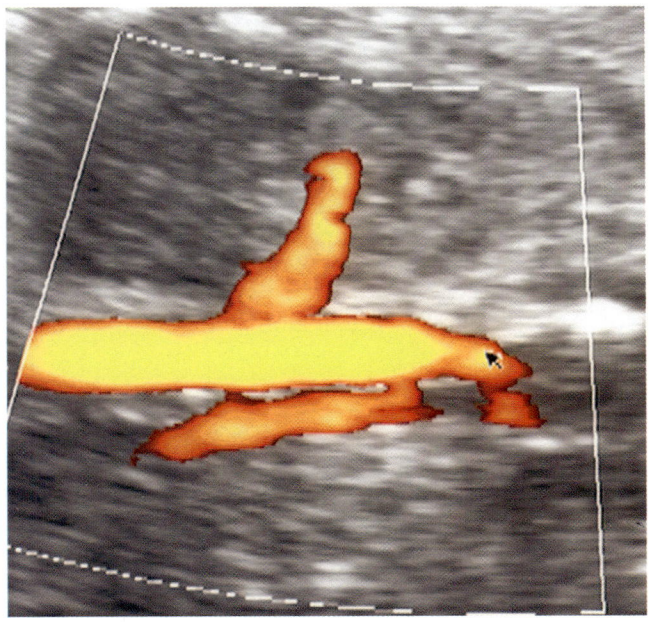

FIGURE 19. Unilateral renal agenesis. A color-flow Doppler image demonstrates a single renal artery, indicating unilateral renal agenesis. The arrow indicates the aorta.

duces oligohydramnios. The two main other causes are severe early intrauterine growth restriction (either secondary to early uteroplacental insufficiency or chromosomal disease such as triploidy) and spontaneous rupture of the membranes.

Making a correct diagnosis in the setting of severe oligohydramnios can be a challenge and depends on meticulous scanning technique. As described earlier absence of the kidneys with the adrenals lying within the renal fossae and an absent bladder confirms bilateral renal agenesis. Bilateral multicystic dysplastic kidneys should be evident by the presence of distinct cysts of varying size within both renal fossae and absence of the bladder. The kidneys in infantile polycystic renal disease are usually enlarged and echogenic if oligohydramnios is present. In severe bladder outlet obstructions the bladder is usually massively distended and fills the uterine cavity. In this situation it can be difficult to demonstrate the anatomy of the fetus.

In severe early growth restriction both kidneys and the bladder should be present and an abnormal umbilical artery Doppler waveform is seen. In spontaneous rupture of the membranes, both kidneys and the bladder are present and there is usually a history of fluid loss per vaginam.

Occasionally no cause can be found for second-trimester oligohydramnios, and the author has seen a number of cases of unexplained or idiopathic oligohydramnios.[46] In most cases liquor volume increases as the pregnancy continues and the outcome is good in the majority of fetuses. When the oligohydramnios persists, however, the outcome is likely to be poor.[35]

Associated Anomalies

Associated anomalies are seen in more than 50% of fetuses with bilateral renal agenesis. All fetuses with bilateral renal agenesis demonstrate the typical Potter facies of low-set ears, a beaked nose, and receding chin in association with limb deformities and pulmonary hypoplasia. These findings are a consequence of the severe oligohydramnios and not considered true associated anomalies.

The major associated anomalies are cardiac, seen in approximately 25%, cardiac defects and the VATER (*ve*rtebral defects, *a*nal atresia, *t*racheo-*e*sophageal, *r*adial and renal anomalies) association seen in 27%, digital anomalies (15%), and mullerian anomalies (20%).[35] Other less common associations are neural tube defects, hydrocephalus, microcephaly, and gastrointestinal tract anomalies such as anal atresia, duodenal atresia, and omphalocele.[47] Diaphragmatic hernia and facial clefting have also been reported.[36]

In addition, there are a number of rare genetic syndromes in which bilateral renal agenesis may be a feature; these are outlined in Table 2.

In unilateral renal agenesis there is a high incidence of contralateral renal abnormalities. Postnatal studies have shown that up to 48% of neonates have associated renal anomalies, the most common being vesicoureteric reflux (28%), vesicoureteric junction obstruction (11%), and pelviureteric junction obstruction (7%).[33,48,49]

Prognosis

In bilateral renal agenesis the outcome is extremely poor, with all babies dying within the first few hours or days of life from pulmonary hypoplasia. Unilateral renal agenesis has a good outcome with normal life expectancy. However, long-term follow-up of patients with unilateral renal agenesis has shown an increased risk of proteinuria (19%), hypertension (47%), and renal insufficiency.[50]

Management

Due to the uniformly lethal nature of bilateral renal agenesis, termination of pregnancy can be offered to the mother.

TABLE 2. SYNDROMES ASSOCIATED WITH RENAL AGENESIS

Syndrome	Clinical findings
Fraser syndrome	Autosomal recessive, cryptophthalmos, syndactyly, cleft palate, laryngeal atresia
Cerebro-oculo-facial skeletal syndrome	Autosomal recessive, microcephaly, micrognathia, kyphosis, rockerbottom feet, contractions of extremities
Acrorenal-mandibular syndrome	Autosomal recessive, split hand, split foot, genital malformations
Branchiootorenal syndrome	Autosomal dominant, preauricular pits, branchial fistulas

As bilateral renal agenesis is a rare finding in the common chromosomal defects, one would not routinely offer a karyotyping procedure in this setting. When the mother does not wish to undergo a termination of pregnancy, conservative management is appropriate.

Fetuses with unilateral renal agenesis require follow-up in the neonatal period with a view to excluding reflux and other contralateral renal abnormalities.[33]

Recurrence Risk

The overall recurrence risk for bilateral renal agenesis is between 3% and 6%.[34,51,52] Up to 9% of parents and siblings of patients with unilateral renal agenesis have asymptomatic renal malformations, compared to a normal adult frequency of 0.3%.[27]

In cases of autosomal dominant and recessive conditions the recurrence risk is 50% and 25%, respectively. Rarely the recurrence rate is even higher; the author has seen one couple with four consecutive fetuses with bilateral renal agenesis.

Renal Ectopia

An ectopic kidney lies outside its normal position in the renal fossa. The most common position is the pelvis in 55%, followed by crossed fused ectopia in 27%, lumbar in 12%, and nonfused ectopia in 5%. Very rarely, an ectopic kidney is thoracic.[53] Ectopic kidney has an incidence of approximately 1 in 1,200.[54]

Pelvic Kidney

Pelvic kidney is a kidney that is situated within the pelvis.

Incidence
The true incidence of pelvic kidney is unknown because the vast majority are asymptomatic. The most likely figure is in the region of 1 in 700.[53,54]

Etiology
A pelvic kidney occurs when the definitive kidney fails to ascend to the lumbar region during the sixth to ninth weeks.

Diagnosis
Scanning the renal fossa reveals absence of the kidney and the presence of the adrenal gland (Fig. 20). The kidney is seen within the pelvis lying superior to the bladder (Fig. 21).

Differential Diagnosis
The differential diagnosis includes unilateral renal agenesis, and in practice it can be quite difficult to visualize the pelvic kidney because its acoustic density is similar to that of the surrounding bowel.

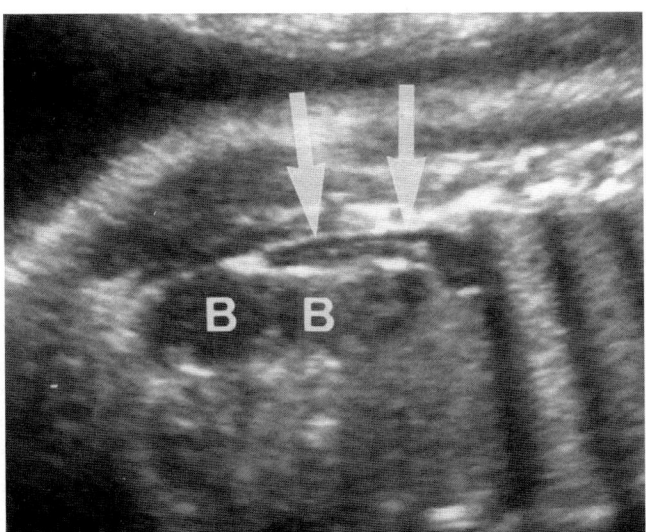

FIGURE 20. Empty renal fossa. A sagittal scan of renal fossa shows absent kidney and flattened adrenal glands (*arrows*). B, bowel.

Associated Anomalies

There is no specific pattern of anomalies; however, intracranial abnormalities have been reported[54] as well as multiple congenital anomalies involving the skeletal, cardiovascular, and gastrointestinal systems.[55] There is also an association with gynecologic abnormalities.[56]

Prognosis

The outlook for an isolated pelvic kidney is excellent; however, postnatal follow-up is probably indicated because the incidence of vesicoureteric reflux is higher than usual.

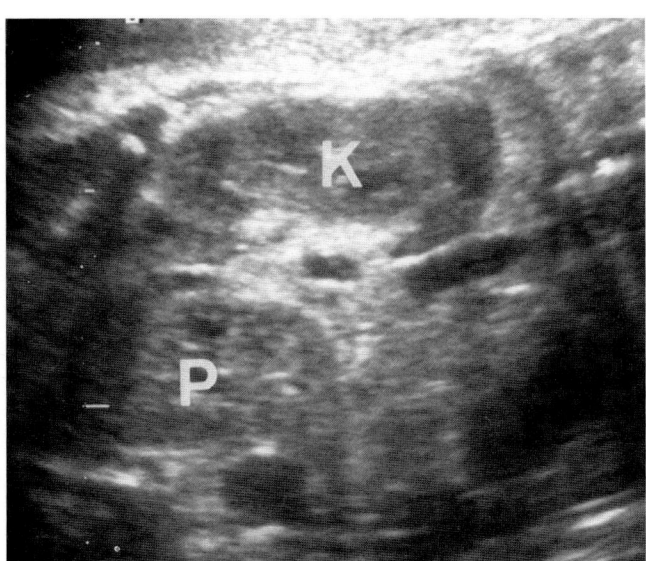

FIGURE 21. Pelvic kidney (*P*). Coronal scan through the lower abdomen. K, normal kidney.

Crossed Renal Ectopia

In crossed renal ectopia, the ectopic kidney lies entirely on the opposite side of the abdomen relative to its ureteral insertion into the bladder. In the majority of cases the crossed kidney fuses with its partner.

Incidence

Crossed renal ectopia is an uncommon condition occurring in 1 in 7,000 autopsies.[57] There is a slight male predominance of this condition.

Etiology

There are a number of hypotheses regarding the etiology, but the two most likely are that the developing kidney crosses from one side completely over to the other during its ascent or alternately the ureteral bud crosses to the contralateral side, inducing development of the metanephric blastema on the side opposite its trigonal insertion.[53] The left kidney crossing to the right is the most common appearance.

Diagnosis

As in pelvic kidney, one renal fossa is empty and an enlarged bilobed kidney is seen, usually in the right side of the abdomen.

Differential Diagnosis

The differential diagnosis should include unilateral renal agenesis with compensatory enlargement of the contralateral kidney. In this situation, however, the contralateral kidney is only slightly enlarged and does not have a bilobed appearance. A renal tumor is another possibility, but renal tumors have a density and texture different from that of normal renal tissue. In addition, it may be possible to detect a collecting system in a crossed kidney; if a renal tumor is present there should be a normal contralateral kidney, which is not the case in crossed renal ectopia.[57]

Associated Anomalies

Vertebral anomalies, especially myelomeningocele and sacral agenesis, have been described as has anal atresia. Urinary anomalies such as the development of hydronephrosis, infection, stone formation, and vesicoureteric reflux are long-term complications.[57]

Prognosis

The outcome for crossed renal ectopia is excellent if isolated. As with pelvic kidney, postnatal follow-up is probably indicated due to the higher incidence of vesicoureteric reflux.

Horseshoe Kidney

Horseshoe kidney is a fusion of the lower poles of both kidneys.

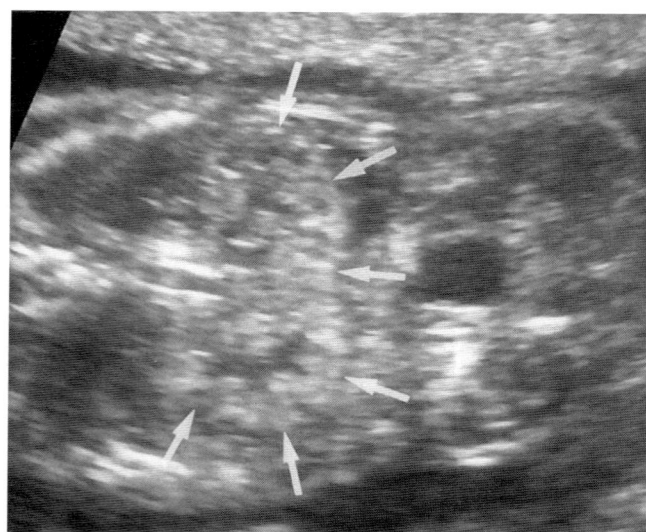

FIGURE 22. Horseshoe kidney (*arrows*) on coronal scan.

Incidence

Horseshoe kidney is a common abnormality with an incidence of 1 in 400 live births. It is more common in boys.[53]

Etiology

Both metanephric blastemas are in close proximity before their ascent from the embryonic pelvis. A disturbance in the separation of the closely approximated renal blastemas may result in a horseshoe kidney. This could be caused by an abnormality of renal blood flow, disordered unfolding of the tail of the embryo, or a teratogenic agent.[53]

Diagnosis

Sonographically, horseshoe kidney is best demonstrated in transverse or coronal planes through the isthmus as it crosses the midline and connects the lower poles of both kidneys (Fig. 22). The isthmus of renal tissue lies anterior to the aorta, and below the inferior mesenteric artery, the ureters course anteriorly.[58,59]

Associated Anomalies

Horseshoe kidney is associated with many other abnormalities. Urogenital anomalies include hypospadias, undescended testicles, and duplex collecting systems. Vesicoureteric reflux is seen in up to 50% of cases.[53] Central nervous system anomalies include hydrocephalus and neural tube defects. Cardiovascular, gastrointestinal, and musculoskeletal defects have also been reported.[60] The main associated chromosomal abnormalities are trisomy 18 and Turner syndrome.

Although horseshoe kidney is at no greater risk for malignancy than normal kidneys, the type of tumor affecting a horseshoe kidney is different. In children Wilms tumors predominate, whereas in adults transitional cell carcinoma is the most common type.[53]

Prognosis

The outlook is excellent for horseshoe kidney. As for other renal fusion anomalies, however, with higher incidences of reflux, infection, and stone formation, postnatal follow-up is probably indicated.

Renal Cystic Disease

Renal cystic disease comprises a mixed group of heritable, developmental, and acquired disorders. Because of their diverse etiology, histology, and clinical presentation, no single scheme of classification has gained acceptance.[61] The Potter classification, although incomplete, does cover the most important conditions seen prenatally (Table 3). In addition, a number of rare syndromes are associated with renal cystic disease; these are outlined in Table 4.

TABLE 3. POTTER CLASSIFICATION OF CYSTIC RENAL DISEASE

Type I	Autosomal recessive (infantile) polycystic renal disease
Type II	Multicystic renal dysplasia
Type III	Autosomal dominant (adult) polycystic renal disease
Type IV	Obstructive cystic dysplasia

TABLE 4. SYNDROMES ASSOCIATED WITH CYSTIC RENAL DISEASE

Syndrome	Clinical findings
Meckel-Gruber syndrome	Large echogenic kidneys, polydactyly, encephalocele
Patau syndrome (trisomy 13)	Large echogenic kidneys, polydactyly, holoprosencephaly, facial clefting
Beckwith-Wiedemann syndrome	Large echogenic kidneys, macrosomia, hepatosplenomegaly, macroglossia, omphalocele
Jeune syndrome	Echogenic kidneys, dwarfism, small thorax
Short rib polydactyly syndrome (Majewski type)	Large echogenic kidneys, dwarfism, polydactyly, small thorax
Laurence-Moon syndrome (Bardet-Biedl syndrome)	Renal cysts, retinal dystrophy, polydactyly, mental deficiency, hypogonadism
Zellweger syndrome	Cystic kidneys, hypotonicity, limb contractures, congenital cataracts, hypoplastic corpus callosum, heterotopias
Perlman syndrome	Macrosomia, hepatosplenomegaly, ascites, micrognathia, depressed nasal bridge
Tuberous sclerosis	Epilepsy, mental retardation, cutaneous lesions, cardiac rhabdomyomas (*in utero*)

Reproduced with permission from Twining P. Urinary tract abnormalities. In: Twining P, McHugo JM, Pilling DW, eds. *Textbook of fetal abnormalities.* London: Churchill Livingstone, 2000.

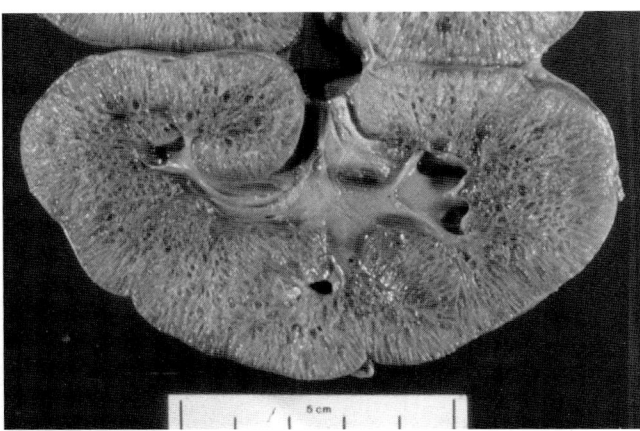

FIGURE 23. Autosomal recessive (infantile) polycystic kidney disease. This section through an affected kidney shows cystic dilatations of the collecting tubules arranged radially throughout the renal parenchyma. (Reproduced with permission from Twining P, McHugo J, Pilling D. *Textbook of fetal abnormalities.* London: Churchill Livingstone, 2000.)

Potter Type I: Autosomal Recessive (Infantile) Polycystic Renal Disease

The condition is characterized by symmetric enlargement of both kidneys secondary to renal collecting tube dilation. This is associated with varying degrees of hepatic fibrosis and biliary ectasia.[62]

Incidence

It is an autosomal recessive condition with an incidence of 1 in 40,000 to 50,000 live births.[63]

Etiology

The etiology is unclear but is likely to be a defect of the collecting ducts resulting in the formation of cystic dilatations of the collecting tubules.[64] The cause of the hepatic fibrosis is also unclear but could be due to overgrowth of the biliary epithelium.

Pathology

The kidneys are symmetrically enlarged, and this is produced by cystic dilatations of the collecting tubules, which are arranged radially throughout the renal parenchyma[64] (Fig. 23). The earlier-forming distal collecting tubules are more severely affected than the proximal collecting tubules.[55] There is no proliferation of the connective tissue, which is seen in some other forms of renal dysplasia.

The hepatic component comprises proliferation and ectasia of the bile ducts, which leads to periportal fibrosis and portal hypertension.[65]

Clinically the disease has been classified into four subtypes depending on the clinical presentation and the degrees of renal and hepatic involvement[65] (Table 5). In general the earlier the disease presents (perinatal type), the greater the renal involvement and the poorer the outlook.

TABLE 5. MANIFESTATIONS OF AUTOSOMAL RECESSIVE INFANTILE POLYCYSTIC RENAL DISEASE ACCORDING TO THE SUBCLASSIFICATION OF BLYTHE AND OCKENDEN

Type	Proportion of dilated renal tubules (%)	Extent of portal fibrosis	Lifespan
Perinatal	90	Minimal	Hours
Neonatal	60	Mild	Months
Infantile	20	Moderate	10 yr
Juvenile	<10	Gross	50 yr

Reproduced with permission from Deget F, Rudnik-Schoneborn S, Zerres K. Course of autosomal recessive polycystic kidney disease (ARPKD) in siblings: a clinical comparison of 20 sibships. *Clin Genet* 1995;47:248–253.

The later the disease occurs (juvenile type), the greater the hepatic involvement and the better the outlook. The degree of renal involvement, therefore, is inversely proportional to the degree of hepatic disease.

Diagnosis

In practice it is usually the most severe perinatal form that is detected prenatally. The typical appearance is of enlarged kidneys showing increased echogenicity associated with a small or absent bladder and oligohydramnios[66,67] (Fig. 24).

These sonographic features may not be present until the third trimester, however, and it is well documented that fetuses with their condition may look absolutely normal at the 20-week scan.[68–70] Thus, this condition cannot be excluded until well into the third trimester and patients should be carefully counseled to that effect. Follow-up scans later in pregnancy should always be arranged for patients at risk for this condition.

Although the appearance may be normal at midtrimester, a few first-trimester diagnoses have been reported.[71] These are based on demonstrating renal enlargement and renal hyperechogenicity, using transvaginal scanning at 12 to 14 weeks' gestation.[71] Careful measurements of renal size are important to the diagnosis because affected kidneys have a faster growth profile than normal kidneys (Fig. 25). Although most kidneys are symmetrically enlarged, occasionally one kidney is of normal size.[72] However, the normal-sized kidney should also show increased echogenicity (Fig. 26).

Differential Diagnosis

The differential diagnosis for enlarged echogenic kidneys is quite large. However, one important consideration is autosomal dominant (adult) polycystic renal disease, which can look identical except that liquor volume is usually normal. In addition, there may be a family history of the disease.

The other main diagnoses are outlined in Table 6, many of which have associated abnormalities that can be detected on ultrasound. With oligohydramnios, some of these abnormalities may be difficult to detect and careful scanning is essential.

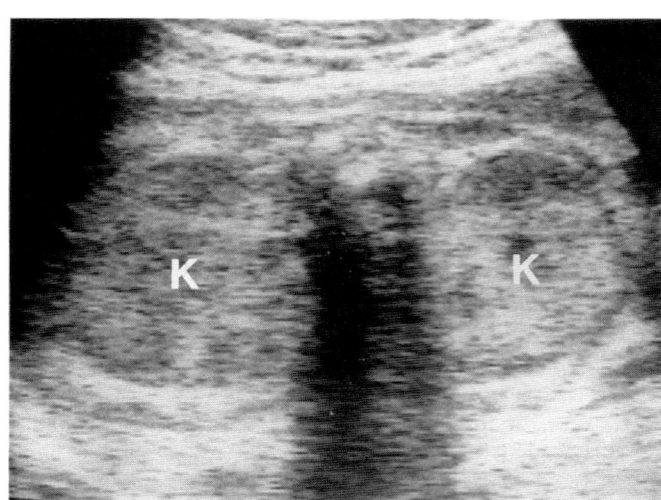

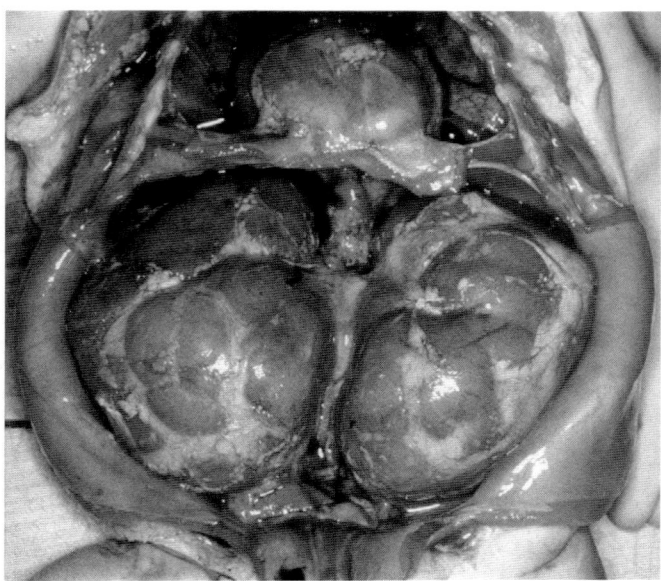

A   B

FIGURE 24. Autosomal recessive (infantile) polycystic kidney disease. **A:** A transverse scan through the fetal abdomen shows enlarged echogenic kidneys (*K*). Oligohydramnios is associated. **B:** A postmortem photograph of the same fetus shows massively enlarged kidneys. (Reproduced with permission from Twining P, McHugo J, Pilling D. *Textbook of fetal abnormalities.* London: Churchill Livingstone, 2000.)

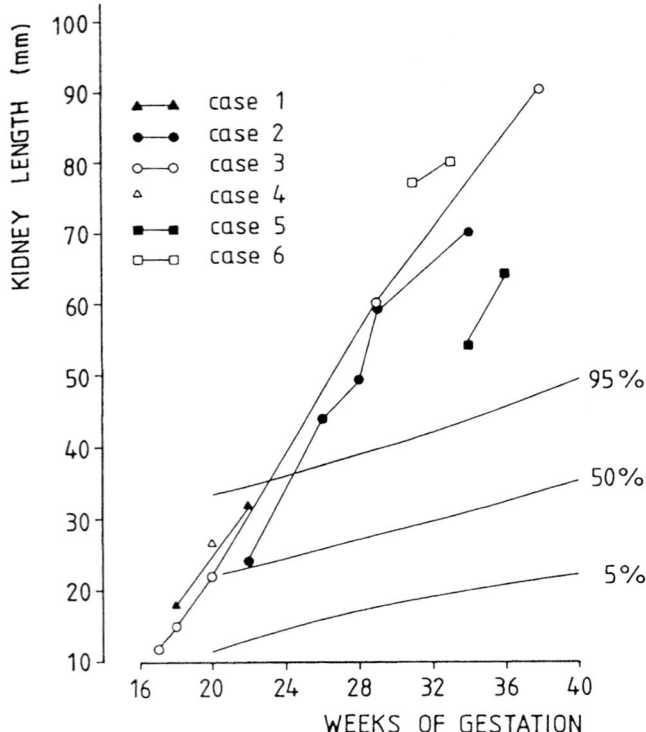

FIGURE 25. Renal lengths versus gestational age in six cases of autosomal recessive polycystic kidney disease. Renal size may be normal early in gestation, but the kidneys typically become enlarged later in gestation. (Reproduced with permission from Zerres K, Hansmann M, Mallmann R. Autosomal recessive polycystic kidney disease—problems of prenatal diagnosis. *Prenat Diagn* 1988;8:215–229.)

Associated Anomalies

The main association is hepatic fibrosis, the severity of which is inversely proportional to that of the renal disease (Table 5).

Genetic Markers

The gene for autosomal recessive polycystic renal disease is located on chromosome 6p.[73]

Prognosis

The outcome is predicted from the severity of the renal disease, with the poorest outlook for the perinatal type, in which most babies succumb in the neonatal period to renal and respiratory failure. The outcome is progressively better with later presentation and decreasing severity of renal involvement. Long-term complications include hypertension, urinary tract infection, and portal hypertension.[62]

Management

When scanning demonstrates bilaterally enlarged echogenic kidneys with oligohydramnios and there is a family history of autosomal recessive polycystic renal disease, the outlook is likely to be very poor. In that setting a termination of pregnancy could be offered to the mother before viability. After 24 weeks' gestation a feticide procedure would have to be considered or expectant management of the pregnancy could be allowed, in the knowledge that the baby would not survive the neonatal period.

When there is no family history of autosomal recessive polycystic disease and liquor volume is normal, other con-

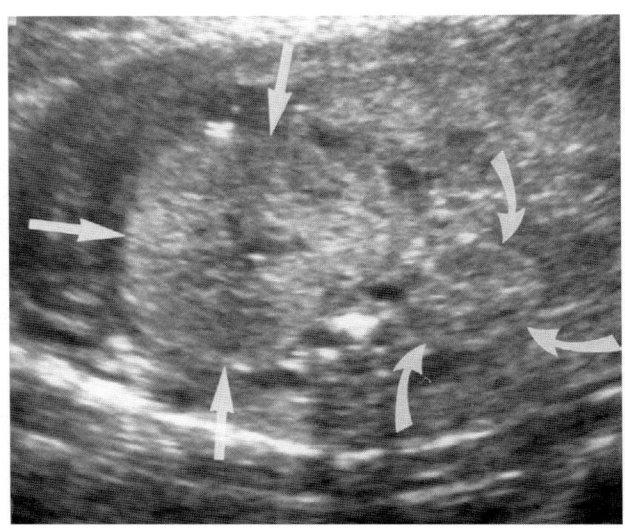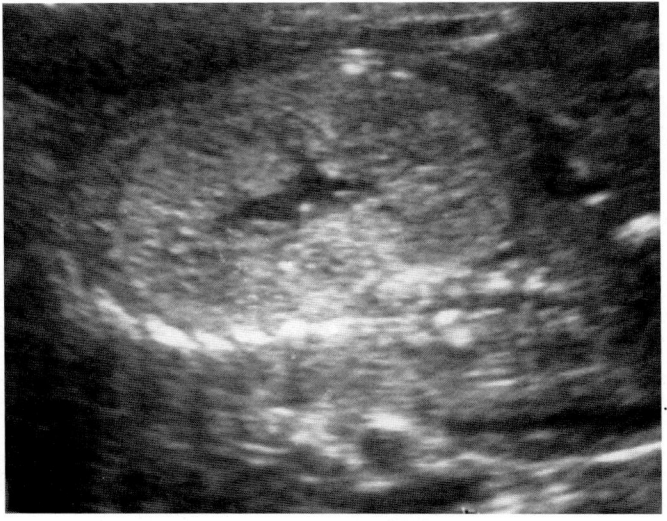

FIGURE 26. Autosomal recessive (infantile) polycystic renal disease with asymmetric involvement. **A:** A transverse scan shows an enlarged echogenic kidney (*straight arrows*) and a normal-sized echogenic kidney (*curved arrows*). **B:** Note the oligohydramnios in a longitudinal scan through the enlarged echogenic kidney.

TABLE 6. ECHOGENIC KIDNEYS: ANTENATAL ULTRASOUND APPEARANCES AND CLINICAL FINDINGS

Condition	Renal size	Cysts present?	Hydro-nephrosis?	Liquor volume	Cysts in parents' kidneys?	Family history	Associated findings
Infantile polycystic kidneys	Large	No	No	Reduced	No	Yes in sibling	Hepatic fibrosis in later life
Adult polycystic kidney disease	Large	Sometimes	No	Normal	Yes >20 yr age	Yes in parent	Occasionally cysts in parents' liver, spleen
Obstructive cystic dysplasia	Small	Often	Yes	Depends on degree of renal obstruction	No	No	Hydronephrosis usually urethral obstruction
Finnish type nephrotic syndrome	Large	No	No	Normal	No	Yes in sibling	Raised serum AFP
Beckwith-Wiedemann syndrome	Large	No	No	Normal or increased	No	Occasionally	Macrosomia, large liver, large spleen, macroglossia, omphalocele
Perlman syndrome	Large	No	Sometimes	Normal or increased	No	Yes in sibling	Macrosomia, hepatosplenomegaly, ascites, micrognathia, depressed nasal bridge
Meckel-Gruber syndrome	Large	Sometimes	No	Reduced	No	Yes in sibling	Polydactyly, encephalocele
Trisomy 13	Large	Sometimes	No	Normal	No	No	Facial clefting, holoprosencephaly cardiac defects, polydactyly
Cytomegalovirus infection	Large	No	No	Normal	No	No	Microcephaly, hydrocephaly intracranial calcification, large liver and spleen, hydrops
Renal vein thrombosis	Large, usually unilateral	No	No	Normal	No	No	Maternal diabetes, maternal pyelonephritis
Normal	Normal	No	No	Normal	No	No	—

AFP, alpha-fetoprotein.
Reproduced with permission from Twining P. Urinary tract abnormalities. In: Twining P, McHugo JM, Pilling DW, eds. *Textbook of fetal abnormalities*. London: Churchill Livingstone, 2000.

ditions, such as autosomal dominant polycystic renal disease, that have a better prognosis need to be considered. In those cases, conservative management is more appropriate.

The presence of other abnormalities should prompt a karyotype. Specific features may indicate a particular syndrome (Table 6).

Follow-up scans are of value to assess liquor volume later in pregnancy.

Recurrence Risk

There is a 25% risk of recurrence.

Potter Type II: Multicystic Renal Dysplasia

The multicystic dysplastic kidney is composed of multiple, smooth-walled, nonfunctioning, noncommunicating cysts of variable size and number. There is little or no normal renal parenchyma.[61]

Incidence

Multicystic renal dysplasia is the most common form of renal cystic disease in childhood and represents one of the most common abdominal masses in the neonate.[74] It has an incidence of 1 in 3,000 live births and is more common in boys.[75,76] The majority are unilateral, but it can be bilateral in up to 23% of cases.[75]

Etiology

The underlying cause is failed coordination and development of the metanephros and the branching ureteric bud, and this may be related to incomplete but severe obstruction to the kidney early in nephrogenesis.[61]

Pathology

Macroscopically the kidney is replaced by multiple smooth-walled cysts of varying size. Between the cysts is a dense stroma but usually no normal renal tissue.[77,78] Typically, atresia of the ureter and renal pelvis is seen and the renal artery is either absent or very small.

Diagnosis

The diagnosis of a multicystic dysplastic kidney is usually straightforward at the midtrimester scan. Multiple cysts of varying size are seen in one renal fossa (Fig. 27). The bladder and liquor volume are usually normal.[75,76] When the condition is bilateral there is oligohydramnios and absence of the bladder (Fig. 28). Multicystic dysplasia usually affects the whole kidney; however, occasionally only part of a kidney is involved, usually the upper pole of a duplex kidney[79] (Fig. 29). Similar findings have been noted in a crossed renal ectopic kidney.[80]

Careful attention should be given to assessment of the contralateral kidney because the incidence of contralateral renal anomalies is high (up to 39%).[48] A search should also be made for nonrenal anomalies.

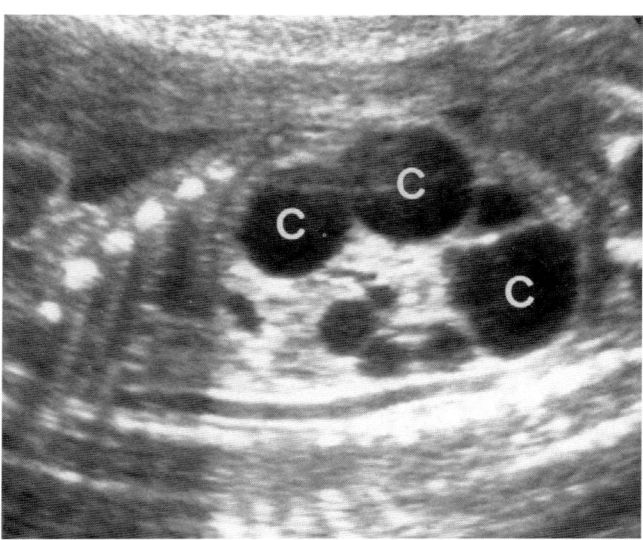

FIGURE 27. Multicystic dysplastic kidney. A sagittal scan through a multicystic dysplastic kidney shows multiple cysts (*C*).

Multicystic kidneys can increase or decrease in size with gestation, and follow-up scans are useful to assess the dysplastic kidney and to reassess the contralateral kidney.

Differential Diagnosis

The differential diagnosis should include hydronephrosis because occasionally a multicystic dysplastic kidney with a large central cyst and small peripheral cysts can mimic a pelviureteric junction obstruction. Careful evaluation of the kidney and demonstration that the cysts do not communicate excludes hydronephrosis.

Occasionally a multicystic dysplastic kidney is ectopic, usually within the pelvis (Fig. 30), producing a confusing appearance simulating an ovarian or other form of pelvic cyst. Careful scanning of both renal fossae reveals an absent finding on one side in this setting.

Very rarely in the case of bilateral multicystic dysplastic kidneys an eccentrically positioned cyst can descend into the fetal pelvis, simulating a normal bladder. This can be difficult to reconcile if severe oligohydramnios is present. Once again meticulous scanning with either high-resolution transabdominal or transvaginal probes usually resolves the problem, particularly if color-flow Doppler imaging is used. In the case of an extraneous pelvic cyst, the umbilical arteries are separate from the cyst and not split around it as seen around the bladder (Fig. 12).

Associated Anomalies

Associated anomalies are seen in the contralateral kidney in up to 39% of cases. Vesicoureteric reflux is the most common, followed by renal agenesis, renal hypoplasia, and pelviureteric junction obstruction.[48,81,82]

Extrarenal abnormalities may also be seen, including cardiac, gastrointestinal, central nervous system, cleft palate, and limb anomalies.[81]

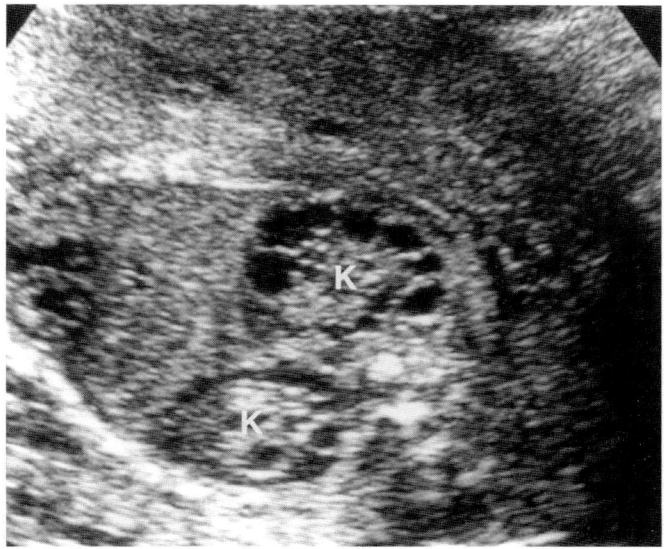

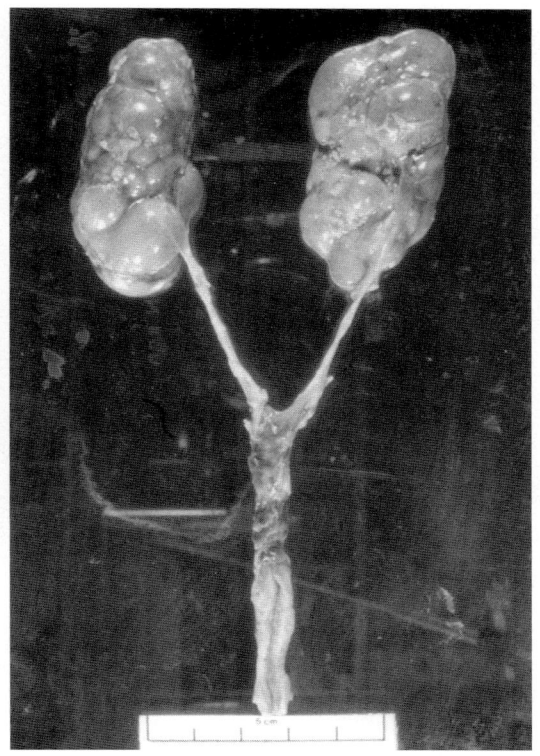

FIGURE 28. Bilateral multicystic dysplastic kidneys. **A:** In a coronal scan through a fetus with bilateral multicystic kidneys, both kidneys (*K*) show multiple peripheral cysts with a dense central stroma. Note also the severe oligohydramnios. **B:** A postmortem specimen shows bilateral multicystic kidneys with multiple cysts of varying sizes. (Reproduced with permission from Twining P, McHugo J, Pilling D. *Textbook of fetal abnormalities*. London: Churchill Livingstone, 2000.)

Prognosis

Unilateral multicystic dysplastic kidney has a good outcome provided the contralateral kidney is normal. If an associated renal anomaly is present, the prognosis depends on the severity of the associated abnormality. The presence of multiple anomalies confers a poorer prognosis.

Bilateral multicystic kidneys have a very poor prognosis, and all babies succumb in the early neonatal period to pulmonary hypoplasia.

Management

Unilateral multicystic kidney can be managed conservatively with follow-up scans in the third trimester to assess both the

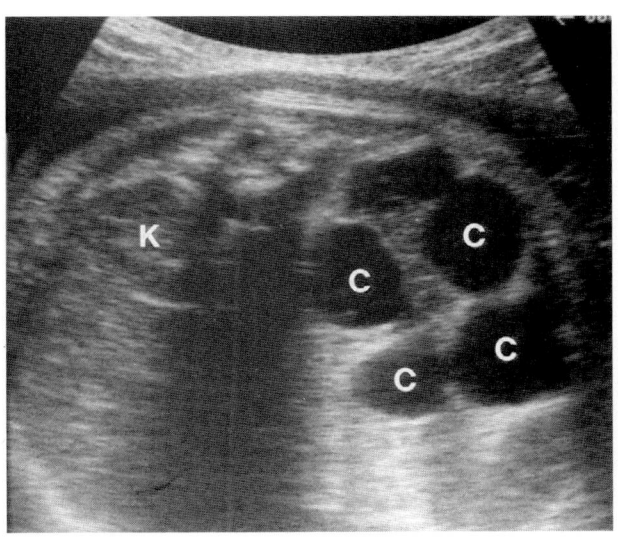

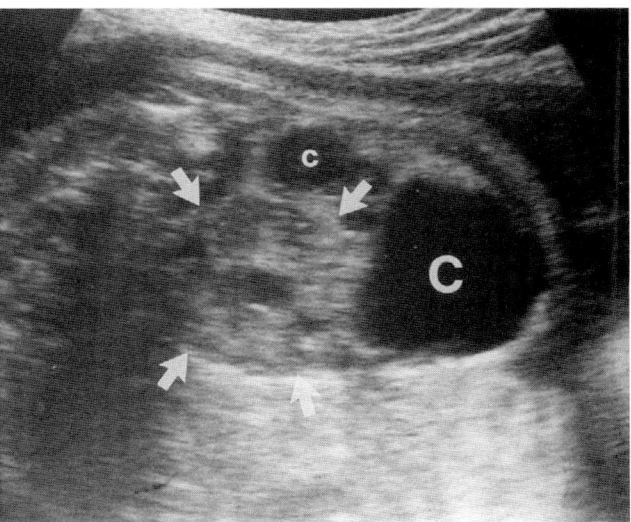

FIGURE 29. Multicystic dysplastic kidney affecting only part of a kidney. **A:** Multicystic kidney with multiple cysts (*C*). K, normal contralateral kidney. **B:** In the same fetus, a portion of normal renal tissue (*arrows*) is seen in the lower pole of the kidney. (Reproduced with permission from Twining P, McHugo J, Pilling D. *Textbook of fetal abnormalities*. London: Churchill Livingstone, 2000.)

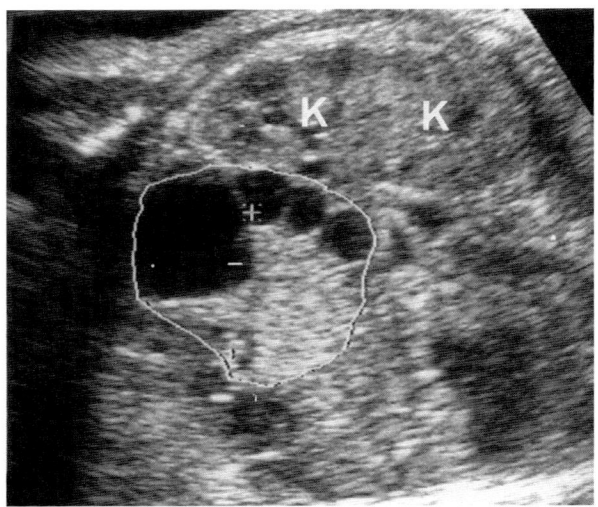

FIGURE 30. Pelvic multicystic dysplastic kidney. A coronal scan demonstrates the hypertrophied normal kidney (*K*) and pelvic multicystic kidney (*outline*).

multicystic and contralateral kidney. These babies also need to be followed carefully in the neonatal period. Starting with a renal scan to confirm the diagnosis, a micturating cystourethrogram (with antibiotic cover) should be carried out within the first month and dimercaptosuccinic acid (DMSA) isotope scan within the first 3 months.[52] Follow-up ultrasound examinations should be carried out every 6 months for the first year and then annually thereafter.

The natural history of multicystic kidneys is toward involution, and a number of studies have looked at the long-term follow-up of multicystic dysplastic kidneys. Wacksman and Phipps[83] found that 18% disappear within the first year of life, 13% during the next 2 years, and a further 23% in the following 2 years up to the age of 5 years. This left 54% present after 5 years of age, and it has been calculated that it may take as long as 20 years for all cases to resolve.[83]

Rarely, cases of sepsis, hypertension, and malignant change have been reported,[84–87] but these complications do not appear in most large follow-up studies.[83,88] The accepted policy at present, therefore, is conservative management, but long-term follow-up is indicated.[88]

Bilateral multicystic kidney has a very poor prognosis, and a termination of pregnancy is an appropriate management strategy.

Recurrence Risk
The condition is sporadic.

Potter Type III: Autosomal Dominant (Adult) Polycystic Renal Disease

Both kidneys show cystic dilatation of the nephrons. In the established adult disease, the kidneys are enlarged and contain multiple cysts of varying sizes.[89]

Incidence
The condition is autosomal dominant and has an incidence of 1 in 1,000 live births.[90] It is the most common of the hereditary renal cystic diseases.

Etiology
The condition is caused by a mutation near the telomere of chromosome 16 in 90% of cases.[91] Five percent of cases are caused by an abnormality on chromosome 4.[92]

Pathology
Autosomal dominant polycystic renal disease is a systemic disorder characterized by cyst formation in ductal organs, particularly the kidneys and liver. Cysts may also be present within the pancreas, spleen, and central nervous system.[61] In the kidneys only 5% of nephrons are cystic in the early part of the disease. It is not known whether more nephrons are recruited into the cystic process over time or whether existing cysts simply enlarge. Whichever process occurs, it results in enlarged kidneys replaced by cysts. The kidneys can enlarge considerably before renal function decreases.[61]

Diagnosis
The sonographic appearance is similar to autosomal recessive polycystic renal disease with symmetrically enlarged echogenic kidneys (Fig. 31). The bladder is usually present, and liquor volume may be normal.[93–98] The corticomedullary junction may appear accentuated[96] or be indistinct,[99] and several reports have described the presence of macroscopic cysts within the echogenic kidneys.[3,94,100]

Similar to autosomal recessive polycystic renal disease, the kidneys can look normal in the second trimester, so follow-up scans are essential in the group with a family history.

Very rarely, the condition can be unilateral.[101,102]

Differential Diagnosis
The main differential diagnosis is autosomal recessive polycystic renal disease; however, in this condition liquor volume is usually reduced and there may be a family history of the condition.

In autosomal dominant polycystic renal disease there may also be a family history, and scanning the parents may reveal renal cysts. In an adult below the age of 30 years the presence of two renal cysts (unilateral or bilateral) indicates a high likelihood of the condition. In patients over 30 years of age at least two cysts must be present in each kidney to confirm the diagnosis.[103]

A number of other conditions exhibit enlarged echogenic kidneys; these are outlined in Table 6. Many of these conditions exhibit other fetal anomalies and thus are amenable to prenatal diagnosis.[104–106] The presence of associated anomalies should always prompt the offer of a karyotype procedure.

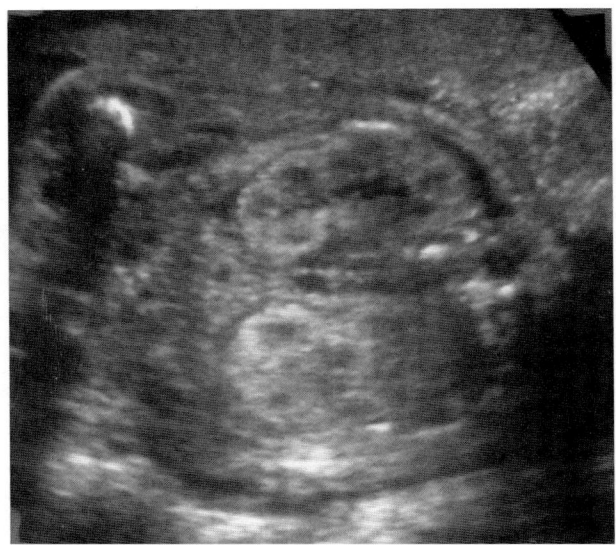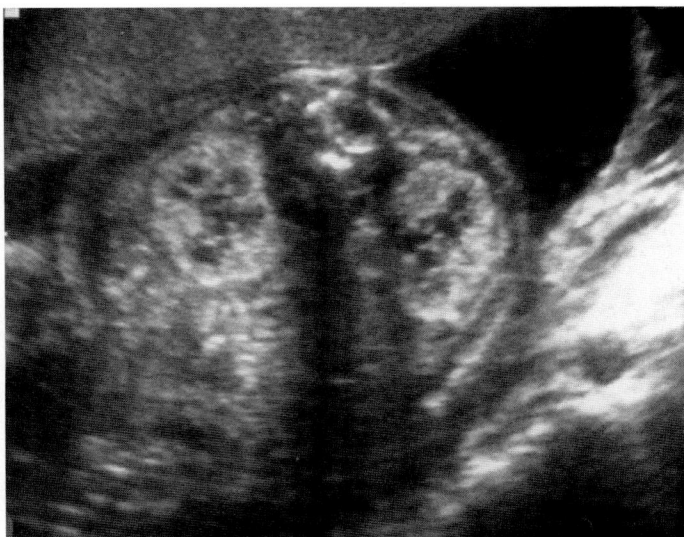

A   B

FIGURE 31. Autosomal dominant (adult) polycystic renal disease. **A:** A coronal scan through a 24-week fetus shows bilaterally enlarged echogenic kidneys. **B:** Normal liquor volume is apparent on this transverse scan.

Associated Anomalies

The most important associated anomalies are cysts in the liver, spleen, and pancreas, although these are only seen in the adult. Noncystic anomalies include cardiac disease (particularly mitral valve prolapse), skeletal anomalies, pyloric stenosis, and intracranial aneurysms.[61,95,107]

Genetic Markers

The condition is known to display genetic heterogeneity; however, 90% of cases are linked to the *PKD1* gene on the short arm of chromosome 16.[91] A further 5% are linked to the *PKD2* gene on chromosome 4.[92] Prenatal diagnosis is, therefore, possible by gene probes from chorion sampling.[93]

Prognosis

The condition is often asymptomatic and usually presents in the fifth decade with hypertension and end-stage renal failure.[90] It accounts for 10% to 15% of all patients requiring renal dialysis or transplantation.

The outlook for those cases diagnosed *in utero* is difficult to determine because to date only 83 cases of adult-type polycystic renal disease presenting prenatally or in the first few months of life have been reported. The best indicator of outcome is from previously affected siblings, as subsequent pregnancies will have a similar outlook.[93]

In the absence of a previously affected pregnancy, it has been estimated that in prenatal cases 43% of babies die within the first year of life and 67% of survivors develop hypertension. Approximately 3% develop end-stage renal failure by the age of 3 years.[93]

Management

Management of the pregnancy depends in large part on the parents' knowledge of the condition. The parents may not be aware that one or the other may have the condition. Alternately they may be under urologic follow-up with a strong family history and a previously affected child. Whatever the setting, the diagnosis of this condition requires very careful counseling as to both the short-term and long-term outlook. It is only after acquiring this knowledge that the parents can make a decision whether to continue with the pregnancy.

Follow-up scans in the third trimester are of value to assess liquor volume.

Recurrence Risk

There is a 50% risk of recurrence.

Potter Type IV: Obstructive Cystic Dysplasia

In obstructive cystic dysplasia, renal dysplasia occurs secondary to obstruction in the first or early second trimester of pregnancy.[108]

Incidence

The incidence of this condition is difficult to determine because only a small proportion of obstructed kidneys progress to renal dysplasia. This probably depends on the timing and severity of obstruction. Analyzing data from a large fetal registry gives an approximate incidence of 1 in 8,000 live births, with 40% being bilateral dysplasia.[3]

Etiology

The condition is caused by early renal obstruction. Unilateral disease can be caused by a pelviureteral or vesicoureteric junction obstruction. Severe obstruction from a ureterocele can cause dysplasia in an upper pole moiety of a duplex kidney.

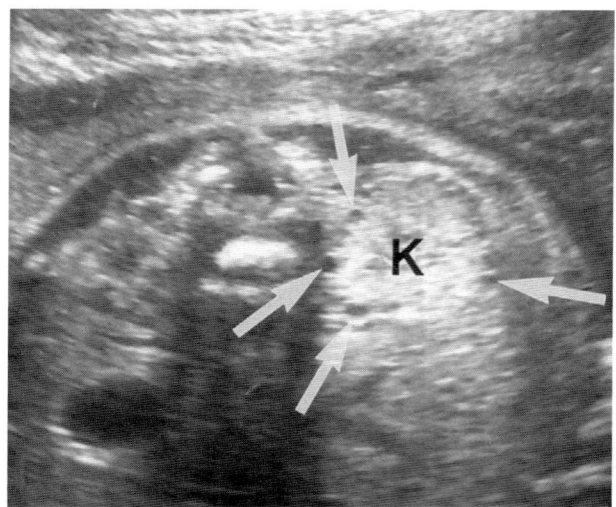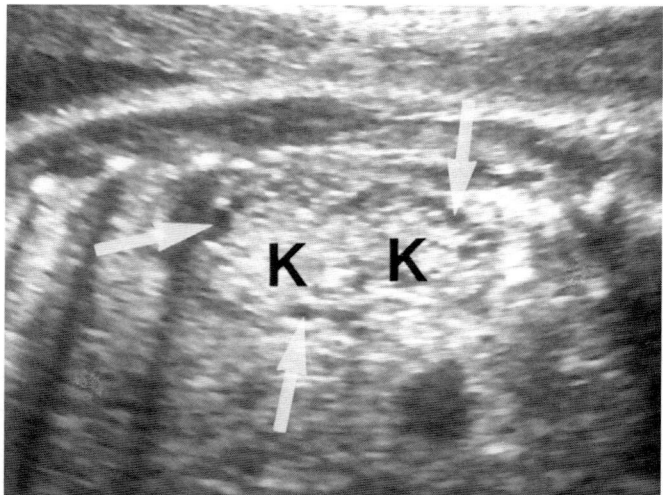

FIGURE 32. Obstructive cystic dysplasia. **A:** A transverse scan shows the echogenic kidney (*K*) with peripheral cortical cysts (*arrows*). **B:** Sagittal scan.

Bilateral obstructive dysplasia is caused by severe bladder outlet obstruction, usually urethral atresia or posterior urethral valves.

Pathology
The kidney is usually small and contains conglomerates of disorganized epithelial structures surrounded by abundant fibrous tissue. Cortical cysts are often present.[109]

Diagnosis
The characteristic appearance is of a small echogenic kidney containing peripheral cortical cysts (Fig. 32). In the case of bilateral disease, this is usually caused by severe

early bladder outlet obstruction, and there may also be bilateral hydronephrosis, a thick-walled bladder that is usually flaccid or collapsing, and severe oligohydramnios (Fig. 33).

Assessment of the renal cortex is important because the presence of cortical cysts with hydronephrosis is indicative of dysplasia.[109] Although increased echogenicity is a good sign of renal dysplasia, normal renal echogenicity does not exclude the condition.[108]

A number of cases have been described in which renal obstruction produces rupture of a calyx and a perinephric urinoma. These kidneys often progress to renal dysplasia[110,111] (Fig. 34).

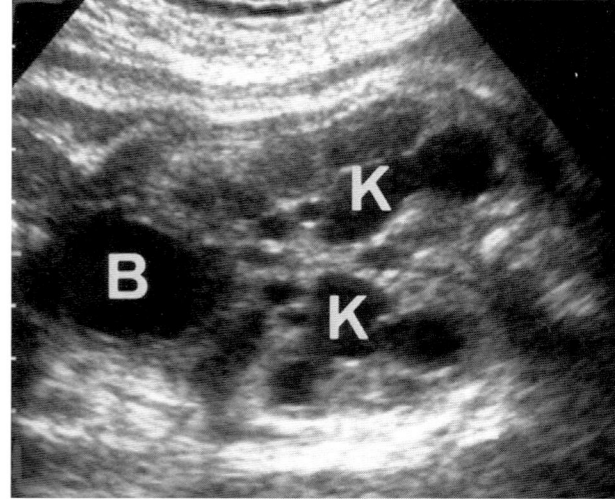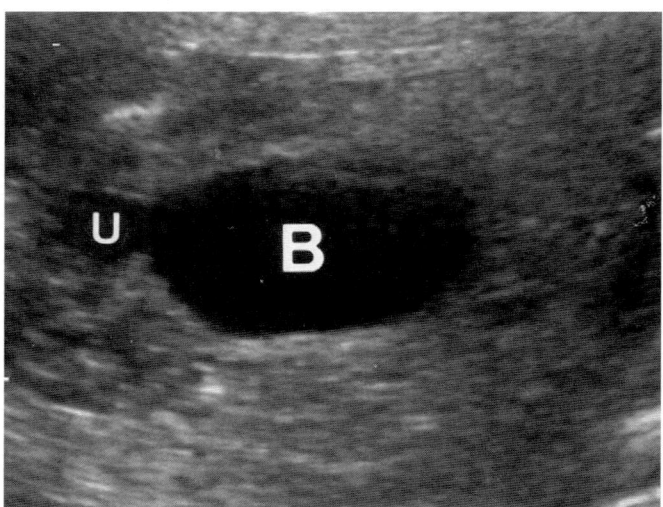

FIGURE 33. Obstructive cystic dysplasia. **A:** A coronal section through a fetus with posterior urethral valves demonstrates the thick-walled bladder (*B*), bilateral hydronephrosis (*K*), and the echogenic cortex. Oligohydramnios is severe. **B:** Distended bladder (*B*) and dilatation of the posterior urethra (*U*).

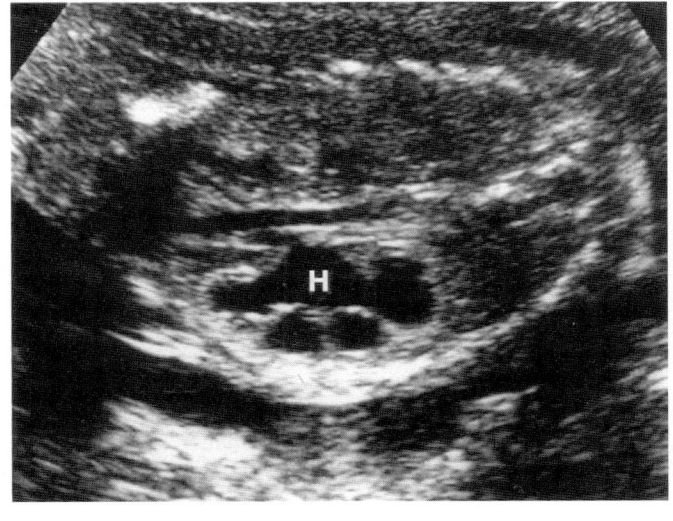

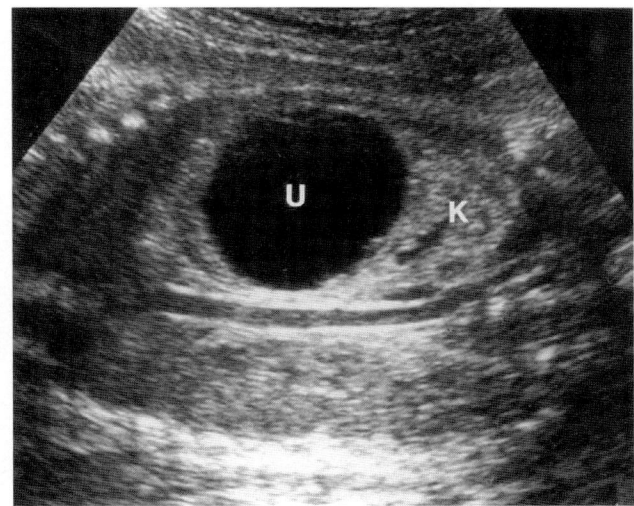

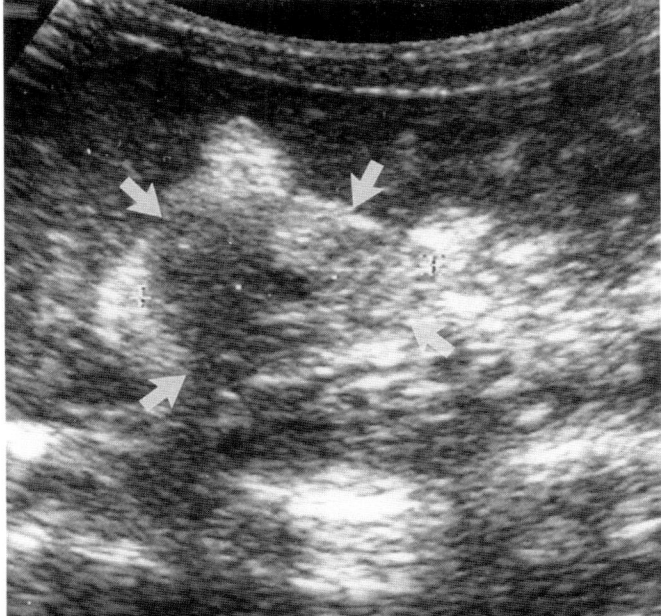

FIGURE 34. Renal dysplasia. **A:** A coronal scan at 20 weeks shows moderate hydronephrosis (*H*). **B:** In the same fetus at 26 weeks' gestation, a large urinoma (*U*) is demonstrated. The kidney (*K*) is compressed by the urinoma. **C:** A follow-up scan in the neonatal period shows a small dysplastic kidney (*arrows*). (Reproduced with permission from Twining P, McHugo J, Pilling D. *Textbook of fetal abnormalities.* London: Churchill Livingstone, 2000.)

Very occasionally the obstructive dysplasia can affect part of a kidney, particularly the upper pole moiety of a duplex system.[112]

Differential Diagnosis

The differential diagnosis is rather limited but does include other causes of small or normal-sized echogenic kidneys (Table 6). Other conditions associated with cystic renal disease also need to be considered (Table 4).

Associated Anomalies

As this group is a rather heterogeneous one depending on the form of obstruction, the associated anomalies also tend to be variable. The main anomalies seen, however, are cardiac anomalies and the VACTERL association (*v*ertebral anomalies, *a*norectal atresia, *c*ardiac anomalies, *t*racheo-*e*sophageal fistula, *r*enal anomalies, and *l*imb abnormalities). Other less common associations are hydrocephalus, cloacal malformation, malrotation, and ambiguous genitalia.[113]

Prognosis

The prognosis depends on whether the condition is unilateral or bilateral. Bilateral disease has a poor prognosis, with most babies succumbing in the neonatal period to pulmonary hypoplasia. In unilateral disease the outcome depends on the presence of renal anomalies affecting the contralateral kidney and the presence or absence of associated abnormalities.

Management

Bilateral disease carries a poor prognosis and in this setting the offer of a termination of pregnancy seems appropriate.

Unilateral disease can be managed conservatively in the absence of contralateral renal disease and associated abnormalities.

Recurrence Risk
The condition is sporadic.

Echogenic Kidneys

As can be seen from the previous descriptions, renal cystic disease encompasses a heterogeneous group of disorders with different clinical and pathologic presentations. These may be inherited, developmental, or acquired. A common finding in most of these conditions is increased echogenicity of the renal parenchyma; however, the differential diagnosis is wide, as demonstrated in Table 6.

To make as precise a diagnosis as possible it is important to have a logical approach to a fetus presenting with echogenic kidneys[114,115] (Fig. 15).

Symmetric enlargement of both kidneys in an otherwise normal-appearing fetus should raise the possibility of autosomal recessive or autosomal dominant polycystic renal disease. Normal liquor tends to favor the autosomal dominant form, particularly if there is a family history. Careful questioning of both parents is useful because either parent may be unaware of the significance of the family history. Another important factor is the appearance of the parents' kidneys, as the presence of cysts confirms the diagnosis.

In the autosomal recessive form there is usually absent or reduced liquor and there may be a previously affected sibling.

The Finnish-type nephrotic syndrome may have similar appearances to the autosomal dominant form of polycystic renal disease with enlarged, echogenic kidneys and normal liquor. There may be a finding of raised serum alpha-fetoprotein, which is a feature of this condition. Because the condition is autosomal recessive there may also be a previously affected sibling.[105]

Two conditions present with enlarged echogenic kidneys and macrosomia: Beckwith-Wiedemann syndrome and Perlman syndrome.[115] In both conditions liquor volume may be normal or increased and there is generalized organomegaly. The main differentiating features are in the face and abdomen. In Beckwith-Wiedemann syndrome there may be macroglossia,[116,117] whereas in Perlman syndrome there may be micrognathia[118,119] and depression of the nasal bridge.

In the abdomen Beckwith-Wiedemann syndrome may show an omphalocele,[116] whereas in Perlman syndrome hydronephrosis or ascites may be seen.[120] In practice, however, it may not be possible to differentiate these two syndromes until the neonatal period.[115]

Two other syndromes with a degree of phenotypic overlap are the Meckel-Gruber syndrome and trisomy 13. Both syndromes demonstrate enlarged echogenic kidneys. Liquor volume may be normal in trisomy 13, but it may be

reduced in Meckel-Gruber syndrome. Both syndromes show major intracranial anomalies; however, they differ in nature, as holoprosencephaly with facial clefting is seen in trisomy 13 and encephalocele in Meckel-Gruber syndrome. This latter anomaly can be missed if oligohydramnios is present. Both syndromes also show postaxial polydactyly. The nature of the specific associated anomalies means that these conditions can usually be diagnosed *in utero*. Karyotyping is indicated to make a precise diagnosis, as Meckel-Gruber syndrome is autosomal recessive and has a 25% risk of recurrence.

Less common causes of enlarged echogenic kidneys include infection with cytomegalovirus and renal vein thrombosis. In the former condition there may be other signs of infection, such as microcephaly, ventriculomegaly, intracranial calcification, and hydrops.[104] Renal vein thrombosis is usually unilateral and can be associated with maternal diabetes or pyelonephritis.[106]

All of the previous conditions produce enlarged echogenic kidneys. When the kidney is of normal size or small, obstructive cystic dysplasia is a possibility, particularly if there is mild hydronephrosis and peripheral cortical cysts.

Renal cystic disease may also be a component of several rare genetic syndromes; some of these are outlined in Table 4.

Finally, it should always be remembered that normal-sized echogenic kidneys may be a normal variant (Fig. 35).

Simple Renal Cyst

Incidence

Simple renal cysts have been reported in the fetus with an incidence that varies with gestational age. Scanning at 14 to 16 weeks' gestation, the incidence is 1 in 1,100.[121] Most sim-

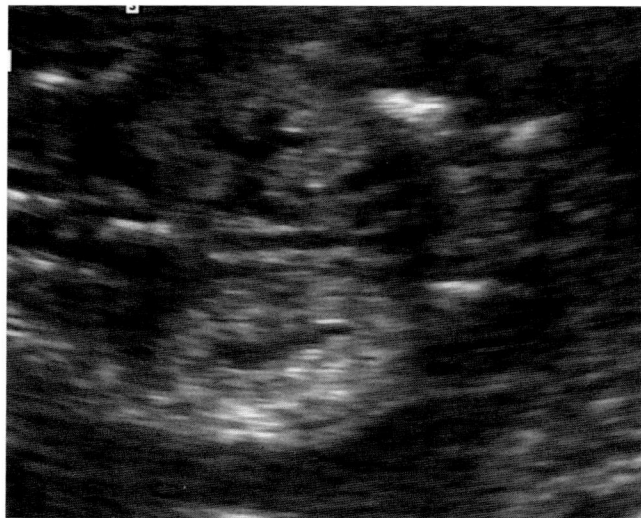

FIGURE 35. Echogenic kidney. This fetus showed echogenic kidneys of normal size throughout pregnancy with normal liquor volume. Follow-up at 5 years showed normal renal function.

ple renal cysts resolve by 20 to 24 weeks' gestation, so that at routine midtrimester scanning the incidence is approximately 1 in 2,400.[122] In childhood simple renal cysts are uncommon, with an incidence ranging from 1 in 500 to 1,000.[123,124]

Etiology

The etiology is unclear but there are two main theories. The most widely held view is that they are retention cysts resulting from the obstruction of renal tubules secondary to local vascular damage or inflammation.[125] The other theory is that the second to fourth generations of uriniferous tubules fail to degenerate or unite with later generations of collecting tubules, persisting as cystic collections.[125]

Pathology

The cysts are usually solitary and unilocular with no communication with the renal pelvis. The rest of the kidney is normal, and the cyst is lined with a single layer of epithelium with a fibrous wall containing no renal elements.[121]

Diagnosis

The cyst appears as a unilocular round or oval anechoic structure with well-defined borders, usually near the periphery of the kidney (Fig. 36). Cysts vary in size from 2.0 to 4.0 mm.[121]

Differential Diagnosis

Cysts at the upper pole of a kidney should be differentiated from hydronephrosis of the upper pole moiety of a duplex

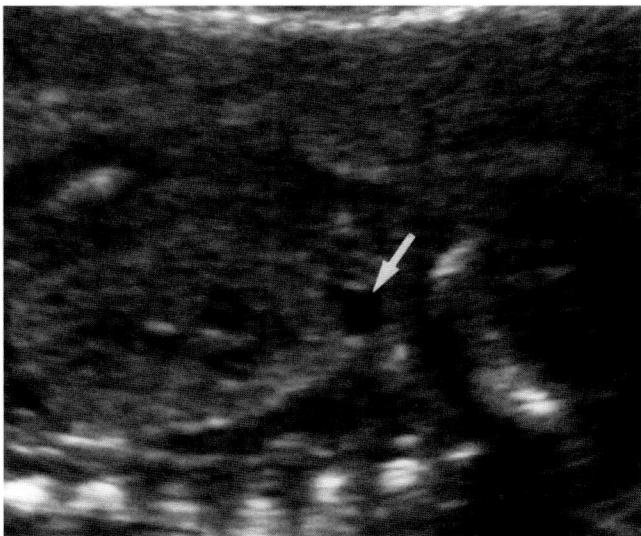

FIGURE 36. Simple renal cyst. A coronal scan through a 20-week fetus shows a single peripheral renal cyst (*arrow*). This cyst was resolved on follow-up scan.

kidney. In this condition the calyceal dilatation can usually be seen and the cyst communicates with the renal pelvis. In addition, the ureter may be dilated and a ureterocele may be visible within the bladder.[126] Another possibility is a perinephric urinoma (Fig. 34).

The other main diagnoses are cysts arising from structures close to the kidneys, usually duplication or mesenteric cysts. Scanning during fetal breathing movements should reveal whether the cyst is renal (moves with the kidney) or extrarenal (the cyst slides over the kidney).

Associated Anomalies

Most simple cysts in children are asymptomatic and rarely associated with structural or other abnormalities. They have occasionally been reported in association with pelviureteric junction obstruction and posterior urethral valves.[121] Simple cysts have also been seen in association with chromosomal abnormalities, particularly Turner syndrome,[127] trisomy 13, trisomy 18, and trisomy 21.[121] In one pathologic study simple renal cysts were seen in 5% of trisomy 21 fetuses and children.[128]

One study documented a simple renal cyst seen at 14 weeks' gestation that developed into a multicystic dysplastic kidney at 18 weeks' gestation,[121] so further follow-up scans are indicated if simple cysts are seen in either the first or second trimester.

Prognosis

The outcome is very good for fetuses with simple cysts: The vast majority resolve by 20 to 24 weeks' gestation, and those that persist stay the same size or only increase slightly.[121] Cysts can persist into the neonatal period and early childhood but are asymptomatic and do not cause complication unless they are large.[123,125] When cysts do become symptomatic, simple aspiration under ultrasound control is the treatment of choice.[126]

Management

Simple cysts seen in the first half of pregnancy can be followed up with scans in the third trimester. The majority resolve, and those that persist do not need any postnatal investigations apart from assessment by ultrasound.

Renal Obstruction

The fetal kidney responds in different ways to obstruction depending on the gestational age at which the obstruction occurs. Very early obstruction produces a multicystic dysplastic kidney, whereas obstruction in the first or early second trimester can produce obstructive cystic dysplasia. Obstruction later in pregnancy can produce hydronephrosis; however, the fetal kidney in the late second trimester

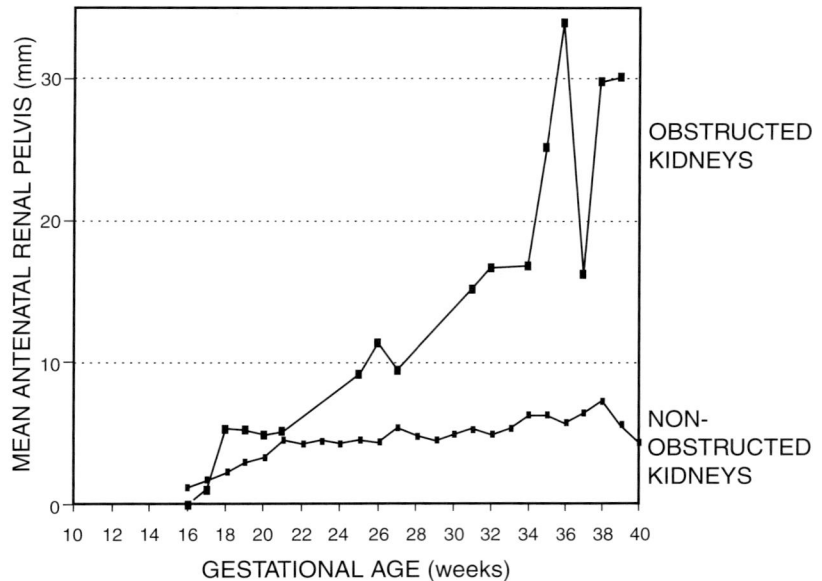

FIGURE 37. A graph of mean renal pelvic diameters of obstructed and nonobstructed fetal kidneys in relation to gestational age. The curves overlap at 16 to 21 weeks' gestation before beginning to diverge. (Reproduced with permission from Anderson N, Clautice-Engle T, Allen R, Abbott G, Wells JE. Detection of obstructive uropathy in the fetus: predictive value of sonographic measurements of renal pelvic diameter at various gestational ages. *Am J Radiol* 1995;164:719–723.)

responds differently to obstruction than does an adult kidney. Comparison of renal pelvic diameter measurements in obstructed and nonobstructed kidneys throughout gestation shows that up to 22 weeks the measurements are very similar (Fig. 37). After 22 weeks obstructed kidneys produce increased renal pelvic diameters and true hydronephrosis.[129] The reason for this is unclear but is likely due to a combination of the low compliance of the fetal renal parenchyma, which is unable to allow dilatation of the collecting system, and the relatively low level of urine production during the first half of pregnancy.[130] The practical consequence of this is that follow-up scans are required in

the third trimester when there is a suspicion of obstruction at the midtrimester scan.[129]

Another major difficulty in the diagnosis of renal obstruction is the high false-positive rate, estimated to be between 36% and 81%[3,29,129,131,132] (Table 7). This is due to so-called transient or mild hydronephrosis, which resolves either in late pregnancy or in the neonatal period.[14] In an attempt to overcome this problem many researchers have defined cutoff values for the anteroposterior diameter of the renal pelvis, above which level obstruction should be suspected (Table 8). It is unfortunate that most of the cutoff values are different, varying between 4 and 10 mm in

TABLE 7. DETECTION RATES AND FINAL DIAGNOSIS IN FETUSES WITH ANTENATAL DIAGNOSIS OF HYDRONEPHROSIS

Study	Population scanned (n)	Abnormal on scan (n)	Significant renal disease [n (%)]	Pelviureteric junction obstruction	Vesicoureteric junction obstruction	Posterior urethral valves	Duplex kidney	Vesicoureteric reflux
				Final diagnosis (n)				
Arger et al.[136]	3,530	30	6 (20)	2	1	2	—	—
Grignon et al.[18]	34,592	92	47 (51)	29	8	4	—	3
Livera et al.[4]	6,292	79	29 (37)	12	4	2	2	2
Mandell et al.[17]	—	154	87 (56)	45	6	2	3	8
Corteville et al.[29]	—	63	45 (71)	23	3	1	1	—
Johnson et al.[133]	7,500	47	17 (36)	7	1	1	—	3
Tam et al.[12]	—	105	63 (60)	43	7	3	8	13
Anderson et al.[129]	12,100	257	24 (9)	23	3	1	1	—
Adra et al.[131]	—	84	30 (36)	11	2	—	2	10
Ouzounian et al.[132]	—	84	48 (57)	—	—	—	—	—
Dudley et al.[134]	18,766	100	21 (21)	3	3	—	1	6
James et al.[14]	105,542	154	97 (63)	52	16	3	12	14
Dillon et al.[13]	25,382	125	80 (64)	14	15	5	2	9

Reproduced with permission from Twining P. Urinary tract abnormalities. In: Twining P, McHugo JM, Pilling DW, eds. *Textbook of fetal abnormalities*. London: Churchill Livingstone, 2000.

TABLE 8. CUTOFF VALUES FOR ANTEROPOSTERIOR DIAMETERS OF THE RENAL PELVIS IN DIFFERENT STUDIES

Study	Cutoff values
Arger et al.[136]	>5 mm (16 wk to term)
Grignon et al.[18]	>10 mm (16 wk to term)
Scott et al.[138]	>5 mm (16 wk to term)
Livera et al.[4]	>10 mm (28 wk to term)
Mandell et al.[17]	>5 mm (16–20 wk)
	>8 mm (20–30 wk)
	>10 mm (30 wk to term)
Corteville et al.[29]	>4 mm (16–33 wk)
	>7 mm (33 wk to term)
Johnson et al.[133]	>10 mm (16 wk to term)
Lam et al.[137]	>10 mm (16 wk to term)
Tam et al.[12]	>4 mm (16 wk to term)
Anderson et al.[129]	>4 mm (16–23 wk)
	>6 mm (23–30 wk)
	>8 mm (30 wk to term)
Adra et al.[131]	>8 mm (28 wk to term)
Barker et al.[135]	>5 mm (16 wk to term)
Ouzounian et al.[132]	>5 mm (16 wk to term)
Dudley et al.[134]	>5 mm (16 wk to term)
James et al.[14]	>5 mm (16–28 wk)
	>7 mm (28 wk to term)

Reproduced with permission from Twining P. Urinary tract abnormalities. In: Twining P, McHugo JM, Pilling DW, eds. *Textbook of fetal abnormalities*. London: Churchill Livingstone, 2000.

the second trimester and 7 and 10 mm in the third trimester.[1,4,12,18,29,129,131–138] Although this makes comparison of results very difficult, important trends are emerging. Studies comparing prenatal renal pelvic diameters with postnatal renal function do show a correlation. Renal pelvic diameters greater than 15 mm have a mean differential function of only 27% and renal pelvic diameters of 10 to 15 mm, 37%[135] (Table 9). It is, therefore, clear that renal pelvic diameters greater than 10 mm require postnatal follow-up investigations.[12,14,29,135,136]

The group that creates the most difficulty are fetuses with renal pelvic diameters between 4 and 10 mm because

TABLE 9. THE MEAN DIFFERENTIAL FUNCTION SHOWN FOR EACH GRADE OF EARLY PRENATAL ANTEROPOSTERIOR RENAL PELVIC DILATATION

Dilatation at median of 19 wk (mm)	Mean differential function (%)
Normal: <4	48.2
Mild: 5–8	42.7
Moderate: 10–15	37.3
Severe: >15	26.6

Reproduced with permission from Barker AP, Case MM, Thomas DSM, et al. Pelviureteric junction obstruction: predictors of outcome. *Br J Urol* 1995;76:649–652.

although postnatal studies show mean differential renal function of 43% (Table 9), which is not a significant reduction, a proportion of these babies later have renal pathology. One of the most important findings in this group is vesicoureteric reflux, which can occur in up to 12%.[12,13,139–141] Indeed, major renal pathology may occur in up to 4% of cases.[142] In terms of a lower limit of normal, most workers consider 4 mm or less a normal finding.[131–136]

Although absolute measurements of renal pelvic diameters are important, many workers have stressed the assessment of calyceal dilatation as an additional sign in the evaluation of renal obstruction. Grignon et al.[18] noted that the presence of calicectasis doubled the rates of surgery for hydronephrotic kidneys, and other reports show that calicectasis is more likely to indicate a significant hydronephrosis than if only renal pelvic dilatation is seen.[29,143]

One further important issue is the association of hydronephrosis with chromosomal disease. A number of workers have reported an association; however, in most cases other abnormalities are present and in that setting the risk is approximately 30%.[144–147] More problematic, however, is the link between mild renal pelvic dilatation and trisomy 21.[145–150] Please see the discussion in Chapter 21.

To summarize, the antenatal diagnosis of renal obstruction can be difficult. By assessing renal pelvic diameters and the degree of calicectasis, however, a logical approach can be developed. Renal pelvic diameters greater than 10 mm are usually associated with calicectasis and always warrant follow-up scans *in utero* and full postnatal assessment including a DMSA scan and a micturating cystourethrogram. It is probably wise to commence prophylactic antibiotic therapy until vesicoureteric reflux has been excluded.

Fetuses with renal pelvic diameters between 5 and 10 mm may have associated calicectasis and require further follow-up scans in the third trimester. Postnatal follow-up is also recommended with scans in the early neonatal period and at 3 to 6 months. When definite hydronephrosis is seen postnatally, further investigation is indicated. Fetuses with renal pelvic diameters of 4 mm or less are likely to be normal.

The importance of diagnosing hydronephrosis prenatally is highlighted by the fact that the clinical diagnosis of renal abnormalities is relatively low, ranging from 15% to 27%, so the majority of renal anomalies are missed clinically.[151–153] In the case of severe bilateral renal disease, the patient may be offered a termination of pregnancy, and when unilateral disease is seen the pregnancy can be monitored and appropriate postnatal investigations instituted. Mild to moderate bilateral renal disease can also be monitored *in utero* and the timing and place of delivery determined depending on the sonographic findings. Rarely, intervention *in utero* may need to be considered in worsening bilateral renal obstruction.[154]

TABLE 10. CAUSES OF HYDRONEPHROSIS

Bilateral hydronephrosis
  Bilateral pelviureteric junction obstruction
  Bilateral vesicoureteric junction obstruction
  Bilateral vesicoureteric reflux
  Megacystis megaureter syndrome
  Posterior urethral valves
  Urethral atresia
  Obstructing ureterocele
  Megacystis-microcolon syndrome
  Congenital megalourethra
  Persistent cloaca
  Hydrometrocolpos
Unilateral hydronephrosis
  Pelviureteric junction obstruction
  Vesicoureteric junction obstruction
  Duplex kidney with ureterocele
  Normal kidney with ureterocele
  Megaureter

The various causes of fetal hydronephrosis are outlined in Table 10; the common causes are pelviureteric junction obstruction, vesicoureteric junction obstruction, vesicoureteric reflux, posterior urethral valves, and obstruction in duplex kidneys (Table 11). These conditions are discussed in the next section.

Pelviureteric Junction Obstruction

In pelviureteric junction obstruction, the kidney is obstructed at the junction between the renal pelvis and ureter.

Incidence

Pelviureteric junction obstruction is the most common form of fetal renal obstruction (Table 11), with an incidence of approximately 1 in 2,000 live births.[14] The condition is more common in boys and is unilateral in 90% of cases.[155]

TABLE 11. FINAL UROLOGIC DIAGNOSIS IN INFANTS WITH SIGNIFICANT PRENATALLY DETECTED UROPATHY

Diagnosis	Percentage
Pelviureteric junction obstruction	35
Vesicoureteric reflux	20
Multicystic dysplastic kidney	15
Vesicoureteric junction obstruction	10
Posterior urethral valves	9
Duplex systems	8
Renal agenesis	3

Reproduced with permission from Thomas DFM. Prenatally detected uropathies: epidemiological considerations. *Br J Urol* 1998;81(Suppl 2):8–12.

Etiology

The etiology of this condition is unknown, and anatomic causes are only seen in a fraction of cases. In most instances the junction is anatomically patent, and the problem is likely to be of a functional nature. Abnormal development of the interwoven muscularis of the ureter could impair bolus formation and propulsion of urine, thus predisposing to obstruction.[156]

Diagnosis

The classic appearance is of a dilated renal pelvis and collecting system without ureteric or bladder dilatation (Fig. 38). Severe obstruction leads to effacement of the calyces and thinning of the overlying cortex (Fig. 39). On rare occasions the renal pelvis can enlarge to massive proportions and produce an abdominal cyst[157] or can rupture with the development of a perinephric urinoma. The outcome for such kidneys is poor[110,111,155] (Fig. 34).

Liquor volume is usually normal but can be increased even with bilateral obstruction. Prenatal series have reported increased liquor with unilateral pelviureteric junction obstruction in 29% to 36% of cases and in 26% to 50% of cases of bilateral disease.[130,155,156] This is thought to be caused by the obstruction impairing renal concentrating ability, resulting in a state of high urine output.[155]

Both kidneys need to be assessed carefully. In particular the affected kidney should be assessed for renal dysplasia, the signs of which are increased renal echogenicity and cortical cysts. The contralateral kidney also needs to be assessed carefully to look for associated renal anomalies.

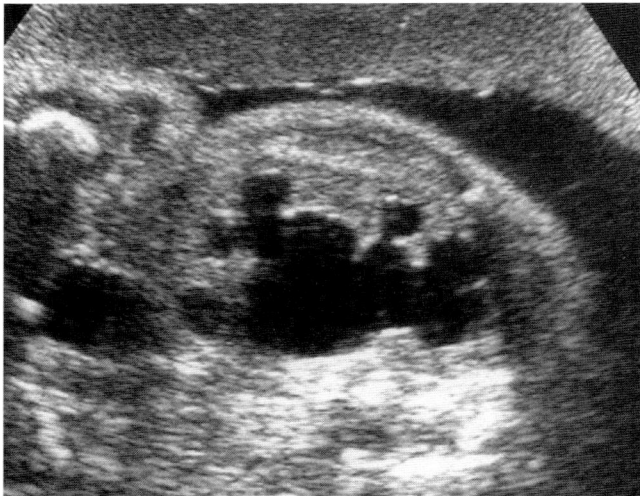

FIGURE 38. Pelviureteric junction obstruction. A coronal section shows moderate dilatation of the collecting system and renal pelvis. The condition was unilateral; note the normal liquor volume.

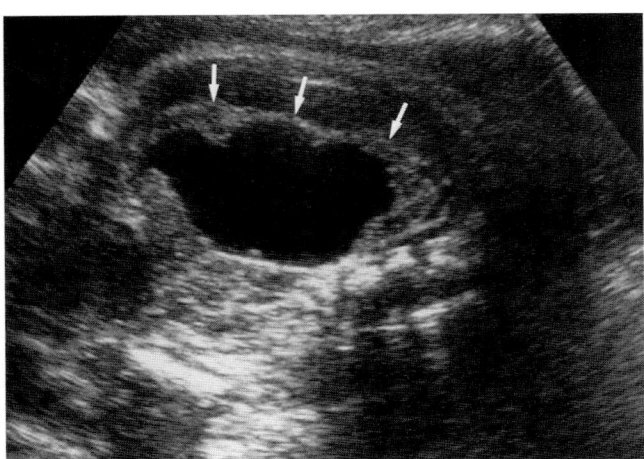

FIGURE 39. Pelviureteric junction obstruction. A coronal scan through the kidney shows hydronephrosis with thinning of the cortex (*arrows*). (Reproduced with permission from Twining P, McHugo J, Pilling D. *Textbook of fetal abnormalities.* London: Churchill Livingstone, 2000.)

Finally, as in all cases of fetal abnormality, a careful search should be made for any extrarenal abnormalities.

Differential Diagnosis

The differential diagnosis includes other causes of renal obstruction such as vesicoureteric junction obstruction and, in bilateral disease, bladder outlet obstruction and bilateral vesicoureteric reflux. In low obstruction the ureters are usually dilated, which is not the case in true pelviureteric junction obstruction.

Other conditions that can mimic a pelviureteric obstruction are multicystic kidney if there is a large central cyst with multiple peripheral cysts, large simple cysts, or a perinephric urinoma.

Associated Anomalies

Associated anomalies may be renal or extrarenal. Renal anomalies in the contralateral kidney are common and seen in up to 25% of cases. The main anomalies are renal agenesis, multicystic renal dysplasia, and vesicoureteric reflux.[158]

Extrarenal anomalies have no specific pattern and are seen in approximately 12% of affected fetuses.[156]

Prognosis

The outcome for a baby with either unilateral or bilateral pelviureteric junction obstruction is usually good. The degree of renal impairment of an affected kidney does relate to a certain extent to the degree of dilatation of the collecting system seen prenatally. The more severe the hydronephrosis the poorer the mean differential renal function seen in the neonatal period (Table 9).

Management

The diagnosis is usually suspected at the time of the midtrimester scan; follow-up scans in the third trimester are usually carried out to assess the degree of hydronephrosis and liquor volume.

Babies are usually begun on prophylactic antibiotics, and a full evaluation is required, including a neonatal ultrasound scan, DMSA scan, and a micturating cystourethrogram. Most cases are managed conservatively unless there is increasing hydronephrosis or poor differential renal function,[159–162] in which case a pyeloplasty is the surgery of choice. The main aim of surgery is to prevent any further deterioration in renal function.[163,164]

Recurrence Risk

The majority of cases are sporadic and so the recurrence risk is low. A few familial cases have been reported.[165,166]

Vesicoureteric Junction Obstruction (Nonrefluxing Megaureter)

In vesicoureteric junction obstruction, hydronephrosis occurs secondary to obstruction at the lower end of the ureter.

Incidence

The incidence is approximately 1 in 6,500 live births and is more common in boys, with a male-to-female ratio of 2:1. The condition may be bilateral in up to 25% of cases.[167]

Etiology

The obstruction is generally thought to be due to a localized region of dysfunction or physiologic obstruction in the distal ureter, which is often narrowed.[168] There should be no evidence of vesicoureteric reflux or bladder outlet obstruction.

Diagnosis

The affected kidney shows dilatation of the renal pelvis and ureter, which often has a very tortuous course (Fig. 40). The dilated ureter can easily be differentiated from bowel, as urine is echogenic-free, whereas the bowel contains low-level echoes. The bladder and liquor volume are usually normal when the condition is unilateral. Liquor volume may be reduced in bilateral disease depending on the severity of the obstruction.[169]

In unilateral cases the contralateral kidney should always be assessed for associated abnormalities.

Differential Diagnosis

The differential diagnosis includes vesicoureteric reflux, which can have an identical appearance and, thus, cannot

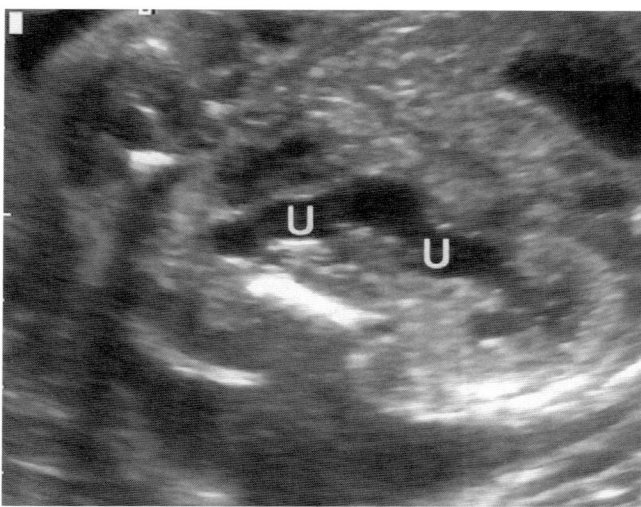

FIGURE 40. Vesicoureteric junction obstruction. Hydronephrosis and dilatation of the ureter (*U*) are present.

be completely excluded until a micturating cystourethrogram is carried out in the neonatal period. Rarely, severe bladder outlet obstruction produces massive reflux into one ureter and kidney with relative sparing of the contralateral kidney, producing vesicoureteric reflux dysplasia in the affected kidney.[170] The clue to this diagnosis is a thick-walled, distended bladder in a male fetus and probably reduced liquor. It is also likely that bladder emptying is incomplete.

The other important cause of a dilated ureter is obstruction caused by a ureterocele in a duplex kidney. In this situation it is usually the upper pole moiety that is hydronephrotic, and the ureterocele is usually visible within the bladder (see Fig. 43).The ureterocele may not be visible if the ureter is ectopically inserted.

Associated Anomalies

The main associated anomalies are seen in the contralateral kidney and are present in up to 16% of cases. These include pelviureteric junction obstruction, multicystic renal dysplasia, pelvic kidney, renal agenesis, and vesicoureteric reflux.[169]

Prognosis

The outlook is generally good even for bilateral involvement, and long-term studies have shown that up to 83% of cases can be managed conservatively.[167,171] Correlation of prenatal findings with outcome has revealed that kidneys with ureteric diameters of 6 mm or less have a good outcome and a low incidence of surgery. Ureters greater than 10 mm, however, have a poorer outcome with a high incidence of surgical correction.[167]

Management

Follow-up scans are indicated to assess the degree of renal tract dilatation and the liquor volume. Postnatal assessment includes DMSA scan and a micturating cystourethrogram. Prophylactic antibiotic therapy is commenced until reflux is excluded. Those with poor or deteriorating renal function are candidates for surgery with reimplantation of the ureter. Surgery prevents any further loss of renal function.[167] Patients with good renal function who are managed conservatively have a good outcome.[171]

Recurrence Risk

The condition is sporadic, with a low risk of recurrence.

Obstruction Secondary to Ureterocele and Ectopic Ureter

A ureterocele is a cystic dilatation of the intravesical segment of the distal ureter.[172] An ectopic ureter is one that does not insert near the posterolateral angle of the normal trigone. In females the ectopic ureter may insert in the vagina, vestibule, or uterus; in males it may insert in the seminal vesicle, vas deferens, or ejaculatory ducts. In both sexes the ureter may insert in the bladder away from the normal location in the trigone, usually in the urethra or bladder neck. Rarely, it can insert into the rectum.[173]

Incidence

The true incidence of ureterocele and ectopic ureter is not easy to determine, but large prenatal studies suggest an incidence of approximately 1 in 9,000 live births.[14] The majority of ureteroceles arise from duplex kidneys, usually the upper pole moiety; however, it has been estimated that 10% to 20% are associated with a solitary renal pelvis[173] (Fig. 41). Ureteroceles associated with duplex kidneys are more common in girls, whereas those associated with a solitary renal pelvis are more common in boys.[2] They are bilateral in 10% to 15% of cases.

Etiology

The development of a duplex kidney is thought to result from an additional ureteral bud arising from the mesonephric duct and meeting the renal blastema at a separate site from the original bud.[174]

Pathology

The distal orifice of the affected ureter is stenotic, resulting in ballooning of the intravesical segment of the ureter, which results in a ureterocele. It consists of bladder and ureteral epithelium separated by varying amounts of connective tissue and smooth muscle.[174] In a duplex system,

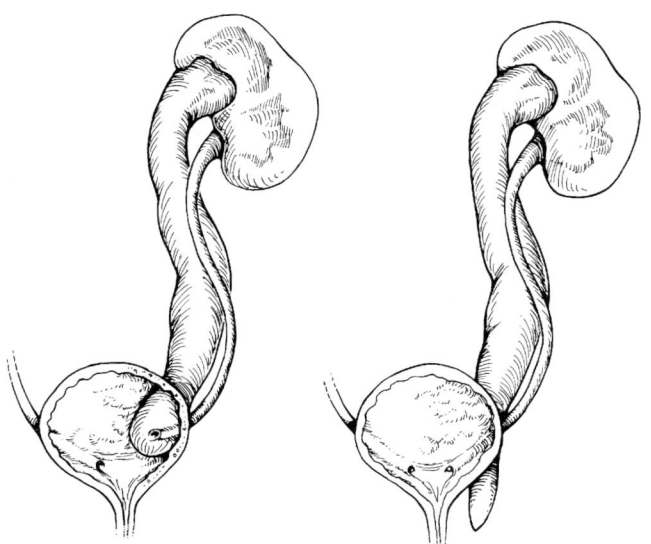

FIGURE 41. Diagram of two duplex kidneys. Both have hydronephrosis of the upper pole; one with and one without an ectopic ureterocele. (Reproduced with permission from Winters WD, Lebowitz RL. Importance of prenatal detection of hydronephrosis of the upper pole. *Am J Radiol* 1990;155:125–129.)

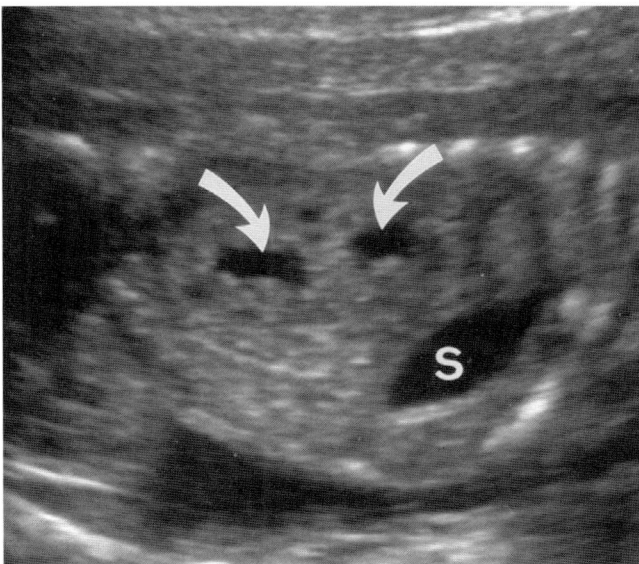

FIGURE 42. Duplex kidney. A sagittal scan through a duplex kidney shows two collecting systems (*arrows*). S, stomach. (Reproduced with permission from Twining P, McHugo J, Pilling D. *Textbook of fetal abnormalities*. London: Churchill Livingstone, 2000.)

the two ureteral orifices are characteristically inverted to the collecting systems they drain. The ureter to the upper pole moiety inserts at a lower and more medial position, and that of the lower pole moiety inserts at a higher and more lateral position. Approximately one-third of the renal parenchyma is drained by the upper collecting system and two-thirds by the lower collecting system.[174]

The presence of a ureterocele, therefore, is liable to produce hydronephrosis in the upper pole moiety. It is also well documented that the lower pole moiety is prone to hydronephrosis, but in this case it is usually due to vesicoureteric reflux.

Hydronephrosis of either the upper or lower pole moiety can lead to renal dysplasia and subsequent poor function of the affected moiety. In the upper pole this is usually caused by an ectopic ureter inserting at a level beyond the bladder neck and in the lower pole by severe vesicoureteric reflux.[174]

Diagnosis

In the absence of a complication, such as a ureterocele producing hydronephrosis, a duplex kidney can be difficult to detect *in utero*. The main clue to the diagnosis is a large kidney with two collecting systems (Fig. 42). The most common appearance prenatally is hydronephrosis of the upper pole moiety associated with a dilated ureter and a ureterocele within the bladder[174–179] (Fig. 43). If the ureter is dilated and appears to insert at a level below the bladder base and there is no ureterocele present, an ectopic ureter should be considered.[173]

If large, ureteroceles can produce obstruction to the contralateral kidney and may also herniate into the urethra, producing bladder outlet obstruction.[177] Ureteroceles may also drain a solitary renal pelvis and produce hydronephrosis of the whole kidney. Ureteroceles can be bilateral in 10% to 15% of cases.[180,181]

The most important sign in the diagnosis is the demonstration of a ureterocele within the bladder; however, there are a number of reasons a ureterocele may not be present or may be misinterpreted. If the bladder is full, the ureterocele can be compressed, resulting in effacement of the ureterocele. Conversely, if the bladder is empty, the ureterocele itself can be mistaken for the bladder. In the presence of dysplasia of the upper pole moiety, urine production may be insufficient to distend the ureterocele.[178] Further difficulties can arise if the ureterocele drains a solitary collecting system because in that setting the whole kidney—not just the upper pole moiety—may become hydronephrotic.

Liquor volume is usually normal in unilateral cases.

Differential Diagnosis

The major elements of the differential diagnosis are those conditions producing hydronephrosis and a dilated ureter: These include vesicoureteric junction obstruction and vesicoureteric reflux. The presence of a ureterocele should confirm the diagnosis.

A large ureterocele producing bladder outlet obstruction should be visible but can resemble obstruction due to urethral valves. Demonstration of the fetal sex can be useful in

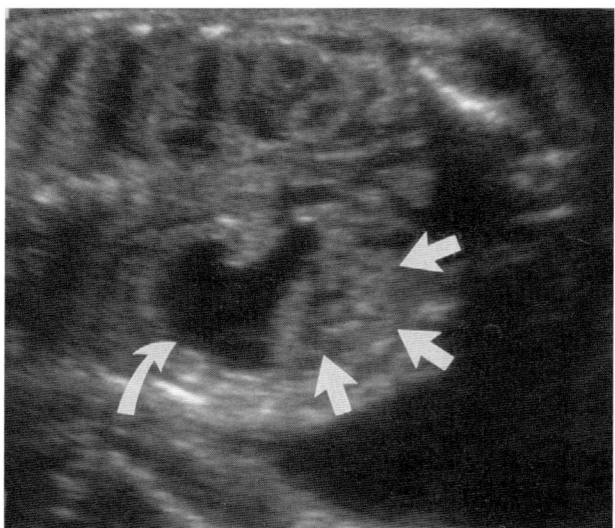
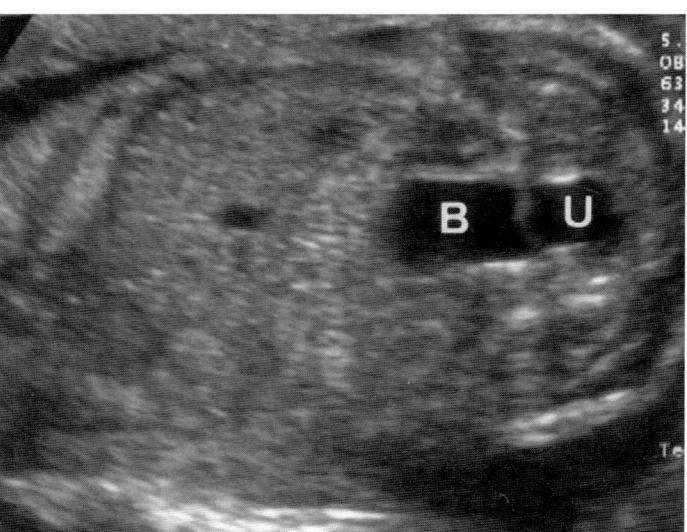

A   B

FIGURE 43. Duplex kidney with hydronephrosis in the upper pole moiety secondary to a ureterocele. **A:** A coronal scan through the duplex kidney shows hydronephrosis of the upper pole moiety (*curved arrow*). The lower pole (*straight arrows*) is normal. **B:** An image of the same fetus shows a ureterocele (*U*) within the bladder (*B*).

differentiating these two conditions: Ureteroceles are more common in girls, whereas urethral valves are seen in boys.

Associated Anomalies

Vesicoureteric reflux into the lower pole moiety is a common finding, occurring in up to 50% of cases. Reflux is more frequent when a ureterocele is present (63%), compared to 33% when the ureter is ectopically inserted,[178] and is probably due to distortion of the ipsilateral lower pole orifice by the ureterocele. Pelviureteric junction

obstruction has also been reported in the lower pole moiety[176] (Fig. 44).

Prognosis

The outcome is generally good. The function of the affected kidney depends on the degree of dysplasia affecting the upper pole moiety, and this tends to be more severe in ectopic ureters than in ureteroceles.[176] In the lower pole moiety severe vesicoureteric reflux also tends to produce more dysplasia and subsequently poorer function.

Management

Follow-up scans later in pregnancy are useful to reevaluate the renal tract and assess the degree of hydronephrosis.

In the postnatal period, a full evaluation is required with neonatal ultrasound scan, DMSA scan, and micturating cystourethrogram. Cystoscopy with puncture of the ureterocele is the treatment of choice for those patients with good function in the upper pole moiety, but it does predispose to a 30% risk of reflux.[2,182] In those neonates with nonfunctioning upper poles, prophylactic antibiotics are usually maintained and an upper pole heminephrectomy can be considered at around 6 months of age if it remains hydronephrotic.[2]

Recurrence Risk

The condition is sporadic, so the recurrence risk is low.

Posterior Urethral Valves

Bladder outlet obstruction is produced by a membrane within the posterior urethra.

FIGURE 44. Duplex kidney with a pelviureteric junction obstruction to lower pole moiety. A coronal scan at 22 weeks shows pelviureteric junction obstruction at the lower pole (*P*). Arrows point to the upper pole moiety. B, bladder.

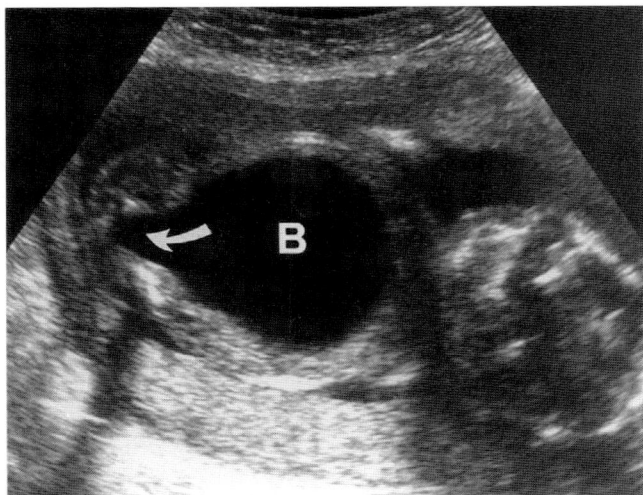

FIGURE 45. Posterior urethral valves. A sagittal section through the fetal abdomen shows a distended bladder (*B*). Arrow points to the dilated posterior urethra.

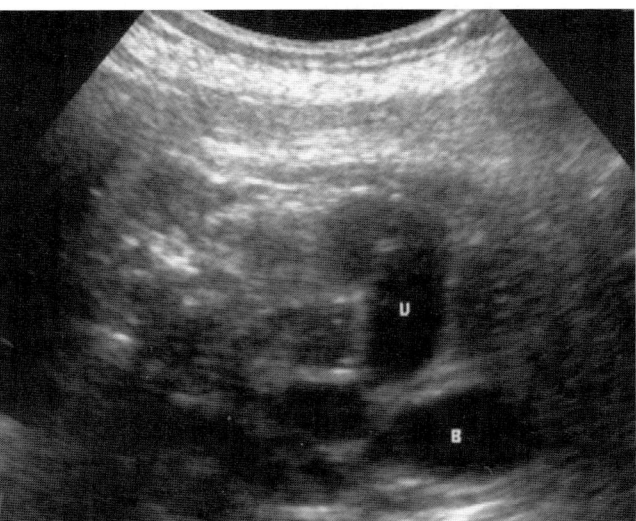

FIGURE 46. Posterior urethral valves. The bladder is distended (*B*), and there is dilatation of the ureters (*U*). Note associated oligohydramnios.

Incidence

The incidence is 1 in 5,000 to 8,000 boys.[154] It is the most common cause of severe obstructive uropathy in childhood. The condition only affects males.

Etiology

The etiology is unknown but may be related to failure of complete disintegration of the urogenital membrane leaving membranous tissue within the posterior urethra.[183]

Pathology

The true nature of the obstruction appears to be a diaphragmatic membrane with a small eccentric opening situated within the posterior urethra. The membrane is a simple mucosal membrane with a scanty fibrous stroma. A fusiform dilatation of the prostatic urethra occurs between the obstructing membrane and the bladder neck.[184]

Diagnosis

The characteristic findings are of a distended, thick-walled bladder with a dilated posterior urethra (Fig. 45). The ureters are also dilated with bilateral hydronephrosis[185,186] (Fig. 46). Liquor volume is variable. The presence of increased cortical echogenicity with or without cysts always raises the possibility of renal dysplasia and a poor prognosis and is usually associated with oligohydramnios.[108,109]

Asymmetric hydronephrosis, with a very marked hydronephrosis on one side and a minimal hydronephrosis on the other, suggests vesicoureteric reflux dysplasia, in which massive reflux essentially destroys one kidney, producing decompression of the bladder with relative sparing of the contralateral kidney.[170,187,188] The bladder can also decom-

press by rupturing to produce urinary ascites[189] (Fig. 47). Like the vesicoureteric reflux dysplasia syndrome, this is thought to be a good prognostic feature.[2] In addition, the presence of a patent urachus can produce relief of the bladder obstruction.

The calyceal system may rupture to produce perinephric urinomas (Fig. 34), but unlike urinary ascites, which may have a good prognosis, this condition leads to renal dysplasia.[110,111]

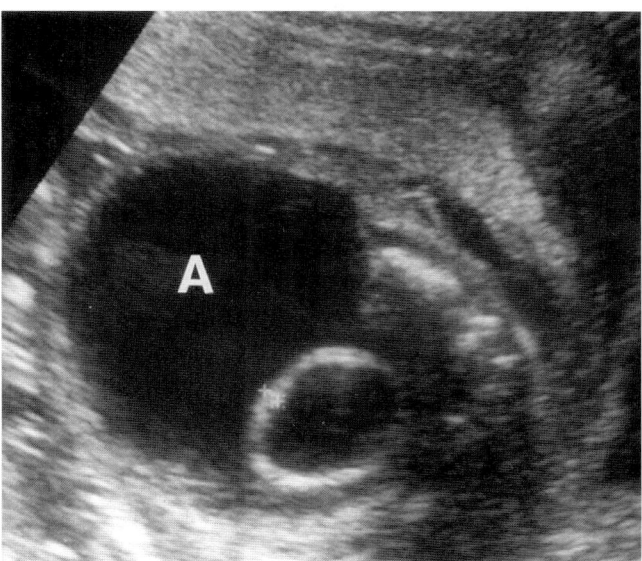

FIGURE 47. Urinary ascites. A thick-walled bladder is noted, surrounded by urinary ascites (*A*). Note associated oligohydramnios. (Reproduced with permission from Twining P, McHugo J, Pilling D. *Textbook of fetal abnormalities*. London: Churchill Livingstone, 2000.)

Differential Diagnosis

The differential diagnosis includes a number of conditions that produce the appearance of bladder outlet obstruction. Severe bilateral vesicoureteric reflux can produce a distended bladder with bilateral hydronephrosis and dilated ureters. The important features in this condition are that liquor volume is usually normal and the bladder, although distended, is often thin-walled, as opposed to the thick-walled bladder of posterior urethral valve obstruction.[143] In addition, there is no dilatation of the posterior urethra, which is the hallmark of posterior urethral valves, and if the fetus is female, this reliably excludes urethral valves as a cause for the dilatation.

Assessment of the renal cortex is important because, although increased echogenicity is associated with renal dysplasia and often oligohydramnios, one report[190] suggests that increased renal echogenicity can predate the development of oligohydramnios and in that setting is a good indicator of an obstructive cause of the hydronephrosis.

Urethral atresia causes severe bladder outlet obstruction and usually presents in the late first or early second trimester with severe oligohydramnios. It is often difficult to visualize the other fetal organs because massive dilatation of the bladder usually completely fills the uterine cavity.

There are a number of rarer causes of bladder outlet obstruction, such as congenital megalourethra, in which the obstruction is at the distal end of the penile urethra. In this condition a cystic mass is demonstrable between the legs of the fetus.[191] Other rarer causes include persistent cloaca and hydrometrocolpos secondary to a urogenital sinus. These diagnoses are difficult to make due to the complexity of the conditions; however, abnormal midline cystic masses within the pelvis that produce bladder compression may be clues to the diagnosis. The megacystis-microcolon syndrome can produce dilatation of the bladder and ureters and bilateral hydronephrosis. In this condition, there may be polyhydramnios,[192] and the condition is more common in female fetuses, which is a useful differentiating factor.

Very rarely, a ureterocele may prolapse into the bladder neck, producing bladder outlet obstruction. In this situation it may be possible to demonstrate the ureterocele within the bladder.

Associated Anomalies

Associated anomalies are seen in up to 43% of cases and include cardiac anomalies, malrotation, anal atresia, the VATER syndrome, and vesicoureteric fistula.[185,193] Chromosomal disease may also be seen in 8% of fetuses, but no specific syndrome is associated.[194]

Severe obstruction is associated with bilateral renal dysplasia, oligohydramnios, and the development of Potter's syndrome. Pulmonary hypoplasia is the rule with the typical Potter's facies of low-set ears, hypertelorism, micrognathia, and limb contractures and talipes.

The condition may also be a cause of the prune-belly syndrome, which is the triad of thinned or absent abdominal wall muscles, cryptorchidism, and urinary tract defects.[195]

There are many other causes of the prune-belly syndrome, including severe vesicoureteric reflux, urethral atresia, ascites, visceromegaly from Beckwith-Wiedemann syndrome, and polycystic renal disease.[195,196] In a number of cases, however, no obstruction can be demonstrated.[195]

Prognosis

The outcome is variable and depends on the severity of the obstruction. Overall mortality in postnatal studies is approximately 8%[197]; however, prenatal series reveal a much higher mortality ranging between 23% and 54%.[198,199] In postnatal studies the proportion of patients developing renal failure increases with age so that at 10 years of age end-stage renal failure is seen in 10% and chronic renal failure in 34%. At the age of 20 years, 38% have end-stage renal failure and 51% have chronic renal failure.[197] Prenatal studies show a higher incidence of renal failure on follow-up, with rates of 64% at 3 years,[200] 20% at 4 years,[201] and 46% at 5 years.[198] Combining the prenatal series produces an overall renal failure rate of 44% at 4 to 5 years of age.[198–203]

There are, however, a number of poor prognostic factors, including diagnosis before 24 weeks' gestation,[203] oligohydramnios,[202] increased cortical echogenicity with cysts indicating renal dysplasia,[190] and marked hydronephrosis[198] (Table 12).

The fetus that presents with all of the above features has a very poor prognosis, and these babies die in the neonatal

TABLE 12. PROGNOSTIC FACTORS IN FETUSES WITH POSTERIOR URETHRAL VALVES

Factors	Good prognostic indicators	Poor prognostic indicators
Sonographic signs	Normal liquor Diagnosis after 24 wk Asymmetric hydronephrosis Urinary ascites Isolated	Oligohydramnios Diagnosis before 24 wk Echogenic kidneys with cysts Perinephric urinoma Associated abnormalities
Urine biochemistry		
Sodium	<100 mEq/L	>100 mEq/L
Chlorine	<90 mEq/L	>90 mEq/L
Osmolality	<210 mOsm/L	>210 mOsm/L
Calcium	<2 mmol/L	>2 mmol/L
Phosphate	<2 mmol/L	>2 mmol/L
β_2-Microglobulins	<2 mg/L	>2 mg/L

Reproduced with permission from Twining P. Urinary tract abnormalities. In: Twining P, McHugo JM, Pilling DW, eds. *Textbook of fetal abnormalities.* London: Churchill Livingstone, 2000.

period from severe pulmonary hypoplasia. Normal liquor with stable hydronephrosis presenting in the third trimester may have a better outcome, but normal renal cortical echogenicity does not exclude renal dysplasia. Up to 23% of kidneys that appear normal prenatally may have renal dysplasia.[204]

The above figures relate to isolated posterior urethral valves; if there are associated abnormalities the outcome is likely to be much poorer.

Management

In the poor prognosis group diagnosed at midtrimester with severe oligohydramnios, marked bladder distension, and bilateral hydronephrotic echogenic kidneys, it seems appropriate to offer termination of pregnancy because these babies ultimately die in the neonatal period from pulmonary hypoplasia.

At the other end of the spectrum, a fetus with normal liquor volume and stable hydronephrosis can probably be monitored by scanning every 2 weeks until 38 to 40 weeks' gestation, when delivery can be carried out.

Difficulties occur when liquor volume starts to decrease together with increasing bladder distension or hydronephrosis. It is in this setting that fetal intervention has been proposed to decompress the bladder and, it is hoped, prevent further renal damage and improve liquor volume and, hence, reduce the risk of pulmonary hypoplasia.[2,154,170] Early animal experimental work has certainly shown that decompressing renal obstruction at an appropriate time can prevent renal dysplasia,[205] and so it is based on this evidence that intervention for worsening fetal obstruction has been developed. It has been estimated that intervention for fetal renal obstruction is rare, indicated in only 1 in 60,000 fetuses; thus, these procedures should be carried out in a small number of tertiary referral centers.[206]

It appears that the best means of assessing renal function *in utero* is to carry out serial aspirations of urine from the fetal bladder over 3 to 4 days. Analyses of the urine biochemistry are made and, depending on the results, the fetus can be assigned to either a good or poor prognostic group[21–23,204,207] (Table 12). In the poor prognostic group, conservative management is recommended because these babies are likely to have severe renal dysplasia and a poor outcome postnatally. Fetuses in the good prognostic group in whom intervention is considered should have detailed scanning to exclude associated anomalies and a fetal karyotype. If detected before 32 weeks' gestation, placement of a vesicoamniotic shunt could be carried out to decompress the urinary system. After 32 weeks, early delivery with postnatal surgery, usually valve ablation, is the recommended management.[154]

There are a number of complications of shunt placement, including chorioamnionitis, shunt malplacement, anterior abdominal wall defects, preterm labor, and fetal

demise.[154,208,209] The outcome for fetuses with urethral valves that have been shunted is difficult to evaluate due to the small numbers of cases involved, but recent work tends to suggest that renal failure rates are similar to those cases diagnosed postnatally.[199]

The exact role of fetal intervention in obstruction uropathy has not been fully determined, but with improvements in techniques and urine biochemistry, prognosis can be predicted more accurately. Another improvement is the introduction of multidisciplinary teams of obstetricians, radiologists, pediatricians, and pediatric urologists in the assessment of each case on an individual basis. In this way knowledge of the natural history and outcomes of treatments can be appreciated by all relevant clinicians and subsequently improve the counseling and prenatal management of fetal obstructive uropathy.[210]

Urethral Atresia

Urethral atresia consists of complete obstruction of the urethra secondary to obliteration of the membranous urethra.

Incidence

The exact incidence is unknown; however, it accounts for 10% to 62% of causes of bladder outlet obstruction in prenatal series.[211,212] Pathologic series report urethral atresia in up to 44% of fetuses with obstructive uropathy.[35] It is more common in boys.

Etiology

The etiology is unknown.

Embryology

The anomaly is thought to result from incomplete canalization of the distal urogenital sinus that forms the membranous urethra.

Diagnosis

Sonographically there is usually massive dilatation of the bladder with bilateral hydronephrosis and oligohydramnios. In severe cases the bladder can completely fill the uterine cavity and make assessment of the remainder of the fetus extremely difficult.[213] Rarely, there may be a communication between the bladder and amniotic cavity, such as a spontaneous vesicocutaneous fistula, and then liquor volume may be normal.[213]

Differential Diagnosis

The differential diagnosis includes other causes of bladder outlet obstruction, such as posterior urethral valves, megacystis-microcolon syndrome, megalourethra, persistent cloaca, and severe vesicoureteric reflux.

Associated Anomalies

Associated anomalies occur in 52% to 66% but may be difficult to demonstrate due to the associated oligohydramnios.[212,213] In one series associated anomalies were seen in only one-half of the affected fetuses.[212]

Abnormalities associated include cardiac defects, diaphragmatic hernia, anal atresia, esophageal atresia, unilateral renal agenesis, polydactyly, cleft lip and palate, and the VATER syndrome.

Chromosomal defects include trisomy 13, 18, and 21.[212,213] The condition is also a cause of the prune-belly syndrome.

Prognosis

Prognosis is poor, with most babies dying in the neonatal period from pulmonary hypoplasia. The development of a vesicocutaneous fistula can decompress the urinary tract and lead to neonatal survival. Those babies who do survive the neonatal period usually develop end-stage renal failure requiring dialysis or transplantation and major reconstructive surgery.[213,214]

Management

In view of the universally poor outlook for this condition, a termination of pregnancy is an appropriate option. If the patient wishes to continue with the pregnancy, a conservative management policy may be adopted.

Recurrence Risk

The condition is sporadic and so the recurrence risk is low.

Megacystis-Microcolon–Intestinal Hypoperistalsis Syndrome

Megacystis-microcolon–intestinal hypoperistalsis syndrome consists of functional small bowel obstruction, intestinal malrotation, microcolon, and an enlarged nonobstructed urinary bladder often associated with bilateral hydronephrosis.[215]

Incidence

The condition is rare, with approximately 80 cases having been reported in the literature.[216] It is more common in females, with a female-to-male ratio of 4 to 1,[217] but has an autosomal recessive inheritance.[145,218,219] The reason for the marked skewing of the sex ratio in reported cases is unclear, but it has been postulated that the disease process in males may be more severe, resulting in spontaneous midpreg-

nancy loss, or that male cases may be misdiagnosed as the prune-belly syndrome.[220]

Etiology

It is the most severe form of functional intestinal obstruction in the neonate, but the etiology remains unclear. Myogenic, neurogenic, and hormonal influences have all been proposed.[221]

Pathology

The pathologic findings vary considerably and include changes to neural tissue and muscle within bowel wall. Several authors have reported increases or decreases in the number of ganglion cells in the submucosal and myenteric plexus, whereas others have reported normal numbers.[217,221,222] Axonal fibers have been reported as prominent or increased, and vacuolar degeneration of smooth muscle is also a common finding.[217] The diverse range of pathologic findings may be due to the focal nature of some of these appearances or may represent pathologic heterogeneity within the syndrome.[217]

Macroscopically there is a dilated, thick-walled bladder that is nonobstructed, functional small bowel obstruction, and a malrotated microcolon.

Diagnosis

Sonographically there is marked dilatation of the bladder, which is thick-walled and usually associated with bilateral hydronephrosis.[215,217,218] Liquor volume is usually normal, and in the third trimester, polyhydramnios may be present in almost 60% of cases. One of the most important factors in the diagnosis is the sex of the fetus as a female fetus with apparent bladder outlet obstruction, and polyhydramnios should always raise the possibility of megacystis-microcolon syndrome.[215,217]

Prenatally, dilatation of the bowel is rare and has only been reported four times: In two cases, the small bowel was dilated,[215,223] in one the stomach,[219] and in one the esophagus.[216]

The diagnosis may be made easier if a previous sibling has been affected.

Differential Diagnosis

The differential diagnosis includes posterior urethral valves and urethral atresia, both of which are more common in male fetuses. Other possibilities include severe vesicoureteric reflux, persistent cloaca, and megalourethra.[224]

Associated Anomalies

Associated anomalies are seen in approximately 14% of cases and include omphalocele, cardiac defects, and cleft palate.[215]

Prognosis

The prognosis is extremely poor, with 80% of infants dying within the first year of life and 90% within 2 years.[215] Although prokinetic agents and parenteral alimentation have prolonged life in several cases, the long-term outlook remains poor. In many cases, families elect not to embark on parenteral feeding in infancy.[217] The main cause of death is sepsis in the majority of infants.

Management

Management of this condition is difficult to dictate because it is extremely difficult to make a definitive diagnosis in the absence of a previously affected sibling.[217] If a family history is available and the sonographic findings are consistent with the diagnosis, a termination of pregnancy is an appropriate option. If there is no family history, the situation is much more complex.

Although bladder outlet obstruction is unusual in female fetuses, urethral stenosis or severe vesicoureteric reflux can produce similar appearances. In a male, posterior urethral valve is the main alternative diagnosis. All of these diagnoses are more frequent and have a better prognosis than megacystis-microcolon syndrome, and so in the absence of an affected sibling the offer of a termination of pregnancy would be difficult to justify given the diagnostic uncertainty. In addition, the vast majority of reported cases have been managed conservatively. In that setting, a conservative approach is likely to be the most appropriate management strategy.

Recurrence Risk

The condition is autosomal recessive, so there is a 25% risk of recurrence.

Congenital Megalourethra

Megalourethra is a rare congenital malformation characterized by dilatation of the penile urethra.

Incidence

This is a rare disorder only affecting males.[225]

Etiology

The etiology is unknown, but an *in utero* vascular accident has been suggested as a possible cause.[225]

Embryology and Pathology

Megalourethra is thought to result from an arrest in the embryogenesis of the corpus spongiosum and less commonly the corpora cavernosum as well at approximately 7 weeks'

gestation.[226] The condition is usually subdivided into the scaphoid type, which is more common (75% of cases), and the fusiform type (25%).[227] The scaphoid type is caused by absence of the corpus spongiosum in the anterior urethra so that the urethra balloons out inferiorly during micturition. The fusiform type is caused by absence of the corpus spongiosum and corpora cavernosum so that the urethra balloons out in a fusiform manner. Although there is normally no evidence of a distal urethral obstruction, it has been postulated that a transient distal obstruction, possibly at the level of the meatus, produces the urethra dilatation and the often-associated signs of bladder outlet obstruction.[227,228]

Diagnosis

The diagnosis is made by demonstrating a pear- or sausage-shaped cystic mass arising from the perineum and extending between the legs.[229,230] In addition, it may be possible to demonstrate continuity of the cystic mass (dilated penile urethra) with the bladder, thus confirming the diagnosis.[229]

There are often signs of bladder outlet obstruction with a distended, thick-walled bladder and bilateral hydronephrosis.[229–231] Liquor volume is variable depending on the degree of obstruction and consequently the degree of renal dysplasia. In some cases liquor volume has been noted to be increased.[228] The presence of an associated anal atresia or rectovesical fistula may produce dilatation of the bowel later in pregnancy.

Differential Diagnosis

The differential includes other causes of bladder outlet obstruction, such as posterior urethral valves, urethral atresia, and severe vesicoureteric reflux. Megacystis-microcolon syndrome is also possible but is more common in females. A urethral diverticulum could produce a focal dilatation of the urethra, but it does not usually produce bladder outlet obstruction.

Associated Anomalies

Associated renal anomalies are seen in the majority of the fusiform type[225,230,231] and include renal agenesis, pelvi-ureteric junction obstruction, megaureter, and a dilated bladder with bilateral hydronephrosis. Renal anomalies are seen in approximately 70% of the scaphoid type.

Extrarenal anomalies are seen in approximately 50% of both types of megalourethra. The anomalies appear to be more severe in the fusiform type and include anal atresia, rectovesical fistula, and the VATER syndrome. Less common findings include cleft lip and palate, talipes, scoliosis, cardiac defects, and a single case of trisomy 21.[225,232]

Prognosis

The presence of associated anomalies contributes to the high perinatal mortality rate for megalourethra, which has been reported to be as high as 60.0% for the fusiform type and 22.5% for the scaphoid type.[228] The main causes of death in postnatal series are renal failure and septicemia secondary to urinary tract infection. Neonatal death from pulmonary hypoplasia due to severe oligohydramnios has also been reported.[229]

Long-term survivors require reconstructive surgery and may have chronic renal failure, impotence, and infertility.[229]

Management

In the case of severe bladder outlet obstruction with oligohydramnios and associated anomalies, a termination of pregnancy seems an appropriate management option due to the anticipated poor outcome. When liquor volume is normal and associated anomalies are absent, the pregnancy may be managed conservatively.

Vesicoureteric Reflux

Vesicoureteric reflux is the retrograde flow of urine from the bladder into the ureter and usually the pelvicalyceal system.[233]

Incidence

It is estimated that reflux occurs in 1% of all children and in 30% to 50% of those who present with a urinary tract infection.[234] In addition, reflux nephropathy is the cause of end-stage renal failure in 3% to 25% of children and 10% to 15% of adults.[235] In the neonatal period reflux is more common in boys, but at the age of 4 to 5 years, girls predominate.[236] Vesicoureteric reflux has been estimated to account for up to 10% of cases of fetal hydronephrosis.[237]

Etiology

The etiology is likely to be multifactorial, as there appear to be two distinct groups: neonatal reflux, which is more common in boys, and reflux seen in older children, which is more common in girls. Delayed maturity of the vesicoureteric junction and dysfunctional voiding[237,238] are two possible causes of reflux in older children. In the neonate it is thought that the high voiding pressures seen in some babies could distort the vesicoureteric junction *in utero* and lead to reflux.[237]

Another possibility is the development of a transient bladder outlet obstruction that resolves before birth.[239] There is some evidence for this with the finding of bladder-wall thickening in boys with neonatal reflux.[236] In addition, there is a very strong familial tendency with high recurrence rates in children of patients with reflux.[240]

Pathology

It is well established that when associated with urinary infection, vesicoureteric reflux can lead to renal scarring

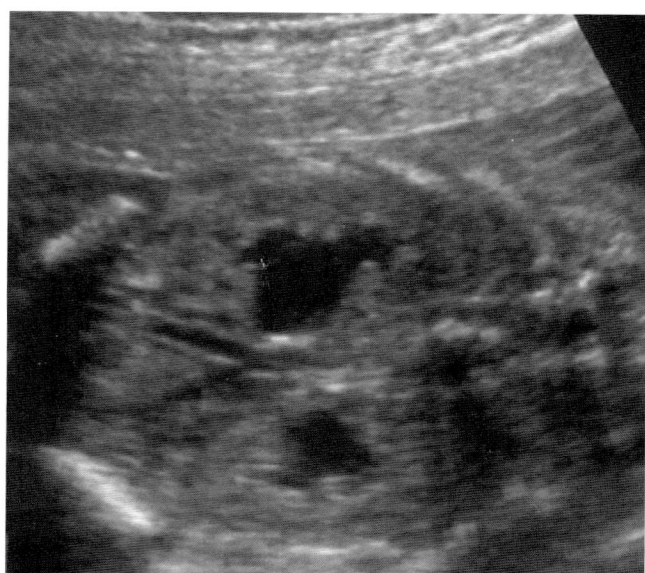

FIGURE 48. Vesicoureteric reflux. A coronal scan at 20 weeks shows mild bilateral hydronephrosis. Bladder and liquor volume are normal. Follow-up scans showed no change. Postnatal investigations revealed bilateral reflux.

and reflux nephropathy.[241] What has also become apparent over the last few years is that in 30% to 40% of baby boys with neonatal reflux there is also focal scarring or small globally damaged kidneys.[236,237,242,243] It is, therefore, likely that this damage occurred *in utero*, before the baby could have been exposed to infection. This type of renal scarring occurs predominantly in boys and is associated with high-grade bilateral reflux.[236]

Diagnosis

The main sonographic features are of hydronephrosis, which may be unilateral or bilateral. The degree of hydronephrosis does not necessarily correlate with the grade of vesicoureteric reflux postnatally; however, severe cases may show marked bilateral hydronephrosis, hydroureters, and a dilated thin-walled bladder—the so-called megacystis-megaureter association—and this can look very similar to posterior urethral valves[244] (Fig. 48). Liquor volume is usually normal throughout gestation.[245,246] There have been reports of the demonstration of vesicoureteric reflux *in utero*, and this finding is pathognomonic of the condition[247] (Fig. 49). Some reports have revealed that up to 14% of fetuses with mild renal pelvic dilatation (between 4 and 10 mm) have vesicoureteric reflux.[248]

Differential Diagnosis

The differential diagnosis includes many of the other causes of hydronephrosis. If unilateral, pelviureteric junction and vesicoureteric junction obstruction are possible. If bilateral,

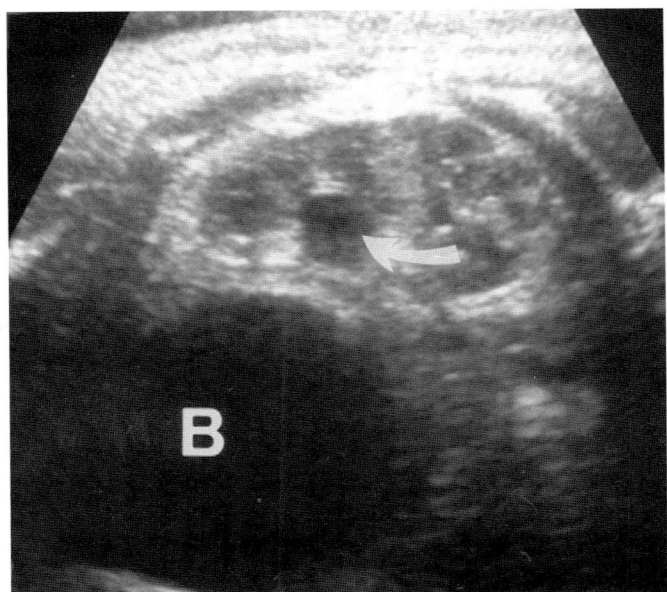 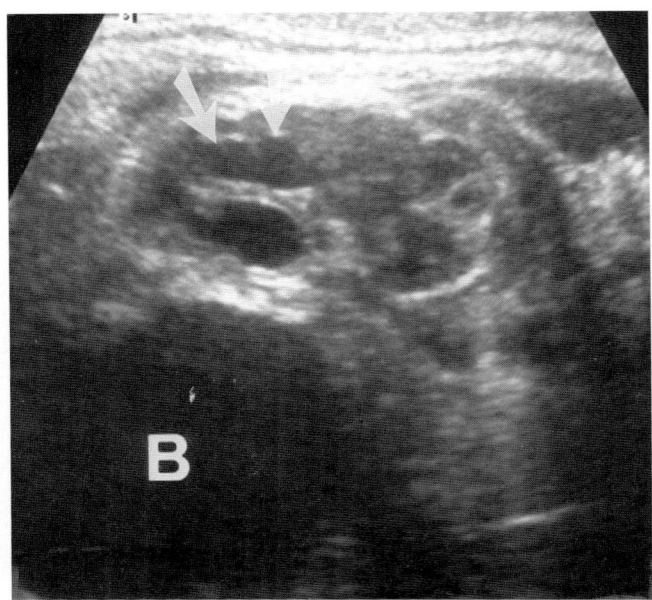

A   B

FIGURE 49. *In utero* vesicoureteric reflux. Coronal scans at 28 weeks' gestation. **A:** Duplex kidney with mild dilatation of the renal pelvis of the lower pole moiety (*curved arrow*). **B:** After reflux, there is dilatation of the collecting system (*arrows*). Note the full bladder (*B*).

posterior urethral valves are possible, as are the other causes of bladder outlet obstruction. A definite diagnosis of vesicoureteric reflux cannot be made until a micturating cystourethrogram is carried out in the neonatal period.

Associated Anomalies

Vesicoureteric reflux can be associated with a large number of contralateral renal anomalies, including pelviureteric junction obstruction, multicystic kidney, duplex kidney, and renal agenesis.[140] Extrarenal anomalies are rare.

Genetic Markers

Familial clustering of vesicoureteric reflux has long been recognized, suggesting a genetic basis. Some workers have proposed a dominantly inherited allele, whereas others hypothesize a multifactorial or polygenic front.[235] Mutations in the *PAX2* gene cause the rare coloboma-ureteral-renal syndrome, but family studies have shown no link with primary vesicoureteric reflux.[235]

Prognosis

Recent studies have shown a remarkably constant incidence of 12% to 14% for vesicoureteric reflux in series of antenatal hydronephrosis.[248–250] Of these babies with neonatal reflux, 27% to 33% show renal scarring, two-thirds of which takes the form of generalized renal damage.[236,250] In addition, reflux nephropathy probably accounts for up to 25% of childhood renal failure and 15% in adults,[235] so

vesicoureteric reflux is a potentially serious disease with long-term sequelae. Fortunately these cases are in the minority as greater than 36% of vesicoureteric reflux cases resolve by the age of 2 years.[245,249] In a large series, Yeung et al.[236] reported resolution in 70% of mild reflux cases and 43% of severe reflux cases at 15 months of age.

Management

When hydronephrosis is demonstrated *in utero*, follow-up scans are indicated in the third trimester to reassess the degree of hydronephrosis and the liquor volume. In most cases of reflux, even when bilateral and severe, liquor volume is normal.

In the postnatal period, ultrasound assessment is indicated but should be delayed for at least 48 hours after delivery. The significance of postnatal ultrasound has been questioned because 25% to 42% of babies subsequently documented with vesicoureteric reflux have normal postnatal appearances.[236,247,249] It is probably wise, therefore, with a prenatal diagnosis of hydronephrosis to commence prophylactic antibiotics and proceed to a micturating cystourethrogram irrespective of the postnatal ultrasound findings.[251]

In the situation of mild renal pelvic dilatation there is no consensus at present, but these babies certainly require postnatal ultrasound and urologic follow-up with repeat ultrasound at 3 months.

Surgery is usually reserved for babies with breakthrough infection, the development of new scars, high-grade reflux, and progression of reflux.[234] In patients with mild to moderate reflux, there appears to be no major advantage over medical treatment.[252]

Recurrence Risk

There is a strong familial tendency, and the risk of reflux in babies of mothers who reflux is 66%.[253] The risk for siblings is 35%.[254]

Persistent Cloaca (Cloacal Malformation)

Persistent cloaca is a complex abnormality in which the urinary, genital, and intestinal tracts converge into a common outflow structure, the cloaca (Latin for "sewer").[162]

Incidence

The condition typically affects females and has an incidence of 1 in 50,000.[163,255]

Etiology

The etiology is unknown, but in two case reports there was an association with maternal narcotics abuse.[256,257]

Embryology

Persistent cloaca results from a failure in the development of the urorectal fold, which separates the rectum from the uterovaginal tract. Normally at 7 weeks the urorectal septum arises between the allantois and hindgut and gradually grows caudally, dividing the cloaca into the anterior portion (urogenital sinus) and posterior portion (anorectal canal). Failure or maldevelopment of the urorectal septum produces persistent cloaca.[258] The cloaca is a single channel into which the urinary, genital, and intestinal tracts converge, with a single opening on the perineum.

It has been classified into two types: (a) the urethral type, in which the perineal opening is a continuation of the urethra, and (b) the vaginal type, in which the opening is a continuation of the vagina[255] (Fig. 50).

The communications of the urethra, vagina, and rectum can be complex and lead to bladder outlet obstruction, hydrometrocolpos, or colonic dilatation.

Diagnosis

The diagnosis may be very difficult due to the complex nature of the anomaly and variable appearances. The most common sonographic findings are ascites, intraabdominal cystic structures (hydrometrocolpos), and associated malformations.[258–260] It has been postulated that the ascites may be transient and occur early due to urine entering the abdominal cavity via the fallopian tubes. Later in pregnancy occlusion of the tubal mucosa occurs, probably because of

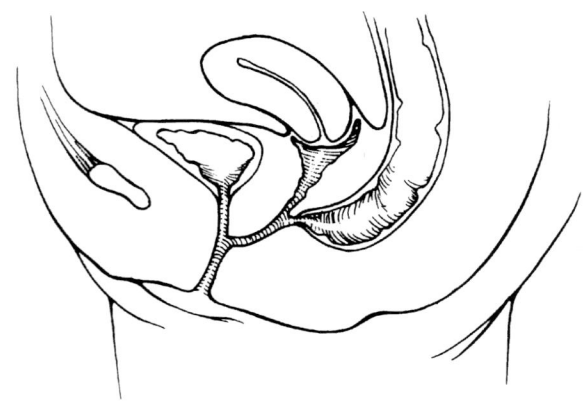

A

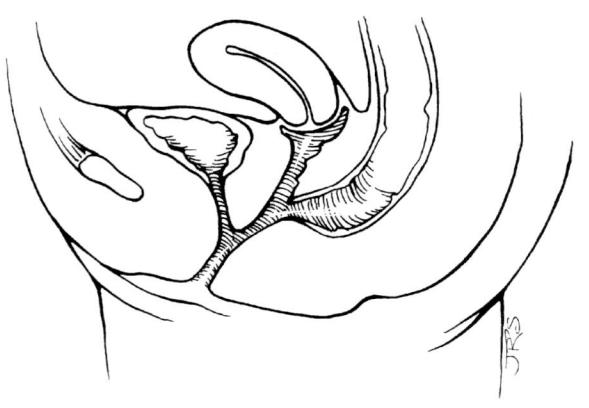

B

FIGURE 50. Persistent cloaca. Diagram outlining the two types of cloacal malformation: the urethral **(A)** and vaginal **(B)** configurations.

irritation by urine and meconium. As there is commonly a degree of obstruction through the cloacal channel, backward pressure is built up, producing a hydrometrocolpos (the midline cystic structure). The midline cystic structure may be bicystic and may show debris or fluid-fluid levels.[258,259] The hydrometrocolpos can compress the bladder to produce bladder outlet obstruction and bilateral hydronephrosis. Similarly, narrowing of the rectal communication or direct compression can lead to colonic dilatation.[260]

Liquor volume is variable and depends on the degree of bladder outlet obstruction. Growth retardation may also be seen. Meconium peritonitis with peritoneal calcification has also been reported,[261] as have colonic calcifications.[262]

The presence of transient ascites followed by the development of a cystic midline pelvic mass with or without bilateral hydronephrosis or colonic dilatation is highly suggestive of persistent cloaca.

Differential Diagnosis

The differential diagnosis includes other causes of bladder outlet obstruction, such as posterior urethral valves and

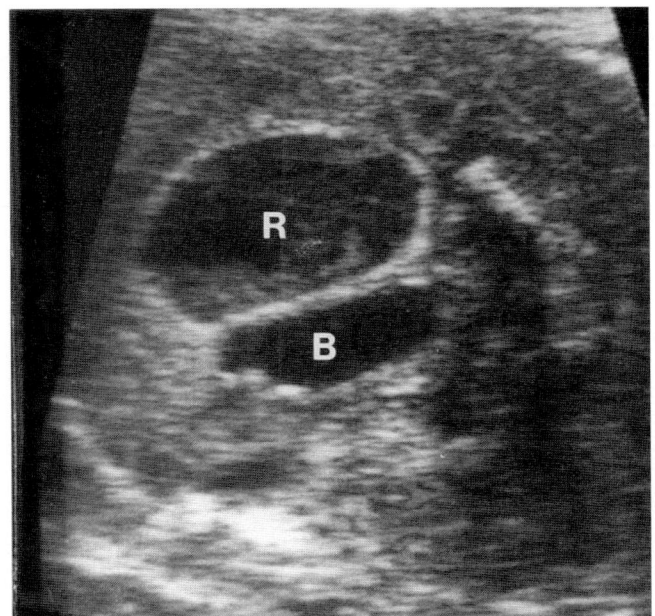
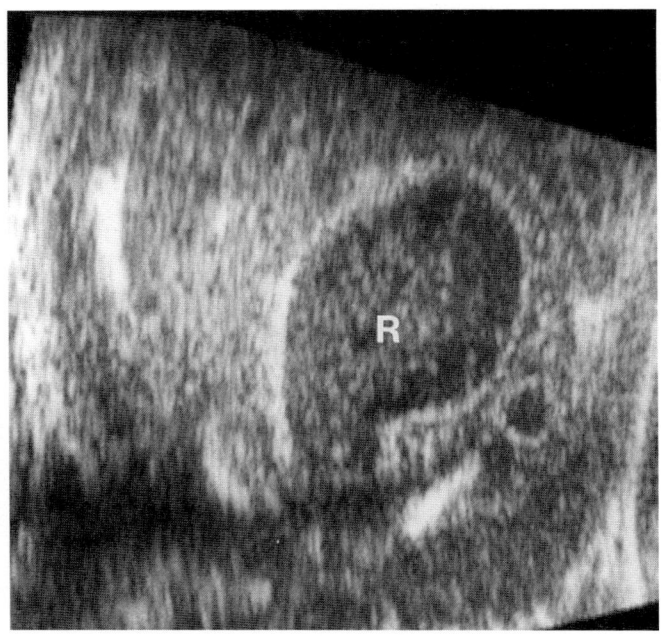

A

B

FIGURE 51. Anal atresia with rectovesical fistula. **A:** A transverse scan through the fetal pelvis shows a normal bladder (*B*) and a dilated fluid-filled rectum (*R*). **B:** A coronal scan through the pelvis shows a distended rectum (*R*) filled with fluid and meconium. During micturition, urine passes directly into the rectum due to the large fistulous communication from which it is absorbed. No urine passes through the urethra, so there is oligohydramnios. Both kidneys, however, are normal.

megacystis-microcolon syndrome.[258] Colonic dilatation can be seen in anal atresia and can be associated with oligohydramnios if there is a retrovesical fistula[263] (Fig. 51). A hydrometrocolpos may also be seen in association with a urogenital sinus.[264] The presence of ascites requires the consideration of other diagnoses, such as urinary ascites, meconium peritonitis, and hydrops.

Associated Anomalies

There is a high incidence of associated malformations, including bladder duplication, uterine duplication, vaginal duplication, hydrometrocolpos, ambiguous genitalia, sacral agenesis, spina bifida, and tethered cord.[255] Extrapelvic anomalies include horseshoe kidney, duplex kidneys, hydronephrosis, renal dysplasia, esophageal and intestinal atresia, and meconium peritonitis. Other anomalies seen are ventricular septal defects, tetralogy of Fallot, craniofacial anomalies, vertebral anomalies, and hydrocephalus.[162]

Prognosis

The presence of oligohydramnios is a poor prognostic sign and usually indicates severe bladder outlet obstruction and pulmonary hypoplasia.[258] Fetuses with normal amniotic fluid levels have a better outcome.

The prognosis for survivors has improved dramatically in recent years, with reasonably good functional outcome after surgical repair.

Management

When the diagnosis is suspected antenatally, meticulous scanning is indicated to assess the severity of the condition and associated anomalies. Careful counseling by a pediatric urologic surgeon who is experienced with the condition is also essential to outline for the parents the likely outcome for the baby. Counseling with regard to a termination of pregnancy should also be considered in view of the severity and complexity of the condition. If the parents elect to continue with the pregnancy, the mother needs to deliver in a tertiary referral center with access to pediatric urologic surgery because prompt surgical intervention is the key to a good outcome. The initial step in the surgical management is a defunctioning colostomy to prevent fecal contamination of the urinary tract. After this, extensive radiologic investigation is required to define the anatomy of the malformation before corrective reconstructive surgery.[255,260]

Recurrence Risk

The condition is sporadic, with low recurrence risk.

Persistent Urogenital Sinus and Hydrometrocolpos

The persistent urogenital sinus is a single-exit chamber for the bladder and vagina, association with an enlarged phallus-like clitoris and a normal anus.[265] Less severe forms may present as an imperforate hymen or vaginal septum. Vaginal atresia may also form part of the spectrum.[266] All of these conditions can produce hydrometrocolpos, which is distension of the uterus and vagina secondary to obstruction.

Incidence

The condition commonly affects females and is rare. The exact incidence is unknown.

Etiology

The condition is most commonly seen in female pseudohermaphroditism resulting from adrenogenital syndrome or other *in utero* exposure to androgenic stimuli.[266] In some cases there is no obvious hormonal basis.[264]

Embryology

The anomaly is the result of abnormal development of the lower vagina from the urogenital sinus (insufficient vaginal urogenital sinus separation). The urogenital sinus often becomes obstructed, producing a pelvic mass that represents a hydrometrocolpos. This can compress the bladder to produce bladder outlet obstruction.

Diagnosis

The diagnosis is based on the demonstration of a midline cystic mass (hydrometrocolpos) that may be compressing the bladder and producing bilateral hydronephrosis. The cystic mass may contain low-level echoes and can be large. Severe bladder outlet obstruction can lead to cystic renal dysplasia and oligohydramnios.[264]

Sonographically, hydrometrocolpos secondary to imperforate hymen presents as a midline cystic mass extending caudally into the perineum with spreading of the labia majora.[267,268]

Differential Diagnosis

The differential diagnosis includes persistent cloaca and other causes of bladder outlet obstruction.

Associated Anomalies

Associated anomalies include ambiguous genitalia, duplex genital tract, and bilateral hydronephrosis. Severe hydronephrosis can lead to renal dysplasia. Hydrometrocolpos secondary to imperforate hymen is usually isolated.

Prognosis

The prognosis depends on the severity of the hydronephrosis and subsequent renal dysplasia. Oligohydramnios is a poor prognostic sign, with most babies dying from pulmonary hypoplasia in the neonatal period. In survivors, the long-term outlook is reasonably good after reconstructive surgery.

Management

When hydrometrocolpos is suspected, careful counseling from a pediatric urologic surgeon is essential and delivery in a tertiary center with access to pediatric surgery is indicated.

Recurrence Risk

The persistent urogenital sinus is a sporadic condition, so recurrence risk is low. Imperforate hymen is also sporadic, but a few familial cases have been reported.[268]

Cloacal Exstrophy (Omphalocele, Vesical Exstrophy, Imperforate Anus, Spinal Abnormalities, OEIS Complex)

Cloacal exstrophy is a complex malformation consisting of bladder exstrophy and externalization of the small and large bowel onto the lower abdominal wall. The phallus is usually bifid, anal atresia is also present, and an omphalocele may be associated[266] (Fig. 52).

Incidence

The incidence is approximately 1 in 250,000 live births. The condition is more common in males and in twin pregnancies.[269]

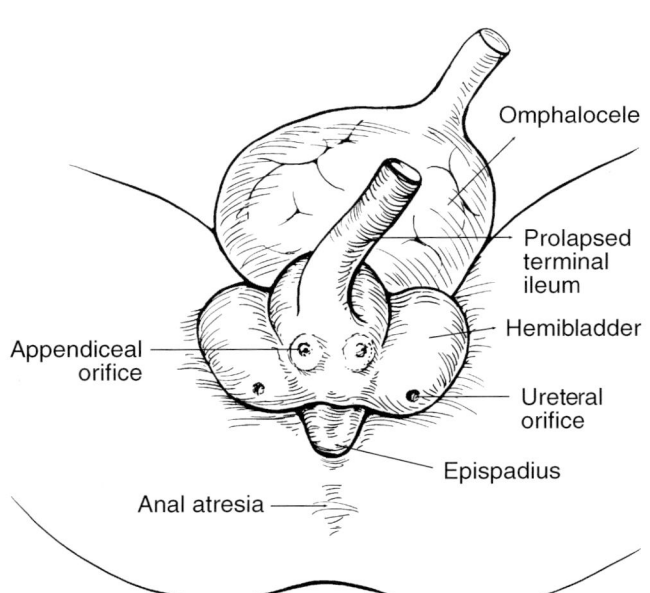

FIGURE 52. Diagram showing the major findings on the anterior abdominal wall in cloacal exstrophy. (Reproduced with permission from Hurwitz RS, Manzoni GA, Ransley PG, Stephens FD. Cloacal exstrophy: a report of 34 cases. *J Urol* 1987;138:1060–1064.)

Etiology

The etiology remains unknown but multifactorial inheritance appears probable.[269]

Embryology

Cloacal exstrophy results from rupture of the cloacal membrane prior to completion of the caudal growth of the urorectal septum. The result is the persistence of a common cloaca where through an inverted vesical mucous membrane, rudimentary elements from the allantois, terminal ileum, and right colon open. Diastasis of the pubic rami and abnormalities of the spine, commonly a closed neural tube defect, are also seen. Imperforate anus with absent or duplicate external genitalia may also be seen.[269]

Diagnosis

Reports have emphasized four major criteria for the diagnosis of cloacal exstrophy: nonvisualization of the bladder, a large midline infraumbilical anterior wall defect or cystic anterior wall structure (persistent cloacal membrane) (Figs. 53 and 54), omphalocele, and lumbosacral meningomyelocele.[270–272]

The midline abdominal wall defect is always situated below the level of the umbilicus, unlike omphalocele, in which the cord inserts into the defect. This low abdominal wall defect represents the everted bladder and bowel. Occasionally the everted terminal ileum can resemble an elephant's trunk, which has been proposed as a further sign of cloacal exstrophy[273,274] (Fig. 52). The cystic anterior wall structure (persistent cloacal membrane) appears to be present in the first trimester but can persist up to 22 weeks' gestation, after which time it usually ruptures and can no longer be visualized.[270,272]

Several minor criteria have also been proposed in the diagnosis of cloacal exstrophy and refer mainly to some of the less common associated anomalies. These minor criteria include talipes, renal anomalies, ascites, widened pubic arches, narrow thorax, hydrocephalus, and a single umbilical artery.[270]

Liquor volume is variable and can be normal or show polyhydramnios.[271]

Differential Diagnosis

The differential diagnosis includes other forms of anterior abdominal wall defect, such as omphalocele and gastroschisis. In the case of cloacal exstrophy the defect is always below the level of the umbilicus and the bladder is always absent. In bladder exstrophy the appearances may be similar but there is a much lower incidence of associated anomalies, particularly neural tube defects, and the lower abdominal wall defect is more of a bulge due to the atrophied bladder rather than the large defect secondary to everted bowel. The limb-body wall complex or amniotic band syndrome could produce similar appearances to cloacal exstrophy with large abdominal wall defects and associated anomalies; however, typical anomalies such as scoliosis, encephalocele, facial clefting, and amputation defects are uncommon in cloacal exstrophy.[275]

Associated Anomalies

Associated anomalies occur in up to 85% of cases.[274] Renal anomalies occur in 66%, the most common being pelvic kidney, unilateral renal agenesis, crossed fused ectopia, and multicystic kidney. Lumbosacral neural tube defects, which are often closed, occur in 70%. Gastrointestinal defects are also common, seen in 46%, and include malrotation, duplication, short small bowel, and duodenal atresia.[274]

Bilateral talipes and a single umbilical artery are also frequent findings.[275]

Prognosis

Before 1960 cloacal exstrophy was believed to be incompatible with life and there were no survivors. With improvements in surgical management and neonatal intensive care, survival rates are now in the range of 70% to 90%.[274] Multiple surgical procedures are required to create a colostomy, close the atrophied bladder, and bring together the widely separated pubic rami. After a variety of bladder reconstruction and urethral and bladder neck continence procedures, urinary continence may be possible, although intermittent catheterization is required.[274,276] Due to the difficulties in creating functioning male genitalia, it is usually recommended that genetic males undergo gender reassignment and be raised as females.[274]

Management

In view of the severity of the condition and the major surgical involvement required, it is a reasonable option to offer the parents a termination of pregnancy if a firm prenatal diagnosis is made. If the parents elect to continue with the

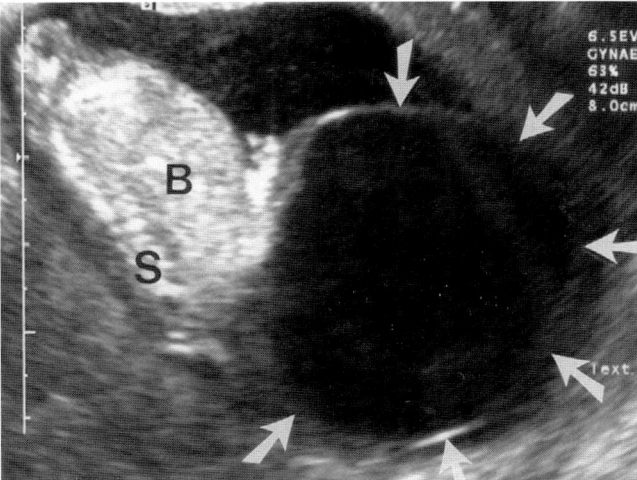

FIGURE 53. Cloacal exstrophy. Transvaginal scan of a 14-week fetus. A sagittal scan through the lower abdomen shows the cloacal membrane (*arrows*). B, body; S, spine.

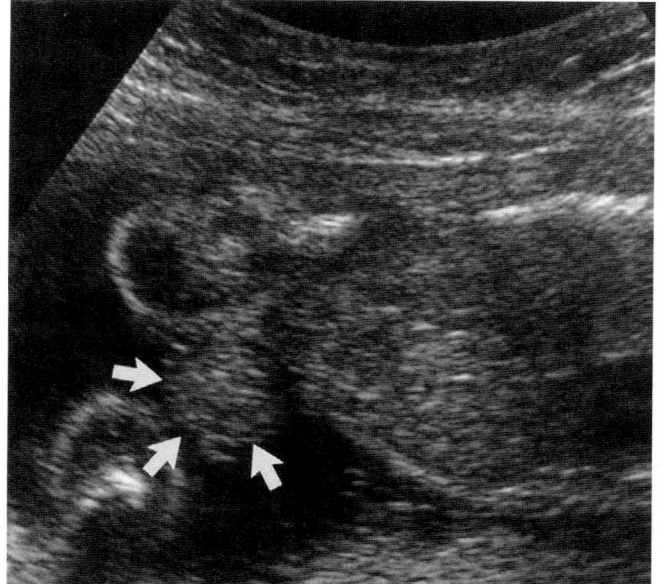

A

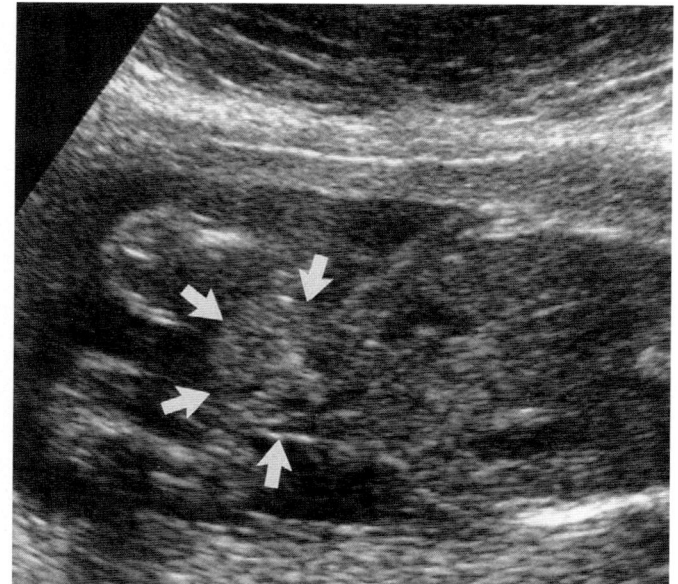

B

FIGURE 54. Cloacal exstrophy. **A:** A sagittal scan through the fetal abdomen at 22 weeks' gestation shows a low anterior abdominal wall defect (*arrows*), which represents the everted bladder and short externalized hindgut. **B:** A transverse section through the lower abdomen demonstrates the low cloacal defect (*arrows*). **C:** A coronal section through the lower spine demonstrates a closed neural tube defect (*arrows*).

C

pregnancy then delivery by cesarean section at a tertiary care center with access to pediatric urologic surgery is essential. In this way the initial surgical management can be carried out as soon as is appropriate.

Recurrence Risk

The condition is sporadic, so the recurrence risk is low.

Bladder Exstrophy

Bladder exstrophy consists of externalization of the bladder onto the anterior abdominal wall.

Incidence

The incidence is approximately 1 in 30,000 live births and is more common in males.[277]

Etiology

The etiology remains unclear, but as in cloacal exstrophy, multifactorial inheritance appears probable.

Embryology

Bladder exstrophy results from rupture of the cloacal membrane after completion of the caudal growth of the urorectal septum. The result is exstrophy of the bladder, which bulges outward at birth. Bladder size varies considerably from normal to a small trigonal plaque. The umbilicus is low lying and there is separation of the pubic bones. The anus is normal but anteriorly positioned. In males the testes are undescended and the penis is small with epispadias. In females the clitoris is cleft.[276]

Diagnosis

A number of important findings are associated with the diagnosis of bladder exstrophy, including absence of the bladder, a lower abdominal bulge representing the atrophied bladder, a small penis with anteriorly displaced scrotum, low insertion of the umbilical cord, and abnormal widening of the iliac crests.[278–280] In at least one reported case the bulge of the atrophied bladder was not present and color-flow Doppler imaging was useful in demonstrating absence of the bladder.[281]

The kidneys and liquor volume are usually normal,[103] and the incidence of associated anomalies is low.

Differential Diagnosis

The differential diagnosis includes cloacal exstrophy; however, there is a high incidence of associated anomalies with cloacal exstrophy particularly omphalocele and spina bifida, which are rare in bladder extrophy.[282] In addition, the abdominal bulge in cloacal exstrophy may be large and show the elephant's trunk appearance.[273]

Omphalocele and gastroschisis also need to be considered, but they are easily differentiated because the former is at the level of the umbilicus and the latter is just to the right of the umbilicus.

Associated Anomalies

Associated anomalies are uncommon but include unilateral renal agenesis, horseshoe kidney, and hydronephrosis.[276] If present, spinal anomalies are minor and are usually spina bifida occulta or lumbarization and sacralization of vertebrae.[282]

Prognosis

After initial bladder closure, major reconstructive surgery is required. Long-term follow-up suggests that overall outcome is relatively good, with expected normal urinary and genital function in many patients.[266] The psychological effects have also been studied, and the condition has a major impact on children and parents alike. Despite multiple operations, urinary leakage, and deviant genitalia, most children have good self-esteem.[283]

Recurrence Risk

The recurrence risk is approximately 1 in 275 for siblings. Children of parents with bladder exstrophy have a much higher incidence—approximately 1 in 70 live births.[277]

Renal Tumors

Renal tumors are those arising from the fetal kidney.

Incidence

Fetal renal tumors are rare. The incidence of all renal tumors in childhood is 1 in 125,000 live births.[284]

Etiology

The etiology is unknown.

Pathology

The most common fetal renal tumor is mesoblastic nephroma, which is benign. Pathologically the features are similar to a hamartoma, with elongated spindle-shaped mesenchymal cells. The tumor is contiguous with the normal nephrons and does not have a well-defined capsule.[285,286] Less commonly, Wilms tumor (nephroblastoma) may be seen antenatally.[287,288] This tumor is a triphasic embryonal neoplasm consisting of blastemal, stromal, and epithelial elements. Wilms tumor does have a well-defined capsule.[288]

Diagnosis

The tumor usually presents as a fairly homogeneous mass in the paraspinal region. The margins of a mesoblastic nephroma may be indistinct because it does not have a true capsule. The tumor may be large and compress other intra-abdominal organs[285,286] (Fig. 55).

Polyhydramnios may be seen in up to 70% of cases and is thought to be related to hypercalcemia with resulting fetal polyuria.[289]

Differential Diagnosis

The differential diagnosis includes adrenal neuroblastoma, which tends to displace the kidneys inferiorly (Fig. 56), and adrenal hemorrhage. Other less common conditions are retroperitoneal teratoma and subdiaphragmatic extralobar pulmonary sequestration. Teratomas tend to be predominantly cystic with areas of calcification and separate from the kidney. Similarly, a subdiaphragmatic sequestration is always situated just below the diaphragm and shows increased echogenicity. It is superior to the kidney and adrenal.

Associated Anomalies

Mesoblastic nephroma is an isolated tumor with no associated anomalies. Wilms tumor is associated with other anomalies in 15% of cases; these include aniridia, genitourinary anomalies, and hemihypertrophy.[288]

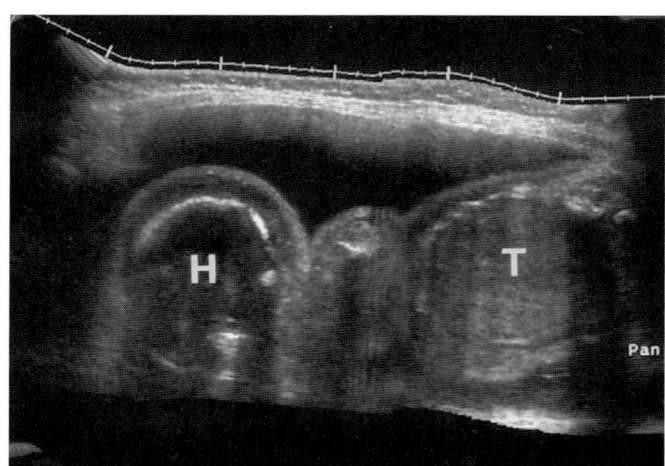

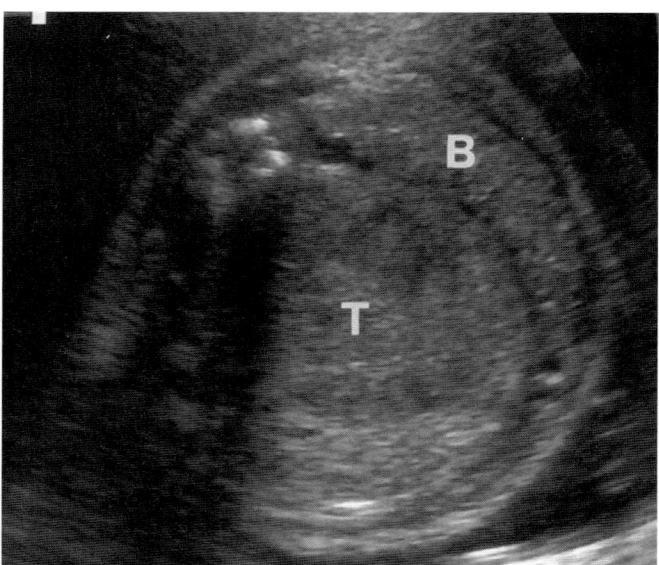

FIGURE 55. Renal tumor. **A:** An extended field of view scan shows a hydropic fetus with a renal tumor (*T*). H, head. **B:** A transverse scan through the fetal abdomen shows a massive renal tumor (*T*) compressing the bowel (*B*). (Reproduced with permission from Twining P, McHugo J, Pilling D. *Textbook of fetal abnormalities.* London: Churchill Livingstone, 2000.)

Genetic Markers

The *WT1* and *WT2* genes located on chromosome 11 and the *WT3* gene on chromosome 16q have been implicated in the development of Wilms tumors in syndromes such as the Beckwith-Wiedemann syndrome and Denys-Drash syndrome.[288]

Prognosis

The outcome is usually good and surgical resection is curative. Tumor rupture in the neonatal period has been

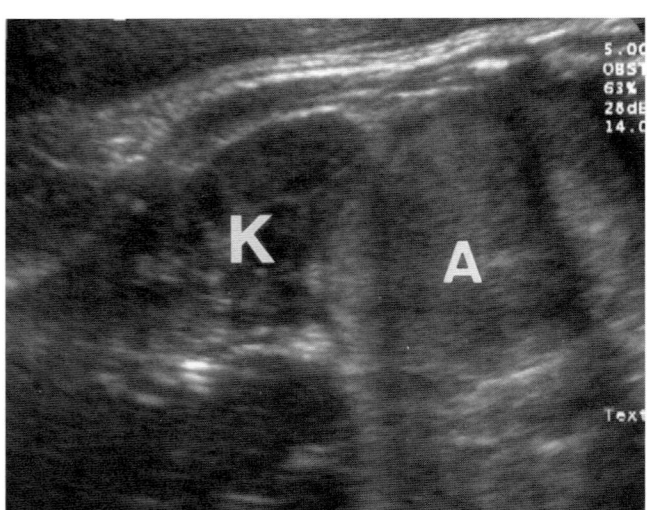

FIGURE 56. Adrenal neuroblastoma. A coronal scan in a 34-week fetus shows an adrenal tumor (*A*) displacing the kidney (*K*).

described, but this is a rare implication.[286] The association of hydrops, although also rare, is a poor prognostic sign.[288]

Management

Delivery at a tertiary care facility is indicated because neonatal surgery is likely to be required.

Recurrence Risk

The condition is sporadic, so the recurrence risk is low.

Fetal Gender

Diagnosis

A number of reports have assessed the accuracy of diagnosis of fetal gender in the second and third trimesters.[290–293] Accuracies range from 93% to 100% of cases. In the female, positive identification of the labia is as essential to the diagnosis as demonstration of the penis and scrotum is in the male (Fig. 57).

In more recent years attention has turned to the diagnosis of fetal gender in the first trimester.[294,295] Up to the eleventh week of gestation, male and female genitalia are identical, so sex determination is not possible prior to 11 weeks.[296]

The most useful scanning plane in the first trimester appears to be the sagittal plane, where the clitoris is represented by a caudally directed phallus. In males, the penis is

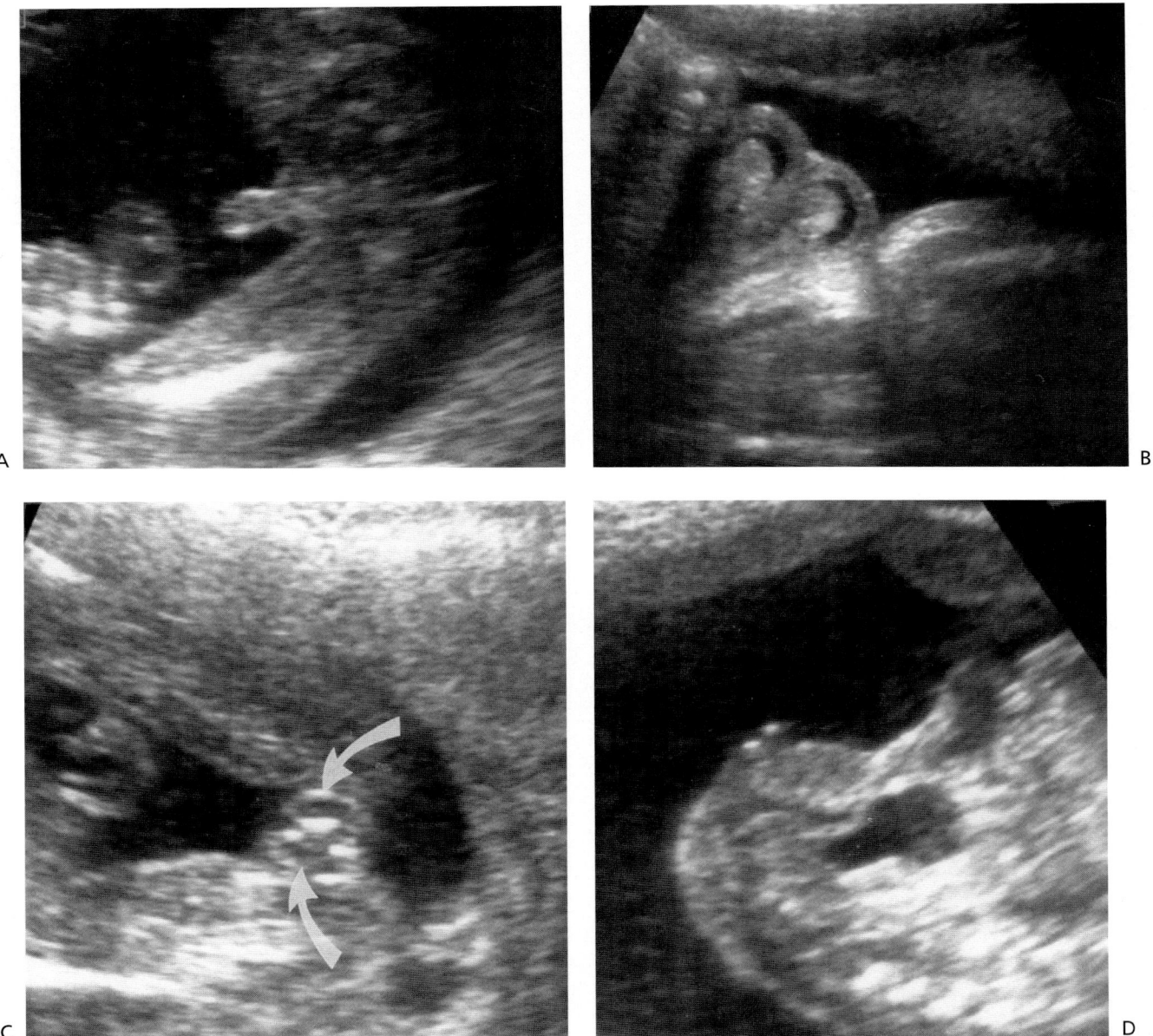

FIGURE 57. **A:** Normal male genitalia. A transverse scan at 20 weeks shows the penis and scrotum. **B:** In a scan through the scrotum of a male fetus at 32 weeks, both testes are present. Small bilateral hydroceles are also present. These are common in the third trimester and are of no significance. **C:** A coronal scan of normal female genitalia. Arrows point to labial folds. **D:** A sagittal scan of normal female genitalia.

seen as a cranially/vertically directed phallus (Fig. 58). Accuracy rates range from 46% to 70% at 11 weeks and 79% to 100% at 13 weeks.[294,295]

The most important aspect of fetal sex determination is in cases of a positive family history of X-linked disorders such as hemophilia, Duchenne's muscular dystrophy, and chronic granulomatous disease. In female fetuses an invasive procedure may be avoided, whereas in males a procedure could be considered to confirm the ultrasound diagnosis.[295]

Ambiguous Genitalia

Ambiguous genitalia is the term used when the appearances of the external genitalia are different from the genetic sex or when on examination there is doubt as to whether the patient is phenotypically male or female.

Incidence

This is a rare group of disorders with incidences in the range of 1 in 50,000 to 70,000.[297]

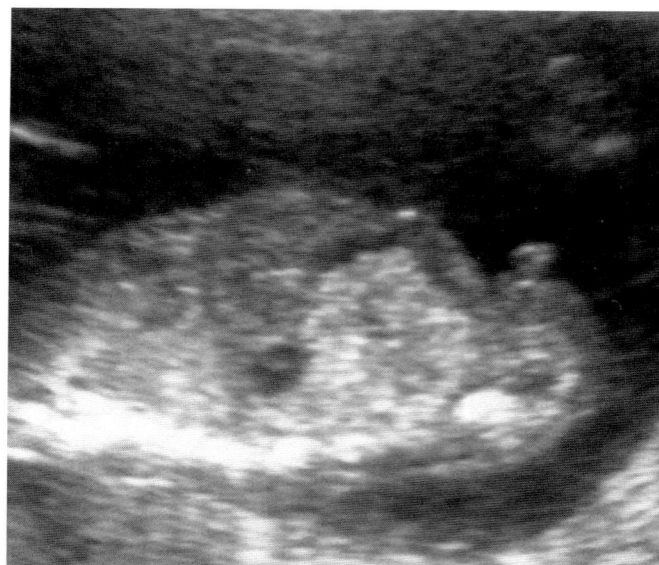

A

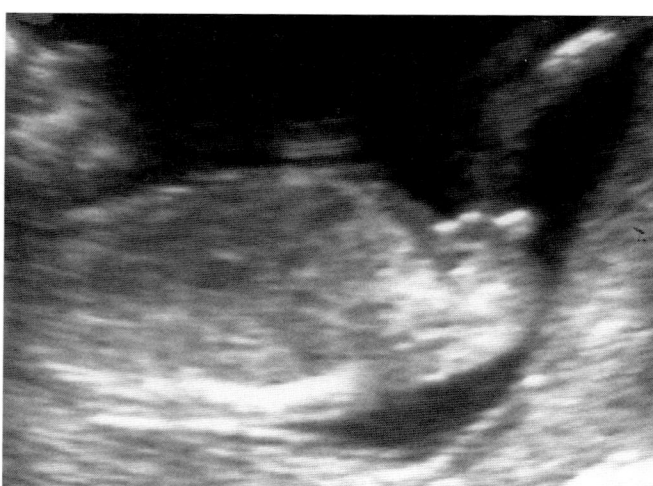

B

FIGURE 58. First-trimester sexing. **A:** A sagittal scan through a 13-week male fetus shows the vertically oriented phallus. **B:** A sagittal scan through a 13-week female fetus shows the horizontally oriented phallus.

Etiology

Ambiguous genitalia are made up of a heterogeneous group of disorders of differing etiologies but that are usually related to either chromosomal defects or an abnormal hormonal influence.

Five main conditions need to be considered when faced with a potential case of ambiguous genitalia: female pseudohermaphroditism, male pseudohermaphroditism, mixed gonadal dysgenesis, pure gonadal dysgenesis, and true hermaphroditism.[276] In addition, ambiguous genitalia may be a feature of a number of conditions, such as cloacal exstrophy, Smith-Lemli-Opitz syndrome, the CHARGE association, and aneuploidy.[298]

The main chromosomal defects include trisomy 13, triploidy, 13q syndrome, Xp21 duplication, 9p23 deletion, and 10q26 deletion.

In female pseudohermaphroditism the karyotype is female (46,XX) and patients have normal ovaries. The external genitalia are masculinized to a variable degree ranging from mild clitoral enlargement to normal male phenotype with an empty scrotum. These findings are secondary to excess androgenesis either from maternal ingestion or endogenous production due to the congenital adrenal hyperplasia (adrenogenital syndrome). In congenital adrenal hyperplasia, enzymatic defects, commonly deficiency of 21-hydroxylase, lead to elevated serum levels of 17-hydroxyprogesterone, and this affects the development of the genitalia in females. Babies with this condition are at risk for dehydration and hypotension due to loss of salt, which occurs due to decreased production of deoxycortisone.[276]

In male pseudohermaphroditism the karyotype is male (46,XY) and patients have two testes. The external genitalia

may appear female with a blind-ending vagina, or there may be a micropenis, alone or associated with cryptorchidism. The main cause is an abnormal response to testosterone (80%) and deficient testosterone production in the rest. Chromosomal anomalies may also be present, such as Klinefelter's syndrome (47,XXY) or the sex reversal male (46,XX).

In mixed gonadal dysgenesis there is chromosomal mosaicism (45,XO/46,XY); this is one of the more common forms of ambiguous genitalia. These patients may have the classic Turner syndrome phenotype or show ambiguous genitalia. Internal findings include a streak ovary on one side and a dysgenetic testis on the other side.[299,300]

In pure gonadal dysgenesis the karyotype is variable (46,XO; 46,XX; 46,XY) and normal external female genitalia and streak ovaries are present. They often present at puberty with amenorrhea and streak gonads.[299]

True hermaphroditism is extremely rare; most are genetic females (46,XX) who have some Y-chromatin material. Less commonly they are mosaic (46,XX/46,XY) or male genotype (46,XY). External genitalia are variable.

Embryology

The external genitalia remain in an undifferentiated state until 7 to 8 weeks' gestation. The presence of testis-determining factor on the Y chromosome is responsible for testicular development; in its absence the ovaries form. In males the gonad differentiates into a testis after the seventh week, the mullerian ducts regress, and the wolffian ducts form the seminal vesicles, vas deferens, and epididymis. The formation of the penis, scrotum, and prostate is dependent on the influence of dihydrotestosterone converted from testosterone by 5-reductase. Absence of the testis-

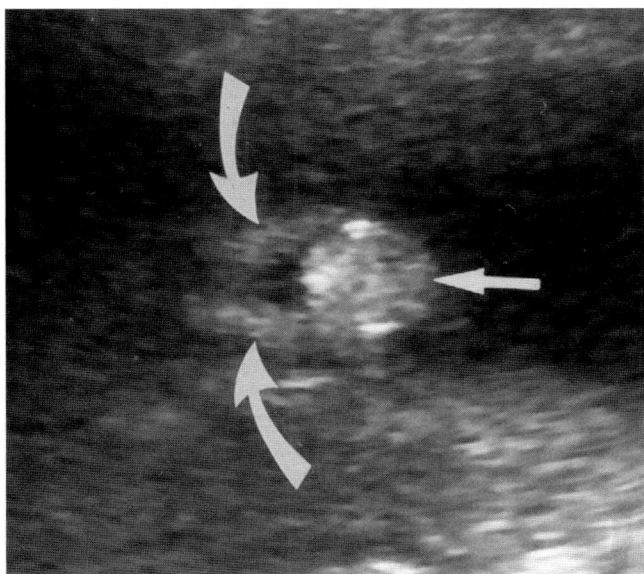

FIGURE 59. Ambiguous genitalia. A coronal scan of a 32-week fetus shows a micropenis (*straight arrow*) and shawl-type scrotum (*curved arrows*).

determining factor and the influence of dihydrotestosterone allows the passive formation of the female genitalia.[171] At 11 to 12 weeks the external genitalia have formed; however, in males, testicular descent does not occur until after 26 weeks, with 62% occurring between 28 and 30 weeks and 93% by 32 weeks.[301]

Diagnosis

The accurate diagnosis of genital abnormalities can be extremely difficult. In the case of sex reversal (i.e., the phenotypic appearances are opposite to the genetic makeup), the diagnosis may be fairly straightforward. Ambiguous genitalia, however, can be rather hard to define accurately because a micropenis with cryptorchidism (Fig. 59) may be impossible to differentiate from an enlarged clitoris with normal labia.[300–302] In this setting it seems wise to be circumspect in the diagnosis and maintain a diagnosis of ambiguous genitalia or genitalia unclear, as the postnatal diagnosis and final gender reassignment are dependent on a number of differing factors.

The main findings on scan in a male are micropenis, penile chordae (ventral curvature of the penis), undescended testes, a shawl or bifid scrotum, and hypospadias. In a female, clitoromegaly is the most common finding. Clearly sex reversal may be seen in either sex.

If ambiguous genitalia are suspected, a karyotype is of value in order to attempt a prenatal diagnosis. In a genetic male with ambiguous genitalia or sex reversal, male pseudohermaphroditism or pure gonadal dysgenesis is likely. Other possibilities include Denys-Drash syndrome and Swyer syndrome.[303,304]

When the ultrasound findings suggest male genitalia and the fetus is genetically female, congenital adrenal hyperplasia is the most likely cause.[302,303] This condition can be confirmed by estimating 17-hydroxyprogesterone levels in amniotic fluid, which are elevated in this condition, and by HLA typing of amniotic cells or chorionic villus sampling. When a diagnosis is made early enough, fetal therapy can be started with dexamethasone to suppress fetal adrenal function and reverse or reduce the masculinizing effects.[303,305] The condition is autosomal recessive, so there may be a previously affected sibling.

The diagnosis of the cause of ambiguous genitalia is fraught with problems, and a recent paper reported that almost 40% of diagnoses were either missed or were false-positives.[300] Follow-up sonograms are particularly useful later in gestation to reassess the fetal genitalia.[300]

Differential Diagnosis

The differential diagnosis is wide and includes many rare genetic and chromosomal conditions.

Prognosis

The prognosis is variable depending on the specific syndrome. Some of the chromosomal abnormalities have a poor outcome due to the associated anomalies. As a rule isolated anomalies have a good prognosis.

Management

It is probably wise not to place a diagnostic label on a fetus prenatally because an accurate diagnosis can only really be made postnatally in most cases. Careful assessment in the neonatal period by a pediatric endocrinologist is the management of choice.

Recurrence Risk

The risk of recurrence depends on the specific diagnosis.

Urachal Anomalies

The urachus is the normal embryonic remnant of the primitive bladder dome. Disorders of the urachus are manifestations of its incomplete regression.[306]

Incidence

Urachal anomalies are uncommon. Patent urachus is estimated to affect 1 in 50,000 to 100,000 live births, with a male-to-female ratio of 2 to 1.[307,308] A postmortem study revealed the incidence of urachal cysts to be 1 in 5,000; however, clinically significant cysts are likely to have a much lower incidence.[309]

Etiology

The etiology is unknown but a few cases of patent urachus have been described in association with posterior urethral valves and prune-belly syndrome.[310,311] In this setting the patent urachus allows decompression of the distended bladder.

Embryology

At approximately 16 days after conception, the allantois forms from a diverticulum off the yolk sac. As the embryo grows, the allantois becomes incorporated into the abdomen of the fetus to form a hollow tube that connects the superior aspect of the urogenital sinus (apex of the bladder) with the anterior abdominal wall at the umbilicus.[307] Eventually, the lumen of this tube becomes obliterated, resulting in a thick fibromuscular cord that connects the bladder with the umbilicus. This cord is the urachus and is also known as the *median umbilical ligament*.[308]

Histologically, the lumen of the urachus is derived from transitional epithelium and as such retains some secretory ability. Incomplete closure of the urachus results in the various types of anomalies that are seen clinically: patent urachus, urachal cyst, and urachal sinus.[309]

Diagnosis

A patent urachus is diagnosed when a cyst is seen within the base of the cord that communicates with the bladder. The cyst is known as an *allantoic* or *vesico-allantoic* cyst. The cyst may persist until delivery,[312] but more often it ruptures, either into the cord[313] or into the amniotic fluid.[307,308,313] After rupture, it is often difficult to see any abnormality apart from an enlarged cord.[313]

Urachal cysts appear as midline cystic masses situated anterior to the bladder.[309,314]

Differential Diagnosis

The differential diagnosis of an allantoic cyst associated with a patent urachus includes an omphalocele, an umbilical cord cyst, varix of the umbilical vein, and an umbilical artery aneurysm. Color-flow Doppler imaging is useful in the diagnosis of the last two conditions.

The differential diagnosis of a urachal cyst includes ovarian cysts, mesenteric cysts, and intraabdominal varix of the umbilical vein.

Associated Anomalies

Associated anomalies are uncommon but include omphalocele, hypospadias, crossed renal ectopia, and vesicoureteric reflux.[306,313]

Prognosis

Clinically, babies with a patent urachus present with discharge or urinary drainage from the umbilicus. Urachal cysts can become infected and rarely can form calculi.[306]

Management

Surgery is indicated for a patent urachus. The urachal remnant is removed together with a cuff of bladder due to the possible risk of malignancy developing in the urachal remnant.[306]

Recurrence Risk

Recurrence risk is low, as the condition is sporadic.

REFERENCES

1. Garrett WJ, Grunwald G, Robinson DE. Prenatal diagnosis of fetal polycystic kidney by ultrasound. *Aust N Z J Obstet Gynecol* 1970;10:7–9.
2. Elder JS. Antenatal hydronephrosis fetal and neonatal management. *Pediatr Clin North Am* 1997;44:1299–1321.
3. Scott JE, Renwick M. Urological anomalies in the northern region fetal abnormality survey. *Arch Dis Child* 1993;68:22–26.
4. Livera LN, Brookfield DSK, Egginton JA, Hawnaur JM. Antenatal ultrasonography to detect fetal renal abnormalities, a prospective screening programme. *BMJ* 1989;298:1421–1423.
5. Gunn TR, Mora JD, Pease P. Antenatal diagnosis of urinary tract abnormalities by ultrasonography after 28 weeks gestation: incidence and outcome. *Am J Obstet Gynecol* 1995;172:479–486.
6. Fugelseth D, Lindemann R, Sande HA, Refsum S, Nordshus T. Prenatal diagnosis of urinary tract anomalies. The value of two ultrasound examinations. *Acta Obstet Gynecol Scand* 1994;73:290–293.
7. Kullendorf CM, Larson LT, Jorgenson. The advantage of antenatal diagnosis of intestinal and urinary tract malformation. *Br J Obstet Gynecol* 1984;91:144–147.
8. Helen I, Personn PH. Prenatal diagnosis of urinary tract abnormalities by ultrasound. *Pediatrics* 1986;78:879–883.
9. Watson AR, Readett D, Nelson CS. Dilemmas associated with antenatally detected urinary tract abnormalities. *Arch Dis Child* 1988;63:719–722.
10. Arthur RJ, Irving MC, Thomas DFM. Bilateral fetal uropathy: what is the outlook? *BMJ* 1989;298:1419–1420.
11. Rosendahl H. Ultrasound screening for fetal urinary tract malformations. A prospective study in the general population. *Eur J Obstet Gynecol Reprod Biol* 1990;36:27–33.
12. Tam JC, Hodson EM, Choong KL, Cass DT, Cohen RC. Postnatal diagnosis and outcome of urinary tract abnormalities detected by antenatal ultrasound. *Med J Aust* 1994;160:633–637.
13. Dillon E, Ryall A. A 10 year audit of antenatal ultrasound detection of renal disease. *Br J Radiol* 1998;71:497–500.
14. James CA, Watson AR, Twining P, Rance CH. Antenatally detected urinary tract abnormalities: changing incidence and management. *Eur J Pediatr* 1998;157:508–511.
15. Greig JD, Raine PA, Young DG, Azmy AF, MacKenzie JF, et al. Value of antenatal diagnosis of the urinary tract. *BMJ* 1989;298:1417–1419.

16. Brand IR, Kaminopatros P, Cave M, Irving HC, Lilford RJ. Specificity of antenatal ultrasound in the Yorkshire region: a prospective study of 2261 ultrasound detected anomalies. *Br J Obstet Gynecol* 1994;101:392–397.

17. Mandell J, Blyth B, Peters C, Retik A, Estroff J, Benacerraf B. Structural genitourinary defects, detected *in utero*. *Radiology* 1991;178:193–196.

18. Grignon A, Fillon R, Filitrault D. Urinary tract dilatation *in utero*—classification and clinical applications. *Radiology* 1986;160:645–647.

19. Thomas DFM. Fetal uropathy. *Br J Urol* 1990;66:225–231.

20. Elder JS, Duckett JW Jr, Synder HM. Intervention for fetal obstructive uropathy: has it been effective? *Lancet* 1987;2:1007–1010.

21. Nicolaides KH, Cheng HH, Snijders RJM, Moniz CF. Fetal urine biochemistry in the assessment of obstructive uropathy. *Am J Obstet Gynecol* 1992;166:932–937.

22. Johnson M, Bukowski TP, Reitleman C, Isada NB, Pryde PG, Evans MI. *In utero* surgical treatment of fetal obstructive uropathy: a new comprehensive approach to identify appropriate candidates for vesico amniotic shunt therapy. *Am J Obstet Gynecol* 1994;170:1770–1779.

23. Crombleholme TM, Harrison MR, Golbus MS, Longaker MT, Langer JC, et al. Fetal intervention in obstructive uropathy: prognostic indicators and efficiency of intervention. *Am J Obstet Gynecol* 1990;162:1239–1244.

24. Larson WJ. *Human embryology.* London: Churchill Livingstone, 1993.

25. Wendell Smith CP, Williams PL, Treadgold S. *Basic human embryology.* London: Pitman Publishing, 1984.

26. Bronshtein M, Yoffe N, Brandes JM, Blumenfeld Z. First and early second-trimester diagnosis of fetal urinary tract anomalies using transvaginal sonography. *Prenat Diagn* 1990;10:653–666.

27. Whitlow BJ, Economides DL. The optimal gestational age to examine fetal anatomy and measure nuchal translucency in the first trimester. *Ultrasound Obstet Gynecol* 1998;11:258–261.

28. Rosati P, Guariglia L. Transvaginal sonographic assessment of the fetal urinary tract in early pregnancy. *Ultrasound Obstet Gynecol* 1996;7:95–100.

29. Corteville JE, Crane JP, Gray DL. Congenital hydronephrosis: correlation of fetal ultrasonographic findings with infant outcome. *Am J Obstet Gynecol* 1991;165:384–388.

30. Nwosu EC, Welch CR, Manasse PR, Walkinshaw SA. Longitudinal assessment of amniotic fluid index. *Br J Obstet Gynaecol* 1993;100:816–819.

31. Hitchcock R, Burge DM. Renal agenesis: an acquired condition? *J Pediatr Surg* 1994;29:454–455.

32. Bronshtein M, Amil A, Achiron R, Noy I, Blumenfeld Z. The early prenatal diagnosis of renal agenesis: techniques and possible pitfalls. *Prenat Diagn* 1994;14:291–297.

33. Cascio S, Paran S, Puri P. Associated urological anomalies in children with unilateral renal agenesis. *J Urol* 1999;162:1081–1083.

34. Bankier A, De Campo M, Newell R, Rogers JG, Danks DM. A pedigree study of perinatally lethal renal disease. *J Med Genet* 1985;22:104–111.

35. Newbould MJ, Lendon M, Barson AJ. Oligohydramnios sequence: the spectrum of renal malformations. *Br J Obstet Gynaecol* 1994;101:598–604.

36. Potter EL. Bilateral absence of ureters and kidneys: report of fifty cases. *Obstet Gynecol* 1965;25:3–12.

37. Mesrobian HG, Rushton HG, Bulas D. Unilateral renal agenesis may result from *in utero* regression of multicystic renal dysplasia. *J Urol* 1993;150:793–796.

38. Hoffman CIT, Filly RA, Callen PW. The lying down adrenal sign: a sonographic indicator of renal agenesis or ectopia in fetuses and neonates. *J Ultrasound Med* 1992;11:533–536.

39. DeVore GR. The value of color Doppler sonography in the diagnosis of renal agenesis. *J Ultrasound Med* 1995;14:443–449.

40. Twining P. The value of transvaginal scanning in the assessment of second trimester oligohydramnios. *Br J Radiol* 1992;65:455–457.

41. Benacerraf B. Examination of the second trimester fetus with severe oligohydramnios using transvaginal scanning. *Obstet Gynecol* 1990;75:491–493.

42. Gembruch U, Hansmann M. Artificial installation of amniotic fluid as a new technique for the diagnostic evaluation of cases of oligohydramnios. *Prenat Diagn* 1988;8:33–45.

43. Nicolini U, Santolaya J, Hubinost C, Fisk N, Maxwell D, Rodeck C. Visualization of fetal intra-abdominal organs in second trimester severe oligohydramnios by intra-perinatal infusion. *Prenat Diagn* 1989;9:191–194.

44. Hackett G, Nicolaides KH, Campbell S. Doppler ultrasound assessment of fetal and uteroplacental circulation in severe second trimester oligohydramnios. *Br J Obstet Gynecol* 1987;94:1074–1077.

45. Jeanty P, Romero R, Kepple D, Stoney D, Coggins T, Fleischer A. Prenatal diagnosis in unilateral empty renal fossa. *J Ultrasound Med* 1990;9:651–654.

46. Twining P. Oligohydramnios—current thoughts and a diagnostic review. *Br Med Ultrasound Soc Bull* May 1995:30–32.

47. Romero R, Cullen M, Graunum P. Antenatal diagnosis of renal anomalies with ultrasound III bilateral renal agenesis. *Am J Obstet Gynecol* 1985;151:38–43.

48. Atiyeh B, Husmann D, Baum M. Contralateral renal abnormalities in patients with renal agenesis and non cystic renal dysplasia. *Pediatrics* 1993;91:4–7.

49. Song JT, Ritchey ML, Zerin M, Bloom D. Incidence of vesicoureteric reflux in children with unilateral renal agenesis. *J Urol* 1995;153:1249–1251.

50. Argueso LR, Ritchey ML, Boyle ET, Milliner DS, Bergstralh EJ, Kramer SA. Progress of patients with unilateral renal agenesis. *Pediatr Nephrol* 1992;6:412–414.

51. Roodhooft AM, Birnholz JC, Holmes LB. Familial nature of congenital absence and severe dysplasia of both kidneys. *N Engl J Med* 1984;310:1341–1345.

52. Carter CO, Evans K, Pescia G. A family study of renal agenesis. *J Med Genet* 1979;16:176–188.

53. Decter RM. Renal duplication and fusion anomalies. *Pediatr Clin North Am* 1997;44:1336–1341.

54. Hill L, Peterson CS. Antenatal diagnosis of fetal pelvic kidneys. *J Ultrasound Med* 1987;6:393–396.

55. Malek RS, Kelalis PP, Burke CC. Ectopic kidney in children and frequency of association with other malformations. *Mayo Clin Proc* 1970;46:461–465.

56. Thompson GJ, Page JM. Ectopic kidney—a review of 97 cases. *Surg Gynaecol Obstet* 1937;64:935–939.

57. Greenblatt AM, Beretsky I, Lankin DH, Phelans L. *In utero*

diagnosis of crossed renal ectopia using high resolution real time ultrasound. *J Ultrasound Med* 1985;4:105–107.

58. Sherer DM, Cullen JBH, Thompson HO, Metlay LA, Woods JR. Prenatal sonographic findings associated with a fetal horseshoe kidney. *J Ultrasound Med* 1990;9:477–479.

59. King KL, Kofinas AD, Simon NV, Clay D. Antenatal ultrasound diagnosis of fetal horseshoe kidney. *J Ultrasound Med* 1991;10:643–644.

60. Boatman DL, Kolln CP, Flocks RH. Congenital anomalies associated with horseshoe kidney. *J Urol* 1972;107:205–207.

61. Thomsen MS, Levine E, Meilstrup JW, Van Slyke MA, Edgar KA, et al. Renal cystic diseases. *Eur Radiol* 1997;7:1267–1275.

62. Zerres K. Autosomal recessive polycystic kidney disease. *Clin Invest* 1992;70:794–901.

63. Tsuda H, Matsumota M, Imanaka M, Ogita S. Measurement of fetal urine production in mild infantile polycystic kidney disease—a case report. *Prenat Diagn* 1994;14:1083–1085.

64. Osathanondh V, Potter EL. Pathogenesis of polycystic kidneys. Type I due to hypoplasia of interstitial portions of collecting tubules. *Arch Pathol* 1964;77:466–473.

65. Blyth H, Ockenden BG. Polycystic disease of kidneys and liver presenting in childhood. *J Med Genet* 1971;8:257–284.

66. Romero R, Cullen M, Jeanty P, Grannum P, Reece EA, et al. The diagnosis of congenital renal anomalies with ultrasound. II. Infantile polycystic kidney disease. *Am J Obstet Gynecol* 1984;150:259–262.

67. Wisser J, Hebisch G, Froster U, Zerres K, Stallmach T, et al. Prenatal sonographic diagnosis of autosomal recessive polycystic kidney disease during the early second trimester. *Prenat Diagn* 1995;15:868–871.

68. Mahony B, Cullen PW, Filly R, Golbus M. Progression of infantile polycystic kidney disease in early pregnancy. *J Ultrasound Med* 1984;3:277–279.

69. Barth R, Guillot A, Capeless E, Clemmons J. Prenatal diagnosis of autosomal recessive polycystic kidney disease: variable outcome in one family. *Am J Obstet Gynecol* 1992;166:560–567.

70. Zerres K, Hansmann M, Mallmann R, Gembruch U. Autosomal recessive polycystic kidney disease. Problems of prenatal diagnosis. *Prenat Diagn* 1988;8:215–229.

71. Bronshtein M, Bar-Hava I, Blumenfeld Z. Clues and pitfalls in the early prenatal diagnosis of "late onset" infantile polycystic kidney. *Prenat Diagn* 1992;12:293–298.

72. Kogutt MS, Robichaux W, Boineau F, Drake G, Simonton S. Asymmetric renal size in autosomal recessive polycystic kidney disease: a unique presentation. *Am J Radiol* 1993;160:835–836.

73. Guay-Woodford LM, Meucher G, Hopkins SD, Avner ED, Germino GG, Guillot AP. The severe form of autosomal recessive polycystic kidney disease maps to chromosome 6p21.1–p12: implications for genetic counseling. *Am J Hum Genet* 1995;56:1101–1107.

74. Al-Khaldi N, Watson AR, Zuccollo J, Twining P, Rose DH. Outcome of antenatally detected cystic dysplastic kidney disease. *Arch Dis Child* 1994;70:520–522.

75. Gough DCS, Postlethwaite RJ, Lewis MA, Bruce J. Multicystic renal dysplasia diagnosed in the antenatal period: a note of caution. *Br J Urol* 1995;76:244–248.

76. Rickwood AMK, Anderson PAM, Williams MPL. Multicystic renal dysplasia detected by prenatal ultrasonography. Natural history and results of conservative management. *Br J Urol* 1992;69:538–540.

77. D'Alton M, Romero R, Grannum P, Jeanty P. Antenatal diagnosis of renal anomalies with ultrasound IV: bilateral multicystic kidney disease. *Am J Obstet Gynecol* 1986;54:532–537.

78. Hashimoto B, Filly R, Callen P. Multicystic dysplastic kidney *in utero*: changing appearance on ultrasound. *Radiology* 1986;159:107–109.

79. Diard F, le Dosseur P, Cadier L, Calabet A, Bondionny JM. Multicystic dysplasia in the upper component of the complete duplex kidney. *Pediatr Radiol* 1984;14:310–313.

80. Siegel RL, Rosenfeld DL, Leiman S. Complete regression of a multicystic dysplastic kidney in the setting of renal crossed fused ectopia. *J Clin Ultrasound* 1992;20:466–469.

81. De Klerk DF, Marshall FF, Jeffs RD. Multicystic dysplastic kidney. *J Urol* 1977;118:306–308.

82. Karmazyn B, Zerin J. Lower urinary tract abnormalities in children with multicystic dysplastic kidney. *Radiology* 1997;203:223–226.

83. Wacksman J, Phipps L. Report of the multicystic kidney registry: preliminary findings. *J Urol* 1993;150:1870–1872.

84. Hartman GE, Smolik LM, Shocat SJ. The dilemma of the multicystic dysplastic kidney. *Am J Dis Child* 1986;140:925–928.

85. Chen YH, Stapleton FB, Roy S, Noe HN. Neonatal hypertension from a unilateral multicystic dysplastic kidney. *J Urol* 1985;133:664.

86. Homsy YL, Anderson JH, Oudjhane K, Russo P. Wilms tumor and multicystic dysplastic kidney disease. *J Urol* 1997;158:2256–2260.

87. de Oliveira-Filho AG, Carvalho MH, Sbragia-Neto L, Miranda ML, Bustorff-Silva JM, de Oliveira ER. Wilms tumor in a prenatally diagnosed multicystic kidney. *J Urol* 1997;158:1926–1927.

88. Strife J, Souza AS, Kirks D, Strife CF, Gelfand MJ, Wacksman J. Multicystic dysplastic kidney in children: US follow up. *Radiology* 1993;186:785–788.

89. Michaud J, Russo P, Grignon A, et al. Autosomal dominant polycystic disease in the fetus. *Am J Med Genet* 1994;51:240–246.

90. Parfrey PS, Bear JC, Morgan J, Cramer BC, McManamon PJ, et al. The diagnosis and prognosis of autosomal dominant polycystic kidney disease. *N Engl J Med* 1990;323:1085–1090.

91. Reeders ST, Breuning MH, Davies KE, et al. A highly polymorphic DNA marker linked to adult type polycystic kidney disease on chromosome 16. *Nature* 1985;317:542–544.

92. Kimberling WJ, Kumar S, Gabow P. Autosomal dominant polycystic kidney disease: localization of the second gene to chromosome 4q13–q23. *Genomics* 1995;18:467–472.

93. MacDermot KD, Saggar-Malik AK, Economides SJ. Prenatal diagnosis of autosomal dominant polycystic kidney disease (PDK 1) presenting *in utero* and prognosis for very early onset disease. *J Med Genet* 1998;35:13–16.

94. Zerres K, Weis H, Bulla M, Roth B. Prenatal diagnosis of an early manifestation of autosomal dominant adult type polycystic kidney disease. *Lancet* 1982;2:988.

95. Pretorius D, Lee M, Manco-Johnson M, Weingast G, Sed-

man A, Gabour P. Diagnosis of autosomal dominant poly-cystic kidney disease *in utero* and in the young infant. *J Ultrasound Med* 1987;6:249–255.

96. McHugo J, Shafi MI, Rowlands D, Weaver JB. Prenatal diagnosis of adult polycystic kidney disease. *Br J Radiol* 1988;61:1072–1074.

97. Fick GM, Johnson AM, Strain JD, Kimberling WJ, Kumar S, Manco-Johnson ML. Characteristics of very early onset autosomal dominant polycystic kidney disease. *J Am Soc Nephrol* 1993;3:1863–1870.

98. Sinibaldi D, Malena S, Mingarelli R, Rizzoni G. Prenatal ultrasonographic findings of dominant polycystic kidney dis-ease and postnatal evolution. *Am J Med Genet* 1996;65:337–341.

99. Turco AE, Padovani EM, Chiaffoni GP, Peissel B, Rossetti S, Marcolongo A. Molecular genetics of autosomal domi-nant polycystic kidney disease in a newborn with bilateral cystic kidneys detected prenatally and multiple skeletal mal-formations. *J Med Genet* 1993;30:419–422.

100. Main D, Mennuti MT, Cornfield D, Coleman B. Prenatal diagnosis of adult polycystic kidney disease. *Lancet* 1983;2:337–338.

101. Hartman SS. Unilateral adult polycystic kidney. *J Ultra-sound Med* 1982;1:371–374.

102. Middlebrook PF, Nizalik E, Schillinger JF. Unilateral renal cys-tic disease; a case presentation. *J Urol* 1992;148:1221–1223.

103. Ravine D, Gibson RN, Walker RG, Sheffield LJ, Kincard-Smith P, Danks DM. Evaluation of ultrasonographic diag-nostic criteria for autosomal dominant polycystic kidney disease 1. *Lancet* 1994;343:824–827.

104. Choong KL, Gruenwald SM, Hodson E. Echogenic fetal kidneys in cytomegalovirus infection. *J Clin Ultrasound* 1993;21:138–142.

105. Moore BS, Pretorius D, Scioscia A, Reznik V. Sonographic findings in a fetus with congenital nephrotic syndrome of the Finnish type. *J Ultrasound Med* 1992;11:113–116.

106. Fishman JE, Joseph RC. Renal vein thrombosis *in utero*: duplex sonography in diagnosis and follow up. *Pediatr Radiol* 1994;24:135–136.

107. Lok JP, Hailer JO, Kassner EG, Aloni A, Glassberg K. Dominantly inherited polycystic kidneys in infants: associ-ated with hypertrophic pyloric stenosis. *Pediatr Radiol* 1977;6:27–30.

108. Saunders RC, Nassbaum AR, Solez K. Renal dysplasia: sonographic findings. *Radiology* 1988;167:623–626.

109. Mahony BS, Filly R, Callen PW, Hricak H, Golbus M, Harrison MR. Fetal renal dysplasia: sonographic evaluation. *Radiology* 1984;152:143–146.

110. Benacerraf B, Peters C, Mandell J. The prenatal evolution of a nonfunctioning kidney in the setting of obstructive hydro-nephrosis. *J Clin Ultrasound* 1991;19:446–450.

111. Avni EF, Thoua Y, Van Gansbeke D, Matos C, Didier F, et al. Development of the hypodysplastic kidney: contribution of antenatal US diagnosis. *Radiology* 1987;164:123–125.

112. Newman LB, McAlister WH, Kissane J. Segmental renal dysplasia associated with ectopic ureteroceles in childhood. *Urology* 1974;3:23–26.

113. Blane CE, Barr M, Dipietro MA, Sedman AB, Bloom DA. Renal obstructive dysplasia: ultrasound diagnosis and thera-peutic implications. *Pediatr Radiol* 1991;21:274–277.

114. Estroff JA, Mandell J, Benacerraf BR. Increased renal paren-chymal echogenicity in the fetus: importance and clinical outcome. *Radiology* 1991;181:135–139.

115. Chitty LS, Griffin DR, Johnson P. The differential diagnosis of enlarged hyperechogenic kidneys with normal or increased liquor: report of five cases and review of the litera-ture. *Ultrasound Obstet Gynecol* 1991;1:115–119.

116. Weinstein L, Anderson C. *In utero* diagnosis of Beckwith-Wiedemann syndrome. *Radiology* 1980;134:473–475.

117. Cobellis G, Iannoto P, Stabile M, Lonardo F, Bruna MD, et al. Prenatal ultrasound diagnosis of macroglossia in the Beck-with-Wiedemann syndrome. *Prenat Diagn* 1988;8:79–81.

118. Greenberg F, Stein F, Gresik MV, Finegold MJ, Carpenter RJ, et al. The Perlman familiar nephroblastomatosis syn-drome. *Am J Med Genet* 1986;24:101–110.

119. Perlman M, Goldberg GM, Bar-Ziu J, Danovitch G. Renal hamartomas and nephroblastomatosis with fetal gigantism: a familiar syndrome. *J Pediatr* 1973;83:414–418.

120. Van Der Stege JG, Van Eyck J, Arabin B. Prenatal ultra-sound observations in subsequent pregnancies with Perlman syndrome. *Ultrasound Obstet Gynecol* 1998;11:149–151.

121. Blazer S, Zimmer E, Bumenfeld Z, Zelikovic I, Bronshtein M. Natural history of fetal simple renal cysts detected in early pregnancy. *J Urol* 1999;162:812–814.

122. Paduano L, Giglio L, Bembi B, Peratoner L, D'Ottavio G, Benussi G. Clinical outcome of fetal uropathy. I. Predictive value of prenatal echography positive for obstructive uropa-thy. *J Urol* 1991;146:1094–1096.

123. McHugh K, Stringer D, Hebert D, Babiak CA. Simple renal cysts in children: diagnosis and follow-up with US. *Radiology* 1991;178:383–385.

124. Mir S, Rapola J, Koskimies O. Renal cysts in pediatric autopsy material. *Nephron* 1983;33:189–195.

125. Siegel MJ, McAlister WH. Simple cysts of the kidney in children. *J Urol* 1980;123:75–78.

126. Steinhardt GF, Slovis TL, Perlmutter AD. Simple renal cysts in infants. *Radiology* 1985;155:349–350.

127. Herman TE, Siegel MJ. Renal cysts associated with Turner's syndrome. *Pediatr Radiol* 1994;24:139–140.

128. Ariel I, Wells TR, Landing BH, Singer DB. The urinary sys-tem in Down syndrome: a study of 124 autopsy cases. *Pedi-atr Pathol* 1991;11:879–888.

129. Anderson N, Clautice-Engle T, Allan R, Abbott G, Wells JE. Detection of obstructive uropathy in the fetus: predic-tive value of sonographic measurements of renal pelvic diameter at various gestational ages. *Am J Radiol* 1995;164:719–723.

130. Takeuchi H, Koyanagi T, Yoshizato T, Takashima T, Satoh S, Nakano H. Fetal urine production at different gestational ages: correlation to various compromised fetuses *in utero*. *Early Hum Dev* 1994;40:1–11.

131. Adra AM, Mejides AA, Dennoui MS, Beydown SN. Fetal pyelectasis: is it always physiologic? *Am J Obstet Gynecol* 1995;173:1263–1266.

132. Ouzounian JG, Cantro MA, Fresquez M, Al-Sulyman OM, Kovacs BW. Diagnostic significance of antenatally detected fetal pyelectasis. *Ultrasound Obstet Gynecol* 1996;7:424–428.

133. Johnson CE, Elder J, Judge NE, Adeeb FN, Grisoni ER, Fattlar DC. The accuracy of antenatal ultrasonography in

identifying renal abnormalities. *Am J Dis Child* 1992;146:1181–1184.

134. Dudley JA, Haworth JA, McGraw ME, Frank JD, Tizard EJ. Clinical relevance and implications of antenatal hydronephrosis. *Arch Dis Child* 1997;76:F31–F34.

135. Barker AF, Cave MM, Thomas DFM, Lilford RJ, et al. Fetal pelvi-ureteric junction obstruction: predictions of outcome. *Br J Urol* 1995;76:649–652.

136. Arger PH, Coleman BG, Mintz MC, Snyder HP, Camardise T, et al. Routine fetal genitourinary tract screening. *Radiology* 1985;156:485–489.

137. Lam CC, Wong SK, Yeung CY, Tang MHY, Ghosh A. Outcome and management of babies with prenatal ultrasonographic renal abnormalities. *Am J Perinatol* 1993;10:263–268.

138. Scott JE, Renwick M. Antenatal diagnosis of congenital abnormalities of the urinary tract. Results from the Northern Region Fetal Abnormality Survey, 1988. *Br J Urol* 1988;62:255–300.

139. Stocks A, Richards D, Frentzen B, Richard G. Correlation of prenatal renal pelvic anteroposterior diameter with outcome in infancy. *J Urol* 1996;155:1050–1052.

140. Zerin MJ, Richey ML, Chang ACH. Incidental vesico-ureteral reflux in neonates with antenatally detected hydronephrosis and other renal anomalies. *Radiology* 1993;187:157–160.

141. Marra G, Barbieri G, Moioli C, Assael BM, Grumieri G, Caccamo ML. Mild fetal hydronephrosis indicating vesicoureteric reflux. *Arch Dis Child* 1994;70:F147–149.

142. Morin L, Cendron M, Crombleholme TM, Garmel S, Klauber GT, D'Alton ME. Minimal hydronephrosis in the fetus: clinical significance and implications for management. *J Urol* 1996;155:2047–2049.

143. Newell SJ, Morgan ME, McHugo JM, White RH, Taylor CM, et al. Clinical significance of antenatal calyceal dilatation detected by ultrasound. *Lancet* 1990;336:372.

144. Nicolaides KH, Cheng HH, Abbas A, Snijders RJM, Gosden C. Fetal renal defects: associated malformations and chromosomal defects. *Fetal Diagn Ther* 1992;7:1–11.

145. Corteville JE, Dicke JM, Crane JP. Fetal pyelectasis and Down's syndrome: is genetic amniocentesis warranted? *Obstet Gynecol* 1992;79:770–772.

146. Wickstrom EA, Thangavelu M, Parilla BV, Tamura RK, Sabbagha R. A prospective study of the association between isolated fetal pyelectasis and chromosomal abnormality. *Obstet Gynecol* 1996;88:379–382.

147. Chitty L, Chudleigh T, Campbell S, Pembray M. Incidence, natural history and clinical significance of fetal pyelectasis. *Br J Radiol* 1992;65:636.

148. Wickstrom E, Maizels M, Sabbagha RE, Tamura RK, Cohen LC, Pergament E. Isolated fetal pyelectasis: assessment of risk for postnatal uropathy and Down's syndrome. *Ultrasound Obstet Gynecol* 1996;8:236–240.

149. Benacerraf B, Mandell J, Estroff JA, Harlow BL, Frigoletto F. Fetal pyelectasis: a possible association with Down's syndrome. *Obstet Gynecol* 1990;76:58–60.

150. Snijders RJM, Nicolaides KH. *Ultrasound marker for fetal chromosomal defects.* Frontiers in Medicine Series. London: Parthenon Publishing, 1996.

151. Thomas DFM, Gordon AC. The management of prenatally diagnosed uropathies. *Arch Dis Child* 1989;64:58–63.

152. Reznick VM, Kaplan GW, Murphy JL. Follow up of infants with bilateral renal disease detected *in utero*. *Am J Dis Child* 1988;142:453–456.

153. Thomas DFM. Prenatally detected uropathy: epidemiological considerations. *Br J Urol* 1998;81(Suppl 2):8–12.

154. Cendron M, D'Alton ME, Crombleholme TM. Prenatal diagnosis and management of the fetus with hydronephrosis. *Semin Perinatol* 1994;18:163–181.

155. Kleiner B, Callen PW, Filly FA. Sonographic analysis of the fetus with uretero-pelvic junction obstruction. *Am J Radiol* 1987;148:359–363.

156. Bosman G, Reuss A, Nijman JM, Wladimiroff JW. Prenatal diagnosis, management and outcome of fetal uretero-pelvic junction obstruction. *Ultrasound Med Biol* 1991;17:117–120.

157. Jaffe R, Abramowicz J, Fejgin M, Ben-Aderet N. Giant fetal abdominal cyst. Ultrasonic diagnosis and management. *J Ultrasound Med* 1987;6:45–47.

158. Drake DP, Stevens P, Eckstein HB. Hydronephrosis secondary to uretero-pelvic obstruction in children: a review of 14 years' experience. *J Urol* 1978;119:649–651.

159. Gordon I, Dhillon HH, Peters AM. Antenatal diagnosis of renal pelvic dilatation—the natural history of conservative management. *Pediatr Radiol* 1991;21:272–275.

160. Madden NP, Thomas DFM, Gordon AC, Arthur RJ, Irving HC, Smith SEW. Antenatally detected pelvic–ureteric junction obstruction. Is nonoperation safe? *Br J Urol* 1991;68:305–310.

161. Arnold AJ, Rickwood AMK. Natural history of pelvic-ureteric obstruction detected by prenatal sonography. *Br J Urol* 1990;65:91–96.

162. O'Flynn KJ, Gough DCS, Gupta S, Lewis MA, Postlethwaite RJ. Prediction of recovery in antenatally diagnosed hydronephrosis. *Br J Urol* 1993;71:478–480.

163. Capolicchio G, Leonard MP, Wong C, Jednak R, Brozezinski A, Pippi Saile JL. Prenatal diagnosis of hydronephrosis: impact on renal function and its recovery after pyeloplasty. *J Urol* 1999;162:1029–1032.

164. McAleer IM, Kaplan GW. Renal function before and after pyeloplasty: does it improve? *J Urol* 1999;162:1041–1044.

165. Atwell JD. Familial pelvic-ureteric junction obstruction and its association with a duplex pelvicalyceal system and vesicoureteric reflux. A family study. *Br J Urol* 1985;57:365–369.

166. Buscemi M, Shanke A, Mallet E. Dominantly inherited ureteropelvic junction obstruction. *Urology* 1985;24:568–571.

167. Liu HYA, Dhillon HK, Yeung CK, Diamond DA, Duffy P, Ransley PG. Clinical outcome and management of prenatally diagnosed primary megaureters. *J Urol* 1994;152:614–617.

168. Dunn V, Glasier CM. Ultrasonographic antenatal demonstration of primary megaureters. *J Ultrasound Med* 1985;4:101–103.

169. Rickwood AMK, Jee LD, Williams MPL, Anderson PAM. Natural history of obstructed and pseudo-obstructed megaureters detected by prenatal ultrasonography. *Br J Urol* 1992;70:322–325.

170. Peters CA. Lower urinary tract obstruction: clinical and experimental aspects. *Br J Urol* 1998;81(Suppl 2):22–32.

171. Baskin LS, Zderic SA, Snyder HM, Duckett JW. Primary dilated megaureter: long term follow up. *J Urol* 1994;152:618–621.

172. Cremin BJ. A review of the ultrasonic appearances of poste-

rior urethral valve and ureteroceles. *Pediatr Radiol* 1986; 16:357–364.

173. Nussbaum AR, Dorst JP, Jeffs RD, Gearhart JP, Sanders RC. Ectopic ureter and ureterocele: their varied sonographic manifestations. *Radiology* 1986;159:227–235.

174. Abuhamad AZ, Horton CE, Evans AT. Renal duplication anomalies in the fetus: clues for prenatal diagnosis. *Ultrasound Obstet Gynecol* 1996;7:174–177.

175. Vergani P, Ceruti P, Locatelli A, Mariani E, Paterlini G, et al. Accuracy of prenatal ultrasonographic diagnosis of duplex renal system. *J Ultrasound Med* 1999;18:463–467.

176. Jee LD, Rickwood AMK, Williams MPL, Anderson PAM. Experience with duplex system anomalies detected by prenatal ultrasonography. *J Urol* 1993;149:808–810.

177. Sherer DM, Menashe M, Lebensort P, Matoth I, Basel D. Sonographic diagnosis of unilateral fetal renal duplication with associated ectopic ureterocele. *J Clin Ultrasound* 1989; 17:371–373.

178. Winters WD, Lebowitz RL. Importance of prenatal detection of hydronephrosis of the upper pole. *Am J Radiol* 1990;155:125–129.

179. Fitzsimmons PJ, Frost RA, Millward S, De Marcia J, Toi A. Prenatal and immediate postnatal ultrasonographic diagnosis of ureterocele. *J Can Assoc Radiol* 1986;37:189–191.

180. Sherer DM, Hulbert WC. Prenatal sonographic diagnosis and subsequent conservative surgical management of bilateral ureteroceles. *Am J Perinatol* 1995;12:174–177.

181. Kang AH, Bruner JP. Antenatal ultrasonographic development of ureteroceles. Implications for management. *Fetal Diagn Ther* 1998;13:157–159.

182. Cuplen DE, Duckett JW. The modern approach to ureteroceles. *J Urol* 1995;153:166–169.

183. Dinneen MD, Dhilwn HK, Ward HC, Duffy PG, Ransley PG. Antenatal diagnosis of posterior urethral valves. *Br J Urol* 1993;72:364–369.

184. Dinneen MD, Duffy PG. Posterior urethral valves. *Br J Urol* 1996;78:275–281.

185. Hayden SA, Russ PD, Pretorius DH, Manco-Johnson ML, Clewell WH. Posterior urethral obstruction. Prenatal sonographic findings and clinical outcome in fourteen cases. *J Ultrasound Med* 1988;7:371–375.

186. Glazer GM, Filly RA, Callen PW. The varied sonographic appearance of the urinary tract in the fetus and newborn with urethral obstruction. *Radiology* 1982;144:563–568.

187. Rittenberg MH, Hulbert WC, Snyder HM, Duckett JW. Protective factors in posterior urethral valves. *J Urol* 1988;140:993–996.

188. Cuckow PM, Dinneen MD, Risdon FA, Ransley PG, Duffy PG. Long-term renal function in the posterior urethral valves, unilateral reflux and renal dysplasia syndrome. *J Urol* 1997;158:1004–1007.

189. Hatjis CG. In utero diagnosis of spontaneous fetal urinary bladder rupture. *J Clin Ultrasound* 1993;21:645–647.

190. Kaefer M, Peters C, Retik AB, Benacerraf B. Increased renal echogenicity: a sonographic sign for differentiating between obstructive and nonobstructive etiologies of *in utero* bladder distension. *J Urol* 1997;158:1026–1029.

191. Simma B, Gabner I, Brezinka C, Ellemunter H, Kreiczy A. Complete prenatal obstruction caused by congenital megalourethra. *J Clin Ultrasound* 1992;20:197–199.

192. McNamara HM, Onwude JL, Thornton JG. Megacystis-microcolon–intestinal hypoperistalsis syndrome: a case report supporting autosomal recessive inheritance. *Prenat Diagn* 1994;14:153–154.

193. Hobbins JC, Romero R, Grannum P, Berkowitz RL, Cullen M, Mahoney M. Antenatal diagnosis of renal anomalies with ultrasound. I. Obstructive uropathy. *Am J Obstet Gynecol* 1984;148:868–877.

194. Manning FA, Harrison MR, Rodeck C. Catheter shunts for fetal hydronephrosis and hydrocephalus. Report of the International Fetal Surgery Registry. *N Engl J Med* 1986;315:336–340.

195. Velden DJ, de Jong G, Van Der Walt JJ. Fetal bilateral obstructive uropathy, a series of nine cases. *Pediatr Pathol* 1995;15:245–258.

196. Smythe AR. Ultrasonic detection of fetal ascites and bladder dilatation with resulting prune belly. *J Pediatr* 1981;98:978–982.

197. Smith GM, Canning D, Schulman S, Snyder H, Dukett J. The long term outcome of posterior urethral valves treated with primary valve ablation and observation. *J Urol* 1996;155:1730–1734.

198. Hutton K, Thomas D, Davies B. Prenatally detected posterior urethral valves: qualitative assessment of second trimester scans and prediction of outcome. *J Urol* 1997;158:1022–1025.

199. Freedman AL, Bukowski T, Smith C, Evans M, Johnson MP, Gonzalez R. Fetal therapy for obstructive uropathy: specific outcomes diagnosis. *J Urol* 1996;156:720–724.

200. Reinberg Y, De Castano I, Gonzalez R. Prognosis for patients with prenatally diagnosed posterior urethral valves. *J Urol* 1992;148:125–126.

201. El-Ghoneimi A, Desgrippes A, Luton D, Macher MA, Guibourdenche J, et al. Outcome of posterior urethral valves: to what extent is it improved by prenatal diagnosis? *J Urol* 1999;162:849–853.

202. Jee LD, Rickwood AM, Turnock RR. Posterior urethral valves. Does prenatal diagnosis influence prognosis? *Br J Urol* 1993;72:830–833.

203. Hutton KAR, Thomas PFM, Arthur RJ, Irving HC, Smith SEW. Prenatally detected posterior urethra valves: is gestational age at detection a predictor of outcome? *J Urol* 1994;152:698–701.

204. Muller F, Dommergues M, Mandelbrot L, Aubry M, Nihoui-Fekete C, Dumez Y. Fetal urinary biochemistry predicts postnatal function in children with bilateral obstructive uropathies. *Obstet Gynecol* 1993;82:813–820.

205. Glick PL, Harrison MR, Adzick NS, Noall RA, Villa RL. Correction of congenital hydronephrosis in utero IV: in utero decompression prevents renal dysplasia. *J Pediatr Surg* 1984;19:649–657.

206. Herndon A, Ferrer F, Freedman A, McKenna P. Consensus on the prenatal management of antenatally detected urological abnormalities, 2000. *J Urol* 2000;164:1052–1056.

207. Lun A, Lenz F, Priem F, Brux B, Gross J, et al. Biochemical diagnosis in prenatal uropathy. *Clin Biochem* 1994;27:283–287.

208. Irwin BH, Vane DW. Complications of intrauterine intervention for treatment of fetal obstructive uropathy. *Urology* 2000;55:774–775.

209. Lewis KM, Pinchert TL, Cain MP, Ghidini A. Complications of intrauterine placement of vesicoamniotic shunt. *Obstet Gynecol* 1998;91:825–827.

210. Crombleholme TM, D'Alton M, Cendron M, Alman B, Goldberg MD, et al. Prenatal diagnosis and the pediatric surgeon: the impact of prenatal consultation on perinatal management. *J Pediatr Surg* 1996;31:156–162.

211. Reece EA, Hobbins JC. *Medicine of the fetus and mother.* Philadelphia: Lippincott–Raven, 1999:592–593.

212. Reuss A, Wladimiroff JW, Stewart PA, Scholtmeijer RJ. Non-invasive management of fetal obstructive uropathy. *Lancet* 1988;2(8617):949–950.

213. Reinberg Y, Chelimsky G, Gonzalez R. Urethral atresia and the prune-belly syndrome. Report of 6 cases. *Br J Urol* 1993;72:112–114.

214. Steinhardt G, Hogan W, Wood E, Weber T, Lynch R. Long-term survival in an infant with urethral atresia. *J Urol* 1990;143:336–337.

215. Stamm E, King G, Thickman D. Megacystis-microcolon–intestinal hypoperistalsis syndrome: prenatal identification in siblings and review of the literature. *J Ultrasound Med* 1991;10:599–602.

216. Alharbi A, Tawil K, Crankson SJ. Megacystis-microcolon intestinal hypoperistalsis syndrome associated with mega-esophagus. *J Pediatr Surg* 1999;15:272–274.

217. White SM, Chamberlain P, Hitchcock R, Sullivan PB, Boyd P. Megacystis-microcolon–intestinal hypoperistalsis syndrome: the difficulties with antenatal diagnosis. Case report and review of the literature. *Prenat Diagn* 2000;20:697–700.

218. Redman JF, Timenez JF, Golladay ES, Seibert J. Megacystis-microcolon–intestinal hypoperistalsis syndrome: case report and review of the literature. *J Urol* 1984;131:981–983.

219. Chen C, Wang T, Chuang C. Sonographic findings with megacystis-microcolon–intestinal hypoperistalsis syndrome. *J Clin Ultrasound* 1997;26:217–220.

220. Young ID, McKeever PA, Brown LA, Lang GD. Prenatal diagnosis of the megacystis-microcolon–intestinal hypoperistalsis syndrome. *J Med Genet* 1988;26:403–406.

221. Ciftci AO, Cook R, Van Velzen D. Megacystis-microcolon–intestinal hypoperistalsis syndrome: evidence of a primary myocellular defect of contractile fiber synthesis. *J Pediatr Surg* 1996;31:1706–1711.

222. Young L, Yunis E, Girdany B, Sieber W. Megacystis-microcolon–intestinal hypoperistalsis syndrome: additional clinical, radiological and histopathological aspects. *Am J Radiol* 1981;137:749–755.

223. Penman DG, Lilford RJ. The megacystis-microcolon–intestinal hypoperistalsis syndrome. A fatal autosomal recessive condition. *J Med Genet* 1989;26:66–68.

224. Manco L, Osterdahl P. The antenatal sonographic features of megacystis-microcolon–intestinal hypoperistalsis syndrome. *J Clin Ultrasound* 1984;12:595–598.

225. Appel R, Kaplan G, Brock W, Streit D. Megalourethra. *J Urol* 1986;135:747–751.

226. Reissigl A, Eberle J, Bartsch G. Megalourethra. *Br J Urol* 1991;68:435–438.

227. Stephens D, Fortune D. Pathogenesis of megalourethra. *J Urol* 1993;149:1512–1516.

228. Sepulveda W, Berry SM, Romero R, King ME, Johnson MP, Cotton DB. Prenatal diagnosis of megalourethra. *J Ultrasound Med* 1993;12:761–766.

229. Fisk NM, Dhillon HK, Ellis CE, Nicolini U, Tannirandorn Y, Rodeck CH. Antenatal diagnosis of megalourethra in a fetus with the prune belly syndrome. *J Clin Ultrasound* 1990;18:124–128.

230. Dillon E, Rose PG, Scott J. Case report. The antenatal ultrasound diagnosis of megalourethra. *Clin Radiol* 1994;49:354–355.

231. Simma B, Gabner I, Brezinka C, Ellemunter H, Kreczy A. Complete prenatal urinary tract obstruction caused by congenital megalourethra. *J Clin Ultrasound* 1992;20:197–199.

232. Kester R, Moopan U, Ohm H, Kim H. Congenital megalourethra. *J Urol* 1990;143:1212–1215.

233. Lebowitz R. The detection and characterization of vesicoureteral reflux in the child. *J Urol* 1992;148:1640–1642.

234. Ferrer F, McKenna P, Hochman H, Herndon A. Results of vesicoureteral reflux pattern survey among American Academy of Pediatrics section on pediatric urology members. *J Urol* 1998;160:1031–1037.

235. Puri P, Cascio S, Lakshmandass G, Colhoun E. Urinary tract infection and renal damage in sibling vesicoureteral reflux. *J Urol* 1998;160:1028–1030.

236. Yeung C, Godley M, Dhillon H, Gordon I, Duffy P, Ransley P. The characteristics of primary vesico-ureteric reflux in male and female infants with prenatal hydronephrosis. *Br J Urol* 1997;80:319–327.

237. Elder JS. Commentary: importance of antenatal diagnosis of vesico-ureteric reflux. *J Urol* 1992;148:1750–1754.

238. Koff SA. Relationship between dysfunctional voiding and reflux. *J Urol* 1992;148:1703–1705.

239. Avni EF, Sopulman CC. The origin of vesico-ureteric reflux in male newborns: further evidence in favour of a transient fetal urethral obstruction. *Br J Urol* 1996;78:454–457.

240. Hellstrom M, Jacobsson B. Diagnosis of vesico-ureteric reflux. *Acta Pediatr Suppl* 1999;431:3–12.

241. Allen T, Arant B, Roberts J. Commentary: vesicoureteral reflux. *J Urol* 1992;148:1758–1760.

242. Marra G, Barbieri G, Dell'Agnola CA, Caccamo ML, Castellani MR, Assael BM. Congenital renal damage associated with primary vesicoureteral reflux detected prenatally in male infants. *J Pediatr* 1994;124:726–730.

243. Anderson PAM, Rickwood AMK. Features of primary vesico-ureteric reflux detected by prenatal sonography. *Br J Urol* 1991;67:267–271.

244. Mandell J, Lebowitz RL, Peters GA, Estroff J, Retik AB, Benacerraf BC. Prenatal diagnosis of the megacystis-megaureter association. *J Urol* 1992;148:720–723.

245. Scott JES. Fetal ureteric reflux: a follow up study. *Br J Urol* 1993;71:481–483.

246. Stewart GD, Abluwalia A, Gowland M. Case report: diagnosis of fetal vesico-ureteric reflux as the cause of pelvicalyceal dilatation on antenatal ultrasound. *Clin Radiol* 1995;50:192–194.

247. Herndon C, McKenna P, Kolon T, Gonzalez E, Baker L. A multicentre outcomes analysis of patients with neonatal reflux presenting with prenatal hydronephrosis. *J Urol* 1999;162:1203–1208.

248. Persutte W, Koyle M, Lewke R, Klas J, Ryan C, Hobbins J. Mild pyelectasis ascertained with prenatal ultrasonography

is pediatrically significant. *Ultrasound Obstet Gynecol* 1997;10:12–18.

249. Farhat W, McLorie G, Geary D, Capolicchio G, Bagli D, et al. The natural history of neonatal vesicoureteral reflux associated with antenatal hydronephrosis. *J Urol* 2000;164:1057–1060.

250. Anderson NG, Abbott GD, Mogridge N, Allan RB, Maling TM, Wells JE. Vesicoureteric reflux in the newborn: relationship to fetal renal pelvic diameter. *Pediatr Nephrol* 1997;11:610–616.

251. Tibballs JM, De Bruyn R. Primary vesicoureteric reflux—how useful is postnatal ultrasound? *Arch Dis Child* 1996;75:444–447.

252. Weiss R, Duckett J, Spitzer A. Results of a randomized clinical trial of medical versus surgical management of infants and children with grades III and IV primary vesico-ureteral reflux. *J Urol* 1992;148:1667–1673.

253. Noe N, Wyatt R, Peeden J, Rinas M. The transmission of vesicoureteral reflux from parent to child. *J Urol* 1992;148:1869–1871.

254. Noe N. The long term results of prospective sibling reflux screening. *J Urol* 1992;148:1739–1742.

255. Jaramillo D, Lebowitz RL, Hendren WH. The cloacal malformation: radiologic findings and imaging recommendations. *Radiology* 1990;177:441–448.

256. Odibo AO, Turner GW, Borgida A, Rodis J, Campbell W. Late prenatal ultrasound features of hydrometrocolpos secondary to cloacal anomaly: case reports and review of the literature. *Ultrasound Obstet Gynecol* 1997;9:419–421.

257. Cilento BG, Benacerraf BR, Mandell J. Prenatal diagnosis of cloacal malformation. *Urology* 1994;43:386–388.

258. Petrikovsky B, Walzak M, Addario P. Fetal cloacal anomalies: prenatal sonographic findings and differential diagnosis. *Obstet Gynecol* 1988;72:464–469.

259. Shalev E, Feldman E, Weiner E, Zuckerman H. Prenatal sonographic appearance of persistent cloaca. *Acta Obstet Gynecol Scand* 1986;65:517–518.

260. Adams M, Ludlow J, Brock J, Rink R. Prenatal urinary ascites and persistent cloaca: risk factors for poor drainage of urine or meconium. *J Urol* 1998;160:2179–2181.

261. Bear JW, Gilsanz V. Calcified meconium and persistent cloaca. *Am J Radiol* 1981;137:867–869.

262. Qureshi F, Jacques SM, Yaron Y, Kramer RI, Evans M, Johnson MP. Prenatal diagnosis of cloacal dysgenesis sequence: differential diagnosis from other forms of fetal obstructive uropathy. *Fetal Diagn Ther* 1998;13:69–72.

263. Arulkumaran S, Nicolini V, Fisk NN, Rodeck CH. Fetal vesicorectal fistula causing oligohydramnios in the second trimester. *Br J Obstet Gynecol* 1990;97:449–451.

264. Blask AR, Saunders RC, Gearhart JP. Obstructed uterovaginal anomalies: demonstration with sonography. Part I. Neonates and infants. *Radiology* 1991;179:79–83.

265. Geifman-Holtzman O, Crane S, Winderl L, Holmes M. Persistent urogenital sinus: prenatal diagnosis and pregnancy complications. *Am J Obstet Gynecol* 1997;176:709–711.

266. Wood BP. Cloacal malformations and exstrophy syndromes. *Radiology* 1990;177:326–327.

267. Davis GH, Wapner RJ, Kurtz AB, Chibber G, FitzSimmons J, Blocklinger AJ. Antenatal diagnosis of hydrometrocolpos by ultrasound examination. *J Ultrasound Med* 1984;3:371–374.

268. Winderl L, Silverman R. Prenatal diagnosis of congenital imperforate hymen. *Obstet Gynecol* 1995;85:857–860.

269. Chitril Y, Zorn B, Filidori M, Robert E, Chasseray JE. Cloacal exstrophy in monozygotic twins detected through antenatal ultrasound scanning. *J Clin Ultrasound* 1993;21:339–342.

270. Austin PF, Homsy YL, Gearhart JP, Porter K, Guidi C, et al. The prenatal diagnosis of cloacal exstrophy. *J Urol* 1998;160:1179–1181.

271. Meizner I, Levi A, Barnhard Y. Cloacal exstrophy sequence: an exceptional ultrasound diagnosis. *Obstet Gynecol* 1995;86:446–450.

272. Kaya A, Oral B, Dittrich R, Ozkaya O. Prenatal diagnosis of cloacal exstrophy before rupture of the cloacal membrane. *Arch Gynecol Obstet* 2000;263:142–144.

273. Hamada H, Takano K, Shina M, Sakai T, Sohda S, Kubo T. New ultrasonographic criterion for the prenatal diagnosis of cloacal exstrophy: elephant trunk-like image. *J Urol* 1999;162:2123–2124.

274. Hurwitz RS, Manzoni GA, Ransley PG, Stephens FD. Cloacal exstrophy: a report of 34 cases. *J Urol* 1987;138:1060–1064.

275. Richards DS, Langham MR, Mahaffey SM. The prenatal ultrasonographic diagnosis of cloacal exstrophy. *J Ultrasound Med* 1992;11:507–510.

276. Zaontz MR, Packer MG. Abnormalities of the external genitalia. *Pediatr Clin North Am* 1997;44:1277–1283.

277. Shapiro E, Lepor H, Jeffs R. The inheritance of the exstrophy-epispadias complex. *J Urol* 1984;132:308–310.

278. Mirk P, Calisti A, Fileni A. Prenatal sonographic diagnosis of bladder exstrophy. *J Ultrasound Med* 1986;5:291–293.

279. Gearhart J, Ben-Chaim J, Jeffs R, Sanders R. Criteria for the prenatal diagnosis of classic bladder exstrophy. *Obstet Gynecol* 1995;85:961–964.

280. Jaffe R, Schoenfield A, Ovadia J. Sonographic findings in the prenatal diagnosis of bladder exstrophy. *Am J Obstet Gynecol* 1990;162:675–678.

281. Barth RA, Filly RA, Sondheimer FK. Prenatal sonographic findings in bladder exstrophy. *J Ultrasound Med* 1990;9:359–361.

282. Cadeddu JA, Benson JE, Silver RI, Lakshmanan Y, Jeffs RD, Gearhart JP. Spinal abnormalities in classic bladder exstrophy. *Br J Urol* 1997;79:975–978.

283. Stjernqvist K, Kockum CC. Bladder exstrophy: psychological impact during childhood. *J Urol* 1999;162:2125–2129.

284. Apuzzio JJ, Unwin W, Adhate A, Nichols R. Prenatal diagnosis of fetal renal mesoblastic nephroma. *Am J Obstet Gynecol* 1986;154:636–637.

285. Geirsson RT, Ricketts NEM, Taylor DJ, Coghill S. Prenatal appearance of a mesoblastic nephroma associated with polyhydramnios. *J Clin Ultrasound* 1985;13:488–490.

286. Matsumura M, Nishi T, Sasaki Y, Yamada R, Yamamoto H, et al. Prenatal diagnosis and treatment strategy for congenital mesoblastic nephroma. *J Pediatr Surg* 1993;28:1607–1609.

287. Suresh I, Suresh S, Arumugam R, Govindarajan M, Reddy MP, Sulochana NV. Antenatal diagnosis of Wilms tumor. *J Ultrasound Med* 1997;16:69–72.

288. Vadeyar S, Ramsay M, James D, O'Neill D. Prenatal diagnosis of congenital Wilms tumor (nephroblastoma) pre-

senting as fetal hydrops. *Ultrasound Obstet Gynecol* 2000; 16:80–83.

289. Fung TY, Fung YM, Ng PC, Yeung CK, Chang MZ. Poly-hydramnios and hypercalcemia associated with congenital mesoblastic nephroma: case report and a new appraisal. *Obstet Gynecol* 1995;85:815–817.

290. Elejalde BR, Mercedes de Elejalde M, Keitman T. Visualization of the fetal genitalia, by ultrasonography. A review of the literature and ethical implication. *J Ultrasound Med* 1985;4:633–639.

291. Stephens JD, Sherman S. Determination of fetal sex by ultrasound. *N Engl J Med* 1983;309:984.

292. Meagher S, Davison G. Early second-trimester determination of fetal gender by ultrasound. *Ultrasound Obstet Gynecol* 1996;8:322–324.

293. Harrington K, Armstrong V, Freeman J, Acquilina J, Campbell S. Fetal sexing by ultrasound in the second trimester: maternal preference and professional ability. *Ultrasound Obstet Gynecol* 1996;8:318–321.

294. Efrat Z, Akinfenwa O, Nicolaides KH. First-trimester determination of fetal gender by ultrasound. *Ultrasound Obstet Gynecol* 1999;13:305–307.

295. Whitlow B, Lakanakis M, Economides D. The sonographic identification of fetal gender from 11–14 weeks of gestation. *Ultrasound Obstet Gynecol* 1999;13:301–304.

296. Benoit B. Opinion: early fetal gender determination. *Ultrasound Obstet Gynecol* 1999;13:299–300.

297. Warkany J. *Congenital malformations*. Chicago: Medical YearBook, 1981.

298. Mandell J, Bromley B, Peters CA, Benacerraf BR. Prenatal sonographic detection of genital malformations. *J Urol* 1995;153:1994–1996.

299. Lazebnik N, Filkins KA, Jackson CL, Linn HB, Doshi N, Hogge W. 45,X/46,XY mosaicism: the role of ultrasound in prenatal diagnosis and counseling. *Ultrasound Obstet Gynecol* 1996;8:325–328.

300. Cheikhelard A, Luton D, Philippe-Chomette P, Leger J, Vuillard E, et al. How accurate is the prenatal diagnosis of abnormal genitalia? *J Urol* 2000;164:984–987.

301. Smith P, Felker R, Noe N, Emerson D, Mercer B. Prenatal diagnosis of genital anomalies. *Urology* 1996;47:114–117.

302. Bronshtein M, Riechler A, Zimmer E. Prenatal sonographic signs of possible fetal genital anomalies. *Prenat Diagn* 1995;15:215–219.

303. Shapiro E. The sonographic appearance of normal and abnormal fetal genitalia. *J Urol* 1999;162:530–533.

304. Neri G, Opitz J. Syndromal (and non-syndromal) forms of male pseudohermaphroditism. *Am J Med Genet* 1999;89:201–209.

305. Dumic M, Brkljacic L, Plavsic V, Zunec R, Ille J, et al. Prenatal diagnosis of congenital adrenal hyperplasia (21-hydroxylase deficiency) in Croatia. *Am J Med Genet* 1997;73:302–306.

306. Cilento B, Bauer S, Retiu A, Peters C, Atala A. Urachal anomalies: defining the best diagnostic modality. *Urology* 1998;52:120–122.

307. Persutte W, Lenke R. Disappearing fetal umbilical cord masses. Are these findings suggestive of urachal anomalies? *J Ultrasound Med* 1990;9:547–551.

308. Sepulveda W, Bower S, Dhillon H, Fisk N. Prenatal diagnosis of congenital patent urachus and allantoic cyst: the value of color flow imaging. *J Ultrasound Med* 1995;14:47–51.

309. Hill L, Kislak S, Belfar H. The sonographic diagnosis of urachal cysts *in utero*. *J Clin Ultrasound* 1990;18:434–437.

310. Kaefer M, Keating M, Adams M, Rink R. Posterior urethral valves. Pressure pop offs and bladder function. *J Urol* 1995;154:708–711.

311. Montemarano H, Bulas D, Rushton G, Selby D. Bladder distension and pyelectasis in the male fetus: causes comparisons and contrasts. *J Ultrasound Med* 1998;17:743–749.

312. Frazier H, Guerrieri J, Thomas R, Christenson P. The detection of a patent urachus and allantoic cyst of the umbilical cord on prenatal ultrasonography. *J Ultrasound Med* 1992;11:117–120.

313. Yoo SJ, Lee YH, Ryu HM, Joo MS, Cheon CK, Park KW. Unusual fate of vesicoallantoic cyst with non-visualization of fetal urinary bladder in a case of patent urachus. *Ultrasound Obstet Gynecol* 1997;9:422–424.

314. Awwad J, Azar G, Soubra M. Sonographic diagnosis of a urachal cyst *in utero*. *Acta Obstet Gynecol Scand* 1994;73:156–157.

SKELETAL DYSPLASIAS*

The skeletal dysplasias are a large heterogeneous group of genetic conditions characterized by abnormal shape, growth, or integrity of bones, with different forms of inheritance, presentation, natural history, management, treatment, and prognosis. Although more than 271 skeletal dysplasias have been described, and more will probably be identified as distinct entities, the number that can be recognized with the use of sonography in the antepartum period is considerably small. Because skeletal dysplasias are uncommon, acquiring a large experience takes time. This chapter reviews the birth prevalence and classification of skeletal dysplasias and provides a frame to approach the diagnoses of conditions identifiable at birth.[1]

Patients with skeletal dysplasia have existed in all societies, and we should make effort to allow them to function as normally as possible in the society. For example, Henri de Toulouse-Lautrec is considered to have experienced a disorder called *pyknodysostosis*.[2–5] Pyknodysostosis is an autosomal recessive skeletal disorder characterized by short stature, increased bone density, delayed closure of cranial sutures, loss of the mandibular angle, dysplastic clavicles, dissolution of the terminal phalanges of the hands and feet, dental abnormalities, and increased bone fragility. The defect links to a narrow region on band 21 of the long arm of chromosome 1.

One person with achondroplasia was relating her anxiety when taking an elevator once in a big city. When the door closed behind her, there was no button she could reach and she was trapped in the elevator until someone else came in. The passage in the United States of the Americans with Disabilities Act has contributed to the adaptation of these special people in society. Hopefully, this will be more widespread around the globe.

Many organizations assist patients with skeletal dysplasia. A vibrant example is the Little People of America (http://www.lpaonline.org) that assists patients with achondroplasia and similar disorders. Physicians should be aware of these resources and help their patients take advantage of the support they provide.

EMBRYOLOGIC DEVELOPMENT OF THE SKELETON

The skeleton undergoes development and growth throughout pregnancy with the most rapid development occurring during the first trimester (Fig. 1). The vertebra develops during the sixth menstrual week, the skull begins to form during the seventh menstrual week, and the clavicle and mandible begin to develop at 8 weeks.[6] Hyaline cartilage of the future appendicular skeleton also begins to appear during the eighth menstrual week. The primary ossification centers of the long bones appear in the center of the shaft, called the *diaphysis*, between the seventh and twelfth menstrual week. By the twelfth menstrual week, fetal long bone measurements of the femur, tibia, fibula, humerus, radius, and ulna can be accurately measured.

Ossification of the metacarpals and metatarsal occurs between 12 and 16 weeks, and the pubis, talus, and calcaneus ossify during the fifth and sixth months. Ossification of the carpal bones and the remaining tarsal bones does not occur until after birth. Secondary ossification centers within the epiphyseal cartilage of the distal femur, proximal tibia, and occasionally the proximal humerus may be seen during the third trimester, whereas the remaining secondary epiphyseal centers do not ossify until after birth.

The process of ossification is categorized into membranous and cartilaginous ossification. Some of the axial skeleton, such as the flat bones of the skull, undergoes membranous ossification. In this process, the mesenchymal cells are directly transferred into osteoblasts, which then develop into membranous bone. In contrast, the appendicular skeleton is formed by cartilaginous ossification in which cartilage is first formed. Parts of the axial skeleton

---

*This chapter discusses skeletal dysplasias and other major abnormalities of the skeleton. It does not include a discussion of amputated, missing, or malformed limbs, which are usually isolated. Amputated, missing, or malformed limbs are also typically unilateral, although clubfeet may be bilateral. The practicing sonographer is encouraged to include views of all four extremities, including both hands and feet, whenever possible, during an anatomic fetal survey to detect these common defects of the extremities.

This chapter is adapted from and copyrighted by http://www.TheFetus.net.

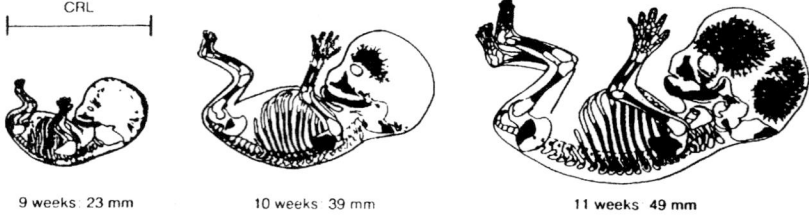

FIGURE 1. Formation of ossification centers at 9, 10, and 11 weeks' gestation. CRL, crown-rump length. (Reproduced with permission from Hansmann M, Hackeloer B-J, Staudach A. *Ultrasound diagnosis in obstetrics and gynecology.* New York: Springer-Verlag New York, 1985:47.)

such as portions of the skull undergo membranous and cartilaginous ossification.

OVERVIEW OF SKELETAL DYSPLASIA

The birth prevalence of skeletal dysplasias, excluding limb amputations, recognizable in the neonatal period has been estimated to be 2.4 per 10,000 births.[7] In a large series, 23% of affected infants were stillbirths and 32% died during the first week of life. The overall frequency of skeletal dysplasias among perinatal deaths was 9.1 per 1,000. The relative frequencies of the different skeletal dysplasias are shown in Figure 2.

The four most common skeletal dysplasias are thanatophoric dysplasia, achondroplasia, osteogenesis imperfecta, and achondrogenesis. Thanatophoric dysplasia and achondrogenesis accounted for 62% of all lethal skeletal dysplasias.[7] The most common nonlethal skeletal dysplasia is achondroplasia.

In another large series, reporting the prevalence and classification of lethal neonatal skeletal dysplasias in West Scotland, the prevalence was 1.1 per 10,000 births, and the most frequently diagnosed conditions were thanatophoric dysplasia (0.24 per 10,000); osteogenesis imperfecta (0.18 per 10,000); rhizomelic chondrodysplasia punctata (0.12 per 10,000); camptomelic syndrome (0.1 per 10,000); and achondrogenesis (0.1 per 10,000).[8]

Figure 3 shows the prevalence of selected skeletal dysplasias in the studies of Anderson and Camera.

CLASSIFICATION OF SKELETAL DYSPLASIAS

The classification of skeletal dysplasia has been hampered by the rarity of the condition and the lack of understanding of the etiologies. Thus, disorders that look the same were assimilated and then separated under new entities. This lack of understanding resulted in classifications that were mainly descriptive, and the technique most likely to identify the findings was predominantly used to categorize the anomalies. Many definitions, therefore, were based on radiologic criteria, with a few based on histologic or clinical criteria. This, in turn, further complicated matters because the nomenclature of the disorder was then either a description of the clinical outcome (e.g., thanatophoric dysplasia, meaning, "carrying death"); clinical description (e.g., diastrophic dysplasia referred to the twisted joints, cleidocranial dysplasia, referring to the affected bones); or possible pathogenesis (e.g., osteogenesis imperfecta, achondrogenesis). Those disorders too uncertain or with too many features were given eponyms (e.g., Ellis-van Creveld syndrome).

This situation has been greatly clarified by the progresses of molecular genetics.

GENETIC AND MOLECULAR ASPECTS OF SKELETAL DYSPLASIAS

Identification of genetic defects represents major landmarks in the knowledge about skeletal dysplasias. Before these

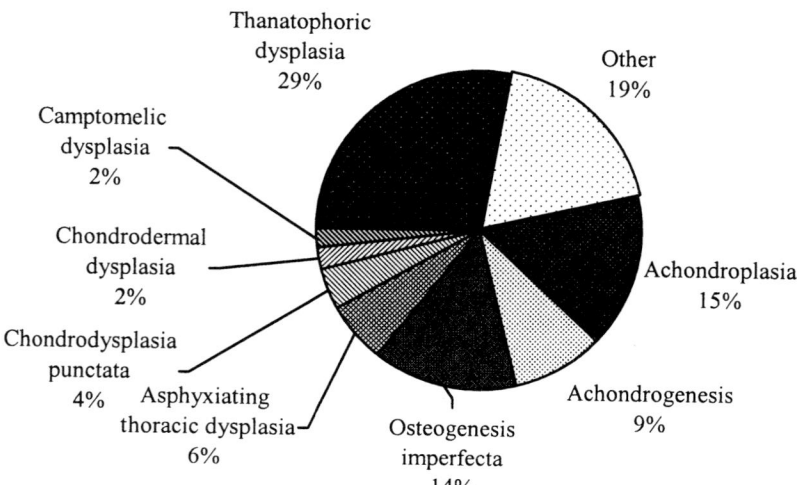

FIGURE 2. The relative frequencies of the different skeletal dysplasias.

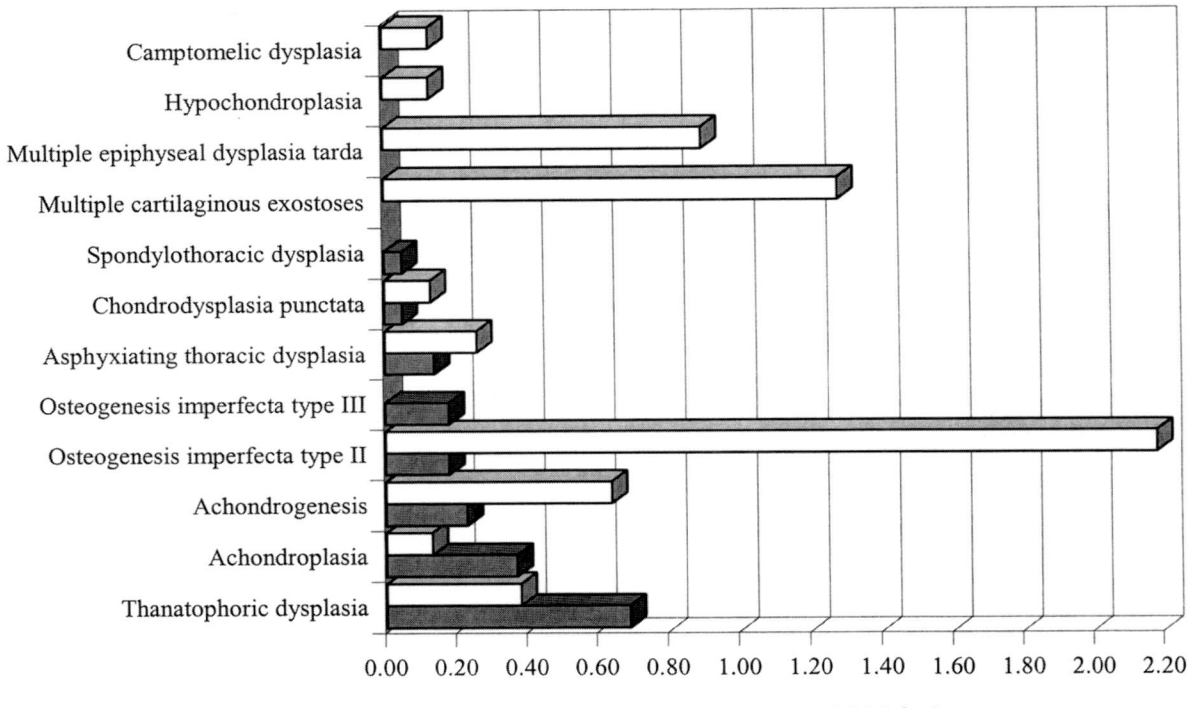

Prevalence per 10,000 births

FIGURE 3. Prevalence of major skeletal dysplasias. (Reproduced with permission from Andersen P, Hauge M. Congenital generalized bone dysplasia: a clinical, radiological, and epidemiological survey. *J Med Genet* 1989;26:37–44; and Camera G, Mastroiacovo P. Birth prevalence of skeletal dysplasias in the Italian multicentric study. In: Papadatos C, Bartsocas C, eds. *Skeletal dysplasias*. Proceedings of the Third International Clinical Genetics Seminar. New York: Liss, 1982:441–449.)

papers, skeletal dysplasias were almost strictly classified by radiologic criteria. These papers marked the beginning of an intense and successful search for gene mapping of skeletal dysplasia. Many of these were found to result from alterations of the fibroblast growth factors (I through III).

It is very difficult to locate the *primary defect* of a skeletal alteration versus the *secondary and/or in cascade effect* of a genetic defect that has repercussions on the skeleton. Numerous genetic and chromosomal syndromes affect the development of the skeleton, making it necessary to locate the primary defect.

For instance, connective tissue alterations are responsible for the skeletal alterations in Gorlin syndrome; Marfan syndrome; neurofibromatosis 1; fragile X syndrome; trisomies 18, 21, and 13; and growth hormone deficiency for those of Cockayne, Rubinstein-Taybi, and Silver-Russell syndromes. Others result from mutations that may affect all chromosomes (aside the 13 and Y) and the mitochondrial DNA.

In an attempt to bring some order to the classification, an *International Nomenclature for Skeletal Dysplasias* was proposed by a group of experts in Paris in 1977. This classification was revised in Germany in 1992 and in Los Angeles in 1998. The current version has been renamed *International Nomenclature of Constitutional Disorders of Bone* and is available online at http://www.csmc.edu/genetics/skeldys/nomenclature.html.

The original five categories have been enlarged into 32 groups in Table 1.

Embryogenesis

The differentiation of the mesodermal tissue into bone and cartilaginous tissue requires genetic-environmental interactions that give rise to normal morphogenesis, before the seventh week of the embryonic development. The ossification begins on the forty-fourth day. The genes direct the synthesis of extracellular or intracellular molecular components, such as matrix proteins, transporting molecules, growth factors, or cellular surface receptors that can serve as signals for genetic transcription and cellular processes inherent to the differentiation and morphogenesis.

Molecular Aspects

Cells and extracellular matrix form the connective tissue. They interact with each other to create its biology and function. There are four groups of fundamental major proteins in the extracellular matrix: collagens, elastin, proteoglycans, and glycoproteins.

TABLE 1. INTERNATIONAL NOMENCLATURE OF CONSTITUTIONAL DISORDERS OF BONE

	Mode of inheritance	OMIM syndrome	Present at birth	Chromosomal locus	Gene	Protein	OMIM gene/protein
1. Achondroplasia group							
Thanatophoric dysplasia, type I	AD	187600	+	4p16.3	FGFR3	FGFR3	134934
Thanatophoric dysplasia, type II	AD	187601	+	4p16.3	FGFR3	FGFR3	134934
Achondroplasia	AD	100800	+	4p16.3	FGFR3	FGFR3	134934
Hypochondroplasia	AD	146000	–	4p16.3	FGFR3	FGFR3	134934
Other FGFR3 disorders	—	—	—	—	—	—	—
2. Spondylodysplastic and other perinatally lethal groups							
Lethal platyspondylic skeletal dys-	SP	270230	+	—	—	—	—
plasias (San Diego type, Tor-		151210	+	—	—	—	—
rance type, Luton type)		151210	+	—	—	—	—
Achondrogenesis type IA	AR	200600	+	—	—	—	—
3. Metatropic dysplasia group							
Fibrochondrogenesis	AR	228520	+	—	—	—	—
Schneckenbecken dysplasia	AR	269250	+	—	—	—	—
Metatropic dysplasia (various forms)	AD	156530	+	—	—	—	—
4. Short-rib dysplasia (SRP) (with or without polydactyly) group							
SRP type I, Saldino-Noonan	AR	263530	+	—	—	—	—
SRP type II, Majewski	AR	263520	+	—	—	—	—
SRP type III, Verma-Naumoff	AR	263510	+	—	—	—	—
SRP type IV, Beemer-Langer	AR	269860	+	—	—	—	—
Asphyxiating thoracic dysplasia (Jeune)	AR	208500	+	—	—	—	—
Chondroectodermal dysplasia (Ellis-van Creveld dysplasia)	AR	225500	+	4p16	—	—	—
5. Atelosteogenesis-omodysplasia group							
Atelosteogenesis type I (includes "Boomerang dysplasia")	SP	108720	+	—	—	—	—
Omodysplasia I (Maroteaux)	AD	164745	+	—	—	—	—
Omodysplasia II (Borochowitz)	AR	258315	+	—	—	—	—
Otopalatodigital syndrome type II	XLR	304120	+	—	—	—	—
Atelosteogenesis type III	SP	108721	+	—	—	—	—
de la Chapelle dysplasia	AR	256050	+	—	—	—	—
6. Diastrophic dysplasia group							
Diastrophic dysplasia	AR	222600	+	5q32-q33	DTDST	Sul. Transporter	—
Achondrogenesis IB	AR	600972	+	5q32-q33	DTDST	Sul. Transporter	—
Atelosteogenesis type II	AR	256050	+	5q32-q33	DTDST	Sul. Transporter	—
7. Dyssegmental dysplasia group							
Dyssegmental dysplasia, Silverman-Handmaker type	AR	224410	+	—	—	—	—
Dyssegmental dysplasia, Rolland-Desbuquois type	AR	224400	+	—	—	—	—
8. Type II collagenopathies							
Achondrogenesis II (Langer-Saldino)	AD	200610	+	12q13.1-q13.3	COL2A1	Type II collagen	120140
Hypochondrogenesis	AD	200610	+	12q13.1-q13.3	COL2A1	Type II collagen	120140
Kniest dysplasia	AD	156550	+	12q13.1-q13.3	COL2A1	Type II collagen	120140
Spondyloepiphyseal dysplasia (SED) congenita	AD	183900	+	12q13.1-q13.3	COL2A1	Type II collagen	120140
Spondyloepimetaphyseal dysplasia (SEMD) Strudwick type	AD	184250	+	12q13.1-q13.3	COL2A1	Type II collagen	120140
SED with brachydactyly	AD	—	—	12q13.1-q13.3	COL2A1	Type II collagen	120140
Mild SED with premature onset arthrosis	AD	—	–	12q13.1-q13.3	COL2A1	Type II collagen	120140
Stickler dysplasia (heterogeneous, some not linked to COL2A1)	AD	108300	+	12q13.1-q13.3	COL2A1	Type II collagen	120140
9. Type XI collagenopathies							
Stickler dysplasia (heterogeneous)	AD	184840	+	6p21	COL11A1	Type XI collagen	120280
Otospondylomegaepiphyseal dys-	AR	215150	+	6p21.3	COL11A2	Type XI collagen	120290
plasia (OSMED)	AD	—	+	6p21.3	COL11A2	Type XI collagen	120290

(*continued*)

TABLE 1. *CONTINUED*

	Mode of inheri- tance	OMIM syndrome	Present at birth	Chromosomal locus	Gene	Protein	OMIM gene/ protein
10. Other SEMDs							
X-linked spondyloepiphyseal dys- plasia tarda	XLD	313400	−	Xp22.2-p22.1	—	—	—
Other late-onset spondyloepimeta- physeal dysplasias (Irapa) (Nama- qualand, et al.)	AR	271650	−	—	—	—	—
Progressive pseudorheumatoid dysplasia	AR	208230	−	—	—	—	—
Dyggve-Melchior-Clausen dysplasia	AR	223800	+	—	—	—	—
Wolcott-Rallison dysplasia	AR	226980	−	—	—	—	—
Immuno-osseous dysplasia-Schimke	AR	242900	+	—	—	—	—
Opsismodysplasia	AR	258480	+	—	—	—	—
Chondrodystrophic myotonia (Schwartz Jampel), type 1, type 2	AR	258480 255800	+ +	— 1q36-34	— —	— —	— —
Spondyloepiphyseal dysplasia with joint laxity	AR	271640	+	—	—	—	—
SPONASTRIME dysplasia	AR	271510	−	—	—	—	—
SEMD short limb—abnormal calci- fication	AR	271665	+	—	—	—	—
11. Multiple epiphyseal dysplasias and pseudoachondroplasia							
Pseudoachondroplasia	AD	177170	−	19p12-13.1	COMP	COMP	600310
Multiple epiphyseal dysplasia (MED)	AD	132400	−	—	—	—	—
(Fairbanks and Ribbing types)	AD	600204	−	19p12-13.1	COMP	COMP	600310
Other MEDs	?	600969	−	1p32.2-33	COL9A2	Type IX collagen	120260
12. Chondrodysplasia punctata (stippled epiphyses group)							
Rhizomelic type	AR	215100	+	4p16-p14	PEX7	Peroxin-7	601757
Zellweger syndrome	AR	214100	+	7q11.23	PEX1	—	—
	AR	214100	+	6p21.1	PEX6	Peroxin-6	601498
	AR	214100	+	7q11.23	PEX1	Peroxin-1	602136
	AR	214100	+	12	PEX5	Peroxin-5	—
	AR	214100	+	8q21.1	PEX2	Peroxin-2	170993
Conradi-Hünermann type	XLD	302950	+	Xq28	CPXD	—	—
X-linked recessive type	XLR	302940	+	Xp22.3	CPXR	—	—
Brachytelephalangic type	XLR	302940	+	Xp22.32	ARSE	Arylsulfatase E	302950
Tibial-metacarpal type	AD	118651	+	—	—	—	—
Vitamin K–dependent coagula- tion defect	AR	277450	+	—	—	—	—
Other acquired and genetic disor- ders, including Warfarin embry- opathy	—	—	—	—	—	—	—
13. Metaphyseal dysplasias							
Jansen type	AD	156400	+	3p22-p21.1	PTHR	PTHR/PTHRP	168468
Schmid type	AD	156500	−	6q21-q22.3	COL10A1	COL10 alpha chain	120110
McKusick type (cartilage-hair hypoplasia)	AR	250250	+	9p13	—	—	—
Metaphyseal anadysplasia	XLR?	309645	−	—	—	—	—
Metaphyseal dysplasia with pancre- atic insufficiency and cyclic neu- tropenia (Shwachman Diamond)	AR	260400	−	—	—	—	—
Adenosine deaminase deficiency	AD	102700	−	20q-13.11	ADA	Adenosine deaminase	102700
Metaphyseal chondrodysplasia (Spahr type)	AR	250400	−	—	—	—	—
Acroscyphodysplasia (various types)	AR	250215	−	—	—	—	—
14. Spondylometaphyseal dysplasias (SMD)							
Spondylometaphyseal dysplasia (Kozlowski type)	AD	184252	+	—	—	—	—
Spondylometaphyseal dysplasia (Sutcliffe type)	AD	184255	+	—	—	—	—

(continued)

TABLE 1. *CONTINUED*

	Mode of inheritance	OMIM syndrome	Present at birth	Chromosomal locus	Gene	Protein	OMIM gene/protein
SMD with severe genu valgum (includes Schmidt and Algerian types)	AD	184253	+	—	—	—	—
SMD Sedaghatian type	AR	—	+	—	—	—	—
Mild SMD different types that have not been well delineated	—	—	–	—	—	—	—
15. Brachyolmia spondylodysplasias							
Hobaek (includes Toledo type)	AR	271530–271630	–	—	—	—	—
Maroteaux type	AR	—	–	—	—	—	—
Autosomal dominant type	AD	113500	–	—	—	—	—
16. Mesomelic dysplasias							
Dyschondrosteosis (Leri-Weill)	AD	127300	–	—	—	—	—
Langer type (homozygous dyschondrosteosis)	AR	249700	+	—	—	—	—
Nievergelt type	AD	163400	+	—	—	—	—
Kozlowski-Reardon type	AR	—	+	—	—	—	—
Reinhardt-Pfeiffer type	AD	191400	+	—	—	—	—
Werner type	AD	—	+	—	—	—	—
Robinow type, dominant	AD	180700	–	—	—	—	—
Robinow type, recessive	AR	268310	–	—	—	—	—
Mesomelic dysplasia with synostoses	AD	600383	+	—	—	—	—
17. Acromelic and acromesomelic dysplasias							
Acromicric dysplasia	AD	102370	+	—	—	—	—
Geleophysic dysplasia	AR	231050	+	—	—	—	—
Weill-Marchesani dysplasia	AR	277600	+	—	—	—	—
Cranioectodermal dysplasia	AR	218330	+	—	—	—	—
Trichorhinophalangeal dysplasia, type I	AD	190350	+	8q24.12	TRPS1	—	—
Trichorhinophalangeal dysplasia, type II (Langer-Giedion)	AD	150230	+	8q24.11-q24.13	TRPS1 + EXT1	—	—
Trichorhinophalangeal dysplasia, type III	AD	190351	+	—	—	—	—
Grebe dysplasia	AR	200700	+	20q11.2	CDMP1	Cartilage-derived morphogenic protein 1	601146
Hunter-Thompson dysplasia	AR	201250	+	20q11.2	CDMP1	Cartilage-derived morphogenic protein 1	601146
Brachydactyly type A1-A4	AD	112500–112800	+	—	—	—	—
Brachydactyly type B	AD	113000	+	—	—	—	—
Brachydactyly type C	AD	133100	+	21q11	CDMP1	Cartilage-derived morphogenic protein 1	601196
	AD			12q24			
Brachydactyly type D	AD	113200	+	—	—	—	—
Brachydactyly type E	AD	113000	–	—	—	—	—
Pseudohypoparathyroidism (Albright hereditary osteodystrophy), various types, see OMIM	—	—	—	20q13	GNAS1	Quanine nucleotide binding protein of adenylate cyclase alpha-subunit	139320
Acrodysostosis	SP(AD)	101800	–	—	—	—	—
Saldino-Mainzer dysplasia	AR	266920	–	—	—	—	—
Brachydactyly-hypertension dysplasia (Bilginturan)	AD	112410	+	12p	—	—	—
Craniofacial conodysplasia	AD	—	+	—	—	—	—
Angel-shaped phalango-epiphyseal dysplasia (ASPED)	AD	105835	+	—	—	—	—
Acromesomelic dysplasia	AR	201250	+	—	—	—	—
Other acromesomelic dysplasias	—	—	–	—	—	—	—

(continued)

TABLE 1. *CONTINUED*

	Mode of inheritance	OMIM syndrome	Present at birth	Chromosomal locus	Gene	Protein	OMIM gene/protein
18. Dysplasias with prominent membranous bone involvement							
Cleidocranial dysplasia	AD	119600	+	6p21	CBFA1	Core binding factor alpha-subunit	600211
Osteodysplasty, Melnick-Needles	XLD	309350	–	—	—	—	—
Precocious osteodysplasty (ter Haar dysplasia)	AR	—	+	—	—	—	—
19. Bent-bone dysplasia group							
Camptomelic dysplasia	AD	114290	+	17q24.3-q25.1	SOX9	SRY-box 9	211970
Kyphomelic dysplasia	?AR	211350	+	—	—	—	—
Stüve-Wiedemann dysplasia	AR	601559	+	—	—	—	—
20. Multiple dislocations with dysplasias							
Larsen syndrome	AD	150250	+	3p21.1-p14.1	LARI	—	—
Larsen-like syndromes (including La Reunion Island)	AR	245600	+	—	—	—	—
Desbuquois dysplasia	AR	251450	+	—	—	—	—
Pseudodiastrophic dysplasia	AR	264180	+	—	—	—	—
21. Dysostosis multiplex group							
Mucopolysaccharidosis IH	AR	252800	–	4p16.3	IDA	Alpha-1-iduronidase	—
Mucopolysaccharidosis IS	AR	252800	–	4p16.3	IDA	Alpha-1-iduronidase	—
Mucopolysaccharidosis II	XLR	309900	–	Xq27.3-q28	IDS	Iduronate-2-sulfatase	—
Mucopolysaccharidosis IIIA	AR	252900	–	17q25.3	HSS	Heparan sulfate sulfatase	—
Mucopolysaccharidosis IIIB	AR	252920	—	17q21	—	N-Ac-alpha-D-gluco-saminidase	—
Mucopolysaccharidosis IIIC	AR	252930	–	—	—	Ac-CoA:alpha-gluco-saminidase-N-acetyl-transferase	—
Mucopolysaccharidosis IIID	AR	252940	–	12q14	GNS	N-Ac-glucosamine-6-sulfatase	—
Mucopolysaccharidosis IVA	AR	230500	–	16q24.3	GALNS	Galactose-6-sulfatase	—
Mucopolysaccharidosis IVB	AR	230500	–	3p21.33	GLBI	Beta-galactosidase	—
Mucopolysaccharidosis VI	AR	253200	–	5q13.3	ARSB	Arylsulfatase B	—
Mucopolysaccharidosis VII	AR	253200	–	7q21.11	GUSB	Beta-glucuronidase	—
Fucosidosis	AR	230000	–	1p34	FUCA	Alpha-fucosidase	—
α-Mannosidosis	AR	248500	–	19p13.2-q12	MAN	Alpha-mannosidase	—
β-Mannosidosis	AR	248510	–	4	MANB	Beta-mannosidase	—
Aspartylglucosaminuria	AR	208400	–	4q23-q27	AgA	Aspartylglucosaminidase	—
GM1 gangliosidosis, several forms	AR	230500	+	3p21-p14.2	GLB1	Beta-galactosidase	—
Sialidosis, several forms	AR	256550	+/–	6p21.3	NEU	Alpha-neuraminidase	—
Sialic acid storage disease	AR	269920	+/–	6q14-q15	SIASD	—	—
Galactosialidosis, several forms	AR	256540	—	20q13.1	PPGB	Beta-galactosidase protective protein	—
Multiple sulfatase deficiency	AR	272200	+/–	—	—	Multiple sulfatases	—
Mucolipidosis II	AR	252500	+	4q21-23	GNPTA	N-Ac-glucosamine-phosphotransferase	—
Mucolipidosis III	AR	252600	–	4q21-23	GNPTA	N-Ac-glucosamine-phosphotransferase	—
Yunis-Varon dysplasia	AR	216340	+	—	—	—	—
22. Osteodysplastic slender bone group							
Type I osteodysplastic dysplasia	AR	210710	+	—	—	—	—
Type II osteodysplastic dysplasia	AR	210720	+	—	—	—	—
Microcephalic osteodysplastic dysplasia	AR	—	—	—	—	—	—
23. Dysplasias with decreased bone density							
Osteogenesis imperfecta I (without opalescent teeth)	AD	166200	+/–	17q21	COL1A1	Alpha (1)I procollagen	120150
Osteogenesis imperfecta I (with opalescent teeth)	AD	166240	+/–	17q21	COL1A1	Alpha (1)I procollagen	120150
	AD	166240	+/–	7q22.1	COL1A2	Alpha (2)I procollagen	120160
Osteogenesis imperfecta II	AD	166210	+	17q21	COL1A1	Alpha (1)I procollagen	120150
	AD	166210	+	7q22.1	COL1A2	Alpha (2)I procollagen	120160
	AR	259400	+	17q21	COL1A1	Alpha (1)I procollagen	120150

(continued)

TABLE 1. *CONTINUED*

	Mode of inheri-tance	OMIM syndrome	Present at birth	Chromosomal locus	Gene	Protein	OMIM gene/protein
Multicentric predominantly carpal, tarsal, and interphalangeal							
Francois syndrome	AR	221800	–	—	—	—	—
Winchester syndrome	AR	277950	–	—	—	—	—
Torg syndrome	AR	259600	–	—	—	—	—
Whyte Hemingway carpal-tarsal phalangeal osteolyses	AD	—	–	—	—	—	—
Predominantly distal phalanges							
Hadju-Cheney syndrome	AD	102500	–	—	—	—	—
Giacci familial neurogenic acroosteolysis	AR	201300	–	—	—	—	—
Mandibulosacral syndrome	AR	248370	–	—	—	—	—
Predominantly involving diaphyses and metaphyses							
Familial expansile osteolysis	AD	174810	–	18q21.1-q22	—	—	—
Juvenile hyaline fibromatosis	AR	228600	+	—	—	—	—
32. Patella dysplasias							
Nail patella dysplasia	AD	161200	–	9q34.1	NPS1	—	—
Scypho-patellar dysplasia	AD	—	+	—	—	—	—

+, present; –, absent; AD, autosomal dominant; AR, autosomal recessive; FGFR, fibroblast growth factor receptor; SP, sporadic; SPONASTRIME, spondylar changes-nasal anomaly-striated-metaphyses; XLD, X-linked dominant; XLR, X-linked recessive.
Reproduced with permission from Skeletal Dysplasia Registry. Cedars-Sinai Medical Center. William.Wilcox@cshs.org.

The collagen family of genes includes more than 25 genes. They are dispersed in more than 12 chromosomes (Table 2). As a family, the collagens are the most abundant protein in the body. Most of the collagens are the main protein in bone, skin, tendon, ligament, sclera, cornea, blood vessels, and many hollow organs. Most collagens have a tissue-limited distribution. For instance, collagen types II, IX, X, and XI are found in hyaline cartilage and the vitreous of the eye. Type IV collagens are limited to basal membranes. Only certain types of differentiated cells synthesize most collagens, but a single cell type may synthesize several collagens. Chondrocytes, for instance, synthesize collagen types II, IX, X, and XI, but not collagen types I or III.

The reason for the rapid revision of the nomenclature has been the explosion of knowledge brought in by the discoveries of the genetic defect underlying many of the conditions. In 1994, two groups (Le Merrer at the INSERM in Paris, France, and Velinov in Farmington, Connecticut) independently concluded that the gene responsible for achondroplasia was located in the telomeric region of the 16.3 band of the short arm of chromosome 4. The next year, Bellus at Johns Hopkins demonstrated that a glycine to arginine at codon 380 of the fibroblast growth factor receptor (FGFR) 3 was responsible for achondroplasia. Fibroblast growth factors regulate cell proliferation, differentiation, and migration by a transmembrane tyrosine-

TABLE 2. GENE AND CHROMOSOME PROTEIN STRUCTURE RELATED TO CLINICAL DISORDERS

Chromosome location	Collagen symbol	Type	Disorder
2q31	COL11A2	Collagen, III, α-1 polypeptide	Ehlers-Danlos syndrome type IV
6p21.3	COL11A2	Collagen, XI, α-2 polypeptide	Stickler syndrome type II
6q21-q22.3	COL10A1	Collagen, X, α-1 polypeptide	Metaphyseal chondrodysplasia, Schmid type
7q22.1	COL1A2	Collagen, I, α-2 polypeptide	Osteogenesis imperfecta, four clinical forms
9q34.2-q34.3	COL5A1	Collagen, V, α-1 polypeptide	Ehlers-Danlos syndrome type II, one form
12q13.11-q13.2	COL2A1	Collagen, II, α-1 polypeptide	Stickler syndrome type I
			Spondyloepiphyseal congenita
			Kniest dysplasia
			Achondrogenesis-hypochondrogenesis type II
			Osteoarthrosis, precocious
			Wagner syndrome type II
			Spondyloepimetaphysial dysplasia Strudwick type
17q21.31-q22.05	COL1A1	Collagen, I, α-1 polypeptide	Osteogenesis imperfecta, four clinical forms

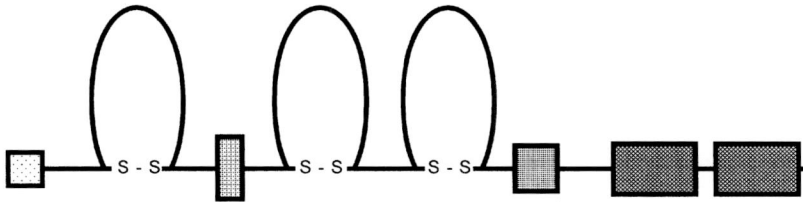

FIGURE 4. Schematic representation of the fibroblast growth factor receptor. On the **left**, the molecule starts with a signal peptide. The extracellular component is composed of three immunoglobulin-like domains (the three arches). On the **right** side of the molecule are the transmembrane domains. (Copyright, Phillippe Jeanty, reproduced with permission from http://www.TheFetus.net.)

kinase receptor called *FGFR*. These molecules contain transmembrane domain components and an extracellular component composed of three immunoglobulin-like domains (Fig. 4).

TABLE 3. MOLECULAR DEFECTS IN THE MOST COMMON CHONDRODYSPLASIAS

Gene	Disorder
Structural proteins of cartilage	
COL2A1	Achondrogenesis II
	Hypochondroplasia
	Spondyloepiphyseal dysplasia
	Spondyloepimetaphyseal dysplasia
	Kniest dysplasia
COL9A2	Multiple epiphyseal dysplasia
COL10A1	Metaphyseal dysplasia Schmit type
	Otospondylomegaepiphyseal dysplasia
Cartilage oligomeric matrix protein	Pseudoachondroplasia
	Multiple epiphyseal dysplasia
Inborn errors of cartilage metabolism	
DTST	Achondrogenesis IB
	Atelosteogenesis II
	Diastrophic dysplasia
Arylsulfatase	Chondrodysplasia punctata XR
Lysosomal enzymes	Mucopolysaccharidoses
	Mucolipidoses
Local regulators of cartilage growth	
FGFR3	Achondroplasia
	Hypochondroplasia
	Thanatophoric I and II
Parathyroid hormone–related peptide PTHr receptor	Metaphyseal dysplasia Jensen type
Systemic defect influencing cartilage development	
Peroxisomal defects	Rhizomelic chondrodysplasia punctata
Adenosine deaminase deficiency	Combined immunodeficiency
Gene identified, unknown mechanism	
SOX9[a]	Camptomelia dysplasia
EXT1[b]	Multiple exostoses 1
Gene mapped, not yet identified	
	Cleidocranial dysplasia
	Ellis-van Creveld syndrome
	Trichorhinophalangeal 1 and 2
	Pyknodysostosis
	Multiple exostoses 2 and 3

FGFR, fibroblast growth factor receptor.
[a]Gene factor transcriptions.
[b]Multiple exostoses.
Reproduced with permission from Rimoin David L. Molecular defect in chondrodysplasias. *Am J Med Genet* 1996;63:106–110.

Over the next few months and years a literal explosion of knowledge occurred thanks to the Human Genome Project and the advances of developmental biology. The loci for Pfeiffer syndrome, Apert syndrome, Crouzon disease, Jackson-Weiss syndrome, thanatophoric dysplasia, achondroplasia, hypochondroplasia, and many others have been identified.

Several other deficient proteins were subsequently discovered. Mutation in the diastrophic dysplasia sulfate transporter gene (DTDST) results in diastrophic dysplasia. Mutation in type II collagen causes the type II collagenopathies and mutations in the cartilage-oligomeric matrix protein in the type XI collagenopathies. Table 3 summarizes known molecular defects for recognized chondrodysplasias.

SONOGRAPHIC APPROACH TO SKELETAL DYSPLASIAS

Many, but certainly not all, conditions can be detected by an abnormally shortened femur length during the course of standard fetal biometry. For this reason, the sonographer is encouraged to obtain views of all four extremities including both hands and feet, when possible, as part of a standard anatomic survey. A growing number of laboratories now include measurements of the humerus length in addition to the femur length as part of standard fetal biometry. Ideally, views are also obtained of each arm, forearm, and distal leg.

Whereas detection of skeletal dysplasias is usually possible by prenatal ultrasound, an accurate specific diagnosis is more difficult. A specific diagnosis may require radiologic, pathologic, and molecular genetic examination. Nevertheless, careful assessment by prenatal ultrasound can usually suggest the correct diagnosis or a limited differential diagnosis in the majority of cases.[9] This evaluation requires a complete and thorough assessment of the fetus.

Assessment of the affected bone may provide important information about the type of skeletal dysplasia. Assessment of the severity and the type of limb shortening limits the differential diagnosis (see Table 4). The bone shape may also provide important clues. Bone curvature suggests osteogenesis imperfecta, camptomelic dysplasia, and hypophosphatasia, whereas *telephone receiver* shape suggests thanatophoric dysplasia and a *dumb-bell* appearance of the long bones is typical of metatropic dysplasia.[10] The mineralization of bones can also be assessed by its echogenicity;

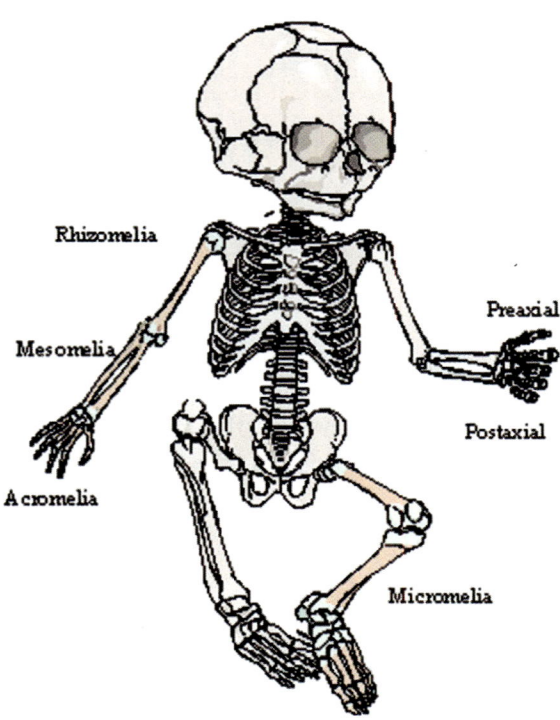

FIGURE 5. Shortening of the extremities can involve the entire limb (micromelia), the proximal segment (rhizomelia), the intermediate segment (mesomelia), or the distal segment (acromelia). Extra digits on the ulnar or fibular side are postaxial and preaxial if they are located on the radial or tibial side. (Copyright, Phillippe Jeanty, reproduced with permission from http://www.TheFetus.net.)

hypomineralization occurs in hypophosphatasia, achondrogenesis, and osteogenesis imperfecta. Detection of aplasia or hypoplasia of certain bones can also provide diagnostic information. Detection of short clavicles may be the initial sign of cleidocranial dysplasia[11] and camptomelic dysplasia is characterized by hypoplastic scapula.

Increased nuchal translucency or cystic hygroma may be the initial manifestation of a variety of skeletal dysplasias during the first trimester and early second trimester (see Chapters 19 and 20).

Type of Limb Shortening

When limb shortening is identified, it can be characterized as involving the entire limb (micromelia), the proximal segment (rhizomelia), the intermediate segment (mesomelia), or the distal segment (acromelia) (Fig. 5). This requires the comparison of the dimensions of the bones of the legs and forearm with those of the thigh and arm. A differential diagnosis can be suggested based on the type of shortening (Table 4).

Abnormalities of the Hands and Feet

Abnormalities of the hands and feet are important clues to the type of skeletal dysplasia (Table 5). *Polydactyly* refers to

TABLE 4. DIFFERENTIAL DIAGNOSIS OF SKELETAL DYSPLASIA BASED ON TYPE OF LIMB SHORTENING

Type of limb shortening	Differential diagnosis
Rhizomelia	Achondroplasia
	Atelosteogenesis
	Chondrodysplasia punctata (rhizomelic type)
	Congenital short femur
	Diastrophic dysplasia
	Thanatophoric dysplasia
Mesomelia	Acromelia
	Ellis-van Creveld syndrome
	Mesomelic dysplasia
Micromelia	Achondrogenesis
	Atelosteogenesis
	Diastrophic dysplasia
	Dyssegmental dysplasia
	Fibrochondrogenesis
	Kniest dysplasia
	Osteogenesis imperfecta (type II)
	Short rib–polydactyly syndrome (types I and III)

the presence of more than five digits. It is classified as postaxial if the extra digits are on the ulnar or fibular side and preaxial if they are located on the radial or tibial side (Fig. 6). Most commonly, the extra digit is a simple skin tag, difficult to see by ultrasound, but occasionally bones may be present, too.

TABLE 5. DIFFERENTIAL DIAGNOSIS OF SKELETAL DYSPLASIAS BASED ON ABNORMALITIES OF HANDS AND FEET

Hand and foot abnormalities	Differential diagnosis
Postaxial polydactyly	Asphyxiating thoracic dysplasia
	Chondroectodermal dysplasia (typical)
	Mesomelic dysplasia Werner syndrome type (associated with absence of thumbs)
	Otopalatodigital syndrome
	Short rib–polydactyly syndrome (type I, type III)
Preaxial polydactyly	Carpenter syndrome
	Chondroectodermal dysplasia
	Short rib–polydactyly syndrome type II
Syndactyly	Apert syndrome
	Carpenter syndrome
	Jarcho-Levin syndrome
	Mesomelic dysplasia Werner syndrome type
	Otopalatodigital syndrome (type II)
	Poland syndrome
	Roberts syndrome
	Thrombocytopenia–absent radius syndrome
Brachydactyly	Mesomelic dysplasia Robinow syndrome type
	Otopalatodigital syndrome
Hitchhiker thumb	Diastrophic dysplasia
Clubfeet deformity	Diastrophic dysplasia
	Kniest dysplasia
	Osteogenesis imperfecta
	Spondyloepiphyseal dysplasia congenita

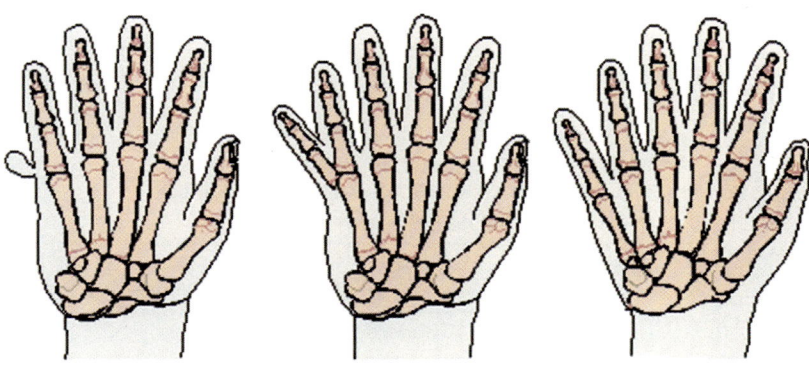

FIGURE 6. *Polydactyly* refers to the presence of extra digits. Most commonly, the extra digit is a simple skin tag, difficult to see by ultrasound, but occasionally bones or a completely duplicated but nonfunctional digit may be present, too. In this illustration, postaxial polydactylies have been represented. (Copyright, Phillippe Jeanty, reproduced with permission from http://www.TheFetus.net.)

Syndactyly refers to soft tissue or bony fusion of adjacent digits and is difficult to recognize in the less-severe forms (Fig. 7).

Clinodactyly consists of deviation of a finger(s). It may result from an abnormal middle fifth phalanx such as in brachymesophalangia (Fig. 8).

Clubbing of the hand is very suggestive of *radial ray* anomalies. Radial ray anomalies (Fig. 9) range from abnormal thumbs (sometimes triphalangeal as in Holt-Oram syndrome) to hypoplasia or absence of the thumb and sometimes absence of the radius or even the radius and the hand. The three most likely diagnoses include Holt-Oram syndrome, thrombocytopenia–absent radius syndrome, and trisomy 18.

The foot length is very close to the femoral length and can be used to compare the two.[12,13] At the level of the feet, a rockerbottom foot (abnormal vertical position of the talus and calcaneus) or a clubfoot should also be sought (Fig. 10).

Abnormalities of the Head and Face

Abnormalities of the head and face are also important in identifying the type of skeletal dysplasia (Table 6). At the level of the head, deviations from the normal shape of the head should be observed. These include brachycephaly, scaphocephaly, and the craniosynostoses (Figs. 11 and 12).

Brachycephaly occurs in many acrocephalopolysyndactylies. Scaphocephaly is more common and is associated with premature rupture of the membranes, growth restriction, *in utero* crowding, and acromesomelic dysplasia.

Craniosynostoses result from premature fusions of the suture. The expanding brain deforms the adjacent bones resulting in specific anomalies. One of the common ones is the cloverleaf shape (or kleeblattschädel) that occurs in thanatophoric dysplasia type II. Other conditions with craniosynostosis are Carpenter syndrome, hypophosphatasia, acrocephalosyndactyly, Crouzon disease, Apert syndrome, acrodysostosis, trimethadione sequence, and many others.

Frontal bossing is a deformity of the forehead that may be associated with achondroplasia and the craniosynostosis but also may be due to increased intracranial size with large hydrocephalus. The diagnosis is often suspected in a section of the lips of the fetus (the section used to assess the presence of a cleft lip) and made or confirmed in a sagittal facial

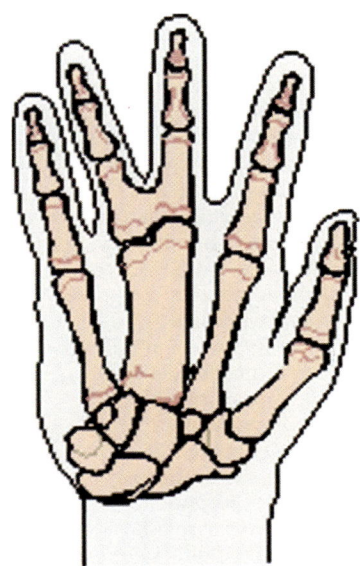

FIGURE 7. Bony syndactyly. (Copyright, Phillippe Jeanty, reproduced with permission from http://www.TheFetus.net.)

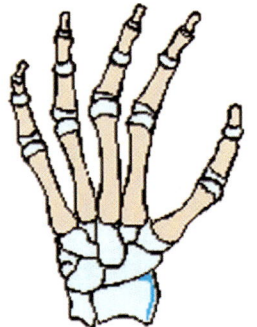 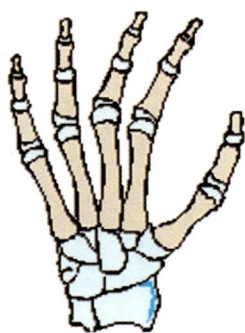

A,B

FIGURE 8. A: An abnormal middle fifth phalanx can be responsible for clinodactyly. **B:** Normal condition. (Copyright, Phillippe Jeanty, reproduced with permission from http://www.TheFetus.net.)

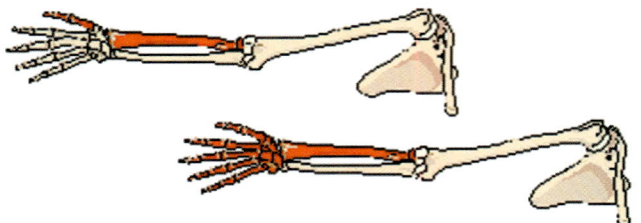

FIGURE 9. Radial ray anomalies range from abnormal thumbs to hypoplasia or absence of the thumb and sometimes absence of the radius, or even the radius and the hand. (Copyright, Phillippe Jeanty, reproduced with permission from http://www.TheFetus.net.)

section. At the same time, a low nasal bridge may be present (Fig. 13).

Wormian bones (Fig. 14) are small bones in the fontanels, and they may be associated with cleidocranial dysplasia, osteogenesis imperfecta, trisomy 21, hypothyroidism, pyknodysostosis, and progeria.

While looking at the head, note the distance between the eyes. A decreased distance (hypotelorism) or increased distance (hypertelorism) may also be present in skeletal dysplasias (Fig. 15).

A smaller jaw (micrognathia, which affected Henri de Toulouse-Lautrec) should also be sought at this time of the examination (Fig. 16).[14]

Abnormalities of the Thorax

At the level of the chest, look for abnormal rib size resulting in a chest that is too narrow. This is a typical finding of most of the lethal skeletal dysplasias (Table 7). These conditions are not lethal because the bones are abnormal, but because the ribs are too short and thus prevent the normal growth of the lungs. The resulting pulmonary hypoplasia is lethal. In practice one does not need to measure the chest or the ribs. It is sufficient to know that the chest diameter should be 80% to 100% of the abdominal diameter (Fig. 17). Lethal skeletal dysplasias often have a chest size around 50%, and thus the anomaly is not subtle.

Abnormalities of the Spine

The most common spinal abnormality seen in skeletal dysplasias is platyspondyly, which consists of flattening of the

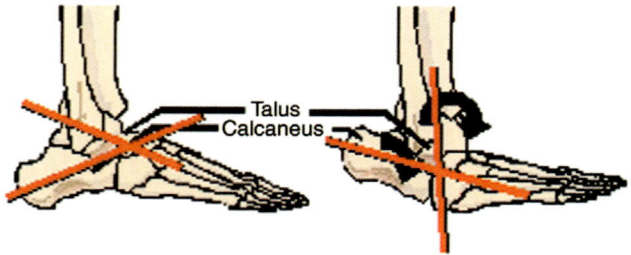

FIGURE 10. An abnormal vertical position of the talus and calcaneus causes a rockerbottom foot. (Copyright, Phillippe Jeanty, reproduced with permission from http://www.TheFetus.net.)

vertebrae. This sign is typical of thanatophoric dysplasia. Achondroplasia shows absence of normal widening of the lumbar spine. Achondrogenesis type I is characterized

TABLE 6. DIFFERENTIAL DIAGNOSIS OF SKELETAL DYSPLASIAS BASED ON HEAD AND FACE ABNORMALITIES

Head and face deformities	Differential diagnosis
Large head	Achondrogenesis
	Achondroplasia
	Camptomelic syndrome
	Cleidocranial dysplasia
	Hypophosphatasia
	Osteogenesis imperfecta
	Otopalatodigital syndrome
	Mesomelic dysplasia Robinow syndrome type
	Short rib–polydactyly syndrome (type III)
	Thanatophoric dysplasia
Cloverleaf skull	Thanatophoric dysplasia (type II)
	Camptomelic syndrome (unusual)
Other cranio-synostoses	Acrocephalosyndactyly
	Acrodysostosis
	Antley-Bixler syndrome
	Apert syndrome
	Carpenter syndrome
	Hypophosphatasia
Cataracts	Chondrodysplasia punctata
Cleft palate	Asphyxiating thoracic dysplasia
	Camptomelic syndrome
	Chondroectodermal dysplasia
	Diastrophic dysplasia
	Dyssegmental dysplasia
	Jarcho-Levin syndrome
	Kniest dysplasia
	Metatropic dysplasia
	Otopalatodigital syndrome (type II)
	Roberts syndrome
	Short rib–polydactyly syndrome (type II)
	Spondyloepiphyseal syndrome
Micrognathia	Achondrogenesis
	Arthrogryposis multiplex congenita
	Atelosteogenesis
	Camptomelic dysplasia
	Diastrophic dysplasia
	Mesomelic dysplasia
	Nager acrofacial dysostosis
	Oromandibular limb hypogenesis
	Otopalatodigital syndrome
Hypertelorism	Achondroplasia
	Apert syndrome
	Arthrogryposis multiplex congenita
	Camptomelic dysplasia
	Cleidocranial dysplasia
	Coffin syndrome
	Holt-Oram syndrome
	Klippel-Feil syndrome
	Larsen syndrome
	Mesomelic dysplasia
	Otopalatodigital syndrome
	Roberts syndrome
	Sprengel deformity

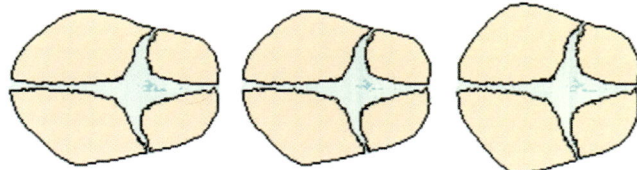

A–C

FIGURE 11. Normal appearance of the skull in cross-section **(B)** should be compared to scaphocephaly (the lateral flattening, **A**) and brachycephaly (the anteroposterior shortening, **C**). (Copyright, Phillippe Jeanty, reproduced with permission from http://www.TheFetus.net.)

radiographically by poor ossification of the spine. Spondyloepiphyseal dysplasia shows multiple vertebral anomalies.

The prenatal diagnosis of congenital hemivertebra has also been reported.[15] Kyphosis and scoliosis can also be identified *in utero*.

BIOMETRY IN THE DIAGNOSIS OF BONE DYSPLASIAS

Long bone biometry has been used extensively in the prediction of gestational age. Nomograms available for this purpose use the long bone as the independent variable and the estimated fetal age as the dependent variable. However, the type of nomogram required to assess the normality of bone dimensions uses the gestational age as the independent variable and the long bone as the dependent variable. For the proper use of these nomograms, the clinician must accurately know the gestational age of the fetus. Therefore, patients at risk for skeletal dysplasias should be advised to seek prenatal care at an early gestational age to assess all clinical estimators of gestational age. Table 8 presents nomograms for the assessment of limb biometry for the upper and lower extremities and the clavicle.

For those patients presenting with uncertain gestational age, comparisons between limb dimensions and the head perimeter can be used. The head perimeter has the advantage of being shape independent. A limitation of this approach is that it assumes that the cranium is not involved in the dysplastic process, and this may not be the case in some skeletal

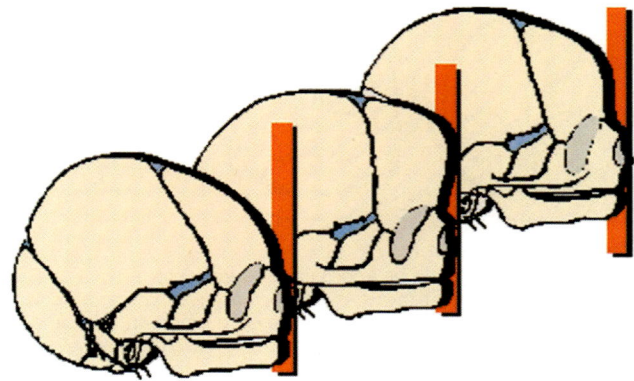

FIGURE 13. The section used to assess the presence of a cleft lip is just in front of the forehead **(right)**. In frontal bossing **(middle)** the forehead appears in the section, and in frontal slanting **(left)** it is further away. (Copyright, Phillippe Jeanty, reproduced with permission from http://www.TheFetus.net.)

dysplasias. The table uses the fifth percentile, and thus a fair number of normal fetuses fall outside these boundaries.

Figure 18[16] illustrates the femoral lengths of several fetuses with skeletal dysplasias. The three upper percentiles are the ninety-fifth, fiftieth, and fifth percentiles and the three lower red lines are the three-fourths, one-half, and one-fourth of the mean, respectively, from top to bottom. From this chart it is clear that most short-limb skeletal dysplasias fall significantly below the fifth percentile. The only exceptions are hypochondroplasia and achondroplasia.

Figure 19[16] is useful in suggesting what might the differential diagnosis be according to femur lengths compared with gestational age. Although this table is based on one of the largest prenatal series, be aware that many skeletal dysplasias are not represented. Simply place a measurement in the graph and see what are the differential diagnoses in that slice. The percentages indicate the percent of the disorder in that category. Of course, when a differential diagnosis is suggested, one should search for findings to confirm or infirm it.

Clinical Presentation

The assessment of skeletal dysplasias occurs either because of a familial history or because of the incidental discovery

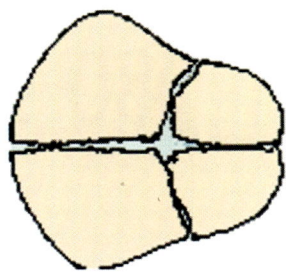

FIGURE 12. Craniosynostosis results from premature fusions of the suture. (Copyright, Phillippe Jeanty, reproduced with permission from http://www.TheFetus.net.)

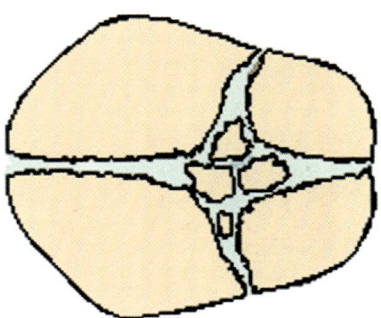

FIGURE 14. Wormian bones are small bones in the fontanels. (Copyright, Phillippe Jeanty, reproduced with permission from http://www.TheFetus.net.)

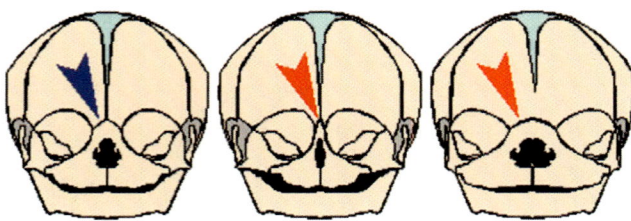

FIGURE 15. The normal distance between the eyes in a cross section of the eyes should be approximately equal to the ocular diameter. Thus, the rule of thirds: the binocular distance can be divided in almost three equal thirds, with one each being an orbit and the third being the distance between the eyes. A decrease of the interocular distance is hypotelorism, whereas an increased distance represents hypertelorism. (Copyright, Phillippe Jeanty, reproduced with permission from http://www.TheFetus.net.)

of an abnormally shaped or too short bone during an examination. When a familial history is present, the task is often limited to assessing whether the same findings are present.

In practice one should look at all long bones and measure all that are not obviously within normal limits.

After the Delivery

Despite all efforts to establish an accurate prenatal diagnosis, a careful study of the newborn is required in all instances. The evaluation should include a detailed physical examination performed by a geneticist or an individual with experience in the field of skeletal dysplasias and radiograms of the skeleton. The latter should include anterior, posterior, lateral, and Towne's views of the skull and anteroposterior views of the spine and extremities, with separate films of hands and feet. Examination of the skeletal radiographs permits precise diagnoses in the overwhelming majority of cases, since the classification of skeletal dysplasias is largely based on radiographic findings. In lethal skeletal dysplasias, histologic examination of the chondroosseous tissue should be included, as this information may help reach a specific diagnosis. Chromosomal studies should be included, as there is a specific group of constitutional bone disorders associated with cytogenetic abnormalities. Biochemical studies are helpful in rare instances (e.g., hypophosphatasia). DNA restrictions and enzymatic activity assays should be considered in

TABLE 7. DIFFERENTIAL DIAGNOSIS OF SKELETAL DYSPLASIAS BASED ON SMALL THORAX

Achondrogenesis
Asphyxiating thoracic dysplasia (Jeune syndrome)
Atelosteogenesis
Camptomelic dysplasia
Chondroectodermal dysplasia (Ellis-van Creveld syndrome)
Cleidocranial dysostosis syndrome
Fibrochondrogenesis
Hypophosphatasia
Jarcho-Levin syndrome
Kniest dysplasia
Melnick-Needles syndrome (osteodysplasty)
Metatropic dysplasia
Osteogenesis imperfecta (type II)
Otopalatodigital syndrome (type II)
Pena-Shokeir syndrome
Short rib–polydactyly syndrome (types I and II)
Thanatophoric dysplasia

those cases in which the phenotype suggests a metabolic disorder such as a mucopolysaccharidosis.

COMMON SKELETAL DYSPLASIAS

A growing number of skeletal dysplasias have been recognized *in utero*. A complete account of each disorder is beyond the scope of this chapter, and the reader is referred to texts on the subject for further details. A few of the most common disorders relevant to prenatal diagnosis are discussed here. Other specific syndromes are discussed in Chapter 5.

Achondrogenesis

Synonyms for achondrogenesis are lethal achondrogenesis, Houston-Harris type (type IA); lethal achondrogenesis, Parenti-Fraccaro type (type IB); and lethal achondrogenesis-hypochondrogenesis, Langer-Saldino type (type II), also

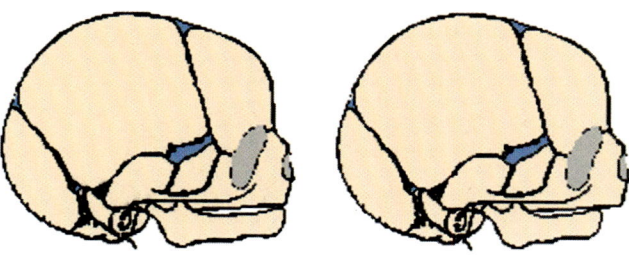

FIGURE 16. Micrognathia is a smaller-than-normal mandible and is associated with many conditions. (Copyright, Phillippe Jeanty, reproduced with permission from http://www.TheFetus.net.)

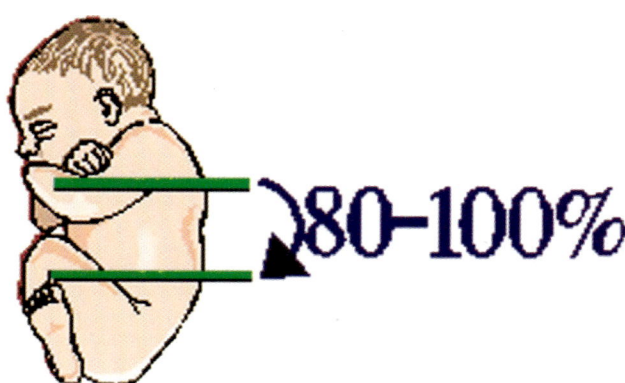

FIGURE 17. The chest diameter should be between 80% to 100% of the abdominal diameter. (Copyright, Phillippe Jeanty, reproduced with permission from http://www.TheFetus.net.)

TABLE 8. NOMOGRAMS FOR NORMAL LIMB BIOMETRY OF THE UPPER AND LOWER EXTREMITIES AND THE CLAVICLE

Age	Femur			Humerus			Tibia			Fibula			Ulna			Radius			Clavicle		
	5th	50th	95th	5th	50th	95th	5th	50th	95th	5th	50th	95th	5th	50th	95th	5th	50th	95th	5th	50th	95th
12	4	9	14	5	9	13	3	7	11	—	5	—	—	8	—	—	7	—	8	13	18
13	7	12	17	9	13	17	6	10	14	—	8	—	—	11	—	—	10	—	10	15	20
14	10	15	20	12	16	20	9	13	17	—	11	17	9	13	17	—	13	—	11	16	21
15	14	19	24	14	18	22	12	16	20	—	14	—	12	16	20	6	15	24	12	17	22
16	17	22	27	17	21	25	15	19	23	—	17	—	15	19	23	9	18	27	13	18	23
17	20	25	30	20	24	28	18	22	26	8	19	30	17	21	25	11	20	29	14	19	24
18	23	28	33	23	27	31	20	24	28	11	22	33	20	24	28	13	22	31	15	20	25
19	26	31	36	25	29	33	23	27	31	13	24	35	22	26	30	15	24	33	16	21	26
20	28	33	38	28	32	36	25	29	33	16	27	38	25	29	33	18	27	36	17	22	27
21	31	36	41	30	34	38	28	32	36	18	29	40	27	31	35	20	29	38	18	23	28
22	34	39	44	32	36	40	30	34	38	20	31	42	29	33	37	22	31	40	20	25	30
23	36	41	46	34	38	42	32	36	40	22	33	44	31	35	39	23	32	41	21	26	31
24	39	44	49	37	41	45	35	39	43	24	35	46	33	37	41	25	34	43	22	27	32
25	41	46	51	39	43	47	37	41	45	26	37	48	35	39	43	27	36	45	23	28	33
26	44	49	54	41	45	49	39	43	47	28	39	50	37	41	45	28	37	46	24	29	34
27	46	51	56	42	46	50	41	45	49	30	41	52	39	43	47	30	39	48	25	30	35
28	48	53	58	44	48	52	43	47	51	32	43	54	40	44	48	31	40	49	26	31	36
29	51	56	61	46	50	54	45	49	53	34	45	56	42	46	50	33	42	51	27	32	37
30	53	58	63	48	52	56	47	51	55	36	47	58	43	47	51	34	43	52	29	34	39
31	55	60	65	49	53	57	48	52	56	37	48	59	45	49	53	35	44	53	30	35	40
32	57	62	67	51	55	59	50	54	58	39	50	61	46	50	54	36	45	54	31	36	41
33	59	64	69	52	56	60	52	56	60	40	51	62	48	52	56	37	46	55	32	37	42
34	60	65	70	53	57	61	53	57	61	41	52	63	49	53	57	38	47	56	33	38	43
35	62	67	72	54	58	62	55	59	63	43	54	65	50	54	58	39	48	57	34	39	44
36	64	69	74	56	60	64	56	60	64	44	55	66	51	55	59	39	48	57	35	40	45
37	66	71	76	57	61	65	57	61	65	45	56	67	52	56	60	40	49	58	36	41	46
38	67	72	77	57	61	65	58	62	66	46	57	68	53	57	61	40	49	58	37	42	47
39	69	74	79	58	62	66	60	64	68	47	58	69	53	57	61	41	50	59	39	44	49
40	70	75	80	59	63	67	61	65	69	48	59	70	54	58	62	41	50	59	40	45	50

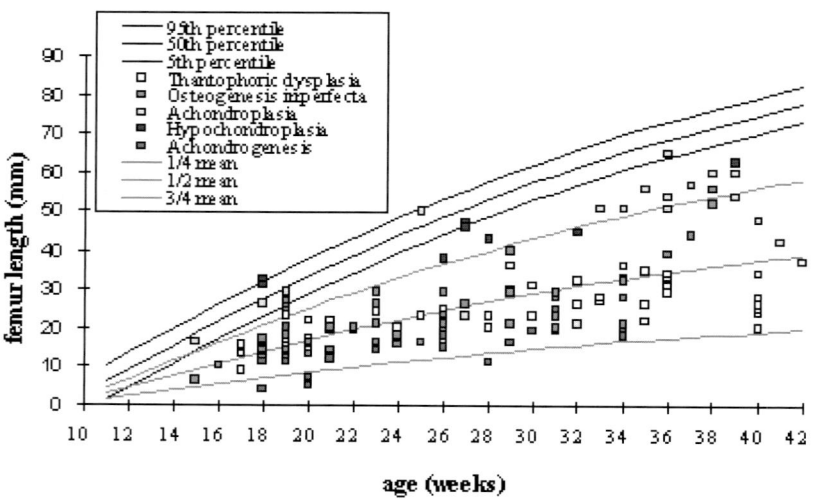

FIGURE 18. Scatter plot of femur length measurements compared with gestational age for five types of skeletal dysplasia: thanatophoric dysplasia, osteogenesis imperfecta, achondroplasia, hypochondroplasia, and achondrogenesis. (Reproduced with permission from Goncalves L, Jeanty P. Fetal biometry of skeletal dysplasias: a multicentric study. *J Ultrasound Med* 1994;13:977–985.)

referred to as chondrogenesis imperfecta, achondrogenesis-hypochondrogenesis, type II.[17]

Achondrogenesis (Figs. 20 through 22) has been categorized into two primary types: types I and II. The less common types III and IV have been questioned, with type III probably representing type II and type IV probably representing hypochondrogenesis.

Incidence

Achondrogenesis is rare, with probably less than 100 cases reported.

Genetic Defect

The genetic defect of achondrogenesis type IA is unknown. Type IB is associated with mutation in the gene for DTDST gene on the long arm (locus 32-33) of chromosome 5.[18–20] Achondrogenesis type II is caused by a new mutation in the type II collagen gene (COL2A1 gene) on chromosome 12.[21] This defect is related to hypochondroplasia, spondyloepiphyseal dysplasia, and the Kniest-Stickler syndrome.[22] These may be allelic variants, with hypochondrogenesis[23] related to achondrogenesis as hypochondroplasia is related to achondroplasia.

Pathologic and Clinical Features

Achondrogenesis type I is a severe chondrodystrophy characterized radiographically by poor ossification of the spine (Fig. 20) and pelvis bones, which results in stillbirth or early death.[24–27]

Achondrogenesis type II presents with the same findings, but the mineralization deficit is less severe and the long bones are less short.

Diagnosis

Ultrasound

The ultrasound manifestation includes very short limbs (Fig. 20) and short thin ribs that may have fractures. The short ribs are responsible for the lethal pulmonary hypoplasia and the polyhydramnios from esophageal compression. The abnormal mineralization may or may not be manifested sonographically as bones that are either very echopenic or in which both cortical margins can be imaged (Fig. 20B). Normally, only the proximal cortical side is imaged, and the distal side is shadowed by the proximal side.

Laboratory

The diagnosis of type IA can be made by chorionic villus sampling in at-risk couples.

Differential Diagnosis

Osteogenesis imperfecta (type II and occasionally IIIC) and hypophosphatasia also present with demineralization but the limb shortening is not usually as severe.

Prognosis and Management

Achondrogenesis is lethal. Termination of pregnancy can be offered before viability. Standard prenatal care is not altered when continuation of the pregnancy is opted. Confirmation of diagnosis after birth is important for genetic counseling.

Recurrence Risk

Achondrogenesis is autosomal recessive (IB) and dominant (II). Because these are lethal disorders, type II autosomal dominant involves a new mutation. It, therefore, carries a much lower recurrence risk than the 25% risk of type IB.

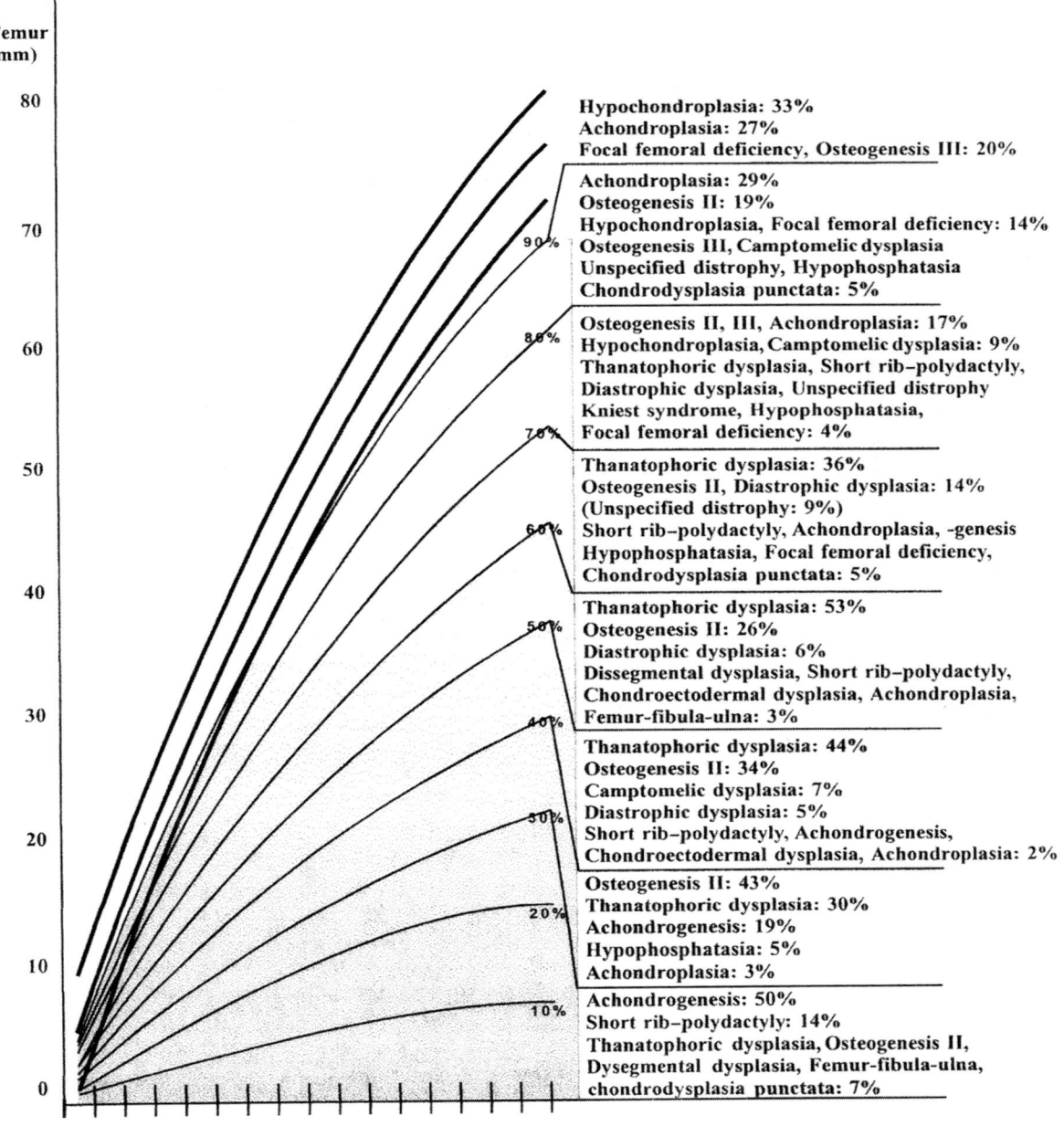

FIGURE 19. Differential diagnosis of selected skeletal dysplasias based on the degree of femur length shortening. The percentages indicate the percent of the disorder in that category. (Reproduced with permission from Goncalves L, Jeanty P. Fetal biometry of skeletal dysplasias: a multicentric study. *J Ultrasound Med* 1994;13:977–985.)

Achondroplasia

There are no synonyms for achondroplasia. Achondroplasia includes rhizomelic micromelia associated with frontal bossing and low nasal bridge.[17]

Incidence

Achondroplasia is common: 0.5 to 1.5 out of 10,000.

Genetic Defect

Achondroplasia results from a mutation in the FGFR3 gene, which is located on the short arm of chromosome 4 at the 16.3 locus.[28,29] Bellus has demonstrated that the anomaly was due to a glycine to arginine substitution at codon 380.[30] These papers are landmarks in the knowledge about skeletal dysplasias. Before these papers, skeletal dysplasias were almost strictly classified by radiologic criteria. These papers marked the beginning of an

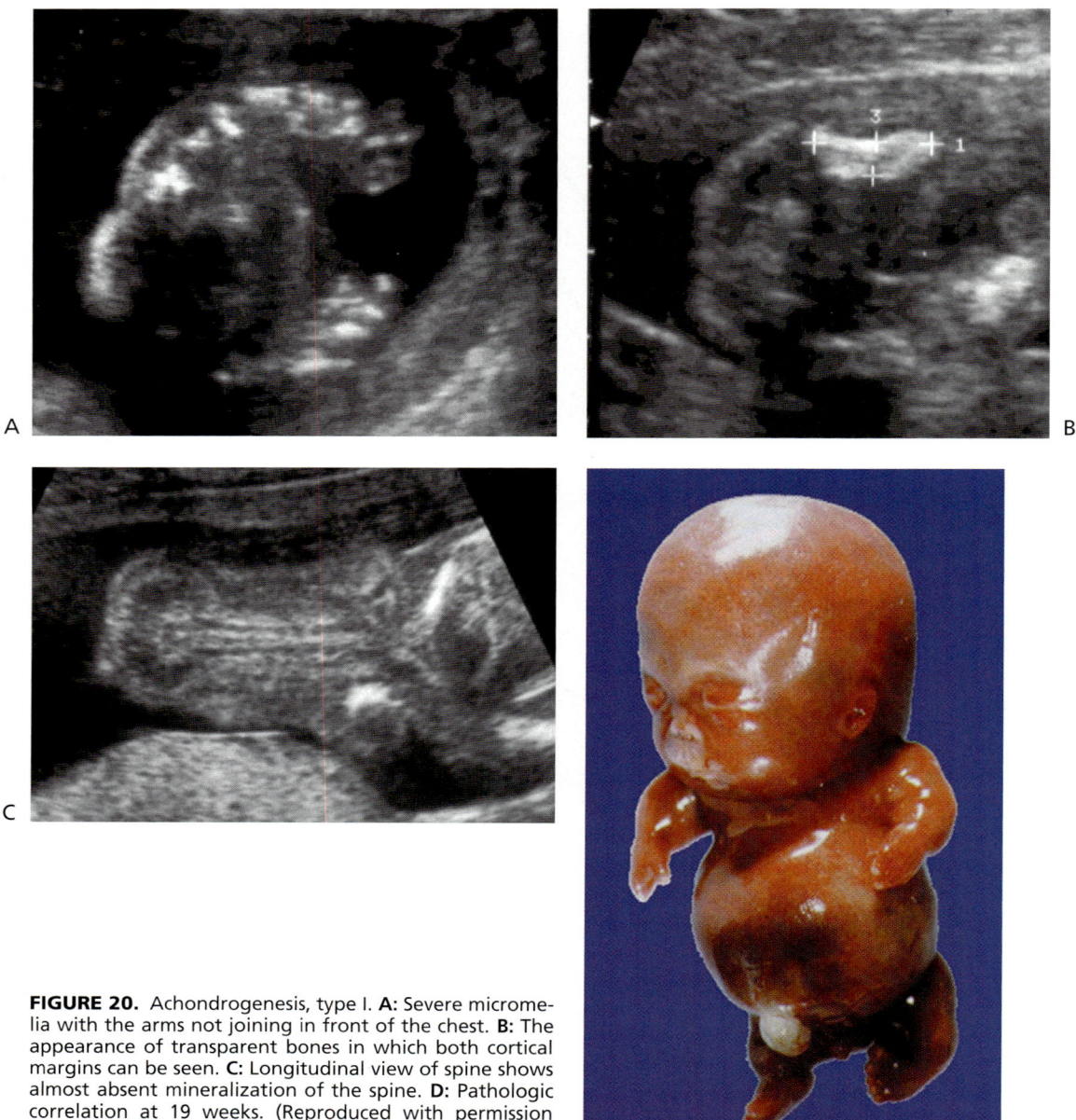

FIGURE 20. Achondrogenesis, type I. **A:** Severe micromelia with the arms not joining in front of the chest. **B:** The appearance of transparent bones in which both cortical margins can be seen. **C:** Longitudinal view of spine shows almost absent mineralization of the spine. **D:** Pathologic correlation at 19 weeks. (Reproduced with permission from http://TheFetus.com.)

intense and successful search for gene mapping of skeletal dysplasia, many of which where subsequently recognized to result from alterations of the fibroblast growth factors (I through III).

Pathologic and Clinical Features

Achondroplasia involves defective cartilaginous molding of the bone precursor.

Diagnosis

The micromelia is the most obvious finding with limbs shorter than the fifth percentile after 20 weeks and below the first percentile after approximately 27 weeks (Fig. 23). The frontal bossing and depressed nasal bridge can also be recognized (Fig. 24). Occasionally, more subtle anomalies such as the trident hand (i.e., an increased interspace between the third and fourth digit) can be recognized (Fig. 25), or the lack of widening of the lumbar canal can also be detected (Fig. 26). Three-dimensional ultrasound may be useful in showing some of these features.[31]

Molecular genetic studies can confirm the diagnosis of achondroplasia. In one case, analysis was performed of fetal DNA from maternal plasma using polymerase chain reaction.[32]

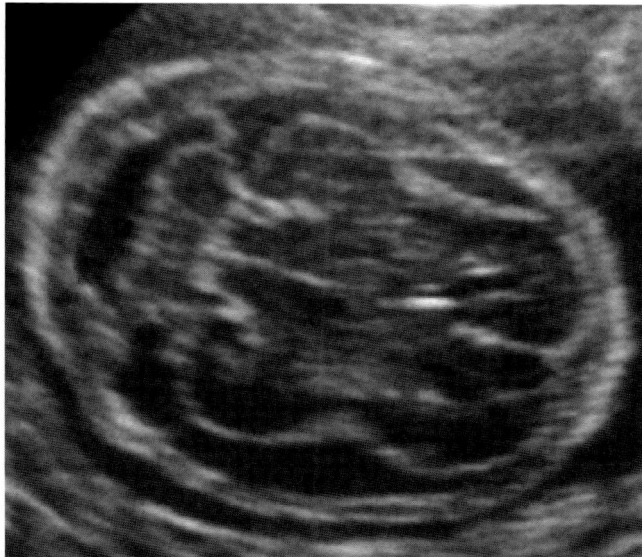

FIGURE 21. Achondrogenesis. Hypomineralization of calvaria results in soft skull (caput membranaceum) and unusually clear visualization of the brain. (Reproduced with permission from http://TheFetus.com.)

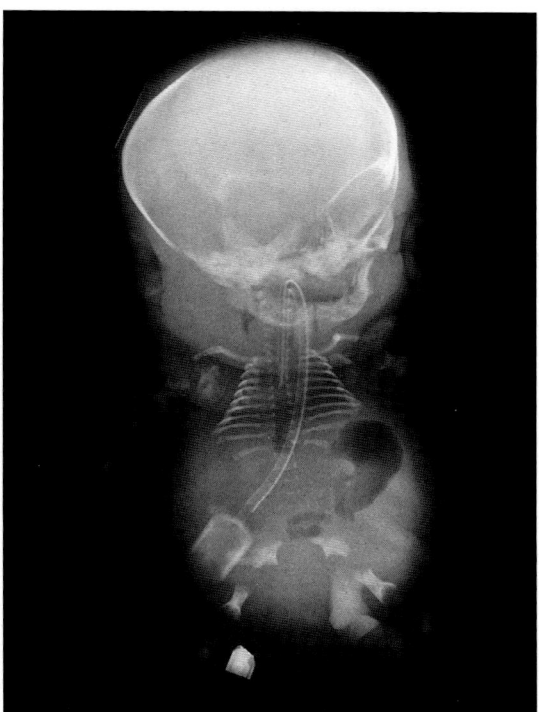

FIGURE 22. Postnatal radiograph showing absent mineralization of spine with achondrogenesis, type II. (Courtesy of Beverly Spirt, MD.)

Differential Diagnosis

The differential diagnosis is with multiple conditions such as

- Thanatophoric dysplasia (narrower chest, platyspondyly, more severe micromelia, no trident hand, more severe polyhydramnios).
- Achondrogenesis (very poor mineralization, with lack of echogenicity of the bones; more severe micromelia; more severe polyhydramnios).
- Osteogenesis imperfecta type II (poor mineralization, in which often the proximal aspect of the brain is well seen through the *transparent* skull; variable micromelia; sometimes visible bone angulations from fractures; bell-shaped chest).
- Diastrophic dysplasias in which the micromelia is associated with joint contractures and, in particular, abnormal finger and toes position.
- Intrauterine growth restriction may present primarily with limb shortening, and it may be difficult to distinguish it from achondroplasia by ultrasound alone initially.
- Hypochondroplasia is a relatively common, milder form of achondroplasia, which varies within and between families. An accurate prenatal ultrasonographic diagnosis is rare.

Prognosis and Management

Children with achondroplasia have normal intellectual achievements. The major problems are orthopedic problems (narrow spinal canal and foramen magnum). There is a vibrant support group (The Little People of America[33]) that is very active in resolving the problems of affected indi-

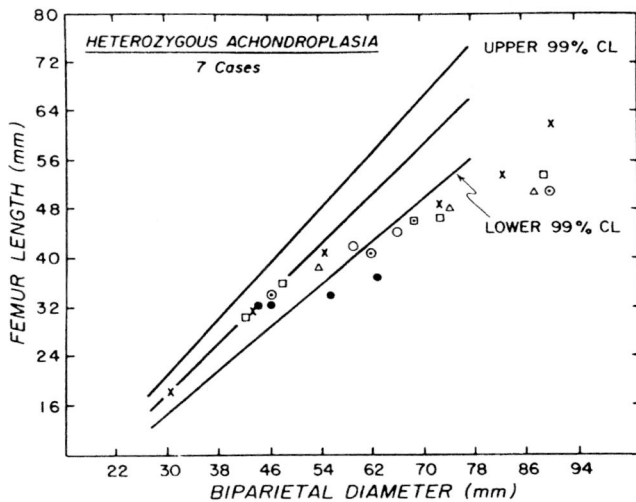

FIGURE 23. Femur length versus biparietal diameter in seven cases of recurrent heterozygous achondroplasia (symbols on graph indicate individual cases). Progressive shortening of femur length occurs during the second and third trimesters. The femur length falls below the fifth percentile after 20 weeks and below the first percentile at approximately 27 weeks. (Reproduced with permission from Kurtz AB, Filly RA, Wapner RJ, et al. In utero analysis of heterozygous achondroplasia: variable time of onset as detected by femur length measurements. *J Ultrasound Med* 1986;5:137–140.)

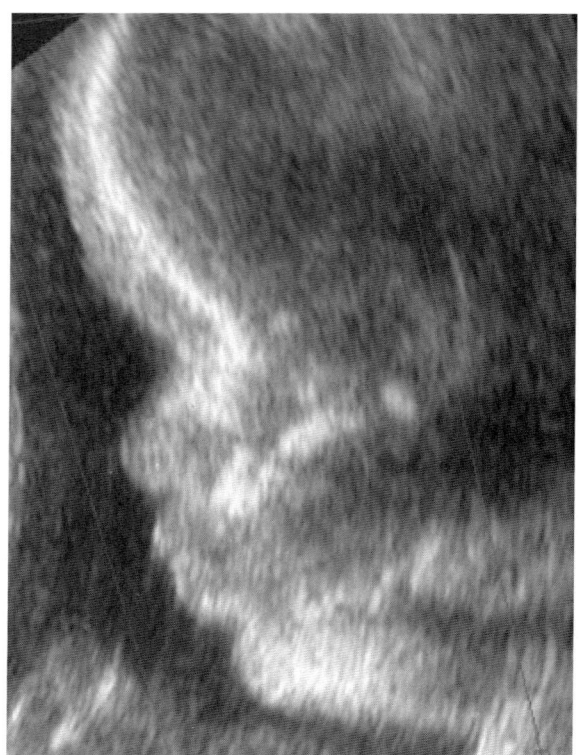

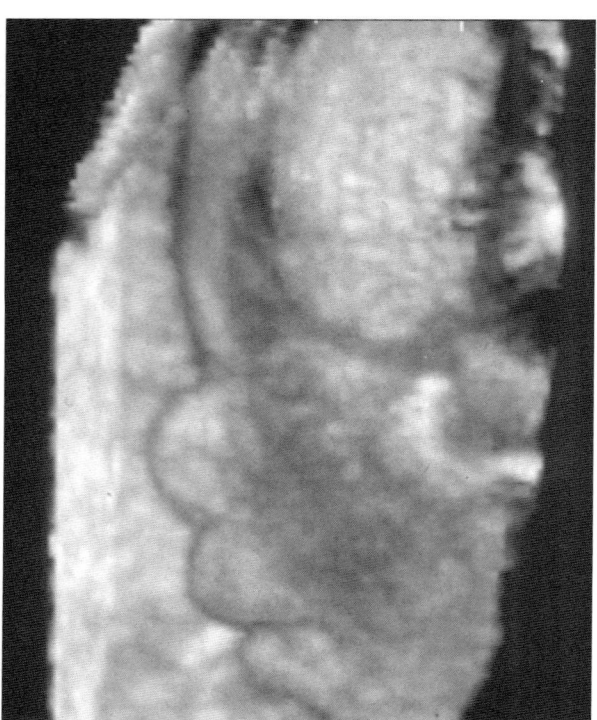

A

B

FIGURE 24. Achondroplasia. **A:** Facial profile at 32 weeks in fetus with rhizomelic limb shortening shows frontal bossing. **B:** Three-dimensional image of another achondroplasia case. (Part **B** courtesy of Beryl Benacerraf, MD, Boston, MA.)

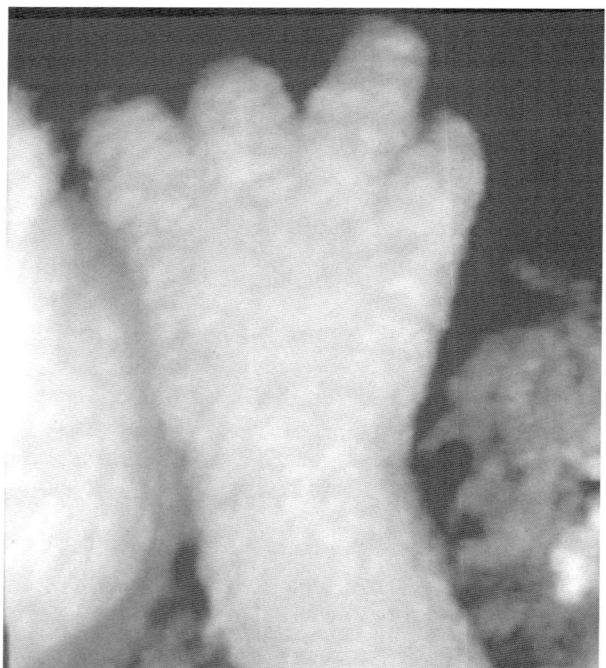

viduals. Although termination of pregnancy can be offered before viability, a majority of these children adapt well in society and lead productive lives.

Recurrence Risk

Achondroplasia is an autosomal dominant skeletal dysplasia caused by a defect in the short arm of chromosome 4.

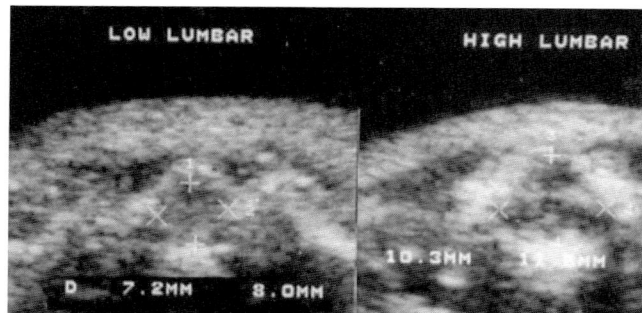

A,B

FIGURE 25. Achondroplasia. Three-dimensional ultrasound shows trident hand with widening between third and fourth digits. (Courtesy of Dru Carlson, MD, Los Angeles, CA.)

FIGURE 26. Lack of widening of the spinal canal with achondroplasia. Transverse views of the low lumbar spine **(A)** measures 8 mm in transverse dimension, whereas the high lumbar spine **(B)** measures 11 mm. This is the reverse of the normal relationship. (Copyright, Phillippe Jeanty, reproduced with permission from http://www.TheFetus.net.)

Acrofacial Dysostosis Syndromes

See Nager Syndrome in Chapter 5.[34]

Acromesomelic Dysplasia

There are no synonyms for acromesomelic dysplasia.[35] Acromesomelic dysplasia is a nonlethal short stature and short limbs dysplasia that, as implied by the name, affects the forearms, hands, and feet. The radius is bowed. The wrist bones and phalanges are particularly short and square.[36–39]

Incidence

Acromesomelic dysplasia is rare.

Genetic Defect

Acromesomelic dysplasia is caused by mutation in cartilage-derived morphogenetic protein-1 (CDMP-1) on chromosome 20. The severe form of acromesomelic dysplasia is the Hunter-Thompson type (AMDH),[40] which is caused by a different CDMP.[41,42]

Diagnosis

The diagnosis is suggested by the finding for abnormal forearms and lower legs, and abnormal hands and feet. The rest of the skeleton is not affected.

Differential Diagnosis

Differential diagnoses include mesomelic dwarfism; Grebe chondrodysplasia (only in a specific group of patients from a certain region of Brazil); and Nager syndrome (but these have micrognathia).

Prognosis and Management

Intellectual development has been reported as being normal, and the orthopedic handicap is the major concern in these children.[38,43] Confirmation of diagnosis after birth is important for genetic counseling.

Recurrence Risk

Acromesomelic dysplasia is autosomal recessive.[44]

Amelia

A synonym for amelia is limb reduction abnormality.[45]

Amelia involves the absence of one or more limbs. Amelia is the complete absence of the skeletal parts of the upper or lower limbs with no bony structure distal to the defect. Total amelia affects all four limbs.[46] This malformation generally is a random event, but is occasionally seen in specific syndromes associated with other congenital anomalies.[46,47]

Incidence

Amelia occurs in 0.04 to 0.15 per 10,000 births.[46]

Embryology and Pathogenesis

Amelia results from the arrest of formation of the primordium in the very early stages of embryo development (before the eighth week of gestation).[46] Failure of formation of the limb primordia during early embryogenesis may be secondary to vascular, mechanical, or teratogenic exposure,[48,49] with complete absence of one or more limbs occurring before the eighth week of gestation.[46] Although the teratogenic potential of thalidomide has been well documented, the spontaneous occurrence of amelia and limb reduction defects in the general population is rare.[2] Most cases have no specific etiology, but some are seen in association with genetically transmitted disorders, such as Roberts syndrome, and in families.

Diagnosis

Ultrasound shows gross absence of the fetal limbs (Fig. 27).[50] Multiple organ system defects have been associated with amelia, including cardiovascular, gastrointestinal, urogenital, skeletal, neural tube, and respiratory.[46,47]

Differential Diagnosis

Differential diagnoses include other limb reduction defects and sirenomelia.

Prognosis and Management

The prognosis is dependent on the presence or absence of other associated anomalies. Infant death is reported to occur in up to 61% of cases complicated by amelia.[46] Cesarean delivery should be performed only for obstetric indications.

Recurrence Risk

The recurrence risk for amelia is not increased.

Apert Syndrome

See Apert Syndrome in Chapter 5.

Arthrogryposis Multiplex Congenita

Synonyms for arthrogryposis multiplex congenita include congenital contractures, fetal akinesia sequence, and Pena-

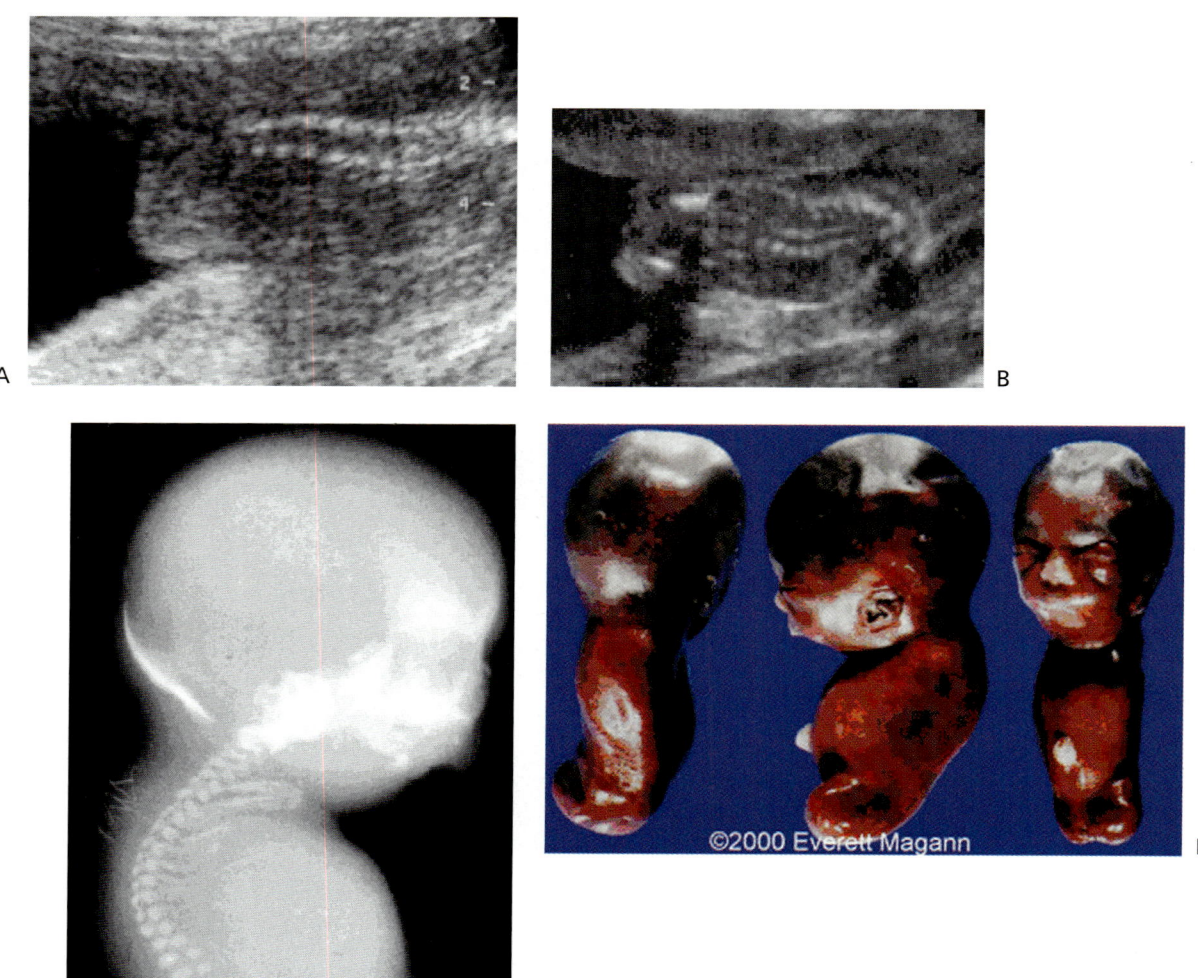

FIGURE 27. Amelia. **A:** Longitudinal scan of the fetal trunk shows absence of extremities. **B:** Longitudinal scan shows scoliosis of the spine. **C:** Postmortem radiograph. **D:** Posterior, lateral, and anterior views of the fetus at postmortem examination.

Shokeir syndrome.[51] This heterogeneous set of conditions shares limitation of movements and joint ankylosis as main findings (Fig. 28). See also Arthrogryposis/Akinesia Sequence in Chapter 5.

Incidence

The incidence for arthrogryposis multiplex congenita is 1 to 3 per 10,000 births.

Genetic Anomalies

Several anomalies have been linked to the following site: 5q35, 9p21-q21, 11p15.5.

Pathogenesis

Arthrogryposis results from decreased *in utero* motion, either from neural,[52] muscular, connective tissue, or infectious origin.

Diagnosis

Although the anomalies are obvious when recognized and in particular when the baby is born, the prenatal diagnosis may be challenging when fluid is decreased and the abnormal limb position appears attributable to the oligohydramnios. Some forms are associated with polyhydramnios, and then the abnormal limb position [knocked knee (Fig. 29), genu

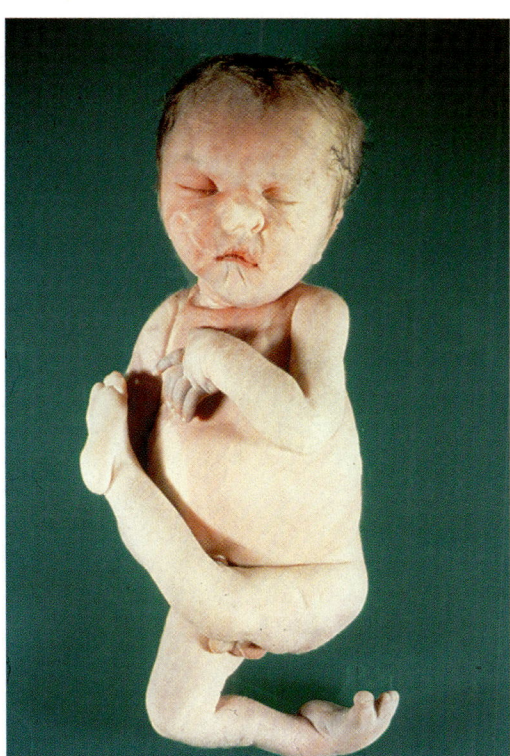

FIGURE 28. Newborn with arthrogryposis multiplex congenita. Note the pronounced anomalies of the limbs that are very rigid. Also note the linear fingers with lack of visible flexion joints. The newborn died of respiratory failure.

recurvatum, clubfeet and hand] makes the diagnosis easy. Polyhydramnios is often a manifestation of decreased swallowing, which may be part of the same pathogenesis as the arthrogryposis itself (muscular or neuronal deficit). An increase in nuchal lucency[53] as well as the characteristic decreased movement[54] can also be seen in the first trimester.

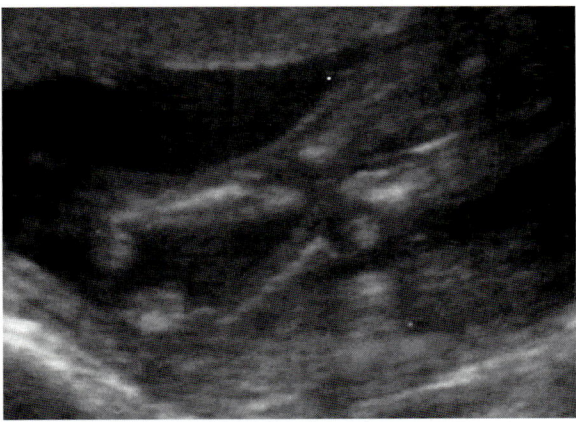

FIGURE 29. Arthrogryposis multiplex congenita. A different fetus with abnormal and rigid position of the knee. The distance between the knees is less than that between the hips. Also note that both feet are inverted.

Differential Diagnosis

Trisomy 18, renal agenesis, and myotonic dystrophy may present with some similar findings.

Associated Anomalies

Because of the heterogeneity of the conditions, numerous associated anomalies have been described including scoliosis, central nervous system anomalies, and even seizures.[55]

Prognosis and Management

The prognosis depends on associated anomalies such as respiratory limitations and scoliosis. Confirmation of diagnosis after birth is important for genetic counseling.

Recurrence Risk

Arthrogryposis is possibly autosomal dominant.

Asphyxiating Thoracic Dysplasia

A synonym for asphyxiating thoracic dysplasia is Jeune syndrome.[56]

Asphyxiating thoracic dysplasia is an autosomal recessive chondrodysplasia characterized by a small thorax, varying degrees of rhizomelic brachymelia, polydactyly, pelvic abnormalities, and renal anomalies.

Incidence

The incidence is unknown, usually affecting white babies.

Genetic Defect

The genetic defect is probably located on the short arm of chromosome 12.

Diagnosis

The most striking ultrasound finding is a very narrow chest with short limbs (Fig. 30).[57–61] The limbs, however, are not as short as those of other lethal conditions such as thanatophoric dysplasia, achondrogenesis, osteogenesis imperfecta type 2, and the short rib–polydactyly syndromes. The increased iliac wing angle, reported in the radiographic literature, has not been reported yet with ultrasound. Pancreatic cysts have been recognized in one case.[62]

Differential Diagnosis

The differential diagnosis for asphyxiating thoracic dysplasia is Ellis-van Creveld syndrome (short arm of chromosome 4) that presents mainly with cardiac anomalies instead of renal anomalies.

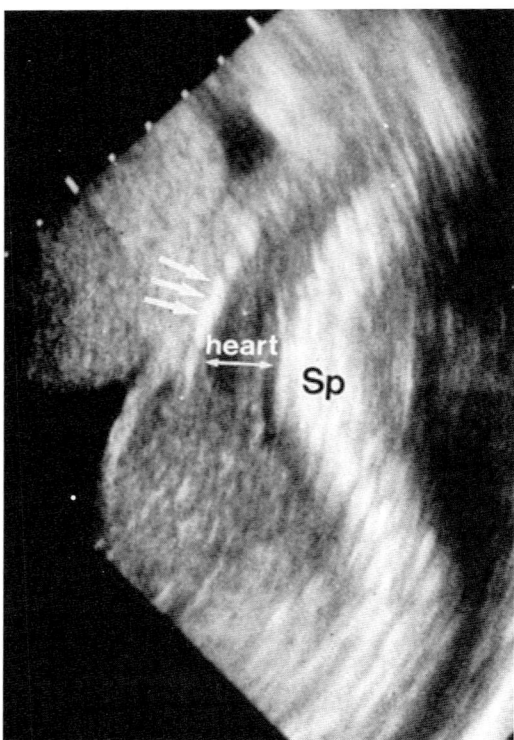

FIGURE 30. Longitudinal view of the chest and abdomen of a fetus with asphyxiating thoracic dysplasia. Note the constriction of the chest (*arrows*). Sp, spine. (Courtesy of Gianluigi Pilu, Bologna, Italy.)

Prognosis and Management

In spite of the name, not all newborns are asphyxiated, and some patients have had a fairly normal outcome after corrective surgery of the chest. Confirmation of diagnosis after birth is important for genetic counseling.

Recurrence Risk

Asphyxiating thoracic dysplasia is autosomal recessive.

Camptomelic Dysplasia

Synonyms for camptomelic dysplasia are camptomelic dysplasia, camptomelic dwarfism, and congenital bowing of the limbs.[63,64]

Camptomelic dysplasia is a congenital disorder characterized by development of abnormal curvature of the long bones, particularly from lower extremities such as femur and tibiae.[65] Some authors have classified the disease into two varieties: *long limbed* and *short limbed*, depending on the type of limbs involved in the pathologic process.[66]

Incidence

The disorder affects 0.02 per 10,000 live births.[67] Sex reversal occurs in some genotypic males that lack the H-Y

antigen. Phenotypic sex ratio is approximately M1:F2.3; karyotypic sex ratio is approximately M2:F1.[64]

Genetic Anomaly

A mutation in SOX9, a sex-determining region of Y-related gene, located at 17q24 seems to be associated with the occurrence of camptomelic dysplasia and sex reversal.[68]

Pathogenesis

Although many theories have been proposed to explain the development of the anomalies present in this syndrome (in particular, the bowing of the bones), the precise mechanism is not known. Some of the theories are

1. Mechanical stress owing to faulty fetal position within the uterus[69]
2. Primary muscle imbalance and shortening, particularly of the calf muscles, causing secondary bending of the tibia[70]
3. Intrauterine fracture with subsequent healing[71]
4. Abnormal vascular and cellular elements of perichondrium[72]
5. Developmental disturbance in the cartilaginous phase of bone formation[73]

Diagnosis

The most characteristic sign of camptomelic dysplasia is the marked anterior bowing of the long bones, particularly of femur and tibia (Fig. 31). The abnormality may be unilateral, and severe angulation may mimic fractures. Other sonographic features that are commonly present include growth restriction; bell-shaped narrow chest; eleven pairs of ribs; hypoplasia of the midthoracic vertebral bodies, fibula, and scapula; scoliosis; shortness of the limbs; talipes equinovarus; tracheobronchomalacia; flat and small face; high forehead with prominent occiput; low nasal bridge; micrognathia; cleft of the soft palate; hypertelorism; low-set and malformed ears; hydrocephalus; and ambiguous genitalia.[74] Three-dimensional ultrasound may be used to identify the hypoplastic scapula (Fig. 32).

Nuchal thickening and increased nuchal translucency may also be seen, as with other types of skeletal dysplasias (Fig. 31A). Polyhydramnios, and various anomalies of the central nervous, cardiac, and renal systems, have been described prenatally. After birth, hearing loss may occur.

Differential Diagnosis

Osteogenesis imperfecta and camptomelic dysplasia may show overlapping findings. Camptomelic dysplasia is characterized by a hypoplastic scapula and is more likely to show renal abnormalities, including mild hydronephrosis (Fig. 31B). Osteogenesis imperfecta type II shows *beaded*

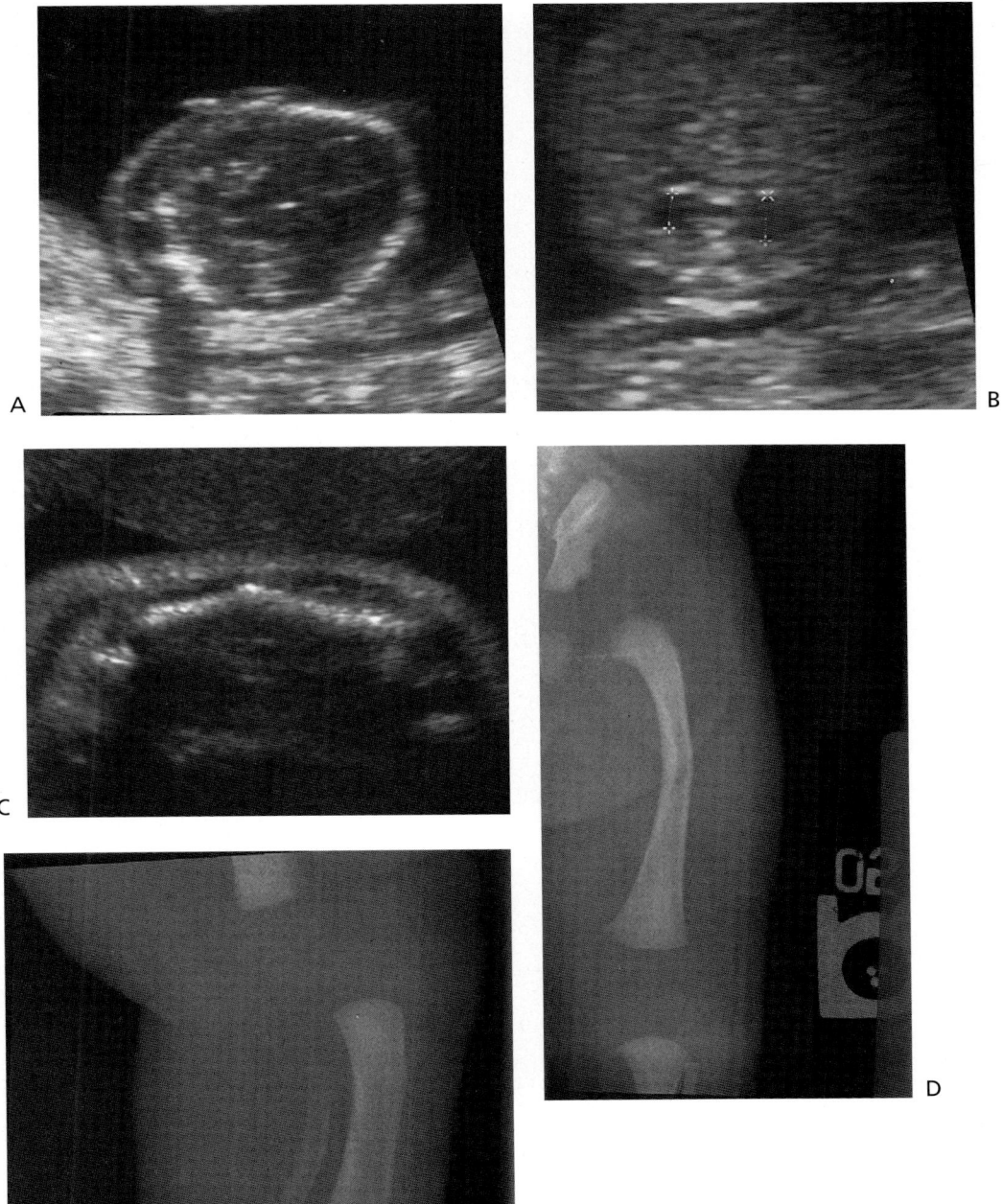

FIGURE 31. Camptomelic dysplasia. **A:** Scan of calvaria at 16 weeks shows nuchal thickening with translucency. **B:** Transverse view of kidneys shows mild bilateral renal pyelectasis (4 mm). The nuchal thickening resolved on follow-up, and renal pyelectasis improved. A single umbilical artery and limb shortening were also identified. **C:** Scan at 32 weeks shows bowing of left femur. The right femur appeared normal. **D:** Postnatal radiograph shows bowing of femur and **(E)** tibia.

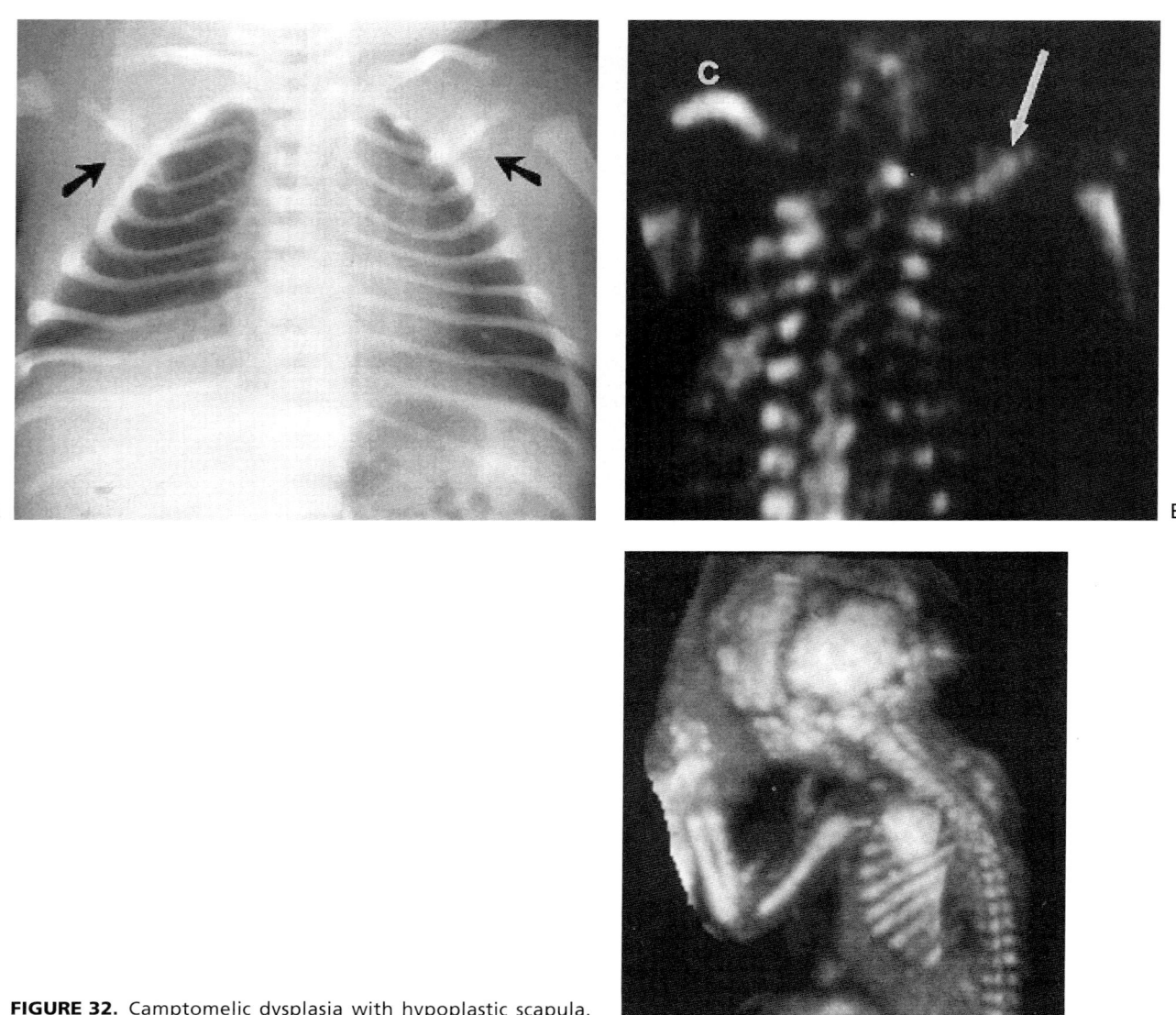

FIGURE 32. Camptomelic dysplasia with hypoplastic scapula. **A:** Postnatal radiograph shows hypoplastic scapula (*arrows*). **B:** Three-dimensional ultrasound shows hypoplastic scapula (*arrow*). C, clavicle. **C:** Three-dimensional ultrasound of a normal fetus for comparison shows well-formed scapula and ribs.

ribs secondary to multiple rib fractures and additional fractures. Other considerations include hypophosphatasia, unclassifiable varieties of congenital bowing of the long bones,[75] thanatophoric dysplasia, mesomelic dysplasia (Reinhart variety),[76] Roberts syndrome, and diastrophic dysplasia.

Prognosis and Management

Almost all cases result in neonatal or infant death, due to respiratory complications. Some survivors, including a boy alive at 17 years, have been reported.[77] Respiratory function in the newborn must be supported.

Recurrence Risk

Most cases are new mutations. Autosomal recessive and sporadic autosomal dominant cases have been described.[78]

Caudal Regression Syndrome

Synonyms for caudal regression syndrome are caudal dysplasia sequence and sacral agenesis.[79]

Caudal regression syndrome is a rare congenital defect, characterized by the absence of the sacrum and defects of variable portions of lumbar spine, associated with anomalies from different systems.

Incidence

The incidence for caudal regression syndrome is 0.1 to 0.25 per 10,000 in normal pregnancies and 200 to 250 times higher in diabetic pregnancies.[80]

Genetic Anomaly

The genetic anomaly is unknown.

Pathogenesis

Disruption of the maturation of the caudal portion of the spinal cord complex before 4 weeks' gestation, leading to motoricity deficits and neurologic impairment varying from incontinence of urine and feces to complete neurologic loss. Maternal diabetes is strongly associated with caudal regression syndrome.[81]

Diagnosis

The sonographic findings are variable and depend on the extent and severity of the defect. The defect ranges from complete absence of the sacrum associated with abnormalities of the lumbar spine (Fig. 33) and lower extremities (such as clubbed feet and contractions of the knees and hips) to abnormalities of the sacrum without associated defects.[82] The most typical findings are the absence of a few vertebrae, the shield-like appearance of the fused or approximated iliac wings (Fig. 33C), and the decreased interspace between the femoral heads. Some sections intersect the fetus at such an angle that no spine is visible, a very striking and probably pathognomonic finding (Fig. 33D). Decreased movement of the legs is frequently observed. First-trimester diagnosis may be hard to accomplish because of the incomplete ossification of the sacrum at that time. A short crown–rump length and abnormal appearance of the yolk sac have been proposed as early sonographic signs of caudal regression syndromes.[82]

Associated Anomalies

Anomalies of the central nervous, musculoskeletal, genitourinary, cardiac, respiratory, and gastrointestinal systems may be found in association with caudal regression syndrome. Less common, associated intraspinal archnoid cyst has been reported.[83]

Differential Diagnosis

Sirenomelia, which was thought to be the most severe form of caudal regression syndrome (it is now considered a different entity),[82] is the main differential diagnosis. Fusion of the lower extremities is a typical finding of sirenomelia.

Prognosis and Management

Prognosis depends on the severity of the spinal defect and associated anomalies, but the vast majority of survivals require urologic and orthopedic interventions. Severe forms are commonly associated with cardiac, renal, and respiratory problems, which are responsible for early neonatal death. If born alive, extensive surgery in a tertiary center is usually needed to repair the defects.

Recurrence Risk

This anomaly is not thought to be hereditary, and the recurrence risk is very small, although higher in diabetics.

Chondroectodermal Dysplasia

A synonym for chondroectodermal dysplasia is Ellis-van Creveld syndrome.

This disorder was described by Richard W. B. Ellis and Simon van Creveld.[84] It is an autosomal recessive disorder characterized by a tetrad of chondrodysplasia, ectodermal dysplasia, postaxial polydactyly, and heart defects (common atrium or atrioventricular septal defect).

Incidence

The incidence is 1 per 60,000 in the general population. Chondroectodermal dysplasia is most prevalent in the Amish population of Lancaster, Pennsylvania, where it occurs in 1 per 5,000 births.

Genetic Defect

Ellis-van Creveld syndrome is a generalized disorder of the maturation of enchondral ossification.[85] The responsible gene has been localized.[86]

Diagnosis

Ellis-van Creveld syndrome is characterized by short limbs, short ribs, postaxial polydactyly, and dysplastic nails and teeth.[87] Anomalies of the central nervous system and urinary tract are rarely reported.

The prenatal sonographic findings include shortened extremities, postaxial polydactyly of the hands (Fig. 34), narrow chest, short ribs, and cardiac defects.[88,89] The diagnosis has been made as early as the first trimester in affected families.[90]

Molecular diagnosis has also been established using markers adjacent to the EvC locus.[91]

Differential Diagnosis

Considerations include asphyxiating thoracic dysplasia (Jeune syndrome) and Verma-Naumoff type or Saldino-Noonan

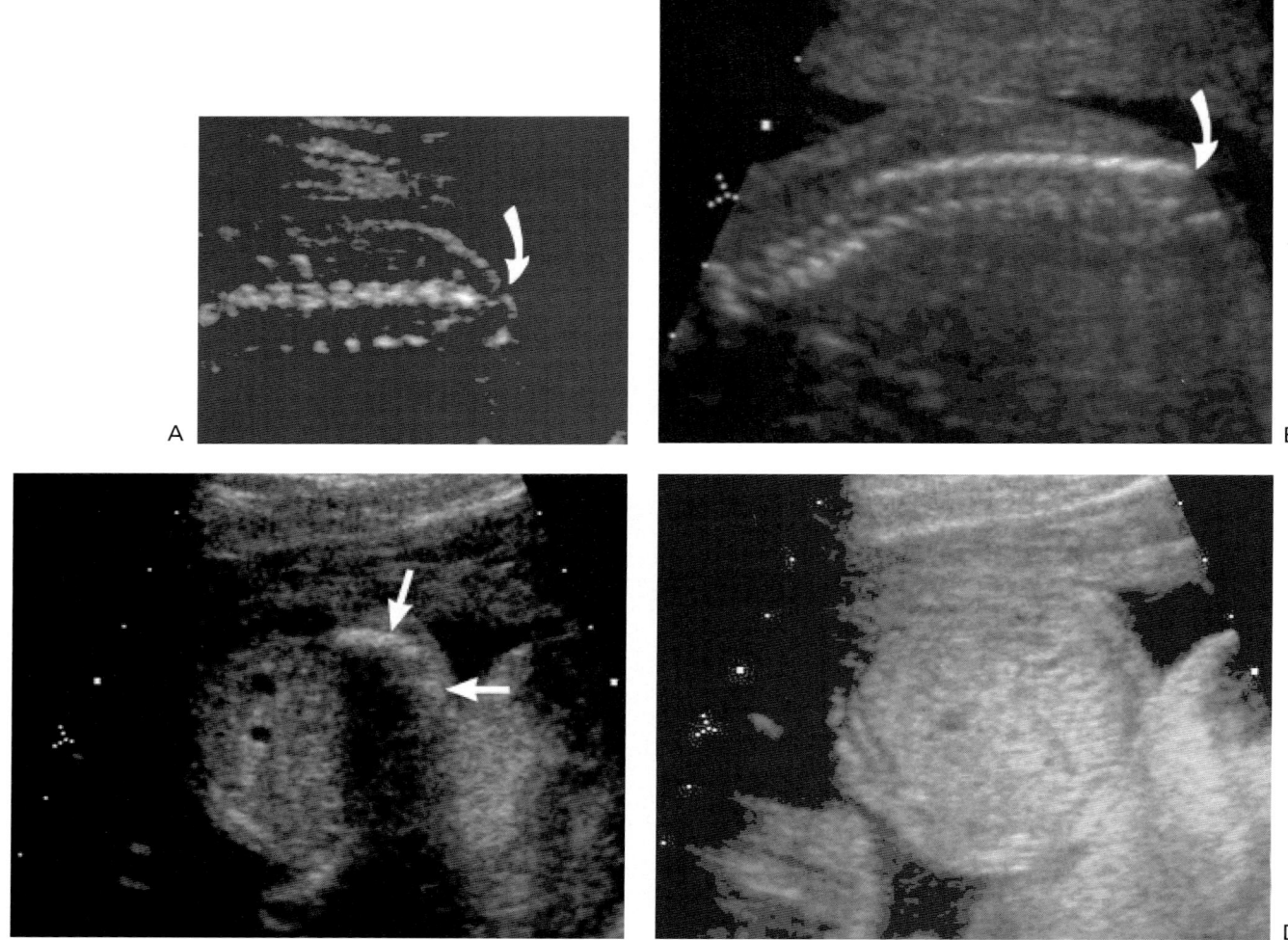

FIGURE 33. Caudal regression syndrome. **A:** Although on superficial examination this image might pass for normal, note that on the caudal side of the image (on the **right**, because the ribs can be seen on the left side of the image) the spine terminates (*arrow*) without the usual landmark of the iliac wings and sacrum. **B:** This same finding is even more striking on the sagittal view of the spine, in which the distal end appears to have been erased (*arrow*). This is actually the finding that caught the eye of an astute sonographer; she was puzzled by the spine "looking too short." **C:** The lack of sacrum allows the iliac wings to be approximated, giving them a shield-like appearance (*arrows*). **D:** Caudal regression syndrome with absent spine. Transverse view of abdomen fails to show normal spine (the spine is approximately at the 2:00 position). Other differential diagnoses, such as achondrogenesis and the severest forms of osteogenesis imperfecta, would not present with the localized anomaly seen here.

types of short rib–polydactyly syndrome.[92] McKusick-Kaufman syndrome can also be considered.[93]

Prognosis and Management

Prognosis and management vary with the specific anomalies, including cardiac defects. In general, the prognosis is good. Oral problems are common in children.

Recurrence Risk

Chondroectodermal dysplasia is autosomal recessive (25% recurrence).

Chondrodysplasia Punctata

Synonyms for chondrodysplasia punctata are Conradi-Hünermann syndrome and chondrodystrophia calcificans congenita.[94]

Related anomalies for chondrodysplasia punctata are chondrodysplasia punctata (X-linked dominant type), dysplasia epiphysealis punctata, and rhizomelic chondrodysplasia punctata.

Description

Chondrodysplasia punctata consists of a depressed nasal bridge and mild stippling of the epiphysis (premature calci-

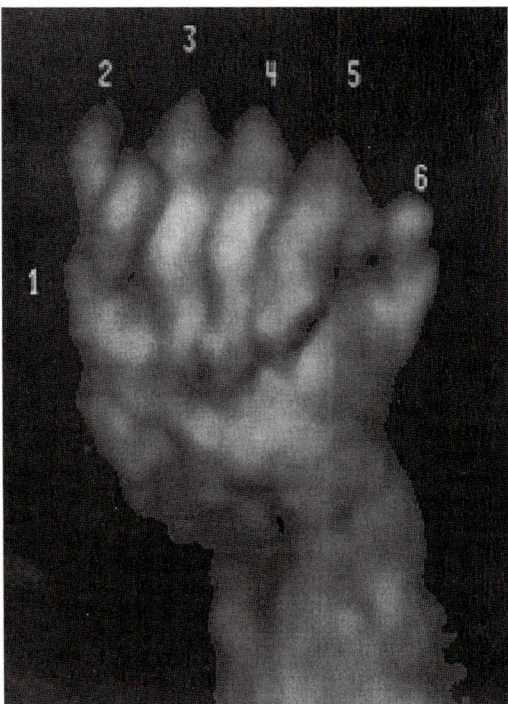 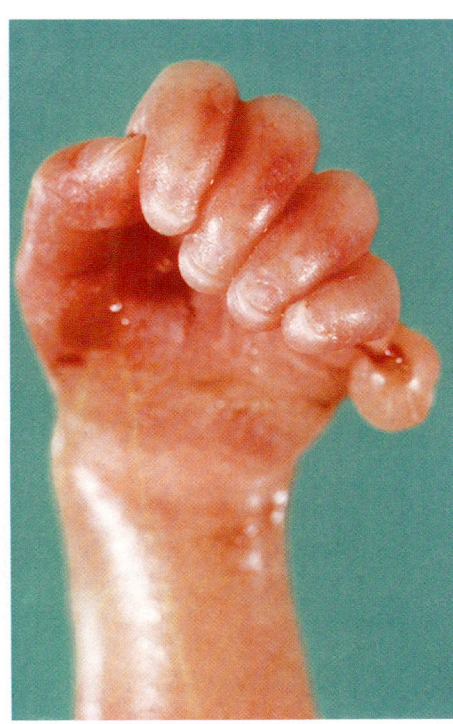

A,B

FIGURE 34. Polydactyly. **A:** Three-dimensional ultrasound showing postaxial polydactyly, as may be seen with chondroectodermal dysplasia. **B:** Pathologic correlation of another fetus with polydactyly.

fications in ultrasound), which affects the vertebrae, tarsal, and carpal bones. This condition results from disruption of the physis with abnormal calcification.

The *rhizomelic type*[95] (an autosomal recessive disorder of peroxisomal function) is usually lethal in infancy and consists of proximal limb shortening, short stature, flat facies, cataracts, mental retardation, and ichthyosiform skin rash.

The *X-linked dominant type*,[96] thought to be lethal in males, is characterized by asymmetrical skeletal abnormalities with short stature; shortening of the long bones; dysplasia and contracture of joints; and scoliosis together with flat nasal bridge, congenital ichthyosiform erythroderma, cicatricial alopecia of the scalp, abnormal hair, and cataracts.

An *X-linked recessive form* has been described[97] in association with a deletion of the terminal short arm of an X chromosome, in brothers with epiphyseal stippling, nasal hypoplasia, ichthyosis, and mental retardation.

The term *Conradi-Hünermann syndrome* has been applied to an apparently heterogeneous group of conditions whose features include asymmetrical short stature, scoliosis, cataracts, ichthyotic skin, and flat facies with nasal hypoplasia.[98] The patients included some with X-linked dominant, autosomal dominant,[99] and sporadic forms[100] and can be quite mildly affected. Patients with the mildest clinical features have been diagnosed in mid-childhood to have *Binder syndrome* (maxillonasal dysplasia).[101]

Incidence

More than 100 cases of chondrodysplasia punctata have been reported, many in Australia.

Diagnosis

Chondrodysplasia punctata has been occasionally diagnosed with rhizomelic shortening and stippled calcification of the epiphysis (Fig. 35).[102] Calcification of the heel and coccyx may also be detected (Fig. 36). Radiographically visible ossification begins in the calcaneum and talus between 22 and 24 weeks of menstrual age.[103] Ossification in the first coccygeal segment usually begins after term but may occasionally be seen in the mid-third trimester.

An association with fetal ascites and polyhydramnios has also been reported.[104]

Associated Anomalies

Chondrodysplasia punctata is associated with postaxial polydactyly (occasional).

Differential Diagnosis

Differential diagnoses of abnormal coccygeal and talar calcifications include warfarin embryopathy, aneuploidy (trisomies 18, 21, triploidy), anencephaly, alcohol and phenytoin exposure, peroxisomal disorders, Smith-Lemli-Opitz syndrome, and GM_1 gangliosidosis.

Prognosis

Bone changes improve in the mild form; the lifespan and intelligence are normal. The only marker in adults is the nasal anomaly.

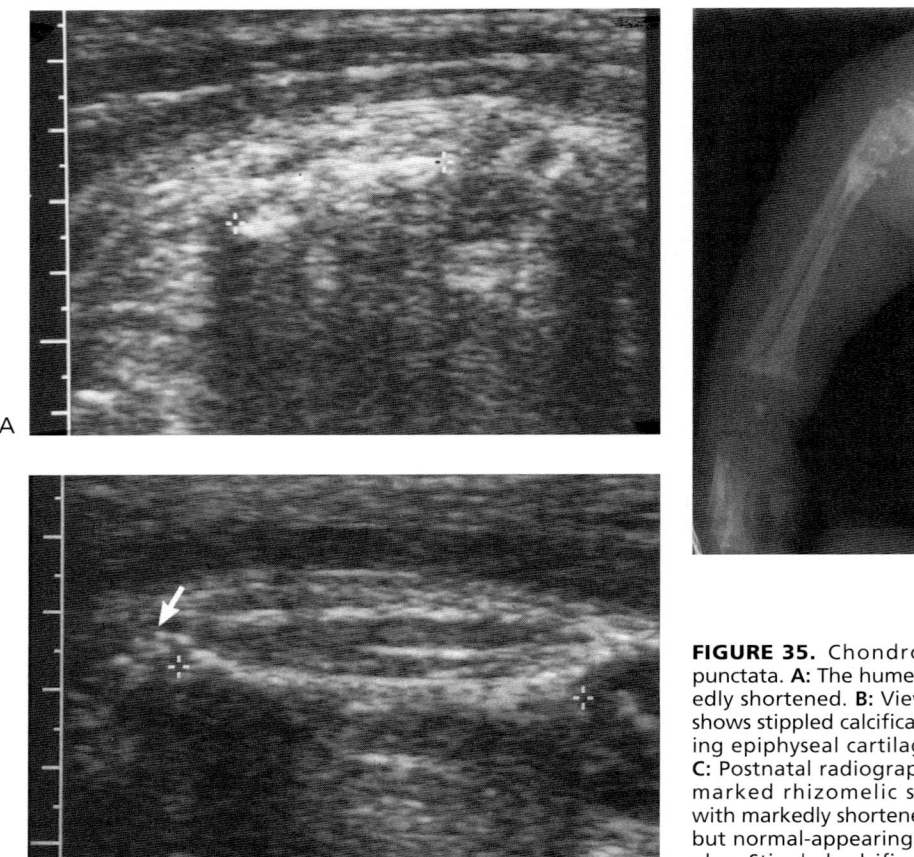

FIGURE 35. Chondrodysplasia punctata. **A:** The humerus is markedly shortened. **B:** View of femur shows stippled calcification involving epiphyseal cartilage (*arrow*). **C:** Postnatal radiograph confirms marked rhizomelic shortening with markedly shortened humerus but normal-appearing radius and ulna. Stippled calcification is also seen at distal end of humerus.

Recurrence Risk

The recurrence risk varies with the type of disorder.

Craniosynostosis

The craniosynostoses are etiologically and pathogenetically heterogeneous. More than 90 syndromes with craniosynostoses have been delineated. Most cases of simple craniosynostoses are sporadic. Sagittal synostosis is most common, accounting for more than one-half the cases.

Incidence

Overall birth prevalence is approximately 1 per 3,000.[105]

Genetic Defect

The FGFR-related conditions result from defects of fibroblast growth factor (see full description of FGFR-related conditions in Chapter 5).

Pathologic and Clinical Features

Head shape depends on which sutures are involved and the developmental stage at which fusion occurs. When the coronal suture is involved, brachycephaly results. Premature closure of the sagittal suture results in dolichocephaly. Unilateral involvement of the coronal or lambdoidal suture produces plagiocephaly. Metopic fusion produces trigonocephaly.

Other anomalies are uncommon with sagittal craniosynostosis but common with coronal synostosis. The cloverleaf skull (kleeblattschädel) may occur as an isolated anomaly or as part of a syndromic pattern, most commonly thanatophoric dysplasia or Pfeiffer syndrome.

Diagnosis

The earliest diagnosis of craniosynostosis has been made at 20 to 23 weeks' gestation. Abnormal skull shape is the first clue to craniosynostosis (Fig. 37), and this has been reported as early as 19 weeks.[106] Sonographic demonstration is difficult before that time and may even be absent

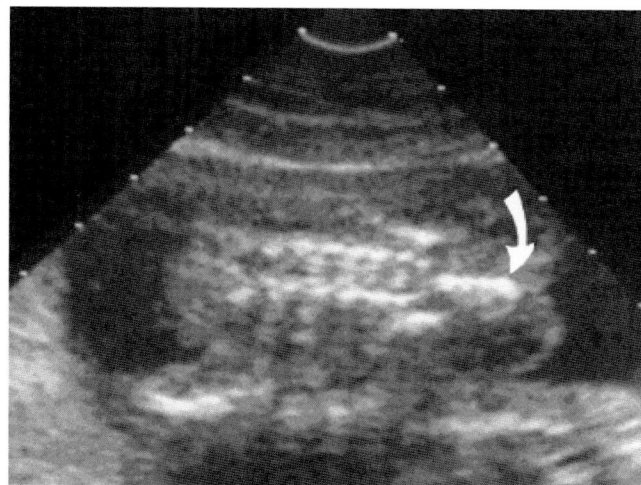

FIGURE 36. Chondrodysplasia punctata. **A:** Coronal scan of distal fetal trunk at 15 weeks, showing echogenic coccyx (*arrow*). **B:** Anteroposterior radiograph showing calcification in coccyx and heel, 29 weeks. **C:** Lateral radiograph of distal spine showing stippled calcification of coccyx. (Courtesy of Margaret Furness, MD, Adelaide, Australia.)

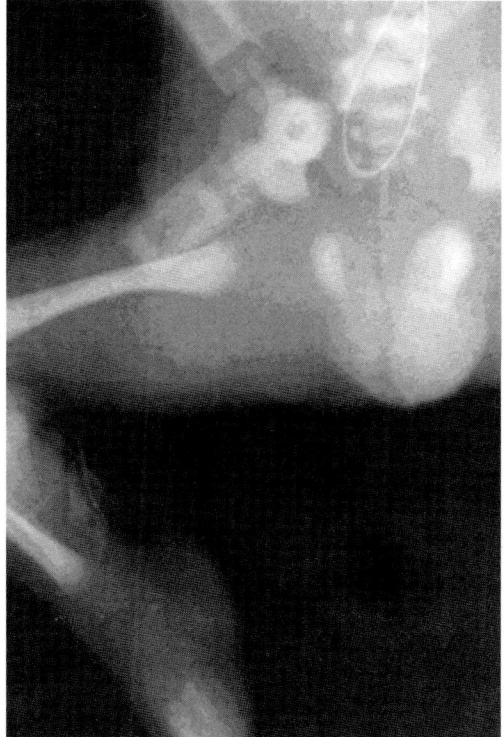

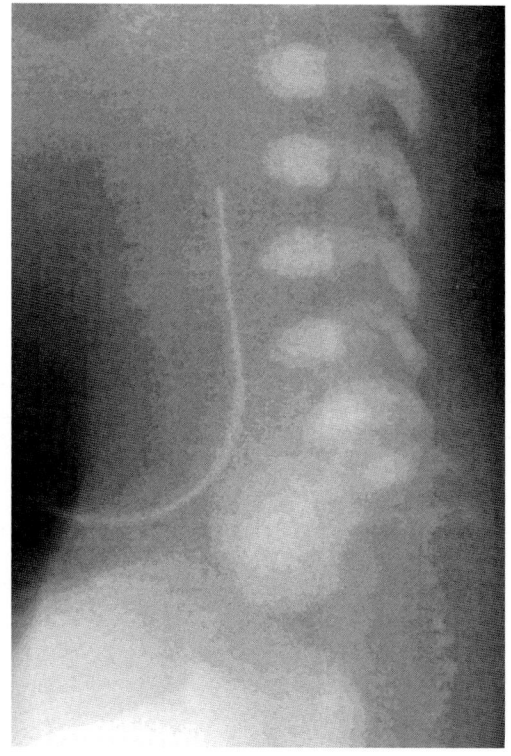

pathologically.[107] These lines of evidence suggest that craniosynostoses is not present during early pregnancy, but develops after the mid-trimester in most cases.

The sutures of fetuses with craniosynostosis can be best evaluated using three-dimensional ultrasound, with which open and closed sutures are easily distinguishable.[108]

Differential Diagnosis

Cranial features of craniosynostosis are nonspecific. Possibilities include trisomy 18, Jacobsen syndrome, thanato-phoric dysplasia, camptomelic dysplasia, Antley-Bixler syndrome, and Carpenter syndrome.

Prognosis and Management

Most patients have intellectual impairment; however, some patients have normal intelligence.[109,110] Surgical correction for nonsyndromic craniosynostosis is usually performed between 6 months and 1 year of age, whereas patients with syndromic craniosynostosis often have multiple surgical procedures, with the first surgery as early as 3 months of age.

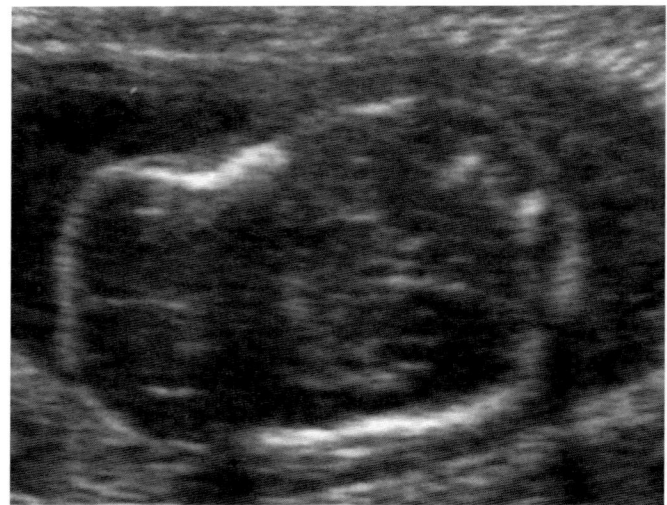
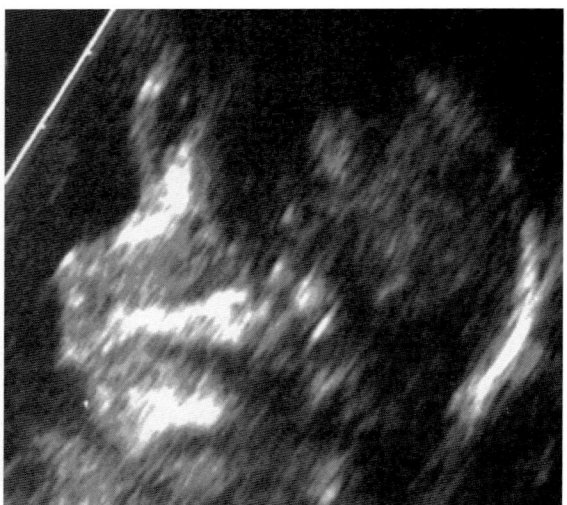

FIGURE 37. Craniosynostosis. **A:** Axial view of the brain and calvarium. Note the narrowing at the level of the coronal suture and the poor mineralization of the frontal area. **B:** Frontal bossing, low nasal bridge, and micrognathia (sagittal view). (Copyright, Phillippe Jeanty, reproduced with permission from http://www.TheFetus.net.)

Recurrence Risk

The recurrence risk varies with the underlying etiology.

Fibrochondrogenesis and Atelosteogenesis

Fibrochondrogenesis and atelosteogenesis have a clinical presentation similar to that of thanatophoric dysplasia,[1] and it may be extremely difficult to distinguish these disorders prenatally. Fibrochondrogenesis is a lethal chondrodysplasia inherited with an autosomal recessive pattern and characterized by rhizomelia, with significant metaphyseal flaring and clefting of the vertebral bodies. Metaphyseal flaring is not a feature of thanatophoric dysplasia.[111] Atelosteogenesis is also a lethal chondrodysplasia characterized by severe micromelia (with hypoplasia of the distal segments of the humerus and femur), bowing of long bones, and dislocation at the level of the elbow and knee. Clubfoot deformities may also be present.[112] Fibrochondrogenesis and atelosteogenesis are extremely rare, and only a few cases of each have been reported.

Hypophosphatasia

A synonym for hypophosphatasia is phosphoethanolaminuria.[113]

Hypophosphatasia is an anomaly due to defective bone mineralization and deficiency of serum and tissue liver/bone/kidney alkaline phosphatase with three subtypes: a lethal *type 1* with prenatal manifestations of short demineralized long bones, craniosynostosis, and neonatal hypercalcemia; a *type 2* with rickets-like skeletal changes, fractures, and premature loss of teeth; and a *type 3* with only metabolic anomalies detected on biochemical screening.

Incidence

Hypophosphatasia is rare.

Genetic Defect

Hypophosphatasia is an anomaly of tissue-nonspecific alkaline phosphatase gene. Types 1 and 2 are different disorders. There are numerous variant tissue-nonspecific alkaline phosphatase genes.[114]

Diagnosis

The diagnosis should be suspected in fetuses with micromelia and demineralization of the bones (Fig. 38).[115] Spurs have been diagnosed postnatally that might be typical. These occur along the midshaft of long bones and at the knees and elbows.[116–118]

Cordocentesis has been successfully performed as early as 15 weeks' gestation, showing undetectable levels of fetal alkaline phosphatase in an affected fetus with hypophosphatasia.[119]

Differential Diagnosis

Hypophosphatasia is probably indistinguishable on ultrasound criteria only from osteogenesis imperfecta type II and achondrogenesis type IA.

Prognosis

Hypophosphatasia is lethal for type I.

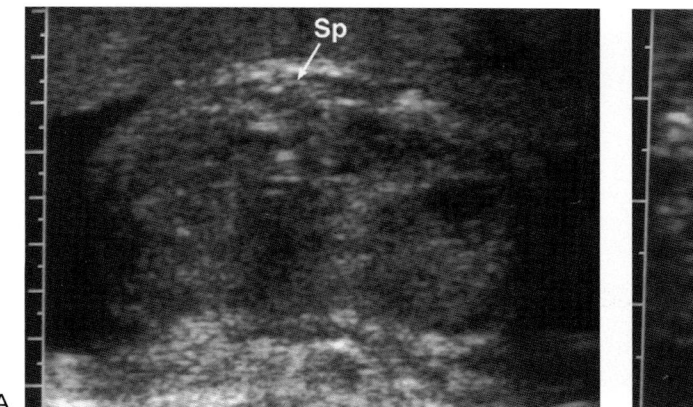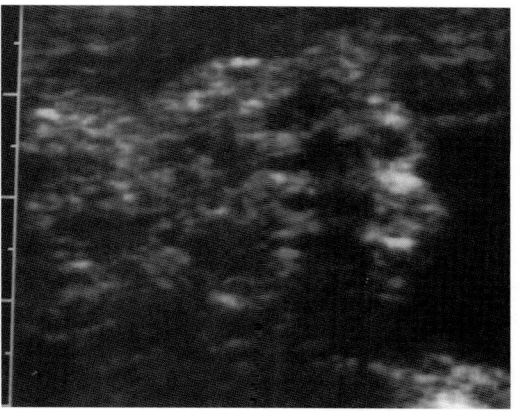

FIGURE 38. Hypophosphatasia. **A:** Transverse view of spine and kidneys shows marked hypomineralization of spine, seen in transverse view (*Sp*). **B:** Magnified view of hand shows marked hypomineralization. (Courtesy of Glen Rouse, MD, CA.)

Recurrence Risk

The recurrence risk is 25%. Carriers can be recognized by their low levels of serum alkaline phosphatase[120] and urinary phosphoethanolamine.

Mesomelic Dysplasia

Synonyms for mesomelic dysplasia are Langer type mesomelic dwarfism; dyschondrosteosis, homozygous.[121]

As implied by its name, mesomelic dysplasia is a skeletal disorder with anomalies of the ulna-radius and tibia-fibula. These anomalies are predominantly hypoplasia and shortening, but these bones can also be malformed or fused. A large number of associated anomalies exist such as hypoplasia of the mandible; ulnar deviation of hands; talipes equinovarus; distal tapering of the humeri; hypoplastic fibulae, radii, and ulnae[122]; bony spurs of the diaphyses[123]; carpal/tarsal synostosis; and dorsolateral foot deviation.[124,125] The most typical form (Langer type) is considered to be the homozygote form of the Leri-Weill dyschondrosteosis.[126]

Incidence

Mesomelic dysplasia is rare.

Diagnosis

The mesomelic findings have been recognized as early as the first trimester in an at-risk propositus[127] and in a routine examination in the second trimester.[128,129]

Genetic Defect

The genetic defect is a nonsense mutation of the gene for the short stature homeobox (SHOX), which is involved in idiopathic growth retardation and possibly Turner syndrome short stature.[130] The gene for one form of mesomelic dysplasia (the Kantaputra type[124]) is mapped to chromosome 2q24-q32.[125] The Leri-Weill dyschondrosteosis has been linked to the marker DXYS6814 in the pseudoautosomal region (PAR1) of the X and Y chromosomes (more severe in females)[126] and to the DCS gene to a microsatellite DNA marker at the DXYS233 locus.[130]

Associated Anomalies

See previous Description section. Aside from the mesomelic dysplasia most other anomalies are skeletal, and the most striking is micrognathia.

Differential Diagnosis

Many other skeletal dysplasias present with mesomelic anomalies, and these include chondrodysplasia punctata (look for stippled calcifications in the sacrum),[131] brachymesomelia,[132] and chondroectodermal dysplasia[133] among many.

Prognosis

The prognosis involves disproportionate short stature. Some forms have normal intellectual capacity.

Recurrence Risk

Mesomelic dysplasia has an autosomal recessive inheritance of 25%.

Microcephalic Osteodysplastic Primordial Dwarfism, Types I through III

Synonyms for microcephalic osteodysplastic primordial dwarfism include osteodysplastic primordial dwarfism, type I; brachymelic primordial dwarfism; Taybi-Linder syndrome; cephaloskeletal dysplasia; and low-birth-weight dwarfism with skeletal dysplasia.[134]

These syndromes associate growth retardation with microcephaly and various facial anomalies.[135–140] The number of reported cases is small, and the difference between the subtypes probably is not identifiable by prenatal ultrasound.

Incidence

Less than 50 cases have been reported.

Genetic Defect

The genetic anomaly is unknown.

Diagnosis

The findings include growth retardation with microcephaly, micrencephaly, lissencephaly, micrognathia, and moderately short limbs.[141] Types II and III may have platyspondyly.

Associated Anomalies

Associated anomalies include beaked nose, large eyes, dysplastic ears, clinodactyly, dysgenesis of the corpus callosum, focal renal medullary dysplasia, small iliac wings with flat acetabular angles, coxa vara, V-shaped distal femoral metaphyses, triangular distal femoral epiphyses, pseudoepiphyses of metacarpals, short first metacarpals, and brachymesophalangy of the fifth digit.[142,143]

Differential Diagnosis

Differential diagnosis includes aneuploidies (trisomy 13, 18).

Prognosis

The prognosis is not known. Most children die within the first year of life.

Recurrence Risk

The recurrence risk is sporadic, with possible autosomal recessive inheritance.[136]

Osteogenesis Imperfecta

Synonyms for osteogenesis imperfecta are osteogenesis imperfecta congenital, van der Hoeve syndrome, Lobstein disease, trias fragilitas osseum, brittle bone disease, and Vrolik disease.[144,145]

Osteogenesis imperfecta is a heterogeneous group of genetic disorders (classically divided in four types assessed by Sillence: I, II or congenital, III, and IV) characterized by severe bone fragility, leading to abnormal ossification and multiple fractures.[146] The four types are described below.

- Type I does not present prenatal deformities, and the diagnosis is made after birth when the limb deformities start to develop.
- Type II is the most severe form, which presents with multiple skeletal malformations such as bone shortening and angulation due to multiple fractures, demineralization of the skull, narrow and bell-shaped chest caused by fractures of the ribs, decreased fetal movement, and wrinkling of the surface of the bones due to multiple fractures.
- Type III is a less severe form than type II that usually presents multiple fractures at birth, with development of progressive bone deformities from neonatal period to adolescence. It is detectable as early as second trimester in the type IIIC.
- Type IV is the mildest presentation of the disorder, not detectable prenatally. It usually involves premature osteoporosis in the fourth or fifth decades of life.

Incidence

The incidence is 0.4 per 10,000 live births, and approximately one-half (0.19 per 10,000) represents type II.[147]

Genetic Defect

A disorder in one of the two genes responsible for the type I collagen production (COLIA1 and COLIA2) is the cause of the disease.[148] A defect of formation, organization, and chemical composition in type I collagen (which is found in skin, ligaments, tendons, demineralized bone, and dentine) is responsible for decreased mineralization and bone fragility.[148]

Diagnosis

The sonographic findings that may be present (particularly in type II) include broad, short, fractured long bones (Fig. 39), with a wrinkled appearance caused by callus formation; decreased ossification of the skull (Fig. 40), with increased visualization of the intracranial structures; small bell-shaped chest (Fig. 41); irregular ribs due to rib fractures (Fig. 41C); abnormal skull shape; broad irregular ribs; angulation of the long bones; and abnormal face. Multiple fractures are present by birth (Fig. 42).

A typical finding of osteogenesis imperfecta type II is the ability to see both cortical margins of a bone. Normally the distal cortical is shadowed out by the proximal but not in the severe demineralization of osteogenesis imperfecta (achondrogenesis and hypophosphatasia may present the same finding). Most of the anomalies can be detected *in utero* by ultrasound in the early second trimester. A normal ultrasound for a high-risk patient does not exclude the disorder. In general, if the fractures do not occur *in utero*, the diagnosis is made only after birth.[146,149]

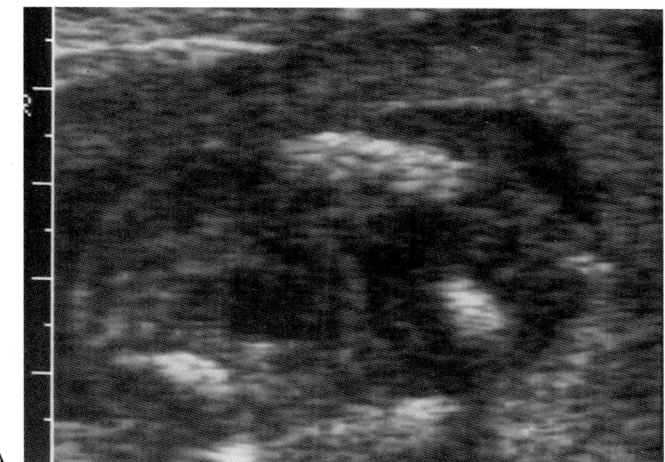

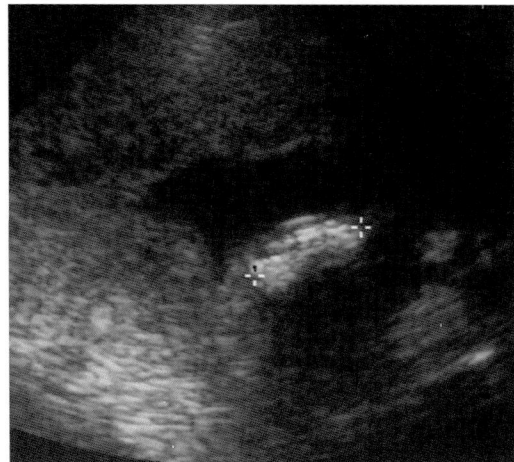

FIGURE 39. Osteogenesis imperfecta. Scans at 20 weeks show markedly shortened femur **(A)** and tibia **(B)**, which correspond in length to 16-week size.

Associated Anomalies

Associated anomalies are kyphoscoliosis, deafness, hypotonia, inguinal hernias, hydrocephalus, hydrops, and prenatal growth deficiency.[150]

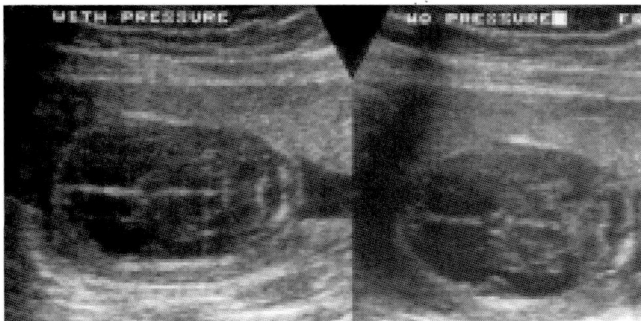

FIGURE 40. Osteogenesis imperfecta. The skull demonstrates markedly decreased echogenicity and is readily compressible even with moderate transducer pressure **(left)**.

Differential Diagnosis

Camptomelic dysplasia should always be considered when osteogenesis imperfecta is suspected. Osteogenesis imperfecta shows multiple fractures, although severe bowing of

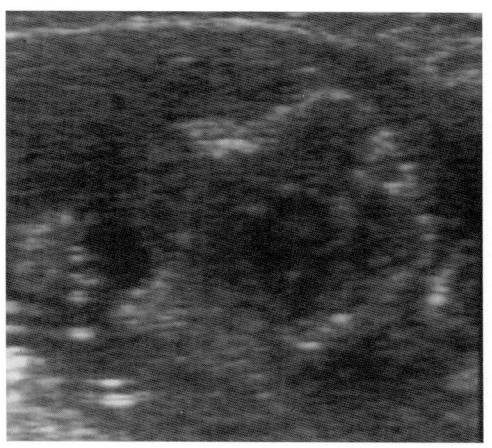

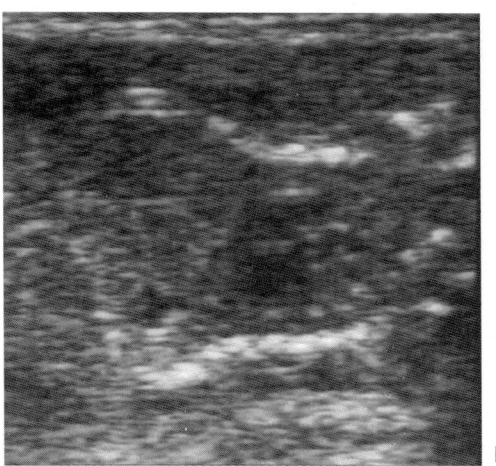

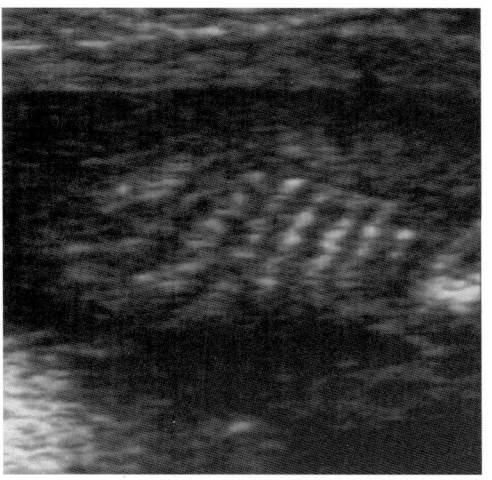

FIGURE 41. Osteogenesis imperfecta, type II. **A:** Transverse view of thorax shows collapsed-appearing ribs. **B:** Longitudinal view shows bell-shaped thorax. **C:** Magnified coronal view of ribs shows beaded appearance due to multiple rib fractures.

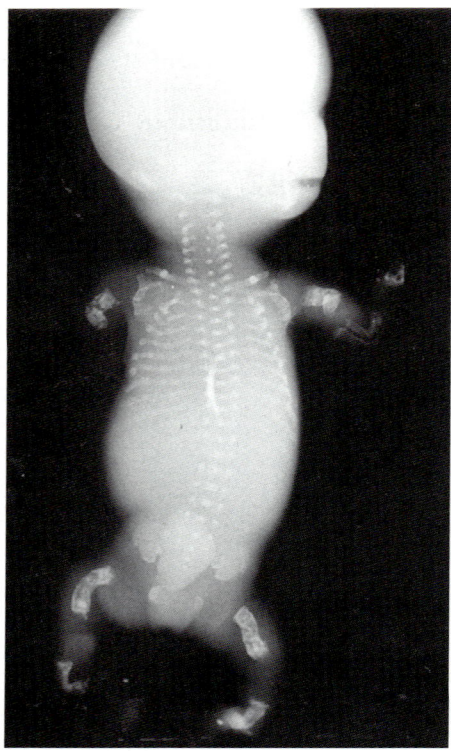
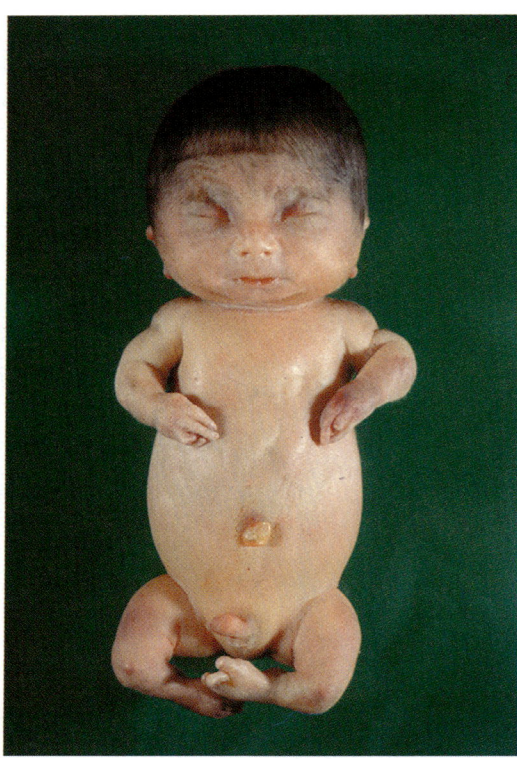

A,B

FIGURE 42. Osteogenesis imperfecta. **A:** Frontal radiograph shows poor marked limb shortening, bone deformities, and numerous fractures. **B:** Postmortem photograph of another case of osteogenesis imperfecta.

camptomelic dysplasia may simulate fractures. Rib fractures with a beaded appearance are characteristic for osteogenesis imperfecta, whereas camptomelic dysplasia is more likely to show renal anomalies. A hypoplastic scapula is also characteristic for camptomelic dysplasia. Other considerations include hypophosphatasia (infantile form), achondrogenesis, and other short-limbed dwarfisms.[146]

Prognosis

Type II osteogenesis imperfecta is uniformly lethal, and the most frequent causes are cerebral hemorrhage and respiratory failure. The other forms develop after birth, progressive deformities of the long bones, and short stature.[146,149]

Management

Because of the uniformly fatal outcome, termination of pregnancy could be offered at any stage of the gestation when type II is diagnosed. For the other forms, termination could be offered before viability. If continuing the pregnancy is opted, standard prenatal care should not be altered.

Recurrence Risk

In the majority of cases of types I and IV, an autosomal dominant pattern is involved. Type II is a *de novo* dominant mutation (with a few reports of autosomal recessive pattern), and type III is either autosomal recessive or domi-

nant.[150] In general, the recurrence risk ranges from 2% to 5% for type II.[146]

Poland Syndrome

Synonyms for Poland syndrome are Poland-Moebius syndrome and subclavian artery supply disruption sequence.[151]

Poland syndrome is a unilateral symbrachydactyly and ipsilateral aplasia of the sternal head of the pectoralis major muscle. Ipsilateral aplasia of the breast exists in females. Dextrocardia has been reported in several cases.[152,153]

Incidence

The incidence is 0.2 per 10,000.[154] Maternal smoking during pregnancy can increase the risk for Poland syndrome by approximately twofold.[155]

Genetic Defect

The genetic defect is not established. Poland syndrome probably results from interruption of the early embryonic blood supply in the subclavian arteries.[156]

Diagnosis

The chest asymmetry and symbrachydactyly can be recognized, but the long bones are probably too normal to be recognized.[157,158]

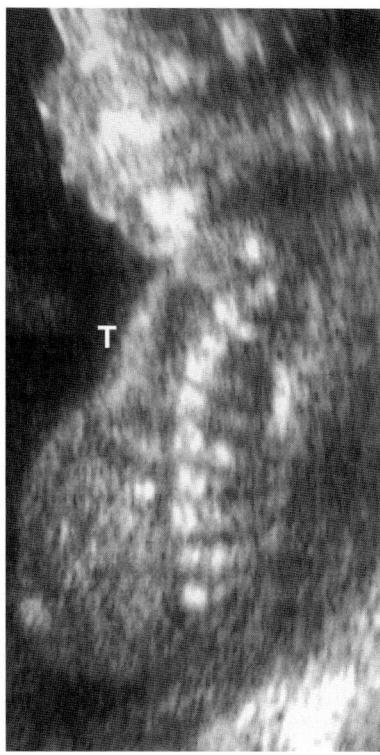
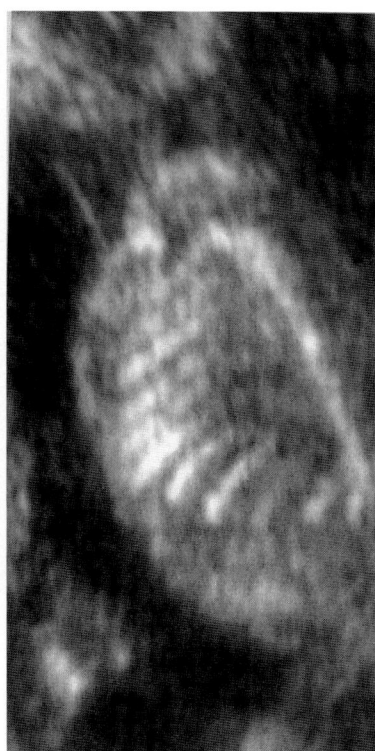

A,B

FIGURE 43. Short rib–polydactyly syndrome. **A:** Parasagittal scan shows short ribs and hypoplastic thorax (*T*). **B:** Normal fetus for comparison.

Associated Anomalies

Association with Moebius syndrome has been reported.[159,160]

Differential Diagnosis

When the unilaterality of the anomalies is recognized, few differential diagnoses exist.

Prognosis and Management

Aside from the anomalies of the extremity, the prognosis is excellent. Confirmation of diagnosis after birth is important for genetic counseling.

Recurrence Risk

Poland syndrome is usually sporadic. Several familial cases have been described.

Roberts SC Syndrome

See Chapter 5.

Short Rib–Polydactyly Syndromes

Short rib–polydactyly syndromes are lethal forms of skeletal dysplasia, characterized by thoracic hypoplasia, polydac-

tyly, and shortening of the long bones. Three types of the disorder were described[161]:

- Type I was described by Saldino and Noonan in 1972.[162]
- Type II was described by Majewski in 1971.[163]
- Type III was described by Naumoff in 1977.[164]

Clinical, radiographic, and morphologic studies suggest that types I and III just represent phenotypic variations of the same disorder.

Incidence

Because of the rarity of the condition, the incidence is not precisely known. No sex preference has been observed.[165]

Genetic Defect

There is a probable gene defect involving either 4q13 or 4p16.

Diagnosis

Prenatal diagnosis by ultrasound can be accomplished by finding the characteristic triad, which includes micromelic dwarfism, short and horizontal ribs with narrow thorax (Fig. 43), and polydactyly.

Some typical features, more frequently seen after birth, differentiate type I from type II:

Type I (Saldino-Noonan): Short stature, postaxial polydactyly of hands and feet, syndactyly, under ossified phalanges, notch-like ossification defect of vertebral bodies, small iliac bones, and triangular ossification defects above the acetabulum. Cardiac, gastrointestinal, and urogenital malformations can also be found. Occasionally preaxial polydactyly and sex-reversal (46,XY with female phenotype) can occur.[166]

Type II (Majewski): Short stature with extremely short limbs, midline cleft lip, cleft palate, short flat nose, low-set and malformed ears, preaxial and postaxial polysyndactyly of hands and feet, premature ossification of proximal epiphyses of femur, humerus and lateral cuboids, under ossified phalanges, high clavicles, and ambiguous genitalia. Less frequently, hydrops and polyhydramnios can also be found.[167]

Differential Diagnosis

The differential diagnosis includes all skeletal dysplasias associated with micromelia and short ribs such as thanatophoric dwarfism, chondrodysplasia punctata, osteogenesis imperfecta, and camptomelic dysplasia.[168] Orofaciodigital syndrome type II is another differential diagnosis of the Majewski type.[167] Most of these conditions are excluded only after birth, by radiographic and morphologic studies.

Prognosis and Management

Short rib–polydactyly syndromes are lethal conditions. Affected neonates usually die within a few hours after birth from respiratory insufficiency due to severe pulmonary hypoplasia.[166,167] Confirmation of diagnosis after birth is important for genetic counseling.

Recurrence Risk

Short rib–polydactyly syndromes are autosomal recessive (25% recurrence).[165]

Sirenomelia

A synonym for sirenomelia is mermaid syndrome, sirenomelia sequence.[169] Tritonmelia is the male variant of sirenomelia.[170]

Sirenomelia is a congenital anomaly caused by a disruptive vascular defect, characterized by fusion of the lower extremities, associated with renal agenesis, absence of the sacrum, rectum, and bladder. It was considered in the past to represent a severe form of caudal regression syndrome.

Pathogenesis

An alteration in early vascular development leads to a *vitelline arterial steal,* in which blood flow is diverted from the caudal region of the embryo to the placenta, resulting in multiple defects of the lower extremities.[171] Many of these fetuses have an aberrant vasculature with the umbilical arteries connected to the old vitelline arteries (the superior mesenteric arteries). There is no known genetic defect.

Diagnosis

The diagnosis of sirenomelia is based on the presence of fusion of the lower extremities (Fig. 44), associated with other skeletal and lumbar spine deformities, bilateral renal agenesis (which leads to severe oligohydramnios and lung hypoplasia), and heart and abdominal wall defects.[172,173] The defect varies from simple cutaneous fusion of the limbs to absence of all long bones but one femur. The defect of the feet is proportional with the defect of the long bones, with cutaneous defect commonly presenting with a double-fused foot with ten toes and more severe defect presenting with a more rudimentary foot and ectromelia. Because the legs are fused, the rotation of the legs does not occur, and they remain in their fetal position. Thus, the fibulas, when present, are between the tibia, and the sole of the foot is oriented *ventrally* instead of *dorsally.*

The fused extremity and the flipper-like deformity of the foot are characteristic of sirenomelia.

Associated Anomalies

Cardiac, renal, abdominal wall, chest, and lower spine defects are frequently seen. Single umbilical artery, imperforate anus, and absence of the genitals are commonly found.

Differential Diagnosis

Caudal regression syndrome is the main differential diagnosis, and it usually presents with milder deformities compared to sirenomelia and normal amniotic fluid volume. Due to the bilateral renal agenesis, fetuses affected by sirenomelia frequently have Potter's facies. Power Doppler can help in assessing the absence of distal branching of the main abdominal vessel, which is a characteristic feature of sirenomelia.[174] The fusion of the lower extremities, present in sirenomelia, makes the differential diagnosis. Other conditions that should be excluded are Fraser's syndrome and VATER complex (*v*ertebral defects, imperforate *a*nus, *t*rache*oe*sophageal fistula, *r*enal defects).

Prognosis

Sirenomelia is a lethal condition due to the associated renal agenesis and its complications. Exceptional cases present without renal agenesis and may survive.

Recurrence Risk

Sirenomelia is sporadic. The recurrence risk is unknown.

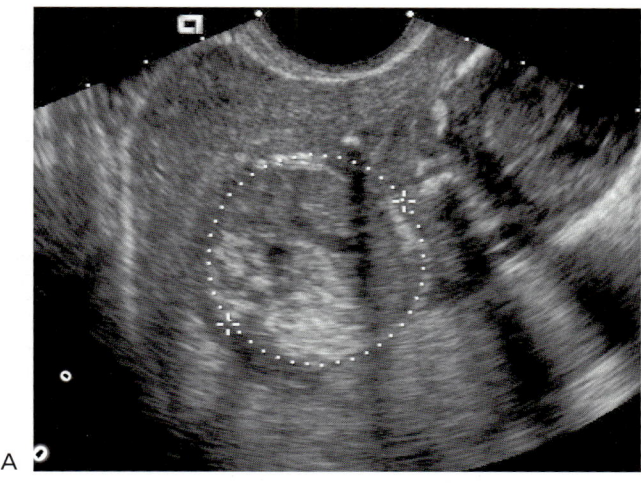
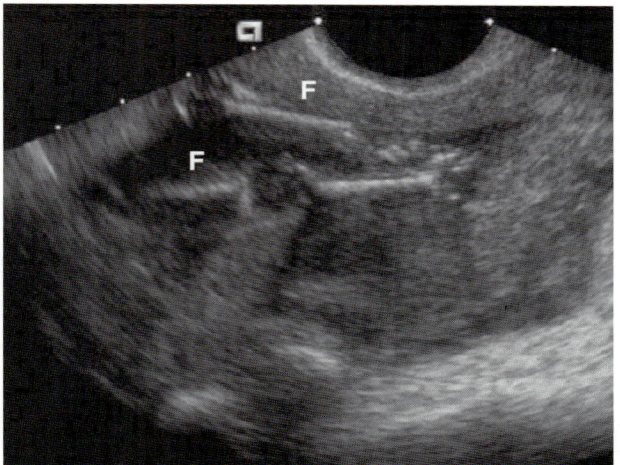
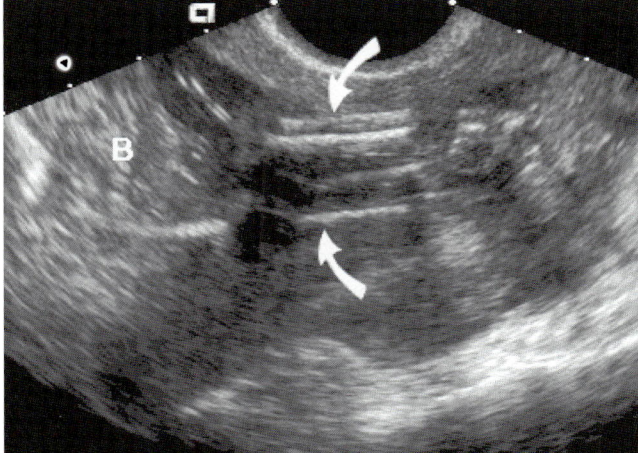
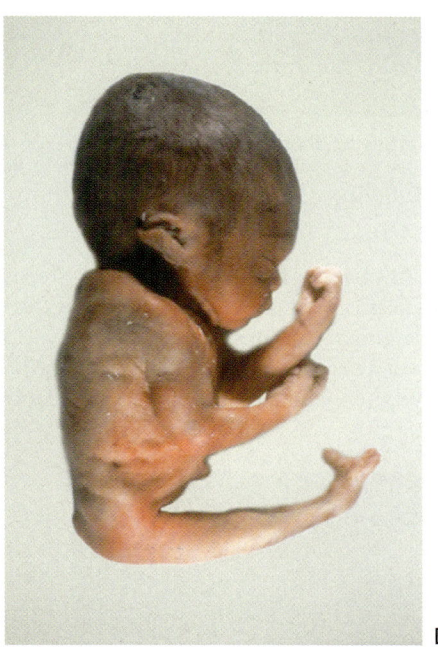

FIGURE 44. Sirenomelia. **A:** Transverse view of abdomen shows marked oligohydramnios secondary to renal agenesis. **B:** The femurs (*F*) are apposed to one another, and the knees are extended. **C:** View of lower leg shows tibias and fibulas are close to one another (*arrows*). Some cases show absence of one or more bones. B, body. **D:** Pathologic correlation. (Copyright, Phillippe Jeanty, reproduced with permission from http://www.TheFetus.net.)

Thanatophoric Dysplasia

A synonym for thanatophoric dysplasia is thanatophoric dwarfism.[174]

Thanatophoric dysplasia is a lethal congenital form of short-limbed chondrodysplasia, divided into two subtypes (Figs. 45 and 46)[175]:

- *Type I* is characterized by extreme rhizomelia, bowed long bones, narrow thorax, a relatively large head, normal trunk length, and absent cloverleaf skull. The spine shows platyspondyly, the cranium has a short base, and, frequently, the foramen magnum is decreased in size. The forehead is prominent, and hypertelorism and a saddle nose may be present. Hands and feet are normal, but fingers are short.
- *Type II* is characterized by short, straight long bones and cloverleaf skull.[176]

Incidence

The incidence is 0.69 per 10,000; M2:F1.[1]

Genetic Defect

Thanatophoric dysplasia results from mutations of the FGFR3.[177]

Pathogenesis

Thanatophoric dysplasia involves characteristic generalized disruption of growth plate with persistent mesenchymal-like tissue.[178]

Diagnosis

Sonographic measurement of fetal femur length, especially when correlated with biparietal diameter, is a reliable

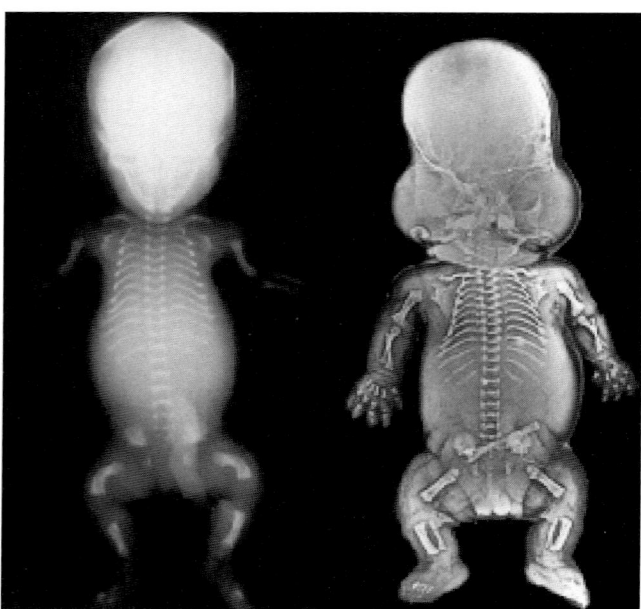

FIGURE 45. The two types of thanatophoric dysplasia. Type I **(A)** shows bowed femurs, and type II **(B)** shows straight femurs and cloverleaf skull deformity.

method in the identification of certain forms of short-limbed skeletal dysplasias, including thanatophoric dysplasia.[179] Sonographic diagnosis can be suspected on the basis of severe short-limbed dwarfism and a narrow thorax.[175] Femur bowing and redundant soft tissues (Fig. 47) become

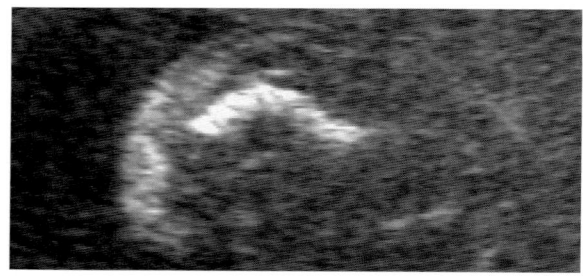

A

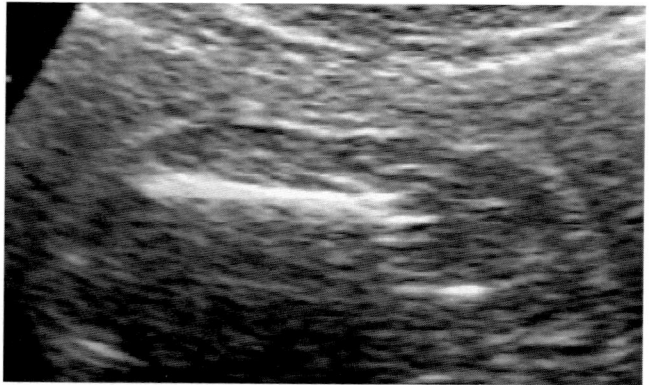

B

FIGURE 46. Thanatophoric dysplasia. Sonographic appearance of femur in type I **(A)** and type II **(B)**.

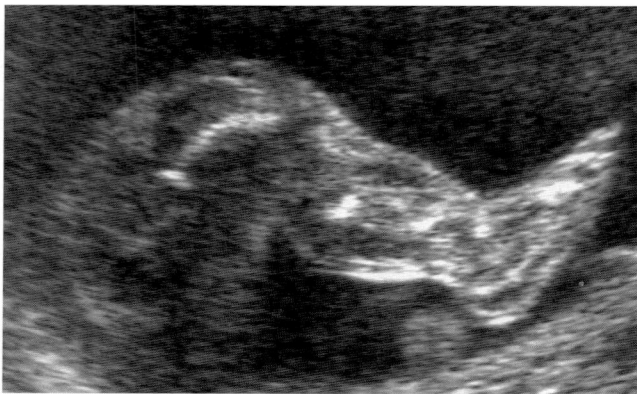

FIGURE 47. Thanatophoric dysplasia, type I. View of lower leg shows bowed femur and redundant soft tissue.

more pronounced with advancing gestation and may not be present in midtrimester.

Cloverleaf skull deformity (Figs. 48 and 49) is characteristic of type II thanatophoric dysplasia. The cloverleaf skull deformity becomes more pronounced with advancing gestational age. Progressive hydrocephalus is often present with cloverleaf skull deformity secondary to obstruction. In either type, the head is elongated, the forehead prominent, and frontal bossing is evident (Fig. 50). The hypoplastic thorax (Fig. 51) is typically obvious. Platyspondyly may also be evident (Fig. 52).

Polyhydramnios frequently develops during the third trimester, and it may precipitate premature labor. Fetal movements do not seem to be affected by the disease, but a decrease in motion during the third trimester has been reported. Decreased hand flexure is probably responsible for the presence of simian crease. A trident appearance of the hand with separation of the third and fourth digits with thanatophoric dysplasia has been observed in several cases (Fig. 48C).

Associated Anomalies

Hydrocephalus, renal abnormalities, atrial septal defect, defective tricuspid valve, imperforate anus, and radioulnar synostosis are associated anomalies.

Differential Diagnosis

Differential diagnoses include chondroectodermal dysplasia (Ellis-van Creveld syndrome), asphyxiating thoracic dysplasia, short rib–polydactyly syndrome, and homozygous achondroplasia. All short-limbed dwarfism should be considered. If type II is suspected, conditions that have association with craniosynostosis and cloverleaf skull should be excluded (Apert syndrome, Crouzon disease, Pfeiffer syndrome, Carpenter syndrome, and kleeblattschädel syndrome).

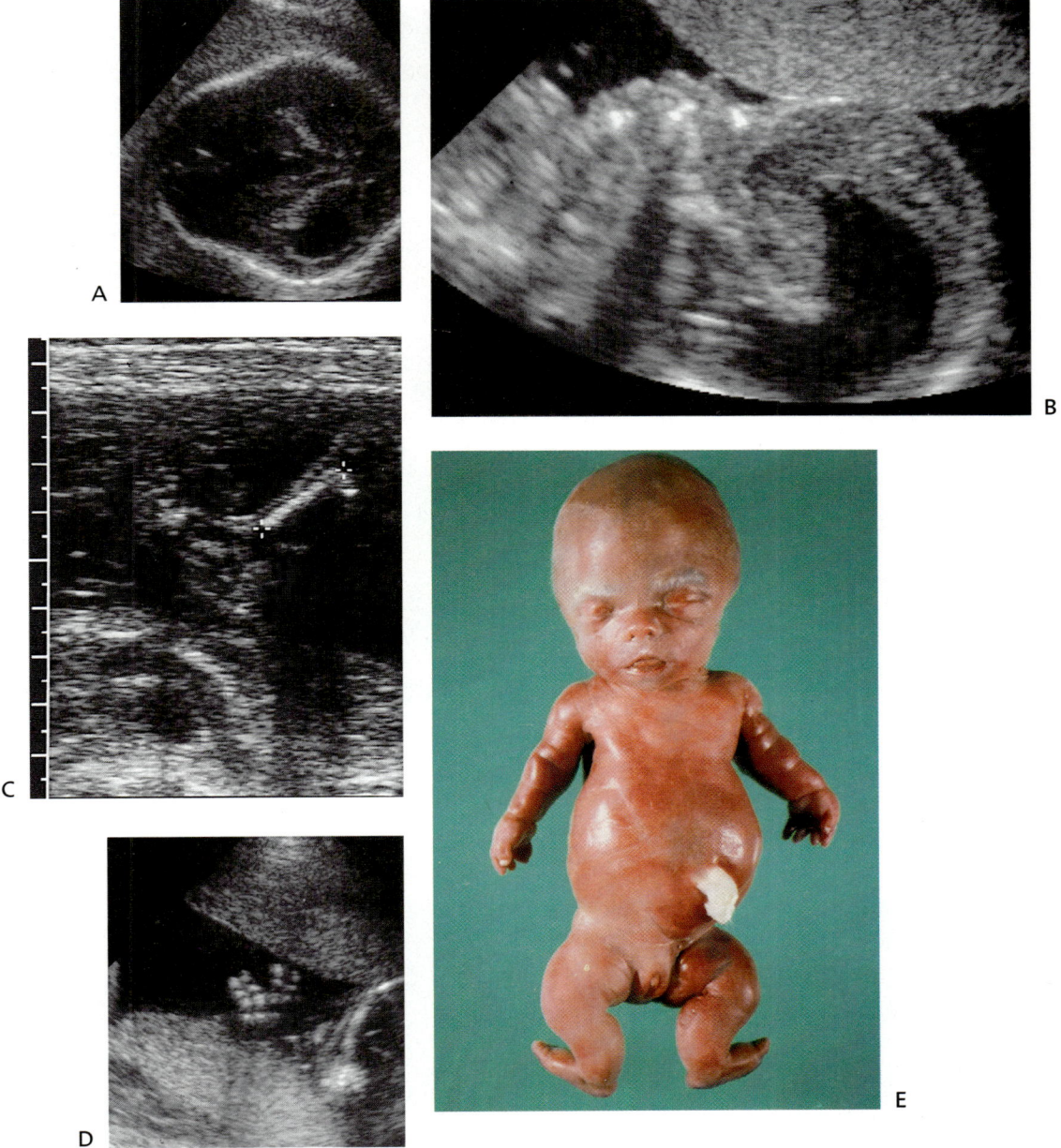

FIGURE 48. Thanatophoric dysplasia, type II. **A:** Transverse view of head shows hydrocephalus and unusual head shape. **B:** Profile view shows vertical elongation of calvaria, bulging forehead, and frontal bossing. **C:** The tibia is short but straight. Note that the foot is longer than the tibia. **D:** View of hand shows separation of digits. **E:** Pathologic correlation.

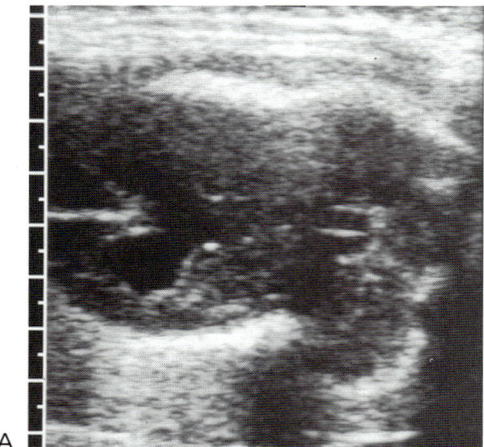

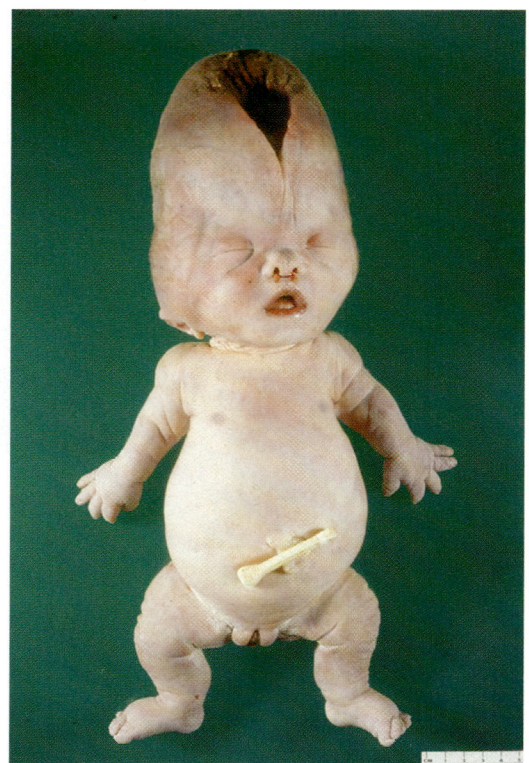

FIGURE 49. Thanatophoric dysplasia with cloverleaf skull. **A:** Transverse view of head shows markedly abnormal head shape with hydrocephalus. **B:** Pathologic correlation shows severe cloverleaf skull deformity.

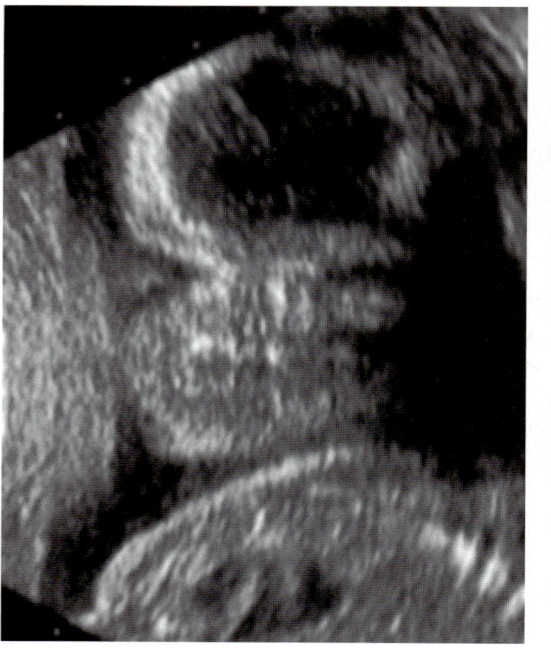

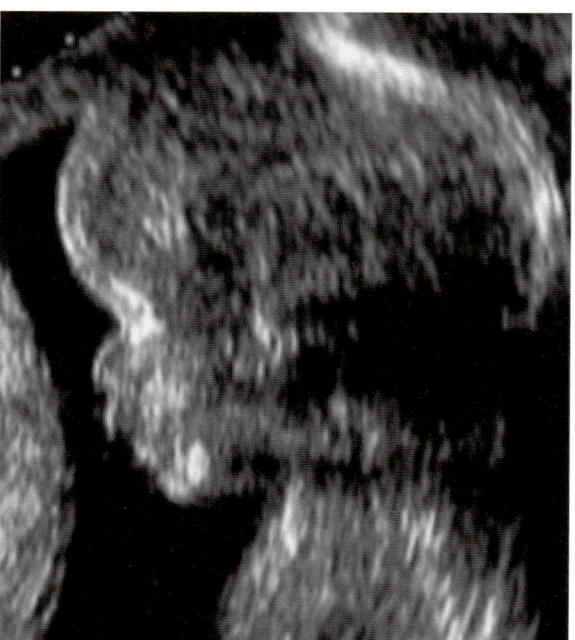

FIGURE 50. Thanatophoric dysplasia with frontal bossing. Coronal **(A)** and profile **(B)** views show frontal bossing in an affected fetus.

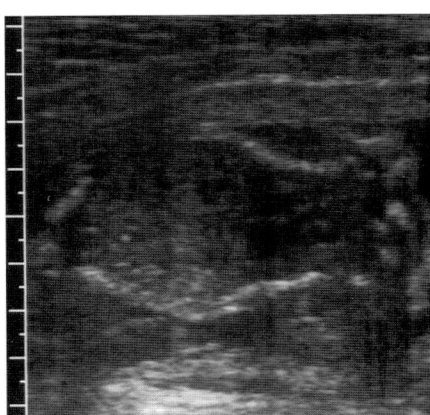

FIGURE 51. Thanatophoric dysplasia with hypoplastic thorax. Longitudinal view shows small chest compared to the abdomen, with a diameter approximately half as large as that of the abdomen. This results from the short ribs and is the cause of pulmonary hypoplasia.

Prognosis and Management

Thanatophoric dysplasia is a uniformly lethal condition, and, in general, affected fetuses die shortly after birth.[178] The cause of death is respiratory failure owing to hypoplastic lungs. If massive hydrocephalus is developed, cephalocentesis and/or elective cesarean section should be considered to avoid maternal trauma.[175]

Recurrence Risk

Thanatophoric dysplasia is possibly autosomal dominant, but the majority of cases result from new mutations. A general empiric risk was estimated in 2%.[180]

Thrombocytopenia–Absent Radius Syndrome

Synonyms for thrombocytopenia–absent radius syndrome are TAR syndrome, megakaryocytopenia–absent radius, and radial aplasia–thrombocytopenia syndrome.[181]

Thrombocytopenia–absent radius syndrome is a congenital disorder described by Gross in 1956,[182] although Hall et al.[183] gave the name and acronym to this syndrome. Characterized by bilateral radial aplasia (Fig. 53) with normal thumbs and thrombocytopenia at a level less than 100,000 per mm³. Other anomalies may include skeletal defects of upper and lower extremities such as ulnar, humeral, and femoral hypoplasia; congenital hip dislocation; toe syndactyly; talipes equinovarus; and genu varum.[184] Cardiac (30% of the cases) and renal defects may be found. Thrombocytopenia, anemia, and eosinophilia may be found.

Incidence

Thrombocytopenia–absent radius syndrome is uncommon.

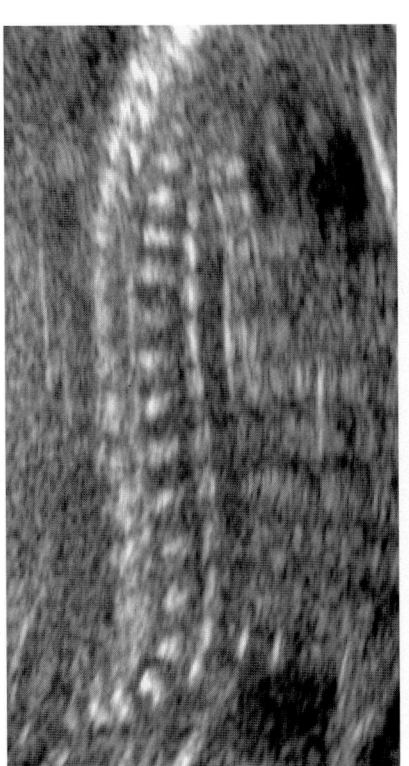
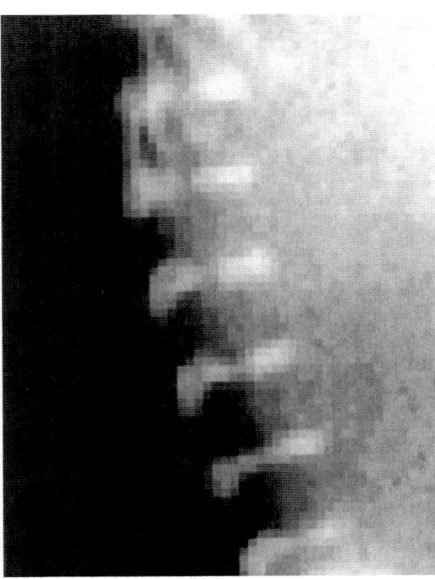

A,B

FIGURE 52. Thanatophoric dysplasia with platyspondyly. **A:** Longitudinal scan of spine shows that the disk interspace is larger than the height of the vertebral bodies. **B:** Radiograph of spine at 19 weeks shows flattened vertebral bodies.

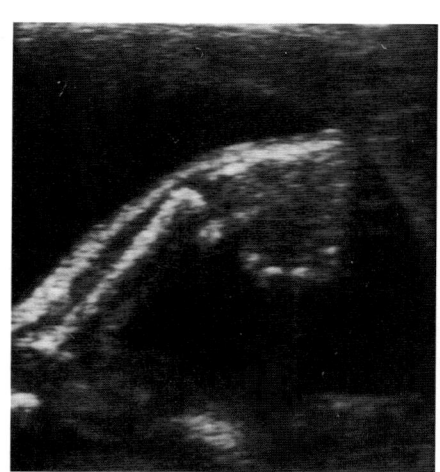
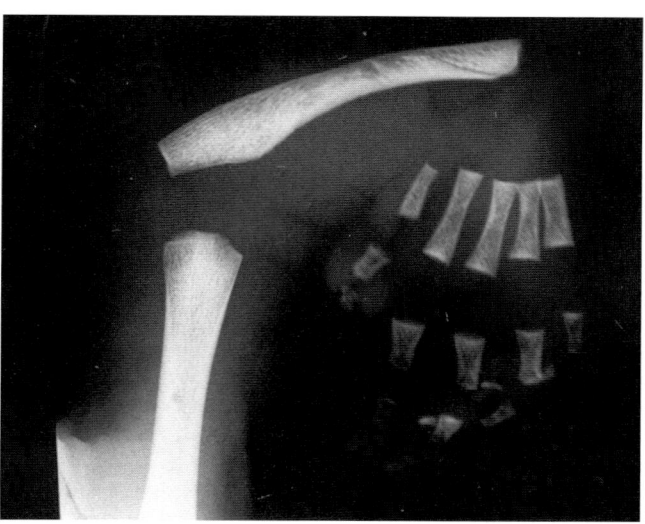

FIGURE 53. Radial aplasia. **A:** View of upper extremity shows characteristic features of radial aplasia with marked medial rotation of the hand and wrist, as may be seen with thrombocytopenia–absent radius syndrome. **B:** Correlation with radiograph after birth.

Genetic Defect

The genetic defect is not known.

Diagnosis

The major finding is that of bilateral club hand due to missing radii (see Fig. 12 in Chapter 20). In some cases the abnormal position of the hands has been detected in the first trimester.[185] When cardiac and renal anomalies are present, oligohydramnios may develop during the second trimester, making the evaluation of the limbs more difficult. Three-dimensional ultrasound has been used.[186]

Thrombocytopenia can be confirmed using cordocentesis.[187–189] Fetoscopy has also been used.[190]

Differential Diagnosis

The primary differential diagnoses of radial ray defect are listed in Table 9. Trisomies must be excluded, especially trisomy 18. There is wide overlap between thrombocytopenia–absent radius syndrome and Roberts syndrome. Other differential diagnoses include Holt-Oram syndrome, Fanconi pancytopenia, and VATER association among others (Table 9).

Prognosis

Forty percent of the affected live births die during early infancy.[191] Hemorrhage and heart disease are the main causes of death. Seven percent have mental impairment. Motor developmental retardation is expected due to the skeletal defects. Hematologic profile improves with age. The prognosis improves after the first year of age. An increased susceptibility to infections is also observed.

Management

Termination of pregnancy can be offered before viability. The infusion of platelet has been advocated before delivery to prevent hemorrhages at this time.[192] Cesarean section is recommended to prevent intracranial hemorrhage of the fetus. Postnatally, transplantation of allogeneic bone marrow from histocompatible sibling may correct persistently low platelet count.[193] The use of adaptive devices for feeding, dressing, and using the toilet, as well as powered mobility aids, is usually better for the function than surgical interventions.[194]

TABLE 9. MAJOR DIFFERENTIAL DIAGNOSIS OF RADIAL RAY DEFECTS

Cornelia de Lange syndrome	Facial defects, growth restriction, and mental retardation
Fanconi syndrome	Absent thumbs, tendency for leukemia
Holt-Oram syndrome	Upper extremity abnormalities, heart defects
Nager syndrome	Mandibular hypoplasia, malformed ears
Roberts syndrome	Severe shortening of limbs, facial anomalies
Thrombocytopenia–absent radius syndrome	Thrombocytopenia, thumb always present
Trisomy 18	Multiple anomalies, clenched hand, craniofacial defects, growth restriction and mental retardation, abnormal hands and feet
Trisomy 13	Multiple malformations, facial defects, vertebral defects, anal atresia
VATER association	Vertebral defects, anal atresia, tracheoesophageal fistula, radial and renal dysplasias

Reproduced with permission from Tongsong T, Sirichotiyakul S, Chanprapaph P. Prenatal diagnosis of thrombocytopenia-absent-radius (TAR) syndrome. *Ultrasound Obstet Gynecol* 2000;15:256–258.

Recurrence Risk

Thrombocytopenia-absent radius is autosomal recessive (recurrence risk, 25%).

REFERENCES

1. Romero R, Pilu G, Jeanty P, et al. *Prenatal diagnosis of congenital anomalies.* Norwalk: Appleton & Lange, 1988:311–384.
2. Trnavsky K. Pyknodysostosis (Maroteaux-Lamy)—disease of the painter Toulouse-Lautrec 1864–1901. *Cas Lek Cesk* 1974;113:1493–1494.
3. Czeizel E. The Toulouse-Lautrec syndrome. *Orv Hetil* 1974;115:2135–2138.
4. Maroteaux P. Toulouse-Lautrec's diagnosis. *Nat Genet* 1995;11:362–363.
5. Polymeropoulos MH, Ortiz De Luna RI, Ide SE, Torres R, Rubenstein J, et al. The gene for pyknodysostosis maps to human chromosome 1cen-q21. *Nat Genet* 1995;10:238–239.
6. Sadler TW. Skeletal system (skull, limbs, vertebral column). In: *Langman's medical embryology*, text ed. Baltimore: Williams & Wilkins, 1990:139–156.
7. Camera G, Mastroiacovo P. Birth prevalence of skeletal dysplasias in the Italian multicentric monitoring system for birth defects. In: Papadatos CJ, Bartsocas CS, eds. *Skeletal dysplasias.* New York: Alan R. Liss, 1982:441–449.
8. Connor JM, Connor RAC, Sweet EM, et al. Lethal neonatal chondrodysplasias in the West of Scotland 1970–1983 with a description of a thanatophoric, dysplasialike, autosomal recessive disorder, Glasgow variant. *Am J Med Genet* 1985;22:243–253.
9. Doray B, Favre R, Viville B, Langer B, Dreyfus M, et al. Prenatal sonographic diagnosis of skeletal dysplasias. A report of 47 cases. *Ann Genet* 2000;43:163–169.
10. Manouvrier-Hanu S, Devisme L, Zelasko MC, Bourgeot P, Vincent-Delorme C, et al. Prenatal diagnosis of metatropic dwarfism. *Prenat Diagn* 1995;15:753–756.
11. Stewart PA, Wallerstein R, Moran E, Lee MJ. Early prenatal ultrasound diagnosis of cleidocranial dysplasia. *Ultrasound Obstet Gynecol* 2000;15:154–156.
12. Campbell J, Henderson A, Campbell S. The fetal femur/foot length ratio: a new parameter to assess dysplastic limb reduction. *Obstet Gynecol* 1989;72:181.
13. Hershey DW. The fetal femur/foot length ratio: a new parameter to assess dysplastic limb reduction. *Obstet Gynecol* 1989;73:682.
14. Pilu G, Romero R, Reece EA, et al. The prenatal diagnosis of Robin anomalad. *Am J Obstet Gynecol* 1986;154:630.
15. Benacerraf BR, Greene MF, Barss VA. Prenatal sonographic diagnosis of congenital hemivertebra. *J Ultrasound Med* 1986;5:257.
16. Goncalves L, Jeanty P. Fetal biometry of skeletal dysplasias: a multicentric study. *J Ultrasound Med* 1994;13:977–985.
17. Reprinted with permission from Silva and Jeanty at http://www.TheFetus.net.
18. Superti-Furga A. A defect in the metabolic activation of sulfate in a patient with achondrogenesis type IB. *Am J Hum Genet* 1994;55:1137–1145.
19. Superti-Furga A, Hastbacka J, Cohn DH, Wilcox W, van der Harten HJ, et al. Defective sulfation of proteoglycans in achondrogenesis type IB is caused by mutations in the DTDST gene: the disorder is allelic to diastrophic dysplasia. *Am J Hum Genet* 1995;57:A48(abst).
20. Superti-Furga A, Hastbacka J, Wilcox WR, Cohn DH, van der Harten HJ, et al. Achondrogenesis type IB is caused by mutations in the diastrophic dysplasia sulphate transporter gene. *Nat Genet* 1996;12:100–102.
21. Rittler M, Orioli IM. Achondrogenesis type II with polydactyly. *Am J Med Genet* 1995;59:157–160.
22. Spranger J. Pattern recognition in bone dysplasias. In: Papadatos CJ, Bartsocas CS, Spranger J, eds. *Endocrine genetics and genetics of growth.* New York: Alan R. Liss, 1985:315–342.
23. Stanescu V, Stanescu R, Maroteaux P. Etude morphologique et biochimique du cartilage de croissance dans les osteochondrodysplasies. *Arch Fr Pediatr* 1977;34:1–80.
24. Parenti GC. La anosteogenesi (una varieta della osteogenesi imperfetta). *Pathologica* 1936;28:447–462.
25. Fraccaro M. Contributo allo studio delle malattie del mesenchima osteopoietico: l'acondrogenesi. *Folia Hered Path* 1952;1:190–208.
26. Maroteaux P, Lamy M. Le diagnostic des nanismes chondro-dystrophiques chez les nouveau-nes. *Arch Fr Pediatr* 1968;25:241–262.
27. Langer LO Jr, Spranger JW, Greinacher I, Herdman RC. Thanatophoric dwarfism: a condition confused with achondroplasia in the neonate, with brief comments on achondrogenesis and homozygous achondroplasia. *Radiology* 1969;92:285–294.
28. Velinov M, Slaugenhaupt SA, Stoilov I, Scott CI Jr, Gusella JF, et al. The gene for achondroplasia maps to the telomeric region of chromosome 4p. *Nat Genet* 1994;6:318–321.
29. Le Merrer M, Rousseau F, Legeai-Mallet L, Landais J-C, Pelet A, et al. A gene for achondroplasia—hypochondroplasia maps to chromosome 4p. *Nat Genet* 1994;6:314–317.
30. Bellus GA, Hefferon TW, Ortiz de Luna RI, Hecht JT, Horton WA, et al. Achondroplasia is defined by recurrent G380R mutations of FGFR3. *Am J Hum Genet* 1995;56:368–373.
31. Moeglin D, Benoit B. Three-dimensional sonographic aspects in the antenatal diagnosis of achondroplasia. *Ultrasound Obstet Gynecol* 2001;18:81–83.
32. Saito H, Sekizawa A, Morimoto T, Suzuki M, Yanaihara T. Prenatal DNA diagnosis of a single-gene disorder from maternal plasma. *Lancet* 2000;356:1170.
33. http://www.lpaonline.org/welcome.html.
34. Reprinted with permission from Silva and Jeanty at http://www.TheFetus.net.
35. Reprinted with permission from Silva and Jeanty at www.TheFetus.net.
36. Ferraz FG, Maroteaux P, Sousa JP, Alves T, Dias I, et al. Acromesomelic dwarfism: a new variation. *J Pediatr Orthop B* 1997;6:27–32.
37. Campailla E, Maroteaux P. Acromesomelic dwarfism: Maroteaux-Martinelli-Campailla type. *Basic Life Sci* 1988;48:177–178.
38. Stichelbout P, Pratz R, Lemaitre G, Wemeau-Jacquemont C, Maroteaux P, et al. Acromesomelic dysplasia. Apropos of a new case. *Arch Fr Pediatr* 1984;41:487–489.

39. Hall CM, Stoker DJ, Robinson DC, Wilkinson DJ. Acromesomelic dwarfism. *Br J Radiol* 1980;53:999–1003.

40. Hunter AG, Thompson MW. Acromesomelic dwarfism: description of a patient and comparison with previously reported cases. *Hum Genet* 1976;34:107–113.

41. Danda S, Phadke SR, Agarwal SS. Acromesomelic dwarfism: report of a family with two affected siblings. *Indian Pediatr* 1997;34:1127–1130.

42. Borrelli P, Fasanelli S, Marini R. Acromesomelic dwarfism in a child with an interesting family history. *Pediatr Radiol* 1983;13:165–158.

43. Pallister PD. A 59-year-old multiparous woman with acromesomelic dwarfism. *Am J Med Genet* 1978;1:343–346.

44. Langer LO Jr, Beals RK, Solomon IL, Bard PA, Bard LA, et al. Acromesomelic dwarfism: manifestations in childhood. *Am J Med Genet* 1977;1:87–100.

45. Magann EF, Ray MA, Shenefelt RE, Chauhan SP, Roberts WE, et al. Amelia. *The Fetus* 1993;3:6.

46. Froster-Iskenius UG, Baird PA. Amelia: incidence and associated defects in a large population. *Teratology* 1990;41:23–31.

47. Ohdo-S, Madokoro-H, Sonoda-T, et al. Association of tetraamelia, ectodermal dysplasia, hypoplastic lacrimal ducts and sacs opening towards the exterior, peculiar face, and developmental retardation. *J Med Genet* 1987;24:609–612.

48. Pauli-RM, Feldman-PF. Major limb malformations following intrauterine exposure to ethanol: two additional cases and literature review. *Teratology* 1986;33:273–280.

49. Milaire J. Histological changes induced in developing limb buds of C57BL mouse embryos submitted in utero to the combined influence of acetazolamide and cadmium sulphate. *Teratology* 1985;32:433–451.

50. Rijhsinghani A, Yankowitz J, Mazursky J, Williamson R. Prenatal ultrasound diagnosis of amelia. *Prenat Diagn* 1995;15:655–659.

51. Modified with permission from Silva and Jeanty at http://www.TheFetus.net.

52. Lammens M, Moerman P, Fryns JP, Lemmens F, van de Kamp GM, et al. Fetal akinesia sequence caused by nemaline myopathy. *Neuropediatrics* 1997;28:116–119.

53. Hyett J, Noble P, Sebire NJ, Snijders R, Nicolaides KH. Lethal congenital arthrogryposis presents with increased nuchal translucency at 10–14 weeks of gestation. *Ultrasound Obstet Gynecol* 1997;9:310–313.

54. Ajayi RA, Keen CE, Knott PD. Ultrasound diagnosis of the Pena Shokeir phenotype at 14 weeks of pregnancy. *Prenat Diagn* 1995;15:762–764.

55. Skupski DW, Sepulveda W, Udom-Rice I, Leo MV, Lescale KB, et al. Fetal seizures: further observations. *Obstet Gynecol* 1996;88:663–665.

56. Modified with permission from Silva and Jeanty at http://www.TheFetus.net.

57. Ben Ami M, Perlitz Y, Haddad S, Matilsky M. Increased nuchal translucency is associated with asphyxiating thoracic dysplasia. *Ultrasound Obstet Gynecol* 1997;10:297–298.

58. Chen CP, Lin SP, Liu FF, Jan SW, Lin SY, et al. Prenatal diagnosis of asphyxiating thoracic dysplasia (Jeune syndrome). *Am J Perinatol* 1996;13:495–498.

59. Skiptunas SM, Weiner S. Early prenatal diagnosis of asphyxiating thoracic dysplasia (Jeune's syndrome). Value of fetal thoracic measurement. *J Ultrasound Med* 1987;6:41–43.

60. Meinel K, Himmel D. Status of ultrasound and roentgen diagnosis in prenatal detection of osteochondrodysplasias. *Zentralbl Gynakol* 1987;109:1303–1313.

61. Schinzel A, Savoldelli G, Briner J, Schubiger G. Prenatal sonographic diagnosis of Jeune syndrome. *Radiology* 1985;154:777–778.

62. Hopper MS, Boultbee JE, Watson AR. Polyhydramnios associated with congenital pancreatic cysts and asphyxiating thoracic dysplasia. A case report. *S Afr Med J* 1979;56:32–33.

63. Modified with permission from Silva and Jeanty at http://www.TheFetus.net.

64. Buyse ML. *Birth defects encyclopedia.* Dover, MA: Blackwell Science, 1990:252–253.

65. Valcamonico A, Jeanty P. Camptomelic dysplasia. *The Fetus* 2000;5:7544–7551.

66. Khajavi A, Lachman R, Rimoin N, et al. Heterogeneity in the camptomelic syndromes. Long and short bone varieties. *Radiology* 1976;120:641–647.

67. Urioste M, Arroyo A, Martinez-Frias ML. Camptomelia, polycystic dysplasia and cervical lymphocele in two sibs. *Am J Med Genet* 1991;41:475–477.

68. Foster JW, et al. Camptomelic dysplasia and autosomal sex reversal caused by mutations in an SRY-related gene. *Nature* 1994;372:525.

69. Caffey J. Prenatal bowing and thickening of tubular bones with multiple cutaneous dimples in arms and legs: a congenital syndrome of mechanical origin. *Am J Dis Child* 1947;74:543–562.

70. Middleton DS. Studies of prenatal lesions of striated muscle as a cause of congenital deformities. *Edinburgh Med J* 1934;41:401–442.

71. Snure H. Intrauterine fracture. *Radiology* 1929;13:362–365.

72. Bain AD, Barrett HS. Congenital bowing of the long bones: report of a case. *Arch Dis Child* 1959;34:516–524.

73. Lee FA, Isaacs H, Strauss J. The "camptomelic" syndrome. *Am J Dis Child* 1972;124:485–496.

74. Huston CS, Opiz JM, Spranger JW, et al. The camptomelic syndrome: review, report of 17 cases, and follow-up on the currently 17-year-old boy first reported by Maroteaux et al. in 1971. *Am J Med Genet* 1983;15:3–28.

75. Cordone M, Lituania M, Zampatti C, et al. In utero ultrasonographic features of camptomelic dysplasia. *Prenat Diagn* 1989;9:745–750.

76. Romero R, Pilu G, Jeanty P, et al. *Prenatal diagnosis of congenital anomalies.* Norwalk: Appleton & Lange, 1988.

77. Maroteaux P, Spranger J, Opiz JM, et al. Le syndrome camptomelique. *Presse Med* 1971;79:1157–1162.

78. Benacerraf BR. *Camptomelic dysplasia in ultrasound of fetal syndromes.* New York: Churchill Livingstone, 1998:168–169.

79. Silva S, Jeanty P. Caudal regression syndrome. http://www.TheFetus.net.

80. Jaffe R, Zeituni M, Fejgin M. Caudal regression syndrome. *Fetus, Spinal Anomalies* 1991;7561:1–3.

81. Jones KL. Caudal dysplasia sequence. In: *Smith's recognizable patterns of human malformation.* Philadelphia: WB Saunders, 1998:635.

82. Benacerraf BR. *Caudal regression syndrome and sirenomelia in ultrasound of fetal syndromes.* New York: Churchill Livingstone, 1998:250–254.

83. Tsugu H, Fukushima T, Oshiro S, Tomonaga M, Utsunomiya H, et al. A case report of caudal regression syndrome associated with an intraspinal arachnoid cyst. *Pediatr Neurosurg* 1999;31:207–212.

84. Ellis RWB, van Creveld S. A syndrome characterized by ectodermal dysplasia, polydactyly, chondro-dysplasia and congenital morbus cordis: report of three cases. *Arch Dis Child* 1940;15:65–84.

85. Sergi C, Voigtlander T, Zoubaa S, Hentze S, Meyberg-Solomeyer G, et al. Ellis-van Creveld syndrome: a generalized dysplasia of enchondral ossification. *Pediatr Radiol* 2001;31:289–293.

86. Polymeropoulos MH, Ide SE, Wright M, Goodship J, Weissenbach J, et al. The gene for the Ellis-van Creveld syndrome is located on chromosome 4p16. *Genomics* 1996;35:1–5.

87. Ruiz-Perez VL, Ide SE, Strom TM, Lorenz B, Wilson D, et al. Mutations in a new gene in Ellis-van Creveld syndrome and Weyers acrodental dysostosis. *Nat Genet* 2000;24:283–286. Erratum: *Nat Genet* 25:125.

88. Tongsong T, Chanprapaph P. Prenatal sonographic diagnosis of Ellis-van Creveld syndrome. *J Clin Ultrasound* 2000;28:38–41.

89. Horigome H, Hamada H, Sohda S, Oyake Y, Kurosaki Y. Prenatal ultrasonic diagnosis of a case of Ellis-van Creveld syndrome with a single atrium. *Pediatr Radiol* 1997;27:942–944.

90. Dugoff L, Thieme G, Hobbins JC. First trimester prenatal diagnosis of chondroectodermal dysplasia (Ellis-van Creveld syndrome) with ultrasound. *Ultrasound Obstet Gynecol* 2001;17:86–88.

91. Torrente I, Mangino M, De Luca A, Mingarelli R, Gennarelli M, et al. First-trimester prenatal diagnosis of Ellis-van Creveld syndrome using linked microsatellite markers. *Prenat Diagn* 1998;18:504–506.

92. Yang SS, Langer LO Jr, Cacciarelli A, Dahms BB, Unger ER, et al. Three conditions in neonatal asphyxiating thoracic dysplasia (Jeune) and short rib-polydactyly syndrome spectrum: a clinicopathologic study. *Am J Med Genet* 1987;3[Suppl]:191–207.

93. Yapar EG, Ekici E, Aydogdu T, Senses E, Gokmen O. Diagnostic problems in a case with mucometrocolpos, polydactyly, congenital heart disease, and skeletal dysplasia. *Am J Med Genet* 1996;66:343–346.

94. Furness ME, Haan EA, Hopkins PB, Chambers HM. Chondrodysplasia punctata, mild symmetric type with echogenic coccyx in a 15 week fetus. Available at: http://www.TheFetus.net. Accessed September 14, 2002.

95. Schutgens RBH, Heymans HSA, Wanders RJA, et al. Peroxisomal disorders: a newly recognized group of genetic diseases. *Eur J Pediatr* 1986;144:430–440.

96. Manzke H, Christophers E, Wiedemann HR. Dominant sex-linked inherited chondrodysplasia punctata. *Clin Genet* 1980;17:97–107.

97. Curry CJR, Magenis RE, Brown M, et al. Inherited chondrodysplasia punctata due to a deletion of the terminal short arm of an X chromosome. *N Engl J Med* 1984;311:1010–1015.

98. Spranger JW, Opitz JM, Bidder U. Heterogeneity of chondrodysplasia punctata. *Humangenetik* 1971;11:190–212.

99. Silengo MC, Luzzatti L, Silverman FN. Clinical and genetic aspects of Conradi-Hunermann disease: a report of three familial cases and review of the literature. *J Pediatr* 1980;97:911–917.

100. Sheffield LJ, Danks DM, Mayne V, et al. Chondrodysplasia punctata—23 cases of a mild and relatively common variety. *J Pediatr* 1976;89:916–923.

101. Maxillo-nasal dysplasia (Binder syndrome). In: Gorlin RJ, Pindborg JJ, Cohen MM, eds. *Syndromes of the head and neck*, 2nd ed. New York: McGraw-Hill, 1976:463–464.

102. Duff P, Harlass FE, Milligan DA. Prenatal diagnosis of chondrodysplasia punctata by sonography. *Obstet Gynecol* 1990;76:497–500.

103. Romero R, Pilu G, Jeanty P, et al. Prenatal diagnosis of congenital anomalies. Norwalk: Appleton & Lange, 1988:311–351.

104. Straub W, Zarabi M, Mazer J. Fetal ascites associated with Conradi's disease (chondrodysplasia punctata): report of a case. *J Clin Ultrasound* 1983;11:234–236.

105. Lammer EJ, Cordero JF, Wilson MJ, et al. *Investigation of a suspected increased prevalence of craniosynostosis—Colorado, 1978–1982.* Proc. Greenwood Genet. Ctr. 6, 126–127; Document EPI-83-56-2, Public Health Service, Centers for Disease Control and Prevention, Atlanta 1987 Apr 8:7.

106. Pooh RK, Nakagawa Y, Pooh KH, Nakagawa Y, Nagamachi N. Fetal craniofacial structure and intracranial morphology in a case of Apert syndrome. *Ultrasound Obstet Gynecol* 1999;13:274–280.

107. Lyu KJ, Ko TM. Prenatal diagnosis of Apert syndrome with widely separated cranial sutures. *Prenat Diagn* 2000;20:254–256.

108. Benacerraf BR, Spiro R, Mitchell A. Using three-dimensional ultrasound to detect craniosynostosis in a fetus with Pfeiffer syndrome. *Ultrasound Obstet Gynecol* 2000;16:391–394.

109. Patton MA, Goodship J, Hayward R, et al. Intellectual development in Aperts syndrome: a long-term follow up of 29 patients. *Med Genet* 1988;25:164–167.

110. Gershoni-Baruch R. Carpenter syndrome: marked variability of expression to include the Summitt and Goodman syndromes. *Am J Med Genet* 1990;35:236–240.

111. Whitley CB, Langer LO, Ophoven J, et al. Fibrochondrogenesis: lethal, autosomal recessive chondrodysplasia with distinctive cartilage histopathology. *Am J Med Genet* 1984;19:265.

112. Chevernak FA, Isaacson G, Rosenberg JC, et al. Antenatal diagnosis of frontal cephalocele in a fetus with atelosteogenesis. *J Ultrasound Med* 1986;5:111.

113. Modified with permission from Silva and Jeanty at http://www.TheFetus.net.

114. Mornet E, Taillandier A, Peyramaure S, Kaper F, Muller F, et al. Identification of fifteen novel mutations in the tissue-nonspecific alkaline phosphatase (TNSALP) gene in European patients with severe hypophosphatasia. *Eur J Hum Genet* 1998;6:308–314.

115. DeLange M, Rouse GA. Prenatal diagnosis of hypophosphatasia. *J Ultrasound Med* 1990;9:115–117.

116. Goldstein DJ, Nichols WC, Mirkin LD. Short-limbed osteochondrodysplasia with osteochondral spurs of knee and elbow joints (spur-limbed dwarfism). *Dysmorph Clin Genet* 1987;1:12–16.

117. Spranger J. 'Spur-limbed' dwarfism identified as hypophosphatasia [Letter]. *Dysmorph Clin Genet* 1988;2:123.

118. Vandevijver N, De Die-Smulders CEM, Offermans JPM, Van Der Linden ES, Arends JW, et al. Lethal hypophosphatasia, spur type: case report and fetopathological study. *Genet Counsel* 1998;9:205–209.

119. Tongsong T, Pongsatha S. Early prenatal sonographic diagnosis of congenital hypophosphatasia. *Ultrasound Obstet Gynecol* 2000;15:252–255.

120. Rathbun JC, MacDonald JW, Robinson HMC, Wanklin JM. Hypophosphatasia: a genetic study. *Arch Dis Child* 1961;36:540–542.

121. Modified with permission from Silva and Jeanty at http://www.TheFetus.net.

122. Brodie SG, Lachman RS, Crandall BF, Fox MA, Rimoin DL, et al. Radiographic and morphologic findings in a previously undescribed type of mesomelic dysplasia resembling atelosteogenesis type II. *Am J Med Genet* 1998;80:247–251.

123. Kerner B, Rimoin DL, Lachman RS. Mesomelic shortening of the upper extremities with spur formation and cutaneous dimpling. *Pediatr Radiol* 1998;28:794–797.

124. Kantaputra PN, Gorlin RJ, Langer LO Jr. Dominant mesomelic dysplasia, ankle, carpal, and tarsal synostosis type: a new autosomal dominant bone disorder. *Am J Med Genet* 1992;44:730–737.

125. Fujimoto M, Kantaputra PN, Ikegawa S, Fukushima Y, Sonta S, et al. The gene for mesomelic dysplasia Kantaputra type is mapped to chromosome 2q24-q32. *J Hum Genet* 1998;43:32–36.

126. Shears DJ, Vassal HJ, Goodman FR, Palmer RW, Reardon W, et al. Mutation and deletion of the pseudoautosomal gene SHOX cause Leri-Weill dyschondrosteosis. *Nat Genet* 1998;19:70–73.

127. den Hollander NS, van der Harten HJ, Vermeij-Keers C, Niermeijer MF, Wladimiroff JW. First-trimester diagnosis of Blomstrand lethal osteochondrodysplasia. *Am J Med Genet* 1997;73:345–350.

128. Roth P, Agnani G, Arbez-Gindre F, Maillet R, Colette C. Langer mesomelic dwarfism: ultrasonographic diagnosis of two cases in early mid-trimester. *Prenat Diagn* 1996;16:247–251.

129. Evans MI, Zador IE, Qureshi F, Budev H, Quigg MH, et al. Ultrasonographic prenatal diagnosis and fetal pathology of Langer mesomelic dwarfism. *Am J Med Genet* 1988;31:915–920.

130. Belin V, Cusin V, Viot G, Girlich D, Toutain A, et al. SHOX mutations in dyschondrosteosis (Leri-Weill syndrome). *Nat Genet* 1998;19:67–69.

131. Argo KM, Toriello HV, Jelsema RD, Zuidema LJ. Prenatal findings in chondrodysplasia punctata, tibia-metacarpal type. *Ultrasound Obstet Gynecol* 1996;8:350–354.

132. Kivlin JD, Carey JC, Richey MA. Brachymesomelia and Peters anomaly: a new syndrome. *Am J Med Genet* 1993;45:416–419.

133. Qureshi F, Jacques SM, Evans MI, Johnson MP, Isada NB, et al. Skeletal histopathology in fetuses with chondroectodermal dysplasia (Ellis-van Creveld syndrome). *Am J Med Genet* 1993;45:471–476.

134. Reprinted with permission from Silva and Jeanty at http://www.TheFetus.net.

135. Majewski F, Goecke TO. Microcephalic osteodysplastic primordial dwarfism type II: report of three cases and review. *Am J Med Genet* 1998;80:25–31.

136. Sigaudy S, Toutain A, Moncla A, Fredouille C, Bourliere B, et al. Microcephalic osteodysplastic primordial dwarfism Taybi-Linder type: report of four cases and review of the literature. *Am J Med Genet* 1998;80:16–24.

137. al Gazali LI, Hamada M, Lytle W. Microcephalic osteodysplastic primordial dwarfism type II. *Clin Dysmorphol* 1995;4:234–238.

138. Haan EA, Furness ME, Knowles S, Morris LL, Scott G, et al. Osteodysplastic primordial dwarfism: report of a further case with manifestations similar to those of types I and III. *Am J Med Genet* 1989;33:224–227.

139. Majewski F, Stoeckenius M, Kemperdick H. Studies of microcephalic primordial dwarfism III: an intrauterine dwarf with platyspondyly and anomalies of pelvis and clavicles—osteodysplastic primordial dwarfism type III. *Am J Med Genet* 1982;12:37–42.

140. Majewski F, Ranke M, Schinzel A. Studies of microcephalic primordial dwarfism II: the osteodysplastic type II of primordial dwarfism. *Am J Med Genet* 1982;12:23–35.

141. Kozlowski K, Donovan T, Masel J, Wright RG. Microcephalic, osteodysplastic, primordial dwarfism. *Australas Radiol* 1993;37:111–114.

142. Berger A, Haschke N, Kohlhauser C, Amman G, Unterberger U, et al. Neonatal cholestasis and focal medullary dysplasia of the kidneys in a case of microcephalic osteodysplastic primordial dwarfism. *J Med Genet* 1998;35:61–64.

143. Spranger S, Tariverdian G, Albert FK, Sontheimer D, Zoller J, et al. Case report. Microcephalic osteodysplastic primordial dwarfism type II: a child with unusual symptoms and clinical course. *Eur J Pediatr* 1996;155:796–799.

144. Reprinted with permission from Silva and Jeanty at http://www.TheFetus.net.

145. Hale AV, Medford E, Izquierdo LA, Curet L. Osteogenesis imperfecta. *Fetus* 1992;2:5–10.

146. Kennon JC, Vitsky JL, Tiller GE, Jeanty P. Osteogenesis imperfecta. *Fetus* 1994;4:11–14.

147. Romero R, Pilu GL, Jeanty P. *Prenatal diagnosis of congenital anomalies*. Norwalk: Appleton & Lange, 1988.

148. Prockop DJ. Mutations in collagen genes as a cause of connective tissue diseases. *N Engl J Med* 1992;326:8.

149. Benacerraf BR. *Osteogenesis imperfecta in ultrasound of fetal syndromes*. New York: Churchill Livingstone, 1998:229–235.

150. Jones KL. Osteogenesis imperfecta syndrome, type I. In: *Smith's recognizable patterns of human malformation*. Philadelphia: WB Saunders, 1997:486–487.

151. Jeanty P, Silva S. Poland syndrome. Available at: http://www.TheFetus.net. Accessed September 14, 2002.

152. Hazir T, Malik MS. Poland anomaly with dextrocardia: a case report. *JPMA J Pak Med Assoc* 1996;46:181–182.

153. Burkhardt H, Buss J. Dextrocardia and Poland syndrome in a 59-year-old patient. *Z Kardiol* 1997;86:639–643.

154. Czeizel A, Vitez M, Lenz W. Birth prevalence of Poland sequence and proportion of its familial cases [Letter]. *Am J Med Genet* 1990;36:524.

155. Martinez-Frias ML, Czeizel AE, Rodriguez-Pinilla E, Bermejo E. Smoking during pregnancy and Poland sequence: results of a population-based registry and a case-control registry. *Teratology* 1999;59:35–38.

156. Bouwes Bavinck JN, Weaver DD. Subclavian artery supply disruption sequence: hypothesis of a vascular etiology for Poland, Klippel-Feil, and Moebius anomalies. *Am J Med Genet* 1986;23:903–918.

157. Sferlazza SJ, Cohen MA. Poland's syndrome: a sonographic sign. *AJR Am J Roentgenol* 1996;167:1597.

158. Risseeuw GA, Janevski B, Meradji M, Maertzdorf W, Sanches H, et al. Poland's syndrome. Including ultrasonography of the pectoralis muscle as a new diagnostic modality. *J Belge Radiol* 1985;68:231–236.

159. Farina D, Gatto G, Leonessa L, Sala U, Gomirato G. Poland syndrome: a case with a combination of síndromes. *Panminerva Med* 1999;41:259–260.

160. Larrandaburu M, Schuler L, Ehlers JA, Reis AM, Silveira EL. The occurrence of Poland and Poland-Moebius syndromes in the same family: further evidence of their genetic component. *Clin Dysmorphol* 1999;8:93–99.

161. Reprinted with permission from Silva and Jeanty at http://www.TheFetus.net.

162. Saldino RM, Noonan CD. Severe thoracic dystrophy with striking micromelia, abnormal osseous development, including the spine, and multiple visceral anomalies. *AJR Am J Roentgenol* 1972;114:257–263.

163. Majewski F, Pfeiffer RA, Lenz W, Muller R, Feil G, et al. Polydactyly, short limbs, and genital malformations—a new syndrome? *Z Kinderheilkd* 1971;111:118–138.

164. Naumoff P, Young LW, Maser J, Amortegui AJ. Short rib polydactyly syndrome type 3. *Radiology* 1977;122:443–447.

165. Meng HW, Pao LK, Shio JL. Prenatal diagnosis of recurrence of short rib polydactyly syndrome. *Am J Med Genet* 1995;55:279–284.

166. Jones KL. Short rib polydactyly syndrome type I (Saldino-Noonan type). In: *Smith's recognizable patterns of human malformation*, 5th ed. Philadelphia: WB Saunders, 1997.

167. Jones KL. Short rib polydactyly syndrome type II (Majewski type). In: *Smith's recognizable patterns of human malformation*, 5th ed. Philadelphia: WB Saunders, 1997.

168. Gembruch U, Hansmann M, Fodisch HJ. Early prenatal diagnosis of short rib polydactyly (SRP) syndrome type I (Majewski) by ultrasound in a case at risk. *Prenat Diagn* 1985;5:357–362.

169. Silva S, Jeanty P. Sirenomelia. Available at: http://www.TheFetus.net. Accessed September 14, 2002.

170. Cortes D, Thorup JM, Beck BL, Visfeldt J. Cryptorchidism as a caudal developmental field defect. A new description of cryptorchidism associated with malformations and dysplasias of the kidneys, the ureters and the spine from T10 to S5. *APMIS* 1998;106:953–958.

171. Stevenson RE, et al. Vascular steal: the pathogenic mechanism producing sirenomelia and associated defects of the viscera and soft tissues. *Pediatrics* 1986;78:451.

172. Benacerraf BR. *Caudal regression syndrome and sirenomelia in ultrasound of fetal syndromes.* New York: Churchill Livingstone, 1998:250–254.

173. Jones KL. Sirenomelia sequence. In: *Smith's recognizable patterns of human malformation*. Philadelphia: WB Saunders, 1998:634.

174. Sepulveda W, Corral E, Sanchez J, Carstens E, Schnapp C. Sirenomelia sequence versus renal agenesis: prenatal differentiation with power Doppler ultrasound. *Ultrasound Obstet Gynecol* 1998;11:445–449.

175. Norris CD, Tiller G, Jeanty P, Malini S. Thanatophoric dysplasia in monozygotic twins. *The Fetus* 1994;4:27–32.

176. Fleischer AC, Romero R, Manning FA, et al. *The principles and practice of ultrasonography in obstetrics and gynecology*, 5th ed. Norwalk: Appleton & Lange, 1995:295–297.

177. Tavormina PL, Shiang R, Thompson LM, et al. Thanatophoric dysplasia (types I and II) caused by distinct mutations in fibroblast growth factor receptor 3. *Nat Genet* 1995;9:321–328.

178. Buyse ML. *Birth defects encyclopedia.* Cambridge: Blackwell Science, 1990:1661–1662.

179. Burrows PE, Stannard MW, Pearrow J, et al. Early antenatal sonographic recognition of thanatophoric dysplasia with cloverleaf skull deformity. *AJR Am J Roentgenol* 1984;143:841–843.

180. Chemke J, Graff G, Lancet M. Familial thanatophoric dwarfism. *Lancet* 1971;1:1358.

181. Jeanty P, Silva S. Thrombocytopenia-absent radius syndromes. Available at: http://www.TheFetus.net. Accessed September 14, 2002.

182. Gross H, Groh C, Weippl G. Congenitale hypoplastische thrombopenie mit radialaplasie. *Neue Osterr Z Kinderheilkd* 1956;1:574.

183. Hall JG, Levin J, Kuhn JP, Ottenheimer EJ, Van Berkum KAP, et al. Thrombocytopenia with absent radius (TAR). *Medicine* 1969;48:411–439.

184. Hedberg VA, Lipton JM. Thrombocytopenia with absent radii. A review of 100 cases. *Am J Pediatr Hematol Oncol* 1988;10:51–64.

185. Boute O, Depret-Mosser S, Vinatier D, Manouvrier S, Martin de Lassale E, et al. Prenatal diagnosis of thrombocytopenia–absent radius syndrome. *Fetal Diagn Ther* 1996;11:224–230.

186. Lee A, Kratochwil A, Deutinger J, Bernaschek G. Three-dimensional ultrasound in diagnosing phocomelia. *Ultrasound Obstet Gynecol* 1995;5:238–240.

187. Tongsong T, Sirichotiyakul S, Chanprapaph P. Prenatal diagnosis of thrombocytopenia-absent-radius (TAR) syndrome. *Ultrasound Obstet Gynecol* 2000;15:256–258.

188. Ergur AR, Yergok YZ, Ertekin A, Tayyar M, Yilmazturk A. Prenatal diagnosis of an uncommon syndrome: thrombocytopenia absent radius (TAR). *Zentralbl Gynakol* 1998;120:75–78.

189. Donnenfeld AE, Wiseman B, Lavi E, Weiner S. Prenatal diagnosis of thrombocytopenia absent radius syndrome by ultrasound and cordocentesis. *Prenat Diagn* 1990;10:29–35.

190. Filkins K, Russo J, Bilinki I, Diamond N, Searle B. Prenatal diagnosis of thrombocytopenia absent radius syndrome using ultrasound and fetoscopy. *Prenat Diagn* 1984;4:139–142.

191. Jones KL. Radial aplasia-thrombocytopenia syndrome. In: *Smith's recognizable patterns of human malformation*. Philadelphia: WB Saunders, 1998:322–323.

192. Weinblatt M, Petrikovsky B, Bialer M, Kochen J, Harper R. Prenatal evaluation and in utero platelet transfusion for thrombocytopenia absent radii syndrome. *Prenat Diagn* 1994;14:892–896.

193. Brochstein JA, Shank B, Kernan NA, Terwilliger JW, O'Reilly RJ. Marrow transplantation for thrombocytopenia-absent radii syndrome. *J Pediatr* 1992;121:587–589.

194. McLaurin TM, Bukrey CD, Lovett RJ, Mochel DM. Management of thrombocytopenia-absent radius (TAR) syndrome. *J Pediatr Orthop* 1999;19:289–296.

16

FETAL HYDROPS AND ASCITES

HYDROPS

Fetal hydrops is defined as an excess of total body water. Hydrops occurs when the production of interstitial fluid by capillary ultrafiltration is in excess of the rate of return of this same interstitial fluid to the circulation via lymphatic vessels. The term *hydrops* or *hydrops fetalis* should be used when fluid is present within two body cavities (i.e., pleural effusion, pericardial effusion, ascites) or within one cavity in the presence of anasarca (skin and subcutaneous tissue thickening). The terms *isolated ascites, pericardial effusion*, and *pleural effusion* imply more specific etiologies, and the prognosis and management differ. Prenatal ultrasound and Doppler have a major role in detecting hydrops, monitoring the fetus, and guiding therapy. In this chapter, fetal hydrops due to immune and nonimmune causes and isolated ascites are discussed.

Immune Hydrops

Immune hydrops results from hemolytic disease of the fetus, often called *erythroblastosis fetalis*. Hydrops arises from incompatibility between maternal and fetal red blood cells. Binding of maternal antibodies to fetal red cell membrane causes hemolysis, fetal anemia, hepatosplenomegaly, and hypoproteinemia that can lead to an increase in total body water.

Immune hydrops is less common than nonimmune hydrops today due to prophylaxis against rhesus (RhD) immunization. Prophylaxis first became available in 1968, and the decline in the incidence of immune hydrops has been constant since then. Other advances that have reduced the incidence of immune hydrops include the recognition of and screening for atypical antibodies, improved monitoring of the fetus at risk by prenatal sonography, the ability to determine fetal Rh status from cells in amniotic fluid, and further experience with methods of fetal therapy.

The Rh blood group system was first discovered in 1940 by Landsteiner and Weiner.[1] Major antigenic loci determining Rh status are D, C, E, c, and e and are encoded by two genes localized on chromosome 1p36.13-p34.3. An opposite epitope to D has not been found (i.e., d does not exist); thus it is the lack of D, possibly from gene deletion, that leads to a D-negative individual, whereas the presence of D results in D-positive status. In the United States, 15% to 16% of whites and 8% of African-Americans are D-negative.[2] Asiatic groups and American Indians are virtually all D-positive.

Although the Rh blood group system is the most common one leading to immunization and hemolytic disease, atypical (non-D) antibodies are assuming a greater role (Table 1). They develop in 1% to 2% of individuals after blood transfusion and are responsible for 2% of cases of hemolytic disease of the fetus.[3] Examples include K of the Kell system and c of the rhesus system. Anti-c is one of the atypical antibodies more likely to cause severe hemolysis.[4] Maternal screening for atypical antibodies is now routine.

Maternal Rh sensitization can occur from fetal-maternal transplacental hemorrhage (during or after delivery of a previous pregnancy, spontaneous or therapeutic abortion, amniocentesis, placental abruption, or intervillous hemorrhage) or incompatible blood transfusions (now uncommon). Transplacental hemorrhage occurs in 75% of gravidas during pregnancy or delivery. The amount of fetal blood transferred to the maternal circulation is less than 0.1 mL in 60% of cases with a risk of sensitization of a D-negative woman of only 3%.[3] However, the potential for sensitization even as early as during the first trimester cannot be overlooked given the fact that as few as 0.2 mL of fetal cells have been shown to be sufficient to lead to maternal antibody (anti-D) formation.[5]

Pathogenesis

After maternal exposure to D-positive fetal red cells, the synthesis of immunoglobulin M (IgM) by the mother is triggered. This is a weak and slow response and by itself has no influence on the fetus, as IgMs have a high molecular weight, which prevents them from crossing the placenta.

A second maternal exposure, however, leads to an IgG response, which, given its low molecular weight, easily crosses the placenta. Surprisingly, however, in certain instances, even though maternal exposure to D-positive cells has occurred, sensitization is not induced or is weak.

TABLE 1. INCIDENCE OF ASSOCIATION OF HEMOLYTIC DISEASE OF THE NEWBORN (HDN) WITH ATYPICAL MATERNAL BLOOD GROUP ANTIBODIES

Frequency of HDN	Antibody
Common	c
	Kell
	E
Uncommon	e
	Cw
	C
	Ce
	Kp^a, Kp^b
	cE
	k
	s
	Wr^a
	Fy^a
Very rare	S
	U
	M
	Fy^b
	N
	Do^a
	Co^a
	Di^a, Di^b
	Lu^a
	Yt^a
	Jk^a, Jk^b
No occurrence	Le^a, Le^b
	P

Reproduced with permission from Bowman JM. Hemolytic disease (erythroblastosis fetalis). In: Creasy RK, Resnik R, eds. *Maternal-fetal medicine: principles and practice.* Philadelphia: W.B. Saunders, 1994.

This, in some cases, may be explained by the apparent protection conferred by ABO incompatibility. In this particular situation, destruction of ABO-incompatible fetal red cells in the maternal circulation occurs even before an immune response to D antigen can be elicited. Furthermore, A and B antigens are sparingly distributed on the surface of red cells, and this may partly explain the milder degree of hemolysis observed. The risk of Rh isoimmunization in the presence of ABO incompatibility is therefore reduced from 16% to 2%.[6] Other factors thought to be involved in the modulation of the maternal response to exposure to D-positive fetal red cells include the presence of inhibitory antibodies in the maternal serum, such as HLA-DR.[7] After crossing the placenta, these form a complex on the membrane of macrophages, thereby resulting in receptor blockade and inhibition of fetal red cell destruction. Other modulators worth mentioning are related to the characteristics of the antibody produced, such as its subclass (IgG3 more phagocytic than IgG1),[8] concentration, and specificity. Finally, antigen density and maturation of expression also influence the disease process. Indeed, antigens such as D, known to be present on the surface of the fetal red cells as early as 4 to 6 weeks of gestation and to be distributed in high den-sity on the cell membranes, are associated with a much greater hemolytic potential.

In most cases, however, once a significant maternal immune response has been triggered, transplacental immunoglobulin transport is initiated. This appears particularly facilitated after 22 weeks as evidenced by the exponential rise in fetal IgG levels that follows.[9] Once in the fetal circulation, IgG then binds to the D antigens present on the fetal red cell surface. The antibody-coated red cells subsequently adhere to macrophages, resulting in their hemolysis.

In response to this immunologic red cell destruction, fetal extramedullary erythropoiesis is stimulated. This is manifested by the appearance of a greater number of reticulocytes and immature red cells in the fetal circulation. When the degree of hemolysis cannot be matched by the increases in erythropoiesis, fetal anemia develops, eventually leading to the development of hydrops.

In an effort to compensate for the severe anemia, the fetus responds with an increase in cardiac output, which allows maintenance of normal blood gas status until a hemoglobin value of less than 0.5 times the median of gestational age is reached and lactic acidosis develops.[10] At this point, compensatory mechanisms are insufficient and hydrops may develop. Although the precise pathophysiologic mechanism responsible for the development of hydrops is still debated, there is evidence to support a role for high-output cardiac failure, liver damage with portal and umbilical venous hypertension, and fetal hypoxemia. It is postulated that as hemodynamic demands exceed cardiac reserves, heart failure ensues, leading to high systemic venous pressures and fetal hypoxemia. This subsequently damages the vascular endothelium, allowing protein leakage and thereby facilitating fluid accumulation in various body cavities. Of note is the normally increased susceptibility to fluid accumulation during fetal life. This is on the basis of the greater capillary permeability and compliance of the interstitial compartment as well as the greater influence of venous pressures on lymphatic circulation present during fetal life.[11]

In addition to these changes, areas of extramedullary erythropoiesis develop in the liver and distort the normal architecture, thereby contributing to hepatic dysfunction.[3] The cords of hepatocytes become compressed, leading to obstruction of the hepatic circulation. Portal and umbilical venous hypertension results in ascites and placental edema. Albumin synthesis by the diseased liver decreases, and placental edema impairs transfer of amino acids, which are precursors required for protein synthesis.[12] Hypoalbuminemia contributes to generalized edema and anasarca.

Although the sequence of events outlined above is widely accepted, the interaction of contributing factors is complex, and clinical manifestations of fetal hydrops are not always predictable.[12–14] Nevertheless, this process provides a basis for understanding and interpreting sono-

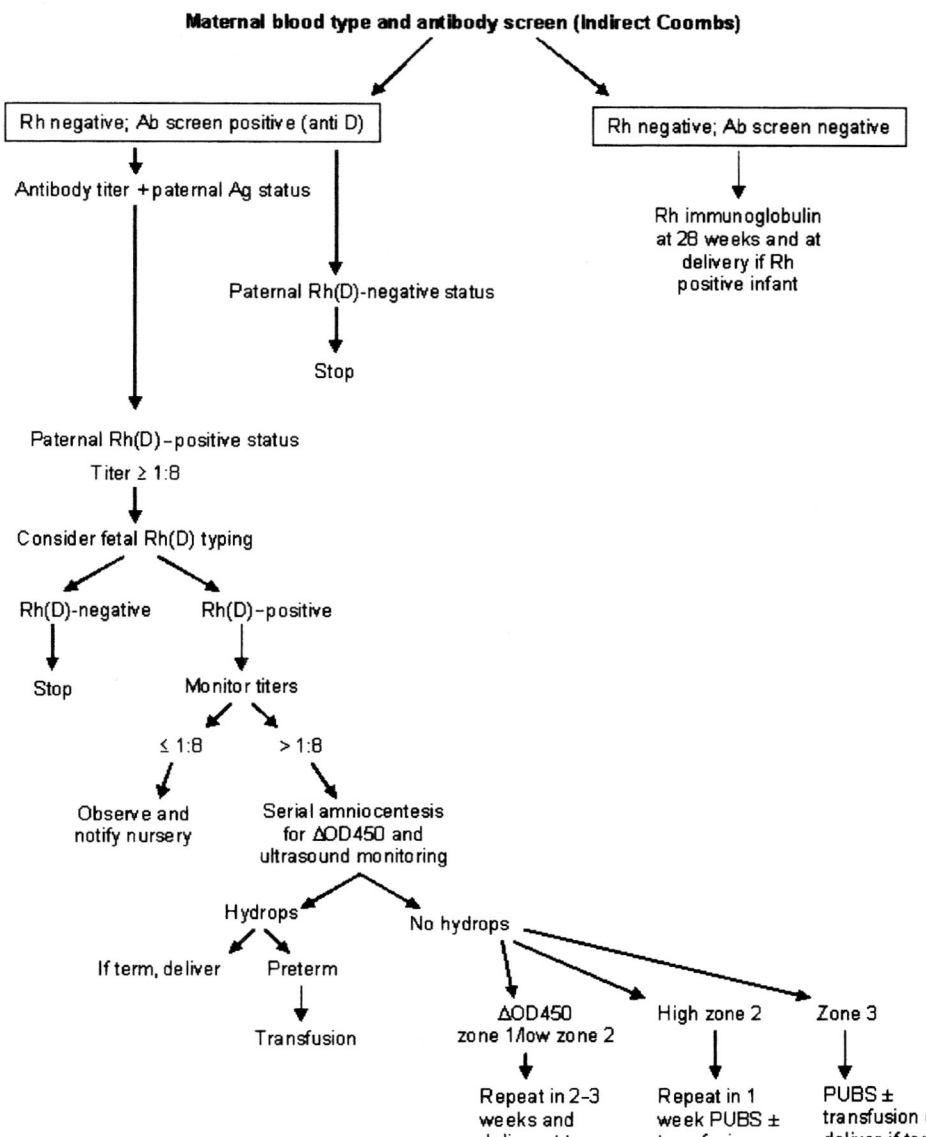

FIGURE 1. General guidelines for evaluation and treatment of rhesus (*Rh*) isoimmunization. Ab, antibody; Ag, antigen; PUBS, percutaneous umbilical blood sampling.

graphic findings of immune hydrops, as well as some types of nonimmune hydrops.

Clinical Approach

The risk of fetal hydrops is related to the severity of hemolytic disease. A prediction of the severity of fetal hemolysis can be made based on prior history and maternal antibody titers. Prenatal sonography immediately identifies the fetus with hydrops, and amniotic fluid spectrophotometric measurements (ΔOD 450) estimate the degree of severity of hemolysis. Cordocentesis (also known as *percutaneous umbilical blood sampling*)[15] determines fetal blood type and hematocrit. Figure 1 outlines a clinical approach to D isoimmunization.

At the first antenatal visit, maternal Rh grouping and antibody screening is performed. A D-positive mother with a negative antibody screen is unlikely to develop severe atypical immunization; however, some centers send a second blood sample at 28 weeks to check for atypical blood group antibodies.[15]

If the mother is D-negative, the father's Rh status is determined. If the father is D-negative, the fetus will have the same genotype and there should be no risk of immunization. If the father is D-positive, his likely zygosity for D is determined based on his Rh genotype. A D-positive father who is heterozygous for D has a 50% chance that his fetus is D-negative, and this halves the risk of Rh immunization. Otherwise, paternal homozygosity will obviously lead to a D-positive fetal genotype.

Once paternal genotype has been assessed, maternal titers, generally reflecting the degree of sensitization, need to be monitored. Each laboratory should set clinical guidelines based on local experience, but as a general rule, antibody titers of 1:16 or less rarely if ever lead to significant fetal disease. Following the demonstration of maternal sensitization, titers should be obtained from a reliable laboratory on a monthly basis.

Subsequently, timing of intervention such as amniocentesis or cordocentesis is determined by both the maternal titer and the obstetric history. Indeed, if a mother has had a previous hydropic fetus, stillbirth (from isoimmunization), or an infant needing exchange transfusion, her risk is further increased. Therefore, it may be appropriate to perform a first amniocentesis at 26 weeks or later in a patient with low titers (1:8 to 1:16) in the context of a first sensitized pregnancy. Otherwise, investigations may be required as early as 22 weeks.

Although maternal anti-D titers are widely used in the management of isoimmunized pregnancies, the predictability of these measurements as it relates to fetal disease has been put in question by the discrepancies that continue to occur. These may be related to the lack of correlation between antibody titration and biologic activity. This has led to the design of new assays that can be classified as quantitative or functional.

Quantitative assays include enzyme-linked immunosorbent assays, radioimmunoassays, and flow cytometry. By measuring anti-D–IgG binding, these assays may help better discriminate affected from unaffected fetuses. At present, the quantification of antibodies using AutoAnalyser (Technicon Instruments Corp., Tarrytown, NY) (in the United Kingdom) appears promising, although a threshold beyond which severe hemolysis will occur has not been established.

Functional assays are designed to measure the biologic activity of these same antibodies. They do so by determining the antibodies' ability to promote interactions between D-positive red cells and effector cells. Such assays include the chemiluminescence test, monocyte monolayer assay, and the antibody-dependent cellular cytotoxicity assay. So far, studies have demonstrated the usefulness of the chemiluminescence assay in predicting the need for invasive testing, although its role in the identification of unaffected fetuses is limited.[16] On the other hand, more information is available on antibody-dependent cellular cytotoxicity assays and they are now routinely used in the management of Rh isoimmunization in the Netherlands given their ability to identify unaffected fetuses.[17] As more data emerge on the usefulness of these testing methods, it is likely that they will gradually be incorporated into standard management in North America.

Preimplantation/Prenatal Diagnosis

With the advances in our understanding of the molecular genetics of the Rh system, it has been possible to design accurate and efficient ways of determining fetal genotype as early as the first trimester. This has also been extended to preimplantation diagnosis with selective D-negative embryo transfer, thereby completely preventing erythroblastosis.[18]

At present, fetal Rh typing can be performed using polymerase chain reaction (PCR) and amplifying DNA sequences found on amniotic cells. A review of 500 cases has shown that this approach carries a 98.7% sensitivity and 100% specificity.[19] The benefits of the information obtained in such a way include the availability of options such as termination, the more accurate determination of adequate timing for intervention, and, important in cases of D-positive genotype, the avoidance of all further testing and the reassurance given to the parents.

To eliminate the need for invasive testing—particularly given its potential association with fetomaternal hemorrhage—efforts have been made to isolate fetal cells from the maternal circulation. Sekizawa et al.[20] have successfully retrieved 101 fetal nucleated erythrocytes from the sera of four mothers and using fluorescence *in situ* hybridization and PCR, subsequently correctly diagnosed fetal gender and Rh status. Although at present this approach remains investigational, it appears promising and warrants further evaluation.

Sonographic Findings

Sonographic findings for immune hydrops are nonspecific. They include serous cavity effusions (peritoneal, scrotal, pleural, and/or pericardial effusions), polyhydramnios, placental edema, and skin and subcutaneous tissue edema (anasarca). Other findings include hepatosplenomegaly, cardiomegaly, and alterations in fetal or umbilical vessel size or Doppler flow. In cases of isoimmunized pregnancies, these findings may occur alone or in combination.

The cause of fetal hydrops often cannot be determined based on the sonographic appearance alone. However, Doppler imaging of the middle cerebral artery may be able to identify anemia as the underlying cause (discussed later in this section). The fetus who is anemic, but not yet hydropic, has the highest likelihood of successful treatment outcome. The most accurate method of determining the severity of fetal anemia is fetal blood sampling.

Sonographic evidence of hydrops generally reflects severe fetal hemolysis. Hydropic fetuses usually have a hematocrit at least 0.5 times below the median for gestational age[10] and total protein levels below 3 g per dL.[15,21] Nicolaides et al.[22] found a hemoglobin level less than 5 g per dL in all hydropic fetuses. However, this relationship is inconsistent and severe anemia (hematocrit below 15%) can be present without sonographic features of hydrops[15,13]; alternately, a hydropic fetus can have only mild anemia, with a hemoglobin level above 7 g per dL.[8] This is partly related to the gestational age differences in hematocrit. A study of 111 fetuses at risk of anemia dem-

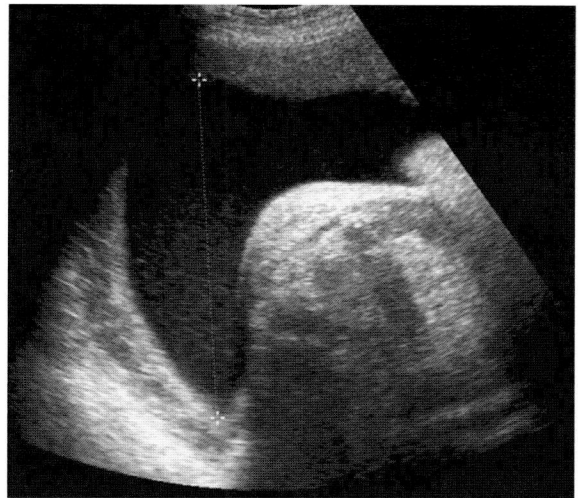
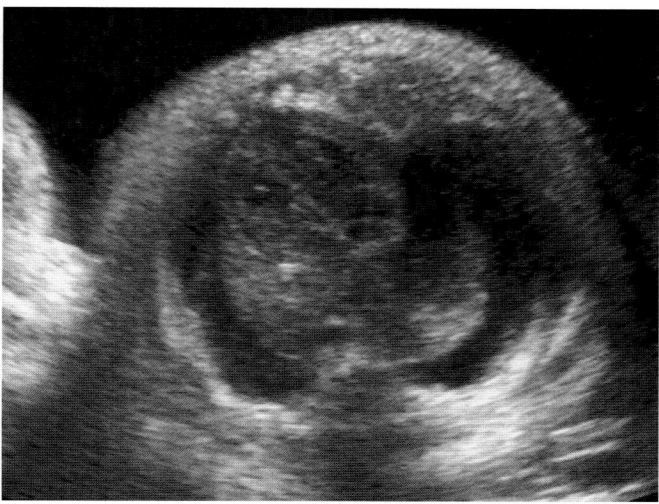

FIGURE 2. Polyhydramnios and hydrops. **A:** Single pocket of fluid measures 8 cm in vertical diameter. **B:** Transverse view of the thorax shows bilateral pleural effusions and body wall edema.

onstrated gradual increases in hemoglobin with advancing gestational age.[10] Given the significant variations present, it is suggested that hemoglobin deficit should be interpreted carefully and in relation to gestational age. In the absence of hydrops, other sonographic parameters (e.g., placental thickness or umbilical vein diameter) cannot reliably distinguish mild from severe fetal hemolytic disease.[22]

Polyhydramnios (Fig. 2) usually accompanies immune hydrops. It is an early sonographic sign and can be seen before other abnormalities develop.[13] Polyhydramnios was associated with a fetal hematocrit of 26% or less in all cases studied by Chitkara et al.[13] Either subjective or semiquantitative methods can be used for evaluation of polyhydramnios (see Chapter 3).

Placental edema can be seen on sonography as placental enlargement, recognized as increased placental thickness (Fig. 3). However, this is an inconstant finding and does not reliably identify severely anemic fetuses.[22] The normal thickness of the placenta increases with gestational age, but it should be less than 4 cm at any stage.[23] Thickness varies depending on the surface area covered within the uterus; a thicker placenta may be associated with smaller surface area. Also, an abnormally thickened placenta compressed by severe polyhydramnios can falsely appear to be of normal thickness.

Ascites is an early sonographic finding in immune hydrops[13] (Fig. 4). Early development of ascites supports the importance attributed to portal hypertension in the pathogenesis of immune hydrops.[12] A small amount of ascites is identified on sonography as fluid between bowel loops, fluid along the abdominal flanks or surrounding the posterior aspect of the liver, outlining the umbilical vessels,

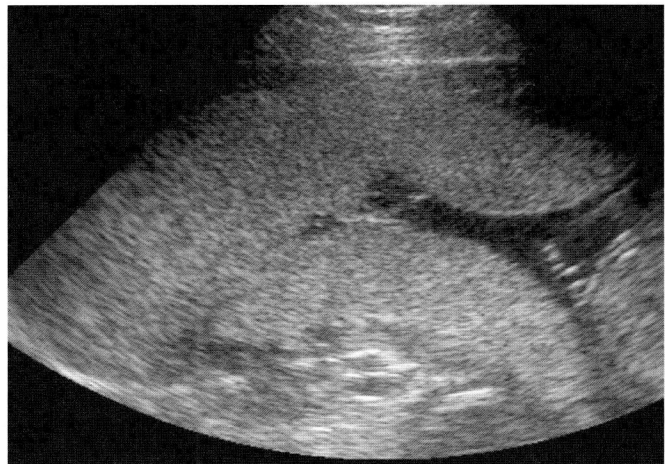
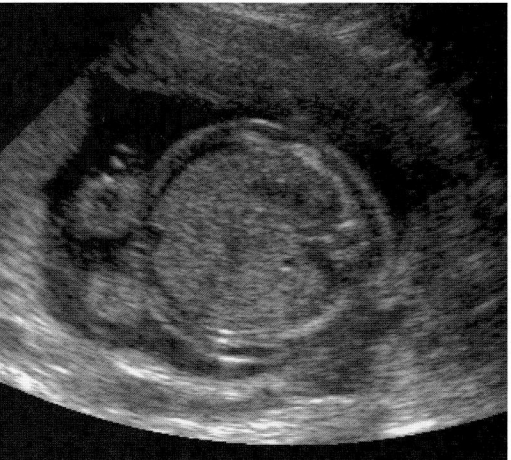

FIGURE 3. Placental edema. **A:** This view of the placenta shows placental thickening. **B:** This view of abdomen shows moderate ascites.

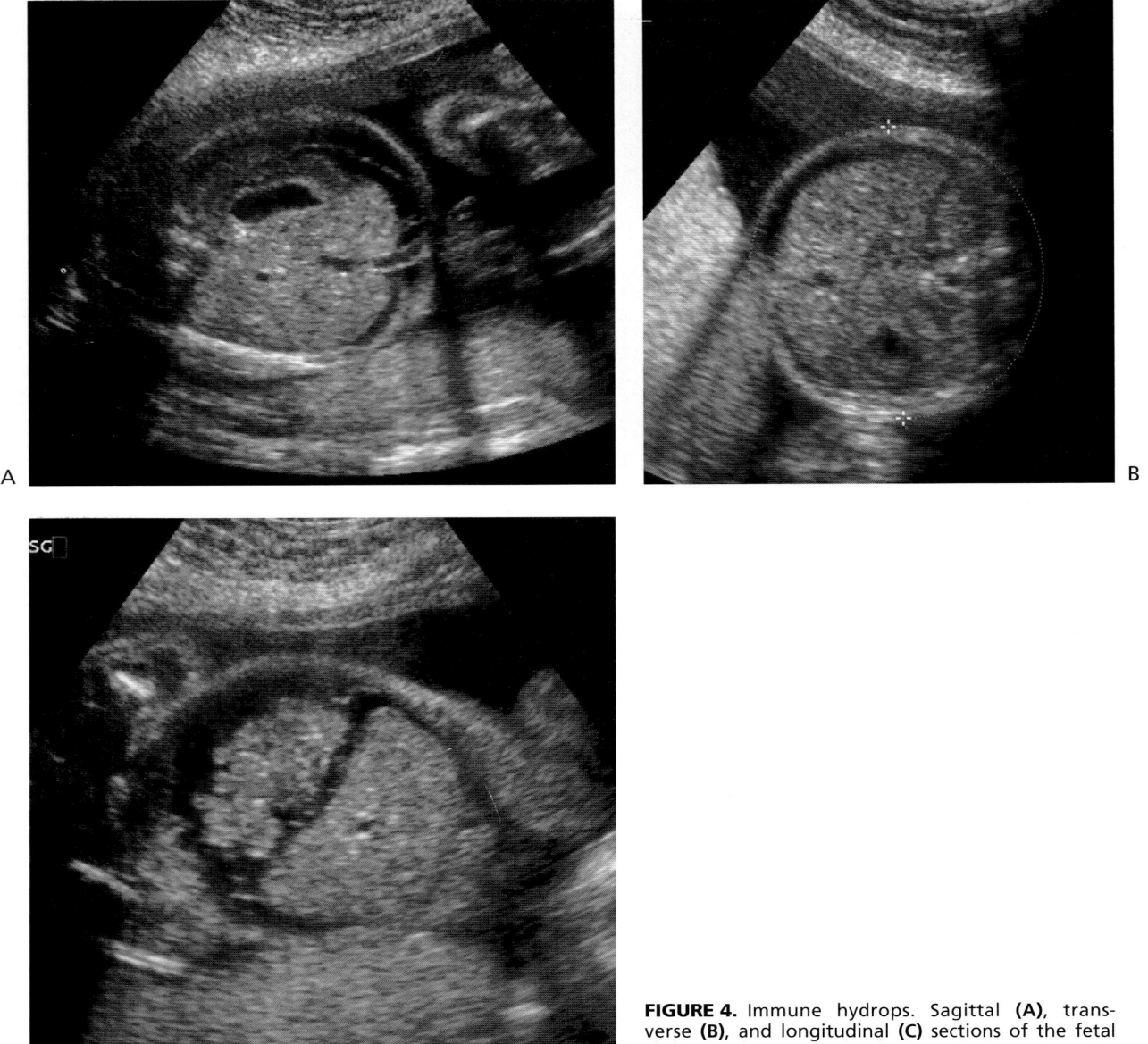

FIGURE 4. Immune hydrops. Sagittal **(A)**, transverse **(B)**, and longitudinal **(C)** sections of the fetal abdomen demonstrate ascites.

or within the pelvis (Fig. 4). Normal abdominal wall muscles, which are observed as a hypoechoic band along the anterior and lateral aspects of the fetal abdomen, can be mistaken for a small amount of ascites. This pitfall is known as *pseudoascites*.[24,25] Care also should be taken to distinguish a true pericardial effusion from the normal hypoechoic fetal myocardium.

Ascites that accompanies fetal hydrops should be distinguished from isolated ascites (discussed in the section Isolated Fetal Ascites). The latter is associated with more local etiologies, such as urinary or gastrointestinal obstruction, and has a more favorable prognosis. The distinction between early hydrops manifest as ascites and isolated ascites can be difficult, and these fetuses require

follow-up to observe for the development of generalized hydrops and thus a poorer prognosis.

Pleural effusions (Figs. 5 and 6) and pericardial effusions are characteristic of more severe immune hydrops.[13,26] Pleural effusions, if large, can lead to pulmonary hypoplasia (Fig. 5). A small amount of pericardial fluid can be normal; greater than 2 mm thickness of pericardial fluid is considered abnormal. Congestive heart failure usually does not occur until late in immune hydrops.[27]

Skin and subcutaneous tissue edema are commonly seen with hydrops. Scalp edema may be a prominent feature of subcutaneous edema (Figs. 7 and 8) and may be seen before abdominal or thoracic edema (Fig. 9). Ascites may distend the abdominal wall so much that edema may be difficult to

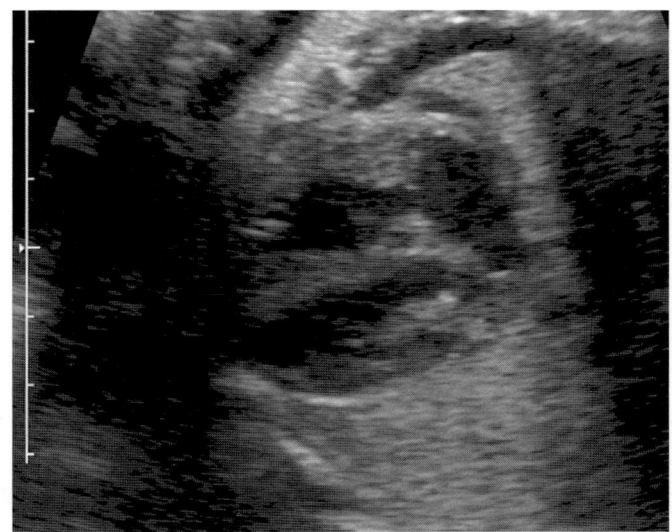 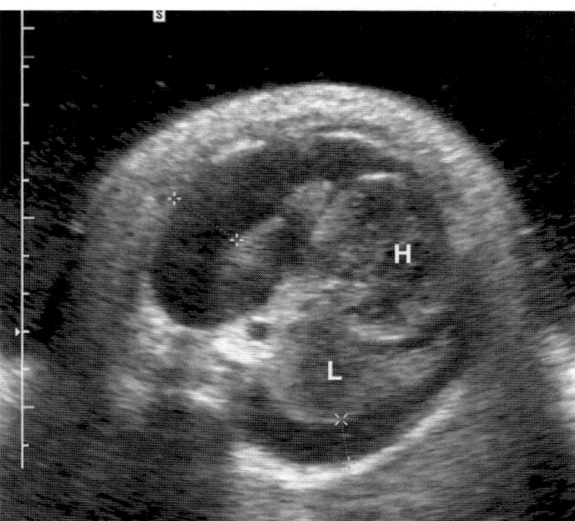

FIGURE 5. Pleural effusion. **A:** This transverse scan at 31 weeks shows small right pleural effusion. **B:** A follow-up scan at 35 weeks shows large bilateral pleural effusions, body wall edema, and polyhydramnios. The lungs (*L*) are compressed. H, heart.

see. Anasarca is a seen as diffuse body wall edema and is a manifestation of fetal hydrops.[13,28] Anasarca may be associated with a cystic hygroma with nonimmune hydrops.

Hepatosplenomegaly, secondary to extramedullary hematopoiesis, is a pathologic hallmark of immune hydrops. Vintzileos and Campbell[29] measured the sagittal length of the right lobe of liver on serial sonograms and found that the liver grew more than 5 mm per week in all fetuses with

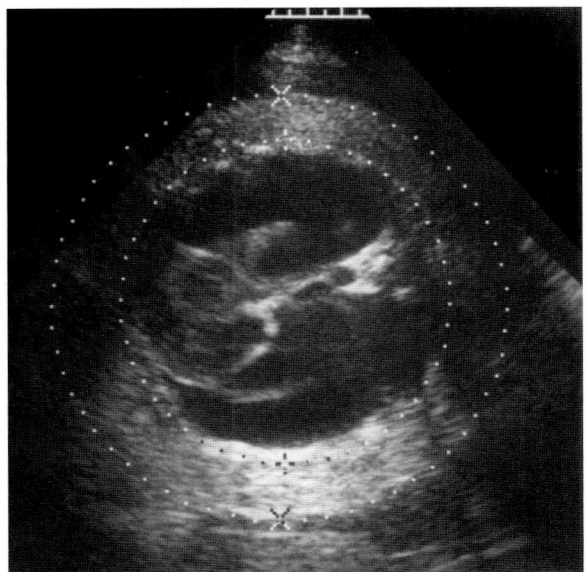

FIGURE 6. Pleural effusion. A transverse view of the thorax shows large bilateral pleural effusions in association with hydrops. The lungs are collapsed. Body wall edema is seen between measurements of outer and inner thoracic circumference.

severe immune hydrops who required transfusion or delivery within 2 weeks of the sonogram. By contrast, Nicolaides et al.[22] found that liver size measurements were of no value in predicting the severity of anemia.

Cardiomegaly (Fig. 10) due to congestive heart failure can develop in immune hydrops, although it is usually a late finding.[30] Cardiac biventricular outer dimensions have been identified as an indicator of perinatal prognosis in nonimmune fetal hydrops. Real-time M-mode echocardiographic measurement of biventricular outer dimensions is made in diastole (Fig. 11). Carlson et al.[31] found that all hydropic fetuses (12 of 12) with biventricular outer dimensions above the 95% confidence interval for gestational age died.

Alterations in fetal and umbilical vessels have been evaluated as a means for monitoring both immune and nonimmune hydrops (Figs. 12 and 13). DeVore et al.[32] suggested that the diameter of the umbilical vein increases (greater than 1 cm) in Rh-hemolytic anemia and that enlargement can be identified before other manifestations of hydrops.[32] However, Chitkara et al.[13] concluded that measurements of umbilical vein diameter were an unreliable predictor of worsening fetal disease; the umbilical vein did not dilate in some instances of severe disease.

The ductus venosus, which may be difficult to visualize in normal fetuses, may become more prominent with developing portal hypertension (Fig. 13). This observation can be explained by increased blood flow through the ductus venosus; the blood flow is directed into the left atrium and thereby circumvents passage through the liver parenchyma.[33] The ductus venosus can be difficult to identify in a hydropic fetus, although improvements in sonographic equipment make it easier to identify the ductus in a normal

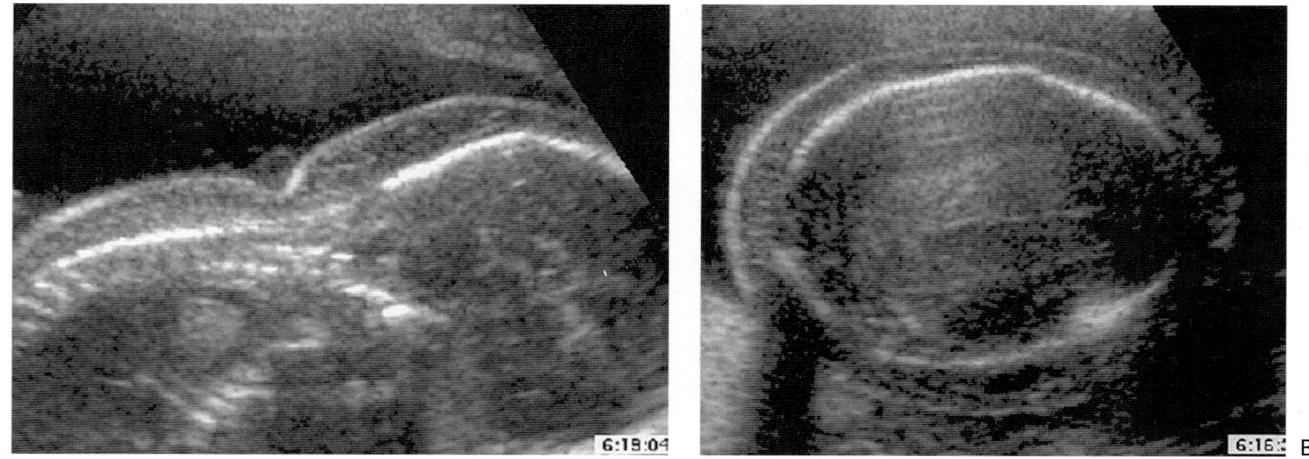

FIGURE 7. Scalp edema. Sagittal **(A)** and transverse **(B)** views of a fetus with rhesus isoimmunization show moderate subcutaneous edema of the scalp.

FIGURE 8. Scalp edema. Transverse **(A)** and longitudinal **(B)** views show scalp edema; view of the abdomen **(C)** shows ascites.

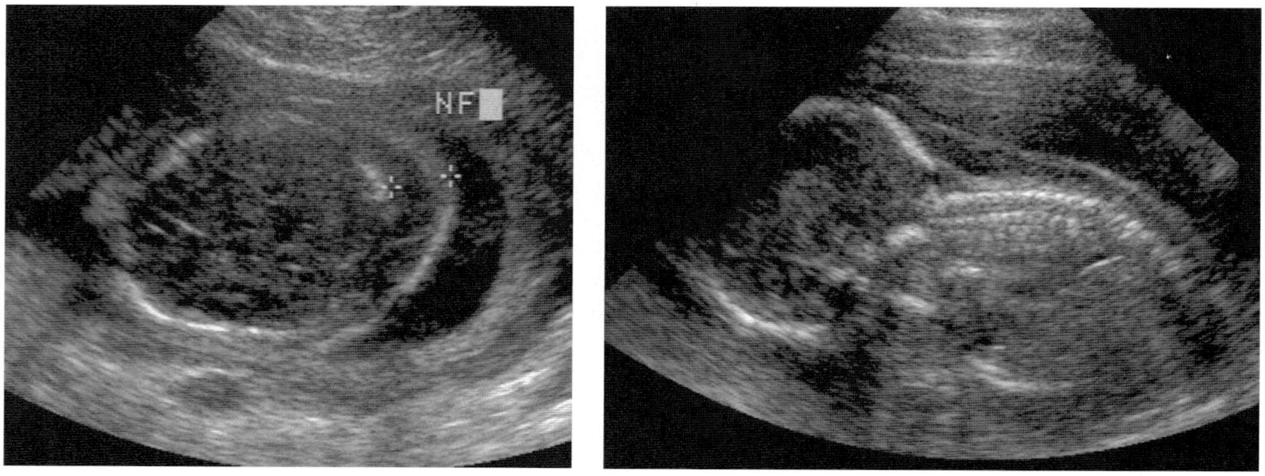

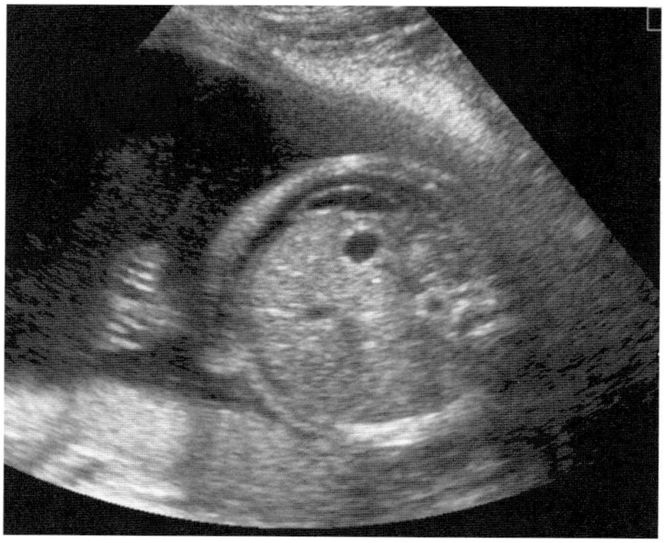

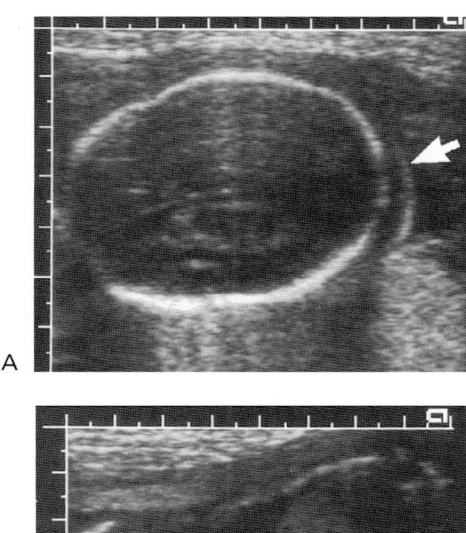

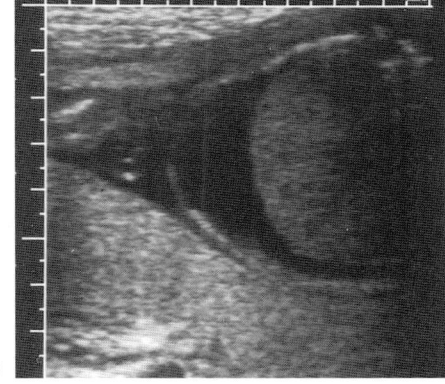

FIGURE 9. A: Rhesus-sensitized patient exhibits mild scalp edema (*arrow*). **B:** A scan of the abdomen shows a large amount of ascites but no body wall edema. Umbilical vein sampling showed a hematocrit of 7.

fetus. Interrogation of this vessel using Doppler imaging also helps further characterize blood flow.

Much interest has been raised over the possible role of Doppler sonography in the evaluation of erythroblastosis,

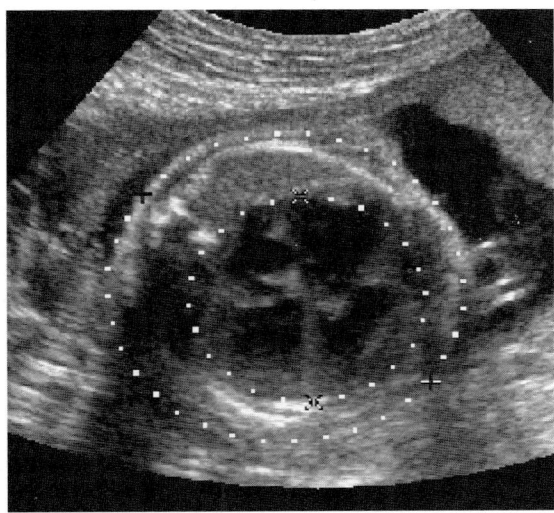

FIGURE 10. A transverse scan of the fetal heart demonstrates marked cardiac enlargement as evidenced by the abnormal cardiothoracic ratio.

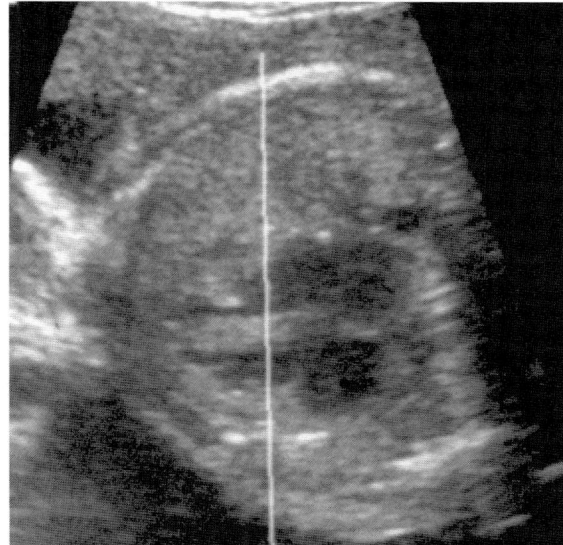

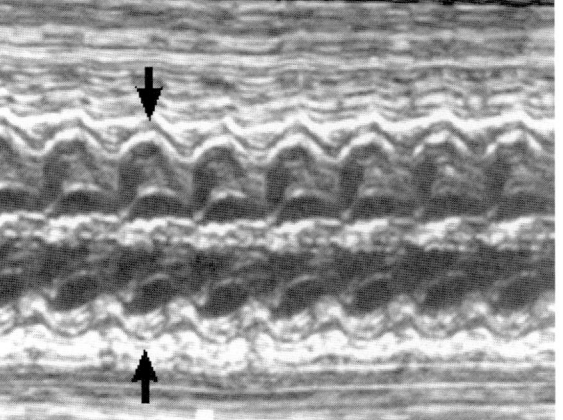

FIGURE 11. A: This real-time image shows the M-mode cursor in perpendicular transection of a four-chamber view. **B:** M-mode tracing and cursor placement for biventricular outer diameter measurement (BVOD). Distance between arrows represents BVOD in diastole.

particularly given the pathophysiologic changes observed in affected fetuses (Fig. 14). Specifically, it has been shown that fetal cardiac output rises as hematocrit falls and that fetal cerebral arteries respond rapidly to hypoxemia by an increase in blood flow velocity. Using these physiologic observations, the Collaborative Group for Doppler Assessment of the Blood Velocity in Anemic Fetuses reported on their peak velocity measurements of middle cerebral arteries in 111 fetuses at risk of anemia from maternal red cell isoimmunization[10] (Fig. 15). When comparing the middle cerebral artery peak velocity to the severity of anemia, investigators were able to correctly identify all fetuses with moderate and severe anemia by using a cut-off value of 1.5 times above the median peak velocity value for the given gestational age. Reference values of peak systolic velocity with gestational age are shown in Table 2.

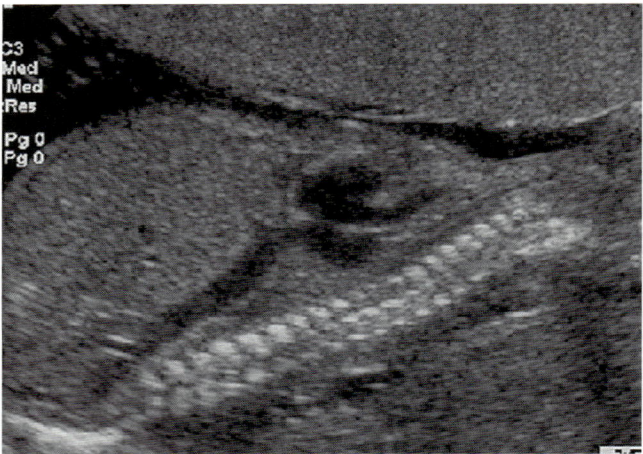

FIGURE 12. This sagittal view of a rhesus-isoimmunized fetus shows hepatomegaly and prominence of the inferior vena cava.

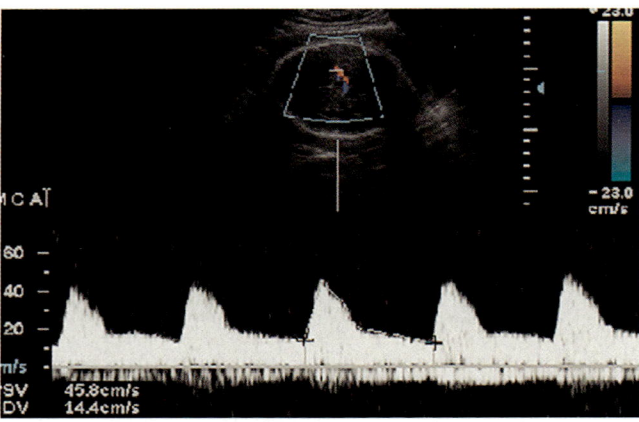

FIGURE 14. Doppler imaging of the middle cerebral artery. A transverse view of the fetal head shows Doppler sampling of the middle cerebral artery in an isoimmunized fetus. Peak velocity (systolic) of 46 cm per second is in the upper limits of normal for 28 weeks.

Although other vessels have been interrogated in the hope the information would provide further accuracy in the identification of the at-risk fetus, so far, none other than middle cerebral arteries has shown to be of value. Specifically, umbilical blood flow maximum velocity has been shown to relate to some degree with fetal hematocrit by predicting the need for postnatal transfusion in a very limited study of seven cases.[34] Splenic artery Doppler velocimetry has also been examined.[35] Results showed that in the presence of a normal Doppler angle in the main splenic artery, a decreased risk of severe anemia was present, whereas a smaller angle might be more reflective of a rapid deceleration phase of the hyperdynamic status of the anemic fetus. Although sensitivity of 100% with a false-positive rate of 8.8% was reported, these results have not yet been reproduced and the small number of fetuses studied limit possible conclusions.

Prognosis

The severity of fetal anemia is determined by the amount of maternal IgG anti-D, its avidity for the Rh antigen, and the ability of the fetus to respond to anemia with increased erythropoiesis. Hydrops develops when the fetal response to hemolysis is unable to compensate adequately. This situation arises in 20% to 25% of untreated D-incompatible pregnancies, and one-half of these fetuses become hydropic

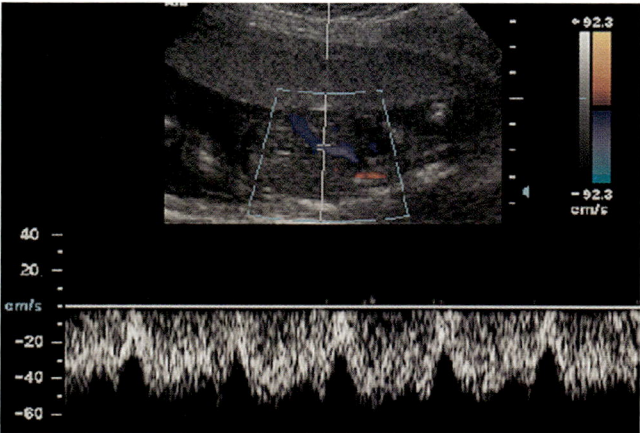

FIGURE 13. Prominent ductus venosus in fetus with immune hydrops. Doppler interrogation reveals high velocity flow that is consistent with the hyperdynamic state of the anemic fetus.

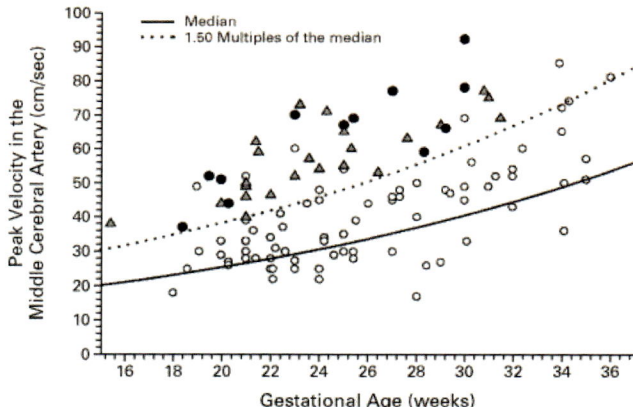

FIGURE 15. Peak velocity of systolic blood flow in the middle cerebral artery in 111 fetuses at risk for anemia due to maternal red-cell alloimmunization. Open circles indicate fetuses with either no anemia or mild anemia (≥0.65 multiples of the median hemoglobin concentration). Triangles indicate fetuses with moderate or severe anemia (<0.65 multiples of the median hemoglobin concentration). Solid circles indicate the fetuses with hydrops. The solid curve indicates the median peak systolic velocity in the middle cerebral artery, and the dotted curve indicates 1.5 multiples of the median. [Reproduced with permission from Mari G, Deter RL, Carpenter RL, Rahman F, Zimmerman R, et al. Noninvasive diagnosis by Doppler ultrasonography of fetal anemia due to maternal red-cell alloimmunization. Collaborative Group for Doppler Assessment of the Blood Velocity in Anemic Fetuses. *N Engl J Med* 2000;342(1):9–14.]

TABLE 2. REFERENCE VALUES OF PEAK SYSTOLIC VELOCITY OF MIDDLE CEREBRAL ARTERY

| Gestational age (wk) | Peak systolic velocity[a] of middle cerebral artery | | | | |
| | Multiples of the median | | | | |
	1	1.3	1.5	1.7	2
15	20	26	30	34	40
16	21	27	32	36	42
17	22	29	33	37	44
18	23	30	35	39	46
19	24	31	36	41	48
20	25	33	38	43	50
21	26	34	39	44	52
22	28	36	42	48	56
23	29	38	44	49	58
24	30	39	45	51	60
25	32	42	48	54	64
26	33	43	50	56	66
27	35	46	53	60	70
28	37	48	56	63	74
29	38	49	57	65	76
30	40	52	60	68	80
31	42	55	63	71	84
32	44	57	66	75	88
33	46	60	69	78	92
34	48	62	72	82	96
35	50	65	75	85	100
36	53	69	80	90	106
37	55	72	83	94	110
38	58	75	87	99	116
39	61	79	92	104	122
40	63	82	95	107	126

[a]Peak systolic velocity (cm/sec) = $e^{(2.31 + 0.046*GA)}$, where GA = gestational age.
Data from Mari G, Deter RL, Carpenter RL, Rahman F, Zimmerman R, et al. Noninvasive diagnosis by Doppler ultrasonography of fetal anemia due to maternal red-cell alloimmunization. Collaborative Group for Doppler Assessment of the Blood Velocity in Anemic Fetuses. *N Engl J Med* 2000;342(1):9–14.

before 34 weeks.[15] Hemoglobin levels of 4 to 6 g per dL or lower and hematocrit levels of less than 15% are typically found in hydropic fetuses.[36] Hydrops has been observed to resolve when the hematocrit rises above 20%.[37]

Fetal blood sampling and intrauterine treatment of fetal anemia by intravascular transfusion (IVT) have significantly improved the prognosis for anemic fetuses.[38] Accurate identification and monitoring of the severely anemic fetus are now possible in tertiary care centers. Overall survival rates of 85% have been reported after intravascular blood transfusion in fetuses with erythroblastosis.[39,40] Important, however, is the influence that hydrops plays in the prognosis. Indeed, survival rates after IVT in nonhydropic fetuses are close to 94% but decrease to 74% in the presence of hydrops.[41] Improved perinatal outcome has been observed with the increased use of fetal IVT in place of intraperitoneal transfusion.[42] The intraperitoneal route may, however, still be reserved for cases when it is technically not feasible to perform IVT.[37] Alternately, some clinicians also advocate its use in the creation of

a "reservoir" of red cells. Indeed, since intraperitoneal transfusion is associated with a slower posttransfusion decline in hematocrit, its use concomitant with IVT may lead to greater intervals between procedures.

Obstetric history helps predict the prognosis for future pregnancies. The risk of hydrops in a first sensitized pregnancy is 8% to 10%. A history of a previous hydropic fetus increases to 90% the likelihood of hydrops in a subsequent D-positive pregnancy. Hydrops tends to develop in the next affected fetus at the same time or earlier in gestation, although this is variable.[15]

Management

Prophylaxis

The management of women with rhesus isoimmunization begins with prophylaxis against Rh sensitization. Major advances have been made due to the availability of Rh immune globulin (RhoGAM) in 1968. The number of sensitized women in the time period 1950 to 1970 was decreased by 70% in the years 1970 to 1976.[43] Rh immune globulin acts by blocking antigenic sites on fetal red blood cells. Subsequently, these immunoglobulin-bound erythrocytes are lysed by complement fixation. In addition, the sequestration of IgG-coated red blood cells in the spleen and lymph nodes may further contribute to antibody suppression. Rh immune globulin, 300 μg, given at 28 weeks' gestation to D-negative women reduces the risk of isoimmunization to 0.2%.[44] This dose is sufficient to protect against 30 mL fetal blood or 15 mL packed fetal red cells. Therefore, if a greater degree of fetomaternal hemorrhage is suspected, a Kleihauer-Betke test must be performed to quantify the fetal blood present in the maternal circulation. This will then guide the dose of Rh IgG that must be administered. Rh immune globulin is also administered after spontaneous or therapeutic abortion, amniocentesis, or any obstetric procedure that may result in fetomaternal hemorrhage. Once a patient is sensitized, there is no benefit in administering Rh immune globulin again. At present, Rh IgG is obtained from pooled donors' sera. Fortunately, the technique used in isolation, cold alcohol fractionation, appears to destroy the human immunodeficiency virus. This, along with universal testing of donors, likely accounts for the fact that there are no reported cases of human immunodeficiency virus transmission through the use of Rh IgG. However, cases of hepatitis C transmission have been reported in Europe before universal donor screening.[45] To circumvent the potential for viral transmission and supply problems, the development of an effective combination of recombinant immunoglobulin for the prevention of Rh(D) sensitization is being investigated. So far, phase I trials using a combination of IgG1 and IgG3 have shown promising results.[46]

Fetal Surveillance and Spectrophotometry

Management of fetal hemolytic disease depends on the severity of hemolysis. Techniques to guide management

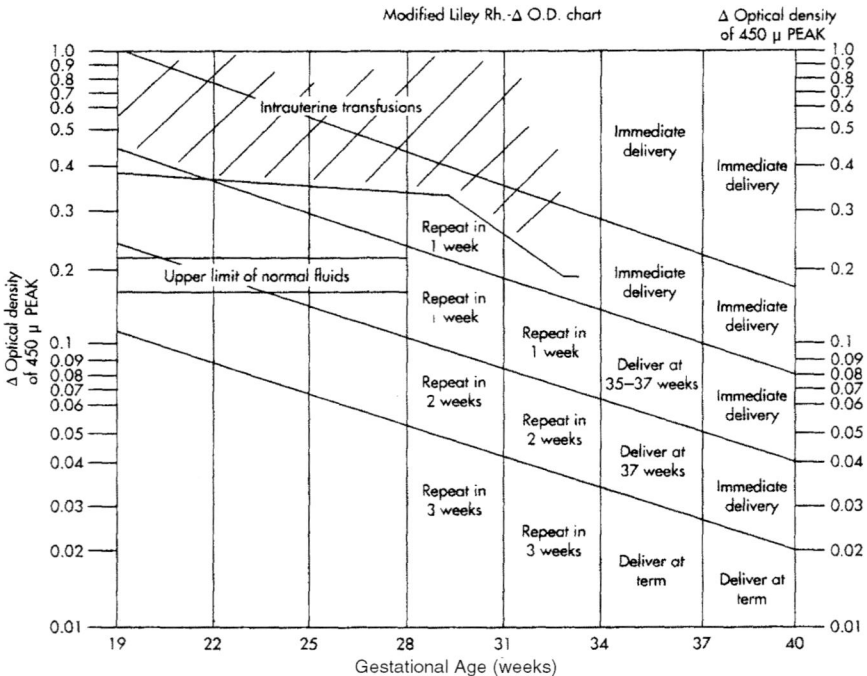

FIGURE 16. Normal Liley curves. Modification of Liley ΔOD 450 reading zone boundaries before 24 weeks' gestation is the same as the zone boundary angle of inclination after 24 weeks' gestation.

include serial maternal titer determination, monitoring by ultrasound and Doppler, serial amniocenteses for amniotic fluid bilirubin optical density readings, and fetal blood sampling to determine hemoglobin and hematocrit levels. Of these, once dictated by elevations in maternal titers (greater than 1:16 to 1:32), amniotic fluid bilirubin optical density measurement (ΔOD 450) is routinely performed to evaluate the severity of fetal hemolysis. Fetal red cell destruction leads to an increase in hemoglobin breakdown products including bilirubin, which is then excreted into the amniotic fluid via the fetal trachea and pulmonary secretions. Therefore, measurements of the concentration of bilirubin in amniotic fluid are reflective of the degree of fetal red cell hemolysis. This measurement is accomplished by performing an amniocentesis under ultrasound guidance, trying to avoid the placenta, an event that might worsen maternal sensitization. The amniotic fluid sample obtained is then immediately protected from light to prevent degradation of bilirubin and then processed by spectrophotometry. This technique allows measurement of the change in amniotic fluid optical density at 450 nm, which reflects the bilirubin concentration. The value obtained is then plotted on a graph as established by Liley[47] in 1961. By collecting optical density readings from 101 D-isoimmunized fetuses between 27 and 41 weeks, he discovered that the deviation from linearity at 450 nm correlated with the severity of hemolytic disease. Using this information, a graph, divided in three zones, was then constructed. Each zone is associated with an increasing degree of severity of fetal anemia.[48] Zone 1 predicts a 10% risk of the need for postnatal exchange transfusion. Zone 2 is subdivided into two areas to further discriminate the severity of the disease.

High zone 2 is associated with moderate disease. Finally, zone 3 is usually indicative of the need for delivery if near term or otherwise of fetal blood sampling for determination of hematocrit and likely *in utero* transfusion. These zones also help guide the frequency of invasive testing. For example, readings in zone 1 or low zone 2 should be repeated in 2 to 4 weeks, whereas a high zone 2 reading warrants a repeat amniocentesis in 1 week (Fig. 16). More recently, with advances and refinements in the diagnostic and therapeutic approaches for erythroblastosis, more immature fetuses have been identified as at risk and have been subjected to investigations and therapy. However, inaccuracies in the ΔOD 450 readings at these earlier gestational ages have been reported. In general, meconium or blood contamination has been shown to preclude an accurate measurement. More important, the predictability of ΔOD 450 before 27 weeks has been questioned, and it has become clear that retrograde linear extension of the Liley curve to those early gestational ages was not appropriate. Nicolaides et al.[48] have demonstrated the very poor predictability of ΔOD 450 in the severity of fetal anemia between 18 and 25 weeks. Furthermore, no cutoff ΔOD 450 level could discriminate severely from mildly affected fetuses. This has led to their recommendation to use fetal blood sampling as opposed to ΔOD 450 during the second trimester. However, as this procedure in itself carries a significant risk of pregnancy loss (1% to 2%) and of worsening maternal sensitization (50% risk fetomaternal hemorrhage), other approaches have been designed. One commonly used approach relies on the modification of the initial Liley curve. By flattening the curve between 18 and 27 weeks, the upper limit of normal is lowered significantly, thereby improving the predictability (Fig. 16). However, in selected cases in which the risk of severe anemia is particularly high, fetal blood sampling may be preferred. As a general rule, the convenience and accuracy of fetal blood sampling must be weighed against the risks of worsening maternal sensitization and procedure-related fetal loss.[41]

In an isoimmunized pregnancy, remote from term, once evidence of severe disease has been obtained, either by sonographic findings described above or by measurement of ΔOD 450, direct hemoglobin determination via fetal blood sampling must be performed and followed by intrauterine transfusion as appropriate.

In Utero Transfusion

The concept of intrauterine transfusion as introduced by Liley in 1963 represented one of the most significant advances in the management of erythroblastosis. By puncturing the fetal abdomen, he performed an intraperitoneal transfusion and subsequently red cells were absorbed via the subdiaphragmatic lymphatics to then enter the venous circulation. Unfortunately, because of impairment in red cell absorption, hydropic fetuses generally did not recover well, thereby explaining their survival rate of only approximately 25%.[3] It is only later in 1984 that Rodeck et al. introduced the technique of IVT.[49] This procedure, now performed under ultrasound guidance, is associated with a loss rate of approximately 2%.[41]

Ultrasonography is indeed a key element in the IVT technique. It is used to localize the optimal access site (usually at level of cord insertion into the placenta), to monitor the fetal heart rate, and to observe the cord for complications such as bleeding. In addition, it allows visualization of flow turbulence (an indicator of flow continuity) within the transfused vessel during the procedure. Once the access site has been determined, a 20- or 22-gauge needle is introduced via the maternal abdomen into the appropriate vessel. Ideally this should be the umbilical vessels, but other sites have been used such as the hepatic portion of the umbilical vein or even the heart directly. Once the needle is in place, depolarizing agents may be used to paralyze the fetus, and a sample of fetal blood is obtained for determination of hematocrit and blood type. The fetal source of the sample obtained can be ascertained by determining the mean corpuscular volume, which should be above 100 μm³ (adult maternal value, 90 μm³).

Generally, a hematocrit of less than 30% is indicative of the need for transfusion as this value is below the 2.5th percentile for fetuses beyond 20 weeks. Blood to be transfused must be packed to a hematocrit of at least 90% to minimize increases in viscosity. In addition, group O-negative, cytomegalovirus (CMV)-negative, irradiated blood is preferred. The volume to be transfused can be estimated either by the help of formulas and nomograms or simply by obtaining pre- and posttransfusion hematocrits. In most cases a posttransfusion hematocrit of 40% is the goal, particularly

TABLE 3. COMPLICATIONS ASSOCIATED WITH INTRAVASCULAR TRANSFUSION (IVT)

Complication	Percentage of IVTs
Fetomaternal hemorrhage	40
Fetal loss	2
Bradycardia	8
Infection	<1
Cord hematoma	0.5
Bleeding from venipuncture site	0.5
Cardiac overload	<1
Premature labor	3–4

because this represents a closer physiologic value (hematocrit is 47% at term). Physiologic changes known to occur during fetal IVT include an increase in umbilical venous pressure and a 25% decrease in cardiac output as a result of an increased afterload due to the greater blood viscosity.[41] These changes are only transient and return to normal within 24 hours. Complications related to IVT include a 50% risk of fetomaternal hemorrhage (thereby potentially worsening maternal sensitization), bleeding at the site of vessel puncture, cord accident (hematoma), cardiac overload, bradycardia, and infection (Table 3).

The timing of the subsequent transfusion depends mostly on the final hematocrit reached at the end of the procedure. As the daily attrition rate of fetal hematocrit is approximately 1%,[50] a repeat procedure may be needed within 2 to 4 weeks. Obviously, during intervals between transfusions, fetal surveillance must be instituted. Therefore, serial biophysical profiles are recommended along with monitoring for any evidence of deterioration. Doppler velocimetry of the middle cerebral artery may also serve as a useful adjunct.

Timing of Delivery and Outcome

Generally, these fetuses should be delivered by 36 weeks because pregnancy beyond this stage will not be of benefit and in fact could be detrimental. The last transfusion to be performed will often be at 35 weeks, and at that time, an amniotic fluid sample can also be obtained for lung maturity assessment by lecithin-to-sphingomyelin ratio and determination of phosphatidylglycerol levels.

The long-term outcome of these infants has generally been reported as favorable. Although the information is still limited, it appears that most children will achieve a normal neurodevelopmental outcome.[51,52] The risk of neurologic abnormalities appears to be correlated to the cord blood hemoglobin levels and the presence of perinatal asphyxia but not to the presence of hydrops. These encouraging results further justify the use of IVTs for the *in utero* treatment of hemolytic disease.

Other Therapeutic Approaches

At this time, other management options are very limited. However, the literature suggests that maternal suppressive therapy may be a useful adjunct, particularly in cases of early and severe sensitization. Indeed, in one review, authors reported that in small series, maternal intravenous immune globulin administration tended to be associated with improved outcomes in index pregnancies compared to previous ones.[53] One advantage was in the delay of the need for intrauterine transfusion until technically easier and therefore likely of less risk to the fetus. At this time, these data remain preliminary and the costs of intravenous immune globulin prohibitive. However, these results warrant future investigation.

Atypical Antigens

Although most isoimmunizations will be related to D antigen, a significant proportion arises from exposure to atypical antigens. Fortunately, in most cases, such as Le and P, antibodies produced are of the IgM type and therefore do not affect the fetal cells. Other antibodies, such as J^K and Fy, cause only mild hemolytic disease. Antibodies associated with moderate to severe disease include Kell, Diego, Duffy, C, c, E, Kid, and MNS. Of these, one of the most severe in its manifestation is Kell. This is partly because Kell antibodies are associated with suppression of erythropoiesis through destruction of erythroid progenitor cells.[54] Therefore, the degree of hemolysis is not reflective of the severity of anemia, and amniotic fluid ΔOD 450 measurements may be misleading. This has led several authors to suggest using direct fetal blood sampling in these particular situations.[54a,54b]

Nonimmune Hydrops

Nonimmune hydrops fetalis was first distinguished from immune hydrops by Edith Potter in 1943.[55] When first described, nonimmune hydrops represented less than 20% of all cases of fetal hydrops. However, with effective prophylaxis against Rh immunization, nonimmune hydrops now constitutes approximately 90% of cases of fetal hydrops.[56–58]

The prevalence of nonimmune hydrops is approximately 1 in 3,000 births.[59] Reported frequencies vary in the literature depending on the definition of nonimmune hydrops. We define nonimmune hydrops as two or more serous body cavity effusions, or one effusion plus anasarca, in a fetus immunologically compatible with the mother. The perinatal death rate from nonimmune hydrops is 30% to 90%.[58–62]

Pathogenesis

Nonimmune hydrops results from a wide variety of underlying causes.[57,63] Success in identifying an underlying cause requires a systematic clinical approach and a targeted effort during sonography. Various studies have reported that an underlying cause can be identified in 50% to 80% of cases of nonimmune hydrops.[58,60–62] The word *cause* is used with some caution because a definite cause and effect relation-

TABLE 4. PATHOPHYSIOLOGIC CLASSIFICATION OF HYDROPS FETALIS

Increased intravascular hydrostatic pressure (due to hemodynamic disturbances)
  Primary myocardial failure
    Arrhythmia
    Severe anemia (e.g., glucose-6-phosphate dehydrogenase deficiency, alpha thalassemia)
    Twin transfusion syndrome
    Myocarditis (e.g., coxsackievirus, TORCH)
    Cardiac malformation
  High-output failure
    Parabiotic syndrome
    Arteriovenous shunt
  Obstruction of venous return: congenital neoplasm/other space-occupying lesions (e.g., cystic adenomatoid malformation)
Decreased plasma oncotic pressure
  Decreased albumin formation (e.g., congenital cirrhosis, hepatitis)
  Increased albumin excretion (e.g., congenital nephrotic syndrome of Finnish type)
Increased capillary permeability: anoxia (e.g., congenital infection, placental edema)
Obstruction of lymph flow (e.g., Turner syndrome)

TORCH, *toxoplasmosis, other agents, rubella, cytomegalovirus, herpes simplex.*
Modified from Im SS, Rizos N, Joutsi P, Shime J, Benzie RJ. Nonimmunologic hydrops fetalis. *Am J Obstet Gynecol* 1984;148:566–569.

ship with the fetal anomaly may be lacking. It may be more appropriate to classify some of these relationships with nonimmune hydrops as *associations*.

Theoretically, development of edema can be attributed to one of six principal factors[64] (Table 4):

1. Primary myocardial failure
2. High-output cardiac failure
3. Decreased plasma oncotic pressure
4. Increased capillary permeability
5. Obstruction of venous return
6. Obstruction of lymphatic flow

One or more of these mechanisms may be responsible in individual cases.

Table 5 outlines a list of possible causes and associations of nonimmune hydrops categorized by the general site of involvement.[65] In many cases, the pathophysiologic mechanism leading to fetal hydrops can be explained, although in other cases the cause of hydrops is uncertain.

Primary myocardial failure can occur in cases of intrauterine infection resulting from myocarditis (e.g., parvovirus), coxsackie pancarditis, or subendocardial fibroelastosis. Disorders that may result in high-output cardiac failure include vascular malformations of the cranium (vein of Galen aneurysm), placenta (chorioangioma), umbilical cord (hemangioma), liver (hemangioendothelioma), or coccyx (sacrococcygeal teratoma). High-output cardiac failure also occurs in twin-twin transfusion due to volume overload in the recipient twin or anemia in the donor twin.

TABLE 5. CONDITIONS ASSOCIATED WITH NONIMMUNE HYDROPS FETALIS

Categories	Individual Conditions	Categories	Individual Conditions
Cardiovascular	Tachyarrhythmia	Respiratory	Diaphragmatic hernia
	Complex dysrhythmia		Cystic adenomatoic malformation
	Congenital heart block		Pulmonary lymphangiectasia
	Anatomic defects (atrial septal defect, ventricular septal defect, hypoplastic, left heart, pulmonary valve insufficiency, Ebstein subaortic stenosis, aortic valve stenosis, subaortic stenosis, atrioventricular canal defect with mitral regurgitation, single ventricle, tetralogy of Fallot, premature closure of the foramen ovale or of the ductus arteriosus, dextrocardia in combination with pulmonic stenosis)		Hamartoma of the lung
			Pulmonary hypoplasia
			Extralobar pulmonary sequestration
		Maternal	Severe anemia
			Severe diabetes mellitus
			Hypoproteinemia
	Subendocardial fibroelastosis	Placenta-umbilical cord	Chorioangioma
	Calcified aortic valve		Chorionic vein thrombosis
	Coronary artery embolus		Fetal-maternal transfusion
	Cardiomyopathy		Aneurysm of the umbilical artery
	Heat block		True cord knots
	Heterotaxy syndromes		Umbilical cord torsion
	Myocarditis (coxsackievirus or cytomegalovirus)		Angiomyxoma of the umbilical cord
	Atrial hemangioma		Placental and umbilical vein thrombosis
	Rhabdomyoma		
	Teratoma		
	Arteriovenous shunts		
	Agenesis of the ductus venosus	Chromosomal	Down syndrome (trisomy 21)
Gastrointestinal	Jejunal atresia		Other trisomies
	Midgut volvulus		Turner syndrome
	Biliary atresia		XX/XY mosaicism
	Metabolic storage disease		Triploidy
	Meconium peritonitis	Infections	Cytomegalovirus
	Hepatic fibrosis		Toxoplasmosis
	Familial cirrhosis		Syphilis
Skeletal malformation	Thanatophoric dwarfism		Herpes simplex type I
	Arthogryposis multiplex congenita		Rubella
	Asphyxiating thoracic dystrophy		Leptospirosis
	Hypophosphatasia		Chagas disease
	Osteogenesis imperfecta		Parvovirus B19
	Achondrogenesis		Adenovirus
	Recessive cystic hygroma	Twin pregnancy	Twin-twin transfusion syndrome
	Francois syndrome, type 3		Acardiac twinning
	Saldino-Noonan syndrome	Genitourinary	Urinary obstruction
	Neu-Laxova syndrome		Congenital nephrosis (Finnish type)
	Pena-Shokier syndrome, type 1		
Medications	Antepartum indomethacin (taken to stop premature labor, causing fetal ductus closure and secondary nonimmune hydrops fetalis)	Tumors	Neuroblastoma
			Sacrococcygeal teratoma
			Teratoma, other locations
Hematologic	Alpha thalassemia		Mesoblastic nephroma
	Anemia, any cause		Wilms tumor
	Fetal Kasabach-Merritt syndrome		Unknown
	In utero closed space hemorrhage		
	Vena cava, portal vein, or renal vein obstruction (e.g., thrombosis)		
	Congenital leukemia		
	Hemochromatosis		
	Erythrocyte enzymopathy (G6PD)		
	Rhesus sensitization		
	Hemophilia A		
Miscellaneous	Congenital lymphedema		
	Congenital hydrothorax or chylothorax deficiency		
	Tuberous sclerosis		
	Multiple pterygium syndrome		
	Familial pulmonary lyumphatic hypoplasia		

Modified from Holzgreve W, Holzgreve B, Curry JR. Nonimmune hydrops fetalis: diagnosis and management. *Semin Perinatol* 1985;9:52.

Obstruction of venous or lymphatic flow may result from hydrothorax, thoracic or cardiac tumors, cystic adenomatoid malformation of the lung, diaphragmatic hernia, or venous thrombosis. Abnormal or delayed development of the lymphatic system is thought to contribute to hydrops in chromosomal disorders.

Fetal anemia may result from decreased production of red blood cells, defective hemoglobin, fetal hemorrhage, or increased hemolysis. Subsequent hydrops may develop from a combination of high output cardiac failure and portal hypertension due to extramedullary hematopoiesis in the liver, resulting in compression of the hepatic vasculature.

In a review of 600 cases of nonimmune hydrops reported since 1982, Jauniaux et al. reported the following causes and associations with nonimmune hydrops: cardiac abnormalities, 22%; chromosome abnormalities, 16%; alpha thalassemia, 10%; twin-twin transfusion, 6%; congenital infections, 4.5%; skeletal dysplasia, 4%; thoracic abnormalities, 6%; placental and cord abnormalities, 3%; idiopathic, 15.5%.[63] A larger percentage of idiopathic cases, approximately 30%, has been reported in other studies.[57,58,62,66]

Clinical Approach

Unlike immune hydrops, no single laboratory test is available to screen pregnancies at risk for nonimmune hydrops. In the great majority of patients, therefore, prenatal sonography represents the sole means for detecting this disorder. Patient history is a very important and common reason for referral to ultrasound to rule out hydrops. Size-date discrepancy resulting from polyhydramnios is another common reason for referral to sonography. Second-trimester maternal serum screening may demonstrate raised human chorionic gonadotropin.[67] Hutchison et al.[68] reported that when polyhydramnios, maternal anemia, and hypertension were used as clinical indications for sonographic evaluation, 80% or more of fetuses with nonimmune hydrops would be detected after 28 weeks' gestation.

The diagnostic approach to nonimmune hydrops is outlined in Table 6.[65,69,70] Immune hydrops can be excluded by the indirect Coombs' test. Clinical history and laboratory studies of maternal serum may identify other maternal causes for nonimmune hydrops, including thalassemia, metabolic disease, anemia, and certain intrauterine infections. Most cases, however, require more invasive methods, including amniocentesis, placental biopsy, or cordocentesis. Cordocentesis provides the most rapid and direct means of evaluating hematologic disorders, serum protein level, metabolic abnormalities, and fetal karyotype.[71]

Sonographic Findings

Sonographic features of nonimmune hydrops resemble those of immune hydrops. Two or more body cavity fluid collections, or one cavity effusion in association with anasarca, provide the diagnosis of hydrops. If maternal red cell antibodies are negative, immune hydrops is excluded. The differential diagnosis then includes an extensive list of possible causes of nonimmune hydrops (Table 5).

TABLE 6. DIAGNOSTIC STEPS IN THE PRENATAL EVALUATION OF NONIMMUNE HYDROPS FETALIS (NIHF)

Levels of diagnosis/invasiveness	Diagnostic test	Possible etiology
Maternal	Complete blood cell count and indices	Hematologic disorders
Noninvasive	Hemoglobin electrophoresis	Alpha thalassemia
	Blood chemistry (e.g., maternal G6PD, pyruvate kinase carrier status)	Possibility of fetal red blood cell enzyme deficiency
	Kleihauer-Betke test	Fetal-maternal transfusion
	Viral titers (coxsackievirus, parvovirus)	Fetal infection
	Syphilis (VDRL) and TORCH titers	
	Ultrasonography	Assessment of NIHF and its progression, exclude multiple pregnancy and congenital malformations
	Fetal echocardiography	Congenital heart defects
		Rhythm disturbances of the fetal heart
	Oral glucose tolerance test	Maternal diabetes mellitus
Amniocentesis	Fetal karyotype	Chromosomal abnormalities
	Amniotic fluid culture	Cytomegalovirus
	Alpha-fetoprotein	Congenital nephrosis, sacrococcygeal teratomas
	Specific metabolic tests	Gaucher disease, Tay-Sachs, GM gangliosidosis, etc.
	Restriction endonuclease tests	Alpha thalassemia
Fetal blood aspiration	Rapid karyotype and metabolic tests	Chromosomal or metabolic abnormalities
	Hemoglobin chain analysis	Thalassemias
	Fetal plasma analysis for specific IgM	Intrauterine infection
	Fetal plasma albumin	Hypoalbuminemia
	Complete blood cell count	Fetal anemia

G6PD, glucose-6-phosphate dehydrogenase; IgM, immunoglobulin M; TORCH, *toxoplasmosis, other agents, rubella, cytomegalovirus, herpes simplex.*
From Holzgreve W, Holzgreve B, Curry JR. Nonimmune hydrops fetalis: diagnosis and management. *Semin Perinatol* 1985;9:52.

TABLE 7. POSSIBLE SONOGRAPHIC FINDINGS IN THE EVALUATION OF NONIMMUNE HYDROPS

Anatomy	Sonographic findings	Possible diagnosis
Head	Intracranial mass	Vein of Galen aneurysm
	Cystic intracranial mass	Porencephalic cyst
	Intracranial bleeding	Thrombocytopenia
	Microcephaly	Cytomegalovirus, toxoplasmosis
	Cranial defect with mass	Encephalocele
Neck	Mass	Cystic hygroma, paratracheal hemangioma, hemangioendothelioma
	Nuchal thickening	Chromosomal abnormality (trisomy 21)
Thorax	Small thorax	Pulmonary hypoplasia, dwarfism, Pena-Shokeir syndrome
	Chest mass	Cystic adenomatoid malformation, pulmonary leiomyosarcoma, extralobar pulmonary sequestration, diaphragmatic hernia
Heart	Mass	Tumor
	Poorly contracting heart	Heart failure
	Irregular heart rhythm	Cardiac dysrhythmia
	Structural cardiac abnormalities	Congenital cardiac malformation
	Pericardial effusion with mass	Pericardial teratoma
	Pericardial calcification	Intrauterine infections
Abdomen	Dilated bowel loops	Gastrointestinal obstruction, atresia, volvulus
	Calcification	Meconium peritonitis
	Hepatic mass	Hemangioma, hemangioendothelioma, hepatoblastoma
	Hepatosplenomegaly	Intrauterine infection, extramedullary hematopoiesis
Genitourinary	Retroperitoneal mass	Neuroblastoma
	Hydronephrosis	Obstructive uropathy
	Echogenic kidneys	Cystic kidney disease
	Thickened urinary bladder wall	Obstructive uropathy
Extremities	Short extremities	Dysplasia
	Fractures	Osteogenesis imperfecta
	Contractures	Arthrogryposis
Placenta	Thick	Intrauterine infections, extramedullary hematopoiesis, anemia
	Mass	Chorioangioma
Amniotic cavity	Umbilical cord abnormalities	Torsion knot, angiomyxoma, hemangioma, umbilical artery aneurysm
	Twin gestation	Twin-twin transfusion

Modified from Fleischer AC, Killam AP, Boehm FH, Hutchison AA, Jones TB, et al. Hydrops fetalis: sonographic evaluation and clinical implications. *Radiology* 1981;141:163–168.

A search for specific fetal structural abnormalities may lead to a diagnosis of the underlying cause. A system-oriented approach to the fetus is helpful (Table 7).[69] Structural abnormalities may involve nearly any organ system and can be identified in approximately 40% of fetuses. Specific disorders that are associated most commonly with nonimmune hydrops are discussed later in this chapter under separate headings. In the absence of any specific fetal organ system abnormality, a precise diagnosis of the underlying cause of hydrops is difficult.

Emphasis should be placed on a detailed cardiac evaluation, as cardiac abnormality is the most common underlying factor in nonimmune hydrops (approximately 20% of cases). Cardiac rhythm disturbances are especially important to recognize. Many tachyarrhythmias respond to appropriate pharmacologic treatment *in utero*, and the prognosis is much improved.[72,73]

Individual fetuses with nonimmune hydrops reveal various patterns in the distribution of fluid collections and sonographic features. Ascites, pleural effusions, pericardial effusion, anasarca, cardiomegaly, polyhydramnios, and placental edema may occur together or in different combinations.[68,69,74] Fluid in only one body space warrants close sonographic follow-up, as this may be the first sign of impending hydrops. Early hydrops in the first-trimester fetus manifests as increased nuchal translucency thickness[75] or generalized skin edema.

The sonographic findings of nonimmune hydrops essentially do not differ from those of immune hydrops; however, some additional points are worth discussing. Skin thickening may be seen in association with conditions other than nonimmune hydrops, including macrosomia, redundant skin folds of short-limb dysplasias, or lymphangiectasia. Numerous septations within subcutaneous tissue fluid collections are seen in lymphangiectasia with cystic hygroma (Figs. 17 and 18). Skin thickening is easiest to visualize over the chest wall and scalp.

Pericardial effusions have been reported as the earliest sign of nonimmune hydrops associated with cardiac abnormalities.[76,77] Pericardial fluid greater than 2 mm is considered abnormal.[77] Increased cardiac biventricular outer dimension indicates cardiomegaly and has been reported as predictive of poor survival.[59]

Pleural effusions can be unilateral or bilateral and, if large, may lead to pulmonary hypoplasia by compressing

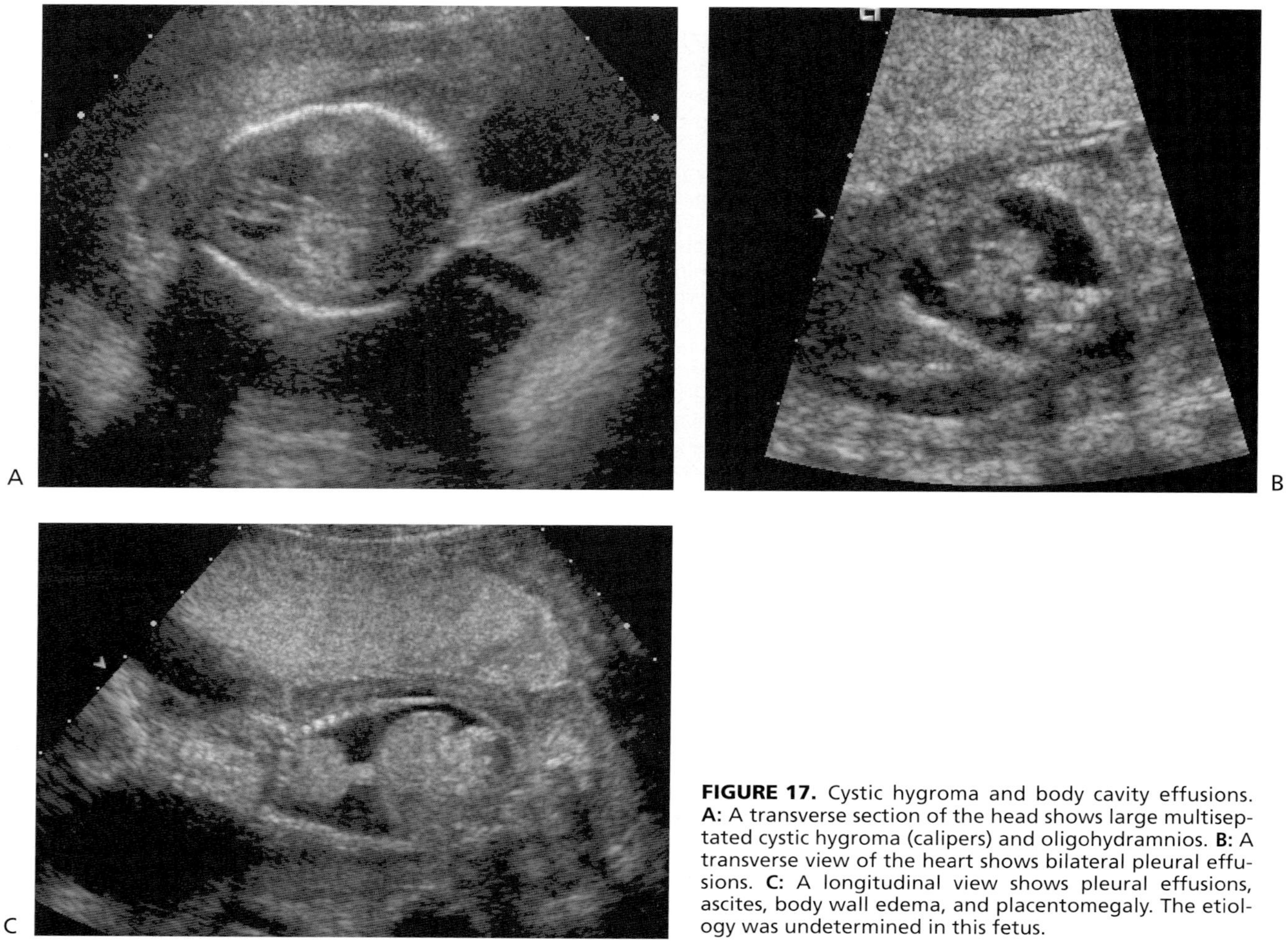

FIGURE 17. Cystic hygroma and body cavity effusions. **A:** A transverse section of the head shows large multiseptated cystic hygroma (calipers) and oligohydramnios. **B:** A transverse view of the heart shows bilateral pleural effusions. **C:** A longitudinal view shows pleural effusions, ascites, body wall edema, and placentomegaly. The etiology was undetermined in this fetus.

the developing lungs. A unilateral effusion typically does not shift the mediastinum; the presence of a space-occupying mass, such as a diaphragmatic hernia, should be considered if there is marked mediastinal shift.[78] Pleural effusions are

rarely seen in hydrops before 15 weeks' gestation, except in cases of Turner syndrome.[75]

Polyhydramnios has been reported in up to 75% of pregnancies with nonimmune hydrops and is a common

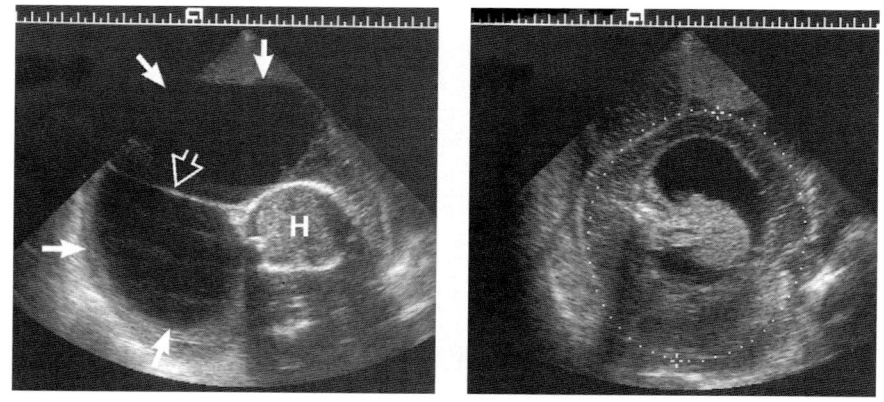

FIGURE 18. Cystic hygroma with hydrops in Turner syndrome. **A:** A transverse view of the head (*H*) shows a massive cystic hygroma (*solid arrows*) containing midline internal septation (*open arrow*). **B:** A view of the abdomen shows a large amount of ascites and marked body wall edema. Oligohydramnios is also evident.

reason for initial referral to sonography. Polyhydramnios contributes to premature labor, uterine atony, postpartum hemorrhage, and retained placental material. Oligohydramnios also can occur and suggests a poor prognosis, although the true prognosis depends on the underlying cause of low amniotic fluid volume.[78]

Placental edema indicated by placental thickening (Fig. 3) is more likely to develop in a hydropic fetus with anemia than in a hydropic fetus without anemia.[79] Measurement of placental thickness (greater than 3 cm at 18 to 21 weeks' gestation) assists in the identification of pregnancies affected by alpha-thalassemia before the onset of hydrops.[80]

Investigators have attempted to derive information from the pattern of sonographic features in nonimmune hydrops. Skoll et al.[66] found that pleural effusions and ascites were less common in fetuses with cardiac causes of nonimmune hydrops, in comparison to fetuses with hydrops unrelated to cardiac conditions. In contrast, Mahony et al.[74] were unable to delineate any characteristic patterns of fluid distribution in nonimmune hydropic fetuses.

Prognosis

The overall prognosis for nonimmune hydrops is poor, with mortality rates higher than 70%.[64,68,74,75] This rate approaches 100% when a fetal structural abnormality is identified sonographically.[64,75] The presence of oligohydramnios in association with hydrops also is associated with a poor prognosis, although this depends on the cause of the oligohydramnios.

Recognition of a treatable cause of nonimmune hydrops, such as a cardiac tachyarrhythmia, provides a good prognosis. Conversion to fetal sinus rhythm is possible with maternal or fetal administration of pharmacologic agents.[73] Other correctable causes of hydrops are few. Hydrops can resolve if severe fetal anemia is corrected by intrauterine transfusion. Spontaneous resolution of hydrops has been observed coincident with infarction of a placental chorioangioma,[81] and in cases of parvovirus and CMV[82] infection.

Despite more aggressive fetal therapy, Wy et al.[58] concluded that overall survival outcome for fetal hydrops has not improved in the 1990s.

Management

Optimal obstetric management of nonimmune hydrops relies on early prenatal diagnosis of the cause of hydrops, detailed sonographic evaluation or monitoring, preterm delivery when appropriate, and prompt postpartum management of the infant in a high-risk perinatal center. Commonly, invasive approaches such as cordocentesis are needed to help establish diagnosis, but the risk of pregnancy loss associated with it is much higher given the hydropic status of the fetus. Occasionally, specific therapy can be administered

in utero, for example, antiarrhythmic therapy for fetal tachycardia, or transfusion to correct fetal anemia due to fetomaternal hemorrhage, glucose-6-phosphate dehydrogenase deficiency, or parvovirus infection.[83,84] Fetal thoracentesis or placement of a thoracoamniotic shunt can be performed to drain pleural effusion. Fetal surgery for sacrococcygeal teratoma[85] and cystic adenomatoid malformation of the lung[86] has been reported. Autopsy and assessment of the fetus by a geneticist or pediatric dysmorphologist in terminated pregnancies or after stillbirth may provide further clues to the diagnosis and thus assist with counseling of recurrence risks and monitoring of future pregnancies.

Conditions Associated with Nonimmune Hydrops

Cardiac Anomalies

Cardiac anomalies are among the most common causes of nonimmune hydrops in white populations, accounting for 22% to 40% of cases.[56,61,87,88] They include arrhythmias or dysrhythmias, structural defects, myocarditis, and tumors.

Obstruction of venous return or arterial outflow, abnormal shunting of blood, or interference with myocardial contractility or function can lead to nonimmune hydrops. However, mechanisms leading to hydrops are not always clear and not all types of cardiac anomalies lead to hydrops. The reasons hydrops develops in association with some types of cardiac structural defects are unclear.[89]

Cardiac arrhythmias are an important cause of nonimmune hydrops. They are easiest to recognize on M-mode sonography. Tachyarrhythmias, bradyarrhythmias, or dysrhythmias can occur. Tachyarrhythmia is one of the few treatable causes of nonimmune hydrops and thus is most important to recognize. Treatments include pharmacologic therapy administered to the mother or direct fetal treatment, which in the appropriate settings can be successful in reverting the fetal heart rate to sinus rhythm.[73,88,90]

Structural cardiac anomalies associated with hydrops include valvular abnormalities, septal defects, or more complex anomalies. Detailed echocardiographic examination is essential and may be possible as early as 14 to 16 weeks.[91] A fetus with structural cardiac anomalies and nonimmune hydrops has a poor prognosis; perinatal mortality approaches 100%.[75,87,92] Thirty percent of fetuses with structural cardiac lesions have an abnormal karyotype[93] and this knowledge may significantly alter management. Careful sonographic search for extracardiac abnormalities also should be made.

The sonographic findings due to cardiac anomalies are generally indistinguishable from those of hydrops from other causes. A few specific patterns exist that can be helpful, such as the finding of right atrial enlargement, which should prompt a search for tricuspid valve abnormalities with tricuspid regurgitation or for pulmonary atresia or stenosis.[94] Devore et al.[95] have suggested that isolated pericardial effusion is the earliest sonographic finding of developing hydrops in fetuses with structural cardiac anomalies, although this observation has not been confirmed by other investigators.

Cardiac failure and hydrops from myocarditis can develop in fetuses with intrauterine infections, such as those related to parvovirus.[96,97] High-output cardiac failure can occur in association with large vascular tumors (arteriovenous shunting or sequestration of red blood cells) or adrenal neuroblastoma (high levels of catecholamines).[78]

Cardiac masses such as atrial hemangioma, atrial rhabdomyoma, or intrapericardial teratoma may lead to hydrops by obstructing blood flow.[98,99] Atrial rhabdomyoma is seen with increased frequency in tuberous sclerosis, which can be inherited as an autosomal dominant condition.

Anemia and Hematologic Disorders

Hematologic disorders may account for approximately 10% of cases of nonimmune hydrops.[100] The pathogenesis of hydrops from these disorders is thought to relate to fetal anemia. Fetal anemia may result from fetal hemorrhage, defective red blood cell production, production of abnormal hemoglobin (thalassemia), or increased hemolysis.[101,102] Intrauterine infection with parvovirus may lead to anemia and fetal hydrops secondary to red cell hemolysis.[96,103,104]

Homozygous alpha-1 thalassemia (Bart hemoglobinopathy) is inherited as an autosomal recessive disorder with a 25% recurrence rate for subsequent pregnancies. Alpha thalassemia is a common cause of hydrops among Southeast Asians.[61,105] An abnormal tetramer of hemoglobin (Bart hemoglobin) is formed as a result of deficient α chain synthesis. Bart hemoglobin has such a high affinity for oxygen that it does not release enough oxygen to fetal tissues. This leads to hypoxia, high-output cardiac failure, and nonimmune hydrops.

Nonimmune hydrops due to homozygous alpha thalassemia is almost universally fatal to the fetus and produces significant maternal morbidity. Women carrying a fetus affected with homozygous alpha thalassemia may experience hypertension and edema (preeclampsia), mild microcytic anemia (non–iron-deficient and unresponsive to therapy), congestive cardiac failure, and polyhydramnios.[105] There have been case reports of fetuses with Bart hemoglobinopathy surviving after intensive therapy.[106]

Beta thalassemias are not a cause of hydrops. Hemoglobin F production is maintained during the fetal period, and reliance on hemoglobin A does not occur prenatally.

Twin-Twin Transfusion

In multiple gestations, fetal hydrops may be secondary to either congenital anomalies or twin-twin transfusion syndrome. Congenital anomalies occur with increased frequency in monozygotic pregnancies. Acardiac twinning is characterized by hydropic changes of the acardiac twin (Fig. 19). Heart failure with hydrops may also complicate the "pump" twin.

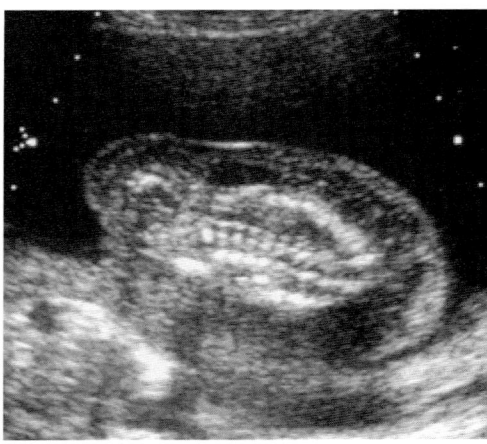

FIGURE 19. Acardiac twin with hydrops. A longitudinal image through the body of a hydropic acardiac twin at 17 weeks' gestational age shows marked anasarca.

The twin-twin transfusion syndrome, unique to monozygotic, monochorionic multiple pregnancies, may account for up to 8% of cases of nonimmune hydrops.[100] Transplacental vascular communications result in alterations of the dynamics of blood flow. The fetus receiving excessive blood flow is plethoric and hydropic and displays features of cardiac decompensation as a result of overload (i.e., large heart and hypertrophy) due to volume overload (Fig. 20). The fetus receiving less blood flow usually shows signs of intrauterine growth retardation, but also may become hydropic as a result of severe anemia.[74] Twin-twin transfusion syndrome should be suspected if the fetal weight is less than 20% of that of the other fetus (or fetuses) or if hydrops develops. Discrepancy in amniotic fluid volume with polyhydramnios developing in the larger fetus is the single most common finding of the twin-twin

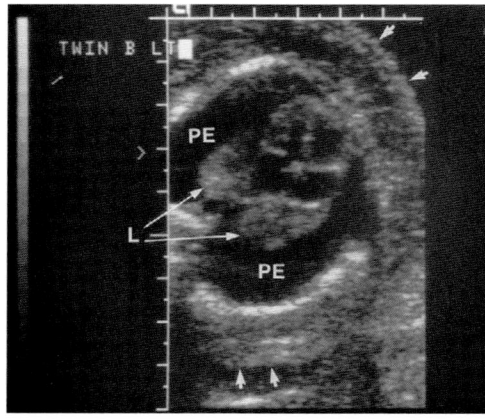

FIGURE 20. Hydrops with twin-twin transfusion syndrome. A transverse view of the thorax in this twin pregnancy shows bilateral pleural effusion (*PE*) and collapsed lungs (*L*). Body wall edema is marked (*small arrows*). This was the recipient twin of the twin-twin transfusion syndrome.

transfusion syndrome.[107] Further discussion of this topic is found in Chapter 18.

Chromosome Abnormalities

Chromosome abnormalities are a relatively common cause of nonimmune hydrops, accounting for up to 16% of cases.[61,63] Nonimmune hydrops diagnosed before 18 weeks' gestation is associated with a higher incidence of chromosome abnormalities than nonimmune hydrops diagnosed during the second half of pregnancy.[108] The most common chromosome abnormalities associated with hydrops include Turner syndrome; trisomies 13, 18, and 21; and triploidy.[68,100,108] Triploidy may be associated with molar changes in the placenta.[75] Fetuses with otherwise unexplained causes of hydrops should be considered for chromosome analysis by amniocentesis, placental biopsy, or cordocentesis. The etiologic mechanism of hydrops is uncertain but involves lymphatic dysplasia or congestive heart failure.

Generalized fetal hydrops with cystic hygroma is commonly called *lymphangiectasia*. The presence of septations within the subcutaneous cystic spaces suggests lymphangiectasia rather than anasarca, which tends to lack septations. Lymphangiectasia often accompanies cystic hygroma. Cystic hygromas are observed most commonly as localized thickening of the skin and subcutaneous tissues in the neck, axillary, or thoracic regions. Isolated cystic hygromas have been observed to resolve over the course of gestation; they do not always go on to generalized lymphangiectasia.[109]

Lymphangiectasia has a universally fatal outcome and is associated with chromosome abnormalities in 66% of cases, particularly Turner syndrome (XO). Thus, it should be distinguished from cases of nonimmune hydrops without cystic hygroma. Amniotic fluid volume may be normal or decreased when the cystic hygroma replaces the amniotic fluid space.[110] It is important not to mistake a large cystic hygroma for the amniotic cavity.

Hereditary and Metabolic Disorders

Hereditary and metabolic disorders may account for up to 12% of cases of nonimmune hydrops.[100] New causes are being recognized and added to the list. Autosomal dominant conditions include congenital myotonic dystrophy,[111] Noonan's syndrome, tuberous sclerosis, and de Lange's syndrome.[112] These syndromes rarely are diagnosed with certainty on the basis of prenatal sonographic findings unless there is a family history of disease. Various metabolic disorders also have been associated with nonimmune hydrops, although it is uncertain how many of these present with isolated ascites that may be induced by hepatomegaly and liver dysfunction. These include Gaucher's disease, gangliosidosis type I, Hurler's syndrome, mucolipidosis type I, Niemann-Pick disease,[113] and carnitine deficiency.[114] Prenatal diagnosis of such metabolic disorders may be possible by enzymatic assay of cultured fibroblasts from amniocentesis or cordocentesis. Also, a history of parental consanguinity should be sought as this is another etiology for nonimmune hydrops.

Thoracic Abnormalities

Thoracic abnormalities account for approximately 6% of nonimmune hydrops.[100] Examples of intrathoracic masses include cystic adenomatoid malformation of the lung, diaphragmatic hernia, pulmonary sequestration, and neoplasms (cardiac, pericardial, mediastinal, or lung neoplasms).[86,115–117] Most of these involve space-occupying lesions that produce hydrops by obstructing venous return to the heart or interfering with cardiac function by compression of the heart.[118] Compression of the esophagus (and impaired fetal swallowing) due to an intrathoracic mass can lead to polyhydramnios. Hydrops in association with intrathoracic masses denotes a poor prognosis.[117]

Although pleural effusions are a common manifestation of severe hydrops, unilateral or bilateral hydrothorax also may be an isolated finding. Chylothorax does not occur in the fetus, because chylomicrons are not produced prenatally.[119] Like isolated ascites, isolated hydrothorax has its own list of etiologic factors and should be distinguished from generalized hydrops (see Chapter 19).

Infections

A variety of infectious agents have been associated with nonimmune hydrops and ascites, including *Toxoplasma*, parvovirus, *Treponema pallidum*, CMV, and coxsackievirus.[103,120,121] Infectious causes are responsible for some of the cases of nonimmune hydrops that have been observed to resolve spontaneously.[122,123] Other abnormal sonographic findings also may be present (see Chapter 17).

Parvovirus B19 causes nonimmune hydrops by (a) stimulating bone marrow aplasia with subsequent anemia[124] and (b) causing myocarditis.[97] Fetal hydrops can be transient and reversible. In most cases of maternal parvovirus infection, the fetus is not affected adversely and the fetal death rate ranges from less than 5% to 9%.[125,126]

The diagnosis of *in utero* parvovirus infection can be established by PCR identification of a portion of the parvovirus genome in amniotic fluid or fetal blood samples.[127] Fetal anemia and increased numbers of nucleated red blood cells may be seen in the fetal blood obtained by cordocentesis.[104] Fetal blood transfusion may be extremely helpful in treating the severe anemia induced by parvovirus.[128,129]

In most cases, infectious causes of nonimmune hydrops are indistinguishable sonographically from other causes. Occasionally, however, unusual calcifications in the pericardium or brain or cerebral ventriculomegaly may suggest an infectious cause.

Neoplasms

Various neoplasms or masses may be associated with nonimmune hydrops, including neuroblastoma, sacrococcygeal teratoma, congenital leukemia, hemangioma of the liver,[130] hemangioendothelioma of the liver[131] or neck,[132] and cardiac or pericardial tumors.[98,99] Possible pathogenetic mechanisms include high-output cardiac failure from shunting through vascular tumors, vascular compression, or development of fetal anemia secondary to sequestration of red cells from intratumor hemorrhage. Most fetal tumors are identified on sonography from an anatomic survey of the fetus.

Placental Abnormalities

Placental abnormalities that have been associated with nonimmune hydrops include tumors of the placenta, hemorrhagic endovasculitis,[84] fetomaternal hemorrhage,[133] umbilical vein thrombosis, umbilical cord knot, or tumors of the umbilical cord.

Chorioangioma of the placenta, a benign hamartomatous tumor, can lead to hydrops by various suggested mechanisms: (a) arteriovenous shunting of blood through the placental chorioangioma and subsequent high-output cardiac failure in the fetus; (b) chronic fetal hypoxia arising from the return to the fetal circulation of arteriovenously shunted, unoxygenated blood from the chorioangioma; (c) microangiopathic hemolytic anemia of the fetus in large, vascular chorioangiomas. The angiomatous vascular subtype of chorioangioma is more likely to be associated with hydrops than is the cellular avascular subtype of chorioangioma.[134] Increasing echogenicity of the chorioangioma has been suggested as a good prognostic indicator related to fibrotic degeneration and reduced shunting of blood.[134] Regression of fetal hydrops has been observed after transfusion to correct anemia[135] and also in association with spontaneous infarction of a chorioangioma.[81]

Miscellaneous Conditions

Various skeletal disorders and dysplasias have been associated with nonimmune hydrops. These include achondroplasia, achondrogenesis, osteogenesis imperfecta type II, thanatophoric dysplasia, asphyxiating thoracic dysplasia, and short rib-polydactyly syndromes.[100,112] The pathogenesis leading to hydrops is unclear in these cases. Perhaps hypoplasia of the thorax is a contributing factor because of interference with amniotic fluid transfer through the lung. Altered composition of the extracellular matrix may play a role in early hydrops. At times it is difficult to differentiate anasarca of hydrops from redundant skin in these fetuses.

Various gastrointestinal and genitourinary abnormalities have been associated with "hydrops" in the literature.[136,137] Often isolated ascites is present in these cases, rather than generalized hydrops.

Summary

Hydrops fetalis is diagnosed easily and confidently with sonography. Testing maternal blood will establish whether isoimmunization is the cause of hydrops. Nonimmune hydrops accounts for the large majority of cases of hydrops. Sonography plays an important role in searching for the underlying causative lesions, particularly those that are correctable. Owing to the extensive list of causes and associations of nonimmune hydrops, a system-oriented approach to the fetus is helpful during sonography. No cause for hydrops is found in 15% to 30% of cases. Sonography is useful for observing the progress of fetal hydrops over time, in guiding needle placement for amniocentesis or umbilical cord blood sampling, and for monitoring response to therapy. Despite advances in fetal therapy, fetal mortality remains high.

ISOLATED FETAL ASCITES

Fetal ascites is most often seen in association with fetal hydrops or as one of the early manifestations of hydropic decompensation. When ascites is first identified, it is important to determine whether it is isolated or whether there are other signs of hydrops, including skin edema, scalp edema, pleural effusions, pericardial effusion, or tricuspid regurgitation. The prognosis and therapy for the fetus with hydrops depend on the etiology of hydrops. However, when fetal ascites is seen in isolation (i.e., without other signs of hydrops), it may represent a separate problem with different management and outcomes. It is important to note the distinction between these disorders; in the literature it is not always clear, and previous studies have frequently classified isolated ascites as fetal hydrops.

Pathogenesis

Isolated ascites is most often secondary to an intraabdominal disorder, rather than to a generalized condition (Table 8). Genitourinary anomalies account for the greatest number of cases, with obstructive uropathy as the most frequently cited cause.[151,161,179,181] In this situation, ascites develops from transudation, rupture, or leakage of urine into the peritoneal cavity. Spontaneous fetal urinary bladder rupture has even presented with isolated ascites.[148,152] Other genitourinary anomalies that may be associated with isolated ascites include renal hypoplasia, polycystic kidneys, hydrometrocolpos, ruptured ovarian cyst, cloacal anomalies, and congenital nephrotic syndrome.[74,164,185]

Gastrointestinal causes of ascites are second in frequency, accounting for approximately 20% of all cases.[147] Meconium peritonitis represents the majority of these and is usually the result of bowel obstruction with subsequent perforation. This can occur in association with meconium ileus[138,144,176,180] (Fig. 21), malrotation and midgut volvulus, small bowel atresia, intussusception, internal bowel hernia, Meckel's diverticulum, intestinal duplication, or vascular insufficiency.[136,137,165,170,171] The extruded meconium, digestive enzymes, or both are thought to incite an inflammatory

TABLE 8. CAUSES OF ASCITES

Immune hydrops
Nonimmune hydrops
Genitourinary (urine ascites)
  Urethrovesical obstruction (most common)
  Ureteropelvic obstruction
  Spontaneous bladder perforation
  Renal hypoplasia
  Cystic dysplastic kidney
  Congenital nephrotic syndrome
  Hydrometrocolpos
  Cloacal anomalies
  Ovarian cyst with torsion and/or rupture
Gastrointestinal
  Meconium peritonitis
  Midgut volvulus
  Intussusception
  Jejunoileal atresia
  Diaphragmatic hernia
  Omphalocele
Liver
  Idiopathic hepatitis/cytomegalovirus hepatitis
  Familial cirrhosis
  Fibrosis
  Biliary atresia
  Spontaneous extrahepatic biliary perforation
  Hepatic necrosis
  Budd-Chiari syndrome
  α_1-Antitrypsin deficiency
  Tumors
Cardiac
  Arrhythmias
  Restrictive foramen ovale
  Restrictive ductus arteriosus
  Ebstein anomaly
  Arteriovenous canal with or without trisomy 21
Infections
  Cytomegalovirus
  Toxoplasmosis
  Congenital syphilis
  Parvovirus
  Varicella
Metabolic storage disorders
  Wolman disease
  Gaucher disease
  Niemann-Pick disease
  GM gangliosidosis
  Sialidosis
  Mucopolysaccharidosis type IVA (Morquio syndrome, type A)
Other
  Congenital chyloperitoneum
  Generalized intestinal lymphangiectasia
Idiopathic

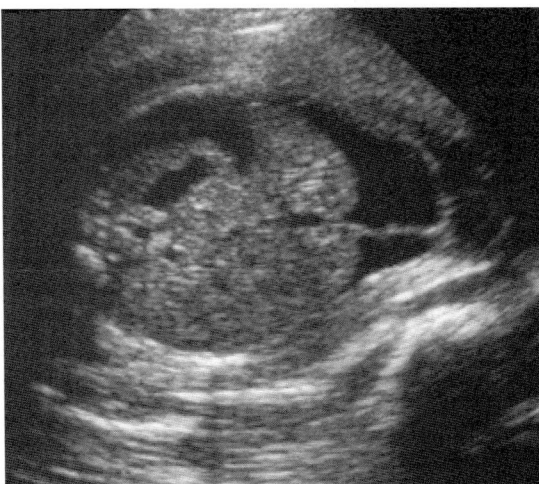

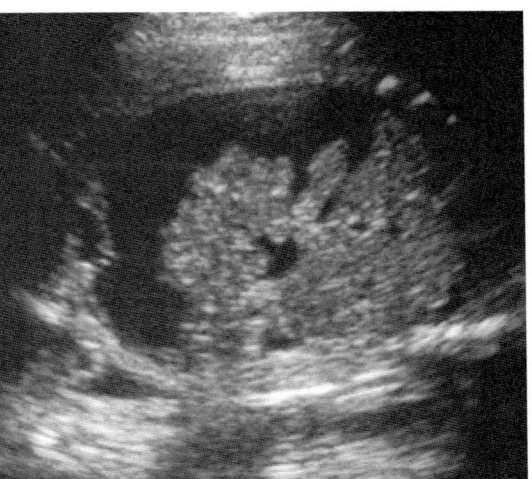

FIGURE 21. Massive fetal ascites secondary to meconium peritonitis from meconium ileus (i.e., cystic fibrosis) in a 28-week gestational age fetus. **A:** A transverse scan through the fetal abdomen shows severe ascites surrounding the liver. **B:** An oblique image through the fetal pelvis shows bowel loops floating in the ascitic fluid.

response with inflammation of serosal surfaces and transudation of fluid into the abdominal cavity causing ascites. Often, peritoneal calcifications are seen in association with the ascites. Venous and/or lymphatic obstruction may also play a role.

Infections such as congenital syphilis,[160,182] CMV,[138,139] varicella, toxoplasmosis,[146] and hepatitis A[145,157] can uncommonly cause fetal ascites. One of the proposed etiologies of ascites secondary to syphilis is the development of an enterocolitis, which impairs intestinal motility, leading to mechanical obstruction or meconium ileus.[182] Infections such as CMV may also cause hepatic fibrosis and subsequent ascites.[150,184] In the literature, parvovirus and varicella-zoster infection have more commonly been associated with fetal hydrops, but isolated ascites may be the first sign.

Finally, ascites may be seen in association with omphalocele and rarely with gastroschisis.[177]

Various liver disorders may cause isolated ascites including hepatitis, familial cirrhosis, hepatic fibrosis, and liver masses. These probably cause ascites in a manner similar to adults with obstruction of venous flow through the liver. Arteriovenous shunting probably is also a factor in the case of certain liver masses, such as cavernous hemangiomas and hemangioendotheliomas.[156] Hypoproteinemia secondary to hepatocellular injury may also be a factor in some cases. Spontaneous perforation of the extrahepatic bile duct has been associated with isolated fetal ascites.[154]

Chylous ascites can occur and is thought to be secondary to increased pressure within the lacteals or congenital deficiencies in lacteal formation. Generalized intestinal lymphangiectasia associated with Turner syndrome has been reported with isolated ascites, although it generally presents with severe hydrops.[140]

In utero heart failure may present as isolated fetal ascites, often as an early presentation of hydrops.[141,163] Cardiac pathology leading to heart failure includes both structural abnormalities and arrhythmias. Lesions that restrict flow from the right heart are particularly prone to produce heart failure. These include restrictive foramen ovale[159] and restrictive ductus arteriosus. Cardiac anomalies that cause severe tricuspid valve regurgitation such as Ebstein's anomaly and arteriovenous canal can also cause cardiac decompensation. Fetal cardiac arrhythmias may also present with ascites.

Metabolic storage disorders are important causes of ascites to consider, since they are inheritable disorders.[183] These include Wolman disease, Gaucher disease, GM_1 gangliosidosis, sialidosis, Morquio syndrome,[172] and Niemann-Pick disease.[178] The cause of ascites in these cases is uncertain but may be related to hypoproteinemia or hepatic filtration leading to sinusoidal obstruction. Another theory is that the infiltrative process damages blood and lymphatic vessels, causing enhanced permeability and leakage of fluid into the peritoneal cavity.

In the respiratory tract, isolated ascites has been associated with laryngeal atresia, stenosis, or both.[166] Lung enlargement, which may be identified by second-trimester ultrasound in these cases, is thought to account for the development of ascites. Marked intrathoracic compression by the enlarged lungs creates pressure on the right atrium and great veins, impeding venous return and subsequently causing congestive heart failure and ascites.

Other rare causes of fetal ascites include Günther disease[167] (congenital erythropoietic porphyria), xerocytosis,[168] and cutis marmorata telangiectatica congenital.[169] The latter rare, benign cutaneous disorder also presents with a markedly elevated maternal serum human chorionic gonadotropin and hepatomegaly at birth.

Idiopathic fetal ascites may be a transient phenomena.[123,189] It usually resolves in the fetal or neonatal period. Transient congestive heart failure, infection, and lymphatic obstruction have been suggested as possible causes; however, the pathogenesis remains unclear.

Other potential causes for isolated fetal ascites include maternal/fetal abuse and maternal electroconvulsive therapy.[173,174]

Sonographic Findings

Fetal ascites is generally identified by demonstrating fluid surrounding the liver, spleen, bowel, extrahepatic portion

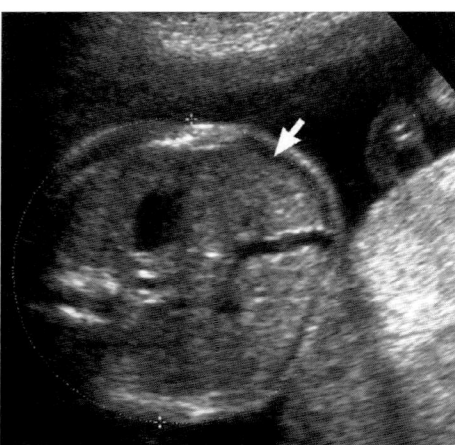

FIGURE 22. Pseudoascites. A transverse scan through the abdomen at 28 weeks demonstrates an anechoic rim (*arrow*) surrounding the abdomen that represents abdominal wall musculature. This should not be confused with true ascites.

of the umbilical vein, falciform ligament, or greater omentum. A small amount of ascites may be difficult to detect, and the absolute quantity of fluid detected is related to fetal size. In a retrospective review, as little as 12 to 14 mL of fluid was seen easily in fetuses at 18 to 20 weeks, whereas 30 to 40 mL of fluid was necessary for detection in fetuses older than 30 weeks.[24] Difficulty may also arise in identifying a large amount of ascites, which may be misinterpreted as amniotic fluid outside the fetus.

Caution must be taken in differentiating true ascites from pseudoascites.[190] A sonolucent layer representing the normal abdominal musculature may be seen immediately beneath the outer margin of the fetal abdomen and may be misinterpreted as ascites (Fig. 22). The muscular layer can sometimes be traced to the muscular insertions on the rib endings. This extraperitoneal tissue remains confined to the anterior or anterolateral aspect of the fetal abdomen, distinguishing it from true ascitic fluid.

Once generalized hydrops has been excluded, a systematic sonographic search to determine the underlying etiology of isolated ascites should be undertaken, with special attention to the genitourinary, gastrointestinal, and cardiovascular systems. Chylous ascites and ascites due to infection are primarily diagnoses of exclusion.[191] Occasionally, as already mentioned, an underlying cause may not be identified by ultrasound, and serial studies are necessary to determine whether additional abnormalities develop or the ascites increases or decreases.

Management

Isolated fetal ascites discovered on an initial sonogram should be followed by an ultrasound approximately 1 week later to determine whether progression to fetal hydrops has occurred. If the ascites remains isolated to the fetal abdomen, then progression to hydrops becomes much less likely.

TABLE 9. TESTS TO CONSIDER IN THE EVALUATION OF ASCITES

Maternal serum screening
  Alpha-fetoprotein
  Cytomegalovirus (CMV)
  Toxoplasmosis
  Syphilis
  Varicella zoster
  Parvovirus
Amniocentesis
  Fetal karyotype
  TORCH titers
  Antigen-specific IgM/IgG
  Polymerase chain reaction (PCR) (i.e., CMV, other viruses)
  Testing for metabolic storage disorders/α_1-antitrypsin deficiency
Percutaneous umbilical blood sampling
  Fetal karyotype
  TORCH titers
  Antigen-specific IgM/IgG
  PCR (i.e., CMV, other viruses)
  Testing for metabolic storage disorders/α_1-antitrypsin deficiency
    Fetal liver function tests
    Blood urea nitrogen/creatinine/electrolytes
Fetal paracentesis
  Fetal karyotype
  TORCH titers
  Antigen-specific IgG/IgM
  PCR (i.e., CMV, other viruses)
  Protein/lymphocyte counts
  Blood urea nitrogen/creatinine
  Meconium

IgG, immunoglobulin G; IgM, immunoglobulin M; TORCH, toxoplasmosis, other agents, rubella, cytomegalovirus, herpes simplex.

Various tests should be considered in the evaluation of the fetus with isolated ascites (Table 9).

If a structural anomaly is discovered by ultrasound, an amniocentesis for fetal karyotyping should be considered. When a definite cause for ascites cannot be determined, the need for fetal karyotyping becomes less certain. Amniocentesis may still be considered under other circumstances, such as in the evaluation of possible fetal infection or in the prenatal diagnosis of inherited metabolic diseases. Fetal blood sampling and evaluation of fetal ascitic fluid are other options. The choice of procedure is based on multiple factors, including maternal serum screening, familial genetic history and risk factors, ultrasound findings (or lack of findings), gestational age, risk versus benefit ratios for each procedure, and maternal preference.

The presence of fetal infection relies on either the identification of the organism itself (from amniotic fluid, fetal blood, or ascitic fluid) or by indirect evidence of infection such as detection of the antigen-specific IgM/IgG antibodies. The application of PCR, in which the replication of short sequences of a viral genome are utilized to identify a specific virus, is an important diagnostic tool used today.[193] This technique may be attempted on any virus from any body fluid. At the present time the most success has been achieved with CMV[195] and parvovirus[127] detected from amniotic fluid,

ascitic fluid, and the placenta. Ascitic fluid may be more useful for PCR analysis as it is not as time-sensitive as amniotic fluid. It takes time for a significant amount of a virus first to pass from the maternal system to the fetus and then to be excreted by the fetal kidneys into the amniotic fluid.

Virtually all the information that can be obtained from amniotic fluid can also be obtained from fetal blood. Cordocentesis has been used to evaluate fetal liver function tests and to assess fetal well-being by measuring blood urea nitrogen, creatinine, and electrolytes.[196,197] It is important to remember when comparing amniocentesis and cordocentesis that the latter is associated with increased risk of perinatal loss compared to amniocentesis, and that risks versus benefits must be evaluated carefully when deciding which sampling method to use.

Fetal paracentesis is rarely considered in the diagnostic workup of fetal ascites. In the event that a tap is done for therapeutic reasons, however, the ascitic fluid might then be useful diagnostically. The ascitic fluid can be evaluated to determine whether it is a transudate or an exudate, to quantitate urea and creatinine if indicated, and in the case of meconium peritonitis, to assess for granulocytes, leukocytes, lanugo hairs, and meconium. Cultures [primarily TORCH (*t*oxoplasmosis, *o*ther agents, *r*ubella, CMV, *h*erpes simplex) titers] can be obtained if necessary. If the cultures are negative, the protein count is low, and the lymphocyte count is over 90%, a presumptive diagnosis of chylous ascites can be made.[189] This can be confirmed postnatally by the finding of chylomicrons in the ascitic fluid. Ascitic fluid also contains lymphocytes that permit rapid karyotyping within 96 hours.[199]

If the cause of fetal ascites remains elusive, a fetal echocardiogram is warranted to rule out a cardiac anomaly or arrhythmia.

Serial ultrasound examinations should be obtained to assess fetal growth and follow the progression of the ascites. These may include serial abdominal circumference and thoracic circumference measurements if the ascites is severe. Massive compression of the chest before 24 weeks' gestation often leads to pulmonary hypoplasia.[200,201] Whether therapeutic paracentesis can be helpful in this situation is not certain, as not enough is known at this time about the natural history of isolated fetal ascites, which can be self-limiting or transitory. Certainly, however, as one approaches term, if the fetal abdomen is greater than 350 mm in circumference, a therapeutic paracentesis could be beneficial to allow for a vaginal delivery and to decrease the risk of abdominal dystocia.[203] Abdomino-amniotic shunting has also been attempted *in utero* but is generally reserved for only complicated cases as it can precipitate preterm labor.

Summary

The recognition of fetal ascites as a separate entity from fetal hydrops is an important distinction. Overall, the perinatal outcome for isolated ascites is much better and the clinical course often more benign, compared with hydrops.[187] Sonographic evaluation is extremely helpful in establishing a diagnosis, monitoring progression, and guiding interventional procedures when indicated.

REFERENCES

1. Landsteiner K, Weiner AS. Agglutinable factor in human blood recognized by immune serum for rhesus blood. *Proc Soc Exper Biol Med* 1940;43:223.
2. Grannum AJ, Copel JA. Prevention of Rh isoimmunization and treatment of the compromised fetus. *Semin Perinatol* 1988;12:324.
3. Duerbeck NB, Seeds JW. Rhesus immunization in pregnancy: a review. *Obstet Gynecol Survey* 1993;48(12):801–810.
4. Bowman JM. Treatment options for the fetus with alloimmune hemolytic disease. *Transfus Med Rev* 1990;4:191.
5. Copel JA, Gollin YG, Grannum PA. Alloimmune disorders and pregnancy. *Semin Perinatol* 1991;15(3):251–256.
6. Nevanlinna HR, et al. The influence of mother-child ABO compatibility on Rh immunization. *Vox Sang* 1965;1:26.
7. Shepard SL, Noble AL, Filbey D, Hadley AG. Inhibition of the monocyte chemiluminescent response to anti-D-sensitized red cells by Fc gamma RI-blocking antibodies which ameliorate the severity of haemolytic disease of the newborn. *Vox Sang* 1996;70(3):157–163.
8. Kumpel BM, Hadley AG. Functional interactions of red cells sensitized by IgG1 and IgG3 human monoclonal anti-D with enzyme-modified human monocytes and FcR-bearing cell lines. *Mol Immunol* 1990;27(3):247–256.
9. Palfi M, Hilden JO, Gottvall T, Selbing A. Placental transport of maternal immunoglobulin G in pregnancies at risk of Rh (D) hemolytic disease of the newborn. *Am J Reprod Immunol* 1998;39(5):323–328.
10. Mari G, Deter RL, Carpenter RL, Rahman F, Zimmerman R, et al. Noninvasive diagnosis by Doppler ultrasonography of fetal anemia due to maternal red-cell alloimmunization. Collaborative Group for Doppler Assessment of the Blood Velocity in Anemic Fetuses. *N Engl J Med* 2000;342(1):9–14.
11. Apkon M. Pathophysiology of hydrops fetalis. *Semin Perinatol* 1995;19(6):437–446.
12. Bowman JM. The management of Rh-isoimmunization. *Obstet Gynecol* 1978;52:1.
13. Chitkara U, Wilkins I, Lynch L. The role of sonography in assessing severity of fetal anemia in Rh and Kell isoimmunized pregnancies. *Obstet Gynecol* 1988;71:393–398.
14. Nicolaides KH, Rodeck CH, Mibashan RD. Have Liley charts outlived their usefulness? *Am J Obstet Gynecol* 1986;155:90–94.
15. Bowman JM. Hemolytic disease (erythroblastosis fetalis). In: Creasy RK, Resnik R, eds. *Maternal-fetal medicine: principles and practice.* Philadelphia: WB Saunders, 1994: 711–743.
16. Hadley AG, Wilkes A, Goodrick J, Penman D, Soothill P, Lucas G. The ability of the chemiluminescence test to predict clinical outcome and the necessity for amniocenteses in pregnancies at risk of haemolytic disease of the newborn. *Br J Obstet Gynaecol* 1998;105:231–234.
17. International Forum. Laboratory procedures for the prediction of the severity of hemolytic disease of the newborn. *Vox Sang* 1995;69:61–69.
18. Avner R, Reubinoff BE, Simon A, Zentner BS, Friedmann A, et al. Management of rhesus isoimmunization by preimplantation genetic diagnosis. *Mol Hum Reprod* 1996;2(1):60–62.
19. Van de Veyver IB, Moise KJ Jr. Fetal RhD typing by polymerase chain reaction in pregnancies complicated by rhesus alloimmunization. *Obstet Gynecol* 1996;88(6):1061–1067.
20. Sekizawa A, Samura O, Zhen DK, Falco V, Bianchi DW. Fetal cell recycling: diagnosis of gender and RhD genotype in the same fetal cell retrieved from maternal blood. *Am J Obstet Gynecol* 1999;181:1237–1242.
21. Ware Branch D, Scott JR. Isoimmunization in pregnancy. In: Gabbe SG, Niebyl JR, Leigh Simpson J, eds. *Obstetrics: normal and problem pregnancies.* London: Churchill Livingstone, 1986:805.
22. Nicolaides KH, Fontanarosa FD, Gabbe SG, Rodeck CH. Failure of ultrasonographic parameters to predict the severity of fetal anemia in rhesus isoimmunization. *Am J Obstet Gynecol* 1988;158:920–926.
23. Hoddick WK, Mahony BS, Callen PW. Placental thickness. *J Ultrasound Med* 1985;4:479–482.
24. Hashimoto B, Filly RA, Callen PW. Sonographic detection of fetal intraperitoneal fluid. *J Ultrasound Med* 1986;5:203–204.
25. Rosenthal SJ, Filly RA, Callen PW. Fetal pseudoascites. *Radiology* 1979;131:195–197.
26. Benacerraf BB, Frigoletto FD. Sonographic sign for the detection of early fetal ascites in the management of severe isoimmune disease without intrauterine transfusion. *Am J Obstet Gynecol* 1985;152:1039–1041.
27. DeVore GR, Donnerstein RL, Kleinman CS, Platt LD, Hobbins JC. Fetal echocardiography. II. The diagnosis and significance of pericardial effusion in the fetus using real-time–directed M-mode ultrasound. *Am J Obstet Gynecol* 1982;144(6):693–700.
28. Warsof SL, Nicolaides KH, Rodeck KC. Immune and nonimmune hydrops. *Clin Obstet Gynecol* 1986;29:533–542.
29. Vintzileos A, Campbell W. Fetal liver ultrasound measurements in isoimmunized pregnancies. *Obstet Gynecol* 1986; 68:162–167.
30. DeVore GR, Donnerstein RL, Kleinman CS, Platt LD, Hobbins JC. Fetal echocardiography. I. Normal anatomy as determined by real-time–directed M-mode ultrasound. *Am J Obstet Gynecol* 1982;144:249.
31. Carlson DE, Platt LD, Medearis AL, Horenstein J. Prognostic indicators of the resolution of nonimmune hydrops fetalis and survival of the fetus. *Am J Obstet Gynecol* 1990;163:1785–1787.
32. DeVore GR, Mayden K, Tortora M, Berkowitz RL, Hobbins JC. Dilation of the fetal umbilical vein in rhesus hemolytic anemia: a predictor of severe disease. *Am J Obstet Gynecol* 1981;141:464–466.
33. Oepkes D, Vandenbussche FP, Van Bel F, Kanhai HH. Fetal ductus venosus blood flow velocities before and after transfusion in red-cell alloimmunized pregnancies. *Obstet Gynecol* 1993;82:237–241.

34. Iskaros J, Kingdom J, Morrison JJ, Rodeck C. Prospective non-invasive monitoring of pregnancies complicated by red cell alloimmunization. *Ultrasound Obstet Gynecol* 1998; 11(6):432–437.

35. Bahado-Singh R, Ozi U, Deren O. A new splenic artery Doppler velocimetric index for prediction of severe fetal anemia associated with Rh alloimmunization. *Am J Obstet Gynecol* 1999;180(1 Pt 1):49–54.

36. Nicolaides KH, Rodeck CH, Millar DS. Fetal haematology in rhesus isoimmunization. *BMJ* 1985;290:661.

37. Barss VA, Benacerraf BB, Frigoletto FD. Management of isoimmunized pregnancy by use of intravascular techniques. *Am J Obstet Gynecol* 1988;159:932–937.

38. Grannum PAT, Copel JA, Moya FR. The reversal of hydrops fetalis by intravascular intrauterine transfusion in severe isoimmune fetal anemia. *Am J Obstet Gynecol* 1988;158:914–919.

39. Ney JA, Socol ML, Dooley SN. Perinatal outcome following intravascular transfusion in severely isoimmunized fetuses. *Int J Gynecol Obstet* 1991;35:41–46.

40. Weiner CP, Williamson RA, Wenstrom KD. Management of fetal hemolytic disease by cordocentesis. II. Outcome of treatment. *Am J Obstet Gynecol* 1991;165:1302–1307.

41. Schumacher B, Moise KJ Jr. Fetal transfusion for red blood cell alloimmunization in pregnancy. *Obstet Gynecol* 1996;88(1):137–150.

42. Harman CR, Bowman JM, Manning FA, Mentiglou SM. Intrauterine transfusion—intraperitoneal versus intravascular approach: a case-control comparison. *Am J Obstet Gynecol* 1990;162:1053–1059.

43. Tovey LAD. Haemolytic disease of the newborn—the changing scene. *Br J Obstet Gynecol* 1986;93:960–966.

44. Bowman JM, Pollock JM. Failures of intravenous Rh immune globulin prophylaxis: an analysis of the reasons for such failures. *Transfus Med Rev* 1987;1:101.

45. Power JP, Lawlor E, Davidson F, Yap PL, Kenny-Walsh E, et al. Hepatitis C viraemia in recipients of Irish intravenous anti-D immunoglobulin. *Lancet* 1994;344:1166–1167.

46. Kumpel BM. Monoclonal anti-D for prophylaxis of RhD haemolytic disease of the newborn. *Transfus Clin Biol* 1997;4(4):351–356.

47. Liley AW. Liquor amnii analysis in the management of pregnancy complicated by rhesus sensitization. *Am J Obstet Gynecol* 1961;82:1359–1370.

48. Nicolaides KH, Rodeck CH, Mibashan RS, Kemp JR. Have Liley charts outlived their usefulness? *Am J Obstet Gynecol* 1986;155(1):90–94.

49. Rodeck CH, Nicolaides KH, Warsof SL, Fysh WJ, Gamsu HR, Kemp JR. The management of severe rhesus isoimmunization by fetoscopic intravascular transfusions. *Am J Obstet Gynecol* 1984;150:769–774.

50. Grannum PA, Copel J. Prevention of Rh isoimmunization and treatment of the compromised fetus. *Semin Perinatol* 1988;12(4):324–335.

51. Hudon L, Moise KJ Jr, Hegemier SE, Hill RM, Moise AA, et al. Long term neurodevelopmental outcome after intrauterine transfusion for the treatment of fetal hemolytic disease. *Am J Obstet Gynecol* 1998;179(4):858–863.

52. Janssens HM, de Haan MJ, van Kamp IL, Brand R, Kanhai HH, Veen S. Outcome for children treated with fetal intravascular transfusions because of severe blood group antagonism. *J Pediatr* 1997;131(3):373–380.

53. Porter FT, Silver RM, Jackson MG, Branch WD, Scott JR. Intravenous immune globulin in the management of severe Rh(D) hemolytic disease. *Obstet Gynecol Surv* 1997;52(3):193–197.

54. Vaughan JL, Manning M, Warwick RM, Letsky EA, Murray NA, Roberts IA. Inhibition of erythroid progenitor cells by anti-Kell antibodies in fetal alloimmune anemia. *N Engl J Med* 1998;338(12):798–803.

54a. Babinski A, Lapinski RH, Berkowitz R. Prognostic factors and management in pregnancies complicated with severe Kell isoimmunization: experiences of the last 13 years. *Am J Perinatol* 1998;15:695–701.

54b. Caine ME, Mueller-Heubach E. Kell sensitization in pregnancy. *Am J Obstet Gynecol* 1986;154:85–90.

55. Potter EL. Universal edema of fetus unassociated with erythroblastosis. *Am J Obstet Gynecol* 1943;46:130–134.

56. Warsof SL, Nicolaides KH, Rodeck KC. Immune and nonimmune hydrops. *Clin Obstet Gynecol* 1986;29:533.

57. Santolaya J, Alley D, Jaffe R, Warsof SL. Antenatal classification of hydrops fetalis. *Obstet Gynecol* 1992;79:256–259.

58. Wy CA, Sajous CH, Loberiza F, Weiss MG. Outcome of infants with a diagnosis of hydrops fetalis in the 1990s. *Am J Perinatol* 1999;16(10):561–567.

59. Carlson DE, Platt LD, Medearis AL, Horenstein J. Prognostic indicators of the resolution of nonimmune hydrops fetalis and survival of the fetus. *Am J Obstet Gynecol* 1990;163;1785.

60. McCoy MC, Katz VL, Gould N, Kuller JA. Non-immune hydrops after 20 weeks' gestation: review of 10 years' experience with suggestions for management. *Obstet Gynecol* 1995;85:578–582.

61. Anandakumar C, Biswas A, Wong YC, Chia D, Annapoorna V, et al. Management of non-immune hydrops: 8 years' experience. *Ultrasound Obstet Gynecol* 1996;8(3):196–200.

62. Swain S, Cameron AD, McNay MB, Howatson AG. Prenatal diagnosis and management of nonimmune hydrops fetalis. *Aust N Z J Obstet Gynecol* 1999;39(3):285–290.

63. Jauniaux E, Van Maldergem L, De Munter C, Moscoso G, Gillerot Y. Non-immune hydrops fetalis associated with genetic abnormalities. *Obstet Gynecol* 1990;75:568–572.

64. Im SS, Rizos N, Joutsi P, Shime J, Benzie RJ. Nonimmunologic hydrops fetalis. *Am J Obstet Gynecol* 1984;148:566–569.

65. Holzgreve W, Holzgreve B, Curry JR. Nonimmune hydrops fetalis: diagnosis and management. *Semin Perinatol* 1985;9:52–67.

66. Skoll MA, Sharland GK, Allan LD. Is the ultrasound definition of fluid collections in non-immune hydrops fetalis helpful in defining the underlying cause or predicting outcome? *Ultrasound Obstet Gynecol* 1991;1:309–312.

67. Saller D, Canick J, Oyer C. The detection of non-immune hydrops through second trimester maternal serum screening. *Prenat Diagn* 1996;16:431–435.

68. Hutchison AA, Drew JH, Yu VY, Williams ML, Fortune DW, Beischer NA. Nonimmunologic hydrops fetalis: a review of 61 cases. *Obstet Gynecol* 1982;59:347–352.

69. Fleischer AC, Killam AP, Boehm FH, Hutchison AA, Jones TB, et al. Hydrops fetalis: sonographic evaluation and clinical implications. *Radiology* 1981;141:163–168.

70. Gough JD, Keeling JW, Castle B, Iliff PJ. The obstetric management of non-immunological hydrops. *Br J Obstet Gynecol* 1986;93:226–234.

71. Horibe S, Imai A, Kawabata I, Tamaya T. Fetal blood sampling in the assessment of acute nonimmune hydrops fetalis. *J Med* 1995;26(3–4):183–188.

72. Maxwell DJ, Crawford DC, Curry PV, Tynan MJ, Allan LD. Obstetric importance, diagnosis and management of fetal tachycardias. *BMJ* 1988;297:107–110.

73. Simpson JM, Sharland GK. Fetal tachycardias: management and outcome of 127 consecutive cases. *Heart* 1998; 79(6):576–581.

74. Mahony BS, Filly RA, Callen PW, Chinn DH, Golbus MS. Severe nonimmune hydrops fetalis: sonographic evaluation. *Radiology* 1984;151:757–761.

75. Jauniaux E. Diagnosis and management of early nonimmune hydrops fetalis. *Prenat Diagn* 1997;17(13)1261–1268.

76. Platt LD, DeVore GR. In utero diagnosis of hydrops fetalis: ultrasound methods. *Clin Perinatol* 1982;9:627.

77. Shenker L, Reed K, Anderson CF. Fetal pericardial effusion. *Am J Obstet Gynecol* 1989;160:1505.

78. Wilkins I. Nonimmune hydrops. In: Creasy RK, Resnik R, eds. *Maternal-fetal medicine*, 3rd ed. Philadelphia: WB Saunders, 1994:744–757.

79. Saltzman DH, Frigoletto FD, Harlow BL. Sonographic evaluation of hydrops fetalis. *Obstet Gynecol* 1989;74;106–111.

80. Tongsong T, Wanapirak C, Sirichotiyakul S. Placental thickness at mid-pregnancy as a predictor of Hb Bart's disease. *Prenat Diagn* 1999;19(11):1027–1030.

81. Chazotte C, Girz B, Koenigsberg M, Cohen WR. Spontaneous infarction of placental chorioangioma and associated regression of hydrops fetalis. *Am J Obstet Gynecol* 1990;163:1180–1181.

82. Fadel HE, Ruedrich DA. Intrauterine resolution of nonimmune hydrops associated with cytomegalovirus infection. *Obstet Gynecol* 1988;71:1003.

83. Bousquet F, Segondy M, Faure JM, Deschamps F, Boulot P. B19 parvovirus-induced fetal hydrops: good outcome after intrauterine blood transfusion at 18 weeks of gestation. *Fetal Diagn Ther* 15(3):132–133.

84. Novak PM, Sander M, Yang SS, von Oeyen PT. Report of fourteen cases of non-immune hydrops fetalis in association with hemorrhagic endovasculitis of the placenta. *Am J Obstet Gynecol* 1991;165:945–950.

85. Langer JC, Harrison MR, Schmidt KG. Fetal hydrops and death from sacrococcygeal teratoma: rationale for fetal surgery. *Am J Obstet Gynecol* 1989;160:1145–1150.

86. Adzick NS, Harrison MR, Crombleholme TM, Flake AW, Howell LJ. Fetal lung lesions: management and outcome. *Am J Obstet Gynecol* 1998;179:884–889.

87. Allan LD, Crawford DC, Sheridan R, Chapman MG. Etiology of non-immune hydrops: the value of echocardiography. *Br J Obstet Gynecol* 1986;93:223–225.

88. Kleinman C, Donnerstein, DeVore G. Fetal echocardiography for evaluation of in utero congestive heart failure. *N Engl J Med* 1982;306:568.

89. Simpson JM, Sharland GK. Nuchal translucency and congenital heart defects: heart failure or not? *Ultrasound Obstet Gynecol* 2000;16:30–36.

90. Oudijk MA, Michon MM, Kleinman CS, Kapusta L, Stoutenbeek P, et al. Sotalol in the treatment of fetal dysrhythmias. *Circulation* 2000;101(23):2721–2726.

91. Sharland GK. First trimester transabdominal fetal echocardiography. *Lancet* 1998;351:1662.

92. Crawford DC, Sunder KC, Allan LD. Prenatal detection of congenital heart disease: factors affecting obstetric management and survival. *Am J Obstet Gynecol* 1988;159:352–356.

93. Copel JA, Cullen M, Green JJ, Mahoney MJ, Hobbins MC, Kleinman CS. The frequency of aneuploidy in prenatally diagnosed congenital heart disease: an indication for fetal karyotyping. *Am J Obstet Gynecol* 1988;158:409–413.

94. Hornberger LK, Sahn DJ, Kleinman CS, Copel JA, Reed KL. Tricuspid valve disease with significant tricuspid insufficiency in the fetus: diagnosis and outcome. *J Am Coll Cardiol* 1991;17:167–173.

95. DeVore G, Donnerstein R, Kleinman C, Platt LD, Hobbins JC. Fetal echocardiography: II. The diagnosis and significance of a pericardial effusion in the fetus using real-time directed M-mode ultrasound. *Am J Obstet Gynecol* 1982;144:693.

96. Moore L, Chambers HM, Foreman AR, Khong TY. A report of human parvovirus B19 infection in hydrops fetalis. *Med J Aust* 1993;159:344–345.

97. Naides SJ, Weiner CP. Antenatal diagnosis and palliative treatment of non-immune hydrops fetalis secondary to fetal parvovirus B19 infection. *Prenat Diagn* 1989;9:105–114.

98. Platt LD, Geierman CA, Turkel SB, Young F, Keegan KA. Atrial hemangioma and hydrops fetalis. *Am J Obstet Gynecol* 1981;141:107–109.

99. Rasmussen SL, Hwang WS, Harder J. Intrapericardial teratoma. Ultrasonic and pathologic features. *J Ultrasound Med* 1987;6:159–162.

100. Holzgreve W, Curry CJR, Golbus MS, Callen PW, Filly RA, Smith JC. Investigation of nonimmune hydrops fetalis. *Am J Obstet Gynecol* 1984;150:805–812.

101. Mentzer WC, Collier E. Hydrops fetalis associated with erythrocyte G-6-PD deficiency and maternal ingestion of fava beans and ascorbic acid. *J Pediatr* 1975;86:565–567.

102. Masson P, Rigot A, Cecile W. Hydrops fetalis and G-6-PD deficiency. *Arch Pediatr* 1995;2(6)541–544.

103. Anand A, Gray ES, Brown T, Clewley JP, Cohen BJ. Human parvovirus infection in pregnancy and hydrops fetalis. *N Engl J Med* 1987;316:183–186.

104. Brown T, Anard A, Ritchie LD. Intrauterine parvovirus infection associated with hydrops fetalis. *Lancet* 1989;ii:1033–1034.

105. Nakayama R, Yamada D, Steinmiller V, Hsia E, Hale RW. Hydrops fetalis secondary to Bart hemoglobinopathy. *Obstet Gynecol* 1986;67:176–180.

106. Ng PC, Fok TF, Lee CH, Cheung KL, Li CK, et al. Is homozygous alpha-thalassaemia a lethal condition in the 1990s? *Acta Paediatr* 1998;87:1197–1199.

107. Brown DL, Benson CB, Driscoll SG, Doubilet PM. Twin-twin transfusion syndrome: sonographic findings. *Radiology* 1989;170(1 Pt 1):61–63.

108. Iskaros J, Jauniaux E, Rodeck C. Outcome of nonimmune hydrops fetalis diagnosed during the first half of pregnancy. *Obstet Gynecol* 1997;90(3):321–325.

109. Bronhstein M, Rottem S, Yoffe N. First-trimester and early second-trimester diagnosis of nuchal cystic hygroma by

transvaginal sonography: diverse prognosis of the septated from the non-septated lesion. *Am J Obstet Gynecol* 1989; 61:78–82.

110. Robinow M, Spisso K, Buschi A. Turner syndrome: sonography showing fetal hydrops simulating hydramnios. *AJR Am J Roentgenol* 1980;135:846–848.

111. Affi AM, Bhatia AR, Eyal F. Hydrops fetalis associated with congenital myotonic dystrophy. *Am J Obstet Gynecol* 1992;166:929.

112. Maldergem L, Jauniaux E, Fourneau C, Gillerot Y. Genetic causes of hydrops fetalis. *Pediatrics* 1992;89:81–86.

113. Meizner I, Levy A, Carmi R, Robinsin C. Niemann-Pick disease associated with non-immune hydrops fetalis. *Am J Obstet Gynecol* 1990;163:128–129.

114. Steenhout P, Elmer C, Clercx A. Carnitine deficiency with cardiomyopathy presenting as neonatal hydrops and successful response to carnitine therapy. *J Inherited Metab Dis* 1990;13:69–75.

115. Benacerraf BR, Frigoletto FD. In utero treatment of a fetus with diaphragmatic hernia complicated by hydrops. *Am J Obstet Gynecol* 1986;155:817–818.

116. Thomas CS, Leopold GR, Hilton S. Fetal hydrops associated with extralobar pulmonary sequestration. *J Ultrasound Med* 1986;68:275–280.

117. Bunduki V, Ruano R, Marques da Silva M, Miguelez J, Miyadahira S, et al. Prognostic factors associated with congenital cystic adenomatoid malformation of the lung. *Prenat Diagn* 2000;20:459–464.

118. Sherer DM, Abramowicz JS, Metlay LA, Roberts M, Woods JR. Non-immune fetal hydrops caused by bilateral type III congenital cystic adenomatoid malformation on the lung at 17 weeks' gestation. *Am J Obstet Gynecol* 1992;167:503–505.

119. Rodeck CH, Fisk NM, Fraser DI. Long-term in utero drainage of fetal hydrothorax. *N Engl J Med* 1988; 319:1135.

120. Bates HR. Coxsackie virus B3 calcified pancarditis and hydrops fetalis. *Am J Obstet Gynecol* 1970;106:629–630.

121. Price JM, Fisch AE, Jacobson J. Ultrasonic findings in fetal cytomegalovirus infection. *J Clin Ultrasound* 1978;6:268.

122. Kirkinen P, Jouppila P, Leisti J. Transient fetal ascites and hydrops with a favorable outcome. *J Reprod Med* 1987; 32:379.

123. Mueller-Heubach E, Mazer J. Sonographically documented disappearance of fetal ascites. *Obstet Gynecol* 1983;61:253–257.

124. Humphrey W, Magoon M, O'Shaughnessy R. Severe non-immune hydrops secondary to parvovirus B-19 infection: spontaneous reversal in utero and survival of a term infant. *Obstet Gynecol* 1991;78:900.

125. Public Health Lab Service Working Party on Fifth Disease. Prospective study of human parvovirus (B19) infection in pregnancy. *BMJ* 1990;300:1166–1170.

126. Rodis JF, Quinn DL, Gary W. Management and outcomes of pregnancies complicated by human B19 parvovirus infection: a prospective study. *Am J Obstet Gynecol* 1990;163: 1168–1171.

127. Kovacs BW, Carlson DE, Shahbahrami B, Platt LD. Prenatal diagnosis of human parvovirus B19 in non-immune hydrops fetalis by polymerase chain reaction. *Am J Obstet Gynecol* 1992;167:461–466.

128. Peters M, Nicolaides K. Cordocentesis for the diagnosis and treatment of human fetal parvovirus infection. *Obstet Gynecol* 1990;75:501–504.

129. Schild RL, Bald R, Plath H, Eis-Hubinger AM, Enders G, Hansmann M. Intrauterine management of fetal parvovirus B19 infection. *Ultrasound Obstet Gynecol* 1999;13(3):161–166.

130. Albano G, Pugliese A, Stabile M, Sirimarco F, Arsieri R. Hydrops foetalis caused by hepatic haemangioma. *Acta Paediatr* 1998;87(12):1307–1309.

131. Gonen R, Fong K, Chiasson DA. Prenatal sonographic diagnosis of hepatic hemangioendothelioma with secondary non-immune hydrops fetalis. *Obstet Gynecol* 1989;73:485–487.

132. McGahan JP, Schneider JM. Fetal neck hemangioendothelioma with secondary hydrops fetalis: sonographic diagnosis. *J Clin Ultrasound* 1986;14:384–388.

133. Thorp JA, Cohen GR, Yeast JD. Non-immune hydrops caused by massive fetomaternal hemorrhage and treated by intravascular transfusion. *Am J Perinatol* 1992;9(1):22–24.

134. Jauniaux E, Ogle R. Color Doppler imaging in the diagnosis and management of chorioangiomas. *Ultrasound Obstet Gynecol* 2000;15(6):463–467.

135. Hirata GI, Masaki DI, O'Toole M, Mederaris AL, Platt LD. Color flow mapping and Doppler velocimetry in the diagnosis and management of a placental chorioangioma associated with non-immune fetal hydrops. *Obstet Gynecol* 1993;81:850–852.

136. Dillard JP, Edwards DU, Leopold GR. Meconium peritonitis masquerading as fetal hydrops. *J Ultrasound Med* 1987;6:49–57.

137. Seward JF, Zusman J. Hydrops fetalis associated with small bowel volvulus. *Lancet* 1978;2:52–53.

138. Pletcher BA, Williams MK, Mulivor RA, Barth D, Linder C, Rawlinson K. Intrauterine cytomegalovirus infection presenting as fetal meconium peritonitis. *Obstet Gynecol* 1991;78:903–904.

139. Binder ND, Buckmaster JW, Benda GI. Outcome for fetus with ascites and cytomegalovirus infection. *Pediatr* 1988;82: 100–103.

140. Wax JR, Blakemore KJ, Baser I, Stretten G. Isolated fetal ascites detected by sonography: an unusual presentation of Turner syndrome. *Obstet Gynecol* 1992;79:862–863.

141. Allan LD. *Manual of fetal echocardiography.* Lancaster, UK: MTP Press Ltd., 1986:156.

142. Nicolaides KH, Snijders RJM, Sebire N. The 11–14-week scan: the diagnosis of fetal abnormalities. London: Parthenon Publishing, 1999:107.

143. Chitayat D, Grisaru-Granovsky S, Ryan G, Toi A, Filler R, et al. Familial ileal perforation: prenatal diagnosis and postnatal follow-up. *Prenat Diagn* 1998;18(1):78–82.

144. Estroff JA, Bromley B, Benaceraff BR. Fetal meconium peritonitis without sequelae. *Pediatr Radiol* 1992;22:277–278.

145. McDuffie RS, Bader T. Fetal meconium peritonitis after maternal hepatitis A. *Am J Obstet Gynecol* 1999;180(4):1031–1032.

146. Blaakaer J. Ultrasonic diagnosis of fetal ascites and toxoplasmosis. *Acta Obstet Gynecol Scand* 1986;65:653–654.

147. Ohno Y, Koyama N, Tsuda M, Arii Y. Antenatal ultrasound appearance of a cloacal anomaly. *Obstet Gynecol* 2000;95(6 Pt 2):1013–1015.

148. Blessed WB, Sepulveda W, Romero R, Berry SM, King ME, Cotton DB. Prenatal diagnosis of spontaneous rupture of the fetal bladder with color Doppler ultrasonography. *Am J Obstet Gynecol* 1993;169(6):1629–1631.

149. Jacquemyn Y, De Catte L, Vaerenberg M. Fetal ascites associated with an imperforate hymen: sonographic observation. *Ultrasound Obstet Gynecol* 1998;12(1):67–69.

150. Sun CJ, Keene CL, Nasey DA. Hepatic fibrosis in congenital cytomegalovirus infection: with fetal ascites and pulmonary hypoplasia. *Pediatr Pathol* 1990;10:641–646.

151. Persutte WH, Lenke RL, Kropp KA. Atypical presentation of fetal obstructive uropathy. *J Diagn Med Sonogr* 1989;1:12–15.

152. Hatjis C. In utero diagnosis of spontaneous fetal urinary bladder rupture. *J Clin Ultrasound* 1993;21:645–647.

153. Degani S, Lewinsky RM. Transient ascites associated with a fetal ovarian cyst. Case report. *Fetal Diagn Ther* 1995;10(3):200–203.

154. Chilukuri S, Bonet V, Cobb M. Antenatal spontaneous perforation of the extrahepatic biliary tree. *Am J Obstet Gynecol* 1990;4:1201–1202.

155. Dirkes K, Crombleholme TM, Craigo SD, et al. The natural history of meconium peritonitis diagnosed in utero. *J Pediatr Surg* 1995;30(7):979–982.

156. Nakamoto SK, Dreilinger A, Dattel B, Mattrey RF, Key TC. The sonographic appearance of hepatic hemangioma in utero. *J Ultrasound Med* 1983;2:239–241.

157. Leiken E, Lysikiewicz A, Garry D, Tejani N. Intrauterine transmission of hepatitis A virus. *Obstet Gynecol* 1996;88(4 Pt 2):690–691.

158. Bagolan P, Bilancioni E, Spina V, Nahom A, Trucchi A, et al. Fetal tachycardia and chylous ascites. *Br J Obstet Gynaecol* 1999;106(4):376–378.

159. Phillipos EF, Robertson MA, Still DK. Prenatal detection of foramen ovale obstruction without hydrops fetalis. *J Am Soc Echo* 1990;3:495–498.

160. Hill LM, Maloney JB. An unusual constellation of sonographic findings associated with congenital syphilis. *Obstet Gynecol* 1991;78:895–897.

161. Mahony BS, Callen PW, Filly RA. Fetal urethral obstruction: US evaluation. *Radiology* 1985;157:221–224.

162. Tasso MJ, Martinez-Guiterrez A, Carrascosa C, Vasques S, Tebar R. GM1-gangliosidosis presenting as nonimmune hydrops fetalis: a case report. *J Perinat Med* 1996;24(5): 445–449.

163. Snider RA, Serwer GA. Echocardiography in pediatric heart disease. St. Louis, MO: Mosby Year Book, 1990:70.

164. Holzgreve W, Curry CJR, Golbus MS, Callen PW, Filly RA, Smith JC. Investigation of non-immune hydrops fetalis. *Am J Obstet Gynecol* 1984;150:805–812.

165. Blumenthal DH, Rushovich AM, Williams RK, Rochester D. Prenatal sonographic findings of meconium peritonitis with pathologic correlation. *J Clin Ultrasound* 1982;10:350–352.

166. Morrison PJ, Macphail S, Williams D, McCusker G, McKeever P, et al. Laryngeal atresia or stenosis presenting as second-trimester fetal ascites—diagnosis and pathology in three independent cases. *Prenat Diagn* 1998;18(9):963–967.

167. Lienhardt A, Aubard Y, Laroche C, Gilbert B, Bernard P, et al. A rare cause of fetal ascites: a case report of Gunther's disease. *Fetal Diagn Ther* 1999;14(5):257–261.

168. Entezami M, Becker R, Menssen HD, Marcinkowski M, Versmold HT. Xerocytosis with concomitant intrauterine ascites: first description and therapeutic approach (letter). *Blood* 1996;87(12):5392–5393.

169. Chen CP, Chen HC, Liu FF, Jan SW, Chern SR, et al. Cutis marmorata telangiectatica congenita associated with elevated serum maternal serum human chorionic gonadotropin level and transitory isolated fetal ascites. *Br J Dermatol* 1997;136(2):267–271.

170. Foster MA, Nyberg DA, Mahony BS, Mack LA, Marks WM, Raabe RD. Meconium peritonitis: prenatal sonographic findings and their clinical significance. *Radiology* 1987;165:661–665.

171. Garb M, Rad FF, Roseborough J. Meconium peritonitis presenting as fetal ascites on ultrasound. *Br J Radiol* 1980;53:602–604.

172. Beck M, Braun S, Coerdt W, Mere E, Young E. Fetal presentation of Morquio disease type A. *Prenat Diagn* 1992;12(12):1019–1029.

173. Akduman EI, Luisiri A, Launius GD. Fetal abuse: a cause of fetal ascites. *AJR Am J Roentgenol* 1997;169:1035–1036.

174. Gilot B, Gonzalez D, Bournazeau JA, Barriere A, Van Lieferinghen P. Case report: electroconvulsive therapy 142 during pregnancy. *Encephale* 1999;25(6):590–594.

175. Griscom NT, Colodny AH, Rosenberg HK, Fliegel CP, Hardy BE. Diagnostic aspects of neonatal ascites: report of 27 cases. *AJR Am J Roentgenol* 1977;128:961–970.

176. Chalubinski K, Deutinger J, Bernaschek G. Meconium peritonitis: extrusion of meconium and different sonographical appearances in relation to the stage of diseases. *Prenat Diagn* 1992;12:631–636.

177. Bair JH, Russ PD, Pretorius DH, Manchester D, Manco-Johnson ML. Fetal omphalocele and gastroschisis: a review of 24 cases. *AJR Am J Roentgenol* 1986;147:1047–1052.

178. Manning DJ, Price WI, Pearse RB. Fetal ascites: an unusual presentation of Niemann-Pick disease type C. *Arch Dis Child* 1990;65(3):335–336.

179. Shweni PM, Kamberan SR, Ramdial K. Fetal ascites. A report of 6 cases. *S Afr Med J* 1984;66:616–618.

180. Goldstein RB, Filly RA, Callen PW. Sonographic diagnosis of meconium ileus in utero. *J Ultrasound Med* 1987;6:663–666.

181. Shalev J, Ben-Rafel Z, Goldman B, Engleberg I, Mashiach S. Mid-trimester diagnosis of bladder neck obstruction by ultrasound and paracentesis. *J Med Genet* 1983;20:223–230.

182. Satin AJ, Twickler DM, Wendel GD Jr. Congenital syphilis associated with dilation of fetal small bowel: a case report. *J Ultrasound Med* 1992;11:49–52.

183. Guillan JE, Lowden JA, Gaskin K, Cutz E. Congenital ascites as a presenting sign of lysosomal storage disease. *J Pediatr* 1984;104:225–231.

184. Szeifert G, Gsecsei K, Toth Z, Papp Z. Prenatal diagnosis of ascites caused by cytomegalovirus hepatitis. *Acta Paediatr Hung* 1985;26:311–316.

185. Petrovsky BM, Walzak MP Jr, D'Addario PF. Fetal cloacal anomalies: prenatal sonographic findings and differential diagnosis. *Obstet Gynecol* 1988;72(3):464–469.

186. Fung TY, Fung HY, Lau TK, Chang AM. Abdomino-amniotic shunting in isolated fetal ascites with polyhydramnios. *Acta Obstet Gynecol Scand* 1997;76(7):706–707.

187. Zelop C, Benaceraff BR. The causes and natural history of fetal ascites. *Prenat Diagn* 1994;14(10):941–946.

188. Mueller-Heubach E, Majer J. Sonographically documented disappearance of fetal ascites. *Obstet Gynecol* 1983;61:253–257.

189. Winn HN, Stillen R, Grannum PAT, Crane JC, Coster B, Romero R. Isolated fetal ascites: prenatal diagnosis and management. *Am J Perinatol* 1990;7:370–373.

190. Hashimoto BE, Filly RA, Gillen PW. Fetal pseudoascites: further anatomic observations. *J Ultrasound Med* 1986;5:151–152.

191. Sarno AP Jr, Bruner JP, Southgate WM. Congenital chyloperitoneum as a cause of isolated fetal ascites *Obstet Gynecol* 1990;76:955–957.

192. Yang YH, Cho JS, Min HW, Lee CH, Song CH. Rapid chromosome analysis and prenatal diagnosis using fluid from the cystic hygroma, hydrothorax and isolated ascites: new source for chromosome analysis. *J Obstet Gynaecol* 1995;21(5):443–450.

193. Wright PA, Wynford-Thomas D. The polymerase chain reaction: miracle or mirage? A critical review of its uses and limitations in diagnosis and research. *J Pathol* 1990;162:99–117.

194. Chen CP, Chern SR, Chuang CY, Chen BF. Prenatal detection of human cytomegalovirus DNA in fetal ascites by the polymerase chain reaction. *Acta Obstet Gynecol Scand* 1998;77(4):446–447.

195. Donner C, Liesnard C, Content J, Busine A, Aderca J, Rodesch F. Prenatal diagnosis of 52 pregnancies at risk for congenital cytomegalovirus infection. *Obstet Gynecol* 1993, 82(4):481–486.

196. Diummick JE, Kalousek DK. *Developmental pathology of the embryo and fetus.* New York: JB Lippincott Co, 1992:535–539.

197. Nelson NM. *Current therapy in neonatal-perinatal medicine.* Toronto: B.C. Decker, 1990:120–124.

198. Durand B, Doyen C, Guibaud S, Calvet AM, Thoulon JM, et al. Ascites with "activated" lymphocytes in a case of hydrops fetalis related to a parvovirus B19 infection. *J Gynecol Obstet Biol Reprod* (Paris) 1997;26(8):828–830.

199. Wax JR, Blakemore KJ, Soloski MJ, Gibson M, Stetten G. Fetal ascitic fluid: a new source of lymphocytes for rapid chromosomal analysis. *Obstet Gynecol* 1992;80:533–535.

200. Benaceraff BR, Frigoletto FD Jr. Mid-trimester fetal thoracentesis. *J Clin Ultrasound* 1985;13:202–204.

201. Benaceroff BR, Frigoletto FD Jr, Wilson M. Successful midtrimester thoracentesis with analysis of the lymphocyte population in the pleural effusion. *Am J Obstet Gynecol* 1986;155:398–399.

202. Reece EA, Hobbins JC, Mahoney MJ, Petrie RH. *Medicine of the fetus and mother.* Philadelphia: JB Lippincott Co., 1992.

203. Haidir P, Korejo R, Jafarey S. Fetal ascites as a cause of dystocia in labor. *J Pakistan Med Assoc* 1991;41(8):195–197.

17

FETAL INFECTIONS

Infections commonly affect pregnancy and are an important cause of fetal/neonatal mortality and morbidity. At least 5% of women are affected by a symptomatic viral illness during pregnancy, and many more are affected by clinically silent infections.[1] Bacterial and parasitic infections may be even more common.

The fetus is normally protected from infection by the placental barrier and maternal mucous membranes. In addition, microbicidal and bacteriostatic agents are present in the amniotic fluid.[2] The first embryonic defenses occur at 8 to 10 weeks' gestation and consist of macrophage precursors and the complement system. Synthesis of B and T lymphocytes and immunoglobulin (Ig)G begins around 14 weeks. IgA and IgM are present in low levels until after birth, as there is usually not much fetal stimulation by antigens *in utero.*

Despite these protective barriers, and even with intact placental membranes, fetal infections are not uncommon and their effects may be devastating. Infections of the embryo and fetus may cause spontaneous abortion, congenital anomalies, premature birth, intrauterine growth restriction (IUGR), and neonatal mortality and morbidity. It is estimated that infections account for as much as 20% of fetal and neonatal diseases.

With intact membranes, many infectious agents may spread hematogenously to the placenta, where they may then proceed to infect the fetus. Other agents may cross the placental barrier directly. Factors that enable fetal infection are variable and include the specific infecting agent, portal of entry, severity of infection, maternal immune status, gestational age of the fetus, and placental and fetal defenses.

Cytomegalovirus (CMV) infections occur in 1% to 2% of all pregnancies and are the most common *in utero* infections. Toxoplasmosis, very common in France, may infect 0.4% of women in the United States. Rubella, a highly teratogenic virus, has significantly decreased in prevalence since the vaccine was developed in 1969, but there have been occasional outbreaks of congenital rubella syndrome (CRS) in the United States. Parvovirus is a relatively uncommon infection, but it may result in nonimmune hydrops and lead to *in utero* demise. Most females are immune to the varicella-zoster virus, but 2% of women infected during pregnancy may

have a fetus with the devastating congenital varicella syndrome. Herpes simplex virus type 2 (HSV-2) most commonly affects infants during vaginal delivery, but in some instances may cause *in utero* infection. Congenital syphilis should be preventable with proper prenatal care, but maternal treatment does not always protect the fetus from infection. Although human immunodeficiency virus type 1 (HIV-1) is not thought to be teratogenic, the increased prevalence of HIV infections in women of childbearing age with potential transmission of the virus to the fetus makes it an important virus in perinatology.

If fetal infection is suspected, it is not appropriate to simply wait until delivery to discover what the infection is, because postnatal serologic studies may not confirm infection. More important, diagnosis *in utero* may alter prenatal care and lead to fetal treatment. Prenatal diagnosis of fetal infection also allows postnatal caretakers to use appropriate infection precaution measures to prevent spread.[3]

When fetal infection is suspected, the mother may undergo a series of serologic tests. However, a specific infectious agent must be suspected, an accurate and sensitive test must be available, and the mother should respond in a predictive fashion to the infection, which does not always occur.

Evaluation and treatment of fetal infection require a logical, coordinated team approach of the obstetrician/perinatologist, sonologist, sonographer, and laboratory personnel. Many of the necessary tests are specialized and should be performed by a reference laboratory to obtain accurate results. Referral to an experienced fetal diagnosis and treatment center optimizes management.

Concern for fetal infection includes evaluation of the mother and the fetus. A thorough maternal history should be obtained; specifically, to evaluate factors such as lifestyle, clinical symptoms, symptomatic family members or coworkers, and geographic locale. Maternal serologic studies are performed to detect any possible acute maternal infections.

Direct and indirect tests may be performed on the fetus to evaluate for infection. Direct testing includes cordocentesis with serologic testing, amniotic fluid culturing, electron microscopy, and polymerase chain reaction (PCR). Indirect tests for infection may also be performed on the fetus. Hematologic profiles may show anemia—abnormalities of white blood cells and platelets—which can be consistent with infection. Hepatic enzymes are also commonly abnormal with viral infections.

Prenatal detection of fetal infection has been greatly aided by the development of PCR (see Chapter 23). It has been particularly useful for diagnosing toxoplasmosis but has also been used for a number of other infectious agents. Studies using PCR have identified agents (adenovirus and enterovirus) not commonly considered to be a cause of fetal infection[4] and have also helped identify the infectious agent in undiagnosed cases of fetal disease, such as hydrops.[5]

Ultrasound is commonly used during pregnancy, and, thus, it is important to recognize sonographic findings that may be indicative of fetal infection. If fetal infection is suspected, suggestive sonographic findings should be sought. Although not specific, common sonographic findings of fetal infection include ventriculomegaly, intracranial calcification, hydranencephaly, microcephaly, cardiac anomalies, hepatosplenomegaly, echogenic bowel, intraabdominal calcifications, hydrops, placentomegaly, IUGR, and abnormal amniotic fluid volume.

It is important to note that most affected fetuses with infection appear sonographically normal. Although a normal anatomic survey can be reassuring, it cannot predict a normal outcome. Findings also change or resolve over time so serial scanning can be very important. When abnormalities are detected on ultrasound, about one-half the cases will show multiorgan involvement. The importance of a thorough sonogram cannot be overemphasized (Table 1).

This chapter discusses a variety of specific agents that may produce fetal infection with an emphasis on associated sonographic findings. Streptococcal infections or infections caused by ascending spread after ruptured membranes are not discussed here.

VIRAL INFECTIONS

Cytomegalovirus

Definition and Prevalence

CMV, a member of the herpesvirus family, is a double-stranded DNA virus. It is the most common cause of infections in the fetus and neonate. Approximately 50% of females in the United States are susceptible to CMV by the time they reach reproductive age, and the highest rate of seroconversion is between the ages of 15 and 35 years. Susceptibility varies with socioeconomic class; 50% of higher-income women are susceptible, compared to 15% of low-income women.[6]

Overall, congenital CMV infections occur in 0.2% to 2.2% of live births,[7,8] affecting 33,000 infants born in the United States annually.[9] An additional 3% to 5% of liveborn infants acquire CMV in the perinatal period, presumably as a result of exposure to infected cervical secretions, blood, or breast milk.

Perinatal transmission does not have serious implications for development of the infant except in cases of very-low-birth-weight infants.

Pathogenesis and Pathology

CMV is transmitted by contact with infected blood, saliva, or urine or by sexual contact. Infection in mothers may spread to the placenta and hence to the fetus. It is suspected that transmission occurs hematogenously via the umbilical vessels when infected leukocytes traverse the placenta to the fetus.[10] If fetal infection occurs, a major site of CMV replication is the tubular epithelium of the kidney, so the fetus excretes virus in the urine.

The incubation period of CMV is 28 to 60 days, with a mean of 40 days. Viremia can be detected 2 to 3 weeks after primary infection. Primary CMV infection in adults is usually asymptomatic, although some patients report a mild, mononucleosis-like syndrome. With primary maternal CMV infection, the risk of transmission to the fetus is 30% to 40%,[7] whereas with recurrent infection the risk is no more than 2%.[9,11] Of those infected *in utero* after a primary infection, 10% exhibit signs and symptoms of CMV infection at birth and develop sequelae.[12]

Approximately 3% of women with antibodies to CMV in the serum (who thus had been thought to be immune) develop recurrent infection during pregnancy.[13] Indeed, recurrent infections are more prevalent than primary infections in women of childbearing age given the greater number of immune women.[13] In contrast to other viral diseases, both primary and recurrent infections can cause damage to the fetus, but the incidence and severity of congenital CMV infections are lower in cases of recurrent infection.[11]

In later infancy, siblings usually are the sources of infections; the main reservoir of CMV is children younger than 2 years.[14] Studies have documented a higher annual seroconversion rate (11% vs. 2%) among day care workers than among other women.[15] It may be advisable, therefore, for susceptible women to avoid such settings if they are pregnant or contemplating pregnancy.

CMV causes cell destruction. A characteristic nuclear inclusion forms after infection, composed of chromatin aggregates and viral particles. In fetal infections, most cell damage takes place after the second month of gestation, peaking later in pregnancy. Although CMV infections usually do not lead to abortions, stillbirth and neonatal death can result from fulminant infection. Some infants fare better than others, which may be related to virulence and the maturity of the humoral system of the infant or fetus.[13]

Congenital CMV in the neonate is diagnosed by one of the following: positive cultures of body fluids, CMV-specific IgM in serum, or intranuclear inclusions and small intracytoplasmic inclusions in CMV-infected visceral cells.

TABLE 1. FETAL INFECTIONS AND EVALUATION, TREATMENT, AND OUTCOME

Infecting agent	Transmission rate	Sonographic findings	Other prenatal diagnostic tests	Treatment	Associated abnormalities/outcome
Cytomegalovirus	Primary infection: 30–40% throughout pregnancy Recurrent infection: <2%	Ascites/hydrops, ventriculomegaly, microcephaly, intracranial calcifications, linear striations of basal ganglia, echogenic bowel, IUGR	Maternal seroconversion, amniocentesis with monoclonal antibody, PCR testing, or culture	None	90% are asymptomatic at birth, 5–15% have long-term neurologic sequelae including sensorineural hearing loss, mental retardation Other complications: low birth weight, jaundice, hepatosplenomegaly, microcephaly, thrombocytopenic purpura, death Prognosis worse for earlier, primary infection
Herpes simplex virus	Transplacental is rare—most infections occur during vaginal delivery	Ventriculomegaly, echogenic bowel	Culture, PCR	Acyclovir for maternal indications; adenosine, arabinoside postnatally	Skin lesions, chorioretinitis, blindness, microphthalmos, microcephaly, seizures, mental retardation, skin lesions, death
Human immunodeficiency virus	13–32% after 13–15 wk	IUGR?	Usually not attempted, as procedures increase risk of fetal infection	Zidovudine after first trimester	20% (transplacental), poor prognosis with short incubation period; 80% (perinatal), better prognosis with long incubation period; pneumonitis; recurrent bacterial infection
Parvovirus	Fetal transmission 33% throughout gestation	Hydrops, cardiomegaly, placentomegaly, polyhydramnios, increased nuchal translucency, elevated Doppler velocities of the middle cerebral artery, echogenic bowel	Maternal seroconversion, cultures not helpful, amniocentesis for IgM and PCR, PUBS: IgM and hematologic indices	Observation, fetal red blood cell transfusion	SAB (stillbirth or live birth), hydrops, normal; spontaneous resolution of hydrops may occur
Rubella	90% first trimester; 25% second trimester; 95–100% third trimester	Cardiac defects, microcephaly, IUGR	Maternal seroconversion; cordocentesis after 20 wk; amniotic fluid culture, PCR; PCR on CVS specimen	None	Hearing loss; mental retardation; cardiac disease: PDA, ASD, VSD, pulmonary artery stenosis; ocular anomalies: cataracts, microphthalmos, glaucoma, chorioretinitis
Syphilis	30–100%; varies with maternal stage and treatment and gestational age	Hydrops, hepatomegaly, placentomegaly, bowel dilatation, IUGR	Maternal serology, amniocentesis, PUBS	Antibiotics with close follow-up for treatment failure/reinfection	Stillbirth, prematurity, osteochondritis, periostitis, saddle nose, Hutchinson teeth; mental retardation, hearing loss, hydrocephalus; hemolytic anemia, petechiae
Toxoplasma	5% first trimester; 17% second trimester; 60% third trimester; overall risk, 40%	Ventriculomegaly, intracranial calcifications, hyperechoic foci within the liver, ascites/hydrops, placentomegaly	Maternal seroconversion; amniocentesis with PCR testing, parasite isolation; PUBS	Spiramycin, pyrimethamine, sulfonamide	Chorioretinitis, seizures, mental retardation, hydrocephalus, hepatosplenomegaly
Varicella	24%; embryopathy, 2% with first- and second-trimester infections	Hyperechoic foci within the liver, hydrops, hypoplastic limbs, IUGR, ventriculomegaly, microcephaly, microphthalmos, cataracts, echogenic bowel	Maternal seroconversion; amniocentesis, PCR	VZIG within 72 h of exposure; acyclovir for maternal indications	Varicella embryopathy: limb hypoplasia, contractures, skin lesions, chorioretinitis, microphthalmos, cataracts, seizures, microcephaly, hydrocephalus, mental retardation

ASD, atrial septal defect; CVS, chorionic villus sampling; IgM, immunoglobulin M; IUGR, intrauterine growth restriction; PCR, polymerase chain reaction; PDA, patent ductus arteriosus; PUBS, percutaneous umbilical blood sampling; SAB, spontaneous abortion; VSD, ventricular septal defect; VZIG, varicella-zoster immune globulin.

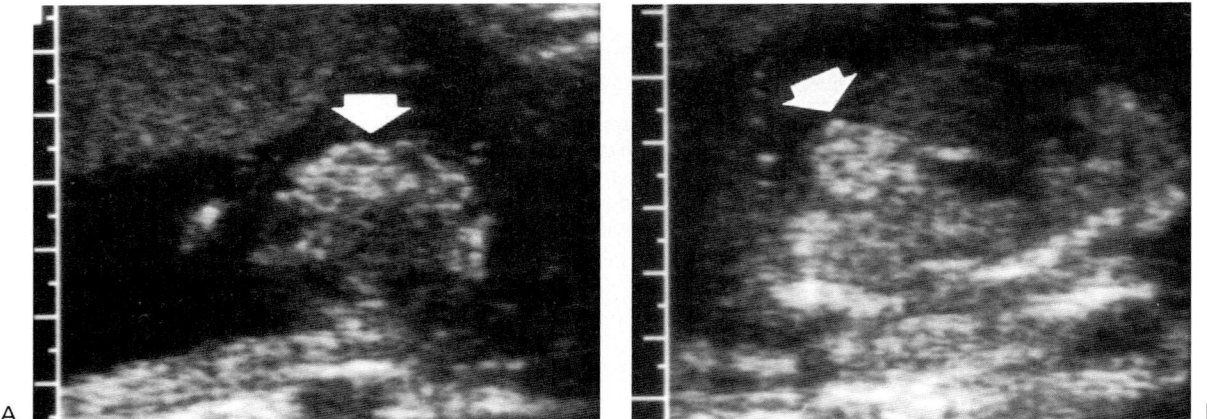

FIGURE 1. Cytomegalovirus. Transverse **(A)** and longitudinal **(B)** scans of the abdomen at 16 weeks demonstrate echogenic bowel (*arrows*) in a fetus with cytomegalovirus infection. Alpha-fetoprotein level was 4.76 multiples of the median.

Typical findings in symptomatic neonates are hepatosplenomegaly, jaundice, chorioretinitis, microcephaly, intracranial calcifications, and petechiae. Most infants with petechiae have thrombocytopenia. More than 90% of affected infants have positive urine viral cultures. A disseminated form of CMV that affects predominantly the kidneys, liver, and lungs is much less common.

The most significant manifestations of CMV infection occur in the brain and may include necrosis, atrophy, and microcephaly. Microcephaly may not be as strongly associated with CMV as originally thought. A study by Ahlfors et al.[16] in an unselected population in Sweden showed that none of 56 infants with congenital CMV infection was born with or developed microcephaly (a head circumference less than 3 standard deviations) within 7 years, but 3.5% of these infants had a head circumference of approximately 2 standard deviations less than normal. Of the 12 children in the population of 10,000 who had microcephaly, only one of these may have been related to CMV. Although seen in only approximately 1% of infected infants, periventricular calcifications have been noted as a consequence of the predilection of CMV to involve the germinal matrix.[17] If lesions occur in the wall of the fourth ventricle, hydrocephalus may occur. Optic defects including chorioretinitis, microphthalmos, cataracts, and optic atrophy may be present.

Diagnosis

Ultrasound

The sonographic appearance of intrauterine CMV infection may consist of increased bowel echogenicity (Figs. 1 and 2), ventriculomegaly, intracranial calcification (Figs. 3 through 5), nonimmune hydrops, ascites, and growth delay. The cause for hyperechoic bowel with infection is unclear but has been well documented.[18–22] Hepatomegaly and liver calcifications may also be seen with CMV infection, although this is more typical of toxoplasmosis or varicella infections. Splenomegaly may be noted close to term.

The intracranial calcifications may appear as periventricular or cortical foci without definite shadowing.[23] The location and multiplicity should lead one to suspect calcifications even if shadowing is not present. CMV infection tends to occur in a more periventricular location than toxoplasmosis, which involves a more diffusely scattered area. Bilateral periventricular calcifications preceded by hypoechoic periventricular ringlike zones were noted in three cases of *in utero* CMV infections.[24] Although no pathologic

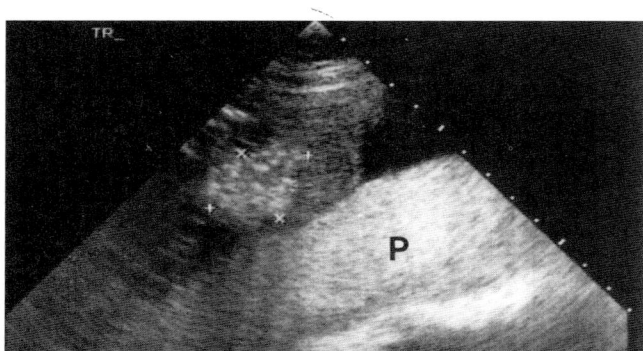

FIGURE 2. Cytomegalovirus. A transverse view of the fetal abdomen at 19 weeks' gestational age demonstrates midabdominal irregularity with an intraperitoneal echogenic area consistent with echogenic bowel (*cursors*). The infant was cytomegalovirus-positive at birth. P, placenta. (Reproduced with permission from Pletcher BA, Williams MIC, Mulivor RA, et al. Intrauterine cytomegalovirus infection presenting as fetal meconium peritonitis. *Obstet Gynecol* 1991;78:903–905.)

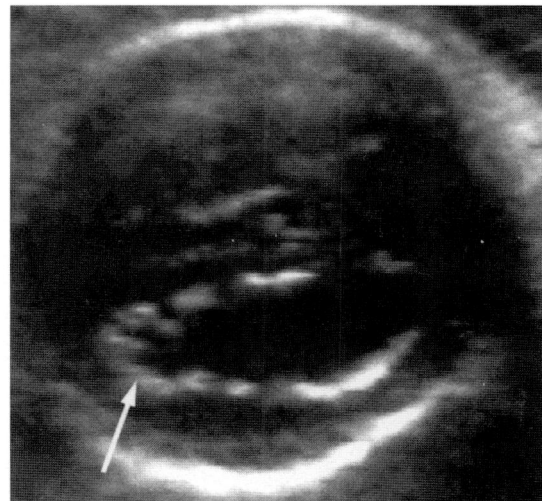
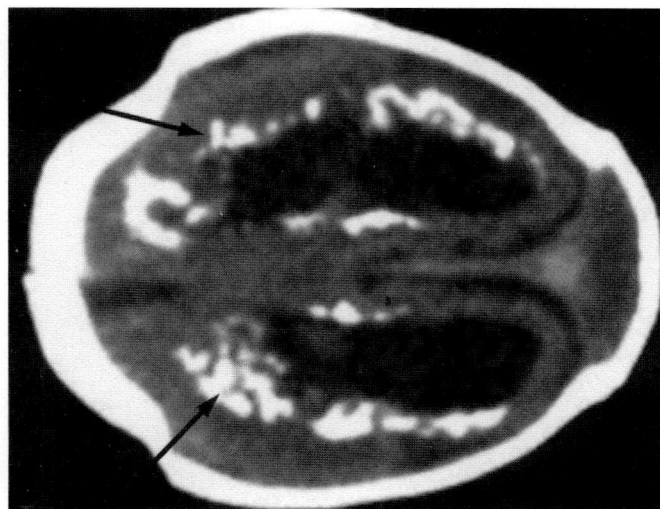

FIGURE 3. Cytomegalovirus. **A:** Transverse view of head shows ventricular dilatation and periventricular echogenic nodules (*arrow*). **B:** Computed tomography scan (oriented to correspond with ultrasound image) after birth confirms hydrocephalus and marked periventricular calcifications (*arrows*). (Courtesy of Luis Izquierdo, MD, Miami, FL.)

proof was available, the authors suspected cellular necrosis and inflammatory edema as a cause.

Linear or branching hyperechoic areas in the basal ganglia or thalami have been noted postnatally in infants with a variety of disorders, including CMV infection, trisomy 21, and trisomy 13.[25,26] These linear or branching calcifications have also been noted on fetal ultrasonograms.[27,28] Prenatal magnetic resonance imaging may also show brain findings in fetuses with suspected CMV infection.[28]

A variety of insults may affect the eyes, including chorioretinitis, optic neuritis, cataract, strabismus, microphthalmos, and colobomata. Ultrasound of the fetal eyes can identify some of these lesions.[29]

Hydrops may be related to hepatic dysfunction and portal hypertension from liver congestion. Isolated fetal ascites may occur with CMV infection and may not always imply a poor prognosis. A case report exists of a fetus with CMV infection and ascites at 27 weeks that resolved over 4 weeks with good interval growth. The infant was born with hepatomegaly and some petechiae. Follow-up at 6 months showed normal eye and ear development.[30] Supraventricular tachycardia also has been reported in association with CMV infection. Weiner and Grose[31] reported a case of pericardial effusion at 23 weeks in association with CMV infection that resolved within 1 week. The child was born without congenital CMV infection, but no long-term follow-up was available.

Drose et al.[32] examined the sonographic findings of *in utero* infections in 19 fetuses. Ten of the 11 confirmed with culture were caused by CMV. Multiple organ anomalies were seen in 47%, intracranial calcifications in 42%, cardiac anomalies in 37%, and parenchymal calcifications in 32%. Large placentas were noted in 32%. Only one had normal amniotic fluid volume, three had polyhydramnios,

and six had oligohydramnios. All of the 37% of fetuses who were not aborted and did not die at birth were developmentally impaired, indicating a grave prognosis when sonographic findings are present.

Laboratory

Several maternal antibody tests are available for CMV infection,[33–36] and this is part of the TORCH (*t*oxoplasmosis, *o*ther agents, *r*ubella, *C*MV, *H*SV) screen. Seroconversion from negative to positive or a significant increase [greater than fourfold rise in antibodies (e.g., 1:4 to 1:16) in IgG] titers over a 3- to 4-week interval is evidence of recent infection. IgG antibodies persist indefinitely. IgM is less reliable but, when present, usually indicates an acute infection that disappears within 30 to 60 days. Unfortunately, IgM is not detectable in the first half of pregnancy, presumably because of the immaturity of the developing fetal immune system. A small number of women with recurrent infection also demonstrate anti-CMV IgM.[35] The reported sensitivity of serology ranges from 50% to 90%.[35]

If a pregnant woman does seroconvert during pregnancy, amniocentesis should be offered to identify fetal infection. Amniotic fluid studies may include culture of amniotic fluid or PCR amplification of viral DNA.[37–39] The reported sensitivity ranges from 77% to 100% for PCR, compared to 50% to 70% for amniotic fluid culture, and both together may have a sensitivity of 80% to 100%.[35] However, sensitivity of amniotic fluid testing is much lower before 21 weeks.[35,40,41] PCR is more sensitive than cordocentesis after 21 weeks' gestation.[39,42] Higher viral loads are more likely to be associated with clinical sequelae.[43] Viral load is associated with higher rates of fetal transmission and symptomatic infection.[44]

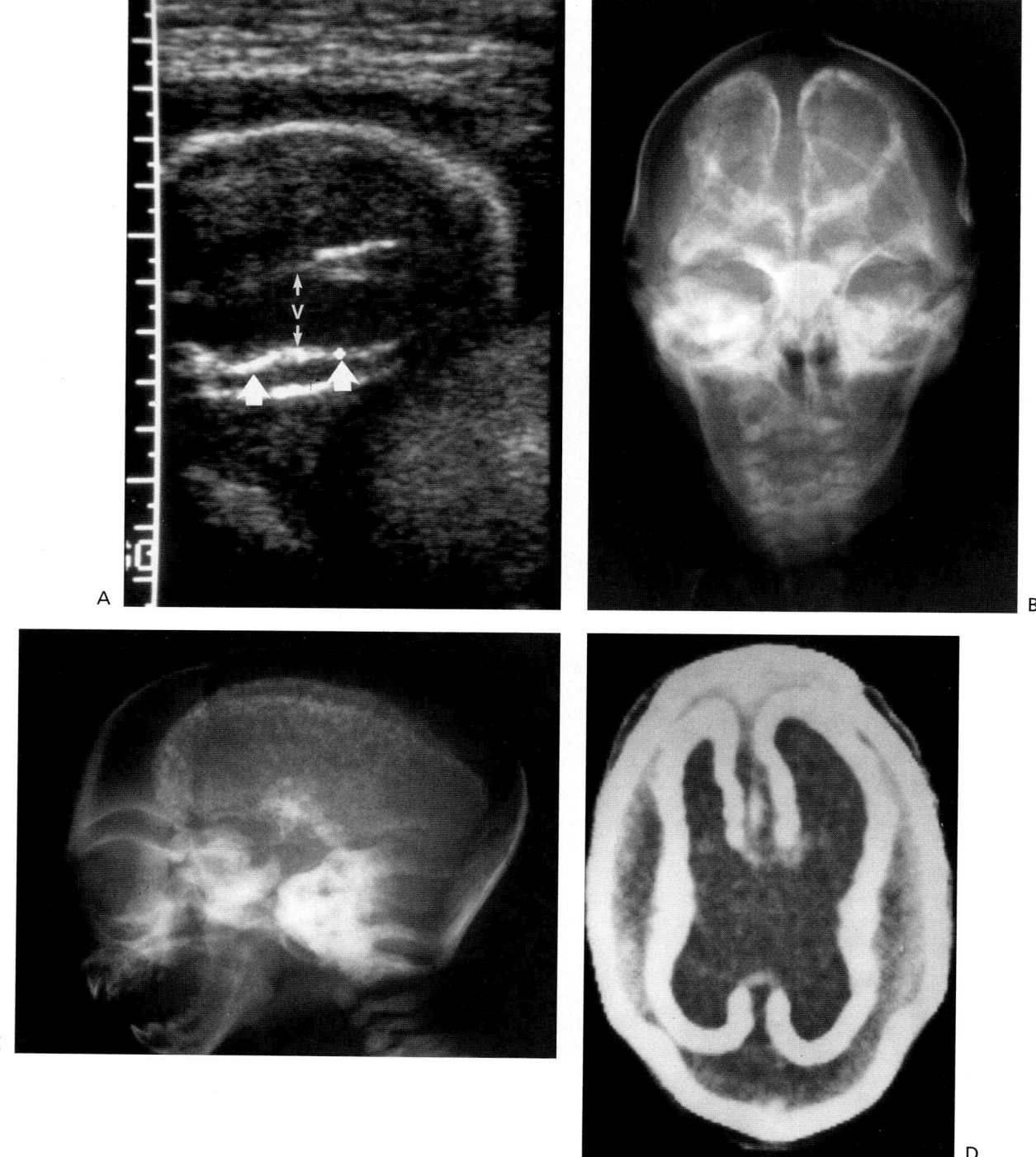

FIGURE 4. Cytomegalovirus. **A:** An axial sonogram through the fetal head at 35 weeks' gestation shows echogenic walls (*large arrows*) of the dilated lateral ventricle (*V*) indicating calcification. The head was also microcephalic, consistent with biparietal diameter at 23 weeks. Frontal **(B)** and lateral **(C)** skull radiographs after delivery show dense periventricular calcifications. **D:** A computed tomographic scan of the head after delivery also demonstrates dense periventricular calcifications. (Reproduced with permission from Nyberg DA, Pretorius DH. Cerebral malformations. In: Nyberg DA, Mahony BS, Pretorius DH, eds. *Diagnostic ultrasound of fetal anomalies. Text and atlas.* Chicago: Yearbook Medical Publishers, 1990.)

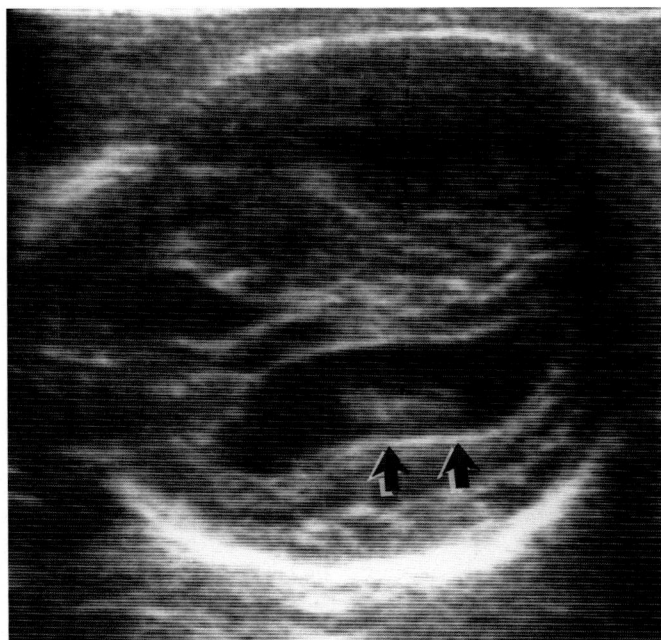 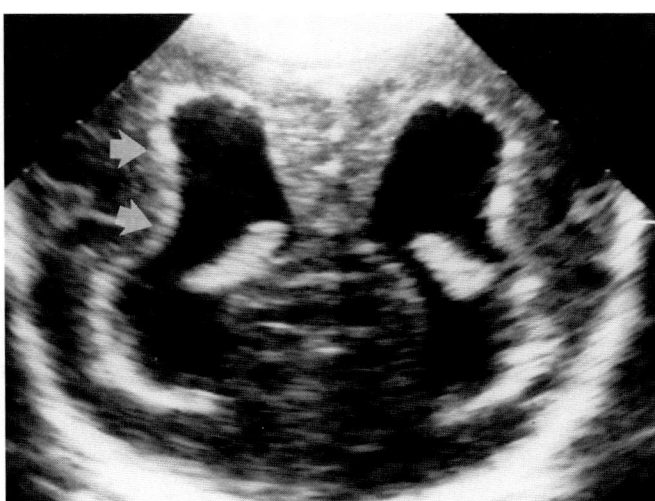

FIGURE 5. Cytomegalovirus. **A:** An axial image through the fetal head at 25 weeks demonstrates ventriculomegaly and increased echogenicity in the periventricular region (*arrows*). **B:** The cranial ultrasound performed on day 1 of life demonstrates increasing ventriculomegaly and periventricular calcification (*arrows*). (Reproduced with permission from Tassin GB, Maklad NF, Stewart RR, et al. Cytomegalic inclusion disease: intrauterine sonographic diagnosis using findings involving the brain. *AJNR Am J Neuroradiol* 1991;12:117–122.)

Screening

Despite the health hazards posed by congenital CMV infection, the general consensus holds that antepartum screening for CMV infection is not indicated. This is partly based on the fact that the overwhelming majority of infected fetuses remains asymptomatic. Maternal screening would require testing of maternal antibodies early and retesting seronegative women for conversion on subsequent visits. It is also difficult to justify screening given the lack of effective therapy, although it is hoped that more effective therapies will be developed.

A live CMV vaccine has been developed. Although the vaccine appears to be safe, there are concerns about the ability of the vaccine to reactivate, as well as a possible oncogenic potential of the vaccine virus. It is hoped that continued developments will produce a commercially available vaccine in the future, at which time screening for CMV should be reassessed.[35]

Differential Diagnosis

In utero infections may have similar sonographic findings or may have no sonographic abnormalities at all. Sonographic findings can include hydrops/ascites, ventriculomegaly, intracranial calcifications, echogenic bowel, or fetal growth retardation. Some infections have specific abnormalities such as dilated loops of bowel or abdominal calcifications.

Hydrops fetalis is characterized by fetal fluid collections in at least two of several body compartments. These fluid collections can collect in the pleural space, pericardial space, or abdominal space (ascites). Hydrops can also produce skin edema, placental thickening, or polyhydramnios. Hydrops is the result of a number of etiologies, including immune hydrops from maternal antibodies or nonimmune hydrops. Nonimmune hydrops may be secondary to abnormalities including fetal infection, cardiac failure, high output failure, placental abnormalities with arteriovenous shunting, and defects that can occur in almost any anatomic region of the fetus. Ultrasound is used to detect hydrops and the specific etiology. For instance, a cardiac abnormality or congenital defect such as a sacrococcygeal teratoma causing high output failure may be identified with ultrasound. Hydrops fetalis is discussed in detail in Chapter 16.

Detection of other *in utero* abnormalities such as intracranial calcifications or ventriculomegaly may help establish an *in utero* infection as the etiology of hydrops.

Fetal ventriculomegaly strictly defines enlargement of the cerebral ventricles without addressing the specific etiology. Ventriculomegaly may be secondary to hydrocephalus, abnormal development of the brain, or brain atrophy. *In utero* infection usually causes ventriculomegaly due to brain destruction, which results in atrophy. Thus, the head circumference may be normal or small (microcephaly). Concomitant intracranial calcifications can also be present and usually appear as periventricular echogenicities. Most commonly, *in utero* ventriculomegaly is secondary to hydrocephalus due to obstruction of flow of the cerebrospinal fluid (CSF) with resultant increased ventricular size. Head circumference may increase depending on the amount of hydrocephalus. Ultrasound often shows a specific etiology of dilated ventricles such as a Dandy-Walker or Chiari malformation. When these findings are identified sonographically, they are distinct from those of *in utero* infection. Additional causes of ventriculomegaly are discussed in detail in Chapter 6.

Besides ascites, other abdominal findings that can occur with *in utero* infections include echogenic bowel, dilated bowel, or focal liver calcifications. Each of these findings may occur in isolation or in combination with other abnormalities with an *in utero* infection. Echogenic bowel is more common with CMV infection than with other *in utero* infections. It also may be a marker for trisomy 21 or cystic fibrosis or may be secondary to the fetus swallowing echogenic (bloody) amniotic fluid. Care must be taken not to overcall echogenic bowel. Some higher-frequency ultrasound transducers may cause the bowel to appear more echogenic than lower-frequency transducers do. Similarly, tissue harmonics may falsely create the impression of echogenic bowel.

Dilated bowel occurs less frequently with *in utero* infections but may be seen with congenital syphilis. Atresias may also cause bowel dilatation secondary to obstruction. Echogenic foci in the liver are seen in varicella infection. Echogenic calcifications in the abdomen or the liver may not have a specific etiology or adverse sequelae. Alternately, uncommon intraabdominal masses such as tumors may calcify and should be considered in the differential diagnosis.

IUGR may occur with CMV, rubella, and possibly HIV infection. Chromosomal abnormalities and placental insufficiency should also be considered in the differential diagnosis of IUGR.

Intracranial calcification is suspicious for infection but not diagnostic. An unusual autosomal recessive disorder has also been associated with intracranial calcification and microcephaly.[45] Intracranial tumors should also be considered.

Prognosis

Only 10% of infected fetuses are symptomatic at birth, but the effects can be devastating. Affected infants may have prematurity, low birth weight, jaundice, hepatosplenomegaly, microcephaly, and thrombocytopenic purpura. Approximately 30% of severely infected infants die, and 80% of survivors have severe neurologic morbidity,[14,46] usually mental retardation, hearing loss, neuromuscular disorders, and chorioretinitis.[47] The incidence of severe fetal infection is much lower after recurrent maternal infection than after primary infection. Infections acquired during the neonatal period are typically asymptomatic and not associated with severe neonatal sequelae.

Among the 90% of infected infants who are asymptomatic at birth, 5% to 15% have long-term neurologic sequelae that develop later in childhood. Unilateral or bilateral sensorineural hearing loss is the most common problem. As a result, CMV is the leading cause of congenital hearing loss. Chorioretinitis, other neurologic defects, and dental enamel dysplasia may also occur as late sequelae.[13]

The poorest outcomes occur with primary infection early in pregnancy. Fowler et al.[11] compared the outcomes for 125 CMV-infected infants whose mothers had primary infection during pregnancy with those for 64 infants born to mothers with recurrent infection during pregnancy. Eighteen percent in the primary infection group were symptomatic at birth versus none in the recurrent group. After follow-up of approximately 4 years, 25% of the initially asymptomatic infants in the primary group showed one or more sequelae, compared with 8% in the recurrent infection group. Mental retardation and hearing loss were the defects noted most commonly.

Management

Although infection can be recognized with amniocentesis, no tests are available to predict whether the fetus will be symptomatic. In the absence of sonographic findings, affected fetuses cannot be identified *in utero*. The risk of fetal morbidity is relatively low and no therapy exists at this time for fetal infections. It is possible that evidence of *in utero* infection may assist physicians later in identifying those 10% to 15% of infants who demonstrate delayed sequelae from CMV infection and, it is hoped, expedite treatment of these infants.

Ganciclovir has been used to treat CMV infections in the neonate and immunocompromised adults, but larger trials are needed to establish its efficacy before *in utero* treatment is attempted.[48] Given the toxicity of ganciclovir, it may never be useful for *in utero* infection. At this time, there is no treatment or vaccine for fetal CMV infection.

As noted, the main reservoir of CMV is small children younger than 2 years,[49] and it may be advisable to keep susceptible women out of day care or child care settings if they are pregnant or are contemplating pregnancy. For a woman who is contemplating pregnancy and who has recently had a primary CMV infection, there are no good recommendations for how long conception should be delayed. Viral shedding is not a useful indicator as the virus is shed into saliva for weeks and months and into the urine and cervix for months and years.

Parvovirus

Definition and Prevalence

Human parvovirus B19 is a small, single-stranded DNA virus discovered in 1975 by Cossart et al.[50] Also known as

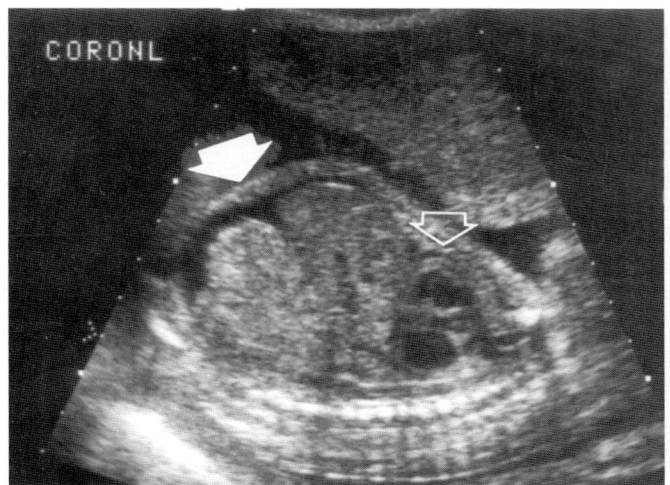
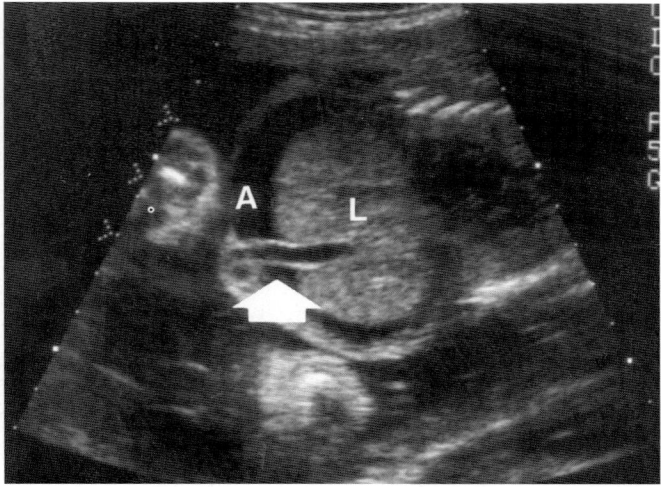

FIGURE 6. Parvovirus. **A:** A coronal image of the abdomen at 23 weeks' estimated gestational age shows ascites (*solid arrow*) and pericardial effusion (*open arrow*). **B:** A second coronal image demonstrates the umbilical vein (*arrow*) suspended within ascites (*A*). By 27 weeks, the hydrops resolved. Mother had a positive immunoglobulin M titer for parvovirus and a history of a rash during the first trimester of pregnancy. L, liver.

fifth disease in children, parvovirus B19 infection is such a common childhood virus among 5- to 15-year-olds that 50% of women of childbearing age are immune to it. Among susceptible individuals, approximately 50% of household contacts and 20% of schoolteachers develop an infection during a community epidemic.[51] The incidence of B19 infection in pregnancy is low unless there is an outbreak in the community.[52]

Pathogenesis and Pathology

Human parvovirus is transmitted via respiratory droplets from infected persons. B19 incubates for approximately 7 days, and viremia ensues for 5 days. Exposure to a household member infected with parvovirus B19 is associated with an approximate 50% risk of seroconversion.[53,54] The risk of transmission in a child-care setting or classroom is lower, ranging from 20% to 50%.[55]

Malaise, myalgias, and low-grade fevers may occur at the time of viremia, and 7 days after viremia, symptoms such as rash (erythema infectiosum), arthralgia, and arthritis may occur.[56] Approximately 20% of adults may be asymptomatic during an infection. The infected person generally is no longer infectious with the onset of the rash.[57]

Transplacental transmission of B19 is estimated to occur in 33% of pregnancies when the mother has the virus. The virus has been found in all fetal tissues, but most notably in erythroid precursors. Cytopathic effects are seen mainly in bone marrow but also occur in sites of extramedullary hematopoiesis such as the liver and spleen. Between 6 weeks and 4 months of gestation, erythrocytes are predominantly in the liver, and early infection affects the liver. Later infections involve the bone marrow.

Parvovirus has been recognized as a cause of nonimmune hydrops and intrauterine fetal death.[58–60] This virus is a lytic virus that affects the hematopoietic system, preventing maturation of erythrocytes and leading to an aplastic crisis of approximately 10 days' duration. Adults with chronic hemolytic anemias may develop an aplastic crisis, but normal adults tolerate this event well with minimal anemia. However, a rapid turnover of red blood cells occurs in the fetus, such that the red blood cell life is half that of adults. Thus, a profound anemia may occur in the fetus infected with parvovirus B19. Hydrops may be due to anemia, high output failure, and myocarditis.

Diagnosis

Ultrasound

Parvovirus may show various manifestations of hydrops including ascites (Fig. 6), pleural and pericardial effusions, cardiomegaly, skin thickening, placentomegaly, and polyhydramnios. Hydropic changes may spontaneously resolve; parvovirus infection should be considered when transient ascites is seen (Fig. 6). Hydrops changes usually appear 4 weeks after symptomatic maternal infection and are unusual after 8 weeks, but they can be seen as late as 12 weeks after symptoms.[61] Serial sonograms now are advised after documented maternal infection to detect early signs of hydrops. However, the optimal frequency of sonograms among patients exposed to parvovirus remains uncertain.

Doppler velocimetry of the middle cerebral artery also appears be helpful in predicting anemia (Fig. 7). Delle Chiaie et al.[62] found 100% sensitivity for detecting fetal anemia when the middle cerebral artery Doppler peak velocity was greater than 1.29 of that expected (1.29 multiples of

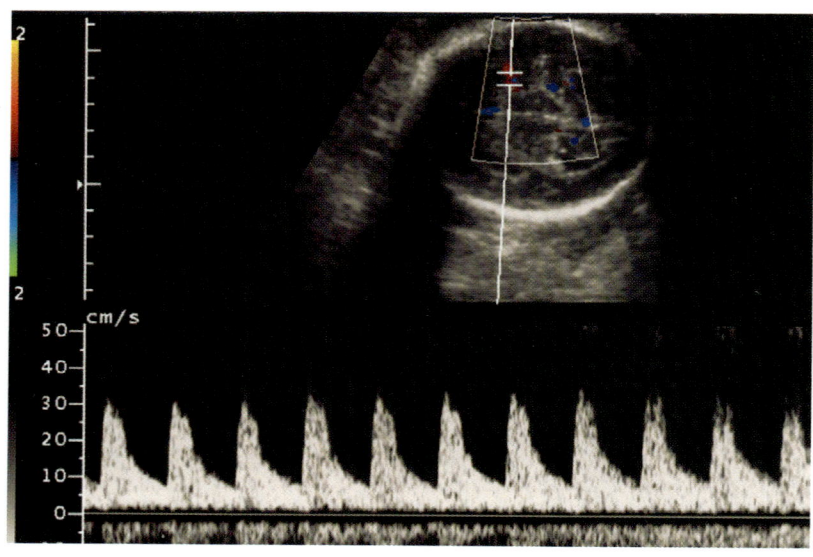

FIGURE 7. Middle cerebral artery. Duplex Doppler imaging in a patient exposed to parvovirus shows normal systolic velocity of 30 cm per second.

median) among 10 fetuses with intrauterine parvovirus infection (Fig. 8).

During the first trimester, sonography may show hydrops[63–65] or increased nuchal translucency.[66] In the absence of karyotype abnormality, fetal B19 infection should be considered in these instances.

Another finding reported with parvovirus infection is meconium peritonitis.[67] Zerbini et al.[68] report four cases of meconium peritonitis in hydropic fetuses with laboratory-diagnosed B19 infection. All four pregnancies had a preterm

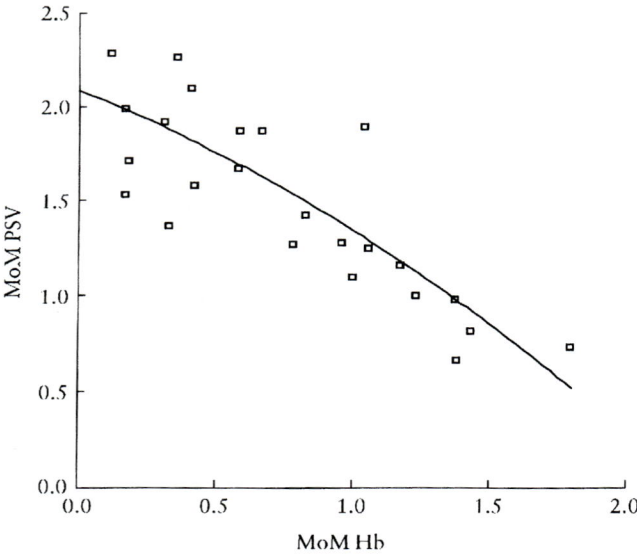

FIGURE 8. The correlation between peak systolic velocity (*PSV*) of the middle cerebral artery, expressed as a multiple of the median (*MoM*), and hemoglobin (*Hb*) concentration, expressed as MoM of Hb. Data were obtained from 25 samples taken from ten fetuses at risk for anemia due to parvovirus B19 infection. Samples were taken before and after transfusion in some cases.

outcome: Two infants recovered after surgery, one recovered spontaneously, and another was stillborn. Ileal atresia was noted in all, but one infant canalized spontaneously.

Laboratory

Unlike other viruses, B19 cannot be cultured on standard tissue culture media. It usually is diagnosed by serologic detection of specific IgM antibodies. The specific IgM antibodies appear 3 days after infection starts but disappear within 1 to 2 months. However, as with other intrauterine infections, IgM antibodies are of limited value before 22 weeks.[35] IgG antibodies persist indefinitely and, in the absence of IgM, indicate prior infection. Cord blood sampling[69] and amniocentesis can yield specific IgM antibodies.[70]

Viral DNA in the fetus has been identified by *in situ* hybridization or Southern blot techniques in autopsy specimens.[71] DNA probes are most useful during acute viremia. PCR amplification has been used for detection of parvovirus in amniotic fluid,[72–74] fetal blood,[75] and chorionic villi.[76]

Maternal serum alpha-fetoprotein (AFP) levels have been noted to rise as early as 4 weeks before development of hydrops.[77] However, other reports indicate that maternal serum AFP and human chorionic gonadotropin levels are ineffective in predicting outcome of pregnancies with known infection.[78]

Differential Diagnosis

See Cytomegalovirus, Differential Diagnosis.

Prognosis

Fetal infection may result in a normal infant, spontaneous abortion in the first trimester, stillbirth with hydrops,[79] or live birth with hydrops. The estimated risk of subsequent fetal demise is less than 9%.[52] A prospective cohort study in the United Kingdom of 193 pregnant women with positive IgM titers showed 84% had normal live infants and 16% had fetal demise.[52] Fetal loss was 17% before 20 weeks' gestation and 6% after 20 weeks' gestation. Analysis of fetal tissues suggested that an estimated 9% of all fetal losses in the study may have been related to B19. Tolfvenstam et al.[59] suggest that parvovirus infection may be a common cause of unexplained fetal death during the late second and third trimesters, and most of these are nonhydropic. They found that 15% of intrauterine fetal deaths had positive fetal or placental DNA for parvovirus B19. On the other hand, Kinney et al.[80] studied pregnant women not selected for parvovirus and noted a similar infection rate (1%) in normal women and women with fetal deaths, suggesting that B19 does not account for a significant number of fetal deaths in the general population.

Torok[81] suggests a 2% to 3% increase in fetal deaths in infected women compared with controls, occurring primarily during the first 20 weeks of pregnancy. Rodis et al.[82] prospectively followed 39 pregnant women who had serologic evidence of B19 infection during an outbreak of fifth disease in Connecticut in 1988. These women were exposed to the virus primarily in the first trimester. Thirty-seven were delivered of healthy infants and two had miscarriages (none with hydrops), for an overall pregnancy loss rate of 5%. Finally, Harger et al.[83] followed 259 susceptible women who were exposed to B19. Fifty-two (16.7%) developed infection, and none of the fetuses developed hydrops or died.

Hydrops can resolve spontaneously (Fig. 6).[84–86] In some of these cases of spontaneous resolution, growth lag during the acute phase with subsequent catch-up growth has been described.

Parvovirus B19 is not believed to be a teratogenic virus, but case reports have described ocular anomalies similar to rubella embryopathy with unilateral microphthalmos; absent irises and lenses; and thick corneas, sclerae, and choroids.[87–89] Most documented infections, however, have occurred in the second trimester or later, after organogenesis. Although malformations have been noted in animals infected with animal parvovirus, human parvovirus appears to target only the red blood cells.[90] Neonatal anemia has been noted as a result of third-trimester parvovirus infection.[90]

Management

Because a variety of outcomes are possible after fetal infection with parvovirus, no consensus on management exists. Nonhydropic fetuses possibly exposed to parvovirus are followed by ultrasound (Fig. 7) including Doppler velocimetry of the middle cerebral artery.

No vaccines are available against B19, and prophylactic administration of Ig to a mother after exposure is not recommended, as its efficacy has not been determined. Hydrops from parvovirus may be treated after 20 weeks'

gestation via cordocentesis and blood transfusion.[91] If the fetus is older than 32 weeks, delivery may be indicated.

Rubella

Definition and Prevalence

Since the rubella vaccine became available in 1969, reported cases of rubella and CRS in the United States are at all-time lows with an incidence of fewer than 1 per 100,000 live births even in epidemic times.[92] From 1969 to 1989, there was a 99.6% decrease in rubella and a 97.4% decrease in CRS in the United States. However, 10% to 20% of women of childbearing age are still susceptible to rubella, and, although uncommon, CRS continues to cause devastating problems—both teratogenic and nonteratogenic—in the fetus and neonate.[93]

Centers for Disease Control and Prevention (CDC) estimates show that in 1984, only 745 cases of rubella and two cases of CRS were reported.[93] In 1990, 1,093 cases of rubella were reported, the highest since 1982,[94] and 23 cases of CRS were reported in Southern California alone.[95] The most recent statistics show that in 1992, there were 160 cases of rubella and 11 cases of CRS in the United States.[96]

CRS was very common in the United States before the availability of vaccine in 1969. Before 1969, epidemics occurred every 6 to 9 years and major pandemics every 10 to 30 years. The last pandemic, in 1964 to 1965, led to approximately 11,000 miscarriages, abortions, and stillbirths as well as the birth of 20,000 infants with CRS.[97] The economic impact of this pandemic was approximately $1.5 billion.[98] Although the vaccine has precipitated an all-time low incidence, the prevalence of the disease may be slightly underestimated because of the existence of mild cases and delayed onset of anomalies. A new vaccine was developed in 1979 to replace the old vaccine; this new vaccine has resulted in higher antibody titers and an immune response that closely parallels natural infection. In general, immunity lasts for at least 14 to 16 years and probably for life.

Pathogenesis and Pathology

Rubella is an RNA virus spread principally via nasopharyngeal secretions. Symptoms occur 2 to 3 weeks after exposure, and a mild prodrome of malaise, fever, and headache may precede the rash by 1 to 5 days. A macular rash begins on the face, spreads downward, and disappears in about 3 days. Transient arthralgias may occur in one-third of infected adult women. Infection is subclinical in 25% to 50% of patients. However, risk of fetal damage from infection in these cases is believed to be very small.[99–101]

Maternal viremia is necessary for placental and fetal rubella infection. Fetal infection is unlikely when maternal infection is not clinically apparent.[102] Reinfections are uncommon and the risk of fetal damage is very small with reinfection, even early in pregnancy. Viral particles infect the decidua and vessels in the placental villi; the fetus then becomes infected via shed endothelial cells and maternal leukocytes.[103] Organ damage is the result of a direct cytotoxic action as well as immunologic mechanisms and obliterative angiitis. The angiitis that occurs in rubella decreases blood supply to fetal tissues, and a mitotic inhibitor released from infected cells leads to growth retardation. As viremia is present about 1 week before a rash is present in the mother, the fetus usually is infected by the time maternal infection is recognized.

Vertical transmission (fetal infection rate) is 90% in the first trimester, 25% at the end of the second trimester, and 95% to 100% in the third trimester.[104,105] Patients shed the virus from the nasopharynx for 1 week before and 1 week after the onset of the rash.[197] If a maternal rash appears within 12 days of the last menstrual period, fetal infection is virtually nonexistent. If the rash appears within 12 to 21 days, the fetal infection rate is 31%, which increases to 100% if maternal infection occurs 3 to 6 weeks from the last period.[106]

The various mechanisms of the disease may result in fetal or neonatal demise as well as transient, persistent, or delayed-onset abnormalities. Transient lesions are the result of inflammation followed by repair. Mitotic inhibition and necrosis result in permanent sequelae. Continuing viral activity and uncovering of early subclinical abnormalities may lead to delayed-onset findings.[47] CRS commonly affects the following organ systems: optic (cataracts, microphthalmos, glaucoma, chorioretinitis), cardiac (patent ductus arteriosus, pulmonary artery stenosis, atrial septal defect, ventricular septal defect, myocarditis), and neurologic (deafness, microcephaly, mental retardation). Retarded growth, hepatosplenomegaly, and thrombocytopenia also are commonly noted, but over one-half of infants with CRS appear normal at birth.

The severity of disease is related to the onset of infection. All fetuses infected during the first trimester are affected, primarily from deafness and cardiovascular disease, such as patent ductus arteriosus, pulmonic stenosis, systemic arterial lesions, and myocarditis. The frequency of anomalies decreases to 35% in the early second trimester.[104] Fetuses infected after the seventeenth week do not incur severe damage.[107,108] Cardiac defects are also rare with infections after the first trimester.[107] Cataracts are another common effect of CRS, presenting at the time of birth or up to several months of age. They are usually subtotal and may involve one or both eyes.

Although pregnant women usually are not vaccinated against rubella during pregnancy, no cases of fetal damage have been reported in these instances.

Diagnosis

Ultrasound

Rubella infection in the first trimester may result in embryonic and fetal demise as well as severe anomalies. Sono-grams may identify some of the cardiac defects associated with rubella: atrial septal defect, ventricular septal defect, and pulmonic stenosis. Microcephaly and growth delay can also be seen.

Laboratory

Rubella stimulates a variety of antibody responses that are used for maternal screening. Hemagglutinin inhibition antibody usually remains positive for life after infection. Specific IgM antibodies, which can be detected shortly after the onset of illness, peak at 7 to 10 days and persist for up to 4 weeks after appearance of the rash. While helpful in some cases, it is not widely available. Also, false-positive results may occur from reinfection, secondary to other viruses, or for unknown reasons.[109] IgG antibody titers show a fourfold increase over a 2-week period with detection of IgM-specific rubella antibodies.

Rubella virus has been isolated from amniotic fluid and grown in cell cultures, but this method is relatively insensitive, must be performed at 16 weeks, and can take up to 6 weeks to get results.[110] Terry et al.[111] have identified specific viral specific antigens or RNA sequences with monoclonal antibodies and cloned complementary DNA probes from chorionic villus sampling specimens. This procedure allows diagnosis within 3 days in the first trimester, but it is specialized and cannot be performed by diagnostic laboratories that are only capable of performing routine tests. Reverse-transcription PCR can be performed from placental tissue obtained by chorionic villus sampling or amniocentesis.[112–114] However, detection of rubella virus in chorionic villus samples by this technique may not always correctly predict fetal rubella virus infection.[115]

Differential Diagnosis

See Cytomegalovirus, Differential Diagnosis.

Prognosis

As noted, the prognosis varies with gestational age at time of infection. The prognosis for a fetus infected with rubella in the first trimester is dismal. Although the prevalence of congenital anomalies decreases in the second trimester, severe defects may still occur. Perhaps the most disturbing feature of CRS is the possibility of delayed occurrence of anomalies.

CRS results in the following anomalies, in decreasing frequency: deafness, mental retardation, cardiac anomalies, and ocular anomalies. One-fourth of infants with CRS demonstrate central nervous system anomalies within the first few months of life: delayed motor development, irritability, meningitis, seizures, growth retardation, and hypotonia.[47] Growth delay is more common with early infection. Panencephalitis may occur in the second decade as a late manifestation.

Cirrhosis, cholestasis, and pancreatitis have all been described, and delayed-onset diabetes has been reported in 20% of CRS cases.[116] Thyroid disease and glaucoma also are delayed manifestations of CRS.

Management

Termination of pregnancy should be offered in cases in which maternal infection occurs between 3 and 10 weeks' gestation. Fetal infection and birth defect rates decrease between 11 and 18 weeks, and prenatal diagnosis can be offered to these patients as an alternative to termination. Prenatal diagnosis of rubella is used more extensively in Europe, where rubella continues to be a problem.

Cordocentesis has been used to detect rubella-specific IgM antibodies consistent with fetal infection. Synthesis of fetal IgM begins after week 12, but in cases of rubella infection is found consistently only after 22 weeks. Thus, this test can only be used between 19 and 25 weeks when the fetus is able to produce adequate IgM. False-negative results have been noted as late as 22 weeks' gestation.[117] Enders and Jonatha[118] found that, in 28 of 31 cases, prenatal diagnosis helped determine correct management of the pregnancy. However, two fetuses tested negative and later proved to have CRS. Another fetus tested positive and was born infected but apparently healthy.

Immune globulin given after early pregnancy exposure to rubella does not prevent fetal infection or defects and therefore has no use. No antiviral treatment for rubella is available at this time. One-third to one-half of CRS cases can be prevented by postpartum vaccination of women who are susceptible to rubella.[98] Susceptible women who do not contact rubella during pregnancy should be immunized in the postpartum period. Although there have been reports of the development of acute arthritis and arthropathies as well as shedding of virus particles into the breast milk,[119] not enough data are available to change the practice of postpartum immunization in susceptible women.[120]

Given the existence of 10% to 20% of women of childbearing age who remain susceptible to rubella, the best strategy at this time is to continue to enforce policies for immunization, especially in school-aged children and women of childbearing age.[121] The goal of rubella immunization is to prevent rubella infection in a future pregnancy.

Varicella-Zoster Virus

Definition and Prevalence

The varicella-zoster virus, a member of the herpesvirus family, is the cause of two disparate diseases: a common childhood illness, chickenpox, and herpes zoster. Infection with this virus in pregnancy may result in a devastating embryopathy. Fortunately, however, as a result of childhood exposure, 95% of adults are immune to the virus. The prevalence of

varicella infection in pregnancy is approximately 1 in 2,000 pregnancies. Only 2% of these cases result in congenital varicella syndrome and this is limited to exposure during the first 20 weeks.[122–124] Herpes zoster in pregnancy is even less common (1 in 10,000, or 0.1%), and the risk of congenital varicella syndrome is negligible with herpes zoster.[125]

Pathogenesis and Pathology

The varicella-zoster virus spreads by water droplets and is highly contagious. Varicella is very common among children in schools and day care centers.[126] It incubates for an average of 15 days and is communicable 2 days before and 5 days after onset of the rash. The virus may persist in a latent state in the posterior root ganglia of the spinal cord for years and become reactivated later, resulting in herpes zoster. Characteristic clinical symptoms consist of skin lesions in dermatomal distribution (76%), neurologic defects (60%), eye diseases (51%), and skeletal anomalies (49%).[127]

Vertical transmission occurs in 24% of cases.[128] Fetal infections after herpes zoster are rare because antibodies in the maternal blood during a zoster infection prevent the virus from crossing the placenta and infecting the fetus.[47]

Varicella embryopathy consists of limb hypoplasia and contractures, cicatricial skin lesions in a dermatomal distribution, chorioretinitis, microphthalmos, cataracts, seizures, microcephaly, hydrocephalus, mental retardation, and paralysis. Skin lesions are the hallmark of varicella embryopathy but are not always present.[129] Polymicrogyria also has been seen in association with varicella embryopathy.[130] Anomalies of the autonomic nervous system, such as loss of bowel and urinary sphincter control, likewise are noted.[131,132] Higa et al.[133] have speculated that these abnormalities are a result of *in utero* reactivation of infection and subsequent fetal herpes zoster rather than direct damage from the varicella virus. These authors propose that both acquisition and reactivation of the virus occur in the fetus and only a small percentage of exposed fetuses develop congenital varicella syndrome.

Most women of uncertain immune status are indeed immune, but those who are truly seronegative have a high likelihood (89%) of contracting chickenpox after an exposure.[123] Varicella-zoster immune globulin (VZIG) also protects most nonimmune women from varicella-zoster, and the remainder only developed mild disease.[134]

Diagnosis

Ultrasound
Sonography is valuable in detecting anomalies compatible with varicella embryopathy. Multiple hyperechoic foci within the liver (Figs. 9 through 11) have been commonly seen. The hyperechoic foci within the liver represent dystrophic calcification on autopsy. Other findings include polyhydramnios, hydrops, IUGR, limb hypoplasia, hydrocephalus, micro-

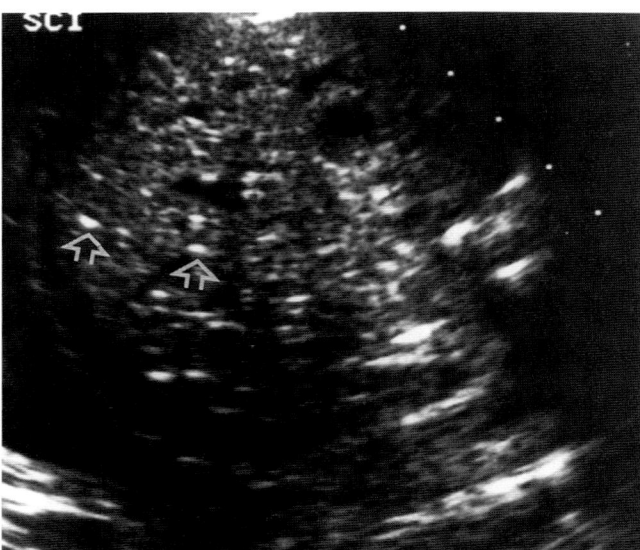

FIGURE 9. Varicella. A transverse view of the abdomen at 24 weeks demonstrates multiple hyperechoic foci within the liver (*arrows*). A small rim of ascites is also evident. Maternal infection occurred at 16 weeks. (Reproduced with permission from Pretorius DH, Hayward I, Jones KL, et al. Sonographic evaluation of pregnancies with maternal varicella infection. *J Ultrasound Med* 1992;11:459–463.)

cephaly, porencephaly, and microphthalmia.[135–137] When performing screening sonography in pregnant women with varicella infection, all fetal long bones should be evaluated due to the risk of limb hypoplasia, and the orbits should be evaluated.

There appears to be a latency period of 5 weeks or more between maternal infection and sonographic identification

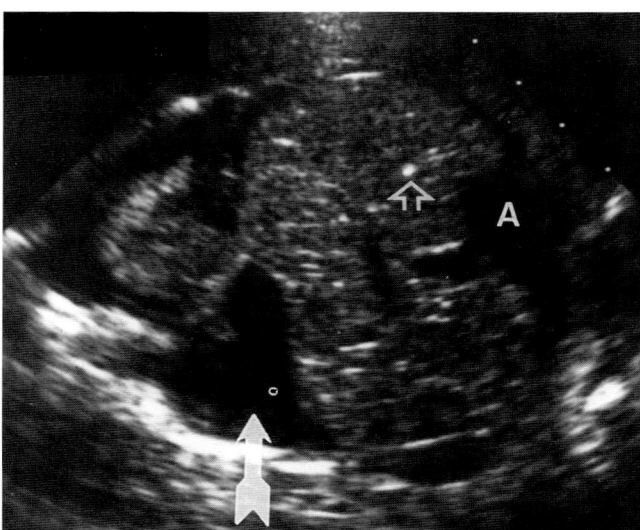

FIGURE 10. Varicella. A coronal view of the fetal abdomen and chest at 24 weeks demonstrates pleural effusions (*solid white arrow*), ascites (*A*), and echogenic foci (*open arrow*) within the liver in a fetus with congenital varicella.

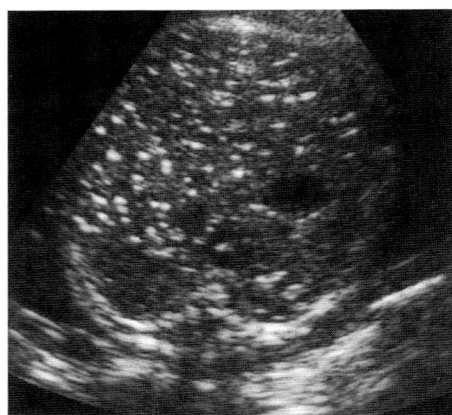

FIGURE 11. Toxoplasmosis. A transverse view of the abdomen shows innumerable echogenic foci within the liver.

of fetal anomalies. Thus, serial sonograms are appropriate. A review of 37 cases of varicella-zoster infections by Pretorius et al.[138] showed sonographic abnormalities in all five fetuses with congenital varicella syndrome and none in the 32 fetuses who were not affected. Sonographic abnormalities in affected fetuses were apparent 5 to 19 weeks after initial maternal infection.

The first case report of prenatal diagnosis of congenital varicella syndrome occurred at 32 weeks, after maternal infection at 20 weeks. The fetus was initially identified as abnormal on sonography, having hydrocephalus and polyhydramnios; IgM antibody was identified after cordocentesis. Specific IgM was not noted within 2 weeks of birth, emphasizing the difficulty of postnatal diagnosis of an *in utero* infection.[139]

Laboratory

A number of serologic assays can detect antibodies to varicella-zoster virus. However, less than one-half of infected neonates have specific IgM.

Fetal infection has been demonstrated by detection of varicella-zoster virus DNA in fetal blood and amniotic fluid by PCR.[140] PCR is more sensitive than cell culture for the detection of varicella-zoster virus in amniotic fluid.[141] Umbilical blood sampling is not very useful as viremia exists only for a short period.

Differential Diagnosis

See Cytomegalovirus, Differential Diagnosis.

Prognosis

Most infants born to mothers infected with varicella-zoster virus during pregnancy are unaffected and well.[142–144] Infection during the second trimester usually does not result in congenital varicella syndrome.[145] If an infant is one of the fewer than 2% expected to develop varicella embryopathy, the outlook is grim. About one-third of infants with congenital varicella syndrome die within the neonatal period, and survivors have severe abnormalities.[146] It is unclear whether delayed symptoms can occur after *in utero* infection, such as is seen with CMV infection.

Perinatal maternal infection does not cause structural abnormalities in the fetus, but it may result in fulminant neonatal infection (varicella of the newborn). The neonate is vulnerable from 5 days before delivery up to 48 hours postpartum as a result of the relative immaturity of the neonatal immune system and the lack of protective maternal antibody.[147] When maternal infection develops during this time, 17% of infants become infected. Infants develop a confluent hemorrhagic rash and respiratory distress syndrome. They may develop necrotic lesions within the liver, lungs, adrenals, and brain. Up to 14% to 31% die,[148] although current mortality rates are probably lower than documented in the 1970s.

Fetuses exposed to maternal varicella-zoster virus *in utero* are at risk for herpes zoster in early childhood.[133] They also may have an increased risk for malignancies, especially leukemia.[149] *In vitro* studies have shown an increase in chromosomal abnormalities in infected cells 20 times greater than in control cells.

Management

Varicella vaccine is now available and is approved for use in healthy susceptible individuals 1 year or older. This can be administered to nonpregnant patients with no history or previous varicella infection, but it is not advised for pregnant patients. Conception should be delayed until 1 month after the second vaccination dose.[35]

When given within 72 hours of exposure, VZIG reduces the severity of maternal infection, although it does not prevent fetal infection. Because most women with questionable or negative history of varicella actually have seroevidence of past infection[150] and given the high cost of VZIG, screening for varicella-zoster virus membrane antigen may help target the population that would benefit from VZIG therapy.[35]

If maternal infection occurs several days before delivery, the neonate should receive VZIG at birth as neonatal mortality in this setting can be high. Transplacental passage of IgG would not have had time to occur. The neonate also should be passively immunized because incomplete uptake of VZIG and transplacental transmission of the virus may have occurred.[151] Infants who develop varicella within the first 2 weeks after delivery should be treated with intravenous acyclovir.

Oral acyclovir ameliorates clinical symptoms in patients who develop chickenpox, if administered within 24 hours of onset of the rash. Acyclovir has been shown to be safe to administer in cases of severe maternal infection with no adverse effects on the fetus.[152,153] VZIG and acyclovir, however, do not appear to prevent fetal infection.

Herpes zoster in pregnancy poses almost no risk to the fetus. However, it may be a sign of another clinical problem in the mother, such as presence of HIV, and an appropriate workup for potential immunocompromise in the mother should be undertaken.

Herpes Simplex Virus Type 2

Definition and Prevalence

HSV-2 infection of the fetus and neonate is devastating. The CDC estimates that 450,000 new cases of HSV occur per year in the United States in adults, with a concomitant increase in fetal and neonatal infections.[154] The prevalence of HSV-2 is approximately 25% in the United States and 4% to 18% in Western Europe.[155] Neonatal infection is estimated to occur at a rate of 1 in 2,000 to 5,000 deliveries.[156] Thus, management of the pregnant woman with this virus poses many problems.

Pathogenesis and Pathology

HSV-2 is a sexually transmitted virus that most commonly involves the genitalia in adults. It can be transmitted *in utero* and in the perinatal period to the fetus and neonate. HSV-2 is a DNA virus that replicates in the cell nucleus but can establish latency for varying periods. The virus can then be reactivated with the proper, as yet undefined, stimulus. Primary infections with herpesvirus are highly cytopathic and cause much cell damage. After the primary infection, the virus replicates at the oral or genital portal of entry, entering the sensory nerve endings and remaining in the dorsal root ganglia (latency).

Eighty-five percent of cases of neonatal herpes simplex are transmitted at birth during passage through the vaginal canal, and less than 5% of cases are estimated to result from transplacental spread *in utero*.[157] Approximately 10% are acquired postnatally either from the mother, from a genital or nongenital site, or from other environmental sources of the virus.[158] HSV infection is diagnosed primarily by cultures; cytologic examination with a Tsanck smear also may be performed, although it is less accurate. A newly developed enzyme-linked immunosorbent assay for HSV may be useful, but further testing is still required. PCR likewise has been used to evaluate neonatal CSF and serum for the presence of HSV.[159]

Two classifications of herpes simplex infections have been described: primary and nonprimary. Primary genital herpes, constituting approximately 2% of cases, occurs in the absence of prior HSV antibodies and causes systemic symptoms such as headache, fever, malaise, and myalgia, in addition to painful genital lesions, and lesions of the fingers, buttocks, and mouth. Nonprimary herpes simplex may demonstrate first-time or recurrent genital lesions. Nonprimary herpes simplex with first-time genital lesions (approximately

7% of cases) occurs in the presence of prior HSV IgG antibodies, usually to HSV-1, indicating that a previous infection has occurred. Most patients, approximately 91%, have HSV IgG antibodies with recurrent genital lesions. The frequency of herpesvirus infection is underestimated, as signs and symptoms occur in fewer than 40% of serologically detected infections. One study estimated the prevalence of HSV-2 infection was 16.4% in the U.S. population aged 15 to 74 years during the late 1970s.[160]

Significant differences are seen between primary and recurrent HSV infections and, accordingly, fetal and neonatal infection varies with the type of HSV infection of the mother. Primary HSV infection results in a higher asymptomatic shedding of virus from the cervix (10.6% vs. 0.5%) and greater amounts of viral excretion for a longer period.[161] In recurrent HSV infection, viral particles are shed mainly from the labia. A prospective study by Brown et al.[161] showed that 40% of patients with primary genital HSV had serious perinatal morbidity, whereas none was found in the 14 patients with nonprimary HSV infection. The number and severity of complications increased with the estimated gestational age at the time of primary infection. A first-trimester infection resulted in a spontaneous abortion at 19 weeks with herpetic chorioamnionitis on pathologic examination. A second-trimester infection led to a premature birth at 32 weeks. Four in five women infected in the third trimester had significant infant morbidity: prematurity, IUGR, and neonatal HSV infection.[161]

Studies also have shown a significant increase in neonatal HSV infection in women with first episode HSV infection versus reactivation. In their study population, Brown et al.[161] noted a ten times greater prevalence of neonatal HSV in infants born to women with a primary infection during pregnancy, 33% prevalence of neonatal HSV. They also noted an increase in neonatal HSV with cervical shedding of virus and use of scalp electrodes. When maternal antibodies to HSV were present (recurrent infection), a decrease in neonatal infection was seen.[162] In their population, 30% of patients with first-time genital lesions had a primary infection. Prober et al.[163] found that none of 34 infants exposed inadvertently to HSV during vaginal delivery developed infection in mothers with recurrent vaginal herpes, and these authors concluded that empiric antiviral therapy is not indicated in all infants of mothers with HSV in the birth canal. The lack of neonatal infection with recurrent HSV infections was thought to be related to several factors: infrequent cervical involvement, the shorter time in which HSV was in the genital canal in lower titers, and the presence of transplacentally acquired antibodies to HSV.

One case report raises the possibility of congenital infection acquired via an ascending route in a woman with intact membranes until the time of cesarean section.[164] A small-for-gestational-age (SGA) infant was born with congenital neurologic defects and developed skin vesicles at 4 days; brain parenchymal abnormalities

also were present at this time. The mother had a history of primary HSV infection at 24 weeks. Pathologic examination showed viral immunostaining in cells in the subamniotic mesenchyme away from the perivascular central portion of the cord.

Diagnosis

Ultrasound

Neonatal HSV is much more common than *in utero* HSV. *In utero* HSV is estimated to occur in 1 in 200,000 deliveries in patients with either primary or recurrent herpes simplex. *In utero* HSV has been reported to cause skin lesions and scars at birth, chorioretinitis, microcephaly, hydranencephaly, and microphthalmos. Death, severe neurologic sequelae, mental retardation, seizures, and blindness have also been noted.[165] *In utero* these findings are not distinct on ultrasound from the rest of the TORCH agents, and the role of ultrasonography in identifying infected fetuses is limited. A case report in a patient with HSV-2 infection and an elevated AFP at 14 multiples of the median showed 9-mm ventricles, echogenic bowel, persistent leg flexion, and a 1-cm calcification in an enlarged liver. Subsequent pathology confirmed evidence of disseminated disease in the fetus.[166] The characteristic skin lesions are identified at birth. These findings are consistent with the tissue tropism typical of HSV infection in adults: neuronal, ocular, and skin findings. Viremia and transplacental transmission are the suspected causes in cases of primary infection. An ascending mode may also occur as 1 of 13 cases documented by Hutto et al.[165] was in a woman with recurrent disease. Overall, the risk of *in utero* transmission is felt to be quite low.[161,165]

Laboratory

As with other infectious agents, herpesvirus can now be detected by PCR and this appears to be more sensitive than standard culture techniques.

Differential Diagnosis

See Cytomegalovirus, Differential Diagnosis.

Prognosis

Fetal and neonatal infections with HSV-2 are serious. Fetal infections, although rare, can lead to skin lesions, chorioretinitis, microcephaly, hydranencephaly, and microphthalmos. Death, seizures, mental retardation, blindness, and other neurologic sequelae also may result. Spontaneous abortions may occur with increased frequency in first-trimester infections. Prematurity has been noted in mothers with primary infections that develop after 20 weeks' gestation. The prognosis in cases of neonatal infection depends on rapid diagnosis and administration of antiviral treatment so disseminated disease does not occur.

Management

Without antiviral treatment, 70% of cases of localized HSV infection progress to disseminated disease, which has a grave prognosis. Acyclovir and adenosine arabinoside are shown to be effective in neonatal HSV, but even with treatment, mortality in cases of disseminated disease is 50% to 60%.[167] The role of acyclovir in treating primary HSV infections in pregnancy is still debatable. There are no established indications for use during pregnancy, but reasonable uses for acyclovir in maternal infections such as disseminated herpes simplex and severe primary genital herpes have been advocated.[168] Other authors believe the data on safety are insufficient to advise giving acyclovir to pregnant women with HSV infection.[158] Acyclovir has been demonstrated to be beneficial in cases of extreme prematurity with rupture of membranes or preterm labor in the presence of HSV lesions. Delay in delivery with concomitant use of acyclovir has been associated with good outcome.[169] Arguments also have been made against acyclovir usage in pregnancy. In nonpregnant adults, acyclovir therapy for primary genital HSV infections is known to delay the humoral antibody response. It is speculated that this delay after an episode of primary genital herpes in late pregnancy could theoretically delay transfer of Igs to the fetus, thereby making the fetus more vulnerable to the HSV harbored asymptomatically in the genital tract during labor. Since transplacentally acquired antibody is known to protect neonates exposed to HSV during vaginal delivery, this decrease in maternally acquired antibodies in the fetus could increase the risk of neonatal HSV infection.[163]

Repetitive culturing for HSV frequently leads to cesarean section, with an estimated ratio of 50 cesarean sections performed to one case of neonatal herpes simplex infection prevented, which seems unacceptable considering that HSV is the most infrequently occurring infection of the newborn for any of the TORCH pathogens.[169] If genital lesions are present at the time of delivery, cesarean section is advocated because vaginal delivery is associated with a 50% rate of neonatal infection when genital lesions are present. If cesarean section is performed within 4 hours of membrane rupture, the prevalence decreases to 15% to 20%. In general, screening cultures are believed not to be cost-effective or necessary in all cases. If genital lesions are present in the perinatal period, cultures are recommended. If cultures are positive at the time of delivery, a cesarean section is recommended. If cultures are negative, vaginal delivery is advised. If no genital lesions are evident, cultures are unnecessary and vaginal delivery is recommended.[170,171] Postpartum cultures of the oropharynx, conjunctiva, and umbilicus of the newborn infant are recommended to determine whether acyclovir treatment is indicated.

Human Immunodeficiency Virus

Definition and Prevalence

Acquired immunodeficiency syndrome (AIDS) is caused by an RNA retrovirus—HIV—that was first described in 1981. In pregnant women and their offspring, HIV infection has become an important issue as the prevalence of AIDS increases worldwide. The World Health Organization has estimated that three million women worldwide were infected with HIV in 1990; most of these were of childbearing age. An estimated half-million children worldwide had positive HIV titers. In most of these children, the virus was transmitted from mother to child (vertical transmission).[172] In the United States, approximately 7,000 HIV positive women give birth each year,[173] a figure that has remained stable from 1988 through 1994.[174]

Pathogenesis and Pathology

HIV attaches to the CD4 molecule on T lymphocytes to gain entry into the cell. Inside the cells, its replication is mediated by reverse transcriptase and the viral DNA becomes incorporated into the host genome. The virus continues to multiply and ultimately T-lymphocyte lysis ensues, leading to a decrease in the number of T-helper cells. When the number of T-helper cells becomes insufficient, AIDS develops. The virus is spread by contact with blood products, sexual intercourse, and intravenous drug use. The standard screening test is the enzyme-linked immunosorbent assay to detect HIV-specific IgG antibodies. Positive tests must be confirmed with a Western blot assay.

Pediatric AIDS, first reported in 1982,[175] is the result of vertical transmission in approximately 80% of cases, and most of the remainder are related to blood transfusions with contaminated blood. Perspective studies estimate that 13% to 32% of pregnant women with AIDS transmit the virus to the fetus[176]; transmission may be as high as 48% in undeveloped countries.[177] These transmission rates seem to be highest in mothers with advanced infection (CD4 counts less than 200 per µL), although pregnancy does not appear to accelerate the disease in the mother.[178] A decline in transmission rates in the United States has been noted since 1994, mostly attributed to use of zidovudine (AZT) and changes in obstetric practices.[174]

HIV may be transmitted from mother to child in three ways: transplacentally, during birth, and via breast milk. One study showed that the first-born twin is more likely to be infected with HIV than the second-born twin for both vaginal deliveries and cesarean sections,[179] indicating infection more likely occurs during delivery rather than transplacentally, as originally suspected.[56] Prenatal diagnostic techniques such as amniocentesis, cordocentesis, and CVS are usually not recommended as they may increase the risk of transmission to the fetus. Although HIV antigens have been demonstrated in amniotic fluid and fetal and placental tissues as early as the first trimester,[180,181] when transplacental transmission does occur, it is after 13 weeks' gestation, which is when CD4-positive cells first begin to appear in the fetus.[71] Rare reports exist of infants with signs of infection at birth.[182]

In 1986, several case reports suggested an AIDS embryopathy that resulted in dysmorphic features: severe IUGR, microcephaly, ocular hypertelorism, boxlike forehead, flat nasal bridge, short nose, and patulous lips.[183,184] This syndrome was disproved as there are many confounding variables in AIDS patients, such as poor socioeconomic class, infectious diseases, malnutrition, intravenous drug abuse, and ethanol abuse.[159,185,186] Additionally, some of the facial characteristics are related to race. More important, HIV virus cannot grow in cells that do not have CD4 receptors, and these do not appear in the fetus until 13 to 15 weeks, which is after the period of embryogenesis. Neurodevelopmental[187,188] and cardiac[189] abnormalities have been described in infants who are HIV positive, but none has been noted *in utero*.

Diagnosis

No specific anomalies are definitely associated with HIV infection. Given the prevalence of low-birth-weight and SGA infants, however, it is not unreasonable to follow HIV patients with serial sonograms to assess for growth disturbances. Additionally, a significant number of HIV patients abuse drugs and alcohol, and sonograms may detect any adverse affects of these substances on the fetus.

Laboratory

Mothers with HIV show positive antibodies.

Differential Diagnosis

See Cytomegalovirus, Differential Diagnosis.

Prognosis

Two clinical types of congenital AIDS are described. Twenty percent of infants with vertically transmitted HIV have a short incubation period of 4 months followed by an increased prevalence of *Pneumocystis carinii* pneumonia and a poor prognosis. Eighty percent have an incubation period of 6 years with subsequent interstitial pneumonitis, recurrent bacterial infection, and a better prognosis. These patterns suggest two different routes of transmission: (a) transplacental spread with early onset of AIDS, and (b) peripartum infection in infants with a more mature immune system that can fight infection, which has a better prognosis.[190]

Studies of AIDS patients in Africa demonstrate IUGR associated with HIV positivity, which may reflect more advanced disease in the mothers.[191] A prospective study showed no difference in pregnancy outcomes between HIV-positive and HIV-negative intravenous drug abusers with regard to abortion, stillbirth, prematurity, and birth weight, but none of the patients had advanced disease.[192] A study of 134 infants born to HIV-positive mothers in the United States demonstrated 48% to have low birth weight, 16% to

be SGA, and 13% to have neonatal bacterial infections associated with vertical transmission of HIV.[176] Minkoff et al.[193] reported low birth weights and premature rupture of membranes in HIV-positive pregnant women, but Alger et al.[178] found no difference in obstetric outcomes in HIV-positive women compared to seronegative women.

Management

Management of the pregnant woman with HIV is a complex issue. Invasive diagnostic procedures to detect infection in the fetus are not advisable as they may actually introduce the infection into the fetus or may initially yield negative results, even though the fetus develops HIV infection later in pregnancy. Moreover, many pregnant women with AIDS do not wish to terminate their pregnancies. As stated previously, pregnancy does not exacerbate AIDS but pregnant women with CD4 counts less than 200 per μL are at much greater risk for opportunistic infections, especially *P. carinii* pneumonia. CD4 counts are usually obtained each trimester. When CD4 counts are low, *P. carinii* pneumonia prophylaxis with trimethoprim-sulfamethoxazole is appropriate. Although studies show no deleterious effect on the fetus, it seems wise to avoid usage in the first trimester if possible.

AZT has unknown effects on the fetus but has been shown to decrease the vertical transmission rate of HIV.[194] In a prospective study of HIV-positive pregnant women, vertical transmission was decreased from 25.5% to 8.3% when AZT was orally administered five times daily antepartum and intravenously during the intrapartum period. The infants also received AZT for 6 weeks. The effects on the fetus are not known, but infants in the AZT group had significantly lower hemoglobin at birth than the control group. However, the anemia resolved by 1 year of age.

A European Collaborative Study has shown that cesarean section was estimated to halve the rate of transmission of HIV to the infant.[195] It is theorized that avoiding direct contact with contaminated blood and cervical secretions in the birth canal decreases the rate of vertical transmission. The study had a number of confounding factors, and the women who had cesarean sections were more advanced in their disease. A randomized controlled trial is necessary before cesarean sections are advised for all gravid women with HIV.

Kass et al.[196] suggest balancing clinical decisions between the woman and the fetus, understanding that the health needs of the pregnant woman are usually whatever is in the best interest of the developing fetus.

Other Viral Infections

Coxsackieviruses B1 and B5 have been associated with anomalies of the genitourinary, gastrointestinal, and cardiovascular systems when infection occurs during the first trimester. There may be generalized fetal infection with focal necrosis of the heart (myocarditis) or central nervous system. Lesions can also occur in the liver, kidneys, or adrenals. Tachycardia and severe heart failure have been described. Neonatal disease usually results from fetal infection in the third trimester of pregnancy.

PARASITIC INFECTIONS

Toxoplasmosis

Definition and Prevalence

Toxoplasmosis is caused by a protozoan, *Toxoplasma gondii*. It infects approximately 4 in 1,000 susceptible pregnant women in the United States, resulting in 1 to 2 congenitally infected infants per 1,000 live births each year.[70] The seroprevalence in the United States is roughly 20%.[197] Treatment of infected gravid women has been shown to decrease fetal infection rate and anomalies, emphasizing the impact of prenatal diagnosis.

Pathogenesis and Pathology

T. gondii is a parasite with a life cycle of three stages: oocyst, tachyzoite, and tissue cyst. The domestic cat is the reservoir for human infection. Infected cats excrete oocysts, which produce sporozoites, the form that infects humans. Oocysts may be ingested by humans from contact with infected raw meat, cat feces, or soil. Sporozoites penetrate the gastrointestinal mucosa and then develop into tachyzoites, which are released into the circulation where they may infect the placenta and, ultimately, fetal tissues.[198] Rapid spread through fetal tissues stops as IgM is produced, suggesting why early infections cause more tissue damage than later infections.[47] Many organs can be infected, but the eyes and brain are major targets.

Congenital toxoplasmosis is marked by the classic triad of chorioretinitis, intracranial calcifications, and hydrocephalus. Other findings may include lymphadenopathy, hepatosplenomegaly, mental retardation, seizures, and encephalitis. Unfortunately, 90% of infections in healthy, pregnant women are asymptomatic, so toxoplasmosis is not commonly suspected clinically. Mild symptoms similar to mononucleosis may occur: occipital and cervical lymphadenopathy, malaise, arthralgia, and low-grade fever.

Thirty percent to 40% of pregnant women in the United States are immune to toxoplasmosis,[199,200] but of the 0.4% who acquire it during pregnancy, 40% give birth to an infected infant. Vertical transmission occurs during acute infection with maternal parasitemia. The placenta must be infected before fetal infection, but the time between maternal and fetal infection varies significantly, ranging from 4 to 16 weeks.[198]

Fetal infection rates and fetal sequelae vary with congenital age. The overall transmission rate to the fetus after primary infection appears to be in the range of 20% to 35%,[201] but this varies significantly with gestational age.[202,203] The rate of infection in fetuses is approximately 5% before 16 weeks' gestation and increases to 17% and 60% during the second and third trimesters, respectively.[204] However, fetuses infected in early pregnancy are much more likely to show clinical signs of infection. Fetal damage decreases with increasing gestational age, from 75% during first-trimester infection to almost 0% in the third trimester.

Diagnosis

Ultrasound

Sonographic findings of fetal toxoplasmosis include multiple liver calcifications or echogenic foci (Fig. 11), hydrops (Fig. 12), intracranial calcifications (Figs. 13 and 14), and hydrocephalus.[205] Intracranial findings indicate a poor prognosis and severe fetal involvement. Microcephaly does not appear to be common in cases of congenital toxoplasmosis.[206]

Hohlfeld et al.[207] examined 89 cases of fetal toxoplasmosis and found sonographic abnormalities in 32. Ventricular dilatation was most common, usually bilateral and symmetric. Evolution was rapid over a period of several days and initially involved the occipital horns. Also noted were intracranial and intrahepatic echogenicities, thick and echogenic placentas, ascites, and, rarely, pleural and pericardial effusions. IUGR and microcephaly were not seen. Correlation with pathologic findings indicated that although sonograms invariably indicate a poor prognosis with cerebral lesions, ultrasonography was unable to detect brain necrosis in the absence of ventricular dilatation.[207]

In a series that examined postnatal sonographic findings in *Toxoplasma*-infected neonates, the incidence of subependymal cysts and choroid plexus cysts was higher than expected. The incidence of choroid plexus cysts was 24%. These findings were in addition to hepatosplenomegaly, thalamostriate artery calcifications, and fetal ascites.[208]

Laboratory

Toxoplasmosis can be diagnosed in a pregnant woman by seroconversion from negative to positive titers, the presence of specific IgM antibodies, or a fourfold increase in specific IgG titers obtained at 3-week intervals. Serologic diagnosis can be confounded by other factors such as individual variation in titers; IgM may persist in some people for more than a year after infection, and different tests have different sensitivities.[209] The importance of using an established reference laboratory for screening cannot be overemphasized.

For direct testing, PCR testing of amniotic fluid has been found to be extremely useful for identification or exclusion of fetal *T. gondii* infection.[210–214] The specificity of PCR is nearly 100%,[212,215] although sensitivity may be as low as 64%.[216] High parasite counts are more likely to show sonographic abnormalities.[217] Foulon et al.[218] found that congenital toxoplasmosis is best predicted by the com-

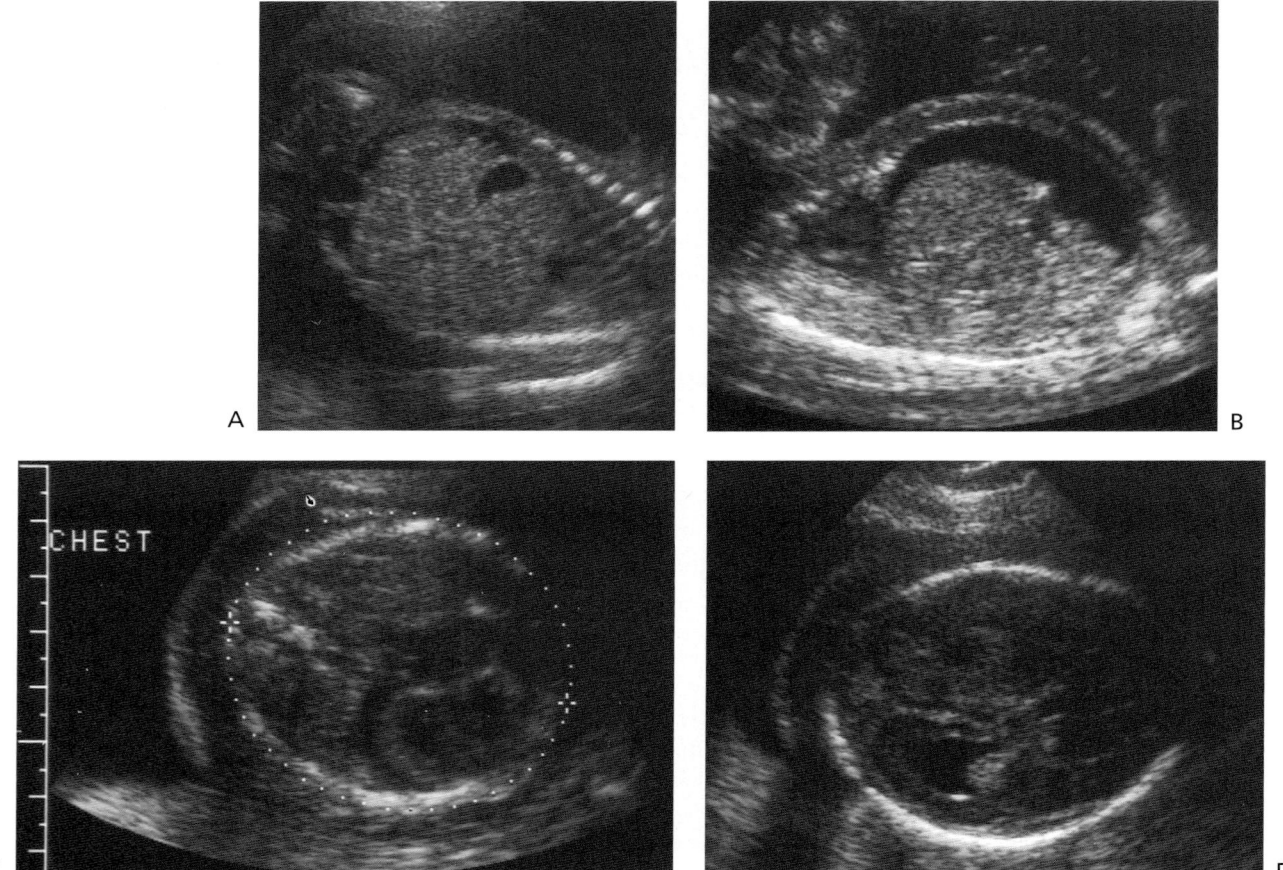

FIGURE 12. Toxoplasmosis. **A:** A longitudinal scan of the abdomen at 22 weeks shows a small amount of ascites. This was the only sonographic abnormality. **B:** Follow-up scan 10 days later shows a large amount of ascites. **C:** A transverse view of the chest shows pericardial effusion and diffuse subcutaneous edema, indicating diffuse hydrops. **D:** The lateral cerebral ventricles are borderline dilated (10 to 11 mm). Diffuse edema is also noted surrounding calvaria.

bination of PCR and mouse inoculation of amniotic fluid, achieving a sensitivity of 91%. Because of development of PCR for amniotic fluid, the role of cordocentesis is now limited.

Screening

Given the relatively low prevalence of congenital toxoplasmosis in the United States, screening is not advised at this time and has not been considered cost-effective. Similar conclusions have been reached in the United Kingdom.[219] The state of Oregon had a screening program for several years that was ultimately discontinued.

Although screening is not considered cost-effective in the United States, it is performed in other countries, notably France. Acute infection is suggested by a rise in titer of IgG antibodies. IgM antibodies become positive within a week and persist for a year, so that a negative IgM antibody virtually excludes recent infection. A Sabin-Feldman dye test usually is performed, which detects both IgG and IgM antibodies. This test usually is performed in a reference laboratory as live parasites are required. Testing and interpret-

ing results are not always straightforward. Some persons may be serofast (have persistent IgM), which presents a diagnostic problem if no pre-pregnancy titers are available.

Differential Diagnosis

See Cytomegalovirus, Differential Diagnosis.

Prognosis

Early toxoplasmosis, in the first trimester, may result in spontaneous abortion. The prevalence of sequelae decreases as gestational age increases, but long-term sequelae can occur with *in utero* infection. Research in the early 1970s showed intellectual deficits in children with subclinical congenital toxoplasmosis who were not treated.[220]

Up to 30% of untreated infected infants are symptomatic at birth, with seizures, chorioretinitis, encephalitis, and hydrocephalus. Of the asymptomatic neonates, most develop chorioretinitis by adulthood, and one-half have severe visual impairment.[221] Antibiotic treatment is recom-

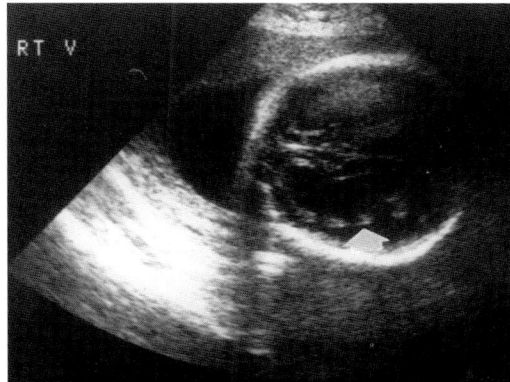

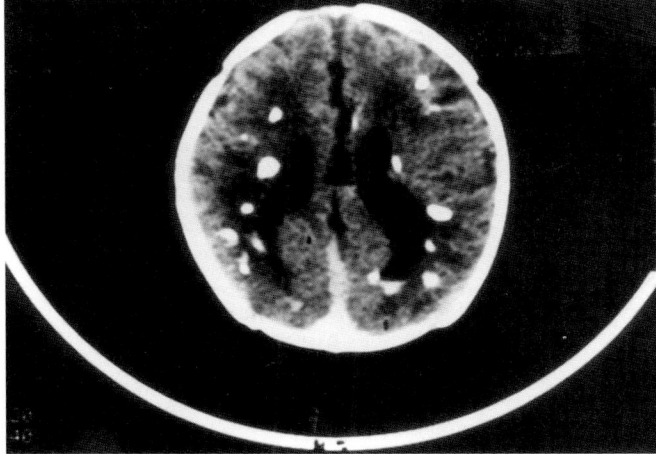

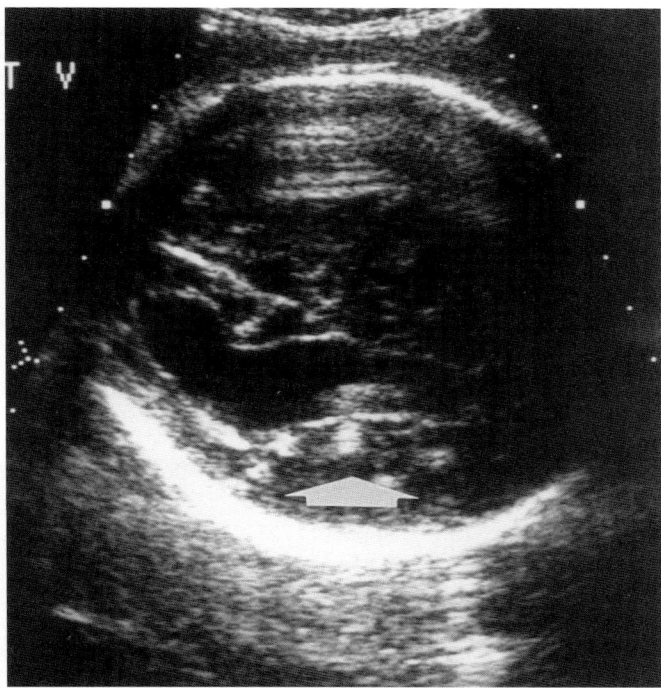

FIGURE 13. Toxoplasmosis. **A:** A transaxial image of the head at 30 weeks shows ventriculomegaly with subtle periventricular hyperechoic areas (*arrow*). **B:** A transaxial image of the head at 33 weeks' gestation demonstrates an increase in the size and number of periventricular hyperechoic areas with intraparenchymal hyperechoic foci as well (*arrow*). **C:** A computed tomographic scan of the head performed postpartum at estimated gestational age of 38 weeks demonstrates periventricular and parenchymal calcifications with ventriculomegaly in infant with known toxoplasmosis. (Reproduced with permission from Desai MB, Kurtz AB, Martin ME, et al. Characteristic findings of toxoplasmosis *in utero*: a case report. *J Ultrasound Med* 1994;13:60–62.)

mended for 1 year after birth to decrease tissue damage rather than to cure disease.

Foulon et al.[222] followed 50 pregnant women at risk for giving birth to a child with congenital toxoplasmosis due to seroconversion or high antibody levels in the first serum sample. Fetal infection was diagnosed in six fetuses by positive *Toxoplasma* culture in amniotic fluid or fetal blood and positive test for IgM in fetal blood. Two fetuses died *in utero* from infection. Two of the four that were born had marked anomalies: hydrocephalus and chorioretinitis in one, and only chorioretinitis in the other. Thirty-five of the 44 infants without evidence of congenital infection demonstrated no specific antibodies at 1 year of age, and in the other nine, specific antibody levels were declining.

A prospective study of maternal and pediatric findings related to toxoplasmosis was performed in 23,000 cases with follow-up to 7 years.[200] From among the 15 pregnancies that were defined as high risk, two infants had congenital toxoplasmosis and three were stillborn. Approximately 39% of women in the study demonstrated

antibodies to *Toxoplasma*, although they did not necessarily have acute infection, and follow-up of their children at 7 years of age showed an increased incidence of bilateral deafness, microcephaly, and low IQ. These findings raise questions about management of all women with antibodies to *Toxoplasma*.

Management

As soon as toxoplasmosis is diagnosed in a pregnant woman, treatment with spiramycin should be started to diminish the possibility of fetal infection. Spiramycin, a macrolide antibiotic with a spectrum similar to that of erythromycin, currently is not licensed in the United States; however, it may be obtained from Europe with special U.S. Food and Drug Administration approval. It is administered at a dosage of 3 g per day when maternal infection is documented. Spiramycin does not cross the placenta but appears to prevent passage of *Toxoplasma* to the fetus via the placenta. Spiramycin has never been tested

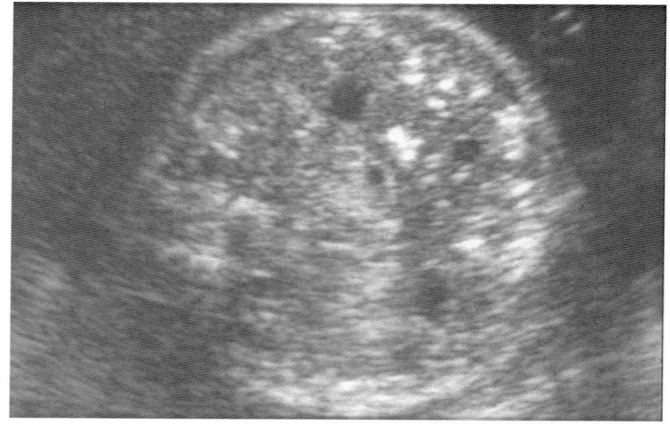

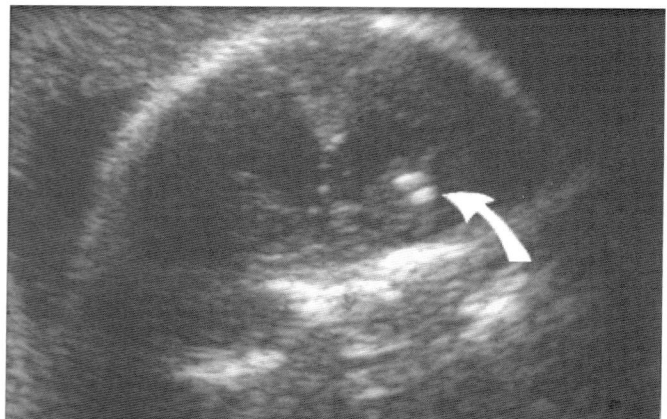

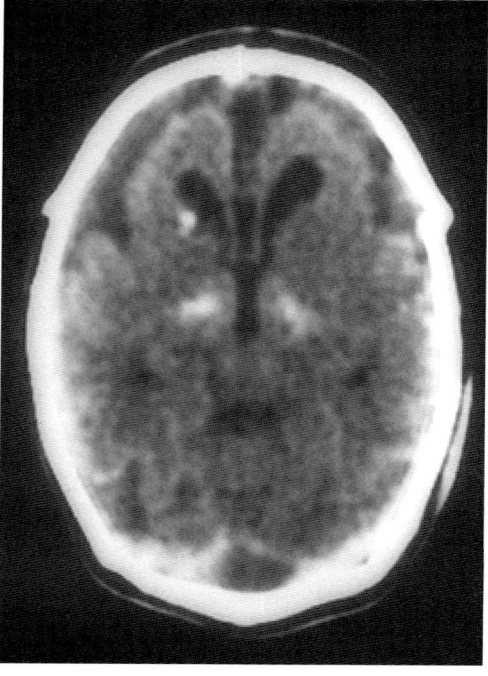

FIGURE 14. Toxoplasmosis. **A:** A transverse view of the abdomen shows multiple bright echogenic foci of liver. **B:** A coronal view of the brain shows bright echogenic area consistent with calcification in the basal ganglia (*arrow*). **C:** A postnatal computed tomogram shows calcification of the basal ganglia.

in a randomized, controlled clinical trial because its efficacy is considered quite high on the basis of comparison with historical controls; at this time, a randomized clinical trial would not be considered ethical given its high efficacy.

If tests indicate the fetus is infected and continuation of pregnancy is desired, further treatment with sulfonamide and pyrimethamine, a folic acid inhibitor and bone marrow suppressant, may be started to decrease the severity of infection. This drug combination is commonly used in Europe, especially France. Both drugs are contraindicated in the first trimester, however, because of toxicity and teratogenic effects. In France, these drugs are given alternately with spiramycin, during pregnancy and for up to 1 year postnatally. Because of false-negative testing, Romand et al.[216] suggest presumptive treatment combining pyrimethamine and sulfonamides in case of maternal infection occurring late in pregnancy.

Prenatal treatment has been shown to reduce the frequency of affected infants. Daffos et al.[223] showed a 70% reduction in congenital toxoplasmosis when compared to prior studies using spiramycin, sulfonamide, and pyrimethamine. However, duration of follow-up was only from 3 to 30 months postnatally, which does not allow time for many of the potentially common late sequelae of infection.

Hohlfeld et al.[204] reported 52 pregnancies in treated infected women with follow-up of the infants for 19 months. Forty-one infants had subclinical infections, 12 had benign infection, and one had congenital toxoplasmosis, representing an overall reduction of severe forms and increased number of subclinical cases, supporting *in utero* treatment of toxoplasmosis. Long-term follow-up of these infants is currently under way to exclude later complications, such as chorioretinitis.

A study by Berrebi et al.[224] showed that in mothers who had acute *Toxoplasma* infection before 28 weeks' gestation and received antiparasitic treatment with spiramycin, pyrimethamine, and sulfadiazine, only 27 of 162 live-born infants had proven congenital toxoplasmosis. All 27 infants had normal neurologic development and were free of symptoms at 15 to 71 months of age despite initial findings of clinical signs of congenital toxoplasmosis, intracranial calcifications, chorioretinitis, and ventricular dilatation. The authors suggest that even in first- and second-trimester infection, the pregnancy does not need to be terminated if antiparasitic treatment is given and fetal ultrasound is normal.

Prevention programs for congenital toxoplasmosis that advocate specific hygienic measures may not be useful. A Belgian study found that the number of seroconversions was reduced by 34% when pregnant patients were instructed to adopt prophylactic measures. However, the difference was not statistically significant and suggests that the impact of a primary prevention program is limited.[225]

Other Parasitic Infections

Other parasitic infections include malaria, schistosomiasis, and trypanosomiasis. Most diseases of malaria are secondary to placental involvement and their effect on the fetus (preterm labor and IUGR). Prenatally acquired malaria occurs predominantly in women who contract malaria during pregnancy and is rare among patients indigenous to malarial areas.

Schistosoma haematobium is especially likely to migrate to the pelvic veins. Excretion of eggs in the uterus and placenta can occur with both *S. haematobium* and *Schistosoma mansoni*.[226] Fetal disease results from placental compromise secondary to massive egg deposition and associated inflammatory reaction.

Trypanosoma cruzi produces Chagas' disease. The placenta is commonly infected. Fetal infection may occur through the umbilical cord or amniotic fluid. Fetal infection affects the heart, muscle, brain, skin, gastrointestinal tract, and reticuloendothelial system. Infection leads to hepatosplenomegaly, anemia, jaundice, and encephalitis. The manifestations may resemble erythroblastosis fetalis. Infection may lead to abortion, prematurity, IUGR, or neonatal death. PCR has a clear advantage over conventional techniques for the early detection of congenital transmission of *T. cruzi* infection and for monitoring infants undergoing chemotherapy.[227]

BACTERIAL INFECTION

Syphilis

Definition and Prevalence

Syphilis is caused by a spirochete, *Treponema pallidum*. Congenital syphilis is defined by the CDC as stillbirth at less than 20 weeks in mothers with positive VDRL and fluorescent treponemal antibody tests with inadequate or no treatment, infants with positive CSF VDRL tests or CSF white blood cell counts greater than 5 cells per μL on a clear tap, and infants with radiographic evidence of syphilis in the long bones or on physical examination.

Although in 1991, reported cases of syphilis in the United States declined for the first time since 1985,[228] congenital syphilis continues to challenge clinicians caring for pregnant women. Congenital syphilis should be preventable with proper prenatal care, but gravid women with syphilis frequently receive little or no prenatal care. Penicillin treatment of the mother does not always protect the fetus from infection and, even if they are treated, women may become reinfected or, rarely, treatment may fail.[229]

Pathogenesis and Pathology

T. pallidum readily crosses the placenta and can induce considerable damage in cases of congenital infection. First-trimester infections do occur as *T. pallidum* can gain access to the fetal compartment as early as 9 to 10 weeks,[230] but they are difficult to recognize as syphilitic lesions and are not observed in the fetus until the fifth month of pregnancy as the embryo is unable to mount a sufficient response against spirochetes in the first trimester. Nathan et al.[231] have demonstrated spirochetes in the amniotic fluid, however, as early as 14 weeks' gestation. The fetus is infected during primary and secondary maternal infections but not during tertiary infection. The spirochete spreads rapidly through the fetus, and granulomatous lesions are found in most organs, especially the liver, lungs, and pancreas, as well as in the placenta and amniotic fluid. Fetal damage is the result of the fetus' own immune reaction to the spirochetes. Congenital syphilis often results in fetal or neonatal death or preterm labor. The risk of developing congenital syphilis is greatest in the last trimester of pregnancy. Fetal survival is best when transmission occurs late in the course of the mother's disease.

Congenital syphilis has been divided into early and late stages; early is symptomatic within the first 2 years. These stages show considerable overlap. Neonates with congenital syphilis may initially appear normal at birth, but petechial skin lesions may develop in 1 to 3 weeks. Findings resemble late-stage adult disease with additional features such as osteochondritis, periostitis with painful abnormalities in the metadiaphyseal areas of long bones (over 90% of cases), peg-shaped upper incisors known as *Hutchinson's teeth*, saddle nose, and a high-arched palate. Mental retardation, hydrocephalus, corneal keratitis, and deafness also may be present later. Hemolytic anemia, jaundice, nephrosis, meningitis, and rhinitis may be seen. Mortality is greatest with bullous eruptions or exfoliation of palms and soles at birth.[51]

Diagnosis

Ultrasound
Sonographic findings associated with congenital syphilis include dilated bowel segments (Figs. 15 and 16), hepatomegaly (Fig. 17), nonimmune hydrops (Fig. 18), and placentomegaly. Nathan et al.[232] measured the fetal liver in the longitudinal plane from mid-right hemidiaphragm to right liver edge in patients with syphilis and found hepatomegaly had a significant association with amniotic fluid infection (Fig. 17).

Nonimmune hydrops, fetal hepatomegaly, and placentomegaly should alert the sonographer to the possibility of

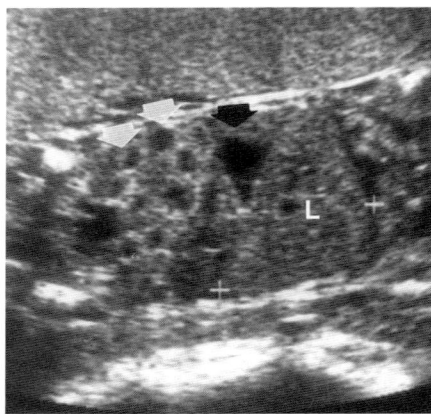

FIGURE 15. Syphilis. A coronal view of the fetal abdomen at 23 weeks demonstrates multiple dilated small bowel loops (*white arrows*) inferior to the stomach bubble (*black arrow*) with associated hepatomegaly (*L*). (Reproduced with permission from Satin AJ, Twickler DM, Wendel GD. Congenital syphilis associated with dilatation of fetal small bowel: a case report. *J Ultrasound Med* 1992;11:49–52.)

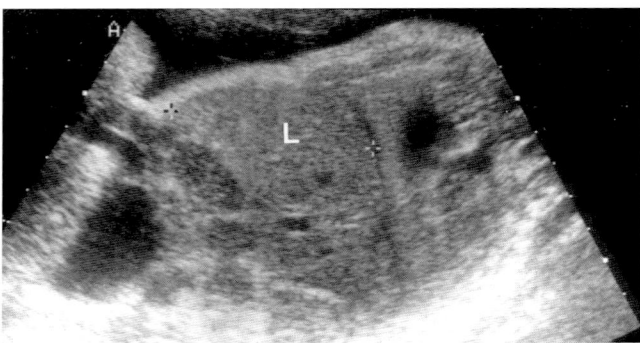

FIGURE 17. Syphilis. A coronal scan of the abdomen (*A*) at 32 weeks demonstrates hepatomegaly. The liver (*L*) measured 51 mm. The mother had secondary syphilis. (Reproduced with permission from Nathan L, Twickler DM, Peters MT, et al. Fetal syphilis: correlation of sonographic findings and rabbit infectivity testing of amniotic fluid. *J Ultrasound Med* 1993;2:97–101.)

congenital syphilis, especially if the mother has a positive history of syphilis. Amniocentesis and percutaneous umbilical blood sampling can be used for confirmation when hydropic changes are identified in a mother with syphilis.[233] Congenital syphilis is a potentially treatable cause of nonimmune hydrops, and Barton et al.[234] have published case reports of nonimmune hydrops in maternal syphilis that was treated aggressively with antibiotics and preterm delivery, resulting in survival of the infants.

Fetal bowel dilatation may develop secondary to syphilitic arteritis, which can lead to stenosis and atresia of the

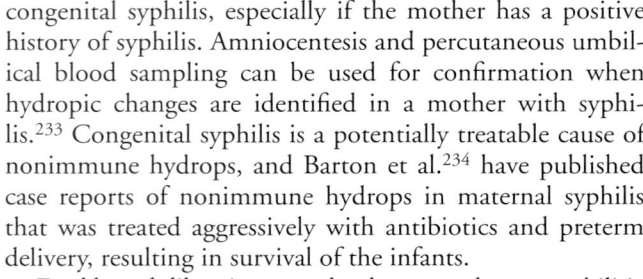

FIGURE 16. Syphilis. A transverse image of the fetal abdomen at 23.5 weeks shows dilated small bowel (*b* = 8 mm) and the spine (*s*). The mother had active syphilis, and the fetus was stillborn 10 days later. (Reproduced with permission from Hill LM, Maloney JB. An unusual constellation of sonographic findings associated with congenital syphilis. *Obstet Gynecol* 1991;78:895–897.)

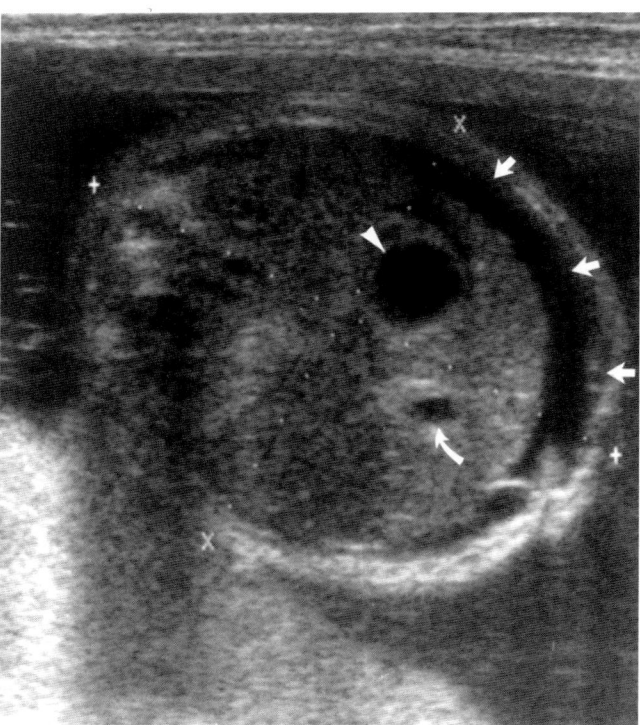

FIGURE 18. Syphilis. A transverse scan of the fetal abdomen in a mother with early latent syphilis at 25 weeks' gestation shows ascites (*arrows*), dilated stomach bubble (*arrowhead*), and the umbilical vein (*curved arrow*). (Reproduced with permission from Nathan L, Twickler DM, Peters MT, et al. Fetal syphilis: correlation of sonographic findings and rabbit infectivity testing of amniotic fluid. *J Ultrasound Med* 1993;2:97–101.)

bowel.[235,236] Pathognomonic mucosal and submucosal mononuclear cell and fibroblast infiltration are present, usually in the small bowel and, less commonly, in the colon and stomach.[237] Syphilitic enterocolitis can impair intestinal motility, leading to meconium ileus or obstruction. Pancreatic fibrosis and hypoplasia of the endocrine glands also may result in this finding. One ultrasound report described dilated small bowel, increased abdominal circumference, and echogenic foci within the abdomen.[235] Another report documented hepatosplenomegaly, placentomegaly, and noncontinuous gastrointestinal tract obstruction associated with congenital syphilis. The gastrointestinal tract obstruction involved both small bowel and stomach.[235]

Although hyperechogenicity of the vasculature in the basal ganglia usually is believed to be related to CMV and rubella virus infection, it has also been noted with syphilis.[239] Pathologically, this finding is thought to represent a mineralizing vasculopathy occurring after a vasculitis of the branching arteries of the basal ganglia and thalami.

Increased resistance of uterine and umbilical arteries with Doppler ultrasound in patients with syphilis was compared with those of uninfected subjects, and both showed a significant increase in patients with syphilis. An even greater association was found when spirochetes were present in the amniotic fluid, indicating these elevated ratios are related to the presence of intrauterine infection. Pathologically, findings are believed to be secondary to the known placental villitis and obliterative arteritis seen with syphilis. Patients followed with serial sonograms during treatment showed normalization of the umbilical systolic/diastolic (S/D) ratios with successful treatment, but in the one case that resulted in fetal death, the umbilical S/D ratio remained elevated. This finding suggests a possible role for Doppler ultrasonography in monitoring treatment success. The numbers of SGA infants in the syphilis group were not large enough to suggest IUGR as an explanation for these abnormal S/D ratios.[238]

Laboratory

The clinical diagnosis of syphilis in pregnant patients is the same as in nonpregnant patients. Primary syphilis can be diagnosed with dark field microscopy of scrapings from a lesion, but these usually are not present in gravid women at the time of prenatal care. Usually, serology is the primary mode of diagnosis. Skin lesions of secondary syphilis are painless, and therefore, most patients do not seek medical attention.

Rapid plasma reagin and VDRL tests are the most common screening tests. Most patients with primary syphilis and essentially all patients with secondary syphilis have positive results. These tests detect nontreponemal antibody, reactive with a titer that is highest in active (secondary) disease.

Specific antitreponemal antibody tests such as microhemagglutination assay–*T. pallidum* and fluorescent treponemal antibody absorption are used to confirm screening tests. Serial titers of nontreponemal tests are used to assess treatment success. With satisfactory treatment, titers decrease to one-fourth of the initial values within 3 months and usually revert to normal within 1 year.[239] In patients with suspected duration of syphilis longer than 1 year, lumbar puncture is required to exclude neurosyphilis, which is not treated in the routine fashion with benzathine penicillin.

PCR is rapidly becoming a useful test for congenital syphilis, early primary syphilis, and neurosyphilis and in distinguishing old versus new infection. Sensitivity is increasing but has not yet equaled that of the rabbit infectivity test.[240]

Screening

Serologic screening has proved cost-effective in pregnant women and is performed at the initial prenatal visit, and again at 28 weeks in high-risk populations.

Differential Diagnosis

See Cytomegalovirus, Differential Diagnosis.

Prognosis

McFarlin et al.[241] prospectively reviewed 253 cases of maternal syphilis and found that single-dose therapy had a significantly decreased rate of congenital syphilis in disease with duration of less than 1 year. Patients with an unknown duration of disease had rates of congenital syphilis of 68% for one-dose treatment and 49% for three-dose treatment. In general, a 28% rate of prematurity was noted in all patients with syphilis even when treated. Findings show an alarming failure rate in the prevention of congenital syphilis. Among the entire group of patients with syphilis (treated and untreated), 14% had stillborn infants, but 66% of untreated patients had stillbirths. VDRL titers at the time of diagnosis were highest in women with stillbirths and lowest in women with babies without congenital syphilis.[241]

Rawston et al.[242] looked at factors associated with congenital syphilis in 403 pregnancies with positive serologic test results for syphilis. Eighteen percent had congenital syphilis, which was strongly associated with lack of prenatal care, no antibiotic treatment, and increased rapid plasma reagin titer. Sixty-six percent of live-born infants with congenital syphilis lacked rash, hepatosplenomegaly, or lymphadenopathy and were identified only by laboratory tests: radiographs, CSF VDRL, bilirubin, or liver function studies. Fifty-three percent of infants with congenital syphilis were stillborn. Congenital syphilis was more likely to result in SGA and premature babies. A history of maternal treatment did not exclude congenital syphilis, so all neonates should be evaluated for congenital syphilis if there is a maternal history of syphilis.[242]

Management

CDC guidelines for syphilis treatment are based on clinical judgment with no scientific data to support efficacy.

Women with syphilis are treated with penicillin according to the CDC guidelines; however, there have been no widespread clinical trials to assess efficacy of this treatment in pregnant women, so serologic follow-up is important. Treatment failures are rare but have been documented and usually occur late in pregnancy.[243] Reinfection occurs more commonly, so that treatment of the patient's partner(s) is crucial. HIV-positive patients have been noted to be refractory to syphilis treatment, and follow-up should be especially vigilant in this group.[244] Hollier et al.[245] found that treatment failure was significantly greater when hepatomegaly and ascites were identified by ultrasound.

Pregnant patients being treated for syphilis, especially early syphilis, must be monitored carefully as a Jarisch-Herxheimer reaction occurs in 60% shortly after antibiotic therapy begins and may lead to fetal demise. The Jarisch-Herxheimer reaction is characterized by fever, headaches, myalgia, tachycardia, malaise, and hypertension with uterine contractions, decreased fetal activity, and fetal heart rate abnormalities. It is thought to be related to a change in prostaglandins, which may result from endotoxin release leading to cardiovascular changes, uterine contractions, and, possibly, fetal compromise.[246]

Other Bacterial Infections

Other bacteria that may cause fetal infection include *Listeria*, *Chlamydia*, *Mycoplasma*, and *Mycobacterium*. *Listeria monocytogenes* is associated with prematurity and low birth weight. It may cause widespread granulomatous lesions, microabscesses, septicemia, meningitis, and hydrops. Maternal infection is characterized by an acute febrile illness that may be followed by spontaneous abortion or delivery of an unaffected baby.

Mycoplasmas and *Chlamydia* may cause intrauterine infection and may be associated with IUGR, prematurity, and low birth weight.

Mycobacterium tuberculosis has an excellent prognosis if treated at an early stage but high mortality for untreated diseases. The liver is the principal site of fetal infection. The lungs may be infected by hematogenous spread or after inhalation of infected amniotic fluid. The bones, kidneys, spleen, gastrointestinal tract, skin, and lymph nodes may be affected. Hepatic granulomata may be detectable with ultrasound.

Q fever is caused by *Coxiella burnetii*. It has been implicated as a significant cause of morbidity and mortality in pregnancy.[247]

REFERENCES

1. Crino JP. Ultrasound and fetal diagnosis of perinatal infection. *Clin Obstet Gynecol* 1999;42:71–80.
2. Tafari N, Ross SM, Naeye RL, Galask RP, Zaar B. Failure of bacterial growth inhibition by amniotic fluid. *Am J Obstet Gynecol* 1977;128:187–189.
3. Weiner CP, Grose CS, Naides SJ. Diagnosis of fetal infection in the patient with an ultrasonographically detected abnormality, but a negative clinical history. *Am J Obstet Gynecol* 1993;168:6–11.
4. Van den Veyver IB, Ni J, Bowles N, Carpenter RJ Jr, Weiner CP, et al. Detection of intrauterine viral infection using the polymerase chain reaction. *Mol Genet Metab* 1998;63:85–95.
5. Ranucci-Weiss D, Uerpairojkit B, Bowles N, Towbin JA, Chan L. Intrauterine adenoviral infection associated with fetal non-immune hydrops. *Prenat Diagn* 1998;18:182–185.
6. Walmus BF, Yow MD, Lester JW, Leeds L, Thompson PK, Woodward RM. Factors predictive of cytomegalovirus immune status in pregnant women. *J Infect Dis* 1988;157:172–177.
7. Stagno S, Pass RF, Cloud G, Britt WJ, Henderson RE, et al. Primary cytomegalovirus infection in pregnancy. Incidence, transmission to fetus, and clinical outcome. *JAMA* 1986;256:1904–1908.
8. Halwach S, Baumann G, Genser B, et al. Screening and diagnosis of congenital cytomegalovirus infection: a 5 year study. *Scand J Infect Dis* 2000;32:137–142.
9. Stagno S, Whitley RJ. Herpesvirus infections of pregnancy, Part 1: cytomegalovirus and Epstein-Barr virus infections. *N Engl J Med* 1985;313:1270–1274.
10. Grose C, Weiner CP. Prenatal diagnosis of congenital cytomegalovirus infection: two decades later. *Am J Obstet Gynecol* 1990;163:447–450.
11. Fowler KB, Stagno S, Pass RF, Britt WJ, Boll TJ, Alford CA. The outcome of congenital cytomegalovirus infection in relation to maternal antibody status. *N Engl J Med* 1992;326:663–667.
12. Hagay ZJ, Biran G, Ornoy A, Reece EA. Congenital cytomegalovirus infection: a long-standing problem still seeking a solution. *Am J Obstet Gynecol* 1996;174:241–245.
13. Stagno S, Reynolds DW, Huang ES, Thames SD, Smith RJ, Alford CA. Congenital cytomegalovirus infection. Occurrence in an immune population. *N Engl J Med* 1977;296:1254–1258.
14. Pass RF, Stagno S, Myers GJ, Alford CA. Outcome of symptomatic congenital cytomegalovirus infection: results of long-term longitudinal follow-up. *Pediatrics* 1980;66:758–762.
15. Adler SP. Cytomegalovirus and child day care. Evidence for an increased infection rate among day-care workers. *N Engl J Med* 1989;321:1290–1296.
16. Ahlfors K, Ivarsson SA, Bjerre I. Microcephaly and congenital cytomegalovirus infection: a combined prospective and retrospective study of a Swedish infant population. *Pediatrics* 1986;78:1058–1063.
17. Ghidini A, Sirtori M, Vergani P, Mariani S, Tucci E, Scola GC. Fetal intracranial calcifications. *Am J Obstet Gynecol* 1989;160:86–87.
18. Nyberg DA. Intraabdominal abnormalities. In: Nyberg DA, Mahony B, Pretorius DH, eds. *Diagnostic ultrasound of fetal anomalies*. St. Louis: Year Book, 1990.
19. Pletcher BA, Williams MK, Mulivor RA, Barth D, Linder C, Rawlinson K. Intrauterine cytomegalovirus, infection presenting as fetal meconium peritonitis. *Obstet Gynecol* 1991;78:903–906.
20. Forouzan I. Fetal abdominal echogenic mass: an early sign of intrauterine cytomegalovirus infection. *Obstet Gynecol* 1992;80:535–537.

21. Nyberg DA, Dubinsky T, Resta RG, Mahony BS, Hickok DE, Luthy DA. Echogenic fetal bowel during the second trimester: clinical importance. *Radiology* 1993;188:527–531.
22. Yaron Y, Hassan S, Geva E, Kupferminc MJ, Yavetz H, Evans MI. Evaluation of fetal echogenic bowel in the second trimester. *Fetal Diagn Ther* 1999;14:176–180.
23. Graham D, Guidi SM, Sanders RC. Sonographic features of in utero periventricular calcification due to cytomegalovirus infection. *J Ultrasound Med* 1982;1:171–172.
24. Tassin GB, Maklad NF, Stewart RR, Bell ME. Cytomegalic inclusion disease: intrauterine sonographic diagnosis using findings involving the brain. *AJNR Am J Neuroradiol* 1991;12:117–122.
25. Teele RL, Hernanz-Schulman M, Sotrel A. Echogenic vasculature in the basal ganglia of neonates: a sonographic sign of vasculopathy. *Radiology* 1988;169:423–427.
26. Hughes P, Weinberger E, Shaw DWW. Linear areas of echogenicity in the thalami and basal ganglia of neonates: an expanded association. *Radiology* 1991;179:103–105.
27. Estroff JA, Parad RB, Teele RL, Benacerraf BR. Echogenic vessels in the fetal thalami and basal ganglia associated with cytomegalovirus, infection. *J Ultrasound Med* 1992;11:686–688.
28. Soussotte C, Maugey-Laulom B, Carles D, Diard F. Contribution of transvaginal ultrasonography and fetal cerebral MRI in a case of congenital cytomegalovirus infection. *Fetal Diagn Ther* 2000;15:219–223.
29. Bailao LA, Rizzi MC, Bonilaaa-Musoles F, Osborne NG. Ultrasound markers of fetal infection: an update. *Ultrasound Q* 2000;16:221–233.
30. Binder ND, Buckmaster JW, Benda GI. Outcome for fetus with ascites and cytomegalovirus infection. *Pediatrics* 1988;82:100–103.
31. Weiner CP, Grose C. Prenatal diagnosis of congenital cytomegalovirus infection by virus isolation from amniotic fluid. *Am J Obstet Gynecol* 1990;163:1253–1255.
32. Drose JA, Dennis MA, Thickman D. Infection in utero: US findings in 19 cases. *Radiology* 1991;178:369–374.
33. Donner C, Liesnard C, Content J, Busine A, Aderca J, Rodesch F. Prenatal diagnosis of 52 pregnancies at risk for congenital cytomegalovirus infection. *Obstet Gynecol* 1993;82:481–486.
34. Gibbs RS, Sweet RL. Maternal and fetal infectious disorders. In: Creasy RK, Resnik R, eds. *Maternal-fetal medicine*, 4th ed. Philadelphia: WB Saunders, 1999:659–724.
35. ACOG practice bulletin. Perinatal viral and parasitic infections. Number 20, September 2000.
36. Lamy ME, Mulongo KN, Gadisseux JF, Lyon G, Gaudy V, Van Lierde MI. Prenatal diagnosis of fetal cytomegalovirus infection. *Am J Obstet Gynecol* 1992;166:91–94.
37. Davis LE, Tweed GV, Chin TDY, Miller GL. Intrauterine diagnosis of cytomegalovirus, infection: viral recovery from amniocentesis fluid. *Am J Obstet Gynecol* 1971;109:1217–1219.
38. Hohlfeld P, Vial Y, Maillard-Brignon C, Vaudau XB, Fawer CL. Cytomegalovirus fetal infection: prenatal diagnosis. *Obstet Gynecol* 1991;78:615–618.
39. Liesnard C, Donner C, Brancart F, Gosselin F, Delforge M, Rodesch F. Prenatal diagnosis of congenital cytomegalovirus: prospective study of 237 pregnancies at risk. *Obstet Gynecol* 2000;95:881–888.
40. Catanzarite V, Dankner WM. Prenatal diagnosis of congenital cytomegalovirus infection: false-negative amniocentesis at 20 weeks' gestation. *Prenat Diagn* 1993;13:1–5.
41. Antsaklis A, Daskalakis GJ, Mesogitis SA, Koutra PT, Michalas SS. Prenatal diagnosis of fetal primary cytomegalovirus infection. *Br J Obstet Gynaecol* 2000;107:84–88.
42. Jones RN, Neale ML, Beattie B, Westmoreland D, Fox JD. Development and application of a PCR-based method including an internal control for diagnosis of congenital cytomegalovirus infection. *J Clin Microbiol* 2000;38(1):1–6.
43. Lazzarotto T, Varani S, Guerra B, Nicolosi A, Lanari M, Landini MP. Prenatal indicators of congenital cytomegalovirus infection. *J Pediatr* 2001;137:90–95.
44. Guerra B, Lazzarotto T, Quarta S, Lanari M, Bovicelli L, et al. Prenatal diagnosis of symptomatic congenital cytomegalovirus infection. *Am J Obstet Gynecol* 2000;183:476–482.
45. Reardon W, Hockey A, Silberstein P, Kendall B, Farag TI, et al. Autosomal recessive congenital intrauterine infection-like syndrome of microcephaly, intracranial calcification, and CNS disease. *Am J Med Genet* 1994;52:58–65.
46. Stagno S, Pass RF, Dworsky ME, Alford CA Jr. Maternal cytomegalovirus infection and perinatal transmission. *Clin Obstet Gynecol* 1982;25:563–576.
47. Naeye R, Tafari N. Antenatal infections. In: Risk factors in pregnancy and diseases of the fetus and newborn. Baltimore: Williams & Wilkins, 1983:77–143.
48. Havard-Fan P, Nahata MC, Brady MT. Gancyclovir—a review of pharmacology, therapeutic efficacy and potential use for treatment of congenital cytomegalovirus infections. *J Clin Pharm Ther* 1989;14:329–340.
49. Pass RF, Little EA, Stagno S, Britt WJ, Alford CA. Young children as a probable source of maternal and congenital cytomegalovirus infection. *N Engl J Med* 1987;316:1366–1370.
50. Cossart YE, Field AM, Cant B, Widdows D. Parvovirus-like particles in human sera. *Lancet* 1975;1:72–73.
51. CDC. Risks associated with human parvovirus B19 infection. *MMWR Morb Mortal Wkly Rep* 1989;38:81–97.
52. Public health laboratory service working party on fifth disease. Prospective study of human parvovirus (B19) infection in pregnancy. *BMJ* 1990;300:1166–1170.
53. *Cytomegalovirus (CMV) infection and prevention.* Atlanta, GA: Centers for Disease Control and Prevention, 1998.
54. Rice PS, Cohen BJ. A school outbreak of parvovirus B19 infection investigated using salivary antibody assays. *Epidemiol Infect* 1996;116:331–338.
55. Valeur-Jensen AK, Pedersen CB, Westergaard T, Jensen IP, Lebech M, et al. Risk factors for parvovirus B19 infection in pregnancy. *JAMA* 1999;281:1099–1105.
56. Grose C, Itani O. Pathogenesis of congenital infection with three diverse viruses: varicella-zoster virus, human parvovirus, and human immunodeficiency virus. *Semin Perinatol* 1989;13(4):278–293.
57. Thurn J. Human parvovirus B19: historical and clinical review. *Rev Infect Dis* 1988;10:1005–1011.
58. Rodis JF, Hovick TJ Jr, Quinn DI, Rosengren SS, Tattersall P. Human parvovirus infection in pregnancy. *Obstet Gynecol* 1988;72:733–738.
59. Tolfvenstam T, Papadogiannakis N, Norbeck O, Petersson K, Broliden K. Frequency of human parvovirus B19 infection in intrauterine fetal death. *Lancet* 2001;357(9267):1494–1497.
60. Anand A, Gray ES, Brown T, Clewley JP, Cohen BJ.

Human parvovirus infection in pregnancy and hydrops fetalis. *N Engl J Med* 1987;316:183–186.

61. Yaegashi N, Okamura K, Yajima A, Murai C, Sugamura K. The frequency of human parvovirus B19 infection in non-immune hydrops fetalis. *J Perinat Med* 1994;22:159–163.

62. Delle Chiaie L, Buck G, Grab D, Terinde R. Prediction of fetal anemia with Doppler measurement of the middle cerebral artery peak systolic velocity in pregnancies complicated by maternal blood group alloimmunization or parvovirus B19 infection. *Ultrasound Obstet Gynecol* 2001;18:232–236.

63. Sohan K, Carroll S, Byrne D, Ashworth M, Soothill P. Parvovirus as a differential diagnosis of hydrops fetalis in the first trimester. *Fetal Diagn* 2000;15:234–236.

64. Smulian JC, Egan JF, Rodis JF. Fetal hydrops in the first trimester associated with maternal parvovirus infection. *J Clin Ultrasound* 1998;26:314–316.

65. Petrikovsky BM, Baker D, Schneider E. Fetal hydrops secondary to human parvovirus infection in early pregnancy. *Prenat Diagn* 1996;16:242–244.

66. Markenson G, Correia LA, Cohn G, Bayer L, Kanaan C. Parvoviral infection associated with increased nuchal translucency: a case report. *J Perinatol* 2000;2:129–131.

67. Schild RL, Plath H, Thomas P, Schulte-Wissermann H, Eis-Hubinger AM, Hansmann M. Fetal parvovirus B19 infection and meconium peritonitis. *Fetal Diagn Ther* 1998;13(1):15–18.

68. Zerbini M, Gentilomi GA, Gallinella G, Morandi R, Calvi S, et al. Intrauterine parvovirus B19 infection and meconium peritonitis. *Prenat Diagn* 1998;18:599–606.

69. Peters MT, Nicolaides KH. Cordocentesis for the diagnosis and treatment of human fetal parvovirus infection. *Obstet Gynecol* 1990;75:501–504.

70. Ghidini A, Lynch L. Prenatal diagnosis and significance of fetal infections in fetal medicine (special issue). *West J Med* 1993;159:366–373.

71. Grose C, Itani O, Weiner CP. Prenatal diagnosis of fetal infection: advances from amniocentesis to cordocentesis—congenital toxoplasmosis, rubella, cytomegalovirus, varicella virus, parvovirus and human immunodeficiency virus. *Pediatr Infect Dis J* 1989;8:459–468.

72. Rogers BB, Singer DB, Mak SK, Gary GW, Fikrig MK, McMillan PN. Detection of human parvovirus B19 in early spontaneous abortuses using serology, histology, electron microscopy, in situ hybridization, and the polymerase chain reaction. *Obstet Gynecol* 1993;81:402–408.

73. Kovacs BW, Carlson DE, Shahbahrami B, Platt LD. Prenatal diagnosis of human parvovirus B19 in nonimmune hydrops fetalis by polymerase chain reaction. *Am J Obstet Gynecol* 1992;167:461–466.

74. Torok TJ, Wang QY, Gary GV, Yang CF, Finch TM, Anderson LJ. Prenatal diagnosis of intrauterine infection with parvovirus B19 by the polymerase chain reaction technique. *J Clin Infect Dis* 1992;14:149–155.

75. Schild RL, Bald R, Plath H, Eis-Hubinger AM, Enders G, Hansmann M. Intrauterine management of fetal parvovirus B19 infection. *Ultrasound Obstet Gynecol* 1999;13:161–166.

76. Dong ZW, Zhou SY, Li Y, Liu RM. Detection of a human parvovirus intrauterine infection with the polymerase chain reaction. *J Reprod Med* 2000;45:410–412.

77. Carrington D, Gilmore DH, Whittle MJ, Aitken D, Gibson AA, et al. Maternal serum alpha-fetoprotein—A marker

78. Komischke K, Searle K, Enders G. Maternal serum alphafetoprotein and human chorionic gonadotropin in pregnant women with acute parvovirus B19 infection with and without fetal complications. *Prenat Diagn* 1997;17:1039–1046.

79. Samra JS, Obhrai MS, Constantine G. Parvovirus infection in pregnancy. *Obstet Gynecol* 1989;73:832–834.

80. Kinney JS, Anderson LJ, Farrar J, Strikas RA, Kumar ML, et al. Risk of adverse outcomes of pregnancy after human parvovirus B19 infection. *J Infect Dis* 1988;157(4):663–667.

81. Torok TJ. Human parvovirus B19 infections in pregnancy. *Pediatr Infect Dis J* 1990;9:772–776.

82. Rodis JF, Quinn DL, Gary GW Jr, Anderson LJ, Rosengren S, et al. Management and outcomes of pregnancies complicated by human B19 parvovirus infection: a prospective study. *Am J Obstet Gynecol* 1990;163:1168–1171.

83. Harger JH, Adler SP, Koch W, Harger GF. Prospective evaluation of 618 pregnant women exposed to parvovirus B19: risks and symptoms. *Obstet Gynecol* 1998;91:413–420.

84. Sheikh AU, Ernest JM, O'Shea M. Long-term outcome in fetal hydrops from parvovirus B19 infection. *Am J Obstet Gynecol* 1992;167:337–341.

85. Humphrey W, Magoon M, O'Shaughnessy R. Severe nonimmune hydrops secondary to parvovirus B-19 infection: spontaneous reversal in utero and survival of a term infant. *Obstet Gynecol* 1991;78(5):900–902.

86. Pryde PG, Nugent CE, Pridjian G, Barr M, Faix RG. Spontaneous resolution of nonimmune hydrops fetalis secondary to human parvovirus B19 infection. *Obstet Gynecol* 1992;79:859–861.

87. Van Elsacker-Niele AMW, Salimans MMM, Weiland HT, Vermey-Keers C, Anderson MJ, Versteeg J. Fetal pathology in human parvovirus, B19 infection. *Br J Obstet Gynecol* 1989;96:768–775.

88. Hartwig NG, Vermeij-Keers C, Van Elsacker-Niele AMW, Fleurer GJ. Embryonic malformations in a case of intrauterine parvovirus B19 infection. *Teratology* 1989;39:295–302.

89. Plachouras N, Stefanidis K, Andronikou S, Lolis D. Severe nonimmune hydrops fetalis and congenital corneal opacification secondary to human parvovirus B19 infection. *J Reprod Med* 1999;44:377–380.

90. Shmoys S, Kaplan C. Parvovirus and pregnancy. *Clin Obstet Gynecol* 1990;33:268–275.

91. Sahakian V, Weiner CP, Naides SJ, Williamson RA, Scharosch LL. Intrauterine transfusion treatment of nonimmune hydrops fetalis secondary to human parvovirus B19 infection. *Am J Obstet Gynecol* 1991;164:1090–1091.

92. Cooper LZ, Preblud SR, Alford CA. Rubella. In: Remington JS, Klein JO, eds. *Infectious diseases of the fetus and newborn infant*, 4th ed. Philadelphia: WB Saunders, 1995:268–311.

93. CDC. Elimination of rubella and congenital rubella syndrome—United States. *MMWR Morb Mortal Wkly Rep* 1985;34:65–66.

94. CDC. Increase in rubella and congenital rubella syndrome—United States, 1988–1990. *MMWR Morb Mortal Wkly Rep* 1991;40:93–99.

95. Lee SH, Ewert DP, Frederick PD, Mascola L. Resurgence of congenital rubella syndrome in the 1990s. *JAMA* 1992;267:2616–2620.

96. CDC. Summary of notifiable diseases, United States 1992. *MMWR Morb Mortal Wkly Rep* 1993;41:50–73.

97. Freij BJ, South MA, Sever JL. Maternal rubella and the congenital rubella syndrome. *Clin Perinatol* 1988;15:247–257.

98. Orenstein WA, Bart KJ, Hinman AR, et al. The opportunity and obligation to eliminate rubella from the United States. *JAMA* 1984;251:1988–1994.

99. Enders G, Calm A, Schaub J. Rubella embryopathy after previous maternal rubella vaccination. *Infection* 1984;12:96–98.

100. Forsgren M, Carlstrom G, Strangert K. Congenital rubella after maternal re-infection. *Scand J Infect Dis* 1979;11:81–83.

101. Forsgren M, Soren L. Subclinical rubella reinfection in vaccinated women with rubella specific IgM response during pregnancy and transmission of virus to the fetus. *Scand J Infect Dis* 1985;17:337–341.

102. Katow S. Rubella virus genome diagnosis during pregnancy and mechanism of congenital rubella. *Intervirology* 1998;41(4–5):163–169.

103. Ornoy A, Segal S, Nishmi M, Simcha A, Polishuk WZ. Fetal and placental pathology in gestational rubella. *Am J Obstet Gynecol* 1973;116:949–956.

104. Miller E, Cradock-Watson JE, Pollock TM. Consequences of confirmed maternal rubella at successive stages of pregnancy. *Lancet* 1982;2:781–784.

105. Cradock-Watson JE, Ridehalgh MKS, Anderson MJ, Pattison JR, Kangro HO. Fetal infection resulting from maternal rubella after first trimester pregnancy. *J Hyg (Camb)* 1980;85:381–391.

106. Enders G, Nickerl-Pacher U, Miller E, Cradock-Watson JE. Outcome of confirmed periconceptional maternal rubella. *Lancet* 1988;1:1445–1447.

107. Grillner L, Forsgren M, Barr B, Bettinger M, Danielsson L, De Verdier C. Outcome of rubella during pregnancy with special reference to the 17th–24th weeks of gestation. *Scand J Infect Dis* 1983;15:321–325.

108. Munro ND, Sheppard S, Smithells RW, Holzel RW, Jones G. Temporal relationship between maternal rubella and congenital defects. *Lancet* 1987;2:201–204.

109. Grangeot-Keros L. Rubella and pregnancy. *Pathol Biol (Paris)* 1992;40(7):706–710.

110. Levin MJ, Oxman MN, Moore MG, Daniels JB, Scheer K. Diagnosis of congenital rubella in utero. *N Engl J Med* 1974;290:1187–1188.

111. Terry GM, Ho-Terry L, Warren RC, Rodeck CH, Cohen A, Rees KR. First trimester prenatal diagnosis of congenital rubella: a laboratory investigation. *BMJ* 1986;292:930–933.

112. Holzgreve W, Helftenbein E, Evans M, Enders G. Early prenatal diagnosis of rubella transmission by cDNA analysis of chorionic villi using polymerase chain reaction. *Am J Obstet Gynecol* 1991;164:350.

113. Eggerding FA, Peters J, Lee RK , Inderlied CB. Detection of rubella virus gene sequences by enzymatic amplification and direct sequencing of amplified DNA. *J Clin Microbiol* 1991;29:945–952.

114. Tanemura M, Suzumori K, Yagami Y, Katow S. Diagnosis of fetal rubella infection with reverse transcription and nested polymerase chain reaction: a study of 34 cases diagnosed in fetuses. *Am J Obstet Gynecol* 1996;174(2):578–582.

115. Bosma TJ, Corbett KM, Eckstein MB, O'Shea S, Vijayalakshmi P, et al. Use of PCR for prenatal and postnatal diagnosis of congenital rubella. *J Clin Microbiol* 1995;33(11): 2881–2887.

116. Menser MA, Forrest JM, Bransby RD. Rubella infection and diabetes mellitus. *Lancet* 1978;1:57–63.

117. Daffos F, Grangeot-Keros L, Lebon P, et al. Prenatal diagnosis of congenital rubella. *Lancet* 1984;2:1–3.

118. Enders G, Jonatha W. Prenatal diagnosis of intrauterine rubella. *Infection* 1987;15:162–164.

119. Tingle AJ, Chantler JK, Pot KH. Postpartum rubella immunization: association with development of prolonged arthritis, neurological sequelae and chronic rubella viremia. *J Infect Dis* 1985;152:606–612.

120. Preblud SR, Orenstein WA, Lopez C, Herrmann KL, Hinman AR. Correspondence: postpartum rubella immunization. *J Infect Dis* 1986;154:367–369.

121. Bart KJ, Orenstein WA, Preblud SR, Hinman AR. Universal immunization to interrupt rubella. *Rev Infect Dis* 1985;7:S177–S184.

122. Pastuszak AL, Levy M, Schick B, et al. Outcome after maternal varicella infection in the first 20 weeks of pregnancy. *N Engl J Med* 1994;330:901–905.

123. Enders G, Miller E, Craddock-Watson J, Bolley I, Ridehalgh M. Consequences of varicella and herpes zoster in pregnancy: prospective study of 1739 cases. *Lancet* 1994;343:1547–1550.

124. Jones KL, Johnson KA, Chambers CD. Offspring of women infected with varicella during pregnancy: a prospective study. *Teratology* 1994;49:29–32.

125. Webster MH, Smith CS. Congenital abnormalities and maternal herpes zoster. *BMJ* 1977;2:1193.

126. Gershon AA. Chickenpox, measles, and mumps. In: Remington JS, Klein JO, eds. *Infectious diseases of the fetus and newborn infant,* 4th ed. Philadelphia: WB Saunders, 1995:565–618.

127. Sauerbrei A, Wutzler P. The congenital varicella syndrome. *J Perinatol* 2000;20(8 Pt 1):548–554.

128. Paryani SG, Arvin AM. Intrauterine infection with varicella-zoster virus after maternal varicella. *N Engl J Med* 1986;314:1542–1546.

129. Hammad E, Helin I, Pacsa A. Case report: early pregnancy varicella and associated congenital anomalies. *Acta Paediatr Scand* 1989;78:963–964.

130. Harding B, Baumer JA. Congenital varicella-zoster: a serologically proven case with necrotizing encephalitis and malformation. *Acta Neuropathol* 1988;76:311–315.

131. Srabstein JC, Morris N, Bryce Larke RP, De Sa DJ, Castelino BB, Sum E. Is there a congenital varicella syndrome? *J Pediatr* 1974;84:239–243.

132. Katz G, Pfau A. Congenital varicella causing neurogenic bladder and anal dysfunction. *Urology* 1986;28:424–425.

133. Higa K, Dan K, Manabe H. Varicella-zoster virus infections during pregnancy: hypothesis concerning the mechanisms of congenital malformations. *Obstet Gynecol* 1987;69:214–222.

134. Enders G. Management of varicella-zoster contact and infection in pregnancy using a standardized varicella-zoster ELISA test. *Postgrad Med J* 1985;61:23–30.

135. Ong CL, Daniel ML. Antenatal diagnosis of a porencephalic cyst in congenital varicella-zoster virus infection. *Pediatr Radiol* 1998;28(2):94.

136. Hofmeyr GJ, Moolla S, Lawrie T. Prenatal sonographic

diagnosis of congenital varicella infection—a case report. *Prenat Diagn* 1996;16(12):1148–1151.

137. Petignat P, Vial Y, Laurini R, Hohlfeld P. Fetal varicella-herpes zoster syndrome in early pregnancy: ultrasonographic and morphological correlation. *Prenat Diagn* 2001;21(2):121–124.

138. Pretorius DH, Hayward I, Jones KL, Stamm E. Sonographic evaluation of pregnancies with maternal varicella infection. *J Ultrasound Med* 1992;11:459–463.

139. Cuthbertson G, Weiner CP, Giller RH, Grose C. Prenatal diagnosis of second–trimester congenital varicella syndrome by virus-specific immunoglobulin M. *J Pediatr* 1987;111:592–595.

140. Hartung J, Enders G, Chaoui R, Arents A, Tennstedt C, Bollmann R. Prenatal diagnosis of congenital varicella syndrome and detection of varicella-zoster virus in the fetus: a case report. *Prenat Diagn* 1999;19(2):163–166.

141. Mouly F, Mirlesse V, Meritet JF, Rozenberg F, Poissonier MH, et al. Prenatal diagnosis of fetal varicella-zoster virus infection with polymerase chain reaction of amniotic fluid in 107 cases. *Am J Obstet Gynecol* 1997;177(4):894–898.

142. Balducci J, Rodis JF, Rosengren S, Vintzileos AM, Spivey G, Vosseller C. Pregnancy outcome following first-trimester varicella infection. *Obstet Gynecol* 1992;79:5–6.

143. Siegel M. Congenital malformations following chickenpox, measles, mumps, and hepatitis. *JAMA* 1973;226:1521–1524.

144. Dufour P, de Bievre P, Vinatier N, et al. Varicella and pregnancy. *Eur J Obstet Gynecol Reprod Biol* 1996;66:119–123.

145. Michie CA, Acolet D, Charlton R, et al. Varicella-zoster contracted in the second trimester of pregnancy. *Pediatr Infect Dis J* 1992;11:1050–1053.

146. Bale JF Jr, Murph JR. Congenital infections and the nervous system. *Pediatr Clin North Am* 1992;39:669–690.

147. Brunell PA. Placental transfer of varicella-zoster antibody. *Pediatrics* 1966;38:1034–1038.

148. Meyers JD. Congenital varicella in term infants: risk reconsidered. *J Infect Dis* 1974;129:215–217.

149. Fine PEM, Adelstein AM, Snowman J, Clarkson JA, Evans SM. Long term effects of exposure to viral infections in utero. *BMJ* 1985;290:509–511.

150. McGregor JA, Mark S, Crawford GP, Levin MJ. Varicella zoster antibody testing in the care of pregnant women exposed to varicella. *Am J Obstet Gynecol* 1987;157:281–284.

151. Committee on Infectious Diseases. Expanded guidelines for use of varicella-zoster immune globulin. *Pediatrics* 1983;72:886–889.

152. Anderson H, Sutton RNP, Scarffe JH. Cytotoxic chemotherapy and viral infections: the role of acyclovir. *J R Coll Physicians Lond* 1984;18:51–55.

153. Eder SE, Apuzzio JJ, Weiss G. Varicella pneumonia during pregnancy. Treatment of two cases with acyclovir. *Am J Perinatol* 1988;5:16–17.

154. CDC. Genital herpes simplex virus infections: sexually transmitted disease statistics. *MMWR Morb Mortal Wkly Rep* 1988;136:53.

155. Wald A, Zeh J, Selke S, Warren T, Ryncorz AJ, et al. Reaction of genital herpes simplex type 2 infection in asymptomatic seropositive persons. *N Engl J Med* 2000;342:844–850.

156. Whitley RJ. Herpes simplex virus infection. In: Remington JS, Klein JO, eds. *Infectious diseases of the fetus and newborn infant,* 3rd ed. Philadelphia: WB Saunders, 1990:282–305.

157. Baldwin S, Whitley RJ. Teratogen update: intrauterine herpes simplex virus infection. *Teratology* 1989;39:1–10.

158. McIntosh D, Isaacs D. Herpes simplex virus infection in pregnancy. *Arch Dis Child* 1992;67:1137–1138.

159. Isada NB, Paar DP, Grossman JH, Straus SE. TORCH infections: diagnosis in the molecular age. *J Reprod Med* 1992;37:499–507.

160. Johnson RE, Nahmias AJ, Magder LS, Lee FK, Brooks CA, Snowden CB. A seroepidemiologic survey of the prevalence of herpes simplex virus type 2 infection in the United States. *N Engl J Med* 1989;321:7–12.

161. Brown ZA, Vontver LA, Benedetti J, Critchlow CW, Sells CJ, et al. Effects on infants of a first episode of genital herpes during pregnancy. *N Engl J Med* 1987;317:1246–1251.

162. Brown ZA, Benedetti J, Ashley R, Burchett S, Selke S, et al. Neonatal herpes simplex virus infection in relation to asymptomatic maternal infection at the time of labor. *N Engl J Med* 1991;324:1247–1252.

163. Prober CG, Sullender WM, Yasukawa LL, Au DS, Yeager AS, Arvin AM. Low risk of herpes simplex virus infections in neonates exposed to the virus at the time of vaginal delivery to mothers with recurrent genital herpes simplex virus infections. *N Engl J Med* 1987;316:240–244.

164. Hyde SR, Giacoia GP. Congenital herpes infection: placental and umbilical cord findings. *Obstet Gynecol* 1993;81:852–855.

165. Hutto C, Arvin A, Jacobs R, et al. Intrauterine herpes simplex virus infections. *J Pediatr* 1987;10:97–101.

166. Lanouette JM, Duquette DA, Jacques SM, Qureshi F, Johnson MP, Berry SM. Prenatal diagnosis of fetal herpes simplex infection. *Fetal Diagn Ther* 1996;11:414–416.

167. Whitley RJ, Arvin A, Prober C, et al. A controlled trial comparing vidarabine with acyclovir in neonatal HSV infection. *N Engl J Med* 1991;324:444–449.

168. Brown ZA, Baker DA. Acyclovir therapy during pregnancy. *Obstet Gynecol* 1989;73:526–531.

169. Martens MG. Herpes simplex in pregnancy. In: Gillstrap LC, Faro S, eds. *Infections in pregnancy.* New York: Alan R. Liss, 1990:143–150.

170. Baker DA. Herpes and pregnancy: new management. *Clin Obstet Gynecol* 1990;33:253–257.

171. Kohl S. Neonatal herpes simplex virus infection. *Clin Perinatol* 1997;24:129–150.

172. Kesson A, Sorrell T. Human immunodeficiency virus infection in pregnancy. *Baillieres Clin Obstet Gynaecol* 1993;7:45–74.

173. Davis SF, Byers RH Jr, Lindegren ML, Caldwell MB, Karon JM, Gwinn M. Prevalence and incidence of vertically acquired HIV infection in the United States. *JAMA* 1995;274(12):952.

174. Lindsay MK, Nesheim SR. Human immunodeficiency virus infection in pregnant women and their newborns. *Clin Perinatol* 1997;24:161–181.

175. CDC. Unexplained immunodeficiency in infants—New York, New Jersey, California. *MMWR Morb Mortal Wkly Rep* 1982;31:665–667.

176. Nair P, Alger L, Hines S, Seiden S, Hebel R, Johnson JP. Maternal and neonatal characteristics associated with HIV infection in infants of seropositive women. *J Acquir Immune Defic Syndr* 1993;6:298–302.

177. Dabis F, Msellati P, Dunn D, Lepage P, Newell ML, et al. Estimating the rate of mother-to-child transmission of HIV. Report of a workshop on methodological issues Ghent (Belgium), 17–20 February 1992. *AIDS* 1993;7:1139–1148.

178. Alger LS, Farley JJ, Robinson BA, Hines SE, Berchin JM, Johnson JP. Interactions of human immunodeficiency virus infection and pregnancy. *Obstet Gynecol* 1993;82:787–796.

179. Goedert JJ, Duliege AM, Amos CI, Felton S, Biggar RI. High risk of HIV-1 infection for first born twins. *Lancet* 1991;338:1471–1475.

180. Sprecher S, Soumenkoff G, Puissant F, Degueldre M. Vertical transmission of HIV in 15 week fetus. *Lancet* 1986;2:288–289.

181. Maury W, Potts BJ, Rabson AB. HIV-1 infection of first trimester and term human placental tissue: a possible mode of maternal-fetal transmission. *J Infect Dis* 1989;160:583–588.

182. Rudin C, Meier D, Pavic N, et al. Intrauterine onset of symptomatic human immunodeficiency virus disease. *Pediatr Infect Dis J* 1993;12:411–415.

183. Marion RW, Wiznia A, Hutcheon RG, Rubenstein A. Human T-cell lymphotropic virus, type III (HTLV-III) embryopathy. A new dysmorphic syndrome associated with intrauterine HTLV-IIII infection. *Am J Dis Child* 1986;140:638–640.

184. Iosub S, Bamji M, Stone RY, Gromisch DS, Wasserman E. More on human immunodeficiency virus embryopathy. *Pediatrics* 1987;80:512–516.

185. Qazi QH, Sheikh TM, Fikrig S, Menikoff H. Lack of evidence for cranial facial dysmorphism in perinatal human immunodeficiency virus infection. *J Pediatr* 1988;112:7–11.

186. Menez-Bautista R, Fikrig SM, Pahwa S, Sarangadharan MG, Stoneburner RL. Monozygotic twins discordant for the acquired immunodeficiency syndrome. *Am J Dis Child* 1986;140:678–679.

187. Curless RG. Congenital AIDS: review of neurologic problems. *Childs Nerv Syst* 1989;5:9–11.

188. Diamond GW, Gurdin P, Wiznia AA, Belman AL, Rubenstein A, Cohen HJ. Effects of congenital HIV infection on neurodevelopmental status of babies in foster care. *Dev Med Child Neurol* 1990;32:999–1005.

189. Steinherz LJ, Brochstein JA, Robins J. Cardiac involvement in congenital acquired immunodeficiency syndrome. *Am J Dis Child* 1986;140:1241–1244.

190. Auger I, Thomas P, DeGruttola V, et al. Incubation periods for pediatric AIDS. *Nature* 1988;336:575–577.

191. Johnstone FD, Willox L, Brettle RP. Survival time after AIDS in pregnancy. *Br J Obstet Gynaecol* 1992;99(8):633–636.

192. Selwyn PA, Schoenbaum EE, Davenny K, Robertson VJ, Feingold AR, et al. Prospective study of human immunodeficiency virus infection and pregnancy outcomes in intravenous drug users. *JAMA* 1989;261:1289–1294.

193. Minkoff H, Nanda D, Menez R, Fikrig S. Pregnancies resulting in infants with acquired immunodeficiency syndrome or AIDS-related complex. *Obstet Gynecol* 1987;69:285–287.

194. Connor EM, Sperling RS, Gelber R, et al. Reduction of maternal-infant transmission of human immunodeficiency virus type 1 with zidovudine treatment. *N Engl J Med* 1994;331:1173–1180.

195. European Collaborative Study. Caesarian section and risk of vertical transmission of HIV-1 infection. *Lancet* 1994;343:1464–1467.

196. Kass NE, Taylor HA, Anderson J. Treatment of human immunodeficiency virus during pregnancy: the shift from an exclusive focus on fetal protection to a more balanced approach. *Am J Obstet Gynecol* 2000;182:856–859.

197. Alger LS. Toxoplasmosis and parvovirus B19. *Infect Dis Clin North Am* 1997;11:55–57.

198. Remington JS, McLeod R, Desmonts G. Toxoplasmosis. In: Remington JS, Klein JO, eds. *Infectious diseases of the fetus and newborn infant*, 4th ed. Philadelphia: WB Saunders, 1995:140–267.

199. Kimball AC, Kean BH, Fuchs F. Congenital toxoplasmosis: a prospective study of 4,048 obstetric patients. *Am J Obstet Gynecol* 1971;111:211–218.

200. Sever JL, Ellenberg JH, Ley AC, et al. Toxoplasmosis: maternal and pediatric findings in 23,000 pregnancies. *Pediatrics* 1988;82:181–192.

201. Enders G, Bader U, Lindemann L, Schalasta G, Daiminger A. Prenatal diagnosis of congenital cytomegalovirus infection in 189 pregnancies with known outcome. *Prenat Diagn* 2001;21(5):362–377.

202. Desmonts G, Couvreur J. Congenital toxoplasmosis. A prospective study of 378 pregnancies. *N Engl J Med* 1974;290(20):1110–1116.

203. Dunn D, Wallon M, Peyron F, Petersen E, Peckham C, Gilbert R. Mother-to-child transmission of toxoplasmosis: risk estimates for clinical counselling. *Lancet* 1999;353(9167):1829–1833.

204. Hohlfeld P, Daffos F, Thulliez P, et al. Fetal toxoplasmosis: outcome of pregnancy and infant follow-up after in utero treatment. *J Pediatr* 1989;115:765–769.

205. Desai MB, Kurtz AB, Martin ME, Wapner RJ. Characteristic findings of toxoplasmosis in utero: a case report. *J Ultrasound Med* 1994;13:60–62.

206. Baron J, Youngblood L, Siewers CMF, Medearis DM. The incidence of cytomegalovirus, herpes simplex, rubella and toxoplasma antibodies in microcephalic, mentally retarded and normocephalic children. *Pediatrics* 1969;44:932–939.

207. Hohlfeld P, MacAleese J, Capella-Pavlovski M, et al. Fetal toxoplasmosis: ultrasonographic signs. *Ultrasound Obstet Gynecol* 1991;1:241–244.

208. Virkola K, Lappalainen M, Valanne L, Koskiniemi M. Radiological signs in newborns exposed to primary toxoplasma infection in utero. *Pediatr Radiol* 1997;27:133–138.

209. Ades AE. Evaluating the sensitivity and predictive value of tests of recent infection: toxoplasmosis in pregnancy. *Epidemiol Infect* 1991;107:527–535.

210. Grangeot-Keros L, Forestier F. Diagnostic des embryofoetopathies infectieuses. In: Forestier F, Schorderet D, eds. *Diagnostics prenatals et biologie moleculaire*. Paris: Lavoisier, 1997:253–272.

211. Forestier F, Hohfield P, Sole Y, Daffos F. Prenatal diagnosis of congenital toxoplasmosis by PCR: extended experience. *Prenat Diagn* 1998;18:405–415.

212. Grover CM, Thulliez P, Remington JS, Boothroyd JC. Rapid prenatal diagnosis of congenital *Toxoplasma* infection by using polymerase chain reaction and amniotic fluid. *J Clin Microbiol* 1990;28(10):2297–2301.

213. Hohlfeld P, Daffos F, Costa JM, Thulliez P, Forestier F, Vidaud M. Prenatal diagnosis of congenital toxoplasmosis with a polymerase-chain-reaction test on amniotic fluid. *N Engl J Med* 1994;331(11):695–699.

214. Gratzl R, Hayde M, Kohlhauser C, Hermon M, Burda G, et al. Follow-up of infants with congenital toxoplasmosis detected by polymerase chain reaction analysis of amniotic fluid. *Eur J Clin Microbiol Infect Dis* 1998;17(12):853–858.

215. Cazenave J, Forestier F, Bessieres MH, Broussin B, Begueret J. Contribution of a new PCR assay to the prenatal diagnosis of congenital toxoplasmosis. *Prenat Diagn* 1992;12:119–127.

216. Romand S, Wallon M, Franck J, Thulliez P, Peyron F, Dumon H. Prenatal diagnosis using polymerase chain reaction on amniotic fluid for congenital toxoplasmosis. *Obstet Gynecol* 2001;97(2):296–300.

217. Costa JM, Ernault P, Gautier E, Bretagne S. Prenatal diagnosis of congenital toxoplasmosis by duplex real-time PCR using fluorescence resonance energy transfer hybridization probes. *Prenat Diagn* 2001;21(2):85–88.

218. Foulon W, Pinon JM, Stray-Pedersen B, Pollak A, Lappalainen M, et al. Prenatal diagnosis of congenital toxoplasmosis: a multicenter evaluation of different diagnostic parameters. *Am J Obstet Gynecol* 1999;181(4):843–847.

219. Peckham CS, Logan S. Screening for toxoplasmosis during pregnancy. *Arch Dis Child* 1993;68:3–5.

220. Saxon SA, Knight W, Reynolds DW, Stagno S, Alford CA. Intellectual deficits in children born with subclinical congenital toxoplasmosis: a preliminary report. *J Pediatr* 1973;82:792–797.

221. Koppe JG, Loewer-Sieger DH, de Roever-Bonnet H. Results of 20-year followup of congenital toxoplasmosis. *Lancet* 1986;1:254–256.

222. Foulon W, Naessens A, Mahler T, de Waile M, de Catte L, de Meuter F. Prenatal diagnosis of congenital toxoplasmosis. *Obstet Gynecol* 1990;76:769–772.

223. Daffos F, Forestier F, Capella-Pavlovsky M, et al. Prenatal management of 746 pregnancies at risk for congenital toxoplasmosis. *N Engl J Med* 1988;318:271–275.

224. Berrebi A, Kobuch WE, Bessieres MH, et al. Termination of pregnancy for maternal toxoplasmosis. *Lancet* 1994;344:36–39.

225. Foulon W, Naessens A, Lauwers S, de Meuter F, Amy JJ. Impact of primary prevention on the incidence of toxoplasmosis during pregnancy. *Obstet Gynecol* 1988;72:363–366.

226. Bittencourt AL, Cardoso de Almeida MA, Iunes MA, Casulari da Motta LD. Placental involvement in schistosomiasis mansoni. Report of four cases. *Am J Trop Med Hyg* 1980;29(4):571–575.

227. Russomando G, de Tomassone MM, de Guillen I, Acosta N, Vera N, et al. Treatment of congenital Chagas' disease diagnosed and followed up by the polymerase chain reaction. *Am J Trop Med Hyg* 1998;59(3):487–491.

228. Webster LA, Rolfs RT. Surveillance for primary and secondary syphilis—United States, 1991. *MMWR Morb Mortal Wkly Rep* 1993;42:13–19.

229. Rawstron SA, Bromberg K. Failure of recommended maternal therapy to prevent congenital syphilis. *Sex Transm Dis* 1991;18:102–106.

230. Genc M, Ledger WJ. Syphilis in pregnancy. *Sex Transm Inf* 2000;76:73–79.

231. Nathan L, Bohman VR, Sanchez PJ, Leos NK, Twickler DM, Wendel GD. In utero infection with *Treponema pallidum* in early pregnancy. *Prenat Diagn* 1997;17:119–123.

232. Nathan L, Twickler DM, Peters MT, Sanchez PJ, Wendel GD. Fetal syphilis: correlation of sonographic findings and rabbit infectivity testing of amniotic fluid. *J Ultrasound Med* 1993;2:97–101.

233. Wendel GD, Sanchez PJ, Peters MT, Harstad TW, Potter LL, Norgard MV. Identification of *Treponema pallidum* in amniotic fluid and fetal blood from pregnancies complicated by congenital syphilis. *Obstet Gynecol* 1991;78:890–895.

234. Barton JR, Thorpe EM Jr, Shaver DC, Hager WD, Sibai BM. Nonimmune hydrops fetalis associated with maternal infection with syphilis. *Am J Obstet Gynecol* 1992;167:56–58.

235. Hill LM, Maloney JB. An unusual constellation of sonographic findings associated with congenital syphilis. *Obstet Gynecol* 1991;78:895–897.

236. Satin AJ, Twickler DM, Wendel GD Jr. Congenital syphilis associated with dilation of fetal small bowel: a case report. *J Ultrasound Med* 1992;11:49–52.

237. Ingall D, Sanchez PJ, Musher D. Syphilis. In: Remington JS, Klein JO, eds. *Infectious diseases of the fetus and newborn infant*, 4th ed. Philadelphia: WB Saunders Co, 1995:529–564.

238. Lucas MJ, Theriot SK, Wendel GD Jr. Doppler systolic-diastolic ratios in pregnancies complicated by syphilis. *Obstet Gynecol* 1991;77:217–222.

239. Wendel GD, Gilstrap LC. Syphilis during pregnancy. In: Gillstrap LC, Faro S, eds. *Infections in pregnancy.* New York: Alan R. Liss, 1990:115–125.

240. Sheffield JS, Wendel GD. Syphilis in pregnancy. *Clin Obstet Gynecol* 1999;41:97–106.

241. McFarlin BL, Bottoms SF, Dock BS, Isada NB. Epidemic syphilis: maternal factors associated with congenital infection. *Am J Obstet Gynecol* 1994;170:535–540.

242. Rawstron SA, Jenkins S, Blanchard S, Li PW, Bromberg K. Maternal and congenital syphilis in Brooklyn, NY: epidemiology, transmission, and diagnosis. *Am J Dis Child* 1993;147;727–731.

243. CDC. Guidelines for the prevention and control of congenital syphilis. *MMWR Morb Mortal Wkly Rep* 1988;37:1–13.

244. Musher DM. Syphilis, neurosyphilis, penicillin in AIDS. *J Infect Dis* 1991;163:1201.

245. Hollier LM, Harstad TW, Sanchez PJ, Twickler DM, Wendel GD Jr. Fetal syphilis: clinical and laboratory characteristics. *Obstet Gynecol* 2001;97(6):947–953.

246. Klein VR, Cox SM, Mitchell MD, Wendel GD. The Jarisch-Herxheimer reaction complicating syphilis therapy in pregnancy. *Obstet Gynecol* 1990;75:375–380.

247. Jover-Diaz F, Robert-Gates J, Andreu-Gimenez L, Merino-Sanchez J. Q fever during pregnancy: an emerging cause of prematurity and abortion. *Infect Dis Obstet Gynecol* 2001;9(1):47–49.

18

MULTIPLE GESTATIONS*

Twins occur in 1.1% to 1.2% of spontaneously conceived pregnancies, although the frequency varies with type of twinning. Higher multiples are rare in natural pregnancies, with triplets occurring in approximately 1 in 8,000 pregnancies delivered, quadruplets in 1 in 729,000 pregnancies, and quintuplets 1 in 65,610,000.[1] This rate of spontaneous higher order multiple gestations can be estimated by Hellins' hypothesis, which states that when the frequency of twinning is n, than the rate of triplets is n^2, quadruplets is n^3, and so on.[2]

Twin pregnancies may be categorized as either monozygotic ("identical") or dizygotic ("fraternal") (Fig. 1). Approximately 30% of spontaneous twins are monozygotic and 70% are dizygotic. Monozygotic twins, arising from a single fertilized ovum, occur in approximately 3.5 per 1,000 pregnancies. This rate is remarkably constant throughout the world and over time, suggesting that it is a sporadic "accident of nature." On the other hand, dizygotic twins result from two different ova fertilized separately. The frequency of dizygotic twinning varies with maternal age, race (blacks > whites > Japanese), and families and has also shown temporal variations, suggesting that environmental factors play a role in this condition. It has been suggested that the ratio of dizygotic to monozygotic gestations may be an overall measure of fertility for a population.[3]

Assisted reproduction greatly increases the frequency of twins and multiple gestations.[4] Ovulation induction increases the rate of twin births approximately fourfold (95% confidence interval = 2, 7) and increases triplet or higher order births approximately 72-fold (95% confidence interval = 26, 203).[5] In vitro fertilization with insertion of multiple embryos increases the risk of multiple gestations even more, so that approximately 25% of pregnancies resulting from in vitro fertilization are multiple pregnancies. Although these increased rates largely reflect an increased chance of dizygotic twins, fertility treatment also increases the rate of monozygotic twinning, estimated as 3.8-fold.[6] Although the reason for this is not entirely clear, fertility treatment may make subtle changes in the zona

pellucida, promoting subsequent division. Whatever the mechanism, multiple gestations of more than two fetuses cannot be assumed to be multizygotic but may comprise a combination of dizygotic and monozygotic conceptions.

Ultrasound plays an important role in all aspects of management of multiple pregnancies including their detection, determination of chorionicity, screening for chromosomal defects and structural abnormalities, monitoring of fetal growth and well-being, planning of delivery, and identification of patients at high risk for preterm delivery. This chapter discusses the types and incidence of multiple gestations with description of zygosity and chorionicity, complications or conditions related to multiple gestations, and procedures that are unique to, or require special consideration in, multiple gestations.

PLACENTATION AND CHORIONICITY

Placentation varies with the type of twinning. Because dizygotic twins implant separately, all zygotic twins form dichorionic placentation. The placentas may either be separate or confluent (Fig. 2). Monozygotic twins, on the other hand, may have one of three placentation types depending on the time of separation[7] (Figs. 1 and 2). Division of the zygote within the first 3 to 4 days after fertilization results in separation implantations and *dichorionic-diamniotic* placentation; division of the zygote 4 to 7 days after conception results in a single chorion and placenta and two amniotic cavities, termed a *monochorionic-diamniotic* gestation; and division 8 or more days after fertilization leads to a *monochorionic-monoamniotic* gestation, with both fetuses in a single amniotic cavity, sharing a common placenta. Among all monozygotic twins, nearly one-third have dichorionic-diamniotic placentation and two-thirds have monochorionic-diamniotic placentation. Monochorionic-monoamniotic placentation is rare, occurring in approximately 1% of monozygotic twin pregnancies.

All cases of monochorionic placentation result from monozygotic twinning, and all dizygotic twins form dichorionic placentation. Because 30% of twins are monozygotic, and two-thirds of these form monochorionic-diamniotic placentas, monochorionic placentation com-

*Jacqueline Reyes, MD; Luís Flávio de Andrade Gonçalves, MD; Sandra Rejane Silva, MD; and Fernando Heredia, MD, also contributed to this chapter.

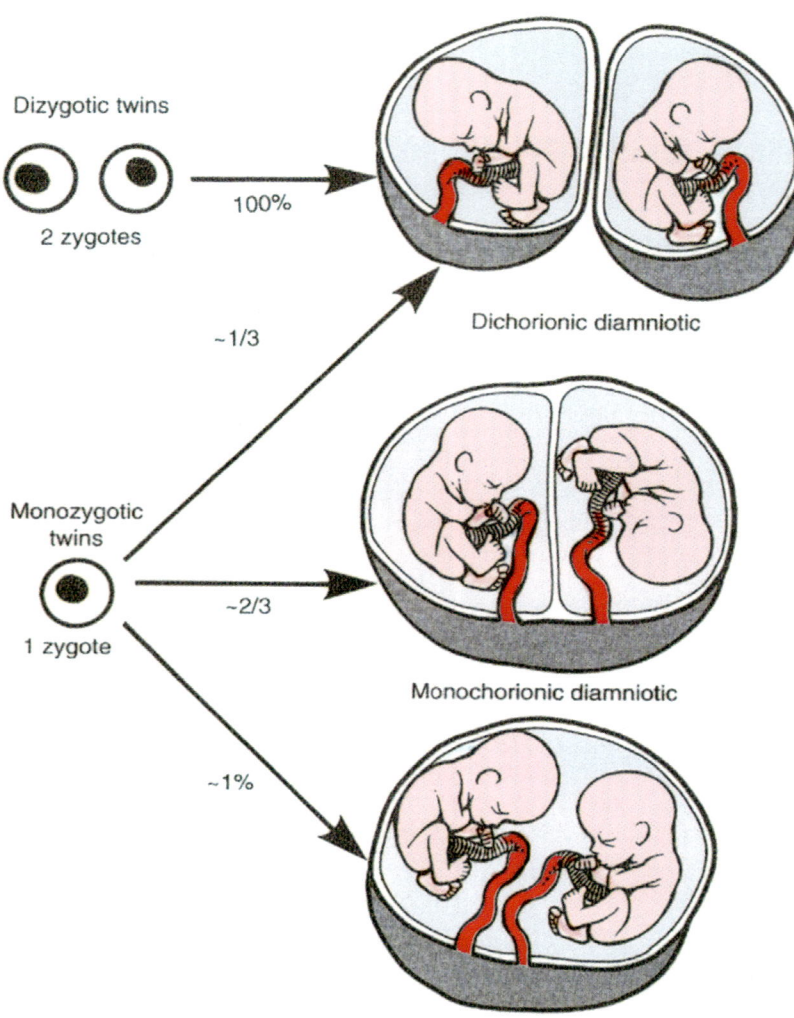

Dizygotic twins

2 zygotes

100%

Dichorionic diamniotic

~1/3

Monozygotic twins

1 zygote

~2/3

Monochorionic diamniotic

~1%

Monochorionic monoamniotic

FIGURE 1. Monozygotic versus dizygotic twins. All dizygotic twins have dichorionic-diamniotic placentation. Monozygotic twins may form dichorionic-diamniotic, monochorionic-diamniotic, or monochorionic-monoamniotic placentation. (Modified from McGahan JP, Porto M. *Diagnostic obstetrical ultrasound.* Philadelphia: JB Lippincott Co, 1994: 434.)

prises approximately 20% of twin pregnancies. Conversely, approximately 80% of twin pregnancies are dichorionic and this includes 10% of twins resulting from monozygotic conceptions.[8,9]

All monozygotic pregnancies result in same-sex twins, and approximately one-half of dizygotic pregnancies result in same sex twins. Definitive diagnosis of a dizygotic gestation can be made in 35% of twins by demonstrating discordant sex. Assuming that monochorionic gestations account for 30% of twins, then without reference to chorionicity, approximately 46% of same-sex twins are monozygotic. A more practical situation arises, however, in the setting of a known dichorionic pregnancy in which case 22% of twins with concordant sex are from monozygotic conceptions and the remaining 78% are from dizygotic conceptions (Fig. 3). These values are very similar to that obtained from Birmingham twin survey[10] although that study reported a slightly lower composition of monochorionic gestations.

Implications of Early Chorionicity Determination

Prenatal diagnosis of chorionicity is important in all multiple pregnancies for a number of reasons.

1. Chorionicity, rather than zygosity, is the main factor determining pregnancy outcome. In monochorionic twins the rates of miscarriage and perinatal death are much higher than in dichorionic twins[11,12] (see Complications and Conditions of Multiple Gestations).

2. Death of a monochorionic fetus is associated with a high chance of sudden death or severe neurologic impairment in the co-twin,[13] which is important for parental counseling should this occur spontaneously as well as for management of discordant fetal abnormality.

3. Diagnostic testing of patients at high-risk for genetic disorders and chromosomal abnormalities is dependent on chorionicity. In monochorionic twin pregnancies, when undertaking invasive diagnostic tests such as amniocentesis

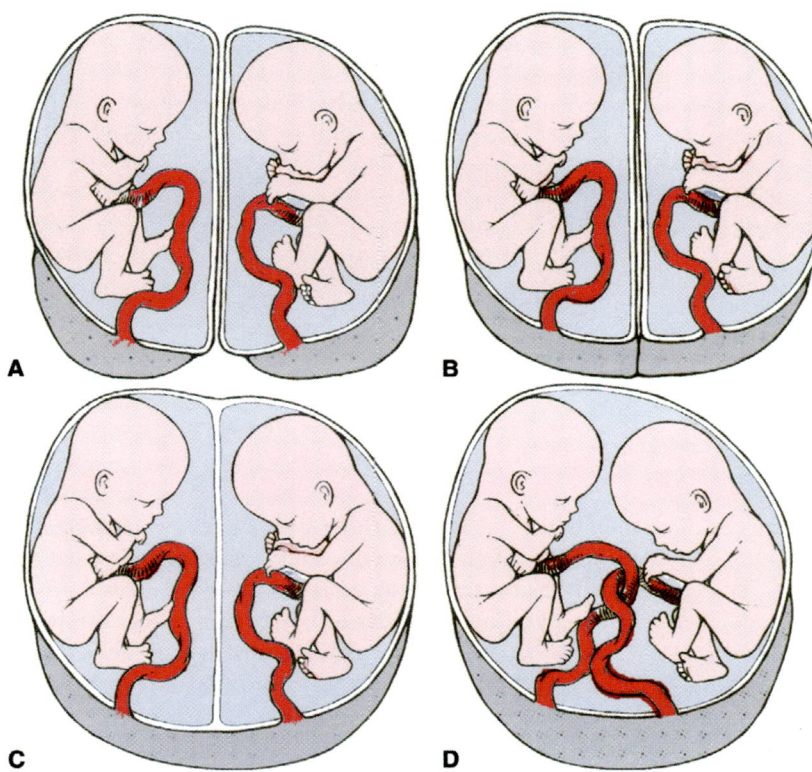

FIGURE 2. Schematic illustrating the position of the placenta in dichorionic and monochorionic placentation. **A:** Dichorionic-diamniotic placentation with two separate placentas. **B:** Dichorionic-diamniotic placentation with a fused placenta. **C:** Monochorionic-diamniotic placentation with a single placenta. **D:** Monochorionic-monoamniotic placentation with a single placenta. (Modified from McGahan JP, Porto M. *Diagnostic obstetrical ultrasound.* Philadelphia: JB Lippincott Co, 1994:434.)

or chorionic villus sampling (CVS), it may be unnecessary to sample both fetuses since they are monozygotic and, therefore, have identical genetic compositions.

4. In the management of twin pregnancy discordant for a major fetal defect, one of the options is selective feticide, but in monochorionic twins this procedure should be avoided, otherwise both fetuses could die or the survivor could suffer severe neurologic impairment.

5. Knowledge of chorionicity allows rational management decisions in multiple pregnancies affected by obstetric complications such as severe intrauterine growth restriction.

Determination of Chorionicity

Prenatal determination of chorionicity by ultrasonography has traditionally been performed in the second and third trimesters when it relies on assessment of fetal gender, number of placentas, and characteristics of the dividing membrane.[14–19] Different-sex twins are always dizygotic and therefore dichorionic, but in approximately two-thirds of twin pregnancies the fetuses are of the same sex; these may be either monozygotic or dizygotic. Similarly, if there are two separate placentas the pregnancy must be dichorionic, but in the majority of cases the two placentas are adjacent to each other and it is often difficult to distinguish between dichorionic-fused and monochorionic placentas.

The intertwin membrane is thicker and more echogenic in dichorionic compared to monochorionic pregnancies (Fig. 4). However, this may be a subjective criterion and is less reliable with advancing gestational age.[20] As pregnancy progresses, the distinction between thin and thick membranes becomes progressively less accurate, from greater than 98% accuracy in the first trimester to 83% accuracy

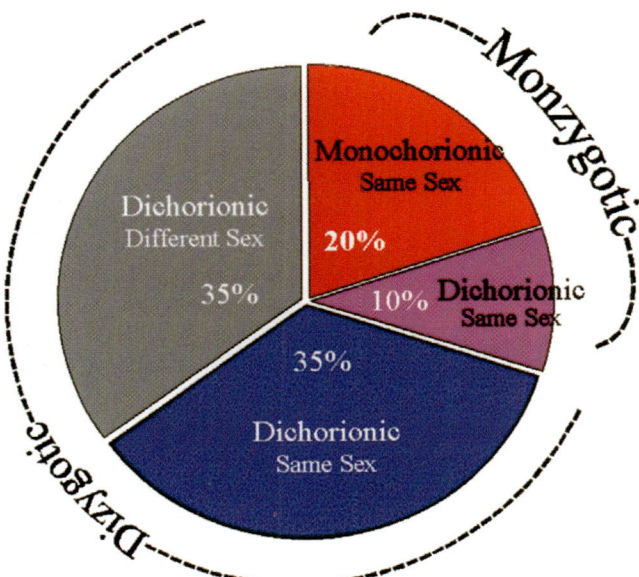

FIGURE 3. Frequency of dichorionic and monochorionic placentation with regard to zygosity and fetal sex.

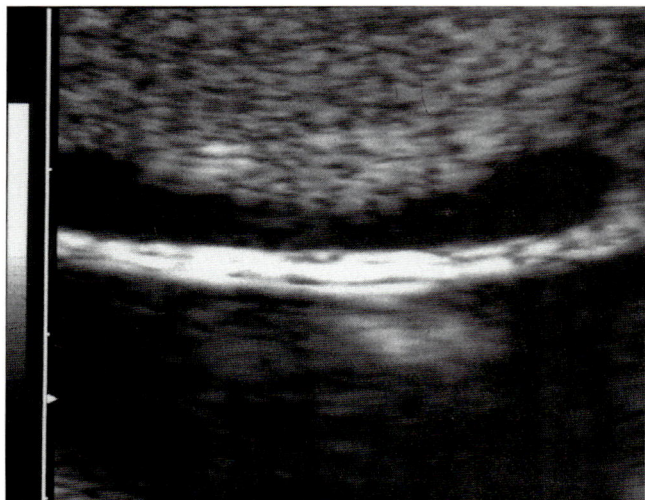

FIGURE 4. Dichorionic twin. In this ultrasound photograph of a section of intertwin membrane in a dichorionic twin pregnancy, the intertwin membrane is thick and echogenic and three layers are seen, confirming dichorionicity.

later in gestation.[15–17] Counting the layers of the intertwin membrane may also be possible because dichorionic pregnancies have more than two layers[21] (Fig. 4), but this is impractical for routine use. Jiggling the membrane could potentially make the layers more visible. However, this is susceptible to motion artifact, in which the same membrane can be imaged in different positions on the same image, giving a false impression of multiple layers.

A defining histologic feature of dichorionicity is the extension of placental tissue into the base of the intertwin

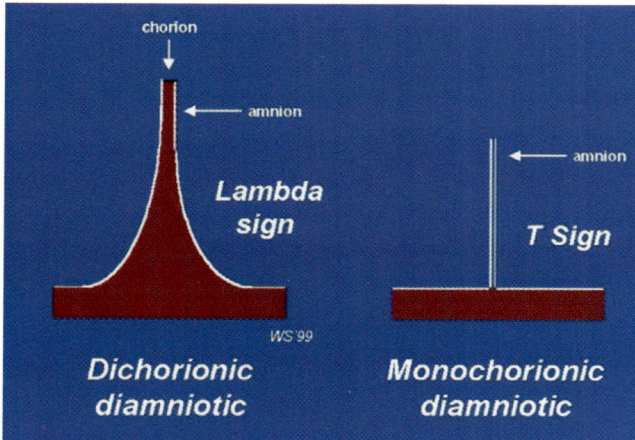

FIGURE 5. Schematic illustrating the lambda, or twin peak, and T signs observed in dichorionic and monochorionic twin pregnancies, respectively. Drawing illustrates how the twin peak sign is reliable evidence of dichorionicity. In a dichorionic pregnancy with fused placentas, both the amnions and the chorions reflect away from the placental surface, creating a potential space into which villi can grow. This is called the *lambda* or *twin peak sign*. Monochorionic-diamniotic pregnancies have a single layer of continuous chorion limiting villous growth. This is called the *T sign*.

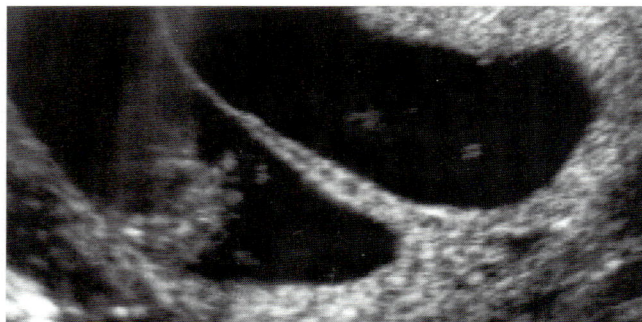

FIGURE 6. Dichorionic placentation. Ultrasound image of intertwin membrane-placental junction in a dichorionic twin pregnancy at 12 weeks' gestation shows extension of the placental tissue into the base of the intertwin membrane (the lambda sign).

membrane, known as the *twin peak* or *lambda sign*[22,23] (Figs. 5 through 7). In contrast, monochorionic placentation is characterized as a single placental mass and the thin separating membrane is best seen when the membrane is oriented perpendicular to the ultrasound beam. This membrane intersects the placental junction with a "T" sign (Fig. 8).

In the first trimester, dichorionic pregnancies have separate gestational sacs with intervening chorion, whereas monochorionic pregnancies have a single gestational sac containing both embryos (Fig. 9). Monochorionic pregnancies are further characterized as diamniotic or, rarely, monoamniotic. A diamniotic gestation can be determined by the presence of a thin separating membrane or two yolk sacs (Fig. 10). As noted, multiple pregnancies may be a combination of multichorionic and monochorionic placentations (Fig. 11).

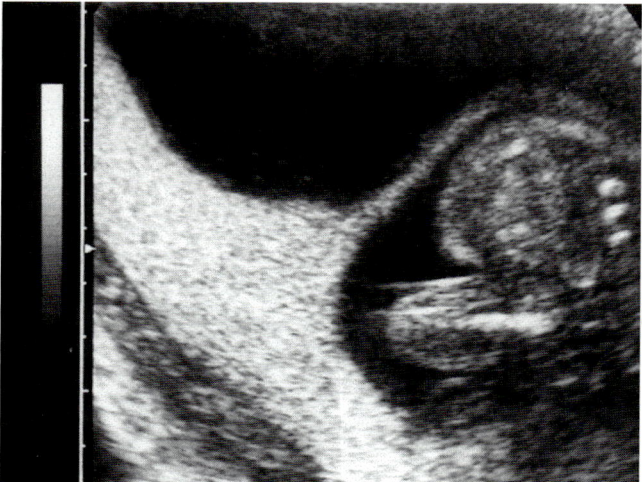

FIGURE 7. Dichorionic placentation. Ultrasound of the intertwin membrane-placental junction in a dichorionic twin pregnancy at 16 weeks of gestation. In this case, the lambda sign is still clearly present.

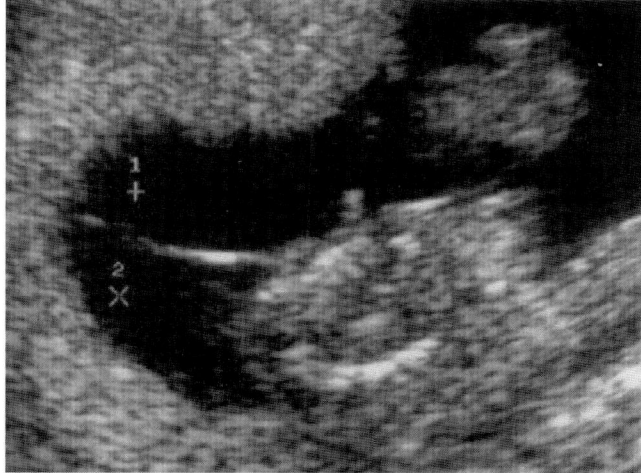

FIGURE 8. Monochorionic placentation. Transabdominal ultrasound of a 12-week monochorionic twin pregnancy shows absence of the lambda sign and the presence of the T sign with the intertwin membrane abruptly joining the placental surface with no intervening chorion.

At 10 to 14 weeks of gestation, pregnancies can be classified as monochorionic if there is a single placental mass in the absence of the lambda sign at the intertwin membrane-placental junction (T sign) and as dichorionic if there is a single placental mass but the lambda sign is present or the placentas are not adjacent to each other.[24] With advancing gestation, the lambda sign becomes progressively more difficult to identify, necessitating a systematic search of the intertwin membrane at the placental attachment throughout its

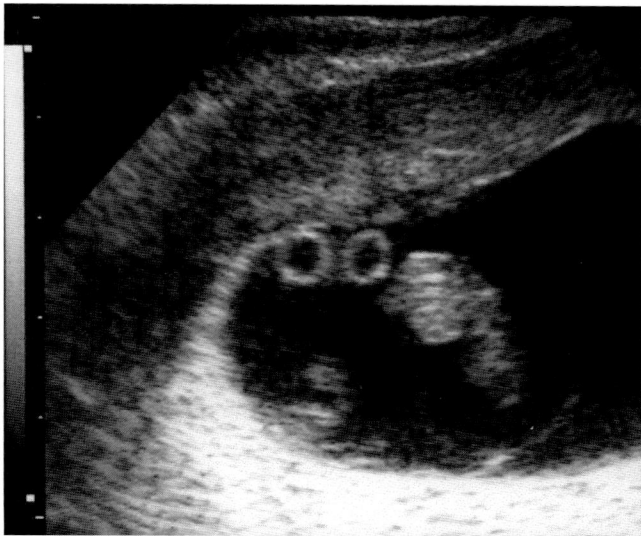

FIGURE 10. Monochorionic-diamniotic placentation with two yolk sacs. Ultrasound image of a monochorionic twin pregnancy in which there was difficulty in identification of the intertwin membrane shows two discrete yolk sacs, confirming a diamniotic gestation.

length. At 20 weeks' gestation, it is identified in approximately 90% of dichorionic pregnancies with fused placentas and approximately 75% with separate placentas. Thus, absence of the lambda sign at 20 weeks and thereafter does not constitute evidence of monochorionicity, but identifica-

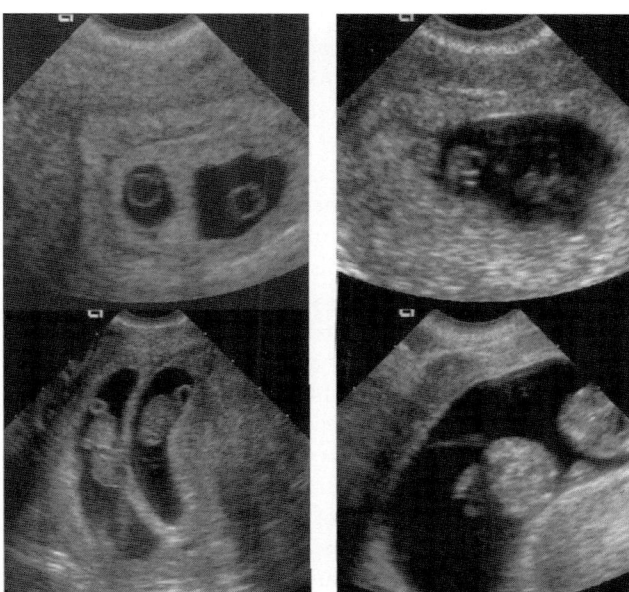

A,B

FIGURE 9. Dichorionic and monochorionic twins, first trimester. First-trimester examples of dichorionic **(A)** and monochorionic **(B)** twin gestations. Note the thick separating membranes of dichorionic placentation.

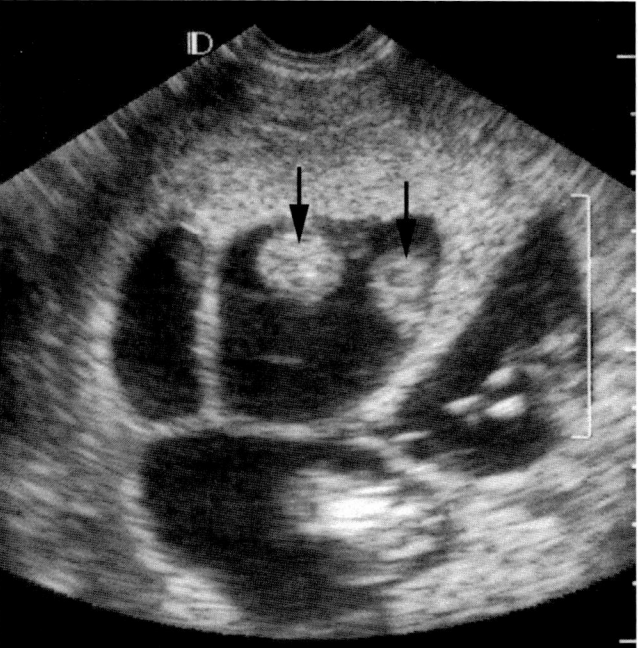

FIGURE 11. Mixed multichorionic and monochorionic quintuplet pregnancy at 10 weeks. Quintuplet, tetrachorionic gestation shows four separate chorionic sacs, including one sac containing a set of monochorionic twin embryos (*arrows*).

tion of this feature at any stage of pregnancy should be considered as evidence of dichorionicity.[25] Similarly, chorionicity in triplet, and higher order, pregnancies may be determined by ultrasonographically examining the membranes at the *ipsilon zone*, where the three amniotic cavities meet.[26]

COMPLICATIONS AND CONDITIONS OF MULTIPLE GESTATIONS

Complications related to twin and multiple pregnancies represent a significant contribution to fetal mortality and morbidity. Handicap rates in twins are approximately 1.5-fold higher than in singletons, and for severe handicap the increase is twofold.[27] The perinatal mortality rate for twins is around sixfold higher than in singletons, mainly because approximately 40% of twin pregnancies spontaneously deliver prematurely.[28] As noted, chorionicity is a major factor in perinatal outcome with a higher rate of complications associated with monochorionic pregnancies compared to dichorionic pregnancies. The fetal loss rate before 24 weeks is approximately 12% in monochorionic compared to approximately 2% in dichorionic pregnancies, and perinatal loss rates are 3% and 1.5%, respectively[9] (Fig. 12). Most early losses are presumably the consequence of the underlying chorioangiopagus and severe early-onset twin-twin transfusion syndrome (TTS).

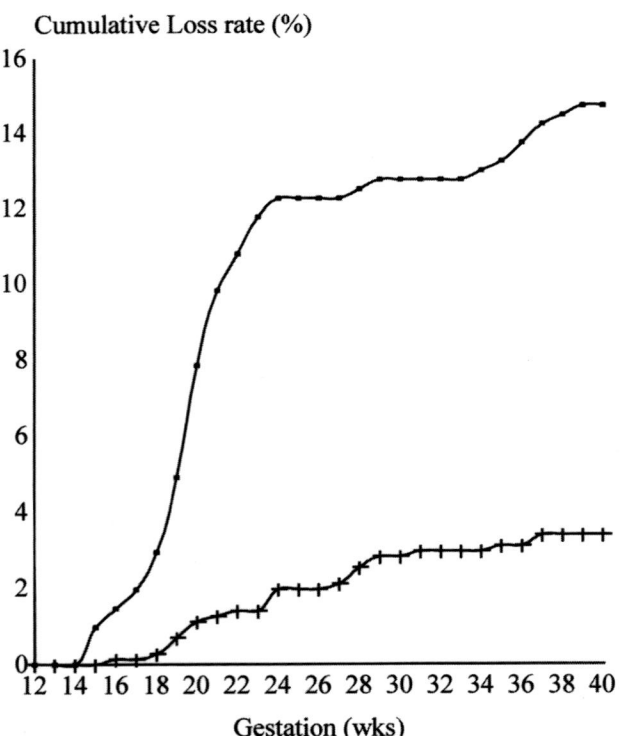

FIGURE 12. Cumulative fetal loss rates in monochorionic (*top line*) and dichorionic (*lower line*) twin pregnancies, from 14 weeks of gestation. (Adapted from Sebire et al. 1997.)

TABLE 1. CONDITIONS UNIQUE TO MONOCHORIONIC (MONOZYGOTIC) GESTATIONS

Anomaly	Description
Monochorionic-diamniotic	
"Embolization" syndrome	Embolization or ischemic injury after demise of a co-twin
Twin-twin transfusion syndrome	Unequal shunting of blood secondary to anastomotic placental vessels
Monochorionic-monoamniotic	
Acardiac twin (twin reversed arterial perfusion sequence)	Twin with absent or rudimentary, nonfunctional heart whose circulation is supplied by donor twin
Conjoined twins	Partial fusion of twins

Multiple pregnancies are at greater risk of delivering low birth weight and growth restricted babies with the degree of prematurity or growth retardation being the main determinants of mortality and morbidity in most cases.[29] Monochorionic twin gestations are at further risk of a variety of conditions, including those unique to monochorionic pregnancies (Table 1). Monochorionic gestations also have an elevated risk of fetal anomalies, three to seven times higher than the risk in dizygotic twins or singletons. Monochorionic-monoamniotic gestations have the added risk of cord accidents from cord entanglement. These complications are discussed in greater detail in the sections that follow.

Considerations in Screening of Twin Pregnancies for Chromosomal Abnormalities

In monozygotic twins, the risk for chromosomal abnormalities is the same as in singleton pregnancies, and both fetuses will be affected. In dizygotic pregnancies, the maternal age–related risk for chromosomal abnormalities for each twin is probably the same as in singleton pregnancies and therefore the chance that at least one fetus is affected by a chromosomal defect is twice as high as in singleton pregnancies. Furthermore, because the rate of dizygotic twinning increases with maternal age and because the mean maternal age in dizygotic twins is increasing (with the more widespread availability of assisted reproductive techniques), the prevalence of chromosomal defects in dizygotic twins is higher than in singleton pregnancies. Determination of chorionicity by ultrasonography allows parents of monochorionic twins to be counseled that both fetuses would be affected and this risk is similar to that in singleton pregnancies. If the pregnancy is dichorionic, then the parents can be counseled that the risk of discordance for a chromosomal abnormality is about twice that in singleton pregnancies; the risk that both fetuses will be affected can be determined by squaring the singleton risk ratio.

Although monozygotic twins should theoretically have the same karyotype, many genetic forms of discordance have been described within monozygotic twin pairs and may even play a role in causing monozygotic twinning.[30] Rarely, a monozygotic pregnancy is found with discordant fetal sex, that is, one apparent male and one apparent female.[31–33] When the karyotypes are discordant, this is known as *heterokaryotypic monozygotic pregnancy.* This may occur with Turner syndrome in a female fetus in whom the Y chromosome was "dropped" and fetal mosaicism with unequal distribution of cell lines. Discordant external genitalia may also occur with a variety of conditions associated with ambiguous genitalia or sex reversal.

In the first trimester, measurement of fetal nuchal translucency (NT)[34] is the most effective method of screening for chromosomal abnormality in multiple pregnancies. The fetal NT is above the ninety-fifth percentile for crown-rump length in approximately 7% of cases, including approximately 85% of those cases with trisomy 21 (see Chapter 20). In chromosomally normal twin pregnancies, increased NT has been found to be higher in fetuses from monochorionic pregnancies than in fetuses from dichorionic pregnancies in one study (8% vs. 5%)[35] but not in another.[36] Increased NT has been observed as a risk factor for TTS in monochorionic pregnancies (see Twin-Twin Transfusion Syndrome, later).

Second-trimester screening with maternal serum is also not as effective in screening for trisomy 21 in multiple pregnancies as it is in singleton pregnancies. Second-trimester ultrasound may be more effective than serum screening for multiple gestations (see Chapter 21).

Anomalies

Multiple pregnancies are at greater risk for chromosomal and fetal anomalies, not only because of the larger number of fetuses present, but also because of an increased risk of anomalies associated with monozygotic gestations. The overall prevalence of structural defects is 1.2 to 2.0 times higher in fetuses from twin pregnancies compared to singletons, with most of the excess risk due to increased rates in monochorionic twins.[37] Anomalies that occur with increased frequency in monozygotic twins include hydrocephalus, anencephaly, holoprosencephaly, and sacrococcygeal teratoma.

For any given defect the pregnancy may be concordant or discordant in terms of the presence, type, and severity of the abnormality. However, the majority (80% to 90%) of structural defects are discordant regardless of zygosity.

In addition to the increased frequency of anomalies seen with monozygotic twins, certain twin-related conditions are seen only in monozygotic twins, including anomalies of acardiac and conjoined twins.

Spontaneous Fetal Death in a Twin Pregnancy

Intrauterine death of a fetus in a twin pregnancy may be associated with adverse outcome for the co-twin, but the type and degree of risk depend on the chorionicity of the pregnancy. Second- or third-trimester intrauterine death of one fetus may be associated with the onset of labor in dichorionic twins and acute hypotensive episodes in monochorionic twins leading to death or handicap of the co-twin. In dichorionic pregnancies, associated cases of cerebral palsy are primarily related to complications of severe preterm delivery, whereas for monochorionic twins there is at least a 25% risk of death or neurologic damage to the co-twin.[38] In neurologically damaged twin infants, compared to normal twin infants, the co-twin dies later in gestation, the duration between the death of the co-twin and delivery is shorter, and the twins are delivered earlier in gestation.[39] Porencephaly and ischemia can be detected with magnetic resonance imaging.[40]

In the first trimester, there is less evidence regarding the implications of single fetal death in a twin pregnancy according to chorionicity. The "vanishing twin" phenomenon has been commonly reported in presumed dichorionic twins from the early first trimester,[41] with little apparent effect on the subsequent outcome of the pregnancy, although it is possible that the reported frequency of this occurrence is an underestimate. However, in a study on twin pregnancies examined at 10 to 14 weeks of gestation, one or both fetuses were dead at the initial scan in significantly more dichorionic twin pregnancies (6%) compared to singleton pregnancies, whereas in monochorionic twin pregnancies there were only 3% with one or both dead fetuses. Furthermore, in the cases with one fetal death, 24% of the pregnancies resulted in miscarriage, including all cases of monochorionic twins.[42] Single intrauterine death in early pregnancy in monochorionic twins is probably highly uncommon because most cases will result in death of both fetuses; a hypothesis supported by combined experience of attempted selective feticide of monochorionic twins in early pregnancy. In contrast, in dichorionic twins, spontaneous death of one fetus is common but this is associated with an increased risk for subsequent miscarriage or severe preterm delivery depending on the gestational age at fetal death.

Preterm Delivery

Approximately 10% of preterm deliveries are from twin gestations. The median gestational age of delivery is approximately 36 weeks for twins, 33 weeks for triplets, and 29 weeks for quadruplets.[43–45] Hence, preterm delivery at 36 weeks or earlier affects approximately one-half of twin gestations and the majority of higher-order multiple gestations (Fig. 13). Multiple gestations result in greater uterine distention, which can initiate labor, and promote earlier cervical changes compared to singleton pregnancies.

Ultrasound assessment of the cervix has been found to be a more reliable measure of cervical changes than digital examination, and these changes help to identify patients at risk for preterm delivery.[46–48] A shortened cervix (Fig. 14)

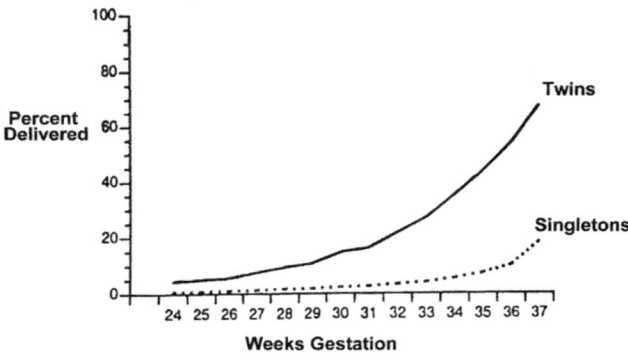

FIGURE 13. Distribution of birth age of twin deliveries compared with singletons. More than one-half of twins are delivered by 36 weeks. (Reproduced with permission from Gardner MD, Goldenberg RL, Oliver SP, et al. The origin and outcome of preterm twin pregnancies. *Obstet Gynecol* 1995;85:553; the American College of Obstetricians and Gynecologists.)

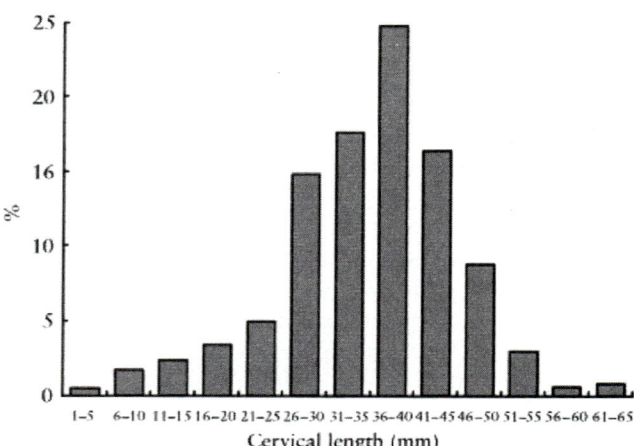

FIGURE 15. Distribution of cervical length in twin pregnancies at 23 weeks. [Reproduced with permission from Skentou C, Souka AP, To MS, Liao AW, Nicolaides KH. Prediction of preterm delivery in twins by cervical assessment at 23 weeks. *Ultrasound Obstet Gynecol* 2001;17(1):7–10.]

also correlates with positive fetal fibronectin levels.[49] Although some studies suggest that cervical funneling and cervical length are independently correlated with preterm delivery,[50] To et al.[51] found that funneling did not provide additional information to closed cervical length among singleton pregnancies.[48]

Among 464 twin pregnancies seen for routine care, Skentou et al.[52] found that the median cervical length at 23 weeks was 36 mm (Fig. 15). The rate of spontaneous delivery before 33 weeks was inversely related to cervical length at 23 weeks. It increased gradually from approximately 2.5% at 60 mm, to 5% at 40 mm, and 12% at 25 mm, and exponentially below this length to 17% at 20 mm and 80% at 8 mm (Fig. 16). A cervical length of 20 mm or less iden-

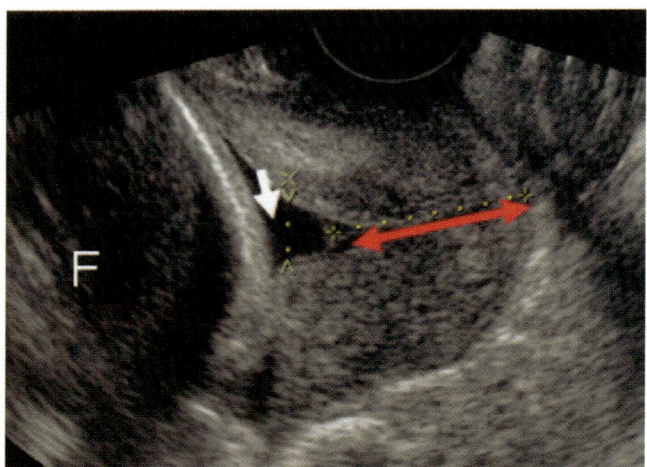

FIGURE 14. Cervical shortening. A transvaginal scan at 23 weeks in twin pregnancy shows mild dilatation with funneling of the internal cervical os (*short arrow*). The closed cervical length measures 2.5 cm (*red arrow*). The closed cervical length is an important variable in prediction of preterm delivery; the degree of funneling may not provide additional predictive information. F, fetus.

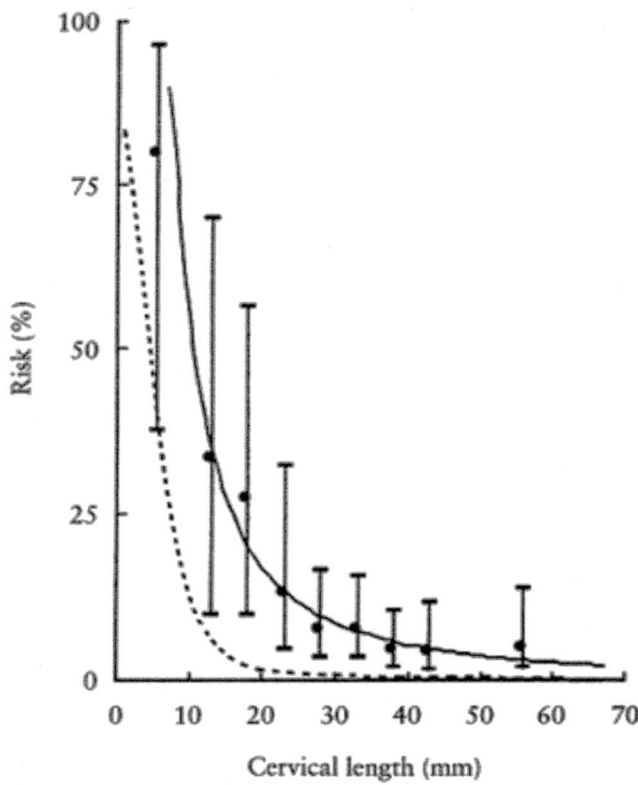

FIGURE 16. Risk of preterm delivery before 33 weeks' gestation compared to closed cervical length at 23 weeks in twin pregnancies. The rate of spontaneous delivery before 33 weeks is inversely related to cervical length measured at 23 weeks. It increased gradually from approximately 2.5% at 6 cm, to 5% at 4 cm, and 12% at 2.5 cm. [Reproduced with permission from Skentou C, Souka AP, To MS, Liao AW, Nicolaides KH. Prediction of preterm delivery in twins by cervical assessment at 23 weeks. *Ultrasound Obstet Gynecol* 2001;17(1):7–10.]

tified 40% of women delivering before 33 weeks and was found in 8% of twin pregnancies. Conversely, a cervical length of at least 35 mm identified a low-risk group of patients for preterm delivery among twin pregnancies.[50]

Similar analysis has been performed for triplet gestations. The rate of spontaneous delivery before 33 weeks increased exponentially with decreasing cervical length at 23 weeks from 8% at 36 to 48 mm, to 11% at 26 to 35 mm, 33% at 16 to 25 mm, and 67% at 15 mm or less. A cervical length of 25 mm or less at 23 weeks was found in 16% of triplet gestations and identified 50% of preterm deliveries.[51]

Growth Restriction

Growth restriction is common in multiple gestations. The majority of infants born of a multiple gestation will be of low birth weight, less than 2,500 g. These infants are at substantial risk of short-term and long-term handicaps.

The sensitivity of fundal height measurements to detect growth restriction in twins is only approximately 20%,[53] and serial ultrasound assessment is therefore essential. The growth of twins parallels that of singletons until approximately 30 weeks, after which time growth rates tend to decline compared to singletons.

Using standardized measurements of the fetal head, abdomen, and femur, the estimated weights of each fetus of a multiple gestation should be calculated, using any one of a variety of published tables or formulas. There is no difference in accuracy of estimated fetal weight prediction between twins and singletons,[54–56] and most centers do not use different growth charts for twins. Once the weights have been calculated, the size of each fetus should be assessed with respect to gestational age by determining its weight percentile for its age. The likelihood of growth restriction varies inversely with the estimated weight percentile and can be further supported by assessment of amniotic fluid and Doppler studies.[57–63] In addition to evaluating the size of each fetus separately for gestational age, the fetal weights should be compared to one another. A common classification suggests discordance when the estimated weight of the larger fetus is 20% or greater than that of the smaller fetus.[64]

In singleton pregnancies with fetal growth retardation due to presumed uteroplacental insufficiency, the main aims of antenatal care are to predict the severity of impaired fetal oxygenation and select the appropriate time for delivery by balancing the relative risks of intrauterine death with expectant management and the risk of neonatal death or handicap from preterm delivery. In dichorionic twin pregnancies discordant for intrauterine growth restriction, the condition of both fetuses needs to be considered to avoid iatrogenic preterm delivery of the normally grown twin while maximizing the survival changes of the growth-restricted co-twin. The minimum gestation at which the growth-retarded fetus can potentially survive is 26 weeks, but iatrogenic delivery at this gestation is associated with an estimated risk of death in 40% of the appropriately grown and 70% of the small-for-gestational-age (SGA) neonates. Furthermore, approximately 25% of the appropriate for gestational age and approximately 70% of the SGA survivors would potentially be severely handicapped. Similarly, at 28 weeks and with the maximum expected weight for the SGA fetus of 700 to 800 g, iatrogenic delivery at this gestation would be associated with an estimated risk of death in 20% of the appropriate for gestational age and 45% of the SGA neonates. Furthermore, approximately 10% of the appropriate for gestational age and approximately 40% of the SGA survivors would be severely handicapped.[65,66] Irrespective of the obstetricians' and parents' preferred policy, accurate data are critical to estimate the chances of survival and risks of handicap for each fetus.

Twin "Embolization" Syndrome

Twin "embolization" syndrome refers to tissue necrosis or death of a living twin following *in utero* demise of a co-twin in a monochorionic pregnancy.[67]

Incidence

The incidence is unknown but is estimated as 2% of survivors following death of the co-twin, most commonly between 16 and 20 weeks' gestation.[68]

Pathology

Tissue damage affects predominantly highly vascularized organs such as the brain and kidneys but can affect almost all organ systems.[69–71] Fetal injury was originally thought to occur from embolization of placental and fetal thromboplastins or from the direct embolization of necrosed fragments of the placenta from the dead fetus, disseminated intravascular coagulation causing embolization, or even an endarteritis.[72,73] However, the mechanism of death or neurologic damage in monochorionic pregnancies is likely to be acute hemodynamic shifts from the live to the dead fetus and reverse blood flow from the live fetus to the dead twin through large superficial intertwin anastomoses.[74–77]

This transient reversal of flow has been documented with Doppler sonography immediately following death of one fetus.[78,79]

Diagnosis

Evidence of tissue damage in the brain may be observed by ultrasound or magnetic resonance imaging. These sonographic findings are not apparent until weeks after the insult[80] but are probably apparent earlier with magnetic resonance imaging. Evidence for brain injury includes ventriculomegaly, porencephaly (Fig. 17), cerebral atrophy, cystic encephalomalacia, and microcephaly. Less likely,

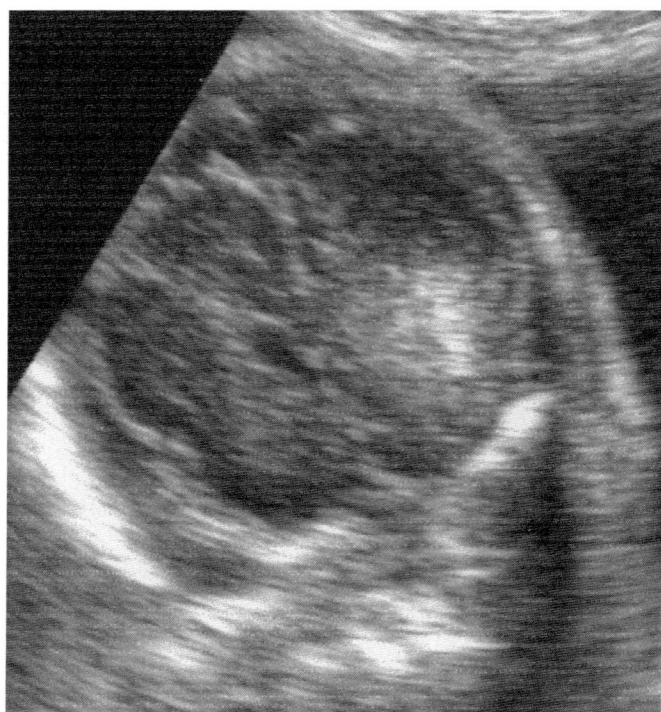
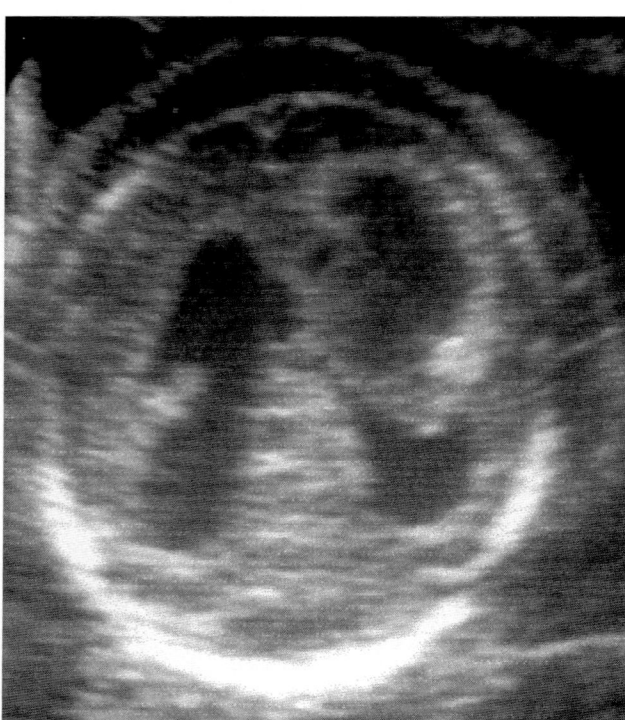

A   B

FIGURE 17. Porencephaly from twin embolization syndrome. **A:** After the demise of a co-twin, the survivor developed an intraparenchymal hemorrhage in the brain, seen as an echogenic area. **B:** A follow-up scan several weeks later shows evolution of the hemorrhage into an area of porencephaly with ventriculomegaly. The mechanism of injury is likely to be secondary to acute hemodynamic shifts away from the live fetus at the time of the co-twin's demise through inter-twin anastomoses.

extracranial abnormalities that may be detected include small bowel atresia, gastroschisis, hydrothorax, and renal abnormality. Only fetal death occurring during the second and third terms of pregnancy is considered.[81]

Unfortunately, there is no way to predict this occurrence following death of a twin. Also, it is likely that any tissue injury has already occurred by the time the twin demise is recognized.

Differential Diagnosis

The presence of any of the anomalies described above in the surviving twin with a dead co-twin should raise suspicion of this condition.[82] The primary differential diagnosis is a congenital birth defect as opposed to acquired tissue injury resulting from this condition.

Prognosis and Management

In general, the prognosis for the surviving fetus is poor but varies with the location and extent of tissue injury. There is no evidence that active management alters the natural outcome.

Management of the monochorionic pregnancy presenting with a dead co-twin, when the exact time of intrauterine demise is usually not known, remains a dilemma. The options are essentially induced delivery, which may result in iatrogenic complications of prematurity without prevention of neurologic damage, or conservative management with serial ultrasound scans for early detection of cerebral lesions. Maternal complications such as disseminated intravascular coagulation have been reported following intrauterine death and retention of the fetus in singleton pregnancies. There is a potential risk of similar complications occurring in a twin pregnancy with the intrauterine death of one fetus with expectant management; however, no such confirmed cases have been reported and the true incidence, if not zero, must be very low.[38,83,84]

Twin-Twin Transfusion Syndrome

TTS is a complication of monochorionic twin pregnancies in which there is imbalance in the net flow of blood across the placental vascular communications from one fetus, the donor, to the other, the recipient (Fig. 18). This has also been described as a subset of the twin oligohydramnios-polydramnios sequence.[85]

Incidence

TTS may occur in as many as 25% of monochorionic pregnancies, but severe TTS occurs in 15%.

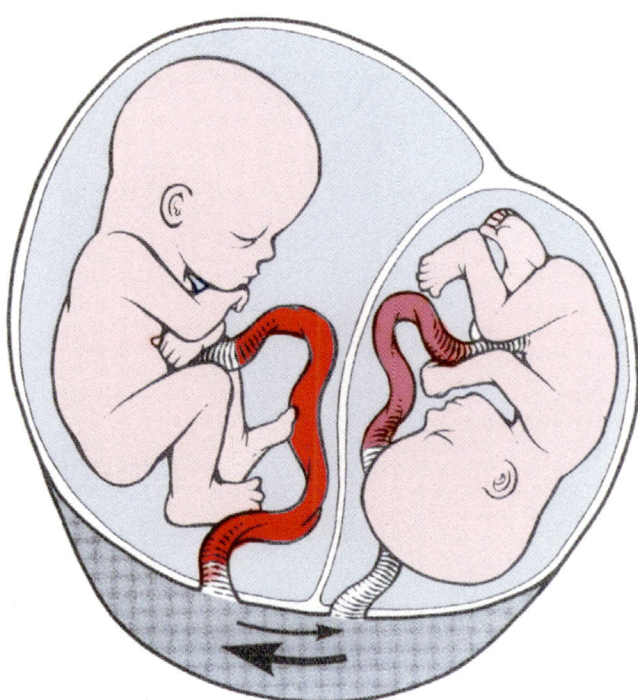

FIGURE 18. Diagram illustrates monochorionic gestation with twin-twin transfusion syndrome. The recipient twin is larger and in a polyhydramniotic sac. The donor twin is smaller and in a oligohydramniotic sac. (Modified from McGahan JP, Porto M. *Diagnostic obstetrical ultrasound*. Philadelphia: JB Lippincott Co, 1994:434.)

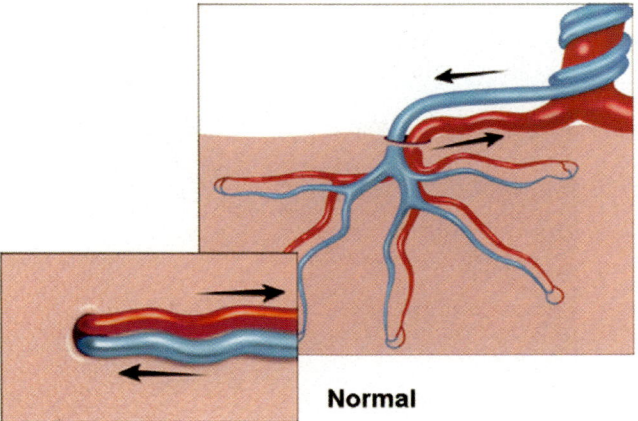

Normal
A

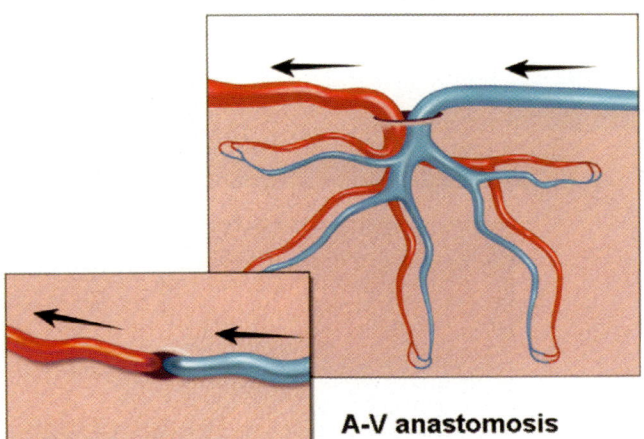

A-V anastomosis
B

FIGURE 19. Placental anastomoses. Schematic representation of placental vessels shows the artery depicted in blue and the vein in red. Arrows indicate the direction of blood flow. The superimposed drawing, at the lower left of each diagram, shows the vascular structures as viewed from the fetal surface of the placenta. **A:** Normal artery and vein pair emanating from and returning to the fetal cord insertion site. **B:** Arteriovenous (*A-V*) anastomosis. As shown, the artery and vein each travel unaccompanied along the placental surface and traverse a common, shared foramen to perfuse the placenta. (Reproduced with permission from Machin GA, Feldstein VA, Van Gemert MJC, Keith LG, Hecher K. Doppler sonographic demonstrations of arteriovenous anastomosis in monochorionic twin gestation. *Ultrasound Obstet Gynecol* 2000;16:214–217.)

Pathology

Interfetal vascular anastomoses are present in almost all monochorionic twin pregnancies[86–90] (Figs. 19 and 20). Anastomosis may be artery to artery, vein to vein, or vein to artery. The most important anastomosis is the arteriovenous shunt. An artery from the donor twin dives into the placenta adjacent to a vein from the recipient twin; the artery and vein connect via anastomoses at the villous level.[91]

TTS is variable in clinical manifestations as mild, moderate, or severe. The underlying mechanism appears to be shunting of blood from the donor to the recipient. The donor suffers from both hypovolemia and hypoxia.[92,93] The recipient fetus compensates for its expanded blood volume with polyuria,[94] but protein and cellular components in its circulation increase the colloid oncotic pressure, which draws water from the maternal compartment across the placenta. A vicious cycle of hypervolemia, polyuria, and hyperosmolality is established leading to high-output heart failure and polyhydramnios. The clinical severity depends on the net flow between these anastomoses, which are common and variable in size, number, and direction.

A characteristic feature of TTS is polyuria in the recipient twin. Increased urinary output is mediated by atrial natriuretic peptide in the distal renal tubules.[95] Polyuria leads to polyhydramnios.

Twins have six to nine times higher incidence of velamentous cord insertion,[2] and an even higher frequency is found in higher-order births. This finding is explained by greater lateral growth of the placenta when embryos are initially most closely apposed, the theory of trophotropism.[96] Velamentous insertion of the umbilical cord in one of the twins is a significant risk factor for TTS.[97,98] Velamentous or marginal insertion of the umbilical cord could lead to a

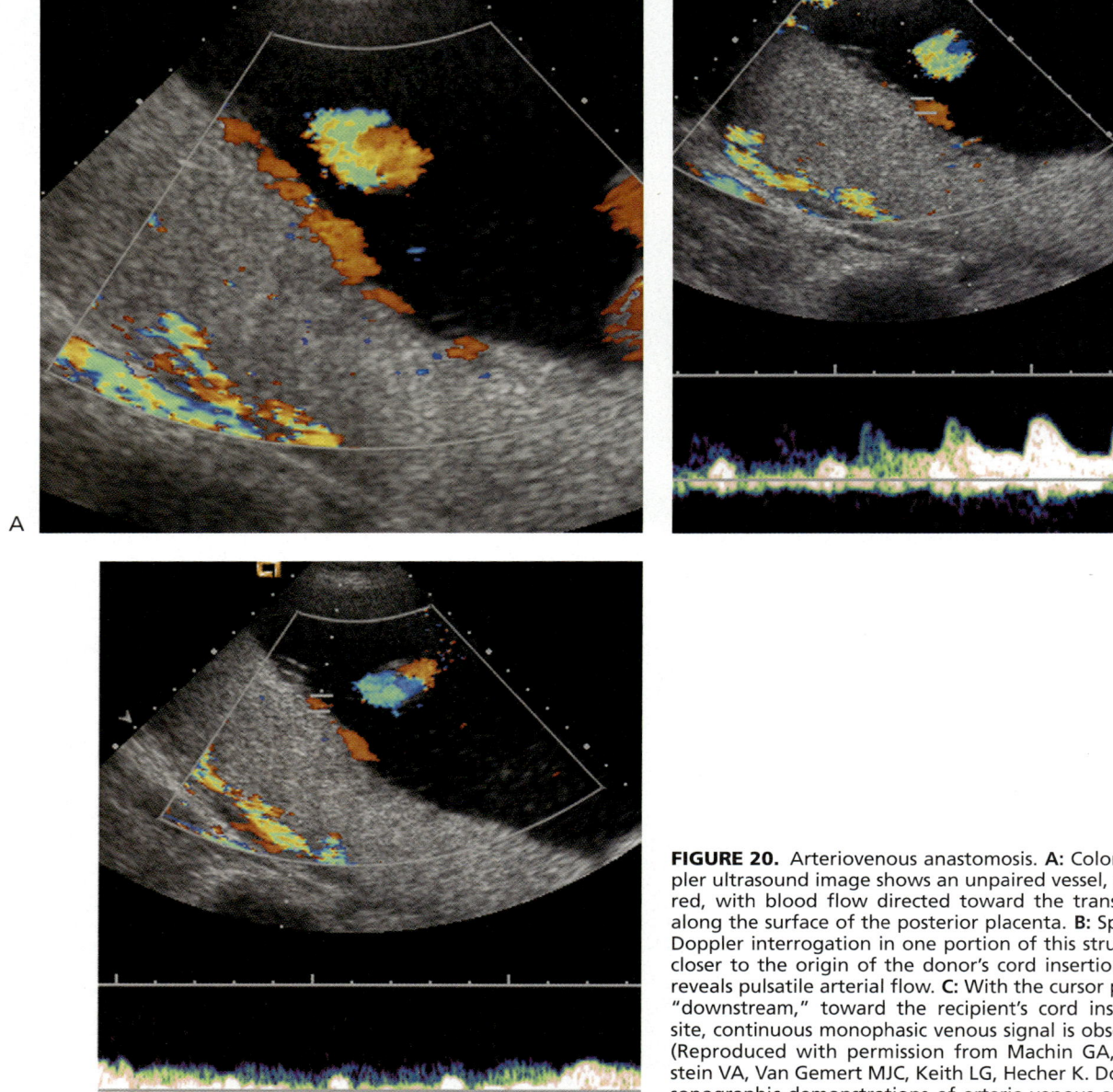

FIGURE 20. Arteriovenous anastomosis. **A:** Color Doppler ultrasound image shows an unpaired vessel, coded red, with blood flow directed toward the transducer along the surface of the posterior placenta. **B:** Spectral Doppler interrogation in one portion of this structure, closer to the origin of the donor's cord insertion site, reveals pulsatile arterial flow. **C:** With the cursor placed "downstream," toward the recipient's cord insertion site, continuous monophasic venous signal is observed. (Reproduced with permission from Machin GA, Feldstein VA, Van Gemert MJC, Keith LG, Hecher K. Doppler sonographic demonstrations of arterio-venous anastomosis in monochorionic twin gestation. *Ultrasound Obstet Gynecol* 2000;16:214–217.)

greater number of feeding vessels that could then anastamose with vessels of the co-twin.

Diagnosis

Although the diagnosis of TTS cannot be made until the second trimester, sonographic clues indicating an at-risk pregnancy may be identified as early as the first trimester. Increased NT measurements and heart rates at 10 to 14 weeks may identify monochorionic gestations at risk for TTS, whereas size discordance is not significantly different at this time. For fetal NT above the ninety-fifth percentile, the positive and negative predictive values for the development of TTS are approximately 40% and 90%, respectively; the likelihood ratios of NT above or below the ninety-fifth percentile for development of TTS are approximately 4.0 and 0.7, respectively.[99]

Mild discrepancy in the amount of amniotic fluid is typically the first sign of TTS. Another typical early finding is the "folding membrane" stage, in which the redundant membrane progressively folds as it wraps itself around the donor, reflecting development of oligohydramnios. At 15

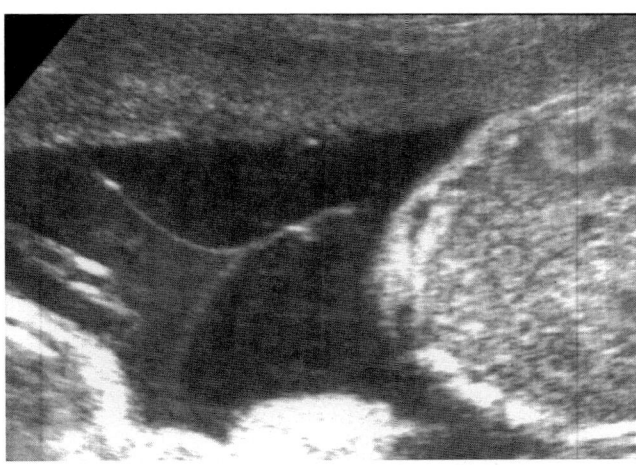

FIGURE 21. Early twin transfusion syndrome. A transabdominal ultrasound photograph of a 16-week monochorionic twin pregnancy affected by early twin-to-twin transfusion syndrome shows folding of the intertwin membrane pointing toward the recipient amniotic sac and the increased echogenicity of the amniotic fluid in the donor sac.

to 17 weeks, intertwin membrane folding (Figs. 21 and 22) is present in approximately one-fourth of monochorionic pregnancies, with subsequent severe TTS developing in about one-half of the cases.[100]

The umbilical cord commonly shows discrepant size with enlargement of the recipient cord and a small or nor-

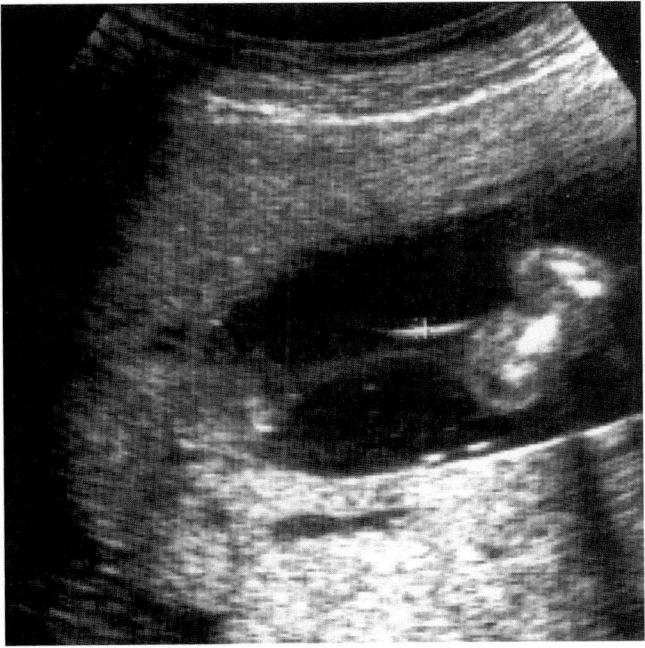

FIGURE 22. Early twin transfusion syndrome. A transabdominal ultrasound photograph of an 18-week monochorionic twin pregnancy affected by twin-to-twin transfusion syndrome shows folding of the intertwin membrane around the limb of the donor fetus, with the two layers of the intertwin membrane seen.

TABLE 2. SONOGRAPHIC FEATURES OF TWIN-TWIN TRANSFUSION SYNDROME

	Donor Twin	Recipient Twin
Size	Small	Large
Fluid	Decreased	Increased
Mobility	Increased	Decreased
Urinary bladder	Small	Distended
Umbilical cord	Small to normal	Enlarged
Blood volume	Decreased	Increased
Complications	Stuck twin phenomenon, intrauterine growth restriction, hypoxia, death	Cardiomyopathy, hydrops, death

mal size cord of the donor twin. Velamentous insertion of the umbilical cord is also common with TTS and may occur with either the donor or recipient twin.

The following summarizes some of the commonly recognized findings of TTS:

- Monochorionic placentation with visualization of a separating membrane
- Midtrimester polyhydramnios-oligohydramnios sequence in the absence of other causes of abnormal amniotic fluid volume
- Size discordance, abdominal circumference difference, or weight discrepancy greater than 20%[101–105]
- Nonvisualization of the donor's bladder with enlarged recipient's bladder
- Velamentous cord insertion[106,107]
- Abnormal Doppler systolic/diastolic ratio of the umbilical cord
- Hydrops or evidence of congestive heart failure[108–110]

Table 2 summarizes some of the more specific sonographic features of the donor and recipient twins in moderate-severe disease. Severe disease usually becomes apparent in the early second trimester of pregnancy, with tense polyhydramnios, discordance in fetal size, and a large bladder in the polyuric recipient fetus (Fig. 23) and oligohydramnios and absent bladder in the anuric donor. In the extreme condition, the donor twin is "stuck" and immobile at an edge of the placenta or the uterine wall, where it is held fixed by the collapsed membranes of the anhydramniotic sac (Figs. 24 and 25).

The recipient twin often develops a hypertrophic, dilated, and dyskinetic heart. The donor may show a dilated heart and hyperechogenic bowel; these features are commonly seen in hypoxemic fetuses in pregnancies with severe uteroplacental insufficiency. The donor fetus may also demonstrate ventriculomegaly, microcephaly, or both.[111,112]

Doppler studies are commonly abnormal. Critically abnormal Doppler studies may include absent/reverse end-diastolic velocity in the umbilical artery, reverse flow in the ductus venosus, or pulsatile flow in the umbilical vein[113–120]

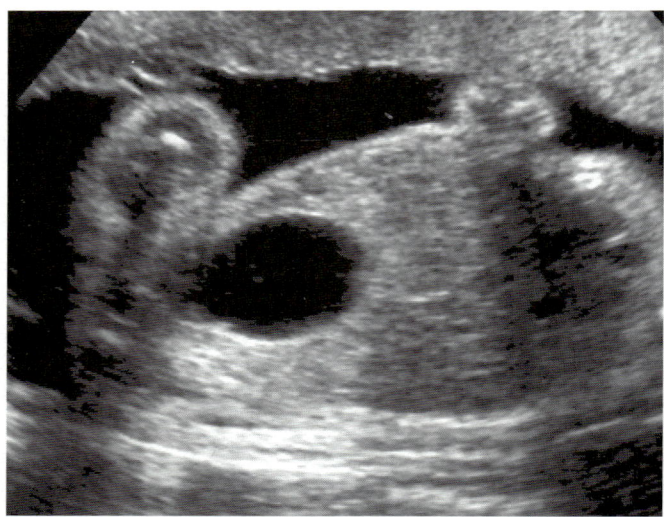
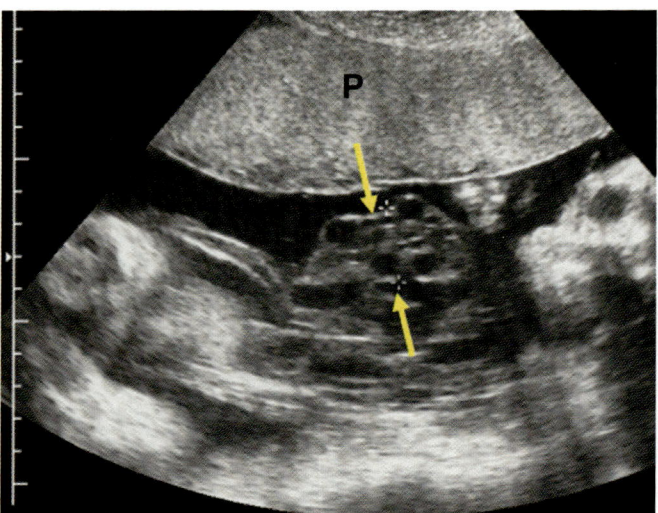

A

B

FIGURE 23. Enlarged urinary bladder and umbilical cord in recipient twin of twin-twin transfusion syndrome. **A:** A longitudinal view of the recipient twin shows the distended urinary bladder, which remained constant throughout the examination. The bladder of the donor twin was small but visible. **B:** A view of the umbilical cord of the recipient twin shows enlarged umbilical cord (*arrows*). The umbilical cord of the donor twin was approximately one-half this diameter. Note that the placenta (*P*) also appears thickened.

(Fig. 26). As an ominous finding frequently leading to death, hydrops may develop in the recipient twin from fluid overload and heart failure (Fig. 27).

FIGURE 24. Stuck twin phenomenon. A scan at 18 weeks shows the "stuck" twin (*solid arrow*) anteriorly, confined within an oligohydramniotic sac. The recipient twin (*open arrow*), posteriorly, is in a polyhydramniotic sac.

Color Doppler imaging can demonstrate the vessels on the surface of the placenta, which connect to the anastomoses deep in the placenta[121,122] (Fig. 20).

Prognosis and Management

Once the oligohydramnios-polyhydramnios sequence is present, the untreated mortality of both fetuses is high. In a review of the literature of 136 fetuses identified before 28 weeks and managed expectantly, the survival rate was 27%.[123] However, it is difficult to compare studies because those managed expectantly may have preferentially included those with a more favorable outcome. There is clearly a range in the severity of TTS, and there is good evidence that earlier onset with more severe polyhydramnios carries a worse outcome.[124]

With active management, the survival rate is improved for severe cases of TTS. Active management may include (a) serial therapeutic amniocentesis, (b) laser coagulation of anastomotic vessels, or (c) cord ligation when death of one of the fetuses appears imminent. Cord coagulation and ligation require considerably more expertise and training than amniocentesis and should only be performed at tertiary centers experienced with these techniques. Each of these techniques are described further under Procedures Related to Multiple Gestations.

Twins affected with TTS are also at risk for brain injury. This may occur from either a prenatal event or as a result of prematurity. Among 40 survivors of monochorionic twin pregnancies complicated by TTS and followed until 24 months of age, Haverkamp et al.[125] found that 24% had severe psychomotor retardation in combination with cerebral palsy. Major neurologic sequelae were more common in recipients than in donors.

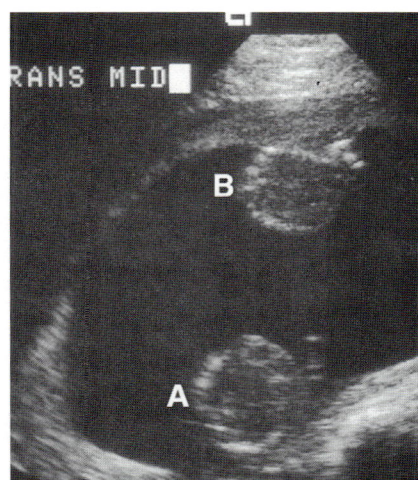

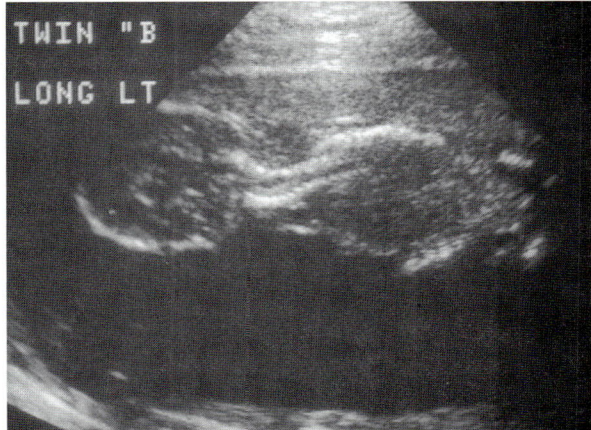

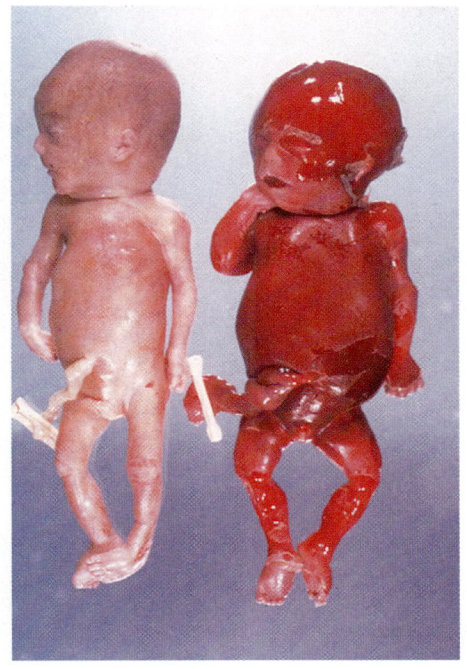

FIGURE 25. Stuck twin phenomenon at 17 weeks. **A:** Twin B is "stuck" (*B*) along the anterior uterine wall in an oligohydramniotic sac, while twin A (*A*) lies in the dependent portion of a polyhydramniotic sac. **B:** A longitudinal view of donor twin B, stuck along the anterior uterine wall. Twin B measured approximately 1 week behind twin A. **C:** Photograph of specimens after twin demise shows plethoric but smaller twin B on the right. This degree of plethora is thought to result from initial death of twin B (note maceration) resulting in return of blood through vascular shunts with secondary anemia and demise of the co-twin.

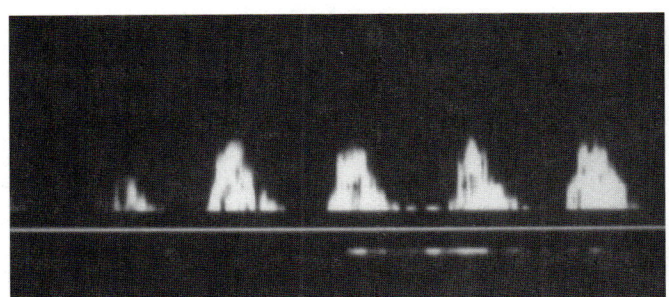

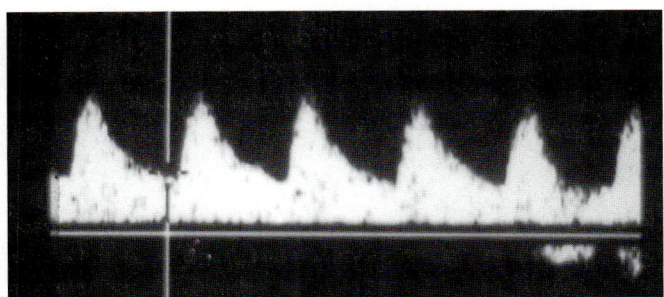

FIGURE 26. Twin transfusion syndrome with abnormal Doppler studies. At 20 weeks, the umbilical artery Doppler waveform shows absent end-diastolic flow in the small donor twin **(A)** and normal diastolic flow in the larger recipient twin **(B)**.

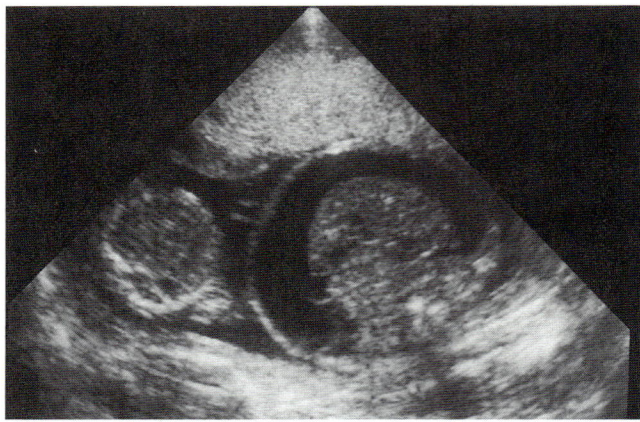

FIGURE 27. Twin transfusion syndrome with hydrops. Ultrasound shows the small donor twin on the left and the hydropic recipient twin with a large amount of ascites on the right.

Monoamniotic Twins

Monoamniotic twins are a subset of monochorionic gestation with a single amnion.

Incidence

The incidence is approximately 1% of twin pregnancies or 2% to 3% of monochorionic twins.

Pathology

Splitting of the embryonic mass after day nine of fertilization results in monoamniotic twins.

The umbilical cords of monoamniotic twins usually insert near one another on the surface of the placenta. The placental vessels typically have large-caliber anastomoses between them.[126] As a result, TTS is less common in monoamniotic twins because imbalance in the two circulations could not be sustained for long periods.

Diagnosis

The sonographic diagnosis depends on demonstration of a single amniotic cavity with a single placenta. Care must be taken not to miss the thin membrane of a monochorionic-diamniotic gestation. Fetal parts are seen to touch and may be intertwined. Cord entanglement is diagnostic of monoamniotic twin gestation[127] (Fig. 28) and is observed in most, if not all, cases of monoamniotic twins at some point. This is usually present from the first trimester.[128,129] The two umbilical cords may insert close to one another, although this may also be seen with monochorionic-diamniotic gestations.

In the first trimester, identification of two yolk sacs in monochorionic twins permits the diagnosis of diamniotic twins even before the amniotic membrane can be imaged (Fig. 10), whereas a single yolk sac is seen with monoamniotic or conjoined twins (Fig. 29). However, a single yolk sac

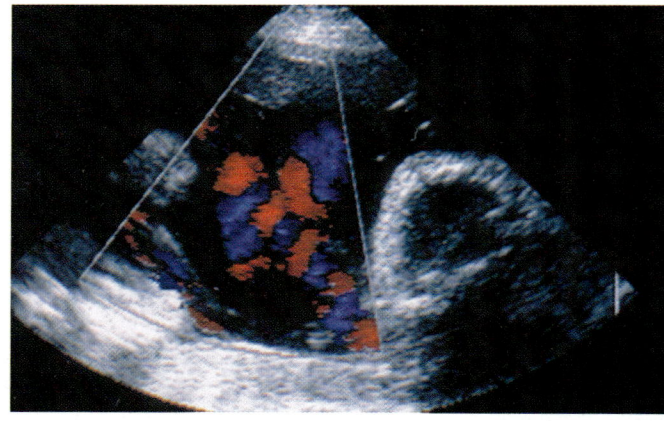

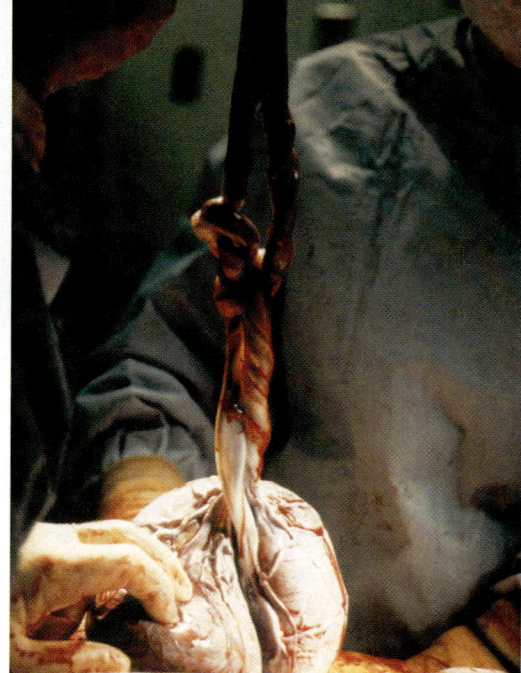

FIGURE 28. Cord entanglement, monoamniotic twins. **A:** Color-flow Doppler image shows entangled umbilical cords. **B:** Photograph at delivery. Both twins were delivered without complication.

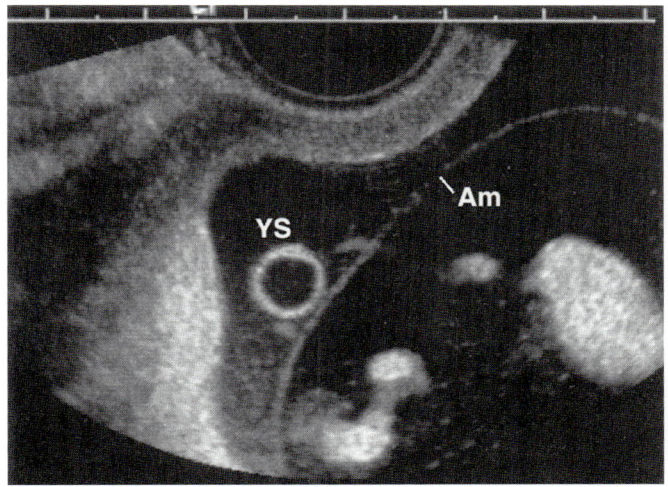

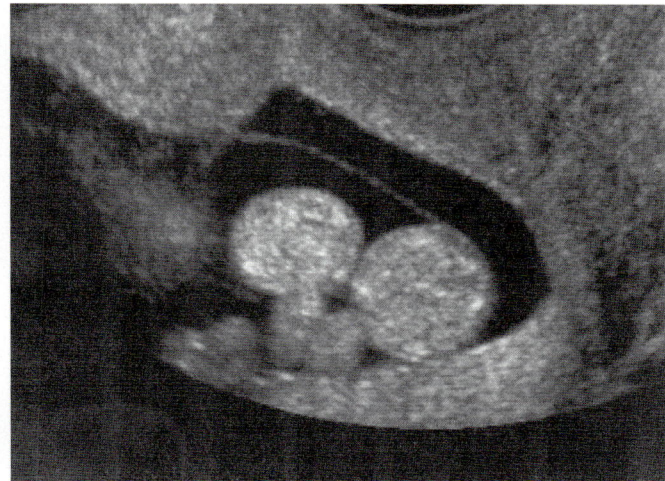

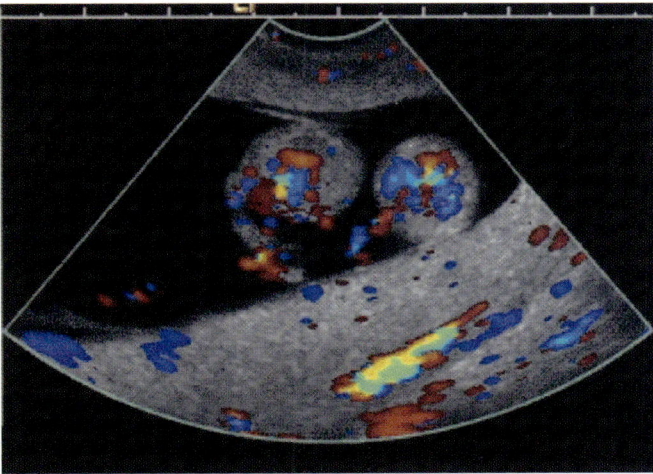

FIGURE 29. Monoamniotic gestation with single yolk sac at 10.5 weeks. **A:** Yolk sac (*YS*) and single amnion (*Am*). **B:** Two adjacent fetuses are nearly touching. **C:** Color-flow Doppler image shows two adjacent umbilical cords. (Courtesy of Gerald Mulligan, MD.)

is not specific during early pregnancy since a second yolk sac may be appreciated on a later scan.[130]

Differential Diagnosis

The primary consideration is diamniotic gestation in which case the dividing membrane is simply not visualized, especially when the membrane is oriented parallel to the ultrasound beam. Further scanning in multiple planes and transvaginal scans should show the dividing membrane perpendicular to the ultrasound beam. The stuck twin phenomenon could be mistaken for a monoamniotic gestation because if the amnion is closely applied to the stuck twin, it may be impossible to visualize. In this case, however, the affected fetus is clearly constrained and immobile. Finally, conjoined twins should be considered whenever monoamniotic twins are diagnosed.

Associated Anomalies

Monoamniotic gestations are at risk for conjoined twinning in addition to the increased risk of anomalies seen with monochorionic gestations. TTS is rare in monoamniotic twins.

Prognosis and Management

The fetal loss rate is as high as 50% due to fetal malformations, preterm delivery, and complications arising from the close proximity of the two umbilical cords. However, there is some evidence that current survival rates may be improving. Rodis et al.[131] noted a 70% survival rate for monoamniotic twins with accurate prenatal diagnosis and intensive fetal surveillance. Patients should be counseled of the high risk of sudden, unexpected, and unpreventable fetal death, at the same time noting the more favorable outcomes experienced with modern management.

Cord entanglement is thought to be the underlying mechanism for the majority of fetal losses, and attempts have been made to prevent this complication by the administration to the mother of nonsteroidal antiinflammatory-type therapy during the second trimester to stabilize the fetal lie by reducing the amniotic fluid volume. However, because some degree of cord entanglement probably occurs in all monoamniotic gestations, a more likely cause of fetal death that is sudden and unpredictable is acute hemodynamic imbalance. Serial growth scans and Doppler examinations of the umbilical cords do not seem able to predict or prevent such intrauterine deaths.

Conjoined Twins

Conjoined twins are monochorionic-monoamniotic twins who are fused or partially fused.

Incidence

The reported frequency varies from 1 in 50,000 to 200,000.[132] There is a female predominance as high as 3:1. No association with maternal age, race, parity, or heredity has been observed. The recurrence risk is negligible.[133,134]

Pathology

The traditional theory is that conjoined twins represent delayed separation of the embryonic mass after day 12 of fertilization. However, an alternate theory is that it represents partial fusion of two separate embryos.[135] This theory may better explain the pathologic spectrum of conjoined twinning. Furthermore, the types of fusion can be explained by fusion of the embryonic disks on the surface of a single sphere (yolk sac).

Classification of Conjoined Twins

A variety of terms have been used to describe the pathologic features of conjoined twinning:

- *Duplicata incompleta*: duplication occurring in only one part or region of the body. Examples include diprosopus (one body, one head, two faces),[136,137] dicephalus (one body, two heads), and dipygus (one head, thorax, and abdomen with two pelvises and/or external genitalia).[138]
- *Duplicata completa*: two relatively complete conjoined twins.
- *Terata catadidyma*: fusion in the lower part of the body. Examples include ischiopagus (fusion of the inferior portion of the coccyx and sacrum) and pygopagus (fusion of the lateral and posterior portions of the coccyx and sacrum).
- *Terata anadidyma*: fusion in the upper part of the body. Examples include syncephalus (fusion of the face) and craniopagus (fusion at homologous portion of the cranial vault).
- *Terata anacatadidyma*: fusion in the midpart of the body. Examples include thoracopagus (fusion of the thoracic wall), xiphopagus (fusion at the xiphoid process),[139] omphalopagus (fusion between the xiphoid and umbilicus), and rachipagus (fusion of spines above the sacrum).

In one attempt to universalize the current nomenclature, a modified classification was proposed, based on the theoretic site of union[140] (Fig. 30):

Ventral union: twins united along the ventral aspect.
  Cephalopagus: fused from the top of the head down to the umbilicus. Two rudimentary (fused) faces, four arms, and four legs. Lower abdomen and pelvis are separated.[141] The cephalothoracopagus Janiceps type is a rare variety of conjoined twins in which the fetuses are joined face to face, the face of each fetus being split in the midline with half turned outward, so that each observed face is made up of the right face of one fetus and the left face of the other. The name originates from Janus, in Roman mythology, the god of gates and doorways, his statue with two faces, facing east and west for the beginning and ending of the day; and caput, head.[142,143]
  Omphalopagus: joined face-to-face primarily in the area of the umbilicus and sometimes involving the lower thorax, but always preserving two distinct hearts. There is not even a cardiac vessel in common. Two pelvises, four arms, and four legs.[144,145]
  Ischiopagus: united ventrally from the umbilicus to a large conjoined pelvis with two sacrums and two symphyses pubis. They appear more frequently joined end-to-end with the spine in a straight line, but they can also present face-to-face with a joined abdomen. Four arms, four legs, and, in general, single external genitalia and a single anus.
Lateral union: twins joined side-by-side with shared umbilicus, abdomen, and pelvis.
  Parapagus: twins that share a conjoined pelvis, one symphysis pubis, and one or two sacrums. When the union is limited to the abdomen and pelvis (does not involve the thorax), it is called *dithoracic parapagus*. If there is one trunk with two heads, it is called *dicephalic parapagus*. If there is a single trunk and a single head with two faces, they are *diprosopic parapagus*. Two, three, or four arms and two or three legs.
Dorsal union: twins joined at the dorsal aspect of the primitive embryonic disc, with no involvement of thorax and abdomen.
  Craniopagus: united on any portion of the skull except the face or foramen magnum. They share bones of the cranium, meninges, and occasionally brain surface. Two trunks, four arms, and four legs.[146]
  Pygopagus: share dorsally the sacrococcygeal and perineal regions and occasionally the spinal cord. One anus, two rectums, four arms, and four legs.
  Rachipagus: twins fused dorsally above the sacrum, involving different segments of the column. This type is extremely rare.

Diagnosis

The diagnosis of conjoined twins can be made as early as the first trimester, and three-dimensional ultrasound has

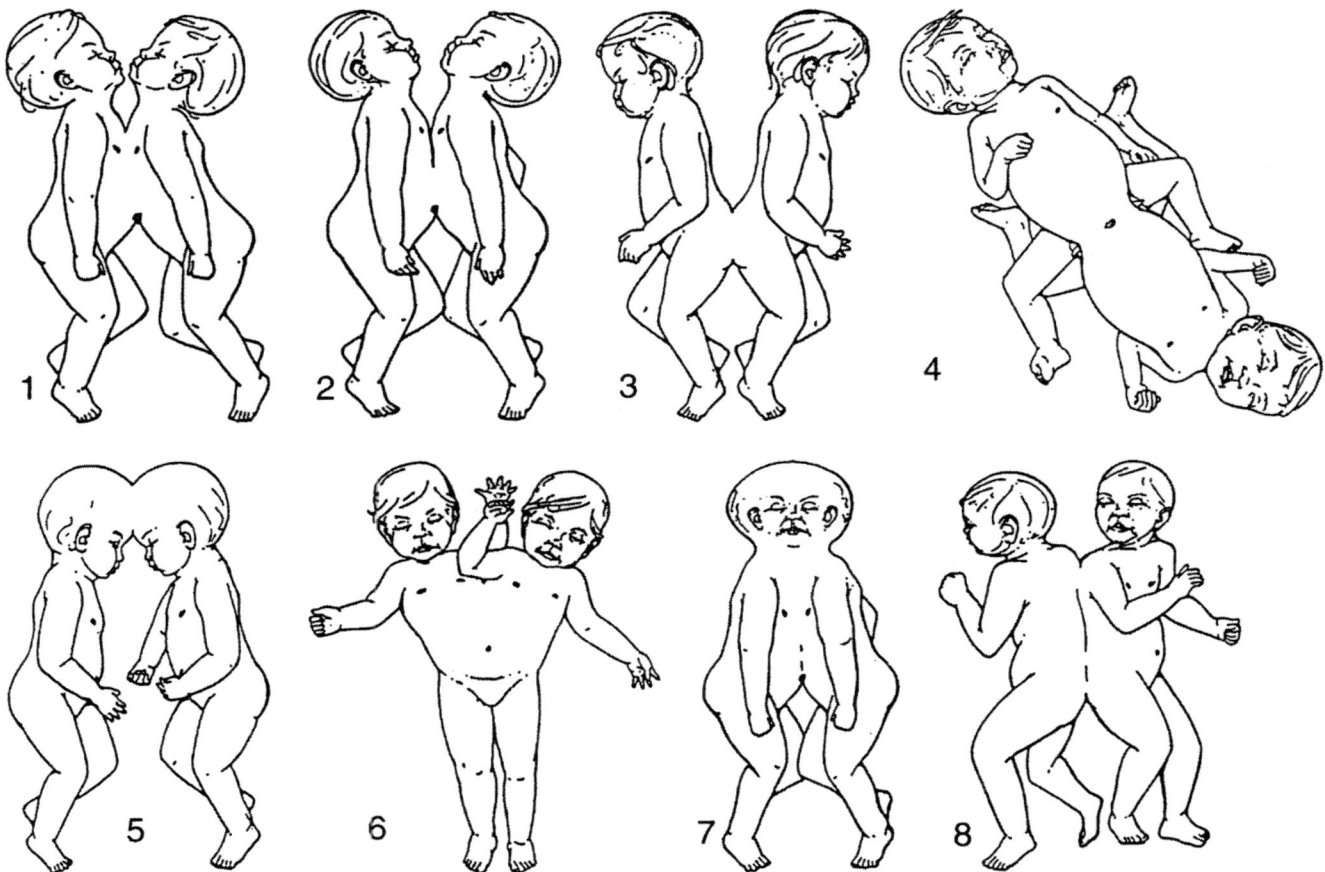

FIGURE 30. Different types of conjoined twins. 1, thoracopagus; 2, omphalopagus; 3, pygopagus; 4, ischiopagus; 5, craniopagus; 6, parapagus; 7, cephalopagus; 8, rachipagus. (Adapted from Spencer.)

also been used at this time.[147–149] Sonographic findings are a monoamniotic twin pregnancy in which the fetal bodies are in an unusual close apposition with fusion at some site[150] (Fig. 31). Various clues that may be seen with conjoined twins include visualization of the heads and bodies of both twins at the same level[151] (Figs. 31 through 33), unusual extension of the spines (Fig. 32), or the presence of a single heart. An abnormal number of vessels (more than three) in the umbilical cord is also seen only with conjoined twins (Fig. 34).

Once conjoined twins have been diagnosed, characterization of the type and severity of the abnormality can be performed with ultrasound, include three-dimensional ultrasound,[152–155] computed tomography, or magnetic resonance imaging[156,157] (Fig. 35).

Differential Diagnosis

Conjoined twins have a unique presentation, and the differential diagnosis can include teratoma or fetus *in fetu*.

Monochorionic-monoamniotic twins are in close proximity to one another but are not fused at any site.

Associated Syndromes

Despite genetic identity, conjoined twins often have discordant anomalies and these more commonly affect the right twin than the left.[135] Congenital anomalies of organs other than the shared ones are present in 50% of cases of conjoined twins. Cardiac defects are the most common association (20% to 30%), and thus echocardiography is recommended in all cases. Neural tube defects and midline fusion defects, orofacial clefts, imperforate anus, and diaphragmatic hernia are also frequently seen. Polyhydramnios is observed in 50% to 75% of cases.

Prognosis

Most conjoined twins are born prematurely, 40% are stillborn, and 35% die within 24 hours.[158] Among the survivors, the

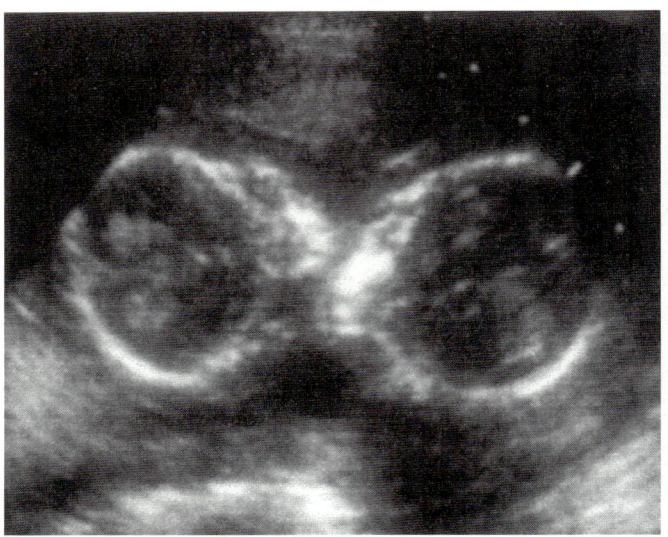

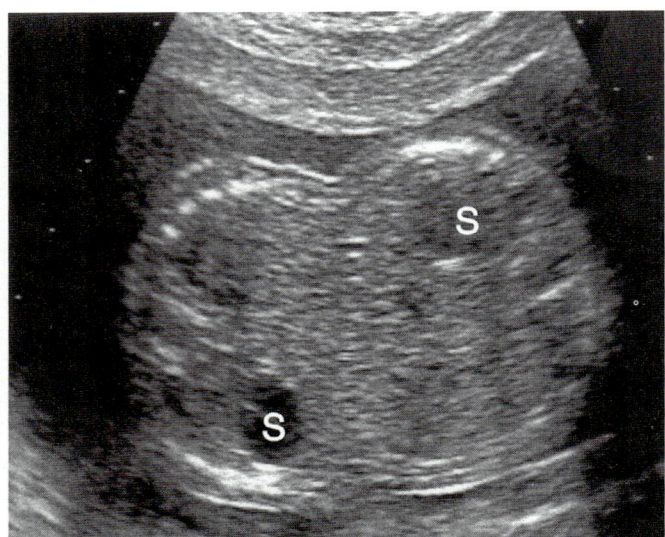

A   B

FIGURE 31. Omphalopagus conjoined twins. **A:** The faces are turned toward each other and are seen at the same level. **B:** Fusion of the abdomen is noted. Note the stomach (*S*) bubbles in diagonal positions.

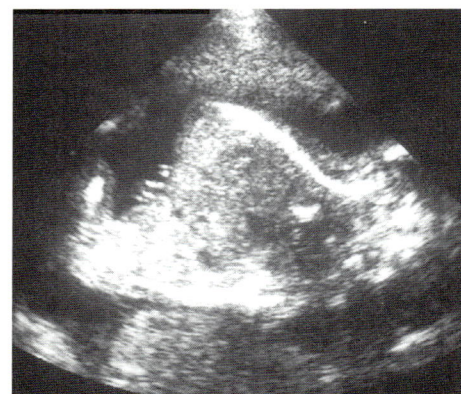

A

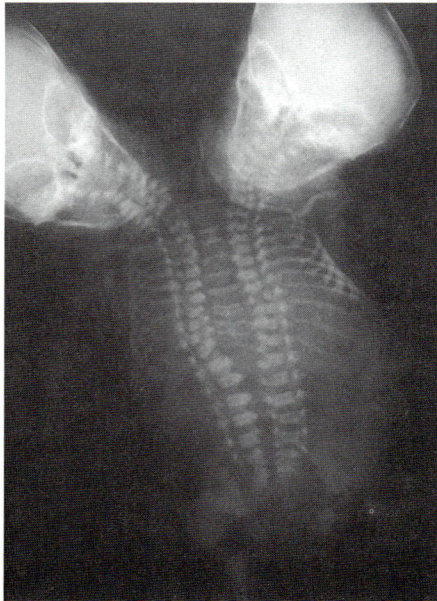

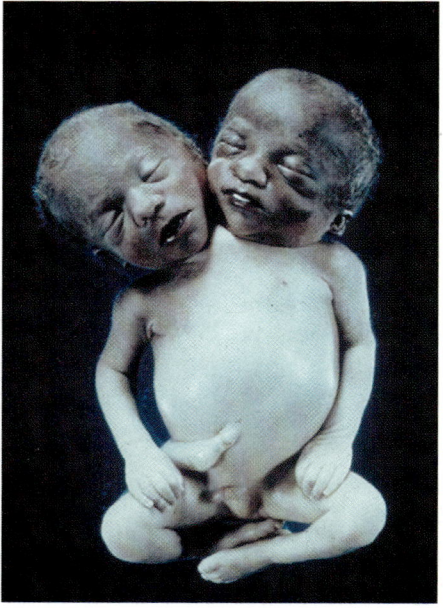

B,C

FIGURE 32. Conjoined twins at the thorax and abdomen. **A:** A coronal scan through the twins shows that they are conjoined at the thorax and abdomen. **B:** Radiograph of the conjoined twins after delivery. **C:** Pathologic photograph correlates with sonographic findings.

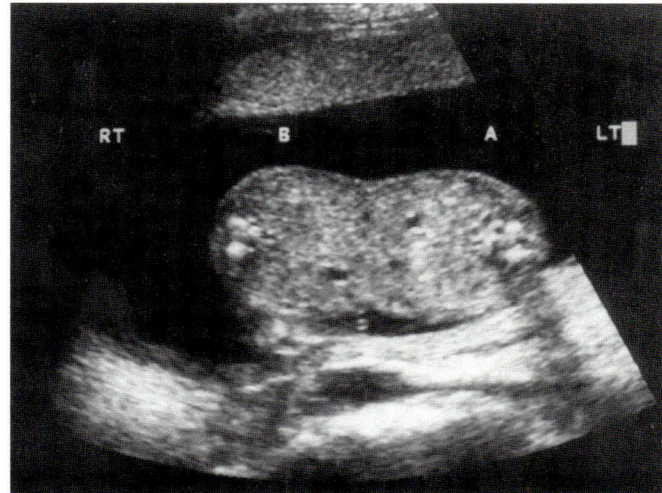

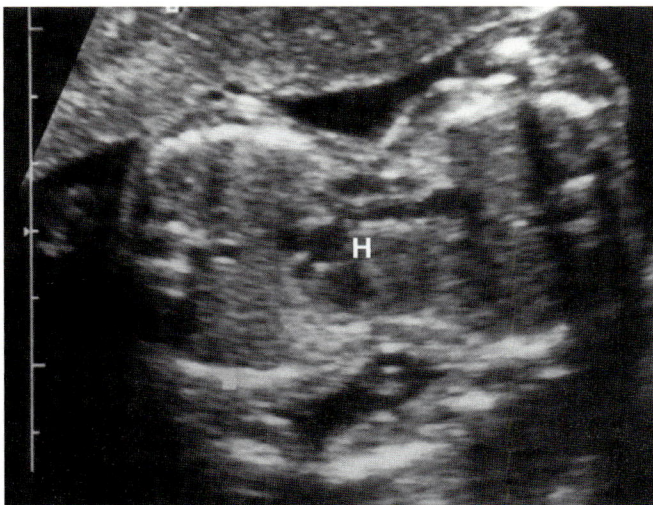

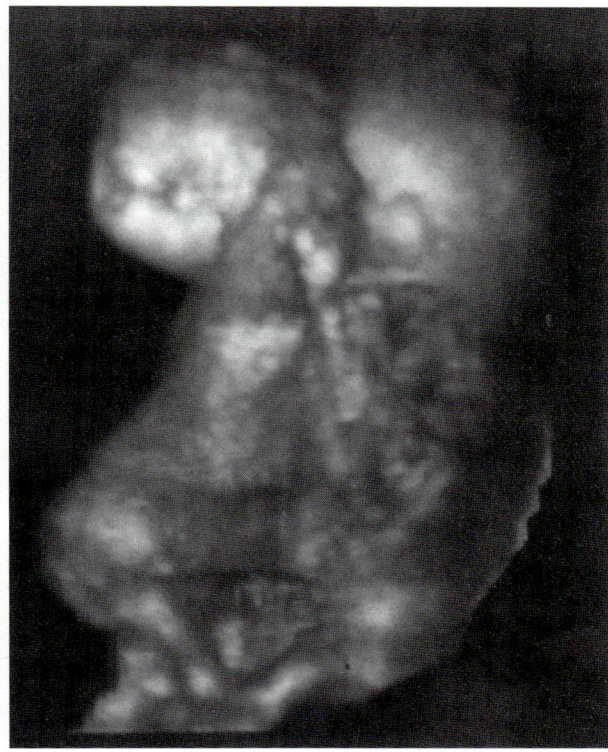

FIGURE 33. Conjoined twins at 19 weeks. The twins (*A, B*) are conjoined in the abdomen **(A)** and in the heart **(B)**. A shared heart (*H*) in conjoined twins is a sign of nonoperability. Three-dimensional ultrasound imaging **(C)** is helpful in demonstrating the twins to the parents. The twins can be seen facing each other in this image. LT, left; RT, right.

prognosis as well as attempts of surgical separation depend on the type of conjunction, degree of involvement of the shared organs, and the presence of associated anomalies.[159] One-third of those born alive have severe defects for which surgery is not possible. In liveborn cases in whom planned surgery is carried out, approximately 60% of infants survive.[160,161]

The most ominous prognosis is among those twins who share a liver or heart, or both. Attempts of separation in cases of a common liver can be undertaken as long as two biliary tracts are seen. In the presence of a shared heart, separation is only attempted if two normal hearts coexist in a single pericardium.[162,163]

Management

Termination of pregnancy can be offered.[147,164–167] The method of choice for delivery is cesarean to maximize survival and prevent maternal and fetal trauma.[168,169] The ideal is elective surgery at 6–12 months of age to allow time for growth, tissue expansion, and accurate imaging demonstra-

tion of the anatomic union and associated anomalies to aid surgical planning.[161] The goal of separation is the survival of one or both twins with a reasonable quality of life.

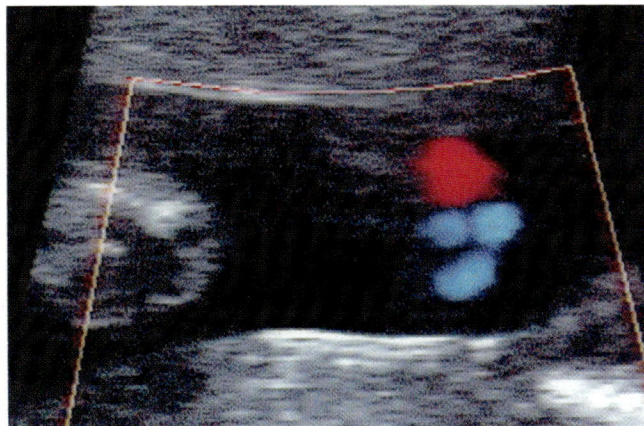

FIGURE 34. The presence of more than three vessels in a cord is a strong marker of conjoined twins.

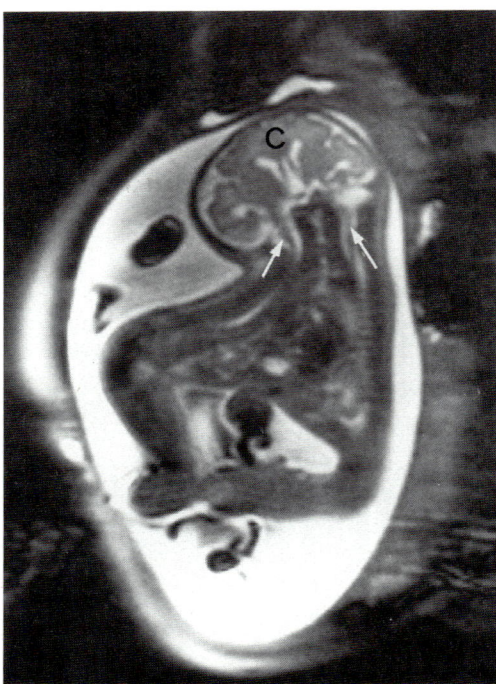

FIGURE 35. Magnetic resonance imaging (MRI) of conjoined twins. The twins are conjoined at the head, thorax, and abdomen. MRI can assist in defining the conjoined anatomy. Separate spinal cords (*arrows*) are identified with a single cerebrum (*C*). (Reproduced with permission from Poutamo J, Vanninen R, Partanen K, Ryynanen, Kirkinen P. Magnetic resonance imaging supplements ultrasonographic imaging of the posterior fossa, pharynx and neck in malformed fetuses. *Ultrasound Obstet Gynecol* 1999;13:327–334.)

Twin-Reversed Arterial Perfusion Sequence/Acardiac Twin

The most extreme manifestation of TTS is acardiac twinning (acardius chorioangiopagus parasiticus). This twin disorder has also been named *twin-reversed arterial perfusion* sequence to explain the underlying mechanism (Fig. 36).

Incidence

Twin-reversed arterial perfusion occurs in 1% of monochorionic twin pregnancies, or 1 in 35,000 pregnancies.[170]

Pathology

The acardiac twin may be considered a parasite[171,172] because it requires blood pumped from the normal twin to keep developing, putting the pump fetus at risk for high-output cardiac failure.[173] The mechanism that has been proposed is the association of paired artery-to-artery and vein-to-vein anastomoses through the placenta combined

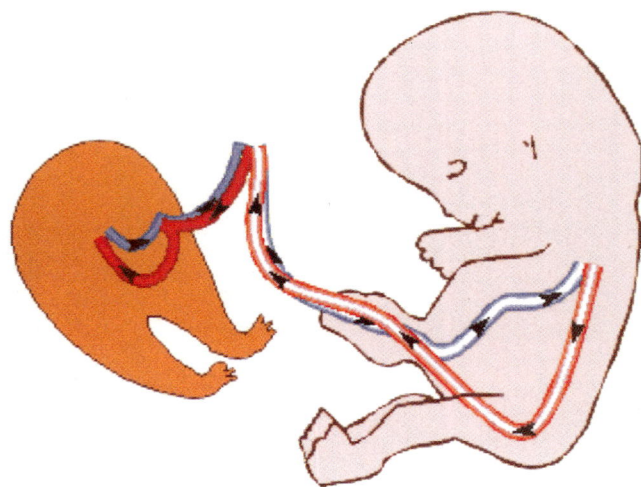

FIGURE 36. In the twin-reversed arterial perfusion syndrome, the acardiac twin receives retrograde perfusion with poorly oxygenated blood.

with delayed cardiac function of one of the twins early in pregnancy.[41,170,174–179]

If one twin develops more slowly, the imbalance in the blood pressure of the twins will result in a retrograde transfer of blood from the healthy twin to the abnormal twin. The retrograde flow of poorly oxygenated blood through the developing heart of the abnormal twin further interferes with development of the heart so that it rarely progresses beyond a rudimentary stage of development.

The pathologic appearance of acardiac twins varies considerably[180] (Figs. 37 and 38) and has been categorized by various terms (Table 3).

In general, the upper half of the body of an acardiac twin is extremely poorly developed and, sometimes, not developed at all. The head, cervical spine, and upper limbs are usually absent. Edema and sonolucent areas in the upper body, consistent with cystic hygroma, are common. In contrast, the lower half of the body, although malformed, is better developed. This pattern of development may be explained by the mechanism of perfusion of the acardiac twin. Blood that enters the abdomen of the fetus is deoxygenated blood from the normal pump twin. The morphologic abnormalities in the acardiac twin are consistent with perfusion of tissues supplied by the common iliac and lower branches of the aorta with deoxygenated blood. Most of the oxygen available is extracted when the blood enters the acardiac twin, allowing for some development of the lower body and extremities. Lower pressure in the upper half of the body due to retrograde perfusion, combined with low oxygen saturation, impairs the development of this area.

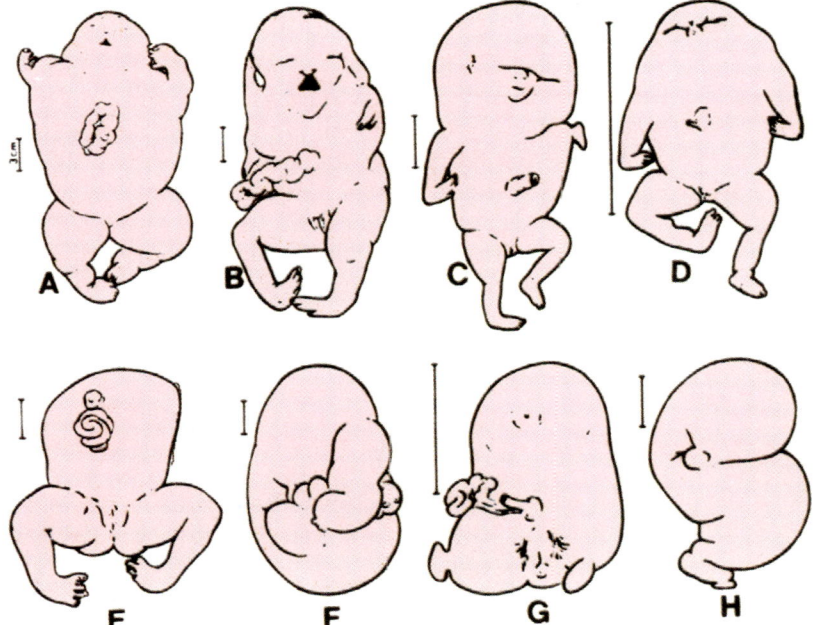

FIGURE 37. Representative examples of acardiac twins with gradation of loss of normal form and relative sparing of the lower body. **A:** Anencephaly, midline cleft lip and palate, microphthalmos, radial aplasia, limb reductions, oligodactyly, and syndactyly. **B:** Anencephaly, midline cleft lip and palate, microphthalmos, gastroschisis, phocomelia, and oligodactyly. **C:** Microphthalmos, radial aplasia, phocomelia, and oligodactyly. **D:** Cyclopia, omphalocele, radial aplasia, oligodactyly, absent cranial vault, clubfeet, and marked edema. **E:** Absent head, thorax, and arms with omphalocele, clubfeet, and oligodactyly. **F:** Absent cranial end with partial abdominal cavity, omphalocele, reduced lower limbs, oligodactyly, and syndactyly. **G:** Absent cranium, minimal thorax, omphalocele, herniation of the gut from the umbilicus, cloacal exstrophy, and skin tags suggestive of limbs. **H:** Hemipelvis, single leg with single toe, omphalocele, and complete absence of thoracic and cranial structures. [Adapted from Van Allen MI, Smith DW, Shepard TH. Twin reversed arterial perfusion (TRAP) sequence: a study of 14 twin pregnancies with acardius. *Semin Perinatol* 1983;7:285–293.]

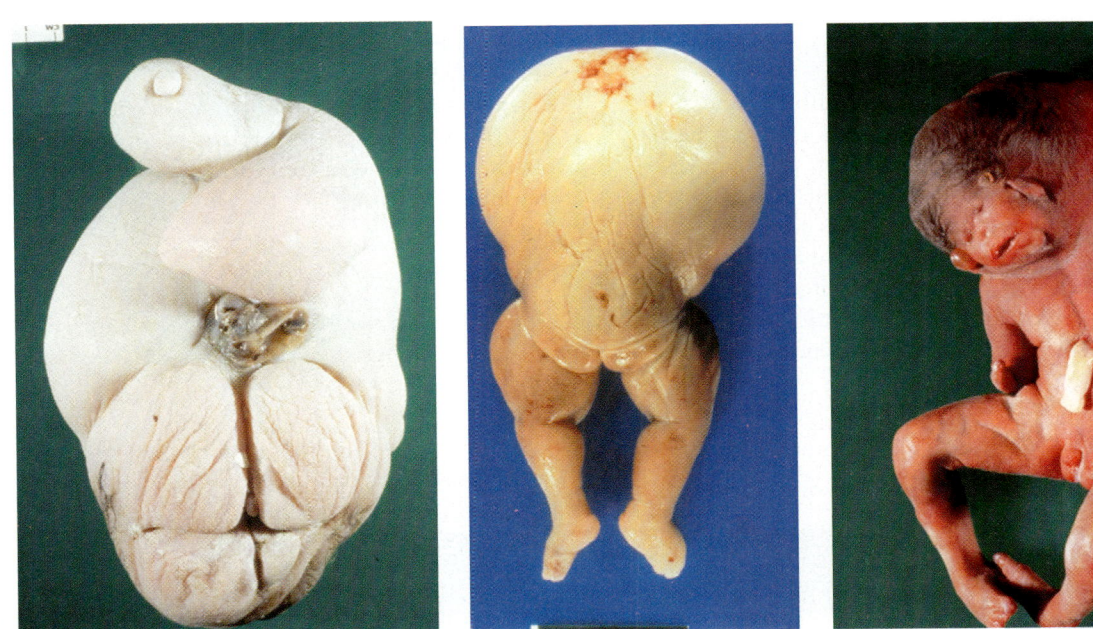

FIGURE 38. **A–C:** Pathologic photographs showing variable development of acardiac twins.

TABLE 3. DESCRIPTION OF ACARDIAC TWINS

Malformation	Description
Acephalus	No cephalic structure present[255]
Anceps	Some cranial structure and or neural tissue present[256]
Acormus	Cephalic structure but no truncal structures
Amorphus	No distinguishable rostral or caudal structure[257]

Some believe the underlying mechanism for development of acardiac twinning is separate fertilization of the polar body and subsequent development as a separate cell mass.[181] Although this might occur rarely, this proposed mechanism does not adequately explain the vast majority of cases. Using DNA fingerprinting patterns, Fisk et al.[182] concluded that affected twins are truly monozygous and calculated the probability of polar body fertilization as the underlying etiology as less than 0.001%.

The reason for discordant chromosomal abnormalities in this subset of monozygotic twins is uncertain. Although fertilization of the polar body could explain some cases, chromosome abnormalities could also be explained postfertilization by nondisjunction.

Diagnosis

The sonographic diagnosis is characterized by a fetus that moves and grows (Fig. 39) but has no effective heart motion of its own. The abnormal fetus presents with impaired or absent development of the cephalic pole, heart, upper limbs, and many viscera. The lower limbs are relatively well preserved, although clubbing and abnormal toes are common. Marked skin thickening, hydrops, and cystic hygroma may be present, and these tend to worsen as the pregnancy progresses (Fig. 40). The appearance is so

pathognomonic that the diagnosis has been made as early as 10 weeks.[183]

Doppler studies show pathognomonic features of reversed arterial perfusion (Fig. 41). Arterial blood flows toward the acardiac twin within the umbilical artery, usually entering the hypogastric artery but occasionally the superior mesenteric artery. Venous blood flow takes the opposite direction, exiting the acardiac twin.[115,184–188] Therefore, the flow direction of both the umbilical artery and vein are reversed from the normal situation.

The pump twin may appear normal or may show signs of congestive heart failure, including hydrops and polyhydramnios.

Differential Diagnosis

TTS can be distinguished by cardiac activity in the smaller fetus. The acardiac twin can be mistaken for fetal demise,[189] although observation reveals fetal activity and growth in the acardiac twin.

Associated Anomalies

The umbilical cord of the acardiac fetus has a single umbilical artery in most cases (66%).[190] Velamentous cord insertions are more common in acardiac twins, as in all monochorionic pregnancies.

Chromosomal abnormalities have been found in 33% of acardiac twins.[191–193] This supports as a possible etiologic factor that aneuploidies could lead to slower development of the abnormal twin.[194]

Prognosis

Acardiac twins have 100% mortality,[41] and the pump twin is also at high risk of demise secondary to congestive

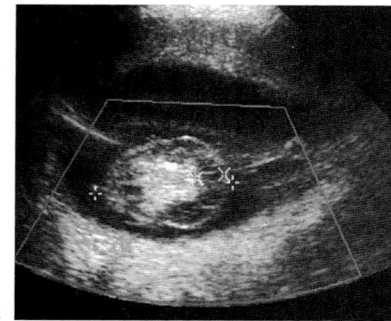
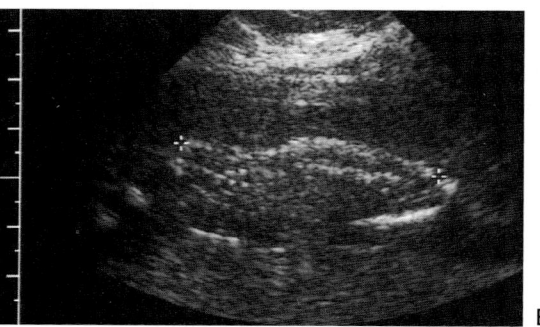

FIGURE 39. Acardiac twin. **A:** A scan at 14 weeks shows amorphous acardiac fetus measuring 2.9 cm in length. **B:** In a follow-up scan 5 weeks later, the acardiac fetus measures 5 cm in length. A well-defined spine is also apparent.

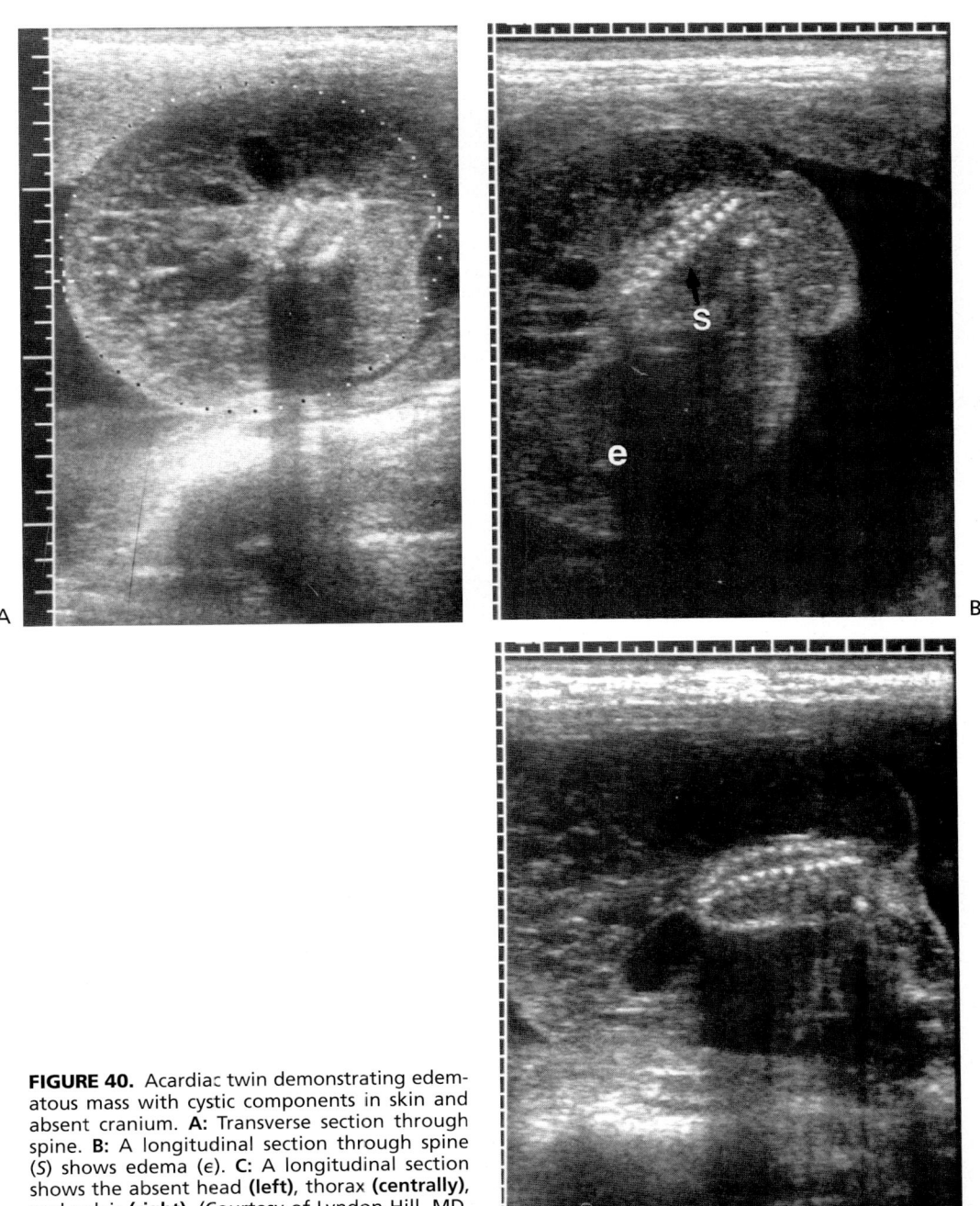

FIGURE 40. Acardiac twin demonstrating edematous mass with cystic components in skin and absent cranium. **A:** Transverse section through spine. **B:** A longitudinal section through spine (*S*) shows edema (*e*). **C:** A longitudinal section shows the absent head **(left)**, thorax **(centrally)**, and pelvis **(right)**. (Courtesy of Lyndon Hill, MD, Pittsburgh, PA.)

heart failure or severe preterm delivery, the consequence of polyhydramnios.[195–198] The risk is directly dependent on the size of the acardiac twin: the higher the weight of the acardiac twin, the higher the risk of cardiac failure and death for the normal twin.

Management

Management includes conservative and invasive therapies. Conservative management includes serial cardiotocography, ultrasonography, and echocardiography and opportune delivery. Noninvasive therapies may be used to support the cardiac function of the pump twin with digoxin and indomethacin. The more invasive form of management consists of termination of pregnancy or interruption of flow to the acardiac fetus by surgical extraction (hysterotomy with selective delivery of the acardiac twin) and ligation of the acardiac twin's umbilical cord,[199,200] ultrasound-guided embolization of the cardiac twin's umbilical artery with absolute alcohol,[201,202] platinum or thrombogenic coils, and laser vaporization.[203,204] Large numbers are not available to compare the various techniques.

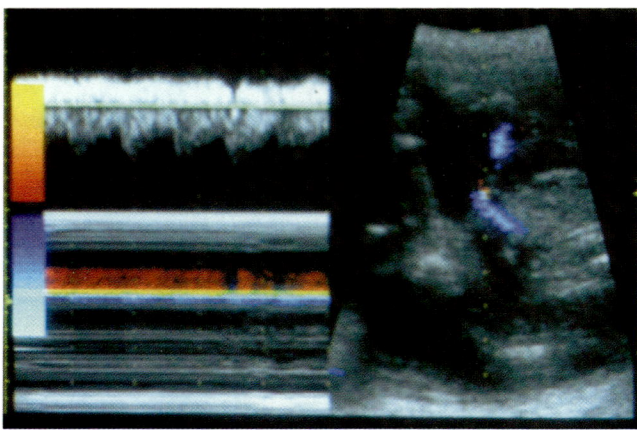

FIGURE 41. Reverse flow on pulsed/color Doppler image: arterial flow in the vessel going in (under the baseline) and venous flow in the vessel going out (above the baseline) in an acardiac twin.

Fetus *In Fetu*

In fetus *in fetu*, a nearly intact but malformed, demised fetus is located within a normal live fetus.

Incidence

Fetus *in fetu* is rare.

Pathology

The fetus *in fetu* contains well-organized fetal structures and all three somatic lines and may be difficult to distinguish from a well-formed teratoma. However, accepted criteria for fetus *in fetu* include the presence of a vertebral axis. Fetus *in fetu* and teratoma may also coexist.[205] Some cases have a surrounding sac and even an umbilical cord.[206] Associated anomalies are routine.

The most common location is within the abdomen. However, multiple other sites have been reported, including intracranial, sacral, and gonadal locations.[207]

Diagnosis

May present prenatally or after birth.[208–213] A number of cases have been diagnosed. The most common description has been an intraabdominal mass, but other sites including intracranial masses have also been described (Fig. 42). Jones et al.[214] described a highly developed case that showed spontaneous movement of the extremities.

Differential Diagnosis

The primary consideration is a teratoma, and it may be impossible to distinguish the two.[215] This includes sacrococcygeal teratoma when it extends to the presacral area.[216] It has also been mistaken for meconium pseudocyst when in the abdomen.[217]

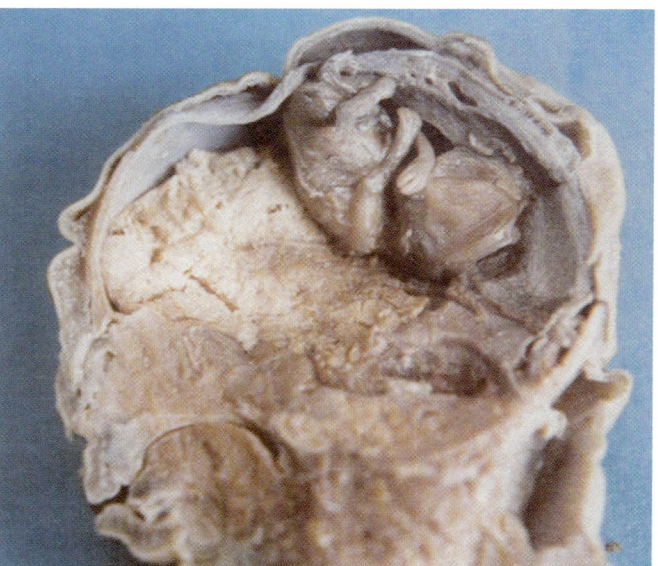

FIGURE 42. Fetus *in fetu*. **A:** A scan of the cranium at 17 weeks shows no normal anatomy. The echogenic area (*arrow*) was observed to have a heartbeat of 70 beats per minute. **B:** A pathologic photograph shows a small, well-formed fetus in the posterior head. [Reproduced with permission from Ianniruberto A, Rossi P, Ianniruberto M, Rella G, Ciminelli V. Sonographic prenatal diagnosis of intracranial fetus *in fetu. Ultrasound Obstet Gynecol* 2001;18(1):67–68.]

Prognosis and Management

The prognosis is highly variable, depending on the location and rate of growth. Many cases are discovered in children or even adults as slowly growing masses.[218–220] Management is surgical resection whenever possible. Malignant recurrence has been reported following resection.[221]

PROCEDURES RELATED TO MULTIPLE GESTATIONS

Procedures that require special consideration in multiple pregnancies include genetic amniocentesis, chorionic villous sampling, multifetal pregnancy reduction, therapeutic amniocentesis for TTS, and more specialized procedures such as laser coagulation of anastomotic vessels.

Genetic Testing

Prenatal genetic testing in twin pregnancies requires special considerations (see also Considerations in Screening of Twin Pregnancies for Chromosomal Abnormalities). When deciding between amniocentesis and CVS in twin pregnancies, the relative safety of the procedures, certainty of sampling both fetuses, and likely subsequent management affect the choice of technique. These procedures in twin pregnancies should be performed in a specialist center. When genetic amniocentesis of a twin pregnancy includes sampling of each fetus, it is important to ensure that amniotic fluid from each sac corresponds to the appropriate fetus and that each sample is appropriately labeled. Amniocentesis is most commonly performed by two uterine insertions of the needle with or without intraamniotic dye injection, but it can also be performed with a single-needle technique in some cases.[222–224]

CVS has been carried out in multiple pregnancies with similar loss rates to those in singletons.[225–229] However, with CVS there is a risk of sampling the same placenta twice, especially when the placentas are on the same side of the uterus, and CVS in twins requires an extremely high degree of expertise in ultrasonography and invasive procedures. In twin pregnancies midtrimester amniocentesis has the advantage that both amniotic sacs can be safely sampled through a single uterine entry; however, when there is discordance for a chromosomal abnormality, selective feticide must be carried out after 18 to 20 weeks, when the risk of procedure-related miscarriage is higher than in early pregnancy.[230,231] Therefore, CVS may be the preferred option for pregnancies at high risk of chromosomal defects since if selective feticide is required it can be carried out in the first trimester, whereas amniocentesis would be preferable if the risk was low and feticide would therefore be unlikely. In pregnancies discordant for fetal trisomy, management options include either selective feticide or expectant management, the decision being based on the relative risk of selective feticide causing miscarriage and hence death of the normal baby, compared to the potential burden of caring for a handicapped child. Selective feticide may be the option of choice in most pregnancies discordant for fetal trisomy 21, whereas with trisomy 18, expectant management is more common since babies with trisomy 18 inevitably die either *in utero* or within the first year of life.

Multifetal Pregnancy Reduction

Assisted reproduction techniques rely on inducing multiple ovulations with or without the transfer of more than one embryo into the uterine cavity; therefore the multiple pregnancy rate with such techniques is increased to approximately 20%.[4] The number of transferred embryos is not the only factor significantly related to the risk of multiple pregnancy: Male infertility, cleavage rates over 50%, and the woman's age (at young ages multiple pregnancy rates are higher) were also significant in assisted reproduction programs. The proportion of multiple births attributable to ovulation induction is approximately 10% overall, 5% of twin births, and greater than 70% for triplet or higher-order births.[232,233] Follow-up studies report no significant differences in mortality or morbidity between babies born by assisted reproduction techniques once confounding factors are taken into account, the additional risks being the consequence of multiple pregnancy.[234] Assisted reproductive techniques have therefore been associated with an exponential increase in the prevalence of multifetal pregnancies and therefore risks of both miscarriage and perinatal death.[235] One option of management in such cases is iatrogenic embryo reduction, which attempts to improve pregnancy outcome by reducing these risks and is now a well-recognized intervention in such cases. Multifetal reduction is an efficient and safe way of improving outcome in multifetal pregnancies, unambiguously for quadruplets or higher orders.[231,236–239]

Iatrogenic fetal death is achieved by the ultrasound-guided puncture of the fetal heart and injection of potassium chloride. The needle can be introduced transabdominally or transvaginally, but the latter may be associated with a higher rate of miscarriage,[230] although some series suggest that in appropriately trained centers the risk may be similar for the two techniques.[231] During the 3 to 4 months after reduction the dead fetuses and their placentas are gradually resorbed.

It is technically feasible to perform reduction from as early as 7 weeks of gestation, and the earlier the gestation the smaller the dead fetoplacental tissue mass, with the theoretic advantage of a lower rate of miscarriage. However, it is preferable to delay the procedure until 11 to 13 weeks to allow for spontaneous reduction. Furthermore, at this gestational age it is possible to diagnose major fetal abnormalities and, through measurement of NT thickness, to screen for chromosomal defects. If all fetuses appear to be normal, the ones chosen for reduction are those farthest away from the cervix to avoid the potential risk of amniorrhexis and ascending infection from the lower genital tract. Overall results report that miscarriage occurs before 24 weeks in approximately 12% of cases, severe preterm delivery at 24 to 32 weeks is seen in 13%, and delivery is after 32 weeks in 75%, but the miscarriage rate and severe preterm delivery rate are related to both the starting and finishing number of fetuses.[231] There are essentially two mechanisms by which embryo reduction can result in miscarriage. First, early loss, within 2 weeks of the procedure, may be as a direct result of intrauterine needling in a similar way to loss following other invasive intrauterine procedures such as early amniocentesis.[240] A more likely explanation for the majority of spontaneous miscarriages, which occur weeks or even months after reduction, and severe preterm delivery, is the development of an inflammatory response to the resorbing dead fetoplacental tissue with release of cytokines and subsequent stimulation of prostaglandins. A final hypothesis is that the pregnancy losses following reduction are the result of placental endocrine disturbances. It is possible that in the human the maximum capacity of the endometrium/decidua to maintain a pregnancy is achieved with twins; in multifetal pregnancies there is crowding and each fetal-placental-endometrial unit has less potential for growth and development than in twin pregnancies. After embryo reduction the surviving twins have smaller placental units and therefore remain at a disadvantage compared to natural twins, and this manifests as spontaneous abortion or severe preterm delivery.

Although in higher-order multifetal pregnancies there is evidence that embryo reduction to twins is associated with a decrease in the background risk of miscarriage and perinatal death, the situation for triplet pregnancies is less clear. Reduction is associated with an upward shift of the gestational age at delivery but is also associated with a procedure-related loss rate (Fig. 43).

From the combined data of 19 studies, it was estimated that fetal reduction from trichorionic triplets to twins is associated with a significantly higher rate of miscarriage (8% vs. 4%) but a threefold reduction in the rate of severe preterm delivery and consequent death and handicap. Thus, the chances of survival are similar with or without reduction, but there may be a small reduction in the risk of severe handicap in reduced pregnancies.[241]

Chorionicity determination is of vital importance before discussion regarding fetal reduction since in dichorionic triplets, for example, selective feticide of one of the monochorionic pair may lead to death or neurologic sequelae in the co-twin (see Twin "Embolization" Syndrome), whereas iatrogenic death of the fetus with a separate placenta results in a monochorionic twin pregnancy that is associated with a much higher risk of miscarriage or severe preterm delivery than dichorionic twins (see Twin "Embolization" Syndrome).

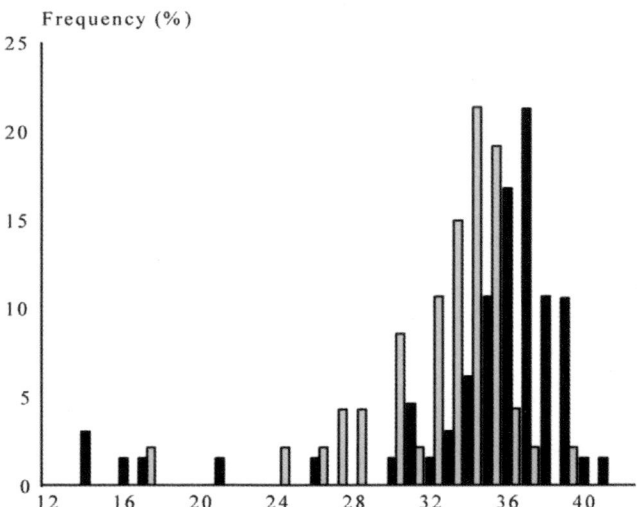

FIGURE 43. Gestational age distribution at delivery of trichorionic triplet pregnancies managed expectantly (*blue bars*) and those reduced to twins (*black bars*). (Adapted from Sebire et al.)

Selective Feticide for Anomalies

Multiple pregnancies discordant for a fetal abnormality can essentially be managed expectantly or by selective feticide of the abnormal twin. In cases in which the abnormality is nonlethal but may well result in handicap, the parents need to decide whether the potential burden of a handicapped child is enough to risk loss of the normal twin from feticide-related complications. In cases in which the abnormality is lethal it may be best to avoid such risk to the normal fetus, unless the condition itself threatens the survival of the normal twin. This management dilemma is exemplified by pregnancies discordant for anencephaly, which is always lethal but may be associated with the development of polyhydramnios, which places the normal co-twin at risk of neonatal death from severe preterm delivery.

Selective feticide is contraindicated in monochorionic twin gestations because vascular anastomoses across the common placenta lead to increased risk of death or twin embolization syndrome in the normal co-twin. When the procedure is performed, it is carried out in the same manner as for multifetal pregnancy reduction, with intracardiac or intrathoracic injection of potassium chloride.

Therapeutic Amnioreduction

Serial amnioreduction is the most widely used therapy for pregnancies complicated by TTS. Amnioreduction not only improves polyhydramnios in the polyhydramniotic sac, it commonly improves amniotic fluid in the oligohydramniotic sac.[242] This can be explained by relief of the pressure of polyhydramnios, which may compress placental vessels and further reduce fetal circulation of the oligohydramniotic sac. This compressive effect is particularly likely for velamentous cord insertions.[107]

The amount of amniotic fluid removed and the number of sessions required vary markedly. Using serial amnioreduction, a multicenter study showed that both fetuses survived in nearly one-half of cases and 70% had survival of at least one twin.[243] However, among survivors, abnormalities on neonatal cranial scan were diagnosed in 24% of recipients and in 25% of donors. The survival rate was related to a number of factors including gestational age at diagnosis, gestational age at delivery, larger birth weight, presence of hydrops, mean volume of amniotic fluid removed per week, and presence of end-diastolic blood flow in the umbilical artery velocity waveforms. The hemoglobin level difference at birth was the only factor associated with abnormal cranial ultrasonography in newborns. Jauniaux et al.[244] suggest that good results, with need for fewer procedures, can be achieved by using a vacuum bottle to drain the polyhydramniotic sac completely. The average volume of fluid drained is 3,252 mL. Ninety-three percent of pregnancies have at least one survivor.

Laser Coagulation

Laser coagulation is the alternative method of treating TTS.[245] Proponents of laser coagulation suggest that it should used for more severe cases presenting before 26 weeks and that amnioreduction be reserved for milder cases or cases presenting later. Certainly, encouraging results have been reported, particularly in reduction of brain injury among survivors.[246] Ongoing randomized trials comparing laser coagulation with therapeutic amnioreduction are not yet available.[247] Laser coagulation may include selection of all vessels crossing the membrane (nonselective) or only specific vessels thought to be anastomotic (selective)[248,249] (Table 4). Anterior placentas present a greater challenge than posterior placentas.[250]

Cord Ligation

Umbilical cord ligation is used to transect the umbilical cord of an anomalous twin. This technique may be used in the setting of a monochorionic twin pregnancy when death

TABLE 4. MANAGEMENT OF TWIN-TWIN TRANSFUSION SYNDROME BY LASER COAGULATION

Study	Study design	Number of cases	Technique	Outcome (n)		Death of both twins	Neurologic handicap in survivors
				Intact survival of twins			
				Both	One		
De Lia et al. 1995[258]	Case series	26	Nd:YAG laser coagulation of the placental vessels crossing the interamniotic membrane	34.6% (9/26)[a]	34.6% (9/26)	30.8% (8/26)	4% (1/28)
Ville et al. 1998[259]	Case series	132	Nd:YAG laser coagulation of the placental vessels crossing the interamniotic membrane	—	—	—	4.2%
Hecher et al. 1999[260]	Comparative study	73	Nd:YAG laser coagulation of the placental vessels crossing the interamniotic membrane	42.5% (31/73)	37.0% (27/73)	20.5% (15/73)	5.6% (5/89)
		43	Serial amniocentesis	41.9% (18/43)	18.6% (8/43)	39.5% (17/43)	18.2% (8/44)[b]
De Lia et al. 1999[261]	Case series	67	Nd:YAG laser coagulation of the placental vessels crossing the interamniotic membrane	56.7% (38/67)	25.4% (17/76)	17.9% (12/76)	4.3% (4/93)
Quintero et al. 2000[262]	Case series	74[c]	Nd:YAG laser coagulation of selected placental vessels appearing as anastomoses by fetoscopy	39.4% (28/71)	43.7% (31/71)	16.9% (12/71)	0.8% (1/128)
Thilaganathan et al. 2000[263]	Case series	10	Nd:YAG laser coagulation of selected placental vessels appearing as anastomoses by fetoscopy and ultrasound	40.0% (4/10)	30.0% (3/10)	30.0% (3/10)[d]	Unknown

Nd:YAG, neodymium:yttrium-aluminum-garnet.
[a]One triplet pregnancy.
[b]Abnormal brain scan in surviving neonates.
[c]Three elective terminations of pregnancy after intervention.
[d]One case of intrauterine death of both twins and two cases of neonatal death of both twins.

appears likely in one fetus. This is most likely in the setting of TTS with hydropic changes in one of the twins. Spontaneous death would produce marked hemodynamic changes in the co-twin through anastomotic vessels, commonly resulting in death or brain injury. The goal of cord ligation is to avoid these complications by completely separating the two circulations.

Cord ligation might also be considered in the setting of a monochorionic or monoamniotic twin pregnancy with lethal anomalies affecting one of the fetuses.[251–254] This has been used most commonly for acardiac twinning. This might help avoid other complications of pregnancy such as polyhydramnios, preterm delivery for monochorionic twins, and cord entanglement for monoamniotic twins.

REFERENCES

1. Benirschke K, Kim CK. Multiple pregnancy, part I. *N Engl J Med* 1973;288:1276–1284.
2. Benirschke K. Multiple gestation: incidence, etiology, and inheritance. In: Creasy RK, Resnik R, eds. *Maternal-fetal medicine. Principles and practice*, 3rd ed. Philadelphia: WB Saunders, 1994:575–588.
3. Tong S, Short RV. Dizygotic twinning as a measure of human fertility. *Hum Reprod* 1998;13(1):95–98.
4. Logerot-Lebrun H, Nicollet B, de Mouzon J, Bachelot A, Pauchard MS, Rufat P. Multiple pregnancy risk factors in medically assisted reproduction. *Contracept Fertil Sex* 1993;21(5):362–366.
5. Sills ES, Tucker MJ, Palermo GD. Assisted reproductive technologies and monozygous twins: implications for future study and clinical practice. *Twin Res* 2000;3(4):217–223.
6. Schieve LA, Meikle SF, Peterson HB, Jeng G, Burnett NM, Wilcox LS. Does assisted hatching pose a risk for monozygotic twinning in pregnancies conceived through in vitro fertilization? *Fertil Steril* 2000;74(2):288–294.
7. Derom C, Derom R, Vlietinck R, Maes H, van den Berghe H. Placentation. In: Keith LG, Papiernik E, Keith DM, Luke B, eds. *Multiple pregnancy*. London: Parthenon Press, 1995:113–128.
8. Botting BJ, Davies IM, Macfarlane AJ. Recent trends in the incidence of multiple births and associated mortality. *Arch Dis Child* 1987;62(9):941–950.
9. Sebire NJ, Snijders RJ, Hughes K, Sepulveda W, Nicolaides KH. The hidden mortality of monochorionic twin pregnancies. *Br J Obstet Gynaecol* 1997;104(10):1203–1207.
10. Cameron AH. The Birmingham twin survey. *Proc R Soc Med* 1968;61(3):229–234.
11. Derom R, Vlietinck R, Derom C, Thiery M, Van Maele G, Van den BH. Perinatal mortality in the East Flanders Prospective Twin Survey (preliminary results). *Eur J Obstet Gynecol Reprod Biol* 1991;41(1):25–26.
12. Machin G, Bamforth F, Innes M, McNichol K. Some perinatal characteristics of monozygotic twins who are dichorionic. *Am J Med Genet* 1995;55(1):71–76.
13. Liu S, Benirschke K, Scioscia AL, Mannino FL. Intrauterine death in multiple gestation. *Acta Genet Med Gemellol* 1992;41:5–26.
14. Mahoney BS, Filly RA, Callen PW. Amnionicity and chorionicity in twin pregnancies: prediction using ultrasound. *Radiology* 1995;155:205–209.
15. Barss VA, Benacerraf BR, Frigoletto FD Jr. Ultrasonographic determination of chorion type in twin gestation. *Obstet Gynecol* 1985;66(6):779–783.
16. Hertzberg BS, Kurtz AB, Choi HY, Kaczmarczyk JM, Warren W, et al. Significance of membrane thickness in the sonographic evaluation of twin gestations. *AJR Am J Roentgenol* 1987;148(1):151–153.
17. Townsend RR, Simpson GF, Filly RA. Membrane thickness in ultrasound prediction of chorionicity of twin gestations. *J Ultrasound Med* 1988;7(6):327–332.
18. D'Alton ME, Dudley DK. The ultrasonographic prediction of chorionicity in twin gestation. *Am J Obstet Gynecol* 1989;160(3):557–561.
19. Winn HN, Gabrielli S, Reece EA, Roberts JA, Salafia C, Hobbins JC. Ultrasonographic criteria for the prenatal diagnosis of placental chorionicity in twin gestations. *Am J Obstet Gynecol* 1989;161(6 Pt 1):1540–1542.
20. Stagiannis KD, Sepulveda W, Southwell D, Price DA, Fisk NM. Ultrasonographic measurement of the dividing membrane in twin pregnancy during the second and third trimesters: a reproducibility study. *Am J Obstet Gynecol* 1995;173(5):1546–1550.
21. Vayssiere CF, Heim N, Camus EP, Hillion YE, Nisand IF. Determination of chorionicity in twin gestations by high-frequency abdominal ultrasonography: counting the layers of the dividing membrane. *Am J Obstet Gynecol* 1996; 175(6):1529–1533.
22. Bessis R, Papiernik E. Echographic imagery of amniotic membranes in twin pregnancies. In: Gedda L, Parisi P, eds. *Twin research 3: twin biology and multiple pregnancy*. New York: Alan R. Liss, 1981:183–187.
23. Finberg HJ. The "twin peak" sign: reliable evidence of dichorionic twinning. *J Ultrasound Med* 1992;11(11):571–577.
24. Sepulveda W, Sebire NJ, Hughes K, Odibo A, Nicolaides KH. The lambda sign at 10–14 weeks of gestation as a predictor of chorionicity in twin pregnancies. *Ultrasound Obstet Gynecol* 1996;7(6):421–423.
25. Sepulveda W, Sebire NJ, Hughes K, Kalogeropoulos A, Nicolaides KH. Evolution of the lambda or twin-chorionic peak sign in dichorionic twin pregnancies. *Obstet Gynecol* 1997;89(3):439–441.
26. Sepulveda W, Sebire NJ, Odibo A, Psarra A, Nicolaides KH. Prenatal determination of chorionicity in triplet pregnancy by ultrasonographic examination of the ipsilon zone. *Obstet Gynecol* 1996;88(5):855–858.
27. Luke B, Keith LG. The contribution of singletons, twins and triplets to low birth weight, infant mortality and handicap in the United States. *J Reprod Med* 1992;37(8):661–666.
28. U.S. Department of Health. USA Department of Health Statistics and Research (SR28). Annual summaries of LHS 27/1 returns. Volume 1: Natality. 1993.
29. Taffel SM. Demographic trends in twin birth, USA. In: Keith LG, Papiernik E, Keith DM, Luke B, eds. *Multiple pregnancy*. London: Parthenon Press, 1995.
30. Hall JG. Twinning: mechanisms and genetic implications. *Curr Opin Genet Dev* 1996;6(3):343–347.

31. Wachtel SS, Somkuti SG, Schinfeld JS. Monozygotic twins of opposite sex. *Cytogenet Cell Genet* 2000;91(1–4):293–295.

32. Somkuti SG, Wachtel SS, Schinfeld JS, Jackson L, Tharapel AT, DiGeorge AM. 46,XY monozygotic twins with discordant sex phenotype. *Fertil Steril* 2000;74(6):1254–1256.

33. Schmid O, Trautmann U, Ashour H, Ulmer R, Pfeiffer RA, Beinder E. Prenatal diagnosis of heterokaryotypic mosaic twins discordant for fetal sex. *Prenat Diagn* 2000;20(12):999–1003.

34. Snijders RJ, Noble P, Sebire N, Souka A, Nicolaides KH. UK multicentre project on assessment of risk of trisomy 21 by maternal age and fetal nuchal-translucency thickness at 10–14 weeks of gestation. Fetal Medicine Foundation First Trimester Screening Group [see comments]. *Lancet* 1998;352(9125):343–346.

35. Sebire NJ, Snijders RJ, Hughes K, Sepulveda W, Nicolaides KH. Screening for trisomy 21 in twin pregnancies by maternal age and fetal nuchal translucency thickness at 10–14 weeks of gestation. *Br J Obstet Gynaecol* 1996;103(10):999–1003.

36. Spencer K. Screening for trisomy 21 in twin pregnancies in the first trimester: does chorionicity impact on maternal serum free beta-hCG or PAPP-A levels? *Prenat Diagn* 2001;21(9):715–717.

37. Baldwin VJ. Anomalous development of twins. In: Baldwin VJ, ed. *Pathology of multiple pregnancy*. New York: Springer-Verlag, 1994:169–197.

38. Sebire NJ, D'Ercole C, Hughes K, Rennie J, Nicolaides KH. Dichorionic twins discordant for intrauterine growth retardation. *Arch Dis Child Fetal Neonatal Ed* 1997;77(3):F235–F236.

39. Murphy KW. Intrauterine death in a twin: implications for the survivor. In: Ward RH, Whittle MJ, eds. *Multiple pregnancy*. London: RCOG Press, 1995:218–230.

40. de Laveaucoupet J, Audibert F, Guis F, Rambaud C, Suarez B, et al. Fetal magnetic resonance imaging (MRI) of ischemic brain injury. *Prenat Diagn* 2001;21(9):729–736.

41. Baldwin VJ. *Pathology of multiple pregnancy*. New York: Springer-Verlag, 1994.

42. Sebire NJ, Thornton S, Hughes K, Snijders RJ, Nicolaides KH. The prevalence and consequences of missed abortion in twin pregnancies at 10 to 14 weeks of gestation. *Br J Obstet Gynaecol* 1997;104(7):847–848.

43. Buscher U, Horstkamp B, Wessel J, Chen FC, Dudenhausen JW. Frequency and significance of preterm delivery in twin pregnancies. *Int J Gynaecol Obstet* 2000;69(1):1–7.

44. Ziadeh SM. The outcome of triplet versus twin pregnancies. *Gynecol Obstet Invest* 2000;50(2):96–99.

45. MacLennan AH. Multiple gestation: clinical characteristics and management. In: Creasy RK, Resnik R, eds. *Maternal-fetal medicine. Principles and practice*, 3rd ed. Philadelphia: WB Saunders, 1994:589–601.

46. Guzman ER, Walters C, O'Reilly-Green C, Kinzler WL, Waldron R, et al. Use of cervical ultrasonography in prediction of spontaneous preterm birth in twin gestations. *Am J Obstet Gynecol* 2000;183(5):1103–1107.

47. Shapiro JL, Kung R, Barrett JF. Cervical length as a predictor of pre-term birth in twin gestations. *Twin Res* 2000;3(4):213–216.

48. To MS, Skentou C, Liao AW, Cacho A, Nicolaides KH. Cervical length and funneling at 23 weeks of gestation in the prediction of spontaneous early preterm delivery. *Ultrasound Obstet Gynecol* 2001;18(3):200–203.

49. Goldenberg RL, Iams JD, Das A, Mercer BM, Meis PJ, et al. The Preterm Prediction Study: sequential cervical length and fetal fibronectin testing for the prediction of spontaneous preterm birth. National Institute of Child Health and Human Development Maternal-Fetal Medicine Units Network. *Am J Obstet Gynecol* 2000;182(3):636–643.

50. Yang JH, Kuhlman K, Daly S, Berghella V. Prediction of preterm birth by second trimester cervical sonography in twin pregnancies. *Ultrasound Obstet Gynecol* 2000;15(4):288–291.

51. To MS, Skentou C, Cicero S, Liao AW, Nicolaides KH. Cervical length at 23 weeks in triplets: prediction of spontaneous preterm delivery. *Ultrasound Obstet Gynecol* 2000;16(6):515–518.

52. Skentou C, Souka AP, To MS, Liao AW, Nicolaides KH. Prediction of preterm delivery in twins by cervical assessment at 23 weeks. *Ultrasound Obstet Gynecol* 2001;17(1):7–10.

53. Egan JF, Vintzileos AM, Turner G, Fleming A, Scorza W, et al. Correlation of uterine fundal height with ultrasonic measurements in twin gestations. *J Mat Fet Invest* 1994;3:18–22.

54. Jensen OH, Jenssen H. Prediction of fetal weights in twins. *Acta Obstet Gynecol Scand* 1995;74(3):177–180.

55. Chauhan SP, Hendrix NW, Magann EF, Morrison JC, Kenney SP, Devoe LD. Limitations of clinical and sonographic estimates of birth weight: experience with 1034 parturients. *Obstet Gynecol* 1998;91(1):72–77.

56. Lynch L, Lapinski R, Alvarez M, Lockwood CJ. Accuracy of ultrasound estimation of fetal weight in multiple pregnancies. *Ultrasound Obstet Gynecol* 1995;6(5):349–352.

57. Degani S, Paltiely J, Lewinsky R, Shapiro I, Sharf M. Fetal internal carotid artery flow velocity time waveforms in twin pregnancies. *J Perinat Med* 1988;16(5–6):405–409.

58. Divon MY, Girz BA, Sklar A, Guidetti DA, Langer O. Discordant twins—a prospective study of the diagnostic value of real-time ultrasonography combined with umbilical artery velocimetry [see comments]. *Am J Obstet Gynecol* 1989;161(3):757–760.

59. Gaziano EP, Knox GE, Bendel RP, Calvin S, Brandt D. Is pulsed Doppler velocimetry useful in the management of multiple-gestation pregnancies? *Am J Obstet Gynecol* 1991;164(6 Pt 1):1426–1431.

60. Degani S, Gonen R, Shapiro I, Paltiely Y, Sharf M. Doppler flow velocity waveforms in fetal surveillance of twins: a prospective longitudinal study. *J Ultrasound Med* 1992;11(10):537–541.

61. Shah YG, Gragg LA, Moodley S, Williams GW. Doppler velocimetry in concordant and discordant twin gestations. *Obstet Gynecol* 1992;80(2):272–276.

62. Hastie SJ, Danskin F, Neilson JP, Whittle MJ. Prediction of the small for gestational age twin fetus by Doppler umbilical artery waveform analysis. *Obstet Gynecol* 1989;74(5):730–733.

63. Rafla NM. Surveillance of triplets with umbilical artery velocimetry waveforms. *Acta Genet Med Gemellol (Roma)* 1989;38(3–4):301–304.

64. Rode ME, Jackson M. Sonographic considerations with multiple gestation. *Semin Roentgenol* 1999;34(1):29–34.

65. Giles WB, Trudinger BJ, Cook CM, Connelly AJ. Umbilical artery waveforms in triplet pregnancy. *Obstet Gynecol* 1990;75(5):813–816.

66. Rennie JM. Perinatal management at the lower margin of viability [see comments]. *Arch Dis Child Fetal Neonatal Ed* 1996;74(3):F214–F218.

67. Patten R, Mack L, Nyberg D, Filly R. Twin embolization syndrome: prenatal sonographic detection and significance. *Radiology* 1989;173(3):685–689.

68. Samuels P. Ultrasound in the management of the twin gestation. *Clin Obstet Gynecol* 1988;31:110–122.

69. Caballero P, Del Campo L, Ocon E. Cystic encephalomalacia in twin embolization syndrome. *Radiology* 1991;178(3):892–893.

70. Fuents A, Porter KB, Torres BA, Saadeh S, Duesenberg K, O'Brien WF. A twin gestation complicated by gastroschisis in both twins. *J Clin Ultrasound* 1996;24(1):48–50.

71. Yancey MK, Brady K, Read JA. Sonographic evidence of fetal hydrothorax after in-utero death of monozygotic twin. *J Clin Ultrasound* 1991;19(3):162–166.

72. Dallay D, Soumireu-Mourat J. Problems posed by the death of one fetus in a twin pregnancy. *Rev Fr Gynecol Obstet* 1985;80(12):877–879.

73. Schinzel A, Smith DW, Miller Jr. Monozygotic twinning and structural defects. *J Pediatr* 1979;95(6):921–930.

74. Liu S, Benirshke K, Scioscia AL, Mannino FI. Intrauterine death in multiple gestation. *Acta Genet Med Gemellol* 1992;41:5–26.

75. Donnenfeld AE, Glazerman LR, Cutillo DM, Librizzi RJ, Weiner S. Fetal exsanguinations following intrauterine angiographic assessment and selective termination of a hydrocephalic, monozygotic co-twin. *Prenat Diagn* 1989;9:301–308.

76. Benirschke K, Kaufman P. *Pathology of the human placenta*, 2nd ed. New York: Springer-Verlag, 1990:672.

77. Fusi L, McParland P, Fisk N, Nicolini U, Wigglesworth J. Acute twin-twin transfusion: a possible mechanism for brain-damaged survivors after intrauterine death of a monochorionic twin. *Obstet Gynecol* 1991;78(3 Pt 2):517–520.

78. Jou HJ, Ng KY, Teng RJ, Hsieh FJ. Doppler sonographic detection of reverse twin-twin transfusion after intrauterine death of the donor. *J Ultrasound Med* 1993;12(5):307–309.

79. Gembruch U, Viski S, Bagamery K, Berg C, Germer U. Twin reversed arterial perfusion sequence in twin-to-twin transfusion syndrome after the death of the donor co-twin in the second trimester. *Ultrasound Obstet Gynecol* 2001;17(2):153–156.

80. Patten RM, Mack LA, Nyberg DA, Filly RA. Twin embolization syndrome: prenatal sonographic detection and significance. *Radiology* 1989;173(3):685–689.

81. Elchala U, Tanos V, Bar-OZ B, Nadjari M. Early second trimester twin embolization syndrome. *J Ultrasound Med* 1997;16(7):509–512.

82. Harrison SD, Cyr DR, Patten RM, Mack LA. Twin growth problems: causes and sonographic analysis. *Semin Ultrasound CT MR* 1993;14(1):56–67.

83. Fusi L, Gordon H. Twin pregnancy complicated by single intrauterine death. Problems and outcome with conservative management. *Br J Obstet Gynaecol* 1990;97(6):511–516.

84. Kilby MD, Govind A, O'Brien PM. Outcome of twin pregnancies complicated by a single intrauterine death: a comparison with viable twin pregnancies. *Obstet Gynecol* 1994;84(1):107–109.

85. Bruner JP, Anderson TL, Rosemond RL. Placental pathophysiology of the twin oligohydramnios-polyhydramnios sequence and the twin-twin transfusion syndrome. *Placenta* 1998;19(1):81–86.

86. Benirschke K. Twin placenta in perinatal mortality. *N Y State J Med* 1961;61:1499–1508.

87. Arts NF, Lohman AHM. The vascular anatomy of monochorionic diamniotic twin placentas and the transfusion syndrome. *Eur J Obstet Gynaecol* 1971;3:85–93.

88. Sekiya S, Hafez ES. Physiomorphology of twin transfusion syndrome. A study of 86 twin gestations. *Obstet Gynecol* 1977;50(3):288–292.

89. Galea P, Scott JM, Goel KM. Feto-fetal transfusion syndrome. *Arch Dis Child* 1982;57(10):781–783.

90. Machin GA, Still K. The twin-twin transfusion syndrome: vascular anatomy of monochorionic placentas and their clinical outcomes. In: Keith LG, Papiernik E, Keith DM, Luke B, eds. *Multiple pregnancy*. London: Parthenon Press, 1995:367–393.

91. Machin G, Still K, Lalani T. Correlations of placental vascular anatomy and clinical outcome in 69 monochorionic twin pregnancies. *Am J Med Genet* 1996;61:229.

92. Saunders NJ, Snijders RJ, Nicolaides KH. Twin-twin transfusion syndrome during the 2nd trimester is associated with small intertwin hemoglobin differences. *Fetal Diagn Ther* 1991;6(1–2):34–36.

93. Saunders NJ, Snijders RJ, Nicolaides KH. Therapeutic amniocentesis in twin-twin transfusion syndrome appearing in the second trimester of pregnancy. *Am J Obstet Gynecol* 1992;166(3):820–824.

94. Rosen DJ, Rabinowitz R, Beyth Y, Fejgin MD, Nicolaides KH. Fetal urine production in normal twins and in twins with acute polyhydramnios. *Fetal Diagn Ther* 1990;5(2):57–60.

95. Bajoria R, Ward S, Sooranna SR. Atrial natriuretic peptide mediated polyuria: pathogenesis of polyhydramnios in the recipient twin of twin-twin transfusion syndrome. *Placenta* 2001;22(8–9):716–724.

96. Ramos-Arroyo MA, Ulbright TM, Yu PL, Christian JC. Twin study: relationship between birth weight, zygosity, placentation, and pathologic placental changes. *Acta Genet Med Gemellol (Roma)* 1988;37(3–4):229–238.

97. Fries MH, Goldstein RB, Kilpatrick SJ, Golbus MS, Callen PW, Filly RA. The role of velamentous cord insertion in the etiology of twin-twin transfusion syndrome. *Obstet Gynecol* 1993;81(4):569–574.

98. Machin GA. Velamentous cord insertion in monochorionic twin gestation. An added risk factor. *J Reprod Med* 1997;42(12):785–789.

99. Sebire NJ, D'Ercole C, Hughes K, Carvalho M, Nicolaides KH. Increased nuchal translucency thickness at 10–14 weeks of gestation as a predictor of severe twin-to-twin transfusion syndrome. *Ultrasound Obstet Gynecol* 1997;10(2):86–89.

100. Sebire NJ, D'Ercole C, Carvelho M, Sepulveda W, Nicolaides KH. Inter-twin membrane folding in monochorionic pregnancies. *Ultrasound Obstet Gynecol* 1998;11(5):324–327.

101. Mari G, Detti L, Levi-D'Ancona R, Kern L. "Pseudo" twin-to-twin transfusion syndrome and fetal outcome. *J Perinatol* 1998;18(5):399–403.

102. Nores J, Athanassiou A, Elkadry E, Malone FD, Craigo SD, D'Alton ME. Gender differences in twin-twin transfusion syndrome. *Obstet Gynecol* 1997;90(4):580–582.

103. Patten RM, Mack LA, Harvey D, Cyr DR, Pretorius DH. Disparity of amniotic fluid volume and fetal size: problem of the stuck twin-US studies. *Radiology* 1989;172(1):153–157.

104. Brown DL, Benson CB, Driscoll SG, Doubilet PM. Twin-twin transfusion syndrome: sonographic findings. *Radiology* 1989;170(1):61–63.

105. Weiner CP, Ludomirsky A. Diagnosis, pathophysiology and treatment of chronic twin-to-twin transfusion syndrome. *Fetal Diagn Ther* 1994;9(5):283–290.

106. Pretorius DH, Budorick NE, Scioscia AL, Krabbe JK, Ko S, Myhre CM. Twin pregnancies in the second trimester in women in an α-fetoprotein screening program: sonographic evaluation and outcome. *AJR Am J Roentgenol* 1993;161:1007–1013.

107. Fries MH, Goldstein RB, Kilpatrick SJ, et al. The role of velamentous cord insertion in the etiology of twin-twin transfusion syndrome. *Obstet Gynecol* 1993;81:569.

108. Weiner CP, Ludomirski A. Diagnosis, pathophysiology, and treatment of chronic twin-to-twin transfusion syndrome. *Fetal Diagn Ther* 1994;9(5):283–290.

109. Wittman BK, Baldwin VJ, Nichol B. Antenatal diagnosis of twin transfusion syndrome by ultrasound. *Obstet Gynecol* 1981;58:123–126.

110. Brennan JN, Diwan RV, Rosen MG, Bellon EM. Fetofetal transfusion syndrome: prenatal ultrasonographic diagnosis. *Radiology* 1982;143:535–536.

111. Sebire NJ, Nicolaides KH. Screening for fetal abnormalities in multiple pregnancies. *Baillieres Clin Obstet Gynaecol* 1998;12(1):19–36.

112. Duncan KR, Denbow ML, Fisk NM. The aetiology and management of twin-twin transfusion syndrome. *Prenat Diagn* 1997;17(13):1227–1236.

113. Farmakides G, Schulman H, Saldona LR, Bracero LA, Fleischer A, Rochelson B. Surveillance of twin pregnancy with umbilical artery velocimetry. *Am J Obstet Gynecol* 1985;53(7):789–792.

114. Giles WB. Doppler ultrasound in multiple pregnancies. *Baillieres Clin Obstet Gynaecol* 1998;12(1):77–89.

115. Hecher K, Ville Y, Nicolaides KH. Color Doppler ultrasonography in the identification of communicating vessels in twin-twin transfusion syndrome and acardiac twin. *J Ultrasound Med* 1995;14(1):37–40.

116. Hecher K, Ville Y, Nicolaides KH. Fetal arterial Doppler studies in twin-twin transfusion syndrome. *J Ultrasound Med* 1995;14(2):101–108.

117. Hecher K, Ville Y, Snijders R, Nicolaides KH. Doppler studies of the fetal circulation in twin-twin transfusion syndrome. *Ultrasound Obstet Gynecol* 1995;5(5):313–324.

118. Sohl S, David M. Doppler ultrasound study of a twin pregnancy with feto-fetal transfusion syndrome. *Geburtshilfe Frauenheilkd* 1994;54(8):475–477.

119. Donner C, Noel JC, Rypens F, van Kerkem J, Avni F, Rodesch F. Twin-twin transfusion syndrome—possible roles for Doppler ultrasound and amniocentesis. *Prenat Diagn* 1995;15(1):60–63.

120. Quintero RA, Morales WJ, Allen MH, Bornick PW, Johnson PK, Kruger M. Staging of twin-twin transfusion syndrome. *J Perinatol* 1999;19(8 Pt 1):550–555.

121. Machin GA, Feldstein VA, Van Gemert MJC, Keith LG, Hecher K. Doppler sonographic demonstrations of arteriovenous anastomosis in monochorionic twin gestation. *Ultrasound Obstet Gynecol* 2000;16:214–217.

122. Taylor MJO, Farquharson D, Cox PM, Fisk NM. Identification of arterio-venous anastomoses in vivo in monochorionic twin pregnancies: preliminary report *Ultrasound Obstet Gynecol* 2000;16:218.

123. Berghella V, Kaufmann M. Natural history of twin-twin transfusion syndrome. *J Reprod Med* 2001;46(5):480–484.

124. Joa E, Chari R, Mayes D, Demianczuk N, Okun N. Twin-to-twin transfusion syndrome: a review of 27 cases and the relationship between gestational age at diagnosis and serial amniocentesis on outcome. *Obstet Gynecol* 2001;97(4 Suppl 1):S46.

125. Haverkamp F, Lex C, Hanisch C, Fahnenstich H, Zerres K. Neurodevelopmental risks in twin-to-twin transfusion syndrome: preliminary findings. *Europ J Paediatr Neurol* 2001;5(1):21–27.

126. Bajoria R. Abundant vascular anastomoses in monoamniotic versus diamniotic monochorionic placentas. *Am J Obstet Gynecol* 1998;179:788–793.

127. Nyberg DA, Filly RA, Golbus MS, Stephens JD. Entangled umbilical cords: a sign of monoamniotic twins. *J Ultrasound Med* 1984;143:29–32.

128. Overton TG, Denbow ML, Duncan KR, Fisk NM. First-trimester cord entanglement in monoamniotic twins. *Ultrasound Obstet Gynecol* 1999;13(2):140–142.

129. Arabin B, Laurini RN, van Eyck J. Early prenatal diagnosis of cord entanglement in monoamniotic multiple pregnancies. *Ultrasound Obstet Gynecol* 1999;13(181):186.

130. Bromley B, Benacerraf B. Using the number of yolk sacs to determine amnionicity in early first trimester monochorionic twins. *J Ultrasound Med* 1995;14(6):415–419.

131. Rodis JF, McIlveen PF, Egan JF, Borgida AF, Turner GW, Campbell WA. Monoamniotic twins: improved perinatal survival with accurate prenatal diagnosis and antenatal fetal surveillance. *Am J Obstet Gynecol* 1997;177:1046–1049.

132. Edmonds LD, Layde PM. Conjoined twins in the United States, 1970–1977. *Teratology* 1982;25:301–308.

133. Conjoined twins—an epidemiological study based on 312 cases. The International Clearinghouse for Birth Defects Monitoring Systems. *Acta Genet Med Gemellol* 1991;40(3–4):325–335.

134. Abossolo T, Dancoisne P, Tuaillin J, Orvain E, Sommer JC, Riviere JP. Early prenatal diagnosis of asymmetric cephalothoracopagus twins. *J Gynecol Obstet Biol Reprod* 1994;23(1):79–84.

135. Spencer R. Theoretical and analytical embryology of conjoined twins: part I: embryogenesis. *Clin Anat* 2000;13(1):36–53.

136. Al Muti Zaitoun A, Chang J, Booker M. Diprosopus (partially duplicated head) associated with anencephaly: a case report. *Pathol Res Pract* 1999;195(1):45–50.

137. Amr SS, Hammouri MF. Craniofacial duplication (diprosopus): report of a case with a review of the literature. *Eur J Obstet Gynecol Reprod Biol* 1995;58(1):77–80.

138. La Torre R, Fusaro P, Anceschi MM, Montanino-Oliva M, Modesto S, Cosmi EV. Unusual case of caudal duplication (dipygus). *J Clin Ultrasound* 1998;26(3):163–165.

139. Mir E, Sencan A, Karaca I, Gunsar C, Etensel B. Truncal duplication: a case report. *Pediatr Surg Int* 1998;14(3):227–228.

140. Spencer R. Anatomic description of conjoined twins: a plea for standardized terminology. *J Pediatr Surg* 1996;31(7):941–944.

141. Spencer R, Robichaux WH. Prosopo-thoracopagus conjoined twins and other cephalopagus-thoracopagus intermediates: case report and review of literature. *Pediatr Dev Pathol* 1998;1(2):164–171.

142. Chen CP, Lee CC, Liu FF, Jan SW, Lin MH, Chen BF. Prenatal diagnosis of cephalothoracopagus janiceps monosymmetros. *Prenat Diagn* 1997;17(4):384–388.

143. Ramadani HM, Johnshrud N, al Nasser M, Rayes O. The antenatal diagnosis of cephalothoracopagus Janiceps conjoined twins. *Aust N Z J Obstet Gynaecol* 1994;34(1):113–115.

144. Koltuksuz U, Eskicioglu S, Mehmetoglu F. Minimally conjoined omphalopagus twinning: a case report. *Eur J Pediatr Surg* 1998;8(6):368–370.

145. Jain PK, Budhwani KS, Gambhir A, Ghritlaharey R. Omphalopagus parasite: a rare congenital anomaly. *J Pediatr Surg* 1998;33(6):946–947.

146. Sathekge MM, Venkannagari RR, Clauss RP. Scintigraphic evaluation of craniopagus twins. *Br J Radiol* 1998;71(850):1096–1099.

147. Barth RA, Filly RA, Goldberg JD, Moore P, Silverman NH. Conjoined twins: prenatal diagnosis and assessment of associated malformations. *Radiology* 1990;177:201–207.

148. Maymom R, Halperin R, Weinraub Z, Herman A, Schneider D. Three-dimensional transvaginal sonography of conjoined twins at 10 weeks: a case report. *Ultrasound Obstet Gynecol* 1998;11(4):292–294.

149. Bonilla-Musoles F, Raga F, Bonilla F Jr, Blanes J, Osborne NG. Early diagnosis of conjoined twins using two-dimensional color Doppler and three-dimensional ultrasound. *J Natl Med Assoc* 1998;90(9):552–556.

150. Divon MY, Weiner Z. Ultrasound in twin pregnancy. *Semin Perinatol* 1995;19(5):404–412.

151. Koontz WL, Herbert WN, Seeds JW, Cefalo RC. Ultrasonography in the antepartum diagnosis of conjoined twins. A report of two cases. *J Reprod Med* 1983;28(9):627–630.

152. Boulot P, Deschamps F, Hedon B, Laffargue F, Viala JL. Conjoined twins associated with a normal singleton: very early diagnosis and successful selective termination. *J Perinat Med* 1992;20(2):135–137.

153. Demidov VN, Stygar AM, Voevodin SM, Iantovskii IuR. Ultrasonic diagnosis of malformations during the 1st trimester of pregnancy. *Sov Med* 1991;(12):25–28.

154. Lam YH, Sin SY, Lam C, Lee CP, Tang MH, Tse HY. Prenatal sonographic diagnosis of conjoined twins in the first trimester: two case reports. *Ultrasound Obstet Gynecol* 1998;11(4):289–291.

155. Kuroda K, Kamei Y, Kozuma S, Kikuchi A, Fujii T, et al. Prenatal evaluation of cephalopagus conjoined twins by means of three-dimensional ultrasound at 13 weeks of pregnancy. *Ultrasound Obstet Gynecol* 2000;16(3):264–266.

156. Kingston CA, McHugh K, Kumaradevan J, Kiely EM, Spitz L. Imaging in the preoperative assessment of conjoined twins. *Radiographics* 2001;21(5):1187–1208.

157. Casele HL, Meyer JR. Ultrafast magnetic resonance imaging of cephalopagus conjoined twins. *Obstet Gynecol* 2000;95(6 Pt 2):1015–1017.

158. Furuya A, Okawa I, Matsukawa T, Kumazawa T. Anesthetic management of cesarean section for conjoined twins. *Masui* 1999;48(2):195–197.

159. Van der Brand SF, Nijhuis JG, van Dongen PW. Prenatal ultrasound diagnosis of conjoined twins. *Obstet Gynecol Surv* 1994;49(9):656–662.

160. Creinin M. Conjoined twins. In: Keith LG, Papiernik E, Keith DM, Luke B, eds. *Multiple pregnancy.* London: Parthenon Press, 1995:93–112.

161. Spitz L. Conjoined twins. *Br J Surg* 1996;83:1028–1030.

162. Hilfiker ML, Hart M, Holmes R, Cooper M, Kriett J, et al. Expansion and division of conjoined twins. *J Pediatr Surg* 1998;33(5):768–770.

163. Karsdorp VH, van der Linden JC, Sobotka-Plojhar MA, Prins H, van der Harten JJ, van Vugt JM. Ultrasonographic prenatal diagnosis of conjoined thoracopagus twins: a case report. *Eur J Obstet Gynecol Reprod Biol* 1991;39(2):157–161.

164. Hubinont C, Kollman P, Malvaux V, Donnez J, Bernard P. First-trimester diagnosis of conjoined twins. *Fetal Diagn Ther* 1997;12(3):185–187.

165. Cazeneuve C, Nihoul-Fekete C, Adafer M, Yassine B, Boury R, et al. Conjoined omphalopagus twins separated at fifteen days of age. *Arch Pediatr* 1995;2(5):452–455.

166. Yang CC, Wu RC, Juo PL, Yang HB, Chou NH. Prenatal diagnosis of dicephalic conjoined twins: report of a case. *J Formos Med Assoc* 1994;93(7):626–628.

167. Monni G, Useli C, Ibba RM, Lai R, Olla G, Cao A. Early antenatal sonographic diagnosis of conjoined syncephalus-craniothoraco-omphalopagus twins. Case report. *J Perinat Med* 1991;19(6):489–492.

168. Vaughn TC, Powell LC. The obstetrical management of conjoined twins. *Obstet Gynecol* 1979;53(3 Suppl):67S–72S.

169. Stoll-Simona U, Ingold W, Tanner H. A rare increase in the incidence of Siamese twin deliveries. *Geburtshilfe Frauenheilkd* 1979;39(2):147–151.

170. Sogaard K, Skibsted L, Brocks V. Acardiac twins: pathophysiology, diagnosis, outcome and treatment. Six cases and review of the literature. *Fetal Diagn Ther* 1999;14(1):53–59.

171. Pavlova M, Fouron JC, Proulx F, Lessard M. Importance of intrauterine diagnosis of rudimentary autonomic circulation in an acardiac twin. *Arch Mal Coeur Vaiss* 1996;89(5):629–632.

172. Imai A, Hirose R, Kawabata I, Tamaya T. Acardiac acephalic monster extremely larger than its co twin. A case report. *Gynecol Obstet Invest* 1991;32(1):62–64.

173. Pezzati M, Cianciulli D, Danesi G. Acardiac twins. Two case reports. *J Perinat Med* 1997;25(1):119–124.

174. Benirschke K, des Roches Haraper V. The acardiac anomaly. *Teratology* 1977;15(3):311–316.

175. Kaplan C, Benirschke K. The acardiac anomaly new case reports and current status. *Acta Genet Med Gemellol* 1979;28(1):51–59.

176. Zhioua F, Rezigua H, Khouja H, Merian S, Ferchiou M, et al. Acardiac malformation: ultrasonographic diagnosis. A case report. *Rev Fr Gynecol Obstet* 1993;88(4):267–272.

177. Landy HJ, Larsen JW Jr, Schoen M, Larsen ME, Kent SG, Weingold AB. Acardiac fetus in a triplet pregnancy. *Teratology* 1988;37(1):1–6.

178. Gibson JY, D'Cruz CA, Patel RB, Palmer SM. Acardiac anomaly: review of the subject with case report and emphasis on practical sonography. *J Clin Ultrasound* 1986;14(7):541–545.

179. Cardwell MS. The acardiac twin. A case report. *J Reprod Med* 1988;33(3):320–322.

180. Van Allen MI, Smith DW, Shepard TH. Twin reversed arterial perfusion (TRAP) sequence: a study of 14 twin pregnancies with acardius. *Semin Perinatol* 1983;7:285–293.

181. Bieber FR, Nance WE, Morton CC, Brown JA, Redwine FO, et al. Genetic studies of an acardiac monster: evidence of polar body twinning in man. *Science* 1981;213(4509):775–777.

182. Fisk NM, Ware M, Stanier P, Moore G, Bennett P. Molecular genetic etiology of twin reversed arterial perfusion sequence. *Am J Obstet Gynecol* 1996;174(3):891–894.

183. Shalev E, Zalel Y, Ben-Ami M, Weiner E. First trimester ultrasonic diagnosis of twin reversed arterial perfusion sequence. *Prenat Diagn* 1992;12(3):219–222.

184. Schwarzler P, Ville Y, Moscosco G, Tennstedt C, Bollman R, Chaoui R. Diagnosis of twin reversed arterial perfusion sequence in the first trimester by transvaginal color Doppler ultrasound. *Ultrasound Obstet Gynecol* 1999;13(2):143–146.

185. Papa T, Dao A, Bruner JP. Pathognomonic sign of twin reversed arterial perfusion using color Doppler sonography. *J Ultrasound Med* 1997;16(7):501–503.

186. Pretorius DH, Leopold GR, Moore TR, Benirschke K, Sivo JJ. Acardiac twin, report of Doppler sonography. *J Ultrasound Med* 1988;7:413–416.

187. Benson CB, Bieber FR, Genest DR, Doubilet PM. Doppler demonstration of reversed umbilical blood flow in an acardiac twin. *J Clin Ultrasound* 1989;17(4):291–295.

188. Sepulveda WH, Qjuiroz VH, Giuliano A, Henriquez R. Prenatal ultrasonographic diagnosis of acardiac twin. *J Perinat Med* 1993;21(3):241–246.

189. Petersen BL, Broholm H, Skibsted L, Graem N. Acardiac twin with preserved brain. *Fetal Diagn Ther* 2001;16(4):231–233.

190. Hanafy A, Peterson CM. Twin-reversed arterial perfusion (TRAP) sequence: case reports and review of literature. *Aust N Z J Obstet Gynaecol* 1997;37(2):187–191.

191. Chaliha C, Schwarzler P, Booker M, Battash MA, Ville Y. Trisomy 2 in acardiac twin in a triplet in vitro fertilization pregnancy. *Hum Reprod* 1999;14(5):1378–1380.

192. Aguer C, Bonan J, Mulliez N, Migne G. Acardiac fetus. *Presse Med* 1996;25(26):1191–1194.

193. Balicher W, Repa C, Schaller A. Acardiac twin pregnancy: associated with trisomy 2: case report. *Hum Reprod* 2000;15(2):474–475.

194. Moore CA, Buehler BA, McManus BM, Harmon JP, Mirkin LD, Goldstein DJ. Acephalus-acardia in twins with aneuploidy. *Am J Med Genet* 1987;3:139–143.

195. Moore TR, Galoe S, Benirschke K. Perinatal outcome of forty-nine pregnancies complicated by acardiac twinning. *Am J Obstet Gynecol* 1990;163:907–912.

196. Sanjaghsaz H, Bayram MO, Qureshi F. Twin reversed arterial perfusion sequence in conjoined, acardiac, acephalic twins associated with a normal triplet. A case report. *J Reprod Med* 1998;43(12):1046–1050.

197. Cox M, Murphy K, Ryan G, Kindom J, Whittle M, McNay M. Spontaneous cessation of umbilical blood flow in the acardius fetus of a twin pregnancy. *Prenat Diagn* 1992;12(8):689–693.

198. Chang DY, Chang RY, Chen RJ, Chen CK, Cheng WF, Huang SC. Triplet pregnancy complicated by intrauterine fetal death of conjoined twins from an umbilical cord accident of an acardius. A case report. *J Reprod Med* 1996;41(6):459–462.

199. Willcourt RJ, Naughton MJ, Knutzen VK, Fitzpatrick C. Laparoscopic ligation of the umbilical cord of an acardiac fetus. *J Am Assoc Gynecol Laparosc* 1995;2(3):319–321.

200. Quintero R, Munoz H, Hasbun J, Pommer R, Gutierrez J, et al. Fetal endoscopic surgery in a case of twin pregnancy complicated by reversed arterial perfusion sequence. *Rev Chil Obstet Ginecol* 1995;60(2):112–116.

201. Sepulveda W, Bower S, Hassan J, Fisk NM. Ablation of acardiac twin by alcohol injection into the intraabdominal umbilical artery. *Obstet Gynecol* 1995;86(4):680–681.

202. Sepulveda W, Sfeir D, Reyes M, Martinez J. Severe polyhydramnios in twin reversed arterial perfusion sequence: successful management with intrafetal alcohol ablation of acardiac twin and amniodrainage. *Ultrasound Obstet Gynecol* 2000;16(3):260–263.

203. Hecher K, Reinhold U, Gbur K, Hackeloer BJ. Interruption of umbilical blood flow in an acardiac twin by endoscopic laser coagulation. *Geburtshilfe Frauenheilkd* 1996;56(2):97–100.

204. Hecher K, Hackeloer BJ, Ville Y. Umbilical cord coagulation by operative microendoscopy at 16 weeks' gestation in an acardiac twin. *Ultrasound Obstet Gynecol* 1997;10(2):130–132.

205. Hanquinet S, Damry N, Heimann P, Delaet MH, Perlmutter N. Association of a fetus *in fetu* and two teratomas: US and MRI. *Pediatr Radiol* 1997;27(4):336–338.

206. Kang YK, Suh YL, Kim CW, Chi JG. Fetus in fetu: a case with complete umbilical cord and fetal sac. *Pediatr Pathol* 1994;14(3):411–419.

207. Shin JH, Yoon CH, Cho KS, Lim SD, Kim EA, et al. Fetus-in-fetu in the scrotal sac of a newborn infant: imaging, surgical and pathological findings. *Eur Radiol* 1999;9(5):945–947.

208. Mills P, Bornick PW, Morales WJ, Allen M, Gilbert-Barness E, et al. Ultrasound prenatal diagnosis of fetus *in fetu*. *Ultrasound Obstet Gynecol* 2001;18(1):69–71.

209. Ianniruberto A, Rossi P, Ianniruberto M, Rella G, Ciminelli V. Sonographic prenatal diagnosis of intracranial fetus *in fetu*. *Ultrasound Obstet Gynecol* 2001;18(1):67–68.

210. Hoeffel CC, Nguyen KQ, Phan HT, Truong NH, Nguyen TS, et al. Fetus *in fetu*: a case report and literature review. *Pediatrics* 2000;105(6):1335–1344.

211. Chen CP, Chern SR, Liu FF, Jan SW, Lee HC, et al. Prenatal diagnosis, pathology, and genetic study of fetus *in fetu*. *Prenat Diagn* 1997;17(1):13–21.

212. de Lagausie P, de Napoli Cocci S, Stempfle N, Truong QD, Vuillard E, et al. Highly differentiated teratoma and fetus-

in-fetu: a single pathology? *J Pediatr Surg* 1997;32(1):115–116.

213. Goldstein I, Jakobi P, Groisman G, Itskovitz-Eldor J. Intracranial fetus-in-fetu. *Am J Obstet Gynecol* 1996;175(5):1389–1390.

214. Jones DC, Reyes-Mugica M, Gallagher PG, Fricks P, Touloukian RJ, Copel JA. Three-dimensional sonographic imaging of a highly developed fetus *in fetu* with spontaneous movement of the extremities. *J Ultrasound Med* 2001;20(12):1357–1363.

215. Thakral CL, Sajwani MJ. Highly differentiated teratoma and fetus-in-fetu: a single pathology? *J Pediatr Surg* 1998;33(1):153.

216. Montgomery ML, Lillehei C, Acker D, Benacerraf BR. Intra-abdominal sacrococcygeal mature teratoma or fetus *in fetu* in a third-trimester fetus. *Ultrasound Obstet Gynecol* 1998;11(3):219–221.

217. Khadaroo RG, Evans MG, Honore LH, Bhargava R, Phillipos E. Fetus-in-fetu presenting as cystic meconium peritonitis: diagnosis, pathology, and surgical management. *J Pediatr Surg* 2000;35(5):721–723.

218. Thakral CL, Maji DC, Sajwani MJ. Fetus-in-fetu: a case report and review of the literature. *J Pediatr Surg* 1998;33(9):1432–1434.

219. Massad MG, Kong L, Benedetti E, Resnick D, Ghosh L, et al. Dysphagia caused by a fetus-in-fetu in a 27-year-old man. *Ann Thorac Surg* 2001;71(4):1338–1341.

220. Awasthi M, Narlawar R, Hira P, Shah P. Fetus *in fetu*. Rare cause of a lump in an adult's abdomen. *Australas Radiol* 2001;45(3):354–356.

221. Hopkins KL, Dickson PK, Ball TI, Ricketts RR, O'Shea PA, Abramowsky CR. Fetus-in-fetu with malignant recurrence. *J Pediatr Surg* 1997;32(10):1476–1479.

222. Jeanty P, Shah D, Roussis P. Single-needle insertion in twin amniocentesis. *J Ultrasound Med* 1990;9(9):511–517.

223. Van Vugt JM, Nieuwint A, Van Geijn HP. Single–needle insertion: an alternative technique for early second-trimester genetic twin amniocentesis. *Fetal Diagn Ther* 1995;10(3):178–181.

224. Sebire NJ, Noble PL, Odibo A, Malligiannis P, Nicolaides KH. Single uterine entry for genetic amniocentesis in twin pregnancies. *Ultrasound Obstet Gynecol* 1996;7(1):26–31.

225. Brambati B, Tului L, Lanzani A, Simoni G, Travi M. First-trimester genetic diagnosis in multiple pregnancy: principles and potential pitfalls. *Prenat Diagn* 1991;11(10):767–774.

226. Appelman Z, Caspi B. Chorionic villus sampling and selective termination of a chromosomally abnormal fetus in a triplet pregnancy. *Prenat Diagn* 1992;12(3):215–217.

227. Christiaens GC, Oosterwijk JC, Stigter RH, Deutz-Terlouw PP, Kneppers AL, Bakker E. First-trimester prenatal diagnosis in twin pregnancies. *Prenat Diagn* 1994;14(1):51–55.

228. Jorgensen FS, Bang J, Tranebjaerg L, Berge LN, Eik-Nes SH, Schwartz M. Early prenatal direct gene diagnosis of cystic fibrosis in a twin pregnancy and subsequent selective termination. *Prenat Diagn* 1994;14(2):149–152.

229. Brambati B, Tului L, Baldi M, Guercilena S. Genetic analysis prior to selective fetal reduction in multiple pregnancy: technical aspects and clinical outcome. *Hum Reprod* 1995;10(4):818–825.

230. Evans MI, Dommergues M, Wapner RJ, Lynch L, Dumez Y, et al. Efficacy of transabdominal multifetal pregnancy reduction: collaborative experience among the world's largest centers. *Obstet Gynecol* 1993;82(1):61–66.

231. Evans MI, Dommergues M, Wapner RJ, Goldberg JD, Lynch L, et al. International, collaborative experience of 1789 patients having multifetal pregnancy reduction: a plateauing of risks and outcomes [see comments]. *J Soc Gynecol Investig* 1996;3(1):23–26.

232. Corchia C, Mastroiacovo P, Lanni R, Mannazzu R, Curro V, Fabris C. What proportion of multiple births are due to ovulation induction? A register-based study in Italy. *Am J Public Health* 1996;86(6):851–854.

233. Callahan TL, Hall JE, Ettner SL, Christiansen CL, Greene MF, Crowley WF Jr. The economic impact of multiple-gestation pregnancies and the contribution of assisted-reproduction techniques to their incidence [see comments]. *N Engl J Med* 1994;331(4):244–249.

234. Tan SL, Doyle P, Campbell S, Beral V, Rizk B, et al. Obstetric outcome of in vitro fertilization pregnancies compared with normally conceived pregnancies. *Am J Obstet Gynecol* 1992;167(3):778–784.

235. Kiely JL, Kleinman JC, Kiely M. Triplets and higher-order multiple births. Time trends and infant mortality. *Am J Dis Child* 1992;146(7):862–868.

236. Dommergues M, Dumez Y, Evans M. [Assessment of the obstetric risk in multiple pregnancies with and without embryo reduction.] *Rev Fr Gynecol Obstet* 1991;86(2):105–107.

237. Evans MI, Dommergues M, Timor-Tritsch I, Zador IE, Wapner RJ, et al. Transabdominal versus transcervical and transvaginal multifetal pregnancy reduction: international collaborative experience of more than one thousand cases. *Am J Obstet Gynecol* 1994;170(3):902–909.

238. Evans MI, Dommergues M, Johnson MP, Dumez Y. Multifetal pregnancy reduction and selective termination. *Curr Opin Obstet Gynecol* 1995;7(2):126–129.

239. Evans MI, Littman L, Richter R, Richter K, Hume RF Jr. Selective reduction for multifetal pregnancy. Early opinions revisited [published erratum appears in *J Reprod Med* 1998;43(2):93A]. *J Reprod Med* 1997;42(12):771–777.

240. Nicolaides K, Brizot MD, Patel F, Snijders R. Comparison of chorionic villus sampling and amniocentesis for fetal karyotyping at 10–13 weeks' gestation. *Lancet* 1994;344(8920):435–439.

241. Sebire NJ, D'Ercole C, Sepulveda W, Hughes K, Nicolaides KH. Effects of embryo reduction from trichorionic triplets to twins. *Br J Obstet Gynaecol* 1997;104(10):1201–1203.

242. Reisner DP, Mahony BS, Petty CN, Nyberg DA, Porter TF, et al. Stuck twin syndrome: outcome in thirty-seven consecutive cases. *Am J Obstet Gynecol* 1993;169(4):991–995.

243. Mari G, Roberts A, Detti L, Kovanci E, Stefos T, et al. Perinatal morbidity and mortality rates in severe twin-twin transfusion syndrome: results of the International Amnioreduction Registry. *Am J Obstet Gynecol* 2001;185(3):708–715.

244. Jauniaux E, Holmes A, Hyett J, Yates R, Rodeck C. Rapid and radical amniodrainage in the treatment of severe twin-twin transfusion syndrome. *Prenat Diagn* 2001;21(6):471–476.

245. Ville Y, Hyett JA, Vandenbussche F, Nicolaides KH. Endoscopic laser coagulation of umbilical cord vessels in twin

reversed arterial perfusion sequence. *Ultrasound Obstet Gynecol* 1994;4:396–398.

246. van Gemert MJ, Umur A, Tijssen JG, Ross MG. Twin-twin transfusion syndrome: etiology, severity and rational management. *Curr Opin Obstet Gynecol* 2001;13(2):193–206.

247. Roberts D, Neilson JP, Weindling AM. Interventions for the treatment of twin-twin transfusion syndrome (Cochrane Review). *Cochrane Database Syst Rev* 2001;1:CD002073.

248. Quintero R, Morales W, Mendoza G, Allen M, Kalter C, et al. Selective photocoagulation of placental vessels in twin-twin transfusion syndrome: evolution of a surgical technique. *Obstet Gynecol Surv* 1998;53:s97–s103.

249. Thilaganathan B, Gloeb D, Sairam S, Tekay A. Sono-endoscopic delineation of the placental vascular equator prior to selective fetoscopic laser ablation in twin-to-twin transfusion syndrome. *Ultrasound Obstet Gynecol* 2000;16:226.

250. Quintero RA, Bornick PW, Allen MH, Johnson PK. Selective laser photocoagulation of communicating vessels in severe twin-twin transfusion syndrome in women with an anterior placenta. *Obstet Gynecol* 2001;97(3):477–481.

251. Young BK, Roque H, Abdelhak Y, Timor-Tristch I, Rebarber A, Rosen R. Endoscopic ligation of umbilical cord at 19 weeks' gestation in monoamniotic-monochorionic twins discordant for hypoplastic left heart syndrome. *Fetal Diagn Ther* 2001;16(1):61–64.

252. Quintero RA, Romero R, Reich H, Goncalves L, Johnson MP, et al. In utero percutaneous umbilical cord ligation in the management of complicated monochorionic multiple gestations. *Ultrasound Obstet Gynecol* 1996;8(1):16–22.

253. Willcourt RJ, Naughton MJ, Knutzen VK, Fitzpatrick C. Laparoscopic ligation of the umbilical cord of an acardiac fetus. *J Am Assoc Gynecol Laparosc* 1995;2(3):319–321.

254. Arias F, Sunderji S, Gimpelson R, Colton E. Treatment of acardiac twinning. *Obstet Gynecol* 1998;91(5 Pt 2):818–821.

255. Sanchioni L, Presti C, Morotti R, Zulianai G, Kustermann A, et al. Twin pregnancy with acephalic acardiac fetus. Anatomo-clinical description cases. *Ann Obstet Ginecol Med Perinat* 1990;111(3):174–180.

256. Ko TM, Tzeng SJ, Hsieh FJ, Chu JS. Acardius anceps: report of 3 cases. *Asia Oceania J Obstet Gynaecol* 1991;17(1):49–56.

257. Natho W, Kirsch M, Abet L, Bollmann R, Prenzlau P, et al. Perinatal imaging diagnosis in twin pregnancies with humanus amorphus. *Zentralbl Gynakol* 1990;112(11):679–688.

258. De Lia J, Kuhlmann RS, Harstad T, Cruikshank D. Fetoscopic laser ablation of placental vessels in severe previable twin-twin transfusion syndrome. *Am J Obstet Gynecol* 1995;172(4 Pt 1):1208–1211.

259. Ville Y, Hecher K, Gagnon A, Sebire N, Hyett J, Nicolaides K. Endose laser coagulation in the management of severe twin-to-twin transfusion syndrome. *Br J Obstet Gynaecol* 1998;105(4):446–453.

260. Hecher K, Plath H, Bregenzer T, Hansmann M, Hackeloer B. Endosco surgery versus serial amniocenteses in the treatment of severe twin-twin transfusion syndrome. *Am J Obstet Gynecol* 1999;180(3 Pt 1):717.

261. De Lia JE, Kuhlmann R, Lopez K. Treating previable twin-twin trans syndrome with fetoscopic laser surgery: outcomes following the learning. *J Perinatal Med* 1999;27(1):61–67.

262. Quintero R, Comas C, Bornick P, Allen M, Kruger M. Selective versus non-selective laser photocoagulation of placental vessels in twin-to-twin transfusion syndrome. *Ultrasound Obstet Gynecol* 2000;16:230.

263. Thilaganathan B, Gloeb DJ, Sairam S, Tekay A. Sono-endoscopic delineation of the placental vascular equator prior to selective fetoscopic laser ablation in twin-to-twin transfusion syndrome. *Ultrasound Obstet Gynecol* 2000;16(3):226–229.

MALFORMATIONS IN
THE FIRST FIFTEEN WEEKS

Transvaginal sonography (TVS) has revolutionized the way obstetrics and gynecology is practiced. It has opened up a new world in which, for the first time, the process of early human fetal development can be seen unfolding in front of our eyes. Although fetal development proceeds most of the time in a normal fashion, developmental malformations do occur. The reported incidence of major congenital anomalies at birth is 1 to 2 per 100. Although intuitively we expect that during the first two trimesters of pregnancy the rate of major congenital anomalies should be higher than at birth, these figures are not available and are further confounded by the relatively high rate of spontaneous fetal losses that occur during the fetal period.

When scanning in the first trimester of the pregnancy, it is important to be familiar with the normal development of the embryo and then the fetus. Anyone embarking on first- or early second-trimester scanning must be familiarized with the major embryologic landmarks during each postmenstrual week of the gestation. The presence or absence of certain structures may be deemed either normal or abnormal depending on the gestational age of the pregnancy. Dividing the pregnancy into trimesters is an ancient custom, which is not practical and makes the communication between clinicians vague and lacking precision. Instead of using the terms *first* and *second trimester*, the exact postmenstrual age in question is indicated in this chapter.

Since 1980, as the resolution of the ultrasound equipment has improved, the number of anomalies detected in utero has increased. As the ultrasound equipment and technology continue to improve, the number of anomalies that can possibly be detected in the first and early second trimester is expected to continue to multiply. The early detection of certain anomalies or malformations, however, is limited by the time in development that such problems become evident. Since the rather fast introduction of three-dimensional (3-D) ultrasound, most laboratories advocate its use in determining facial anatomy or pathology. An increasing body of informa-tion is now available on the successful application of 3-D ultrasound in diagnosing congenital anomalies.

Before describing such anomalies, a review of the pertinent sonoembryology with emphasis on important milestones of each gestational age is presented.

This chapter discusses mostly the prenatal diagnosis of fetal anomalies up to 14 to 15 postmenstrual weeks and attempts to describe as many of these anomalies that have been encountered in practice or have been reported by others.

NORMAL ANATOMY FROM THE FIFTH TO THE FOURTEENTH WEEK

Embryologists, obstetricians, sonographers, and sonologists use different terms and different starting points to assess gestational age. Embryologists use *conceptual age* to assess gestational age, with conception as the first day of the pregnancy. On the other hand, clinicians use *postmenstrual age* to date the pregnancy, with the first day of the last postmenstrual period as the beginning of the gestation. The main difference between conceptual age and postmenstrual age is a two-week discrepancy with the postmenstrual age being always 2 weeks ahead. In ultrasonography, by convention, gestational age is expressed in postmenstrual weeks. In this chapter, all gestational ages, unless otherwise noted, are expressed in postmenstrual age. At times, therefore, the term *postmenstrual weeks* appears, and, at other times, the *weeks* are only indicated (e.g., sixth week). The meaning, though, is the same.

Another important difference in nomenclature between embryologists and sonologist or sonographers is the term used to refer to the conceptus. The latter group of individuals refers to the conceptus from the first time it is imaged as the *fetus* or *fetal pole*. But, in the strictest embryologic nomenclature for the first 9 postmenstrual weeks, the conceptus is actually an *embryo*.

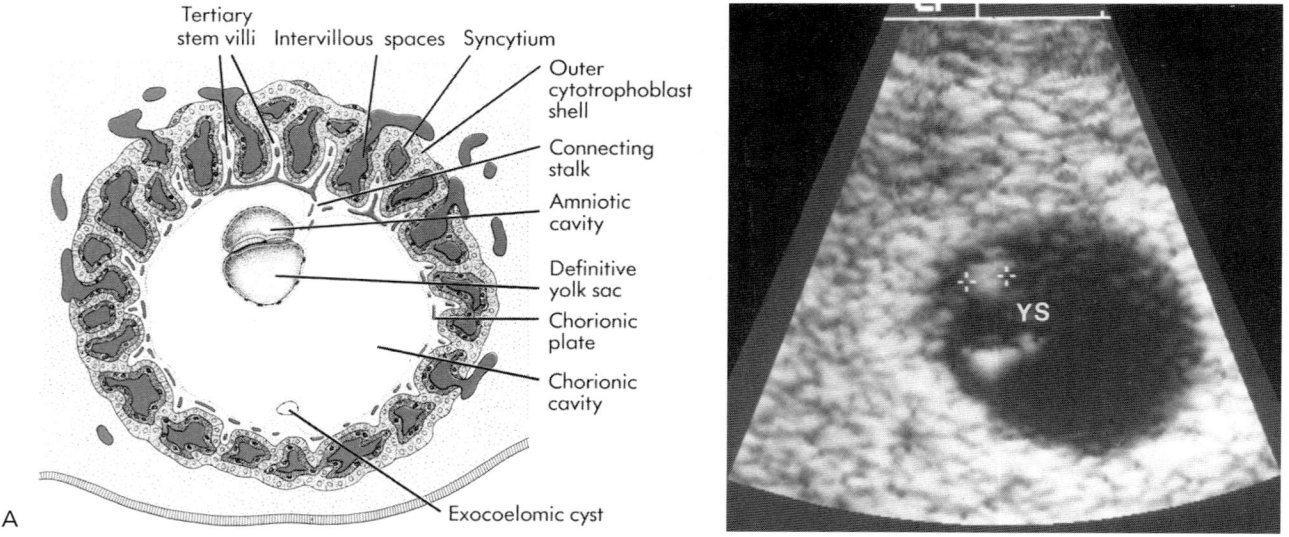

FIGURE 1. Normal embryologic development at 5 to 6 menstrual weeks (3 conceptual weeks). **A:** Diagram illustrating the primitive embryonic disk located between the secondary yolk sac (*YS*) and the amniotic cavity. **B:** Sonogram showing embryonic pole (calipers) at 5.8 menstrual weeks. (Reproduced with permission from Sadler TW. *Langman's medical embryology*, 5th ed. Baltimore: Williams & Wilkins, 1985.)

The gestational or chorionic sac can be imaged consistently from the fifth postmenstrual week. By 6 menstrual weeks, an embryonic pole can be identified adjacent to the yolk sac (Fig. 1).

The embryo/fetus develops rapidly during the first trimester (Fig. 2). The first anatomical structure that becomes sonographically apparent in the embryo during the latter half of the sixth week and early seventh week is the primitive neural tube. The sonographic appearance is that of a hypoechoic longitudinal structure running throughout the length of the embryo. Because of the excessive curling of the embryonic body, only segments of this neural tube (in the shape of two parallel lines) can be imaged at any given time. By the seventh postmenstrual week, the fetal head becomes discernible from the rest of the fetal body, and the primitive ventricular system can be imaged for the first time. Its

appearance, in the coronal and sagittal view, is that of a single round sonolucent cavity, which almost completely fills the fetal head. Although, the entire fetal body can be seen, structural details are hard to image with the presently available equipment. A sagittal view of the fetal head at 8 postmenstrual weeks reveals sonolucencies within the primitive brain. The primitive brain shows three primary brain vesicles, including (a) the prosencephalon or forebrain, (b) the mesencephalon or midbrain, and (c) the rhombencephalon or hindbrain. The portions of the brain further divide. Some of these structures such as the rhombencephalon can be identified by ultrasound (Fig. 3). If a posterior coronal section is obtained, the cerebral aqueduct and future fourth ventricle can also be imaged.

At 9 postmenstrual weeks the most important development within the fetal brain is the appearance of the falx

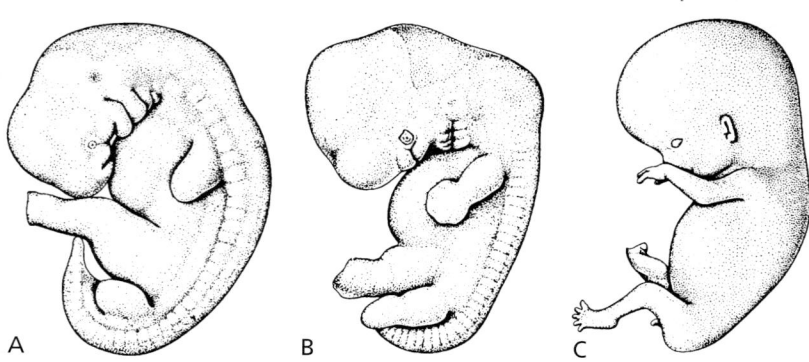

FIGURE 2. Normal embryonic development at 7 menstrual weeks **(A)**, 9 menstrual weeks **(B)**, and 12 menstrual weeks **(C)**. (Reproduced with permission from Sadler TW. *Langman's medical embryology*, 5th ed. Baltimore: Williams and Wilkins, 1985.)

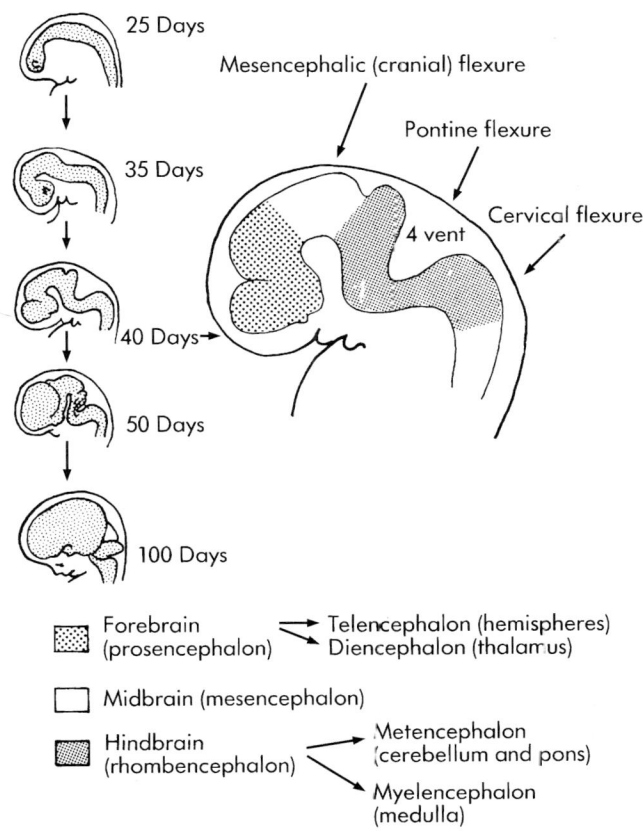

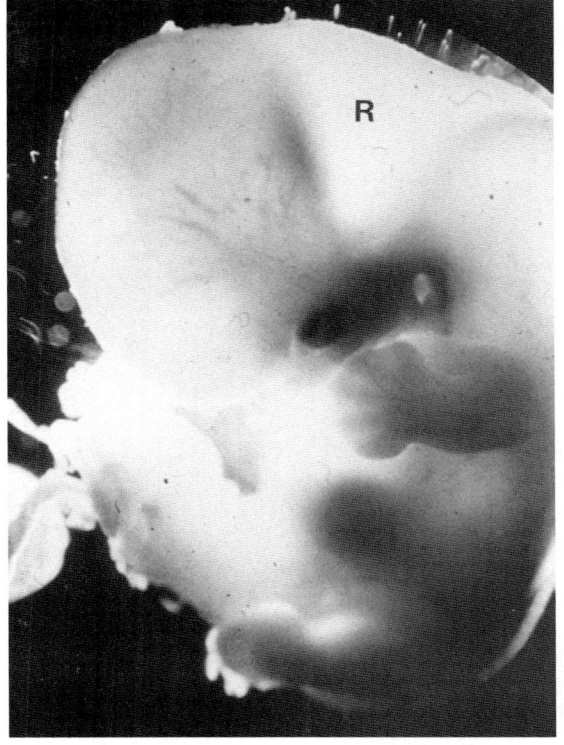

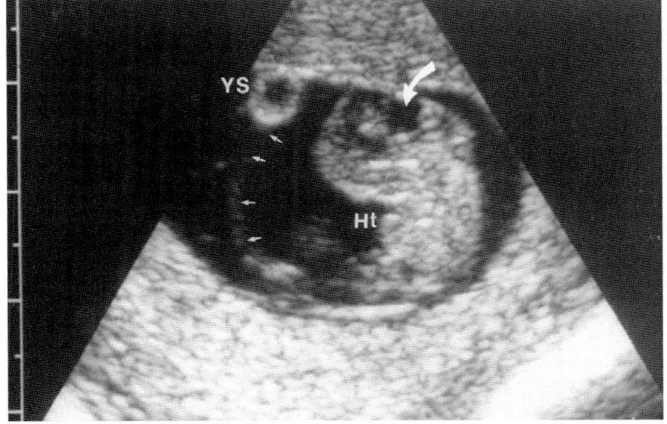

FIGURE 3. A: Normal embryologic development of the brain from 25 to 100 days (6 to 17 menstrual weeks). **B:** Pathologic photograph of embryo at 8 menstrual weeks shows cystic rhombencephalon (*R*). **C:** Corresponding sonogram at 8 menstrual weeks (6 weeks postconception). Note cystic rhombencephalon (*curved arrow*). Small arrows show amnion. Ht, heart; YS, yolk sac. (**A:** Reproduced with permission from Wigglesworth JS. *Perinatal pathology.* Philadelphia: WB Saunders, 1984:262–288. **B, C:** Reproduced with permission from Nyberg DA, Hill LM, Bohm-Velez M, Mendelson EB, eds. *Transvaginal sonography.* Chicago: Mosby–Year Book, 1992.)

cerebri and the choroid plexus (Fig. 4). The embryo becomes easier to scan, and a limited structural evaluation is possible. The long bones and fingers can be imaged at this gestational age for the first time.[1,2] Table 1 summarizes the gestational age at which a variety of fetal organs or structures can be consistently imaged.

From 9 to 14 postmenstrual weeks, few new fetal structures appear, but the previously developed organs or structures become easier to image as the rapid growth of the fetus continues.[3] The brain is now well visualized, and the echogenic choroid plexus should be seen in each cerebral hemisphere (Fig. 4). The cerebellum is first imaged by 10 to 11 menstrual weeks. Also, at this gestational age, the fetal

face and bony components (palate) as well as the fetal foot and toes can be viewed.

The anterior contour of the fetus reveals the physiologic midgut herniation, which returns to the abdomen by 12 menstrual weeks. 3-D ultrasound (Fig. 5) can illustrate this herniation at the umbilical cord insertion site, as well as other external features of the developing fetus.

Although the four-chamber view of the fetal heart can be seen as early as the eleventh postmenstrual week, this view does not become easily imaged until the fourteenth postmenstrual week. It is important to note that although the palate may be imaged from the eleventh postmenstrual week, it is not fully mineralized until 13 to 14 postmenstrual weeks.

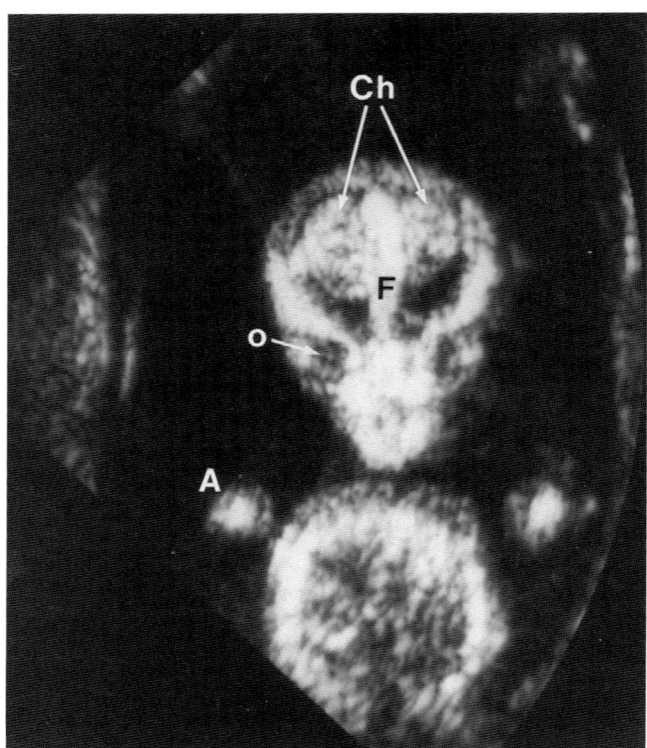

FIGURE 4. Normal brain. Coronal view at 11 menstrual weeks shows normal echogenic choroid plexus (*Ch*) filling much of each hemisphere of the brain. A, arm; F, falx; O, orbit.

Most, but definitely not all, structures may be revealed using a high-frequency transvaginal probe before the fourteenth postmenstrual week (Figs. 6A through C). Therefore, it is becoming increasingly evident that the first fairly comprehensive scan of the fetus could be undertaken at or shortly before 15 postmenstrual weeks. Of course, it is understood that one can scan for individual organs before these arbitrary times in gestation, if the organs in question can be visualized in all or in the overwhelming majority of the normally developing fetuses.[3] Tables 2 through 5 are transvaginally derived biometric measurements of the fetus between 6 and 12 postmenstrual weeks.

ABNORMAL EMBRYO AND FETUS

This chapter is arranged by anomalies that can be identified by transvaginal ultrasound before 15 weeks' gestation. The emphasis of this chapter is on the sonographic features of specific abnormalities and also potential pitfalls that may be encountered during this time. Emphasis is placed on the development and embryology of the embryo and fetus, and focuses on the advantages of transvaginal ultrasound in detecting early fetal abnormalities. Specific abnormalities are covered by their ultrasound features in this chapter. More detailed description of these abnormalities, however, is detailed in other chapters in this book that deal on specific organ systems.

TABLE 1. SUMMARY OF EMBRYONIC STRUCTURES AND THE GESTATIONAL AGE IN POSTMENSTRUAL WEEKS AT WHICH THEY BECOME CONSISTENTLY IMAGED USING HIGH-FREQUENCY TRANSVAGINAL SONOGRAPHY

	Postmenstrual wk										
Embryonic structure	4	5	6	7	8	9	10	11	12	13	14
Gestational sac	x	x	x	x	x	x	x	x	x	x	x
Yolk sac	—	x	x	x	x	x	x	x	x	x	x
Fetal heart rate	—	—	x	x	x	x	x	x	x	x	x
Neural tube	—	—	—	x	x	x	x	x	x	x	x
Fetal head	—	—	—	x	x	x	x	x	x	x	x
Single lateral ventricle	—	—	—	x	x	x	—	—	—	—	—
Midgut herniation	—	—	—	—	x	x	x	x	—	—	—
Falx cerebri	—	—	—	—	—	x	x	x	x	x	x
Choroid plexus	—	—	—	—	—	x	x	x	x	x	x
Thalamus	—	—	—	—	—	x	x	x	x	x	x
Anterior and posterior contour	—	—	—	—	—	x	x	x	x	x	x
Humerus and femur	—	—	—	—	—	x	x	x	x	x	x
Finger	—	—	—	—	—	x	x	x	x	x	x
Tibia and radius	—	—	—	—	—	—	x	x	x	x	x
Toes	—	—	—	—	—	—	—	x	x	x	x
Cerebellum	—	—	—	—	—	—	—	x	x	x	x
Face	—	—	—	—	—	—	—	x	x	x	x
Lens	—	—	—	—	—	—	—	—	x	x	x
Palate	—	—	—	—	—	—	—	x	x	x	x
Heart, four chambers	—	—	—	—	—	—	—	x	x	x	x
Stomach	—	—	—	—	—	—	—	—	—	x	x

Modified from Warren WB, Timor-Tritsch I, Peisner DB, Raju S, Rosen MG. Dating the early pregnancy by sequential appearance of embryonic structures. *Am J Obstet Gynecol* 1989;161:747–753.

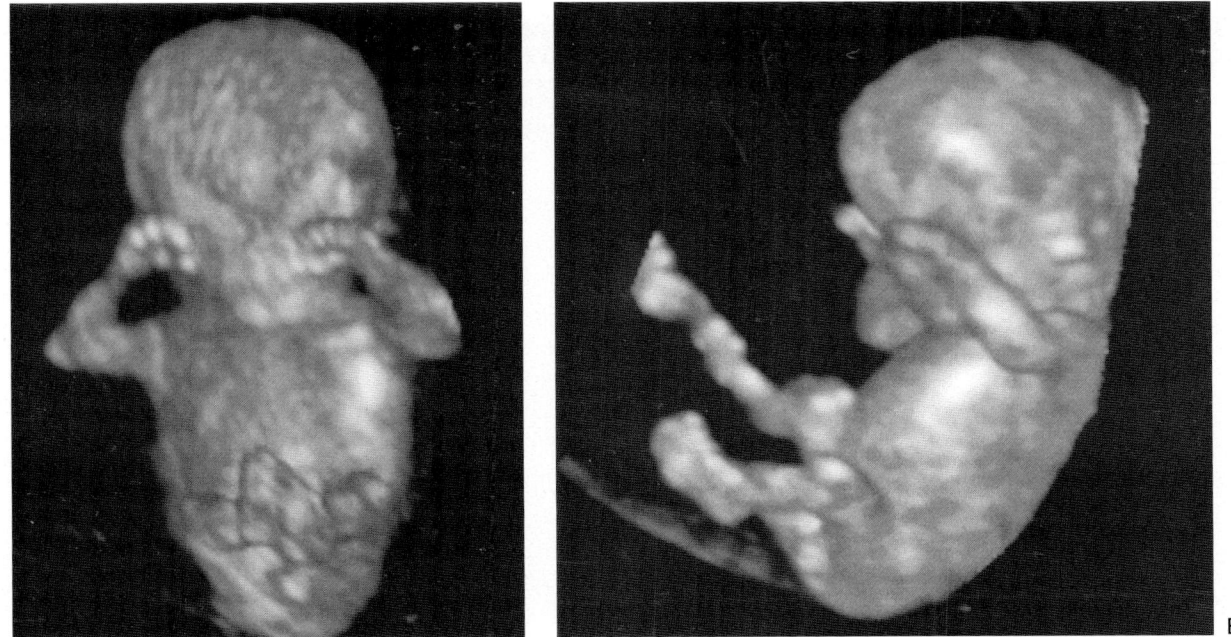

A
B

FIGURE 5. Three-dimensional ultrasound. Frontal **(A)** and side **(B)** views show a normal fetus at 10 weeks' gestational age. (Courtesy of David A. Nyberg, MD.)

Common Malformations of the Fetal Head, Neck, and Spine

Head and Brain

Acrania or Exencephaly

Acrania or exencephaly refers to a malformation in which there is absence of the entire or a significant portion of the cranium in the presence of the brain. This entity is theorized to be the embryologic predecessor of anencephaly in man.[4–10] Using TVS, the integrity of the cranium can be assessed during the first trimester, because the ossification of the fetal cranium begins and accelerates after 9 weeks.[11,12] Abnormal mineralization of the skull bones can

be sonographically determined by the early second trimester by assessing the degree of echogenicity of the bone.[13] Well-mineralized bone is highly echogenic. In addition to determining if calcification or mineralization is occurring normally, the sonographic appearance of the brain for the gestational age must be taken into account. An abnormal appearance of the brain can aid in the diagnosis of these two entities. Acrania has been reported as early as the twelfth postmenstrual week (Fig. 7).[13] The first-trimester exencephalic fetus has an abnormally shaped head with sonolucent spaces within the disintegrating brain. The outer shape of the head may be bilobed, and this has been referred to as a *Mickey Mouse head.*[14–16]

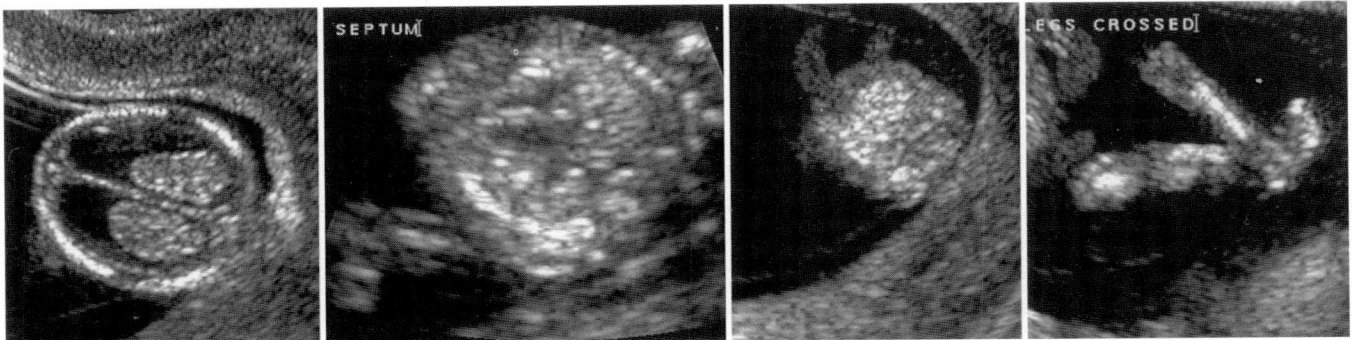

A,B
C,D

FIGURE 6. Early transvaginal anatomy scan of a fetus at 14 weeks, 1 day by menstrual history and 13 weeks, 1 day by crown-rump length. **A:** Axial section through the fetal head demonstrating the normal choroid plexus. **B:** Cross section of the heart showing the intact intraventricular septum. **C:** The fetal abdomen and the lower legs and feet **(D)**.

TABLE 2. CONVERSION TABLE FOR CROWN-RUMP LENGTH MEASUREMENTS (IN CM) TO MENSTRUAL AGE (95% CONFIDENCE INTERVAL IS ± 4 DAYS)

Menstrual age (wk + d)	Crown-rump length	Menstrual age (wk + d)	Crown-rump length
6 + 0	0.23	10 + 1	3.28
6 + 1	0.31	10 + 2	3.41
6 + 2	0.39	10 + 3	3.54
6 + 3	0.47	10 + 4	3.68
6 + 4	0.56	10 + 5	3.82
6 + 5	0.64	10 + 6	3.96
6 + 6	0.73	11 + 0	4.10
7 + 0	0.82	11 + 1	4.25
7 + 1	0.91	11 + 2	4.39
7 + 2	1.01	11 + 3	4.54
7 + 3	1.11	11 + 4	4.69
7 + 4	1.20	11 + 5	4.84
7 + 5	1.30	11 + 6	4.94
7 + 6	1.40	12 + 0	5.15
8 + 0	1.51	12 + 1	5.30
8 + 1	1.62	12 + 2	5.46
8 + 2	1.72	12 + 3	5.62
8 + 3	1.83	12 + 4	5.79
8 + 4	1.94	12 + 5	5.95
8 + 5	2.05	12 + 6	6.11
8 + 6	2.17	13 + 0	6.28
9 + 0	2.28	13 + 1	6.45
9 + 1	2.40	13 + 2	6.62
9 + 2	2.52	13 + 3	6.80
9 + 3	2.64	13 + 4	6.97
9 + 4	2.77	13 + 5	7.15
9 + 5	2.89	13 + 6	7.33
9 + 6	3.02	14 + 0	7.51
10 + 0	3.15	14 + 1	7.69

Modified from Warren WB, Timor-Tritsch I, Peisner DB, Raju S, Rosen MG. Dating the early pregnancy by sequential appearance of embryonic structures. *Am J Obstet Gynecol* 1989;161:747–753.

TABLE 3. CONVERSION TABLE FOR BIPARIETAL DIAMETER MEASUREMENTS (IN CM) TO MENSTRUAL AGE (95% CONFIDENCE LIMIT IS ± 5 DAYS)

Menstrual age (wk + d)	Biparietal diameter	Menstrual age (wk + d)	Biparietal diameter
7 + 0	0.47	10 + 4	1.37
7 + 1	0.49	10 + 5	1.43
7 + 2	0.51	10 + 6	1.50
7 + 3	0.53	11 + 0	1.56
7 + 4	0.56	11 + 1	1.63
7 + 5	0.58	11 + 2	1.70
7 + 6	0.61	11 + 3	1.78
8 + 0	0.63	11 + 4	1.86
8 + 1	0.66	11 + 5	1.94
8 + 2	0.69	11 + 6	2.02
8 + 3	0.72	12 + 0	2.11
8 + 4	0.75	12 + 1	2.20
8 + 5	0.79	12 + 2	2.30
8 + 6	0.82	12 + 3	2.40
9 + 0	0.86	12 + 4	2.51
9 + 1	0.89	12 + 5	2.62
9 + 2	0.93	12 + 6	2.73
9 + 3	0.97	13 + 0	2.85
9 + 4	1.02	13 + 1	2.98
9 + 5	1.06	13 + 2	3.11
9 + 6	1.11	13 + 3	3.24
10 + 0	1.16	13 + 4	3.38
10 + 1	1.21	13 + 5	3.53
10 + 2	1.26	13 + 6	3.69
10 + 3	1.32	14 + 0	3.85

Modified from Warren WB, Timor-Tritsch I, Peisner DB, Raju S, Rosen MG. Dating the early pregnancy by sequential appearance of embryonic structures. *Am J Obstet Gynecol* 1989;161:747–753.

Anencephaly

Anencephaly at 17 postmenstrual weeks was the first malformation reported using transabdominal ultrasound, and, subsequently, almost 20 years later was the first malformation reported with TVS at 11 weeks and 5 days postmenstrual.[17,18] Using TVS, the anencephalic fetus can be definitively identified by the twelfth postmenstrual week, although in some cases this diagnosis has been made earlier at 9 to 10 postmenstrual weeks.[19] In the coronal plane, the typical *frog's facies* is identified in which there is absence of the cranium above the prominent orbits with preservation of the base of the skull and facial features.[20] The median view reveals a normal fetal profile up to the area of the orbital ridges beyond which the forehead and calvaria are missing. Variable amounts of remnant brain tissue may be imaged over the area of the skull defect. Craniorachischisis may also be present in up to 10% of the anencephalic fetuses.[21]

Sepulveda et al.[22] described the measurement of the crown-chin length and its ratio to the crown-rump length (CRL) at 10 to 14 postmenstrual weeks as another clue to assist in the early recognition of anencephaly. In 77% of the cases with anencephaly, the fetuses had a crown-chin length measurement below fifth percentile, and, in 62% of the cases, the ratio of the crown-chin length to the CRL was below fifth percentile.

Cephaloceles

Cephaloceles are usually midline cranial defects in which there is herniation of the brain and meninges. The reported incidence is 0.8 to 3.0 per 10,000 live births. The cephalocele may also involve the occipital, frontal parietal, orbital, nasal, or nasopharyngeal region of the head. The prevalence of the different types of cephalocele shows geographic variation. In the Western Hemisphere, 80% of the cephaloceles is occipital, with the other 20% being equally distributed among the frontal and parietal cephaloceles. In the Eastern Hemisphere, sincipital (frontal) cephaloceles are more common.[20,23,24,26–29]

Posterior cephalocele has been diagnosed as early as 12 postmenstrual weeks.[30] Prenatal diagnosis of Meckel-Gruber syndrome has been made in the first and early second trimesters.[28,31–35] Sepulveda et al.[34] correctly diagnosed the four affected fetuses in nine pregnancies at risk for the syndrome. In 1996, van Zalen-Sprock[35] and colleagues reported on nine fetuses at risk for the Meckel-Gruber, Walker-Warburg, and Joubert's syndromes. In five out of nine fetuses, structural anomalies were detected during a first- or early second-

TABLE 4. CONVERSION TABLE FOR HEAD CIRCUMFERENCE MEASUREMENTS (IN CM) TO MENSTRUAL AGE (95% CONFIDENCE INTERVAL IS ± 4.8 DAYS)

Menstrual age (wk + d)	Head circumference	Menstrual age (wk + d)	Head circumference
8 + 5	3.53	11 + 4	6.49
8 + 6	3.68	11 + 5	6.64
9 + 0	3.82	11 + 6	6.78
9 + 1	3.97	12 + 0	6.93
9 + 2	4.12	12 + 1	7 08
9 + 3	4.27	12 + 2	7.23
9 + 4	4.42	12 + 3	7.38
9 + 5	4.56	12 + 4	7.52
9 + 6	4.71	12 + 5	7.67
10 + 0	4.86	12 + 6	7.82
10 + 1	5.00	13 + 0	7.97
10 + 2	5.16	13 + 1	8.12
10 + 3	5.30	13 + 2	8.26
10 + 4	5.45	13 + 3	8.41
10 + 5	5.60	13 + 4	8.56
10 + 6	5.75	13 + 5	8.71
11 + 0	5.90	13 + 6	8.86
11 + 1	6.04	14 + 0	9.00
11 + 2	6.19	14 + 1	9.15
11 + 3	6.34	14 + 2	9.30

Modified from Warren WB, Timor-Tritsch I, Peisner DB, Raju S, Rosen MG. Dating the early pregnancy by sequential appearance of embryonic structures. *Am J Obstet Gynecol* 1989;161:747–753.

TABLE 5. CONVERSION TABLE FOR ABDOMINAL CIRCUMFERENCE MEASUREMENTS (IN CM) TO MENSTRUAL AGE (95% CONFIDENCE LIMIT IS ± 6 DAYS)

Menstrual age (wk + d)	Abdominal circumference	Menstrual age (wk + d)	Abdominal circumference
8 + 5	3.09	11 + 4	4.91
8 + 6	3.17	11 + 5	5.02
9 + 0	3.24	11 + 6	5.14
9 + 1	3.32	12 + 0	5.26
9 + 2	3.40	12 + 1	5.38
9 + 3	3.47	12 + 2	5.51
9 + 4	3.56	12 + 3	5.64
9 + 5	3.64	12 + 4	5.77
9 + 6	3.72	12 + 5	5.90
10 + 0	3.81	12 + 6	6.04
10 + 1	3.90	13 + 0	6.18
10 + 2	3.99	13 + 1	6.32
10 + 3	4.08	13 + 2	6.47
10 + 4	4.18	13 + 3	6.62
10 + 5	4.27	13 + 4	6.78
10 + 6	4.37	13 + 5	6.93
11 + 0	4.48	13 + 6	7.09
11 + 1	4.58	14 + 0	7.26
11 + 2	4.69	14 + 1	7.43
11 + 3	4.80	14 + 2	7.60

Modified from Warren WB, Timor-Tritsch I, Peisner DB, Raju S, Rosen MG. Dating the early pregnancy by sequential appearance of embryonic structures. *Am J Obstet Gynecol* 1989;161:747–753.

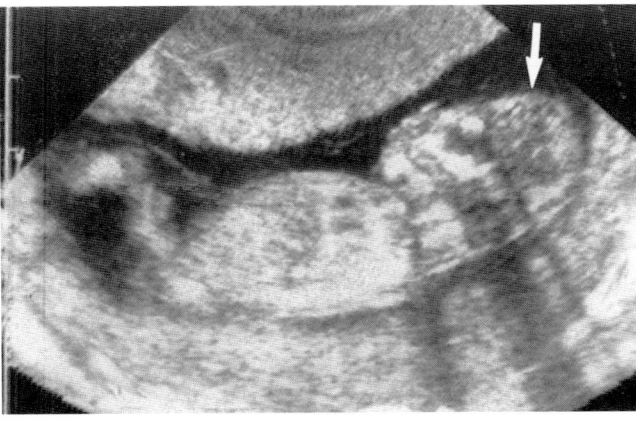

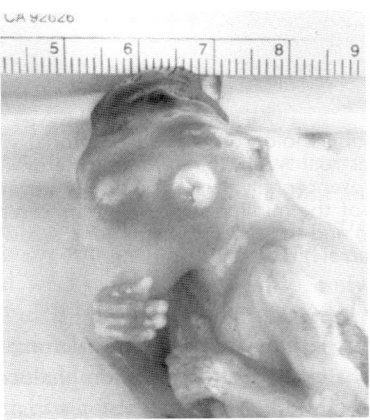

FIGURE 7. Acrania. Sagittal paramedian section of a fetus with acrania at 13 postmenstrual weeks and 3 days. **A:** The arrow points to the fetal head. Note that beyond the fetal orbits no calvaria exists (no hyperechogenic material is imaged covering the fetal brain). Also, note that there is significant amount of abnormal-looking brain present. **B:** Profile view of the abortus demonstrating the absent calvaria and the remnant brain tissue.

trimester ultrasound. In two out of five affected fetuses, sonographic detection of a cephalocele was predated by the visualization of an enlarged rhombencephalon cavity diameter at approximately 9 postmenstrual weeks of gestation.

Iniencephaly

Iniencephaly is a rare, lethal developmental anomaly. Its three main features are (a) a defect in the occiput involving the foramen magnum; (b) retroflexion of the entire spine, which forces the fetus to look upward with its occiput directed toward the lumbar region; and (c) open spinal defects of variable degrees.[36–42] The malformation results from a developmental arrest of the embryo during the third postmenstrual week, resulting in persistence of the embryonic cervical retroflexion, which leads to failure of the neural groove to close in the area of the cervical spine or upper thorax.[36,43,44] Associated malformations occur in up to 84% of the cases and include hydrocephaly, microcephaly, ventricular atresia, holoprosencephaly, polymicrogyria, agenesis of the cerebellar vermis, occipital encephalocele,

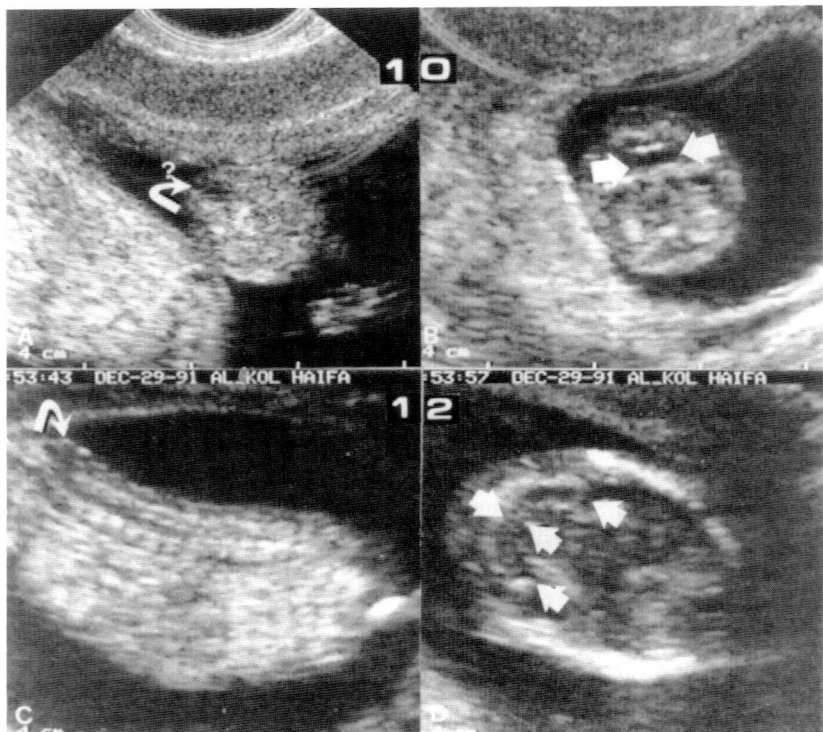

A–D

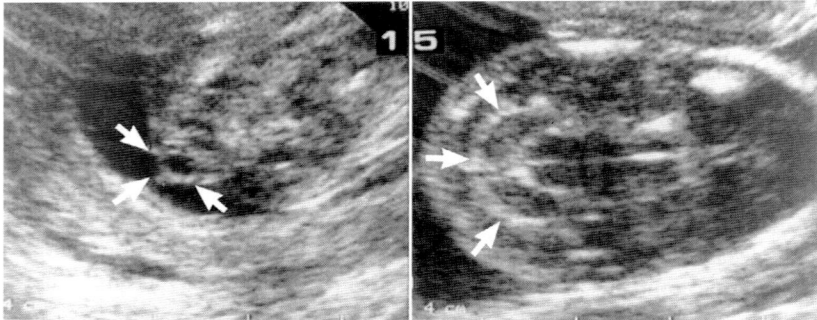

E,F

FIGURE 11. Spina bifida with dynamic development of the banana sign during the first trimester. **A:** Examination of the transverse scan of the low fetal trunk at 10 postmenstrual weeks raised the suspicion of a skin defect (*arrow*). **B:** At the same gestational age, the fetal cerebellum appeared normal (*arrows*). **C:** At 12 postmenstrual weeks, a spinal defect is more clearly suggested in the sacral area (*arrow*). **D:** The cerebellum appeared convex posteriorly (*arrows*). **E:** Follow-up at 15 weeks shows unequivocal meningocele on transvaginal sonography (*arrows*). **F:** Definite banana sign is identified with obliteration of the cisterna magna and loss of normal biconvex shape of cerebellum (*arrows*). (Reproduced with permission from Blumenfeld Z, Siegler E, Bronshtein M. The early diagnosis of neural tube defects. *Prenat Diagn* 1993;13: 863–71.) **G:** Postabortal autopsy showing the herniation of the cerebellum within the foramen magnum, creating the convexity of the banana sign (*arrows*). **H:** Spinal defect (*arrow*). (Parts **G** and **H** courtesy of Zeev Blumenfeld, Rambam Medical Center, Israel.)

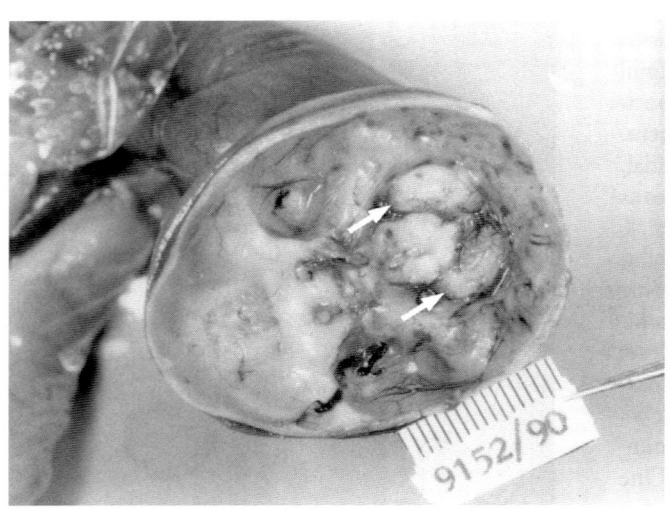

G

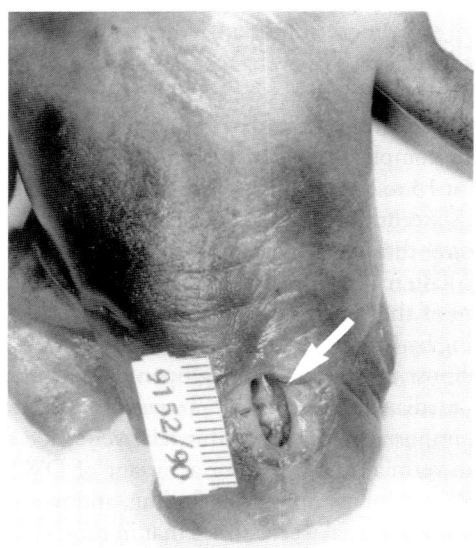

H

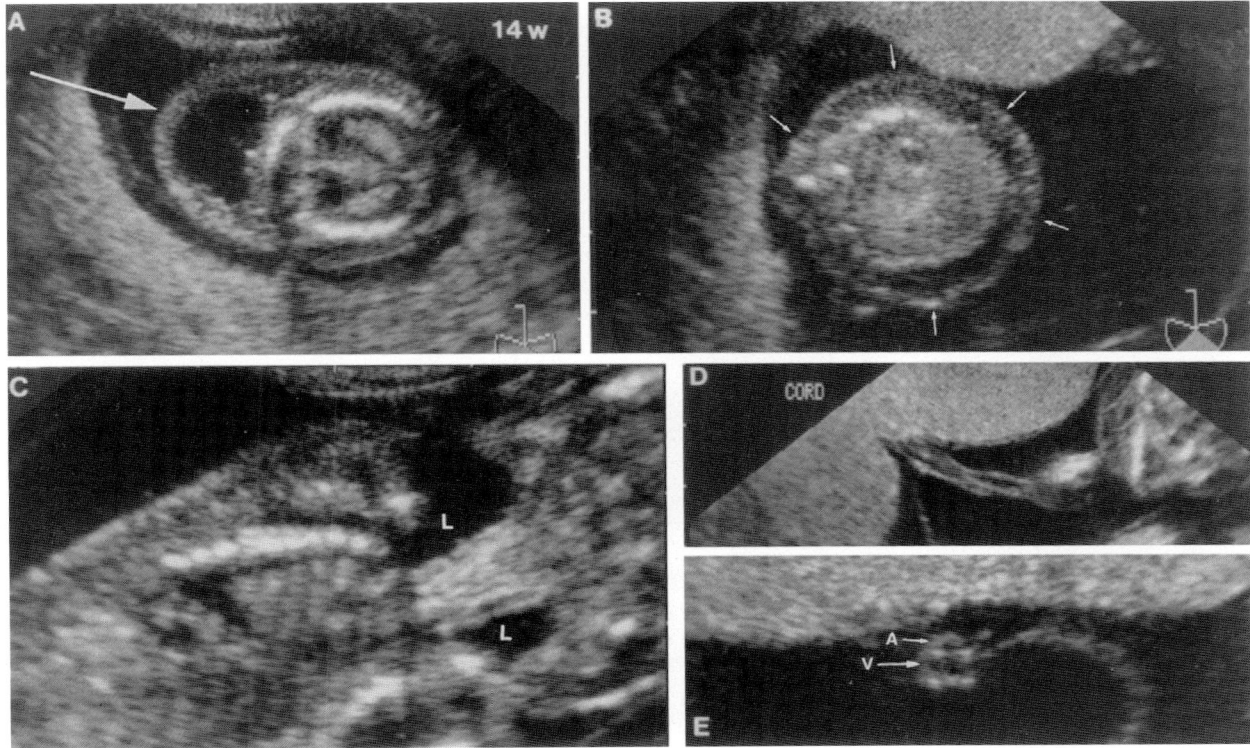

FIGURE 12. Cystic hygroma. Fetus at 14 postmenstrual weeks with a nonseptated cystic hygroma. **A:** Posterior coronal section of the fetal head demonstrates a large nonseptated hygroma (*arrow*). 14 w, 14 postmenstrual weeks. **B:** Cross section of the abdomen demonstrates the body edema (*arrows*). **C:** Within the fetal neck, the jugular lymphatic channels (*L*) are prominent. **D:** A two-vessel cord inserting into the placenta. Note the lack of coiling or braiding of the cord. **E:** Cross section of the cord showing one large vein (*V*) and a single umbilical artery (*A*).

The Neck: Nuchal Translucency and Cystic Hygroma

Two important abnormalities of the fetal neck during the first trimester are increased nuchal translucency and the cystic hygroma. These abnormalities are discussed in greater detail in Chapter 20 and Chapter 8. In cystic hygroma the classical finding is a fluid-filled cystic structure located in the posterior nuchal area of the fetus. At times, generalized fetal edema, pleural and pericardial effusions, and ascites may also be present (Fig. 12A through C).

The Face

The fetal face begins to resemble that of a baby by the end of the embryonic period. Development of the face occurs mostly between the fourth and eighth weeks postconception or the sixth to tenth postmenstrual weeks. During this period, there is transformation of the brachial apparatus into the tongue, face, lips, jaws, palate, pharynx, and neck, eventually resulting in the typical human facies.[80] Anomalies of the face can occur as an isolated finding but are frequently associated with chromosomal aneuploidy, such as trisomy 18

and 13 (Fig. 13), as well as nonchromosomal syndromes. When a facial anomaly is imaged, a targeted scan of the fetus as well as genetic counseling and testing are indicated.

One has to mention here the use of 3-D ultrasound in the targeted imaging of the face. Surface rendering of the face is the most known (not necessarily the most important) feature of 3-D ultrasound. The detection of a large number of facial anomalies was reported in the literature.[81–90] It is true that most of the experience was accumulated in the second and third trimesters, however, it is possible to rely on the analysis of facial structures in the orthogonal planes. This seems to be feasible in the late first and early second trimesters.

Cleft Lip and Palate

Cleft lip and palate (Fig. 14) is not only the most common facial anomaly, but it is also among the most common anomalies affecting the developing fetus, with a reported incidence of 1 per 1,000 live births.[4,81] In up to 80% of the cases, cleft lip is unilateral rather than bilateral, and most of the affected fetuses are male. Unilateral cleft lip is more commonly located on the left side.[4]

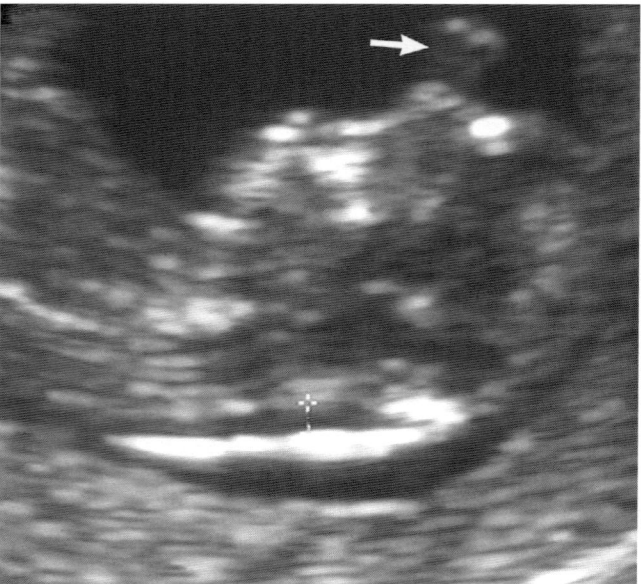

FIGURE 13. Proboscis. Sagittal view of face at 13 weeks shows abnormal facial profile with flattened face and proboscis (*arrow*) above level of orbits. Alobar holoprosencephaly was also identified. The karyotype was trisomy 13.

process to fuse. Clefts may be unilateral or bilateral. Cleft lip and palate have been diagnosed in utero as early as the thirteenth and fourteenth postmenstrual week.[82,83,92]

In the literature, there are several sonographic markers that help in the detection of this anomaly. One marker is the detection of an echogenic median mass, which actually is the premaxillary protrusion. In the case of a bilateral cleft, the mass is made up of soft tissue and, at times, of osseous and dental structures.[84] This mass can be imaged either in the median plane or in the coronal plane and can be especially useful in the second trimester to detect this anomaly. Using this marker, cleft lip and palate has been diagnosed as early as the seventeenth postmenstrual week.[84] A second sonographic marker is pseudoprognathism.[82,83] Pseudoprognathism or prolabium refers to a relative protrusion of the mandible as compared to the maxilla imaged on the sagittal or a paramedian section, which passes through the cleft lip and palate. Using this sign, cleft lip and palate has been diagnosed as early as the thirteenth and fourteenth postmenstrual week.[82,83] In summary, at 13 to 14 postmenstrual weeks using coronal and sagittal view of the fetal face, cleft lip and palate can be reliably diagnosed. When this anomaly is imaged, genetic counseling as well as a search for other anomalies must be undertaken.

Ocular Anomalies

Ocular anomalies affecting the developing fetus have been reported during the twelfth to eighteenth postmenstrual weeks using TVS.[85] Isolated anomalies affecting the developing fetal eye are rare, and in most cases anomalies are associated with other malformations, especially those of the developing brain (alobar holoprosencephaly) as well as with chromosomal aneuploidy (trisomy 13) and nonchromosomal syndromes.[85,93] Stoll et al.[94] found a prevalence of congenital eye malformations in the population that they

Developmentally, a continuous upper lip is formed by 8 weeks when the medial nasal and maxillary processes fuse. Failure of fusion of the medial nasal and maxillary processes results in a cleft lip affecting one or both sides.[91] Cleft palate with or without cleft lip has a reported incidence of 1 in 2,500 live births, and more commonly affects female fetuses.[4,81] The palate develops from the primary and the secondary palate. Its development starts at 7 postmenstrual weeks but is not complete until the fourteenth postmenstrual week.[81] Cleft palate results from failure of the mesenchymal masses in the lateral palatine

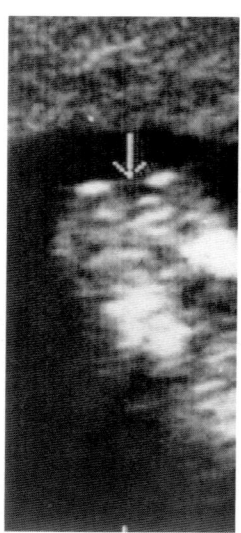
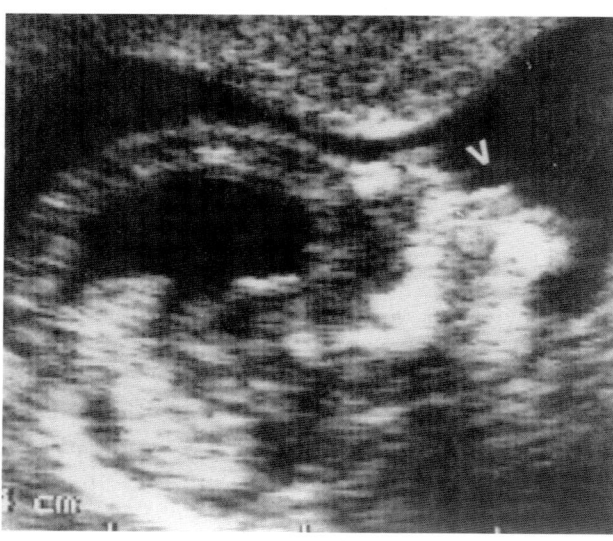

A,B

FIGURE 14. Cleft lip and palate. A: Transverse image shows labial defect (*arrow*). B: Sagittal paramedian view through the lesion demonstrating the pseudoprognathism (*arrowhead*). (Reproduced with permission from Vergani P, Ghidini A, Sirtori M, et al. Antenatal diagnosis of fetal acrania. *J Ultrasound Med* 1987;6:715–717.)

studied to be 7.5 per 10,000 live births. Approximately 54% of the cases had other associated malformations. Included in this group of anomalies were clubfeet, microcephaly, hydrocephaly, and facial dysmorphism.

Conditions such as hyper- and hypotelorism, anophthalmia, and microphthalmia have been diagnosed from 12 to 16 postmenstrual weeks by measuring the interocular distance, ocular diameter, and biocular distance.[85,86,93] All of these measurements can be made in a single transverse section at the plane of the orbits.[85,93] The fetal lens can be imaged consistently from the twelfth postmenstrual week.[85] The sonographic appearance of the normal lens is that of a hyperechogenic ring with a sonolucent core located within the fetal orbits. The lens is best viewed in an anterior coronal section of the face. The hyaloid artery can be seen posterior to the lens as a thin echogenic line between the lens and the posterior aspect of the lens.[85] The hyaloid artery is best imaged in a paramedian section through the orbits.

Fetal Cataracts

Fetal cataracts or opacification of the lens has been diagnosed *in utero*.[95–97] The lens affected with cataracts no longer has its typical sonographic appearance of a hyperechogenic ring with a clear center, but it has a variety of appearances such as thick, irregular, or crenated border, dense homogenous echogenic center, or with clusters of hyperechogenic material.[87,95] Using these sonographic appearances, congenital cataracts have been diagnosed from 14 postmenstrual weeks.[87] In those patients with a history of autosomal dominant cataracts, the cataracts were diagnosed as early as the twelfth postmenstrual week. Congenital cataracts are commonly inherited in an autosomal dominant fashion but are also the result of in utero infections, especially rubella during the sixth to ninth postmenstrual weeks.[87,98,99]

Malformations of the Heart and Diaphragm

Congenital malformations of the heart (Fig. 15) are common and account for approximately 25% of all congenital anomalies.[100] The reported incidence of congenital heart disease is two to eight per 1,000 live births.[101–103] In the literature, the association between congenital heart disease and extracardiac malformations and karyotypic aneuploidy has been well established. Paladini et al.[104] tried to determined the incidence of aneuploidy among fetuses with congenital heart disease scanned between 16 and 38 postmenstrual weeks. In their series of 31 fetuses with heart disease and complete follow-up, 48% also had an abnormal karyotype with trisomy 21 being the most common karyotypic abnormality followed by trisomy 18, trisomy 13, and triploidy. The most commonly encountered congenital heart disease with abnormal karyotype was atrioventricular septal defects and ventricular septal defect.[104] Bronshtein et al.[105] found 47 cases of congenital heart disease among 12,793 fetuses scanned transvag-

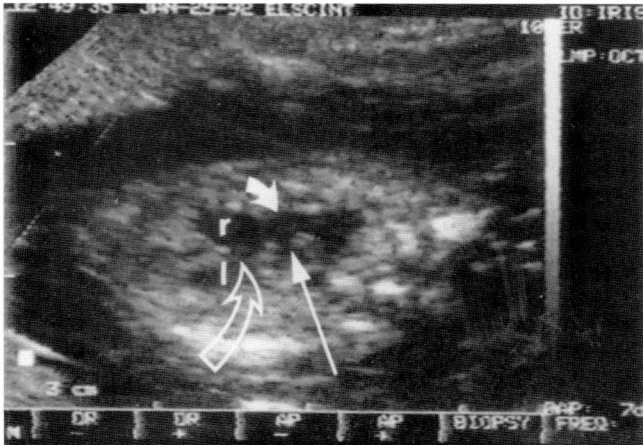

FIGURE 15. Truncus arteriosus. Short-axis view of the fetal heart demonstrates large ventricular septal defect (*open curved arrow*) with only one great artery (*closed curved arrow*), giving rise to the pulmonic artery (*long straight arrow*). This was confirmed pathologically. l, left ventricle; r, right ventricle. (Reproduced with permission from Rosati P, Guariglia L. Transvaginal sonographic assessment of the fetal urinary tract in early pregnancy. *Ultrasound Obstet Gynecol* 1996;7:95–100.)

inally at 12 to 16 postmenstrual weeks. Sixty-two percent of the affected fetuses had extra cardiac anomalies. Among the pregnancies karyotyped, 36% were aneuploidy. The anomalies detected were ventricular septal defect, common atrioventricular canal, hypoplastic left heart, transposition of the great vessels, Ebstein's anomaly, single ventricle, and coarctation of the aorta. Achiron et al.[106] found eight cases of congenital heart disease among approximately 1,000 fetuses scanned transvaginal between 10 and 12 postmenstrual weeks. Only one fetus had an abnormal karyotype (45,XO), but all fetuses showed extra cardiac abnormalities. The most common extra cardiac abnormalities were cystic hygroma and pericardial effusion with or without hydrops. The heart anomalies detected were ventricular septal defect, atrioventricular septal defect, ectopia cordis, giant right atrium, and tachycardia.

Fetal cardiac activity is consistently detected from 6 postmenstrual weeks or from a fetal pole size of 2 to 4 mm. The heart rate of the fetus steadily increases during the first trimester.[107] The mean heart rate increases from approximately 110 bpm at a CRL of 3 to 4 mm to 171 to 178[108–115] bpm at a CRL of 15 to 32 cm.[106] Heart rates in the first trimester outside these ranges have been associated with pregnancy failure.[106,107]

In the literature, there are eight cases reported with reversed end-diastolic umbilical artery (UA) blood flow at 10 to 14 weeks' gestation.[108,109,116,117] In six cases, the reversed-end diastolic flow was associated with chromosomal anomalies, two trisomy 18, trisomy 13, 45,X, triploidy (69,XXX) and trisomy 9 with a ventricular septal defect, and one had congenital heart disease with normal chromosomes.[108,110,116,117] In three cases there was also increased nuchal translucency.[116,118]

Using TVS, the fetal heart, specifically the four-chamber view, can be imaged from 10 weeks. Different authors have reported on the earliest gestational age at which the fetal heart can be consistently imaged and this ranges from 12 to 14 postmenstrual weeks.[3,101,111–114] But all authors agree that by 14 postmenstrual weeks on, the four-chamber view can be imaged in all patients in which this view was attempted. In addition, the great arteries can also be imaged from 11 postmenstrual weeks, and, similarly to the four-chamber view, they can be consistently imaged from 13 to 14 weeks onward.[101,112,114] Bronshtein et al.[105] found that at 12 to 16 postmenstrual weeks, the sensitivity of the four-chamber view to detect a cardiac defect was 77% versus up to 92% sensitivity reported beyond 18 postmenstrual weeks using transabdominal sonography.[113,114,119]

Gembruch et al.[112,114] reported on three major limitations of transvaginal echocardiography, including (a) difficulties in spatial orientation; (b) limitations in obtaining the desired planes as a result of narrow focal range of the probe, fetal position, and limited angles of insonation owing to the restricted mobility of the probe; and (c) the small size of the first-trimester fetal heart. These limitations can be overcome by manipulating the uterus and, in turn, the fetus with the free hand of the sonographer or sonologist.[115]

Similar to the customary echocardiography that takes place beyond 16 postmenstrual weeks, when performing an echo at 12 to 14 postmenstrual weeks the same general guidelines are applicable. For example, the right and left ventricle should be roughly of the same size, the heart should not occupy more than one-third of the thoracic cavity, and at the crux of the heart the tricuspid valve should be located more apically when compared to the mitral valve.[105] It is beyond the scope of this chapter to describe in detail how to perform a fetal echocardiogram. For the reader who is familiar with performing a transabdominal fetal echocardiogram and TVS, it is relatively easy to master the technique of transvaginal echocardiography.

Congenital Diaphragmatic Hernia

Congenital diaphragmatic hernia is the only common congenital abnormality of the diaphragm occurring in approximately 1 of 2,000[120] to 1 in 4, 000[121,122] live-born infants. The defect most commonly affects the left hemidiaphragm compared to the right. The diaphragm develops from four structures: (a) septum transversum, (b) pleuroperitoneal membranes, (c) the dorsal mesentery of the esophagus, and (d) the body wall. Failure of the pleuroperitoneal membrane to fuse with the other diaphragmatic components before the intestines return to abdominal cavity from the physiologic midgut herniation results in the intestines passing into the thoracic cavity.[120] The diagnosis of congenital diaphragmatic hernia is made when in a transverse section of the thorax, the stomach, and the heart are located in the same section. Sebire et al.[121] published on the association of increased nuchal translucency at 10 to 14 postmenstrual weeks and congenital diaphragmatic hernia. They found that at the 10- to 14-week scan, the fetal nuchal translucency was above the 95th percentile for CRL in seven (37%) of the 19 cases of diaphragmatic hernia, which was diagnosed at the initial or subsequent scans or at birth. Fifteen patients continued the pregnancy, which resulted in live births with subsequent repair (nine neonates survived and six died). The translucency was increased in five of the six cases that resulted in neonatal death, compared with two of the nine survivors.

Malformations of the Abdominal Wall and Gastrointestinal Tract

Omphalocele

Omphalocele (Figs. 16 through 18) is a median abdominal wall defect in which the bowel and liver or bowel alone have herniated through into a peritoneal sac. The defect usually occurs at the level of the umbilical cord with the cord inserting at the apex of the defect. There are two types of omphalocele: liver-containing and non–liver-containing omphalocele. The bowel-containing omphalocele can only be reliably diagnosed after 12 postmenstrual weeks, because at this age it is difficult to differentiate it from the physiologic midgut herniation.[123,124] In contrast to the fetal bowel, the liver does not follow a physiologic migration outside the abdominal cavity during development. During the fourth to fifth week of development, the flat embryo begins to fold. Four folds occur: cephalic, caudal, and right and left lateral folds that converge at the site of the umbilicus. Each lateral fold forms one-half of the abdominal wall.[125,126] If normal folding and bowel rotation occur, a physiologic midgut herniation takes place between the eighth and twelfth postmenstrual weeks.[123] If normal folding takes place, but for some reason the extraembryonic gut fails to return to the abdominal cavity, a bowel-containing omphalocele results.[125–127] In this case, as said, the liver is not in the hernia, because during development it does not follow a physiologic migration outside the abdomen. Some authors have called this defect *hernia into the cord.*[127]

In approximately 40% to 60% of the cases, a chromosomal abnormality such as trisomy 18, 21, or 13 is present. In bowel-containing omphalocele, the amount of herniated bowel may be variable, and this type of omphalocele is associated with chromosomal aneuploidy, especially trisomy 18.[128] If, however, the lateral folds fail to close, a large abdominal wall defect is created, through which the abdominal cavity contents, including the liver, can herniate.[125,126] The result is a liver-containing omphalocele. This type of omphalocele is associated with a normal karyotype.[128–130] Sonographically this type of omphalocele can be diagnosed during the first trimester, as early as 9 to 10 postmenstrual weeks, if a mass, with the consistency of

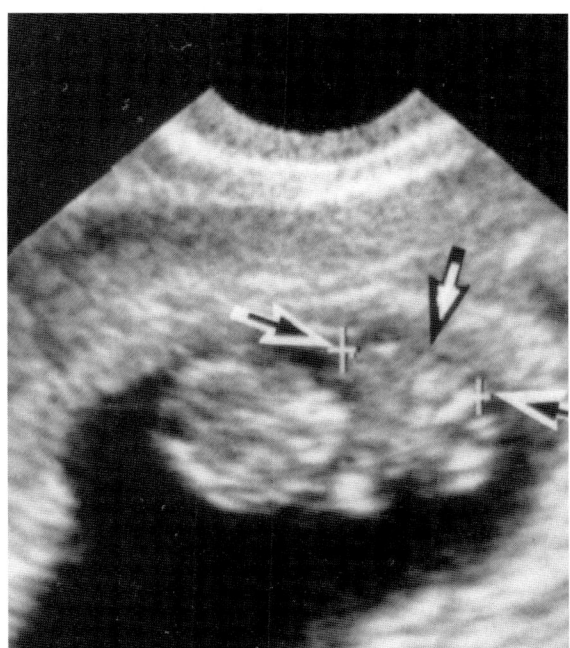
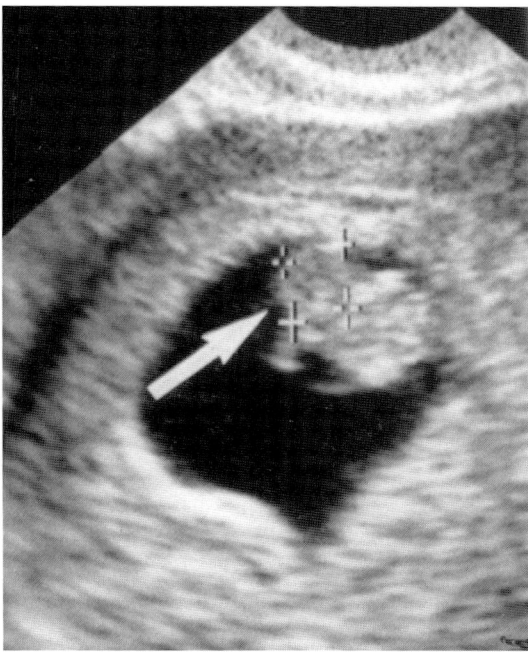

FIGURE 16. Omphalocele. Fetus at 9 postmenstrual weeks and 1 day showing a liver containing omphalocele. **A:** Long view of the fetus showing the large mass measuring 11.0 mm × 7.8 mm × 6.4 mm located anteriorly to the abdominal wall (*black and white arrows*). The mass is located within the area of the physiologic midgut herniation, and the contents have the sonographic appearance similar to that of fetal liver. **B:** Cross section of the abdomen shows that the mass or liver-containing omphalocele is almost as large as the abdominal circumference (*arrow*).

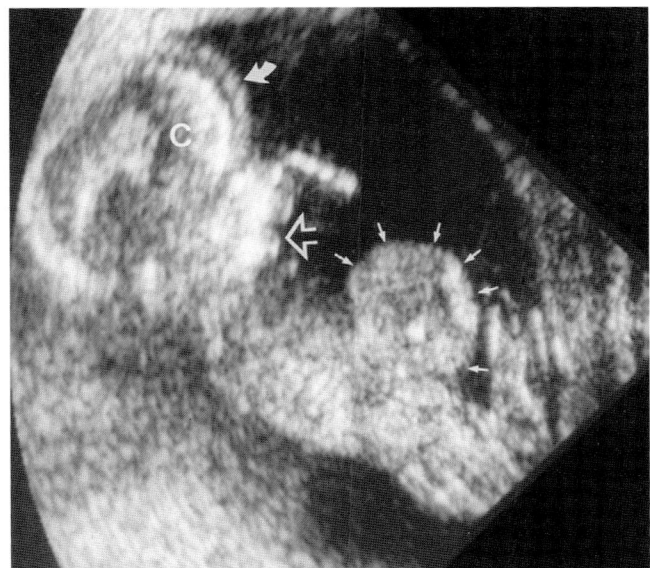

FIGURE 17. Omphalocele with trisomy 13. Transvaginal scan at 13 weeks and 3 days shows omphalocele with extracorporeal liver (*small arrows*). Subcutaneous edema (*curved arrow*) was also noted, and there was suggestion of micrognathia (*open arrow*). The karyotype proved to be trisomy 13. C, cranium.

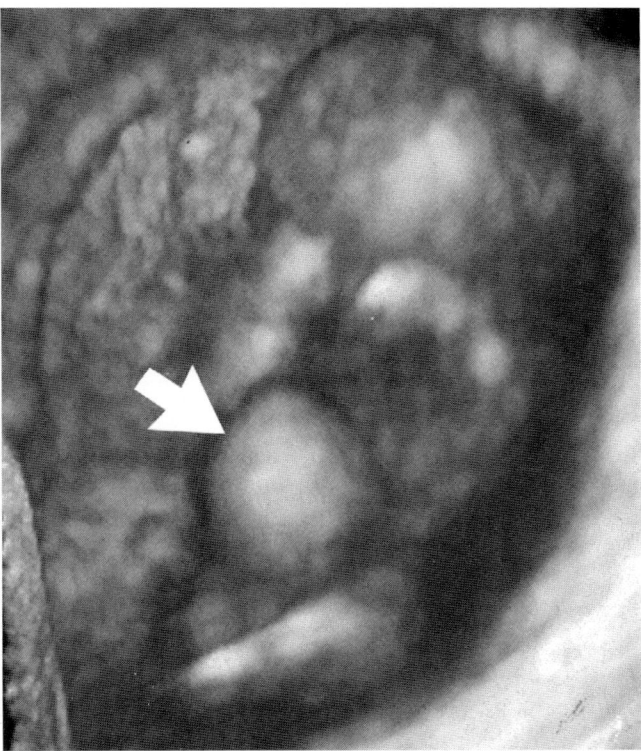

FIGURE 18. Omphalocele (*arrow*) with trisomy 18. Three-dimensional scan in surface-rendered mode at 11 menstrual weeks shows a liver containing omphalocele. A cystic hygroma was also present. Chorionic villus sampling revealed trisomy 18.

liver, measuring greater than 5 to 10 mm in diameter[124,131–135] is imaged within the area of the physiologic midgut herniation. During the first trimester the liver is homogeneous, whereas the bowel is more echogenic. This different sonographic appearance can help differentiate between the liver and the bowel in the first trimester. An omphalocele containing only bowel may be difficult to diagnose before 12 postmenstrual weeks, and, therefore, this diagnosis must likely be reserved to cases beyond 12 weeks. In addition, omphaloceles have been associated with nonchromosomal syndromes such as Turner (45,X), and Beckwith-Wiedemann syndromes.[136–138]

In addition to the chromosomal abnormalities, fetuses with omphalocele have other associated malformations. In as many as 50% of the cases, a congenital heart defect may be present as well as a wide range of anomalies, including gastrointestinal anomalies, genitourinary anomalies, neural tube defects, and intrauterine growth retardation.[134,135] In addition, in fetuses with increased nuchal translucency, even in the presence of normal chromosomes, the prevalence of omphalocele is ten times higher than in the general population.[122]

Gastroschisis

Gastroschisis refers to a defect of the abdominal wall, usually to the right of the umbilicus through which evisceration of the intestinal organs has occurred.[139] It is theorized that gastroschisis is the result of a vascular compromise of either the umbilical vein or the omphalomesenteric artery.[139–141] The anterior abdominal wall can be consistently imaged from 9 postmenstrual weeks.[3] Gastroschisis has been diagnosed as early as the twelfth postmenstrual week.[142,143] Gastroschisis, unlike omphalocele, is not associated with an increased incidence of chromosomal aneuploidy. Gastroschisis has been associated with a number of other malformations such as exstrophy of the urinary bladder, intrauterine growth restriction, and malrotation of the bowel, to name a few.[135,139,144]

Ectopia Cordis

Ectopia cordis (Fig. 19) is a rare defect. The heart is partly or completely exposed on the surface of the thorax. It results from failure of fusion of the lateral folds in the thoracic area during the sixth postmenstrual week.[101] The diagnosis of ectopia cordis has been reported as early as the twelfth to fourteenth postmenstrual weeks.[145,146] Pentalogy of Cantrell is another rare and complex malformation in which ectopia cordis can occur as a result of a thoracoabdominal defect. The five anomalies encompassed in pentalogy of Cantrell are (a) median supraumbilical abdominal defect, (b) defect of the lower sternum, (c) deficiency of the diaphragmatic pericardium, (d) deficiency of the anterior diaphragm, and (e) intracardiac abnormality.[134] This mal-

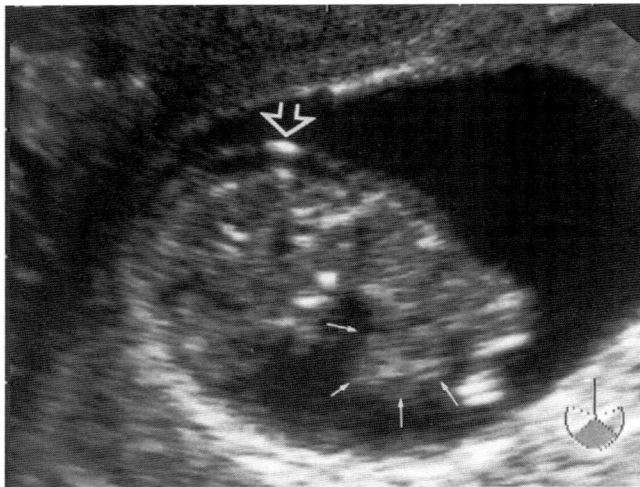

FIGURE 19. Ectopia cordis. A fetus at 10 postmenstrual weeks shows increased nuchal translucency posteriorly (*open arrow*) and an anterior abdominal wall defect. The evicerated mass (*small arrows*) also included the heart, which was observed to be beating on real-time ultrasound.

formation has been diagnosed as early as 11 postmenstrual weeks.[147] Using conventional two-dimensional and 3-D ultrasound, Liang et al.[148] made the diagnosis at the tenth postmenstrual weeks. Pentalogy of Cantrell has been associated with trisomies 18, 13, and 21. In addition, cystic hygroma has also been reported with Pentalogy of Cantrell.

The body stalk anomaly is a lethal malformation, which occurs as a result of failure of fusion of the lateral folds during the sixth postmenstrual week. In a study by Forrester et al.[149] dealing with the epidemiology of abdominal wall defects in Hawaii between 1986–1997, the incidence of this anomaly was 0.32 per 10,000 births. In this malformation, the abdominal organs lie outside the cavity. The organs are contained within a sac, which is covered by a amnioperitoneal membrane and is attached directly to the placenta.[30,150] The umbilical cord in these cases may be totally absent or significantly shortened, and severe kyphoscoliosis may be present. This malformation has been reported in utero as early as 9 postmenstrual weeks.[151] In addition, several case reports exist in the literature dealing with the first- and early second-trimester diagnosis of this anomaly.[147,151–153]

Umbilical Cord Cysts

Umbilical cord cysts and single UA (SUA) are abnormalities involving the umbilical cord that can be diagnosed within the first 14 weeks. The umbilical cord develops when the embryo is 35 mm in length as a result of the folding of the embryo.[154] Umbilical cord cysts can be imaged from around the eighth and ninth postmenstrual weeks.[154,155] Skibo et al.[154] suggested that because of the embryologic features and content of the umbilical cord, six potentially cystic masses can occur. These six masses are (a) amniotic inclusion cyst, (b) omphalomesenteric duct cysts, (c) allantoic cysts, (d) vascular anomalies, (e) neoplasm, and (f) Wharton's jelly abnormalities. Sonographically, the exact nature of the umbilical cord cyst may not be determined. Cysts, which are located close to the fetal body, are most likely derived from the allantois, omphalomesenteric or vitelline duct.[154] Vascular cystic structures can be identified by using color Doppler and visualizing flow within the cystic space.[154] Umbilical cord cysts that are transient during the first trimester do not seem to be associated with either chromosomal or structural anomalies, but persistent cord cysts that are imaged during the second and third trimester have been associated with other fetal anomalies as well as chromosomal aneuploidy.[154–158] Ross et al.[159] reported on the prevalence, morphologic characteristics, and natural history of umbilical cord cysts detected by ultrasound in the first trimester of pregnancy. This was an ultrasound screening study for the presence of umbilical cord cysts in 859 pregnant women with singleton live fetuses at 7 to 13 postmenstrual weeks. The results revealed that umbilical cord cysts were present in 29 (3.4%) of the 859 pregnancies. Fetal abnormalities were found in seven (26%) of the 27 cases with ongoing pregnancies. The fetus was more likely to be abnormal if the cyst was located near the placental or fetal extremity of the cord [relative risk (RR) 3.3; 95% confidence interval (CI) 1.3, 8.5] or paraxially (RR 3.8; 95% CI 1.2, 12.0), or if it persisted beyond 12 weeks' gestation (RR 7.7; 95% CI 3.2, 18.6).

Single Umbilical Artery

SUA is the most common abnormality affecting the umbilical cord. It is estimated that SUA affects 0.2% to 1% of all pregnancies.[160–163] Using TVS, the vessels of the umbilical cord can be imaged and counted starting from 8 to 9 postmenstrual weeks, and SUA has been diagnosed from 13 postmenstrual weeks.[147] Prenatally, the prevalence of SUA is higher during the third trimester than during the first trimester.[164] Blazer et al.[165] followed 46 fetuses with SUA in which the side of the existing artery was identified by TVS at 14 to 16 postmenstrual weeks. A right artery was detected in 25 fetuses (54.3%), and a left artery was detected in 21 cases (45.7%). Six fetuses (13%) had associated anomalies, with five of them in the urinary system. No correlation was found between the type or severity of the malformations and the side of the missing (or existing) UA.

Single umbilical vessel probably results from three possible mechanisms: (a) primary agenesis of one of the umbilical arteries; (b) secondary atrophy or atresia of a previously normal artery; and (c) persistence of the original single allantoic artery of the body stalk.[160,164] Sonographically an SUA can be imaged in the transverse and longitudinal plane. In addition, the cords appear to be less coiled or braided than in the three vessel cords (I. E. Timor-Tritsch, *unpublished observation*). Fetuses with SUA have a higher incidence of congeni-

tal anomalies, intrauterine growth restriction, prematurity, perinatal mortality, and chromosomal aneuploidy.[160,164]

Malformations of the Genitourinary Tract

The fetal kidneys assume their adult position within the renal fossa by 11 postmenstrual weeks.[166] Using TVS the fetal kidneys can be consistently imaged from 12 to 13 postmenstrual weeks.[167–169] Although identification of the kidneys has been reported as early as the ninth postmenstrual week, imaging before 12 to 13 postmenstrual weeks is not reliable.[170] Green et al.,[168] using transabdominal sonography, were able to visualize the kidneys in 60% of cases by 10 postmenstrual weeks; by 11 postmenstrual weeks the kidneys were seen in 98% of cases; and by 12 weeks the kidneys were seen in 100% of cases. The bladder appears later, and by 12 postmenstrual weeks this organ can be identified in 50% of cases. Using TVS Rosati et al.[167] were able to image the fetal kidneys and fetal urinary bladder in 92% of the cases screened by the thirteenth postmenstrual week. It is likely that renal agenesis can be diagnosed (or excluded) reliably in the first trimester. With improving technology, prenatal diagnosis of some fetal anomalies is now possible in the first trimester.

The fetal kidney appears relatively hyperechogenic up to approximately 16 postmenstrual weeks. The echogenicity of the kidney before 16 postmenstrual weeks has been described as similar to that of the fetal lung at a comparable gestational age.[171] Beyond 16 postmenstrual weeks the fetal kidneys assume the well-recognized hypoechogenic appearance.[171] Table 6 is a nomogram of the fetal renal dimensions between 12 and 14 postmenstrual weeks.

The fetal adrenal during the first and early second trimester is relatively large in comparison to the kidneys, but the adrenal-to-kidney length ratio decreases linearly between 12 and 17 postmenstrual weeks.[172] The sonographic appearance of the fetal adrenal gland between the age of 12 and 17 postmenstrual weeks is that of a hypoechoic ellipse. Unlike the fetal kidneys, which change their sonographic appearance during gestation, the adrenal glands remain hypoechoic throughout gestation.[171] Table 7 is a nomogram of the fetal adrenal length from 13 to 17 postmenstrual weeks.

TABLE 6. FETAL KIDNEY DIMENSION BETWEEN 12 AND 14 POSTMENSTRUAL WEEKS

Gestational age (wk)	Kidney diameter (cm)		
	Antero-posterior	Transverse	Longitudinal
12	0.40–0.12	0.40–0.09	0.61–0.06
13	0.53–0.08	0.52–0.06	0.83–0.18
14	0.56–0.09	0.59–0.12	0.92–0.11

Modified from Bronshtein M, Kushnir O, Ben-Rafael Z, et al. Transvaginal sonographic measurement of fetal kidneys in the first trimester of pregnancy. *J Clin Ultrasound* 1990;18:299–301.

TABLE 7. NOMOGRAM OF THE FETAL ADRENAL LENGTH BETWEEN 13 AND 17 POSTMENSTRUAL WEEKS

Gestational age (wk)	Adrenal length (cm)	
	Left	Right
13	2.4–1.4	2.5–1.4
14	2.8–1.4	3.0–1.4
15	3.2–1.4	3.5–1.4
16	3.5–1.4	4.0–1.4
17	4.0–1.4	4.5–1.4

Bronshtein M, Tzidony D, Dimant M, et al. Transvaginal ultrasonographic measurements of the fetal adrenal glands at 12 to 17 weeks. *Am J Obstet Gynecol* 1993;169:1205–1210

Hydronephrosis

Several congenital malformations involving the fetal kidneys have been diagnosed in utero. Some of these have also been detected early using TVS.[170,171,173,174] Hydronephrosis is a relatively common sonographic finding during the second and third trimesters. Between 15 and 20 postmenstrual weeks, an anterior-posterior diameter of the renal pelvis greater than 4 mm has been found to be associated with a risk of congenital hydronephrosis and trisomy 21.[173,174] Scanty information is available regarding the cut-off value below 15 postmenstrual weeks. Bronshtein et al.[170] used a cut-off value of 3 mm between 14 and 16 postmenstrual weeks and found this value to be associated with chromosomal and structural abnormalities. But, in most fetuses, the hydronephrosis disappears between 15 postmenstrual weeks to term.

Bilateral Renal Agenesis

Bilateral renal agenesis (BRA) is usually diagnosed by ultrasound in the (a) absence of the fetal bladder; (b) bilateral absence of the fetal kidneys; and (c) oligohydramnios.[175] BRA is a rare and lethal malformation. The diagnosis has been made before 16 postmenstrual weeks, by assessing the echogenicity of the contents of the renal fossa.[171] If bilateral echogenic structures with the usual shape and size of the fetal kidneys are imaged in the renal fossa, then normal kidneys can be assumed. But if a relatively large hypoechoic structure is imaged without the sonographic signs of an ectopic kidney or a bilateral empty renal fossa is apparent, BRA should be suspected. Before 17 postmenstrual weeks oligohydramnios and absence of the fetal bladder may not be sonographically apparent. Therefore, oligohydramnios and absence of the fetal bladder may not be a reliable sign of BRA before 17 postmenstrual weeks. A follow-up scan after 17 postmenstrual weeks is indicated in these cases.

Multicystic Dysplastic Kidney Disease and Infantile Polycystic Kidney Disease

Multicystic dysplastic kidney disease has been diagnosed as early as the twelfth to fifteenth postmenstrual week.[170] The diagnosis is made when in the renal fossa one or both kidneys are absent, and, instead, cysts of variable sizes are present. Infantile polycystic kidney disease has also been diagnosed at 13 to 16 postmenstrual weeks.[170,173] In infantile polycystic kidney disease, in contrast to multicystic dysplastic kidney disease, the cysts are small and both kidneys are affected. The affected kidneys are echogenic and large, but retained their typical kidney shape. Oligohydramnios, which is always present beyond 16 postmenstrual weeks, may not be present before 16 postmenstrual weeks. The fetal urinary bladder may or may not be imaged. Other renal anomalies diagnosed in utero at 16 postmenstrual weeks include double collecting system and horseshoe kidney.

Congenital kidney disease is associated with an increased risk of fetal chromosomal abnormalities.[176] This association is especially true in the face of other nonrenal malformations. Therefore, when faced with a renal abnormality a fetal karyotype is indicated.

The urinary bladder becomes sonographically apparent at 10 to 12 postmenstrual weeks, but, similarly to the kidney, does not become consistently imaged until the thirteenth week.[170,174,175] Cyclical filling and emptying of the fetal bladder should be imaged by the thirteenth postmenstrual week. This cycle of emptying and filling of the fetal bladder is repeated every 30 to 155 minutes.[174,175,177] Nonvisualization of the fetal bladder between 14 and 16 postmenstrual weeks has been reported to be associated with bladder exstrophy, multicystic dysplastic kidneys, and BRA.[174] In the case of bladder exstrophy, a slightly protruding lower abdominal mass is evident. The differential diagnosis in these cases includes omphalocele and gastroschisis. Imaging the insertion of the umbilical cord helps in the differentiation of bladder exstrophy from omphalocele and gastroschisis.[178] In addition, on two of the reported cases of nonvisualization of the fetal bladder, followed serially, the amniotic fluid volume was normal at 15 postmenstrual weeks, and oligohydramnios only became obvious at 16 postmenstrual weeks. In conclusion, nonvisualization of the fetal bladder at 13 to 16 postmenstrual weeks should trigger a careful evaluation of the fetal kidneys and lower abdominal wall. In addition, even if no other abnormality is imaged initially, a follow-up scan after 16 postmenstrual weeks is indicated to rule out any anomalies, especially those involving the kidneys.

Obstructive Uropathy

Obstructive uropathy (Figs. 20 through 22) especially when it occurs at the level of the urethra results in an enlarged urinary bladder. A dilated bladder may rise out of the pelvis and extend into the fetal abdomen and may present as an intra-abdominal cyst.[179] Bladder outlet obstruction has been diagnosed as early as the eleventh postmenstrual week.[180,181] Favre et al.[181] evaluated the prognostic criteria of early fetal megacystis. In a prospec-

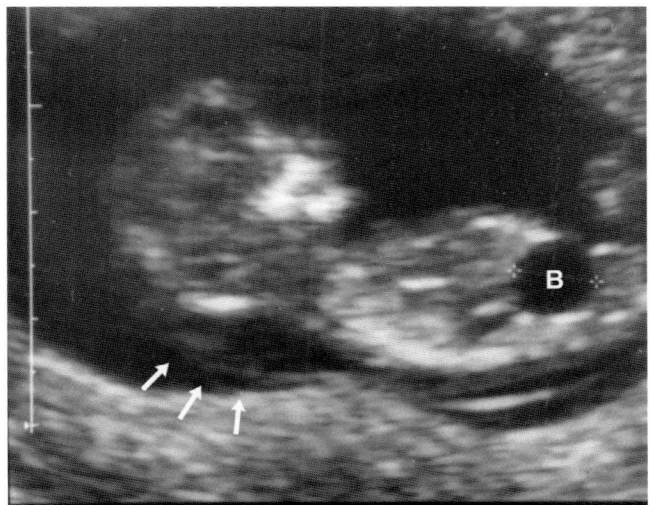

FIGURE 20. Megacystis. Scan at 11 weeks shows distended urinary bladder (*B*) and increased nuchal translucency (*arrows*). The karyotype was trisomy 13.

tive, transvaginal ultrasound, cross-sectional study at 11 to 15 postmenstrual weeks at a tertiary referral fetal medicine unit, 16 pregnancies out of a total of 5,240 were identified with early fetal megacystis. The karyotype was available in 15 cases. Vesicocentesis was performed in six fetuses and three had concomitant cystoscopies. The results revealed that in six fetuses, the megacystis was isolated. In the remaining ten, associated hygroma (n = 5), nuchal translucency (n = 3), omphalocele (n = 1), mild pyelectasis (n = 1),

and bilateral talipes (n = 1) were detected. In three cases the fetuses demonstrated renal hyperechogenicity with cysts, and in two cases oligohydramnios was found. Four cases (25%) had chromosomal abnormalities: 47,XY + 13 (two cases), 47,XY + 18, and 47,XY + 21. Only one fetus from this study survived. The remaining 13 terminated the pregnancy because of the poor prognosis.

The exact mechanism for the formation of amniotic fluid during the first trimester has not been clearly delineated. But the most likely mechanism appears to be an active transport of solutes by the amnion into the amniotic space with water moving across the osmotic gradient.[182] Fetal urine first enters the amniotic cavity at around 8 to 11 postmenstrual weeks.[183] Before the fifteenth postmenstrual week of the gestation, fetal urine does not contribute significantly to the amniotic fluid volume.[184] Oligohydramnios during the second trimester is associated with a poor fetal outcome.[184,185] Associated anomalies reported with early second-trimester oligohydramnios include BRA, congenital heart disease, skeletal dysplasia, and chromosomal aneuploidy. TVS in cases of oligohydramnios can demonstrate fetal anatomy and identify the presence of any structural abnormality.[186,187]

Malformations of the Skeleton

The limbs begin to develop toward the end of the sixth postmenstrual week. The upper limbs develop before the lower limbs.[188] Using TVS the limbs can be imaged by the eighth postmenstrual week.[1] By the ninth postmenstrual

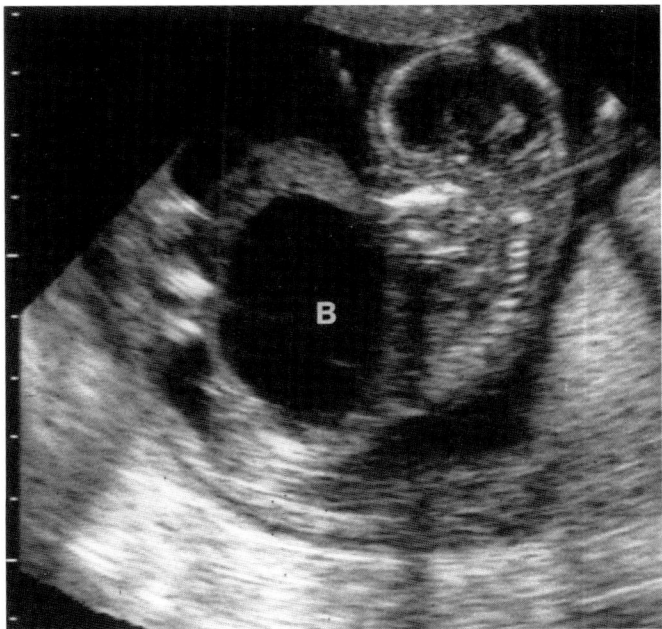
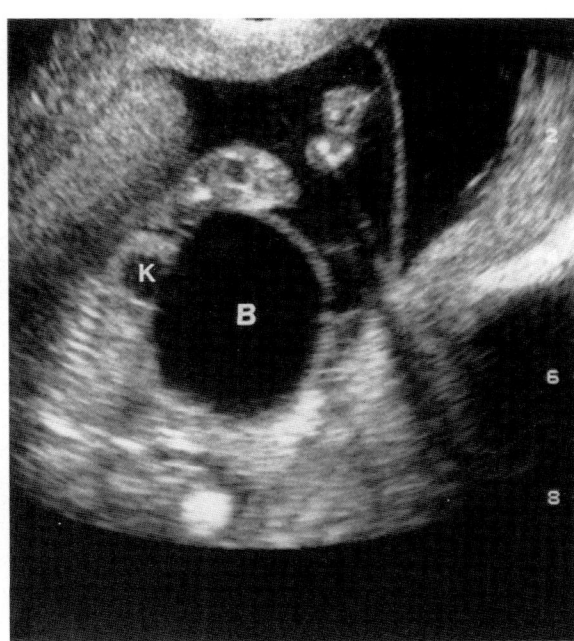

FIGURE 21. Urethral obstruction at 14 menstrual weeks. **A:** Note the large bladder (*B*). **B:** The large bladder rises out of the pelvis. In addition, to the dilated bladder (*B*) the renal pelvis (*K*) is prominent. (Courtesy of Professor Israel Meizner, Beer-Sheba, Israel.)

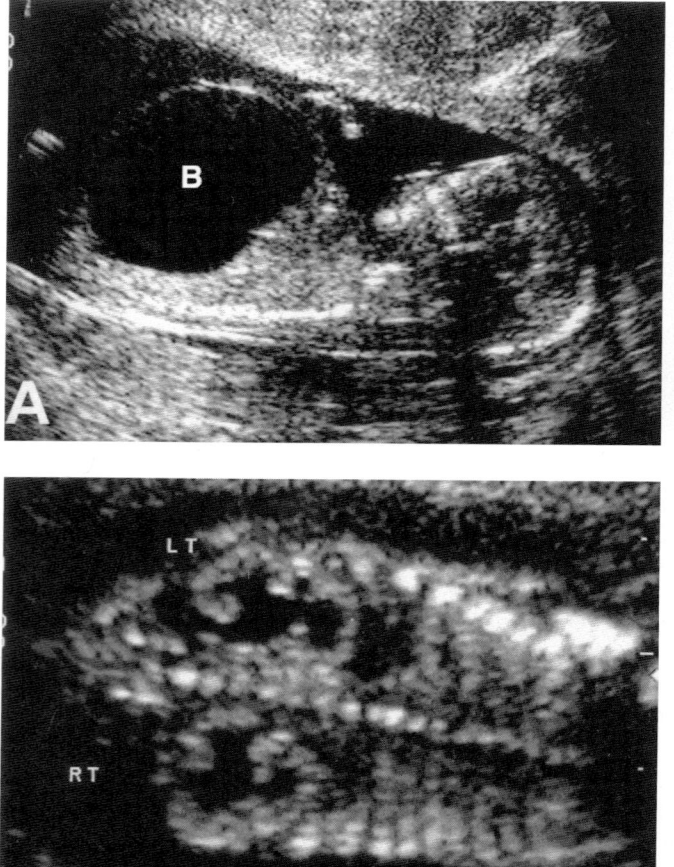

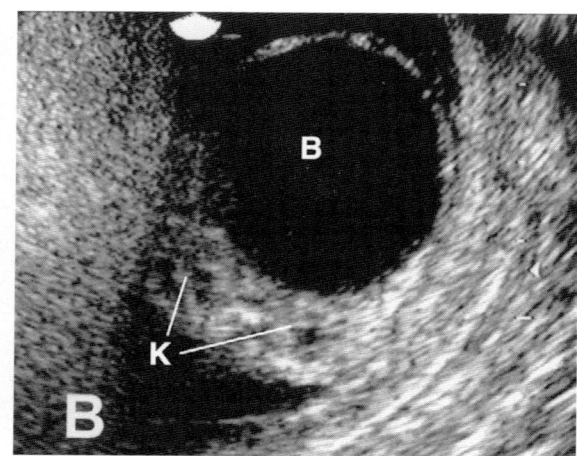

FIGURE 22. Urethral obstruction. **A:** Median view at 14 menstrual weeks shows markedly distended urinary bladder (*B*). **B:** Cross section at the level of the kidneys (*K*) shows markedly enlarged bladder (*B*). **C:** Coronal view of both kidneys shows mild bilateral hydronephrosis. LT, left kidney; RT, right kidney.

week the femur and humerus can be seen, and by the tenth postmenstrual week the shorter and thinner radius-ulna and tibia and fibula can be imaged.[3] The fingers can consistently be imaged by 12 postmenstrual weeks, and not until the thirteenth postmenstrual week are the foot and toes consistently imaged. Active fetal movements can be observed from the tenth postmenstrual week.[3] The clavicle and the mandible are the first bones to begin to ossify by the eighth postmenstrual week. By the twelfth postmenstrual week the long bones, phalanges, ilium, and scapula begin to ossify. The metacarpals and metatarsals ossify by between 12 and 16 postmenstrual weeks.[189]

There is scant literature about the first and early second-trimester diagnoses of skeletal dysplasia, as well as other abnormalities affecting the fetal extremities. A variety of abnormalities of the trunk and extremities, however, can be identified (Figs. 23 through 25).

Osteogenesis Imperfecta

Osteogenesis imperfecta (OI) is one of the lethal skeletal dysplasias that has been diagnosed as early as 13 to 15 postmenstrual weeks using ultrasound.[13,190–193] Prenatal diagnosis of OI type II is made when there are multiple fractures, demineralization of the calvaria (decreased bone echogenicity), and shortened femurs. Femur-length shortening of more than 3 standard deviations below the mean for gestational age by 17 postmenstrual weeks is significant for OI type II.[194–196] In the first trimester, OI type II can also be diagnosed by chorionic villi sampling using biochemical or DNA analysis. OI type III also has been diagnosed as early as 15 weeks.[197,198] Aylsworth et al.[198] followed a case of OI type III serially. At 15.5 postmenstrual weeks only a single fracture was present, but by 19 postmenstrual weeks shortening and deformity of the long bones was noted. OI type IV and I are the nonlethal types. Their diagnosis in utero is difficult because clinical symptoms may take years to develop.[194] The inheritance of OI type IV and I is autosomal dominant, but type I and II may be autosomal recessive, new autosomal dominant mutation, or gonadal mosaicism.[194]

Sirenomelia

Sirenomelia (Fig. 24) is a lethal skeletal anomaly in which the main feature is complete or nearly complete fusion of

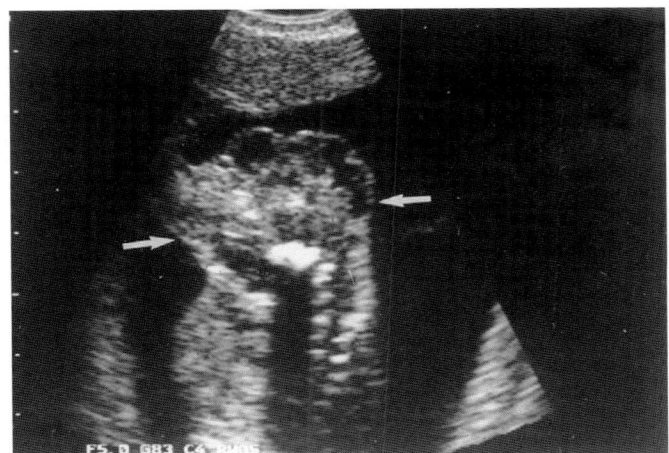

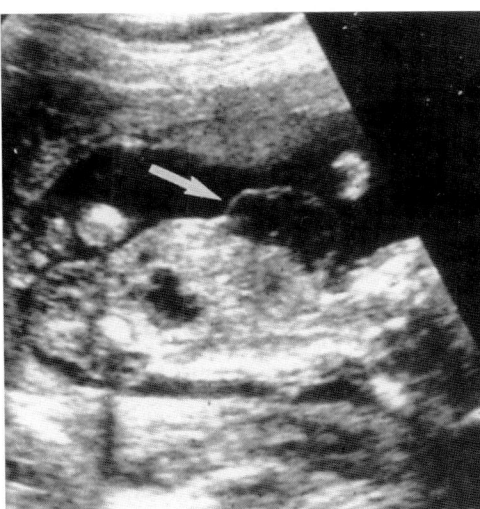

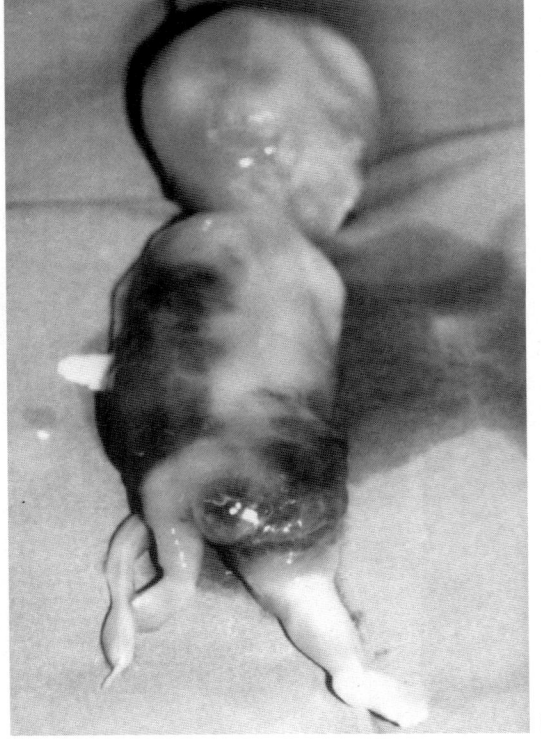

FIGURE 23. Klippel-Trenaunay-Weber syndrome, 14 menstrual weeks. **A:** Longitudinal scan through the lower sacrococcygeal region shows bulging semisolid mass (*arrows*) mimicking a sacrococcygeal teratoma. **B:** Longitudinal scan of the fetus showing huge multicystic sonolucent area arising from the fetal chest (*arrow*). **C:** The abortus showing the semisolid lesions in the sacrococcygeal and thoracic regions. Note the marked differences in size of the legs. (Courtesy of Professor Israel Meizner, Beer Sheba, Israel.)

the lower extremities. In addition, a number of other anomalies may be present, such renal agenesis, renal dysplasia, rudimentary ureters, agenesis of the bladder, abnormalities of the external and internal organs, imperforate anus with a blindly ending colon, and abnormalities of the pelvic bone and spine.[199–202] Sirenomelia has been diagnosed in utero as early as 11 to 14 postmenstrual weeks using TVS (Fig. 24).[201] Sepulveda et al.[200] used color Doppler to aid in the diagnosis of sirenomelia by imaging a single large intraabdominal vessel (the vitelline artery) that does not branch within the fetal pelvis into the iliac vessels and courses ventrally into the umbilical cord.[199]

Bronshtein et al.[203] has the largest reported series on the prenatally diagnosed skeletal abnormalities in the first and early second trimesters. Table 8 is a summary of the cases that the authors have encountered. In this study, the authors were able to detect 96% of the anomalies between 14 and 16 postmenstrual weeks, 3% between 12 and 14 postmenstrual weeks, and 1% at 10 to 12 postmenstrual weeks.

3-D ultrasound can optimally illustrate abnormalities of the extremities during the first trimester because the entire embryo/fetus can be included in the volume of interest (Fig. 25).

COMPLICATIONS OF MULTIFETAL PREGNANCIES

Vanishing Twin Syndrome

Vanishing twin syndrome refers to the phenomenon in which one member of the twin pair is lost. Approximately 20% of twin pregnancies diagnosed by ultrasound are lost during the first trimester resulting in a singleton pregnancy.[204,205]

Twins, in general, have a higher incidence of structural anomalies when compared to singletons (Figs. 26 and 27).[206,207] This is the result of the increased incidence of structural anomalies seen in monozygotic twins.[208] However, neural tube defects are typically discordant in twin pregnancies (Fig. 27). The incidence of malformations is reported to be approximately 2.12%,[209] with a higher rate found in monozygotic twins compared to dizygotic twins.

Complications unique to monochorionic pregnancies, which have been reported up to 14 weeks, include twin

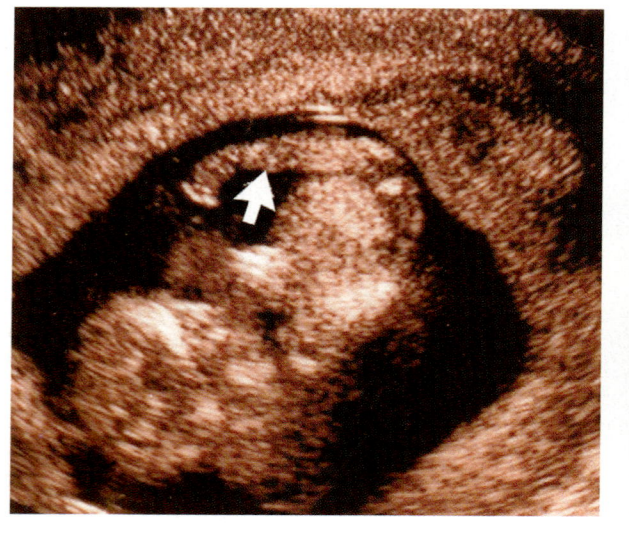

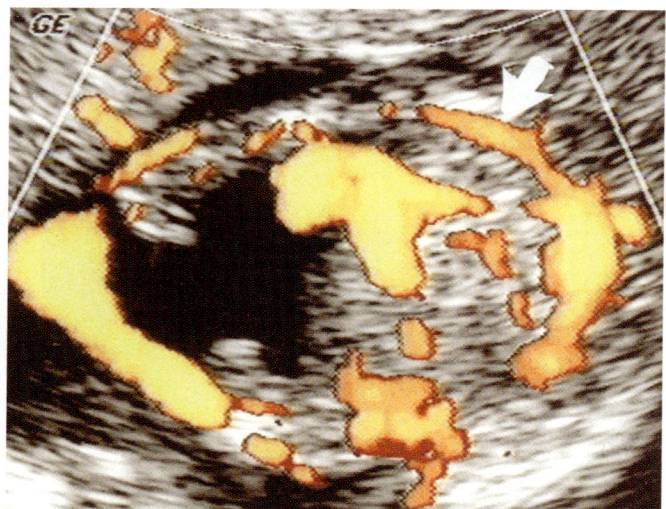

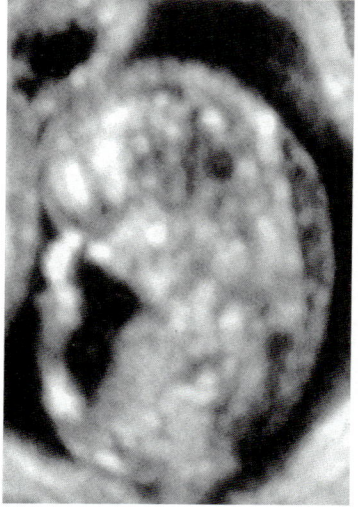

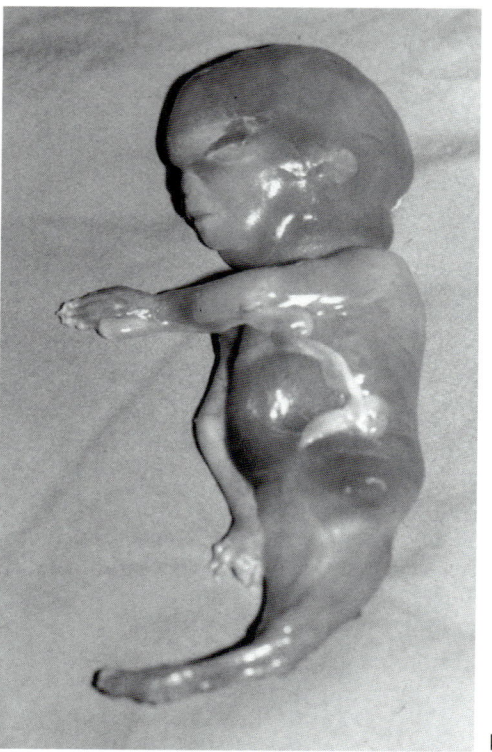

FIGURE 24. Sirenomelia and increased nuchal translucency at 11 menstrual weeks. **A:** In this long axis view of the fetus, a long and single lower extremity is imaged (*arrow*). **B:** Color Doppler image showing the aorta and the single iliac vessel (*arrow*). **C:** The three-dimensional reconstruction shows increased nuchal translucency and the single lower extremity. **D:** Abortus of similar case. (Courtesy of Professor Eliezer Shalev, Emek Hospital, Afula, Israel.)

reversed arterial perfusion syndrome, or acardiac twin, and conjoined twins.

Twin reversed arterial perfusion syndrome or acardiac twin has been reported to occur 1 in 30,000 deliveries or 1 per 100 monozygotic twins.[210] This syndrome is characterized by vascular anastomoses (artery-artery and vein-vein) between the fetuses. The *perfused twin* has multiple abnormalities including absence of the heart, abdominal organs, fetal head, and upper extremities. The *pump twin* is morphologically normal. The reported perinatal mortality for the pump twin is 55%. Approximately 50% of the twins have a chromosomal abnormality. Twin reversed arterial

perfusion has been reported at 10 to 12 postmenstrual weeks using TVS and color Doppler.[211,212] Color Doppler shows that umbilical arterial blood flow is toward the perfused fetus away from the normal or pump twin.[212,213]

Conjoined Twins

Conjoined twins (Fig. 28) occur rarely, with a reported incidence of 1 in 33,000 to 1 in 165,000 births.[210] Thirty-nine percent of the conjoined twins are stillborn and another 34% die shortly after birth.[214] The most common types of conjoined twins are thoracoomphalopagus (28%),

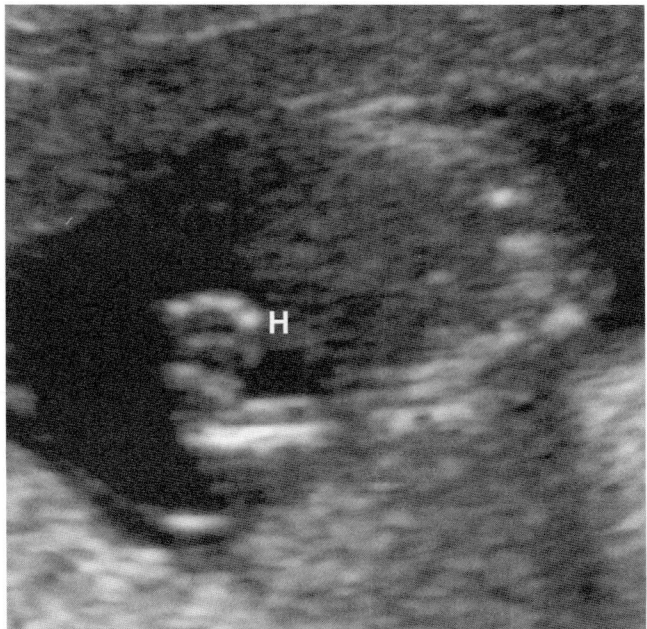

A

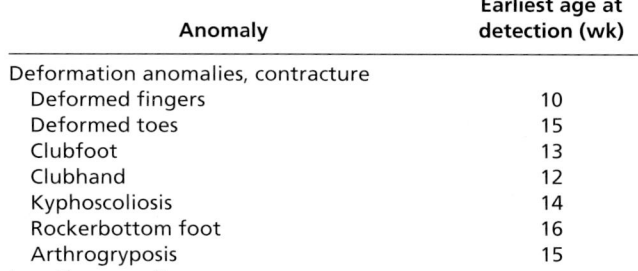

TABLE 8. SKELETAL ANOMALIES DETECTED IN THE FIRST AND EARLY SECOND TRIMESTER

Anomaly	Earliest age at detection (wk)
Deformation anomalies, contracture	
Deformed fingers	10
Deformed toes	15
Clubfoot	13
Clubhand	12
Kyphoscoliosis	14
Rockerbottom foot	16
Arthrogryposis	15
Length anomalies	
Rhizomelia	16
Mesomelia	14
Proximal femoral deficiency	14
Lack of formation	
Amelia	16
Adactyly	16

Modified from Bronshtein M, Keret D, Deutsch M, et al. Transvaginal sonographic detection of skeletal anomalies in the first and early second trimesters. *Prenat Diagn* 1993;13:597–601.

nosis of conjoined twins at 11 postmenstrual weeks and 6 days. Subsequently, Meizner et al.[223] reported on a case of thoracoomphalopagus at 9 weeks. Goldberg et al.[219] reported on the diagnosis of conjoined twins using TVS as early as the eighth postmenstrual week in a triplet pregnancy that was the result of *in vitro* fertilization and intracytoplasmic sperm injection.

B,C

FIGURE 25. Radial aplasia at 13 menstrual weeks. **A:** Scan of left upper extremity shows characteristic features of radial aplasia with markedly shortened forearm and fixed hand (*H*) and wrist deformity. **B:** Three-dimensional ultrasound in surface-rendered mode shows abnormal left arm by trunk (*arrow*). The normal right arm is positioned in front of face. **C:** Frontal view of three-dimensional scan shows the radial aplasia (*arrow*). (Courtesy of David A. Nyberg, MD.)

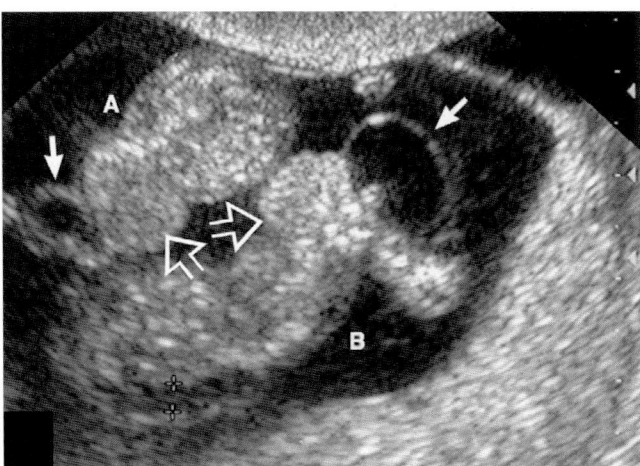

FIGURE 26. Dichorionic-diamniotic triplet pregnancy at 10 postmenstrual weeks and 3 days. Fetuses A and B are monochorionic monoamniotic and are concordant for bladder exstrophy. Abdominal contents are eviscerated (*open arrows*), and the urinary bladder is seen as a cystic structure (*arrows*) and abnormal in shape and echotexture. (Reproduced with permission from Timor-Tritsch IE, Monteagudo A, Horan C, Stangel JJ. Dichorionic triplet pregnancy with the monoamniotic twin pair concordant for omphalocele and bladder exstrophy. *Ultrasound Obstet Gynecol* 2000;16:669–671.)

thoracopagus (18%), omphalopagus (10%), incomplete duplication (10%), and craniopagus (6%).[214] Conjoined twins result from a postimplantation division of the zygote between day 13 and 16 after conception.[210,215] Several authors have reported early prenatal diagnosis of conjoined twins.[216–223] Schmidt et al.[224] in 1981 reported on the diag-

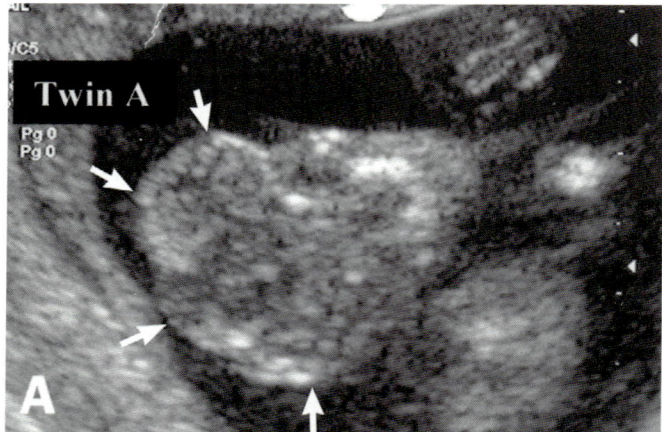

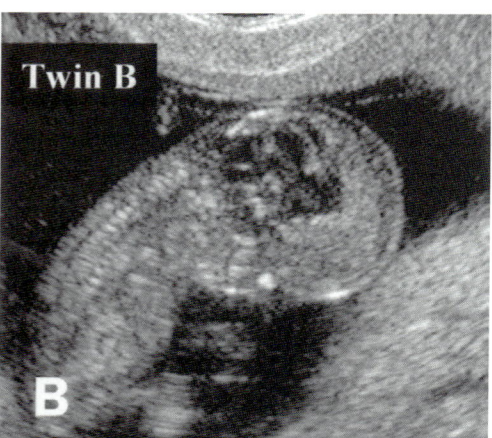

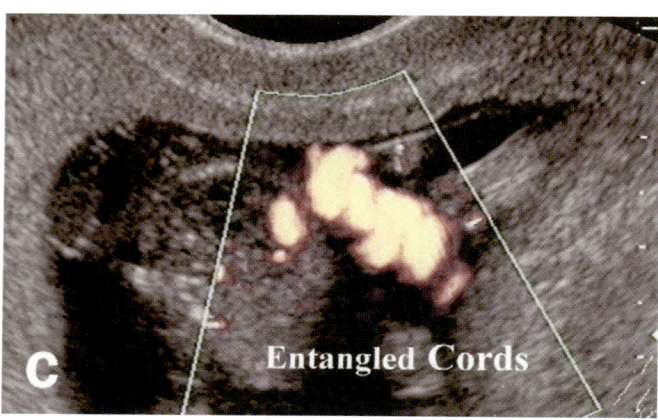

FIGURE 27. Monoamniotic twin pregnancy discordant for neural tube defect. **A:** Coronal view of head at 12 weeks, 2 days shows exencephaly (acrania) of twin A. The brain is eviscerated (*arrows*) and abnormal in shape and echotexture. **B:** The co-twin shows normal anatomy of the head. **C:** Umbilical cord entanglement confirms monoamniotic placentation.

CONCLUSION

Since 1987, with the introduction of TVS, an ever-increasing number of congenital anomalies affecting the developing fetus have been diagnosed. Given the present state of technology, the earliest time to perform a targeted scan for anomalies is 14 to 15 postmenstrual weeks. Because not all anomalies become apparent by 14 to 15 postmenstrual weeks, a later scan at 22 to 23 postmenstrual weeks is still warranted to improve on the detection rate of malformations.

It is clear that all anomalies that develop early or that involve organs, which complete their development early enough, can be imaged at or around 15 postmenstrual weeks and indeed may be imaged better at this gestational age than later in pregnancy. A later scan involves a transabdominal probe, with all of its well-known drawbacks and limitations.

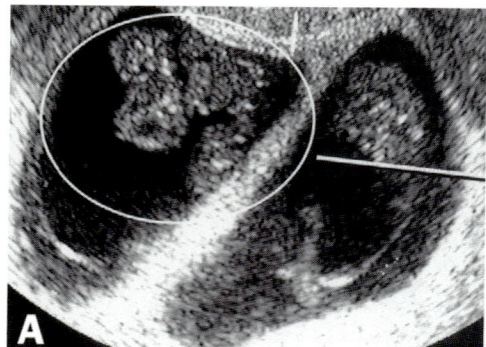

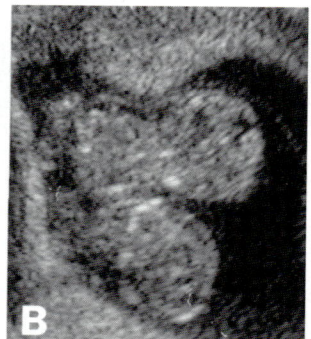

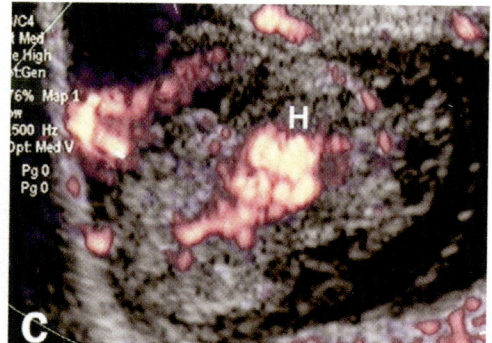

FIGURE 28. Conjoined fetuses. **A:** Triplet pregnancy at 10 postmenstrual weeks. **B, C:** Fetuses are conjoined. Part **C** shows shared heart (*H*). In addition, these fetuses had a rate of 200 bpm and had a cystic hygroma. This twin pair was eventually reduced, and the patient delivered a healthy baby.

Using 5-MHz to 7.5-MHz probes through the vaginal approach enables an early and reliable answer to the question: Does the fetal anatomy look normal? Because a small percentage of anomalies become apparent after 14 to 15 weeks (e.g., agenesis of the corpus callosum), a second scan at 20 to 22 weeks is still warranted. At the present time, it is extremely hard or almost impossible to implement general and routine screening ultrasound at 14 to 15 and at 20 to 22 postmenstrual weeks. This is owing to a multitude of subjective and of objective factors. Some of the main reasons are the lack of an adequate number of skilled operators and a lack of widely available optimal ultrasound equipment (only a very few ultrasound machines indeed answer the strict requirements to produce high-resolution images). The results of the RADIUS study[226] clearly showed some of the shortcomings encountered in the United States on the way to achieve a comprehensive obstetric screening policy.

The authors of this chapter firmly believe that if an experienced sonographer or sonologist with the appropriate equipment is available, TVS can and should be offered to all pregnant women. Adequate patient counseling is important to place unrealistic patient expectations into the correct perspective. In the future, when the financial and the risk-versus-benefit considerations regarding routine scans may be worked out, more than two compulsory routine scans can be expected before the completion of the first half of the pregnancy. Of all these scans, the most important may turn out to be the transvaginal evaluation of the fetal anatomy at 14 to 15 postmenstrual weeks.

In addition, while preparing this manuscript, it became obvious that many, if not most, of the anomalies or malformations that have been described in this text have something in common during the first or early second trimester, and that is increased nuchal translucency. Though this subject was not covered in this chapter because it is extensively covered in Chapter 20, Nuchal Translucency, the impact that screening using this measurement has made in the first-trimester diagnosis of chromosomal and nonchromosomal syndromes as well as abnormalities affecting the developing human is evident.

REFERENCES

1. Timor-Tritsch IE, Farine D, Rosen MG. A close look at early embryonic development with the high-frequency transvaginal transducer. *Am J Obstet Gynecol* 1988;159:676–681.
2. Timor-Tritsch IE, Monteagudo A, Warren WB. Transvaginal ultrasonographic definition of the central nervous system in the first and early second trimesters. *Am J Obstet Gynecol* 1991;164:497–503.
3. Timor-Tritsch IE, Monteagudo A, Peisner DB. High-frequency transvaginal sonographic examination for the potential malformation assessment of the 9-week to 14-week fetus. *J Clin Ultrasound* 1992;20:231–238.
4. O'Rahilly R, Muller F. *Human embryology and teratology.* New York: Wiley-Liss, 1992:253–291.
5. Moore K. The nervous system. In: Moore K, ed. *The developing human. Clinically oriented embryology.* Philadelphia: WB Saunders, 1988:364–401.
6. Vergani P, Ghidini A, Sirtori M, et al. Antenatal diagnosis of fetal acrania. *J Ultrasound Med* 1987;6:715–717.
7. Bronshtein M, Ornoy A. Acrania: anencephaly resulting from secondary degeneration of a closed neural tube: two cases in the same family. *J Clin Ultrasound* 1991;19:230–234.
8. Cox GG, Rosenthal SJ, Holsapple JW. Exencephaly: sonographic findings and radiologic-pathologic correlation. *Radiology* 1985;155:755–756.
9. Ganchrow D, Ornoy A. Possible evidence for secondary degeneration of central nervous system in the pathogenesis of anencephaly and brain dysraphia. A study in young human fetuses. *Virchows Arch A Pathol Anat Histol* 1979;384:285–294.
10. Padmanabhan R. Is exencephaly the forerunner of anencephaly? An experimental study on the effect of prolonged gestation on the exencephaly induced after neural tube closure in the rat. *Acta Anat* 1991;141:182–192.
11. Inman V, Saunders JB de CM. The ossification of the human frontal bone. *J Anat* 1937;71:383–394.
12. Kennedy KA, Flick KJ, Thurmond AS. First-trimester diagnosis of exencephaly. *Am J Obstet Gynecol* 1990;162:461–463.
13. Bronshtein M, Weiner Z. Anencephaly in a fetus with osteogenesis imperfecta: early diagnosis by transvaginal sonography. *Prenat Diagn* 1992;12:831–834.
14. Nishi T, Nakano R. First-trimester diagnosis of exencephaly by transvaginal ultrasonography. *J Ultrasound Med* 1994;13:149–151.
15. Chatzipapas IK, Whitlow BJ, Economides DL. The 'Mickey Mouse' sign and the diagnosis of anencephaly in early pregnancy. *Ultrasound Obstet Gynecol* 1999;13:196–199.
16. Monteagudo A, Timor-Tritsch I. Fetal neurosonography of congenital brain anomalies. In: Timor-Tritsch I, Monteagudo A, Cohen H, eds. *Ultrasonography of the prenatal and neonatal brain.* New York: McGraw-Hill, 2001.
17. Campbell S, Johnstone F, Holt E, et al. Anencephalus: early ultrasonic diagnosis and active management. *Lancet* 1972;2:1226.
18. Rottem S, Bronshtein M, Thaler I, et al. First trimester transvaginal sonographic diagnosis of fetal anomalies [letter]. *Lancet* 1989;1:444–445.
19. Johnson SP, Sebire NJ, Snijders RJ, et al. Ultrasound screening for anencephaly at 10–14 postmenstrual weeks. *Ultrasound Obstet Gynecol* 1997;9:14–16.
20. Hidalgo H, Bowie J, Rosenberg ER, et al. Review. In utero sonographic diagnosis of fetal cerebral anomalies. *AJR Am J Roentgenol* 1982;139:143–148.
21. Salamanca A, Gonzalez-Gomez F, Padilla M. Prenatal ultrasound semiography of anencephaly: sonographic-pathological correlations. *Ultrasound Obstet Gynecol* 1992;2:95–100.
22. Sepulveda W, Sebire NJ, Fung TY, et al. Crown-chin length in normal and anencephalic fetuses at 10 to 14 weeks' gestation. *Am J Obstet Gynecol* 1997;176:852–855.
23. Icenogle DA, Kaplan AM. A review of congenital neurologic malformations. *Clin Pediatr* 1981;20:565–576.
24. Pretorius DH, Russ PD, Rumack CM, et al. Diagnosis of brain neuropathology in utero. *Neuroradiology* 1986;28:386–397.
25. Reference deleted.

26. Chervenak FA, Isaacson G, Mahoney MJ, et al. Diagnosis and management of fetal cephalocele. *Obstet Gynecol* 1984; 64:86–91.

27. Naidich TP, Altman NR, Braffman BH, et al. Cephaloceles and related malformations. *Am J Neurol* 1992;13:655–690.

28. Nyberg DA, Hallesy D, Mahony BS, et al. Meckel-Gruber syndrome. Importance of prenatal diagnosis. *J Ultrasound Med* 1990;9:691–696.

29. Monteagudo A. Cephalocele: anterior. *Fetus* 1992;2:1–4.

30. Bronshtein M, Timor-Tritsch I, Rottem S. Early detection of fetal anomalies. In: Timor-Tritsch I, Rottem S, eds. *Transvaginal sonography*. New York: Chapman & Hall, 1991:327–371.

31. Braithwaite JM, Economides DL. First-trimester diagnosis of Meckel-Gruber syndrome by transabdominal sonography in a low-risk case. *Prenat Diagn* 1995;15:1168–1170.

32. Dumez Y, Dommergues M, Gubler MC, et al. Meckel-Gruber syndrome: prenatal diagnosis at 10 menstrual weeks using embryoscopy. *Prenat Diagn* 1994;14:141–144.

33. Pachi A, Giancotti A, Torcia F, et al. Meckel-Gruber syndrome: ultrasonographic diagnosis at 13 weeks' gestational age in an at-risk case. *Prenat Diagn* 1989;9:187–190.

34. Sepulveda W, Sebire NJ, Souka A, et al. Diagnosis of the Meckel-Gruber syndrome at eleven to fourteen weeks' gestation. *Am J Obstet Gynecol* 1997;176:316–319.

35. van Zalen-Sprock RM, van Vugt JM, van Geijn HP. First-trimester sonographic detection of neurodevelopmental abnormalities in some single-gene disorders. *Prenat Diagn* 1996;16:199–202.

36. Foderaro AE, Abu-Yousef MM, Benda JA, et al. Antenatal ultrasound diagnosis of iniencephaly. *J Clin Ultrasound* 1987;15:550–554.

37. Sherer DM, Hearn-Stebbins B, Harvey W, et al. Endovaginal sonographic diagnosis of iniencephaly apertus and craniorachischisis at 13 weeks, menstrual age. *J Clin Ultrasound* 1993;21:124–127.

38. Shoham Z, Caspi B, Chemke J, et al. Iniencephaly: prenatal ultrasonographic diagnosis—a case report. *J Perinat Med* 1988;16:139–143.

39. Lemire R, Beckwith J, Shepard T. Iniencephaly and anencephaly with spinal retroflexion. A comparative study of eight human specimens. *Birth Defects* 1987;23:225.

40. Nishimura H, Okamoto N. Iniencephaly. In: Vinken P, Bruyn G, eds. *Handbook of clinical neurology*, vol. 30. Amsterdam: Elsevier-North Holland Publishing Co., 1976:257–268.

41. Rodriguez MM, Reik RA, Carreno TD, et al. Cluster of iniencephaly in Miami. *Pediatr Pathol* 1991;11:211–221.

42. Aleksic S, Budzilovich G. Iniencephaly. In: Myrianthopoulos N, ed. *Malformations*, vol. 50. Amsterdam: Elsevier Science, 1987:129–136.

43. Romero R, Pilu G, Jeanty P, et al. Iniencephaly. In: Romero R, Pilu G, Jeanty P, et al., eds. *Prenatal diagnosis of congenital anomalies*. Norwalk: Appleton & Lange, 1988:65–67.

44. Aleksic S, Budzilovich G, Greco MA, et al. Iniencephaly: a neuropathologic study. *Clin Neurol* 1983;2:55–61.

45. Reference deleted.

46. Reference deleted.

47. David TJ, Nixon A. Congenital malformations associated with anencephaly and iniencephaly. *J Med Genet* 1976;13: 263–265.

48. Babcock DS. Sonography of congenital malformations of the brain. *Neuroradiology* 1986;28:428–439.

49. Filly RA, Chinn DH, Callen PW. Alobar holoprosencephaly: ultrasonographic prenatal diagnosis. *Radiology* 1984; 151:455–459.

50. Cohen MM Jr, Sulik KK. Perspectives on holoprosencephaly: part II. Central nervous system, craniofacial anatomy, syndrome commentary, diagnostic approach, and experimental studies. *J Craniofac Genet Dev Biol* 1992;12:196–244.

51. DeMyer W, Zeman W, Palmer CG. The face predicts the brain: diagnostic significance of medial facial anomalies for holoprosencephaly (arrhinencephaly). *Pediatrics* 1964;34: 256–262.

52. Toth Z, Csecsei K, Szeifert G, et al. Early prenatal diagnosis of cyclopia associated with holoprosencephaly. *J Clin Ultrasound* 1986;14:550–553.

53. Icenogle DA, Kaplan AM. A review of congenital neurologic malformations. *Clin Pediatr* 1981;20:565–576.

54. Bronshtein M, Wiener Z. Early transvaginal sonographic diagnosis of alobar holoprosencephaly. *Prenat Diagn* 1991;11:459–462.

55. Gonzalez-Gomez F, Salamanca A, Padilla MC, et al. Alobar holoprosencephalic embryo detected via transvaginal sonography. *Eur J Obstet Gynecol Reprod Biol* 1992;47:266–270.

56. Turner CD, Silva S, Jeanty P. Prenatal diagnosis of alobar holoprosencephaly at 10 postmenstrual weeks. *Ultrasound Obstet Gynecol* 1999;13:360–362.

57. Wong HS, Lam YH, Tang MH, et al. First-trimester ultrasound diagnosis of holoprosencephaly: three case reports. *Ultrasound Obstet Gynecol* 1999;13:356–359.

58. Nelson LH, King M. Early diagnosis of holoprosencephaly. *J Ultrasound Med* 1992;11:57–59.

59. Reference deleted.

60. Turner CD, Silva S, Jeanty P. Prenatal diagnosis of alobar holoprosencephaly at 10 postmenstrual weeks. *Ultrasound Obstet Gynecol* 1999;13:360–362.

61. Habib Z. Genetics and genetic counseling in neonatal hydrocephalus. *Obstet Gynecol Surv* 1981;36:529–534.

62. Chinn DH, Callen PW, Filly RA. The lateral cerebral ventricle in early second trimester. *Radiology* 1983;148:529–531.

63. Benacerraf BR, Birnholz JC. The diagnosis of fetal hydrocephalus prior to 22 weeks. *J Clin Ultrasound* 1987;15:531–536.

64. Cardoza JD, Filly RA, Podrasky AE. The dangling choroid plexus: a sonographic observation of value in excluding ventriculomegaly. *AJR Am J Roentgenol* 1988;151:767–770.

65. Bronshtein M, Ben-Shlomo I. Choroid plexus dysmorphism detected by transvaginal sonography: the earliest sign of fetal hydrocephalus. *J Clin Ultrasound* 1991;19:547–553.

66. Russ PD, Pretorius DH, Johnson MJ. Dandy-Walker syndrome: a review of fifteen cases evaluated by prenatal sonography. *Am J Obstet Gynecol* 1989;161:401–406.

67. Hirsch JF, Pierre-Kahn A, Renier D, et al. The Dandy-Walker malformation. A review of 40 cases. *J Neurosurg* 1984;61:515–522.

68. Nyberg DA, Cyr DR, Mack LA, et al. The Dandy-Walker malformation prenatal sonographic diagnosis and its clinical significance. *J Ultrasound Med* 1988;7:65–71.

69. Taylor GA, Sanders RC. Dandy-Walker syndrome: recognition by sonography. *AJNR Am J Neuroradiol* 1983;4:1203.

70. Fileni A, Colosimo C Jr, Mirk P, et al. Dandy-Walker syn-

drome: diagnosis in utero by means of ultrasound and CT correlations. *Neuroradiology* 1983;24:233–235.

71. Kirkinen P, Jouppila P, Valkeakari T, et al. Ultrasonic evaluation of the Dandy-Walker syndrome. *Obstet Gynecol* 1982;59:18S–21S.

72. Achiron R, Achiron A, Yagel S. First trimester transvaginal sonographic diagnosis of Dandy-Walker malformation. *J Clin Ultrasound* 1993;21:62–64.

73. Bromley B, Nadel AS, Pauker S, Estroff JA, et al. Closure of the cerebellar vermis: evaluation with second trimester US. *Radiology* 1994;193:761–763.

74. Baxi L, Warren W, Collins MH, et al. Early detection of caudal regression syndrome with transvaginal scanning. *Obstet Gynecol* 1990;75:486–489.

75. Nicolaides KH, Campbell S, Gabbe SG, et al. Ultrasound screening for spina bifida: cranial and cerebellar signs. *Lancet* 1986;2:72–74.

76. Campbell J, Gilbert WM, Nicolaides KH, et al. Ultrasound screening for spina bifida: cranial and cerebellar signs in a high-risk population. *Obstet Gynecol* 1987;70:247–250.

77. Blumenfeld Z, Siegler E, Bronshtein M. The early diagnosis of neural tube defects. *Prenat Diagn* 1993;13:863–871.

78. Sebire NJ, Noble PL, Thorpe-Beeston JG, et al. Presence of the 'lemon' sign in fetuses with spina bifida at the 10–14-week scan. *Ultrasound Obstet Gynecol* 1997;10:403–405.

79. Bernard JP, Suarez B, Rambaud C, et al. Prenatal diagnosis of neural tube defect before 12 weeks' gestation: direct and indirect ultrasonographic semeiology. *Ultrasound Obstet Gynecol* 1997;10:406–409.

80. Moore K. The branchial apparatus and the head and neck. In: Moore K, ed. *The developing human. Clinically oriented embryology.* Philadelphia: WB Saunders, 1988:170–206.

81. Bronshtein M, Mashiah N, Blumenfeld I, et al. Pseudoprognathism—an auxiliary ultrasonographic sign for transvaginal ultrasonographic diagnosis of cleft lip and palate in the early second trimester. *Am J Obstet Gynecol* 1991;165.

82. Bronshtein M, Blumenfeld I, Kohn J, et al. Detection of cleft lip by early second-trimester transvaginal sonography. *Obstet Gynecol* 1994;84:73–76.

83. Nyberg D, Mahoney B, Kramer D. Paranasal echogenic mass: sonographic sign of bilateral complete cleft lip and palate before 20 menstrual weeks. *Radiology* 1992;184.

84. Bronshtein M, Zimmer E, Gershoni-Baruch R, et al. First- and second-trimester diagnosis of fetal ocular defects and associated anomalies: report of eight cases. *Obstet Gynecol* 1991;77:443–449.

85. Feldman E, Shalev E, Weiner E, et al. Microphthalmia—prenatal ultrasonic diagnosis: a case report. *Prenat Diagn* 1985;5:205–207.

86. Gaary E, Rawnsley E, Marin-Padilla J, et al. In utero detection of fetal cataracts. *J Ultrasound Med* 1993;4:234–236.

87. Zimmer E, Bronshtein M, Ophir E, et al. Sonographic diagnosis of fetal congenital cataracts. *Prenat Diagn* 1993;13:503–511.

88. Bronshtein M, Blumenfeld I, Zimmer EZ, et al. Prenatal sonographic diagnosis of nasal malformations. *Prenat Diagn* 1998;18:447–454.

89. Drysdale K, Kyle PM, Sepulveda W. Prenatal detection of congenital inherited cataracts. *Ultrasound Obstet Gynecol* 1997;9:62–63.

90. Gull I, Wolman I, Har-Toov J, et al. Antenatal sonographic diagnosis of epignathus at 15 weeks of pregnancy. *Ultrasound Obstet Gynecol* 1999;13:271–273.

91. Reference deleted.

92. Merz E, Weber G, Bahlmann F, et al. Application of transvaginal and abdominal three-dimensional ultrasound for the detection or exclusion of malformations of the fetal face. *Ultrasound Obstet Gynecol* 1997;9:237–243.

93. Jeanty P, Dramaix-Wilmet M, Van Gansbeke D, et al. Fetal ocular biometry by ultrasound. *Radiology* 1982;143:513–516.

94. Stoll C, Alembik Y, Dott B, et al. Epidemiology of congenital eye malformations in 131,760 consecutive births. *Ophthalmic Paediatr Genet* 1992;13:179–186.

95. Monteagudo A, Timor-Tritsch IE, Friedman AH, et al. Autosomal dominant cataracts of the fetus: early detection by transvaginal ultrasound. *Ultrasound Obstet Gynecol* 1996;8:104–108.

96. Rosner M, Bronshtein M, Leikomovitz P, et al. Transvaginal sonographic diagnosis of cataract in a fetus. *Eur J Ophthalmol* 1996;6:90–93.

97. Benacerraf B. *Ultrasound of fetal syndromes.* New York: Churchill Livingstone, 1998:97.

98. Moore K. The eye and ear. In: Moore K, ed. *The developing human. Clinically oriented embryology.* Philadelphia: WB Saunders, 1988:402–420.

99. Jones K. *Smith's recognizable patterns of human malformation.* Philadelphia: WB Saunders, 1997:789–790.

100. Moore K. The cardiovascular system. In: Moore K, ed. *The developing human. Clinically oriented embryology.* Philadelphia: WB Saunders, 1988:286–333.

101. D'Amelio R, Giorlandino C, Masala L, et al. Fetal echocardiography using transvaginal and transabdominal probes during the first period of pregnancy: a comparative study. *Prenat Diagn* 1991;11:69–75.

102. Mitchell SC, Korones SB, Berendes HW. Congenital heart disease in 56,109 births. Incidence and natural history. *Circulation* 1971;43:323–332.

103. Allan LD, Crawford DC, Chita SK, et al. Prenatal screening for congenital heart disease. *BMJ* 1986;292:1717–1719.

104. Paladini D, Calabro R, Palmieri S, et al. Prenatal diagnosis of congenital heart disease and fetal karyotyping. *Obstet Gynecol* 1993;81:679–682.

105. Bronshtein M, Zimmer EZ, Gerlis LM, et al. Early ultrasound diagnosis of fetal congenital heart defects in high-risk and low-risk pregnancies. *Obstet Gynecol* 1993;82:225–229.

106. Achiron R, Rotstein Z, Lipitz S, et al. First-trimester diagnosis of fetal congenital heart disease by transvaginal ultrasonography. *Obstet Gynecol* 1994;84:69–72.

107. Laboda LA, Estroff JA, Benacerraf BR. First trimester bradycardia. A sign of impending fetal loss. *J Ultrasound Med* 1989;8:561–563.

108. Montenegro N, Beires J, Leite LP. Reverse end-diastolic umbilical artery blood flow at 11 weeks' gestation. *Ultrasound Obstet Gynecol* 1995;5:141–142.

109. Ariyuki Y, Hata T, Kitao M. Reverse end-diastolic umbilical artery velocity in a case of intrauterine fetal death at 14 weeks' gestation. *Am J Obstet Gynecol* 1993;169:1621–1622.

110. Borrell A, Costa D, Martinez JM, et al. Reversed end-diastolic umbilical flow in a first-trimester fetus with congenital heart disease. *Prenat Diagn* 1998;18:1001–1005.

111. Murta CG, Moron AF, Avila MA. Reversed diastolic umbilical artery flow in the first trimester associated with chromosomal fetal abnormalities or cardiac defects. *Obstet Gynecol* 2000;95:1011–1013.

112. Gembruch U, Knopfle G, Bald R, et al. Early diagnosis of fetal congenital heart disease by transvaginal echocardiography. *Ultrasound Obstet Gynecol* 1993;3:310–317.

113. Dolkart LA, Reimers FT. Transvaginal fetal echocardiography in early pregnancy: normative data. *Am J Obstet Gynecol* 1991;165:688–691.

114. Gembruch U, Knopfle G, Chatterjee M, et al. First-trimester diagnosis of fetal congenital heart disease by transvaginal two-dimensional and Doppler echocardiography. *Obstet Gynecol* 1990;75:496–498.

115. Bronshtein M, Siegler E, Eshcoli Z, et al. Transvaginal ultrasound measurements of the fetal heart at 11 to 17 weeks. *Am J Perinatol* 1992;9:38–42.

116. Comas C, Carrera M, Devesa R, et al. Early detection of reversed diastolic umbilical flow: should we offer karyotyping? *Ultrasound Obstet Gynecol* 1997;10:400–402.

117. Martinez Crespo JM, Comas C, Borrell A, et al. Reversed end-diastolic umbilical artery velocity in two cases of trisomy 18 at 10 weeks' gestation. *Ultrasound Obstet Gynecol* 1996;7:447–449.

118. Murta CG, Moron AF, Avila MA. Reversed diastolic umbilical artery flow in the first trimester associated with chromosomal fetal abnormalities or cardiac defects. *Obstet Gynecol* 2000;95:1011–1013.

119. Copel JA, Pilu G, Green J, et al. Fetal echocardiographic screening for congenital heart disease: the importance of the four-chamber view. *Am J Obstet Gynecol* 1987;157:648–655.

120. Moore K. Development of body cavities primitive mesenteries, and the diaphragm. In: Moore K, ed. *The developing human. Clinically oriented embryology.* Philadelphia: WB Saunders, 1988:164–166.

121. Sebire NJ, Snijders RJ, Davenport M, et al. Fetal nuchal translucency thickness at 10–14 weeks' gestation and congenital diaphragmatic hernia. *Obstet Gynecol* 1997;90:943–946.

122. Nicolaides K, Sebire N, Snijders R. The 11–14 week scan. The diagnosis of fetal abnormalities. In: Nicolaides K, ed. *Diploma in fetal medicine series.* New York: The Parthenon Publishing Group, 1999:76–77.

123. Cyr DR, Mack LA, Schoenecker SA, et al. Bowel migration in the normal fetus: US detection. *Radiology* 1986;161:119–121.

124. Curtis JA, Watson L. Sonographic diagnosis of omphalocele in the first trimester of fetal gestation. *J Ultrasound Med* 1988;7:97–100.

125. Hutchin P. Somatic anomalies of the umbilicus and anterior abdominal wall. *Surg Gynecol Obstet* 1965;120:1075.

126. Duhamel B. Embryology of exomphalus and allied malformations. *Arch Dis Child* 1963;38:142–143.

127. Margulis L. Omphalocele (amniocele). *Am J Obstet Gynecol* 1945;49:695.

128. van Zalen-Sprock RM, Vugt JM, van Geijn HP. First-trimester sonography of physiological midgut herniation and early diagnosis of omphalocele. *Prenat Diagn* 1997;17:511–518.

129. Nyberg DA, Fitzsimmons J, Mack LA, et al. Chromosomal abnormalities in fetuses with omphalocele. Significance of omphalocele contents. *J Ultrasound Med* 1989;8:299–308.

130. Benacerraf BR, Saltzman DH, Estroff JA, et al. Abnormal karyotype of fetuses with omphalocele: prediction based on omphalocele contents. *Obstet Gynecol* 1990;75:317–319.

131. Pagliano M, Mossetti M, Ragno P. Echographic diagnosis of omphalocele in the first trimester of pregnancy. *J Clin Ultrasound* 1990;18:658–660.

132. Brown DL, Emerson DS, Shulman LP, et al. Sonographic diagnosis of omphalocele during 10th week of gestation. *AJR Am J Roentgenol* 1989;153:825–856.

133. Gray DL, Martin CM, Crane JP. Differential diagnosis of first trimester ventral wall defect. *J Ultrasound Med* 1989;8:255–258.

134. Romero R, Pilu G, Jeanty P, et al. Omphalocele. In: Romero R, Pilu G, Jeanty P, et al., eds. *Prenatal diagnosis of congenital anomalies.* Norwalk: Appleton & Lange, 1988:220–223.

135. Khoury MJ, Erickson JD, Cordero JF, et al. Congenital malformations and intrauterine growth retardation: a population study. *Pediatrics* 1988;82:83–90.

136. Saller DN Jr, Dailey JV, Doyle DL, et al. Turner syndrome associated with an omphalocele [letter]. *Prenat Diagn* 1993;13:424–426.

137. Ranzini AC, Day-Salvatore D, Turner T, et al. Intrauterine growth and ultrasound findings in fetuses with Beckwith-Wiedemann syndrome. *Obstet Gynecol* 1997;89:538–542.

138. Kasznica J, Maldonado NM. Umbilical cord hernia, single umbilical artery, and lung hypoplasia in Ullrich-Turner syndrome [letter]. *Am J Med Genet* 1995;57:496–497.

139. Romero R, Pilu G, Jeanty P, et al. Gastroschisis. In: Romero R, Pilu G, Jeanty P, et al., eds. *Prenatal diagnosis of congenital anomalies.* Norwalk: Appleton & Lange, 1988:224–225.

140. Hoyme HE, Higginbottom MC, Jones KL. The vascular pathogenesis of gastroschisis: intrauterine interruption of the omphalomesenteric artery. *J Pediatr* 1981;98:228–231.

141. Hoyme HE, Jones MC, Jones KL. Gastroschisis: abdominal wall disruption secondary to early gestational interruption of the omphalomesenteric artery. *Semin Perinatol* 1983;7:294–298.

142. Guzman ER. Early prenatal diagnosis of gastroschisis with transvaginal ultrasonography. *Am J Obstet Gynecol* 1990; 162:1253–1254.

143. Kushnir O, Izquierdo L, Vigil D, et al. Early transvaginal sonographic diagnosis of gastroschisis. *J Clin Ultrasound* 1990;18:194–197.

144. Sadler T. *Digestive system. Langman's medical embryology.* Baltimore: Williams & Wilkins, 1990:237–259.

145. Fleming AD, Vintzileos AM, Rodis JF, et al. Diagnosis of fetal ectopia cordis by transvaginal ultrasound. *J Ultrasound Med* 1991;10:413–415.

146. Bennett TL, Burlbaw J, Drake CK, et al. Diagnosis of ectopia cordis at 12 postmenstrual weeks using transabdominal ultrasonography with color flow Doppler. *J Ultrasound Med* 1991;10:695–696.

147. Hiett AK, Devoe LD, Falls DG, et al. Ultrasound diagnosis of a twin gestation with concordant body stalk anomaly. A case report. *J Reprod Med* 1992;37:944–946.

148. Liang RI, Huang SE, Chang FM. Prenatal diagnosis of ectopia cordis at 10 weeks using two-dimensional and three-dimensional ultrasonography. *Ultrasound Obstet Gynecol* 1997;10:137–139.

149. Forrester MB, Merz RD. Epidemiology of abdominal wall defects, Hawaii, 1986–1997. *Teratology* 1999;60:117–123.

150. Romero R, Pilu G, Jeanty P, et al. Body stalk anomaly. In: Romero R, Pilu G, Jeanty P, et al., eds. *Prenatal diagnosis of congenital anomalies.* Norwalk: Appleton & Lange, 1988:226–227.
151. Becker R, Runkel S, Entezami M. Prenatal diagnosis of body stalk anomaly at 9 weeks. Case report. *Fetal Diagn Ther* 2000;15:301–303.
152. Daskalakis G, Sebire NJ, Jurkovic D, et al. Body stalk anomaly at 10–14 weeks. *Ultrasound Obstet Gynecol* 1997;10:416–418.
153. Ginsberg NE, Cadkin A, Strom C. Prenatal diagnosis of body stalk anomaly in the first trimester of pregnancy. *Ultrasound Obstet Gynecol* 1997;10:419–421.
154. Skibo LK, Lyons EA, Levi CS. First-trimester umbilical cord cysts. *Radiology* 1992;182:719–722.
155. Rempen A. Sonographic first-trimester diagnosis of umbilical cord cyst. *J Clin Ultrasound* 1989;17:53–55.
156. Sepulveda W, Pryde P, Greb A, et al. Prenatal diagnosis of umbilical cord pseudocyst. *Ultrasound Obstet Gynecol* 1994;4:147–150.
157. Jauniaux E, Donner C, Thomas C, et al. Umbilical cord pseudocyst in trisomy 18 [see comments]. *Prenat Diagn* 1988;8:557–663.
158. Fink IJ, Filly RA. Omphalocele associated with umbilical cord allantoic cyst: sonographic evaluation in utero. *Radiology* 1983;149:473–476.
159. Ross JA, Jurkovic D, Zosmer N, et al. Umbilical cord cysts in early pregnancy. *Obstet Gynecol* 1997;89:442–445.
160. Nyberg DA, Mahony BS, Luthy D, et al. Single umbilical artery. Prenatal detection of concurrent anomalies. *J Ultrasound Med* 1991;10:247–253.
161. Benirschke K, Bourne G. The incidence and prognostic implication of congenital absence of one umbilical artery. *Am J Obstet Gynecol* 1960;79:251.
162. Benirschke K, Brown W. A vascular anomaly of the umbilical cord. *Obstet Gynecol* 1955;6:399.
163. Bryan EM, Kohler HG. The missing umbilical artery. I. Prospective study based on a maternity unit. *Arch Dis Child* 1974;49:844–852.
164. Romero R, Pilu G, Jeanty P, et al. Single umbilical artery. In: Romero R, Pilu G, Jeanty P, et al., eds. *Prenatal diagnosis of congenital anomalies.* Norwalk: Appleton & Lange, 1988:387–390.
165. Blazer S, Sujov P, Escholi Z, et al. Single umbilical artery—right or left? Does it matter? [see comments]. *Prenat Diagn* 1997;17:5–8.
166. Moore K. The urogenital system. In: Moore K, ed. *The developing human. Clinically oriented embryology.* Philadelphia: WB Saunders, 1988:246–285.
167. Rosati P, Guariglia L. Transvaginal sonographic assessment of the fetal urinary tract in early pregnancy. *Ultrasound Obstet Gynecol* 1996;7:95–100.
168. Green JJ, Hobbins JC. Abdominal ultrasound examination of the first-trimester fetus. *Am J Obstet Gynecol* 1988;159:165–175.
169. Bronshtein M, Kushnir O, Ben-Rafael Z, et al. Transvaginal sonographic measurement of fetal kidneys in the first trimester of pregnancy. *J Clin Ultrasound* 1990;18:299–301.
170. Bronshtein M, Yoffe N, Brandes JM, et al. First and early second-trimester diagnosis of fetal urinary tract anomalies using transvaginal sonography. *Prenat Diagn* 1990;10:653–666.
171. Bronshtein M, Amit A, Achiron R, et al. The early prenatal sonographic diagnosis of renal agenesis: techniques and possible pitfalls. *Prenat Diagn* 1994;14:291–297.
172. Bronshtein M, Tzidony D, Dimant M, et al. Transvaginal ultrasonographic measurements of the fetal adrenal glands at 12 to 17 weeks. *Am J Obstet Gynecol* 1993;169:1205–1210.
173. Bronshtein M, Bar-Hava I, Blumenfeld Z. Clues and pitfalls in the early prenatal diagnosis of 'late onset' infantile polycystic kidney. *Prenat Diagn* 1992;12:293–298.
174. Bronshtein M, Bar-Hava I, Blumenfeld Z. Differential diagnosis of the nonvisualized fetal urinary bladder by transvaginal sonography in the early second trimester. *Obstet Gynecol* 1993;82:490–493.
175. Romero R, Pilu G, Jeanty P, et al. Bilateral renal agenesis. In: Romero R, Pilu G, Jeanty P, et al., eds. *Prenatal diagnosis of congenital anomalies.* Norwalk: Appleton & Lange, 1988:259–266.
176. Nicolaides KH, Cheng HH, Abbas A, et al. Fetal renal defects: associated malformations and chromosomal defects. *Fetal Diagn Ther* 1992;7:1–11.
177. Campbell S, Wladimiroff JW, Dewhurst CJ. The antenatal measurement of fetal urine production. *J Obstet Gynaecol Br Commonw* 1973;80:680–686.
178. Jaffe R, Schoenfeld A, Ovadia J. Sonographic findings in the prenatal diagnosis of bladder exstrophy. *Am J Obstet Gynecol* 1990;162:675–678.
179. Zimmer EZ, Bronshtein M. Fetal intra-abdominal cysts detected in the first and early second trimester by transvaginal sonography. *J Clin Ultrasound* 1991;19:564–567.
180. Stiller RJ. Early ultrasonic appearance of fetal bladder outlet obstruction. *Am J Obstet Gynecol* 1989;160:584–585.
181. Favre R, Kohler M, Gasser B, et al. Early fetal megacystis between 11 and 15 weeks. *Ultrasound Obstet Gynecol* 1999;14:402–406.
182. Brace R. Amniotic fluid dynamics. In: Creasy R, Resnik R, eds. *Maternal-fetal medicine. Principles and practice.* Philadelphia: WB Saunders, 1994:106–114.
183. Abramovich D, Page K. Pathways of water transfer between amnio and the feto-placental unit at term. *Eur J Obstet Gynecol* 1973;3:155.
184. Bronshtein M, Blumenfeld Z. First and early second trimester oligohydramnios—a predictor of poor fetal outcome except in iatrogenic oligohydramnios post chorionic villus sampling. *Ultrasound Obstet Gynecol* 1991;1:245–249.
185. Barss VA, Benacerraf BR, Frigoletto FD, Jr. Second trimester oligohydramnios, a predictor of poor fetal outcome. *Obstet Gynecol* 1984;64:608–610.
186. Twining P. The value of transvaginal scanning in the assessment of second trimester oligohydramnios. *Br J Radiol* 1992;65:455–457.
187. Benacerraf BR. Examination of the second-trimester fetus with severe oligohydramnios using transvaginal scanning. *Obstet Gynecol* 1990;75:491–493.
188. Moore K. The limbs. In: Moore K, ed. *The developing human. Clinically oriented embryology.* Philadelphia: WB Saunders, 1988:355–363.
189. Mahoney B. Ultrasound evaluation of the fetal musculoskeletal system. In: Callen P, ed. *Ultrasonography in obstetrics and gynecology.* Philadelphia: WB Saunders, 1994:254–290.
190. D'Ottavio G, Tamaro LF, Mandruzzato G. Early prenatal

ultrasonographic diagnosis of osteogenesis imperfecta: a case report. *Am J Obstet Gynecol* 1993;169:384–385.

191. DiMaio MS, Barth R, Koprivnikar KE, et al. First-trimester prenatal diagnosis of osteogenesis imperfecta type II by DNA analysis and sonography. *Prenat Diagn* 1993;13:589–596.

192. Brons JT, van der Harten HJ, Wladimiroff JW, et al. Prenatal ultrasonographic diagnosis of osteogenesis imperfecta. *Am J Obstet Gynecol* 1988;159:176–181.

193. Stephens JD, Filly RA, Callen PW, et al. Prenatal diagnosis of osteogenesis imperfecta type II by real-time ultrasound. *Hum Genet* 1983;64:191–193.

194. Bulas DI, Stern HJ, Rosenbaum KN, et al. Variable prenatal appearance of osteogenesis imperfecta. *J Ultrasound Med* 1994;13:419–427.

195. Ghosh A, Woo JS, Wan CW, et al. Simple ultrasonic diagnosis of osteogenesis imperfecta type II in early second trimester. *Prenat Diagn* 1984;4:235–240.

196. Thompson EM. Non-invasive prenatal diagnosis of osteogenesis imperfecta. *Am J Med Genet* 1993;45:201–206.

197. Phillips OP, Shulman LP, Altieri LA, et al. Prenatal counseling and diagnosis in progressively deforming osteogenesis imperfecta: a case of autosomal dominant transmission. *Prenat Diagn* 1991;11:705–710.

198. Aylsworth AS, Seeds JW, Guilford WB, et al. Prenatal diagnosis of a severe deforming type of osteogenesis imperfecta. *Am J Med Genet* 1984;19:707–714.

199. Sepulveda W, Romero R, Pryde PG, et al. Prenatal diagnosis of sirenomelus with color Doppler ultrasonography. *Am J Obstet Gynecol* 1994;170:1377–1379.

200. Sepulveda W, Corral E, Sanchez J, et al. Sirenomelia sequence versus renal agenesis: prenatal differentiation with power Doppler ultrasound. *Ultrasound Obstet Gynecol* 1998;11:445–449.

201. van Zalen-Sprock MM, van Vugt JM, van der Harten JJ, et al. Early second-trimester diagnosis of sirenomelia. *Prenat Diagn* 1995;15:171–117.

202. Valenzano M, Paoletti R, Rossi A, et al. Sirenomelia. Pathological features, antenatal ultrasonographic clues, and a review of current embryogenic theories. *Hum Reprod Update* 1999;5:82–86.

203. Bronshtein M, Keret D, Deutsch M, et al. Transvaginal sonographic detection of skeletal anomalies in the first and early second trimesters. *Prenat Diagn* 1993;13:597–601.

204. Landy HJ, Weiner S, Corson SL, et al. The "vanishing twin": ultrasonographic assessment of fetal disappearance in the first trimester. *Am J Obstet Gynecol* 1986;155:14–19.

205. Jauniaux E, Elkazen N, Leroy F, et al. Clinical and morphologic aspects of the vanishing twin phenomenon. *Obstet Gynecol* 1988;72:577–581.

206. Benirschke K, Kim CK. Multiple pregnancy. 2. *N Engl J Med* 1973;288:1329–1336.

207. Little J, Bryan E. Congenital anomalies in twins. *Semin Perinatol* 1986;10:50–64.

208. Schinzel AA, Smith DW, Miller JR. Monozygotic twinning and structural defects. *J Pediatr* 1979;96:921–930.

209. Kohl S. Twin gestation. *Mt. Sinai J Med* 1975;42.

210. Benirschke K, Kim CK. Multiple pregnancy. 1. *N Engl J Med* 1973;288:1276–1284.

211. Shalev E, Zalele Y, Ben Ami M, et al. First trimester ultrasonic diagnosis of twin reversed arterial perfusion sequence. *Prenat Diagn* 1992;2:21–22.

212. Langlotz H, Sauerbrei E, Murray S. Transvaginal Doppler sonographic diagnosis of an acardiac twin at 12 week gestation. *J Ultrasound Med* 1991;10:175–179.

213. Pretorius DH, Leopold GR, Moore TR, et al. Acardiac twin. Report of Doppler sonography. *J Ultrasound Med* 1988;7:413.

214. Romero R, Pilu G, Jeanty P, et al. Conjoined twins. In: Romero R, Pilu G, Jeanty P, et al., eds. *Prenatal diagnosis of congenital anomalies*. Norwalk: Appleton & Lange, 1988:405–409.

215. Moore K. Multiple pregnancy. In: Moore K, ed. *The developing human*. Philadelphia: WB Saunders, 1988:122–130.

216. van Eyndhoven HW, ter Brugge H. The first-trimester ultrasonographic diagnosis of dicephalus conjoined twins. *Acta Obstet Gynecol Scand* 1998;77:464–466.

217. Tongsong T, Chanprapaph P, Pongsatha S. First-trimester diagnosis of conjoined twins: a report of three cases. *Ultrasound Obstet Gynecol* 1999;14:434–437.

218. Bonilla-Musoles F, Raga F, Bonilla F Jr, et al. Early diagnosis of conjoined twins using two-dimensional color Doppler and three-dimensional ultrasound. *J Natl Med Assoc* 1998; 90:552–556.

219. Goldberg Y, Ben-Shlomo I, Weiner E, et al. First trimester diagnosis of conjoined twins in a triplet pregnancy after IVF and ICSI: case report. *Hum Reprod* 2000;15:1413–1415.

220. Hill LM. The sonographic detection of early first-trimester conjoined twins. *Prenat Diagn* 1997;17:961–963.

221. Lam YH, Sin SY, Lam C, et al. Prenatal sonographic diagnosis of conjoined twins in the first trimester: two case reports. *Ultrasound Obstet Gynecol* 1998;11:289–291.

222. Maymon R, Halperin R, Weinraub Z, et al. Three-dimensional transvaginal sonography of conjoined twins at 10 weeks: a case report. *Ultrasound Obstet Gynecol* 1998;11:292–294.

223. Meizner I, Levy A, Katz M, et al. [Early ultrasonic diagnosis of conjoined twins]. *Harefuah* 1993;124:741–744, 796.

224. Schmidt W, Heberling D, Kubli F. Antepartum ultrasonographic diagnosis of conjoined twins in early pregnancy. *Am J Obstet Gynecol* 1981;139:961–963.

225. Reference deleted.

226. Ewigman BG, Crane JP, Frigoletto FD, et al. Effect of prenatal ultrasound screening on perinatal outcome. RADIUS Study Group [see comments]. *N Engl J Med* 1993;329:821–827.

NUCHAL TRANSLUCENCY

The sonographic abnormality of increased nuchal translucency (NT)* is essentially based on the observation made more than 100 years ago by Dr. Langdon Down, who in 1866 reported that the skin of individuals affected by trisomy 21 appeared to be too large for their bodies.[15] It is now known that the excess skin of individuals with Down syndrome can be visualized by ultrasonography as increased NT in the first 3 months of intrauterine life (Figs. 1 and 2).[12] Indeed, increased NT at 11 to 14 weeks of gestation is a common finding in fetuses affected by other chromosomal defects, cardiac abnormalities, and many genetic syndromes.

MEASUREMENT OF NUCHAL TRANSLUCENCY

The successful use of second-trimester serum screening for chromosomal abnormalities relies on extensive measures of quality control, all of which occur at the laboratory before the result is issued to the clinician. If NT screening is to be adopted and is to achieve uniformity of results, it is important that the method of measurement of NT is standardized and that there is a mechanism for checking the quality

of the ultrasound examination. The following criteria are important:

1. All sonographers performing fetal scans should be appropriately trained and their results subjected to rigorous audit. The Fetal Medicine Foundation, under the auspices of the International Society of Ultrasound in Obstetrics and Gynecology, has introduced a Certificate of Competence in the 11- to 14-week scan, which is awarded to those sonographers who can perform the scan to a high standard and can demonstrate a good knowledge of the diagnostic features and management of the conditions identified by this scan.

2. The ultrasound equipment must be of good quality, it should have a video-loop function, and the calipers should be able to provide measurements to one decimal point.

3. NT can be measured successfully by transabdominal ultrasound examination in approximately 95% of cases; in the other cases, transvaginal sonography is necessary.

4. The ability to measure NT and obtain reproducible results improves with training; good results are achieved after 80 and 100 scans for the transabdominal and the transvaginal routes, respectively.[16] The intraobserver and interobserver differences in measurements are less than 0.5 mm in 95% of cases.[17]

5. The minimum fetal crown–rump length should be 45 mm and the maximum 84 mm. The optimal gestational age for measurement of fetal NT is 11^{+0} to 13^{+6} weeks.

6. Fetal NT increases with crown–rump length, and, therefore, it is essential to take gestation into account when determining whether a given translucency thickness is increased.[14]

7. A good sagittal section of the fetus, as for measurement of fetal crown–rump length, should be obtained, and the NT should be measured with the fetus in the neutral position (Fig. 3). When the fetal neck is hyperextended, the measurement can be increased by 0.6 mm, and, when the neck is flexed, the measurement can be decreased by 0.4 mm.[18]

8. The magnification should be such that each increment in the distance between calipers should be only

---

*Development of nuchal translucency.

During the 1980s, many ultrasound studies described the typical appearance of cystic hygromas in the second trimester and its association with aneuploidy, particularly Turner syndrome.[1–6] At the same time, it was observed that cystic hygromas seen during the first trimester may have different appearances (nonseptated), and different associations (trisomies) than those seen during the second trimester.[7–10] It was also observed that *cystic hygromas* seen during the first trimester can resolve to nuchal thickening alone or even normal nuchal thickness and still be associated with aneuploidy. In a related observation, Benacerraf and colleagues[11] noted that second-trimester nuchal thickening was associated with an increased risk of Down syndrome.

In 1992, Nicolaides and colleagues[12] proposed the term *nuchal translucency* (NT) for the sonographic appearance of fluid under the skin at the back of the fetal neck observed in all fetuses during the first trimester. They further reported an association between the thickness of the translucency and the risk of fetal aneuploidy, especially trisomies. This concept of measuring NT in all fetuses formed the basis for first-trimester screening by ultrasound. By 1995, the first large studies of NT were published.[13] Subsequent studies have confirmed that NT thickness can be reliably measured at 11 to 14 weeks gestation and, combined with maternal age, can produce an effective means of screening for trisomy 21.[14]

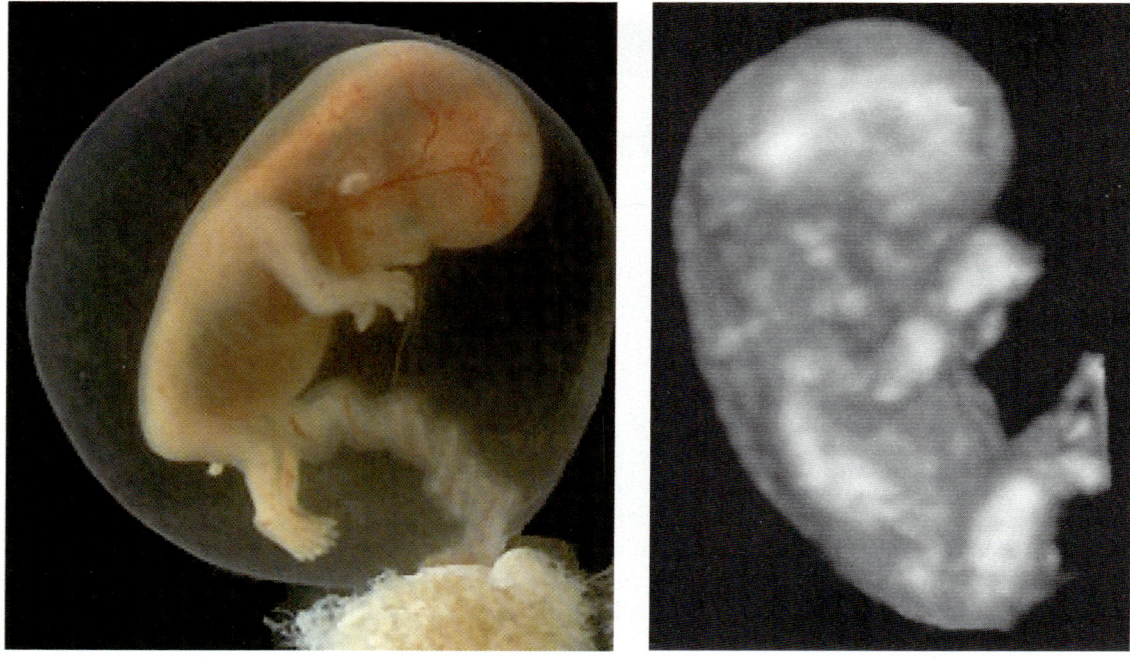

FIGURE 1. Increased nuchal translucency. **A:** Pathologic correlation of increased nuchal translucency (*arrows*) in human fetus at 11 weeks. **B:** Corresponding three-dimensional ultrasound showing increased nuchal translucency. (Part **A** courtesy of Edward C. Klatt, MD, Department of Pathology, Florida State University College of Medicine; Part **B** courtesy of David Nyberg, MD.)

0.1 mm. A study, in which rat heart ventricles were measured initially by ultrasound and then by dissection, has demonstrated that ultrasound measurements can be accurate to the nearest 0.1 to 0.2 mm.[19]

9. Care must be taken to distinguish between fetal skin and amnion, because, at this gestation, both structures appear as thin membranes (Fig. 3).[12] Increased NT can be overlooked unless specifically sought by erroneously assuming the membrane is the amnion, especially when the nuchal region is positioned posteriorly (Fig. 4). This can be avoided by waiting for spontaneous fetal movement away from the amniotic membrane; alternatively, the fetus is bounced off the

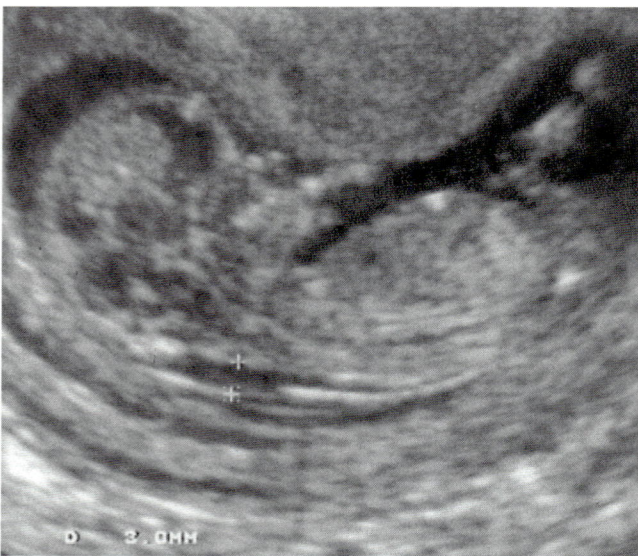

FIGURE 2. Trisomy 21. Scan of an 11-week-old fetus shows increased nuchal translucency thickness of 3 mm. The karyotype proved to be trisomy 21.

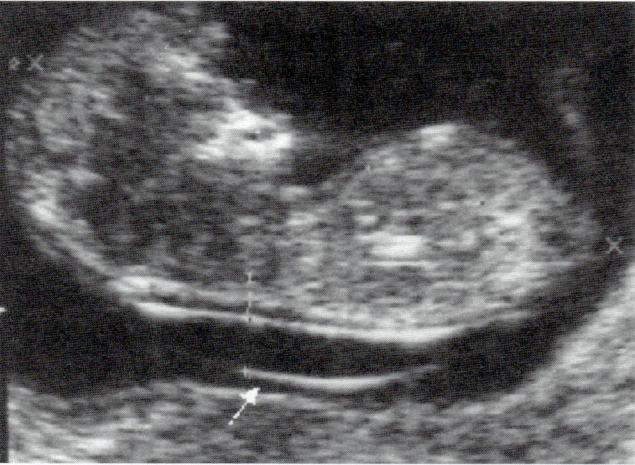

FIGURE 3. Normal nuchal measurement. Scan at 12 weeks demonstrates correct measurement of nuchal translucency. A longitudinal section of the fetus allows measurement of crown-rump length (x) and nuchal translucency (+). The amniotic membrane is clearly visible (*arrow*). The maximum nuchal translucency thickness is measured.

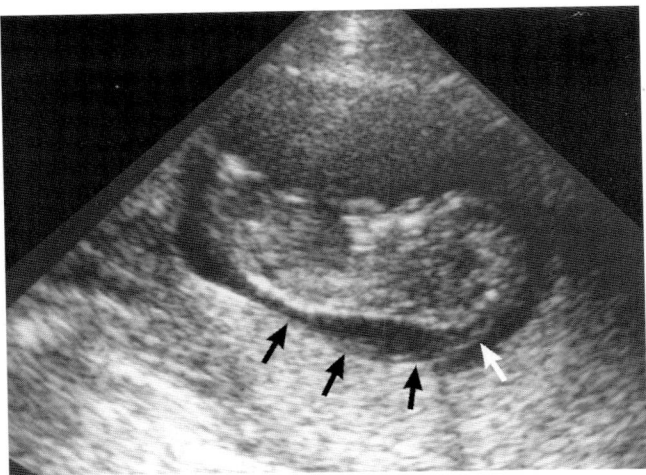

FIGURE 4. Increased nuchal translucency. Increased nuchal translucency (*arrows*) could be overlooked unless specifically sought, especially with nuchal region positioned posteriorly.

amnion by asking the mother to cough or by tapping the maternal abdomen.

10. The maximum thickness of the subcutaneous translucency between the skin and the soft tissue overlying the cervical spine should be measured. The calipers are placed on the inner borders of the echogenic lines representing the fetal skin and subcuticular tissues (Fig. 5). During the scan, more than one measurement must be taken, and the maximum one should be recorded.

11. The umbilical cord may be around the fetal neck in 5% to 10% of cases, and this finding may produce a falsely increased NT, adding approximately 0.8 mm to the measurement.[20] In such cases, the measurements of NT above and below the cord are different, and, in the calculation of risk, it is more appropriate to use the smaller measurement.

The ability to achieve a reliable measurement of NT is dependent on adherence to the criteria previously outlined

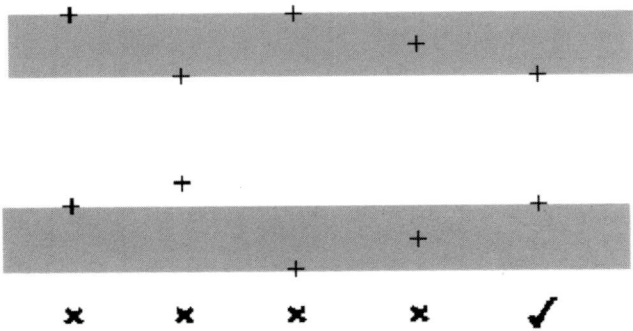

FIGURE 5. Schematic diagram showing the correct placement of the calipers for accurate measurement of nuchal translucency. Both calipers are placed on the inner border of the echogenic line bounding the skin and the subcuticular tissues.

and on the motivation of sonographers. For example, in a screening study in which the time spent in examining patients was less than 3 minutes and in which 54% of cases were examined before 10 weeks, the sonographers were unable to measure NT in 42% of the cases.[21] A study comparing the results obtained from hospitals in which NT was used in clinical practice (interventional) compared to those from hospitals in which they merely recorded the measurements but did not act on the results (observational) reported that in the interventional group successful measurement of NT was achieved in 100% of cases, and the measurement was greater than 2.5 mm in 2.3% of cases; the respective percentages in the observational group were 85% and 12%.[22,23] Appropriate training, high motivation, and adherence to a standard technique for the measurement of NT are essential prerequisites for good clinical practice. Monni et al. reported that after modifying their technique of measuring NT by following the guidelines established by The Fetal Medicine Foundation, their detection rate of trisomy 21 improved from 30% to 84%.[24]

PATHOPHYSIOLOGY OF INCREASED NUCHAL TRANSLUCENCY

Possible mechanisms for increased NT include the following:

1. Cardiac failure in association with abnormalities of the heart and great arteries. Studies involving pathologic examination in chromosomally abnormal and normal fetuses with increased NT at 11 to 14 weeks have demonstrated a high prevalence of abnormalities of the heart and great arteries.[25,26] Doppler ultrasound studies examining ductal flow at 11 to 14 weeks in fetuses with increased NT reported absent or reverse flow during atrial contraction in approximately 90% of chromosomally abnormal fetuses and in chromosomally normal fetuses with cardiac defects.[27,28] In trisomic fetuses with increased NT, there are increased levels of atrial and brain natriuretic peptide mRNA in fetal hearts, suggesting the presence of heart strain.[29]

2. Venous congestion in the head and neck, caused by constriction of the fetal body in amnion rupture sequence or superior mediastinal compression found in diaphragmatic hernia or the narrow chest in skeletal dysplasia.[30–32]

3. Altered composition of the extracellular matrix. Many of the component proteins of the extracellular matrix are encoded on chromosomes 21, 18, or 13. Immunohistochemical studies of the skin of chromosomally abnormal fetuses have demonstrated specific alterations of the extracellular matrix, which may be attributed to gene dosage effects.[33,34] Altered composition of the extracellular matrix may also be the underlying mechanism for increased fetal NT in an expanding number of genetic syndromes, which are associated

with alterations in collagen metabolism (e.g., achondrogenesis type II); abnormalities of fibroblast growth factor receptors (e.g., achondroplasia and thanatophoric dysplasia); or disturbed metabolism of peroxisome biogenesis factor (e.g., Zellweger syndrome).

4. Abnormal or delayed development of the lymphatic system. In normal embryos, the main lymphatics develop from the venous walls, but they subsequently lose their connections with the veins to form a separate lymphatic system, except for the juguloaxillary sacs, which drain the lymph to the venous system. A possible mechanism for increased translucency is dilatation of the jugular lymphatic sacs, because of developmental delay in the connection with the venous system or a primary abnormal dilatation or proliferation of the lymphatic channels interfering with a normal flow between the lymphatic and venous systems. In fetuses with Turner syndrome, there is hypoplasia of lymphatic vessels.[35,36]

5. Failure of lymphatic drainage because of impaired fetal movements in various neuromuscular disorders, such as fetal akinesia deformation sequence.[37]

6. Fetal anemia or hypoproteinemia.[38]

7. Congenital infection, acting through anemia or cardiac dysfunction.[39,40]

SCREENING FOR CHROMOSOMAL DEFECTS

Every woman has a risk that her baby will be affected by a chromosomal abnormality. This background risk depends on maternal and gestational age and whether a history of previous pregnancies affected by chromosomal abnormality exists. The background risk can be modified by applying risk factors derived from screening tests, such as the assessment of NT thickness, undertaken during pregnancy. The new risk is calculated by multiplying the background risk by a factor, known as the *likelihood ratio*, which is determined by the screening test.

Background Risk—Maternal Age, Gestational Age, and Previous Trisomies

The risk for many chromosomal abnormalities increases with maternal age (Fig. 6). Additionally, because fetuses with chromosomal defects are more likely to die in utero than normal fetuses, the risk of chromosomal abnormality decreases with advancing gestation (Fig. 7). Estimates of the maternal age-related risk for trisomy 21 at birth are based on two surveys with almost complete ascertainment of the affected patients.[41] Since 1992, with the introduction of maternal serum biochemistry and ultrasound screening for chromosomal defects at different stages of pregnancy, it has become necessary to establish maternal and gestational age-specific risks for chromosomal

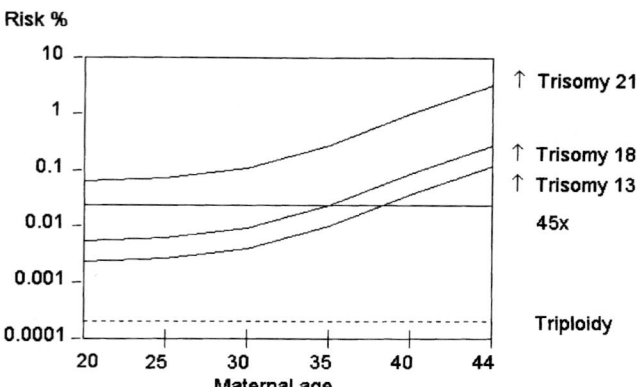

FIGURE 6. Maternal age–related risk for chromosomal abnormalities.

defects.[42–45] Such estimates were derived by comparing the birth prevalence of trisomy 21 to the prevalence in women undergoing second-trimester amniocentesis or first-trimester chorionic villus sampling. Rates of spontaneous fetal death between different gestations and delivery at 40 weeks were estimated on the basis of the observed prevalence in pregnancies that had antenatal fetal karyotyping and the reported prevalence in live births. The rates of fetal death in trisomy 21 between 12 weeks (when NT screening is carried out) and term is 30%. Between 16 weeks (when serum screening is traditionally carried out) and term, the rate of intrauterine lethality is 20%.[42–44]

Similar methods have been used to produce risk estimates for other chromosomal abnormalities.[42] Risks for trisomies 18 and 13 also increase with maternal age and decrease with gestation. The rate of intrauterine lethality for these conditions is as high as 80%. Turner syndrome is not associated with maternal age, but the prevalence of this condition (1 in 1,500 at 12 weeks, 1 in 3,000 at 20 weeks, and 1 in 4,000 at 40 weeks) is affected by the high rate of death *in utero*. The other sex chromosome abnormalities

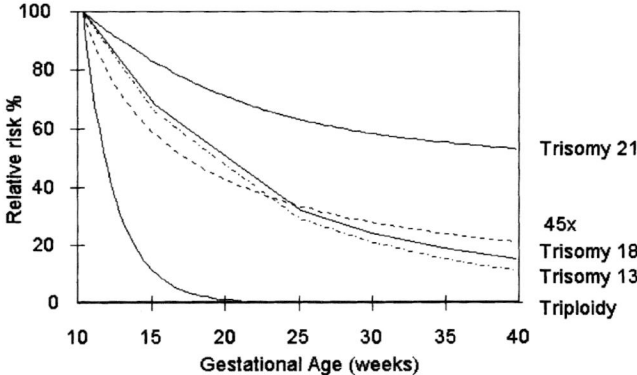

FIGURE 7. Gestational age–related risk for chromosomal abnormalities. The lines represent the relative risk according to the risk at 10 weeks of gestation.

are not affected by either maternal or gestational age, and the overall prevalence (1 in 500) does not change. Polyploidy affects approximately 2% of recognized conceptions but is highly lethal and rarely results in live birth; the prevalence at 12 weeks' gestation and birth is approximately 1 in 2,000 and 1 in 250,000 pregnancies, respectively.[42] The risk for trisomies in women who have had a previous fetus or child with a trisomy is higher than the one expected on the basis of their age alone. In a study of 2,054 women who had a previous pregnancy with trisomy 21, the risk of recurrence in the subsequent pregnancy was 0.75% higher than the maternal and gestational age-related risk for trisomy 21 at the time of testing. A similar increase in risk was found for women who had a previous pregnancy affected by trisomy 18, but whereas the risk increased for a pregnancy affected by trisomy 18, the risk for trisomy 21 did not change.[46] Thus, for a 35-year-old woman at 12 weeks' gestation who has had a previous pregnancy affected by trisomy 21, the risk increases from 1 in 249 (0.40%), based on maternal and gestational age, to 1 in 87 (1.15%), including the previous history.

Adjustment of Risk Based on Nuchal Translucency Thickness

The risk for chromosomal abnormality can be adjusted on the basis of NT thickness by multiplying the background risk by a factor, the likelihood ratio, to derive the new risk. The likelihood ratio is calculated by comparing the distributions of NT thickness in populations of chromosomally normal fetuses and fetuses affected by trisomy 21 (Fig. 8).[47] The likelihood ratio for a given NT thickness is calculated by dividing the percentage of trisomy 21 fetuses with this NT thickness by the percentage of chromosomally normal fetuses with this NT measurement. NT thickness is known to increase with gestation, which needs to be taken into

account to perform the screening test over a wide gestational age range. Comparisons between 11⁺⁰ and 13⁺⁶ weeks' gestation are made by comparing the NT measurement to the normal range for gestational age (based on crown-rump length), and the NT measurement is expressed as a multiple of the median before calculating the appropriate likelihood ratio.

Although it is important for individuals involved in NT screening programs to understand the basis for calculation of risks, these calculations can in fact be made by a computer program that simply requires the mother's date of birth and obstetric history, the fetal crown-rump length, and NT thickness.

Effectiveness in Screening for Trisomy 21

In a multicenter study under the auspices of The Fetal Medicine Foundation, 96,127 singleton pregnancies were examined, including 326 affected by trisomy 21 and 325 with other chromosomal abnormalities.[14] In each pregnancy, the fetal crown-rump length and NT were measured, and the risk of trisomy 21 was calculated by multiplying the background risk based on maternal and gestational age by the likelihood ratio, based on the deviation of NT from normal. The distribution of risks was determined, and the sensitivity of a cutoff risk of 1 in 300 was calculated. The median gestation at the time of screening was 12 weeks (range, 10 to 14 weeks), and the median maternal age was 31 years (range, 14 to 45 years). The fetal NT was above the ninety-fifth percentile for crown-rump length in 72% of the trisomy 21 pregnancies (Fig. 9). The estimated risk for trisomy 21 based on maternal age and fetal NT was more than 1 in 300 in 8.3% of normal pregnancies and 82% of those affected by trisomy

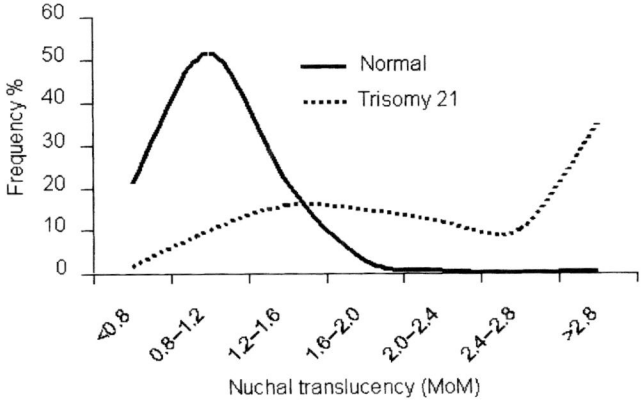

FIGURE 8. Distribution of nuchal translucency thickness expressed as deviation from the median (*MoM*) for crown-rump length in chromosomally normal fetuses and fetuses with trisomy 21.

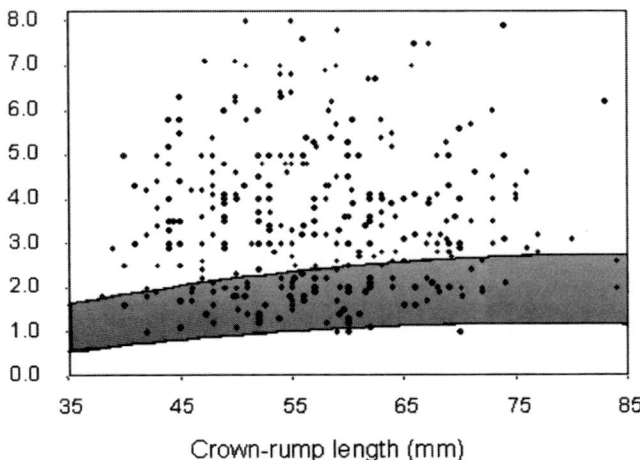

FIGURE 9. Nuchal translucency measurement in 326 trisomy 21 fetuses plotted on the normal range for crown-rump length (fifth and ninety-fifth percentiles).

21. For a screen positive rate of 5%, the sensitivity was 77% (95% CI: 72% to 82%).

Screening for chromosomal defects in the first rather than the second trimester of pregnancy has the advantage of earlier prenatal diagnosis and, consequently, less traumatic termination of pregnancy for those couples who chose this option.[48] A potential disadvantage is that earlier screening preferentially identifies those chromosomally abnormal fetuses that are destined to miscarry. This issue of intrauterine lethality does, of course, apply to all forms of screening for chromosomal abnormality, including second-trimester biochemistry; whereas 30% of fetuses affected by trisomy 21 die between 12 weeks of gestation and term, the rate of intrauterine lethality between 16 weeks and term is 20%.[43] The Fetal Medicine Foundation Multicentre Project estimated that assessment of risk by a combination of maternal age and fetal NT, followed by invasive diagnostic testing for 5% of pregnancies with a screen-positive result and selective termination of affected fetuses, would reduce the livebirth incidence of trisomy 21 by 75%.[14]

In addition to data from The Fetal Medicine Foundation study, ten other studies have reported results from the implementation of NT screening in a total of 44,962 pregnancies. Direct comparison of these studies is complicated by the differing cutoffs used to define the screen-positive group. The combined data demonstrate a sensitivity of 77% for a false-positive rate of 3% (Table 1).[49–58]

Effectiveness in Screening for Other Chromosomal Abnormalities

In The Fetal Medicine Foundation Study there were 325 cases of chromosomal abnormality other than trisomy 21.[5] The NT measurement was above the ninety-fifth percentile for gestational age in 71% of these cases. Furthermore, 78% of these pregnancies were included in the screen-positive group based on a risk of greater than 1 in 300 for trisomy 21. These fetuses often have other characteristic findings.

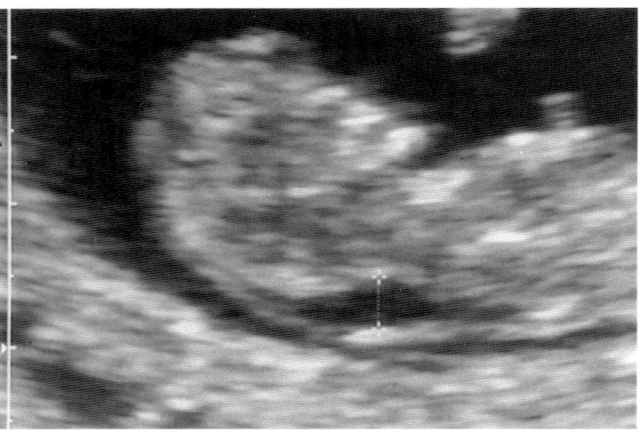

FIGURE 10. Trisomy 18. Increased nuchal translucency is observed. The karyotype proved to be trisomy 18.

For example, trisomy 18 (Fig. 10) is associated with early onset growth retardation (which enhances the deviation on NT thickness from the median); relative bradycardia; and structural abnormalities, such as exomphalos, seen in 30% of cases.[59] Trisomy 13 is similarly characterized by intrauterine growth retardation, fetal tachycardia and holoprosencephaly or exomphalos in 30% of cases.[60] Turner syndrome is associated with extremely large NT measurements, fetal tachycardia, and early onset growth retardation.[61] Fetuses with triploidy have evidence of asymmetrical growth retardation, bradycardia, holoprosencephaly, exomphalos, or a posterior fossa cyst, and molar changes in the placenta can be seen in 30% of cases.[62]

COMBINED SCREENING FOR CHROMOSOMAL DEFECTS

The most effective method of screening for chromosomal defects combines maternal age, fetal NT thickness, and two

TABLE 1. STUDIES EXAMINING THE IMPLEMENTATION OF FETAL NUCHAL TRANSLUCENCY (NT) MEASUREMENT AT 10 TO 14 WEEKS OF GESTATION IN SCREENING FOR TRISOMY 21

Author	N	Screening cutoff	False-positive rate	Detection rate
Pandya et al.[49]	1,763	NT >2.5 mm	3.6%	3 of 4 (75%)
Szabo et al.[50]	3,380	NT >3.0 mm	1.6%	28 of 31 (90%)
Taipale et al.[51]	6,939	NT >3.0 mm	0.8%	4 of 6 (67%)
Hafner et al.[52]	4,233	NT >2.5 mm	1.7%	3 of 7 (43%)
Pajkrt et al.[53]	1,473	NT >3.0 mm	2.2%	6 of 9 (67%)
Economides et al.[54]	2,281	NT >99th percentile	0.4%	6 of 8 (75%)
Zoppi et al.[55]	5,210	Risk >1 in 100	4.2%	33 of 47 (70%)
Thilaganathan et al.[56]	11,398	Risk >1 in 200	4.7%	16 of 21 (76%)
Schwarzler et al.[57]	4,523	Risk >1 in 270	4.7%	10 of 12 (83%)
Theodoropoulos et al.[58]	3,550	Risk >1 in 300	4.9%	10 of 11 (91%)
Total	44,750		3.0%	119 of 156 (76%)

maternal serum proteins at 11 to 14 weeks of gestation. Maternal serum free β-human chorionic gonadotropin (β-hCG) normally decreases with gestation after 10 weeks. Levels are increased in pregnancies affected by trisomy 21, and this difference becomes more marked with advancing gestation.[63] If free β-hCG is used alone to screen for trisomy 21 at 11 to 14 weeks' gestation, for a false-positive rate of 5%, the detection rate is 35%, rising to 45% when combined with maternal age.[64] Maternal serum pregnancy-associated plasma protein A (PAPP-A) levels normally increase with advancing gestation. Levels are decreased in pregnancies affected by trisomy 21, a difference which becomes less marked with advancing gestation.[63] Screening for trisomy 21 using PAPP-A at 11 to 14 weeks' gestation detects 40% of affected pregnancies for a false-positive rate of 5%, rising to 50% when combined with maternal age.[64]

There does not appear to be any correlation between the rise in free β-hCG and fall in PAPP-A seen in trisomy 21 pregnancies, so these markers may be combined for screening purposes.[64] Similarly, these biochemical markers are independent of fetal NT thickness, allowing combination of biochemical and ultrasound tests.[65,66] This combined test involving maternal age, fetal NT thickness, free β-hCG, and PAPP-A gives a detection rate of approximately 90% for a screen-positive rate of 5% (Table 2).[64,67–72]

Whereas NT is increased in other chromosomal abnormalities, the changes seen in first-trimester biochemical markers may differ from those typically associated with trisomy 21. In trisomies 18 and 13, maternal serum free β-hCG and PAPP-A are decreased.[73,74] In cases of sex chromosomal anomalies, maternal serum free β-hCG is normal and PAPP-A is low.[75] Triploidy of paternal origin, which is associated with a partial molar placenta, has greatly increased levels of free β-hCG, whereas PAPP-A is mildly decreased.[76] In contrast, digynic triploidy, characterized by severe asymmetrical fetal growth restriction, is associated with markedly decreased maternal serum free β-hCG and PAPP-A. Screening by a combination of fetal NT, free β-hCG and PAPP-A can identify approximately 90% of these anomalies for a screen positive rate of 1%.

Nuchal Translucency Followed by Second-Trimester Biochemistry

In women having second-trimester biochemical testing following first-trimester NT screening (with or without maternal serum biochemistry), the background risk needs to be adjusted to take into account the first-trimester screening results. Because first-trimester screening identifies almost 90% of trisomy 21 pregnancies, second-trimester biochemistry will identify—at best—6% (60% of the residual 10%) of the affected pregnancies, with doubling of the overall invasive testing rate (from 5% to 10%). It is theoretically possible to use various statistical techniques to combine NT with different components of first-trimester and second-trimester biochemical testing. One such hypothetical model has combined first-trimester nuchal and PAPP-A with second-trimester free β-hCG, estriol, and inhibin A, claiming a potential sensitivity of 94% for a 5% false-positive rate.[77] Even if the assumptions made in this statistical technique are valid, it is unlikely that it will gain widespread clinical acceptability.[78]

Two studies have reported on the impact of first-trimester screening by NT on second-trimester serum biochemical testing. In one study, the proportion of affected pregnancies in the screen-positive group (positive predictive value) of screening by the double test in the second trimester was 1 in 40; after the introduction of screening by NT, 83% of trisomy 21 pregnancies were identified in the first trimester, and the positive predictive value of biochemical screening decreased to 1 in 200.[79] In the second study, first-trimester screening by NT identified 71% of trisomy 21 pregnancies for a screen-positive rate of 2%, and the positive predictive value of second-trimester screening by the quadruple test was only 1 in 150.[80]

Nuchal Translucency Followed by Second-Trimester Ultrasonography

In the mid-trimester scan, minor fetal defects or markers are common and they are not usually associated with any handicap, unless there is an associated chromosomal abnormality. Routine karyotyping of all pregnancies with these markers would have major implications, in terms of miscarriage and in economic costs. It is best to base counseling on an individual estimated risk for a chromosomal abnormality, rather than the arbitrary advice that invasive testing is recommended because the risk is high. The estimated risk can be derived by multiplying the background risk (based on maternal age, gestational age, history of previously affected pregnancies, and, where appropriate, the results of previous screening by NT and biochemistry in the current pregnancy) by the likelihood ratio of the specific defect.[81]

TABLE 2. STUDIES EXAMINING THE IMPLEMENTATION OF A COMBINED FIRST-TRIMESTER TEST USING MATERNAL AGE, FETAL NUCHAL TRANSLUCENCY THICKNESS, FREE β-hCG AND PAPP-A TO SCREEN FOR TRISOMY 21

Author	N	False-positive rate (%)	Detection rate
Orlandi et al.[67]	744	5.0	6 of 7 (87%)
Biagotti et al.[68]	232	5.0	24 of 32 (76%)
Benattar et al.[69]	1,656	5.0	5 of 5 (100%)
De Biasio et al.[70]	1,467	3.3	11 of 13 (85%)
De Graff et al.[71]	300	5.0	31 of 37 (85%)
Spencer et al.[64]	1,156	5.0	187 of 210 (89%)
Krantz et al.[72]	5,718	5.0	30 of 33 (90%)
Total	**11,273**	**4.8**	**294 of 337 (87%)**

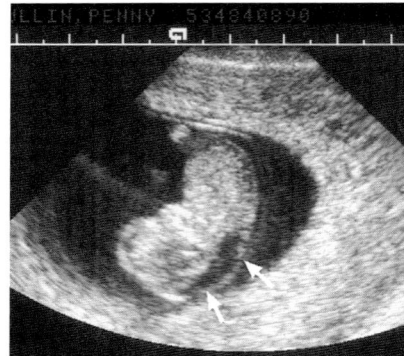 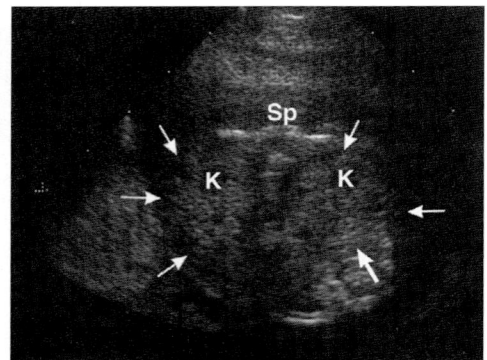

FIGURE 11. Increased nuchal translucency and renal dysplasia. **A:** Transvaginal scan performed at 10 weeks shows increased nuchal translucency (*arrows*). This study was performed for dating purposes and is earlier than recommended for nuchal screening. **B:** Follow-up scan at 17 weeks with transverse view of kidney regions shows enlarged, echogenic kidneys (*K*, *arrows*) consistent with renal dysplasia. Sp, spine. (Courtesy of David Nyberg, MD.)

On the basis of existing publications for apparently isolated markers the estimated likelihood ratio for trisomy 21 is 15 for nuchal edema, 4 for short femur and for echogenic foci in the heart, 3 for hyperechogenic bowel, and 1.5 for choroid plexus cysts and for mild hydronephrosis.[47] These likelihood ratios change as further publications can be added to the analysis. Nyberg et al. have also calculated likelihood ratios for these markers, based on a series of 142 fetuses affected by trisomy 21,[82] and has refined this for single markers.[83]

Little data exist on the interrelation between these second-trimester ultrasound markers and NT at 11 to 14 weeks or first- and second-trimester biochemistry. No obvious physiologic reason exists, however, for such an interrelation, and it is therefore reasonable to assume that they are independent. Consequently, in estimating the risk in a pregnancy with a marker, it is logical to take into account the results of previous screening tests. For example, in a 20-year-old woman at 20 weeks of gestation (background risk of 1 in 1,295), who had an 11 to 14 week assessment by NT measurement that resulted in a 5-fold reduction in risk (to approximately 1 in 6,475), the estimated risk has increased by a factor of 1.5 to 1.0 in 4,317 after the diagnosis of mild hydronephrosis at the 20-week scan. In contrast, for the same ultrasound finding of fetal mild hydronephrosis in a 40-year-old woman (background risk of 1 in 82), who did not have NT or biochemistry screening, the new estimated risk is 1 in 55.

There are some exceptions to this process of sequential screening, which assumes independence between the findings of different screening results. The findings of nuchal edema or a cardiac defect at the mid-trimester scan cannot be considered independently of NT screening at 11 to 14 weeks. Similarly, hyperechogenic bowel (which may be caused by intra-amniotic bleeding) and relative shortening of the femur (which may be caused by placental insufficiency) may well be related to serum biochemistry (high

free β-hCG and inhibin-A and low estriol may be markers of placental damage) and can, therefore, not be considered independently in estimating the risk for trisomy 21.

Nuchal Translucency and Abnormalities in Euploid Fetuses

Extensive studies have now established that, in chromosomally normal fetuses, increased NT is associated with a wide range of fetal defects (Figs. 11 and 12) and genetic syndromes.[97] Furthermore, the prevalence of fetal abnormalities increases with NT thickness (Table 3). Souka et al. reported the overall risk of adverse outcome, including miscarriage and intrauterine death, was 32% for those with NT of 3.5 to 4.4 mm, 49% for NT of 4.5 to 5.4 mm, 67% for NT 5.5 to 6.4 mm, and 89% for those NT of 6.5 mm or more (Fig. 13).[84] Among 1,080 surviving fetuses with NT of 3.5 mm or more, 5.56% had abnormalities requiring medical or surgical treatment or leading to mental handicap. The chance of no defect among live births was 86% for those with NT of 3.5 to 4.4 mm, 77% for those with NT of 4.5 to 5.4 mm, 67% for those with NT of 5.5 to 6.4, and 31% for those with NT of 6.5 mm or more.

It should be emphasized to the parents that increased NT per se does not constitute a fetal abnormality, and, once chromosomal defects have been excluded, nearly 90% of live borns with fetal translucency below 4.5 mm results in healthy live births.

Increased Nuchal Translucency and Cardiac Defects

Abnormalities of the heart and great arteries are the most common congenital defects, and the birth prevalence is 5 to 10 per 1,000. In general, approximately one-half are either lethal or require surgery, and one-half are asymptomatic. The first two groups are referred to as *major*. Specialist

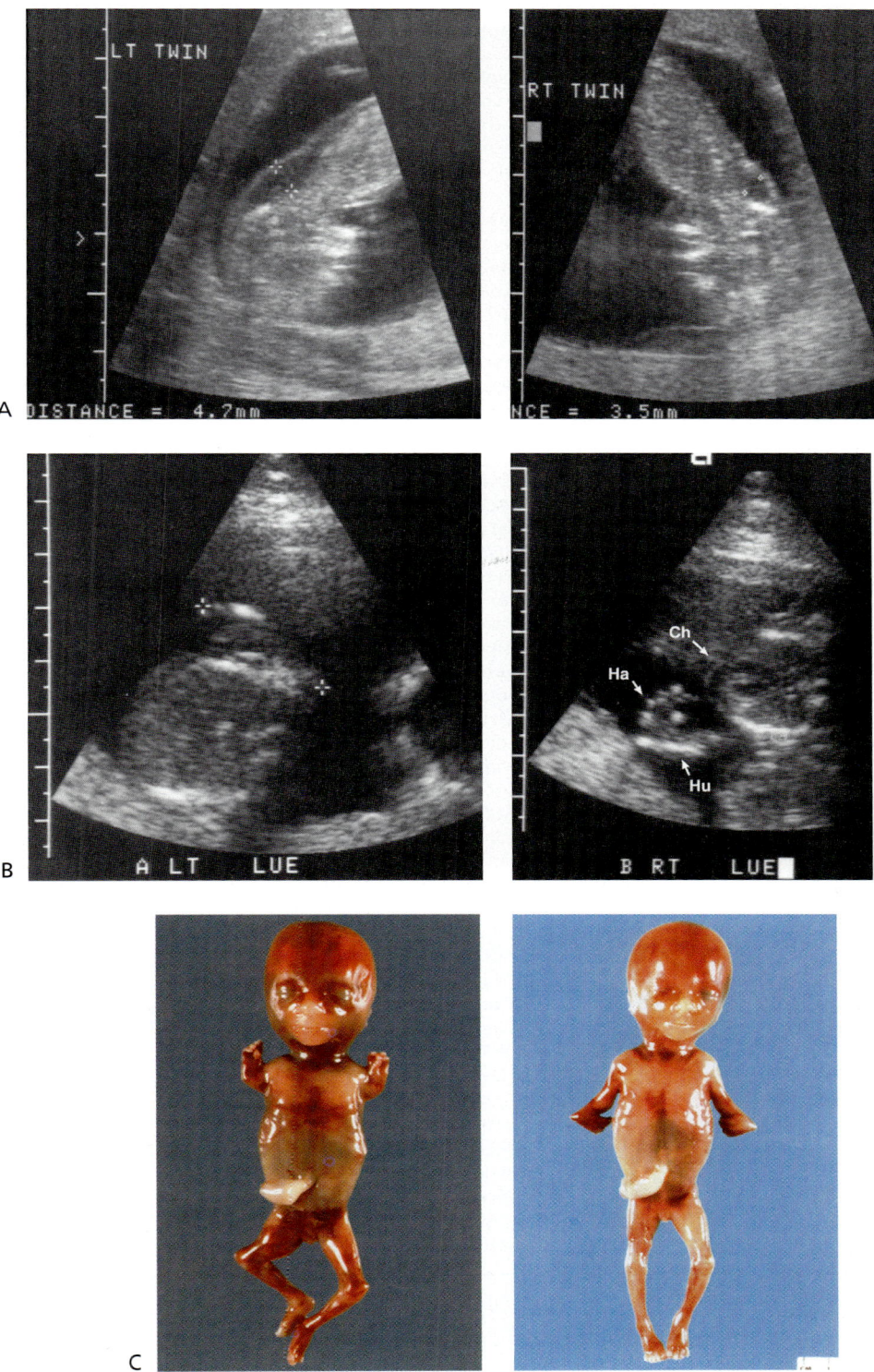

FIGURE 12. Increased nuchal translucency and upper limb phocomelia. **A:** Transvaginal scan performed at 12 weeks in monozygotic twin pregnancy shows increased nuchal translucency in both twins. **B:** Follow-up scan shows shortened upper extremities of each fetus with radial aplasia for twin B. Ch, chest; Ha, hand; Hu, humerus. **C:** Postmortem photographs confirm upper limb phocomelia for each fetus with radial aplasia in twin B. It was not possible to distinguish Roberts syndrome from thrombocytopenia, absent radius syndrome in this case. (Reproduced in part with permission from Souter V, Nyberg D, Siebert JR, Gonzales A, Luthardt F, et al. Upper limb phocomelia associated with increased nuchal translucency in a monochorionic twin pregnancy. *J Ultrasound Med* 2002;21:355–360.)

TABLE 3. ABNORMALITIES AND GENETIC SYNDROMES REPORTED IN ASSOCIATION WITH INCREASED NUCHAL TRANSLUCENCY AND NORMAL KARYOTYPE

Central nervous system defect
  Anencephaly
  Craniosynostosis
  Dandy-Walker malformation
  Diastematomyelia
  Encephalocele
  Holoprosencephaly
  Hydrolethalis syndrome
  Joubert syndrome
  Microcephaly
  Macrocephaly
  Spina bifida
  Iniencephaly
  Trigonocephaly C
  Ventriculomegaly
Facial defect
  Agnathia/micrognathia
  Facial cleft
  Treacher Collins syndrome
Nuchal defect
  Cystic hygroma
  Neck lipoma
Cardiac defect
  DiGeorge syndrome
Pulmonary defects
  Cystic adenomatoid malformation
  Diaphragmatic hernia
  Fryns syndrome
Abdominal wall defect
  Cloacal exstrophy
  Omphalocele
  Gastroschisis
Gastrointestinal defect
  Crohn disease
  Duodenal atresia
  Esophageal atresia
  Small-bowel obstruction
Genitourinary defect
  Ambiguous genitalia
  Congenital nephrotic syndrome
  Hydronephrosis
  Hypospadias
  Infantile polycystic kidney disease
  Meckel-Gruber syndrome
  Megacystis
  Multicystic dysplastic kidney disease
  Renal agenesis

Skeletal defect
  Achondrogenesis
  Achondroplasia
  Asphyxiating thoracic dystrophy
  Blomstrand osteochondrodysplasia
  Camptomelic dwarfism
  Jarcho-Levin syndrome
  Kyphoscoliosis
  Limb reduction defect
  Noonan-Sweeny syndrome
  Osteogenesis imperfecta
  Roberts syndrome
  Robinow syndrome[95]
  Short rib polydactyly
  Sirenomelia
  Talipes equinovarus
  Split hand/foot malformation[96]
  Thanatophoric dwarfism
  VACTERL association
Fetal anemia
  Blackfan-Diamond anemia
  Dyserythropoietic anemia
  Fanconi's anemia
  Parvovirus 19 infection
  Alpha thalassemia
Neuromuscular defect
  Fetal akinesia deformation sequence
  Myotonic dystrophy
  Spinal muscular atrophy
Metabolic defect
  Beckwith-Wiedemann syndrome
  GM_1 gangliosidosis
  Long-chain 3-hydroyacyl-coenzyme A dehydrogenase deficiency
  Mucopolysaccharidosis type VII
  Smith-Lemli-Opitz syndrome
  Vitamin D–resistant rickets
  Zellweger syndrome
Other
  Body stalk anomaly (limb-body wall complex)
  Brachmann-de Lange syndrome
  CHARGE association
  Deficiency of the immune system
  Congenital lymphedema
  Ectrodactyly-ectodermal dysplasia–cleft palate syndrome
  Neonatal myoclonic encephalopathy
  Noonan syndrome
  Perlman syndrome
  Stickler syndrome
  Unspecified syndrome
  Severe developmental delay

CHARGE, *coloboma, heart anomaly, choanal atresia, retardation, and genital and ear abnormalities*; VACTERL, *vertebral, anal, cardiac, tracheal, esophageal, and renal*.
Adapted from Souka AP, Krampl E, Bakalis S, et al. Outcome of pregnancy in chromosomally normal fetuses with increased nuchal translucency in the first trimester. *Ultrasound Obstet Gynecol* 2001;18(1):9–17.

echocardiography at around 20 weeks of gestation can identify most of the major cardiac defects, but the main challenge in prenatal diagnosis is to identify the high-risk group for referral to specialist centers. Currently, screening is based on examination of the four-chamber view of the heart at the 20-week scan, but this identifies only approxi-

mately 25% of the major cardiac defects.[85] Evidence exists that measurement of NT may provide more effective screening for major abnormalities of the heart and great arteries.

Several case reports or small series exist on the sonographic diagnosis of cardiac defects at the 11- to 14-week

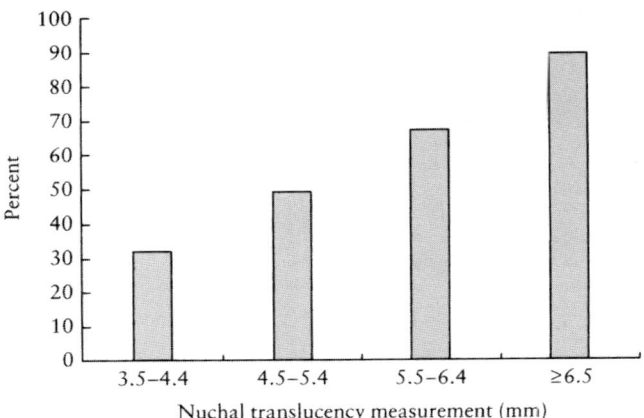

FIGURE 13. Chance of adverse outcome among fetuses with increased nuchal translucency (3.5 mm or more) and normal karyotype. [Adapted from Souka AP, Krampl E, Bakalis S, Heath V, Nicolaides KH. Outcome of pregnancy in chromosomally normal fetuses with increased nuchal translucency in the first trimester. *Ultrasound Obstet Gynecol* 2001;18(1):9–17.]

scan; in a total of 21 fetuses with major cardiac defects, 17 (81%) had increased NT.[86–89] A retrospective study of 29,154 chromosomally normal singleton pregnancies identified major defects of the heart and great arteries in 50 cases.[90] The prevalence of defects increased with NT from 0.8 per 1,000 for those with translucency below the ninety-fifth percentile to 63.5 per 1,000 for translucency above the ninety-ninth percentile (Fig. 14). Approximately 40% of the cardiac defects were in the subgroup with translucency above the ninety-ninth percentile, and 56% were in the subgroup with translucency above the ninety-fifth percentile (Fig. 15).

In a prospective study of 398 chromosomally normal fetuses with an NT measurement above the ninety-ninth percentile (greater than 3.5 mm), specialist fetal echocardiography was carried out.[91] Major cardiac defects were present in 29 (7.6%) cases, and, in 28 of these, the diagnosis was made by antenatal echocardiography. The prevalence of cardiac defects

increased from 3% in those with an NT of 3.5 to 5.4 mm to 15% in those with a measurement of 5.5 mm or more.

The clinical implication of these findings is that increased NT constitutes an indication for specialist fetal echocardiography. Certainly, the overall prevalence of major cardiac defects in such a group of fetuses (approximately 2%) is similar to that found in pregnancies affected by maternal diabetes mellitus or with a history of a previously affected offspring, which are well-accepted indications for fetal echocardiography. At present, there may not be sufficient facilities for specialist fetal echocardiography to accommodate the potential increase in demand if the ninety-fifth percentile of NT is used as the cutoff for referral. In contrast, a cutoff of the ninety-ninth percentile would result in only a small increase in workload, and, in this population, the prevalence of major cardiac defects would be very high (approximately 6%).

Based on the high risk of cardiac and other defects in fetuses with increased NT, the suggested management for affected pregnancies is shown in Figure 16. Patients identified by NT scanning as being at high risk for cardiac defects need not wait until 20 weeks for specialist echocardiography. Improvements in the resolution of ultrasound machines have now made it possible to undertake detailed cardiac scanning in the first trimester of pregnancy.[88,91,92] A specialist scan from 14 weeks can effectively reassure the majority of parents that no major cardiac defect exists. In the cases with a major defect, the early scan can either lead to the correct diagnosis or at least raise suspicions so that follow-up scans are carried out.

NUCHAL TRANSLUCENCY AND MULTIPLE PREGNANCY

Screening for Chromosomal Defects

In dichorionic twin pregnancies, the sensitivity and false-positive rate of fetal NT in screening for trisomy 21 are similar to those in singleton pregnancies.[93] Therefore, effective screening and diagnosis of major chromosomal abnormalities can be achieved in the first trimester, allowing the possibility of earlier and, therefore, safer selective feticide for those parents that choose this option.

In monochorionic pregnancies, the number of cases examined is still too small to draw definite conclusions as to whether, in the calculation of risk of trisomy 21 in monochorionic pregnancies, the NT of the fetus with the largest or the smallest measurement (or the average of the two) should be considered.

Twin-to-Twin Transfusion Syndrome

Ultrasonographic features of the underlying hemodynamic changes in severe twin-to-twin transfusion syndrome may be present from as early as 11 to 14 weeks of gestation and

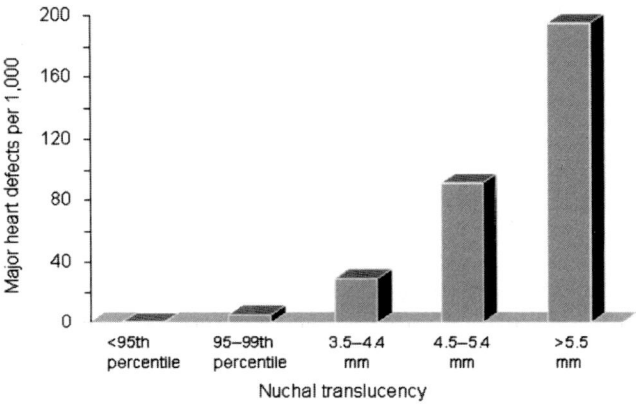

FIGURE 14. Prevalence of major cardiac defects in a series of 29,154 fetuses screened for chromosomal abnormalities using nuchal translucency at 11 to 14 weeks' gestation.

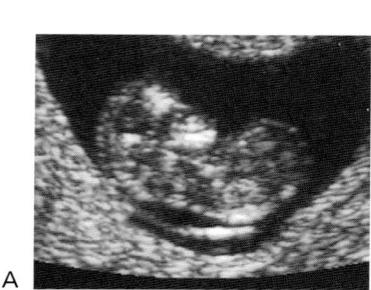
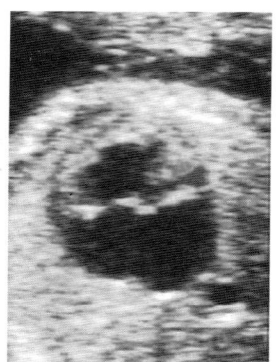

FIGURE 15. Increased nuchal translucency and cardiac defect. **A:** Longitudinal image at 10 weeks. **B:** Transverse images at 10 weeks (earlier than recommended for nuchal translucency screening) shows increased nuchal translucency. A follow-up scan at 19 weeks showed complex cardiac defect with functional single ventricle. (Courtesy of David Nyberg, MD.)

manifest as increased NT thickness in one or both of the fetuses. In a study of 132 monochorionic twin pregnancies, including 16 that developed severe twin-to-twin transfu-

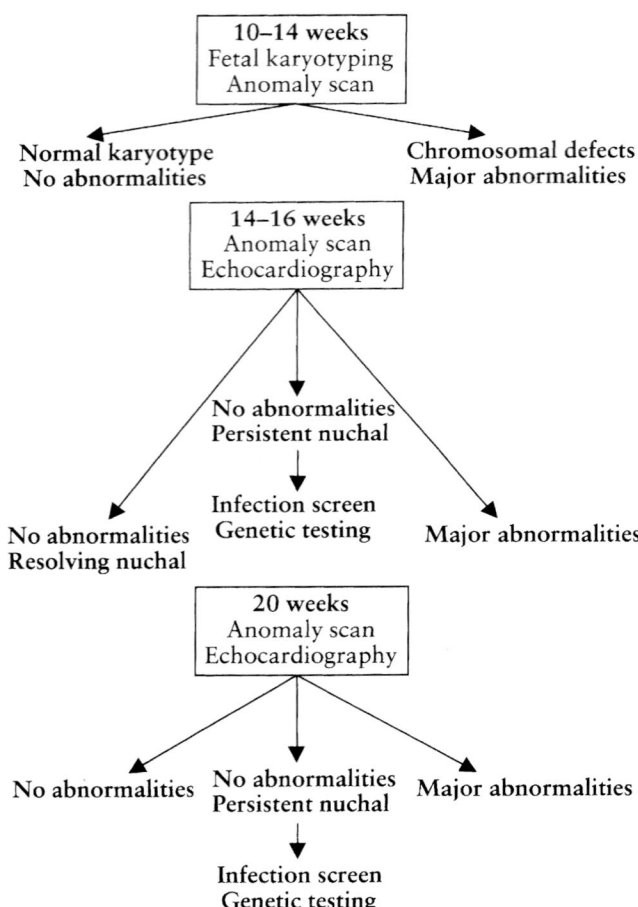

FIGURE 16. Suggested management of pregnancies with increased nuchal translucency.

sion syndrome at 15 to 22 weeks of gestation, increased NT (above the ninety-fifth percentile of the normal range) at the 11- to 14-week scan was associated with a fourfold increase in risk for the subsequent development of severe twin-to-twin transfusion syndrome.[94] It is possible that increased NT thickness in the recipient fetus may be a manifestation of heart failure due to hypervolemic congestion. With advancing gestation and the development of diuresis that would tend to correct the hypervolemia and reduce heart strain, the congestive heart failure and NT resolve.

REFERENCES

1. Phillips HE, McGahan JP. Intrauterine fetal cystic hygromas: sonographic detection. *AJR Am J Roentgenol* 1981;136(4): 799–802.
2. Toftager-Larsen K, Benzie RJ, Doran TA, et al. Alpha-fetoprotein and ultrasound scanning in the prenatal diagnosis of Turner's syndrome. *Prenat Diagn* 1983;3(1):35–40.
3. Chervenak FA, Isaacson G, Blakemore KJ, et al. Fetal cystic hygroma. Cause and natural history. *N Engl J Med* 1983;309(14):822–825.
4. Redford DH, McNay MB, Ferguson-Smith ME, et al. Aneuploidy and cystic hygroma detectable by ultrasound. *Prenat Diagn* 1984;4(5):377–382.
5. Marchese C, Savin E, Dragone E, et al. Cystic hygroma: prenatal diagnosis and genetic counseling. *Prenat Diagn* 1985;5(3):221–227.
6. Garden AS, Benzie RJ, Miskin M, et al. Fetal cystic hygroma colli: antenatal diagnosis, significance, and management. *Am J Obstet Gynecol* 1986;154(2):221–225.
7. Brambati B, Simoni G. Diagnosis of fetal trisomy 21 in first trimester. *Lancet* 1983;1(8324):586.
8. Gustavii B, Edvall H. First trimester diagnosis of cystic nuchal hygroma. *Acta Obstet Gynecol Scand* 1984;4:383–386.
9. Reuss A, Pijpers L, Schampers PTFN, et al. The importance of chorionic villus sampling after first trimester diagnosis of cystic hygroma. *Prenat Diagn* 1987;7:299–301.

10. Bronshtein M, Rottem S, Yoffe N, et al. First-trimester and early second-trimester diagnosis of nuchal cystic hygroma by transvaginal sonography: diverse prognosis of the septated from the nonseptated lesion. *Am J Obstet Gynecol* 1988;161(1):78–82.

11. Benacerraf BR, Barss V, Laboda LA. A sonographic sign for detection in the second trimester of the fetus with Down's syndrome. *Am J Obstet Gynecol* 1985;151:1078–1079.

12. Nicolaides KH, Azar G, Byrne D, et al. Fetal nuchal translucency: ultrasound screening for chromosomal defects in first trimester of pregnancy. *BMJ* 1992;304(6831):867–869.

13. Pandya PP, Kondylios A, Hilbert L, et al. Chromosomal defects and outcome in 1015 fetuses with increased nuchal translucency. *Ultrasound Obstet Gynecol* 1995;5:15–19.

14. Snijders RJM, Noble P, Sebire N, et al. UK multicentre project on assessment of risk of trisomy 21 by maternal age and fetal nuchal-translucency thickness at 10–14 weeks of gestation. *Lancet* 1998;352:343–346.

15. Langdon Down J. *Observations on an ethnic classification of idiots*. Clinical Lectures and Reports, London Hospital 3, 1866:259–262.

16. Braithwaite JM, Kadir RA, Pepera TA, et al. Nuchal translucency measurements: training of potential examiners. *Ultrasound Obstet Gynecol* 1996;8:192–195.

17. Pandya PP, Altman D, Brizot ML, et al. Repeatability of measurement of fetal nuchal translucency thickness. *Ultrasound Obstet Gynecol* 1995;5:334–337.

18. Whitlow BJ, Chatzipapas IK, Economides DL. The effect of fetal neck position on nuchal translucency measurement. *Br J Obstet Gynaecol* 1998;105:872–876.

19. Braithwaite JM, Morris RW, Economides DL. Nuchal translucency measurements: frequency distribution and changes with gestation in a general population. *Br J Obstet Gynaecol* 1996;103:1201–1204.

20. Schaefer M, Laurichesse-Delmas H, Ville Y. The effect of nuchal cord on nuchal translucency measurement at 10–14 weeks. *Ultrasound Obstet Gynecol* 1998;11:271–273.

21. Kornman LH, Morssink LP, Beekhuis JR, et al. Nuchal translucency cannot be used as a screening test for chromosomal abnormalities in the first trimester of pregnancy in a routine ultrasound practice. *Prenat Diagn* 1996;16:797–805.

22. Bower S, Chitty L, Bewley S, et al. *First trimester nuchal translucency screening of the general population: data from three centres* (abst). Presented at the 27th British Congress of Obstetrics and Gynaecology. Dublin: Royal College of Obstetrics and Gynaecology, 1995.

23. Roberts LJ, Bewley S, Mackinson AM, et al. First trimester fetal nuchal translucency: problems with screening the general population. 1. *Br J Obstet Gynaecol* 1995;102:381–385.

24. Monni G, Ibba RM, Zoppi MA. Antenatal screening for Down's syndrome. *Lancet* 1998;352:1631–1632.

25. Hyett JA, Moscoso G, Nicolaides KH. Abnormalities of the heart and great arteries in first trimester chromosomally abnormal fetuses. *Am J Med Genet* 1997;69:207–216.

26. Hyett JA, Perdu M, Sharland GK, et al. Increased nuchal translucency at 10–14 weeks of gestation as a marker for major cardiac defects. *Ultrasound Obstet Gynecol* 1997;10:242–246.

27. Matias A, Gomes C, Flack N, et al. Screening for chromosomal abnormalities at 11–14 weeks: the role of ductus venosus blood flow. *Ultrasound Obstet Gynecol* 1998;12:380–384.

28. Matias A, Huggon I, Areias JC, et al. Cardiac defects in chromosomally normal fetuses with abnormal ductus venosus blood flow at 10–14 weeks. *Ultrasound Obstet Gynecol* 1999;14:307–310.

29. Hyett JA, Brizot ML, von Kaisenberg CS, et al. Cardiac gene expression of atrial natriuretic peptide and brain natriuretic peptide in trisomic fetuses. *Obstet Gynecol* 1996;87:506–510.

30. Souka AP, Snidjers RJM, Novakov A, et al. Defects and syndromes in chromosomally normal fetuses with increased nuchal translucency thickness at 10–14 weeks of gestation. *Ultrasound Obstet Gynecol* 1998;11:391–400.

31. Sebire NJ, Snijders RJ, Davenport M, et al. Fetal nuchal translucency thickness at 10–14 weeks' gestation and congenital diaphragmatic hernia. *Obstet Gynecol* 1997;90:943–946.

32. Daskalakis G, Sebire NJ, Jurkovic D, et al. Body stalk anomaly at 10–14 weeks of gestation. *Ultrasound Obstet Gynecol* 1997;10:416–418.

33. von Kaisenberg CS, Brand-Saberi B, Christ B, et al. Collagen type VI gene expression in the skin of trisomy 21 fetuses. *Obstet Gynecol* 1998;91:319–323.

34. von Kaisenberg CS, Krenn V, Ludwig M, et al. Morphological classification of nuchal skin in fetuses with trisomy 21, 18 and 13 at 12–18 weeks and in a trisomy 16 mouse. *Anat Embryol* 1998;197:105–124.

35. Chitayat D, Kalousek DK, Bamforth JS. Lymphatic abnormalities in fetuses with posterior cervical cystic hygroma. *Am J Med Genet* 1989;33:352–356.

36. von Kaisenberg CS, Nicolaides KH, Brand-Saberi B. Lymphatic vessel hypoplasia in fetuses with Turner syndrome. *Human Reprod* 1999;14:823–826.

37. Hyett J, Noble P, Sebire NJ, et al. Lethal congenital arthrogryposis presents with increased nuchal translucency at 10–14 weeks of gestation. *Ultrasound Obstet Gynecol* 1997;9:310–313.

38. Lam YH, Tang MH, Lee CP, et al. Nuchal translucency in fetuses affected by homozygous α-thalassemia-1 at 12–13 weeks of gestation. *Ultrasound Obstet Gynecol* 1999;13:238–240.

39. Sebire NJ, Bianco D, Snijders RJM, et al. Increased fetal nuchal translucency thickness at 10–14 weeks: is screening for maternal-fetal infection necessary? *Br J Obstet Gynaecol* 1997;104:212–215.

40. Petrikovsky BM, Baker D, Schneider E. Fetal hydrops secondary to human parvovirus infection in early pregnancy. *Prenat Diagn* 1996;16:342–344.

41. Hecht CA, Hook EB. The imprecision in rates of Down syndrome by 1-year maternal age intervals: a critical analysis of rates used in biochemical screening. *Prenat Diagn* 1994;14:729–738.

42. Snijders RJM, Sebire NJ, Cuckle H, et al. Maternal age and gestational age-specific risks for chromosomal defects. *Fetal Diagn Ther* 1995;10:356–367.

43. Snijders RJM, Sundberg K, Holzgreve W, et al. Maternal age and gestation specific risk for trisomy 21. *Ultrasound Obstet Gynecol* 1999;13:167–170.

44. Halliday JL, Watson LF, Lumley J, et al. New estimates of Down syndrome risks at chorionic villus sampling, amniocentesis and live birth in women of advanced maternal age from a uniquely defined population. *Prenat Diagn* 1995;15:455–465.

45. Morris JK, Wald NJ, Watt HC. Fetal loss in Down syndrome pregnancies. *Prenat Diagn* 1999;19:142–145.

46. Snijders RJM, Sundberg K, Holzgreve W, et al. Maternal age and gestation specific risk for trisomy 21: effect of previous affected pregnancy. *Ultrasound Obstet Gynecol* 1999;13: 167–170.

47. Nicolaides KH, Sebire NJ, Snijders RJM. Nuchal translucency and chromosomal defects. In: Nicolaides KH, ed. *The 11–14–week scan; the diagnosis of fetal abnormalities.* London: Parthenon Publishing, 1999:3–65.

48. Spencer JW, Cox DN. A comparison of chorionic villus sampling and amniocentesis: acceptability of procedure and maternal attachment to pregnancy. *Obstet Gynecol* 1988;72:714–718.

49. Pandya PP, Goldberg H, Walton B, et al. The implementation of first-trimester scanning at 10–13 weeks' gestation and the measurement of fetal nuchal translucency thickness in two maternity units. *Ultrasound Obstet Gynecol* 1995;5:20–25.

50. Szabo J, Gellen J, Szemere G. First-trimester ultrasound screening for fetal aneuploidies in women over 35 and under 35 years of age. *Ultrasound Obstet Gynecol* 1995;5:161–163.

51. Taipale P, Hiilesmaa V, Salonen R, et al. Increased nuchal translucency as a marker for fetal chromosomal defects. *N Engl J Med* 1997;337:1654–1658.

52. Hafner E, Schuchter K, Liebhart E, et al. Results of routine fetal nuchal translucency measurement at 10–13 weeks in 4,233 unselected pregnant women. *Prenat Diagn* 1998;18:29–34.

53. Pajkrt E, van Lith JMM, Mol BWJ, et al. Screening for Down's syndrome by fetal nuchal translucency measurement in a general obstetric population. *Ultrasound Obstet Gynecol* 1998;12:163–169.

54. Economides DL, Whitlow BJ, Kadir R, et al. First trimester sonographic detection of chromosomal abnormalities in an unselected population. *Br J Obstet Gynaecol* 1998;105:58–62.

55. Zoppi MA, Ibba RM, Putzolu M, et al. Assessment of risk for chromosomal abnormalities at 10–14 weeks of gestation by nuchal translucency and maternal age in 5,210 fetuses at a single centre. *Fetal Diagn Ther* 2000;15:170–173.

56. Thilaganathan B, Sairam S, Michailidis G, et al. First trimester nuchal translucency: effective routine screening for Down's syndrome. *Br J Radiol* 1999;72:946–948.

57. Schwarzler P, Carvalho JS, Senat MV, et al. Screening for fetal aneuploidies and fetal cardiac abnormalities by nuchal translucency thickness measurement at 10–14 weeks of gestation as part of routine antenatal care in an unselected population. *Br J Obstet Gynaecol* 1999;106:1029–1034.

58. Theodoropoulkos P, Lolis D, Papageorgiou C, et al. Evaluation of first trimester screening by fetal nuchal translucency and maternal age. *Prenat Diagn* 1998;18:133–137.

59. Sherrod C, Sebire NJ, Nayar R, et al. Prenatal diagnosis of trisomy 18 at the 10–14 week ultrasound scan. *Ultrasound Obstet Gynecol* 1997;10:387–390.

60. Snijders RJM, Sebire NJ, Nayar R, et al. Increased nuchal translucency in trisomy 13 fetuses at 10–14 weeks of gestation. *Am J Med Genet* 1999;86:205–207.

61. Sebire NJ, Snijders RJ, Brown R, et al. Detection of sex chromosome abnormalities by nuchal translucency screening at 10–14 weeks. *Prenat Diagn* 1998;18:581–584.

62. Jauniaux E, Brown R, Snijders RJ, et al. Early prenatal diagnosis of triploidy. *Am J Obstet Gynecol* 1997;176:550–554.

63. Cuckle HS, van Lith JM. Appropriate biochemical parameters in first-trimester screening for Down syndrome. *Prenat Diagn* 1999;19:505–512.

64. Spencer K, Souter V, Tul N, et al. A screening program for trisomy 21 at 10–14 weeks using fetal nuchal translucency, maternal serum free β-human chorionic gonadotropin and pregnancy-associated plasma protein-A. *Ultrasound Obstet Gynecol* 1999;13:231–237.

65. Brizot ML, Snijders RJM, Bersinger NA, et al. Maternal serum pregnancy associated placental protein A and fetal nuchal translucency thickness for the prediction of fetal trisomies in early pregnancy. *Obstet Gynecol* 1994;84:918–922.

66. Brizot ML, Snijders RJM, Butler J, et al. Maternal serum hCG and fetal nuchal translucency thickness for the prediction of fetal trisomies in the first trimester of pregnancy. *Br J Obstet Gynaecol* 1995;102:1227–1232.

67. Orlandi F, Damiani G, Hallahan TW, et al. First-trimester screening for fetal aneuploidy: biochemistry and nuchal translucency. *Ultrasound Obstet Gynecol* 1997;10:381–386.

68. Biagiotti R, Brizzi L, Periti E, et al. First trimester screening for Down's syndrome using maternal serum PAPP-A and free beta-hCG in combination with fetal nuchal translucency thickness. *Br J Obstet Gynecol* 1998;105:917–920.

69. Benattar C, Audibert F, Taieb J, et al. Efficiency of ultrasound and biochemical markers for Down's syndrome risk screening. A prospective study. *Fetal Diagn Ther* 1999; 14:112–117.

70. De Biasio P, Siccardi M, Volpe G, et al. First trimester screening for Down syndrome using nuchal translucency measurement with beta-hCG and PAPP-A between 10 and 13 weeks of pregnancy—the combination test. *Prenat Diagn* 1999;19:360–363.

71. De Graaf IM, Parkrt E, Bilardo CM, et al. Early pregnancy screening for fetal aneuploidy with serum markers and nuchal translucency. *Prenat Diagn* 1999;19:458–462.

72. Krantz DA, Hallahan TW, Orlandi F, et al. First-trimester Down syndrome screening using dried blood biochemistry and nuchal translucency. *Obstet Gynecol* 2000;96:207–213.

73. Tul N, Spencer K, Noble P, et al. Screening for trisomy 18 by fetal nuchal translucency and maternal serum free beta hCG and PAPP-A at 10–14 weeks of gestation. *Prenat Diagn* 1999;19:1035–1042.

74. Spencer K, Ong C, Skentou H, et al. Screening for trisomy 13 by fetal nuchal translucency and maternal serum free beta hCG and PAPP-A at 10–14 weeks of gestation. *Prenat Diagn* 2000;20:411–416.

75. Spencer K, Tul N, Nicolaides KH. Maternal serum free beta hCG and PAPP-A in fetal sex chromosome defects in the first trimester. *Prenat Diagn* 2000;20:390–394.

76. Spencer K, Liao A, Skentou H, et al. Screening for triploidy by fetal nuchal translucency and maternal serum free β-hCG and PAPP-A at 10–14 weeks of gestation. *Prenat Diagn* 2000;20:495–499.

77. Wald NJ, Watt HC, Hackshaw AK. Integrated screening for Down's syndrome based on tests performed during the first and second trimesters. *N Engl J Med* 1999;341:461–467.

78. Copel J, Bahado-Singh RO. Prenatal screening for Down's syndrome—a search for the family's values. *N Engl J Med* 1999;341:521–522.

79. Kadir RA, Economides DL. The effect of nuchal translucency measurement on second trimester biochemical screening for Down's syndrome. *Ultrasound Obstet Gynecol* 1997;9:244–247.

80. Thilaganathan B, Slack A, Wathen NC. Effect of first-trimester nuchal translucency on second-trimester maternal serum biochemical screening for Down's syndrome. *Ultrasound Obstet Gynecol* 1997;10:261–264.

81. Snijders, RJM, Nicolaides, KH. Assessment of risks. In: *Ultrasound markers for fetal chromosomal defects*. Carnforth, UK: Parthenon Publishing, 1996:63–120.

82. Nyberg DA, Luthy DA, Resta RG, et al. Age-adjusted ultrasound risk assessment for fetal Down's syndrome during the second trimester: description of the method and analysis of 142 cases. *Ultrasound Obstet Gynaecol* 1998;12:8–14.

83. Nyberg DA, Souter VL, El-Bastawissi A, et al. Isolated sonographic markers for detection of fetal Down syndrome in the second trimester of pregnancy. *J Ultrasound Med* 2001;20(10):1053–1063.

84. Souka AP, Krampl E, Bakalis S, et al. Outcome of pregnancy in chromosomally normal fetuses with increased nuchal translucency in the first trimester. *Ultrasound Obstet Gynecol* 2001;18(1):9–17.

85. Tegnander E, Eik-Nes SH, Johansen OJ, et al. Prenatal detection of heart defects at the routine fetal examination at 18 weeks in a non-selected population. *Ultrasound Obstet Gynecol* 1995;5:372–380.

86. Gembruch U, Knopfle G, Chatterjee M, et al. First-trimester diagnosis of fetal congenital heart disease by transvaginal two-dimensional and Doppler echocardiography. *Obstet Gynecol* 1990;75:496–498.

87. Bronshtein M, Siegler E, Yoffe N, et al. Prenatal diagnosis of ventricular septal defect and overriding aorta at 14 weeks' gestation, using transvaginal sonography. *Prenat Diagn* 1990;10:697–702.

88. Gembruch U, Knopfle G, Bald R, et al. Early diagnosis of fetal congenital heart disease by transvaginal echocardiography. *Ultrasound Obstet Gynecol* 1993;3:310–317.

89. Achiron R, Rotstein Z, Lipitz S, et al. First-trimester diagnosis of fetal congenital heart disease by transvaginal ultrasonography. *Obstet Gynecol* 1994;84:69–72.

90. Hyett JA, Perdu M, Sharland GK, et al. Using fetal nuchal translucency to screen for major congenital cardiac defects at 10–14 weeks of gestation: population based cohort study. *BMJ* 1999;318:81–85.

91. Zosmer N, Souter VL, Chan CSY, et al. Early diagnosis of major cardiac defects in chromosomally normal fetuses with increased nuchal translucency. *Br J Obstet Gynaecol* 1999;106:829–833.

92. Carvahlo JS, Moscoso G, Ville Y. First trimester transabdominal fetal echocardiography. *Lancet* 1998;351:1023–1027.

93. Sebire NJ, Snijders RJM, Hughes K, et al. Screening for trisomy 21 in twin pregnancies by maternal age and fetal nuchal translucency thickness at 10–14 weeks of gestation. *Br J Obstet Gynaecol* 1996;103:999–1003.

94. Sebire NJ, Hughes K, D'Ercole C, et al. Increased fetal nuchal translucency at 10–14 weeks as a predictor of severe twin-to-twin transfusion syndrome. *Ultrasound Obstet Gynecol* 1997;10:86–89.

95. Percin EF, Guvenal T, Cetin A, et al. First-trimester diagnosis of Robinow syndrome. *Fetal Diagn Ther* 2001;16(5):308–311.

96. Haak MC, Cobben JM, van Vugt JM. First trimester diagnosis of split hand/foot by transvaginal ultrasound. *Fetal Diagn Ther* 2001;16(3):146–149.

97. Souter V, Nyberg D, Siebert JR, Gonzales A, Luthardt F, et al. Upper limb phocomelia associated with increased nuchal translucency in a monochorionic twin pregnancy. *J Ultrasound Med* 2002;21:355–360.

CHROMOSOMAL ABNORMALITIES

This chapter discusses chromosomal abnormalities and sonographic findings of chromosomal abnormalities, primarily during the second trimester. Related chapters discuss first-trimester detection of chromosomal abnormalities via increased nuchal translucency (Chapter 20), biochemical screening for chromosomal abnormalities (Chapter 22), and prenatal diagnostic methods of detecting chromosomal abnormalities and other genetic conditions (Chapter 23). Features of specific chromosomal abnormalities are also discussed in Chapter 5.

CLINICAL PERSPECTIVE

Chromosomal abnormalities are a common phenomenon in human development. The prevalence varies with the age of the population as well as the gestational age at the time of ascertainment. In 1977, Hook and Hamerton[1] published a review of seven cytogenetic studies involving a total of 57,000 newborns and calculated an overall prevalence of chromosomal abnormalities of 0.6%. In a more recent Danish study, 0.8% had a chromosomal abnormality at birth.[2] In a collaborative European study of women undergoing amniocentesis because of advanced maternal age (35 years or older), some type of chromosomal abnormality was found in 2.26%.[3]

The prevalence of chromosomal abnormalities increases dramatically with early gestational age and among nonviable pregnancies. Approximately 25% of morphologic embryos conceived through *in vitro* fertilization are associated with numeric chromosomal abnormalities.[4] Aneuploidy is found in 6% of stillborns and 50% of early spontaneous abortuses. These differences reflect the high mortality rate for major chromosomal abnormalities throughout pregnancy. The greatest loss occurs during the first trimester and then slows, so that the prevalence of trisomy 21 is 30% higher at 12 weeks and 21% higher at 16 weeks than at 40 weeks.[5] The mortality rates for trisomies 18 and 13 are substantially higher.

Types of Chromosomal Abnormalities

The main types of chromosomal abnormalities that present problems in the prenatal period may be categorized as abnormal numbers of chromosomes, abnormal structure, mosaicism, uniparental disomy, and microdeletions (Table 1). In this categorization, we have included both aneuploidy (abnormal numbers of whole chromosomes) and marker chromosomes as abnormal numbers of chromosomes.

A marker chromosome is a supernumerary altered chromosome, usually too small to be characterized on G-banding. It may take the form of a ring chromosome and may be composed of euchromatin, heterochromatic centromeric material, or both. Approximately 80% of markers appear to arise as a *de novo* event.[6] Marker chromosomes are observed in 0.4 to 1.5 per 1,000 prenatal samples, and their incidence increases with increasing maternal age.[7] Most marker chromosomes are found in phenotypically normal individuals, although approximately 13% of prenatally detected markers are associated with physical or cognitive impairment.[8] This risk may be as high as 28% when the marker chromosome is derived from a nonacrocentric chromosome (chromosomes 13, 14, 15, 21, and 22 have the centromere near one end of the chromosome and are thus termed *acrocentric*).[9]

A balanced translocation occurs when material is exchanged between different chromosomes but the exchanged material is otherwise intact. Balanced translocations are usually coincidental findings in normal individuals. However, they may produce unbalanced rearrangements in offspring, resulting in phenotypic anomalies. Also, in the case of *de novo* translocations, it is difficult to know with certainty whether a particular translocation is truly balanced because important alterations may be too small to be visible under the microscope using standard cytogenetic techniques.

Robertsonian translocations are a type of balanced translocation in which effectively all of one chromosome is joined end-to-end with another. These involve the acrocentric chromosomes. Two types (13q14q and 14q21q) of robertsonian translocations are relatively common. The translocation involving 13q and 14q is found in approximately 1 in 1,300

TABLE 1. TYPES OF CHROMOSOMAL ABNORMALITIES PRESENTING PRENATALLY

Abnormalities of number
    Trisomies 21, 13, 18, plus others
    Turner syndrome (45,X)
    Triploidy and tetratriploidy
    Marker chromosomes
Abnormalities of structure
    Deletions
    Translocations
    Inversions
Mosaicism
Uniparental disomy
Submicroscopic rearrangements

TABLE 3. CHROMOSOMAL MICRODELETIONS RESULTING IN RECOGNIZED SYNDROMES

Alagille syndrome (20p12)
Angelman syndrome (15q11-q13)
Beckwith-Wiedemann syndrome (11q15)
Hemoglobin H–related mental retardation (16p13.3)
Langer-Giedion syndrome (8q24.11-q24.13)
Miller-Dieker syndrome (17q13.3)
Prader-Willi syndrome (15q11-q13)
Rubinstein-Taybi syndrome (16p13.3)
Velocardiofacial syndrome (22q11)
WAGR syndrome (Wilms tumor, aniridia, genitourinary abnormalities, mental retardation) (11p13)
Williams syndrome (Williams-Beuren syndrome) (7q11.2)

people and is the single most common chromosome rearrangement in humans. Although a carrier of a robertsonian or balanced translocation is phenotypically normal, offspring may be unbalanced. A robertsonian translocation involving chromosome 21 is at risk for producing a fetus with trisomy 21, resulting in Down syndrome.

Mosaicism occurs when two or more chromosomally different cell lines are present. For example, an individual may have cells in some tissues that have a trisomy, such as trisomy 21, while other cells have a normal chromosomal complement. Mosaicism may or may not be associated with phenotypic abnormalities, depending on the degree of mosaicism and the specific chromosomal abnormality. In this situation, a careful fetal survey with targeted ultrasound may be helpful.

In some cases, mosaicism is confined to extraembryonic cell lines. Confined placental mosaicism results when the mosaic cells affect only the placenta. This is a finding in 1% to 2% of late first-trimester chorionic villus samples.[10] Although this would be expected to result in a phenotypically normal fetus, confined placental mosaicism is associated with fetal anomalies in some cases. In one mechanism, both copies of a particular chromosome may belong to one of the parents [uniparental disomy (UPD)]. This has been explained by a trisomic condition with trisomic "rescue" resulting from early loss of one of the chromosomes.[11]

UPD occurs when an individual inherits two copies of a chromosome from the same parent instead of receiving one chromosome from each parent. This is important because some chromosomes are known to be "imprinted," or to act differently depending on whether they are inherited from the mother or the father. A number of clinical syndromes are now known to be associated with UPD (Table 2). For example, maternal origin of UPD for trisomy 15 may result in Prader-Willi syn-

drome, whereas paternal origin of UPD for chromosome 15 may result in Angelman syndrome. Severe intrauterine growth restriction (IUGR) has also been associated with UPD.

Submicroscopic microdeletions are too small to be visible under the microscope using standard cytogenetic techniques. Some of these alterations may be detected using fluorescent *in situ* hybridization probes that are specific for the affected chromosomal region. A number of so-called microdeletion syndromes have been described in association with submicroscopic chromosomal abnormalities (Table 3). Unbalanced submicroscopic chromosomal rearrangements near the ends or telomeres of the chromosomes have been reported in association[12] with mental retardation and birth defects in children[12] and prenatally diagnosed major fetal structural anomalies.[13]

Although patterns of common chromosomal abnormalities are well recognized, many unique or rare chromosomal abnormalities also occur. The frequency and type of chromosomal abnormalities encountered depend largely on the time of assessment, the population evaluated for structural chromosomal abnormalities, and the banding level at which the cytogenetic evaluation is performed.[14–16] Among newborns with chromosomal abnormalities, approximately one-third have autosomal disorders, one-third have sex chromosomal abnormalities, and one-third have translocations or other rearrangements. In comparison, a prenatal study of women undergoing amniocentesis because of maternal age found that, among fetuses with chromosomal abnormalities, 64% were trisomies (including 51% of trisomy 21), 11% were translocations, 17% were sex chromosomal abnormalities, and 8% were other types.[3] This higher frequency of trisomies can be attributed to both the earlier gestational age and the sampling group, since advanced gestational age is associated with some chromosomal abnormalities but not others.

TABLE 2. CONDITIONS THAT MAY BE CAUSED BY UNIPARENTAL DISOMY

Angelman syndrome (15q11-q13, paternal)
Beckwith-Wiedemann syndrome (11p15.5)
Prader-Willi syndrome (chromosome 15, maternal)
Silver-Russell syndrome (chromosome 7)

Prognosis

Chromosomal abnormalities frequently affect large segments of the genome and, as a result, are often associated with multiple congenital anomalies, a high mortality and morbidity rate, and a poor long-term prognosis. Birth defects are the leading cause of infant mortality in the United States, and 13% of these birth defects are associated with chromosomal abnormalities.[17] However, the prognosis varies greatly with the type of chromosomal abnormality and the type of congenital anomalies present. The life expectancy for Down syndrome has also improved so that for live-born infants, survival rates of approximately 90% at 1 year of life and 80% at 10 years have been reported.[18,19] On the other hand, few infants with trisomy 18 or 13 survive to 5 years of age.

Children with major chromosomal abnormalities are usually mentally impaired. Chromosomal abnormalities that are "cryptic," or too small to be visible using standard karyotyping, are also being recognized as an important cause of mental retardation, particularly in the presence of birth defects, dysmorphic features, and a family history of mental retardation.[20]

The clinical phenotypes associated with the common aneuploidies such as trisomy 13, trisomy 18, trisomy 21, and triploidy are well documented. Many of the other chromosomal abnormalities present more complex problems in terms of the implications for the phenotype and long-term outcome for the baby. When such a chromosomal abnormality is detected, it is important to seek advice from a clinical geneticist and a cytogeneticist as soon as possible, because further studies such as parental karyotyping, fluorescent *in situ* hybridization, spectral karyotyping, or studies for UPD may help refine the diagnosis and thus alter the likely prognosis (see Chapter 23).

Confined placental mosaicism has also been associated with adverse outcome. Trisomy 16 mosaicism may be associated with IUGR in approximately 50% of cases and fetal demise in approximately 20%.[21] Fetal structural defects, including cardiac defects, have also been reported. These complications appear to be related to the proportion of trisomic cells within the placenta and have been reported in cases of trisomy 16 placental mosaicism, with and without UPD for chromosome 16.[21]

Even when discovered later in pregnancy, knowledge of a major chromosomal abnormality may influence other obstetric considerations including the place, time, or mode of delivery. Cesarean delivery generally is considered an unnecessary risk to the mother of an affected fetus, although fetal aneuploidy more often leads to intrapartum fetal distress, resulting in higher rate of cesarean deliveries if unrecognized.[22]

Who Is at Risk?

All pregnancies are at risk of fetal aneuploidy. Additional risk factors include advanced maternal age, a history of fetal aneuploidy, a known balanced translocation or other structural rearrangements in one of the parents, abnormal biochemical screening results, and abnormalities detected on a screening ultrasound.

TABLE 4. AGE-RELATED RISKS FOR TRISOMY 21 AT THE TIME OF SECOND-TRIMESTER AMNIOCENTESIS

Maternal age (yr)	Odds (1 in __)
20	1,176
21	1,160
22	1,136
23	1,114
24	1,087
25	1,040
26	990
27	928
28	855
29	760
30	690
31	597
32	508
33	421
34	342
35	274
36	216
37	168
38	129
39	98
40	74
41	56
42	42
43	31
44	23

Data from Snijders RJ, Sundberg K, Holzgreve W, Henry G, Nicolaides KH. Maternal age- and gestation-specific risk for trisomy 21. *Ultrasound Obstet Gynecol* 1999;13(3):167–170.

Maternal and Paternal Age

Maternal age is positively correlated with various chromosomal abnormalities, including trisomies 18, 13, and 21, XXX, and XXY, but not with 45,X.[4] The specific risk of trisomy 21 at the time of second-trimester amniocentesis varies from 1 in 274 for women 35 years old to 1 in 10 for women 48 years old (Table 4). Some studies[23,24] suggest that a lesser effect may also be true for advancing paternal age, with the incidence in fathers older than 39 years being greater than three times that in fathers under 35 years.

A fundamental shift in birth trends has been observed during the last three decades with more births in women aged 35 years and older as family size has decreased.[25] As a result, the general prevalence of Down syndrome during the second trimester has increased from 1 in 740 in 1974 to 1 in 504 in 1997. The proportion of Down syndrome fetuses at 16 weeks' gestation in women termed *advanced maternal age* (35 to 49 years) increased from 28.5% in 1974 to 47.3% in 1997, whereas live births increased more rapidly from 4.7% to 12.6%.

TABLE 5. COMMON FEATURES OF MAJOR TRISOMIES

	Trisomy 21	Trisomy 18	Trisomy 13
Major features	Cardiac defects, duodenal atresia, cystic hygroma, hydrops	Cardiac defects, spina bifida, cerebellar dysgenesis, micrognathia, diaphragmatic hernia, omphalocele, clenched hands/wrists, radial aplasia, clubfeet, cystic hygroma	Cardiac defects, central nervous system abnormalities, facial anomalies, cleft lip/palate, urogenital anomalies/echogenic kidneys, omphalocele, polydactyly, rocker-bottom feet, cystic hygroma
Markers or subtle findings	Nuchal thickening, hyperechoic bowel, EIF, shortened limbs, pyelectasis, mild ventriculomegaly, widened pelvic angle, shortened frontal lobe, clinodactyly, widened sandal gap, hypoplastic or absent nasal bone	Choroid cysts, brachycephaly, shortened limbs, IUGR, single umbilical artery	EIF, mild ventriculomegaly, pyelectasis, IUGR, single umbilical artery

EIF, echogenic intracardiac focus; IUGR, intrauterine growth restriction.

Previous Chromosomal Abnormality

Women with a previous pregnancy affected by trisomy 21 are generally quoted a recurrence risk of approximately 1% above the maternal age–related risk.[26] The limited published data that is available is based on relatively small numbers of cases. Of 842 Japanese women with a previous pregnancy affected with trisomy 21, 1.2% (ten) had another affected fetus diagnosed on second-trimester amniocentesis.[27] In rare cases, recurrence of trisomy 21 has been reported in association with parental mosaicism for trisomy 21.[28,29] It is also possible that in some instances, mosaicism may be confined to the germ cells and therefore be undetected by routine cytogenetic studies.[30]

Biochemical Screening

Biochemical screening has made a major impact on screening for fetal Down syndrome during the second trimester, whereas maternal age alone has become less important. In Wallonia in South Belgium, prenatal detection of Down syndrome increased from 17% to 56% following introduction of the triple test. The authors estimated that this translated to a decrease in the birth prevalence of Down syndrome from 1 in 794 to 1 in 1,606.[31]

Patients 35 years and older, traditionally considered at risk, have questioned whether they really need to undergo invasive procedures since biochemical and ultrasound screening have dramatically improved the detection rates of fetal Down syndrome.[32–35] In evaluating women 35 years and older, Haddow et al.[34] calculated that biochemical screening (risk threshold of 1 in 200, including maternal age and analytes) could detect 89% (48 of 54) of fetuses with Down syndrome with a 25% false-positive rate. Performing amniocentesis in all women would identify another 11% of affected fetuses with a 75% increase in the false-positive rate. Biochemical screening would also have detected 47% (7 of 15) of other trisomies, 44% (11 of 25) of sex aneuploidies, and 11% (one of nine) of miscellaneous chromosomal abnormalities.

Development of ultrasound screening has also affected patients' perceptions of their need for genetic amniocentesis. Many patients seem to rely on ultrasound, which they can see themselves, compared to biochemical screening.

SONOGRAPHIC FINDINGS OF FETAL ANEUPLOIDY

Ultrasound can frequently detect many abnormalities in fetuses with aneuploidy.[36–42] These may include structural defects, nonstructural findings, or sonographic markers of fetal aneuploidy (SMFA) (Table 5). A major abnormality (e.g., cardiac defect, omphalocele) can be confirmed after birth or at autopsy and carries greater risk for fetal mortality and morbidity. Because chromosomal abnormalities may affect all cells of the body, any organ system may be involved.

Available studies suggest a good correlation between prenatal ultrasound findings and pathologic findings in fetuses with chromosomal abnormalities.[43] The prevalence of various structural abnormalities in fetuses with major chromosomal abnormalities can be estimated from postmortem studies or from clinical findings in live births. However, each of these approaches has inherent biases: Pathologic studies tend to be associated with fetuses with major structural anomalies, which lead to their prenatal detection or intrauterine demise, and live-born infants tend to have fewer major anomalies and hence greater potential to survive to term.

Sonographic findings of fetal aneuploidy were originally limited only to major or structural abnormalities. However, a number of less specific sonographic findings have also been described in association with fetal aneuploidy, especially trisomy 21. These have been termed sonographic *markers*. Unlike structural anomalies, SMFAs are nonspecific, most frequently seen in normal fetuses, often transient, and insignificant in regard to outcome. The most common SMFAs in

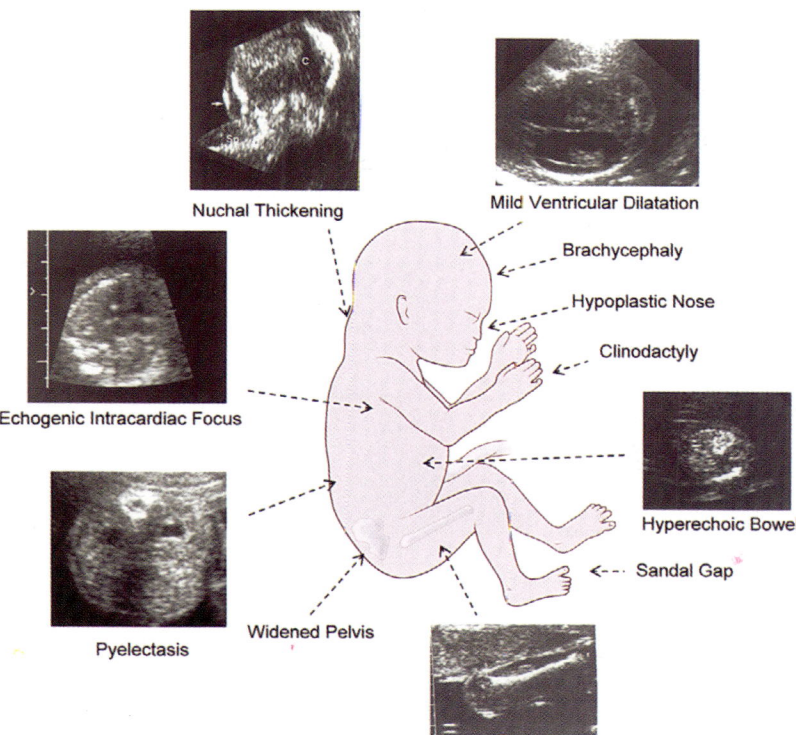

Nuchal Thickening

Mild Ventricular Dilatation

Brachycephaly

Hypoplastic Nose

Clinodactyly

Echogenic Intracardiac Focus

Hyperechoic Bowel

Sandal Gap

Pyelectasis

Widened Pelvis

Shortened Limbs

FIGURE 1. Common sonographic markers of trisomy 21. This does not include major or structural defects such as cardiac defects, cystic hygroma, or duodenal atresia.

the second trimester are nuchal thickening, hyperechoic bowel, shortened extremities, renal pyelectasis, echogenic intracardiac foci (EIF), and choroid plexus cysts (CPCs). In general, the risk of chromosomal abnormality increases as the number of markers present increases. Individual markers are discussed in detail under Sonographic Markers and their use in risk assessment is discussed under Risk Assessment, later in this chapter.

Although the phenotypic expression of major chromosomal abnormalities is highly variable among individuals, certain patterns of anomalies can be recognized. Figures 1 through 3 highlight sonographic markers or subtle abnormalities for trisomies 21, 18, and 13, respectively, and Figures 4 and 5 summarize typical features of Turner syndrome and triploidy, respectively. Table 5 summarizes the common structural anomalies and sonographic markers associated with the three common trisomic conditions (i.e., trisomies 13, 18, and 21). Tables 6 through 9 summarize sonographic findings in fetuses with trisomies 13, 18, and 21 and triploidy from selected papers. Specific pathologic and sonographic features of each of these conditions are also discussed in Chapter 5.

The type and frequency of ultrasound findings vary with gestational age. Reasons for referral, criteria for a positive scan, and the quality of ultrasound also affect reported detection rates. Major or structural abnormalities are seen

in fewer than an estimated 20% of fetuses with trisomy 21 (excluding ventriculomegaly, which probably should be considered a marker) during the second trimester, compared to the majority of fetuses with trisomies 18 and 13. Combined with SMFAs, sonographic findings are identified in 50% to 70% of fetuses with Down syndrome, 80% of fetuses with trisomy 18, and 90% of fetuses with trisomy 13. These findings emphasize the potential importance of nonstructural markers in the detection of fetal trisomy.

Positive ultrasound findings increase the risk of fetal aneuploidy, whereas a normal ultrasound reduces the risk. The degree to which the risk is increased or decreased depends on a variety of factors including the type of chromosomal abnormality, gestational age at the time of ultrasound, criteria for a positive scan, and the quality of ultrasound. Although high sensitivies of detection have been reported for trisomic conditions, low detection rates can be expected from less experienced sonographers of low-risk populations.[44]

Almost any congenital anomaly increases the risk of an underlying chromosomal abnormality with the exception of "acquired" disorders resulting from tissue or vascular disruption. Examples include tumors, hydranencephaly, amniotic band syndrome, limb-body wall complex, tumors, jejunoileal atresia caused by vascular insufficiency, and gastroschisis. Other complex types of anomalies, such as the

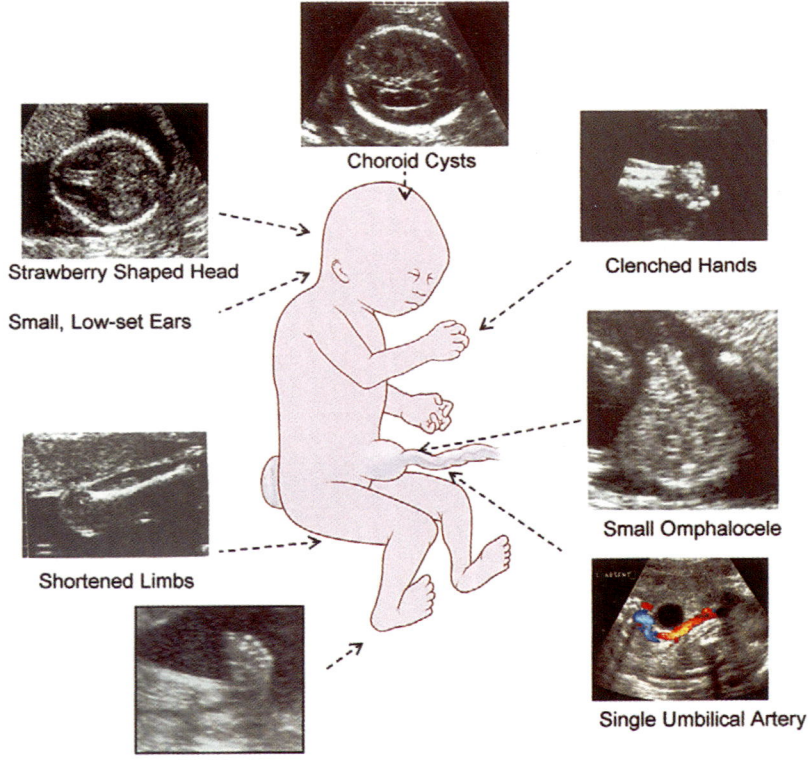

FIGURE 2. Sonographic markers or subtle abnormalities of trisomy 18. This does not include major abnormalities such as cardiac defects, cystic hygroma, radial aplasia, spina bifida, esophageal atresia, or cerebellar anomalies.

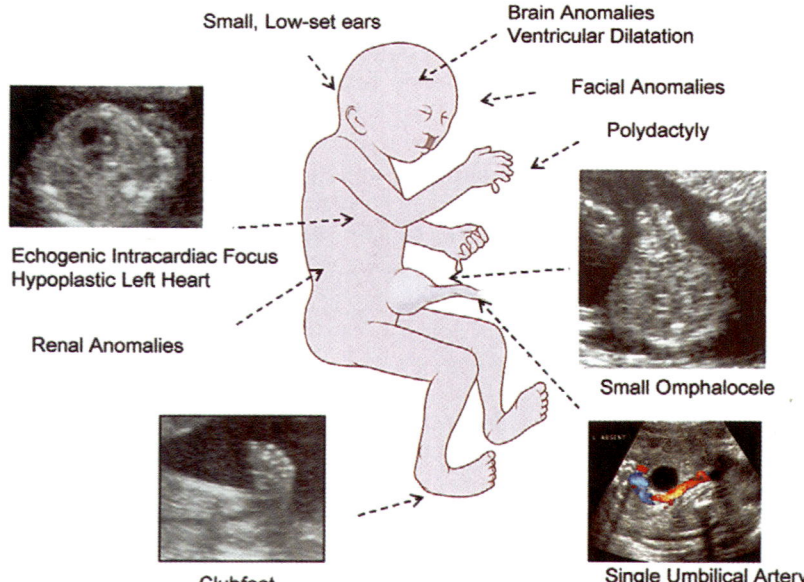

FIGURE 3. Sonographic markers or subtle abnormalities of trisomy 13. This does not include major abnormalities such as holoprosencephaly, cleft lip/palate, cardiac defects, and renal anomalies.

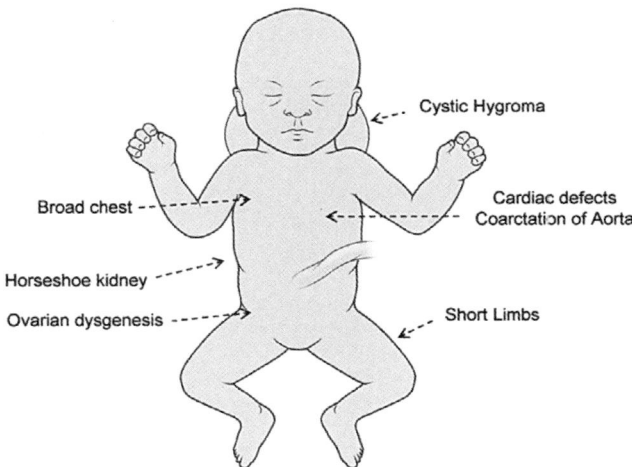

FIGURE 4. Common abnormalities of Turner syndrome.

FIGURE 5. Common abnormalities of triploidy. IUGR, intrauterine growth restriction.

cardiosplenic syndromes, are also universally associated with a normal fetal karyotype for unknown reasons.

Structural Abnormalities

In the following sections, we discuss specific structural or major abnormalities and the association with fetal aneuploidy. When interpreting reported estimates, it should be noted that the frequency of aneuploidy may be underestimated when based on the total number of fetuses with a given malformation because not all fetuses undergo chromosome analysis; the risk may be overestimated when based only on fetuses with known karyotype, because invasive testing is more likely to be requested in higher-risk women or in the setting of additional anomalies.

TABLE 6. PREVALENCE (AS A PERCENTAGE OF ALL CASES) OF SOME OF THE COMMON PRENATAL ULTRASOUND FINDINGS IN FOUR STUDIES OF FETUSES WITH TRISOMY 13

	Nicolaides et al.[40]	Lehman et al.[253]		De Vigan et al.[a]	Tongsong et al.[b]	Combined data[c]
Fetuses (N)	31	18	15	85	15	164
Gestational age (wk)	15–44	12–20	20–32	All ages	16–22	—
Holoprosencephaly	35	22	60	18	47	28
Hypotelorism/cyclopia	—	28	47	—	40	40
Proboscis	—	—	—	—	27	27
Facial cleft	48	17	60	18	33	29
Abnormal extremities	68	17	53	—	40	48
Cardiac defect	45	44	53	20	33	32
Urinary tract anomalies	65	22	47	14	27	29
Ventriculomegaly	10	11	7	3	20	7
Abdominal wall defect	23	17	13	3	13	6
Abnormal posterior fossa	19	11	20	—	7	14
Intrauterine growth restriction	48	22	80	—	27	44
Echogenic intracardiac foci	—	39	20	—	20	27
Nuchal translucency/cystic hygroma	23	33	7	11	7	15
Hyperechoic bowel	—	11	0	—	—	6
Single umbilical artery	—	6	47	—	13	21
≥1 structural abnormality	100	91		68	93	81.1

[a]De Vigan C, Baena N, Cariati E, Clementi M, Stoll C. Contribution of ultrasonographic examination to the prenatal detection of chromosomal abnormalities in 19 centres across Europe. *Ann Genet* 2001;44:209–217.
[b]Tongsong T, Sirichotiyakul S, Wanapirak C, Chanprapah P. Sonographic features of trisomy 13 at midpregnancy. *Int J Gynecol Obstet* 2002;76:143–148.
[c]Combined data consider only those studies reporting that feature.

TABLE 7. PREVALENCE (AS A PERCENTAGE OF ALL CASES) OF SOME OF THE COMMON PRENATAL ULTRASOUND FINDINGS IN FOUR STUDIES OF FETUSES WITH TRISOMY 18 IN THE SECOND TRIMESTER (14 TO 24 WEEKS OF GESTATION)

	Nyberg et al.[a]	Shields et al.[160]	DeVore[b]	Brumfield et al.[189]	Combined data[c]
Fetuses (N)	29	35	30	30	124
Intrauterine growth restriction	28	29	—	10	22
Polyhydramnios	3	9	3	7	6
Choroid plexus cysts	38	43	53	30	41
Nuchal translucency/cystic hygroma	31	17	17	13	19
Clenched hands	17	46	3	10	20
Abnormal feet	21	—	—	—	21
Abdominal wall defect	17	14	—	10	14
Cardiac defect	14	37	80	13	30
Myelomeningocele	14	9	—	—	11
Strawberry-shaped head	14	34	—	3	18
Posterior fossa abnormality	3	3	—	—	3
Cleft lip/palate	3	—	3	—	3
Urinary tract anomalies	17	9	—	7	11
Single umbilical artery	10	40	7	3	16
≥1 ultrasound finding	72	86	97	70	81.6

[a]Nyberg DA, Kramer D, Resta RG, Kapur R, Mahony BS, et al. Prenatal sonographic findings of trisomy 18: review of 47 cases. *J Ultrasound* 1993;12:103–113.
[b]DeVore GR. Second trimester ultrasonography may identify 77% to 97% of fetuses with trisomy 18. *J Ultrasound Med* 2000;19:565–576.
[c]Combined data consider only those studies reporting that feature.

TABLE 8. SUMMARY OF SOME STUDIES USING SECOND-TRIMESTER ULTRASOUND IN TRISOMY 21 SCREENING

Study	Total (N)	Trisomy 21 (N)	Criteria	Gestational age, wk (mean)	Sensitivity (%)	False-positive rate (%)	Likelihood ratio positive[a]	Likelihood ratio normal[b]
Benacerraf et al.[c]	106 controls	45	Ultrasound	14–21	73	4	18.3	0.28
DeVore and Alfi[323]	1,028	15	Ultrasound + fetal echocardiography with color Doppler	(17.4)	87	7.4	11.8	0.14
Nadel et al.[d]	694 controls	71	Ultrasound	14–21	80	4	20	0.2
Bahado-Singh et al.[241]	4,079	40	Ultrasound	15–24 (17.3)	70.6	14	5	0.34
Bromley et al.[318]	177 controls	53	—	—	75	5.7	13.1	0.27
Bahado-Singh et al.[325]	3,278	24	Ultrasound	15–24 (16.7)	60	4.5	13.3	0.41
Nyberg et al.[e]	930 controls	142	Ultrasound + age (AAURA)	14–21 (16.8)	74	14.7	5	0.3
Deren et al.[f]	3,838	44	Ultrasound	15–24	63	12.8	4.9	0.42
Verdin and Economides[322]	459	11	Ultrasound	14–24 (17)	81.8	9.8	8.3	0.2
Vintzileos et al.[g]	1,835	34	Ultrasound	15–24 (19.2)	82	13	6.3	0.2
Sohl et al.[202]	2,743	55	Ultrasound	14–24 (17.3)	67.3	19.4	3.5	0.41
Vergani et al.[h]	920	22	Ultrasound	14–22 (17)	59.2	5.3	11.1	0.43

[a]Likelihood ratio of positive scan = sensitivity/false-positive rate.
[b]Likelihood ratio of normal scan = false-negative rate/specificity.
[c]Benacerraf BR, Nadel AS, Bromley B. Identification of second-trimester fetuses with autosomal trisomy by use of a sonographic scoring index. *Radiology* 1994;193:135–140.
[d]Nadel AS, Bromley B, Frigoletto FD Jr, Benacerraf BR. Can the presumed risk of autosomal trisomy be decreased in fetuses of older women following a normal sonogram? *J Ultrasound Med* 1995;14(4):297–302.
[e]Nyberg DA, Luthy DA, Resta RG, Nyberg BC, Williams MA. Age-adjusted ultrasound risk assessment for fetal Down's syndrome during the second trimester: description of the method and analysis of 142 cases. *Ultrasound Obstet Gynecol* 1998;12:8–14.
[f]Deren O, Mahoney MJ, Copel JA, Bahado-Singh RO. Subtle ultrasonographic anomalies: Do they improve the Down syndrome detection rate? *Am J Obstet Gynecol* 1998;178(3):441–445.
[g]Vintzileos AM, Guzman ER, Smulian JC, Day-Salvatore DL, Knuppel RA. Indication-specific accuracy of second-trimester genetic ultrasonography for the detection of trisomy 21. *Am J Obstet Gynecol* 1999;181(5 Pt 1):1045–1048.
[h]Vergani P, Locatelli A, Piccoli MG, Ceruti P, Mariani E, et al. Best second trimester sonographic markers for the detection of trisomy 21. *J Ultrasound Med* 1999;18:469–473.

TABLE 9. FREQUENTLY REPORTED FINDINGS ON ULTRASOUND EXAMINATION OF FETUSES WITH TRIPLOIDY

	Jauniaux et al.[a]	Rijhsinghani et al.[b]	Mittal et al.[c]	De Vigan et al.[d]	Combined data
Fetuses (N)	70	17	20	44	151
Mean gestation (range) in weeks	20 (13–29)	—	20 (14–25)	—	—
Increased nuchal fold thickness/cystic hygroma	11%	0	5%	7%	9%
Holoprosencephaly	3%	0	0	4%	3%
Ventriculomegaly	34%	23%	25%	21%	23%
Facial cleft	1%	0	0	2%	1%
Micrognathia	24%	—	—	—	24%
Abnormal upper limbs	49%	—	0	—	38%
Clubfeet	7%	—	5%	—	7%
Abdominal wall defect	6%	12%	0	4%	5%
Cardiac defect	31%	6%	5%	11%	20%
Enlarged placenta	—	41%	55%	—	49%
Structural abnormality	93%	71%	80%	—	87%
Central nervous system abnormality	29%	41%	45%	30%	35%
Urinary tract anomalies	11%	23%	15%	7%	13%
Myelomeningocele	7%	0	25%	—	9%
Posterior fossa abnormality	7%	12%	0	—	7%
Intrauterine growth restriction	—	71%	55%	32%	44%
Oligohydramnios	44%	59%	60%	—	50%
Maternal ovarian luteal cysts	9%	—	15%	—	10%
≥1 structural abnormality	100%	94%	85%	79%	91.4%

[a]Jauniaux E, Brown R, Rodeck C, Nicolaides KH. Prenatal diagnosis of triploidy during the second trimester of pregnancy. *Obstet Gynecol* 1996;88(6):983–989.
[b]Rijhsinghani A, Yankowitz J, Strauss RA, Kuller JA, Shivanand P, Williamson RA. Risk of preeclampsia in second-trimester triploid pregnancies. *Obstet Gynecol* 1997;90(6):884–888.
[c]Mittal TK, Vuhanic GM, Morrissey BM, Jones A. Triploidy: antenatal sonographic features with post mortem correlation. *Prenat Diagn* 1998;18:1253–1262.
[d]De Vigan C, Baena N, Cariati E, Clementi M, Stoll C. Contribution of ultrasonographic examination to the prenatal detection of chromosomal abnormalities in 19 centres across Europe. *Ann Genet* 2001;44:209–217.

Central Nervous System Anomalies

Holoprosencephaly

An underlying chromosomal abnormality may be identified in as many as 40% to 60% of fetuses with alobar or semilobar holoprosencephaly (Fig. 6). In one series of 68 cases of holoprosencephaly,[45] 38% were associated with a chromosomal abnormality of which 75% were trisomy 13. Additional nonfacial abnormalities were present in all of the cases with aneuploidy. Of the euploid group, 90% had facial abnormalities and 70% had other abnormalities. The overall prevalence of holoprosencephaly in second-trimester pregnancies was approximately 1 in 8,000.

Trisomy 13 or a variant of trisomy 13 is the most common chromosomal abnormality associated with holoprosencephaly, representing approximately one-half of the cases of aneuploidy. A wide variety of other chromosome disorders have also been associated with holoprosencephaly including trisomy 18, triploidy, 5p+, 13q–, 18p–, and various other karyotypes.[46–48] An underlying chromosomal abnormality carries little recurrence risk, whereas a normal karyotype is more likely to be associated with various inheritable syndromes that may also be expressed as holoprosencephaly.

The presence of facial malformations appears to increase the risk of an underlying chromosomal abnormality in fetuses with holoprosencephaly.[49] In our experience, other extrafacial anomalies, notably omphalocele or renal cystic dysplasia, are strongly predictive of a chromosomal abnormality.

Dandy-Walker Malformation/Cerebellar Hypoplasia

The classic form of Dandy-Walker malformation (DWM) is only the most severe form in a spectrum of abnormalities that may affect the cerebellum. Other abnormalities of the cerebellum include cerebellar hypoplasia and incomplete vermian agenesis, commonly known as *Dandy-Walker variant* (DWV). DWM is recognized as a nonspecific anomaly with a diversity of causes.[50,51] Inheritable syndromes that may express DWM include the Ellis-van Creveld syndrome and the Meckel-Gruber syndrome. Cerebellar abnormalities, including cerebellar hypoplasia or DWM, have also been associated with various chromosomal abnormalities, primarily trisomies 18 and 13.[52–54]

Prenatal detection of cerebellar abnormalities carries a high risk for associated anomalies and aneuploidy.[55] Trisomy 18 is most common (see Fig. 38 in Chapter 5), but other aneuploidies may also be seen with abnormalities of the cerebellum and cerebellar vermis (Figs. 7 and 8). Subtelomeric rearrangements have also been observed in association with brain anomalies including hypoplastic cerebellum and

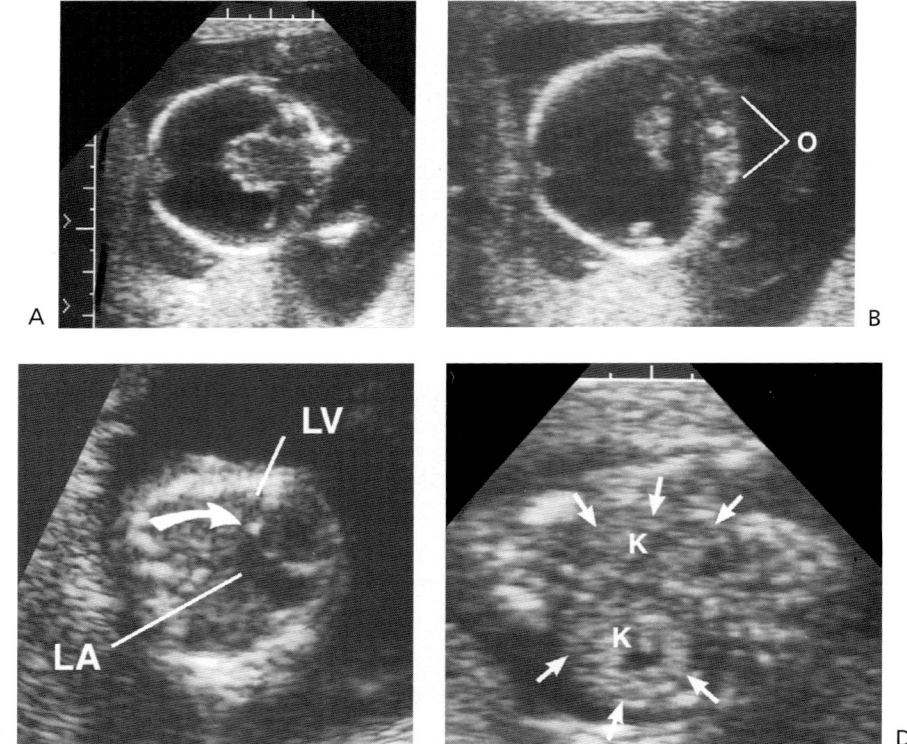

FIGURE 6. Alobar holoprosencephaly and trisomy 13 at 17 weeks. **A:** A transverse view of the head shows alobar holoprosencephaly with a single monoventricle and fused central thalami. **B:** A slightly lower axial view shows microphthalmos and hypotelorism. O, orbits. **C:** A transverse view of the heart shows echogenic intracardiac focus (*arrow*) and cardiac defect with hypoplastic left ventricle (*LV*) and atrium (*LA*). **D:** A longitudinal view shows echogenic kidneys (*arrows; K*) consistent with renal dysplasia.

hydrocephalus (Fig. 8). DWV appears to be more strongly associated with chromosomal abnormalities than the classic DWM, as first suggested by Nyberg et al.,[56,57] even though it is a more subtle abnormality. In one study, Chang et al.[58] found chromosomal abnormalities in 53% (17 of 32) fetuses with DWV compared to 32% (6 of 19) of those with DWM, among those tested. Others have found a high rate of aneuploidy among both groups,[59] although results vary with the criteria of each condition. The risk of chromosomal abnormality may also be higher among fetuses with DWM detected at an early gestational age.[60]

Cerebellar hypoplasia, with enlargement of the cisterna magna, is also associated with aneuploidy in some cases (Fig. 9). Although most commonly observed in normal fetuses, enlargement of the cisterna magna may be a clue to aneuploidy, especially trisomy 18. This is most commonly visualized during the third trimester[61] and is less likely during the second trimester.[62,63] When observed with trisomy 18 during the third trimester, other sonographic findings may include polyhydramnios and IUGR (see sections on Polyhydramnios and Intrauterine Growth Restriction, later in this chapter). In a selected population of fetuses with vermian agenesis or enlarged cisterna magna, Nyberg et al. reported 18 (55%) with a chromosomal abnormality, including trisomy 18 or trisomy 18 variant (12), trisomy 13 (three), Turner syndrome (one), or other rearrangements (two).[57] The presence of associated anomalies and absence of ventricular dilatation correlated most strongly with a chromosomal abnormality. On the other hand, the presence of an enlarged cisterna magna alone, especially after 26 weeks, and in the absence of other structural defects is usually associated with normal outcome and karyotype.[64] Among normal fetuses, enlargement of the cisterna magna may be more common among males.[65] It is our anecdotal observation that many of these fetuses are large, or have disproportionately larger cranial measurements, or both.

Hydrocephalus and Spina Bifida

Hydrocephalus and spina bifida, alone and together, have been associated with various chromosomal abnormalities, primarily trisomies 18 and 13 and triploidy.[66–70] Mild or borderline cerebral ventricular dilatation has also been associated with trisomy 21. Because this finding is not specific,

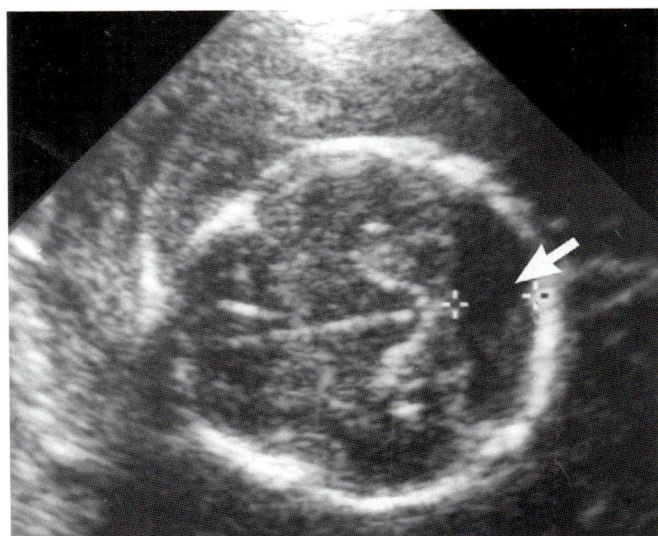

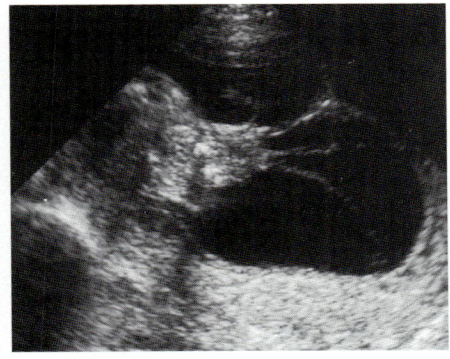

FIGURE 7. Dandy-Walker variant at 18 weeks. **A:** A transverse view of the head shows abnormal fluid in the posterior fossa (*arrow*) with hypoplastic cerebellum and vermis. **B:** A transverse view of the posterior neck shows a massive cystic hygroma with multiple internal septations, including midline septation. The cystic hygroma filled much of the amniotic cavity. Chromosome analysis yielded Turner syndrome (monosomy X).

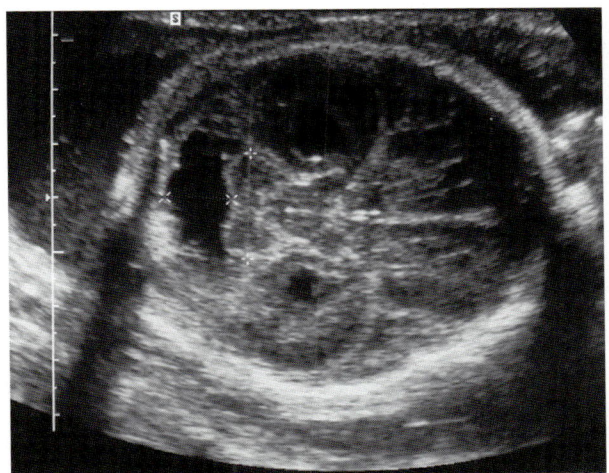

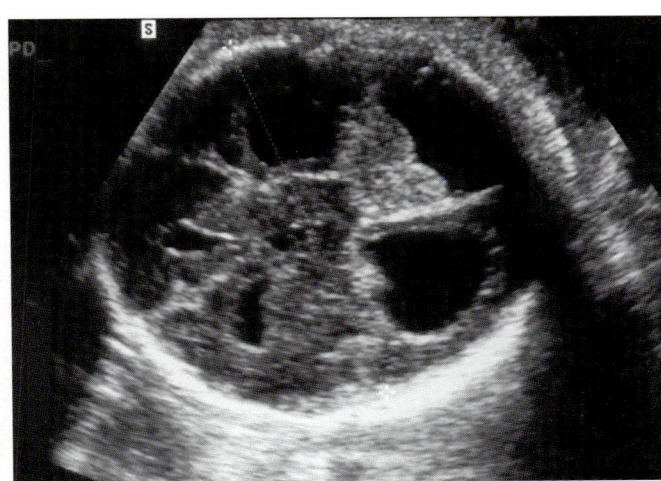

FIGURE 8. Brain abnormalities and microdeletion. **A:** Ultrasound examination at 25 weeks of gestation shows a hypoplastic cerebellum and an enlarged cisterna magna (12 mm anterior-posterior). **B:** Ultrasound examination at 32 weeks shows a hypoplastic cerebellum and hydrocephalus. **C:** Fluorescent *in situ* hybridization analysis showed unbalanced, half cryptic, subtelomeric chromosomal rearrangement resulting in monosomy for the distal long arm of chromosome 6 and trisomy for the distal short arm of chromosome 17. Hybridization of a metaphase cell to a probe for the distal end of the short arm of chromosome 17 (TelVysion 17p, Vysis, Inc., Downers Grove, IL) shows the presence of a yellow signal on the long arm of the derivative chromosome 6 [der(6)] and on both normal chromosomes 17. A control probe for the centromere of chromosome 6 (pink signal) is present on both chromosome 6 homologues. (Part **C** courtesy of C. Disteche, Genetics Department, University of Washington Medical Center, Seattle, WA.)

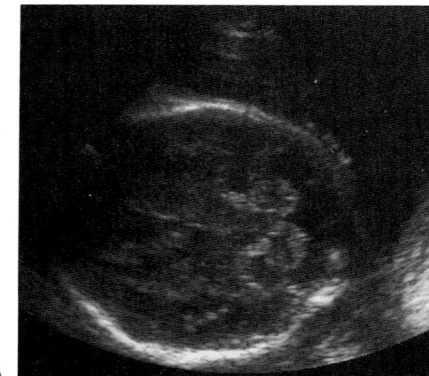
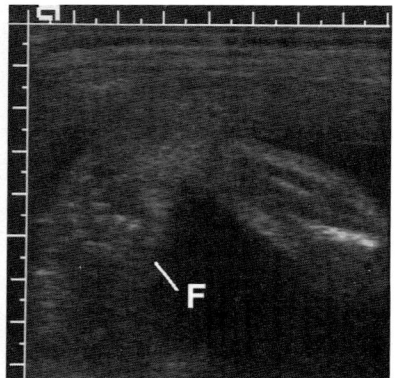

FIGURE 9. Cerebellar hypoplasia and trisomy 18. **A:** A scan at 35 weeks in a fetus shows enlarged cisterna magna and cerebellar hypoplasia. **B:** Clubfoot is shown. The fetus also showed signs of intrauterine growth restriction. F, foot.

however, it is discussed in its own section under Sonographic Markers, later in this chapter.

The precise risk of a chromosomal abnormality undoubtedly varies with the specific malformation present. In a review of 107 fetuses with central nervous system anomalies, chromosomal abnormalities were found in 3% (1 of 30) of fetuses with hydrocephalus, 8% (3 of 38) of fetuses with hydrocephalus and spina bifida, and 33% (three of nine) of fetuses with spina bifida alone.[67] Considering only fetuses who underwent chromosome analysis, these figures are 8%, 15%, and 50%, respectively. Fetal karyotyping is recommended after the sonographic diagnosis of spina bifida if the pregnancy is continued. Babcook et al.[71] evaluated 63 fetuses with spina bifida at a referral center, and aneuploidy was found in 14% (17% of those tested). Karyotype abnormalities included trisomy 18, trisomy 13, triploidy, and translocation. Twenty-two percent of chromosomally abnormal fetuses had no other sonographic anomaly.

Agenesis of the Corpus Callosum

Agenesis of the corpus callosum has been associated with a variety of chromosomal abnormalities including trisomies 8, 11, 13, 14, 15, and 18; triploidy; and translocations.[72] However, the frequency of chromosomal abnormalities remains uncertain due to the small number of cases reported *in utero*.[73,74] Gupta and Lilford[75] reviewed 70 cases of prenatally detected agenesis of the corpus callosum reported in the literature. Of these, 10% were associated with a chromosomal abnormality. Goodyear et al.[76] reviewed 14 prenatally diagnosed and 61 postnatally diagnosed cases of agenesis of the corpus callosum. Chromosomal abnormalities were present in 4.0% of postnatal cases, 8.0% of prenatally diagnosed cases, and 9.3% of cases overall. Prenatal detection of agenesis of the corpus callosum is very difficult before 22 weeks' gestation.[77]

Facial Abnormalities

Cleft Lip/Palate

Cleft lip/palate has been associated with chromosomal abnormalities (trisomies 13 and 18), particularly when central nervous system disorders or other malformations also are present[78–82] (Figs. 10 and 11). Nyberg et al.[83] correlated ultrasound classification of cleft lip/palate with outcome in 65 fetuses diagnosed with cleft by prenatal sonography. Chromosomal abnormalities varied with the type of cleft as follows: cleft lip alone, 0; unilateral cleft lip and palate, 20%; bilateral cleft lip and palate, 30%; median cleft, 52%; and slash type of defect, 0. Similarly, Berge et al.[84] reported aneuploidy in none of three fetuses with unilateral cleft lip, 32% (8 of 25) with unilateral cleft lip and palate, 59% (17 of 29) with bilateral cleft lip and palate, and 82% (9 of 11) with median cleft lip and palate.

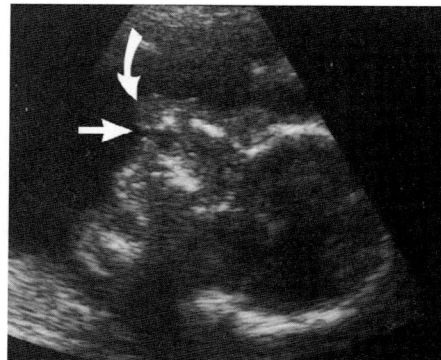

FIGURE 10. Cleft lip and palate, trisomy 13. A parasagittal view of the face shows cleft (*straight arrow*) and premaxillary protrusion (*curved arrow*), suggesting that this represents bilateral cleft lip and palate. Hypotelorism, microphthalmos, and major cardiac defect were also identified. The brain appeared normal, however. Chromosome analysis revealed trisomy 13.

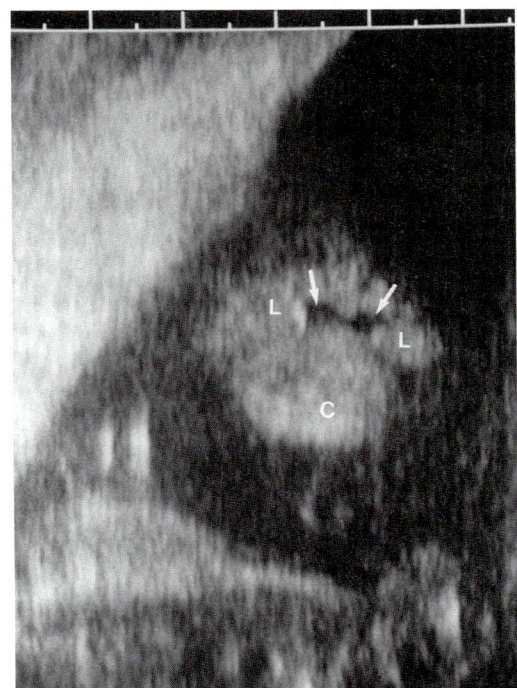

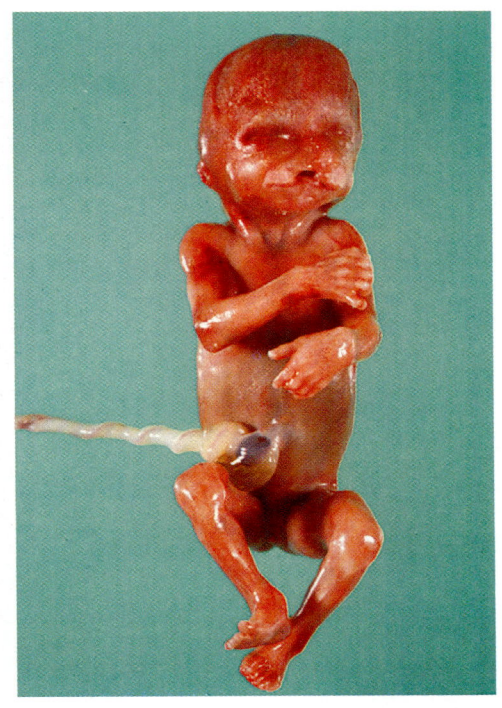

FIGURE 11. Median cleft lip/palate and trisomy 13. **A:** A coronal view shows large midline cleft (*arrows*) of the upper lip (*L*) and palate. Note nonvisualization of the nose, consistent with hypoplastic midface. C, chin. **B:** Postmortem photograph showing median cleft lip.

Prenatal detection of cleft lip/palate is clearly improving for less severe types. This would be expected to lower the reported risk of aneuploidy because less severe types of clefts are less likely to be associated with fetal aneuploidy.[85] Cleft lip alone carries a low risk of aneuploidy and may not always require fetal karyotyping. However, because it is sometimes difficult to distinguish cleft lip alone from cleft lip/palate, it may be prudent to offer genetic amniocentesis for all patients with fetal cleft lip and/or palate. Walker et al.[86] reported aneuploidy among one of 84 (1.2%) infants with cleft lip alone (unilateral or bilateral), 5 of 112 (4.5%) with unilateral cleft lip and palate, and 9 of 67 (13.4%) with bilateral cleft lip and palate.

Ocular Abnormalities

A variety of ocular abnormalities, including cyclopia, hypotelorism, and hypertelorism, may be associated with chromosomal abnormalities. When seen in association with other malformations, particularly holoprosencephaly, ocular abnormalities carry a high risk of aneuploidy.

Other Craniofacial Abnormalities

Facial abnormalities are commonly observed on visual inspection of fetuses or infants with aneuploidy. Micrognathia is present in the majority of fetuses with triploidy or trisomy 18.[87] A facial profile may demonstrate other cranial abnormalities such as a prominent occiput, which is frequently found in fetuses with trisomy 18.

Small, deformed ears have also been associated with chromosome disorders including trisomies 13, 18, and 21.[88] Among newborns, Aase et al.[89] found that, other than hypotonia, short ear length was the most consistent clinical feature suggestive of Down syndrome. Several ultrasound studies have also evaluated the value of measuring ear length in detection of fetal abnormalities.[90–93] In the largest prenatal ultrasound study, Chitkara et al.[94] were able to measure ear lengths in 1,311 of 1,848 (71%) fetuses. Of 34 fetuses with significant chromosomal abnormalities, 11 (32%) had short ear length, and in six of these cases, short ear length was the only detectable abnormality. These included three fetuses with trisomy 21, one fetus with triploidy, and two with other chromosomal abnormality. Overall, shortened ear length was identified in five of 19 (26%) fetuses with trisomy 21 and in three of four (75%) fetuses with trisomy 18. Shimizu et al.[95] also found that short ear length had predictive value similar to that of nuchal thickening in detection of fetal aneuploidy. Despite these encouraging data, ear abnormalities remain difficult to detect, particularly as part of a routine fetal screen during the second trimester. Including it may be useful in patients considered at particularly high risk for fetal aneuploidy. Use of three-dimensional ultrasound may further improve assessment of ear abnormalities.[96]

Nasal abnormalities have also been associated with aneuploidy.[97,98] In the first trimester, sonographic absence of the nasal bone may identify patients at risk for fetal Down syndrome.[99,100] Cicero et al.[99] reported sonographic "absence" of the nasal bone, corresponding to delayed nasal development, in 43 of 59 (72.9%) trisomy 21 fetuses compared to only three of 603 (0.5%) chromosomally normal fetuses at 11 to 14 weeks. Absence or hypoplasia of the nasal bone may also be a useful marker for trisomy 21 after the first trimester. In a postmortem radiographic study, Stempfle et al.[101] found that ossification of the nasal bones was absent in one-fourth of trisomic fetuses, regardless of gestational age.

Cystic Hygroma

Cystic hygromas are often associated with fetal aneuploidy. However, the frequency of aneuploidy varies with gestational age, the appearance, the presence of hydrops and other anomalies, and probably the size of the cystic hygroma. Large cystic hygromas, typically seen during the second trimester (after 14 weeks), also tend to have characteristic septations. When fetal cells are successfully cultured in the second trimester, approximately 75% are associated with a chromosomal abnormality, and Turner syndrome (45,X) accounts for 80% of these.[102–104] Trisomies 18, 13, and 21 are also encountered. A variety of other karyotypic abnormalities have been associated with cystic hygromas including 13q–, 18p–, and triploidy. Of fetuses with normal karyotypes, 46,XX is approximately twice as common as 46,XY.

For cystic hygroma seen during the first trimester, the rate of aneuploidy appears to be lower and the proportion of trisomy 21 and other karyotypic abnormalities is higher. Ville et al.[105] found chromosomal abnormalities in 29%, including trisomy 18 (38%), trisomy 21 (31%), Turner syndrome (25%), and 47,XXX (6%). Malone et al.[106] reported 61 fetuses with cystic hygroma from 20,645 (1 in 338) nonselected patients at 10 to 14 weeks. Karyotype evaluation was performed in 46 cases, and 24 (39% of total) were found to have aneuploidy, including nine with trisomy 21, seven with Turner syndrome, three with trisomy 18, three with triploidy, and two with trisomy 13. Sixteen (26%) fetuses had a good outcome.

Based on available data, chromosome analysis is recommended whenever a cervical cystic hygroma is identified prenatally. Isolated cystic hygromas in an atypical location (noncervical) also do not appear to carry a significant risk of a chromosomal abnormality.

Nonimmune Hydrops

Nonimmune hydrops fetalis, characterized by generalized skin edema, ascites, and pericardial and pleural effusions, is a nonspecific endpoint resulting from a variety of fetal and maternal disorders.[107] Fetuses with nonimmune hydrops should be distinguished from those who also demonstrate cystic hygromas, since the latter group has a higher frequency of chromosomal abnormalities.

Hydrothorax and Ascites

Fetal hydrothorax (pleural effusion, chylothorax) has been associated with various outcomes including chromosomal abnormalities. Chromosomal abnormalities reported include 45,X (Turner syndrome), trisomy 21, and trisomy 13.[108,109] In a review of 82 cases of apparently isolated fetal pleural effusion reported in the literature, Hagay et al.[109] observed trisomy 21 in 4.9% and cardiac defects in another 4.9%. Perinatal mortality was high (36%) and was related to the development of nonimmune hydrops, prematurity, and pulmonary hypoplasia, indicating that pleural effusion may precede generalized hydrops. Because hydrothorax carries a significant risk of aneuploidy, chromosome analysis is encouraged whenever hydrothorax is identified prenatally, particularly when intrauterine drainage of the hydrothorax or other surgical procedure is considered.[110,111]

Ascites may also be seen without generalized hydrops and may have a variable outcome. Zelop and Benacerraf[112] evaluated 18 fetuses with ascites but without hydrops. One fetus proved to have trisomy 21. Other outcomes included intrauterine infections (in four), gastrointestinal processes (seven), genitourinary tract abnormalities (two), and "idiopathic" (four). The authors concluded that chromosomal abnormalities and infection should be considered when ascites is detected without hydrops.

Cardiovascular Malformations

Cardiovascular malformations are found in greater than 90% of fetuses with trisomy 18 and 13, 40% to 50% of fetuses with trisomy 21, and 15% to 20% of those with Turner syndrome.[113] Hence, the presence of a cardiac malformation (Figs. 12 and 13) significantly increases the risk of an underlying chromosomal abnormality.[114–118] Ferencz et al.[117] reported chromosome disorders in 13% of 2,103 live-born infants with a cardiovascular malformation, compared to only 0.1% of infants without a cardiovascular malformation. A much greater frequency of chromosomal abnormalities (22% to 32%) has been observed in fetuses with a sonographically detectable cardiac defect compared to postnatal studies.[119–121] The type of chromosomal abnormalities also differs: Trisomy 21 accounted for nearly 78% of chromosomal abnormalities reported by Ferencz et al.,[117] whereas a greater proportion of other major chromosomal abnormalities (trisomies 18 and 13) has been reported from prenatal studies.

Factors contributing to the frequency of aneuploidy include gestational age, indication for the sonogram, accuracy of ultrasound, and the type of cardiac defect. The risk of aneuploidy is much higher for atrioventricular septal defect (endocardial cushion defect), double-outlet right

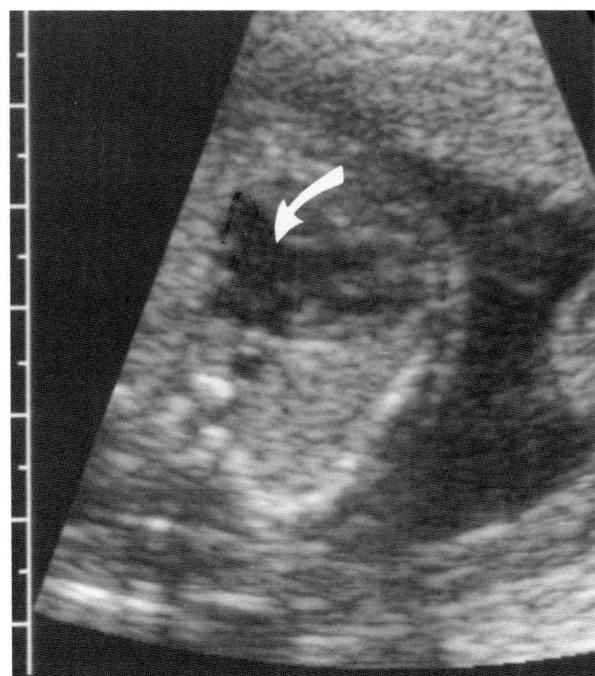

FIGURE 12. Atrioventricular septal defect and trisomy 21. An axial view of the heart at 18 weeks shows central atrioventricular septal defect (*arrow*) with common atrium.

isomerism, transposition of the great arteries, and pulmonary atresia or stenosis had normal chromosomes.

Atrioventricular septal defect (Fig. 12) is important to consider because of the high risk of aneuploidy. Huggon et al.[122] evaluated outcomes in 301 cases of atrioventricular septal defect identified by prenatal ultrasound. A chromosomal abnormality was found in 107 (36%), including 86 (29% of total, or 39% of 218 with known karyotypes) with trisomy 21, and 21 (7% or 10%) had other chromosomal abnormalities. Right isomerism occurred in 37 (12%), left isomerism in 62 (20%), and mirror atrial arrangement in two (1%). Extracardiac abnormalities and nonkaryotypic syndromes were evident in 40 fetuses (13%). In another series of atrioventricular septal defect, Delisle et al.[123] found an abnormal karyotype in 58% (22 of 38): 19 with trisomy 21, one with trisomy 18, one with trisomy 13, and one with mosaicism. The cardiac lesions were isolated in 20 of 38 fetuses (53%).

Uncomplicated atrioventricular septal defect is more likely to be associated with aneuploidy compared to those associated with other cardiac or extracardiac anomalies. This appears to reflect the association of atrioventricular septal defect with cardiosplenic syndrome, especially polysplenia. Cardiosplenic syndromes tend to have more complex cardiac defects and are always associated with a normal karyotype.[124] Delisle et al.[123] found that the odds of trisomy 21 were 16 times higher in fetuses with isolated cardiac lesions compared to those with associated cardiac anomalies and that fetuses with trisomy 21 and this cardiac anomaly may have a better survival rate than fetuses with normal karyotypes.

Diaphragmatic Hernia

Diaphragmatic hernia (Fig. 14) has been associated with various chromosomal abnormalities including trisomies 18, 13, and 21 and Turner syndrome.[125] The reported fre-

ventricle, tetralogy of Fallot, or hypoplastic heart compared to isolated ventricular septal defect or valvular stenosis. From a review of 203 fetuses with cardiac defects evaluated at a referral center, Chaoui et al.[118] reported aneuploidy in 22% with the following specific rates: atrioventricular septal defect, 55%; ventricular septal defect and aortic coarctation, 43% each; and tetralogy of Fallot and double-outlet right ventricle, 36% each. In comparison, fetuses with

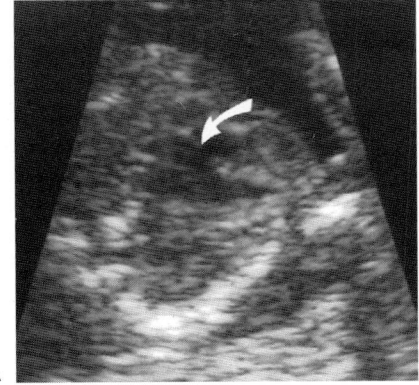
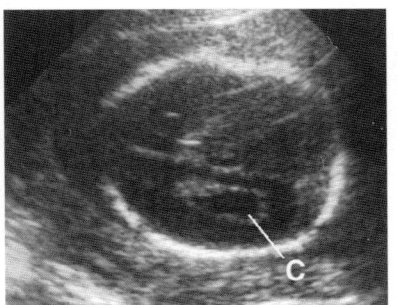

FIGURE 13. Cardiac defect and trisomy 18. **A:** An axial view of the heart at 16 weeks shows a large ventricular septal defect (*curved arrow*). **B:** An axial view of the head shows a large choroid plexus cyst (*C*) of the far ventricle, measuring 10 mm in diameter.

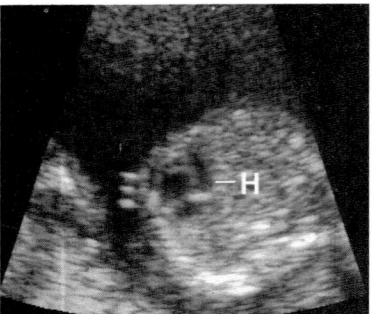

FIGURE 14. Diaphragmatic hernia and trisomy 18. A transverse view of the thorax shows displacement of the heart (*H*) to the right and anteriorly by a large diaphragmatic hernia. Abnormalities of the hands and feet were also demonstrated. The karyotype was trisomy 18.

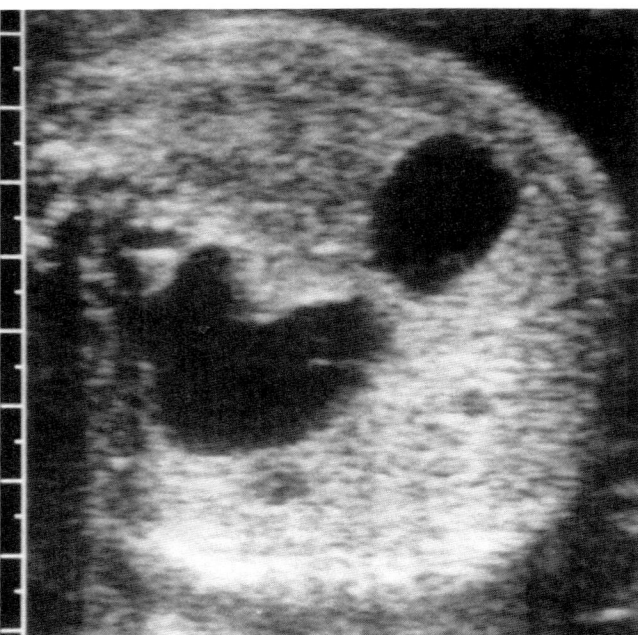

FIGURE 15. Duodenal atresia and trisomy 21. An axial scan of the abdomen at 30 weeks shows the classic double bubble appearance of duodenal atresia. Polyhydramnios was also present. At least one-third of fetuses with duodenal atresia prove to have trisomy 21.

quency of aneuploidy varies markedly between neonatal and prenatal series.[126,127] In a neonatal series, Puri and Gorman[126] reported two chromosomal abnormalities (trisomies 18 and 13) among 36 infants (6%) born with a diaphragmatic hernia. In prenatal series, the frequency of chromosomal abnormality has been reported in the range of 8% to 34%, most commonly 10% to 20%.[128–133] Trisomy 18 is the most common major chromosomal abnormality, but other types may also occur. In a review of 48 fetuses with diaphragmatic hernia, Howe et al.[133] reported that 34% of those tested had a chromosomal abnormality, including three with trisomies and nine with more complex abnormalities (translocations, deletions, and marker chromosomes). As with other anomalies, the specific risk of fetal aneuploidy varies with other factors including maternal age and the presence of other detectable anomalies.

Duodenal Atresia

Trisomy 21 (Down syndrome) is present in approximately one-third of cases of duodenal atresia detected prenatally[134] (Fig. 15). Unfortunately, characteristic sonographic findings of duodenal atresia (the double bubble sign and polyhydramnios) are frequently not apparent until after 20 to 24 weeks. Occasionally, however, duodenal atresia may be seen before 20 weeks as a mildly dilated duodenum.[135,136] Even when duodenal atresia is not detected until the third trimester, knowledge of the fetal karyotype is essential for patient counseling and optimal obstetric management of affected pregnancies. Chromosome analysis is therefore recommended whenever duodenal atresia is identified prenatally.

Omphalocele

Omphalocele carries a high risk of aneuploidy.[137–142] Trisomies 18 and 13 have been reported most often, followed by trisomy 21, 45,X (Turner syndrome), and triploidy. A

higher frequency of chromosomal abnormalities has been observed in most prenatal studies (30% to 40%) than in neonatal studies (combined rate of 12%), probably due to the inclusion of more severely anomalous fetuses who die *in utero* or during the immediate neonatal period. In one study, aneuploidy was present in 61% of fetuses with omphalocele from trisomy 18, trisomy 13, or triploidy, and the corresponding frequencies of omphalocele in fetuses with these chromosomal defects were 22.5%, 9.1%, and 12.5%, respectively.

The actual risk of aneuploidy with omphalocele varies with maternal age, gestational age, associated anomalies, and the contents of the omphalocele (liver vs. no liver).[143,144] Nyberg et al.[144] were the first to suggest that omphaloceles with intracorporeal liver (bowel only) carry a much greater risk for aneuploidy than do omphaloceles that contain liver (Fig. 16). This suggestion has been confirmed by a number of other studies.[145–148] Conversely, we have observed a very low risk of aneuploidy for fetuses with omphalocele and extracorporeal liver with no other anomalies.

Genitourinary Anomalies

Anomalies of the genitourinary tract are among the most commonly detected by prenatal sonography. As in other organ systems, the risk of a chromosomal abnormality in the genitourinary tract appears to vary with the specific

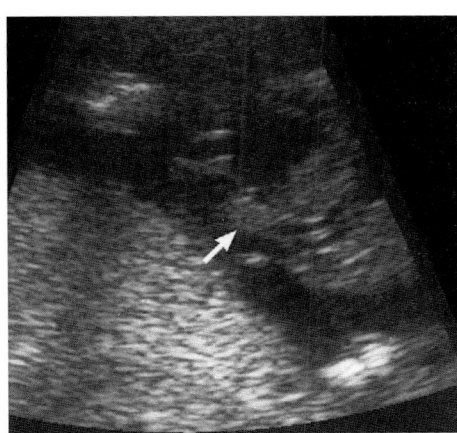

FIGURE 16. Omphalocele and trisomy 18. A transverse view of the anterior abdominal wall at cord insertion shows a small omphalocele (*arrow*) containing only bowel. The karyotype was trisomy 18.

malformation present. The highest frequency of chromosomal abnormalities has been reported in fetuses with bladder outlet obstruction (urethrovesical obstruction), most commonly from trisomy 18 or 13. In a series of 39 fetuses with obstruction at or distal to the urethrovesical junction, Nicolaides et al.[40] reported chromosomal abnormalities in nine (23%). Although it is uncertain whether this estimate represents the true risk, an association between urethrovesical obstruction and chromosomal abnormalities has been noted in many additional case reports.[149–151]

Chromosomal abnormalities have been reported less frequently for more proximal urinary malformations. This risk is considered to be low for unilateral renal abnormalities including ureteropelvic junction obstruction and multicystic dysplastic kidneys.[152]

Based on available evidence, chromosome analysis is recommended for fetuses with bladder outlet obstruction, particularly when *in utero* surgery or drainage procedures are considered.[153] Whether chromosome analysis is indicated for other types of genitourinary malformations when no additional anomalies are identified is not established. We do not currently recommend chromosome analysis when unilateral cystic dysplasia or ureteropelvic junction obstruction is demonstrated.

Clubfoot (Talipes Equinovarus)

Clubfoot (Fig. 17) has been associated with multiple chromosomal abnormalities, including trisomies 18 and 13.[154,155] However, most affected fetuses show other detectable anomalies, in which case the risk of aneuploidy is high. Several studies have now addressed the question of whether isolated clubfoot also justifies genetic amniocentesis. In a review of 51 cases of apparently isolated clubfoot from more than 27,000 targeted prenatal ultrasound examinations (mean age, 21.6 weeks), Malone et al.[156] found no

cases of aneuploidy or additional malformations detected at birth. The authors concluded that isolated unilateral or bilateral clubfoot does not appear to be an indication for fetal karyotyping, provided that a detailed sonographic fetal anatomy survey is normal and the patient is otherwise considered at low risk.

On the other hand, Shipp and Benacerraf[157] evaluated 87 fetuses with apparently isolated clubfoot on prenatal ultrasonography, with follow-up available in 68 cases. Sixty of the 68 fetuses (88%) proved to have clubfoot after delivery (false-positive rate 11.8%). Four fetuses (5.9%) had abnormal karyotypes: 47,XXY, 47,XXX, trisomy 18, and trisomy 21. Nine fetuses had hip or other limb abnormalities noted after birth. Other anomalies were detected after birth: ventricular septal defects (in two), early renal dysplasia, and mild posterior urethral valves. Shipp and Benacerraf[157] recommend fetal karyotyping when isolated clubfoot is identified on prenatal sonogram because other subtle associated malformations may not be detected ultrasonographically in the early second trimester.

Limb Reduction and Other Extremity Malformations

Limb reduction abnormalities have been associated with chromosomal abnormalities, particularly trisomy 18.[158,159] Radial aplasia (Fig. 18) is a relatively common finding of trisomy 18. Indeed, when radial aplasia is demonstrated, the first consideration should be trisomy 18.

Flexion deformities or movement disorders are common with trisomy 18 (Fig. 19). The most characteristic finding is fixed flexion of the hands, often with overlapping fingers. Some fetuses with trisomy 18 also show generalized arthrogryposis. In a postmortem study, clenched hands were present in 35%, clubfeet in 23%, and rocker-bottom feet in 10% of cases.[43] A prenatal sonographic study reported clenched hands in 16 of 35 (46%) fetuses during the second trimester.[160] Paluda et al.[161] showed flexion abnormalities of the hand and wrist in 22 fetuses. Thirteen (59%) had an abnormal karyotype, and among the nine with normal chromosomes, three had evidence of a movement disorder.

Characteristic abnormalities of the hands and fingers may provide important clues to an underlying chromosomal abnormality. Syndactyly of the third and fourth digits is a characteristic feature of triploidy (see Fig. 46 in Chapter 5), and polydactyly (Fig. 20) is present in the majority of fetuses with trisomy 13. Clinodactyly (hypoplasia of the middle phalanx of the fifth digit) is common with trisomy 21 (Fig. 21) and was observed in approximately one-third of cases in a pathologic study.[101]

An association between shortened limb length and aneuploidy has also been observed and is discussed further in the next section, under Shortened Limbs and Other Skeletal Abnormalities.

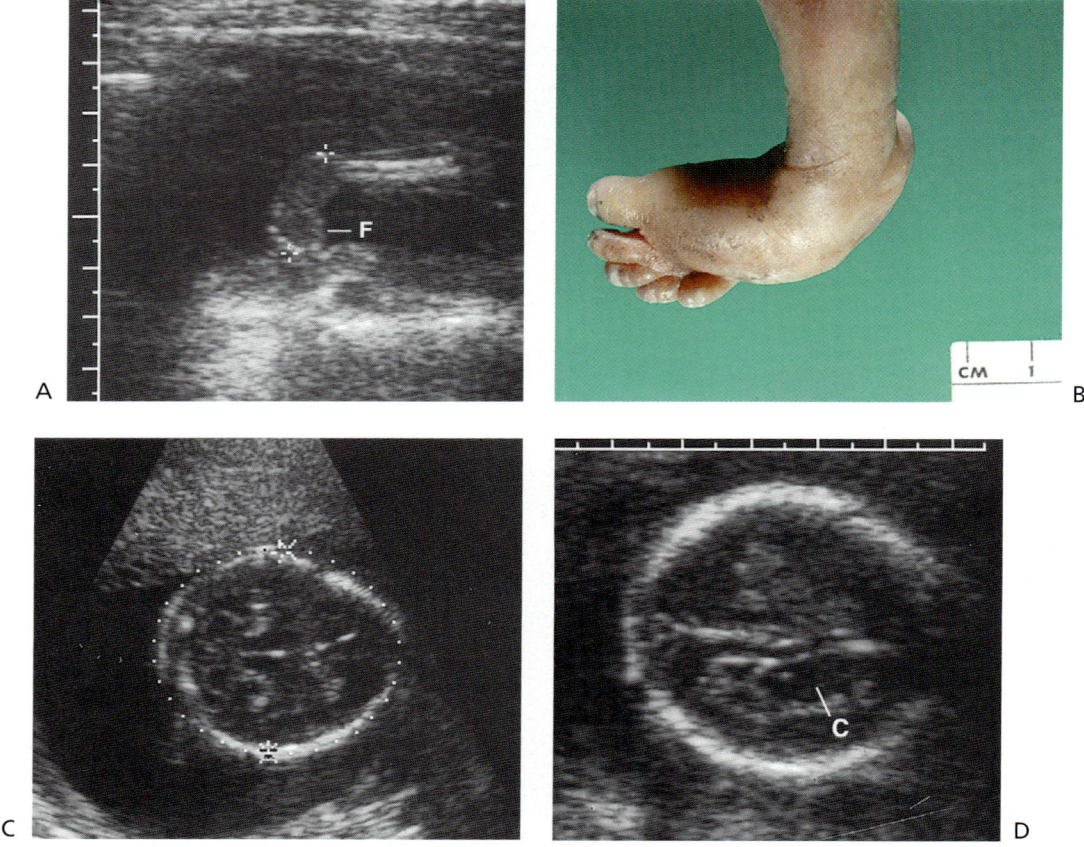

FIGURE 17. Clubfoot and trisomy 18. A scan at 17 weeks shows clubfoot (*F*) **(A)** with pathologic correlation **(B)**. Other abnormalities were identified, including brachycephaly **(C)** and choroid plexus cysts (*C*) **(D)**.

Sonographic Markers

Specific SMFA are discussed in the sections that follow. For a discussion of the use of sonographic markers in quantitative risk assessment of fetal aneuploidy, see Risk Assessment, later in this chapter.

Choroid Plexus Cysts

CPCs are a relatively common variant during the second trimester, are transient, and have no known effect on fetal development. Unlike some of the other SMFAs (nuchal thickening, hyperechoic bowel), there is no known association with other adverse outcome when the karyotype is normal.

Chudleigh et al.[162] first reported detection of CPCs on prenatal sonography as a benign, transient finding in five fetuses examined from 17 to 19 weeks and in whom the cysts resolved by 20 to 23 weeks. Subsequently, an association with aneuploidy was found, specifically with trisomy 18.[163] This initiated considerable interest in CPCs.[164–172] Despite the number of studies reported, variation in the prevalence of CPCs among normal fetuses remains considerable. The reported prevalence ranges from 0.3% to 3.6%.[173–176] Variables that may influence prevalence include gestational age, thoroughness of the ultrasound, size threshold for diagnosis of a choroid cyst, underlying risk factors, and reasons for referral.

Metaanalyses of CPCs have been reported, but they suffer from the same limitation of the original reports[177]: Many of these reports do not take into account important factors such as maternal age and other risk factors when evaluating the potential risk of CPCs. A metaanalysis study by Yoder et al.[178] suggests a likelihood ratio of 13.8 [confidence interval (CI), 7.7 to 25.0] for trisomy 18 and 1.87 (CI, 0.78 to 4.46) for trisomy 21. Among 1,346 fetuses with isolated CPCs, seven had trisomy 18 and five had trisomy 21.

In a detailed analysis from a single center, Snijders et al.[179] observed CPCs in 50% of fetuses with trisomy 18 and 1% of karyotypically normal fetuses. However, the vast majority of affected fetuses showed other abnormalities so the risk of isolated choroid cysts was only marginally increased (likelihood ratio less than 2), whereas the presence of just one other abnormality increased the risk 20 times (Table 10). Snijders et al. suggest that maternal age should be a major factor in deciding whether to offer fetal karyotyping when isolated CPCs are detected.

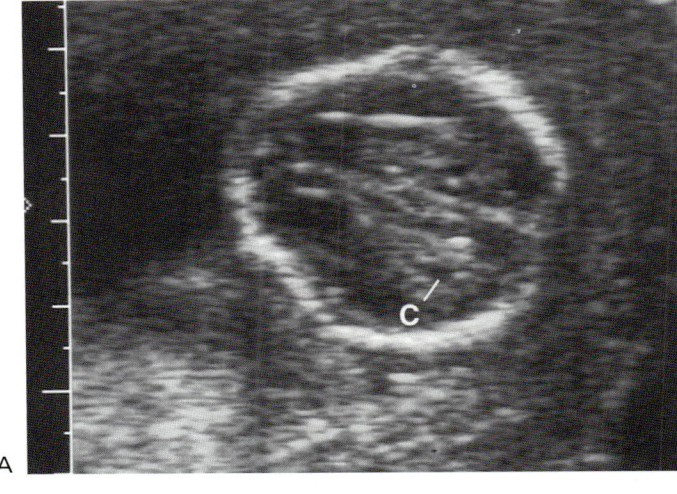

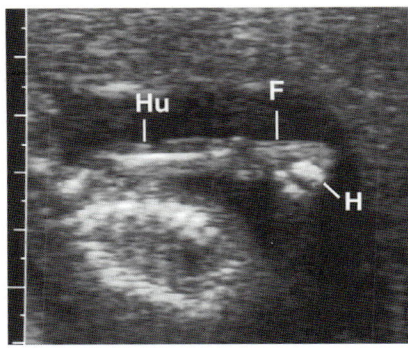

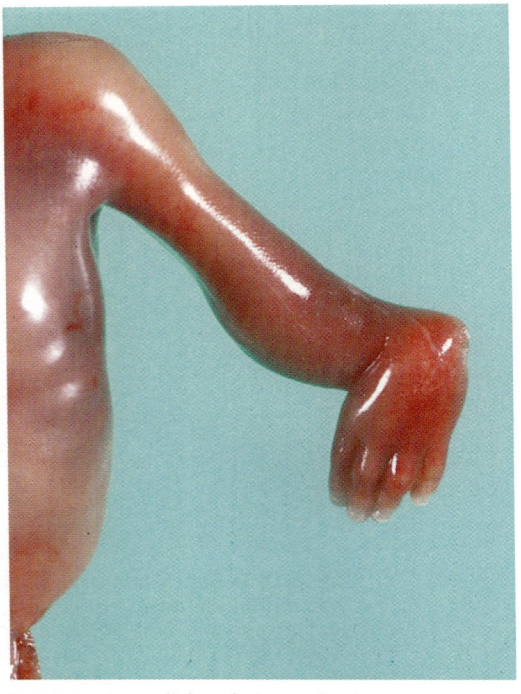

FIGURE 18. Radial aplasia and trisomy 18. **A:** A transverse view of the head at 15 weeks shows brachycephaly and a small choroid plexus cyst (*C*). **B:** A scan of the arm shows the characteristic appearance of radial aplasia. The hand (*H*) is turned inward, and the forearm (*F*) is shortened. Hu, humerus. **C:** Pathologic correlation of radial aplasia.

Among other variables, available evidence suggests that larger cysts (more than 10 mm) further increase the risk of trisomy 18 compared to smaller cysts[180–184] (Figs. 22 and 23). Such large cysts undoubtedly take longer to resolve, supporting observations that delayed resolution of choroid cysts carries an increased risk for trisomy 18. Whether the cysts are unilateral or bilateral does not appear significant, although it is probably true that large cysts also tend to be bilateral.

Although an association between CPCs and trisomy 18 has been clearly established, a possible link with trisomy 21

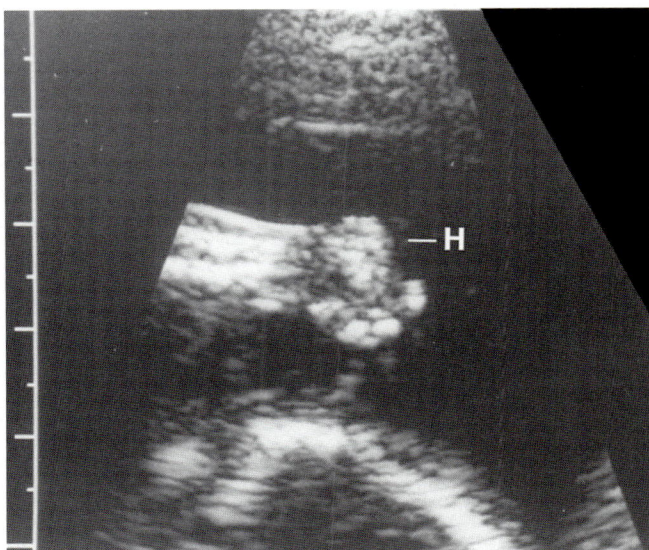

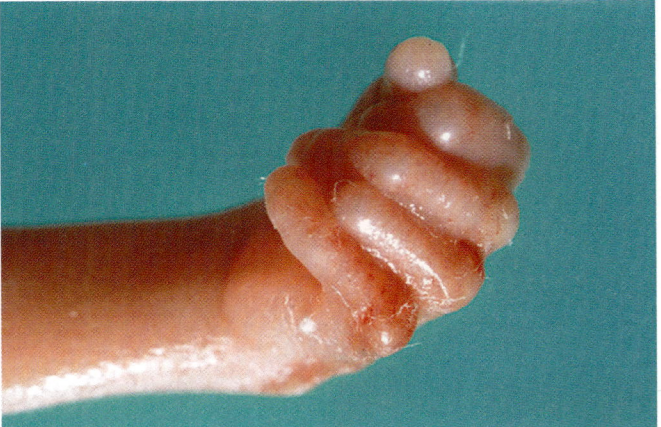

FIGURE 19. Clenched hands and trisomy 18. **A:** A sonogram shows a clenched hand (*H*), which persisted throughout the examination. **B:** Pathologic correlation with overlapping digits.

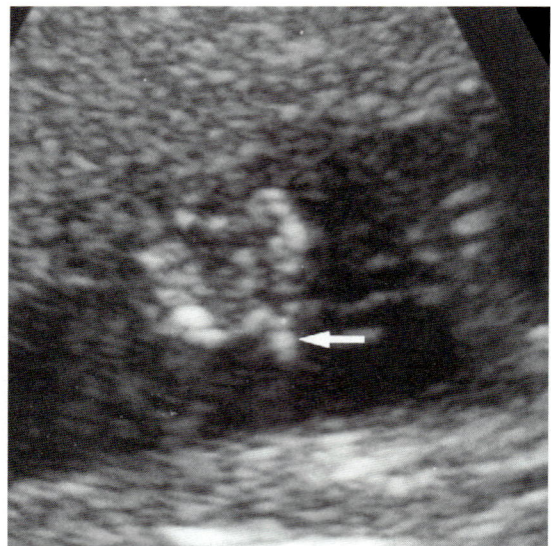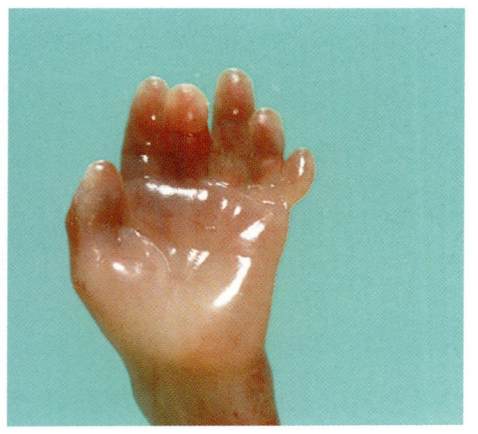

A   B

FIGURE 20. Polydactyly and trisomy 13. **A:** A scan of the hand at 20 weeks shows an extra digit (*arrow*) indicating postaxial polydactyly. Other views showed echogenic intracardiac focus, rocker-bottom feet, and microphthalmos. **B:** Pathologic correlation from a similar case. [Reproduced with permission from Lehman CD, Nyberg DA, Winter TC III, Kapur R, Resta RG, Luthy DA. Trisomy 13 syndrome: prenatal US findings in a review of 33 cases. *Radiology* 1995;194(1):217–222.]

has been controversial. As noted, Yoder et al.[178] suggest a likelihood ratio of 1.87 but this was not statistically significant. Bromley et al.[185] also found that isolated CPCs are not associated with trisomy 21. Our own analysis suggests that CPCs are seen more commonly in fetuses with trisomy 21 but not as an isolated finding.

It is apparent that detection of a CPC, as with any SMFA, should initiate a careful search for additional abnormalities. Furthermore, a CPC can be presumed to be isolated only after a detailed fetal survey fails to show structural abnormalities or other SMFAs. Leonardi et al.[167] found that 18 of 149 (12%) fetuses with CPCs had other

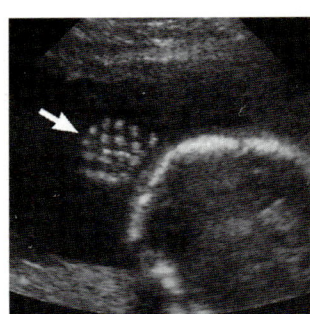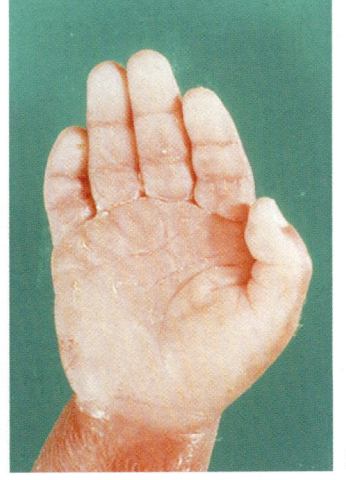

A   B

FIGURE 21. Clinodactyly and trisomy 21. **A:** A view of the hand shows clinodactyly with a curved fifth finger and small middle phalanx (*arrow*). **B:** Corresponding photograph at delivery.

TABLE 10. APPROXIMATE RISK OF TRISOMY 18 IN FETUSES WITH CHOROID PLEXUS CYSTS

Gestational age (wk)	Risk		
	Baseline	Isolated cyst	Other abnormalities
20–24	1:4,500	1:2,950	1:225
25–29	1:3,600	1:2,300	1:175
30–34	1:2,000	1:1,300	1:100
35–39	1:750	1:470	1:35
40–44	1:400	1:100	1:10

Data from Snijders RJ, Shawa L, Nicolaides KH. Fetal choroid plexus cysts and trisomy 18: assessment of risk based on ultrasound findings and maternal age. *Prenat Diagn* 1994;14(12):1119–1127.

sonographic anomalies; in ten they were minor, and two of the ten had abnormal karyotypes. Four of eight fetuses with major anomalies were aneuploid. All 131 fetuses with isolated CPCs had normal karyotypes, and all aneuploid fetuses had additional anomalies.

As an isolated finding following a high-quality ultrasound—assuming the patient is otherwise considered at low risk for fetal aneuploidy—we believe that detection of CPCs should not alter obstetric management. Similar conclusions have been reached by a number of other authorities.[186] Invasive testing based on the presence of isolated CPCs is also not justified from a cost/benefit standpoint.[187,188]

Additional reassurance can be obtained by correlating ultrasound findings with serum biochemical markers.[189,190]

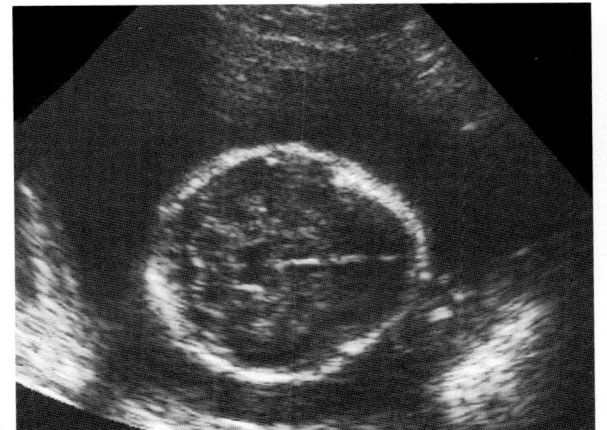
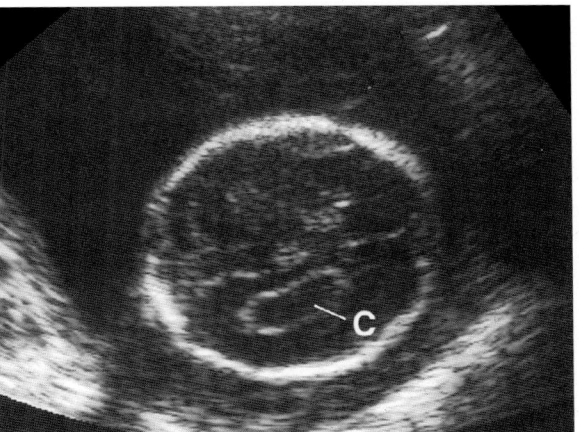

FIGURE 22. Choroid plexus cyst and trisomy 18. **A:** An axial scan of the head shows brachycephaly. **B:** A more cephalad scan through the ventricles shows a large choroid plexus cyst (C) of the far ventricle, measuring 15 mm in length. A cardiac abnormality was also identified.

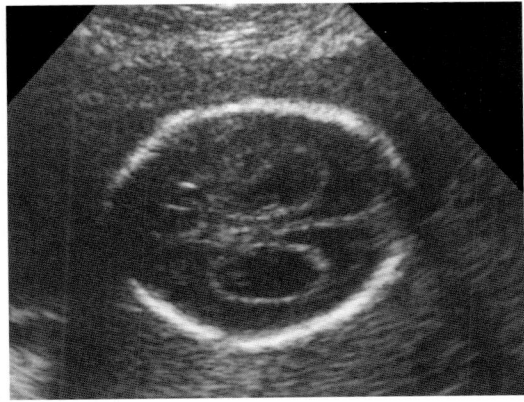
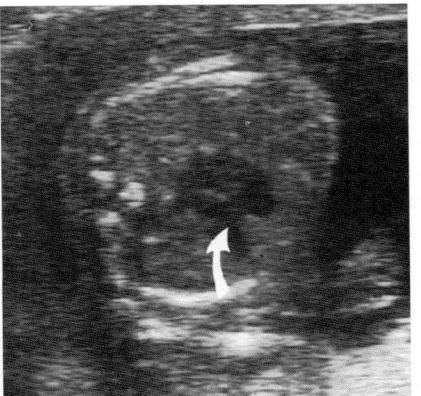

FIGURE 23. Choroid plexus cysts and trisomy 18. **A:** An axial scan of the head shows unusually large choroid plexus cysts measuring 20 mm in diameter. **B:** A view of the heart shows a ventricular septal defect (*arrow*).

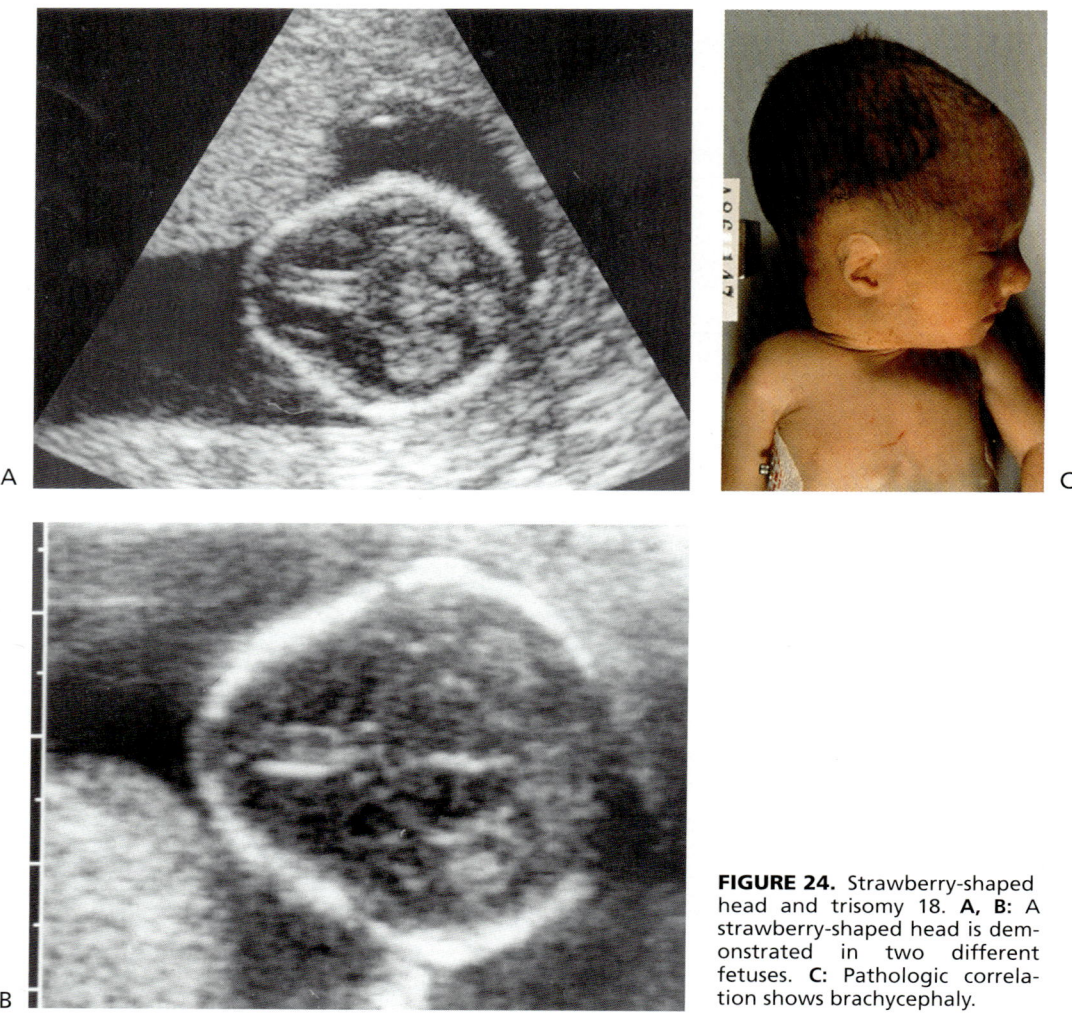

FIGURE 24. Strawberry-shaped head and trisomy 18. **A, B:** A strawberry-shaped head is demonstrated in two different fetuses. **C:** Pathologic correlation shows brachycephaly.

Sullivan et al.[190] conclude that the triple screen is a useful adjunct to targeted ultrasonography in selecting patients with fetal CPCs for amniocentesis; a normal triple-screen result and the absence of additional fetal anomalies on ultrasonography makes the risk of chromosomal abnormality extremely low.

If fetal karyotyping is not performed, we disagree with the common practice of recommending a follow-up ultrasound when CPCs are identified. Because CPCs always resolve, a follow-up ultrasound is also of no value in decision making, unless it is to detect other abnormalities that were missed.

Strawberry-Shaped Head

Brachycephaly is a common pathologic feature of trisomy 18. On ultrasound, brachycephaly sometimes appears as a strawberry-shaped head (Fig. 24), so named by Nicolaides et al.[191] These investigators reported a strawberry-shaped head in 43 of 83 (52%) fetuses with trisomy 18 who had other anomalies seen by ultrasound. Similarly, Shields et

al.[192] reported a strawberry-shaped head in 12 of 35 (34%) fetuses with trisomy 18, and abnormal head shape, including the lemon-shaped head, was found in 43%. The false-positive rate in normal fetuses is uncertain, but it is probably approximately 1% since it may superficially resemble a lemon-shaped head.[193] Therefore, as with other sonographic markers, it is a nonspecific finding that is most commonly seen in normal fetuses. However, as it may be the initial or primary clue to the presence of trisomy 18, other sonographic findings should be specifically sought. The combination of brachycephaly and CPCs, particularly large cysts, indicates a high risk for this condition.

Mild Cerebral Ventricular Dilatation

The size of the lateral cerebral ventricles remains relatively constant throughout gestation at a mean diameter of 6.1 mm ± 1.3 mm, with slightly larger ventricles in males than in females (6.4 mm vs. 5.8 mm).[194] Ventriculomegaly is suspected when the atrial diameter reaches 10 mm,

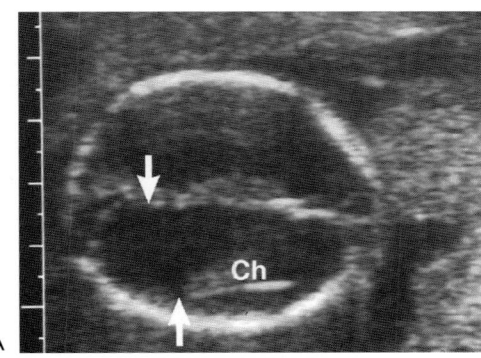
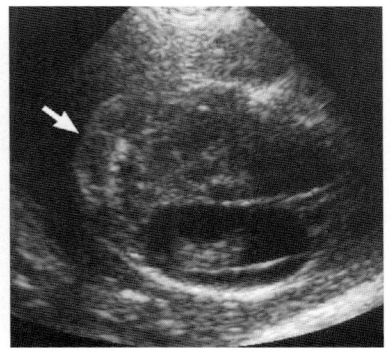
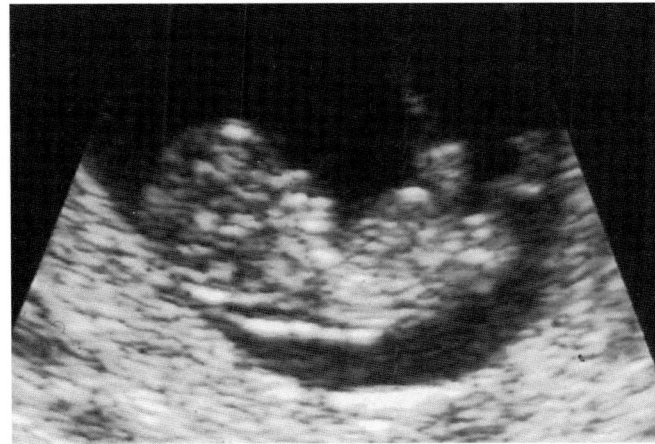

FIGURE 25. Cerebral ventricular dilatation and trisomy 21. **A:** A transverse view of the head shows ventricular dilatation (*arrows*). The choroid plexus (*Ch*) rests on the dependent side of the ventricle. Although ventricular dilatation appears subjectively moderate in degree, transverse ventricular measurement at the level of the ventricular atrium was only 12 mm. **B:** An oblique scan through the posterior fossa shows nuchal thickening (*arrow*). **C:** An earlier scan at 10.5 weeks appeared normal without increased nuchal translucency.

although separation of the dependent choroid from the medial ventricular wall may be visible evidence for early ventricular dilatation.[195]

Mild dilatation of the cerebral ventricles has been associated with trisomy 21 and other aneuploidies[196–199] (Fig. 25). Although some authors have categorized it as a major abnormality, we believe it shares similar characteristics (i.e., nonspecific, common in normal fetuses, often transient)[200] with other minor markers. It is more likely to be seen as a normal variant later in the second trimester (after 20 weeks) and in male fetuses.

In a series by Bromley et al.,[197] 12% (5 of 43) with mild ventriculomegaly (ventricular diameter 10 to 12 mm) had abnormal karyotypes (three with trisomy 21 and two with trisomy 18), although all of these showed other findings. Similarly, in our most recent series of trisomy 21,[214] mild cerebral ventricular dilatation was observed in 4.3% (8 of 186) of affected fetuses, but all had other findings: structural defects in three, three or more soft markers in three, or nuchal thickening alone in two.

On the other hand, Pilu et al.[198] evaluated 31 fetuses with isolated borderline ventricular dilatation (10 to 15 mm) and found three with aneuploidy (two with trisomy 21 and one with trisomy 13). In a review of the literature including their own cases (234 total), chromosomal aberrations, mostly trisomy 21, were observed in 3.8%. Vergani et al.[201] evaluated 82 cases of mild ventriculomegaly (10 to 15 mm) and found aneuploidy in two cases, both associated with advanced maternal age. Seven additional cases of aneuploidy were associated with other anomalies. Sohl et al.[202] reported on 2,743 cases, 3.8% (104) of which were chromosomally abnormal. Trisomy 21 was present in 2% (55). Mild ventriculomegaly was observed in 0.5% of chromosomally normal fetuses and 6.8% of chromosomally abnormal fetuses including 5.5% of fetuses with trisomy 21. The odds ratio of mild ventriculomegaly for chromosomal abnormality was 4.4 (95% CI, 1.3 to 93.4). However, mild ventriculomegaly was not seen as an isolated finding in any case of chromosomal abnormality. Choroid separation, defined as 3-mm or larger separation between the choroid plexus and the medial ventricular wall, was also investigated. Choroid separation had an odds ratio of 4.4 for chromosomal abnormality (95% CI, 0.6 to 34.1) when observed in conjunction with other ultrasound findings. As an isolated finding, the odds ratio was 10.4 (95% CI, 2.9 to 36.7).[180]

Current experience suggests that mild cerebral ventricular dilatation increases the risk for fetal aneuploidy, although this risk remains difficult to determine when it is the only finding in low-risk patients. Certainly, a careful

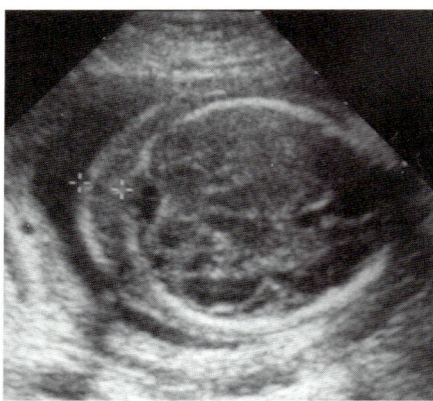

FIGURE 26. Nuchal thickening and trisomy 21. A slightly oblique view through the posterior fossa shows an abnormally thickened nuchal fold, measuring 6 mm.

search for additional anomalies is indicated and fetal echocardiography should also be considered. Further studies are needed, including comparison of ventricular measurements in fetuses with trisomy 21 and normal karyotype.

Nuchal Thickening

Redundant skin at the back of the neck is a characteristic clinical feature of trisomy 21 and was first reported by Dr. Langdon Down in 1866.[203] It is reportedly present in 80% of newborns with trisomy 21, as well as other chromosomal abnormalities (trisomies 13 and 18 and 45,X).[204] It is considered part of the spectrum of nuchal abnormalities that also includes cystic hygroma. Indeed, nuchal thickening may result from resolution of cystic hygromas in some cases.[205]

Benacerraf et al.[206,207] and Benacerraf and Frigoletto[208] were the first to report the sonographic correlate of this clinical feature in terms of nuchal thickening, and thus began the search for other ultrasound markers. Nuchal thickening remains one of the most sensitive and important markers of trisomy 21 during the second trimester (Figs. 26 and 27). Indeed, although centers may vary the other criteria used, virtually all centers use nuchal thickening as a marker for trisomy 21. Although the sensitivity and false-positive rates vary with gestational age and the exact criteria for a positive scan, sensitivities in the range of 20% to 40% are most common. Although transverse scans are typically used to assess nuchal thickening during the second trimester, it is clear that sagittal scans can also demonstrate increased nuchal thickening just as sagittal scans are used to measure nuchal translucency during the first trimester (Fig. 27).

The criteria for increased nuchal thickening vary between centers. Based on early experience, Benacerraf et al.[206] suggested that a threshold of 6 mm or more after 15 weeks indicated a high risk for trisomy 21. However, in a subsequent paper,[207] Benacerraf observed that none of

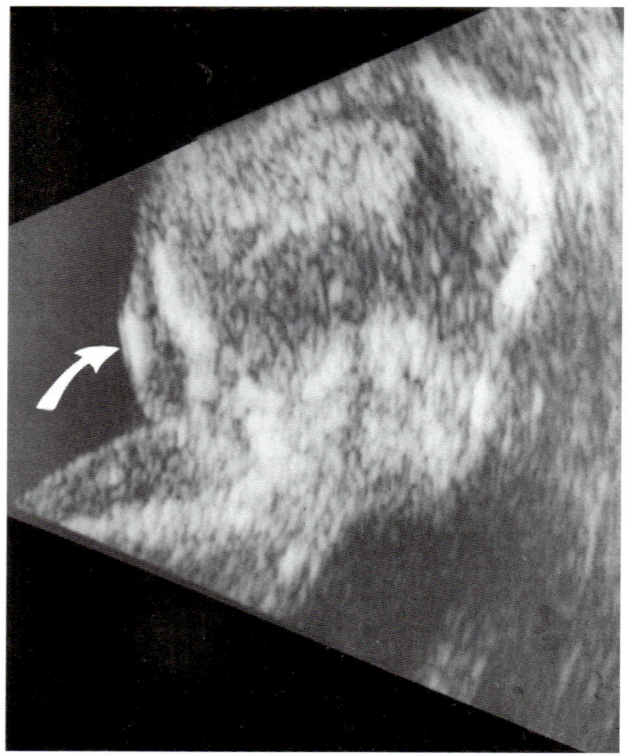

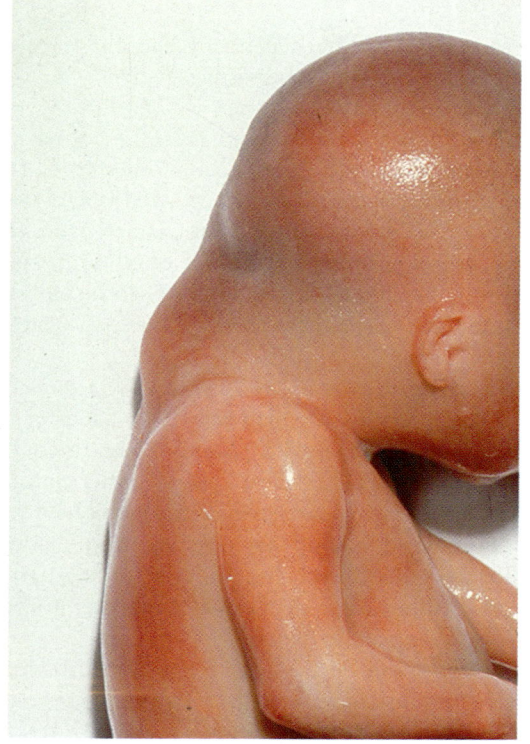

FIGURE 27. Nuchal thickening and trisomy 21. **A:** A sagittal view of the neck shows a thickened nuchal fold that is bulging posteriorly (*arrow*). **B:** Pathologic photograph shows increased nuchal fold.

303 normal fetuses showed nuchal thickening over 5 mm up to 20 weeks. Several prospective studies have suggested that 5 mm is a better threshold and results in improved sensitivity with only a slight increase in the false-positive rate, and we have used a 5-mm cutoff for more than 10 years.[209–211]

As a further refinement, a number of studies have confirmed that normal nuchal thickness varies with gestational age, suggesting that gestational age–specific criteria should be used instead of a single cutoff.[212,213] Use of multiples of the median data, comparing the actual nuchal measurement with the expected measurement, permits calculation of likelihood ratios and integration with maternal serum biochemical markers for a combined risk. Bahado-Singh et al.[213] have reported multiples of the median and associated likelihood ratios for a range of nuchal thickness measurements.

Using a 5-mm cutoff, we have found that isolated nuchal thickening carries a likelihood ratio of approximately 11[214] (see Table 13). This means that patients of any age would be considered at increased risk for fetal aneu-

ploidy when increased nuchal thickening is demonstrated. However, we encourage use of more precise risk estimates using continuous variables and risks associated with multiples of the median when those risk estimates have been better defined.

Hyperechoic Bowel

Like other nonstructural markers, hyperechoic bowel is nonspecific and most commonly observed in normal fetuses. However, it is observed with increased frequency among fetuses with aneuploidy, particularly trisomy 21[215–221] (Figs. 28 and 29). First suggested by Nyberg et al.,[222] this association has been confirmed by many others. Hyperechoic bowel has also been reported in association with bowel atresia, congenital infection, and rarely with meconium ileus secondary to cystic fibrosis.[223] An increased risk of IUGR, fetal demise, and placenta-related complications is also recognized with hyperechoic bowel.[224]

Despite its subjectivity, the prevalence of hyperechoic bowel among normal fetuses (0.5%) has been remarkably

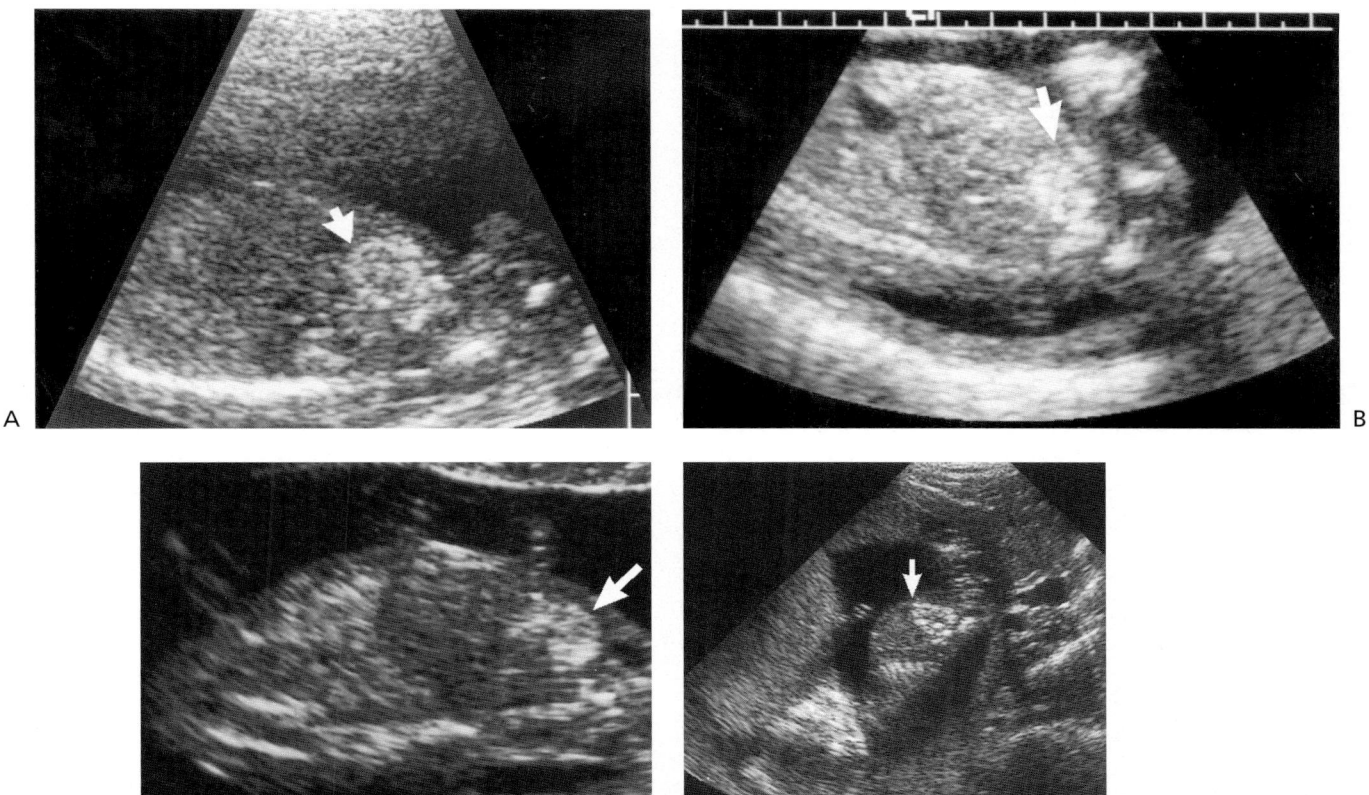

FIGURE 28. Hyperechoic bowel and trisomy 21. Scans from four fetuses **(A, B, C, D)** seen during the second trimester with varying degrees of hyperechoic bowel (*arrows*). The karyotype was trisomy 21 in each case. As with all sonographic markers, hyperechoic bowel is nonspecific and most commonly seen in normal fetuses.

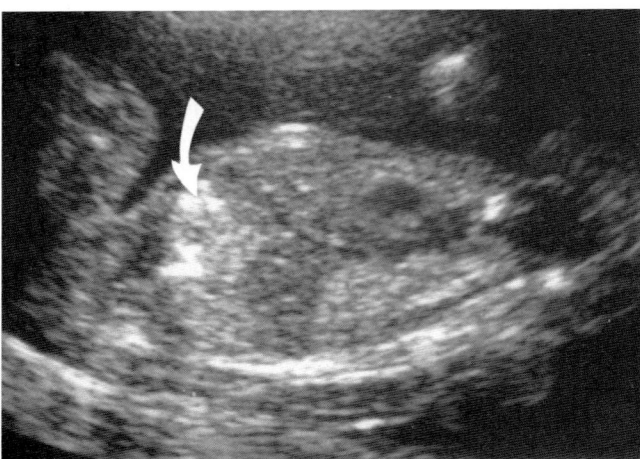

FIGURE 29. Hyperechoic bowel and Turner syndrome. A longitudinal view of the abdomen at 17 weeks shows hyperechoic bowel (*arrow*). A cystic hygroma was also present. The karyotype was 45,X.

consistent at our center in the last decade and is similar to other reports, suggesting that different centers can agree on the presence of hyperechoic bowel. We use a grading system for hyperechoic bowel: Grade 1 is mildly echogenic and typically diffuse, grade 2 is moderately echogenic and typically focal, and grade 3 is very echogenic, similar to that of bone structures.[225] The echogenicity of normal bowel also increases with transducer frequency,[226] although this effect is uniform whereas true hyperechoic bowel tends to be focal. To minimize subjectivity, some authors consider only bowel that is markedly hyperechoic, whereas we and others[227,228] recognize both moderate and markedly hyperechoic bowel (grades 2 and 3) as an increased risk for fetal aneuploidy.

A number of studies have estimated the risk of fetal aneuploidy with hyperechoic bowel. In one study of 171 fetuses (prevalence, 0.7%) with hyperechoic bowel after exclusion of fetuses with major anomalies or those referred for abnormal outside ultrasound, Al-Kouatly et al.[220] reported fetal aneuploidy in five cases (3.6%), including four cases of trisomy 21 and one case of trisomy 18. One of the five cases had a CPC, and the remaining four cases were isolated.

Based on cumulative experience, hyperechoic bowel appears to increase the risk of trisomy 21 by six- to sevenfold.[214] However, a number of these studies are referral centers and may have selection bias or may preferentially see higher-risk or older patients. As always, the precise risk varies with patient age and other risk factors. Nyberg et al.[214] calculated the likelihood ratio of isolated hyperechoic bowel to be 6.7, and a metaanalysis study by Smith-Bindman et al.[229] showed a similar likelihood ratio of 6.1. Based on an approximate likelihood ratio of 6.7 for isolated hyperechoic bowel and assuming an overall risk of Down syndrome of 1 in 500 in the population, isolated hyperechoic bowel would be expected to be associated with a risk

of Down syndrome in the range of 1% to 2% in the general population.

Other Potential Intraabdominal Markers

Intrahepatic calcification (hyperechogenic liver foci) is not uncommon and usually has a normal outcome as an isolated finding. However, adverse outcome including aneuploidy has been occasionally reported.[230] Koopman and Wladimiroff[231] evaluated intrahepatic calcifications in seven fetuses from among 7,260 patients examined at a referral center. One fetus proved to have trisomy 18 but showed other major abnormalities. Another fetus with normal karyotype also showed other major anomalies. In the largest study yet on the subject, Simchen et al.[232] evaluated 61 fetuses with liver calcification. Eleven (18%) fetuses had abnormal karyotype, including four with trisomy 13, two with trisomy 21, and one with trisomy 18. Of 21 cases without other ultrasound findings, one fetus had trisomy 21 and the remainder had normal outcomes. This experience indicates that fetal karyotyping is recommended when additional structural anomalies are present, but the outcome of isolated intrahepatic calcification appears to be excellent.

An enlarged fetal gallbladder has been implicated with fetal aneuploidy in one case.[233] Another case report noted hepatosplenomegaly and oligohydramnios as the only signs of trisomy 21 with a myeloproliferative disorder.[234]

Shortened Limbs and Other Skeletal Abnormalities

A characteristic of children with trisomy 21 is short stature associated with disproportionately short proximal long bones (femur and humerus). Limb shortening can also be detected in some fetuses with trisomy 21 during the second trimester.[235–241] However, there is a large overlap in bone measurements between affected and normal fetuses. Shortened humerus length appears to be a slightly more specific indicator than shortened femur length. Results probably vary with gestational age, ethnic group, possibly fetal gender, and the criteria used, as well as systematic differences in long bone measurements.[242] Despite these variables, this marker is commonly used at screening centers.

The most common method for determination of shortened humerus or femur length is comparison of the actual measurement with the expected measurement, typically based on biparietal diameter or other dating parameters rather than gestational age. However, like nuchal measurements, optimal results would be expected by using multiples of the median data and corresponding likelihood ratios rather than a single cutoff.[243] These methods are best performed with computer calculations.

Other skeletal abnormalities associated with trisomy 21 are clinodactyly (shortened middle phalanx of the fifth finger) and widened pelvic angle. Although both are well-known clinical features of trisomy 21, these can be difficult to assess on second-trimester sonography and thus are not typically included in most screening programs.

Echogenic Intracardiac Focus (Papillary Muscle Calcification)

EIF is a common finding during the second trimester, observed in 3% to 4% of normal fetuses.[244,245] The prevalence appears to be significantly higher among Asian populations: Shipp et al.[246] found EIF three times more often among Asian patients compared to whites. Thus, observations made in white populations may not apply to Asian populations.

Because EIF is a subjective finding, its detection depends on a variety of factors including resolution of the ultrasound equipment, technique, thoroughness of the examination, and the sonographer's experience. Fetal position is also important because EIFs are best visualized when the cardiac apex is oriented toward the transducer.[247] Despite these variable factors, similar detection rates of EIF from different studies suggest that experienced sonographers can largely agree on its presence or absence. Like many sonographic markers, it typically resolves by the third trimester despite the outcome.[248]

Roberts and Genest[249] were the first to suggest an association with aneuploidy and mineralization of the papillary muscle in a pathologic study. Mineralization of the papillary muscle was observed in 2% of normal fetuses compared to 16% (20 of 126) of those with trisomy 21 and 39% (nine of 23) with trisomy 13. Similar but slightly higher rates of EIF have been observed in sonographic studies during the second trimester, possibly because small foci may escape pathologic detection. Comparison of these data, as well as direct correlation by Brown et al.,[250] suggests that EIF correlates with papillary muscle mineralization that can be seen histologically. However, it could also represent coarse intramyocardial calcifications surrounded by myocardial fibrosis.[251]

In the first two ultrasound reports of EIF and aneuploidy, Bromley et al.[252] detected EIF in 4.7% (62 of 1,312) of control subjects compared to 18% (4 of 22) of those with trisomy 21, and Lehman et al.[253] reported EIF in 39% of fetuses with trisomy 13 before 20 weeks (Figs. 30 and 31). A number of studies have confirmed an association between EIF and trisomy 21[254–260] (Figs. 32 and 33), although some other studies have failed to show this association.[261–263] The likelihood ratio of EIF for trisomy 21 is estimated in the range of 1.8 to 4.2.

The risk of aneuploidy from isolated EIF, as well as other SMFAs, may be underestimated among low-risk patients because of incomplete ascertainment. Few patients with an isolated marker undergo chromosome analysis unless they are already considered at high risk. In one of the few studies to address this issue, Simpson et al.[255] evaluated 205 fetuses with isolated EIF from low-risk patients. Clinical follow-up was obtained by way of a standard questionnaire completed by the parents when the infant was 6 weeks old. Two (1%) infants proved to have aneuploidy (one trisomy 21, one unbalanced translocation).

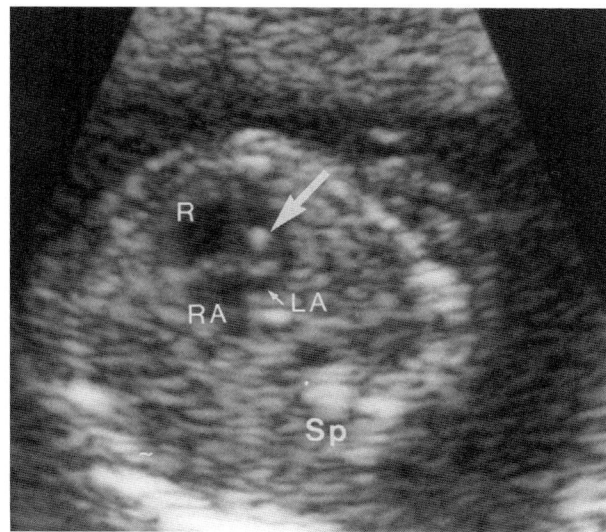

FIGURE 30. Echogenic intracardiac focus (EIF) and trisomy 13. A transverse view of the heart at 20 weeks shows discrete EIF (*arrow*) within the left ventricle. Hypoplastic left ventricle is also present, with a smaller left ventricle compared to the right ventricle (*R*) and a small left atrium (*LA*) compared to the right atrium (*RA*). Other abnormalities included polydactyly and rocker-bottom feet. The combination of EIF with hypoplastic-appearing left heart appears to be strongly associated with trisomy 13. Sp, spine. [Reproduced with permission from Lehman CD, Nyberg DA, Winter TC III, Kapur R, Resta RG, Luthy DA. Trisomy 13 syndrome: prenatal US findings in a review of 33 cases. *Radiology* 1995;194(1):217–222.]

On the other hand, the risk of EIF and other markers is probably overestimated in studies in which the fetal karyotype is known for all patients given that ultrasound findings influence patient decision making. Many high-risk patients

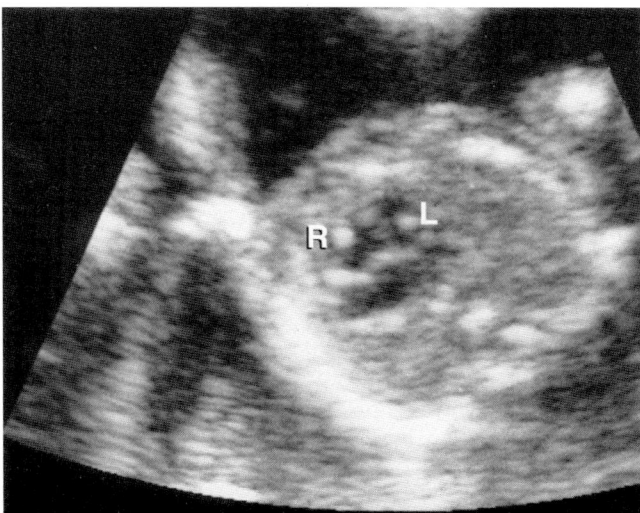

FIGURE 31. Echogenic intracardiac foci and trisomy 13. A four-chamber view of the heart at 16 weeks shows echogenic intracardiac foci in the left (*L*) and right (*R*) ventricles of the heart. These were the only sonographic abnormalities. Karyotypic analysis, performed in part because of advanced maternal age, showed trisomy 13.

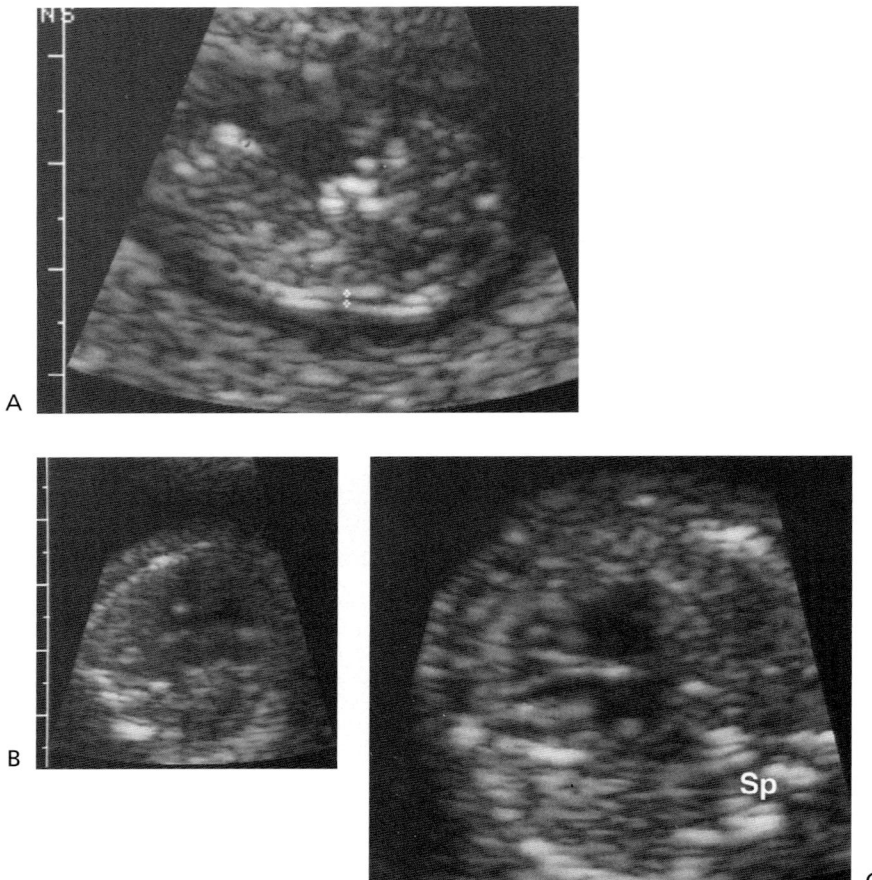

FIGURE 32. Echogenic intracardiac focus (EIF) and trisomy 21. **A:** An initial scan at 10.5 weeks shows normal nuchal translucency, measuring 1 mm. **B:** A follow-up scan at 18 weeks with the apex up shows discrete EIF in the left ventricle of the heart. No other abnormalities were identified. However, serum biochemistry indicated a high risk for trisomy 21, and genetic amniocentesis yielded trisomy 21. **C:** A scan with the apex to the side fails to show the EIF. Sp, spine.

now wait for the results from the second-trimester ultrasound before deciding to undergo genetic amniocentesis, and appropriately, high-risk patients are more likely to undergo genetic amniocentesis than low-risk patients based on the same ultrasound finding. We observed EIF in 5.4% of fetuses with known normal karyotype compared to 3.9% for all consecutive patients who had normal or presumed normal fetal karyotype.[214] Previous studies confined to known karyotype have also shown a higher prevalence of EIF, emphasizing the potential for bias in studies of sonographic markers that restrict patients to known fetal karyotype.

Multiple or large EIF may further increase the risk of aneuploidy (Figs. 31 and 33B). Bettelheim et al.[264] found EIF in the left ventricle in 96% of cases, combined left and right ventricle in 4.3%, and isolated to the right ventricle in just 0.7%. Bromley et al.[257] concluded that right-sided and bilateral EIF combined had approxi-

mately a twofold greater risk for aneuploidy compared to left-sided foci, and others have also found that EIF involving both ventricles are more often associated with aneuploidy. Wax and Philput[260] reported that aneuploidy was more common when EIF involved both ventricles compared to either ventricle alone. Vibhakar et al.[258] found that of 15 fetuses with multiple EIF, ten (67%) had abnormal karyotype and only two of these had other sonographic abnormalities.

Renal Pyelectasis

Mild pyelectasis (hydronephrosis) has been associated with an increased risk of aneuploidy,[265–268] primarily trisomy 21, but is also a relatively common finding during routine obstetric ultrasound. The prevalence of pyelectasis undoubtedly varies with gestational age even during the

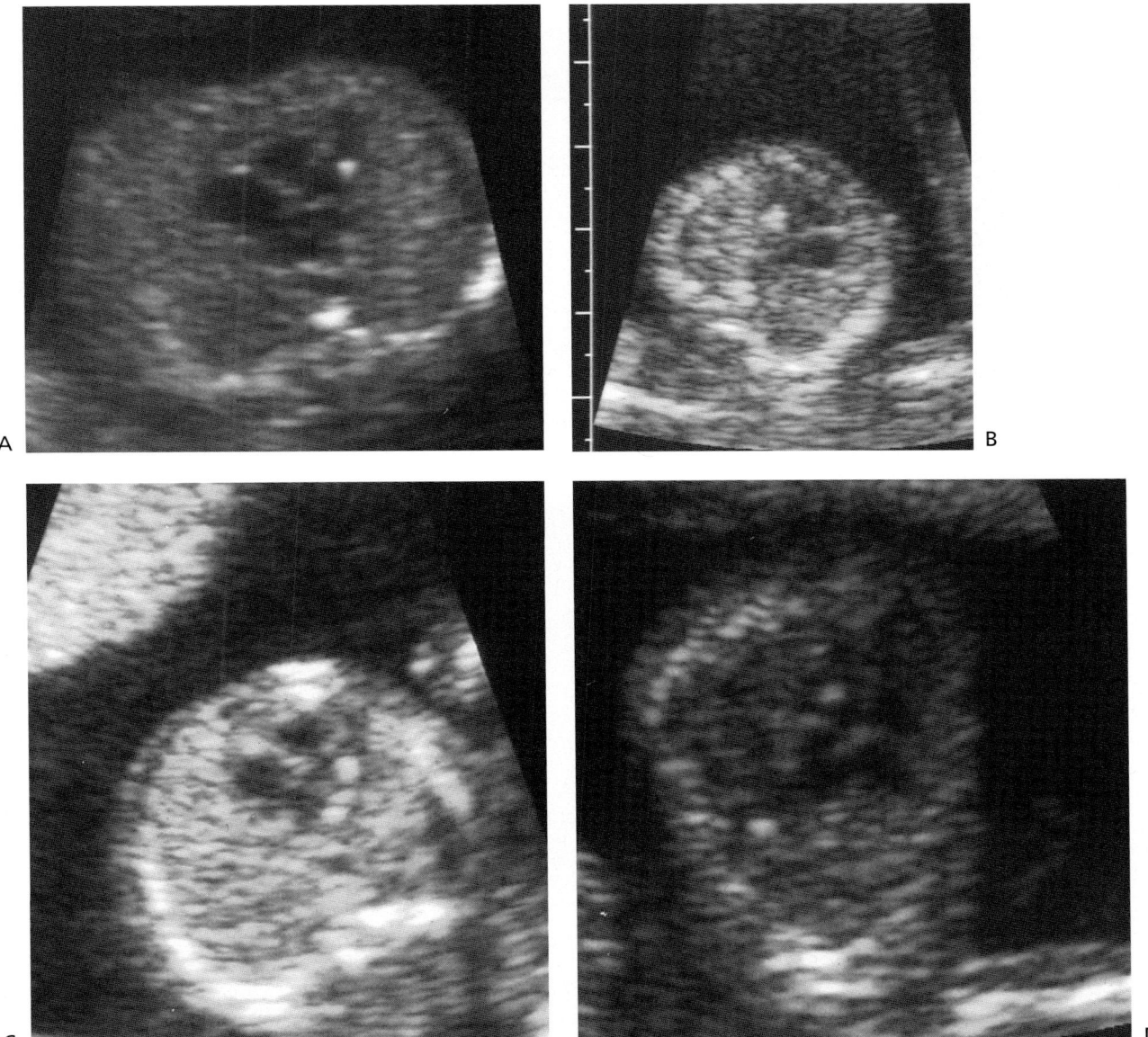

FIGURE 33. Echogenic intracardiac foci (EIF) from four different cases. **A:** A scan at 19 weeks from a twin pregnancy shows EIF in the left ventricle of the heart. Other abnormalities included borderline nuchal thickening (5 mm), shortened femur length, and moderate size bilateral choroid plexus cysts (11 mm). Chromosome analysis yielded trisomy 21. The other twin appeared normal and had normal karyotype. **B:** A scan at 15 weeks from a twin pregnancy shows prominent EIF in the left ventricle of the heart. No other abnormalities were apparent. This fetus proved to have trisomy 21. The other twin appeared normal and had normal karyotype. **C:** Prominent EIF in the left ventricle of the heart at 17 weeks. No other abnormalities were identified. The fetus proved to have trisomy 21. **D:** A transverse image shows EIF in the left ventricle of the heart. The karyotype was normal.

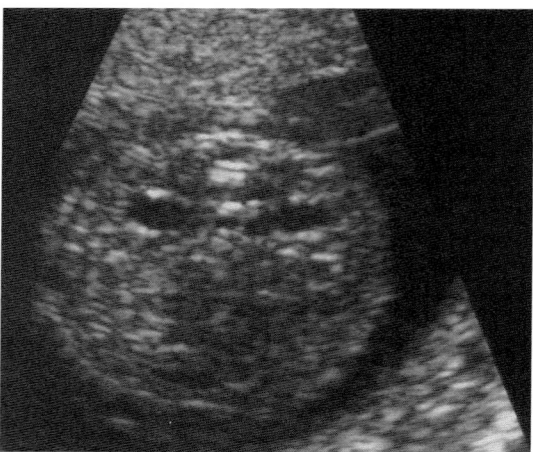

FIGURE 34. Pyelectasis and trisomy 21. A transverse scan at 18 weeks shows mild pyelectasis, with the renal pelvis measuring 4 mm in the anteroposterior direction. This was the only sonographic marker in this case, which is unusual.

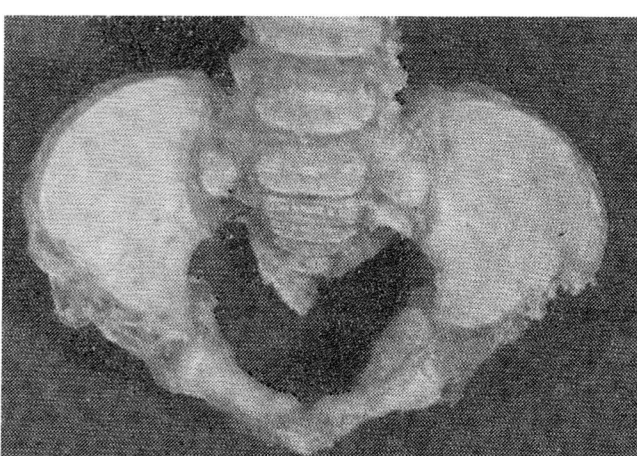

FIGURE 35. Widened pelvic angle and trisomy 21. A three-dimensional reconstructed computed tomographic scan of a pathologic specimen with trisomy 21 shows a widened pelvic angle.

time of second-trimester scans (14 to 22 weeks), although this variable has not been evaluated in detail. Renal pyelectasis is measured as the fluid-filled renal pelvis in an anterior-posterior dimension. We prefer measurement when the kidneys and spine are oriented toward or away from the transducer rather than to the side. The threshold for a positive scan varies among centers, but the most common is 3 to 4 mm. Ideally, gestational age–dependent criteria might be used in the future.

Using a cutoff of more than 3 mm, we observe pyelectasis (Fig. 34) in approximately 3% of normal fetuses at our center. Snijders et al. estimate that mild pyelectasis increases the risk of trisomy 21 by 1.6-fold over the baseline risk. Our own analysis is consistent with this risk, although this risk may not be increased when pyelectasis is isolated. The lack of association as an isolated finding has also been suggested by other studies,[269,270] although one center has shown an association as an isolated finding.[271]

Widened Pelvic Angle

Flaring of the iliac bone ("elephant ears") is a well-known radiographic feature of infants with Down syndrome. It is not surprising that second-trimester fetuses with trisomy 21 also have a significantly greater iliac angle than euploid fetuses[272–275] (Fig. 35). The iliac bone is also longer.[276] However, measurement of the pelvic angle is subject to significant intra- and interobserver variability. A number of factors influence measurement of the pelvic angle including gestational age, axial level, and spine orientation.[277] Kliewer et al.[277] found that the iliac angle decreased by 15.7 degrees from the superior to inferior portion of the pelvis and decreased by as much as 15.6

degrees when the spine is directed to the side. Because of these variables and overlap with normal fetuses, most authorities believe a widened pelvic angle is not a useful marker, particularly when used as part of a screening ultrasound.[278] However, use of standardized axial planes with three-dimensional ultrasound has the potential to better assess pelvic angle, making this approach more reliable.[279]

Intrauterine Growth Restriction

Early onset of IUGR is a common manifestation of major chromosomal abnormalities, particularly trisomies 18 and 13 and triploidy. Snijders et al.[280] evaluated 458 cases of fetuses with IUGR at a highly selective referral center. The fetal karyotype was abnormal in 19% of cases, but 96% of these showed multisystem fetal defects that were characteristic of the type of aneuploidy. The most common chromosomal defect in the group referred earlier than 26 weeks' gestation was triploidy; in those referred at 26 weeks or later, it was trisomy 18.

Early IUGR has been associated with trisomies 18 and 13 and triploidy.[281] Bahado-Singh et al.[282] reported the risk for aneuploidy to be substantially increased (odds ratio of 9.04) when the crown-rump length was shortened by 14 mm or more from that expected for the menstrual age. However, trisomy 21 has not been shown to be associated with significant shortening in the crown-rump length in the first trimester.

"Symmetric" or "asymmetric" types are probably not of value in assessing this risk. Traditionally, symmetric type was considered the highest risk. However, one of the most severe types of aneuploidy, triploidy, is associated with

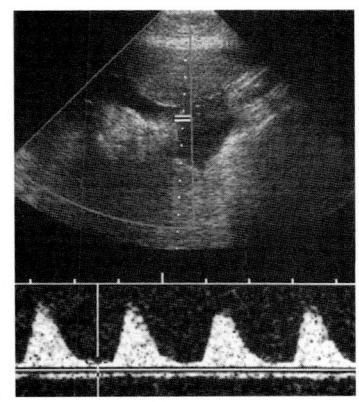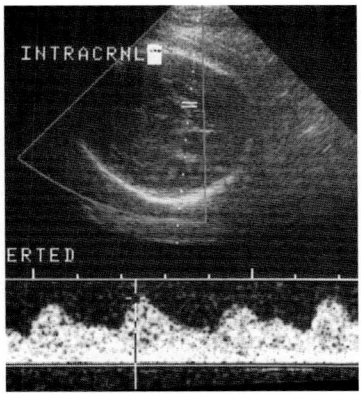

FIGURE 36. Growth restriction and trisomy 21. A 37-year-old patient presents at 36 weeks with significant fetal growth restriction (estimated weight in the first percentile) and normal amniotic fluid. **A:** Umbilical artery Doppler image shows an abnormally high systolic to diastolic ratio of 10. **B:** Intracranial Doppler image of the middle cerebral artery shows an abnormally low ratio of 1.9. No other abnormalities were identified. The infant was found to have trisomy 21 at birth.

characteristic asymmetric IUGR with small body relative to the head.

The onset and severity of IUGR are probably most important in assessing the risk of aneuploidy. Dicke and Crane[283] reported that midtrimester-onset growth delay was evident in 43% of fetuses with trisomy 13 and 59% of fetuses with trisomy 18. We have also encountered fetal trisomy 21 presenting with IUGR and abnormal Doppler studies during the third trimester (Fig. 36).

The combination of IUGR and polyhydramnios also carries a high risk of aneuploidy (see Polyhydramnios, later in this chapter).

Single Umbilical Artery/Umbilical Cord Abnormalities

A single umbilical artery (SUA) has long been of interest because of its association with congenital malformations and chromosomal abnormalities.[284–289] More than 50% of fetuses with trisomy 18 and 10% to 50% of fetuses with trisomy 13 have an SUA. Turner syndrome (45,X), triploidy, and other chromosomal abnormalities also appear to have an increased frequency of SUA over the general population (1%). We have included SUA as a marker because it has no direct significance on the fetus itself and is nonspecific, most commonly seen in normal fetuses.

The risk of a chromosomal abnormality from an SUA clearly depends on the presence of associated anomalies.[290–295] Sohl et al.[202] reported an odds ratio of 10.4 (95% CI, 2.9 to 36.7) for chromosomal abnormality in the presence of an isolated two-vessel cord and 16.4 (95% CI, 1.8 to 150.7) when other anomalies were present. Only those women undergoing amniocentesis were included in this study. As the decision to undergo an invasive test is influenced to some extent by ultrasound findings, this may have introduced bias into the study and produced an elevated prevalence of the markers. As a result, these figures should be interpreted with caution. In another study, Chow et al.[289] evaluated 167 fetuses with SUA and found additional abnormalities in approximately one-third. Five fetuses had abnormal karyotypes and all of these had other anomalies. Among 85 cases with apparently isolated SUA at sonography and known fetal outcome, six (7%) proved to have some anomaly at birth.

Based on available evidence, we believe that identification of an SUA should initiate a search for additional malformations but is not itself an indication for chromosome analysis among low-risk patients. However, patients may be at risk for subtle anomalies at birth.

Umbilical Cord Cysts/Pseudocysts

Umbilical cord pseudocysts have been associated with chromosomal abnormalities.[296] The degree of risk is difficult to determine because of the small number of cases. Smith et al.[296] reviewed 23 reported cases of umbilical cord cysts in the second and third trimesters and found a high association (78%) with lethal chromosomal anomalies, congenital malformations, or both. Among 13 cases reported by Sepulveda et al.[297] additional sonographic findings were noted in 11 and seven had a chromosomal abnormality (five trisomy 18, one trisomy 13, and one inversion).

Placental Abnormalities

Placental abnormalities, such as thickening or cystic changes, may be a clue to an underlying chromosomal

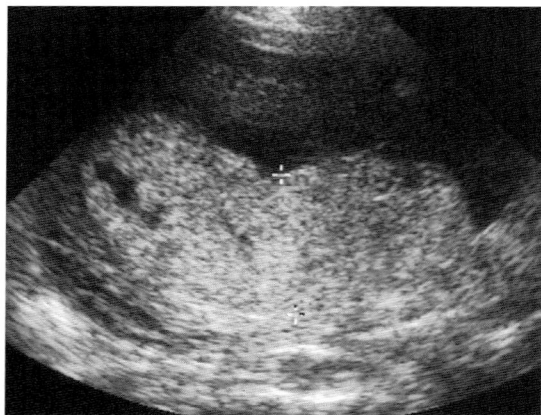

FIGURE 37. Confined placental mosaicism for trisomy 16. A scan at 20 weeks shows mildly thickened (4 cm) and heterogeneous placenta. Intrauterine growth restriction and hyperechoic bowel were also present. The fetus died at 26 weeks.

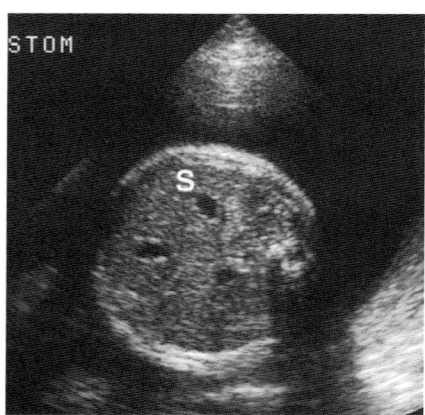

FIGURE 38. Polyhydramnios, growth restriction, and trisomy 18. A scan at 36 weeks showed growth restriction with estimated fetal weight less than the fifth percentile and polyhydramnios. A small fluid-filled stomach (*S*)—thought to reflect decreased fetal swallowing—is also noted. This fetus previously had large choroid plexus cysts, which resolved.

abnormality, particularly triploidy. Placental abnormalities such as intraplacental cystic areas have also been associated with other chromosomal abnormalities, including trisomies 18 and 13 and confined placental mosaicism[298] (Fig. 37). A chromosomal abnormality should therefore be considered when multiple cystic areas are identified in the placenta, especially in association with oligohydramnios or early-onset IUGR. Placental abnormalities also can result in an abnormal systolic/diastolic ratio with umbilical artery Doppler imaging (see Chapter 4).

Nonfusion of the amnion after 14 weeks has been associated with fetal aneuploidy.[299,300]

Abnormal Amniotic Fluid Volume

Polyhydramnios

Polyhydramnios may be the initial or primary manifestation of an underlying fetal disorder, especially during the third trimester.[301–303]

The risk of an underlying anomaly and aneuploidy increases with the severity of polyhydramnios[304,305] (Fig. 38). Barkin et al.[304] reviewed 191 singleton pregnancies complicated by polyhydramnios, including 138 (72%) with mild polyhydramnios and 57 (30%) with severe polyhydramnios. Of the 57 fetuses with severe polyhydramnios, congenital anomalies were found in 43 (75%) and chromosomal abnormalities were found in six (10%). Five of the fetuses with chromosomal abnormalities had other detectable anomalies, and one fetus had ascites only. By comparison, 29% of fetuses with mild polyhydramnios had anomalies, and none of these fetuses had chromosomal abnormalities.

The significance of polyhydramnios is inversely related to fetal size. "Idiopathic" polyhydramnios is most commonly associated with a large-for-gestational-age fetus, with or without maternal diabetes.[306–309] In contrast, fetuses with major chromosomal abnormalities frequently exhibit IUGR. Therefore, it is not surprising that the presence of both polyhydramnios and IUGR has been strongly associated with underlying fetal anomaly and aneuploidy.[310–312] This has been described as an ominous combination by Sickler et al.,[310] who evaluated 39 fetuses with this combination prenatally and found major anomalies after birth in 92%. Among nine fetuses without sonographically detectable prenatal anomalies, six (67%) had one or more anomalies at birth. Chromosomal abnormalities were present in 38% (15 cases) including ten fetuses with trisomy 18 and one with trisomy 13.

The ominous combination of polyhydramnios and IUGR has been confirmed by others. In a series of 67,806 singleton deliveries, Furman et al.[311] reported that 152 neonates had a history of polyhydramnios and were small for gestational age, and 25% of these had anomalies. In a series of 275 singleton pregnancies with polyhydramnios (amniotic fluid index >25), Lazebnik and Many[312] reported anomalies in 54.5% of small-for-gestational-age fetuses compared to 12.7% for average-for-gestational-age fetuses and 10.8% for large-for-gestational-age fetuses (*p* <.001). Multiple logistic analyses confirmed the significance of severe polyhydramnios, small-for-gestational-age status, and preterm delivery as independent contributors to congenital anomalies. In an earlier study that supported genetic amniocentesis based on polyhydramnios, Barnhard et al.[313] reported chromosomal abnormality in two of 49 fetuses with polyhydramnios; however, both of these exhibited IUGR.

TABLE 11. COMPONENTS OF THE SECOND-TRIMESTER "GENETIC SONOGRAM" FOR DETECTION OF FETAL DOWN SYNDROME

Study	Nuchal	Humerus	Femur	Renal	Hyperechoic bowel	Echogenic intracardiac focus	Choroid cysts	Other
Benacerraf et al.[337]	+	+	+	+	+	−	+	−
DeVore[323]	+	−	−	+	+	+	+	+
Nyberg et al.[343]	+	+	+	+	+	+	−	−
Bahado-Singh et al.[325]	+	+	−	−	+	−	+	−
Vergani et al.[239]	+	−	−	−	−	−	−	−
Sohl et al.[202]	+	−	−	−	+	+	+	+
Vintzileos et al.[340]	+	+	+	+	+	+	+	+++

+, utilized; −, not utilized.

Based on available evidence, detection of an associated anomaly or IUGR carries a significant risk for fetal aneuploidy and other anomalies. Marked polyhydramnios should also initiate a careful search for underlying anomalies. We believe that chromosome analysis is not required when "idiopathic" polyhydramnios is present, particularly when the fetus is large for gestational age.

Oligohydramnios

Oligohydramnios may reflect an underlying chromosomal abnormality when seen in association with early-onset IUGR (see Triploidy and Tetraploidy in Chapter 5).

RISK ASSESSMENT

Sonographic Risk Assessment for Down Syndrome

It is clear that ultrasound can modify the risk of fetal aneuploidy based on the presence or absence of ultrasound findings known to be associated with aneuploidy.[335] Detection of even minor markers on second-trimester ultrasonography increases the risk of an abnormal karyotype, whereas the absence of these findings reduces this risk.

The sensitivities of most sonographic markers are low, particularly in comparison to that reported for nuchal translucency in the first trimester. However, the incremental value of each marker improves the overall sensitivity of second-trimester ultrasound so that one or more markers are observed in greater than 50% of fetuses with trisomy 21 (Table 8). When combined with major abnormalities, the overall sensitivity of second-trimester ultrasound at our center is 69%.

The actual sensitivity of a genetic sonogram* depends on various factors including the markers

sought, gestational age, reasons for referral, and quality of the ultrasound. Considering these variables and differences in the types of ultrasound markers used (Table 11), the results from different centers are surprisingly similar (Table 8). Reported detection rates range from 59% to 82%. Detection rates exceeding 90% have even been reported with a high detection rate of cardiac abnormalities.[315]

The risk of fetal trisomy 21 increases exponentially with the number of markers present (Table 12). Two or more markers are detected in nearly one-third of fetuses with trisomy 21 at our center, compared to less than 2% for normal fetuses. In comparison, a single marker is observed in greater than 11% of normal fetuses compared to 22.6% of fetuses with trisomy 21. Similarly, Sohl et al.[202] observed a single marker in 14.6% of normal fetuses. Based on this data, a single marker increases the risk twofold, two markers increase the risk nearly tenfold, and three or more markers increase the risk more than 100-fold. The actual risk depends on the type as well as the number of markers present.

Use of multiple ultrasound markers improves the sensitivity of ultrasound for detection of fetal Down syndrome,

---

*A *genetic sonogram* is defined as an ultrasound that can modify the *a priori* risk of fetal aneuploidy, typically based on a panel of ultrasound markers.

TABLE 12. COMPARISON OF NUMBER OF MARKERS IN FETUSES WITH DOWN SYNDROME AND CONTROL SUBJECTS

Number of markers or major abnormality	Down syndrome, % (186 cases)	Control subjects, % (8,712)	Likelihood ratio[a]
0	31 (58)	86.7 (7,541)	0.36
1	22.6 (42)	11.3 (987)	2.0
2	15.1 (28)	1.5 (136)	9.6
3+	14.5 (27)	0.1 (11)	115
Major abnormality	16.7 (31)	0.4 (37)	39.2

[a]Likelihood ratio = Down syndrome cases (%)/controls (%).

TABLE 13. COMPARISON OF LIKELIHOOD RATIOS REPORTED FOR SONOGRAPHIC MARKERS OF FETAL ANEUPLOIDY

Sonographic marker	Likelihood ratio (95% confidence interval)		
	Nyberg et al.[335]	Bromley et al.[a]	Smith-Bindman et al.[229]
Nuchal thickening	11.0 (5.5–22.0)	12	17 (8–38)
Hyperechoic bowel	6.7 (2.7–16.8)	—	6.1 (3.0–12.6)
Short humerus	5.1 (1.6–16.5)	6	7.5 (4.7–12.0)
Short femur	1.5 (0.8–2.8)	1	2.7 (1.2–6.0)
Echogenic intracardiac focus	1.8 (1.0–3.0)	1.2	2.8 (1.5–5.5)
Pyelectasis	1.5 (0.6–3.6)	1.3	1.9 (0.7–5.1)
Normal ultrasound	0.36	0.2	—

[a]Bromley B, Lieberman E, Shipp T, Benacerraf BR. The genetic sonogram: a method of risk assessment for Down syndrome in the second trimester. *J Ultrasound Med* 2002;21:1087–1096.

but it is also likely to result in a higher false-positive rate. If the presence of any single marker is considered a positive screen, this high false-positive rate can lead to considerable anxiety[316] and inconsistent management[317] among low-risk patients. Sonologists should attempt to minimize these false-positive results among low-risk patients, while maximizing the sensitivity in high-risk patients.

To optimize clinical management of sonographic markers, Benacerraf et al.[336] devised a scoring index system in which 2 points are given for structural abnormalities or nuchal thickening and 1 point is given for other markers. Amniocentesis is offered to those with a score of 2 or more. This approach avoids the false-positive rates from a single marker, except nuchal thickening, which is considered a higher risk, but would lower the sensitivity. The scoring index system has been modified to incorporate maternal age by giving 1 point for maternal age of 35 years or older and 2 points for maternal age of 40 years or more.[318] With this modification, a single sonographic marker is considered a positive screen for higher-risk women aged 35 to 39 years and advanced maternal age alone is a sufficient criterion for women 40 years or older. A primary advantage of the scoring index method is that it is easy to use and understand.

Another method of optimizing ultrasound findings is to integrate the risk of ultrasound markers with the *a priori* risk based on maternal age. This has been termed *age-adjusted ultrasound risk assessment* (AAURA) for Down syndrome. The ultrasound markers are "weighted" by the strength of individual findings, expressed as likelihood ratios. Likelihood ratios have been reported by several authors (Table 13). The *post priori* risk is estimated by the likelihood ratios, and the *a priori* risk is based on maternal age. Table 14 estimates the reduction of risk following a normal ultrasound examination over a wide range of assumed sensitivities of ultrasound for a set false-positive rate. Table 15 estimates the risk of fetal Down syn-

drome based on isolated markers derived from data of Table 13.

Using AAURA, both the sensitivity of fetal Down syndrome detection and the false-positive rate increase with maternal age. This is appropriate because older women desire a high sensitivity, and the clinical alternative is amniocentesis for all women aged 35 years or older (100% false-positive rate). At the same time, AAURA minimizes the false-positive rate for younger women (4% false-positive rate) with a satisfactory sensitivity (61.5%). Very similar results can be obtained with the modified index scoring method, which incorporates maternal age, although AAURA has the advantage of providing a patient-specific risk estimate.[319] Because ultrasound findings appear to be largely independent of both maternal age and biochemical analytes,[320–322] we believe the risk from biochemical screen (serum markers plus maternal age risk) can be substituted for maternal age risk alone, when known.

Reduction of Risk in Women Otherwise Considered High Risk

Increasingly, a normal ultrasound is used to help reduce the risk of Down syndrome for women who otherwise would be considered at risk for fetal trisomy 21.[323–326] Reduction of risk is most useful for women in an intermediate age group, ages 34 to 40 years, or for women with intermediate risk based on biochemical screen (1 in 100 or less). The degree to which the risk is reduced depends on a variety of factors, including the number and type of criteria used, individual thresholds, the gestational age of the scan, and the sensitivity of ultrasound. Despite differences among centers, most recent studies suggest a likelihood ratio in the range of 0.3 to 0.4 after a normal ultrasound. These likelihood ratios correspond to a 60% to 70% reduction of risk. Using a larger number of criteria, or a higher threshold, sensitivity of ultrasound approaching 90% has been

TABLE 14. RISK OF FETAL DOWN SYNDROME, EXPRESSED AS ODDS CATEGORIZED BY MATERNAL AGE AND PRESUMED SENSITIVITY OF ULTRASOUND[a,b]

Maternal age (yr)	Age risk (1:__)	Postultrasound risk (1:__)								
		SU: 10% LR: 1.00	SU: 20% LR: 0.91	SU: 30% LR: 0.80	SU: 40% LR: 0.68	SU: 50% LR: 0.57	SU: 60% LR: 0.45	SU: 70% LR: 0.34	SU: 80% LR: 0.23	SU: 90% LR: 0.11
20	1,176	1,150	1,294	1,478	1,724	2,069	2,586	3,448	5,171	10,341
21	1,160	1,134	1,276	1,458	1,701	2,041	2,551	3,401	5,101	10,200
22	1,136	1,111	1,250	1,428	1,666	1,999	2,498	3,330	4,995	9,989
23	1,114	1,089	1,225	1,400	1,633	1,960	2,450	3,266	4,898	9,795
24	1,087	1,063	1,196	1,366	1,594	1,912	2,390	3,187	4,779	9,558
25	1,040	1,017	1,144	1,307	1,525	1,830	2,287	3,049	4,573	9,144
26	990	968	1,089	1,244	1,452	1,742	2,177	2,902	4,353	8,704
27	928	907	1,021	1,166	1,361	1,633	2,040	2,720	4,080	8,159
28	855	836	940	1,075	1,254	1,504	1,880	2,506	3,759	7,516
29	760	743	836	955	1,114	1,337	1,671	2,227	3,341	6,680
30	690	675	759	867	1,012	1,214	1,517	2,022	3,033	6,064
31	597	584	657	750	875	1,050	1,312	1,749	2,623	5,246
32	508	497	559	638	745	893	1,116	1,488	2,232	4,463
33	421	412	463	529	617	740	925	1,233	1,849	3,697
34	342	334	376	430	501	601	751	1,001	1,501	3,002
35	274	268	301	344	401	481	602	802	1,202	2,403
36	216	211	238	271	316	379	474	632	947	1,893
37	168	164	185	211	246	295	368	491	736	1,471
38	129	126	142	162	189	226	283	376	564	1,127
39	98	96	108	123	143	172	214	286	428	855
40	74	72	81	93	108	129	162	215	322	643
41	56	55	62	70	82	98	122	162	243	485
42	42	41	46	53	61	73	91	121	181	362
43	31	30	34	39	45	54	67	89	133	265
44	23	23	25	29	33	40	49	66	98	195

LR, likelihood ratio; SU, sensitivity of ultrasound.
[a]Note that reduction of risk varies markedly with sensitivity of ultrasound for a set false-positive rate.
[b]Likelihood ratio of normal ultrasound for identification of trisomy 21, calculated as false-negative rate/specificity. False-negative rate = (1 − sensitivity); specificity = (1 − false-positive rate). False-positive rate assumed to be 12% using multiple ultrasound markers.
Adapted from Nyberg DA, Luthy DA, Resta RG, Nyberg BC, Williams MA. Age-adjusted ultrasound risk assessment for fetal Down's syndrome during the second trimester: description of the method and analysis of 142 cases. *Ultrasound Obstet Gynecol* 1998;12:8–14.

reported. Vintzileos et al.[337] use a large number of SMFAs but apply this only to reduce the risk among low-risk patients.

Comparison of Ultrasound and Biochemistry

Surprisingly little data is currently available comparing second-trimester ultrasound with second-trimester biochemistry.[320–322,327,328] The reported sensitivity for Down syndrome at high-risk centers appears to be similar to that of second-trimester biochemistry. Considering the maternal age distribution at the high-risk centers that have reported results, the false-positive results of ultrasound are also similar to biochemistry. One difference is that serum biochemistry can reduce the risk by much more than a normal ultrasound can. Biochemistry is also more widely available than high-quality ultrasound.

A combined risk using both ultrasound and biochemistry could be more effective and less confusing than competing results from each. To date, however, few studies have evaluated the effectiveness of combining ultrasound and biochemistry in the second trimester,[329,330] even though a large number of papers address this combined risk for the first trimester. It now seems clear that the combination of ultrasound and biochemistry is more effective than either one alone. Roberts et al.[331] found that ultrasound improved detection from 65% to 80%. Bahado-Singh et al.[332] have shown that incorporation of humerus length and nuchal thickness measurements improves the receiver operator curves for biochemical risk assessment, and the addition of other markers, especially nuchal thickening, are expected to further improve combined screening. Addition of inhibin to the standard triple test is expected to further increase detection rates during the second trimester.[333,334]

It is anticipated that a sensitivity of at least 85% and false-positive rate of 5% can be achieved with a combination of ultrasound markers and biochemistry. Optimal risk assessment requires computer calculations based on specific measurements (nuchal thickening, limb length, etc.). How first-trimester screening will be integrated with second-trimester screening remains to be determined.

TABLE 15. MATERNAL AGE–SPECIFIC ODDS OF FETAL DOWN SYNDROME DURING THE SECOND TRIMESTER BASED ON SONOGRAPHIC MARKERS OF FETAL ANEUPLOIDY[a]

Maternal age (yr)	Before ultrasound	Normal ultrasound (LR 0.36)	Nuchal thickness (LR 11)	Hyperechoic bowel (LR 6.7)	Short femur length (LR 1.5)	Short humerus length (LR 5.1)	Echogenic intracardiac foci (LR 1.8)	Renal pelvis (LR 1.5)
				Odds[b] (1:___)				
20	1,176	3,265	108	176	784	231	654	784
21	1,160	3,220	106	174	774	228	645	774
22	1,136	3,154	104	170	758	224	632	758
23	1,114	3,093	102	167	743	219	619	743
24	1,087	3,018	100	163	725	214	604	725
25	1,040	2,887	95	156	694	205	578	694
26	990	2,748	91	149	660	195	550	660
27	928	2,576	85	139	619	183	516	619
28	855	2,373	79	128	570	168	475	570
29	760	2,109	70	114	507	150	423	507
30	690	1,915	64	104	460	136	384	460
31	597	1,657	55	90	398	118	332	398
32	508	1,409	47	77	339	100	283	339
33	421	1,168	39	64	281	83	234	281
34	342	948	32	52	228	68	190	228
35	274	759	26	42	183	55	153	183
36	216	598	21	33	144	43	120	144
37	168	465	16	26	112	34	94	112
38	129	357	13	20	86	26	72	86
39	98	270	10	15	66	20	55	66
40	74	204	8	12	50	15	42	50
41	56	154	6	9	38	12	32	38
42	42	115	5	7	28	9	24	28
43	31	84	4	5	21	7	18	21
44	23	62	3	4	16	5	13	16

[a]Using likelihood ratios of Nyberg et al. in Table 8.
[b]Odds ratios based on formula: Odds for Down syndrome = (odds for maternal age)/LR + 1 − 1/LR, where LR is the likelihood ratio.
Data from Nyberg DA, Souter VL, El-Bastawissi A, Young S, Luthhardt F, Luthy DA. Isolated sonographic markers for detection of fetal Down syndrome in the second trimester of pregnancy. *J Ultrasound Med* 2001;20(10):1053–1063.

REFERENCES

1. Hook EB, Hamerton JL. The frequency of chromosome abnormalities detected in consecutive newborn studies—differences between studies—results by sex and severity of phenotypic involvement. In: Hook EB, Porter IH, eds. *Population cytogenetics: studies in humans: proceedings of a Symposium on Human Population Cytogenetics sponsored by the Birth Defects Institute of the New York State Department of Health, held in Albany, New York, October 14–15, 1975.* New York: Academic Press, 1977:63–79.

2. Nielsen J, Wohlert M. Chromosome abnormalities found among 34,910 newborn children: results from a 13-year incidence study in Arhus, Denmark. *Hum Genet* 1991;87:81–83.

3. Ferguson-Smith MA, Yates JRW. Maternal age specific rates for chromosome aberrations and factors influencing them: report of a collaborative European study on 52,965 amniocenteses. *Prenat Diagn* 1984;4:5–44.

4. Munne S, Sultan KM, Weier HU. Assessment of numeric chromosome abnormalities of X, Y, 18 and 16 chromosomes in preimplantation human embryos before transfer. *Am J Obstet Gynecol* 1995;172:1191–1199.

5. Snijders RJ, Sundberg K, Holzgreve W, Henry G, Nicolaides KH. Maternal age– and gestation-specific risk for trisomy 21. *Ultrasound Obstet Gynecol* 1999;13(3):167–170.

6. Hastings RJ, Nisbet DL, Waters K, Spencer T, Chitty LS. Prenatal detection of extra structurally abnormal chromosomes (ESACs): new cases and a review of the literature. *Prenat Diagn* 1999;19:436–445.

7. Li MM, Howard-Peebles PN, Killos LD, Fallon L, Listgarten E, Stanley WS. Characterization and clinical implications of marker chromosomes identified at prenatal diagnosis. *Prenat Diagn* 2000;20:138–143.

8. Warburton D. De novo balanced chromosome rearrangements and extra marker chromosomes identified at prenatal

diagnosis: clinical significance and distribution of breakpoints. *Am J Hum Genet* 1991;49:995–1013.

9. Crolla JA, Long F, Rivera H, Dennis NR. FISH and molecular study of autosomal supernumerary marker chromosomes 15 and 22: I. Results of 26 new cases. *Am J Med Genet* 1998;75:355–366.

10. Hahnemann JM, Vejerslev LO. Accuracy of cytogenetic findings on chorionic villus sampling (CVS)—diagnostic consequences of CVS mosaicism and non-mosaic discrepancy in centres contributing to EUCROMIC 1986–1992. *Prenat Diagn* 1997;17(9):801–820.

11. Kalousek DK. Confined placental mosaicism and genomic imprinting. *Bailliere's Clin Obstet Gynaecol* 2000;14(4):723–730.

12. Knight SJL, Flint J. Perfect endings: a review of subtelomeric probes and their use in clinical diagnosis. *J Med Genet* 2000;37:401–409.

13. Kilby MD, Brackley KJ, Walters JJ, Morton J, Roberts E, Davison EV. First-trimester prenatal diagnosis of a familial subtelomeric translocation. *Ultrasound Obstet Gynecol* 2001; 17:531–533.

14. Hook ES. Chromosome abnormalities and spontaneous fetal death following amniocentesis: further data and associations with maternal age. *Am J Hum Genet* 1983;35:110–116.

15. Hook ES. Spontaneous deaths of fetuses with chromosomal abnormalities diagnosed prenatally. *N Engl J Med* 1978;299:1036–1038.

16. Simpson JL, Golbus MS, Martin AO, et al. *Genetics in obstetrics and gynecology*. Philadelphia: Grune & Stratton, 1982.

17. Petrini J, Damus K, Johnston RB Jr. An overview of infant mortality and birth defects in the United States. *Teratology* 1997;56(1–2):8–10.

18. Hayes C, Johnson Z, Thornton L, Fogarty J, Lyons R, et al. Ten-year survival of Down syndrome births. *Int J Epidemiol* 1997;26(4):822–829.

19. Leonard S, Bower C, Petterson B, Leonard H. Survival of infants born with Down's syndrome: 1980–96. *Paediatr Perinat Epidemiol* 2000;14(2):163–171.

20. Knight SJL, Regan R, Nicod A, Horsley SW, Kearney L, et al. Subtle chromosome rearrangements in children with unexplained mental retardation. *Lancet* 1999;354:1676.

21. Benn P. Trisomy 16 and trisomy 16 mosaicism: a review. *Am J Med Genet* 1998;79:121–133.

22. Schneider AS, Mennuti MT, Zacki EH. High caesarean section rate in trisomy 18 births: a potential indication for late prenatal diagnosis. *Am J Obstet Gynecol* 1981;140:367–370.

23. Jalbert P. Down's syndrome incidence and paternal age. *Down's Screening News* 1995;3:5.

24. Lansac J, Thepot F, Mayaux MJ, Czyglick F, Wack T, et al. Pregnancy outcome after artificial insemination or IVF with frozen semen donor: a collaborative study of the French CECOS Federation on 21597 pregnancies. *Eur J Obstet Gynecol Reprod Biol* 1997;74:223–228.

25. Egan JF, Benn P, Borgida AF, Rodis JF, Campbell WA, Vintzileos AM. Efficacy of screening for fetal Down syndrome in the United States from 1974 to 1997. *Obstet Gynecol* 2000;96(6):979–985.

26. Tolmie JL. Down syndrome and other autosomal trisomies. In: Rimoin DL, Connor MJ, Pyeritz RE, eds. *Emery and Rimoin's principles and practice of medical genetics*, 3rd ed. New York: Churchill Livingstone, 1997:944.

27. Uehara S, Yaegashi N, Maeda T, Hoshi N, Fujimoto S, et al. Risk of recurrence of fetal chromosomal aberrations: analysis of trisomy 21, trisomy 18, trisomy 13, and 45,X in 1,076 Japanese mothers. *J Obstet Gynaecol Res* 1999;25:373–379.

28. Harris DJ, Begleiter ML, Chamberlin J, Hankins L, Magenis RE. Parental trisomy 21 mosaicism. *Am J Hum Genet* 1982;34(1):125–133.

29. James RS, Ellis K, Pettay D, Jacobs PA. Cytogenetic and molecular study of four couples with multiple trisomy 21 pregnancies. *Eur J Hum Genet* 1998;6(3):207–212.

30. Bruyere H, Rupps R, Kuchinka BD, Friedman JM, Robinson WP. Recurrent trisomy 21 in a couple with a child presenting trisomy 21 mosaicism and maternal uniparental disomy for chromosome 21 in the euploid cell line. *Am J Med Genet* 2000;94(1):35–41.

31. Verloes A, Gillerot Y, Van Maldergem L, Schoos R, Herens C, et al. Major decrease in the incidence of trisomy 21 at birth in South Belgium: mass impact of triple test? *Eur J Hum Genet* 2001;9:1–4.

32. Merkatz IR, Nitowsky HM, Macri JN, Johnson WE. An association between low maternal serum alpha-fetoprotein and fetal chromosome abnormalities. *Am J Obstet Gynecol* 1984;148:886–894.

33. Wald NJ, Cuckle HS, Densem JW, Nanchahal K, Royston P, et al. Maternal serum screening for Down's syndrome in early pregnancy. *BMJ* 1988;297:883–887.

34. Haddow JE, Palomaki GE, Knight GJ, Cunningham GC, Lustig LS, Boyd PA. Reducing the need for amniocentesis in women 35 years of age or older with serum markers for screening. *N Engl J Med* 1994;330(16):1114–1118.

35. Kaminsky L, Egan J, Ying J, Borgida A, De Roche M, Benn P. Combined second trimester biochemical and ultrasonographic screening for Down syndrome is highly effective. *Am J Obstet Gynecol* 2001;185(6):S78.

36. Williamson RA, Weiner CP, Patil S, Benda J, Varner MW, Abu-Yousef MM. Abnormal pregnancy sonogram: selective indication for fetal karyotype. *Obstet Gynecol* 1987;69:15–20.

37. Wladimiroff JW, Sachs ES, Reuss A, Stewart PA, Pijpers L, Niermeijer MF. Prenatal diagnosis of chromosome abnormalities in the presence of fetal structural defects. *Am J Med Genet* 1988;29:289–291.

38. Nicolaides KH, Rodeck CH, Gosden CM. Rapid karyotyping in nonlethal fetal malformations. *Lancet* 1986;1:283–287.

39. Hegge FN, Prescott GH, Watson PT. Sonography at the time of genetic amniocentesis to screen for fetal malformations. *Obstet Gynecol* 1988;71:522–525.

40. Nicolaides KH, Snijders RJ, Gosden CM, Berry C, Campbell S. Ultrasonographically detectable markers of fetal chromosomal abnormalities. *Lancet* 1992;340(8821):704–707.

41. Nyberg DA, Souter VL. Ultrasound markers of fetal aneuploidy. In: Clinics in perinatology. Congenital anomalies. Malone F, D'Alton M, eds. 2000;27(4):761–789.

42. Nyberg DA, Souter VL. Sonographic markers of fetal trisomies: second trimester. *J Ultrasound Med* 2001;20(6):655–674.

43. Isaksen CV, Eik-Nes SH, Blaas HG, Torp SH, Van Der Hagen CB, Ormerod E. A correlative study of prenatal ultrasound and post-mortem findings in fetuses and infants with an abnormal karyotype. *Ultrasound Obstet Gynecol* 2000;16(1):37–45.

44. Stoll C, Dott B, Alembik Y, Roth MP. Evaluation of routine prenatal ultrasound examination in detecting fetal chromosomal abnormalities in a low risk population. *Hum Genet* 1993;91(1):37–41.

45. Bullen PJ, Rankin JM, Robson SC. Investigation of the epidemiology and prenatal diagnosis of holoprosencephaly in the North of England. *Am J Obstet Gynecol* 2001;184:1256–1262.

46. Cohen MM. An update on the holoprosencephalic disorders. *J Pediatr* 1982;101:865–869.

47. Nyberg DA, Mack LA, Bronstein A, Hirsch J, Pagon RA. Holoprosencephaly: prenatal sonographic diagnosis. *AJR Am J Roentgenol* 1987;149:1050–1058.

48. Pilu G, Romero R, Rizzo N, Jeanty P, Bovicelli L, Hobbins JC. Criteria for the prenatal diagnosis of holoprosencephaly. *Am J Perinatol* 1987;4:41–49.

49. McGahan JP, Nyberg DA, Mack LA. Sonography of facial features of alobar and semilobar holoprosencephaly. *AJR Am J Roentgenol* 1990;154(1):143–148.

50. Murray J, Johnson J, Bird T. Dandy-Walker malformation: etiologic heterogeneity and empiric recurrence risks. *Clin Genet* 1985;28:272–283.

51. Pilu G, Romero R, De Palma L, Rizzo N, Jeanty P, et al. Antenatal diagnosis and obstetric management of Dandy-Walker syndrome. *J Reprod Med* 1986;31:1017–1022.

52. Norman RM. Neuropathological findings in trisomies 13–15 and 17–18 with special reference to the cerebellum. *Dev Med Child Neurol* 1966;8:170–177.

53. Passarge E, True CW, Sueoka WT, Baumgartner NR, Keer KR. Malformations of the central nervous system in trisomy 18 syndrome. *J Pediatr* 1966;69:771–778.

54. Sumi SM. Brain malformations in the trisomy 18 syndrome. *Brain* 1970;93:821–830.

55. Kolble N, Wisser J, Kurmanavicius J, Bolthauser E, Stallmach T, et al. Dandy-Walker malformation: prenatal diagnosis and outcome. *Prenat Diagn* 2000;20(4):318–327.

56. Nyberg DA, Cyr DR, Mack LA, Fitzsimmons J, Hickok D, Mahony BS. The Dandy-Walker malformation: prenatal sonographic diagnosis and its clinical significance. *J Ultrasound Med* 1988;7:65–71.

57. Nyberg DA, Mahony BS, Hegge FN, Hickok D, Luthy DA, Kapur R. Enlarged cisterna magna and the Dandy-Walker malformation: factors associated with chromosome abnormalities. *Obstet Gynecol* 1991;77(3):436–442.

58. Chang MC, Russell SA, Callen PW, Filly RA, Goldstein RB. Sonographic detection of inferior vermian agenesis in Dandy-Walker malformations: prognostic implications. *Radiology* 1994;193(3):765–770.

59. Ecker JL, Shipp TD, Bromley B, Benacerraf B. The sonographic diagnosis of Dandy-Walker and Dandy-Walker variant: associated findings and outcomes. *Prenat Diagn* 2000;20(4):328–332.

60. Ulm B, Ulm MR, Deutinger J, Bernaschek G. Dandy-Walker malformation diagnosed before 21 weeks of gestation: associated malformations and chromosomal abnormalities. *Ultrasound Obstet Gynecol* 1997;10(3):167–170.

61. Chen CP, Hung TH, Jan SW, Jeng CJ. Enlarged cisterna magna in the third trimester as a clue to fetal trisomy 18. *Fetal Diagn Ther* 1998;13(1):29–34.

62. Watson WJ, Katz VL, Chescheir NC, Miller RC, Menard MK, Hansen WF. The cisterna magna in second-trimester fetuses with abnormal karyotypes. *Obstet Gynecol* 1992;79(5 Pt 1):723–725.

63. Steiger RM, Porto M, Lagrew DC, Randall R. Biometry of the fetal cisterna magna: estimates of the ability to detect trisomy 18. *Ultrasound Obstet Gynecol* 1995;5(6):384–390.

64. Haimovici JA, Doubilet PM, Benson CB, Frates MC. Clinical significance of isolated enlargement of the cisterna magna (>10 mm) on prenatal sonography. *J Ultrasound Med* 1997;16(11):731–734.

65. Ek S, Anadakumar C, Wong YC, Chau TM, Gole LA, Malarvishy G. Enlargement of cisterna magna as an indicator of chromosomal abnormalities in a low-risk Asian population. *J Perinat Med* 1998;26(4):325–327.

66. Chervenak FA, Goldberg JD, Chiu TH, Gilbert F, Berkowitz RL. The importance of karyotype determination in a fetus with ventriculomegaly and spina bifida discovered during the third trimester. *J Ultrasound Med* 1986;5:405–406.

67. Nyberg DA, Mack LA, Hirsch J, Pagon RO, Shepard TH. Fetal hydrocephalus: sonographic detection and clinical significance of associated anomalies. *Radiology* 1987;163:187–191.

68. Williamson RA, Schauberger CW, Varner MW, Aschenbrener CA. Heterogeneity of prenatal onset hydrocephalus: management and counseling implications. *Am J Med Genet* 1984;17:497–508.

69. Levitsky DB, Mack LA, Nyberg DA, Shurtleff DB, Shields LA, et al. Fetal aqueductal stenosis diagnosed sonographically: how grave is the prognosis? *AJR Am J Roentgenol* 1995;164(3):725–730.

70. Nyberg DA, Shepard T, Mack LA, Hirsch J, Luthy D, Fitzsimmons J. Significance of a single umbilical artery in fetuses with central nervous system malformations. *J Ultrasound Med* 1988;7:265–273.

71. Babcook CJ, Goldstein RB, Filly RA. Prenatally detected fetal myelomeningocele: is karyotype analysis warranted? *Radiology* 1995;194(2):491–494.

72. Jeret JS, Serur D, Wisenieski KE, Lubin RA. Clinicopathological findings associated with agenesis of the corpus callosum. *Brain Dev* 1987;9:255–264.

73. Bertino RE, Nyberg DA, Cyr DR, Mack LA. Prenatal diagnosis of agenesis of the corpus callosum. *J Ultrasound Med* 1987;7:251–260.

74. Comstock CH, Culp D, Gonzalez J, Boal DB. Agenesis of the corpus callosum in the fetus: its evolution and significance. *J Ultrasound Med* 1985;4:613–616.

75. Gupta JK, Lilford RJ. Assessment and management of agenesis of the corpus callosum. *Prenat Diagn* 1995;15:301–312.

76. Goodyear PW, Bannister CM, Russel S, Rimmer S. Outcome in prenatally diagnosed fetal agenesis of the corpus callosum. *Fetal Diagn Ther* 2001;16:139–145.

77. Bennett GL, Bromley B, Benacerraf BR. Agenesis of the corpus callosum: prenatal detection usually is not possible before 22 weeks of gestation. *Radiology* 1996;199(2):447–450.

78. Lopoo JB, Hedrick MH, Chasen S, Montgomery L, Chervenak FA, et al. Natural history of fetuses with cleft lip. *Plast Reconstr Surg* 1999;103(1):34–38.

79. Benacerraf BR, Mulliken JB. Fetal cleft lip and palate: sonographic diagnosis and postnatal outcome. *Plast Reconstr Surg* 1993;92(6):1045–1051.

80. Hegge FN, Prescott GH, Watson PT. Fetal facial abnormalities identified during obstetric sonography. *J Ultrasound Med* 1986;5:679–684.

81. Nyberg DA, Mahony BS, Kramer D. Paranasal echogenic mass: sonographic sign of bilateral complete cleft lip and palate before 20 menstrual weeks. *Radiology* 1992;184(3): 757–759.

82. Saltzman DH, Benacerraf BR, Frigoletto FD. Diagnosis and management of fetal facial clefts. *Am J Obstet Gynecol* 1986;155:377–379.

83. Nyberg DA, Sickler GK, Hegge FN, Kramer DJ, Kropp RJ. Fetal cleft lip with and without cleft palate: US classification and correlation with outcome. *Radiology* 1995;195(3):677–684.

84. Berge SJ, Plath H, Van de Vondel PT, Appel T, Niederhagen B, et al. Fetal cleft lip and palate: sonographic diagnosis, chromosomal abnormalities, associated anomalies and postnatal outcome in 70 fetuses. *Ultrasound Obstet Gynecol* 2001;18:422–431.

85. Stoll C, Dott B, Alembik Y, Roth M. Evaluation of prenatal diagnosis of cleft lip/palate by foetal ultrasonographic examination. *Ann Genet* 2000;43(1):11–14.

86. Walker SJ, Ball RH, Babcook CJ, Feldkamp MM. Prevalence of aneuploidy and additional anatomic abnormalities in fetuses and neonates with cleft lip with or without cleft palate. *J Ultrasound Med* 2001;20:1175–1180.

87. Benacerraf BR, Frigoletto FD Jr, Green MF. Abnormal facial features and extremities in human trisomy syndromes: prenatal US appearance. *Radiology* 1986;159:243–246.

88. Lettieri L, Rodis JF, Vintzileos AM, Feeney L, Ciarleglio L, Craffey A. Ear length in second-trimester aneuploid fetuses. *Obstet Gynecol* 1993;81(1):57–60.

89. Aase JM, Wilson AC, Smith DW. Small ears in Down's syndrome: a helpful diagnostic aid. *J Pediatr* 1973;82(5):845–847.

90. Birnholz JC, Farrell EE. Fetal ear length. *Pediatrics* 1988;81:555–558.

91. Lettieri L, Rodis JF, Vintzileos AM, Feeney L, Ciarleglio L, Craffey A. Ear length in second-trimester aneuploid fetuses. *Obstet Gynecol* 1993;81(1):57–60.

92. Awwad JT, Azar GB, Karam KS, Nicolaides KH. Ear length: a potential sonographic marker for Down syndrome. *Int J Gynaecol Obstet* 1994;44(3):233–238.

93. Gill P, Vanhook J, Fitzsimmons J, Pascoe-Mason J, Fantel A. Fetal ear measurements in the prenatal detection of trisomy 21. *Prenat Diagn* 1994;14(8):739–743.

94. Chitkara U, Lee L, Oehlert JW, Block DA, Holbrook RH Jr, et al. Fetal ear length measurement: a useful predictor of aneuploidy? *Ultrasound Obstet Gynecol* 2002;19:131–135.

95. Shimizu T, Salvador L, Hughes-Benzie R, Dawson L, Nimrod C, Allanson J. The role of reduced ear size in the prenatal detection of chromosomal abnormalities. *Prenat Diagn* 1997;17(6):545–549.

96. Shih JC, Shyu MK, Lee CN, Wu CH, Lin GJ, Hsieh FJ. Antenatal depiction of the fetal ear with three-dimensional ultrasonography. *Obstet Gynecol* 1998;91(4):500–505.

97. Bronshtein M, Blumenfeld I, Zimmer EZ, Ben-Ami M, Blumenfeld Z. Prenatal sonographic diagnosis of nasal malformations. *Prenat Diagn* 1998;18(5):447–454.

98. Pinette MG, Blackstone J, Pan Y, Pinette SG. Measurement of fetal nasal width by ultrasonography. *Am J Obstet Gynecol* 1997;177(4):842–845.

99. Cicero S, Curcio P, Papageorghiou A, Sonek J, Nicolaides K. Absence of nasal bone in fetuses with trisomy 21 at 11–14 weeks of gestation: an observational study. *Lancet* 2001;358(9294):1665–1667.

100. Sonek JD, Nicolaides KH. Prenatal ultrasonographic diagnosis of nasal bone abnormalities in fetuses with Down syndrome. *Am J Obstet Gynecol* 2002;186(1):139–141.

101. Stempfle N, Huten Y, Fredoulle C, Brisse H, Nessman C. Skeletal abnormalities in fetuses with Down's syndrome: a radiographic postmortem study. *Pediatr Radiol* 1999;29(9): 682–688.

102. Pearce JM, Griffin D, Campbell S. Cystic hygromata in trisomy 18 and 21. *Prenat Diagn* 1984;4:371–375.

103. Redford DH, McNay MB, Ferguson-Smith ME, Jamieson ME. Aneuploidy and cystic hygroma detectable by ultrasound. *Prenat Diagn* 1984;4:327–328.

104. Carr RF, Ochs RH, Ritter DA, Kenny JD, Fridey JL, Ming PM. Fetal cystic hygroma and Turner's syndrome. *Am J Dis Child* 1986;140:580.

105. Ville Y, Lalondrelle C, Doumerc S, Daffos F, Frydman R, et al. First-trimester diagnosis of nuchal anomalies: significance and outcome. *Ultrasound Obstet Gynecol* 1992;2:314–316.

106. Malone FD, Ball BH, Nyberg DA, Gross SJ, Comstock CH, et al. First trimester cystic hygroma—a population based screening study (the FASTER trial). *Am J Obstet Gynecol* 2001;185(6):S99.

107. Holzgreve W, Curry CJ, Golbus MS, Callen PW, Filly RA, Smith JC. Investigation of nonimmune hydrops fetalis. *Am J Obstet Gynecol* 1984;150:805–812.

108. Petrikovsky BM, Shmoys SM, Baker DA, Monheit AG. Pleural effusion in aneuploidy. *Am J Perinatol* 1991;8(3): 214–216.

109. Hagay Z, Reece A, Roberts A, Hobbins JC. Isolated fetal pleural effusion: a prenatal management dilemma. *Obstet Gynecol* 1993;81(1):147–152.

110. Blott M, Nicolaides KH, Greenough A. Pleuroamniotic shunting for decompression of fetal pleural effusions. *Obstet Gynecol* 1988;71:798–800.

111. Rodeck CH, Fisk NM, Fraser DI, Nicolini U. Long-term in utero drainage of fetal hydrothorax. *N Engl J Med* 1988;310:1135–1138.

112. Zelop C, Benacerraf BR. The causes and natural history of fetal ascites. *Prenat Diagn* 1994;14(10):941–946.

113. Matsuoka R, Misugi K, Goto A, Gilbert EF, Ando M. Congenital heart anomalies in the trisomy 18 syndrome, with reference to congenital polyvalvular disease. *Am J Med Genet* 1983;14:657–668.

114. Wladimiroff JW, Stewart PA, Sachs ES, Niermeijer MF. Prenatal diagnosis and management of congenital heart defect: significance of associated fetal anomalies and prenatal chromosome studies. *Am J Med Genet* 1985;21:285–290.

115. Berg KA, Clark EB, Astemborski JA, Boughman JA. Prenatal detection of cardiovascular malformations by echocardiography: an indication for cytogenetic evaluation. *Am J Obstet Gynecol* 1988;159:477–481.

116. Copel JA, Cullen M, Green JJ, Mahoney MJ, Hobbins JC, Kleinman CS. The frequency of aneuploidy in prenatally diagnosed congenital heart disease: an indication for fetal karyotyping. *Am J Obstet Gynecol* 1988;158:409–413.

117. Ferencz C, Rubin JD, McCarter RJ, Boughman JA, Wilson PD, et al. Cardiac and noncardiac malformations: observations in a population based study. *Teratology* 1987;35:367–378.

118. Chaoui R, Korner H, Bommer C, Goldner B, Bierlich A, Bollmann R. [Prenatal diagnosis of heart defects and associated chromosomal aberrations]. *Ultraschall Med* 1999;20(5):177–184.

119. Benacerraf BR, Pober BR, Sanders SP. Accuracy of fetal echocardiography. *Radiology* 1987;165:847–849.

120. Crawford DC, Chita SK, Allan LD. Prenatal detection of congenital heart disease: factors affecting obstetric management and survival. *Am J Obstet Gynecol* 1988;159:352–356.

121. Copel JA, Pilu G, Kleinman CS. Congenital heart disease and extracardiac anomalies: associations and indications for fetal echocardiography. *Am J Obstet Gynecol* 1986;154:1121–1132.

122. Huggon IC, Cook AC, Smeeton NC, Magee AG, Sharland GK. Atrioventricular septal defects diagnosed in fetal life: associated cardiac and extra-cardiac abnormalities and outcome. *J Am Coll Cardiol* 2000;36(2):593–601.

123. Delisle MF, Sandor GG, Tessier F, Farquharson DF. Outcome of fetuses diagnosed with atrioventricular septal defect. *Obstet Gynecol* 1999;94(5 Pt 1):763–767.

124. Brown DL, Emerson DS, Shulman LP, Doubilet PM, Felker RE, Van Praagh S. Predicting aneuploidy in fetuses with cardiac anomalies: significance of visceral situs and noncardiac anomalies. *J Ultrasound Med* 1993;12(3):153–161.

125. Benjamin DR, Juul S, Siebert JR. Congenital posterolateral diaphragmatic hernia: associated malformations. *J Pediatr Surg* 1988;23:899–903.

126. Puri P, Gorman F. Lethal non-pulmonary anomalies associated with congenital diaphragmatic hernia: implications for early intra-uterine surgery. *J Pediatr Surg* 1984;19:29–32.

127. Benacerraf BR, Adzick NS. Fetal diaphragmatic hernia: ultrasound diagnosis and clinical outcome in 19 cases. *Am J Obstet Gynecol* 1987;156:573–576.

128. Dillon E, Renwick M, Wright C. Congenital diaphragmatic herniation: antenatal detection and outcome. *Br J Radiol* 2000;73(868):360–365.

129. Kaiser JR, Rosenfeld CR. A population-based study of congenital diaphragmatic hernia: impact of associated anomalies and preoperative blood gases on survival. *J Pediatr Surg* 1999;34(8):1196–1202.

130. Hsieh YY, Chang FC, Tsai HD, Hsu TY, Yang TC. Accuracy of sonography in predicting the outcome of fetal congenital diaphragmatic hernia. *Chung Hua I Hsueh Tsa Chih (Taipei)* 2000;63(10):751–757.

131. Thorpe-Beeston JG, Gosden CM, Nicolaides KH. Prenatal diagnosis of congenital diaphragmatic hernia: associated malformations and chromosomal defects. *Fetal Ther* 1989;4(1):21–28.

132. Bollmann R, Kalache K, Mau H, Chaoui R, Tennstedt C. Associated malformations and chromosomal defects in congenital diaphragmatic hernia. *Fetal Diagn Ther* 1995;10(1):52–59.

133. Howe DT, Kilby MD, Sirry H, Barker GM, Roberts E, et al. Structural chromosome anomalies in congenital diaphragmatic hernia. *Prenat Diagn* 1996;16(11):1003–1009.

134. Fonkalsrud EW, DeLorimier AA, Hays DM. Congenital atresia and stenosis of the duodenum. A review compiled from the members of the Surgical Section of the American Academy of Pediatrics. *Pediatrics* 1969;43:79–83.

135. Romero R, Ghidini A, Costigan K, Touloukian R, Hobbins JC. Prenatal diagnosis of duodenal atresia: does it make any difference? *Obstet Gynecol* 1988;71:739–741.

136. Lawrence MJ, Ford WD, Furness ME, Hayward T, Wilson T. Congenital duodenal obstruction: early antenatal ultrasound diagnosis. *Pediatr Surg Int* 2000;16(5–6):342–345.

137. Mabogunje OOA, Mahour GH. Omphalocele and gastroschisis: trends in survival across two decades. *Am J Surg* 1984;148:679–686.

138. Skupski DW. Prenatal diagnosis of gastrointestinal anomalies with ultrasound. What have we learned? *Ann N Y Acad Sci* 1998;847:53–58.

139. Rankin J, Dillon E, Wright C. Congenital anterior abdominal wall defects in the north of England, 1986–1996: occurrence and outcome. *Prenat Diagn* 1999;19(7):662–668.

140. Kilby MD, Lander A, Usher-Somers M. Exomphalos. *Prenat Diagn* 1998;18(12):1283–1288.

141. Gilbert WM, Nicolaides KH. Fetal omphalocele: associated malformations and chromosomal defects. *Obstet Gynecol* 1987;70:633–635.

142. Snijders RJ, Sebire NJ, Souka A, Santiago C, Nicolaides KH. Fetal exomphalos and chromosomal defects: relationship to maternal age and gestation. *Ultrasound Obstet Gynecol* 1995;6(4):250–255.

143. Hughes MD, Nyberg DA, Mack LA, Pretorius DH. Fetal omphalocele: prenatal detection of concurrent anomalies and other predictors of outcome. *Radiology* 1989;173(2):371–376.

144. Nyberg DA, Fitzsimmons J, Mack LA, Hughes M, Pretorius DH, et al. Chromosomal abnormalities in fetuses with omphalocele: the significance of omphalocele contents. *J Ultrasound Med* 1989;8:299–308.

145. Benacerraf BR, Saltzman DH, Estroff JA, Frigoletto FD Jr. Abnormal karyotype of fetuses with omphalocele: prediction based on omphalocele contents. *Obstet Gynecol* 1990;75(3 Pt 1):317–319.

146. Getachew MM, Goldstein RB, Edge V, Goldberg JD, Filly RA. Correlation between omphalocele contents and karyotypic abnormalities: sonographic study in 37 cases. *AJR Am J Roentgenol* 1992;158(1):133–136.

147. De Veciana M, Major CA, Porto M. Prediction of an abnormal karyotype in fetuses with omphalocele. *Prenat Diagn* 1994;14(6):487–492.

148. St-Vil D, Shaw KS, Lallier M, Yazbeck S, Di Lorenzo M, et al. Chromosomal anomalies in newborns with omphalocele. *J Pediatr Surg* 1996;31(6):831–834.

149. Frydman M, Magenis RE, Mohandas TK, Kaback MM. Chromosome abnormalities in infants with prune belly syndrome: association with trisomy 18. *Am J Med Genet* 1983;15:145–148.

150. McKeown CME, Donnai D. Prune belly in trisomy 13. *Prenat Diagn* 1986;6:379–381.

151. Nevin NC, Nevin J, Dunlop JM, et al. Antenatal diagnosis of grossly distended bladder owing to absence of urethra in a fetus with trisomy 18. *J Med Genet* 1983;20:132–133.

152. Rizzo N, Gabrielli S, Pilu G, et al. Prenatal diagnosis and obstetrical management of multicystic dysplastic kidney disease. *Prenat Diagn* 1987;7:109–118.

153. Appleman Z, Golbus MS. The management of fetal urinary tract obstruction. *Clin Obstet Gynecol* 1986;29:483–489.

154. Benacerraf BR. Antenatal sonographic diagnosis of congenital clubfoot: a possible indication for amniocentesis. *J Clin Ultrasound* 1986;14:703–706.

155. Jeanty P, Romero R, D'Alton M, Venus I, Hobbins JC. In utero sonographic detection of hand and foot deformities. *J Ultrasound Med* 1985;4:595–601.

156. Malone FD, Marino T, Bianchi DW, Johnston K, D'Alton ME. Isolated clubfoot diagnosed prenatally: is karyotyping indicated? *Obstet Gynecol* 2000;95(3):437–440.

157. Shipp TD, Benacerraf BR. The significance of prenatally identified isolated clubfoot: Is amniocentesis indicated? *Am J Obstet Gynecol* 1998;178(3):600–602.

158. Pfeiffer RA, Santelmann R. Limb anomalies in chromosomal aberrations. *Birth Defects* 1977;13:319–337.

159. Christianson AL, Nelson MM. Four cases of trisomy 18 syndrome with limb reduction malformation. *J Med Genet* 1984;21:293.

160. Shields LE, Carpenter LA, Smith KM, Nghiem HV. Ultrasonographic diagnosis of trisomy 18: Is it practical in the early second trimester? *J Ultrasound Med* 1998;17(5):327–331.

161. Paluda SM, Comstock CH, Kirk JS, Lee W, Smith RS. The significance of ultrasonographically diagnosed fetal wrist position anomalies. *Am J Obstet Gynecol* 1996;174(6):1834–1837; discussion 1837–1839.

162. Chudleigh P, Pearce JM, Campbell S. The prenatal diagnosis of transient cysts of the fetal choroid plexus. *Prenat Diagn* 1984;4:135–137.

163. Furness ME. Choroid plexus cysts and trisomy 18. *Lancet* 1987;ii:693.

164. Nadel AS, Bromley BS, Frigoletto FD Jr, Estroff JA, Benacerraf BR. Isolated choroid plexus cysts in the second-trimester fetus: is amniocentesis really indicated? *Radiology* 1992;185(2):545–548.

165. Benacerraf BR, Harlow B, Frigoletto FD Jr. Are choroid plexus cysts an indication for second-trimester amniocentesis? *Am J Obstet Gynecol* 1990;162(4):1001–1006.

166. Reinsch RC. Choroid plexus cysts—association with trisomy: prospective review of 16,059 patients. *Am J Obstet Gynecol* 1997;176(6):1381–1383.

167. Leonardi MR, Wolfe HM, Lanouette JM, Landwehr JB, Johnson MP, Evans MI. The apparently isolated choroid plexus cyst: importance of minor abnormalities in predicting the risk for aneuploidy. *Fetal Diagn Ther* 1998;13(1):49–52.

168. Morcos CL, Platt LD, Carlson DE, Gregory KD, Greene NH, Korst LM. The isolated choroid plexus cyst. *Obstet Gynecol* 1998;92(2):232–236.

169. Gross SJ, Shulman LP, Tolley EA, Emerson DS, Felker RE, et al. Isolated fetal choroid plexus cysts and trisomy 18: a review and meta-analysis. *Am J Obstet Gynecol* 1995;172:83–87.

170. Gupta JK, Cave M, Lilford RJ, Farrell TA, Irving HC, et al. Clinical significance of fetal choroid plexus cysts. *Lancet* 1995;346(8977):724–729.

171. Peleg D, Yankowitz J. Choroid plexus cysts and aneuploidy. *J Med Genet* 1998;35(7):554–557.

172. Walkinshaw SA. Fetal choroid plexus cysts: are we there yet? *Prenat Diagn* 2000;20(8):657–662.

173. Chan L, Hixson JL, Laifer SA, Marchese SG, Martin JG, Hill LM. A sonographic karyotypic study of second-trimester fetal choroid plexus cysts. *Obstet Gynecol* 1989;73:703–706.

174. Chinn DH, Miller EI, Worthy LM, Towers CV. Sonographically detected fetal choroid plexus cysts. Frequency and association with aneuploidy. *J Ultrasound Med* 1991;10(5):255–258.

175. DeRoo TR, Harris RD, Sargent SK, Denholm TA, Crow HC. Fetal choroid plexus cysts: prevalence, clinical significance, and sonographic appearance. *AJR Am J Roentgenol* 1988;151:1179–1181.

176. Ostlere SJ, Irving HC, Lilford RJ. A prospective study of the incidence and significance of fetal choroid plexus cysts. *Prenat Diagn* 1989;9:205–211.

177. Ghidini A, Strobelt N, Locatelli A, Mariani E, Piccoli MG, Vergani P. Isolated fetal choroid plexus cysts: role of ultrasonography in establishment of the risk of trisomy 18. *Am J Obstet Gynecol* 2000;182(4):972–977.

178. Yoder PR, Sabbagha RE, Gross SJ, Zelop CM. The second-trimester fetus with isolated choroid plexus cysts: a meta-analysis of risk of trisomies 18 and 21. *Obstet Gynecol* 1999;93(5 Pt 2):869–872.

179. Snijders RJ, Shawa L, Nicolaides KH. Fetal choroid plexus cysts and trisomy 18: assessment of risk based on ultrasound findings and maternal age. *Prenat Diagn* 1994;14(12):1119–1127.

180. Porto M, Murata Y, Warneke LA, Keegan KA Jr. Fetal choroid plexus cysts: an independent risk factor for chromosomal anomalies. *J Clin Ultrasound* 1993;21(2):103–108.

181. Gray DL, Winborn RC, Suessen TL, Crane JP. Is genetic amniocentesis warranted when isolated choroid plexus cysts are found? *Prenat Diagn* 1996;16(11):983–990.

182. Walkinshaw S, Pilling D, Spriggs A. Isolated choroid plexus cysts: the need for routine offer of karyotyping. *Prenat Diagn* 1994;14(8):663.

183. Ostlere SJ, Irving HC, Lilford RJ. Fetal choroid plexus cysts: a report of 100 cases. *Radiology* 1990;175(3):753–755.

184. Twining P, Zuccollo J, Clewes J, Swallow J. Fetal choroid plexus cysts: a prospective study and review of the literature. *Br J Radiol* 1991;64(758):98–102.

185. Bromley B, Lieberman R, Benacerraf BR. Choroid plexus cysts: not associated with Down syndrome. *Ultrasound Obstet Gynecol* 1996;8(4):232–235.

186. Chitty LS, Chudleigh P, Wright E, Campbell S, Pembrey M. The significance of choroid plexus cysts in an unselected population: results of a multicenter study. *Ultrasound Obstet Gynecol* 1998;12(6):391–397.

187. Vintzileos AM, Ananth CV, Fisher AJ, Smulian JC, Day-Salvatore D, et al. An economic evaluation of prenatal strat-

egies for detection of trisomy 18. *Am J Obstet Gynecol* 1998;179(5):1220–1224.

188. Donnenfeld AE. Prenatal sonographic detection of isolated fetal choroid plexus cysts: Should we screen for trisomy 18? *J Med Screen* 1995;2(1):18–21.

189. Brumfield CG, Wenstrom KD, Owen J, Davis RO. Ultrasound findings and multiple marker screening in trisomy 18. *Obstet Gynecol* 2000;95(1):51–54.

190. Sullivan A, Giudice T, Vavelidis F, Thiagarajah S. Choroid plexus cysts: Is biochemical testing a valuable adjunct to targeted ultrasonography? *Am J Obstet Gynecol* 1999;181(2):260–265.

191. Nicolaides KH, Salvesen DR, Snijders RJ, Gosden CM. Strawberry-shaped skull in fetal trisomy 18. *Fetal Diagn Ther* 1992;7(2):132–137.

192. Shields LE, Carpenter LA, Smith KM, Nghiem HV. Ultrasonographic diagnosis of trisomy 18: Is it practical in the early second trimester? *J Ultrasound Med* 1998;17(5):327–331.

193. Nyberg DA, Mack LA, Hirsch J, Mahony BS. Abnormalities of fetal cranial contour in sonographic detection of spina bifida: evaluation of the "lemon" sign. *Radiology* 1988;167:387–392.

194. Patel MD, Goldstein RB, Tung S, Filly RA. Fetal cerebral ventricular atrium: difference in size according to sex. *Radiology* 1995;194(3):713–715.

195. Hertzberg BS, Lile R, Foosaner DE, Kliewer MA, Paine SS, et al. Choroid plexus–ventricular wall separation in fetuses with normal-sized cerebral ventricles at sonography: postnatal outcome. *AJR Am J Roentgenol* 1994;163(2):405–410.

196. Mahony BS, Nyberg DA, Hirsch JH, Petty CN, Hendricks SK, Mack LA. Mild idiopathic lateral cerebral ventricular dilatation in utero: sonographic evaluation. *Radiology* 1988;169:715–721.

197. Bromley B, Frigoletto FD Jr, Benacerraf BR. Mild fetal lateral cerebral ventriculomegaly: clinical course and outcome. *Am J Obstet Gynecol* 1991;164:863–867.

198. Pilu G, Falco P, Gabrielli S, Perolo A, Sandri F, Bovicelli L. The clinical significance of fetal isolated cerebral borderline ventriculomegaly: report of 31 cases and review of the literature. *Ultrasound Obstet Gynecol* 1999;14(5):320–326.

199. Nicolaides KH, Berry S, Snijders RJ, Thorpe-Beeston JG, Gosden C. Fetal lateral cerebral ventriculomegaly: associated malformations and chromosomal defects. *Fetal Diagn Ther* 1990;5(1):5–14.

200. Tomlinson MW, Treadwell MC, Bottoms SF. Isolated mild ventriculomegaly: associated karyotypic abnormalities and in utero observations. *J Matern Fetal Med* 1997;6(4):241–244.

201. Vergani P, Locatelli A, Strobelt N, Cavallone M, Ceruti P, et al. Clinical outcome of mild fetal ventriculomegaly. *Am J Obstet Gynecol* 1998;178(2):218–222.

202. Sohl BD, Scioscia AL, Budorick NE, Moore TR. Utility of minor ultrasonographic markers in the prediction of abnormal fetal karyotype at a prenatal diagnostic center. *Am J Obstet Gynecol* 1999;181(4):898–903.

203. Down LJ. Observations on an ethnic classification of idiots. *Clin Lectures Reports, London Hospital* 1866;3:259–262.

204. Hall B. Mongolism in newborn infants. *Clin Pediatr* 1966;5:12.

205. Chodirker BN, Harman CR, Greenberg CR. Spontaneous resolution of a cystic hygroma in a fetus with Turner syndrome. *Prenat Diagn* 1988;8:291–292.

206. Benacerraf B, Frigoletto F, Laboda L. Sonographic diagnosis of Down syndrome in the second trimester. *Am J Obstet Gynecol* 1985;153:49–52.

207. Benacerraf B, Gelman R, Frigoletto F. Sonographic identification of second trimester fetuses with Down syndrome. *N Engl J Med* 1987;317:1371–1376.

208. Benacerraf BR, Frigoletto FD. Soft tissue nuchal fold in the second trimester fetus: standards for normal measurements compared to the fetus with Down syndrome. *Am J Obstet Gynecol* 1987;157:1146–1149.

209. Gray DL, Crane JP. Optimal nuchal skin-fold thresholds based on gestational age for prenatal detection of Down syndrome. *Am J Obstet Gynecol* 1994;171:1282–1286.

210. Borrell A, Costa D, Martinez JM, Delgado RD, Casals E, et al. Early midtrimester fetal nuchal thickness: effectiveness as a marker of Down syndrome. *Am J Obstet Gynecol* 1996;175(1):45–49.

211. Tannirandorn Y, Manotaya S, Uerpairojkit B, Tanawattanacharoen S, Charoenvidhya D, Phaosavasdi S. Cut-off criteria for second-trimester nuchal skinfold thickness for prenatal detection of Down syndrome in a Thai population. *Int J Gynaecol Obstet* 1999;65(2):137–141.

212. Mahoney MJ. Gestational age standardized nuchal thickness values for estimating mid-trimester Down's syndrome risk. *J Matern Fetal Med* 1999;8(2):37–43.

213. Bahado-Singh RO, Oz UA, Kovanci E, Deren O, Feather M, et al. Gestational age standardized nuchal thickness values for estimating mid-trimester Down's syndrome risk. *J Matern Fetal Med* 1999;8(2):37–43.

214. Nyberg DA, Souter VL, El-Bastawissi A, Young S, Luthardt F, Luthy DA. Isolated sonographic markers for detection of fetal Down syndrome in the second trimester of pregnancy. *J Ultrasound Med* 2001;20(10):1053–1063.

215. Scioscia AL, Pretorius DH, Budorick NE, Cahill TC, Axelrod FT, Leopold GR. Second-trimester echogenic bowel and chromosomal abnormalities. *Am J Obstet Gynecol* 1992;167:889–894.

216. Bromley B, Doubilet P, Frigoletto FD Jr, Krauss C, Estroff JA, Benacerraf BR. Is fetal hyperechogenic bowel on second-trimester sonogram an indication for amniocentesis? *Obstet Gynecol* 1994;83:647–651.

217. Sipes SL, Weiner CP, Wenstrom KD, Williamson RA, Grant SS, Mueller GM. Fetal echogenic bowel on ultrasound: Is there clinical significance? *Fetal Diagn Ther* 1994;9(1):38–43.

218. Bahado-Singh R, Morotti R, Copel JA, Mahoney MJ. Hyperechoic fetal bowel: the perinatal consequences. *Prenat Diagn* 1994;14(10):981–987.

219. Stipoljev F, Sertic J, Kos M, Miskovic B, Obrad-Sabljak R, et al. Incidence of chromosomopathies and cystic fibrosis mutations in second trimester fetuses with isolated hyperechoic bowel. *J Matern Fetal Med* 1999;8(2):44–47.

220. Al-Kouatly HB, Chasen ST, Strelzoff J, Chervenak FA. The clinical significance of echogenic bowel. *Am J Obstet Gynecol* 2001;185:1035–1038.

221. Strocker AM, Snijders RJ, Carlson DE, Greene N, Gregory KD, et al. Fetal echogenic bowel: parameters to be consid-

ered in differential diagnosis. *Ultrasound Obstet Gynecol* 2000;16(6):519–523.

222. Nyberg DA, Resta R, Luthy DA, Hickok DE, Mahony BS, Hirsch JH. Prenatal sonographic findings of Down syndrome: review of 94 cases. *Obstet Gynecol* 1990;76:370–377.

223. Muller F, Dommergues M, Aubry MC, Simon-Bouy B, Gautier E, et al. Hyperechogenic fetal bowel: an ultrasonographic marker for adverse fetal and neonatal outcome. *Am J Obstet Gynecol* 1995;173(2):508–513.

224. Sepulveda W, Reid R, Nicolaidis P, Prendiville O, Chapman RS, Fisk NM. Second-trimester echogenic bowel and intraamniotic bleeding: association between fetal bowel echogenicity and amniotic fluid spectrophotometry at 410 nm. *Am J Obstet Gynecol* 1996;174(3):839–842.

225. Nyberg DA, Resta RG, Luthy DA, Hickok DE, Dubinsky T, et al. Echogenic bowel and Down's syndrome. *Ultrasound Obstet Gynecol* 1993;3:330–333.

226. Vincoff NS, Callen PW, Smith-Bindman R, Goldstein RB. Effect of ultrasound transducer frequency on the appearance of the fetal bowel. *J Ultrasound Med* 1999;18(12):799–803.

227. Hill LM, Fries J, Hecker J, Grzybek P. Second-trimester echogenic small bowel: an increased risk for adverse perinatal outcome. *Prenat Diagn* 1994;14:845–850.

228. Slotnick RN, Abuhamad AZ. Prognostic implications of fetal echogenic bowel. *Lancet* 1996;347(8994):85–87.

229. Smith-Bindman R, Hosmer W, Feldstein VA, Deeks JJ, Goldberg JD. Second-trimester ultrasound to detect fetuses with Down syndrome: a meta-analysis. *JAMA* 2001;285(8):1044–1055.

230. Stein B, Bromley B, Michlewitz H, Miller WA, Benacerraf BR. Fetal liver calcifications: sonographic appearance and postnatal outcome. *Radiology* 1995;197(2):489–492.

231. Koopman E, Wladimiroff JW. Fetal intrahepatic hyperechogenic foci: prenatal ultrasound diagnosis and outcome. *Prenat Diagn* 1998;18(4):339–342.

232. Simchen MJ, Toi A, Bona M, Alkazaleh F, Ryan G, et al. Fetal hepatic calcifications: prenatal diagnosis and outcome. *Am J Obstet Gynecol* (in press).

233. Sepulveda W, Nicolaidis P, Hollingsworth J, Fisk NM. Fetal cholecystomegaly: a prenatal marker of aneuploidy. *Prenat Diagn* 1995;15(2):193–197.

234. Hartung J, Chaoui R, Wauer R, Bollmann R. Fetal hepatosplenomegaly: an isolated sonographic sign of trisomy 21 in a case of myeloproliferative disorder. *Ultrasound Obstet Gynecol* 1998;11(6):453–455.

235. Benacerraf BR, Cnann A, Gelman R, Laboda LA, Frigoletto FD Jr. Can sonographers reliably identify anatomic features associated with Down syndrome in fetuses? *Radiology* 1989;173:377–380.

236. Benacerraf BR, Neuberg D, Frigoletto FD Jr. Humeral shortening in second-trimester fetuses with Down syndrome. *Obstet Gynecol* 1991;77:223–227.

237. Fitzsimmons J, Droste S, Shepard TH, Pascoe-Mason J, Chinn A, Mack LA. Long-bone growth in fetuses with Down syndrome. *Am J Obstet Gynecol* 1989;161:1174–1177.

238. Nyberg DA, Resta RG, Luthy DA, Hickok DE, Williams MA. Humerus and femur length shortening in the detec-

tion of Down's syndrome. *Am J Obstet Gynecol* 1993;168:534–539.

239. Vergani P, Locatelli A, Giiovanna Piccoli M, Mariani E, Strobelt N, et al. Critical reappraisal of the utility of sonographic fetal femur length in the prediction of trisomy 21. *Prenat Diagn* 2000;20:210–214.

240. Johnson MP, Michaelson JE, Barr M Jr, Treadwell MC, Hume RF Jr, et al. Combining humerus and femur length for improved ultrasonographic identification of pregnancies at increased risk for trisomy 21. *Am J Obstet Gynecol* 1995;172:1229–1235.

241. Bahado-Singh RO, Deren O, Tan A, D'Ancona RL, Hunter D, et al. Ultrasonographically adjusted midtrimester risk of trisomy 21 and significant chromosomal defects in advanced maternal age. *Am J Obstet Gynecol* 1996;175(6):1563–1568.

242. Shipp TD, Bromley B, Mascola M, Benacerraf B. Variation in fetal femur length with respect to maternal race. *J Ultrasound Med* 2001;20:141–144.

243. Bahado-Singh RO, Oz AU, Kovanci E, Deren O, Copel J, et al. New Down syndrome screening algorithm: ultrasonographic biometry and multiple serum markers combined with maternal age. *Am J Obstet Gynecol* 1998;179:1627–1631.

244. Schechter AG, Fakhry J, Shapiro LR, Gewitz MH. In utero thickening of the chordae tendinae. A cause of intracardiac echogenic foci. *J Ultrasound Med* 1987;6(12):691–695.

245. Levy DW, Mintz MC. The left ventricular echogenic focus: a normal finding. *AJR Am J Roentgenol* 1988;150(1):85–86.

246. Shipp TD, Bromley B, Liberman EP, Benacerraf BR. The frequency of fetal echogenic intracardiac foci with respect to maternal race. *J Ultrasound Med* 1999;18(3 Suppl):S108.

247. Ranzini AC, McLean DA, Sharma S, Ananth CV. Fetal intracardiac echogenic foci: Does visualization depend on the orientation of the four-chamber view? *J Ultrasound Med* 1999;18(3 Suppl):S108.

248. Petrikovsky BM, Challenger M, Wyse LJ. Natural history of echogenic foci within ventricles of the fetal heart. *Ultrasound Obstet Gynecol* 1995;5(2):92–94.

249. Roberts DJ, Genest D. Cardiac histologic pathology characteristic of trisomies 13 and 21. *Hum Pathol* 1992;23:1130–1140.

250. Brown DL, Roberts DJ, Miller WA. Left ventricular echogenic focus in the fetal heart: pathologic correlation. *J Ultrasound Med* 1994;13(8):613–616.

251. Tennstedt C, Chaoui R, Vogel M, Goldner B, Dietel M. Pathologic correlation of sonographic echogenic foci in the fetal heart. *Prenat Diagn* 2000;20(4):287–292.

252. Bromley B, Lieberman E, Laboda L, Benacerraf BR. Echogenic intracardiac focus: a sonographic sign for fetal Down syndrome. *Obstet Gynecol* 1995;86(6):998–1001.

253. Lehman CD, Nyberg DA, Winter TC III, Kapur R, Resta RG, Luthy DA. Trisomy 13 syndrome: prenatal US findings in a review of 33 cases. *Radiology* 1995;194(1):217–222.

254. Sepulveda W, Cullen S, Nicolaidis P, Hollingsworth J, Fisk NM. Echogenic foci in the fetal heart: a marker of chromosomal abnormality. *Br J Obstet Gynaecol* 1995;102(6):490–492.

255. Simpson JM, Cook A, Sharland G. The significance of echogenic foci in the fetal heart: a prospective study of 228 cases. *Ultrasound Obstet Gynecol* 1996;8(4):225–228.

256. Manning JE, Ragavendra N, Sayre J, Laifer-Narin SL, Melany ML, et al. Significance of fetal intracardiac echogenic foci in relation to trisomy 21: a prospective sonographic study of high-risk pregnant women. *AJR Am J Roentgenol* 1998;170(4):1083–1084.

257. Bromley B, Lieberman E, Shipp TD, Richardson M, Benacerraf BR. Significance of an echogenic intracardiac focus in fetuses at high and low risk for aneuploidy. *J Ultrasound Med* 1998;17(2):127–131.

258. Vibhakar NI, Budorick NE, Scioscia AL, Harby LD, Mullen ML, Sklansky MS. Prevalence of aneuploidy with a cardiac intraventricular echogenic focus in at-risk patient population. *J Ultrasound Med* 1999;18:265–268.

259. Winter TC, Anderson AM, Cheng EY, Komarniski CA, Souter VL, et al. The echogenic intracardiac focus in second trimester fetuses with trisomy 21: usefulness as a US marker. *Radiology* 2000;216:450–456.

260. Wax JR, Philput C. Fetal intracardiac echogenic foci: does it matter which ventricle? *J Ultrasound Med* 1998;17:141–144.

261. Achiron R, Lipitz S, Gabbay U, Yagel S. Prenatal ultrasonographic diagnosis of fetal heart echogenic foci: no correlation with Down syndrome. *Obstet Gynecol* 1997;89(6):945–948.

262. Dildy GA, Judd VE, Clark SL. Prospective evaluation of the antenatal incidence and postnatal significance of the fetal echogenic cardiac focus: a case-control study. *Am J Obstet Gynecol* 1996;175(4 Pt 1):1008–1012.

263. How HY, Villafane J, Parihus RR, Spinnato JA. Small hyperechoic foci of the fetal cardiac ventricle: a benign sonographic finding? *Ultrasound Obstet Gynecol* 1994;4:205–207.

264. Bettelheim D, Deutinger J, Bernaschek G. The value of echogenic foci ("golfballs") in the fetal heart as a marker of chromosomal abnormalities. *Ultrasound Obstet Gynecol* 1999;14(2):98–100.

265. Benacerraf BR, Mandell J, Estroff JA, Harlow BL, Frigoletto FD Jr. Fetal pyelectasis: a possible association with Down syndrome. *Obstet Gynecol* 1990;76:58–60.

266. Corteville JE, Dicke JM, Crane JP. Fetal pyelectasis and Down syndrome: is genetic amniocentesis warranted? *Obstet Gynecol* 1992;79(5 Pt 1):770–772.

267. Wilson RD, Lynch S, Lessoway VA. Fetal pyelectasis: comparison of postnatal renal pathology with unilateral and bilateral pyelectasis. *Prenat Diagn* 1997;17(5):451–455.

268. Wickstrom E, Maizels M, Sabbagha RE, Tamura RK, Cohen LC, Pergament E. Isolated fetal pyelectasis: assessment of risk for postnatal uropathy and Down syndrome. *Ultrasound Obstet Gynecol* 1996;8(4):236–240.

269. Vintzileos AM, Egan JFX. Adjusting the risk for trisomy 21 on the basis of second-trimester ultrasonography. *Am J Obstet Gynecol* 1995;172:837–844.

270. Snijders RJ, Sebire NJ, Faria M, Patel F, Nicolaides KH. Fetal mild hydronephrosis and chromosomal defects: relation to maternal age and gestation. *Fetal Diagn Ther* 1995;10(6):349–355.

271. Wickstrom EA, Thangavelu M, Parilla BV, Tamura RK, Sabbagha RE. A prospective study of the association between isolated fetal pyelectasis and chromosomal abnormality. *Obstet Gynecol* 1996;88(3):379–382.

272. Zook PD, Winter TC 3rd, Nyberg DA. Iliac angle as a marker for Down syndrome in second-trimester fetuses: CT measurement. *Radiology* 1999;211(2):447–451.

273. Bork MD, Egan JF, Cusick W, Borgida AF, Campbell WA, Rodis JF. Iliac wing angle as a marker for trisomy 21 in the second trimester. *Obstet Gynecol* 1997;89(5 Pt 1):734–737.

274. Kliewer MA, Hertzberg BS, Freed KS, DeLong DM, Kay HH, et al. Dysmorphologic features of the fetal pelvis in Down syndrome: prenatal sonographic depiction and diagnostic implications of the iliac angle. *Radiology* 1996;201(3):681–684.

275. Shipp TD, Bromley B, Lieberman E, Benacerraf BR. The iliac angle as a sonographic marker for Down syndrome in second-trimester fetuses. *Obstet Gynecol* 1997;89(3):446–450.

276. Zoppi MA, Ibba RM, Floris M, Monni G. Can fetal iliac bone measurement be used as a marker for Down's syndrome screening? *Ultrasound Obstet Gynecol* 1998;12(1):19–22.

277. Kliewer MA, Hertzberg BS, Freed KS, McNally PJ, DeLong DM. Normal fetal pelvis: important factors for morphometric characterization with US. *Radiology* 2000;215(2):453–457.

278. Grange G, Thoury A, Dupont J, Pannier E, LeRhun F, et al. Sonographic measurement of the fetal iliac angle cannot be used alone as a marker for trisomy 21. *Fetal Diagn Ther* 2000;15(1):41–45.

279. Lee W, Blanckaert K, Bronsteen RA, Huang R, Romero R. Fetal iliac angle measurements by three-dimensional sonography. *Ultrasound Obstet Gynecol* 2001;18(2):150–154.

280. Snijders RJ, Sherrod C, Gosden CM, Nicolaides KH. Fetal growth retardation: associated malformations and chromosomal abnormalities. *Am J Obstet Gynecol* 1993;168(2):547–555.

281. Jauniaux E, Brown R, Snijders RJM, Noble P, Nicolaides KH. Early prenatal diagnosis of triploidy. *Am J Obstet Gynecol* 1997;176:550–554.

282. Bahado-Singh RO, Lynch L, Deren O, Morroti R, Copel JA, et al. First-trimester growth restriction and fetal aneuploidy: the effect of type and gestational age. *Am J Obstet Gynecol* 1997;176:976–980.

283. Dicke JM, Crane JP. Sonographic recognition of major malformations and aberrant fetal growth in trisomic fetuses. *J Ultrasound Med* 1991;10(8):433–438.

284. Bryan EM, Kohler HG. The missing umbilical artery: prospective study based on a maternity unit. *Arch Dis Child* 1974;49:844–852.

285. Byrne J, Blane WA. Malformations and chromosome anomalies in spontaneously aborted fetuses with single umbilical artery. *Am J Obstet Gynecol* 1985;151:340–342.

286. Lenoski EF, Medovy H. Single umbilical artery: incidence, clinical significance and relation to autosomal trisomy. *Can Med Assoc J* 1962;87:1229–1231.

287. Monies IW. Genesis of single umbilical artery. *Am J Obstet Gynecol* 1970;108:400–405.

288. Geipel A, Germer U, Welp T, Schwinger E, Gembruch U. Prenatal diagnosis of single umbilical artery: determination of the absent side, associated anomalies, Doppler findings and perinatal outcome. *Ultrasound Obstet Gynecol* 2000;15(2):114–117.

289. Chow JS, Benson CB, Doubilet PM. Frequency and nature of structural anomalies in fetuses with single umbilical arteries. *J Ultrasound Med* 1998;17(12):765–768.

290. Vlietinck RF, Thiery M, Orye E, De Clercq A, Van Vaerenbergh P. Significance of the single umbilical artery. *Arch Dis Child* 1972;47:639–642.

291. Nyberg DA, Mahony BS, Luthy D, Kapur R. Single umbilical artery. Prenatal detection of concurrent anomalies. *J Ultrasound Med* 1991;10(5):247–253.

292. Lee CN, Cheng WF, Lai HL, Cheng SP, Shih JC, et al. Perinatal management and outcome of fetuses with single umbilical artery diagnosed prenatally. *J Matern Fetal Investig* 1998;8(4):156–159.

293. Sener T, Ozalp S, Hassa H, Zeytinoglu S, Basaran N, Durak B. Ultrasonographic detection of single umbilical artery: a simple marker of fetal anomaly. *Int J Gynaecol Obstet* 1997;58(2):217–221.

294. Abuhamad AZ, Shaffer W, Mari G, Copel JA, Hobbins JC, Evans AT. Single umbilical artery: does it matter which artery is missing? *Am J Obstet Gynecol* 1995;173(3 Pt 1):728–732.

295. Parilla BV, Tamura RK, MacGregor SN, Geibel LJ, Sabbagha RE. The clinical significance of a single umbilical artery as an isolated finding on prenatal ultrasound. *Obstet Gynecol* 1995;85(4):570–572.

296. Smith GN, Walker M, Johnston S, Ash K. The sonographic finding of persistent umbilical cord cystic masses is associated with lethal aneuploidy and/or congenital anomalies. *Prenat Diagn* 1996;16(12):1141–1147.

297. Sepulveda W, Gutierrez J, Sanchez J, Be C, Schnapp C. Pseudocyst of the umbilical cord: prenatal sonographic appearance and clinical significance. *Obstet Gynecol* 1999;93(3):377–381.

298. Astner A, Schwinger E, Caliebe A, Jonat W, Gembruch U. Sonographically detected fetal and placental abnormalities associated with trisomy 16 confined to the placenta. A case report and review of the literature. *Prenat Diagn* 1998;18(12):1308–1315.

299. Ulm B, Ulm MR, Bernaschek G. Unfused amnion and chorion after 14 weeks of gestation: associated fetal structural and chromosomal abnormalities. *Ultrasound Obstet Gynecol* 1999;13(6):392–395.

300. Bromley B, Shipp TD, Benacerraf BR. Amnion-chorion separation after 17 weeks' gestation. *Obstet Gynecol* 1999; 94(6):1024–1026.

301. Liang ST, Yam AW, Tang MH, Ghosh A. Trisomy 18: the value of late prenatal diagnosis. *Eur J Obstet Gynecol Reprod Biol* 1986;22:95–97.

302. Landy HJ, Isada NB, Larsen JW Jr. Genetic implications of idiopathic hydramnios. *Am J Obstet Gynecol* 1987;157:114–117.

303. Brady K, Polzin WJ, Kopelman JN, Read JA. Risk of chromosomal abnormalities in patients with idiopathic polyhydramnios. *Obstet Gynecol* 1992;79(2):234–238.

304. Barkin SZ, Pretorius DH, Beckett MK, Manchester DK, Nelson TR, Manco-Johnson ML. Severe polyhydramnios: incidence of anomalies. *AJR Am J Roentgenol* 1987;148:155–159.

305. Glantz JC, Abramowicz JS, Sherer DM. Significance of idiopathic midtrimester polyhydramnios. *Am J Perinatol* 1994;11(4):305–308.

306. Benson CB, Coughlin BF, Doubilet PM. Amniotic fluid volume in large-for-gestational-age fetuses of nondiabetic mothers. *J Ultrasound Med* 1991;10(3):149–151.

307. Panting-Kemp A, Nguyen T, Chang E, Quillen E, Castro L. Idiopathic polyhydramnios and perinatal outcome. *Am J Obstet Gynecol* 1999;181(5 Pt 1):1079–1082.

308. Maymon E, Ghezzi F, Shoham-Vardi I, Franchi M, Silberstein T, et al. Isolated hydramnios at term gestation and the occurrence of peripartum complications. *Eur J Obstet Gynecol Reprod Biol* 1998;77(2):157–161.

309. Sohaey R, Nyberg DA, Sickler GK, Williams MA. Idiopathic polyhydramnios: association with fetal macrosomia. *Radiology* 1994;190(2):393–396.

310. Sickler GK, Nyberg DA, Sohaey R, Luthy DA. Polyhydramnios and fetal intrauterine growth restriction: ominous combination. *J Ultrasound Med* 1997;16(9):609–614.

311. Furman B, Erez O, Senior L, Shoham-Vardi I, Bar-David J, et al. Hydramnios and small for gestational age: prevalence and clinical significance. *Acta Obstet Gynecol Scand* 2000; 79(1):31–36.

312. Lazebnik N, Many A. The severity of polyhydramnios, estimated fetal weight and preterm delivery are independent risk factors for the presence of congenital malformations. *Gynecol Obstet Invest* 1999;48(1):28–32.

313. Barnhard Y, Bar-Hava I, Divon MY. Is polyhydramnios in an ultrasonographically normal fetus an indication for genetic evaluation? *Am J Obstet Gynecol* 1995;173(5):1523–1527.

314. Drugan A, Johnson MP, Evans MI. Ultrasound screening for fetal chromosome anomalies. *Am J Med Genet* 2000; 90(2):98–107.

315. DeVore GR. Trisomy 21: 91% detection rate using second-trimester ultrasound markers. *Ultrasound Obstet Gynecol* 2000;16(2):133–141.

316. Filly RA. Obstetric sonography: the best way to terrify a pregnant woman. *J Ultrasound Med* 2000;19:1–5.

317. Maclachlan N, Iskaros J, Chitty L. Ultrasound markers of fetal chromosomal abnormality: a survey of policies and practices in UK maternity ultrasound departments. *Ultrasound Obstet Gynecol* 2000;15:387–390.

318. Bromley B, Lieberman E, Benacerraf BR. The incorporation of maternal age into the sonographic scoring index for the detection at 14–20 weeks of fetuses with Down's syndrome. *Ultrasound Obstet Gynecol* 1997;10(5):321–324.

319. Winter TC, Uhrich SB, Souter VL, Nyberg DA. The "genetic sonogram": comparison of the index scoring system with the age-adjusted US risk assessment. *Radiology* 2000;215:775–782.

320. Nyberg DA, Luthy DA, Cheng EY, Sheley RC, Resta RG, Williams MA. Role of prenatal ultrasound in women with positive screen for Down syndrome based on maternal serum markers. *Am J Obstet Gynecol* 1995;173:1030–1035.

321. Drugan A, Reichler A, Bronstein M, Johnson MP, Sokol RJ, Evans MI. Abnormal biochemical serum screening versus 2nd-trimester ultrasound-detected minor anomalies as predictors of aneuploidy in low-risk patients. *Fetal Diagn Ther* 1996;11(5):301–305.

322. Verdin SM, Economides DL. The role of ultrasonographic markers for trisomy 21 in women with positive serum biochemistry. *Br J Obstet Gynaecol* 1998;105(1):63–67.

323. DeVore GR, Alfi O. The use of color Doppler ultrasound to identify fetuses at increased risk for trisomy 21: an alternative for high-risk patients who decline genetic amniocentesis. *Obstet Gynecol* 1995;85(3):378–386.

324. DeVore GR, Romero R. Genetic sonography: a cost-effective method for evaluating women 35 years and older who decline genetic amniocentesis. *J Ultrasound Med* 2002; 21(1):5–13.

325. Bahado-Singh RO, Deren O, Oz U, Tan A, Hunter D, et al. An alternative for women initially declining genetic amniocentesis: individual Down syndrome odds on the basis of maternal age and multiple ultrasonographic markers. *Am J Obstet Gynecol* 1998;179:514–519.

326. DeVore GR. The genetic sonogram: its use in the detection of chromosomal abnormalities in fetuses of women of advanced maternal age. *Prenat Diagn* 2001;21(1):40–45.

327. Yagel S, Anteby EY, Hochner-Celnikier D, Ariel I, Chaap T, Ben Neriah Z. The role of midtrimester targeted fetal organ screening combined with the "triple test" and maternal age in the diagnosis of trisomy 21: a retrospective study. *Am J Obstet Gynecol* 1998;178(1 Pt 1):40–44.

328. Souter VL, Nyberg DA, El-Bastawissi A, Zebelman A, Luthhardt F, Luthy DA. Correlation of ultrasound findings and biochemical markers in the second trimester of pregnancy in fetuses with trisomy 21. *Prenat Diagn* 2002; 22(3):175–182.

329. Owen J, Wenstrom KD, Hardin JM, Boots LR, Hsu CC, et al. The utility of fetal biometry as an adjunct to the multiple-marker screening test for Down syndrome. *Am J Obstet Gynecol* 1994;171(4):1041–1046.

330. Bahado-Singh RO, Goldstein I, Uerpairojkit B, Copel JA, Mahoney MJ, Baumgarten A. Normal nuchal thickness in the midtrimester indicates reduced risk of Down syndrome in pregnancies with abnormal triple-screen results. *Am J Obstet Gynecol* 1995;173(4):1106–1110.

331. Roberts D, Walkinshaw SA, McCormack MJ, Ellis J. Prenatal detection of trisomy 21: combined experience of two British hospitals. *Prenat Diagn* 2000;20(1):17–22.

332. Bahado-Singh RO, Oz AU, Gomez K, Hunter D, Copel J, et al. Combined ultrasound biometry, serum markers and age for Down syndrome risk estimation. *Ultrasound Obstet Gynecol* 2000;15:199–204.

333. Wald NJ, Densem JW, George L, Muttukrishna S, Knight PG. Prenatal screening for Down's syndrome using inhibin-A as a serum marker. *Prenat Diagn* 1996;16(2):143–153.

334. Wald NJ, Huttly WJ. Validation of risk estimation using the quadruple test in prenatal screening for Down syndrome. *Prenat Diagn* 1999;19(11):1083–1084.

335. Nyberg DA, Luthy DA, Resta RG, Nyberg BC, Williams MA. Age-adjusted ultrasound risk assessment for fetal Down's syndrome during the second trimester: description of the method and analysis of 142 cases. *Ultrasound Obstet Gynecol* 1998;12:8–14.

336. Benacerraf BR, Nadel AS, Bromley B. Identification of second-trimester fetuses with autosomal trisomy by use of a sonographic scoring index. *Radiology* 1994;193:135–140.

337. Vintzileos AM, Guzman ER, Smulian JC, Day-Salvatore DL, Knuppel RA. Indication-specific accuracy of second-trimester genetic ultrasonography for the detection of trisomy 21. *Am J Obstet Gynecol* 1999;181(5 Pt 1):1045–1048.

BIOCHEMICAL SCREENING

The last three decades have witnessed major changes in pregnancy screening through the use of biochemical markers. The initial screening method involved offering amniocentesis for determination of amniotic fluid alpha-fetoprotein (AFP) only for patients considered at high risk for spina bifida or neural tube defect (NTD); serum screening is now offered to all pregnant women. Even the primary goal of screening has changed since the original intent of detecting fetal spina bifida has been superseded at many centers with improvements in ultrasound imaging and interpretation by experienced sonographers. Today, detection of fetal aneuploidy is the principal aim of biochemical screening. Dramatic developments in aneuploidy screening have accelerated in recent years so that current options include any combination of second-trimester biochemistry, second-trimester ultrasound (see Chapter 25), first-trimester biochemistry, and first-trimester nuchal translucency (NT) screening (see Chapter 20).

This chapter discusses NTD screening, aneuploidy screening, characteristics of the analytes, and other associations that may be important to screening.

NEURAL TUBE DEFECT SCREENING

Bergstrand and Czar, performing protein electrophoresis on human amniotic fluid, were the first to report a new fraction migrating between albumin and α1-globulin.[1] Its proximity to the peak of albumin is probably at least partially responsible for early detection difficulties. Later, this substance was named alpha-fetoprotein by Gitlin, and this designation was officially adopted by the International Agency for Research on Cancer.

In 1972, Brock and Sutcliffe[2] reported that AFP was elevated in the amniotic fluid in women carrying a fetus with an NTD, thus allowing prenatal diagnosis with amniocentesis. With the advent of radioimmunoassays, many authors quickly reported the ability to detect maternal serum levels as low as 10 ng per mL and it was apparent that serum screening was possible.[3] These developments eventually led to serum screening programs in the United Kingdom by the late 1970s and in the United States by the early 1980s.

AFP is a glycoprotein initially produced in the embryonic yolk sac and subsequently by the fetal gastrointestinal tract and liver (Fig. 1). The exact role of the protein is unknown and normal fetuses that do not make AFP have been identified[4]; thus, it is not essential for survival. AFP in the fetal serum passes through the glomeruli intact and is then reabsorbed in the renal tubules. Normally, only a small amount escapes and appears in the fetal urine and amniotic fluid. Early in gestation AFP also enters the amniotic fluid via transudation across the immature epithelium. Diffusion of AFP from the fetal to maternal compartment is across the fetal membranes and at the placental level. Hence, AFP distributions should be considered in three compartments: fetal serum, amniotic fluid, and maternal serum.

Figure 2 shows mean concentrations of AFP in the fetal serum, amniotic fluid, and maternal serum.[5] The peak fetal serum level is at 13 weeks' gestation at 3 mg per mL, and peak amniotic fluid level is at approximately the same time. Production of AFP actually increases until about 32 weeks of gestation, but concentrations fall because of a dilution effect caused by rapid fetal growth.

Maternal serum levels of AFP (MS-AFP) continue to rise until 32 weeks' gestation simply due to the increasing size of the fetus even though amniotic and fetal levels have declined. Between 16 and 20 weeks' gestation, levels of MS-AFP are approximately 100,000 times smaller than those found in the fetal serum. Radioimmunoassay techniques are necessary for quantitative determinations of such low MS-AFP.

Interpretation

Although it may seem logical to report the results of AFP concentrations in the amniotic fluid and maternal serum as absolute levels, this is impractical. Individual laboratories and different manufacturers kits are often internally standardized, making direct comparisons difficult, if not impossible. It is therefore the custom to report AFP levels in terms of multiples of the median (MoMs). Because the median is the middle value in an array of values, it is not as sensitive as the mean to wide variations at either extreme of

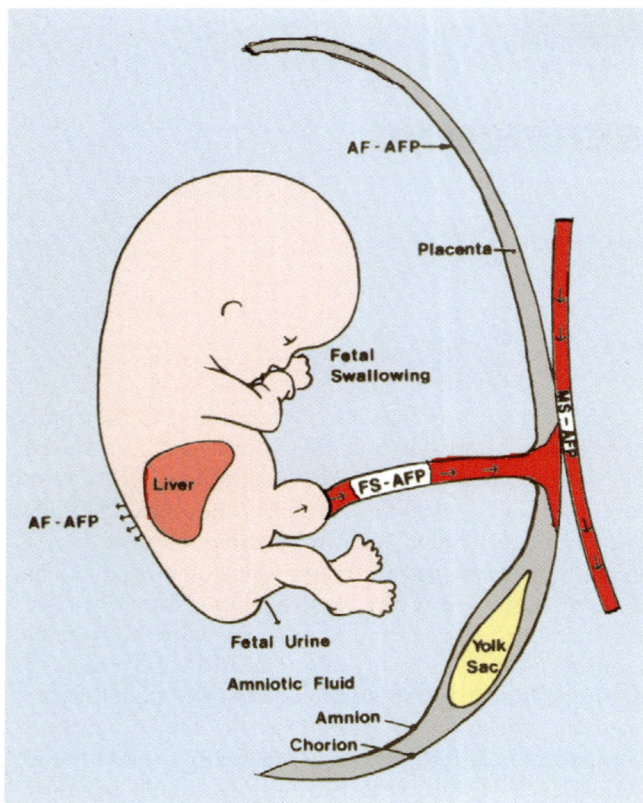

FIGURE 1. Schematic drawing showing the production and distribution of alpha-fetoprotein (*AFP*) into its three compartments: fetal tissues, amniotic fluid (*AF*), and maternal serum (*MS*). FS, fetal serum.

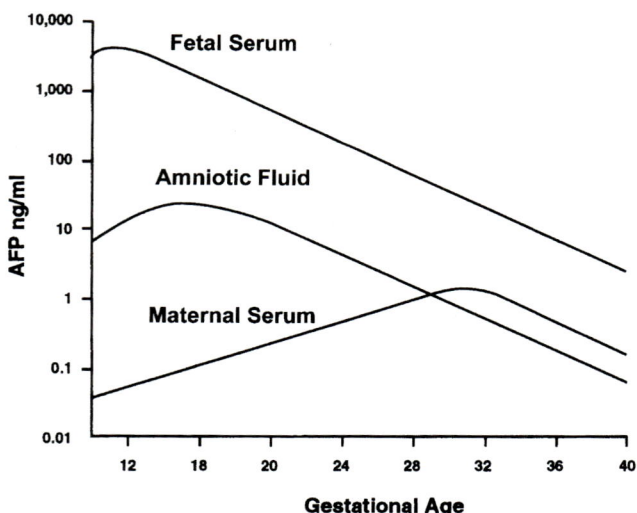

FIGURE 2. Concentrations of alpha-fetoprotein (*AFP*) values in fetal serum, amniotic fluid, and maternal serum. Note the logarithmic scale, indicating much higher levels of AFP in the fetal serum compared to maternal serum. (Reproduced with permission from Haddow JE. Prenatal screening for open neural tube defects, Down's syndrome, and other major fetal disorders. *Semin Perinatol* 1990;14:488.)

the measurement. In addition, because MS-AFP increases with gestation, it allows for this variation of marker level with gestational age. Moreover, this method allows consistent reporting among institutions and different analytic methods. Use of MoM data has now been applied to other screening parameters.

Optimal interpretation of MS-AFP levels takes into account other contributing factors such as maternal weight,[6] diabetes mellitus,[7,8] and ethnicity. The California Expanded AFP program adjusts specifically for the woman's ethnicity to take these subtle variations into account. Twins have twice as much AFP entering the maternal serum, and this has to be taken into account. In California the pregnancy is considered at risk for an NTD in either or both fetuses if the MS-AFP is at least 4.5 MoM. The prevalence of NTDs in the community should also be considered, since this affects the positive predictive value of an abnormal test. All of these factors have led to some elaborate protocols designed to optimize screening.

Some laboratories report AFP results only as positive (increased risk) or negative. Others calculate a numeric risk based on the level of MS-AFP with a positive screen suggested when the value is over a certain threshold.

Incorrect Dates

Less than 5% of patients initially reported as having an elevated test actually carry a fetus with an NTD or other anomaly. Because absolute levels of AFP are highly dependent on the age of gestation, poor obstetric dating is by far the most common reason for elevated levels. If an ultrasound examination has not previously confirmed or established the menstrual dates before the AFP test, approximately 20% of positive tests are due to a more advanced gestation. Recalculation after determination of correct gestational age eliminates the need for further study in this group.

In addition to identifying NTDs, MS-AFP identifies myriad fetal and pregnancy-related disorders (Table 1).[9]

Multiple Gestations

Multiple fetuses account for approximately 10% of high values in screening programs. If amniocentesis is performed and amniotic fluid–AFP is examined, however, it is usually normal, because nearly all fetuses are contained within their own amniotic sac.

Placental Abnormalities

Underlying placental abnormalities with fetal-placental hemorrhage can cause elevated MS-AFP. Because concentrations of AFP in the fetal serum are approximately 100,000 times greater than in the maternal serum during the midtrimester, it is easy to understand how even small amounts of fetal blood may cause major elevations in MS-AFP.

TABLE 1. ASSOCIATIONS WITH ELEVATED MATERNAL SERUM ALPHA-FETOPROTEIN

Fetal anomalies
  Neural tube defects
    Anencephaly
    Encephalocele
    Spina bifida
  Abdominal wall defects
    Gastroschisis
    Omphalocele
    Cloacal exstrophy
    Bladder exstrophy
  Renal anomalies and obstructive uropathy
    Renal agenesis
    Cystic malformations
    Congenital nephrosis
  Skin lesions (cutis aplasia, epidermolysis conditions)
  High fetal bowel obstruction
    Duodenal obstruction
    Esophageal atresia
  Limb body wall complex
  Amniotic bands
  Cystic hygroma
  Epignathus
  Sacrococcygeal teratoma
  Congenital cystic adenomatoid malformation
Other fetal events
  Fetal demise
  Multiple gestation
  Fetal growth restriction
  More advanced gestational age
  Fetal to maternal hemorrhage
  Fetal parvovirus infection
Other pregnancy findings
  Placenta accreta
  Rupture of membranes
  Placental or cord tumors
    Chorioangioma
    Cord hemangioma
  Oligohydramnios
  Increased risk for preeclampsia
Maternal specific disorders
  Maternal liver disease
    Hepatitis
    Hepatocellular carcinoma
  Germ cell ovarian neoplasm

Adapted from Main DM, Mennuti MT. Neural tube defects: issues in prenatal diagnosis and counselling. *Obstet Gynecol* 1986;67(1):1–16.

Vascular tumors of the placenta (chorioangioma) and umbilical cord (hemangioma) have also been associated with elevated MS-AFP levels. Indeed, markedly elevated AFP levels may result from these lesions. In these cases, elevated AFP is thought to be secondary to either hemorrhage in the tumor or increased transudation of fetal proteins to the amniotic fluid. Elevated AFP has been associated with placenta previa and placenta accreta, presumably on the same basis.[10–12] Elevated MS-AFP has also been associated with placental sonolucencies and placental infarct.[13,14] The association with placental abnormalities is linked to observation of a higher likelihood of adverse outcome observed

in women with biochemical alterations (see Pregnancy Complications and Adverse Outcome at the end of this chapter). Further discussion regarding placental abnormalities can be found in Chapter 3.

Fetal Anomalies

A variety of congenital anomalies are associated with elevated MS-AFP levels. Most such anomalies should be easily detected by sonography, although some (e.g., skin defects) are not. These can be categorized by their mechanism of MS-AFP elevation as follows: (a) NTDs, abdominal wall defects, sacrococcygeal teratoma, cystic hygroma, skin defects, and other anomalies resulting in exposure or leakage of fetal tissue into amniotic fluid; (b) renal anomalies; and (c) otherwise unexplained. Unexplained associations include cystic adenomatoid malformation of the lung and upper gastrointestinal obstructions.

Neural Tube Defects

As suggested by Brock and Sutcliffe,[2] elevated MS-AFP apparently reflects high levels of AFP in the amniotic fluid, which results from transudation of AFP across exposed neural tissue. Distribution curves have been generated for populations of normal subjects, anencephaly, and open spina bifida pregnancies (Fig. 3). As might be expected, the highest AFP values occur with anencephaly and the lowest levels occur with closed spinal defects.

Most laboratories use a MoM between 2.0 and 2.5 as the value over which the pregnancy is considered at increased risk for an NTD. Using a cutoff of 2.5 MoM, 80% of open spina bifida cases can be detected with a false-positive rate of 3% to 4%.[3,15–17] The false-positive rate has been further lowered with more precise assays.[18]

Yaron et al.[19] found that the combination of abnormally elevated MS-AFP and low estriol is highly predictive of NTDs, particularly anencephaly. Among 51 patients with this combination, 16 had NTDs, including 14 with anencephaly.

At the same time that screening protocols were being developed in the mid-1980s, second-trimester ultrasound dramatically improved. In the early 1980s, ultrasound was considered inferior to maternal serum screening for identification of NTDs. By the mid to late 1980s, ultrasound had not only surpassed serum screening but also exceeded amniotic fluid testing for identification of NTDs. Sonographic recognition of cranial findings associated with NTDs has been found to be of great value in conjunction with an MS-AFP screening program (see Chapter 7).

Abdominal Wall Defects

After NTDs, abdominal wall defects are the second most common type of anomaly identified in most AFP screening programs. Figure 4 shows the normal distribution of MS-

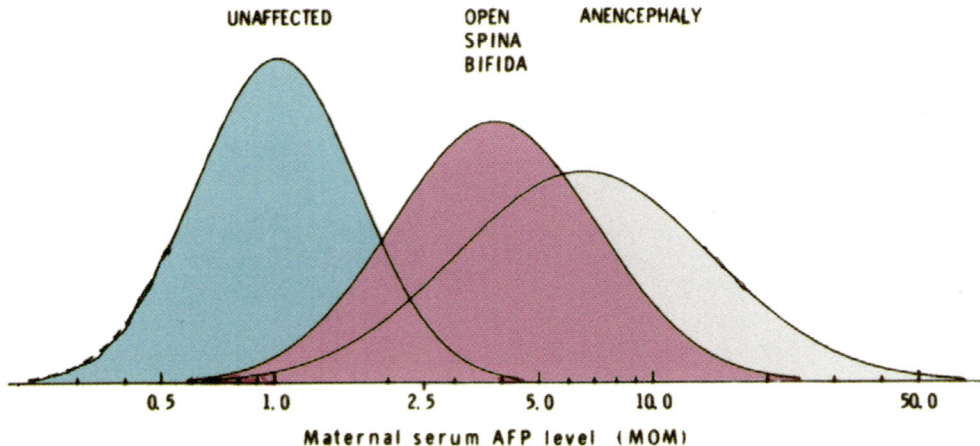

FIGURE 3. Distribution of maternal serum alpha-fetoprotein (*AFP*) values in series of normal patients and in patients carrying a fetus with spina bifida or anencephaly. MoM, multiples of the median. (Modified from Wald NJ, Cuckle HS. Neural tube defects: screening and biochemical diagnosis. *Prenat Diagn* 1983;3:210–241.)

AFP in fetuses with gastroschisis, omphalocele, and normal control subjects.

The majority of fetuses with gastroschisis are now detected before 20 weeks with serum AFP screening and a targeted sonogram. Because eviscerated organs of gastroschisis come into direct contact with the amniotic fluid, AFP levels of gastroschisis tend to be higher than those associated with omphalocele.[20] The limiting membrane presents a relative barrier to leakage of AFP into the amniotic fluid so that MS-AFP levels associated with omphalocele are generally lower and show a broader range than those observed with gastroschisis.[20,21]

MS-AFP screening detects approximately 85% of gastroschisis cases and about one-half of omphaloceles. Limb-body wall complex, an even larger and more complex defect, may produce markedly elevated MS-AFP levels. Abdominal wall defects are discussed in detail in Chapter 12.

Renal Anomalies

Because the kidneys normally resorb AFP, renal disease may allow spillage of more AFP into the amniotic fluid. This is seen with congenital nephrosis, an autosomal recessive disorder.[22,23] In congenital nephrosis, the kidneys may appear normal; however, the MS-AFP is usually quite elevated over 10 MoM.[24] Cystic kidney disorders and obstructive uropathy may also result in elevated MS-AFP levels.

Amniocentesis for Elevated Maternal Serum Alpha-Fetoprotein

Historically, amniocentesis was routinely offered to women with elevated MS-AFP levels. Certainly, analysis of AFP combined with acetylcholinesterase can provide much greater risk assessment for the possibility of NTD or other open defect as shown in the Reports of the Collaborative Acetylcholinesterase Study.[25,26] Today, however, amniotic fluid analysis is no more accurate than a high-quality ultrasound and does not provide information on the location, size, or origin of the defect or on important associated anomalies.

Elaborate protocols have been developed for the management of patients with elevated MS-AFP levels. There is

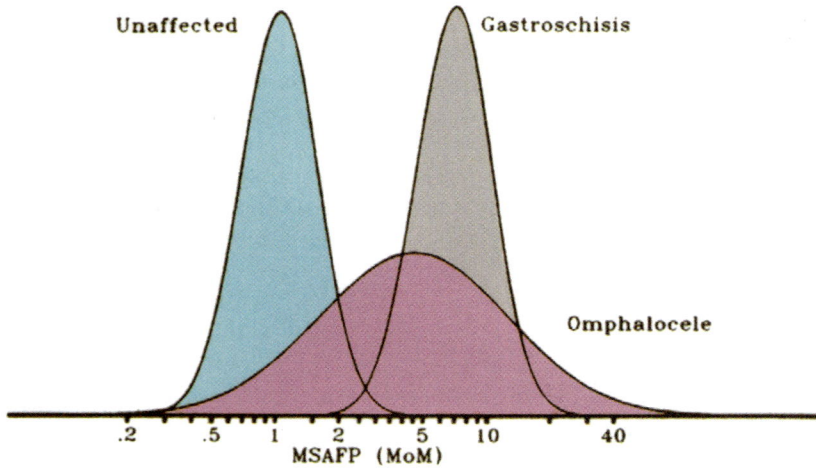

FIGURE 4. Distribution of maternal serum alpha-fetoprotein (*MSAFP*) in patients carrying a fetus with gastroschisis or omphalocele compared to unaffected fetuses. The lower values with omphalocele reflect the covering membrane of omphalocele. MoM, multiples of the median. (Reproduced with permission from Palomaki GE, Hill L, Knight G, et al. *Obstet Gynecol* 1988;71:906–909.)

still surprising variation between centers, and no consensus has been reached. However, several clear trends are established. Fewer patients now accept amniocentesis solely for the indication of elevated MS-AFP levels. This trend has paralleled both an overall trend away from invasive procedures, if possible, and increased awareness of the high accuracy of ultrasound. Indeed, ultrasound is considered more accurate than even amniotic fluid analysis at many centers.[27,28]

Thus, many centers no longer recommend an amniocentesis in this situation, as the risk of miscarriage is greater than the chance of identifying a small NTD.[29–31] The risk of miscarriage may be even higher in women with elevated AFP levels compared to women with normal or reduced levels. Invasive procedures may reasonably be considered if AFP levels are unusually high, the patient is considered at risk for fetal aneuploidy, or ultrasound is not diagnostic.

Because of the accuracy of ultrasound, the primary reason to perform amniocentesis rather than targeted ultrasound in women with elevated MS-AFP is to identify fetal aneuploidy, reported in approximately 1% of patients. The cost-benefit analysis of Nadel et al.[32] showed that protocols of amniocentesis are not cost-effective if fetal chromosome analysis is not performed in addition to measurements of AFP and acetylcholinesterase. Even this practice is questionable, however, since fetuses with major chromosome abnormalities typically show anomalies as the source of the elevated AFP. Also, over one-half of cases of fetal aneuploidy will have sex chromosomal aneuploidies, of which less than one-half will undergo pregnancy termination.[33]

Neural Tube Defect Screening in the First Trimester

MS-AFP is only useful as a marker for NTD after 14 weeks of gestation. The Report of the U.K. Collaborative Study on AFP in relation to NTDs[34] showed that the optimal detection for open spina bifida occurred at 16 to 18 weeks, with a fall to 20% at 10 to 12 weeks. Aitken et al.[35] analyzed MS-AFP in pregnancies with open NTD in the first and second trimesters. In the 14 cases investigated prior to 14 weeks none had AFP levels above 2 MoM, whereas all had elevated levels in the paired second-trimester sample. Sebire et al.[36] found raised MS-AFP levels in seven of nine anencephalic pregnancies at 10 to 14 weeks' gestation, but levels were normal in cases with spina bifida. Clearly, any move away from simultaneous screening for NTD and aneuploidy in the second trimester will need to consider whether to offer an additional screen for NTDs in the second trimester. The increasing successful use of high-resolution ultrasound to detect NTDs at the 20-week anomaly scan, the declining incidence of NTD,[37] and the increasing use of periconceptional folic acid supplementation[38] may make biochemical screening for NTDs unnecessary.

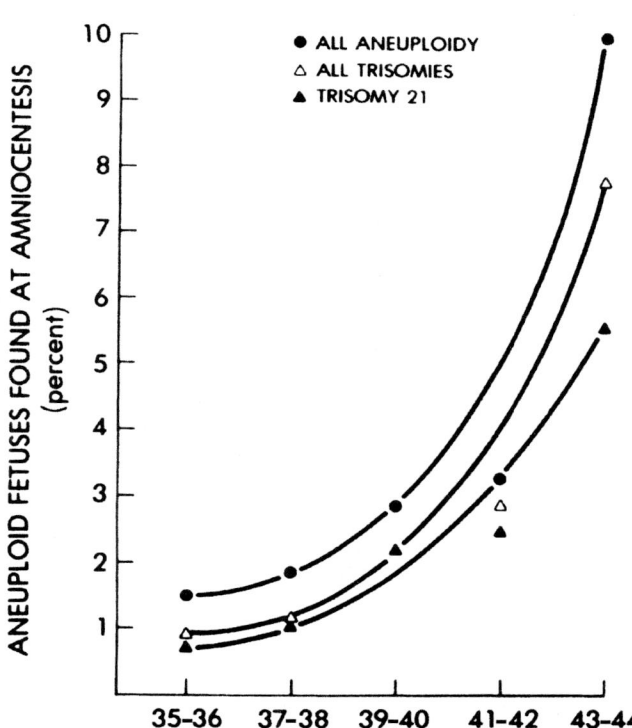

FIGURE 5. Risk of fetal aneuploidy at the time of second-trimester amniocentesis shows exponential risk with trisomies 18, 13, and 21. (Reproduced with permission from Simpson JL, Golbus MS, Martin AO, et al. *Genetics in obstetrics and gynecology.* Philadelphia: Grune & Stratton, 1982.)

FETAL ANEUPLOIDY SCREENING

Frequency and Occurrence

The natural frequency of chromosome abnormalities at birth, in the absence of any prenatal diagnosis, has been estimated at 6 per 1,000 births.[39] The most common of these is the autosomal trisomy 21 (Down syndrome). The risk of fetal Down syndrome varies dramatically with maternal age (Fig. 5). The overall birth prevalence of trisomy 21 has been quoted as 1 in 700,[40] although this varies with the maternal age distribution. In the United States, women in the "advanced maternal age" (35 to 49 years) group contributed 12.6% of live births in 1997 compared to just 4.7% in 1974.[41] As a result, the general prevalence of Down syndrome during the second trimester increased from 1 in 740 in 1974 to 1 in 504 in 1997 (Fig. 6). The impact of changing maternal age patterns for the United Kingdom is shown in Figure 7.

The other common autosomal trisomies include trisomy 18 (Edwards syndrome) and trisomy 13 (Patau syndrome) with birth incidences of 1 in 6,500 and 1 in 12,500, respectively.[40]

Maternal Age Risks

The relationship between advancing maternal age and increased risk of carrying a fetus with trisomy 21 was ini-

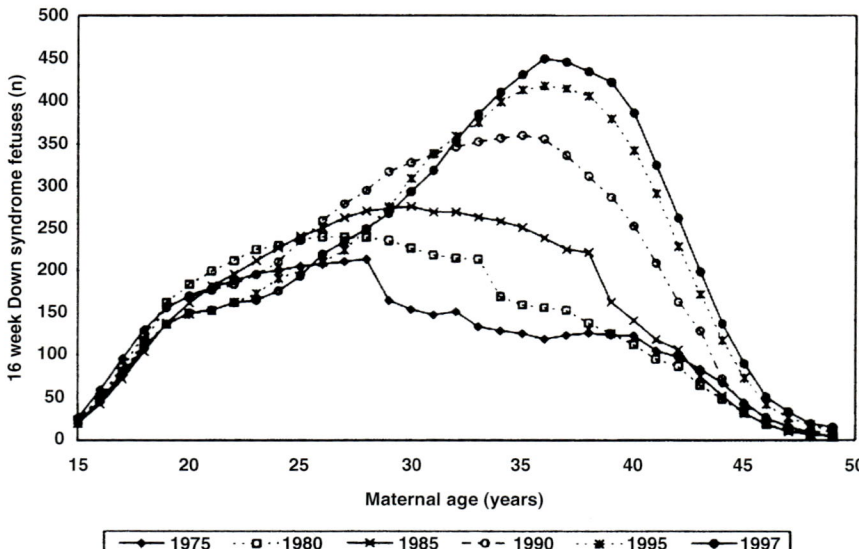

FIGURE 6. Maternal age–specific 16-week prevalence of Down syndrome fetuses in the United States in 5-year intervals from 1975 to 1995 and in 1997. There has been a rightward shift of the curve, reflecting the change in demographics toward delayed childbearing. [Reproduced with permission from Egan JF, Benn P, Borgida AF, Rodis JF, Campbell WA, Vintzileos AM. Efficacy of screening for fetal Down syndrome in the United States from 1974 to 1997. *Obstet Gynecol* 2000;96(6):979–985.]

tially established by Penrose[42] in 1933. Some studies[43,44] suggest that the prevalence also increases with paternal age, with the incidence in fathers older than 39 being more than three times that in fathers younger than 35 (i.e., 4.1 per 1,000 vs. 1.4 per 1,000).

There are numerous published rates of trisomy 21 at different maternal ages. One of the most commonly used in commercial software is that of Cuckle et al.,[45] which provides regressed maternal age risks at individual maternal ages based on data from eight published surveys. Other studies[46–48] on similar data have found higher rates, and considerable discussion continues as to which, if any, of these are correct.[49]

Fetal Loss

Many published rates are expressed as term risks.[45–47] A higher spontaneous loss of affected fetuses occurs across preg-

nancy, resulting in a higher probability of finding an affected fetus at the time of amniocentesis or chorionic villus sampling. Studies of fetal loss rates from various periods in pregnancies with an affected fetus have largely focused on populations of women having chorionic villus sampling or amniocentesis because of increased maternal age. Such studies may provide a biased assessment since, in unaffected pregnancies, fetal loss rates in women over 30 rise exponentially.[50] Morris et al.[51] carried out an investigation of fetal loss rate from data from the U.K. National Down Syndrome Cytogenetic Register, which contains records of cases diagnosed pre- or postnatally in women of all ages. The data from this individual study showed fetal loss rates of 31% between the first trimester and term and 24% between the second trimester and term. Snijders et al.[52] reported very similar results. These data may be more appropriate than the combined data from other series (Table 2).[53]

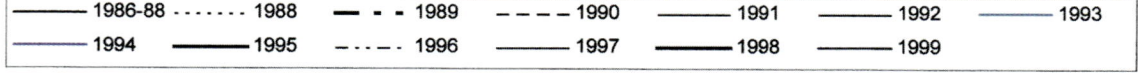

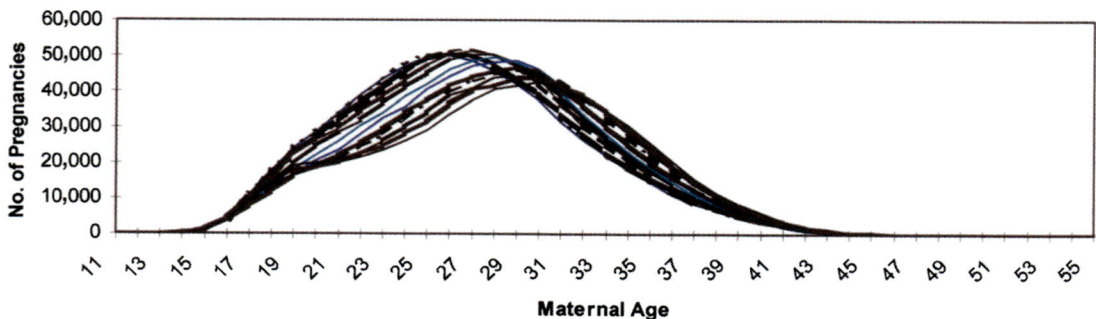

FIGURE 7. Changing pattern of maternal age of maternities in England and Wales from 1986 to 1999.

TABLE 2. ESTIMATES OF FETAL LOSS BETWEEN THE FIRST OR SECOND TRIMESTER AND TERM

Study	Maternal age range (yr)	Fetal loss rate, % (cases) First trimester	Fetal loss rate, % (cases) Second trimester
Hook et al.[306]	16–49	75 (8)	50 (168)
Halliday et al.[323]	36–43	31 (39)	18 (73)
Macintosh et al.[302,303]	35–48	48 (302)	24 (610)
Bray et al.[47]	35–50	31 (341)	12 (1,159)
Morris et al.[51]	16–49	31 (441)	24 (2,035)
Snijders et al.[52]	35–45	31 (221)	21 (317)

Fetal loss rates for other trisomies are thought to be even higher than for trisomy 21, and Snijders et al.[54] have compiled risk estimates for the three most common trisomies depending on the gestational age of the pregnancy being investigated.

Previous Trisomy 21

In women with a previous pregnancy affected by trisomy 21 Cuckle and Wald[55] found an additional risk of 0.34% at term (0.42% in the second trimester). This residual background risk should be added to the age-specific risk, which results in a relatively large risk for young women but risks not significantly different from the maternal age background risk by the age of 35.

Prenatal Screening

Screening by Maternal Age

Before the advent of MS-AFP screening, maternal age was used to select women with a high background risk of trisomy 21 in whom diagnostic testing may be considered appropriate. In the United States and the United Kingdom, women over a chosen cutoff age, commonly 35 years, were offered amniocentesis in the 1970s and early 1980s. Unfortunately, using specific maternal age cutoffs alone is a relatively poor marker for trisomy 21, since in the 1970–1985 period only 25% to 30% of cases of trisomy 21 cases occurred in women over 35 and only 6% to 7% of all pregnant women were over 35. As a result the predictive value of screening by maternal age alone was poor, with about one abnormal case being detected for every 125 invasive diagnostic procedures. Furthermore, the low uptake of amniocentesis among this group resulted in even lower detection rates than the 25% to 30% theoretically expected.

As a result of the changing demographics of pregnant populations in the western world, in which maternity is often delayed until later life, the proportion of pregnant women in the 35 and over group is now 12% to 15%.

Using a maternal age cutoff of 35 to offer amniocentesis in today's populations would result in the detection of one

case for every 178 invasive procedures. Assuming a 1% procedural loss rate, this would mean the loss of two normal unaffected pregnancies for every case of trisomy 21 identified—a loss that cannot be considered acceptable.

Dramatic advances have been made in screening for fetal aneuploidy during the past 2 decades by the use of biochemical markers and antenatal ultrasound. Screening protocols now permit detection of fetal trisomy 21 and other anomalies among younger women who previously would have been considered at low risk based on maternal age alone. Use of such protocols has thrown into question whether routine genetic amniocentesis is necessary only on the basis of maternal age.[56] Women themselves questioned this assumption long before other screening protocols were developed.

Development of Markers

Maternal Serum Markers

Second Trimester. *Alpha-Fetoprotein.* In 1984, Merkatz et al.[57] observed low AFP levels in fetuses with trisomy 18 and trisomy 21 in the second trimester. This was quickly confirmed by Cuckle et al.[58] and subsequently many other studies (Table 3). The initial screening proposal to use specific maternal age–related AFP MoM cutoffs to select women for amniocentesis showed that AFP alone was a poor marker for trisomy 21.[59] This observation led to a search for other markers of fetal aneuploidy, and a larger number of markers has now been investigated, initially in the second trimester and more recently in the first trimester (Table 3).

Human Chorionic Gonadotropin. In what proved to be one of the key developments, Bogart et al.[60,61] reported that levels of human chorionic gonadotropin (hCG) and its free α subunit were altered in pregnancies with fetal aneuploidy in the late second trimester (i.e., 18 to 25 weeks of gestation). Many subsequent studies have confirmed that hCG levels are increased approximately twofold in cases with trisomy 21 in the second trimester (Table 3). For the free α subunit, however, other workers have found only small but significant elevations.[62–64]

Assays for hCG can have varying specificities, which can have considerable clinical consequences not only when screening for chromosomal anomalies but also in monitoring other clinical scenarios.[65–67] Broadly speaking, assays can be categorized into two types, those detecting intact (dimeric) hCG and those detecting total hCG (i.e., dimeric plus free β subunit of hCG) (see Summary of Analytes, Human Chorionic Gonadotropin). In clinical terms, dimeric and total hCG do not appear to behave differently when screening for aneuploid pregnancies.

In regard to other aneuploidies, hCG levels are low in association with trisomy 18,[68,69] unchanged for trisomy 13,[70] and variable for sex aneuploidies and triploidy. For Turner syndrome, hCG levels are increased in the presence of hydrops and decreased in the absence of hydrops.[71]

TABLE 3. MATERNAL SERUM MARKER MEDIAN MULTIPLES OF THE MEDIAN (MoM) IN PREGNANCIES AFFECTED BY TRISOMIES 21 AND 18 IN THE FIRST AND SECOND TRIMESTERS

| | Second trimester | | | | First trimester | | | |
| | Trisomy 21 | | Trisomy 18 | | Trisomy 21 | | Trisomy 18 | |
Maternal serum	N	Median (MoM)	N	Median (MoM)	N	Median (MoM)	N	Median (MoM)
Alpha-fetoprotein	1,328	0.75	519	0.65	611	0.80	53	0.91
Unconjugated estriol	733	0.72	263	0.42	210	0.71	—	—
Total hCG	907	2.06	347	0.32	625	1.33	53	0.38
Free β-hCG	562	2.20	145	0.33	846	1.98	126	0.27
Free α-hCG	239	1.43	12	0.86	162	1.00	—	—
Inhibin A	524	1.92	73	0.87	112	1.59	—	—
SP-1	448	1.46	25	1.13	246	0.86	—	—
CA125	187	1.01	—	—	34	1.14	—	—
HPL	81	1.29	12	0.55	—	—	—	—
α Inhibin	64	1.63	—	—	112	1.59	—	—
Activin-A	82	1.23	—	—	—	—	—	—
PAPP-A	159	0.97	90	0.11	777	0.45	119	0.20
Placental alkaline phosphatase	70	1.07	18	0.94	—	—	—	—

hCG, human chorionic gonadotropin; HPL, human placental lactogen; PAPP-A, pregnancy-associated plasma protein A.

Estriol. The next milestone came in 1988 when Canick and colleagues[72,73] reported that maternal serum unconjugated estriol levels were reduced in pregnancies with trisomy 21 in the second trimester. Although levels of unconjugated estriol are low in cases of trisomy 21 and also in cases of trisomy 18, trisomy 13, and Turner syndrome, the use of this marker in trisomy 21 screening programs has been controversial.[74–79]

In the same year (1988), Wald et al.[80] proposed a method in which many of the individual elements of risk for fetal trisomy 21 could be combined to provide a multimarker risk assessment in which the key components were maternal age, MS-AFP concentrations, total hCG, and unconjugated estriol, all corrected for the gestational age of the pregnancy. This procedure became known as the *triple test* and was widely adopted in the United States during the 1990s. Use of the triple test was much lower in the United Kingdom, where a two-marker screen based on total hCG or free β-hCG and AFP is used by greater than 70% of screening centers.[81]

In 1990 and 1991, Macri et al.[82] and Spencer[83] reported that maternal serum levels of the free β subunit of hCG were elevated in cases of trisomy 21. Although much of the early work related to free β-hCG was challenged in the literature, many subsequent studies have confirmed the greater second-trimester median shift in the median MoM for free β-hCG (2.20) compared to that for intact or total hCG (2.06) (Table 3).

In cases of trisomy 18, very low levels of free β-hCG are found as well as elevated levels in type I triploidy, very low levels in type II triploidy, and raised levels in hydropic Turner syndrome.[84]

Table 4 summarizes the pattern of the principal second-trimester marker changes in the most common aneuploidies.

Inhibin A. In the early 1990s, preliminary studies[85–87] showed that levels of immunoreactive inhibin (α inhibin) were increased in pregnancies affected by trisomy 21. Inhibin, a member of the transforming growth factor–beta superfamily, is a dimer composed of an α subunit and one

TABLE 4. SECOND-TRIMESTER MARKER PATTERNS IN THE MOST COMMON ANEUPLOIDIES

Anomaly	Human chorionic gonadotropin/free β	Alpha-fetoprotein	Unconjugated estriol
Trisomy 21	↑	↓	↓
Trisomy 18	↓	↓	↓
Trisomy 13	Normal	Small ↑	Normal
Turner syndrome	↑ (with hydrops)	Small ↓	Small ↓
Other sex aneuploidies	Normal or ↑	Normal or ↑	Normal
Triploidy			
Type I	↑	Normal or ↑	Little data
Type II	↓	Variable	Little data

↑, increased; ↓, decreased.

TABLE 5. MEDIAN MARKER MULTIPLES OF THE MEDIAN IN DIFFERENT ANEUPLOIDIES IN THE FIRST TRIMESTER AT 10 TO 14 WEEKS OF GESTATION

Aneuploidy	Study	Median NT	Median free β-hCG	Median PAPP-A
Trisomy 21	Spencer et al.[178]	2.27	2.15	0.51
Trisomy 18	Tul et al.[201]	3.27	0.28	0.18
Trisomy 13	Spencer et al.[208]	2.87	0.51	0.25
Turner syndrome	Spencer et al.[229]	4.76	1.11	0.49
Other sex aneuploidies	Spencer et al.[229]	2.07	1.07	0.88
Type I triploidy	Spencer et al.[227]	2.76	8.04	0.75
Type II triploidy	Spencer et al.[227]	0.88	0.18	0.06

hCG, human chorionic gonadotropin; NT, nuchal translucency; PAPP-A, pregnancy-associated plasma protein A.

of two similar but distinguishable β subunits. Early assays for inhibin were nonspecific and measured specifically all forms containing the α subunit. The development of more specific assays to allow measurement of specifically dimeric inhibin A has found potential application as a new second-trimester marker for trisomy 21.[88–92] Although levels are increased to something approaching that of total hCG, there is nevertheless a high degree of correlation between these two markers and between inhibin and free β-hCG. This coupled with an evolutionary assay methodology,[93] variable standardization, lack of stable and robust commercially developed assays, and poor center-to-center comparability[81] has delayed the appearance of any real prospective performance data with this marker (see Summary of Analytes, Inhibin A). What has been published with other trisomies is limited, but it does seem that levels are largely unremarkable in trisomy 18,[94,95] whereas in Turner syndrome hydrops levels are higher than normal.[94]

First Trimester. Alpha-Fetoprotein. In the first trimester a different pattern of maternal serum marker levels has emerged over the past decade. AFP has been shown to be reduced in pregnancies affected by trisomy 21 and trisomy 18 but to a lesser degree than in the second trimester.[96,97]

Human Chorionic Gonadotropin. Initial studies with total hCG[98] showed that levels were only slightly raised in cases of trisomy 21. Haddow et al.[99] later suggested that total hCG levels are sufficiently elevated to be used effectively to screen for trisomy 21 in the first trimester. However, a subsequent larger study[96] has confirmed that this is not the case unless screening is carried out at the very end of the first trimester (13 weeks), when levels of total hCG are increasing to the peak levels seen at 16 weeks in trisomy 21 pregnancies. Table 3 summarizes the literature median for total hCG in the first trimester and indicates a much lower median compared with that observed in the second trimester.

A major development was the observation of Spencer et al.[100] that free β-hCG levels are increased in trisomy 21 pregnancies at a time when total hCG levels are normal. Many other workers have subsequently confirmed elevated levels. The largest series to date[101] of 210 cases of trisomy

21 showed a median MoM of 2.15, and the combined world series totaling 846 cases gives a median MoM of 1.98, which is only slightly lower than that in the second trimester.

Pregnancy-Associated Plasma Protein A. Brambati et al.[102] first observed that pregnancy-associated plasma protein A (PAPP-A) was reduced in cases of aneuploidy including trisomy 21 during the first trimester. This has since been confirmed by many other studies. The largest series to date[101] showed PAPP-A reduced to 0.51 MoM in 210 cases at 10 to 14 weeks of gestation. An accumulative series shows a total of 777 cases with a median MoM 0.45 MoM, although these levels progressively change across the first trimester to reach near normal levels by 17 weeks.[103,104]

Other first-trimester markers of trisomy 21 have been largely unremarkable. In particular, inhibin A, has been found to be of no value in the first trimester even though it is a potentially useful second-trimester marker.[105]

Table 5 summarizes the median marker MoM levels in different aneuploidies in the first trimester.

Urine Markers. Maternal serum hCG is metabolized predominantly through the urine route. Initially hCG follows a deactivation pathway in which the β subunit has the peptide linkage between residues 47 and 48 cleaved (less frequently between 43 and 44 or 44 and 45). This nicked hCG is unstable and dissociates into free α and free β subunits, which may be excreted in the urine. The free β subunit may be degraded further to β-core fragment, and this is the principal hCG β-subunit–related molecule in pregnancy urine.[106,107] It has been hypothesized that the reason maternal serum free β-hCG is more discriminating for trisomy 21 than total hCG is that in fetal trisomy 21 the deactivation or nicking process is accelerated, resulting in elevated maternal serum levels of nicked free β-hCG.[108] Initial studies suggested very high levels of β-core fragment,[109–112] although later studies[113–118] showed median MoMs closer to 3. These studies have questioned the validity of the earlier studies and cast doubt over assay suitability and specificity[119] as well as over sample stability.[120]

TABLE 6. MATERNAL URINE MARKER MEDIAN MULTIPLES OF THE MEDIAN IN FIRST AND SECOND TRIMESTER OF PREGNANCIES AFFECTED BY TRISOMY 21

	N	β-Core fragment hCG	N	Total estriol	N	Free β-hCG
First trimester	50	2.10	22	0.83	36	1.71
Second trimester	280	3.88	151	0.62	127	3.16

hCG, human chorionic gonadotropin.

When β-core fragment has also been measured in first-trimester urines,[121–123] although levels are increased (2.10 MoM), the very wide spread of the data in the trisomy 21 cases and the unaffected population made for poor clinical discrimination. When free β-hCG has been measured in urine (summarized in Hsu et al.[117]) levels approaching that in serum have been found, but in general the discrimination is poorer than with serum because of the wider spread of results in the affected and unaffected populations. In addition to hCG-related molecules, some studies have also measured total estriol and attempted to use this in a ratio form to enhance the detection rate,[106,124] although this is not particularly effective.[117]

Table 6 summarizes the median marker MoM for urine markers studied in the first and second trimesters.

A more recent development measures levels of a hyperglycosylated form of hCG (a form of hCG characterized by a more complex oligosaccharide side chain) initially in the urine, but also in the serum.[107,125–128] Cole et al.[127] extended an original study of 23 cases with a further 18 cases and found even higher results (median MoM 9.5), with 80% of cases above the ninety-fifth percentile.

Despite these encouraging results, commercial assays are not available and question marks exist over the stability of hyperglycosylated hCG[127] and the method of correcting for renal concentrating effects. A further development with perhaps even greater potential is measurement of this analyte in the serum. Shahabi et al.[129] studied ten second-trimester cases with trisomy 21 and found levels to be elevated at a median of 3.9 MoM with 60% of cases above the ninety-fifth percentile of normal. Using a different assay based on lectin affinity immunoassay, Abushoufa et al.[130] studied 39 cases of trisomy 21 in the 16- to 18-week period and found raised levels (median MoM 2.2) and approximately 74% of cases above the ninetieth percentile of normal. Additional studies are currently underway to evaluate urinary and serum hyperglycosylated hCG.

Ultrasound Markers

A number of ultrasound markers of fetal trisomy have been identified during the second trimester.[131] The sensitivities of most sonographic markers are low, particularly in comparison to that reported by NT in the first trimester. However, the incremental value of each marker improves the overall sensitivity of second-trimester ultrasound. When combined with structural anomalies and systematically sought as part of a "genetic sonogram," detection rates exceed 50% at many referral centers.[132–137] Detection rates exceeding 90% have even been reported with a high detection rate of cardiac abnormalities.[138] However, application to low-risk patients would be expected to result in lower detection rates and possibly unacceptably high false-positive rates,[139] unless maternal age and the strength of the ultrasound marker are accounted for.[140–143] Ultrasound markers of fetal aneuploidy during the second trimester are discussed in detail in Chapter 25.

First-trimester (10 to 14 weeks) screening with ultrasound began with the observation that "cystic hygromas" observed during the first trimester were more likely to be associated with trisomies, including trisomy 21, than typical cystic hygromas seen during the second trimester.[144,145] It was further observed that cystic hygromas seen during the first trimester may have a different appearance (nonseptated) than those seen during the second trimester[146] and commonly resolved. In 1992, Nicolaides et al.[147] proposed the term *nuchal translucency* for the sonographic appearance of fluid under the skin at the back of the fetal neck observed in all fetuses during the first trimester. They reported an association between the thickness of the translucency and the risk of fetal aneuploidy, especially trisomies. This concept of measuring NT in all fetuses formed the basis for first-trimester screening by ultrasound. By 1995, the first large studies of NT were published.[148] It has now been shown that NT thickness can be reliably measured using standardized techniques by ultrasound scanning at 11 to 14 weeks' gestation in nine tertiary referral centers, and when combined with maternal age can produce an effective means of screening for trisomy 21.[149] Because of the importance to fetal aneuploidy as well as other anomalies, NT is described in detail in Chapter 20.

Calculation of Risks

Many of the biologic and biophysical observations in pregnancy vary with the duration of the pregnancy, with some values increasing, others decreasing, and others both increasing and decreasing as the pregnancy progresses (see Summary of Analytes and Fig. 13). To remove gestational age variation effects and to allow some degree of standardization from center to center, many biochemical (and some biophysical) parameters have been expressed as MoMs for unaffected pregnancies of the same gestational age. Thus, an MoM of 1 means the result is normal, an MoM of 2 indicates the level is 100% greater than that expected in a normal pregnancy of the same gestation, and an MoM of 0.5 indicates the level is 50% lower than that expected in a normal pregnancy.

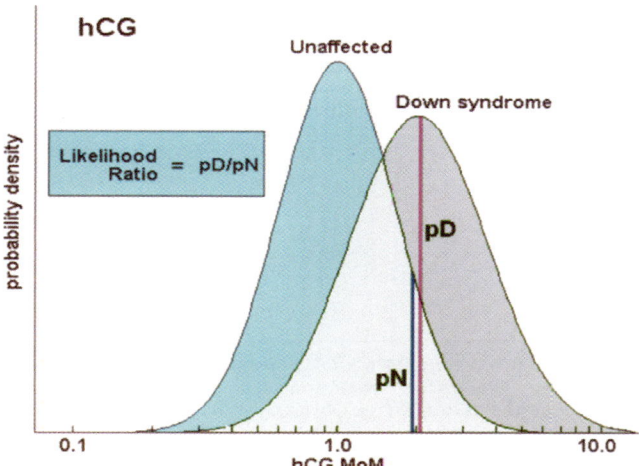

FIGURE 8. Distribution of free β–human chorionic gonadotropin (hCG) in normal pregnancies and pregnancies affected by trisomy 21. MoM, multiples of the median. pD, probability of Down syndrome; pN, probability of normal.

TABLE 7. MAHALANOBIS DISTANCES FOR SELECTED FIRST- AND SECOND-TRIMESTER MARKERS OF TRISOMY 21

Marker	Mahalanobis distance	
	Second trimester	First trimester
Serum		
Alpha-fetoprotein	0.69	0.23
Unconjugated estriol	1.20	0.68
Intact/total hCG	1.86	0.38
Free β-hCG	2.04	1.45
Dimeric inhibin A	1.65	0.35
Pregnancy-associated plasma protein A	—	2.08
Ultrasound		
Nuchal translucency	—	6.46

hCG, human chorionic gonadotropin.

When expressed as MoMs, the majority of biochemical markers (and NT) follow a gaussian distribution in both normal and affected populations only when the MoM is log transformed. Figure 8 shows the distribution of free β-hCG in normal and trisomy 21 pregnancies affected. Even with the best marker there is still significant overlap of the two populations, so to use the marker information Cuckle et al.[45] proposed the use of a gaussian model to derive a probability or likelihood that a particular analyte concentration was associated with an affected pregnancy. In essence, the ratio of the heights of the distributions in the affected and unaffected pregnancies at a given marker MoM, as shown in Figure 8, is the likelihood ratio. This ratio can then be used to modify the *a priori* maternal age-specific risk to produce a patient-specific risk. It follows from Figure 8 that two important features of the marker distribution dictate how good the marker is in discriminating between unaffected and affected populations. The two features are (a) the difference between the median values in the two populations (sometimes called the *median shift*) and (b) the width of the distributions (the standard deviation). Together these two features define the extent of overlap of the unaffected and affected populations. For markers with similar standard deviations, the marker with the largest median shift will have a better predictive value, whereas for markers with similar median shifts, the marker with the smallest spread of values will be the most effective. Using the Mahalanobis distance calculated from

$$\left(\frac{Mean\ Unaffected - Mean\ Affected}{SDU\ Unaffected} \right)^2$$

where the means and SD are in the $\log_{10}$ domain,[150] allows markers to be ranked in a scale of effectiveness. Table 7 shows the Mahalanobis distance for the commonly used markers in the first and second trimesters. Clearly in the second trimester the most effective markers are free β-hCG, followed by total hCG and dimeric inhibin A, whereas in the first trimester NT is the most effective with PAPP-A and free β-hCG being the most effective biochemical markers.

Although of all the markers NT is perhaps the only marker that would have sufficient discrimination to be used alone in conjunction with maternal age, in practice a more efficient method is to combine information from more than one marker. To do this, however, it is necessary to ensure that information from one marker is not duplicated by information from another—that is, we need to make sure they are not correlated or providing the same information. One way to obviate this is to take into account correlation between markers in both affected and unaffected populations. For example, it is imperative to take into account the high correlation between hCG markers and inhibin A and that between AFP and unconjugated estriol.

The mathematic basis behind multimarker risk assessment is an extension of that used for the single-marker case, with the addition of marker correlation information. The detailed mathematics behind this is beyond the scope of this review but has been explained in detail by Reynolds and Penny.[150a]

The expected screening performance using various marker combinations can be modeled from the data obtained in a number of retrospective case-control studies of trisomies 21 and 18. Considerable disparity in estimates of detection and false-positive rates have been reported; this may be as a result of a variety of factors, including variations in sample size, sample selection, assay methodology, analyte stability, risk calculation algorithms, estimation of gestational ages, marker distributions, marker correlations, and correction for covariables.[151] In addition, the modeling uses maternal age distribution of maternities as the baseline, and in some retrospective studies,[18,80] the authors have used the distribution of maternities in the study population (which may not be representative of the total pregnant population) rather than using a standardized maternal age distribution. Even using standardized maternal age distributions is problematic because early retrospective studies[80] used maternity distributions from England and Wales in 1986 to 1988, whereas more recent studies[18] use maternity distributions as of 1996 to 1998, in which the proportion of maternities to older women has increased significantly (see Fetal Aneuploidy Screening, Frequency and Occurrence and Fig. 7). There is therefore little wonder that claims in the literature for detection rates are confusing and controversial.[152]

Theoretical modeling of performance of screening protocols can only be as good as the quality of the data within the model. The models are invariably constructed from very small data sets of affected samples and often equally small series control unaffected pregnancies. In real-life screening, the models may not reflect the reality, and many authors have argued that a better measure of true screening performance should be expected from audits or routine real-life screening programs.

Reporting Risks

Once a risk assessment has been made, screening results categorize women into those at increased risk or those not at increased risk of carrying an affected fetus. This may be expressed in various ways. Commonly a numeric value indicating the calculated risk is given, usually expressed as an odds ratio. Cutoff values for positive screens vary among centers. Some use the risk level of that associated with a woman age 35 years. Other programs set the cutoff at a false-positive rate of 5%. To add more complexity, risk assessment can be based on second-trimester risk or live-born risk for Down syndrome. The risk of a second-trimester fetus having Down syndrome is higher because of intrauterine lethality.

Wald et al.[153] showed how the method of risk screening can be validated in any screening program and provided a methodology for assessing risk accuracy by looking at the reported risk based on maternal age and serum markers and seeing if this was close to the birth prevalence. Such a procedure has been carried out and shown to be accurate for approximately 76,000 pregnancies screened by the three-marker (AFP, total hCG, and estriol) scheme[153] and confirmed by Canick and Rish[154] in approximately 50,000 pregnancies. Also Spencer et al.[155] confirmed this for approximately 60,000 pregnancies screened by the two-marker (AFP and free β-hCG) scheme.

While reporting results with a numeric risk provides patients with a precise risk estimate, this may lead to increased patient anxiety[156] compared to patients given the over simplistic screen positive or screen negative reports, although other studies have found the opposite result.[157] Evidence from studies of patient acceptance of offers of amniocentesis does seem to suggest higher uptake of amniocentesis as the risk increases, suggesting that risk is at least understood to some degree.[158]

TABLE 8. DETECTION RATE AND FALSE-POSITIVE RATE FOR TRISOMY 21 IN THE SECOND TRIMESTER USING THE THREE-MARKER APPROACH

Maternal age (yr)	False-positive rate (%)	Detection rate (%)
20	3.2	44.7
25	3.8	47.5
30	6.1	56.0
35	15.8	73.8
38	28.6	85.5
40	40.9	91.6
44	70.0	98.1

Adapted from Reynolds TM, Nix AB, Dunstan FD, Dawson AJ. Age specific detection and false positive rates: an aid to counselling in Down syndrome risk screening. *Obstet Gynecol* 1993;81:447–450.

One factor that is often overlooked in screening programs is the fact that detection rates and false-positive rates vary dramatically with maternal age. In younger women the detection rate using second-trimester screening falls quite dramatically, as does the false-positive rate. Conversely, in older women the detection rate increases but so does the false-positive rate (Table 8). For example, one study using a dual screen[158] found prospective detection rates and false-positive rates of 63.0% and 2.5% in women under 30, 67.0% and 5.0% in women 31 to 34, and 89.0% and 15.4% in women 35 and older. Screening programs that quote only global detection and false-positive rates could be misleading to patients. These issues need to be considered when counseling women on the test and its results.[159]

Detection Rates for Trisomy 21

Second Trimester

Screening protocols have been in evolution since the initial observation that low AFP levels were associated with trisomies 21 and 18 in 1984.[57] It is currently uncertain which protocol, if any, will ultimately prove to be most effective. Based on changes in protocols since the inception of maternal serum screening, it is likely that protocols will continue to evolve; the ultimate screening protocol has yet to be developed. It is clear though that a variety of approaches have proved to be effective and that different centers may choose to adopt different protocols. We discuss detection rates for the most commonly accepted screening methods here.

Biochemistry

In 1988, Wald et al.[73] proposed addition of hCG and estriol together as a triple-marker combination and the initial study of Wald et al.[80] predicted a detection rate of 61% at a 5% false-positive rate. Using numerous adjustments to the data, based on correction for maternal weight and gestational dating by ultrasound and using more recent maternal age distributions, this model now predicts detection

TABLE 9. REPORTED PROSPECTIVE SCREENING PERFORMANCE USING ALPHA-FETOPROTEIN/TOTAL HUMAN CHORIONIC GONADOTROPIN AND UNCONJUGATED ESTRIOL

Study (number in Fig. 9)	Age group	Patients screened (N)	Trisomy 21 cases (N)	Detected cases (N)	Detection rate (%)	False-positive rate (%)
Haddow et al.[307] (1)	All	25,207	35	21	60	3.8
Phillips et al.[308] (2)	<35	9,530	7	4	70	3.2
Wald et al.[309] (3)	All	12,603	25	12	48	4.1
Cheng et al.[310] (4)	All	7,718	22	20	91	6.0
Burton et al.[311] (5)	All	8,233	12	10	83	5.9
Pescia et al.[312] (6)	All	7,039	16	11	69	5.9
Piggott et al.[313] (7)	All	6,990	11	8	73	3.0
Goodburn et al.[304] (8)	All	25,359	48	36	75	4.1
Mancini et al.[314] (9)	>30	2,892	5	4	80	13.3
Kellner et al.[315] (10)	>34	10,605	16	12	75	7.2
Total		**116,176**	**197**	**138**	**70**	**4.8**

rates as high as 69% for a 5% false-positive rate.[160] However, the data of Wald and colleagues are not necessarily the definitive data set. Much of the data contributing to the model are based on a series of only 77 cases and 385 controls collected during 1973 to 1983 and which have been repeatedly removed from storage to have multiple analytes tested on them and for which there are serious questions of stability.[161] Table 9 summarizes published data on results from prospective screening programs using the three-marker (AFP, total hCG, estriol) screen.

As noted previously, others have proposed a dual test using AFP and total hCG[69] or AFP and free β-hCG,[74,83] and this remains the most common protocol for screening in Great Britain. Table 10 summarizes those studies using AFP and total hCG; Table 11 summarizes those using the AFP and free β-hCG protocol. When results of these studies are compared with triple-screen studies (Fig. 9), it is evident that there is large overlap of the detection and no one protocol can be said to outperform the other.[162]

Inhibin A has been added to the triple-marker test to form a "quadruple test," and this is now commercially available. The additional gain in detection using this marker is again disputed. The general consensus estimate is a 5% to 7% gain when other studies are taken into account.[91,121,163,164]

Predicted 96% detection rates with a 5% false-positive rate for urinary hyperglycosylated hCG in combination

with maternal age and serum AFP need confirmation in much larger studies, as does their performance when combined with ultrasound biometry.[127,165]

Biochemistry and Ultrasound

Due in part to the number of second markers, these have not been closely integrated with biochemical screening. However, it appears clear that incorporation of ultrasound data improves the performance of second-trimester serum screening.[165,166]

Because ultrasound findings appear to be largely independent of both maternal age and biochemical analytes,[167-169] the combination of biochemical and ultrasound markers could further improve second-trimester screening. Improved screening performance has been supported by relatively few studies that have combined biochemistry and ultrasound in the second trimester.[165,166,170-174] This can be most easily done with parameters that can be reported as MoMs, such as nuchal thickening and limb length. Bahado-Singh et al.[173] reported that incorporation of humerus length and nuchal thickness improved the screening performance compared to serum biochemistry alone. Also, using ultrasound measurements of humeral length and nuchal thickness combined with hyperglycosylated hCG, Bahado-Singh et al.[165] reported a 91.3% detection rate with a 3.2% false-positive rate, although this was in a high-risk population. These approaches,

TABLE 10. REPORTED PROSPECTIVE SCREENING PERFORMANCE USING ALPHA-FETOPROTEIN AND TOTAL HUMAN CHORIONIC GONADOTROPIN

Study (number in Fig. 9)	Age	Patients screened (N)	Trisomy 21 cases (N)	Detected cases (N)	Detection rate (%)	False-positive rate (%)
Dawson et al.[316] (11)	All	8,414	14	7	50	3.5
Burn[317] (12)	All	4,898	7	4	57	3.5
Beekhuis[318] (13)	All	2,099	6	5	83	7.3
Crossley et al.[319] (14)	All	30,084	37	26	70	5.1
Mooney et al.[320] (15)	All	12,170	18	10	56	5.6
Total		**57,665**	**82**	**52**	**63**	**4.9**

TABLE 11. REPORTED PROSPECTIVE SCREENING PERFORMANCE USING ALPHA-FETOPROTEIN AND FREE β–HUMAN CHORIONIC GONADOTROPIN

Study (number in Fig. 9)	Age group	Patients screened (N)	Trisomy 21 cases (N)	Detected cases (N)	Detection rate (%)	False-positive rate (%)
(Sheffield) Spencer et al.[321] (16)	All	10,000	12	11	92	4.2
(Portsmouth) Spencer et al.[321] (17)	All	6,080	10	8	80	5.1
Macri et al.[322] (18)	<35	44,272	42	29	69	3.8
Hsu et al.[305] (19)	<34	4,084	6	5	83	4.7
Macri et al.[296] (20)	<35	7,494	8	6	75	2.7
Spencer[58] (21)	All	67,904	107	80	75	5.1
Total		**139,834**	**185**	**139**	**75**	**5.1**

while promising, require further evaluation with larger prospective studies.

First Trimester

Biochemistry

Among biochemical markers, only free β-hCG and PAPP-A have been shown to be of value in numerous retrospective and some prospective series. Detection rates in the range of 55% to 68% have been reported.[175–177] However, detection rates with these markers are very dependent on the gestational age at which samples are taken since the median shifts for free β-hCG and PAPP-A are not constant across the first trimester.[101] This has significant implications for screening algorithms and the parameter sets used.[178,179]

Algorithms that use population parameters from studies over a wide gestational age will inevitably be inaccurate in their risk estimations.

Biochemistry and Ultrasound

Combining maternal serum biochemistry and NT measurement in the first trimester is an effective screening protocol because the two modalities do not appear to be correlated. A retrospective study[101] of 210 cases of trisomy 21 and approximately 1,000 controls reported that this combined approach achieved 89% detection for a 5% false-positive rate. Other studies[180–182] have also found that the combination of first-trimester biochemistry and NT is better than either one alone, with detection rates in excess of 80%. Table 12 summarizes detection rates for various com-

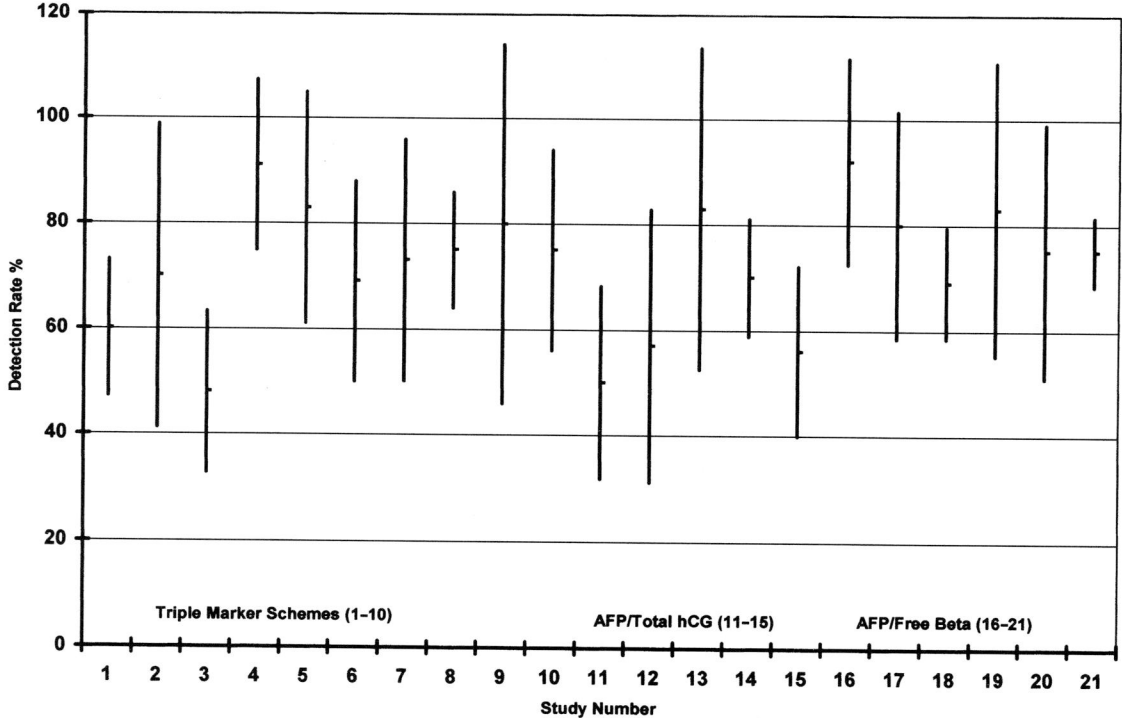

FIGURE 9. Reported sensitivities and confidence intervals for 5% false-positive rate using three different protocols for second-trimester serum screening: triple-marker screen [human chorionic gonadotropin (*hCG*), alpha-fetoprotein (*AFP*), and estriol], AFP and total hCG, and AFP and free β-hCG.

TABLE 12. FALSE-POSITIVE RATES AT FIXED DETECTION RATES FOR COMBINATIONS OF MATERNAL SERUM BIOCHEMICAL MARKERS WITH AND WITHOUT FETAL NUCHAL TRANSLUCENCY (NT)

Detection rate (%)	Free β-hCG and PAPP-A	NT and free β-hCG	NT and PAPP-A	NT, free β-hCG, and PAPP-A
90	23.0	12.0	12.0	6.0
85	16.0	7.0	7.0	3.5
80	11.0	5.0	4.0	2.1
75	8.0	3.0	2.7	1.5
70	6.0	2.2	1.5	1.0

hCG, human chorionic gonadotropin; PAPP-A, pregnancy-associated plasma protein A.

binations of biochemical markers and NT measurements based on the study of Spencer et al.[101]

As with second-trimester screening, detection rates using NT and first-trimester biochemistry vary with maternal age. Spencer[182a] calculated the detection rate and the predictive value of an increased risk result at various maternal ages, the results of which are shown in Table 13.

Comparison of First- and Second-Trimester Screening

To compare detection rates at different periods of gestation allowance needs to be made for the inherent lethality of fetal aneuploidy. Hence, a detection rate of 75% in the first trimester is actually worse than the same detection rate in the second trimester. Dunstan and Nix[183] have provided a methodology to make this comparison. If one assumes that the fetal loss rates observed by Morris et al.[51] in women of all ages is the most accurate, then using this methodology and assuming a detection rate of 75% in the second trimester, detection rates in the first trimester would need to be 3.5% higher to be statistically significantly higher.[183a] In practice this cannot be achieved by maternal serum biochemistry or NT alone but can be achieved by combining the two when following the recommendations of the Royal College of Obstetricians and Gynaecologists.[184]

First-trimester screening presents logistical challenges, particularly the narrow gestational window (11 to 14 weeks) when NT is most effective for screening. Inevitably some women will be too early and some too late. For those who are too late, second-trimester biochemical screening must be available as an alternative; in our experience.[184a] this amounts to approximately 6% of pregnancies.

Inevitably some women, either by accident or design, will have second-trimester biochemical screening or possibly additional ultrasound screening after a first-trimester screen. Results from these subsequent tests should not be considered in isolation, and the first-trimester risk must be combined with the new information to produce accurate risk estimates. Cuckle and Sehmi[185] have shown how this can be achieved for first-trimester NT and second-trimester

biochemistry. Sequential testing of this type is likely to lead to confusion if women are given different risk estimates at different stages. Wald et al.[160] pointed out that sequential

TABLE 13. DETECTION RATE, FALSE-POSITIVE RATE, AND POSITIVE PREDICTIVE VALUE BY MATERNAL AGE WHEN SCREENING IN THE FIRST TRIMESTER USING FETAL NUCHAL TRANSLUCENCY AND MATERNAL SERUM–FREE β–HUMAN CHORIONIC GONADOTROPIN AND PREGNANCY-ASSOCIATED PLASMA PROTEIN A

Maternal age (yr)	Detection rate (%)	False-positive rate (%)	Positive predictive value
15	76.98	1.87	2.92
16	77.34	2.02	2.87
17	77.84	2.17	2.84
18	78.36	2.26	2.89
19	78.61	2.30	2.99
20	78.81	2.34	3.04
21	79.23	2.50	2.99
22	79.50	2.59	2.98
23	79.78	2.68	3.02
24	80.13	2.78	3.04
25	80.65	2.87	3.12
26	81.12	3.00	3.15
27	81.59	3.18	3.20
28	82.19	3.33	3.31
29	82.90	3.66	3.36
30	83.80	3.96	3.50
31	84.88	4.43	3.57
32	85.89	5.14	3.62
33	87.12	6.19	3.63
34	88.37	7.23	3.83
35	89.66	8.71	3.99
36	91.12	10.53	4.24
37	92.56	13.10	4.47
38	93.91	15.93	4.88
39	95.08	19.77	5.27
40	96.07	24.36	5.76
41	96.96	29.77	6.36
42	97.73	35.38	7.18
43	98.26	41.24	8.18
44	98.76	47.12	9.36
45	98.96	52.65	10.68
46	99.14	58.13	12.05
47	99.33	62.38	13.47
48	99.45	65.44	14.75
49	99.60	67.43	15.64

testing was inefficient and further recommended that screening be carried out at one stage of pregnancy only.

Wald et al.[186] have proposed an integrated approach using information from selected first- and second-trimester markers. These authors predicted, based on mathematical modeling of data from many studies, that by integrating information from NT and PAPP-A at 10 to 13 weeks and combining this with AFP, total hCG, unconjugated estriol, and dimeric inhibin A at 15 to 18 weeks, detection rates of 94% for trisomy 21 could be achieved at a 5% false-positive rate. Implementation of this approach in routine screening could be difficult because of the delay following the first-trimester screen. This approach also raises ethical issues,[187–189] especially when 90% of the detected cases of trisomy 21 could have been detected earlier from the first-trimester screen alone.

Other Chromosomal Abnormalities

Although screening performance is based primarily on the detection of trisomy 21, screening protocols can also detect other chromosomal abnormalities. Biochemical associations with other common chromosome abnormalities are discussed further below.

Trisomy 18

Second Trimester

An association with low AFP levels and trisomy 18 was first observed by Merkatz et al.[57] and later confirmed by others.[68] Other associations with trisomy 18 during the second trimester include low levels of estriol, and low levels of hCG, progesterone, inhibin, and PAPP-A.[69,190,191] The tendency toward decreased levels of all analytes with trisomy 18 suggests an overall problem in synthesis or secretion of placental hormones. This may also coincide with the association of trisomy 18 with growth restriction, even at 15 to 20 weeks of gestation.

Based on the profile for trisomy 18, many screening centers now routinely include a separate screening protocol for trisomy 18, based either on a simple fixed cutoff approach when marker MoMs are below certain levels[68] or based on a specific trisomy 18 calculated risk.[63,192,193] Detection rates similar to those achieved for trisomy 21 have been reported for only small additional false-positive rates.

Using a five-marker protocol (estriol, free α-hCG, free β-hCG, estradiol, and human placental lactogen), Staples et al.[191] predicted a 58% detection at a 0.3% false-positive rate. Spencer et al.[63] using a two-marker protocol (AFP and free β-hCG) predicted a 50% detection with a 1% false-positive rate. Using a three-marker protocol (AFP, total hCG, and estriol), Barkai et al.[192] predicted a 67% detection at a 0.3% false-positive rate. Using the same protocol, Palomaki et al.[193] found a detection rate of 60% at a 0.2% false-positive rate. Benn et al.[194] compared the detection

rates using the fixed cutoff method and the risk-based procedure and found the latter to be more efficient.

The use of additional markers such as inhibin does not appear to further increase detection rates.[94] PAPP-A, however, may be one of the most discriminating markers for trisomy 18 in the second trimester,[195,196] although this is unlikely to be used in practice because this marker is of no use in the detection of cases of trisomy 21 at this time.

The occasional association with elevated MS-AFP reflects an underlying anomaly, such as spina bifida or omphalocele, rather than a specific profile for trisomy 18. Ultrasound can also detect various markers of trisomy 18 during the second trimester, including both structural anomalies and markers.[197] Others, however, have found that the sensitivity of ultrasound is too low and recommend amniocentesis whenever the risk for trisomy 18 is considered increased.[198] Correlation of biochemical screen can help risk assessment when ultrasound markers of trisomy 18 are identified, for example, following detection of choroid plexus cysts.[199]

First Trimester

During the first trimester, levels of free β-hCG and PAPP-A are significantly reduced.[200] The largest series of Tul et al.[201] of 50 cases added to the world literature gives a free β-hCG median of 0.27 MoM from 126 cases and a PAPP-A median of 0.20 MoM from 119 cases (Table 3). When total hCG and AFP were examined in the series reported by Tul et al.[201] the AFP median was only slightly reduced (0.91 MoM) and the total hCG was not as low (0.38) as that reported for free β-hCG.[97]

NT measurements are also significantly increased with trisomy 18 and, in fact, tend to be even greater than observed with trisomy 21.[202,203] When combined with maternal age, Tul et al.[201] predicted that 89% of cases of trisomy 18 could be detected at a 1% false-positive rate.

Trisomy 13

Second Trimester

Second-trimester screening with AFP, estriol, and hCG is probably not useful in detecting trisomy 13.[70] However, using a quadruple screen with incorporation of inhibin, Wenstrom et al.[204] reported detection of five in seven (71%) fetuses with trisomy 13 and Cuckle et al.[95] also showed elevated inhibin levels in three of six cases. Trisomy 13 may also present with elevated MS-AFP because of associated spinal or abdominal wall defects.[205]

Ultrasound alone can detect abnormalities in up to 90% of fetuses with trisomy 13 during the second trimester.[206,207]

First Trimester

Detection of trisomy 13 appears to be effective during the first trimester.[208] Free β-hCG and PAPP-A are also reduced with medians of 0.51 and 0.25 MoM, respectively, in a series of 42 cases.[208] When AFP and total hCG were examined in this same series,[97] only total hCG levels were reduced (0.74 MoM) but to a much lesser extent than that seen for free β-hCG.

NT is also increased with trisomy 13. When combined with maternal age, 90% of cases of trisomy 13 could be detected at a 0.5% false-positive rate.

Triploidy

Second Trimester

Biochemical studies of triploid pregnancies during the second trimester have shown that maternal serum hCG can either be very low or high.[209–214] This difference usually reflects the type of triploidy.[215–217] Type I triploidy is characterized by paternal origin (diandric) of the extra chromosome and elevated hCG levels. Type I fetuses with triploidy also often show elevation of AFP from NTD or abdominal wall defect and molar changes of the placenta.[218] This is an example of genomic imprinting in humans with the extra paternal set of chromosomes overexpressing hCG.[219–223] Increased inhibin A has also been reported in association with partial mole.[224] Type II triploidy is characterized by maternal origin (digynic) with low hCG levels, severe growth delay, and a small but otherwise normal appearing placenta. Hence, high hCG is almost always seen with placentas showing molar changes, whereas low hCG is infrequently associated with molar changes.[225]

First Trimester

Jauniaux et al.[226] found elevated hCG levels in 11 of 13 (84.6%) fetuses with triploidy, with a similar distribution in both molar and nonmolar cases. NT thickness was also above the ninety-fifth percentile in 12 (66.7%) cases evaluated. In a series of 25 cases, Spencer et al.[227] also found that free β-hCG follows a similar pattern to that observed in the second trimester with respect to types I and II, with type I having elevated levels (8.04 MoM) and type II having reduced levels (0.18 MoM). PAPP-A is mildly decreased in type I (0.75 MoM) but depressed (0.06 MoM) in type II. Increased NT (2.76 MoM) was also found for type I, and normal nuchal measurements were found for type II.

Turner Syndrome and Other Chromosome Abnormalities

Second Trimester

Various alterations in biochemical markers have been associated with Turner syndrome (45X). Saller et al.[71] reported that both hydropic and nonhydropic cases were associated with markedly decreased levels of estriol and slightly reduced levels of AFP. Total hCG and inhibin levels are also elevated with hydrops but low in the absence of hydrops.[54] Laundon et al.[84] also found free β-hCG increased in cases of Turner syndrome. Using the quadruple screen, Wenstrom et al.[204] reported detection of 9 in 17 (53%) fetuses with Turner syndrome, 10 in 17 (59%) fetuses other sex chromosome aneu-

ploidies, and one case of trisomy 22. Sex chromosome abnormalities or other atypical chromosome abnormalities may also be detected on the basis of elevated AFP.[228]

First Trimester

Spencer et al.[229] observed a significantly higher NT (4.76 MoM) and lower PAPP-A (0.49 MoM) for fetuses with Turner syndrome during the first trimester. For other sex chromosomal anomalies (47XXX, XXY, XYY), NT was also increased (2.07 MoM) but biochemical values were not significantly different from controls. Using a combined first-trimester protocol of NT, PAPP-A, free β-hCG, and maternal age, Spencer et al.[229] estimated that 96% of fetuses with Turner syndrome and 62% of the other sex chromosomal anomalies could be identified.

Confined Placental Mosaicism

Confined placental mosaicism, especially for trisomy 16, is associated with elevated levels of maternal serum hCG.[230] This risk is further increased when both hCG and AFP are elevated. Zimmerman et al.[231] found that elevated AFP and hCG were found in 0.3% of screened patients, and 30% (three of ten) had confined placental mosaicism with trisomy 16. Groli et al.[232] described five cases of trisomy 16 confined to the placenta, all with elevated levels of hCG. Four of five also had elevated MS-AFP levels.

In a group of 12 women with unexplained "dual positivity" (AFP value of 2.5 or greater MoMs and a Down syndrome risk of 1:250 or greater), abnormal karyotypes were found in three fetuses, two triploidies with partial hydatidiform mole and one fetus with Down syndrome.[233] In nine cases the fetal karyotype was normal, but four of these had confined placental mosaicism for trisomy 16.

SUMMARY OF ANALYTES

Alpha-Fetoprotein

AFP is a 69-kDa single-chain glycoprotein initially produced in the embryonic yolk sac and subsequently by the fetal gastrointestinal tract and liver. By the end of the first trimester nearly all AFP is synthesized in the liver. AFP in the fetal serum passes through the glomeruli intact and is then reabsorbed in the renal tubules. Normally, only a small amount escapes and appears in the fetal urine and amniotic fluid. Early in gestation, AFP also enters the amniotic fluid via transudation across the immature epithelium. Diffusion of AFP from the fetal to maternal compartment is across the fetal membranes and at the placental level.

Although much is known about AFP, the exact role of the protein remains uncertain. Before albumin becomes the major protein of the fetus, some believe it serves as the principal oncotic substance of the fetal vascular system.

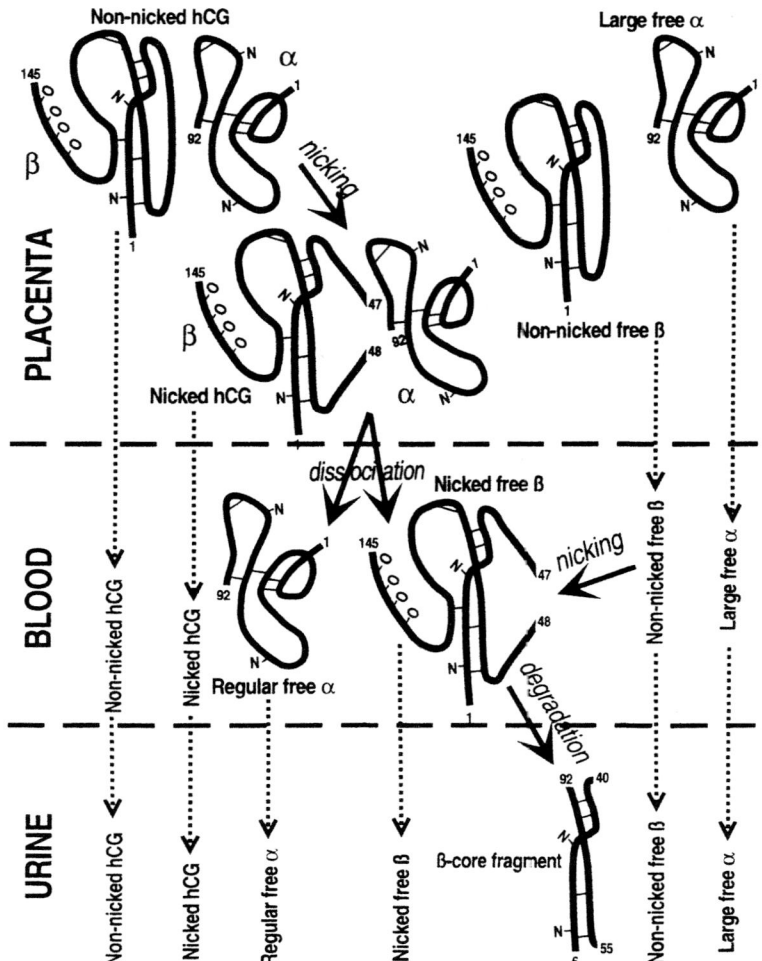

FIGURE 10. Various human chorionic gonadotropin (hCG)–related molecules in placenta, blood, and urine and the proposed degradation pathway. (Reproduced with permission from Cole LA. Immunoassay of human chorionic gonadotropin, its free subunits, and metabolites. *Clin Chem* 1997;43:2233–2243.)

Others have postulated an anti-immune role, preventing the mother from rejecting the fetus as foreign protein.[1]

Human Chorionic Gonadotropin

hCG is a 39.5-kDa dimeric glycoprotein composed of two dissimilar subunits joined noncovalently. The α subunit (15 kDa) is identical to that of the other pituitary glycoprotein hormones: luteinizing hormone, follicle-stimulating hormone, and thyroid-stimulating hormone. The β subunit (23 kDa), however, is unique and confers biological specificity. Approximately 80% sequence homology occurs between the β subunits of luteinizing hormone and hCG. Only the intact dimeric hormone is biologically active. hCG is produced by the syncytiotrophoblast of the placenta. The synthesis involves an independent translation of the respective messenger RNAs for the α and β subunits. At least six genes from chromosome 19 are known to code for the β subunit. One gene on chromosome 6 codes for the α subunit. Posttranslation glycosylation of the subunits occurs before the subunits are released in the form of α-hCG or free β-hCG along with the combined form of intact hCG. Regulation of the synthe-

sis of intact hCG appears to be limited by production of the β subunit. A variety of agents may have a negative or positive effect on the rate of production of the β subunit.

The α subunit of 92 amino acids is linked together by five disulphide bridges. The subunit also has two *N*-linked oligosaccharide side chains at positions 52 and 78. The β subunit of 145 amino acids, linked by six disulphide bridges, contains two *N*-linked oligosaccharide side chains at positions 13 and 30. Additionally four *O*-linked oligosaccharide side chains are found in the C-terminal region. In the placenta, maternal serum, and urine, hCG is present in multiple related forms including degraded hCG molecules, hyper- and hypoglycosylated hCG, free subunits, and fragments. Urine is the major route for clearance of hCG from the circulation, and it is suggested that β-core fragment, the major breakdown product of hCG, is produced within the kidney. Figure 10 shows schematically the various hCG related molecules in placenta, blood, and urine and the proposed degradation pathway. Initially intact hCG (nonnicked) undergoes a single cleavage in the β subunit at peptide linkage 47-48 (less frequently at 43-44 or 44-45) to form nicked hCG. The proportion of nicked

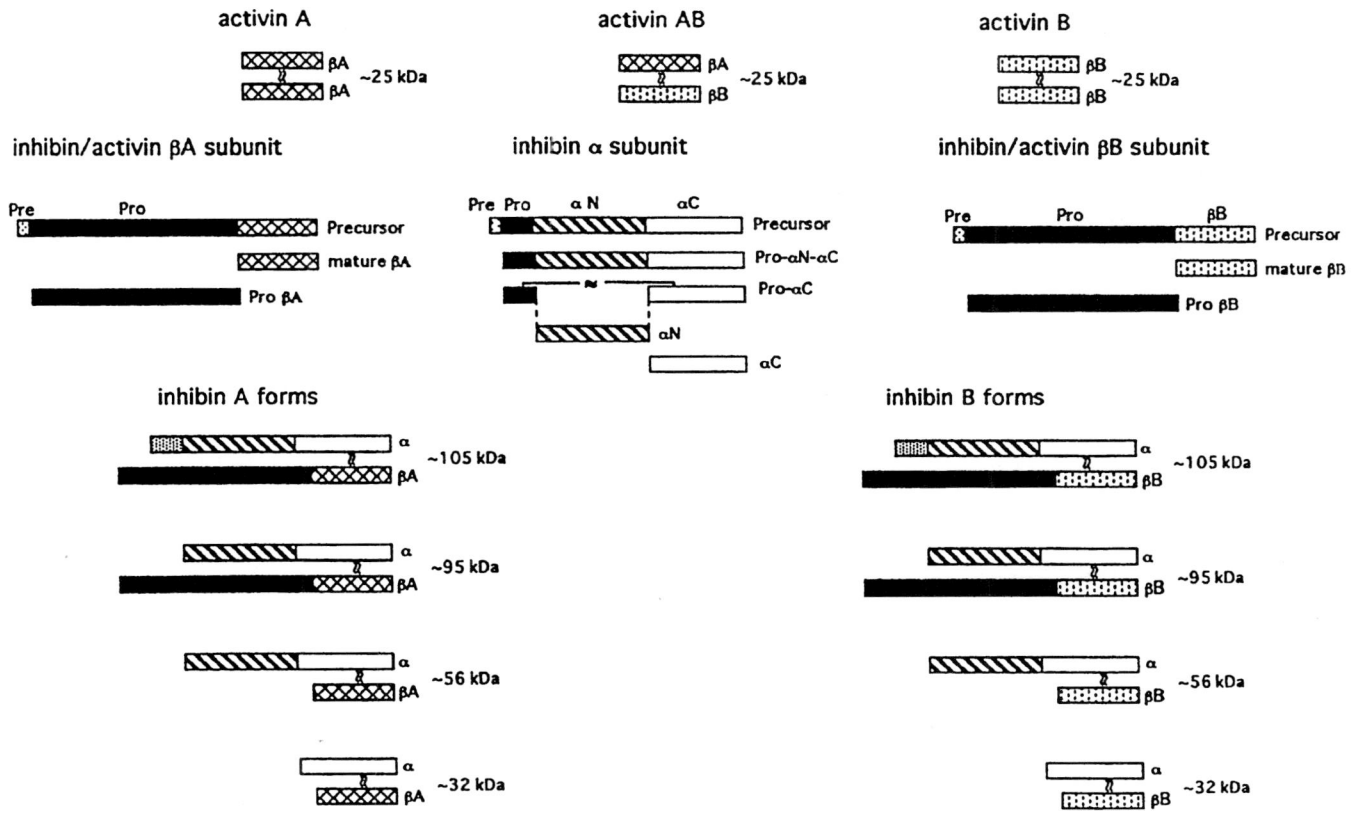

activin A
βA ~25 kDa
βA

activin AB
βA ~25 kDa
βB

activin B
βB ~25 kDa
βB

inhibin/activin βA subunit

Pre   Pro
Precursor
mature βA
Pro βA

inhibin α subunit

Pre Pro   α N   αC
Precursor
Pro-αN-αC
Pro-αC
αN
αC

inhibin/activin βB subunit

Pre   Pro   βB
Precursor
mature βB
Pro βB

inhibin A forms

α
~105 kDa
βA

α
~95 kDa
βA

α
~56 kDa
βA

α
~32 kDa
βA

inhibin B forms

α
~105 kDa
βB

α
~95 kDa
βB

α
~56 kDa
βB

α
~32 kDa
βB

FIGURE 11. Many different molecular forms of unprocessed and partially processed inhibin subunits have been described in follicular fluid, amniotic fluid, and serum. (Reproduced with permission from Knight PG. Roles of inhibins, activins and follistatin in the female reproductive system. *Front Neuroendocrinol* 1996;17:476–509.)

hCG increases during pregnancy from approximately 9% at week 8 to approximately 21% by 38 weeks, although person-to-person variation appears to be significant. Cell culture studies suggest that hCG is nicked after secretion by enzymes produced by macrophages associated with trophoblast cells. Nicked hCG is less stable than nonnicked hCG and rapidly dissociates into free α-hCG and nicked free β-hCG in serum. Nicked free β-hCG is then degraded further in the kidneys to be excreted as β-core fragment.

Two forms of free α seem to exist in blood and urine: (a) the regular free α and (b) a hyperglycosylated form with more complex *N*-linked oligosaccharides. This large free α cannot combine with free β-hCG.

β-Core fragment is the end product of hCG degradation and is undetectable in pregnancy serum. β-Core fragment consists of two peptides from β subunit residues 6-40 and 55-92 linked by five disulphide bridges. In urine, the pattern of β-core concentrations mirror those of serum.

Greater and more variable portions of nicked hCG, free β-hCG, and β-core fragment have been detected, particularly in pregnancies affected by trisomy 21 and also to some extent in those affected by preeclampsia. The peptide *N*-linked and *O*-linked oligosaccharide structures of hCG from normal pregnancies, molar pregnancies, and choriocarcinoma have

revealed the presence of hyperglycosylation. The proportion of hyperglycosylation in pregnancy is highest at 4 to 6 weeks (26%), falling to 11% at 6 to 8 weeks, 3% by 12 weeks, and 2% by 38 weeks. Cole and colleagues[127] have demonstrated that increased proportions of hyperglycosylated hCG occur in pregnancies affected by trisomy 21, and this may form the basis for improved screening programs in the future.

Inhibin A

Inhibins and activins are members of the transforming growth factor–beta superfamily, which are a group of structurally but functionally diverse growth factors. Mature inhibin is a 31- or 32-kDa heterodimeric glycoprotein composed of an α subunit linked by disulphide bridges to one of two possible β subunits, βA or βB. Two possible forms of mature inhibin can exist therefore, inhibin A and inhibin B. The β subunits can combine to form the homodimer activin, of which three possible forms can exist: activin A (βA-βA), activin B (βB-βB), and activin AB (βA-βB). Many different molecular forms of unprocessed and partially processed inhibin subunits have been described in follicular fluid, amniotic fluid, and serum (Fig. 11), but only the dimeric species (either mature or partially processed) are biologically active.

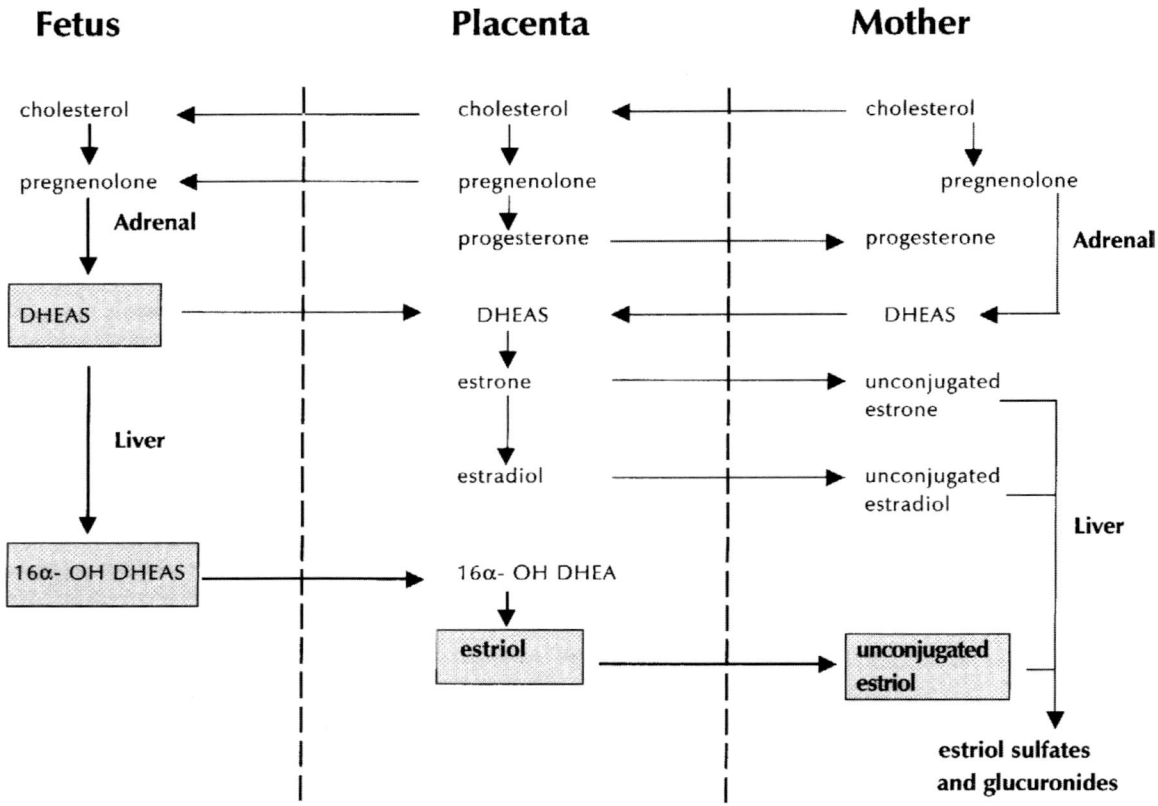

FIGURE 12. Metabolic pathway involved in the synthesis of estrogens, showing that once in the maternal compartment they undergo conjugation with glucuronic acid or sulfate by the liver. DHEAS, dehydroepiandrosterone sulfate.

Considering the complexity of the various molecular forms of inhibin, it is little wonder that specific assays have been developed only recently to measure the major forms; clinical studies using these selective assays are now being reported.[92]

During pregnancy inhibin is produced by the syncytio- and cytotrophoblast cells of the placenta, although smaller amounts are produced by the decidua, fetal membranes, and developing fetus. The control of secretion from the placenta is not fully understood, but *in vitro* studies have shown that hCG stimulates trophoblast secretion of inhibin and conversely inhibin suppresses hCG secretion. This effect is thought to be gestational age–specific, with no inhibin-induced hCG suppression in cell cultures from first-trimester trophoblasts. Activin stimulates hCG secretion from trophoblast cultures, and the two may be involved in the regulation of progesterone and prostaglandin production. Both activin and inhibin levels have been shown to be increased in women with established pre-eclampsia and also before the onset of the disease in the second and even the first trimester.

Estriol

Estrogens are products of the fetoplacental unit and consist of four main molecules: estriol, estradiol, estrone, and estetrol. The relative levels of these steroids are approximately in the ratio 200:20:10:1. Figure 12 shows the metabolic pathway involved in the synthesis of estrogens, showing that once in the maternal compartment they undergo conjugation with glucuronic acid or sulfate by the liver. A small proportion (less than 10%) of total estriol output is not conjugated and remains as unconjugated estriol. Approximately 70% of all estrogens are bound to sex hormone–binding globulin and are thought not to be biologically active. Diurnal variations of both total estriol and unconjugated estriol have been reported, with serum values being 15% lower in the morning than in the afternoon.

In addition to being associated with trisomies 18 and 21, low maternal serum levels are associated with a number of other conditions. Perhaps the most common is the presence of a male fetus affected by placental sulfatase deficiency or X-linked icthyosis.[234–236] All three studies reported cases of confirmed steroid sulfatase deficiency in women presenting with unconjugated estriol levels less than 0.15 MoM. Low estriol levels may also suggest the presence of anencephaly or congenital adrenal hypoplasia. Low estriol has also been reported in cases with Smith-Lemli-Opitz syndrome.[237–239] Increased NT may also be associated with this condition.[240]

Pregnancy-Associated Plasma Protein A

PAPP-A is a large dimeric zinc containing metalloglycoprotein with a molecular weight of 800 kDa. Each subunit consists of 1,547 amino acid residues and is derived from a larger precursor of placental origin. In maternal serum, PAPP-A exists complexed 2:2 with the proform of eosinophil major basis protein (ProMBP).[241] ProMBP also can be complexed with angiotensinogen, and this new complex can also be complexed with complement 3dg. Syncytiotrophoblastic tissue of the placenta is the main source of circulating PAPP-A. The gene for PAPP-A has been localized to the long arch of chromosome 9. Circulating levels are detected 28 days after conception and increased throughout pregnancy. The biologic function of PAPP-A is still unknown although it has recently been identified as an insulin-like growth factor–dependent protease that cleaves insulin-like growth factor–binding protein-4.[242] A noncompetitive inhibition of human granulocytic elastase has been demonstrated, and a possible role in modulating the maternal immune response has been suggested. The clinical usefulness appears to be limited to the first trimester. Very low PAPP-A levels have been observed days or even weeks before fetal demise. This observation indicates a high predictive value of PAPP-A for pregnancy failure.[102] Very low levels have also been observed in association with the Cornelia de Lange syndrome.[243]

MATERNAL AND PREGNANCY VARIABLES

Effect of Covariables

Many factors that influence serum marker levels and therefore the risk estimate derived from them have been recognized. Refinements to multimarker screening that take these factors into account have been introduced, allowing a more accurate estimate of risk and possible improvements to detection rates as a result of reducing the population variance.

Gestation

All maternal serum marker concentrations vary with gestation (Fig. 13). In the second trimester, AFP, PAPP-A, and estriol levels rise with advancing gestation, while total hCG, free β-hCG and inhibin A levels fall. As noted previously, comparison of levels at different gestations is achieved by conversion of marker concentration to MoM, but the precision of this estimate depends on the accuracy of the gestational estimate, whether it be derived from a last menstrual period or (more preferably) from an ultrasound assessment of fetal maturity. The greatest error associated with inaccurate gestational estimates is found for estriol, which has the greatest rate of change with gestation, and the least error with inhibin A, which has a relatively flat concentration profile in the second trimester. An overestimated gestation will result in the calculation of lower MoMs for AFP and estriol (and

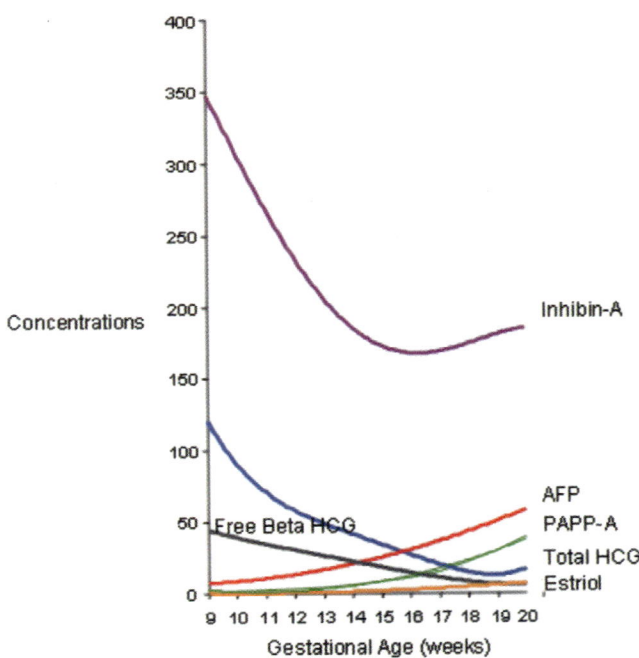

FIGURE 13. Change in concentrations of maternal serum analytes with gestational age. Units of concentration vary for individual serum analytes as follows: inhibin A (pg/mL), alpha-fetoprotein (AFP) (KU/L), pregnancy-associated plasma protein A (PAPP-A) (IU/L), total human chorionic gonadotropin (HCG) (KU/L), and estriol (nmol/L).

therefore greater likelihood ratios) and higher MoMs for total hCG, free β-hCG, and inhibin A (and therefore greater likelihood ratios), leading to the calculation of a higher than appropriate risk for any combination of these markers. An underestimated gestation will have the opposite effect.

In the first trimester, gestational dating errors are probably less likely than in the second trimester since biochemical measurements at this time are normally combined with ultrasound measurement.

Ethnicity

The assessment of the influence of ethnic origin on maternal serum marker levels from published data is often difficult since many earlier studies did not apply maternal weight correction to marker levels. This is an important prerequisite since average maternal weights in black Afro-Caribbean populations are higher than those in white women, while Asian/Oriental women have a much lower maternal weight. When maternal weight is taken into account, significantly higher AFP levels (15%), higher total hCG levels (18%), higher free β-hCG levels (12%), and lower inhibin A levels (8%) are found in black Afro-Caribbean women in the second trimester than in whites. For estriol, no significant difference has been observed. It is reasonably well established that in Asian and Oriental women, weight-corrected second-trimester hCG levels (both total and free β) are also higher than in white women.[244,245] AFP levels are increased in Asian populations. Watt et al.[246] proposed a method of correcting for ethnic origin, but a gain of only 0.5% in detection rate could be expected at the population level.

In the first trimester a study of Afro-Caribbean and Asian women[247] found that weight-corrected free β-hCG and PAPP-A medians were 21% and 57% higher, respectively, in Afro-Caribbean women and 4% and 17% higher, respectively, in Asian women. It was estimated that correcting for ethnicity would increase the overall population detection rate by only 1.4%, but the effect at an individual level could be highly significant. For example, in a 67-kg, 25-year-old Afro-Caribbean woman with an uncorrected free β-hCG of 2.10 MoM and a PAPP-A of 0.65 MoM, the risk before correction would be 1 in 540. After correction, the free β-hCG MoM becomes 1.73 and the PAPP-A MoM becomes 0.41, with a corrected risk of 1 in 260.

Gravidity and Parity

In the second trimester, both maternal serum total hCG and free β-hCG have been shown to decrease with an increasing number of pregnancies (gravidity) or an increasing number of previous births (parity).[247a,247b] The observed effect (after taking into account an increased maternal weight with increasing number of pregnancies) is quite small—less than 6% between primigravid and multigravid women. Correction for such a small change is not considered worthwhile when screening in the second trimester.

In the first trimester, Spencer et al.[248] have shown that gravidity and parity are associated with a small but progressive decrease in fetal NT and a small but progressive increase in both free β-hCG and PAPP-A. None of these changes had statistical significance, and correction for this variable was not considered necessary.

Multiple Pregnancy

Serum markers show increased concentration in maternal serum from multifetal pregnancies in the second trimester. A metaanalysis of published studies gave twin median MoM levels of 2.18 MoM for AFP on 1,638 unaffected twin pregnancies, 1.63 MoM for estriol on 286 pregnancies, 1.89 MoM for total hCG on 559 pregnancies, and 2.11 MoM for free β-hCG on 645 pregnancies.[248a] There are few corresponding data on twin pregnancies affected by Down syndrome. Spencer et al.[79] reported AFP and free β-hCG levels in eight sets of dizygous twin pregnancies discordant for Down syndrome. A twin corrected median MoM of 0.72 MoM was estimated for AFP and 1.54 MoM for free β-hCG. A detection rate for Down syndrome of 51% at a 5% false-positive rate was estimated using AFP, free β-hCG, and maternal age. Estimation of an accurate risk of Down syn-

drome in a twin pregnancy based on a combination of biochemical markers and maternal age is complicated where chorionicity is unknown. The age-related risk of Down syndrome in monozygous twin pregnancies is approximately equivalent to that of singleton pregnancies of women of the same age, whereas for dizygous twins the age-related risk that either fetus will have Down syndrome is double that of a singleton pregnancy.

In a series of 159 first-trimester twin pregnancies compared with 3,466 singleton controls the free β-hCG median was 2.1 times higher and the PAPP-A median 1.86 times higher than in singletons.[96] Although screening for twins in the second trimester is considered by some to be problematic because of the significant clinical, technical, and ethical challenges posed for the diagnosis and management of such pregnancies, correction methods that will produce "pseudo-risks" in such situations have been introduced.[79,248b] These are estimated to allow detection of just greater than 50% of cases in which twins are discordant for trisomy 21. Similar methods have been proposed for correction in the first trimester when detection rates of 52% can be expected in discordant twins.[96] These methods can also be used with NT measurements, when a combination of ultrasound and biochemical measurements can be expected to detect 80% of twins discordant for trisomy 21.[96] Such algorithms are already in use in prospective practice.[249]

Maternal Weight

All the maternal serum markers seem to decrease with increasing maternal weight, due to the dilution effect of the greater blood volume in heavy women diluting a fixed amount of placental product. Conversely, in smaller women the blood volume is decreased and so the effect is to concentrate the placental/fetal product. Correction for maternal weight can be made by dividing either the analyte result in concentration units or in MoM by the expected value for the weight based on a regression curve. In the second trimester this has been done using either a linear regression method[250] or a reciprocal regression method,[251] and the latter has been shown to be more accurate.[252] It is important, however, that each center constructs its own weight correction curve because any difference in median weight between populations will introduce inaccuracies. This is particularly important when considering nonwhite populations such as Asians or Orientals.[244] In the first trimester, the reciprocal regression model gives the best fit at the extremes of the distribution. Weight-correction equations based on data from 5,422 white women have been published.[247]

Fetal Gender

In the second trimester, the presence of a female fetus is known to result in a 7% higher maternal serum free β-hCG

MoM and a 3% lower AFP MoM.[97] These changes lead to a significantly higher false-positive rate in women carrying a female fetus. Although it has been suggested that this effect would lead to a reduced detection rate in female fetuses affected by trisomy 21,[253,254] Spencer et al.[97] could find no evidence for any fetal gender bias in detection rates among large series of pregnancies. When fetal sex was examined in the first trimester[255] in both chromosomally normal fetuses and in the presence of fetuses with trisomy 21, free β-hCG levels were increased by 15% and 11%, respectively, in female fetuses. PAPP-A levels were increased by 10% and 13%, respectively, in female fetuses. In contrast fetal NT was 3% to 4% lower in both chromosomally normal and trisomy 21 female fetuses. The consequence of such changes when screening for trisomy 21 will be a reduction in the detection rate in female fetuses of 1% to 2%.[255]

Smoking

Maternal smoking during pregnancy is a known health problem associated with significant risks to the fetus. Thomsen et al.[256] first reported that second-trimester MS-AFP levels in women who smoked were higher than those in nonsmokers. Bernstein et al.[257] reported that maternal serum levels of hCG and estradiol in early pregnancy were significantly depressed in women who smoked. Cuckle et al.[55] confirmed these findings, noting a 7% increase in AFP, a 5% fall in estriol, and an 11% fall in hCG. This was reinforced by Bartels et al.,[258] who reported a 21% fall in total hCG levels and also produced evidence to suggest that this fall in total hCG was not dependent on the number of cigarettes smoked. They also found a 3% reduction in estriol levels. Palomaki et al.[258a] found a 25% reduction in total hCG but also reported a weak dose-response relationship between nicotine levels and the magnitude of the decrease in hCG levels. The impact of smoking on free β-hCG in the second trimester is a reduction in levels in smokers by 14%.[258b] Ferriman et al.[259] reported that inhibin A levels are increased by 47% in smokers, suggesting a possible underlying cause for the reductions in total hCG and free β-hCG levels. When marker levels were investigated in Down syndrome pregnancies in women who smoked,[55,258b] AFP levels were found to be approximately 10% higher than in nonsmokers, estriol levels were 2% lower, total hCG levels were 27% lower, and free β-hCG levels were 16% lower than in nonsmokers. These changes in marker levels in pregnancies affected by Down syndrome reflect the changes seen in unaffected pregnancies. The consequence is a significantly lower detection rate and a lower false-positive rate in women who smoke.[258b] Although correction for smoking would have a significant impact on any one individual's risk, the overall effect on population screening would be only a modest 1% to 2% improvement in detection rates.[55,258b] These changes in detection rate and false-positive rate will also vary from center to center, being dependent on the incidence of smoking in the population,

which in turn is significantly influenced by age distribution and socioeconomic status.

In the first trimester, Brambati et al.[260] reported a 4% reduction in free β-hCG levels in smokers in a series of 740 pregnancies and a 4% reduction in PAPP-A levels. No reduction in free β-hCG levels in smokers was apparent among a group of 3,111 women with unaffected pregnancies,[260a] whereas for PAPP-A the median weight-corrected level in smokers was significantly reduced to 0.85 MoM. Uncorrected, this 15% reduction was estimated to reduce detection rates for Down syndrome in smokers from 67% to 61%. Analyte levels have also been examined in women who smoked and had a pregnancy affected by trisomy 21,[261] free β-hCG levels were 13% lower than in nonsmokers with affected pregnancies, and PAPP-A levels were 6% higher, although neither change was statistically significant. The implications of this data would be for a decrease in the detection rate and an increase in the false-positive rate when screening for trisomy 21 among women who smoked.

Suggestions have been made that there is a negative association between Down syndrome births and maternal cigarette smoking.[262-265] Other studies[266] that were carefully controlled for maternal age could not confirm a relationship between maternal smoking and a lower rate of Down syndrome births. The prevalence of Down syndrome births increases with advancing maternal age, whereas cigarette smoking decreases with advancing maternal age. Chen et al.[266] demonstrated that it was important to control for maternal age in individual year increments rather than in broad age bands. In two studies, one in the second trimester[258b] and the other[261] in the first trimester, of the effect of maternal smoking on maternal serum markers no deficit of Down syndrome cases was found in the second-trimester study, but in the first trimester there was a reduction of 25% in the Down syndrome cases among smokers. If an association between maternal smoking and Down syndrome rates is confirmed it would require correction to the *a priori* age risks to provide accurate risk estimates for women who smoke.

Previous Screening Results

In women who have an increased second-trimester Down syndrome risk in a first pregnancy there is a five-fold greater chance of them also having an increased Down syndrome risk in a second pregnancy.[267,268] The extent of this is more noticeable in younger women such that at 20 years of age the relative chance is five-fold, reducing to 1.3-fold at age 40. Such a biological association of serum marker levels between pregnancies suggests that additional maternal or genetic factors influence the levels of these serum markers, other than the physiologic factors, which also are poorly understood. Correcting for a previous result has been estimated to have only a small (0.2%) impact on false-positive rates,[268] although others consider correction worthwhile.[269]

In the first trimester, Spencer et al.[178] showed that there was no correlation between NT MoMs in the first or subsequent pregnancy, but for maternal serum free β-hCG and PAPP-A there was a significant correlation between pregnancies of 0.42 and 0.33, respectively. The implication of this association is that women who have an increased first-trimester Down risk in one pregnancy were twice likely to be at increased risk in their next pregnancy.

Assisted Reproduction

In the second trimester, assisted reproduction techniques appear to have an impact on maternal serum marker levels. In women undergoing ovulation induction only, total hCG levels were 9% higher and estriol 8% lower, while AFP was not significantly different.[270] In women having *in vitro* fertilization (IVF), the various studies are inconsistent. Muller et al.[210] reported normal hCG levels in 138 IVF pregnancies, whereas Heionen et al.,[271] Ribbert et al.,[272] Frishman et al.,[273] Lam et al.,[274] and Wald et al.[274a] have reported increases of 52%, 29%, 22%, 22%, and 14%, respectively. In one study,[270] a 7% decrease was reported. For AFP, the general consensus is that in IVF pregnancy levels are no different from controls, and estriol levels are reduced by 6% to 8%. Inhibin A in one small study was not significantly different.[186]

In pregnancies conceived by intrauterine insemination, AFP levels were significantly lower (0.76 MoM) compared with normally conceived pregnancies (1.05 MoM), while the levels of free β-hCG were not significantly different.[117] In pregnancies conceived by intracytoplasmic sperm injection, the median AFP was also significantly reduced (0.76 vs. 0.94 MoM), whereas for total hCG the change was not significant (0.88 vs. 0.94 MoM).[274]

In the first trimester, free β-hCG was increased (14%) in IVF pregnancies while PAPP-A was decreased (8%).[275] In those having intracytoplasmic sperm injection only PAPP-A was significantly decreased (20%), whereas in the group having only ovulation-inducing drug levels were not significantly different from the controls. The difference in free β-hCG and PAPP-A levels in the IVF pregnancies would result in at least a 1% higher false-positive rate in this group, and correction may be worthwhile.[275]

An important point to remember when estimating risks in IVF pregnancies is that in cases in which a donor egg is used the prior risk should be based on the maternal age of the donor rather than on the recipient's maternal age.

Insulin-Dependent Diabetes Mellitus

In women with insulin-dependent diabetes mellitus (IDDM), second-trimester maternal serum marker levels on the whole are reduced, although considerable variation exists in the published literature. This variation is partly due to the fact that maternal weight correction has often not been applied (women with IDDM tend to be approximately 6 kg heavier) and the possibility that the extent of the reduction is dependent upon the adequacy of diabetic control. Early studies reported marked reductions in AFP levels to 0.60 to 0.80 MoM.[7,276,276a] Reese et al.[277] found a median AFP level of 0.91 MoM, which increased to 0.96 MoM when corrected for maternal weight. Canick et al.[277a] reported a median AFP level of 0.97 MoM, and Crossley et al.[277b] found levels of 0.89 MoM (0.98 MoM when corrected for maternal weight). High levels of glycosylated hemoglobin indicate poor control of IDDM during pregnancy, and an inverse relationship has been established between the level of glycosylated hemoglobin and AFP.[277–279] Although an overall estimate of a 10% reduction for AFP might seem reasonable in IDDM women, genuine differences probably exist among different populations reflecting differences in the level of diabetic control. Ideally, correction factors should be established locally, but published data suggest that estriol, total hCG, and free β-hCG all show reductions of less than 10%.[276a,277b,279a,279b] Dimeric inhibin A on the other hand has been reported raised by 17% in one study[280] but reduced by 12% in another.[281]

For first-trimester markers, levels of PAPP-A are reduced in IDDM mothers,[282] and in those with preexisting or gestational diabetes the levels of free β-hCG and PAPP-A are reduced by 20% and 25%, respectively.[283] If such reductions are confirmed in other studies correction of both markers will be necessary in diabetic women.

Vaginal Bleeding

The presence of vaginal bleeding in early pregnancy complicates the interpretation of serum screening for Down syndrome. In one study,[283a] AFP levels were significantly increased in cases of vaginal bleeding (by 9%), but the increases in estriol (5%) and total hCG (12%) levels did not reach significance. Although Cuckle et al.[283a] proposed a method of correcting for vaginal bleeding which was estimated to increase the detection rate by less than 1%, in practice correction is rarely applied as the magnitude of the marker changes is related to the proximity of the bleed to the time of sampling. Correction is also made more difficult by the fact that vaginal bleeding is more common in older women and that it is also a risk factor for Down syndrome.[55]

Pregnancy Complications and Adverse Outcome

In the second trimester conflicting views have been expressed as to the relationship between biochemical marker levels and the incidence of pregnancy complications and adverse outcomes such as preeclampsia, intrauterine growth restriction, low birth weight, preterm delivery, and stillbirth.[208] It would appear that apart from the association of increased free β-hCG (or total hCG) with an increased incidence of preeclampsia, an isolated raised free β-hCG is not associated with adverse outcome in the second trimester. When this was examined in the first trimester, free β-hCG levels were not increased in cases developing preeclampsia[283] and, if anything, values were lower in cases of pregnancy-induced hypertension. Low maternal serum PAPP-A was associated with subsequent miscarriage, development of pregnancy-induced hypertension, and growth restriction. However, the sensitivity and specificity of these tests were low and therefore they are not useful as predictors of subsequent complications of pregnancy.[283] In contrast Morssink et al.[284] in a smaller study could find no association between first-trimester free β-hCG and PAPP-A levels in cases with preterm delivery or intrauterine growth restriction. Cuckle et al.[284a] have also shown that low PAPP-A is associated with poor fetal viability, confirming earlier reports.[102,243]

Increased levels of inhibin A in the second trimester have been reportedly associated with increased risk for preeclampsia,[284b] and this was subsequently confirmed.[285,286] A preliminary study[287] of a small series of cases in the first trimester suggested this was also elevated but this could not be confirmed in a much larger series of 131 cases.[288] Activin however was increased to 1.49 MoM in this series at 10 to 14 weeks of gestation.

Assay Specificity and Sample Stability

Free β-hCG is present in maternal serum in a milieu of hCG-related molecules. Many different forms of hCG exist and include intact hCG (the combined α and β subunits), hyperglycosylated forms of both intact and free β-hCG and the various nicked forms of both intact and free β-hCG.[65,66] The levels of free β-hCG, for example, are 0.5% of the total circulating hCG, thus assays must be very specific and be able to measure the specific free β form against this high background. Since it has also been suggested that nicked free β-hCG production in trisomy 21 may account for the improved specificity of free β-hCG in the second trimester,[65] it may be important that free β-hCG assays also measure the nicked and nonnicked forms. The assays that have been used to generate much of the clinical data with respect to free β-hCG have been thoroughly evaluated and have been shown to be specific for only the free β subunit and to also recognize the nicked form.[289]

Consideration should also be given to sample collection and storage conditions. Free β-hCG stability at room temperature was originally questioned based on anecdotal evidence of the thermal degradation of intact hCG, producing elevated levels of free β-hCG. Scientific studies have shown that intact hCG in serum is stable for up to 70 hours at room temperature (15° to 25°C) although free β-hCG

levels can increase in whole blood after 35 hours at room temperature.[290–292] Others have shown that these limitations have no impact on screening performance.[293,294] Provided samples are in serum form then stability during transport does not become an operational issue. In those situations when shipment of serum is not possible, dried filter paper blood spots provide a reliable alternative with stability in excess of 7 days at 37°C.[295–297]

Assay specificity is also of some concern with respect to PAPP-A. In maternal serum PAPP-A exists complexed 2:2 with ProMBP.[241] ProMBP also can be complexed with angiotensinogen, and this new complex can also be complexed with complement 3dg.[298] Early assays for PAPP-A were either radioimmunoassays employing purified and labeled PAPP-A with a short shelf-life and questionable specificity or enzyme-linked immunosorbent assays employing polyclonal antibodies. The specificity of the polyclonal antibodies has been a source of controversy for some years, and a widely used commercial polyclonal antibody (A0230, DAKO) has been shown to cross-react with SP1, ProMBP, and haptoglobin,[298] which could lead to underestimates of the clinical utility of PAPP-A.[299] Assay systems using dual monoclonal antibodies against PAPP-A[300] have been shown to give lower median MoMs in trisomy 21 samples compared with the dual polyclonal assay.[301] Now that commercial monoclonal assays are available for PAPP-A [e.g., Brahms Diagnostica Kryptor (formerly CIS), Perkin Elmer Delfia, Johnson & Johnson Amerlex-M], it is hoped that the problem of assay specificity is resolved.

On the question of PAPP-A stability, little has been published, but our own studies have shown that up to five freeze/thaw cycles and storage of samples for up to 7 days at room temperature have no effect on measured PAPP-A levels. The only effect noted was that associated with blood collected in ethylenediaminetetraacetic acid, which complexes the zinc moiety at the center of PAPP-A, which results in a conformational change to the molecule, making it invisible in the monoclonal assay system (Spencer, *unpublished observations*, 1998).

REFERENCES

1. Bergstrand CG, Czar B. Demonstration of a new protein fraction in serum from the human fetus. *Scand J Clin Lab Invest* 1956;8:174.
2. Brock DJ, Sutcliffe RG. Alpha-fetoprotein in the antenatal diagnosis of anencephaly and spina bifida. *Lancet* 1972; 2:197–199.
3. Wald NJ, Cuckle H, Brock JH, Peto R, Polani PE, Woodford FP. Maternal serum alpha-fetoprotein measurement in antenatal screening for anencephaly and spina bifida in early pregnancy: report of UK Collaborative Study on Alpha-fetoprotein in Relation to Neural Tube Defects. *Lancet* 1977;i:1323–1332.
4. Greenberg F, Faucett A, Rose E, Bancalari L, Kardon NB,

et al. Congenital deficiency of alpha-fetoprotein. *J Obstet Gynecol* 1992;167:509–511.

5. Haddow JE. Prenatal screening for open neural tube defects, Down's syndrome, and other major fetal disorders. *Semin Perinatol* 1990;14:488–503.

6. Haddow JE, Kloza EM, Knight GJ, Smith DE. Relation between maternal weight and serum alpha-fetoprotein concentration during the second trimester. *Clin Chem* 1981;27(1):133–134.

7. Wald NJ, Cuckle H, Boreham J, Stirrat GM, Turnbull AC. Maternal serum alpha-fetoprotein and diabetes mellitus. *Br J Obstet Gynaecol* 1979;86(2):101–105.

8. Kucera J. Rate and type of congenital anomalies among offspring of diabetic women. *J Reprod Med* 1971;7(2):73–82.

9. Main DM, Mennuti MT. Neural tube defects: issues in prenatal diagnosis and counselling. *Obstet Gynecol* 1986;67(1):1–16.

10. Zelop C, Nadel A, Frigoletto FD Jr, Pauker S, MacMillan M, Benacerraf BR. Placenta accreta/percreta/increta: a cause of elevated maternal serum alpha-fetoprotein. *Obstet Gynecol* 1992;80(4):693–694.

11. Kuperminc MJ, Tamura RK, Wigton TR, Glassenberg R, Socol ML. Placenta accreta is associated with elevated maternal serum alpha-fetoprotein. *Obstet Gynecol* 1993; 82(2):266–269.

12. Butler EL, Dashe JS, Ramus RM. Association between maternal serum alpha-fetoprotein and adverse outcomes in pregnancies with placenta previa. *Obstet Gynecol* 2001;97:35–38.

13. Kelly R, Nyberg DA, Mack LA, et al. Placental abnormalities and oligohydramnios in women with elevated alpha-fetoprotein: comparison with normal controls. *AJR Am J Roentgenol* 1989;152:815–819.

14. Bernstein IM, Barth RA, Miller R, Capeless EL. Elevated maternal serum alpha-fetoprotein: association with placental sonolucencies, fetomaternal hemorrhage, vaginal bleeding, and pregnancy outcome in the absence of fetal anomalies. *Obstet Gynecol* 1992;79:71–74.

15. Macri JN, Weiss RR. Prenatal serum alpha-fetoprotein screening for neural tube defects. *Obstet Gynecol* 1982; 59(5):633–639.

16. Milunsky A. Prenatal detection of neural tube defects. VI. Experience with 20,000 pregnancies. *JAMA* 1980;244(24): 2731–2735.

17. Crandall BF, Matsumoto M. Routine amniotic fluid alphafetoprotein assay: experience with 40,000 pregnancies. *Am J Med Genet* 1986;24(1):143–149.

18. Wald NJ, Hackshaw AK, George LM. Assay precision of serum alpha fetoprotein in antenatal screening for neural tube defects and Down's syndrome. *J Med Screen* 2000;7(2):74–77.

19. Yaron Y, Hamby DD, O'Brien JE, Critchfield G, Leon J, et al. Combination of elevated maternal serum alpha-fetoprotein (MSAFP) and low estriol is highly predictive of anencephaly. *Am J Med Genet* 1998;75(3):297–299.

20. Palomaki GE, Hill LE, Knight GJ, Haddow JE, Carpenter M. Second-trimester maternal serum alpha-fetoprotein levels in pregnancies associated with gastroschisis and omphalocele. *Obstet Gynecol* 1988;71:906–909.

21. Saller DN Jr, Canick JA, Palomaki GE, Knight GJ, Haddow JE. Second-trimester maternal serum alpha-fetoprotein, unconjugated estriol, and hCG levels in pregnancies with ventral wall defects. *Obstet Gynecol* 1994;84:852–855.

22. Albright SG, Warner AA, Seeds JW, Burton BK. Congeni-

tal nephrosis as a cause of elevated alpha-fetoprotein. *Obstet Gynecol* 1990;76(5 Pt 2):969–971.

23. Wiggelinkhuizen J, Nelson MM, et al. Alpha fetoprotein in the antenatal diagnosis of the congenital nephrotic syndrome. *J Pediatr* 1976;89:452–455.

24. Seppala M, Aula P, Rapola J, Karajalainen O, Huttunen NP, Ruoslahti E. Congenital nephrotic syndrome: prenatal diagnosis and genetic counseling by estimation of amniotic fluid and maternal serum alpha-fetoprotein. *Lancet* 1976;ii:123–124.

25. Report of the Collaborative Acetylcholinesterase Study. Amniotic fluid acetylcholinesterase electrophoresis as a secondary test in the diagnosis of anencephaly and open spina bifida in early pregnancy. *Lancet* 1981;ii:321–324.

26. Second Report of the Collaborative Acetylcholinesterase Study. Amniotic fluid acetylcholinesterase measurement in the prenatal diagnosis of open neural tube defects. *Prenat Diagn* 1989;9:813–829.

27. Sepulveda W, Donaldson A, Johnson RD, Davies G, Fisk NM. Are routine alpha-fetoprotein and acetylcholinesterase determination still necessary at second-trimester amniocentesis? Impact of high-resolution ultrasonography. *Obstet Gynecol* 1995;85:107–112.

28. Nadel AS, Green JK, Holmes LB, Frigoletto FD Jr, Benacerraf BR. Absence of need for amniocentesis in patients with elevated levels of maternal serum alpha-fetoprotein and normal ultrasonographic examinations. *N Engl J Med* 1990;30:557–561.

29. Richards DS, Seeds JW, Katz VL, Lingley LH, Albright SG, Cefalo RC. Elevated maternal serum alpha-fetoprotein with normal ultrasound: Is amniocentesis always appropriate? A review of 26,069 screened patients. *Obstet Gynecol* 1988;71: 203–207.

30. Shields LE, Uhrich SB, Komarniski CA, Wener MH, Winter TC. Amniotic fluid alpha-fetoprotein determination at the time of genetic amniocentesis: Has it outlived its usefulness? *J Ultrasound Med* 1996;15:735–739.

31. Manning et al. Life without amniocentesis. *Ultrasound Obstet Gynecol* 1994;4:199–204.

32. Nadel AS, Norton ME, Wilkins-Haug L. Cost-effectiveness of strategies used in the evaluation of pregnancies complicated by elevated maternal serum alpha-fetoprotein levels. *Obstet Gynecol* 1997;89:660–665.

33. Watson WJ, Chescheir NC, Katz VL, Seeds JW. The role of ultrasound in evaluation of patients with elevated maternal serum alpha-fetoprotein: a review. *Obstet Gynecol* 1991;78:123–128.

34. Report of the U.K. Collaborative Study on Alpha-fetoprotein in Relation to Neural-tube Defects. Maternal serum alphafetoprotein measurement in antenatal screening for anencephaly and spina bifida in early pregnancy. *Lancet* 1977;I:1323–1332.

35. Aitken DA, McCaw G, Crossley JA, Berry E, Connor JM, Macri JN. First trimester screening for fetal chromosome abnormalities and neural tube defects. *Prenat Diagn* 1993;13:681–689.

36. Sebire NJ, Spencer K, Noble PL, Hughes K, Nicolaides KH. Maternal serum alpha-fetoprotein in fetal neural tube and abdominal wall defects at 10 to 14 weeks of gestation. *Br J Obstet Gynaecol* 1997;104:849–851.

37. McDonnell RJ, Johnson Z, Delaney V, Dack P. East Ireland 1980–1994: epidemiology of neural tube defects. *J Epidemiol Community Health* 1999;53:782–788.

38. Rose NC, Menutti MT. Periconceptional folic acid supplementation as a social intervention. *Semin Perinatol* 1995; 19:243–254.

39. Hook EB, Hamerton JL. The frequency of chromosome abnormalities detected in consecutive newborn studies— differences between studies—results by sex and severity of phenotypic involvement. In: Hook EB, Porter IH, eds. *Population cytogenetics, studies in humans.* New York: Academic Press, 1977:63–79.

40. Hook EB. Prevalence, risks and recurrence. In: Brock DJH, Rodeck CH, Ferguson-Smith MA, eds. *Prenatal diagnosis and screening.* Edinburgh: Churchill Livingstone, 1992:351–392.

41. Egan JF, Benn P, Borgida AF, Rodis JF, Campbell WA, Vintzileos AM. Efficacy of screening for fetal Down syndrome in the United States from 1974 to 1997. *Obstet Gynecol* 2000;96:979–985.

42. Penrose LS. The relative effects of paternal age and maternal age in mongolism. *J Genet* 1933;27:219–224.

43. Jalbert P. Down's syndrome incidence and paternal age. *Down's Screening News* 1995;3:5.

44. Lansac J, Thepot F, Mayaux MJ, Czyglick F, Wack T, et al. Pregnancy outcome after artificial insemination or IVF with frozen semen donor: a collaborative study of the French CECOS Federation on 21597 pregnancies. *Eur J Obstet Gynecol Reprod Biol* 1997;74:223–228.

45. Cuckle HS, Wald NJ, Thomson SG. Estimating a woman's risk of having a pregnancy associated with Down's syndrome using her age and serum alphafetoprotein level. *Br J Obstet Gynaecol* 1987;94:387–402.

46. Hecht CA, Hook EB. Rates of Down syndrome at livebirth by one-year maternal age intervals in studies with apparent close to complete ascertainment in populations of European origin: a proposed revised rate schedule for use in genetic and prenatal screening. *Am J Med Genet* 1996;62:376–385.

47. Bray I, Wright DE, Davies C, Hook EB. Joint estimation of Down syndrome risk and ascertainment rates: a meta analysis of nine published data sets. *Prenat Diagn* 1998;18:9–20.

48. Hecht CA, Hook EB. The imprecision of rates of Down syndrome by 1 year age intervals—a critical analysis of rate used in biochemical screening. *Prenat Diagn* 1994;14:729–738.

49. Hook EB. Maternal age-specific rates of Down syndrome used in serum screening are biased low. *Prenat Diagn* 2000;20:169.

50. Andersen A-MN, Wohlfahrt J, Christens P, Olsen J, Melbye M. Maternal age and fetal loss: population based register linkage study. *BMJ* 2000;320:1708–1712.

51. Morris JK, Wald NJ, Watt HC. Fetal loss in Down's syndrome pregnancies. *Prenat Diagn* 1999;19:142–145.

52. Snijders RJ, Sundberg K, Holzgreve W, Henry G, Nicolaides KH. Maternal age- and gestation-specific risk for trisomy 21. *Ultrasound Obstet Gynecol* 1999;13:167–170.

53. Spencer K, Liao AW, Ong CY, Geerts L, Nicolaides KH. Maternal serum levels of dimeric inhibin A in pregnancies affected by trisomy 21 in the first trimester. *Prenat Diagn* 2001;21:441–444.

54. Snijders RJ, Holzgreve W, Cuckle H, Nicolaides KH. Maternal age-specific risks for trisomies at 9–14 weeks' gestation. *Prenat Diagn* 1994;14:543–552.

55. Cuckle HS, Wald NJ. Screening for Down syndrome. In: Lilford RJ, ed. *Prenatal diagnosis and prognosis.* Oxford: Heinemann, 1990:67–92.

56. Haddow JE, Palomaki GE, Kight GJ, Cunningham GC, Lustig LS, Boyd PA. Reducing the need for amniocentesis in women 35 years of age or older with serum markers for screening. *N Engl J Med* 1994;330:1114–1118.

57. Merkatz IR, Nitowsky HM, Macri JN, Johnson WE. An association between low maternal serum alpha-fetoprotein and fetal chromosomal abnormalities. *Am J Obstet Gynecol* 1984;148:886–894.

58. Cuckle HS, Wald NJ, Lindenbaum RH. Maternal serum alpha fetoprotein measurements: a screening test for Down's syndrome. *Lancet* 1984;i:926–929.

59. Spencer K, Carpenter P. Screening for Down's syndrome using serum α fetoprotein: a retrospective study indicating caution. *BMJ* 1985;290:1940–1943.

60. Bogart MH, Pandian MR, Jones OW. Abnormal maternal serum chorionic gonadotropin levels in pregnancies with fetal chromosome abnormalities. *Prenat Diagn* 1987;7:623–630.

61. Bogart MH, Golbus MS, Sorg ND, Jones OW. Human chorionic gonadotropin levels in pregnancies with aneuploid fetuses. *Prenat Diagn* 1989;9:379–384.

62. Ryall RG, Staples AJ, Robertson EF, Pollard AC. Improved performance in a prenatal screening programme for Down's syndrome incorporating serum free hCG subunit analyses. *Prenat Diagn* 1992;12:251–261.

63. Spencer K, Mallard AS, Coombes EJ, Macri JN. Prenatal screening for trisomy 18 with free beta human chorionic gonadotrophin as a marker. *BMJ* 1993;307:1455–1458.

64. Spencer K, Aitken DA, Crossley JA, McGaw G, Berry E, et al. First trimester biochemistry screening for trisomy 21: the role of free beta hCG, alpha fetoprotein and pregnancy associated plasma protein A. *Ann Clin Biochem* 1994;31:447–454.

65. Cole LA. Multiple hCG related molecules. In: Grudzinskas JG, Chard T, Chapman M, Cuckle H, eds. *Screening for Down's syndrome.* Cambridge: Cambridge University Press, 1994:119–140.

66. Cole LA. Immunoassay of human chorionic gonadotropin, its free subunits, and metabolites. *Clin Chem* 1997;43:2233–2243.

67. Rotmensch S, Cole LA. False diagnosis and needless therapy of presumed malignant disease in women with false-positive human chorionic gonadotropin concentrations. *Lancet* 2000;355:712–715.

68. Canick JA, Palomaki GE, Osathanondh R. Prenatal screening for trisomy 18 in the second trimester. *Prenat Diagn* 1990;10:546–548.

69. Crossley JA, Aitken DA, Connor JM. Prenatal screening for chromosome abnormalities using maternal serum chorionic gonadotrophin, alphafetoprotein and age. *Prenat Diagn* 1991;11:88–101.

70. Saller DN, Canick JA, Blitzer MG, Palomaki GE, Schwartz S, et al. Second trimester maternal serum analyte levels associated with fetal trisomy 13. *Prenat Diagn* 1999;19:813–816.

71. Saller DN, Canick JA, Schwartz S, Blitzer MG. Multiple-marker screening in pregnancies with hydropic and nonhydropic Turner syndrome. *Am J Obstet Gynecol* 1992;167:1021–1024.

72. Canick JA, Knight GJ, Palomaki GE, Haddow JE, Cuckle HS, et al. Low second trimester maternal serum unconjugated oestriol in pregnancies with Down's syndrome. *Br J Obstet Gynaecol* 1988;95:330–333.

73. Wald NJ, Cuckle HS, Densem JW, Nanchahal K, Canick

JA, et al. Maternal serum unconjugated oestriol as an antenatal screening test for Down's syndrome. *Br J Obstet Gynaecol* 1988;95:334–341.

74. Macri JN, Kasturi RV, Krantz DA, Cook EJ, Sunderji SG, et al. Maternal serum Down screening: unconjugated estriol is not useful. *Am J Obstet Gynecol* 1990;162:672–673.

75. Reynolds T, John R. A comparison of unconjugated oestriol assay kits shows that expression of results as multiples of the median causes unacceptable variation in calculated Down syndrome risk factors. *Clin Chem* 1992;38:1888–1893.

76. Cuckle H. Measuring unconjugated estriol in maternal serum to screen for fetal Down syndrome. *Clin Chem* 1992;38:1687–1689.

77. Reynolds TM, John R, Spencer K. The utility of unconjugated estriol in Down syndrome screening is not proven. *Clin Chem* 1993;39:2023–2025.

78. Crossley JA, Aitken DA, Connor JM. Second trimester unconjugated oestriol in maternal serum from chromosomally abnormal pregnancies using an optimised assay. *Prenat Diagn* 1993;13:271–280.

79. Spencer K, Salonen R, Muller F. Down's syndrome screening in multiple pregnancies using alpha-fetoprotein and free beta hCG. *Prenat Diagn* 1994;14:537–542.

80. Wald NJ, Cuckle HS, Densem JW, Nanchahal K, Royston P, et al. Maternal serum screening for Down's syndrome in early pregnancy. *BMJ* 1988;297:883–887.

81. Seth J, Sturgeon CM, Ellis AR, Al-Sadies R, Logan M. UK NEQAS for peptide hormones and related substances. Annual Review 1999. UK NEQAS, Edinburgh, 2000:65.

82. Macri JN, Kasturi RV, Krantz DA, Cook EJ, Moore ND, et al. Maternal serum Down syndrome screening: free beta protein is a more effective marker than human chorionic gonadotropin. *Am J Obstet Gynecol* 1990;163:1248–1253.

83. Spencer K. Evaluation of an assay of the free beta-subunit of choriogonadotropin and its potential value in screening for Down's syndrome. *Clin Chem* 1991;37:809–814.

84. Laundon CH, Spencer K, Macri JN, Anderson RW, Buchanan PD. Free beta hCG screening of hydropic and non-hydropic Turner syndrome pregnancies. *Prenat Diagn* 1996;16:853–856.

85. Van Lith JM, Pratt JJ, Beekhuis JR, Mantingh A. Second trimester maternal serum immunoreactive inhibin as a marker for fetal Down's syndrome. *Prenat Diagn* 1992;12:801–806.

86. Spencer K, Wood PJ, Anthony FW. Elevated levels of maternal serum inhibin immunoreactivity in second trimester pregnancies affected by Down's syndrome *Ann Clin Biochem* 1993;30:219–220.

87. Cuckle HS. Risk estimation in Down's syndrome screening policy and practice. In: Grudzinskas JG, Chard T, Chapman M, Cuckle H, eds. *Screening for Down's syndrome.* Cambridge: Cambridge University Press, 1994:31–46

88. Cuckle HS, Jones RG. Posting maternal blood samples for free beta-human chorionic gonadotrophin testing. *Prenat Diagn* 1995;15:879–880.

89. Aitken DA, Wallace EM, Crossley JA, Swanston IA, van Pareren Y, et al. Dimeric inhibin A as a marker for Down's syndrome in early pregnancy. *N Engl J Med* 1996;334:1231–1236.

90. Spencer K, Wallace EM, Ritoe S. Second trimester dimeric inhibin-A in Down's syndrome screening. *Prenat Diagn* 1996;16:1101–1110.

91. Wald NJ, Densem JW, George L, Muttukrishna S, Knight PG. Prenatal screening for Down's syndrome using inhibin-A as a serum marker. *Prenat Diagn* 1996;16:143–153.

92. Wallace EM, Healy DL. Inhibins and activins: roles in clinical practice. *Br J Obstet Gynaecol* 1996;103:945–956.

93. Wallace EM, Crossley JA, Ritoe SC, Aitken DA, Spencer K, Groome NP. Evolution of an inhibin-A ELISA method: implications for Down's syndrome screening. *Ann Clin Biochem* 1998;35:656–664.

94. Lambert-Messerlian GM, Saller DN, Tumber MB, French CA, Peterson CJ, Canick JA. Second-trimester maternal serum inhibin A levels in fetal trisomy 18 and Turner syndrome with and without hydrops. *Prenat Diagn* 1998;18:1061–1067.

95. Cuckle HS, Sehmi IK, Jones RG. Inhibin-A and non-Down syndrome aneuploidy. *Prenat Diagn* 1999;19:787–788.

96. Spencer K, Berry E, Crossley JA, Aitken DA, Nicolaides KH. Is maternal serum total hCG a marker of trisomy 21 in the first trimester of pregnancy? *Prenat Diagn* 2000;20:311–317.

97. Spencer K, Heath V, Flack N, Ong C, Nicolaides KH. First trimester maternal serum AFP and total hCG in aneuploides other than trisomy 21. *Prenat Diagn* 2000;20:635–639.

98. Brock DJH, Barron L, Holloway S, Liston WA, Hillier SG, Seppala M. First trimester maternal serum biochemical indicators in Down's syndrome. *Prenat Diagn* 1990;10:245–251.

99. Haddow JE, Palomaki GE, Knight GJ, Williams J, Miller WA, Johnson A. Screening of maternal serum for fetal Down's syndrome in the first trimester. *N Engl J Med* 1998;338:955–961.

100. Spencer K, Macri JN. Early detection of Down's syndrome using free beta human choriogonadotropin. *Ann Clin Biochem* 1992;29:349–350.

101. Spencer K, Souter V, Tul N, Snijders R, Nicolaides KH. A screening program for trisomy 21 at 10–14 weeks using fetal nuchal translucency, maternal serum free β-human chorionic gonadotropin and pregnancy-associated plasma protein-A. *Ultrasound Obstet Gynecol* 1999;13:231–237.

102. Brambati B, Lanzani A, Tului L. Ultrasound and biochemical assessment of first trimester pregnancy. In: Chapman M, Grudzinskas JG, Chard T, eds. *The embryo: normal and abnormal development and growth.* New York: Springer-Verlag, 1991:181–194.

103. Spencer K. The measurement of hCG subunits in screening for Down's syndrome. In: Grudzinskas JG, Chard T, Chapman M, Cuckle H, eds. *Screening for Down's syndrome.* Cambridge: Cambridge University Press, 1994:85–100.

104. Berry E, Aitken DA, Crossley JA, Macri JN, Connor JM. Screening for Down's syndrome: changes in marker levels and detection rates between first and second trimester. *Br J Obstet Gynaecol* 1997;104:811–817.

105. Noble PL, Wallace EM, Snijders RJ, Groome NP, Nicolaides KH. Maternal serum inhibin-A and free beta-hCG concentrations in trisomy 21 pregnancies at 10 to 14 weeks of gestation. *Br J Obstet Gynaecol* 1997;104:367–371.

106. Cole LA, Acuna E, Isozaki T, Palomaki GE, Bahado-Singh RO, Mahoney MJ. Combining beta core fragment and total oestriol measurements to test for Down syndrome pregnancies. *Prenat Diagn* 1997;17:1125–1133.

107. Cole LA, Cermik D, Bahado-Singh RO. Oligosaccharide variants of hCG-related molecules: potential screening markers for Down syndrome. *Prenat Diagn* 1997;17:1188–1190.

108. Rotmensch S, Liberati M, Kardana A, Copel JA, Ben Rafael Z, Cole LA. Nicked free beta-subunit of human chorionic

gonadotropin: a potential new marker for Down syndrome screening. *Am J Obstet Gynecol* 1996;174:609–611.

109. Cuckle HS, Iles RK, Chard T. Urinary β-core human chorionic gonadotrophin: a new approach to Down's syndrome screening. *Prenat Diagn* 1994;14:953–958.

110. Cuckle HS, Iles RK, Sehmi IH, Chard T, Oakey RE, et al. Urinary multiple marker screening for Down's syndrome. *Prenat Diagn* 1995;15:745–751.

111. Canick J, Kellner LH, Saller DN, Palomaki GE, Walker RP, Osathanondh R. Second trimester levels of maternal urinary gonadotropin peptide in Down syndrome pregnancy. *Prenat Diagn* 1995;15:752–759.

112. Canick JA, Kellner LH, Saller DN, Palomaki GE, Tumber MB, et al. A second level evaluation of maternal urinary gonadotropin peptide as a marker for second trimester Down syndrome screening. *Recent Adv Prenat Diagn Aneuploidy* 1996: Abstract 28.

113. Spencer K, Aitken DA, Macri JN, Buchanan PD. Urine free beta hCG and beta core in pregnancies affected by Down's syndrome. *Prenat Diagn* 1996;16:605–613.

114. Isozaki T, Palomaki GE, Bahado-Singh RO, Cole LA. Screening for Down syndrome pregnancy using beta core fragment: prospective study. *Prenat Diagn* 1997;17:407–413.

115. Hallahan TW, Krantz DA, Tului L, Alberti E, Buchanan PD, et al. Comparison of urinary free beta hCG and beta core in prenatal screening for chromosomal abnormalities in the second trimester of pregnancy. *Prenat Diagn* 1998;15:11–16.

116. Lam YH, Tang MH, Tang LC, Lee CP, Ho PK. Second-trimester maternal urinary gonadotrophin peptide screening for fetal Down syndrome in Asian women. *Prenat Diagn* 1997;17:1101–1106.

117. Hsu JJ, Spencer K, Aitken DA, Crossley J, Ozaki M, et al. Urinary free beta hCG, beta core fragment and total oestriol as markers of Down syndrome in the second trimester of pregnancy. *Prenat Diagn* 1999;109:146–158.

118. Cuckle HS, Canick JA, Kellner LH. Collaborative study of maternal urine β core human chorionic gonadotrophin screening for Down syndrome. *Prenat Diagn* 1999;19:911–917.

119. Cole LA. Down's syndrome screening using urine beta core fragment test: choice of immunoassay. *Prenat Diagn* 1995;15:679–682.

120. Cole LA, Rinne KM, Mahajan SM, Oz UA, Shahabi S, et al. Urinary screening tests for fetal Down's syndrome: I. Fresh β-core fragment. *Prenat Diagn* 1999;19:340–350.

121. Cuckle HS, Canick JA, Kellner LH, Van Lith JM, White I, et al. Urinary beta-core-hCG screening in the first trimester. *Prenat Diagn* 1996;16:1057–1059.

122. Spencer K, Noble P, Snijders RJM, Nicolaides KH. First trimester urine free beta hCG, beta core, and total oestriol in pregnancies affected by Down's syndrome: implications for first trimester screening with nuchal translucency and serum free beta hCG. *Prenat Diagn* 1997;17:525–538.

123. Macintosh MCM, Nicolaides KH, Noble P, Chard T, Gunn L, et al. Urinary β-core hCG: screening for aneuploides in early pregnancy (11–14 weeks' gestation). *Prenat Diagn* 1997;17:401–405.

124. Kellner LH, Canick JA, Palomaki GE, Neveux LM, Sallar DN, et al. Levels of urinary beta core fragment, total oestriol and the ratio of the two in second trimester screening for Down syndrome. *Prenat Diagn* 1997;17:1135–1141.

125. Cole LA, Omrani A, Cermik D, Bahado-Singh RO, Mahoney MJ. Hyperglycosylated hCG, a potential alternative to hCG in Down syndrome screening. *Prenat Diagn* 1998;18:926–933.

126. Cole LA, Shahabi S, Oz UA, Rinne KM, Omrani A, et al. Urinary screening tests for fetal Down syndrome: II. Hyperglycosylated hCG. *Prenat Diagn* 1999;19:351–359.

127. Cole LA, Shahabi S, Oz UA, Bahado-Singh RO, Mahoney MJ. Hyperglycosylated human chorionic gonadotropin (invasive trophoblast antigen) immunoassay: a new basis for gestational Down syndrome screening. *Clin Chem* 1999;45:2109–2119.

128. Weinans MJN, Butler SA, Mantingh A, Cole LA. Urinary hyperglycosylated hCG in first trimester screening for chromosomal abnormalities. *Prenat Diagn* 2000;20:976–978.

129. Shahabi S, Oz UA, Bahado-Singh RO, Mahoney MJ, Omrani A, et al. Serum hyperglycosylated hCG: a potential screening test for fetal Down syndrome. *Prenat Diagn* 1999;19:488–489.

130. Abushoufa RA, Talbot JA, Brownbill K, Rafferty B, Kane JW, et al. The development of a sialic acid specific lectin immunoassay for the measurement of human chorionic gonadotrophin glycoforms in serum and its application in normal and Down's syndrome pregnancies. *Clin Endocrinol* 2000;52:499–508.

131. Nyberg DA, Souter VL. Sonographic markers of fetal trisomies: second trimester. *J Ultrasound Med* 2001;20:655–674.

132. Vintzileos AM, Campbell WA, Rodis JF, Guzman ER, Smulian JC, et al. The use of second-trimester genetic sonogram in guiding clinical management of patients at increased risk for fetal trisomy 21. *Obstet Gynecol* 1996;87:948–952.

133. Vintzileos AM, Campbell WA, Guzman ER, Smulian JC, McLean DA, et al. Second-trimester ultrasound markers for detection of trisomy 21: Which markers are best? *Obstet Gynecol* 1997;89:941–944.

134. Vergani P, Locatelli A, Piccoli MG, Ceruti P, Mariani E, et al. Best second trimester sonographic markers for the detection of trisomy 21. *J Ultrasound Med* 1999;18(7):469–473.

135. Benacerraf BR, Neuberg D, Bromley B, Frigoletto FD Jr. Sonographic scoring index for prenatal detection of chromosomal abnormalities. *J Ultrasound Med* 1992;11(9):449–458.

136. Benacerraf BR, Nadel AS, Bromley B. Identification of second-trimester fetuses with autosomal trisomy by use of a sonographic scoring index. *Radiology* 1994;193:135–140.

137. Nyberg DA, Souter VL. Sonographic markers of fetal aneuploidy. *Clin Perinatol* 2000;27:761–789.

138. DeVore GR, Alfi O. The use of color Doppler ultrasound to identify fetuses at increased risk for trisomy 21: an alternative for high-risk patients who decline genetic amniocentesis. *Obstet Gynecol* 1995;85:378–386.

139. Smith-Bindman R, Hosmer W, Feldstein VA, Deeks JJ, Goldberg JD. Second-trimester ultrasound to detect fetuses with Down syndrome: a meta-analysis. *JAMA* 2001;285:1044–1055.

140. Winter TC, Uhrich SB, Souter VL, Nyberg DA. The "Genetic Sonogram": comparison of the index scoring system with the age-adjusted US risk assessment. *Radiology* 2000;215:775–782.

141. Nyberg DA, Luthy DA, Resta RG, Nyberg BC, Williams MA. Age-adjusted ultrasound risk assessment for fetal Down's syndrome during the second trimester: description of the method and analysis of 142 cases. *Ultrasound Obstet Gynecol* 1998;12:8–14.

142. Nyberg DA, Souter VL, El-Bastawissi A, Young S, Luth-

hardt F, Luthy DA. Isolated sonographic markers for detection of fetal Down syndrome in the second trimester of pregnancy. *J Ultrasound Med* 2001;20:1053–1063.

143. Bromley B, Lieberman E, Benacerraf BR. The incorporation of maternal age into the sonographic scoring index for the detection at 14–20 weeks of fetuses with Down's syndrome. *Ultrasound Obstet Gynecol* 1997;10(5):321–324.

144. Gustavii B, Edvall H. First trimester diagnosis of cystic nuchal hygroma. *Acta Obstet Gynecol Scand* 1984;4:383–386.

145. Reuss A, Pijpers L, Schampers PTFN, Wladimiroff JW, Sachs ES. The importance of chorionic villus sampling after first trimester diagnosis of cystic hygroma. *Prenat Diagn* 1987;7:299–301.

146. Bronshtein M, Rottem S, Yoffe N, Blumenfeld Z. First-trimester and early second-trimester diagnosis of nuchal cystic hygroma by transvaginal sonography: diverse prognosis of the septated from the nonseptated lesion. *Am J Obstet Gynecol* 1998;161:78–82.

147. Nicolaides KH, Azar G, Byrne D, Mansur C, Marks K. Fetal nuchal translucency: ultrasound screening for chromosomal defects in first trimester of pregnancy. *BMJ* 1992;304:867–869.

148. Pandya PP, Kondylios A, Hilbert L, Snijders RJM, Nicolaides KH. Chromosomal defects and outcome in 1015 fetuses with increased nuchal translucency. *Ultrasound Obstet Gynecol* 1995;5:15–19.

149. Snijders RJM, Noble P, Sebire N, Souka A, Nicolaides KH. UK multicentre project on assessment of risk of trisomy 21 by maternal age and fetal nuchal translucency thickness at 10–14 weeks of gestation. *Lancet* 1998;352:343–346.

150. Wright D, Reynolds T, Donovan C. Assessment of atypicality: an adjunct to screening for Down syndrome that facilitates detection of other chromosomal defects. *Ann Clin Biochem* 1993;30:578–583.

150a. Reynolds TM, Penney MD. The mathematical basis of multivariate risk screening: with special reference to screening for Down's syndrome associated pregnancy. *Ann Clin Biochem* 1990;27:452–458.

151. Reynolds TM. Screening by test combination: a statistical overview. In: Grudzinskas JG, Chard T, Chapman M, Cuckle H, eds. *Screening for Down's syndrome.* Cambridge: Cambridge University Press, 1994:47–71.

152. Reynolds TM. Down's syndrome screening: a controversial test, with more controversy to come! *J Clin Pathol* 2000;53:893–898.

153. Wald NJ, Hackshaw AK, Huttly W, Kennard A. Empirical validation of risk screening for Down's syndrome. *J Med Screen* 1996;3:185–187.

154. Canick JA, Rish S. The accuracy of assigned risk in maternal serum screening. *Prenat Diagn* 1998;18:413–415.

155. Spencer K, Crossley JA, Green K, Worthington DJ, Brownbill K, et al. Second trimester levels of pregnancy associated plasma protein-A in cases of trisomy 18. *Prenat Diagn* 1999;19:1127–1134.

156. Quaglianni D, Betti S, Brambati B, Nicolini U. Coping with serum screening for Down syndrome when the result is given as a numeric value. *Prenat Diagn* 1998;18:816–821.

157. Marteau TM, Saidi G, Goodburn S, Lawton J, Michie S, et al. Numbers or words? A randomised controlled trial of presenting screen negative results to pregnant women. *Prenat Diagn* 2000;20:719–724.

158. Spencer K. Second trimester prenatal screening for Down's syndrome using alpha-fetoprotein and free beta hCG: a seven year review. *Br J Obstet Gynaecol* 1999;106:1287–1293.

159. Reynolds TM, Nix AB, Dunstan FD, Dawson AJ. Age specific detection and false positive rates: an aid to counselling in Down syndrome risk screening. *Obstet Gynecol* 1993;81:447–450.

160. Wald NJ, Kennard A, Hackshaw A, McGuire A. Antenatal screening for Down's syndrome. *J Med Screen* 1997;4:181–246.

161. Spencer K, Macri JN. The use of free β hCG in antenatal screening for Down's syndrome. *Br J Obstet Gynaecol* 1994;101:175–176.

162. Dunstan F, Gray J, Nix A, Reynolds T. Detection rates and false positive rates for Down's syndrome screening: How precisely can they be estimated and what factors influence their value. *Statist Med* 1997;16:1481–1495.

163. Haddow JE, Palomaki GE, Knight GJ, Foster DL, Neveux LM. Second trimester screening for Down's syndrome using maternal serum dimeric inhibin A. *J Med Screen* 1998;5:115–119.

164. Wenstrom KD, Owen J, Chu DC, Boots L. Elevated second trimester dimeric inhibin A levels identify Down syndrome pregnancies. *Am J Obstet Gynecol* 1997;177:992–996.

165. Bahado-Singh R, Oz U, Shahabi S, Omrani A, Mahoney M, et al. Urine hyperglycosylated hCG plus ultrasound biometry for detection of Down syndrome in the second trimester in a high risk population. *Obstet Gynecol* 2000;95:889–894.

166. Bahado-Singh RO, Oz AU, Kovanci E, Deren O, Copel J, et al. New Down syndrome screening algorithm: ultrasonographic biometry and multiple serum markers combined with maternal age. *Am J Obstet Gynecol* 1998;179:1627–1631.

167. Drugan A, Reichler A, Bronstein M, Johnson MP, Sokol RJ, et al. Abnormal biochemical serum screening versus 2nd-trimester ultrasound-detected minor anomalies as predictors of aneuploidy in low-risk patients. *Fetal Diagn Ther* 1996;11:301–305.

168. Verdin SM, Economides DL. The role of ultrasonographic markers for trisomy 21 in women with positive serum biochemistry. *Br J Obstet Gynaecol* 1998;105(1):63–67.

169. Souter VL, Nyberg DA, El-Bastawissi A, Zebelman A, Luthhardt F, et al. Correlation of ultrasound findings and biochemical markers in the second trimester of pregnancy in trisomy 21. *Prenat Diagn* 2002;22:175–182.

170. Owen J, Wenstrom KD, Hardin JM, Boots LR, Hsu CC, et al. The utility of fetal biometry as an adjunct to the multiple-marker screening test for Down syndrome. *Am J Obstet Gynecol* 1994;171(4):1041–1046.

171. Bahado-Singh RO, Goldstein I, Uerpairojkit B, Copel JA, Mahoney MJ, et al. Normal nuchal thickness in the midtrimester indicates reduced risk of Down syndrome in pregnancies with abnormal triple-screen results. *Am J Obstet Gynecol* 1995;173(4):1106–1110.

172. Roberts D, Walkinshaw SA, McCormack MJ, Ellis J. Prenatal detection of trisomy 21: combined experience of two British hospitals. *Prenat Diagn* 2000;20(1):17–22.

173. Bahado-Singh RO, Oz AU, Gomez K, Hunter D, Copel J, et al. Combined ultrasound biometry, serum markers and age for Down syndrome risk estimation. *Ultrasound Obstet Gynecol* 2000;15:199–204.

174. Nyberg DA, Bahado-Singh R, Souter VL, Oz R, Zebelman A, et al. An algorithm combining second-trimester ultrasound and biochemical markers is superior to the "triple

screen" for detection of fetal Down syndrome. (abs) *J Ultrasound Med* 2001;20:s27.

175. Wald NJ, George L, Smith D, Densem JW, Petterson K, on behalf of the International Prenatal Screening Research Group. Serum screening for Down's syndrome between 8 and 14 weeks of pregnancy. *Br J Obstet Gynecol* 1996;103:407–412.

176. Krantz DA, Larsen JW, Buchanan PD, Macri JN. First-trimester Down syndrome screening: free beta-human chorionic gonadotropin and pregnancy-associated plasma protein A. *Am J Obstet Gynecol* 1996;174:612–616.

177. Forest JC, Masse J, Moutquin JM. Screening for Down syndrome during first trimester: a prospective study using free beta-human chorionic gonadotropin and pregnancy-associated plasma protein A. *Clin Biochem* 1997;30:333–338.

178. Spencer K, Crossley JA, Aitken DA, Nix ABJ, Dunstan FDJ, et al. Temporal changes in maternal serum biochemical markers of trisomy 21 across the first and second trimester of pregnancy. *Ann Clin Biochem* 2002;39:(in press).

179. Spencer K, Crossley JA, Aitken DA, Nix ABJ, Dunstan FDJ, Williams K. Variation in detection rate and individual patient specific risks as a result of temporal variation in biochemical markers of trisomy 21 across the first and second trimester of pregnancy: Implications for screening algorithms *Ann Clin Biochem* 2002;39:(in press).

180. Wald NJ, Hackshaw AK. Combining ultrasound and biochemistry in first-trimester screening for Down's syndrome. *Prenat Diagn* 1997;17:821–829.

181. Cuckle HS, van Lith JMM. Appropriate biochemical parameters in first-trimester screening for Down syndrome. *Prenat Diagn* 1999;19:505–512.

182. De Graaf IM, Pajkrt E, Bilardo CM, Leschot NJ, Cuckle HS, et al. Early pregnancy screening of fetal aneuploidy with serum markers and nuchal translucency. *Prenat Diagn* 1999;19:458–462.

182a. Spencer K. Age related detection and false positive rates when screening for Down's syndrome in the first trimester using nuchal translucency and maternal serum free β-hCG and PAPP-A. *Br J Obstet Gynaecol* 2001;108:1043–1046.

183. Dunstan FDJ, Nix ABJ. Screening for Down's syndrome: the effect of test date on the detection rate. *Ann Clin Biochem* 1998;35:57–61.

183a. Spencer K. What is the true fetal loss rate in pregnancies affected by trisomy 21 and how does this influence when the first trimester detection rates are superior to those in the second trimester. *Prenat Diagn* 2001;21:788–789.

184. RCOG Recommendations arising from the 32nd Study Group: Screening for Down syndrome in the first trimester. In: Grudzinskas JG, Ward RHT, eds. *Screening for Down syndrome in the first trimester.* London: RCOG Press, 1997:353–356.

184a. Spencer K, Spencer CE, Power M, Moakes A, Nicolaides KH. One stop clinic for assessment of risk for fetal anomalies: a report of the first year of prospective screening for chromosomal anomalies in the first trimester. *Br J Obstet Gynaecol* 2000;107:1271–1275.

185. Cuckle H, Sehmi I. Calculating correct Down's syndrome risks. *Br J Obstet Gynaecol* 1999;106:371–372.

186. Wald NJ, Watt HC, Hackshaw AK. Integrated screening for Down's syndrome on the basis of tests performed during the first and second trimesters. *N Engl J Med* 1999;341:461–467.

187. Copel JA, Bahado-Singh RO. Prenatal screening for Down's syndrome—a search for the family's values. *N Engl J Med* 1999;341:521–522.

188. Reynolds T, Zimmerman R, Wright E. Integrated screening for Down syndrome. *N Engl J Med* 1999;341:1935.

189. Down's Syndrome News. Integrated Test. *Down's Screening News* 2000;7:28–29.

190. Barkai G, Chaki R, Sochat M, Goldman B. Human chorionic gonadotrophin and trisomy 18. *Am J Med Genet* 1991;41(1):52–53.

191. Staples AJ, Robertson EF, Ranieri E, Ryall RG, Haan EA. A maternal serum screen for trisomy 18: an extension of maternal serum screening for Down syndrome. *Am J Hum Genet* 1991;49:1025–1033.

192. Barkai G, Goldman B, Ries L, Chaki R, Zer T, et al. Expanding multiple marker screening for Down's syndrome to include Edwards syndrome. *Prenat Diagn* 1993;13:843–850.

193. Palomaki GE, Haddow JE, Knight GJ, Wald NJ, Kennard A, et al. Risk-based prenatal screening for trisomy 18 using alpha-fetoprotein, unconjugated oestriol and human chorionic gonadotropin. *Prenat Diagn* 1995;15:713–723.

194. Benn PA, Leo MV, Rodis JF, Beazoglou T, Collins R, et al. Maternal serum screening for fetal trisomy 18: a comparison of fixed cut off and patient-specific risk protocols. *Obstet Gynecol* 1999;93:707–711.

195. Spencer K. Accuracy of Down's syndrome risks produced in a prenatal screening program. *Ann Clin Biochem* 1999;36: 101–103.

196. Bersinger NA, Leporrier N, Herrou M, Leymarie P. Maternal serum pregnancy-associated plasma protein A (PAPP-A) but not pregnancy-specific beta1-glycoprotein (SP1) is a useful second-trimester marker for fetal trisomy 18. *Prenat Diagn* 1999;19:537–541.

197. Brumfield CG, Wenstrom KD, Owen J, Davis RO. Ultrasound findings and multiple marker screening in trisomy 18. *Obstet Gynecol* 2000;95:51–54.

198. Feuchtbaum LB, Currier RJ, Lorey FW, Cunningham GC. Prenatal ultrasound findings in affected and unaffected pregnancies that are screen-positive for trisomy 18: the California experience. *Prenat Diagn* 2000;20:293–299.

199. Sullivan A, Giudice T, Vavelidis F, Thiagarajah S. Choroid plexus cysts: Is biochemical testing a valuable adjunct to targeted ultrasonography? *Am J Obstet Gynecol* 1999;181:260–265.

200. Brambati B, Macintosh MCM, Teisner B, Maguiness S, Shrimanker K, et al. Low maternal serum levels of pregnancy associated plasma protein A (PAPP-A) in the first trimester in association with abnormal fetal karyotype. *Br J Obstet Gynaecol* 1993;100:324–326.

201. Tul N, Spencer K, Noble P, Chan C, Nicolaides K. Screening for trisomy 18 by fetal nuchal translucency and maternal serum free beta-hCG and PAPP-A at 10–14 weeks of gestation. *Prenat Diagn* 1999;19:1035–1042.

202. Sherod C, Sebire NJ, Soares W, Snijders RJM, Nicolaides KH. Prenatal diagnosis of trisomy 18 at the 10-14 week ultrasound scan. *Ultrasound Obstet Gynecol* 1997;10:387–390.

203. Biagiotti R, Cariati E, Brizzi L, Cappelli G, D'Agata A. Maternal serum screening for trisomy 18 in the first trimester of pregnancy. *Prenat Diagn* 1998;18:907–913.

204. Wenstrom KD, Chu DC, Owen J, Boots L. Maternal serum alpha-fetoprotein and dimeric inhibin A detect ane-

uploidies other than Down syndrome. *Am J Obstet Gynecol* 1998;179(4):966–970.

205. Feuchtbaum LB, Cunningham G, Waller DK, Lustig LS, Tompkinson DG, et al. Fetal karyotyping for chromosome abnormalities after an unexplained elevated maternal serum alpha-fetoprotein screening. *Obstet Gynecol* 1995;86:248–254.

206. Benacerraf BR, Miller WA, Frigoletto FD Jr. Sonographic detection of fetuses with trisomies 13 and 18: accuracy and limitations. *Am J Obstet Gynecol* 1988;158:404–409.

207. Lehman CD, Nyberg DA, Winter TC 3rd, Kapur RP, Resta RG, et al. Trisomy 13 syndrome: prenatal US findings in a review of 33 cases. *Radiology* 1995;194(1):217–222.

208. Spencer K, Ong C, Skentou H, Liao A, Nicolaides K. Screening for trisomy 13 by fetal nuchal translucency and maternal serum free beta-hCG and PAPP-A at 10–14 weeks of gestation. *Prenat Diagn* 2000;20:411–416.

209. Oyer CE, Canick JA. Maternal serum hCG levels in triploidy: variability and need to consider molar tissue. *Prenat Diagn* 1992;12:627–629.

210. Muller F, Aegerter P, Boue A. Prospective maternal serum human chorionic gonadotropin screening for the risk of fetal chromosome anomalies and of subsequent fetal and neonatal deaths. *Prenat Diagn* 1993;13:29–43.

211. Kohn G, Zamir R, Zer T, Amiel A, Fejgin M. Significance of very low maternal serum human chorionic gonadotropin in prenatal diagnosis of triploidy. *Prenat Diagn* 1991;11:277.

212. Mason G, Linton C, Cuckle H, Holding S. Low maternal serum human chorionic gonadotrophin and unconjugated oestriol in a triploidy pregnancy. *Prenat Diagn* 1992;12:545–546.

213. Fejgin MD, Amiel A, Golberger S, Barnes I, Zer T, et al. Placental insufficiency as a possible cause of low maternal serum human chorionic gonadotropin and low maternal serum unconjugated estriol levels in triploidy. *Am J Obstet Gynecol* 1992;167:766–767.

214. Fejgin MD, Amiel A, Kohn G. More about low maternal serum human chorionic gonadotropin and unconjugated estriol values in triploidy. *Am J Obstet Gynecol* 1993;168:1641.

215. Jacobs PA, Szulman AE, Funkhouser J, Matsuura JS, Wilson CC. Human triploidy: relationship between parental origin of the additional haploid complement and development of partial hydatidiform mole. *Ann Hum Genet* 1982;46:223–231.

216. McFadden DE, Kalousek DK. Two different phenotypes of fetuses with chromosomal triploidy: correlation with parental origin of the extra haploid set. *Am J Med Genet* 1991;38:535–538.

217. Schmidt D, Shaffer LG, McCaskill C, Rose E, Greenberg F. Very low maternal serum chorionic gonadotropin levels in association with fetal triploidy. *Am J Obstet Gynecol* 1994;170:77–80.

218. Jauniaux E, Brown R, Rodeck C, Nicolaides KH. Prenatal diagnosis of triploidy during the second trimester of pregnancy. *Obstet Gynecol* 1996;83:616–619.

219. McFadden DE, Lockitch G, Langlois S. Triple screen in triploidy. *Am J Hum Genet* 1998;63[Suppl]:A168 (abstract).

220. McFadden DE, Kwong LC, Yam IYL, Langlois S. Parental origin of triploidy in human fetuses: evidence for genomic imprinting. *Hum Genet* 1993;92:465–469.

221. Dietzsch E, Ramsay M, Christianson AL, Henderson BD, de Ravel TJL. Maternal origin of the extra haploid set of chromosomes in third trimester triploid fetuses. *Am J Med Genet* 1995;58:360–364.

222. Goshen R. The genomic basis of the β subunit of human chorionic gonadotropin diversity in triploidy. *Am J Obstet Gynecol* 1994;170:700–701.

223. Eiben B, Hammans W, Goebel R. Triploidy, imprinting, and hCG levels in maternal serum screening. *Prenat Diagn* 1996;16:377–378.

224. Craig K, Pinetter MG, Blackstone J, Chard R, Cartin A. Highly abnormal maternal inhibin and beta-human gonadotrophin level along with severe HELLP (hemolysis, elevated liver enzymes, and low platelet count) syndrome at 17 weeks' gestation with triploidy. *Am J Obstet Gynecol* 2000;182(3):737–739.

225. Benn PA, Gainey A, Ingardia CJ, Rodis JF, Egan JF. Second trimester maternal serum analytes in triploid pregnancies: correlation with phenotype and sex chromosome complement. *Prenat Diagn* 2001;21:680–686.

226. Jauniaux E, Brown R, Snijders RJ, Noble P, Nicolaides KH. Early prenatal diagnosis of triploidy. *Am J Obstet Gynecol* 1997;176:550–554.

227. Spencer K, Liao AWJ, Skentou H, Cicero S, Nicolaides KH. Screening for triploidy by fetal nuchal translucency and maternal serum free β-hCG and PAPP-A at 10–14 weeks of gestation. *Prenat Diagn* 2000;20:495–499.

228. Hiett AK, Callaghan CM, Brown HL, Golichowski AM, Heerema NA. The association of aneuploidy and unexplained elevated maternal serum alpha-fetoprotein. *J Perinatol* 1998;18:343–346.

229. Spencer K, Tul N, Nicolaides KH. Maternal serum free beta-hCG and PAPP-A in fetal sex chromosome defects in the first trimester. *Prenat Diagn* 2000;20:390–394.

230. Morssink LP, Sikkema-Raddatz B, Beekhuis JR, De Wolf BT, Mantingh A. Placental mosaicism is associated with unexplained second-trimester elevation of MShCG levels, but not with elevation of MSAFP levels. *Prenat Diagn* 1996;16:845–851.

231. Zimmermann R, Lauper U, Streicher A, Huch R, Huch A. Elevated alpha-fetoprotein and human chorionic gonadotropin as a marker for placental trisomy 16 in the second trimester. *Prenat Diagn* 1995;15:1121–1124.

232. Groli C, Cerri V, Tarantini M, Bellotti D, Jacobello C, et al. Maternal serum screening and trisomy 16 confined to the placenta. *Prenat Diagn* 1996;16:685–689.

233. Zanini R, Tarantini M, Cerri V, Jacobello C, Bellotti D, et al. "Dual positivity" for neural tube defects and Down syndrome at maternal serum screening: gestational outcome. *Fetal Diagn Ther* 1998;13:106–110.

234. Raggatt PR, Carr C, Taylor NF, Yates JRW, Goodburn SF. Placental sulphatase deficiency detected in the second trimester by the "triple screening test." Proceedings of the ACB National Meeting, 1992:41.

235. David M, Israel N, Merksamer R, Bar-Nizan N, Borochowitz Z, et al. Very low maternal serum unconjugated estriol and prenatal diagnosis of steroid sulphatase deficiency. *Fetal Diagn Ther* 1995;10:76–79.

236. Keren DF, Canick JA, Johnson MZ, Schaldenbrand JD, Haning RV, et al. Low maternal serum unconjugated estriol during prenatal screening as an indication of placental steroid sulfatase deficiency and X-linked ichthyosis. *Am J Clin Pathol* 1995;103:400–403.

237. Blitzer MG, Kelley RI, Schwartz MF. Abnormal maternal serum marker patterns associated with Smith-Lemli-Opitz syndrome. *Am J Hum Genet* 1994;55:A277.

238. Bradley LA, Palomaki GE, Knight GJ, Haddow JE, Opitz JM, et al. Levels of unconjugated estriol and other maternal serum markers in pregnancies with Smith-Lemli-Opitz (RSH) syndrome fetuses. *Am J Med Genet* 1999;82:355–358.

239. Bick DP, McCorkle D, Stanley WS, Stern HJ, Staszak P, et al. Prenatal diagnosis of Smith-Lemli-Opitz syndrome in a pregnancy with low maternal serum oestriol and a sex-reversed fetus. *Prenat Diagn* 1999;19:68–71.

240. Hyett JA, Clayton PT, Moscoso G, Nicolaides KH. Increased first trimester nuchal translucency as a prenatal manifestation of Smith-Lemli-Opitz syndrome. *Am J Med Genet* 1995;58:374–376.

241. Oxvig C, Sand O, Kristensen T, Kristensen L, Sottrup-Jensen L. Isolation and characterisation of circulating complex between human pregnancy associated plasma protein-A and proform of eosinophil major basic protein. *Biochim Biophys Acta* 1994;1201:415–423.

242. Lawrence JB, Oxvig C, Overgaard MT, Sottrup-Jensen L, Gleich GJ, et al. The insulin-like growth factor (IGF)-dependent IGF binding protein-4 protease secreted by human fibroblasts is pregnancy-associated plasma protein-A. *Proc Natl Acad Sci U S A* 1999;96:3149–3153.

243. Westergaard JG, Chemnitz J, Teisner B, Poulsen HK, Ipsen L, et al. Pregnancy-associated plasma protein A: a possible marker in the classification and prenatal diagnosis of Cornelia de Lange syndrome. *Prenat Diagn* 1983;3:225–232.

244. Hseih TT, Hsu JJ, Chen CP, Tsai MS, Hsieh FJ, et al. Down's syndrome screening with AFP and free Beta hCG: an analysis of the influence of Chinese ethnic origin on screening parameters. *Am J Hum Genet* 1995;57:A281.

245. Onda T, Kitagawa M, Takeda O, Sago H, Kubonoya K, et al. Triple marker screening in native Japanese women. *Prenat Diagn* 1996;16:713–717.

246. Watt HC, Wald NJ, Smith D, Kennard A, Densem J. Effect of allowing for ethnic group in prenatal screening for Down's syndrome. *Prenat Diagn* 1996;16:691–698.

247. Spencer K, Ong CYT, Liao AWJ, Nicolaides KH. The influence of ethnic origin on first trimester biochemical markers of chromosomal abnormalities. *Prenat Diagn* 2000;20:491–494.

247a. Spencer K. The influence of gravidity on Down's syndrome screening with free beta hCG. *Prenat Diagn* 1995;15:87–89.

247b. Haddow JE, Palomaki GE, Knight GJ. Effect of parity on human chorionic gonadotrophin levels and Down's syndrome screening. *J Med Screen* 1995;2:28–30.

248. Spencer K, Ong CY, Liao AW, Nicolaides KH. The influence of parity and gravidity on first trimester markers of chromosomal abnormality. *Prenat Diagn* 2000;20:792–794.

248a. Aitken DA. Biochemical screening in twins. In: Ward RH, Whittle M, eds. *Multiple pregnancy.* London: RCOG Press, 1995:171–185.

248b. Wald N, Cuckle H, Wu TS, George L. Maternal serum unconjugated oestriol and human chorionic gonadotrophin levels in twin pregnancies: implications for screening for Down syndrome. *Br J Obstet Gynaecol* 1991;98:905–908.

249. Spencer K, Nicolaides KH. First trimester prenatal diagnosis of trisomy 21 in discordant twins using fetal nuchal

250. Palomaki GE, Panizza DS, Canick JA. Screening for Down syndrome using AFP, uE3 and hCG: effect of maternal weight. *Am J Hum Genet* 1990;47:245–249.

251. Neveux LM, Palomaki GE, Larrivee DA, Knight GJ, Haddow JE. Refinements in managing maternal weight adjustment for interpreting prenatal screening results. *Prenat Diagn* 1996;16:1115–1119.

252. Kennedy DM, Edwards VM, Worthington DJ. Evaluation of different weight correction methods for antenatal serum screening using data from two multi-centre programmes. *Ann Clin Biochem* 1999;36:359–364.

253. Bazzett LB, Yaron Y, O'Brien JW, Critchfield G, Kramer RL, et al. Fetal gender impact on multiple-marker screening results. *Am J Med Genet* 1998;76:369–371.

254. Ghidini A, Spong CY, Grier RE, Walker CN, Pezzullo JC. Is maternal serum triple screening a better predictor of Down syndrome in female than in male fetuses? *Prenat Diagn* 1998;18:123–126.

255. Spencer K, Ong CYT, Liao AWJ, Papademetriou D, Nicolaides KH. The influence of fetal sex in screening for trisomy 21 by fetal nuchal translucency, maternal serum free β-hCG and PAPP-A at 10–14 weeks of gestation. *Prenat Diagn* 2000;20:673–675.

256. Thomsen SG, Isager-Sally L, Lange AP, Saurbrey N, Schiolier V. Smoking habits and maternal serum alpha-fetoprotein levels during the second trimester of pregnancy. *Br J Obstet Gynaecol* 1983;90:716–717.

257. Bernstein L, Pike MC, Lobo RA, Depue RH, Ross RK, Henderson BE. Cigarette smoking in pregnancy results in marked decrease in maternal hCG and oestradiol levels. *Br J Obstet Gynaecol* 1989;96:92–96.

258. Bartels I, Hoppe-Sievert B, Bockel B, Herold S, Caesar J. Adjustment formulae for maternal serum alpha-fetoprotein, human chorionic gonadotropin, and unconjugated oestriol to maternal weight and smoking. *Prenat Diagn* 1993;13:123–130.

258a. Palomaki GE, Knight GJ, Haddow JE, Canick JA, Wald NJ, et al. Cigarette smoking and levels of maternal serum alpha-fetoprotein, unconjugated estriol and hCG: impact on Down syndrome screening. *Obstet Gynecol* 1993;81:675–678.

258b. Spencer K. The influence of smoking on maternal serum AFP and free beta hCG levels and the impact on screening for Down syndrome. *Prenat Diagn* 1998;18:225–234.

259. Ferriman EL, Sehmi IK, Jones R, Cuckle HS. The effect of smoking in pregnancy on maternal serum inhibin A levels. *Prenat Diagn* 1999;19:372–374.

260. Brambati B, Macri JN, Tului L, Hallahan TW, Krantz DA, Alberti E. First trimester fetal aneuploidy screening: maternal serum PAPP-A and free β hCG. In: Grudzinskas JG, Ward RHT, eds. *Screening for Down's syndrome in the first trimester.* London: RCOG Press, 1997:135–147.

260a. Spencer K. The influence of smoking on maternal serum PAPP-A and free beta hCG levels in the first trimester of pregnancy. *Prenat Diagn* 1999;19:1065–1066.

261. Spencer K, Ong CYT, Liao AWJ, Papademetriou D, Nicolaides KH. First trimester markers of trisomy 21 and the influence of maternal cigarette smoking status. *Prenat Diagn* 2000;20:852–853.

262. Klein J, Stein Z, Susser M, Warburton D. New insights into epidemiology of chromosome disorders; their relevance to

the prevention of Down's syndrome. In: Miterl, ed. *Frontiers in knowledge in mental retardation, Vol 2. Biochemical aspects.* Baltimore; University Park Press, 1981:131–141.

263. Shiono PH, Klebanoff MA, Berendes HW. Congenital malformations and maternal smoking during pregnancy. *Teratology* 1986;34:65–71.

264. Hook EB, Cross PK. Cigarette smoking and Down syndrome. *Am J Hum Genet* 1985;37:1216–1224.

265. Christianson RE, Torfs CP. Maternal smoking and Down syndrome. *Am J Hum Genet* 1988;43:545–547.

266. Chen CL, Gilbert TJ, Daling JR. Maternal smoking and Down syndrome: the confounding effect of maternal age. *Am J Epidemiol* 1999;149:442–446.

267. Holding S, Cuckle H. Maternal serum screening for Down's syndrome taking account of the result in a previous pregnancy. *Prenat Diagn* 1994;14:321–322.

268. Spencer K. Between-pregnancy biological variability of maternal serum alpha-fetoprotein and free beta hCG: implications for Down syndrome screening in subsequent pregnancies. *Prenat Diagn* 1997;17:39–45.

269. Larsen SO, Christiansen M, Norgaard-Pedersen B. Inclusion of serum marker measurements from a previous pregnancy improves Down syndrome screening performance. *Prenat Diagn* 1998;18:706–712.

270. Barkai G, Goldman B, Ries L, Chaki R, Dor J, et al. Down's syndrome screening marker levels following assisted reproduction. *Prenat Diagn* 1996;16:1111–1114.

271. Heionen S, Ryynanen M, Kirkinen P, Hippelainen M, Saarikoski S. Effect of in vitro fertilization on human chorionic gonadotropin serum concentrations and Down's syndrome screening. *Fertil Steril* 1996;66:398–403.

272. Ribbert LS, Kornman LH, De Wolf BT, Simons AH, Jansen CA, et al. Maternal serum screening for fetal Down syndrome in IVF pregnancies. *Prenat Diagn* 1996;16:35–38.

273. Frishman GN, Canick JA, Hogan JW, Hackett RJ, Kellner LH, et al. Serum triple-marker screening in in vitro fertilization and naturally conceived pregnancies. *Obstet Gynecol* 1997;90:98–101.

274. Lam YH, Yeung WS, Tang MH, Ng EH, So WW, et al. Maternal serum alpha-fetoprotein and human chorionic gonadotrophin in pregnancies conceived after intracytoplasmic sperm injection and conventional in-vitro fertilization. *Hum Reprod* 1999;14:2120–2123.

274a. Wald NJ, White N, Morris JK, Huttly WJ, Canick JA. Serum markers for Down's syndrome in women who have had in vitro fertilization: implications for antenatal screening. *Br J Obstet Gynaecol* 1999;106:1304–1306.

275. Liao AW, Heath V, Kametas N, Spencer K, Nicolaides KH. First trimester screening for trisomy 21 in singleton pregnancies achieved by assisted reproduction. *Human Reprod* 2001;16:1501–1504.

276. Milunsky A, Alpert E, Kitzmiller JL, Younger MD, Neff RK. Prenatal diagnosis of neural tube defects. VIII. The importance of serum alpha-fetoprotein screening in diabetic pregnant women. *Am J Obstet Gynecol* 1982;142:1030–1032.

276a. Wald NJ, Cuckle HS, Densem JW, Stone RB. Maternal serum unconjugated oestriol and human chorionic gonadotrophin levels in pregnancies with insulin-dependent diabetes: implication for screening for Down's syndrome. *Br J Obstet Gynaecol* 1992;99:51–53.

277. Reese EA, Davis N, Mahoney MJ, Baumgarten A. Maternal serum alpha-fetoprotein in diabetic pregnancy: correlation with blood glucose control. *Lancet* 1987;ii:275.

277a. Canick JA, Panizza DS, Palomaki GE. Prenatal screening for Down's syndrome using AFP, UE3, and hCG: effect of maternal race, insulin dependent diabetes and twin pregnancy. *Am J Hum Genet* 1990;47:A270.

277b. Crossley JA, Berry E, Aitken DA, Connor JM. Insulin Dependent Diabetes and prenatal screening results: current experience from a regional screening programme. *Prenat Diagn* 1996;16:1039–1042.

278. Baumgarten A, Robinson J. Prospective study of an inverse relationship between maternal glycosylated hemoglobin and serum alpha-fetoprotein concentrations in pregnant women with diabetes. *Am J Obstet Gynecol* 1988;159:77–81.

279. Martin AO, Dempsey LM, Minogue J, Liu K, Keller J, et al. Maternal serum alpha-fetoprotein levels in pregnancies complicated by diabetes: implications for screening programs. *Am J Obstet Gynecol* 1990;63:1209–1216.

279a. Palomaki GE, Knight GJ, Haddow JE. Human chorionic gonadotropin and unconjugated oestriol measurements in insulin dependent diabetic pregnant women being screened for fetal Down syndrome. *Prenat Diagn* 1994;14:65–68.

279b. Wald NJ, Densem JW, Cheng R, Collishaw S. Maternal serum free alpha- and free beta-human chorionic gonadotrophin in pregnancies with insulin-dependent diabetes mellitus: implications for screening for Down syndrome. *Prenat Diagn* 1994;14:835–837.

280. Wallace EM, Crossley JA, Ritoe SC, Groome NP, Aitken DA. Maternal serum inhibin-A in pregnancies complicated by insulin dependent diabetes mellitus. *Br J Obstet Gynaecol* 1997;104:946–948.

281. Wald NJ, Watt HC, George L. Maternal serum inhibin-A in pregnancies with insulin-dependent diabetes mellitus: implications for screening for Down's syndrome. *Prenat Diagn* 1996;16:923–926.

282. Pedersen JF, Sorensen S, Molsted-Pedersen L. Pregnancy-associated plasma protein A in first trimester of diabetic pregnancy and subsequent fetal growth. *Acta Obstet Gynecol Scand* 1998;77:932–934.

283. Ong CYT, Liao AWJ, Spencer K, Nicolaides KH. First trimester maternal serum free-hCG and PAPP-A as predictors of pregnancy complications. *Br J Obstet Gynaecol* 2000;107:1265–1270.

283a. Cuckle H, van Oudgaarden ED, Mason G, Holding S. Taking account of vaginal bleeding in screening for Down's syndrome. *Br J Obstet Gynaecol* 1994;101:948–953.

284. Morssink LP, Kornman LH, Hallahan TW, Kloosterman MD, Beekhuis JR, et al. Maternal serum levels of free β-hCG and PAPP-A in the first trimester of pregnancy are not associated with subsequent fetal growth retardation or preterm delivery. *Prenat Diagn* 1998;18:147–152.

284a. Cuckle HS, Sehmi IK, Jones RG, Mason G. Low maternal serum PAPP-A and fetal viability. *Prenat Diagn* 1999;19:787–790.

284b. Cuckle H, Sehmi I, Jones R. Maternal serum inhibin A can predict pre-eclampsia. *Br J Obstet Gynaecol* 1998;105:1101–1103.

285. Aquilina J, Barnett A, Thompson O, Harrington K. Second-trimester maternal serum inhibin A concentration as

an early marker for preeclampsia. *Am J Obstet Gynecol* 1999; 181:131–136.

286. Muttukrishna S, North RA, Morris J, Schellenberg J-C, Taylor RS, et al. Serum inhibin A and activin A are elevated prior to the onset of pre-eclampsia. *Hum Reprod* 2000;15:1640–1645.

287. Sebire NJ, Roberts L, Noble P, Wallace E, Nicolaides KH. Raised maternal serum inhibin-A concentration at 10 to 14 weeks gestation is associated with pre-eclampsia. *Br J Obstet Gynaecol* 200;107:795–797.

288. Ong CYT, Liao AW, Munim S, Spencer K, Nicolaides KH. First trimester maternal serum activin A and inhibin A in pre-eclampsia and fetal growth restriction. *Br J Obstet Gynaecol* 2002;109:(in press).

289. Macri JN, Spencer K, Anderson R, Cook EJ. Free beta chorionic gonadotropin: a cross reactivity study of two immunometric assays used in prenatal maternal serum screening for Down syndrome. *Ann Clin Biochem* 1993;30:94–98.

290. Spencer K, Macri JN, Carpenter P, Anderson R, Krantz DA. Stability of intact hCG in serum, liquid whole blood and dried whole blood filter paper spots and its impact on free beta hCG Down's syndrome screening. *Clin Chem* 1993;39:1064–1068.

291. Stevenson HP, Leslie H, Sheridan B. Serum free β human chorionic gonadotropin concentrations increase in unseparated blood specimens. *Ann Clin Biochem* 1993;30:99–100.

292. Sancken U, Bahner D. The effects of thermal instability on intact human chorionic gonadotropin (ihCG) on the application of its free β subunit (free β-hCG) as a serum marker in Down syndrome screening. *Prenat Diagn* 1995; 15:731–738.

293. Cuckle HS, Jones RG. Maternal serum free beta human chorionic gonadotrophin level: the effect of sample transportation. *Ann Clin Biochem* 1994;31:97–98.

294. Muller F, Doche C, Ngo S, Faiini S, Charvin M-A, et al. Stability of free β-subunit in routine practice for trisomy 21 maternal serum screening. *Prenat Diagn* 1999;19:85–86.

295. Verloes A, Schoos R, Herens C, Vintens A, Koulischer L. A prenatal trisomy 21 screening program using alpha-fetoprotein, human chorionic gonadotropin, and free estriol assays on maternal dried blood. *Am J Obstet Gynecol* 1995;172:167–174.

296. Macri JN, Anderson RW, Krantz DA, Larsen JW, Buchanan PD. Prenatal maternal dried blood screening with alpha-fetoprotein and free β-human chorionic gonadotropin for open neural tube defect and Down syndrome. *Am J Obstet Gynecol* 1996;174:566–572.

297. Krantz DA, Hallahan TW, Orlandi F, Buchanan P, Larsen JW, Macri JN. First-trimester Down syndrome screening using dried blood biochemistry and nuchal translucency. *Obstet Gynecol* 2000;96:207–213.

298. Christiannsen M, Norgaard-Pedersen B. Maternal serum screening for Down syndrome in first trimester using Schwangerschaftsprotein 1, PAPP-A/proMBP-complex and the proform of eosinophil major basic protein as markers. In: Grudzinskas JG, Ward RHT, eds. *Screening for Down syndrome in the first trimester.* London: RCOG Press, 1997:148–182.

299. Qin QP, Nguyen TK, Christiansen M, Larsen SO, Norgaard-Pedersen B. Time resolved immunofluorometric assay of pregnancy-associated plasma protein-A in maternal serum screening for Down's syndrome in first trimester of pregnancy. *Clin Chim Acta* 1996;253:113–129.

300. Bersinger NA, Meisser A, Bessou T, Seguin P, Birkhauser MH, et al. Production and characterisation of monoclonal antibodies against pregnancy associated plasma protein-A. *Mol Hum Reprod* 1999;5:675–681.

301. Qin QP, Christiansen M, Oxvig C, Pettersson K, Sottrup-Jensen L, et al. Double-monoclonal immunofluorometric assays for pregnancy-associated plasma protein A/proeosinophil major basic protein (PAPP-A/proMBP) complex for first-trimester maternal serum screening for Down syndrome. *Clin Chem* 1997;43:2323–2332.

302. Macintosh MC, Wald NJ, Chard T, Hansen J, Mikkelsen M, et al. Selective miscarriage of Down's syndrome fetuses in women aged 35 years and older. *Br J Obstet Gynaecol* 1995;102:798–801.

303. Macintosh MC, Wald NJ, Chard T, Hansen J, Mikkelsen M, et al. The selective miscarriage of Down's syndrome from 10 weeks of pregnancy. *Br J Obstet Gynaecol* 1996;103: 1172–1173.

304. Goodburn SF, Yates JR, Raggatt PR, Carr C, Ferguson-Smith ME, et al. Second-trimester maternal serum screening using alpha-fetoprotein, human chorionic gonadotrophin, and unconjugated oestriol: experience of a regional programme. *Prenat Diagn* 1994;14:391–402.

305. Hsu JJ, Hseih TT, Liou JD, Hsieh FJ, Spencer K. AFP and free β hCG in prospective screening for Down syndrome in Taiwanese pregnant women under 34 years of age. *Am J Hum Genet* 1995;57:A2003.

306. Hook EB, Mutton DE, Ide R, Alberman E, Bobrow M. The natural history of Down syndrome conceptuses diagnosed prenatally that are not electively terminated. *Am J Hum Genet* 1995;57:875–881.

307. Haddow JE, Palomaki GE, Knight GJ. Prenatal screening for Down's syndrome with use of maternal serum markers. *N Engl J Med* 1992;327:588–593.

308. Phillips OP, Elias S, Schulman LP, Andersen RN, Morgan CD, Simpson JL. Maternal serum screening for fetal Down syndrome in women less than 35 years of age using alpha fetoprotein, hCG and unconjugated oestriol: a prospective 2 year study. *Obstet Gynecol* 1992;80:353–358.

309. Wald NJ, Kennard A, Densem JW, Cuckle HS, Chard T, Butler L. Antenatal maternal serum screening for Down's syndrome: results of a demonstration project. *BMJ* 1992; 305:391–394.

310. Cheng EY, Luthy DA, Zebelman AM, Williams MA, Lieppman RE, Hickok DE. A prospective evaluation of second trimester screening test for Down syndrome using alpha-fetoprotein, hCG and unconjugated estriol. *Obstet Gynecol* 1993;81:72–77.

311. Burton BK, Prins GS, Verp MS. A prospective trial of prenatal screening for Down syndrome by means of maternal serum alpha-fetoprotein, human chorionic gonadotropin and unconjugated estriol. *Am J Obstet Gynecol* 1993;169: 526–530.

312. Pescia G, Dao MH, Wekhs. Le triple depistage del la trisomie 21: resultants prospectifs de 7039 evaluations. *Rev Med Suisse Romande* 1993;113:277–280.

313. Piggott M, Wilkinson P, Bennett J. Implementation of an

antenatal screening programme for Down's syndrome in two districts (Brighton and Eastbourne). *J Med Screen* 1994;1:45–49.

314. Mancini G, Perona A, Dall'Amico D. Maternal serum markers. Estimation of the risk of Down's syndrome: a prospective study. *Int J Clin Lab Res* 1994;14:49–53.

315. Kellner LH, Weiss RR, Weiner Z. The advantages of using triple-marker screening for chromosomal abnormalities. *Am J Obstet Gynecol* 1995;172:831–836.

316. Dawson AJ, Jones G, Mathura MS, et al. Serum screening for Down's syndrome. *Br J Obstet Gynaecol* 1993;100:875–877.

317. Burn J. Maternal serum screening for Down's syndrome: audit of process and outcome in the northern region of England. *Report of the RCOG working party on biochemical markers and detection of Down's syndrome.* London: RCOG Press, 1993.

318. Beekhuis JR. *Maternal serum screening for fetal Down's syndrome and neural tube defects. A prospective study performed in the north of the Netherlands.* The Netherlands: Gronigen University, 1993 (PhD thesis).

319. Crossley JA, Aitken DA, Berry E, Connor JM. Impact of a regional screening programme using maternal serum alpha fetoprotein (AFP) and human chorionic gonadotrophin (hCG) on the birth incidence of Down's syndrome in the west of Scotland. *J Med Screen* 1994;1:180–183.

320. Mooney RA, Peterson J, Franch CA, Saller DN, Arvan DA. Effectiveness of combining maternal serum alpha fetoprotein and hCG in a second trimester screening program for Down syndrome. *Obstet Gynecol* 1994;84:298–303.

321. Spencer K, Macri JN, Coombes EJ, Ward AM. Antenatal screening for Down's syndrome. *BMJ* 1993;30:219–220.

322. Macri JN, Spencer K, Garver K, Buchanan PD, Say B, et al. Maternal serum free beta Down syndrome screening: results of twelve studies including 480 cases of Down syndrome. *Prenat Diagn* 1994;14:97–103.

323. Halliday JL, Watson LF, Lumley J, Danks DM, Sheffield LJ. New estimates of Down syndrome risks at chorionic villus sampling, amniocentesis, and livebirth in women of advanced maternal age from a uniquely defined population. *Prenat Diagn* 1995;15:455–465.

PRENATAL DIAGNOSTIC TECHNIQUES

The objective of prenatal diagnosis is to provide physical, genetic, biochemical, and physiologic information about the fetus. This permits reassurance of normalcy in the vast majority of pregnancies, at the same time detecting important fetal anomalies and assessing the severity of anomalies in affected fetuses. To this end, a number of tools are now available for prenatal diagnosis (Table 1). Common noninvasive procedures using ultrasound and magnetic resonance imaging are described extensively throughout this textbook. This chapter focuses on methods for prenatal diagnosis using genetic and biochemical testing of fetal tissue. Maternal serum biochemical screening is reported separately (see Chapter 22).

Impressive advances in the understanding of genetic conditions and laboratory technical capabilities have occurred over the past century (Table 2), culminating in the virtually complete sequencing of the human genome.[1,2] The contributions and discoveries leading up to this event are beyond the scope of this chapter. It is worthwhile, however, to first review some basic principles of molecular genetics. Following this, the basic genetic tests used for prenatal diagnosis and the procedures for obtaining fetal genetic material for analysis are described.

FUNDAMENTAL PRINCIPLES OF MOLECULAR GENETICS

The nuclei of most human cells contain two sets of chromosomes, one set given by each parent. There are a total of 46 chromosomes consisting of 23 pairs; 22 are called *autosomes* and 1 pair are the *sex chromosomes* (X and Y). Chromosomes consist of tightly coiled threads of DNA and associated protein molecules (Fig. 1).

Each DNA molecule consists of two strands that are held together by weak bonds between the bases on each strand, forming base pairs. Only four base pairs comprise the entire genome, although their sequence determines the order of amino acids that make up complex proteins. The human genome contains roughly three billion base pairs; each strand of DNA contains an average of 150 million bases, making it among the largest molecules known.

A gene is a segment of a DNA molecule ranging from fewer than one thousand base pairs to several million base pairs. Each gene contains the information necessary for protein synthesis. There appear to be approximately 30,000 to 40,000 protein-coding genes in the human genome—or approximately twice as many as in the worm or fly. However, the genes are complex, with more alternative splicing generating a larger number of protein products. Only approximately 10% of DNA is known to include protein-coding sequences (exons). Interspersed between the exons are intron sequences, which have no coding function. The balance of the genome is thought to consist of other noncoding regions such as control sequences and intergenic regions, whose functions are obscure.

Proteins are large, complex molecules made up of long chains of subunits called *amino acids*. Twenty different kinds of amino acids are usually found in proteins. Each amino acid is specified by a sequence of three DNA bases, or a codon. For example, the base sequence ATG codes for the amino acid methionine. The genetic code is thus a series of codons that specify which amino acids are required to make up specific proteins. The protein-coding instructions from the genes are transmitted indirectly through messenger RNA (mRNA), a transient intermediary molecule similar to a single strand of DNA. For the information within a gene to be expressed, a complementary RNA strand is produced (transcription) from the DNA template in the nucleus. This mRNA is moved from the nucleus to the cellular cytoplasm, where it serves as the template for protein synthesis.

The DNA replicates itself through processes of meiosis (gamete formation) and mitosis (cell division) (Fig. 2). Although this process is highly efficient, it can produce errors. Many of these errors are corrected. Errors that are not corrected, however, can lead to abnormalities in embryonic and fetal development.

GENETIC DISORDERS

A genetic disorder indicates that genetic material, on a chromosomal or a gene level, contains one or more muta-

TABLE 1. TYPES AND TIMING OF COMMON PROCEDURES DURING PREGNANCY

Chorionic villus sampling	10–13 wk
Early amniocentesis[a]	10–14 wk
Standard amniocentesis	15 wk–term
	Optimum, 15–20 wk
Maternal biochemical screen	
Second-trimester screen	15–21 wk
First-trimester screen	10–14 wk
Nuchal translucency scan	11–14 wk
Fetal ultrasound for detection of anomalies	9 wk–term
	Optimum, 18–22 wk
Fetal magnetic resonance imaging	12 wk–term
Fetal echocardiography	14 wk–term
	Optimum, 18–22 wk
Percutaneous umbilical blood sampling	18 wk–term

[a]No longer recommended.

tions, which results in clinical abnormalities. *Genetic* does not necessarily mean hereditary, because many genetic abnormalities are not transmitted to a subsequent generation. Genetic conditions are common—as many as 1 in 20 live-born infants is expected to have a condition with an important genetic component by age 25 years.[3,4]

Genetic disorders are generally of four types:

1. Chromosomal disorders. These affect up to 1 in 200 live-born children.[5] They may be subcategorized as

TABLE 2. LANDMARKS IN GENETICS WITH RESPECT TO PRENATAL DIAGNOSIS

1860–1865	Genetic inheritance shown in biologic species (Mendel)
1944	DNA found to transmit genetic information (Avery et al.)[107]
1953	Double helix of DNA (Watson, Crick)
1956	Forty-six human chromosomes discovered (Tijo and Levan)[101] (Ford and Hamerton)[102]
1959	Trisomy 21 discovered as the basis for Down syndrome (Lejeune et al.)[103]
1960–1966	Deciphering genetic code for amino acid bases (Nirenberg)[108]
1966	Amniocentesis performed for fetal karyotyping (Steele and Breg)[104]
1967	Amniocentesis performed for fetal karyotyping of Down syndrome
1975	Method devised to pinpoint a genetic sequence (Southern)[109]
1976	High-resolution banding technique (Yunis)[105]
1978	Discovery of restriction-fragment-length polymorphisms as genetic markers for linkage analysis (Kan and Dozy)[110]
1985–1990	Polymerase chain reaction allows rapidly amplifying DNA sequence (Mullis et al.)[111]
1986	Feasibility of fluorescence *in situ* hybridization (Cremer et al.)[106]
2001	Complete sequencing of human genome (Venter)[1] (International Human Genome Sequencing Consortium)[2]

abnormalities of chromosome number (aneuploidy) and abnormalities of chromosome structure, such as translocations, in which two chromosomes exchange segments. Chromosome disorders are discussed further later (see Cytogenetic Testing).

2. Single gene (*mendelian*) disorders. These are abnormalities that are the result of mutations in single genes, at a specific gene locus. As many as 1 in 300 individuals will experience a monogenic disease within the first two decades of life,[3] but this figure may be as high as 1% if the lifetime probability of manifesting a monogenic disorder is considered. Four patterns of inheritance are observed in single gene disorders caused by nuclear genes: autosomal dominant (one mutated gene of the pair is sufficient to produce symptoms); autosomal recessive (the two alleles in the paired genes must be abnormal to cause the phenotype); and X-linked, which includes recessive (only affecting males); and, less frequently, X-linked dominant gene mutations (females are affected and the condition is usually lethal in males). Only a few genes, particularly those involved in sex determination and fertility, have been localized to the Y chromosome. The transmission of Y-linked traits can only occur from a father to his son.

3. Polygenic or *multifactorial* disorders. These are abnormalities in which strictly chromosomal or monogenic patterns of inheritance are not identified. Polygenic implies that the association of several different genes, each one slightly modified, is necessary to produce the disorder. Multifactorial inheritance implies that genetic and nongenetic (environmental, either pre- or postnatal) factors are associated to produce the pathology.

4. Mitochondrial disorders. Disorders resulting from mutations in the mitochondrial genome have been identified. Each cell contains hundreds or thousands of mitochondria, each containing one or several circular chromosomes. These chromosomes have deletions or contain other types of mutations that interfere with cellular production of adenosine triphosphate. Thus, the energy vital for the cell/organ/organism is decreased. The symptoms depend on the tissues involved and on the proportion of mitochondria mutated, but affect first the central nervous system and muscle, because of their large energy demands.[6,7] The incidence of mitochondrial mutations in human disease is still unknown. In many cases the mutation is *de novo* in an affected individual, but hereditary transmission is purely maternal, because an embryo's mitochondria originate from the maternal germ cell only.

GENETIC TESTING

Genetic abnormalities can be identified by one of three methods:

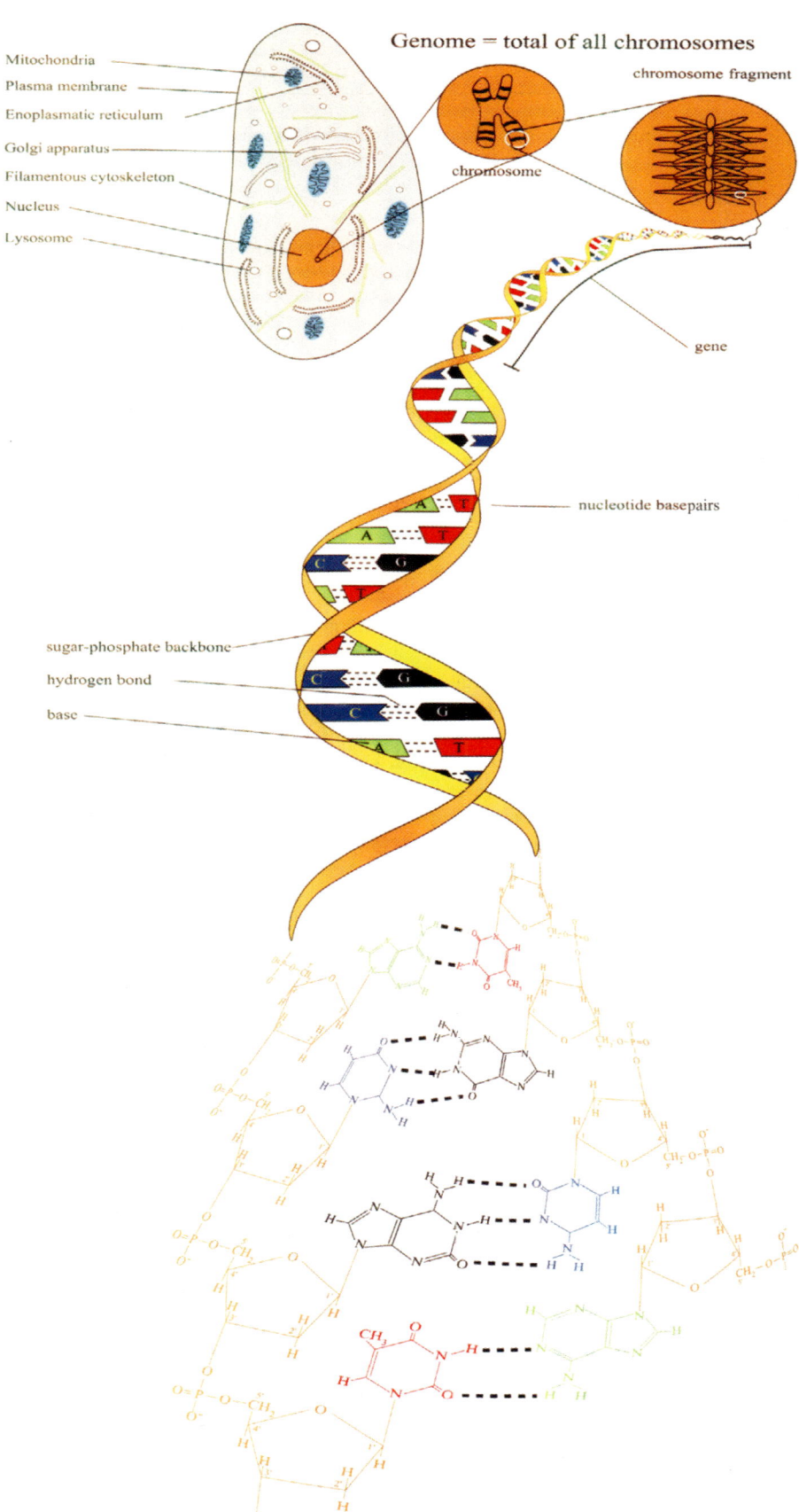

Genome = total of all chromosomes

Mitochondria
Plasma membrane
Enoplasmatic reticulum
Golgi apparatus
Filamentous cytoskeleton
Nucleus
Lysosome

chromosome fragment

chromosome

gene

nucleotide basepairs

sugar-phosphate backbone

hydrogen bond

base

FIGURE 1. Chromosomes consist of tightly coiled threads of DNA and associated protein molecules. (Courtesy of Andy Vierstraete, University of Gent, Department of Biology, http://allserv. rug.ac.be/~avierstr/index.html.)

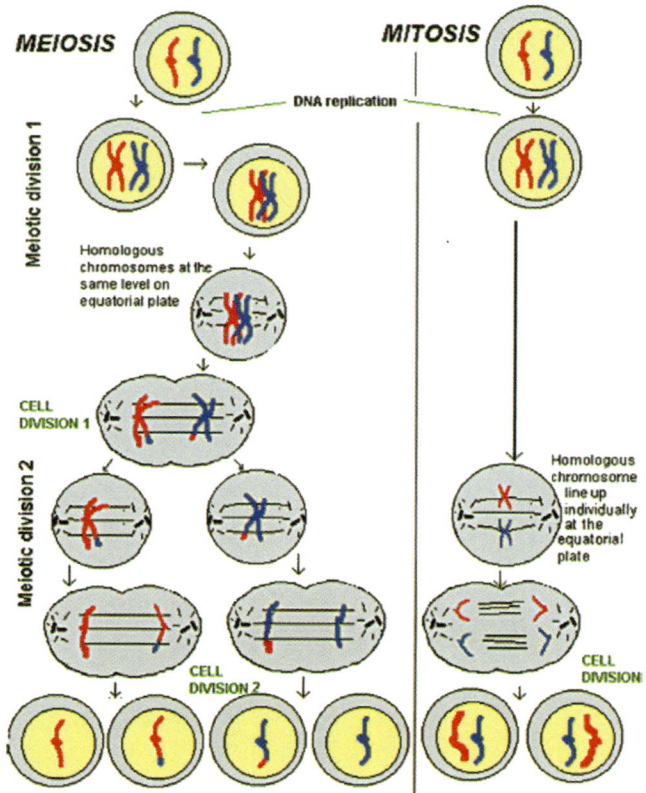

FIGURE 2. The DNA replicates itself through processes of meiosis (gamete formation) and mitosis (cell division).

1. Biochemical tests evaluate protein or other abnormal end products resulting from genetic mutations. Each of these tests is described in greater detail in the Biochemical Testing section.
2. DNA testing evaluates specific genes that are too small to visualize with standard cytogenetic testing.
3. Cytogenetic studies analyze the number of chromosomes present or rearrangements in the chromosome structure.

Biochemical Testing

Biochemical testing involves direct analysis of samples for levels of proteins or other metabolites that are abnormal in some genetic conditions. Cells from chorionic villus sampling (CVS) or cultured amniotic fluid cells may be used in the analysis, particularly of enzyme levels. Amniotic fluid may also be used for the diagnosis of certain conditions (Table 3). These tests often require prior diagnosis of the condition in the family, although testing of phenylketonuria in the newborn is an exception.

DNA Testing

DNA testing involves direct examination of the DNA molecule. The first prenatal diagnosis of a monogenic disorder was

TABLE 3. EXAMPLES OF CONDITIONS THAT CAN BE DIAGNOSED BY BIOCHEMICAL ANALYSIS OF FETAL MATERIAL

Osteogenesis imperfecta (biochemical analysis of collagen and procollagen molecules in chorionic villus samples)
Smith-Lemli-Opitz syndrome (measurement of cholesterol precursors in amniotic fluid)
Tyrosinemia type I (measurement of succinyl acetone in amniotic fluid)
Methylmalonic acidemia (cultured amniocytes for measurement of methylmalonyl-CoA mutase enzyme activity)
Propionic acidemia (cultured amniocytes for measurement of propionyl-CoA carboxylase activity)
Peroxisomal disorders (e.g., Zellweger syndrome, rhizomelic chondrodysplasia punctata) (Immunoblot analysis of peroxisomal acyl-CoA oxidase and peroxisomal thiolase in chorionic villus samples)

CoA, coenzyme A.
Note: Many biochemical disorders are now diagnosed prenatally by deoxyribonucleic acid analysis. The first step in prenatal diagnosis of biochemical disorders is to try to identify the underlying deoxyribonucleic acid mutations in the affected child or the parents.

reported for sickle cell anemia in 1978.[8] Newer techniques, including the development of the polymerase chain reaction (PCR), now permit testing for many monogenic diseases, and more are being added to the list each month. It is no longer meaningful or possible to produce an exhaustive catalogue of diseases for which DNA testing is available. The most common conditions for which DNA testing is used in the prenatal setting are shown in Table 4. Cystic fibrosis is the most common serious genetic disease of childhood in populations of white European origin. Fragile X syndrome is one of the most common causes of mental retardation in males.

Testing of monogenic diseases may be expensive, depending on the techniques involved, and may require a specialized laboratory. Not all laboratories perform all tests. Laboratories testing specific conditions are now published

TABLE 4. THE MOST COMMON DNA TESTS USED IN THE PRENATAL SETTING

Cystic fibrosis
Rhesus D genotyping
Alpha- and beta-thalassemia
Sickle cell anemia
Prader-Willi syndrome and Angelman syndrome (deoxyribonucleic acid methylation test to detect uniparental disomy)
Fragile X-linked mental retardation
Duchenne and Becker muscular dystrophies
Hemophilia A and B
Achondroplasia (fibroblast growth factor receptor 3)
Viral studies (cytomegalovirus)

Note: Up-to-the-minute availability of DNA testing for a specific disorder can be determined by accessing the following World Wide Web sites: Online Mendelian Inheritance in Man (OMIM), http://www3.ncbi.nlm.nih.gov/omim/searchomim.html; GeneTests, http://www.genetests.org/servlet/access.

on Internet-based databases (Table 4) so that samples can be sent anywhere in the world.

For many monogenic diseases, testing is often reserved for families that are known to be at risk. This usually requires prior diagnosis of an affected individual or identification of a carrier couple (for recessively inherited disorders), with molecular investigation performed ideally before pregnancy to define the precise mutation. In some cases, definitive testing may not be possible and linkage analysis may be required, such as in a family affected by Duchenne muscular dystrophy in which no mutation has been defined.

Testing for monogenic conditions may be categorized as direct or indirect. Direct analysis of the mutation responsible for a disease permits a rapid diagnosis, with 100% accuracy, and generally at reasonable cost. Short pieces of DNA or probes are used to identify mutated sequences. In diseases with a mutation common to all affected individuals, such as sickle cell anemia or achondroplasia, the test can be performed without any preliminary family studies. In those diseases with multiple mutations in the causative gene, such as cystic fibrosis, it is necessary to study an affected index patient (or carrier) to identify the particular mutation(s) relevant to the family seeking prenatal diagnosis.

Indirect analysis is performed when direct analysis is not possible, either because the disease gene is not completely characterized or because the exact mutation in a family cannot be identified. In this situation, a linked marker is used, when available. A linked marker is a sequence of DNA that is physically located near the gene of interest and shows individual variation in the DNA sequence, which permits the laboratory to track the inheritance of the chromosome carrying the mutated gene. Indirect analysis carries a small risk of error if the marker is not localized very close to the region of interest. This risk is proportional to the distance between the polymorphic marker and the abnormal gene, and so it is important to use the most closely linked markers available. This risk of error can be nearly eliminated by using more than one marker localized to each side of the gene.

DNA testing can be performed on any nucleated cells from the embryo or fetus. Preimplantation genetic diagnosis, in which single cells from a number of embryos are tested and only nonaffected embryos implanted, has already been successfully used to avoid the birth of an affected infant with cystic fibrosis or chromosome abnormalities.

Cytogenetic Testing

Prenatal indications for cytogenetic evaluation are much more common than testing for biochemical abnormalities or monogenic conditions. These include individuals with

- Increased risk of fetal aneuploidy because of advanced maternal age, abnormal serum biochemistry testing, or ultrasound abnormalities.

- Familial chromosomal aberrations, including autosomal translocations or parental sex chromosome abnormalities.
- Previous history of a fetus or child with a chromosome abnormality.

Cytogenetic disorders can be either numeric, in which there is an abnormal number of chromosomes (aneuploidy), or structural, in which there is an abnormality in the structure of a particular chromosome.

Numeric Abnormalities

Numeric aberrations involve the loss or gain of a part of or an entire chromosome. The most common fetal autosomal numeric chromosome aberration in the live-born infant is trisomy 21 (Down syndrome) (Fig. 3). The risk of Down syndrome, as well as the rarer disorders trisomy 18 and trisomy 13, increases with increasing maternal age. Abnormalities of the sex chromosomes are on the order of 1 in 750 livebirths. The incidence of 47,XXY (Klinefelter syndrome) and 47,XXX (triple X syndrome) also increases with increasing maternal age. Turner syndrome (45,X) occurs in 1 in 2,500 livebirths and is associated with sonographic abnormalities. There is no relationship between Turner syndrome and maternal age.

Structural Abnormalities

Structural aberrations affect a portion of one or several chromosomes; these can be of several types and imply in general that a break has taken place and given rise to one of the following rearrangements (Fig. 4).

Translocations, the most frequent type of rearrangement between two chromosomes or two arms of the same chromosome, involve an exchange of genetic material. Depending on whether the quantity of chromatin is modified, they are either balanced or unbalanced. Insertions refer to the addition of chromosomal material in an unusual location. Inversions refer to a portion of a chromosome being rearranged upside down. Ring chromosomes occur with annealing of the two extremities of a chromosome after loss of their terminal segments. Isochromosomes refer to one arm of a chromosome being present in two copies, separated from each other by a centromere.

Marker chromosomes are structurally altered chromosomes that cannot be identified by international standards of chromosome nomenclature. They occur in approximately 1 per 4,000 newborns but are 10 times more common in patients with mental retardation. Because the phenotype can range from normal to physical and mental abnormalities, marker chromosomes present an enormous challenge when detected prenatally.

For balanced translocations, a normal quantity of chromosomal material is preserved, but in a disorganized fashion, either because of an exchange between two chromosomes (translocation), with no net loss or gain of

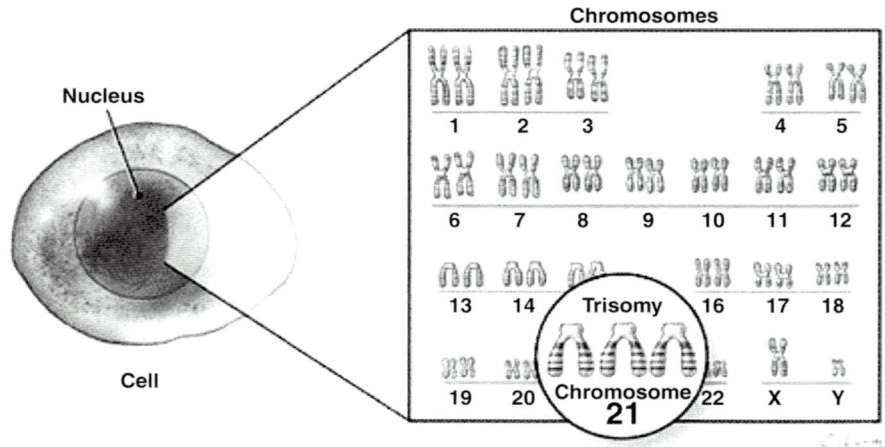

FIGURE 3. Representation of trisomy 21, the most common autosomal abnormality in the number of chromosomes among liveborn infants.

genetic material, or due to a centromeric fusion. Whatever the structural defect, there is rarely a major clinical abnormality, but reproductive problems may arise. In women with balanced translocations, spontaneous abortion is most often seen, whereas in men, spermatogenesis may be impaired, resulting in primary sterility.

TECHNIQUES OF GENETIC TESTING

Cell Culture

Traditional karyotyping assesses chromosome copy number and the presence of any obvious structural abnormalities. Cell culture is performed to provide sufficient material for accurate cytogenetic analysis.

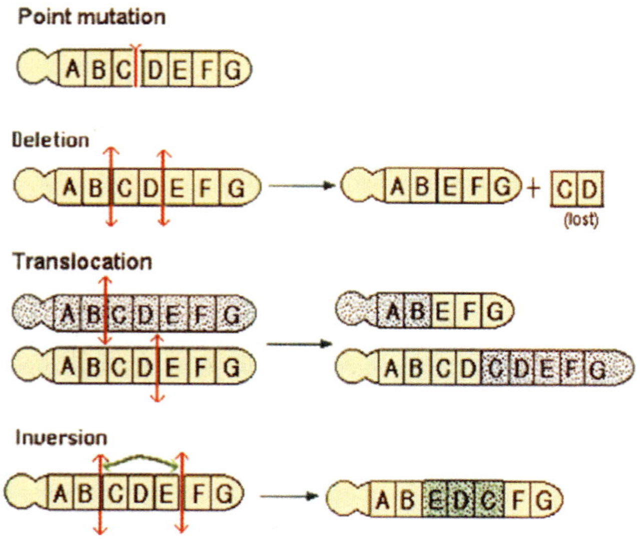

Technique

Cells are cultured and then harvested at the metaphase stage, at which time chromosomes are condensed and display their banded appearance (Fig. 5). Highly trained analysts use high-magnification light microscopy to look for abnormalities of chromosome number and structure. With the introduction of banding in 1971, chromosome identification was markedly improved.[9] The most widely used chromosome banding technique, Giemsa-trypsin banding, produces up to 400 to 500 metaphase bands in a haploid set of human chromosomes.

Cell culture includes quality control measures, such as double-checking names and medical record numbers; splitting each amniotic fluid sample for set-up by two technolo-

Point mutation

Deletion

Translocation

Inversion

FIGURE 4. Representation of genetic mutations, including point mutation, deletion, and translocation.

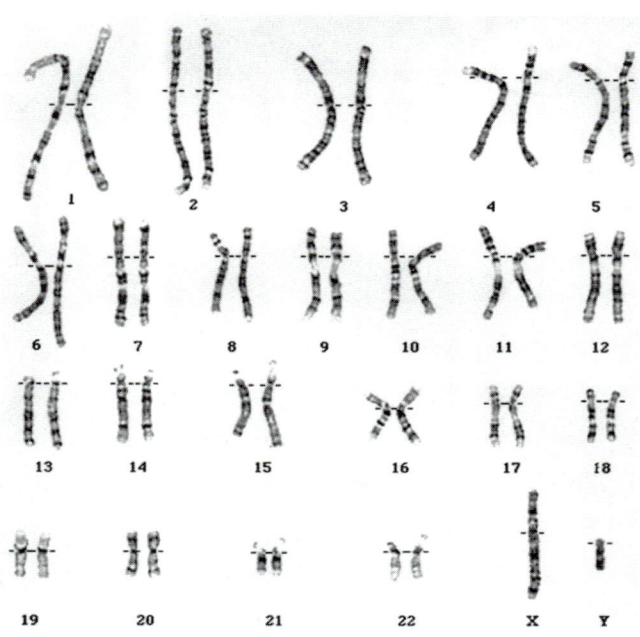

FIGURE 5. Normal male karyotype. Standard cytogenetic preparation shows characteristic banding for each of the 22 paired chromosomes plus the X and Y chromosomes.

gists; and use of at least two different lots of culture flasks, media, and incubators for each specimen.[10]

Advantages

Traditional cytogenetic analysis, when performed on cultured, dividing amniotic fluid cells, is highly accurate and thorough in its detection of all numeric and structural chromosome abnormalities.

In general a culture failure rate of less than 1%, and closer to 0.5%, should be expected from cytogenetics laboratories today.[10] Culture failure may occur because of microbial contamination, poor quality plastic ware and media storage, or incubator failure. Culture failure does not necessarily imply that a result cannot be obtained, as fluorescence *in situ* hybridization (FISH) studies can be used on uncultured cells during interphase to provide numeric information on chromosomes 13, 18, 21, X, and Y.[11] When amniotic fluid culture failure does occur, a chromosomal abnormality is more likely to be present.[12]

Disadvantages

The technique is labor-intensive and requires trained laboratory personnel. However, the major disadvantage, from the patient's perspective, is that the analysis takes 7 to 10 days. The wait for results can be anxiety provoking, especially in the setting of a fetal abnormality detected on ultrasound examination.

Direct Preparation

Direct preparation of genetic material, without culturing, is possible after CVS because the cytotrophoblastic tissue has an extremely high mitotic rate. This permits a provisional interpretation to be provided in as little as 24 to 48 hours. This method also minimizes the risk of maternal cell contamination (MCC), but suffers from poor quality Giemsa banding so that chromosomal resolution is decreased and may result in some structural chromosomal abnormalities being missed. A more common problem is false-positive results from placental mosaicism. Because of these possibilities, it is essential that standard tissue culture always accompany direct analysis. Tissue culture should provide final results in 5 to 7 days, and is less likely to miss a small structural chromosomal abnormality. Tissue culture is, however, more subject to the effects of MCC.

Fluorescence *In Situ* Hybridization

FISH has the power to combine molecular with cytogenetic analysis. In the prenatal setting, it is most commonly used to rapidly (within 24 to 48 hours) diagnose the common aneuploidies. Since the early 1990s, FISH detection of fetal aneuploidy has gone from investigational to an established role in the prenatal diagnosis of fetuses at high risk for abnormality.

By means of recombinant DNA technology, it is possible to generate fluorescently labeled DNA probes that hybridize specifically to known genetic loci and chromosome regions. The ability to visualize single gene loci as well as specific whole chromosomes has revolutionized the clinical and research applications of cytogenetics in furthering the knowledge and understanding of human diseases.

Technique

The technique for FISH relies on the unique ability of a portion of single-stranded DNA, known as a *probe*, to hybridize (bond) with its complementary target DNA sequence. The signal is directly visualized by fluorescent microscopy, and the presence or absence of specific DNA sequence is determined by observing whether a signal is present. For the X, Y, and 18 chromosomes, tandem repeat sequences in the centromeric region are detected. Specific probes can be used to anneal to a single gene loci on chromosomes 13 and 21 (Fig. 6). Using commercially available probes and proper temperatures, the entire FISH process can be completed within 6 to 8 hours and as many as 5 to 7 probes may be used simultaneously, each labeled with a differently colored fluorochrome.

There are three categories of chromosome-specific probes: repetitive probes, painting probes, and locus-specific probes. Repetitive sequences in the centromeres are the same in some chromosomes but differ in others. It is now possible to identify repetitive sequences for the X, Y, and 18 chromosomes. Repetitive probes are useful for rapid determination of the most common chromosomal aberrations. Locus-specific probes are capable of annealing to a single gene locus that ranges in size from less than 1,000 base pairs to as many as 1,000,000 base pairs. Locus-specific probes can be used to localize a gene to a chromosome region or to determine whether deletions and duplications

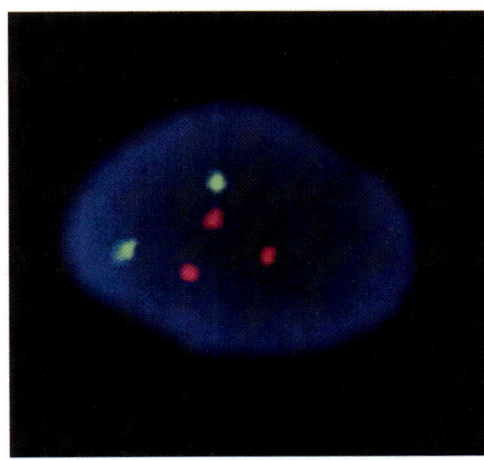

FIGURE 6. Fluorescence *in situ* hybridization of an interphase nucleus. Trisomy 21 is detected by three red dots, each corresponding to a copy of chromosome 21.

at the submicroscopic level are present. They are also useful in addressing problems associated with repetitive probes, for example, shared sequences between chromosomes 13 and 21, target variability, and difficulties in detecting trisomies in the case of Robertsonian translocations.

Interphase cytogenetic analysis is possible because each chromosome occupies a distinct physical space within the nondividing nucleus. This allows a discrete hybridization signal to be obtained for each chromosome.[13] If a highly specific chromosome probe is used, the FISH technique determines the number of copies of a given chromosome that are present within a given nucleus.

Clinical Applications

Rapid Fetal Karyotyping (Interphase Applications)
FISH can be applied to dividing cells (metaphase) and nondividing cells (interphase). Interphase FISH has been successfully applied in uncultured or short-term cultured amniocytes and chorionic villus cells for rapid karyotyping (Table 5). Cremer first demonstrated the general feasibility of detecting chromosome abnormalities in interphase nuclei in 1986[14] whereas Klinger and colleagues were the first to demonstrate the clinical use of FISH for prenatal diagnosis in 1992.[13]

Consistent data are emerging from multiple centers that, even with a test accuracy of 100%, routine use of FISH tests for fetal aneuploidy using probes for chromosomes X, Y, 13, 18, and 21 will miss 25% to 30% of all fetal chromosome abnormalities. Among women with advanced mater-

nal age, sensitivity approaches 80% because of the increased prevalence of aneuploidy due to maternal nondisjunction. Cases in which FISH is performed because of abnormal fetal sonogram or abnormal serum screening results have a lower sensitivity, on the order of 65% to 70%. It is important for physicians to realize there are unavoidable false-negative results with FISH because the test is designed only to look at abnormalities in the number of chromosomes X, Y, 13, 18, and 21.

In 2000, the American College of Medical Genetics and the American Society of Human Genetics revised an earlier policy statement[15] and stated that when a fetus has an abnormal result by FISH, the fetus should be characterized further using traditional chromosome analysis to determine the specific abnormality; but that it is "reasonable" to report interphase FISH results to the patient and physician. Clinical decision making should be based on two of the following three analyses: positive FISH results, confirmatory metaphase chromosome analysis, or consistent clinical information (American College of Medical Genetics and the American Society of Human Genetics, 2000). Interphase applications require reference ranges to report results.[14]

Detection of Chromosome Structural Rearrangements (Metaphase Applications)
FISH probes can be localized to specific chromosome sites, which can assist in detecting or confirming structural rearrangements (Table 5). This has been found to be highly useful and accurate for determining the origin of extra chromosome material (such as in marker chromosomes) and determining whether such a marker chromosome is also present in one of the parents. This technique is also useful in the detection of microdeletions, cryptic translocations, and chromosome mosaicism. Cryptic translocations frequently involve the subtelomeric regions of the chromosomes. It is estimated that 6% to 8% of unexplained mental retardation is caused by cryptic subtelomeric translocations.[17] This allows more accurate risk assessment and counseling.[18,19]

Studies of Fluorescence In Situ Hybridization

Ward et al.[20] reported on the results of the first clinical program that applied FISH to the rapid detection of chromosome aneuploidies in uncultured amniocytes. Region-specific DNA probes to chromosomes 13, 18, 21, X, and Y were used to analyze the number of signals in samples from 4,500 patients. These probes were used because aneuploidies of these chromosomes account for greater than 60% of all chromosome abnormalities detected at amniocentesis and up to 95% of the abnormalities that result in major birth defects.

FISH is highly accurate for detection of specific aneuploidies with targeted probes. Eiben et al.[21] compared FISH on uncultured amniocytes to standard karyotyping in 3,150 prenatal cases. For all of the aneuploidies diagnosable

---

TABLE 5.   CONDITIONS THAT CAN BE DIAGNOSED BY FLUORESCENCE *IN SITU* HYBRIDIZATION

Interphase analysis (count number of signals)
  Trisomy 13
  Trisomy 18
  Trisomy 21
  Klinefelter syndrome (47,XXY)
  Turner syndrome (45,X)
  Triple X (47,XXX)
  Triploidy
  Mosaicism (allows scoring of a larger number of samples)
Metaphase analysis (adjunct to traditional cytogenetics)
Microdeletions—may or may not be observed in karyotype

Cri du chat syndrome	5p15.2
DiGeorge syndrome	22q11.2
Miller-Dieker (lissencephaly) syndrome	17p13.3
Wolf-Hirschhorn syndrome	4p16.3
Williams syndrome	7q11.23
Smith-Magenis syndrome	17p11.2
Prader-Willi syndrome and Angelman syndrome	15q11.2

Marker chromosome identification

by FISH, the results showed 100% agreement with traditional cytogenetics. Feldman et al.[22] summarized the current *real life* clinical use of FISH in a study of 301 high-risk cases using clinical material from CVS, amniotic fluid cells, and umbilical cord blood samples. The only exclusion criterion was the presence of grossly bloody or brown amniotic fluid. Euploidy (a normal number of chromosomes) was diagnosed when at least 85% of the cells were euploid. Aneuploidy (an abnormal number of chromosomes) was diagnosed when at least 85% of the cells were aneuploid. In all 32 cases of aneuploidy, FISH analysis gave the correct results. An additional 10 cases of karyotypic abnormalities were detected that could not have been detected by the FISH probe set, giving an overall sensitivity of 76.2%, specificity of 100%, positive predictive value of 100%, and negative predictive value of 96.3%.

Potential Problems with Fluorescence In Situ *Hybridization*

Uninformative Results

A sample may be uninformative if it is bloody or contains insufficient cells for analysis. Ninety percent of samples were informative in the study of Ward et al. An uninformative result may be more likely in the third trimester compared to the second trimester.[11]

Maternal Cell Contamination

MCC sometimes results in discrepancy between FISH and traditional karyotype results, particularly in the setting of bloody amniotic fluid or oligohydramnios.[23] MCC was noted in as many as 2% of samples submitted for FISH analysis at one center.[24] MCC is more likely with placental penetration of the needle, a greater number of needle passes to obtain fluid, and operator inexperience. MCC is rarely seen in cultured amniotic fluid samples because the majority of contaminating cells are leukocytes, which require suspension cultures in which to grow.[24]

False-Negative Results

Because FISH targets specific chromosome regions, probe sets cannot evaluate all chromosome abnormalities. Rather, current probe sets target only the most common major chromosome abnormalities. This means that 25% to 30% of all fetal cytogenetic abnormalities remain undetected due to a chromosome deletion, inversion, addition, or translocation. The standard prenatal FISH assay is not designed to detect these structural rearrangements. Evans, et al.[25] performed a theoretical analysis of what percentage of abnormalities would be detectable if only interphase FISH using probes for chromosomes 13, 18, 21, X, and Y were used. They compiled a database of 146,128 consecutive metaphase karyotypes from eight centers in five countries over a 4-year period. Among 4,163 abnormalities, only 69% of them would have been detected by FISH using this probe

set, assuming 100% accuracy. Therefore, although a positive FISH result can be very useful, a normal FISH result should be confirmed by traditional metaphase chromosome analysis in cultured cells. Widespread consensus exists that the test is highly accurate but that it should serve as an adjunct to the metaphase karyotype.

Spectral Karyotyping

Spectral karyotyping *paints* each chromosome with complete genomic hybridization (Fig. 7). Each chromosome is represented by a single color, and rearranged chromosomes present two or more colors corresponding to different chromosome rearrangements. This technique is rapid and simple. Because it evaluates the entire genome, it detects larger abnormalities but is not as specific as targeted FISH analysis. A number of reports have shown that spectral karyotyping is useful in identifying chromosomal exchanges and to characterize marker and ring chromosomes. In many cases with supernumerary marker chromosomes, it is impractical to apply FISH probes specific for each individual chromosome to determine marker origin. Spectral karyotyping has been most commonly used in oncology for detection of complex chromosome rearrangements. It is still considered investigational for prenatal diagnostic applications.

Other Hybridization Techniques

New technologies to further analyze chromosomes include comparative genomic hybridization, multicolor FISH, microdissection/FISH, and telomere visualization probes.

Polymerase Chain Reaction

Described as being to genes what Gutenberg's printing press was to the written word, PCR can amplify a desired DNA sequence of any origin (virus, bacteria, plant, or human) hundreds of millions of times in a matter of hours, a task that would have required several days with recombinant technology. PCR is especially valuable because the reaction is highly specific, easily automated, and capable of amplifying minute amounts of sample.

PCR is a process based on a specialized polymerase enzyme, which can synthesize a complementary strand to a given DNA strand in a mixture containing the four DNA bases and two DNA fragments (primers, each approximately 20 bases long) flanking the target sequence (Fig. 8). The mixture is heated to separate the strands of double-stranded DNA containing the target sequence and then cooled to allow (a) the primers to find and bind to their complementary sequences on the separated strands and (b) the polymerase to extend the primers into new complementary strands. Repeated heating and cooling cycles multiply the target DNA exponentially, since each new double strand separates to become two templates for further syn-

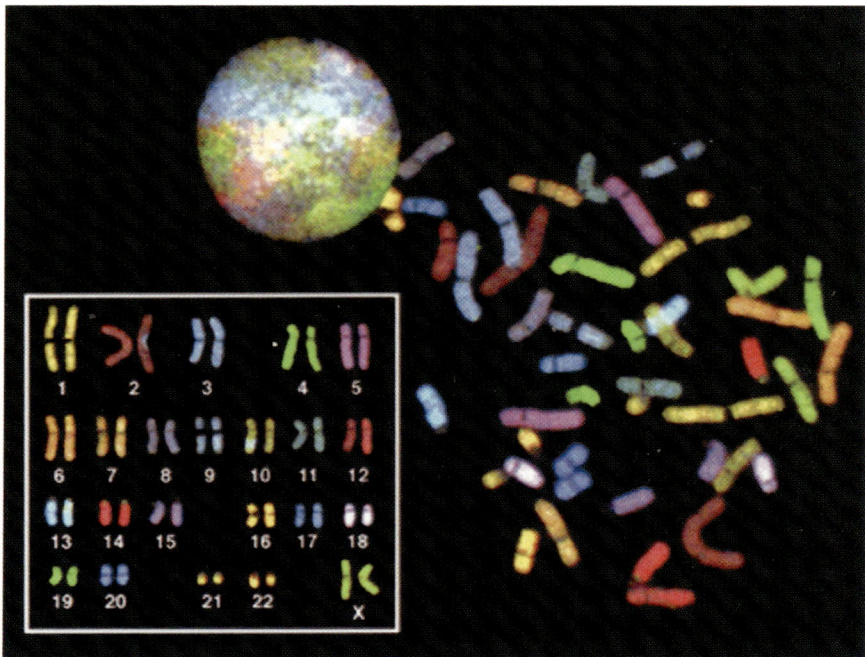

FIGURE 7. Spectral karyotyping paints each chromosome with complete genomic hybridization.

thesis. In approximately 1 hour, 20 PCR cycles can amplify the target by a millionfold (Fig. 9).

PCR permits rapid prenatal diagnosis of major chromosome abnormalities including trisomies 21, 18, 13, and the sex chromosome abnormalities.[26,27] In a series of 4,995 samples, Levett et al. found 89 autosomal abnormalities with no false-positive or false-negative results. Amniocentesis-PCR results can be available an average of 2 days from the time of amniocentesis. Unlike FISH, this technique is feasible on very small volumes of amniotic fluid (0.5 to 1.0 cc). PCR amplifies

30 – 40 cycles of 3 steps :

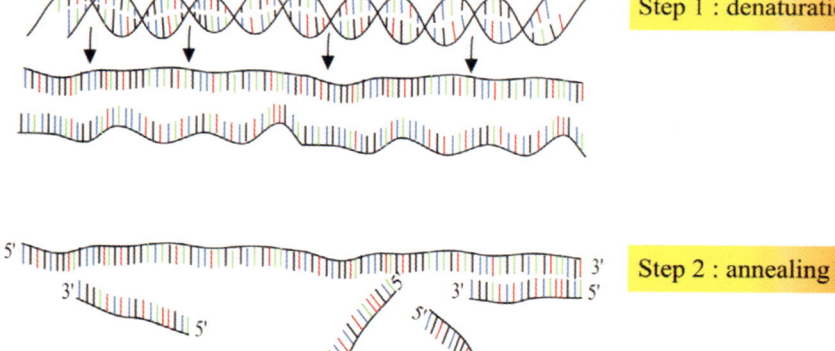

Step 1 : denaturation

Step 2 : annealing

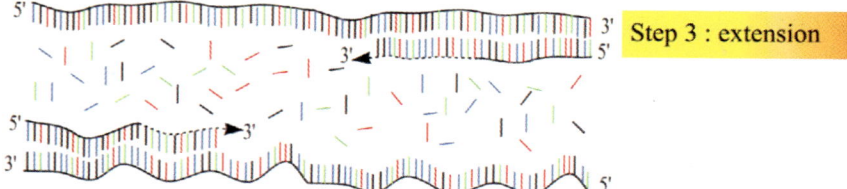

Step 3 : extension

FIGURE 8. Technique of polymerase chain reaction. The mixture is heated in step 1 to separate the paired DNA strands and cooled in steps 2 and 3 to allow DNA fragments and bases to form complementary strands. (Courtesy of Andy Vierstraete, University of Gent, Department of Biology, http://allserv.rug.ac.be/~avierstr/index.html.)

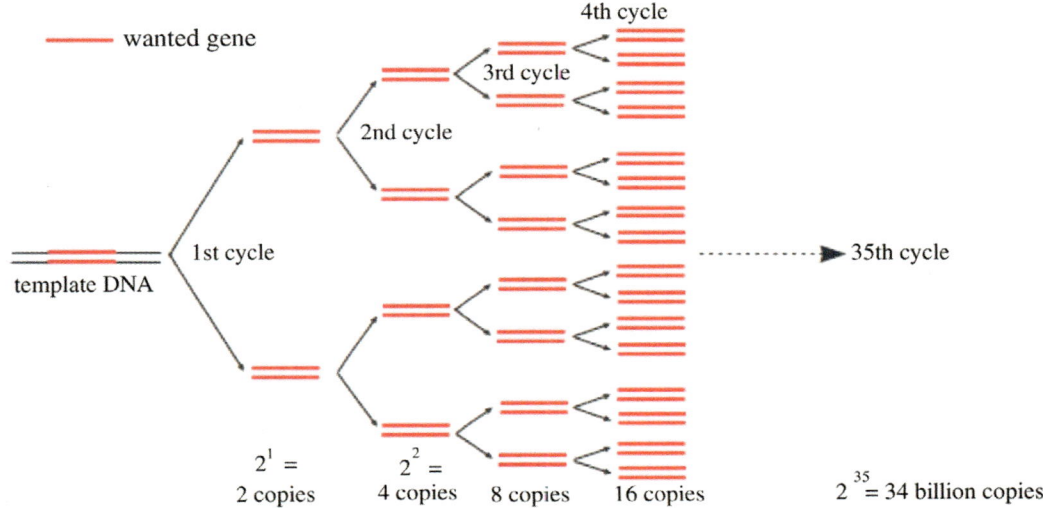

FIGURE 9. Amplification. Polymerase chain reaction results in exponential increase in DNA strands. After the thirty-fifth cycle, polymerase chain reaction has made 34 billion copies of the paired DNA strand. (Courtesy of Andy Vierstraete, University of Gent, Department of Biology, http://allserv.rug.ac.be/~avierstr/index.html.)

DNA from cells and so does not rely on the cells being alive or intact. PCR suffers from the same disadvantages of FISH in that only specific chromosome anomalies are detected.

METHODS OF OBTAINING GENETIC MATERIAL

Genetic material can be obtained from the fetus or from the trophoblast (Table 6). The most common procedures are genetic amniocentesis or CVS. More invasive methods include umbilical vein sampling to obtain fetal blood and fetoscopy for fetal skin biopsy. New methods include pre-implantation diagnosis of the developing blastocyst, cervical lavage for trophoblastic cells, and evaluation of fetal DNA or fetal cells in the maternal circulation. These procedures are used at different times during the pregnancy (Fig. 10).

Invasive Techniques for Obtaining Fetal DNA

Amniocentesis

Genetic amniocentesis is most commonly performed during the second trimester (15 to 20 weeks) but can be per-

formed at any time up to delivery. It accounts for approximately 90% of prenatal tests. A needle is inserted through the woman's abdominal wall and into the amniotic sac around the fetus, under ultrasound guidance, and a sample is collected. The cells in the amniotic fluid have been shed from the surface of the fetus and membranes. These cells are then usually cultured for around 10 days before performing the prenatal diagnostic tests. Testing may involve chromosomal, biochemical, or DNA analysis.

When performed during the second trimester, fetal karyotyping is usually performed with traditional cell culture (see Technique later). The main limitation of amniocentesis is the relatively advanced gestational age at which it is performed and the need to culture cells in the laboratory. This can take up to an additional 2 weeks, leading to a sig-

TABLE 6. MEANS OF OBTAINING FETAL OR TROPHOBLASTIC GENETIC MATERIAL

Invasive
  Amniocentesis
  Chorionic villus sampling
  Placental biopsy
  Umbilical vein sampling
  Fetoscopy or skin biopsy
Noninvasive
  Cervical washing
  Preimplantation diagnosis
  Maternal blood sampling for fetal cells or DNA

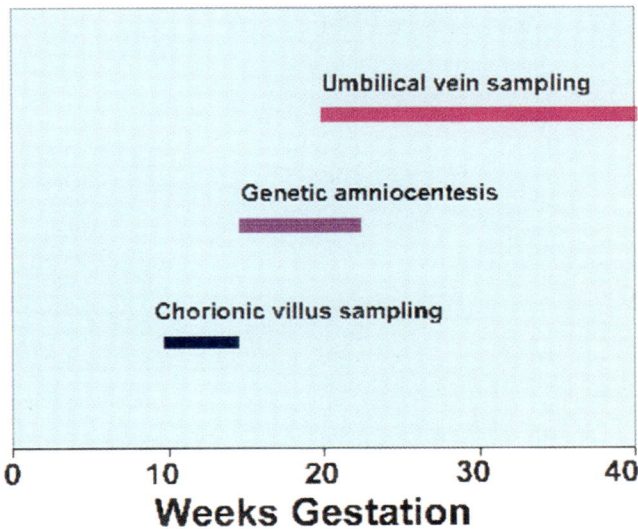

FIGURE 10. Timing of chorionic villus sampling, second-trimester genetic amniocentesis, and umbilical vein sampling during pregnancy.

TABLE 7. INDICATIONS FOR AMNIOCENTESIS RELATED TO PRENATAL DIAGNOSES

Fetal karyotyping
  Advanced maternal age
  Abnormal biochemical screen
  Ultrasound findings
  Family or personal history of trisomy
  Abnormal parental karyotype
Known familial biochemical disorders (see Table 2)
Genetic testing
  Family history of single gene disorder (see Table 3)
Endocrine disorders
  Maternal hypothyroidism
Suspected fetal anemia
  Rhesus sensitization
  Fetal hydrops
Suspected fetal infection

nificant time delay and added anxiety for parents. If the result is abnormal and the parents choose termination of pregnancy, definitive treatment is often not available until after 18 weeks. Pregnancy termination at these gestational ages is more difficult and results in more complications than termination performed toward the end of the first trimester.[28] For these reasons, there is considerable interest in more rapid methods of diagnosis.

Indications

Indications for amniocentesis related to prenatal diagnosis are listed in Table 7. The most common indication for amniocentesis is a perceived increased risk of fetal aneuploidy based on maternal age, abnormal serum screen results, prior medical history, or abnormal prenatal sonographic findings. Table 8 summarizes the age-related risk of Down syndrome and other aneuploidies. For twins and multiple pregnancies, the overall risk to the pregnancy is increased proportionately for dizygotic or multizygotic pregnancies.[29–31]

Amniocentesis can provide fetal genetic material (fetal DNA analysis) that may be useful for certain conditions including rhesus (Rh) disease. This can be used to determine fetal RhD status in pregnancies at risk from Rh isoimmunization (mother Rh negative and father Rh positive). If the fetus is Rh negative, further testing and monitoring are not required.[32] If the pregnancy is considered at risk for Rh disease (fetus is Rh positive and the mother is Rh negative and RhD antibody positive), further monitoring is indicated. This may include serial titers of maternal anti-D antibodies, bilirubin products in amniotic fluid, fetal hematocrit, and fetal Doppler of the middle cerebral artery[33] (see Chapter 16).

Another indication for amniocentesis is in the evaluation of intrauterine infection. In cases of preterm labor,

TABLE 8. ESTIMATED RISKS OF DOWN SYNDROME AND OF ANY CHROMOSOMAL ABNORMALITY, AT THE TIME OF AMNIOCENTESIS AND AT THE EXPECTED DATE OF DELIVERY, BASED ON MATERNAL AGE

	Risk at the time of amniocentesis		Risk at the expected date of delivery	
Maternal age (yr)	Down syndrome	Any chromosomal abnormality	Down syndrome	Any chromosomal abnormality
25	1/885	1/1,533	1/1,250	1/476
26	1/826	1/1,202	1/1,176	1/476
27	1/769	1/943	1/1,111	1/455
28	1/719	1/740	1/1,053	1/435
29	1/680	1/580	1/1,000	1/417
30	1/641	1/455	1/952	1/385
31	1/610	1/357	1/909	1/385
32	1/481	1/280	1/769	1/322
33	1/389	1/219	1/602	1/286
34	1/303	1/172	1/485	1/238
35	1/237	1/135	1/378	1/192
36	1/185	1/106	1/289	1/156
37	1/145	1/83	1/224	1/127
38	1/113	1/65	1/173	1/102
39	1/89	1/51	1/136	1/83
40	1/69	1/40	1/106	1/66
41	1/55	1/31	1/82	1/53
42	1/43	1/25	1/63	1/42
43	1/33	1/19	1/49	1/33
44	1/26	1/15	1/38	1/26
45	1/21	1/12	1/30	1/21
46	1/16	1/9	1/23	1/16
47	1/13	1/7	1/18	1/13
48	1/10	1/6	1/14	1/10
49	1/8	1/4	1/11	1/8

Modified from Hook EB. Rates of chromosomal abnormalities at different maternal ages. *Obstet Gynecol* 1981;58:282–285; and Hook EB, Cross PK, Schreinemachers DM. Chromosomal abnormality rates at amniocentesis and in live-born infants. *JAMA* 1983;249:2034–2038.

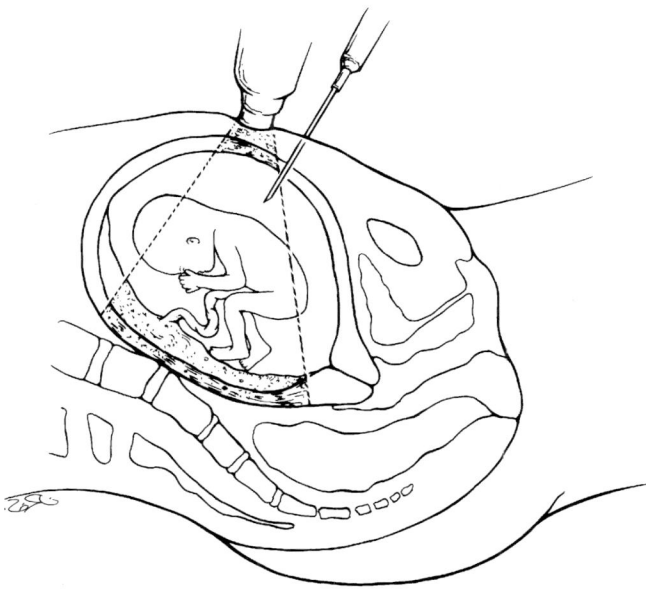

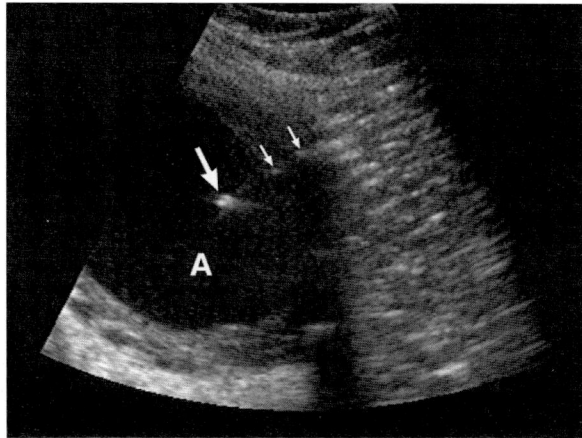

FIGURE 11. Transabdominal amniocentesis. **A:** Illustration showing the procedure of amniocentesis. **B:** Ultrasound demonstrating a 22-gauge spinal needle (*small arrows*) traversing the abdominal and uterine walls, with the needle tip (*large arrow*) clearly visible within the amniotic cavity (*A*).

preterm premature rupture of membranes or chorioamnionitis, amniocentesis can be performed to assay for white cell count, glucose concentration, protein level, Gram stain, bacterial culture, and other markers of infection, such as interleukin 6.[34] The evaluation for infection using amniocentesis might also be indicated in the presence of certain fetal sonographic features, such as echogenic bowel associated with cytomegalovirus infection, or intracranial calcifications associated with toxoplasma infection (see Chapter 17). A range of specific antibodies, both IgG and IgM, can also be assayed for a variety of fetal infections.

Technique

Before performing genetic amniocentesis, all patients should receive appropriate genetic counseling and should give informed consent. Appropriate experience and training of the operator is required (refer to American College of Obstetricians and Gynecologists guidelines). Using continuous sonographic guidance and visualization, the needle is quickly passed through the skin at an appropriate site on the maternal abdomen (Fig. 11). Needle placement can be performed with a *free-hand* technique or with the aid of a needle-guide attached to the transducer. While a transplacental passage of the needle should generally be avoided, at least one study suggests that transplacental amniocentesis is not associated with an increased incidence of adverse fetal outcome.[35]

After correct placement of the needle, an appropriate amount of amniotic fluid is withdrawn. If aspiration is unsuccessful, a common reason is tenting of the amniotic membrane, especially if the procedure is performed at an early gestational age. This is much more likely if amnionchorion separation is visualized sonographically.

Amniocentesis in multiple gestations presents special issues. Although ultrasound is highly reliable for distinguishing monochorionic from dichorionic gestations early in pregnancy, it is less reliable in this distinction during the second trimester. Therefore, caution is advised in sampling a single sac even when monochorionic gestation is suspected. Also, postmeiotic nondisjunction of chromosomes may rarely occur. For these reasons, separate sampling of each amniotic sac is recommended even if the gestation appears to be monochorionic.

If it is not possible to reliably distinguish the needle position within separate sacs, a dye study may be required. This technique involves instillation of a small amount (5 mL) of a blue dye, such as indigo carmine, before withdrawal from the first puncture.[36] Methylene blue should not be used as the dye for this procedure as its use has been associated with fetal hemolytic anemia, small intestinal atresia, and fetal demise.[37] Another technique in twin amniocentesis is sampling of both sacs through a single percutaneous puncture.[38] Theoretically, this method should reduce the loss rate since only a single puncture is required. However, a disadvantage is that it could disrupt the intervening membrane and allow mixing of amniotic fluid between the sacs.

After the procedure, Rh immunoglobulin (RhoGAM) should be given for patients who are Rh negative. While there are no randomized trials confirming the protective effect of Rh immunoglobulin administration for isoimmunization after amniocentesis, it is currently recommended that prophylaxis be given to eligible patients after prenatal diagnostic procedures.[39] There is no value in giving Rh immunoglobulin to a patient who is already Rh sensitized. The amniotic fluid sample should be sent promptly, at room temperature, to a cytogenetics laboratory that has the necessary skill and experience to perform amniotic fluid cell culture.

Complications

Adverse consequences of amniocentesis are rare but are dependent on the gestational age at which the procedure is performed. For example, the implications of procedure-related rupture of membranes or intrauterine infection at 16 weeks are significantly more serious than the same complications at 34 weeks' gestation. These complications are described below.

Amniocentesis Failure

With the universal use of real-time sonographic guidance and the centralization of amniocentesis procedures at expert centers, the success rates of obtaining an adequate fluid sample are maximized. In the Canadian Early and Mid-Trimester Amniocentesis Trial (CEMAT) comparing first- and second-trimester amniocenteses, 99.6% of the 1,775 second-trimester amniocenteses were performed successfully at the initial attempt.[40] By contrast, 96.9% of the 1,916 first-trimester amniocenteses in that trial were performed successfully at the initial attempt. In the Danish randomized trial evaluating the safety of second-trimester amniocentesis, 2% of the 2,264 patients required two needle insertions to complete the procedure.[41] In a recent study of third-trimester amniocenteses, 1.6% of the 913 procedures were unsuccessful.[42]

Pregnancy Loss Rate

While genetic amniocentesis in the second trimester has been performed for many years, there are surprisingly few reliable studies that agree on pregnancy loss rates. In 1976, a prospective registry of 1,040 amniocenteses performed in the United States, together with 992 matched controls, demonstrated a 3.5% overall pregnancy loss rate after amniocentesis compared with 3.2% in the control group.[43] This was not a significant difference and resulted in the conclusion that midtrimester amniocentesis was a highly accurate and safe procedure. In a prospective Canadian study of 1,223 amniocenteses, the overall pregnancy loss rate was 3.2%, although there was no control group available for comparison.[44]

The Medical Research Council in the United Kingdom prospectively compared 2,428 amniocenteses to a similar control group and noted a 1.3% procedure-related pregnancy loss rate, as well as a significant increase in neonatal respiratory difficulties and orthopedic problems in the amniocentesis group.[45] The only randomized trial to assess the safety of amniocentesis was reported from Denmark, in which 4,606 low-risk patients were randomized to amniocentesis or noninvasive prenatal diagnosis.[41] The amniocentesis group had a 1.7% pregnancy loss rate, compared with a 0.7% pregnancy loss rate in the control group, suggesting a 1% procedure-related loss rate. This trial has been criticized as being nonrepresentative of current prenatal diagnostic practice, as it was reported in the paper's methodology that an 18-gauge needle was used for amniocenteses.[41] In a subse-

quent letter clarifying the methodology, the authors stated that the paper was in error and that a 20-gauge needle was actually used for the majority of the procedures.[46]

The explanation for the large discrepancy between the North American and European studies is unclear. The British study had a higher mean maternal age of participants, and this age distribution may be responsible in part for the higher pregnancy loss rate.[45] Additionally, the British and Danish studies contained a higher proportion of amniocenteses for elevated maternal serum alpha fetoprotein, a factor that is known to be independently associated with an increased risk of pregnancy loss.[41,45] The randomized trial from Denmark can also be criticized for the size of the needle used, as, even if the subsequently published erratum is used, both 18- and 20-gauge needles are larger than the traditional 22-gauge needle used today.[41,46] Also, some of these studies included many patients whose amniocenteses were performed without real-time ultrasound guidance, again limiting their applicability to contemporary practice.

More contemporary studies also suggest procedure-related pregnancy loss rates of 0.5% to 1.5%, although none have been randomized or well controlled.[35,47,49,50] It should also be noted that unless close to 100% follow-up is obtained for all procedures performed, the true pregnancy loss rate would most likely be significantly underestimated.[47] While it is reasonable to counsel patients that a 0.5% to 1.0% pregnancy loss rate can be expected with amniocentesis, the most accurate counseling should require maintaining follow-up on each operator's own procedures and quotation of loss rates for one's own center and experience.

Pregnancy Loss Rate for Multiple Gestations

Limited data exist for accurate counseling of patients regarding procedure-related loss rates for amniocentesis in multiple gestations. In one review of amniocentesis in 81 twin pregnancies, there was a 100% success rate in sampling all fetuses, and the pregnancy loss rate before 28 weeks' gestation was 2.9%.[51] In another series of 101 twin pregnancies undergoing amniocentesis, the pregnancy loss rate was 3.5%, which was not significantly different from a 3.2% loss rate in control twin pregnancies.[52] In a further series of 339 multiple gestations undergoing amniocentesis, the loss rate to 28 weeks was 3.6%, compared with a singleton loss rate of 0.6%.[53] It is likely that the apparent increased loss rate for multiple gestations is most likely related to the increased background loss rate of multiple gestations. We currently counsel all patients with singleton or multiple gestations of a 0.5% to 1.0% procedure-related loss rate.

Direct Fetal Injury

Direct fetal injury to the fetus from an amniocentesis needle is an extremely uncommon event in the hands of an experienced operator using continuous sonographic visualization of the needle tip. A review from the 1970s suggesting a 1% to 3% incidence of direct fetal injury at the time of amniocentesis is most likely an overestimate due to the lack of continuous sonographic guidance for procedures performed at that time.[54] Other isolated case reports have cited fetal exsanguination, intestinal atresia, ileocutaneous fistula, gangrene of a fetal limb, uniocular blindness, porencephalic cysts, patellar tendon disruption, skin dimples, and peripheral nerve damage following direct injury by an amniocentesis needle.[36] All should be considered extremely unlikely using today's amniocentesis techniques.

Transient Amniotic Fluid Leakage

The incidence of amniotic fluid leakage after second-trimester genetic amniocentesis varies from 1% to 8%.[41,43] In the original Danish randomized trial of amniocentesis, transient fluid leakage was reported in up to 8.1% of cases, compared with 1.7% of controls.[41] However, there was no reported difference in the incidence of premature rupture of membranes before 37 weeks, occurring in 1.8% of amniocentesis cases compared with 1.5% of controls. This suggests that while transient amniotic fluid leakage can be quite common after amniocentesis, in the majority of cases this is of no clinical significance and resolves as the pregnancy progresses. In the CEMAT study, the incidence of post-amniocentesis fluid leakage was 1.7% for second-trimester procedures, but was as high as 3.5% for first-trimester procedures.[40]

One study compared the outcome of second-trimester membrane rupture owing to amniocentesis with spontaneous second-trimester membrane rupture.[55] The mean latency period between membrane rupture and delivery was 18 weeks for cases following amniocentesis, compared with only 4 weeks for cases of spontaneous rupture, and the overall perinatal survival was 91% and 9%, respectively. This study confirms that the natural history of post-amniocentesis amniotic fluid leakage is very different from cases of spontaneous membrane rupture and is associated with a significantly better overall prognosis.

Mosaicism

Chromosomal mosaicism occurs in approximately 0.3% of amniocentesis cases.[56] A diagnosis of true mosaicism is made when two cell populations with different karyotypes are found in at least two independent culture vessels. Pseudomosaicism is diagnosed when there is only one cell or one region in a colony with abnormal karyotype, or when only one entire colony has an identical abnormal karyotype, or when multiple colonies within only one culture vessel show an identical abnormal karyotype. Depending on which definition is used, between 0.7% and 2.5% of all amniocentesis specimens will show pseudomosaicism.[56] Excluding true mosaicism requires fetal blood sampling, with karyotyping of cultured fetal lymphocytes. All fetuses with apparent mosaicism should also have a targeted fetal sonographic anatomy survey to aid in counseling. In cases of true mosaicism, the actual phenotype of the child is difficult to predict. After birth, the placenta should be sent for careful cytogenetic analysis.

Complications of Third-Trimester Amniocentesis

Considerably less data are available for counseling patients regarding the risks of third-trimester amniocentesis than exist for first- and second-trimester amniocenteses. The largest series available for review is a retrospective study of 913 third-trimester amniocenteses performed for fetal lung maturity assessment over a 7-year period.[42] The success rate for obtaining an adequate fluid sample was 98.4%. The incidence of procedure-related complications that required urgent delivery was 0.7%, which included three fetal heart rate abnormalities, one episode of placental bleeding, one placental abruption, and one uterine rupture.[42] None of the complications was associated with membrane rupture.

Early Amniocentesis

Amniocentesis performed between 11 and zero-sevenths weeks and 13 and six-sevenths weeks is commonly referred to as *early amniocentesis* (EA). Interest in EA grew out of the success of second-trimester amniocentesis and the desire to offer earlier diagnoses. An assumption was made that since amniocentesis had been shown to be safe and effective during the second trimester, it would be equally safe and effective during the first trimester of pregnancy. This assumption, however, has been demonstrated to be false.

In the CEMAT study, 4,374 patients were randomized to either EA (from 11 weeks to 12 and six-sevenths weeks) or to traditional second-trimester amniocentesis (15 weeks to 16 and six-sevenths weeks).[40] The technical aspects of EA were all found to be worse than second-trimester amniocentesis, with a significantly higher chance of the procedure being difficult or unsuccessful (1.6% vs. 0.4%), a second needle insertion being required (5.4% vs. 2.1%), and a significantly higher karyotypic culture failure rate (2.4% vs. 0.25%).[57] Additionally, safety concerns were also documented with EA. This study demonstrated a significantly higher total pregnancy loss rate (7.6% vs. 5.9%), significantly higher post-procedural amniotic fluid loss rate (3.5% vs. 1.7%), and significantly higher incidence of clubfoot (1.3% vs. 0.1%) for first- compared with second-trimester amniocentesis.[40]

The reasons for the increased technical difficulty and the increased risk associated with EA are unclear. At less than 15 weeks' gestation, the amniotic membranes may not be completely fused and the extraembryonic coelom may not yet be obliterated. This may lead to a higher chance of membrane *tenting* during the procedure, which may result in failure to obtain fluid, need for additional needle insertions, and extraamniotic extravasation of amniotic fluid. These may be some of the underlying reasons for the decreased safety of EA. Based on the results of the CEMAT, it is clear that the documented safety of second-trimester amniocentesis cannot be simply extrapolated to the first trimester. There are ample data attesting to the decreased safety of EA between 11 and 12 and six-sevenths weeks. There are insufficient data to comment on the safety of EA between 13 and 14 and six-sevenths weeks. Therefore, it is recommended that genetic amniocentesis not be performed before 15 weeks' gestation, unless additional counseling regarding the specific risks of the procedure are provided to, and accepted by, the patient.

EA also results in a higher frequency of clubfoot. In a randomized trial of amniocentesis performed between 11 and 13 weeks' gestation and transabdominal CVS performed between 10 and 12 weeks' gestation, a significantly higher risk of clubfoot was noted in the amniocentesis group.[58] This trial was stopped early because of the clubfoot findings, and therefore compromised the study's ability to comment on the relative risk of pregnancy loss. A meta-analysis of trials comparing CVS and EA suggests a higher pregnancy loss rate and greater risk of clubfoot for EA compared with CVS.[59]

Chorionic Villus Sampling

Given the significant disadvantages of EA, the best remaining option for first-trimester diagnosis is CVS, in which a biopsy or aspirate of trophoblastic tissue is obtained directly from the placenta. CVS has been performed as early as 6 to 8 weeks' gestation, although it is now extremely rare to perform the procedure before 10 weeks' gestation because of a reported association with fetal limb-reduction defects.[60,61] The optimal time to perform CVS is between 10 and 12 weeks' gestation.[62] At this gestational age, embryonic viability is more easily confirmed, and the borders of the placenta are easily identifiable.

A theoretical upper limit of 13 to 14 weeks' gestation is sometimes placed on performance of transcervical CVS because of concerns that beyond this time the decidua capsularis and the decidua vera (sometimes called the *decidua parietalis*), may have fused.[63] Attempts to insert a CVS catheter between the uterine wall and the chorionic tissue after such fusion may theoretically lead to an increased risk of membrane damage.

Indications

The indications for CVS are similar to those for genetic amniocentesis (Table 9). Patients who are identified as being at increased risk for fetal chromosomal abnormalities during the first trimester of pregnancy include advanced maternal age, abnormal parental karyotype, or a history of a prior affected pregnancy. In addition, much work has been recently performed on the role of first-trimester serum and sonographic screening to identify patients at sufficiently high risk to warrant CVS[64–66] (see Chapters 20 and 22).

TABLE 9. INDICATIONS FOR CHORIONIC VILLUS SAMPLING

Fetal karyotyping
Advanced maternal age
Abnormal first-trimester biochemical screen
Ultrasound findings (first trimester)
Family or personal history of trisomy
Abnormal parental karyotype
Known familial biochemical disorders (see Table 2)
Genetic testing
Family history of single gene disorder (see Table 3)
Cystic fibrosis
Duchenne muscular dystrophy
Osteogenesis imperfecta
Endocrine disorders
Maternal hypothyroidism

In addition to fetal aneuploidy, other indications for CVS include prenatal diagnosis of single gene disorders in at-risk families. A major advantage of CVS is that it provides an abundant sample of fetal-derived tissue for analysis, which is important when DNA analysis and enzymatic diagnostic techniques are needed. The increased tissue volume ensures that adequate material is available to eliminate homozygous and heterozygous enzymatic deficiency states, although care must be taken to distinguish contaminating maternal decidua from trophoblastic villi. Common conditions amenable to CVS diagnosis include cystic fibrosis, Duchenne muscular dystrophy, and osteogenesis imperfecta.

It should be noted that CVS cannot evaluate alpha-fetoprotein levels and therefore cannot be used to diagnose open neural tube defects. Therefore, following first-trimester invasive testing with CVS, further testing is still required in the second trimester to exclude neural tube defects. Additionally, due to different methylation patterns between trophoblastic tissue and fetal tissue, CVS has only a limited role in the prenatal diagnosis of fragile X mental retardation.[62]

Technique

All patients should receive appropriate genetic counseling and should give informed consent. Ultrasound examination should be performed before CVS to identify the number of fetuses, gestational age, fetal position(s), placental location(s), the presence of any obvious fetal abnormalities, the size of the maternal bladder, and the position of the uterus. Chorionic villi can be obtained by either a transcervical (Fig. 12) or transabdominal (Fig. 13) approach. Real-time sonographic guidance is used throughout the procedure.

In our practice, a transcervical sample is obtained with a flexible polyethylene catheter together with a stainless steel malleable stylet to facilitate insertion (Cook Obstetrics/Gynecology, Spencer, IN). The catheter is gently inserted into the cervical canal, and real-time transabdominal sonography is used as the tip is advanced through the chorion frondosum to the distal end of the placenta (Fig.

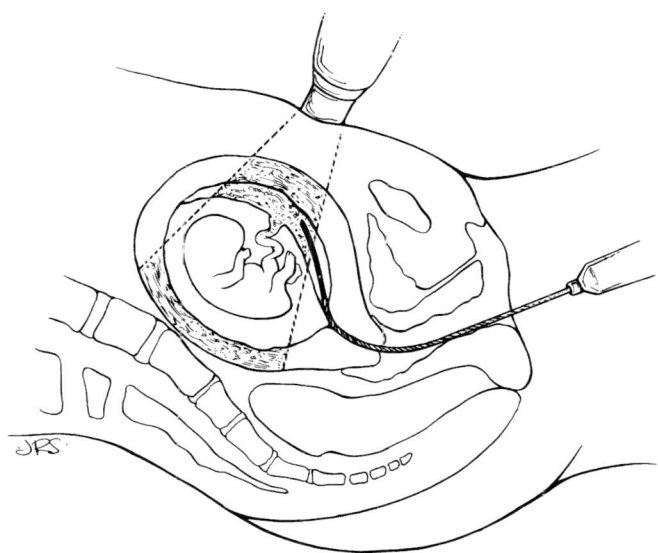

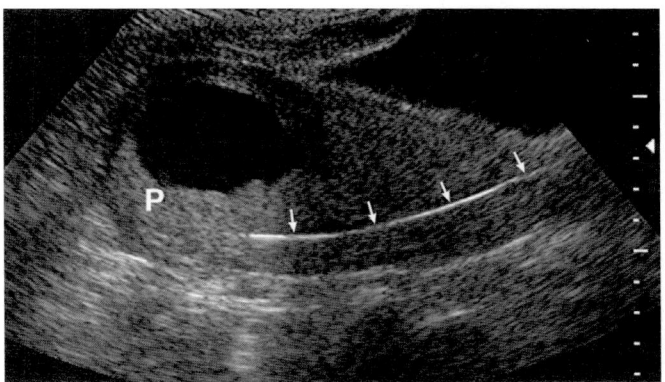

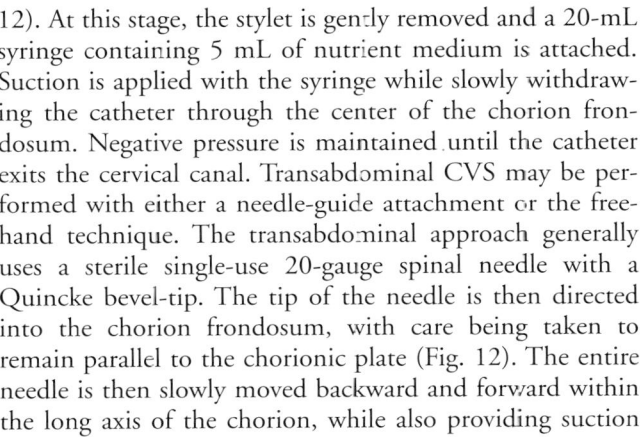

FIGURE 12. Transcervical chorionic villus sampling. **A:** Illustration showing the procedure of transcervical chorionic villus sampling. **B:** Sonogram at 11 weeks' gestation demonstrates a 5.7 French catheter (*small arrows*) traversing the internal cervical os and being placed within the chorion frondosum of a posterior placenta (*P*).

12). At this stage, the stylet is gently removed and a 20-mL syringe containing 5 mL of nutrient medium is attached. Suction is applied with the syringe while slowly withdrawing the catheter through the center of the chorion frondosum. Negative pressure is maintained until the catheter exits the cervical canal. Transabdominal CVS may be performed with either a needle-guide attachment or the free-hand technique. The transabdominal approach generally uses a sterile single-use 20-gauge spinal needle with a Quincke bevel-tip. The tip of the needle is then directed into the chorion frondosum, with care being taken to remain parallel to the chorionic plate (Fig. 12). The entire needle is then slowly moved backward and forward within the long axis of the chorion, while also providing suction

with the syringe. After four or five passes the needle is then slowly withdrawn from the abdomen.

CVS has been successfully used for early prenatal diagnosis in multiple gestations, both twins and higher-order pregnancies.[67] It is essential to perform detailed sonographic mapping of each individual gestational sac and placental location, and create a clear visual record before performing such procedures. The possibility of cross-contamination of samples is greater with CVS than with amniocentesis as there is no intervening membrane to help confirm that separate samples have been obtained. It is essential therefore to sample each placenta at a site that is as distant as possible from the other placenta. This is generally easily achieved with meticulous sonographic guidance

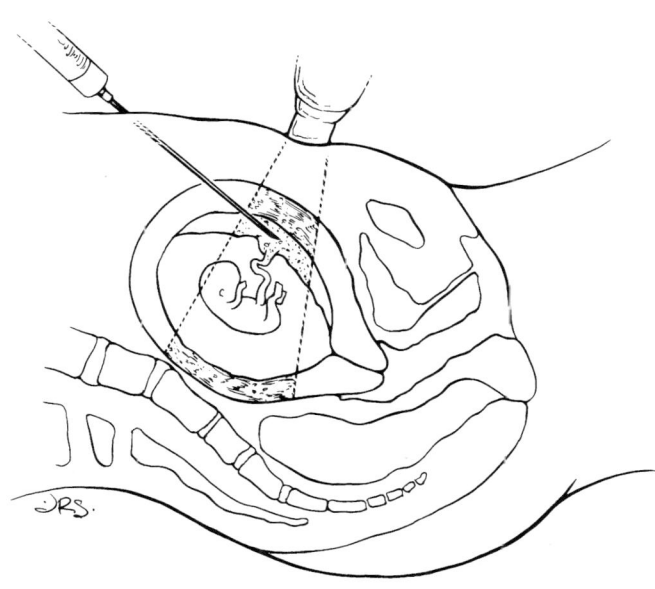

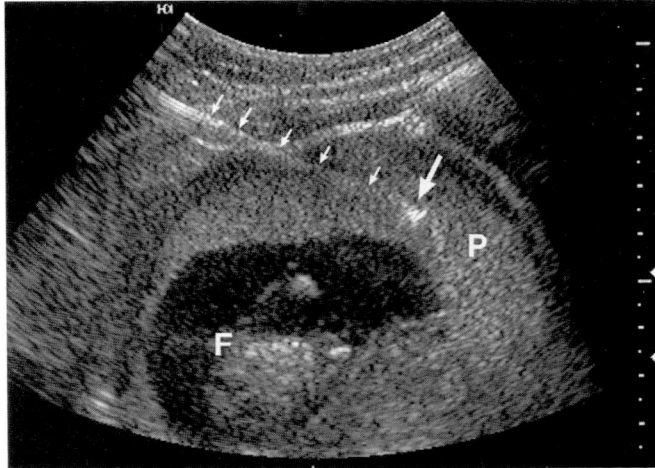

FIGURE 13. Transabdominal chorionic villus sampling procedure. **A:** Illustration showing the procedure of transabdominal chorionic villus sampling. **B:** Sonogram at 12 weeks' gestation shows a 20-gauge spinal needle (*small arrows*) traversing the abdominal and uterine walls and being placed within the chorion frondosum of an anterior placenta (*P*). F, fetus; large arrow, needle tip.

when a dichorionic pregnancy is being sampled. For pregnancies with a confluent single placenta, it may be prudent to independently sample opposite poles.

After aspiration, the contents of the syringe and catheter or needle are flushed into a Petrie dish containing additional nutrient medium. The sample should be carefully examined in strong light to confirm the presence of at least 10 to 30 mg of tissue. Occasionally a dissecting microscope may be needed to distinguish free-floating villus branches from contaminating decidua.

Patients should be advised that it is quite common to expect some light vaginal spotting, especially after transcervical procedures, during the first 24 hours following the procedure. Heavy vaginal bleeding or foul-smelling vaginal discharge more than 24 hours after the procedure is unusual and should warrant a prompt medical evaluation.

Complications

Chorionic Villus Sampling Failure. When performed by a skilled team, it is very unusual to fail to obtain an adequate villus sample. One of the world's most experienced CVS centers in Philadelphia has described a 100% success rate at retrieving an adequate sample in more than 16,000 consecutive patients.[68] Such success rates may not be realistic at all centers performing CVS. In the U.S. nonrandomized trial comparing 2,278 CVS procedures and 671 second-trimester amniocenteses, cytogenetic diagnoses were obtained in 97.8% and 99.4% of cases, respectively.[69] In the three randomized trials comparing transabdominal and transcervical CVS procedures, failure rates of 0.2% to 3.4% were reported.[67,70,71] In the U.S. randomized trial, 6% of transabdominal and 10% of transcervical CVS procedures required more than one insertion of the needle or catheter.[71]

Pregnancy Loss. If pregnancy loss following first-trimester CVS is to be compared with that following second-trimester amniocentesis, the higher background pregnancy loss rate of all first-trimester pregnancies must be considered. Therefore, invasive procedures performed at different gestational ages should be compared based on total pregnancy loss rates, spontaneous and induced, in a group of patients enrolled before any procedure being performed.

In the Canadian Collaborative CVS–Amniocentesis Clinical Trial Group study, almost 2,400 patients were randomized to either first-trimester CVS or second-trimester amniocentesis. The total pregnancy loss rate was 7.6% in the CVS group and 7.0% in the amniocentesis group, representing an excess loss risk of 0.6% for CVS, a difference that was not statistically significant.[72] In the U.S. nonrandomized prospective trial, 2,278 patients chose CVS and were compared with 671 patients who chose second-trimester amniocentesis. The total pregnancy loss rate was 7.2% in the CVS group and 5.7% in the amniocentesis group, which after adjustment, represented an excess loss risk of 0.8% for CVS, a difference that was also not statistically significant.[69] In this trial, however, it was

noted that the CVS loss rate was directly associated with the number of catheter insertions needed to complete the procedure, rising to a 10.8% loss rate for procedures needing three or more attempts, compared with a 2.9% loss rate for procedures completed at the first attempt.[69]

In a prospective trial in Europe, 1,609 patients were randomized to CVS and 1,592 were randomized to second-trimester amniocentesis.[73] This trial revealed a 13.6% loss rate for CVS, compared with a 9.0% loss rate for amniocentesis, which represented a 4.6% excess risk of loss with CVS. This trial has been criticized, as a large number of operators performed the CVS procedures, suggesting that operator inexperience may have explained the unusually high loss rate. In summary, it appears reasonable to conclude that the excess risk of pregnancy loss for CVS compared with second-trimester amniocentesis is between 0.5% and 1.0%, but is unlikely to be any greater than 2.7%.[62]

Controversy exists on whether the two approaches to CVS (transabdominal vs. transcervical) are equally safe. In a randomized trial of 1,194 cases of transabdominal and transcervical CVS performed by a single operator, the rates of pregnancy loss were not significantly different, 16.5% and 15.5%, respectively.[67] A randomized trial comparing 1,944 cases of transcervical CVS and 1,929 cases of transabdominal CVS demonstrated no significant differences between the two procedures, with pregnancy loss rates of 2.5% and 2.3%, respectively.[71] The only study demonstrating an increased risk of pregnancy loss with transcervical CVS was a trial of 3,079 patients in Denmark who were randomized to transcervical CVS, transabdominal CVS, or second-trimester amniocentesis.[70] This study demonstrated a significantly higher risk of pregnancy loss for transcervical CVS compared with either of the other two procedures, with total loss rates of 10.9%, 6.3%, and 6.4%, respectively. Focusing only on the euploid fetuses that underwent CVS, the Danish trial demonstrated a 7.7% loss rate for transcervical CVS compared with a 3.7% loss rate for transabdominal CVS.[70] In summary, it appears that in the hands of operators experienced in both techniques, transcervical and transabdominal CVS are equally safe.[62]

Limb Reduction Defects. A report of five cases of unusual severe limb abnormalities in a series of 289 CVS procedures performed between 8 and 9 weeks' gestation was published in 1991 and resulted in considerable debate on the possible role of CVS in the etiology of oromandibular–limb hypogenesis syndrome and other fetal limb anomalies.[60] This incidence appeared to be significantly higher than the expected incidence of 1 in 175,000 births for oromandibular–limb hypogenesis syndrome and 5 in 10,000 births for all limb reduction defects in the general population. The mechanism by which CVS might cause limb abnormalities is speculative, but the most plausible mechanism is release of vasoactive peptides from the placenta after CVS, which may result in fetal vasospasm and hypoperfusion of the fetal extremities.[36]

Subsequent much larger studies have failed to demonstrate either a causal link or a strong association between CVS and limb reduction defects. In a registry of 216,381 CVS procedures maintained by the World Health Organization, data suggest that the risk of limb abnormalities is greatest after procedures performed early in the first trimester.[74] In a subset of 106,383 procedures, the incidence of limb reduction defects decreased from 11.7 to 4.9, 3.8, 3.4, and 2.3 per 10,000 CVS procedures performed at 8, 9, 10, 11, and greater than 12 weeks' gestation. Grouping diverse abnormalities together may mask an actual real increase in risk of limb abnormalities. In a Centers for Disease Control and Prevention case-control study, while no overall increased risk of limb abnormalities was noted, there was a sixfold increased risk of transverse digital deformity associated with CVS, with an absolute risk of 1 in 3,000 births.[75]

Although there are no conclusive data to link CVS performed at 10 to 12 weeks' gestation with limb abnormalities, it is reasonable to counsel patients of a possible risk as high as 1 in 3,000 births.[62] Genetic counseling for CVS procedures performed before 10 weeks' gestation should be very different, however, with patients being informed that such early procedures may be associated with a risk of limb abnormalities as high as 1% to 2%.[68]

Complications during the Second and Third Trimester. CVS performed after the first trimester, sometimes referred to as *placental biopsy*, has been extensively described in the literature. In one series of 1,000 second- and third-trimester CVS procedures, 2% of patients developed complications, including placental hematoma, fever, and pregnancy loss.[76] In another series of 876 second- and third-trimester CVS procedures it was noted that the incidence of confined placental mosaicism (CPM) increased significantly with advancing gestational age, thereby limiting the usefulness of the test beyond 20 weeks' gestation.[77]

Other Complications. Vaginal bleeding occurs after 7% to 10% of transcervical CVS procedures, but is considerably rarer following transabdominal procedures.[69,73] Infectious complications are also rare following CVS, but are more common after transcervical procedures. In 30% to 50% of cases of transcervical CVS, bacteria and candida species have been isolated from the catheter tip, although this finding has not correlated with risk of adverse pregnancy outcome.[67] In one study, 4.1% of transcervical procedures resulted in maternal bacteremia, compared with 0% of transabdominal procedures.[78] These data underscore the need to adhere to strict aseptic principles when performing invasive prenatal procedures.

Confined Placental Mosaicism. Although not technically a *complication*, a significant laboratory problem with CVS is chromosomal mosaicism in chorionic tissue that is not subsequently found in the fetus. This is termed CPM and is seen in 1% of all CVS specimens.[79] CPM may arise from mutations occurring only in the trophoblast or extraembryonic mesoderm progenitor cells, but not in embryonic tissues. Another mechanism by which CPM can occur is mitotic rescue of an initially trisomic conceptus. With this scenario, in the subsequent mitotic divisions of a trisomic conceptus one cell may lose the extra chromosome; this cell line may give rise to the inner cell mass, resulting in a normal disomic fetus while much of the placenta remains trisomic. One-third of the time, the remaining two chromosomes originate from a single parent. This is known as *uniparental disomy*. It is important to realize that in this scenario, the fetal karyotype will be normal but the fetus will still be at risk for conditions associated with uniparental disomy, such as Prader-Willi syndrome or transient neonatal diabetes.

When placental mosaicism is discovered at CVS, an amniocentesis is generally recommended, and in 60% to 90% of cases this confirms that the fetus is euploid.[68] In certain cases of CPM it may also be necessary to perform fetal blood sampling or tissue biopsy before fetal aneuploidy can be reliably excluded. There is also increasing evidence that in cases of CPM in which the fetal karyotype is confirmed to be normal, the incidence of adverse perinatal outcome is significantly increased. In one series the overall fetal loss rate following CVS was 2.3%, but in the subgroup of patients with CPM, the fetal loss rate ranged from 16.7% to 24.0%.[57] CPM involving trisomy 16 may represent a particularly high-risk group for adverse perinatal outcome. Pregnancies in which CPM has been confirmed should therefore receive careful sonographic surveillance for intrauterine growth restriction and fetal well being.

Umbilical Vein Sampling

Fetal umbilical vein sampling, also known as *percutaneous umbilical blood sampling* (PUBS), refers to the aspiration of fetal blood from the umbilical vein using continuous sonographic guidance. Other terms commonly used for the same procedure include *cordocentesis*, funicentesis, and *fetal blood sampling*. PUBS can be an effective tool for prenatal diagnosis, although the associated pregnancy loss rate and technical difficulties imply that this procedure should be reserved for specific situations in which the risks are justified (Table 10).

PUBS is generally performed between 18 weeks' gestation and term. The limiting factor for PUBS in early pregnancy is the technical challenge of placing a 22-gauge needle accurately into the umbilical vein. Therefore, while PUBS has been performed successfully as early as 12 weeks' gestation, it is much more common to perform it only after 19 to 20 weeks' gestation.[80] The risks also appear higher before 21 weeks than later.[80]

Indications
The indications for PUBS have decreased with advances in alternative methods of diagnosis. DNA technology

TABLE 10. INDICATIONS FOR UMBILICAL VEIN SAMPLING

Fetal karyotyping
   Ultrasound abnormalities suspicious for aneuploidy
Known familial biochemical disorders (see Table 3)
Endocrine disorders
   Maternal hypothyroidism
Hematologic conditions
   Rhesus isoimmunization
   Platelet alloimmunization
   Idiopathic thrombocytopenic purpura
   Hemoglobinopathies
   Congenital coagulopathies

increases the range of genetic diseases that can be diagnosed using chorionic villi or amniocytes, and the range of infectious diseases that can be diagnosed using amniotic fluid. Additionally, advances in sonographic technology have increased the options for noninvasive diagnosis of fetal anemia, a relatively common indication for PUBS.

The most common genetic indication for PUBS is rapid fetal karyotyping. Fetal karyotype can generally be achieved from cultured fetal lymphocytes in 48 to 72 hours. Such a need may arise if a fetal anomaly is diagnosed by sonography in a patient who is close to the upper gestational age limit for pregnancy termination or to assist in deciding mode of delivery in a patient who is close to term. PUBS may also be indicated when chromosomal mosaicism is diagnosed at CVS or amniocentesis.

Hematologic indications for PUBS include assessment of fetal hematocrit in pregnant women with red cell isoimmunization and assessment of fetal platelet count in pregnant women with platelet alloimmunization. Assessment of risk of fetal anemia in red cell isoimmunization has generally been performed using serial amniocenteses and quantification of amniotic fluid bilirubin values. These values are plotted against gestational age on curves, such as the Liley curve, and provide indirect evidence of fetal hemolysis. When the risk appears high, a PUBS procedure is performed to directly measure the fetal hematocrit. If significant anemia is present, a fetal transfusion using packed red blood cells can be performed at the same procedure. Some investigators believe that PUBS should be the procedure of choice in patients with red cell isoimmunization, as serial amniocenteses and quantification of amniotic fluid bilirubin values may not be reliable at earlier gestational ages or in patients with Kell blood group isoimmunization.[81,82]

Alloimmune thrombocytopenia is the platelet equivalent of Rh isoimmunization. Severe fetal thrombocytopenia develops from transplacental passage of maternal antibodies and may lead to intracranial hemorrhage *in utero*. PUBS is indicated in patients with previous pregnancies complicated by alloimmune thrombocytopenia to quantify the fetal platelet count and possibly begin antenatal therapy with maternal administration of intravenous gamma globu-

lin. Idiopathic thrombocytopenic purpura (ITP) is much more common in obstetrics than alloimmune thrombocytopenia. In the setting of ITP, maternal autoantibodies may cross the placenta and cause fetal thrombocytopenia, albeit much less frequently and of much less severity than with alloimmune thrombocytopenia. There is considerable debate as to whether the risks of PUBS are justified by the small risk of adverse fetal outcome from ITP. If PUBS confirms the presence of severe fetal thrombocytopenia in the setting of ITP at term, cesarean delivery may be performed.[83] No evidence exists, however, that such a management strategy improves perinatal outcome. Consequently, PUBS is being used less frequently in the contemporary management of ITP in pregnancy.

PUBS has also been used extensively in the diagnosis of infectious diseases affecting the fetus. In countries such as France, where routine screening for Toxoplasma gondii infection in pregnancy is performed, PUBS is commonly used to culture the organism and confirm fetal infection. PUBS may also be used to evaluate for Toxoplasma-specific IgM antibodies. As advances in PCR techniques continue, it is likely that the role of PUBS in the prenatal diagnosis of fetal Toxoplasmosis and other infections will decrease, in favor of analysis of amniotic fluid samples.

Other indications for PUBS include prenatal diagnosis of inherited hematologic disorders, such as hemoglobinopathies, and congenital coagulopathies. However, most of these conditions can now be diagnosed accurately using fetal DNA obtained from amniocytes or chorionic villi, further reducing the need for PUBS for prenatal genetic diagnosis in contemporary practice.

Technique

Local anesthesia may or may not be administered. There are no data confirming or refuting the need for prophylactic antibiotics for PUBS procedures. Initial sonography should be performed to select the best target for sampling. The most commonly used site is the umbilical vein at its placental insertion, as the cord is relatively immobile at this area. If the placenta is posterior and the placental cord insertion site cannot be reached, it is reasonable to attempt PUBS from the umbilical vein at its entry into the fetal abdomen. If neither end of the umbilical vein can be reached, occasionally a free loop of cord may be sampled, although this is technically more difficult as the mobility of the cord can make needle entry difficult. Rarely it may be necessary to obtain fetal blood from the intrahepatic vein if no other site is accessible. The umbilical artery should not be targeted for aspiration, as this may be associated with extremely high fetal loss rates, as high as 42% in one series.[84]

Needle placement may be performed with either a *freehand* technique or a needle-guide attachment. A sterile 22-gauge needle is used for a PUBS that is intended to be purely diagnostic, and a 20-gauge needle is used for transfusion of packed red cells. Using continuous sonographic

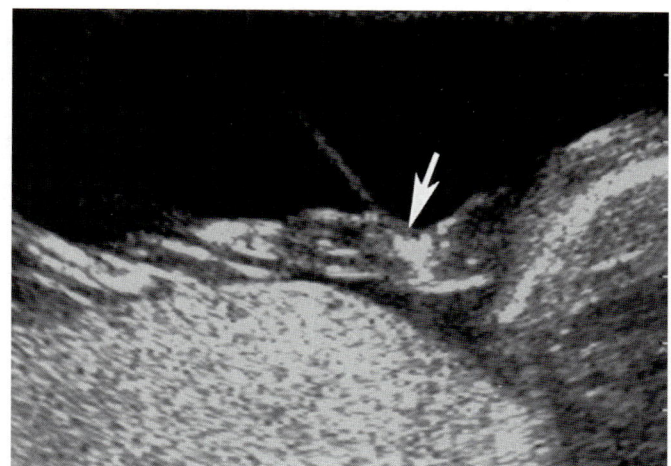
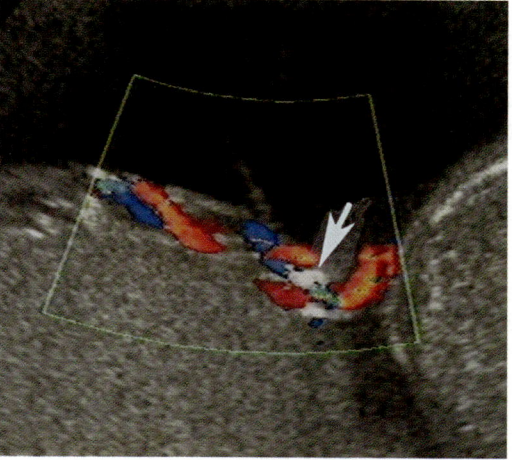

FIGURE 14. Percutaneous umbilical blood sampling procedure at 28 weeks' gestation. Grey scale **(A)** and color-flow **(B)** images show the tip of a 20-gauge needle (*arrows*) within the lumen of the umbilical vein near its placental insertion site.

guidance and visualization, the needle is quickly passed through the skin at an appropriate site on the maternal abdomen toward the umbilical vein (Fig. 14A). Color Doppler sonography may be helpful to confirm the target (Fig. 14B).

Care must be taken after traversing the patient's skin that the needle is not passed through loops of bowel. The umbilical artery should be avoided because puncture of the artery may cause vasospasm and fetal bradycardia. Once free flow of blood is confirmed, a small sample of blood should be aspirated into a heparinized syringe and sent to the laboratory for confirmation of fetal origin (see Confirmation of Fetal Blood Cell Origin). Once confirmed, fetal blood can be aspirated for diagnostic purposes. After sampling is complete, if no transfusion is planned, the needle is withdrawn and the site of the umbilical cord puncture is imaged until blood streaming has ceased. Rh immunoglobulin should be given if the patient is Rh negative. If the procedure is being performed after fetal viability (24 weeks' gestation), a fetal nonstress test is generally also performed after the PUBS is complete.

Confirmation of Fetal Blood Cell Origin

A number of approaches are available to confirm the blood sample is fetal in origin. Placement of a Coulter counter in the prenatal diagnosis center permits immediate confirmation of fetal blood sample by measuring the mean corpuscular volume. The mean corpuscular volume of fetal red cells is significantly larger than that of the adult, with values of 130 fL, 120 fL, and 115 fL expected at 20, 28, and 32 weeks, respectively, compared with adult values of 85 fL or lower. It should be noted, however, that if the fetus has received transfusions of adult packed red blood cells, the ability of mean corpuscular volume to confirm umbilical vein entry is compromised. Other techniques used for dif-

ferentiating fetal and maternal blood samples include performance of a Kleihauer-Betke smear (in which fetal red cells are more stable in an acid elution buffer than adult red cells), or performance of an Apt test (in which centrifuged fetal blood remains pink after addition of base whereas adult blood is less resistant and turns brown), or evaluation for the presence of nucleated red blood cells (which are much more prevalent in fetal than adult blood).

Complications

Failure to Obtain Fetal Blood. Failure to obtain an adequate fetal blood sample is most likely dependent on the skill and experience of the operator, as well as on the gestational age of the procedure. In one series of 1,320 cases performed between 16 and 24 weeks' gestation, 97% of procedures were completed successfully at the first attempt.[85] If the fetal intrahepatic vein is the only target available for sampling, the failure rate to obtain fetal blood may be as high as 8.9%.[86]

Fetal Loss. PUBS is associated with a higher risk of pregnancy loss than other invasive prenatal diagnostic techniques.[86a] However, it should be noted that fetuses selected for PUBS tend to have a higher background rate of adverse pregnancy outcome, mostly because such fetuses are more likely to have structural malformations, aneuploidy, infection, or hematologic disturbance. No studies are available in which pregnancy loss rates have been compared between fetuses undergoing PUBS and an appropriately matched control group.

Various studies have reported fetal loss rates of 0.9% to 3.2%.[52,84,86b] In a review of 7,462 PUBS procedures, the fetal loss rate within 14 days of the procedure was calculated at 1.1% per procedure.[86c] However, this report may underestimate the true risk of PUBS, as it relied on the operator's subjective impression as to whether a pregnancy loss was procedure-related. In a more recent review of 1,320 procedures performed at a single center in Thailand, the total fetal loss rate was 3.2%, with a procedure-related loss rate of 1%.[85] Other complications of the procedure noted included needle site bleeding (20.2%), transient fetal bradycardia (4.3%), chorioamnionitis (0.15%), and umbilical cord hematoma (less than 0.1%). Maxwell et al. found that pregnancy loss rates vary greatly depending on the indication for the procedure, ranging from 1% for fetuses with normal ultrasound findings, 7% for fetuses with structural malformations, and 25% for fetuses with nonimmune hydrops.[87]

Fetoscopy

Sampling of other fetal tissues is sometimes required for prenatal genetic diagnosis where no other tests are available. For example, fetal skin biopsy can be performed with fetoscopy for diagnosis of junctional epidermolysis bullosa, a severe genetic skin disorder. Fetoscopy for diagnostic purposes is infrequently performed today, but has seen a resurgence of interest in therapeutic purposes, specifically for coagulation of communicating vessels in the twin-twin transfusion syndrome.

Noninvasive Techniques for Obtaining Fetal DNA

Cervical Washing

Fetal and trophoblastic cells can be obtained from the cervix and lower uterine segment region.[88–90] Methods for obtaining cells include aspiration, cytobrush, endocervical lavage, or intrauterine lavage. One advantage is that this technique can be performed during the first trimester of pregnancy. Trisomy has been diagnosed with transcervical flushing.[89,90] However, a number of questions remain regarding the reliability of this technique, and it should be considered investigational.

Preimplantation Genetic Diagnosis

Preimplantation genetic diagnosis involves either biopsy of the blastomere at the eight cell stage before embryo transfer or biopsy of a polar body in oocytes before fertilization.[91] Preimplantation diagnosis is now possible for a variety of conditions[92] including single gene disorders and couples at risk for chromosomally unbalanced offspring due to parental translocation or mosaicism. Screening of preimplantation embryos for common aneuploidies has been demonstrated to reduce spontaneous abortions[93] and increase the success of embryo implantation.[94] Although first used for couples of advanced maternal age undergoing *in vitro* fertilization, some authors now suggest that all pre-

implantation embryos should undergo FISH analysis before transfer to enhance pregnancy outcome. If blastomere biopsy is performed, conventional cryopreservation protocols are discouraged.[95]

Intracytoplasmic sperm injection has also been performed to inseminate only those oocytes found to be chromosomally normal.[96] Diagnosis of common chromosome abnormalities is feasible within time limits imposed by intracytoplasmic sperm injection insemination (6 hours or less). Polar body testing of oocytes provides an accurate and reliable approach for prevention of age-related aneuploidies in *in vitro* fertilization patients of advanced maternal age.[97]

Because preimplantation genetic diagnosis of single gene disorders is based on single cell DNA analysis, its accuracy depends mainly on overcoming the major limitations of single cell PCR, which include allele drop out and preferential amplification.

Analysis of Fetal Cells and Fetal DNA Obtained from Maternal Circulation

Techniques are being developed to isolate intact fetal cells[98,99] and fetal cell–free DNA from the maternal circulation to facilitate noninvasive prenatal diagnosis. Most enrichment protocols rely either on magnetic- or fluorescent-activated cell sorting using fetal-specific antibodies. FISH is then performed on interphase fetal cells to diagnose aneuploidy. These techniques are not yet sufficiently developed to have application outside a research setting.

It has become appreciated that large quantities of extracellular fetal DNA are present in maternal serum and plasma.[100] Unlike intact fetal cells that cross the placenta, fetal DNA is quickly cleared from the maternal circulation after delivery. Clinical applications include noninvasive detection of unique fetal gene sequences not shared with the mother and quantitation of fetal DNA in conditions such as preeclampsia. One study has reported the diagnosis of fetal achondroplasia using this technique with PCR and restriction fragment length polymorphism analysis. Other single gene disorders in which fetal DNA has been used for analysis include RhD, myotonic dystrophy, and congenital adrenal hyperplasia.

INTERPRETATION AND COUNSELING

Interpretation and counseling are an essential part of the process of evaluating the risk for fetal genetic disorders. For relatively common disorders, genetic counseling information is often transmitted by the family doctor, the pediatrician, or the obstetrician. However, with the recognition that thousands of problems have a major hereditary component, counseling is increasingly performed in specialized centers for prenatal diagnosis. This is optimally performed by a trained genetic counselor, medical geneticist, or obstetrician with special expertise in genetics, who can obtain a detailed family history and interpret the results of genetic testing. Genetic professionals include board-certified medical geneticists, genetic counselors, and diagnostic laboratory directors.

The process of genetic counseling has changed dramatically over the past two decades. Instead of being based on purely clinical findings, the identity of many disorders can be proven because their genic or chromosomal basis is known. The availability of an ever-increasing number of laboratory tests allows more accurate diagnosis, and often gives the opportunity for presymptomatic or prenatal diagnosis to family members who prefer to use it. However, the availability of such tests also poses psychological and ethical questions that may be difficult to resolve.

Genetic counseling should be, in so far as is possible, impartial and nondirective. The goal is never to make a decision for the couple, whose familial, social, moral, and religious situation is different from that of the counselor, but rather to provide them with the objective information that allows them to make their own informed decisions. Prenatal genetic counseling includes

1. Estimation of risks to develop the disorder and to transmit it to offspring, which includes a detailed family history.
2. Arriving at a specific diagnosis, which is often the most difficult, trying, and time-consuming part of the process. This includes review of medical records, examination of affected individuals, and coordination of diagnostic studies within a family.
3. Practical aid, which includes, for example, recommending doctors for specialized examinations or health care professionals for speech or educational therapy.
4. Supportive role, which is important because many genetic disorders cannot be cured or satisfactorily treated.

REFERENCES

1. Venter JC. The sequence of the human genome. *Science* 2001;291(5507):1304–1351.
2. International Human Genome Sequencing Consortium. Initial sequencing and analysis of the human genome. *Nature* 2001;409(6822):860–921.
3. Baird PA, Anderson TW, Newcombe HB, Lowry RB. Genetic disorders in children and young adults: a population study. *Am J Hum Genet* 1988;42(5):677–593.
4. Czeizel A, Sankaranarayanan K. The load of genetic and partially genetic disorders in man. I. Congenital anomalies: estimates of detriment in terms of years of life lost and years of impaired life. *Mutat Res* 1984;128:73–103.
5. Robinson A, Puck TT. Studies on chromosomal nondisjunction in man. II. *Am J Hum Genet* 1967;19(2):112–129.
6. Morris MA. Mitochondrial mutations in neuro-ophthalmological diseases. A review. *J Clin Neuroophthalmol* 1990;10(3):159–166.
7. Wallace DC, Lott MT, Lezza AM, Seibel P, Voljavec AS, et al. Mitochondrial DNA mutations associated with neuromuscular diseases: analysis and diagnosis using the polymerase chain reaction. *Pediatr Res* 1990;28(5):525–528.
8. Kan YW, Dozy AM. Antenatal diagnosis of sickle-cell anaemia by D.N.A. analysis of amniotic-fluid cells. *Lancet* 1978;ii:910–912.
9. Caspersson T, Lomakka G, Zeck I. 24 fluorescence patterns of human metaphase chromosomes—distinguishing characters and variability. *Hereditas* 1971;67:89–102.
10. Hoehn HW. Fluid cell culture. In: Milunsky A, ed. *Genetic disorders and the fetus: diagnosis, prevention and treatment*, 4th ed. Baltimore: Johns Hopkins University Press, 1998:128–149.
11. D'Alton ME, Malone FD, Chelmow D, Ward BE, Bianchi DW. Defining the role of fluorescence in situ hybridization on uncultured amniocytes for prenatal diagnosis of aneuploidies. *Am J Obstet Gynecol* 1997;176:769–776.
12. Reid R, Sepulveda W, Kyle PM, Davies G. Amniotic fluid culture failure: clinical significance and association with aneuploidy. *Obstet Gynecol* 1996;87:588–592.
13. Klinger K, Landes G, Shook D, Harvey R, Lopez L, et al. Rapid detection of chromosome aneuploidies in uncultured amniocytes by using fluorescence in situ hybridization (FISH). *Am J Hum Genet* 1992;51:55–65.
14. Cremer T, Landegent J, Bruckner A, School HP, Schardin M, et al. Detection of chromosome aberrations in the human interphase nucleus by visualization of specific target DNAs with radioactive and non-radioactive in situ hybridization techniques: diagnosis of trisomy 18 with probe LI.84. *Hum Genet* 1986;74:346–352.
15. American College of Medical Genetics and American Society of Human Genetics. Test and Technology Transfer Committee. Technical and clinical assessment of fluorescence in situ hybridization: an ACMG/ASHG position statement. I. Technical considerations. *Gen Med* 2000;2:356–361.
16. Reference deleted.
17. Flint J, Wildie AOM, Buckel VJ, et al. The detection of subtelomeric chromosomal rearrangements in idiopathic mental retardation. *Nat Gen* 1995;9:132–140.
18. Brondum-Nielsen K, Mikkelsen M. A 10-year survey, 1980–1990, of prenatally diagnosed small supernumerary marker chromosomes, identified by FISH analysis. Outcome and follow-up of 14 cases diagnosed in a series of 12,699 prenatal samples. *Prenat Diagn* 1995;15:615–619.
19. Callen DF, Eyre H, Yip MY, Freemantle J, Haan EA. Molecular cytogenetic and clinical studies of 42 patients with marker chromosomes. *M J Med Genet* 1992;43(4):709–715.
20. Ward BE, Gersen SL, Carelli MP, McGuire NM, Dackowski WR, et al. Rapid prenatal diagnosis of chromosomal aneuploidies by fluorescence in situ hybridization: clinical experience with 4,500 specimens. *Am J Hum Genet* 1993;52:854–865.
21. Eiben B, Trawicki W, Hammans W, et al. Rapid prenatal diagnosis of aneuploidies in uncultured amniocytes by fluorescence in situ hybridization. *Fetal Diagn Ther* 1999;14:193–197.

22. Feldman B, Ebrahim SAD, Hazan SL, Gyi K, Johnson MP, et al. Routine prenatal diagnosis of aneuploidy by FISH studies in high-risk pregnancies. *Am J Med Genet* 2000;90: 233–238.

23. Estabrooks LL, Hanna JS, Lamb AN. Overwhelming maternal cell contamination in amniotic fluid samples from patients with oligohydramnios can lead to false prenatal interphase FISH results. *Prenat Diagn* 1999;19:179–181.

24. Hockstein S, Chen PX, Thangavelu M, Pergament E. Factors associated with maternal cell contamination in amniocentesis samples as evaluated by fluorescent in situ hybridization. *Obstet Gynecol* 1998;92:551–556.

25. Evans MI, Henry GP, Miller WA, Bui TH, Snijders RJ, et al. International, collaborative assessment of 146,000 prenatal karyotypes: expected limitations if only chromosome-specific probes and fluorescent in-situ hybridization are used. *Hum Reprod* 1999;14:1213–1216.

26. Verma L, Macdonald F, Leedham P, McConachie M, Dhanjal S, et al. Rapid and simple prenatal DNA diagnosis of Down's syndrome. *Lancet* 1998;352:9–12.

27. Levett LJ, Liddle S, Meredith R. A large-scale evaluation of amnio-PCR for the rapid prenatal diagnosis of fetal trisomy. *Ultrasound Obstet Gynecol* 2001;17:115–118.

28. Lawson HW, Frye A, Atrash HK, Smith JC, Shulman HB, et al. Abortion mortality, United States, 1972 through 1987. *Am J Obstet Gynecol* 1994;171:1365–1372.

29. Rodis JF, Egan JF, Craffey A, Clarlegio L, Greenstein RM, et al. Calculated risks of chromosomal abnormalities in twin gestations. *Obstet Gynecol* 1990;76:1037–1041.

30. Meyers C, Adam R, Dungan J, Prenger V. Aneuploidy in twin gestations: when is maternal age advanced? *Obstet Gynecol* 1997;89:248–251.

31. Malone FD, D'Alton ME. Multiple gestation: clinical characteristics and management. In: Creasy RK, Resnik R, eds. *Maternal fetal medicine*, 4th ed. Philadelphia: WB Saunders, 1999:598–615.

32. Bennett PR, Le Van Kim C, Colin Y, et al. Prenatal determination of fetal RhD type by DNA amplification. *N Engl J Med* 1993;329:607–610.

33. Mari G, Deter RL, Carpenter RL, et al. Noninvasive diagnosis by Doppler ultrasonography of fetal anemia due to maternal red-cell alloimmunization. Collaborative Group for Doppler Assessment of the Blood Velocity in Anemic Fetuses. *N Engl J Med* 2000;342:9–14.

34. Romero R, Athayde N, Maymon E, Pacora P, Bahado-Singh R. Premature rupture of the membranes. In: Reece EA, Hobbins JC, eds. *Medicine of the fetus and mother*, 2nd ed. Philadelphia: Lippincott 1999:1581–1625.

35. Bombard AT, Powers JF, Carter S, et al. Procedure-related fetal losses in transplacental versus nontransplacental genetic amniocentesis. *Am J Obstet Gynecol* 1995;172:868–872.

36. Bianchi DW, Crombleholme TM, D'Alton ME. Prenatal diagnostic procedures. In: Bianchi DW, Crombleholme TM, D'Alton ME, eds. *Fetology: diagnosis and management of the fetal patient*. New York: McGraw-Hill, 2000:11–33.

37. Kidd SA, Lancaster PA, Anderson JC, et al. Fetal death after exposure to methylene blue dye during mid-trimester amniocentesis in twin pregnancy. *Prenat Diagn* 1996;16: 39–47.

38. Jeanty P, Shah D, Roussis P. Single-needle insertion in twin amniocentesis. *J Ultrasound Med* 1990;9:11–17.

39. American College of Obstetricians and Gynecologists. *Prevention of RhD alloimmunization. American College of Obstetricians and Gynecologists Practice Bulletin. 4.* Washington, DC: The College, May 1999.

40. Canadian Early and Mid-Trimester Amniocentesis Trial Group. Randomized trial to assess safety and fetal outcome of early and mid-trimester amniocentesis. *Lancet* 1998;351:242–247.

41. Tabor A, Philip J, Madsen M, Bang J, Obel EB, et al. Randomized controlled trial of genetic amniocentesis in 4606 low-risk women. *Lancet* 1986;1:1287–1293.

42. Stark CM, Smith RS, Lagrandeur RM, Batton DG, Lorenz RP. Need for urgent delivery after third-trimester amniocentesis. *Obstet Gynecol* 2000;95:48–50.

43. NICHD National Registry for Amniocentesis Study Group. Midtrimester amniocentesis for prenatal diagnosis: safety and accuracy. *JAMA* 1976;236:1471–1476.

44. Simpson NE, Dallaire L, Miller JR, et al. Prenatal diagnosis of genetic disease in Canada: report of a collaborative study. *Can Med Assoc J* 1976;115:739–748.

45. Working Party on Amniocentesis. An assessment of the hazards of amniocentesis. *Br J Obstet Gynaecol* 1978;85[Suppl 2]:1–41.

46. Tabor A, Philip J, Bang J, Madsen M, Obel EB, et al. Needle size and risk of miscarriage after amniocentesis. *Lancet* 1988;1:183–184.

47. Halliday JL, Lumley J, Sheffield LJ, Robinson HP, Renou P, et al. Importance of complete follow-up of spontaneous fetal loss after amniocentesis and chorion villus sampling. *Lancet* 1992;340:886–890.

48. Reference deleted.

49. Antsaklis A, Papantoniou N, Xygakis A, Mesogitis S, Tzortzis E, et al. Genetic amniocentesis in women 20–34 years old: associated risks. *Prenat Diagn* 2000;20:247–250.

50. Reid KP, Guerin LC, Dickinson JE, Newnhan JP, Phillips JM. Pregnancy loss rates following second trimester genetic amniocentesis. *Aust N Z J Obstet Gynaecol* 1999;39:281–285.

51. Wapner RJ, Johnson A, Davis G, Urban A, Morgan P, et al. Prenatal diagnosis in twin gestations: a comparison between second-trimester amniocentesis and first-trimester chorionic villus sampling. *Obstet Gynecol* 1993;82:49–56.

52. Ghidini A, Lynch L, Hicks C, Alvarez M, Lockwood CJ. The risk of second-trimester amniocentesis in twin gestations: a case-control study. *Am J Obstet Gynecol* 1993;169: 1013–1016.

53. Anderson RL, Goldberg JD, Golbus MS. Prenatal diagnosis in multiple gestation: 20 years' experience with amniocentesis. *Prenat Diagn* 1991;11:263–270.

54. Karp LE, Hayden PW. Fetal puncture during mid-trimester amniocentesis. *Obstet Gynecol* 1977;49:115–117.

55. Borgida AF, Mills AA, Feldman AM, Rodis JF, Egan JFX. Outcome of pregnancies complicated by ruptured membranes after genetic amniocentesis. *Am J Obstet Gynecol* 2000;183:937–939.

56. Hsu LY, Perlis TE. United States survey on chromosome mosaicism and pseudomosaicism in prenatal diagnosis. *Prenat Diagn* 1984;4:97–130.

57. Johnson A, Wapner RJ, Davis GH, et al. Mosaicism in chorionic villus sampling: an association with poor perinatal outcome. *Obstet Gynecol* 1990;75:573–577.

58. Sundberg K, Bang J, Smidt-Jensen S, et al. Randomized study of risk of fetal loss related to early amniocentesis versus chorionic villus sampling. *Lancet* 1997;350:697–703.

59. Alfirevic Z. Early amniocentesis versus transabdominal chorionic villus sampling for prenatal diagnosis. *Cochrane Database Syst Rev* 2000;2:CDO00077.

60. Firth HV, Boyd PA, Chamberlain P, MacKenzie IZ, Lindenbaum RH, et al. Limb abnormalities and chorionic villus sampling. *Lancet* 1990;337:762–763.

61. Brambati B, Simoni G, Travi M, et al. Genetic diagnosis by chorionic villus sampling before 8 gestational weeks: efficiency, reliability, and risks in 317 completed pregnancies. *Prenat Diagn* 1992;12:789–799.

62. American College of Obstetricians and Gynecologists. *Chorionic villus sampling. American College of Obstetricians and Gynecologists Committee Opinion. 160.* Washington, DC: The College, October 1995.

63. Brambati B, Tului L. Prenatal diagnosis through chorionic villus sampling. In: Milunsky A, ed. *Genetic disorders and the fetus: diagnosis, prevention and treatment,* 4th ed. Baltimore: Johns Hopkins University Press, 1998:150–178.

64. Malone FD, Berkowitz RL, Canick JA, D'Alton ME. First-trimester screening for aneuploidy: research or standard of care? *Am J Obstet Gynecol* 2000;182:490–496.

65. Canick JA, Kellner LH. First trimester screening for aneuploidy: serum biochemical markers. *Semin Perinatol* 1999;23:359–368.

66. Stewart TL, Malone FD. First trimester screening for aneuploidy: nuchal translucency sonography. *Semin Perinatol* 1999;23:369–381.

67. Brambati B, Terzian E, Tognom G. Randomized clinical trial of transabdominal versus transcervical chorionic villus sampling methods. *Prenat Diagn* 1991;11:285–293.

68. Jenkins TM, Wapner RJ. First trimester prenatal diagnosis: chorionic villus sampling. *Semin Perinatol* 1999;23:403–413.

69. Rhoads GG, Jackson LG, Schlesselman SE, de la Cruz FF, Desnick RJ, et al. The safety and efficacy of chorionic villus sampling for early prenatal diagnosis of cytogenetic abnormalities. *N Engl J Med* 1989;320(10):609–617.

70. Smidt-Jensen S, Permin M, Philip J, et al. Randomized comparison of amniocentesis and transabdominal and transcervical chorionic villus sampling. *Lancet* 1992;340:1237–1244.

71. Jackson LG, Zachary JM, Fowler SE, et al. A randomized comparison of transcervical and transabdominal chorionic-villus sampling. *N Engl J Med* 1992;327:594–598.

72. Canadian Collaborative CVS—Amniocentesis Clinical Trial Group. Multicenter randomised trial of chorion villus sampling and amniocentesis. *Lancet* 1989;1:1–16.

73. MRC Working Party on the Evaluation of Chorion Villus Sampling. Medical Research Council European trial of chorion villus sampling. *Lancet* 1991;337:1491–1499.

74. WHO/PAHO Consultation on CVS. Evaluation of chorionic villus sampling safety. *Prenat Diagn* 1999;19:97–99.

75. Olney RS, Khoury MJ, Alo CJ, et al. Increased risk for transverse digital deficiency after chorionic villus sampling—results of the United States multistate case-control study, 1988–1992. *Teratology* 1995;51:20–29.

76. Podobnik M, Ciglar S, Singer Z, Podobnik-Sarkanji S, Duic Z, et al. Transabdominal chorionic villus sampling in the second and third trimesters of high-risk pregnancies. *Prenat Diagn* 1997;17:125–133.

77. Carroll SG, Davies T, Kyle PM, Abdel-Fattah S, Soothill PW. Fetal karyotyping by chorionic villus sampling after the first trimester. *Br J Obstet Gynaecol* 1999;106:1035–1040.

78. Silverman NS, Sullivan MW, Jungking DL, et al. Incidence of bacteremia associated with chorionic villus sampling. *Obstet Gynecol* 1994;84:1021–1024.

79. Vejerslev LO, Mikkelsen M. The European collaborative study on mosaicism in chorionic villus sampling: data from 1986 to 1987. *Prenat Diagn* 1989;9:575–588.

80. Orlandi F, Damiani G, Jakil C, Lauricella S, Bertolino O, et al. The risks of early cordocentesis (12–21 weeks): analysis of 500 procedures. *Prenat Diagn* 1990;10:425–428.

81. Nicolaides KH, Rodeck CH, Mlbashan RS, et al. Have Liley charts outlived their usefulness? *Am J Obstet Gynecol* 1986;155:90–94.

82. Weiner CP, Widness JA. Decreased fetal erythropoiesis and hemolysis in Kell hemolytic anemia. *Am J Obstet Gynecol* 1996;174:547–551.

83. Garmel SH, Craigo SD, Morin LM, Crowley JM, D'Alton ME. The role of percutaneous umbilical blood sampling in the management of immune thrombocytopenic purpura. *Prenat Diagn* 1995;15:439–445.

84. Weiner CP, Okamura K. Diagnostic fetal blood sampling-technique related losses. *Fetal Diagn Ther* 1996;11:169–175.

85. Tongsong T, Wanapirak C, Kunavikatikul C, Sirirchotiyakul S, Piyarnongkol W, et al. Cordocentesis at 16–24 weeks of gestation: experience of 1,320 cases. *Prenat Diagn* 2000;20:224–228.

86. Nicolini U, Nicolaidis P, Fisk NM, Tannirandorn Y, Rodeck CH. Fetal blood sampling from the intrahepatic vein: analysis of safety and clinical experience with 214 procedures. *Obstet Gynecol* 1990;76:47–53.

86a. D'Alton ME, DeCherney AH. Prenatal diagnosis. *N Engl J Med* 1993;328:114–120.

86b. Buscaglia M, Ghisoni L, Bellotti M, et al. Percutaneous umbilical blood sampling: indication changes and procedure loss rate in nine years' experience. *Fetal Diagn Ther* 1996;11:106–113.

86c. Megerian G, Ludomirsky A. Role of cordocentesis in perinatal medicine. *Curr Opin Obstet Gynecol* 1994;6:30–35.

87. Maxwell DJ, Johnson P, Hurley P, Neales K, Allan L, et al. Fetal blood sampling and pregnancy loss in relation to indication. *Br J Obstet Gynaecol* 1991;98:892–897.

88. Bahado-Singh RO, Kliman H, Feng TY, Hobbins J, Copel JA, et al. First-trimester endocervical irrigation: feasibility of obtaining trophoblast cells for prenatal diagnosis. *Obstet Gynecol* 1995;85(3):461–464.

89. Rodeck C, Tutschek B, Sherlock J, Kingdom J. Methods for the transcervical collection of fetal cells during the first trimester of pregnancy. *Prenat Diagn* 1995;15(10):933–942.

90. Bulmer JN, Rodeck C, Adinolfi M. Immunohistochemical characterization of cells retrieved by transcervical sampling in early pregnancy. *Prenat Diagn* 1995;15(12):1143–1153.

91. Munne S, Magli C, Bahce M, Fung J, Legator M, et al. Preimplantation diagnosis of the aneuploidies most commonly

found in spontaneous abortions and live births: XY, 13, 14, 15, 16, 18, 21, 22. *Prenat Diagn* 1998;18(13):1459–1466.

92. ESHRE PGD Consortium Steering Committee. ESHRE preimplantation genetic diagnosis (PGD) consortium: preliminary assessment of data from January 1997 to September 1998. *Hum Reprod* 1999;14:3138–3148.

93. Munne S, Magli C, Cohen J, Morton P, Sadowy S, et al. Positive outcome after preimplantation diagnosis of aneuploidy in human embryos. *Hum Reprod* 1999;14(9):2191–2199.

94. Gianaroli L, Magli MC, Munne S, Fortini D, Ferraretti AP. Advantages of day 4 embryo transfer in patients undergoing preimplantation genetic diagnosis of aneuploidy. *J Assist Reprod Genet* 1999;16(4):170–175.

95. Magli MC, Glanaroli L, Fortini D, Ferraretti AP, Munne S. Impact of blastomere biopsy and cryopreservation techniques on human embryo viability. *Hum Reprod* 1999;14(3):770–773.

96. Munne S, Sepulveda S, Balmaceda J, Fernandez E, Fabres C, et al. Selection of the most common chromosome abnormalities in oocytes prior to ICSI. *Prenat Diagn* 2000; 20(7):582–586.

97. Verlinsky Y, Cieslak J, Ivakhnenko V, Evsikov S, Wolf G, et al. Prevention of age-related aneuploidies by polar body testing of oocytes. *J Assist Reprod Genet* 1999;16(4):165–169.

98. Simpson JL, Elias S. Isolating fetal cells from maternal blood. Advances in prenatal diagnosis through molecular technology. *JAMA* 1993;270(19):2357–2361.

99. Bianchi DW. Fetal cells in the maternal circulation: feasibility for prenatal diagnosis. *Br J Haematol* 1999;105:574–583.

100. Pertl B, Bianchi DW. Fetal DNA in maternal plasma: emerging clinical applications. *Obstet Gynecol* 2001;98:483–490.

101. Tijo JH, Levan A. The chromosome number of man. *Hereditas* 1956;42:1–6.

102. Ford CE, Hamerton JL. The chromosomes of man. *Nature* 1956;178:1020–1023.

103. Lejeune J, Jautier M, Turpin MR. Etude des chromosomes somatiques de neuf infant mongoliens. *CR Acad Sci (Paris)* 1959:248:1721–1722.

104. Steele MW, Breg WR. Chromosome analysis of human amniotic-fluid cells. *Lancet* 1966;i:7434.

105. Yunis JJ. High resolution of human chromosomes. *Science* 1976;191:1268–1270.

106. Cremer T, Landegent J, Bruckner A, School HP, Schardin M, et al. Detection of chromosome aberrations in the human interphase nucleus by visualization of specific target DNAs with radioactive and non-radioactive in situ hybridization techniques: diagnosis of trisomy 18 with probe L1.84. *Hum Genet* 1986;74:346–352.

107. Avery OT, MacLeod CM, MacCarty M. Studies on the chemical nature of the substance inducing transformation of pneumococcal types. *J Exp Med* 1994;79:136–158.

108. Nirenberg M. Protein synthesis and the RNA code. Harvey lectures. 1965;59:155–185.

109. Southern EM. Detection of specific sequences among DNA fragments separated by gel electrophoresis. *J Molecular Biol* 1975;98:503–517.

110. Kan YW, Dozy AM. Antenatal diagnosis of sickle-cell anemia by DNA analysis of amniotic-fluid cells. *Lancet* 1978;2: 910–912.

111. Mullis K, Faloona F, Schart S, Saiki R, Horn G, et al. Specific enzyme amplification of DNA in vitro: the polymerase chain reaction. 1986. *Biotechnology* 1992;24:17–27.

THREE-DIMENSIONAL ULTRASOUND IN OBSTETRICS

There is no question that fetal ultrasound has revolutionized the field of obstetrics. Before the emergence of ultrasound, clinicians and families had little information about the health of the growing fetus. In the early 1970s, two-dimensional static-scanning ultrasound (2DUS) permitted physicians to view the fetus for the first time. A further advance was real-time B-mode imaging in the early 1980s. Beginning in the late 1980s, ultrasonography underwent a significant improvement when three-dimensional ultrasound (3DUS) was introduced.[1-3] 3DUS provides physicians and expectant families with more accurate information about the developing fetus.[4,5] Data also can be acquired by less-experienced personnel, then evaluated by a trained professional who can adjust and optimize the image quality to see the fetus, uterus, and adnexa in more detail.

Families, obstetricians, and pediatricians benefit from improved prenatal diagnosis, providing better care of newborns, particularly with congenital anomalies. The advantages of three-dimensional ultrasonography are summarized in Table 1.[1]

This chapter reviews applications of 3DUS in obstetric imaging that show promise in providing information not readily available with 2DUS regarding normal and abnormal pregnancy and fetal development. A brief review of 3DUS acquisition and display methods is given. The overall approach is to provide a review of applications to imaging in the first trimester followed by the second- and third-trimester imaging. Within each trimester grouping, the applications of 3DUS to fetal evaluation are reviewed by organ sections. Certainly the improved visualization of the fetus provided by 3DUS continues to enhance the ability to understand and observe fetal development. Future improvements will continue to push back the limits to the ability to evaluate earlier stages of development plus life within the womb.

Data from several centers suggest that 3DUS can provide additional information compared to conventional 2DUS in evaluating fetal anomalies. Merz et al. studied 204 patients with anomalies and found that 3DUS was advantageous in demonstrating fetal defects in 127 (62%), equivalent in 73 (36%), and disadvantageous in 4 (2%).[4] Dyson and Pretorius et al. reported similar results in 63 patients with 103 anomalies: 3DUS was advantageous in 53 (51%), equivalent in 46 (45%), and disadvantageous in 4 (4%).[6] This enhanced imaging had many important implications. Several anomalies were identified only on 3DUS (e.g., cleft lip, abnormal facies), but the majority was better visualized with 3DUS compared with 2DUS.[4,6] Patient management was changed in only 5% of patients, but the improved visualization from multiplanar images as well as rendered images assisted the physicians and families in understanding the anomalies.

ACQUISITION OF VOLUME DATA

In conventional 2DUS a single plane of image information is acquired using conventional transducers. 3DUS acquires a cube or volume of data using a variety of techniques, including a volume probe with a mechanically swept transducer, a conventional 2DUS probe with an attached positional sensor, a conventional 2DUS probe without position sensing, or a 2-D array transducer.[1] Volume data are obtained rapidly and evaluated at the time of the examination and after the patient has left the clinic. When evaluating the fetus, volumes should be acquired during times that the fetus is quiet and repeated if the fetus moves during the acquisition. In general, one or two volumes are needed to evaluate a region. If abnormalities are identified, multiple data sets may be needed.

New technology permits images to be acquired at up to 16 frames per second, which permits viewing of fetal movements and opens the possibility of assessing movement and performing functional studies.

DISPLAY OF VOLUME DATA

2DUS presents a single plane of image information on a monitor or film. In 3DUS a cube or volume of data can be

TABLE 1. ADVANTAGES OF THREE-DIMENSIONAL ULTRASONOGRAPHY IN OBSTETRICS

Rapid acquisition of volume data
Improved identification of suspected or detected anomalies
More accurate identification of the extent and size of anomalies
    not seen with two-dimensional static-scanning ultrasound
    using orientations and planes unobtainable with two-dimen-
    sional static-scanning ultrasound
Improved recognition of anomalies by less experienced physicians
Improved comprehension of fetal anatomy by families
Improved maternal-fetal bonding

viewed as single or multiple planes or in combination with a rendered image, which conveys information from the entire volume in a single image. In rendered images, specific features within the volume may be emphasized to more clearly present anatomy compared to a single planar image. For example, the bones of the skeleton or blood in vessels may be displayed. Perhaps the best-known and compelling rendered images are those of the fetal face, which are immediately recognizable to parents and physicians alike (Fig. 1).

Most equipment vendors show multiplanar images as three orthogonal planes similar to 2DUS images. Rotation of volume data into a standard orientation makes it possible to view longitudinal, transverse, and coronal planes simultaneously, which often improves identification and comprehension of anatomy or pathology (Fig. 2). Furthermore, viewing multiplanar images makes it possible to view planes that are not possible to obtain with 2DUS because of fetal position or restrictions related to anatomy. A cursor showing the point of common intersection provides a reference of the three multiplanar images to each other. Volume data are typically evaluated by rotating the volume to a standard orientation and then scrolling through parallel planes. In some cases it is helpful to rotate the data around the localizing cursor to assess oblique planes. Multiplanar

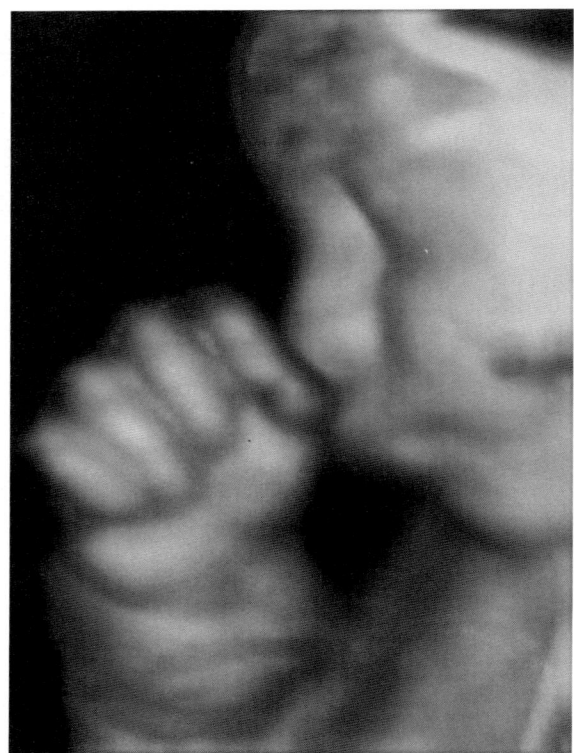

FIGURE 1. Normal face and hand at 32 weeks' gestation.

displays are valuable for assessing anatomy, particularly for internal fetal anatomy such as the anterior palate.

Rendering of volume data permits information from throughout the volume to be projected onto a single image. Various algorithms are used, which vary opacity, transparency, and depth to form the rendered images. An important feature of rendering algorithms is that they provide the physician with interactive control over the rendering parameters to optimize the display. Although some systems

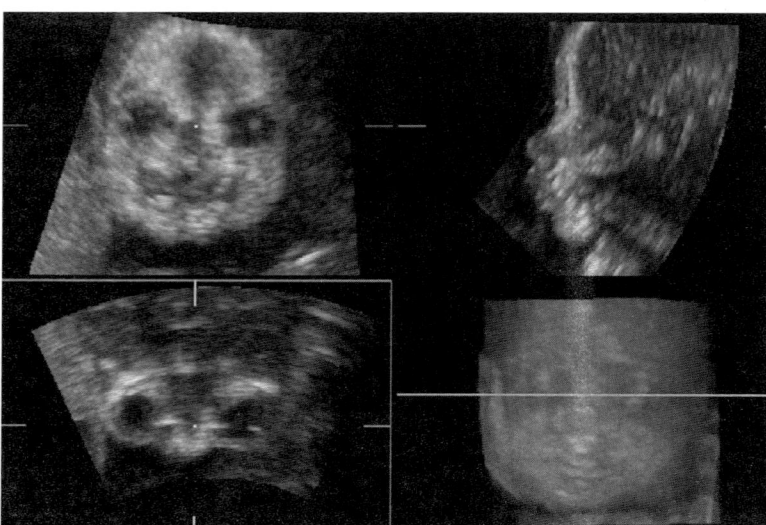

FIGURE 2. Normal face at 24 weeks' gestational age. Multiplanar images of the face in the **upper left** (coronal), **upper right** (sagittal), and **lower left** (axial) boxes. A normal volume-rendered image of the face is seen in the **lower right** image.

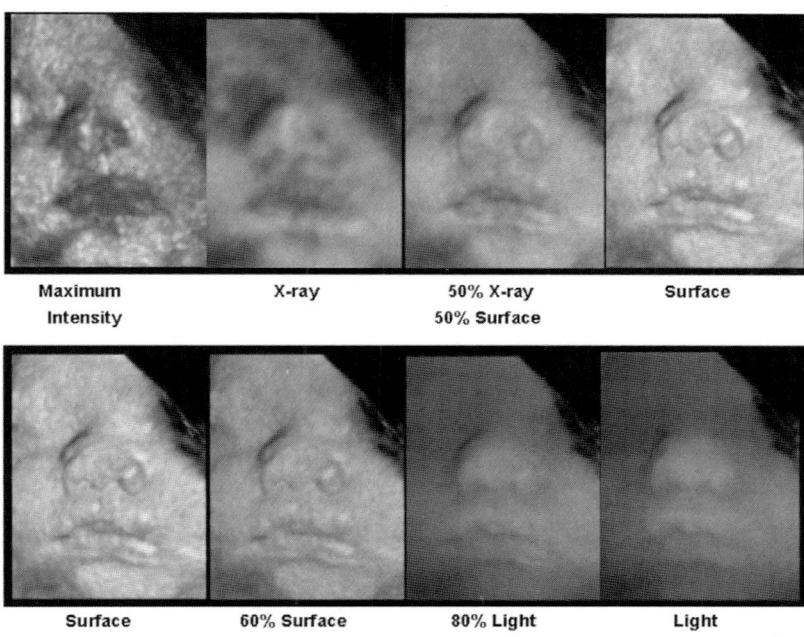

| Maximum Intensity | X-ray | 50% X-ray 50% Surface | Surface |

| Surface | 60% Surface 40% Light | 80% Light 20% Surface | Light |

FIGURE 3. Images of a fetal face showing the effect of different types of rendering. (Reproduced with permission from Nelson TR, Downey DB, Pretorius DH, Fenster A. *Three-dimensional ultrasound.* Philadelphia: Lippincott, Williams & Wilkins, 1999.)

are automated, the physician generally selects the rendering algorithm that is optimal for a particular organ or structure. The quality of the rendered images is directly related to the original 2DUS image quality from the acquisition. High-quality rendered images of fetal surfaces require sufficient amniotic fluid adjacent to the area of interest to clearly differentiate the surface. When combined with multiplanar displays, the rendered image provides a valuable guide for localization of anatomic references. Generally rendering approaches use one or two basic strategies to present anatomic features (Fig. 3). To display the fetal surface or vascular structures, the rendering algorithm is adjusted to emphasize the interface between the amniotic fluid and the fetal skin surface. Shading and blending parameters permit adjustment to emphasize soft-tissue features. Images of the fetal face, limbs, and body appear similar to what is actually seen by fetoscopy or postnatally. Rendering allows the curved surfaces of the fetal face or other structures to be viewed in a single image. When the surface is adjacent to other tissues (e.g., placenta) or in a shadow zone, then image quality is degraded.

To display features of the fetal skeleton, other rendering approaches using some degree of transparency are used, such as maximum intensity projection. Maximum intensity projection methods register the highest gray levels along the projection direction, which tends to enhance hyperechoic structures. The fetal skeleton is well visualized using this mode because the contribution from soft tissues is greatly reduced. In a similar fashion, minimum intensity projection methods can be used to accentuate hypoechoic structures such as cysts or blood vessels.[7]

Because the fetus is surrounded by other structures and tissues, some of which can obscure important diagnostic information, editing tools have been developed to assist in optimizing rendered image presentation. For example, echoes from overlying placenta can be eliminated or erased from the volume to view the fetal structure more clearly. This is often helpful in evaluating the fetal face (removing adjacent placenta, cord, or limbs) or limbs.

THREE-DIMENSIONAL ULTRASOUND IN THE FIRST TRIMESTER

In the first trimester of pregnancy, 3DUS is an excellent tool that permits extensive evaluation of the embryo. Volume data are acquired with transvaginal transducers and rotated to identify the desired structures. Using multiple planar views, the anatomy can be evaluated in standard planes. Hull and colleagues have shown that significantly more anatomic structures were identified with 3DUS than 2DUS (Fig. 4).[8] In this way, a more accurate fetal anomaly survey can be performed, particularly in instances where fetuses are at increased risk for chromosomal abnormalities. Structures such as the limbs, cord insertion, stomach, and bladder can be routinely evaluated. The examiner also may look for nuchal lucency (Fig. 5) or nuchal thickening, which may raise suspicions for chromosome abnormalities as well as other anomalies (Fig. 6).[9,10] 3DUS permits the embryo to be rotated into a sagittal plane easily, irrespective of the plane of acquisition. In addition, the length of time that the patient was scanned with the transducer was signif-

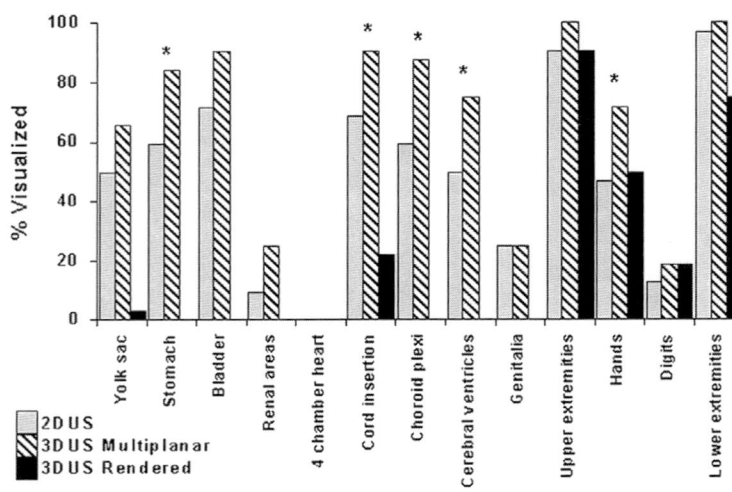

FIGURE 4. Visualization of fetal anatomic structures using two-dimensional static-scanning ultrasound (2DUS), multiplanar three-dimensional ultrasound (3DUS), and rendered 3DUS. Statistically significant differences between 2DUS and multiplanar 3DUS for individual anatomic features are indicated by asterisks placed above the bars. [Reproduced with permission from Hull AD, James G, Salerno C, Nelson T, Pretorius D. Three-dimensional ultrasound and the assessment of the first trimester fetus. *J Ultrasound Med* 2001;20(4):287–293.]

icantly less with 3DUS (2.7 minutes) compared to 2DUS (14.7 minutes).[8]

The embryology of the first 13 weeks of fetal life has also been examined with 3DUS by Blaas et al.[11,12] as well as Benoit. It is possible to see the cavities of the brain as early as 7 weeks' gestational age.[11,12] The cavities of the brain grow and develop with time, and the volume of the cavities can be accurately measured with 3DUS. Lack of identification of cavities (i.e., a dense head) after 8 weeks suggests abnormal brain development, and serial ultrasound examinations are recommended (B. Benoit, *personal communication*, 2000) (Fig. 7).

Manipulation of volume data showing the embryo in the first trimester should allow for improved assessment of congenital anomalies because planes can be examined from transvaginal acquisitions that could not be obtained with 2DUS. Several reports have identified such anomalies, including conjoined twins[13] and cardiac ectopia.[14]

Rendered images of embryos are very lifelike and patients respond to them immediately (Fig. 8). Surface features such as the limbs and cord insertion are generally shown well. Steiner et al. have shown that the volume of the gestational sac can be measured in the first trimester and that it is more predictive of a successful pregnancy outcome than the level of several maternal hormone levels.[15]

THREE-DIMENSIONAL ULTRASOUND IN THE SECOND AND THIRD TRIMESTERS

3DUS is very useful during the second and third trimesters for detecting as well as excluding abnormalities. 3DUS has been used to characterize many anomalies including those

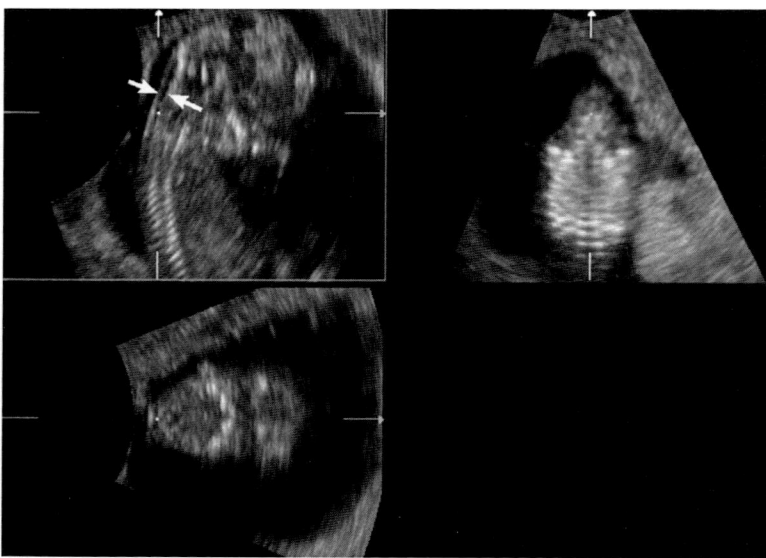

FIGURE 5. Normal nuchal lucency at 12 weeks' gestational age. Multiplanar images show that the embryo has been rotated into a standard orientation for measurement of the nuchal lucency (*arrows*). The embryo is in a midline sagittal plane in the **upper left** image, coronal plane in the **upper right** image, and in the axial plane in the **lower left** image.

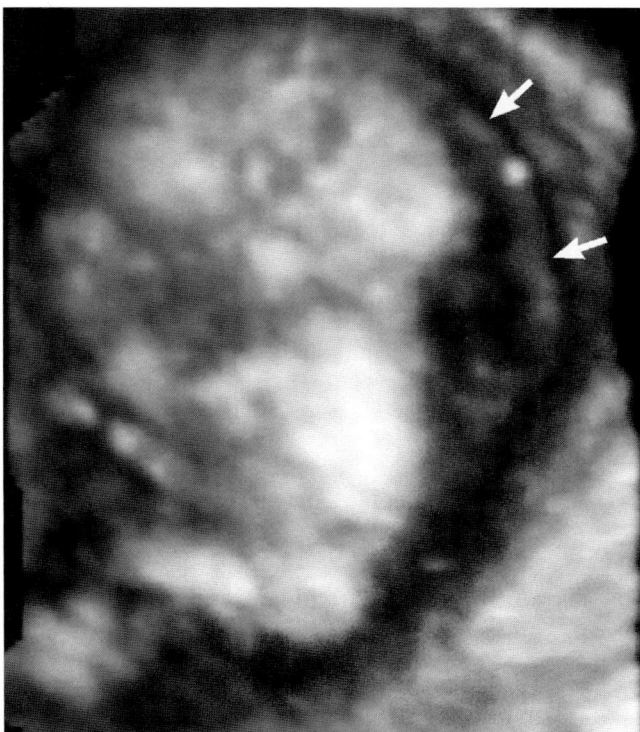

FIGURE 6. Cystic hygroma at 12 weeks' gestational age. Sagittal view of the volume-rendered image of the fetus shows a bulge in the posterior neck consistent with a cystic hygroma (*arrows*).

of the face, skull, brain, spine, heart, limbs, urinary tract, umbilical cord, and placenta. 3DUS has also been used to verify normal anatomy when an abnormality was suspected

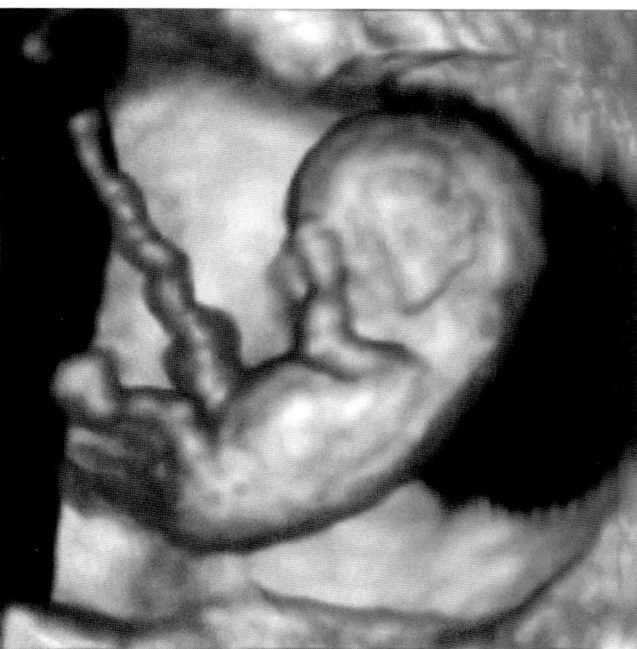

FIGURE 8. Normal embryo at 10 weeks' gestational age. The embryo is seen with the umbilical cord entering the abdomen. The head is to the right of the image, and the legs are to the left.

using conventional imaging and in patients at high risk for anomalies. Additional clinical applications are being identified, such as fetal weight estimation, cerebral anomalies, placenta, cord and cervix evaluation, and identification of uterine anomalies such as bicornuate versus septate uterus in pregnant patients.

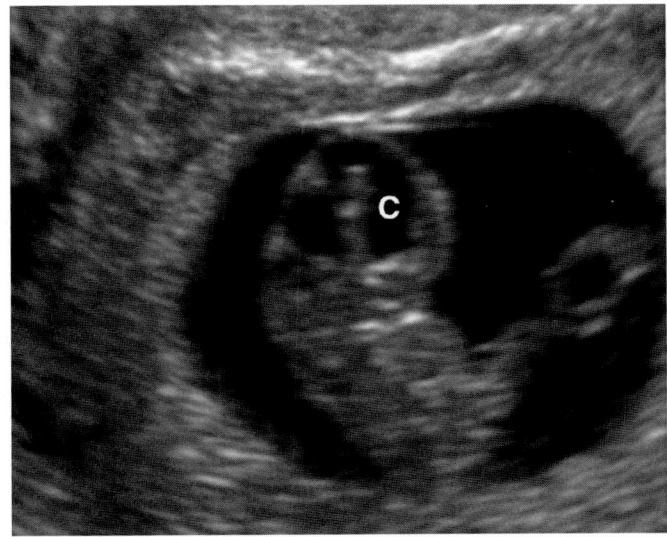

A

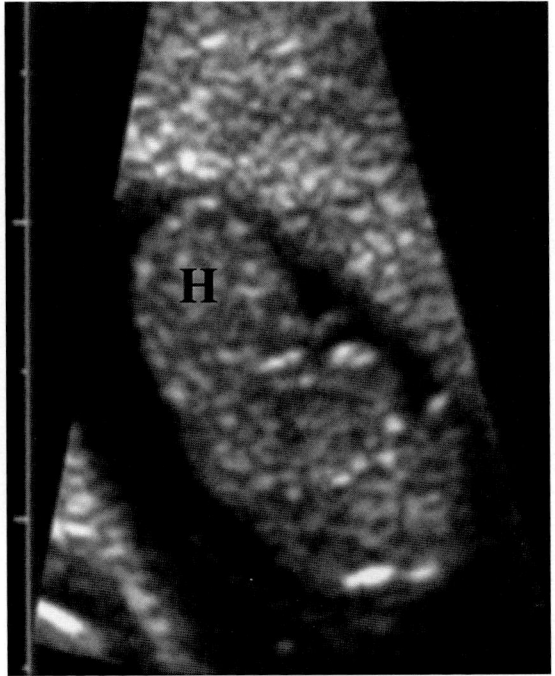

B

FIGURE 7. Embryos at 8 weeks' gestational age. **A:** The normal head has lucent areas, which correspond to the intracerebral ventricular cavities (*C*). **B:** An abnormal head (*H*) appears dense, without lucent areas, at 8 weeks. This fetus developed hydrocephalus several weeks later. (Courtesy of Dr. Bernard Benoit, Nice, France.)

As patients have become aware of 3DUS, requests for studies for reassurance are more frequent. This is a sensitive area with many conflicting opinions within the medical community. Information regarding parental-fetal bonding is discussed later.

FACIAL ANOMALIES

The most valuable aspect of using 3DUS for evaluation of the face lies in the ability of the operator to rotate the face into a standard anatomic orientation such that the examiner looks directly at an upright face (Fig. 2); he or she can then scroll through the face millimeter by millimeter using a reference plane from the orthogonal views or the rendered image to identify accurately the location of the targeted plane. The lip is best evaluated in the coronal plane with the face tipped posteriorly slightly, whereas the palate and chin are best evaluated with the face directly upright in the axial and sagittal planes, respectively. With experience, we have found that the axial plane is also an excellent plane to assess for continuity of the normal lip or clefting of the lip, information that has been translated into improved scanning with conventional 2DUS when 3DUS is unavailable.

Multiplanar views of the face can generally be obtained in most fetuses, whereas surface-rendered displays are obtained successfully in only 70% of patients.[16] Rendered images are very lifelike for patients and physicians; normal images can be very reassuring to families with increased risk for facial anomalies. Editing tools now allow the volume to be modified to optimize the surface-rendered images by erasing or eliminating adjacent structures. Rendered surface images are best acquired between 20 and 35 weeks' gestational age according to Merz et al.[16]; we have found that a shorter window from 24 to 30 weeks is more practical in the clinical setting. However, we expect this window to extend earlier into gestation as the equipment develops. It is necessary to have some amniotic fluid adjacent to the face to obtain adequate rendered images. At times, this can be facilitated by tapping on the maternal abdomen with the examiner's finger at a distance from the transducer, moving the mother into different positions or having her walk or exercise.

In several studies, 3DUS has been shown to be beneficial in detecting facial anomalies such as cleft lip or palate, micrognathia, midface hypoplasia, asymmetric facies, facial masses, hypo/hypertelorism, facial dysmorphia, holoprosencephaly, and deformed ears.[1,4,16–21] Although a few anomalies (e.g., cleft lip or palate, micrognathia, flat facies, unilateral orbital hypoplasia, cranial ossification defect)[14,15,19] have been detected on 3DUS that were not detected on 2DUS, generally, 3DUS has offered an improved understanding of the anomalies detected on 2DUS for the physician and the family, clarification of the extent of anomalies, and a visual image of the reality of the anomaly for the family.

3DUS offers significant advantages in evaluating the face for cleft lip and primary palate. Cleft lip and palate are important for families to be aware of prenatally, because decisions regarding continuation of pregnancy, breast versus bottle-feeding, specialty care, and even insurance options can be discussed before delivery. The primary benefits of 3DUS for cleft lip and palate are in assessing the anterior alveolar ridge (primary or hard palate) for clefting and for showing the rendered image of the cleft to the family (Fig. 9).[17,21–23] Lee et al. reported that the rendered image also assisted in identifying premaxillary protrusion from bilateral cleft lip and palate that was not appreciated on multiplanar imaging. They were also able to tilt the rendered image to visualize a cleft palate defect in one case; this was not possible with 2DUS.[21] Rendered images are rotated from side to side to demonstrate the anatomy to families and consulting physicians.

Multiplanar imaging in a standard orientation allows the examiner to be more confident of his or her interpretation than conventional 2DUS with real-time.[23] The anterior alveolar ridge is best evaluated in the axial plane; the volumes should be acquired in the axial plane if possible to obtain the highest resolution possible. The best-rendered images of the face are generally acquired in the profile up plane or the frontal plane. The localizing cursor should be positioned on the cleft lip in the coronal view and then identified on the axial view to confirm that a suspected lucency seen on the axial view connects to the cleft lip and is a cleft palate rather than a normal nostril. The nostrils frequently are not parallel in fetuses with cleft lip because of the distorted anatomy and thus can be misinterpreted as a cleft palate. In a series of fetuses referred for cleft lip and palate, it was found that 2DUS identified only 10 of 22 cleft palates, whereas 3DUS identified 19.[23] In addition, seven patients had a change of management: four changed their mind about continuation of pregnancy, and three learned that their fetuses had a normal lip. In another study of 63 fetuses, it was found that 3DUS was useful for confirming the presence of normal lips in fetuses less than 24 weeks' gestational age, especially in families with a history of cleft lip and palate.[17] It is still not possible to identify all cleft lips and palates accurately with 3DUS; some fetuses are not in an appropriate position, or scanning parameters may not be optimal. In our experience as well as Lee et al.,[21] fetuses with a suspected unilateral cleft lip and palate were born with bilateral cleft lip and palate.

The fetal tooth germs can be a clue to prenatal diagnosis, as many genetic syndromes and facial abnormalities are associated with oligodontia or anodontia. The most common of these include facial clefts and Down syndrome. Ulm et al. reported that 3DUS was useful in identifying the tooth germs and in characterizing facial clefts.[24] The mineralized, echogenic portions of the fetal tooth buds can be visualized from as early as the 18th week of gestation. Fetuses with cleft palate often lack the tooth germs in the area of the cleft,

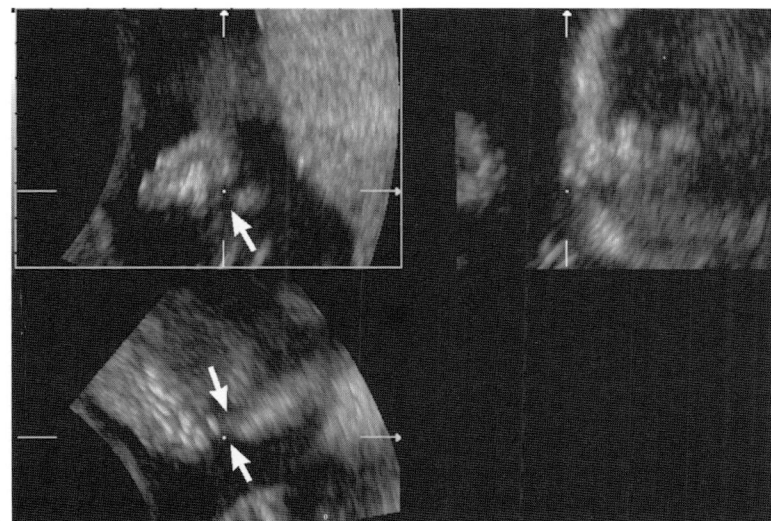

A

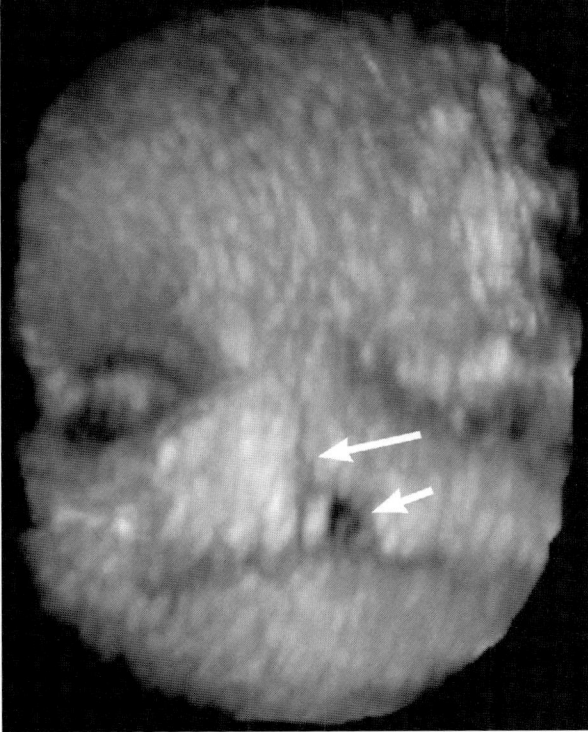

B

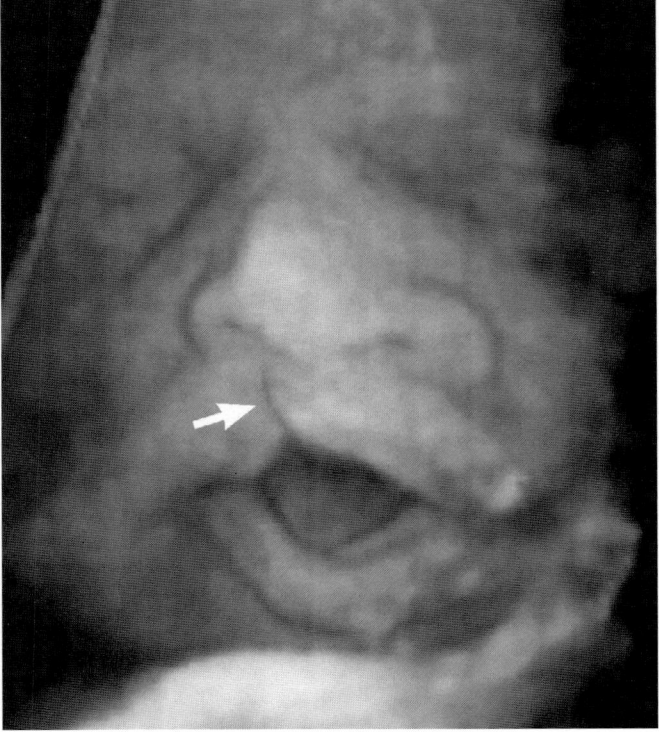

C

FIGURE 9. Cleft lip and palate. **A:** Multiplanar images of the face in the **upper left** image (coronal), **upper right** image (sagittal), and through the palate in the **lower left** image (axial) at 28 weeks' gestational age. **B:** Rendered image of the face in **(A)** showing the cleft lip. Short arrow points to cleft lip and long arrow points to cleft palate. **C:** Rendered image of cleft lip (*arrow*) in another fetus. (Courtesy of Dr. Bernard Benoit, Nice, France.)

which is recognized by seeing an interruption in the continuity of the anterior alveolar ridge. Visualization of fetal tooth buds is often more difficult in fetuses with clefts because of the displacement of the maxillary and mandibular arches and the tongue lying in the area of the cleft. Axial evaluation also permits evaluation of the orbits for hypertelorism, because this is occasionally a component of facial clefting.

Artifacts in 3DUS volumes can also simulate clefting of normal lips. It is important to recognize these artifacts so that accurate diagnoses are made. Artifacts include shadowing from a portion of the umbilical cord lying adjacent to the

fetal face,[18,25] motion during acquisition, shadowing from the nasal bone, and misinterpretation of the nostril as a cleft.

3DUS allows the fetal profile to be examined accurately and in the correct anatomic location. When a volume of the fetal face is acquired, the profile image can be obtained irrespective of the orientation of acquisition. It is often difficult to obtain a profile image on 2DUS scanning but nearly always possible with 3DUS. Rotation of the volume into a standard orientation allows the midsagittal image of the profile to be obtained consistently and accurately. Merz et al. found that without multiplanar imaging, the profile was off

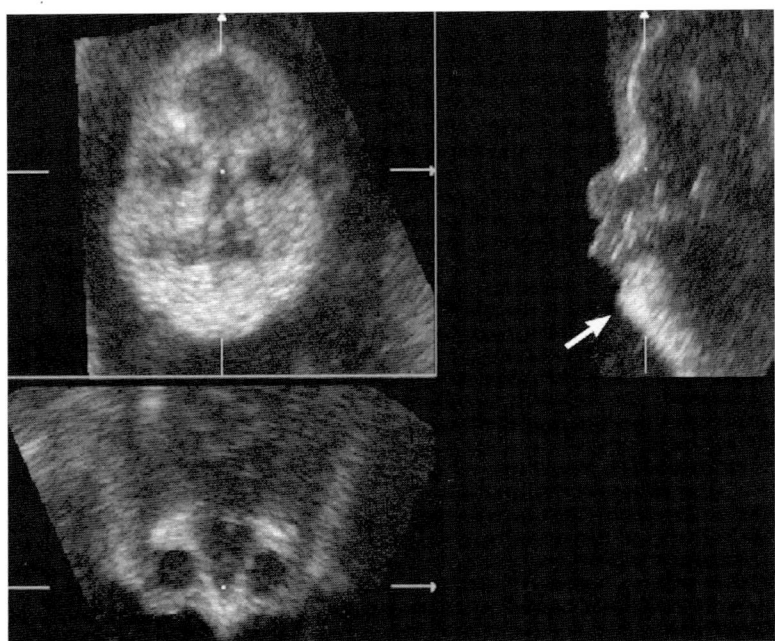

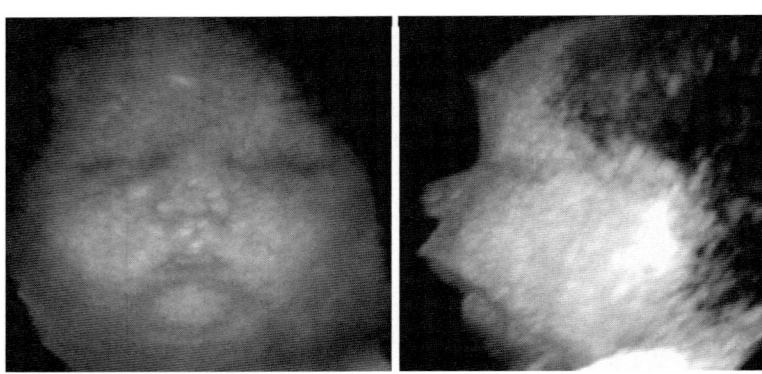

FIGURE 10. Micrognathia at 35 weeks' gestational age. **A:** Multiplanar images of the face in the **upper left** (coronal), **upper right** (sagittal), and **lower left** (axial). The small chin (*arrow*) is seen best on the sagittal view in the **upper right** image. **B:** Volume-rendered image of the face in the frontal and profile projections.

by up to 20 degrees in 30.4% of 125 cases; using 3DUS, the true sagittal plane could be correctly identified immediately.[16] The profile image is useful in diagnosing micrognathia (Fig. 10), midface hypoplasia, sloping forehead, flat facies,[26] and flat noses. 3DUS has been useful in identifying micrognathia when the 2DUS was interpreted as normal.[1,17]

In addition to the face, the ears can also be evaluated with 3DUS. Shih et al. studied 125 fetuses and were able to reconstruct successfully the ears in 105 cases.[27] In their series, 18 had abnormal ears, including microtia, low set position, abnormal orientation, abnormal lobulation, and edema. Many syndromes are associated with abnormal ears and include chromosomal anomalies; pharyngeal arch syndromes; holoprosencephaly; Crouzon's disease; Treacher Collins syndrome; vertebral, anus, cardiac, tracheal, renal, and limb syndrome; and coloboma of the eye, heart anomaly, choanal atresia, retardation, and genital and ear anomalies association.[27]

Limitations to 3DUS of the face are a reality. As indicated, several clinical scenarios make it impossible to obtain an adequate rendered image of the face (e.g., lack of amniotic fluid either positional or in cases of oligohydramnios, a limb obscuring the face (Fig. 11), the face positioned too close to the uterine wall or placenta, and an early gestational age fetus). Although multiplanar images can generally be obtained, occasionally these are not possible either, primarily because of the position of the face in the uterus.

Artifacts of the face are also important limitations of 3DUS and should be recognized by examiners.[25] Overthresholding leads to the appearance of black eyes (Fig. 12) and inappropriate rendering may lead to the appearance of a single nostril (Fig. 13). Artifacts simulating cleft lip and palate are previously discussed within this section.

FETAL HEAD

Mueller et al. reported that 3DUS is useful in demonstrating skull defects, particularly in the multiplanar orthogonal

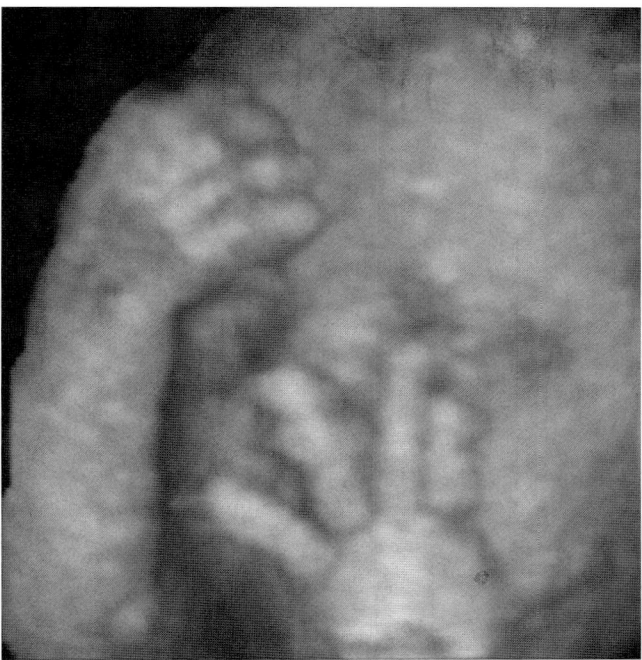

FIGURE 11. Normal face obscured by hands at 30 weeks' gestational age.

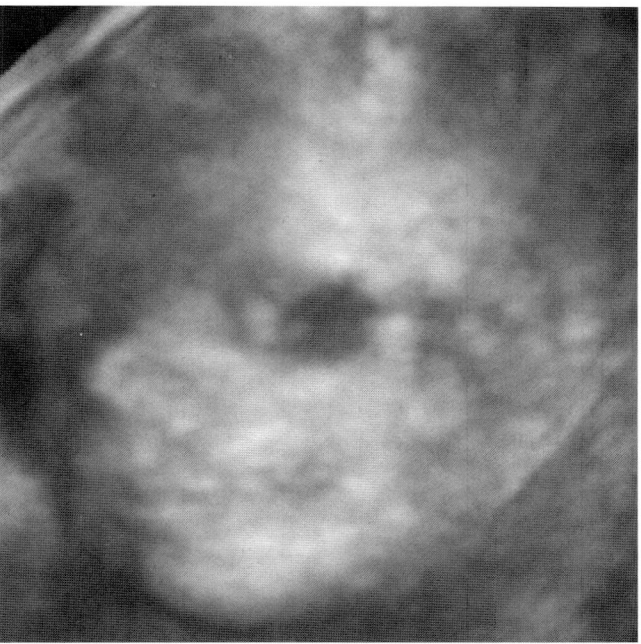

FIGURE 12. Artifact showing black eyes. Oblique volume-rendered view of the face showing black eyes, which are a result of overthresholding.

planes.[28] We have found this to be the case in assessing encephaloceles.

Volume data allow the brain to be evaluated using new views that have been previously used in assessing the neonatal brain. Timor-Tritsch et al. emphasized use of the oblique *three-horn view* to evaluate the lateral ventricles; in this view, the anterior, inferior, and posterior horns are all visualized. The authors note that any fluid in the inferior horn is abnormal and an early sign of ventriculomegaly.[29]

Symmetry of intracranial pathology can be accurately and rapidly assessed with 3DUS. The volume of the brain is rotated into standard orientation to assess asymmetric conditions such as hemorrhage, ventricular dilatation, and parenchymal destruction (Fig. 14).

Location of a marker dot within the volume allows the clinician to navigate through cystic structures, ventricles, parenchyma, and along vascular structures. Monteagudo et al. gave several examples of when this technology was

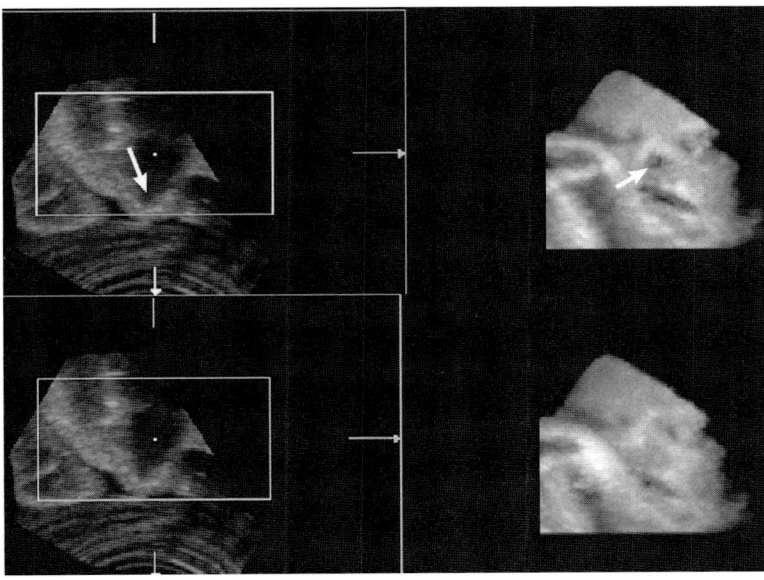

FIGURE 13. Artifact suggesting that the fetus has a single nostril in a volume-rendering image of the face. **Upper left** image shows the rendering line through tip of nose, which results in a pseudo single nostril. Arrow points to the region of shadowing from the nasal bone. **Lower left** image shows the rendering line positioned inferiorly off the nose, and the pseudo single nostril is no longer seen. The images on the **right** are volume-rendered images associated with the planar images on the **left**.

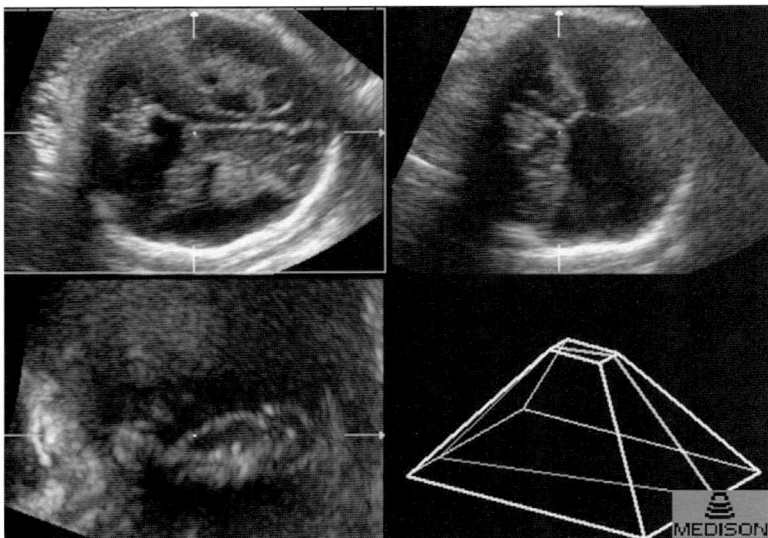

FIGURE 14. Cerebral dysgenesis at 37 weeks' gestational age. Multiplanar images through the fetal brain show asymmetric, abnormal brain parenchyma. **Upper left** (axial), **upper right** (coronal), and **lower left** (sagittal).

extremely beneficial.[30] First, in evaluating agenesis of the corpus callosum, the marker dot allowed the examiner to find the corpus callosum or lack of the callosum in sagittal and coronal planes. It also allowed the pericallosal artery to be followed through serial scans.[29,30] Second, it allowed for accurate localization of an arachnoid cyst. Third, a deviated pericallosal artery could be followed around an arachnoid cyst. The authors also reported that the 3-D volume data were helpful in informing neurosurgeons and pediatric neurologists of abnormal pathology.[30]

Intracranial anomalies have been identified as early as 8 weeks' gestational age using multiplanar, 3-D techniques (B. Benoit, *personal communication*, 2000). The cranium should have cavities seen as lucencies at 8 weeks' gestational age, whereas an abnormal brain (which later developed into hydrocephalus, Dandy Walker cyst, or encephalocele) may have the appearance of a dense brain without lucencies (Fig. 7).

Abnormal sutures and fontanelles of the skull may be a component of multiple abnormality syndromes as well as isolated anomalies. These structures are seen with improved visualization using 3DUS because the curvature can be displayed on the rendered images.[31] Preliminary results suggest that 3DUS assists in identifying craniosynostosis from the shape of the skull, which has been rotated into a symmetrical, standard orientation, as well as the position of the sutures. Some cases of craniosynostosis have normal-appearing sutures because the synostosis may occur only within the cartilage, whereas others have fused sutures as demonstrated by Benacerraf et al. in a case of Pfeiffer syndrome.[32]

An artifact involving the skull, which is common, involves the appearance of a hole in the skull and is related to setting the rendering boundaries through the cranium (Fig. 15). Another artifact occurs when the rendering box is positioned within the cranium and a pseudohydrocephalus picture is created from normal hypoechoic brain parenchyma (Fig. 16).

CENTRAL NERVOUS SYSTEM

The entire fetal spine can be acquired and evaluated from one volume in fetuses less than 13 weeks' gestational age, but in older fetuses multiple volumes are necessary. Visualization techniques allow the spine to be examined in a standard multiplanar orientation as well as along a curved flight path, which permits the vertebral bodies to be studied serially in the transverse plane. Rendering techniques that optimize bone visualization (Fig. 17), including maximum intensity and transparency modes, often provide a better

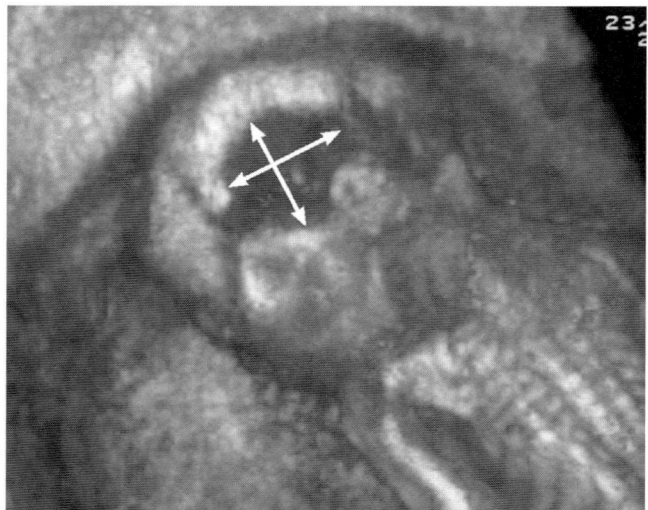

FIGURE 15. Volume-rendered image of a normal fetal cranium with a cranial artifact. An apparent hole (*arrows*) in the skull results from the boundaries of the rendering box traversing the fetal head.

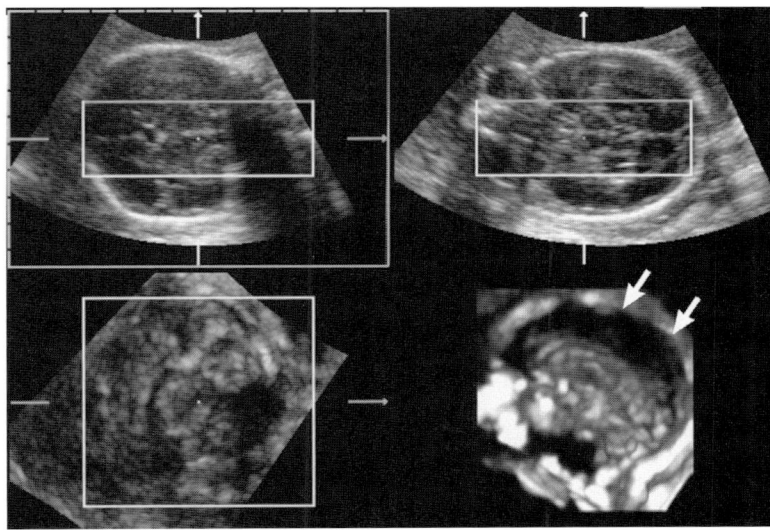

FIGURE 16. Artifact of pseudohydrocephalus. The boundaries of the rendering box are shown on the multiplanar images. The image on the **bottom right** is volume rendered; the lucent area (*arrows*) is the normal hypoechoic brain parenchyma, not dilated ventricles.

overall impression of pathology such as scoliosis and neural tube defects. Rotation of volume data permits the spine to be visualized more clearly. Endovaginal scans of the spine can be rotated to evaluate specific planes as needed—planes that are often not available with 2DUS.

It is important to identify the level of involvement of neural tube defects when evaluating fetuses prenatally, as this information is valuable in counseling families regarding prognosis. Preliminary data from two groups suggests that multiplanar evaluation of these defects allows the level to be more accurately identified with 3DUS because the transverse and coronal images can be viewed simultaneously with the rendered image (Fig. 18).[28,33] The level of the neural tube defect can be identified by counting from the twelfth rib or from the top of the iliac wing (first sacral vertebral body in the second trimester).

Scoliosis and segmentation anomalies such as hemivertebrae can be evaluated more accurately with 3DUS (Fig. 19). Visualization of these anomalies is more clearly understood by the families using the rendered images.

FETAL CARDIAC IMAGING

The fetal heart is a difficult structure to evaluate because of its motion and complexity. Volume imaging offers advantages in evaluating complex heart disease as well as the normal heart. Rotation of the heart into a standard orientation facilitates recognition of structures, normal and abnormal. To capture the rapid motion of the fetal heart, which beats at an average rate of 140 beats per minute, requires specialized equipment and algorithms. Most current clinical 3DUS equipment can only acquire static, nongated volume images of the fetal heart, which makes adequate evaluation of the fetal heart problematic.

Because the heart beats approximately nine times during a routine acquisition, motion artifacts are seen within the volume. Although early preliminary work[34] suggested that valuable information regarding the internal structure of the heart can be obtained from nongated acquisitions, the best images are generally obtained from the acquisition plane and thus are similar to 2-D imaging. The great vessels can often be reconstructed because they are nonmoving. Several studies have shown that cardiac lesions have not been iden-

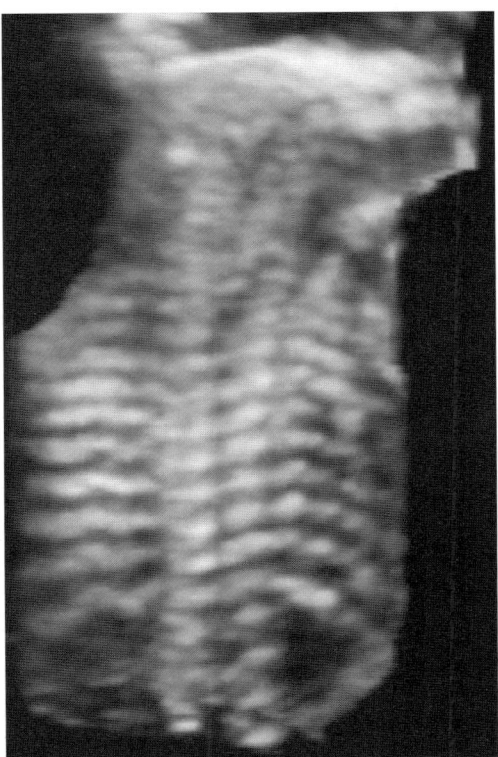

FIGURE 17. Normal spine at 25 weeks' gestational age. Volume-rendered image of the thoracic spine and thorax.

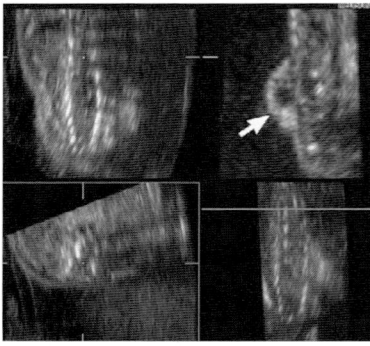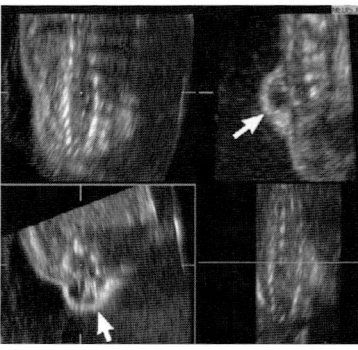

FIGURE 18. Myelocystocele at 18.5 weeks' gestational age. Multiplanar images of the spine **upper left** (coronal), **upper right** (sagittal), and **lower left** (axial). **Left** image shows multiplanar views through the spine at the second lumbar level. Notice the splaying of the spinal elements. **Right** image shows multiplanar views through the spine at the fifth lumbar level. Notice the cystocele (*arrows*).

tified accurately using nongated cardiac acquisitions.[4,35] In general, motion-related artifacts and image blurring in nongated studies degrade image quality inside the heart.

Cardiac gating is generally required to produce adequate image quality to evaluate the fetal heart. Because it is difficult to obtain adequate fetal electrocardiographic signals, other options have been explored to synchronize the cardiac cycle to volume data. Fourier analysis,[36] M-mode,[37] and Doppler[38] techniques have been used to determine the heart rate and create gated fetal cardiac images at each point throughout the cardiac cycle. Fetal cardiac anatomy has been demonstrated more consistently using gated volume

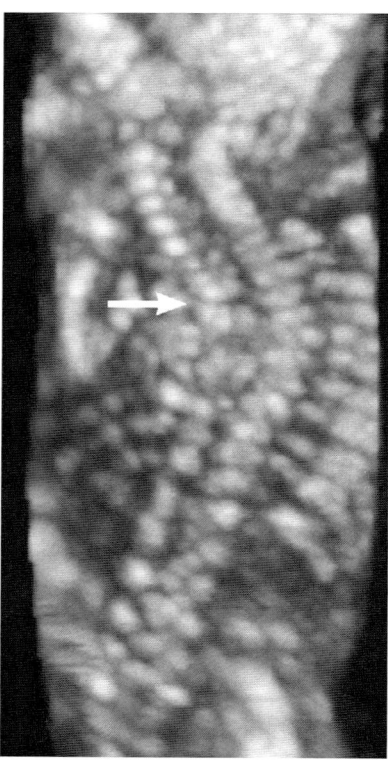

FIGURE 19. Scoliosis at 22 weeks' gestational age. Volume-rendered image of a fetal spine using maximum intensity mode showing scoliosis secondary to segmentation anomaly at the fifth thoracic vertebral level (*arrow*).

data than 2DUS methods and is less dependent on the orientation of the volume acquisition.[39] Display of cardiac gated data permits the reviewer to *slow down* the heart and evaluate the anatomy from various orientations in multiple planes throughout the cardiac cycle (Fig. 20).

Display of cardiac and great vessel anatomy includes multiplanar and volume-rendered images. Multiplanar techniques can be used to identify a specific structure or location in various planes simultaneously. For example, the optimal view of the aorta may be found by identifying a portion of the aorta in one plane, moving the cursor to that point, and rotating the volume until the optimal view is obtained. Volume-rendered images of the cardiac cavities (ventricles, atria, vessels) and valves may be helpful in assessing chamber geometry, valve configuration, and great vessel anatomy. Animation sequences with rotation and gated cine-loop displays throughout the cardiac cycle assist in understanding cardiac anatomy as well as function.

Volume measurements of the chambers can be determined using gated data; it is hopeful that this data is helpful in assessing cardiac function.[40] Several investigators also have shown that 3DUS can be used to determine the overall volume of the fetal heart using nongated techniques.[41,42]

In the future real-time volume imaging may be available for evaluation of the fetal heart. Preliminary studies suggest that this technology is applicable to the fetus[43] but more development is necessary.

FETAL ABDOMEN AND PELVIS

Congenital abnormalities of the abdomen and pelvis such as omphalocele, gastroschisis, bowel obstruction, hydronephrosis, and multicystic kidney can certainly be evaluated with 3DUS. It is unclear at this point if additional information is obtained compared to 2DUS. However, families can often understand 3DUS images of the defects more readily than 2DUS images (Fig. 21). The volume of defects, such as omphalocele and gastroschisis, can be estimated and may be of value in predicting prognosis in the future.

It is often difficult to assess ambiguous genitalia from normal genitalia with 2DUS, and 3DUS may be of bene-

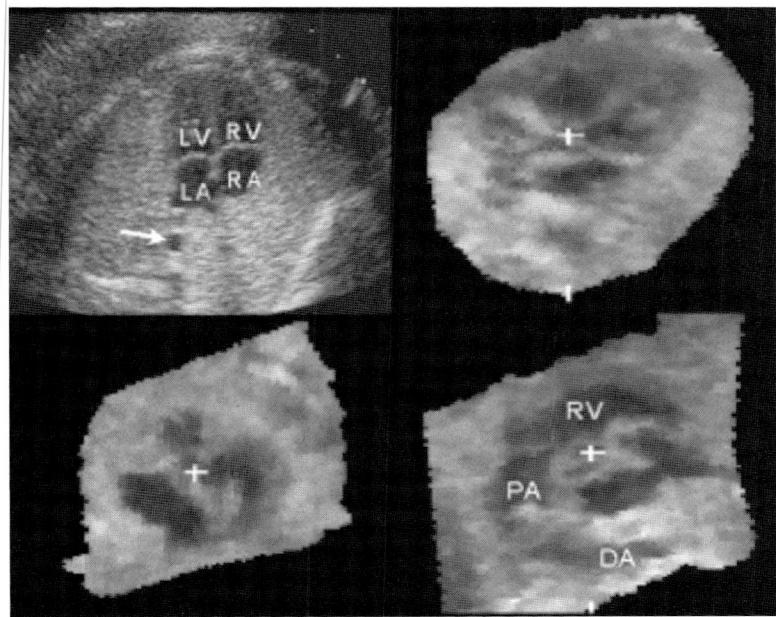

FIGURE 20. Volume rendering of fetal heart. **Upper left** image shows the four-chamber view of the heart in the acquisition plane. **Upper right** image shows the volume-rendered image of the four-chamber view. **Lower left** image shows an axial plane through the heart. **Lower right** image shows the ductal arch (*DA*). Notice that the cursor is the intersecting point in all the images. LA, left atrium; LV, left ventricle; PA, pulmonary artery; RA, right atrium; RV, right ventricle.

fit.[44] Lee and colleagues reported on one case of a bipartite scrotum that was clearly visualized with 3DUS.[45] 3DUS may also be of benefit in differentiating male from female genitalia in fetuses from 11 to 14 weeks' gestation. Lev-Toaff et al. showed that the midsagittal plane of the young fetus can be obtained easily using the multiplanar format with 3DUS and the correct genitalia identified.[46]

FETAL EXTREMITIES

Rapid acquisition techniques now allow most extremities to be assessed with 3DUS. If a limb moves during an acquisition, the volume should be deleted and another one acquired. Once a volume is obtained, the structure can be studied carefully without motion. The extremity can be rotated to a standard orientation (sagittal, axial, and coronal) and evaluated millimeter by millimeter to clearly see the relationship between the long bones and the wrist or ankle.[47–49] It is important to assess the volume for shadowing because when viewing the tibia and fibula or the radius and ulna, shadowing from the adjacent bone may lead to an artifactual shortening of one of the bones.[50] In the late second and third trimesters, the extremities are often remarkably realistic (Fig. 22).

Budorick and coauthors reported on a series of normal and abnormal hands.[48] They found that volume data did not need to be collected in any particular orientation, but rather it could be rotated into a standard position with the radius and ulna positioned vertically. Rendered images using surface and maximum intensity options are optimal for evaluating surface and bony features. 3DUS is valuable in assessing the number of digits as well as the position of loosely curled fingers, as overlapping fingers are usually abnormal.[48]

Polydactyly can be identified on multiplanar and volume-rendered images using 3DUS.[48] The ability to scroll through parallel sections allows the reviewer to count digits accu-

FIGURE 21. Omphalocele at 24 weeks' gestational age. Volume-rendered image of the omphalocele (*arrow*).

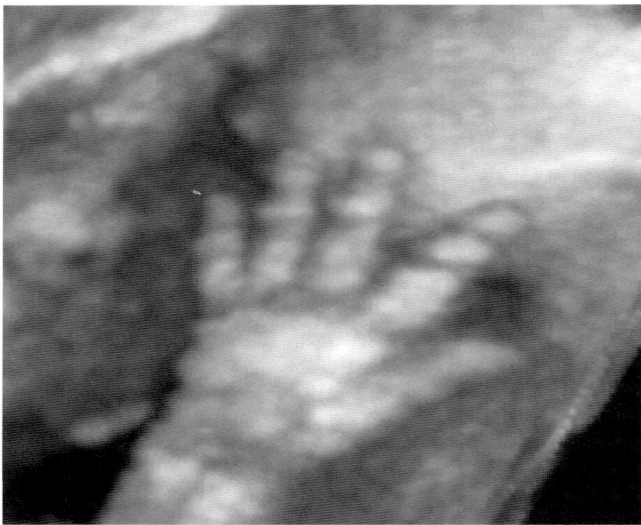

FIGURE 22. Normal fetal hand at 24 weeks' gestational age. Volume-rendered image of the fetal hand.

rately (Fig. 23). The volume-rendered images are helpful for parents to understand what the baby will look like at delivery.

Clubfeet are common anomalies that may be isolated or seen with associated anomalies. The spectrum of pathology ranges from mild to severe deformities. It is often difficult to determine whether abnormal positioning is fixed or transient; in our tertiary center, several false-positive and false-negative cases of clubfoot have occurred. 3DUS has assisted in the evaluation of clubfeet in some but not all cases.[47] Rotation of the leg into a standard orientation permits meticulous review of the relationship between the lower leg, the ankle, and the foot (Fig. 24). Experience in using 3DUS in evaluating the distal extremity has permitted

more confidence in scanning patients with 2DUS because the relationship between the lower leg and the foot are more readily understood.[1] In a normal foot, when the lower leg is optimally rotated, scrolling down a vertical long bone ends with an image of the sole of the foot, the so-called *hang ten* position, whereas with a clubfoot, the sole of the foot cannot be obtained with the lower leg vertical. Live 3-D scanning may be helpful in the future in assessing fixed positioning of extremities in the future.

3DUS offers advantages in studying fetuses with skeletal dysplasias.[26,51,52] The short ribs, abnormal bone shapes, and abnormal facies can be more accurately identified with volume acquisitions. Garjian et al. reported that 3DUS permits identification of abnormalities not seen on 2DUS in three of seven fetuses with skeletal dysplasia.[26] 3DUS permits bones to be evaluated that are generally not a part of the routine evaluation. For example, a hypoplastic scapula was detected on 3DUS that was not initially seen on 2DUS; this observation narrowed the differential diagnosis to a specific entity—camptomelic dysplasia (Fig. 25). Rendered images allow families to comprehend anomalies with shortened limbs more readily than 2-D images.

FETAL WEIGHT

Volume estimations of the fetus near term are desirable, but it has not been possible to obtain volumes through the entire fetus. Estimated fetal weights have been predicted using volume data acquired from the fetal abdomen and extremities.[53–58] Most investigators have measured a fractional volume of an extremity by tracing the circumference of the limb over several slices and then permitting the equipment to calculate the partial volume. These studies are encouraging. Schild et al. found that upper-arm and thigh volumes corre-

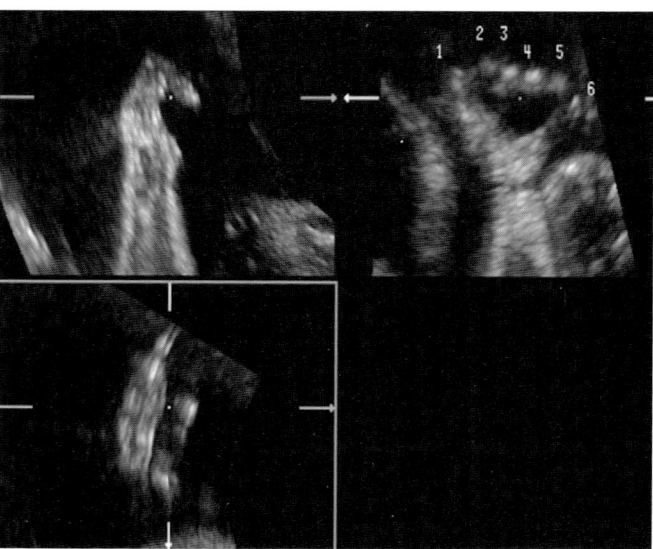

A,B

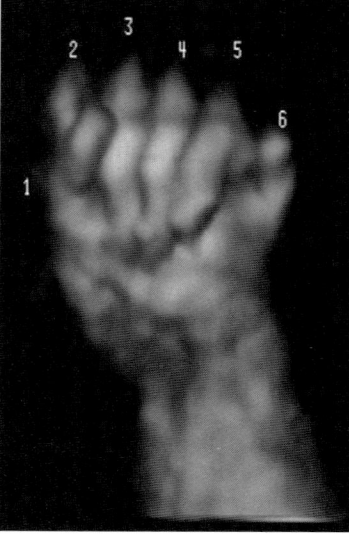

FIGURE 23. Polydactyly at 27 weeks' gestational age. **A:** Image shows multiplanar images of the hand **upper left** (sagittal), **upper right** (coronal), and **lower left** (axial). **B:** Image shows rendered image of the hand showing polydactyly with extra digit (*6*) on lateral aspect of hand.

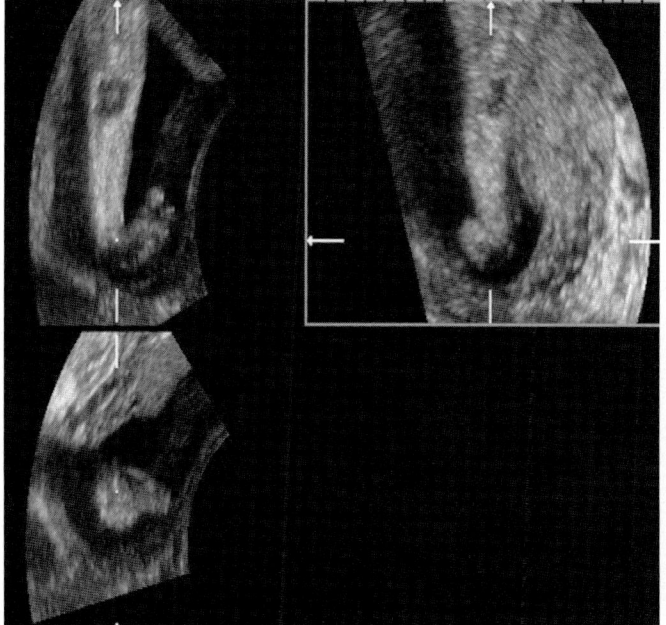

A,B

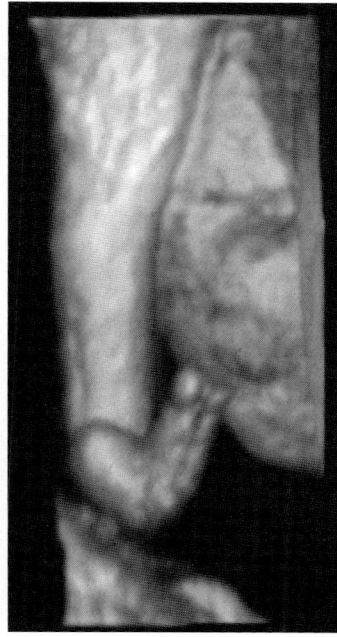

FIGURE 24. Clubfoot at 28 weeks' gestational age. Multiplanar **(A)** and volume-rendered **(B)** images of the leg show a markedly deformed lower extremity.

lated well with birth weight but that the best results were achieved with a combination of standard 2DUS measurements and volume measurements.[59]

Measurements of the liver[60,61] may assist in identifying fetuses at risk for growth restriction, macrosomia, or other abnormalities such as anemia. Chang et al. compared 3DUS to conventional 2DUS measurements of the liver and found that 2DUS underestimated the volume of the liver.[61] It is also hypothesized that volume measurements of

the lung may be helpful in predicting pulmonary hypoplasia. Several investigators have recorded measurements of lung volumes for normal fetuses throughout gestation.[62,63]

CERVIX

Evaluation of the cervix during pregnancy may be assisted by using 3DUS. Volume data obtained through the cervix

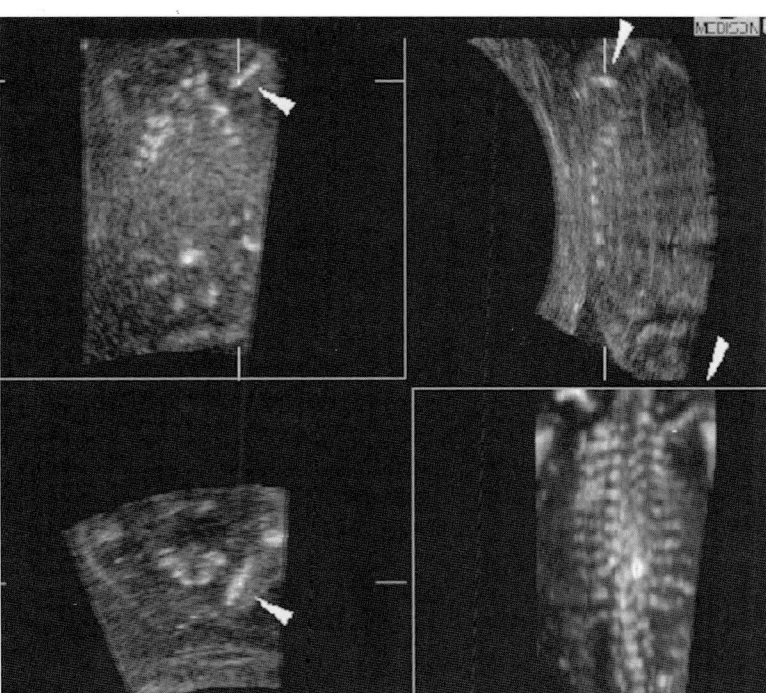

FIGURE 25. Camptomelic dysplasia at 31 weeks' gestational age. Multiplanar and volume-rendered images show a hypoplastic scapula (*arrowheads*), which was seen on three-dimensional ultrasound initially and then confirmed on two-dimensional imaging. **Upper left** is frontal, **upper right** is sagittal, **lower left** is axial, and **lower right** is a rendered image.

allows the clinician to rotate the data into a plane that runs parallel to the cervical canal. Bega et al. showed that the true midsagittal plane of the cervix was not obtained in 27% of the 2DUS examinations.[64] The variable position of the cervix is related to the inherent technical limitations of 2DUS (i.e., the limited mobility of the endovaginal transducer). It is unknown whether obtaining accurate measurements of the cervical length with 3DUS will impact clinical outcome.

Bega et al. also found that 3DUS is helpful in assessing funneling of the cervix. They found in 21 examinations showing funneling that funneling was seen on 2DUS and 3DUS in 15 but was seen only on 3DUS in six. 3DUS was also helpful in imaging an entire cerclage in the axial plane, a plane not available with 2DUS.[64]

VASCULAR

Vascular structures such as the umbilical cord, the placenta, and large fetal vessels can be assessed with 3DUS. The curvature and continuity of vessels is well demonstrated with 3DUS.[65] Acquisition of vascular images can be difficult due to motion, flash artifacts, and the relatively longer time needed to acquire volumes with color and power Doppler techniques.

Rendered images are particularly helpful in understanding the distribution of multiple vessels such as placenta accreta and percreta. Hull and colleagues reported that 3DUS allowed a means to correctly evaluate the extent of invasion of placenta percreta by using the rendered and multiplanar views (Fig. 26).[66,67] The information obtained from the 3DUS study assisted in surgical planning. In another report by the same group, 3DUS was found to be of assistance in evaluating accreta and percreta in seven of eight cases.[67]

Vasa previa can be a difficult diagnosis to make with 2DUS in some cases. 3DUS can assist in the evaluation of the location and proximity of fetal vessels to the cervical os. Vasa previa occurs in the setting of a velamentous cord insertion or a succenturiate lobe with a connecting vessel. Pretorius et al. found 3DUS useful in assessing six of six cases of vasa previa (Fig. 27).[67] They found multiplanar and volume-rendered images helpful. Lee et al. also found that 3DUS was useful in assessing vasa previa in two cases.[68]

The location of the cord insertion, particularly when it is abnormal such as velamentous insertions, can often be

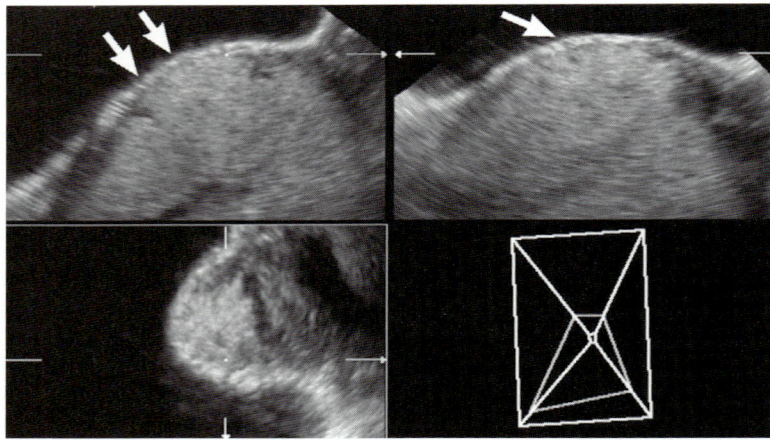

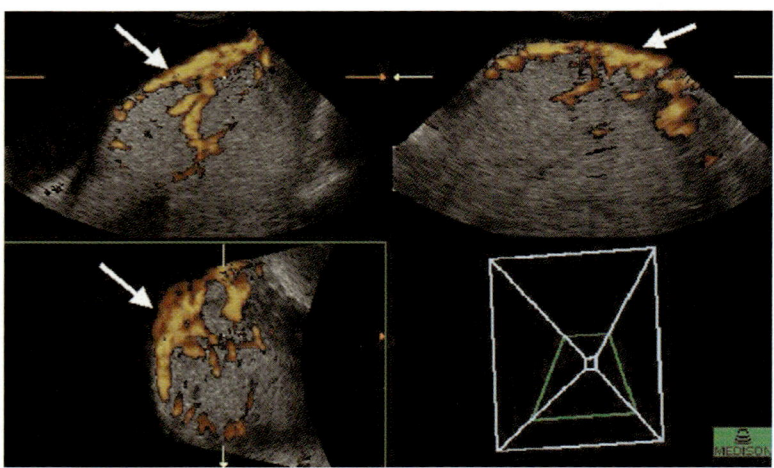

FIGURE 26. Placenta accreta at 26 weeks' gestational age. **A:** Multiplanar endovaginal images **upper left** (sagittal), **upper right** (coronal), and **lower left** (axial) showing invasion of the placenta into the myometrium (*arrows*). **B:** Multiplanar power Doppler endovaginal images **upper left** (sagittal), **upper right** (coronal), and **lower left** (axial) showing vessels extending into the region of invasion (*arrows*).

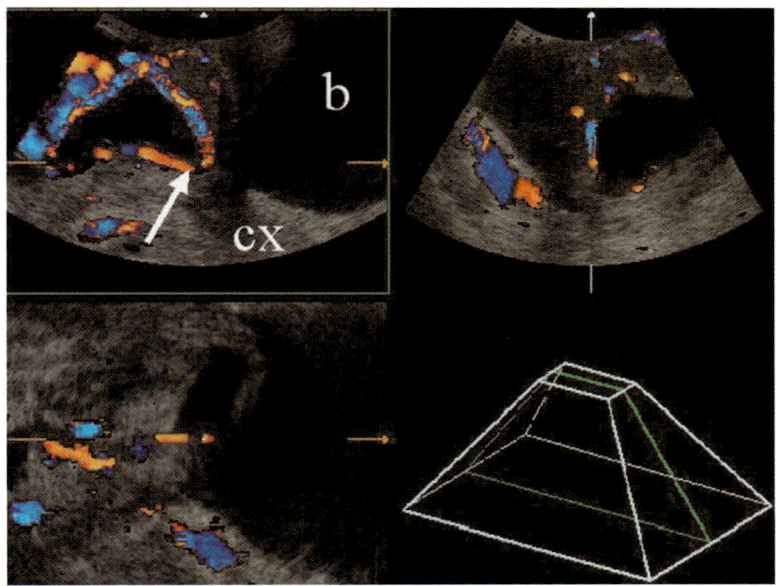

FIGURE 27. Vasa previa at 30 weeks' gestational age. The fetal blood vessel (*arrow*) is seen arising from a velamentous insertion crossing over the cervix (*cx*). b, bladder.

readily displayed with 3DUS. The location of umbilical cord cysts may also be assisted by visualization with 3DUS.[69]

Vascular anomalies such as the aneurysm of the vein of Galen have been shown using 3DUS by several authors.[70–72] 3DUS assisted in mapping the blood supply and the venous drainage and in understanding the spacial orientation of the vessels.

A recent report on blood flow sonoangiography demonstrates remarkable images of vascular structures of the fetus that resemble volume images.[73] This new technology produced by the LOGIQ700 (GE Medical Systems, Milwaukee, WI) uses digitally encoded techniques to suppress tissue clutter and improve sensitivity for the direct visualization of blood reflectors.

MATERNAL- AND PATERNAL-FETAL BONDING

Preliminary data suggest that parents may bond better to the growing fetus when they see a 3DUS image that is easily recognizable.[74] Maier et al. studied 20 high-risk women from 24 to 32 weeks of pregnancy and found that 3DUS had a positive influence on the patient's perception of the fetus. Most of the women in the study found that the 3-D imaging provided a higher degree of security and increased their insight into the psychophysical aspects of their pregnancy.

It has been hypothesized that 3DUS may impact mothers in choosing less abusive behaviors such as smoking, alcohol, and drug use during pregnancy. Preliminary data in a group of mothers who smoked during pregnancy were encouraging.[75]

In a group of patients who underwent 3DUS for reassurance at the University of California, San Diego, we found that certain groups of patients seem to benefit significantly: women with previous fetal/neonatal demise, women with previous congenital anomalies, women carrying fetuses with fatal anomalies (hospice patients) (Fig. 28), infertility couples, and couples with surrogate women carrying their pregnancies.

INTERVENTIONAL PROCEDURES

Interventional procedures may be improved by using a 3DUS approach. Volume scanning permits the needle or

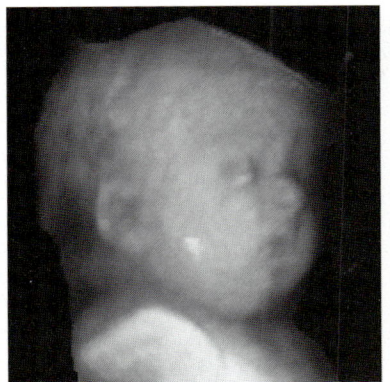
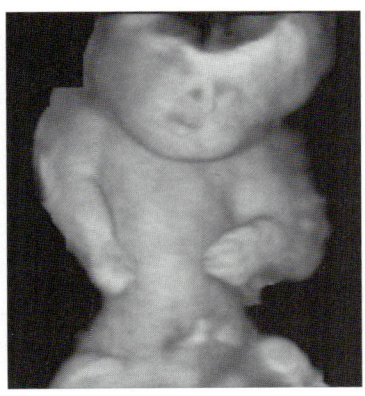

A,B

FIGURE 28. Osteogenesis imperfecta at 34 weeks' gestational age. Volume-rendered images of the face **(A)** and entire body **(B)** in a patient carrying a fetus with a fatal anomaly. The mother felt joy and peace after viewing these images.

catheter to be localized in a volume rather than a plane. The tip of the needle or catheter can be seen in sagittal, coronal, and axial images.[76] This technology has been used in treating ectopic pregnancies, in performing oocyte aspiration, embryo transfer, and laser surgery.[76,77]

LIMITATIONS OF THREE-DIMENSIONAL ULTRASOUND AND THE FUTURE

Clinicians have not accepted 3DUS. Why? First, quality from 3DUS images is generally not quite as good as 2DUS images. The image quality is directly related to image quality of the 2DUS used to acquire volumes, but the multiplanar images vary in resolution, being best in the acquired plane, moderate in the plane perpendicular, and poorest in the plane parallel to the transducer head. It is important to acquire volumes in the appropriate plane when the highest resolution is needed. Second, the beautiful rendered images cannot be obtained on all patients. They are dependent on gestational age and the amount of amniotic fluid adjacent to the area of interest. Optimal rendered images are obtained at 10 to 12 weeks using a transvaginal probe and from 24 to 30 weeks when using the transabdominal probe. If the head is deep in the pelvis or just adjacent to the uterine wall or placenta, then a rendered image of the face cannot be obtained. In addition, in the setting of oligohydramnios, rendered images of the fetal surface cannot be obtained. Third, 3DUS equipment is not readily available. The ultrasound manufacturers have been primarily exploring small aspects of 3DUS without making a full commitment to develop and integrate a user-friendly product into routine clinical equipment. Fourth, the clinical data supporting application of 3DUS to patient care are evolving with much promise but as yet have unproven results. Fifth, it currently takes additional time to perform and learn 3DUS, particularly to obtain optimal rendered images. Sixth, reimbursement for clinical 3-D studies has been challenging to obtain.

3DUS is the way of the future. Volume imaging is gaining an increasingly important place in medical imaging across a range of modalities such as computed tomography, magnetic resonance imaging, interventional fluoroscopic guidance, and even viewing of histologic data. While there are specific areas of diagnostic use in which 3DUS has been proven to have an impact on clinical management, we are only at the tip of the iceberg in exploring the full range of applications. It is expected that clinical research is forthcoming, which will identify additional clinical applications. It is also expected that the ultrasound industry will pursue faster, easier methods to understand and use this new technology.

REFERENCES

1. Nelson TR, Downey DB, Pretorius DH, Fenster A. *Three-dimensional ultrasound.* Philadelphia: Lippincott, Williams & Wilkins, 1999.

2. Baba K, Satoh K, Sakamoto S, Okai T, Ishii S. Development of an ultrasonic system for three-dimensional reconstruction of the fetus. *J Perinat Med* 1989;17:19–24.

3. Baba K, Jurkovic D. *Three-dimensional ultrasound in obstetrics and gynecology.* New York: Parthenon Publishing Group, 1997.

4. Merz E, Bahlmann F, Weber G. Volume scanning in the evaluation of fetal malformations: a new dimension in prenatal diagnosis. *Ultrasound Obstet Gynecol* 1995;5:222–227.

5. Platt L, Santulli T, Dru E, Carlson MD, Greene N, et al. Three-dimensional ultrasonography in obstetrics and gynecology: preliminary experience. *Am J Obstet Gynecol* 1998;178(6):1199–1206.

6. Dyson RL, Pretorius DH, Budorick NE, Johnson DD, Sklansky MS, et al. Three-dimensional ultrasound in the evaluation of fetal anomalies. *Ultrasound Obstet Gynecol* 2000;16:321–328.

7. Brandl H, Gritzky A, Haizinger M. 3D ultrasound: a dedicated system. *Eur Radiol* 1999;9[Suppl 3]:S331–S333.

8. Hull AD, James G, Salerno C, Nelson T, Pretorius D. Three-dimensional ultrasound and the assessment of the first trimester fetus. *J Ultrasound Med* 2001;20(4):287–293.

9. Bonilla-Musoles F, Raga F, Villalobos A, Blanes J, Osborne NG. First-trimester neck abnormalities: three-dimensional evaluation. *J Ultrasound Med* 1998;17(7):419–425.

10. Chung BL. The application of three-dimensional ultrasound to nuchal translucency measurement in early pregnancy (10–14 weeks): a preliminary study. *Ultrasound Obstet Gynecol* 2000;15(2):122–125.

11. Blaas HG, Eik-Nes SH, Kiserud T, Berg S, Angelsen B, et al. Three-dimensional imaging of the brain cavities in human embryos. *Ultrasound Obstet Gynecol* 1995;5(4):228–232.

12. Blass HG, Eik-Nes SH, Berg S, Torp H. In-vivo three-dimensional ultrasound reconstructions of embryos and early fetuses. *Lancet* 1998;352:1182–1186.

13. Bega G, Wapner R, Lev-Toaff L, Kuhlman K. Diagnosis of conjoined twins at 10 weeks using three-dimensional ultrasound: a case report. *Ultrasound Obstet Gynecol* 2000;16:388–390.

14. Liang RI, Huang SE, Chang FM. Prenatal diagnosis of ectopia cordis at 10 weeks of gestation using two-dimensional and three-dimensional ultrasonography. *Ultrasound Obstet Gynecol* 1995;5L:228–232.

15. Steiner H, Gregg AR, Bogner G, Graf AH, Weiner CP. First trimester three-dimensional ultrasound volumetry of the gestational sac. *Arch Gynecol Obstet* 1994;255:165–170.

16. Merz E, Weber G, Bahlmann F, Miric-Tesanic D. Application of transvaginal and abdominal three-dimensional ultrasound for the detection or exclusion of malformations of the fetal face. *Ultrasound Obstet Gynecol* 1997;9:237–243.

17. Pretorius DH, House M, Nelson TR, Hollenbach KA. Evaluation of normal and abnormal lips in fetuses: comparison between three- and two-dimensional sonography. *AJR Am J Roentgenol* 1995;165:1233–1237.

18. Pretorius DH, Nelson TR. Fetal face visualization using three-dimensional ultrasonography. *J Ultrasound Med* 1995;349–356.

19. Hata T, Yonehara T, Aoki S, Manabe A, Hata K, et al. Three-dimensional sonographic visualization of the fetal face. *AJR Am J Roentgenol* 1998;170:481–483.

20. Devonald K, Ellwood DA, Griffiths KA, Kossoff G, Gill RW, et al. Volume imaging: three-dimensional appreciation of the fetal head and face. *J Ultrasound Med* 1995;14:919–925.

21. Lee W, Kirk JS, Shaheen KW, Romero R, Hodges AN, et al. Fetal cleft lip and palate detection by three-dimensional ultrasonography. *Ultrasound Obstet Gynecol* 2000;16(4):314–320.

22. Pretorius DH, Nelson TR. Three-dimensional ultrasound in gynecology and obstetrics, a review. *Ultrasound Quarterly* 1998;14(4):218.

23. Johnson DD, Pretorius DH, Budorick NE, Jones MC, Lou KV, et al. Fetal lip and primary palate: three-dimensional versus two-dimensional US. *Radiology* 2000;217:236–239.

24. Ulm MR, Kratochwil A, Ulm B, Lee A, Betteheim D, et al. Three-dimensional ultrasonographic imaging of fetal tooth buds for characterization of facial clefts. *Early Hum Dev* 1999;55:67.

25. Nelson TR, Pretorius DH, Hull AD, Riccabona M, Sklansky MS, et al. Sources and impact of artifacts on clinical 3DUS imaging. *Ultrasound Obstet Gynecol* 2000;16:374–383.

26. Garjian KV, Pretorius DH, Budorick NE, Cantrell CJ, Johnson DD, et al. Fetal skeletal dysplasia: three-dimensional US—initial experience. *Radiology* 2000;214(3):717–723.

27. Shih JC, Shyu MK, Lee CN, Wu CH, Lin GJ, et al. Antenatal depiction of the fetal ear with three-dimensional ultrasonography. *Ultrasound Obstet Gynecol* 1998;91(4):500.

28. Mueller GM, Weiner CP, Yankowitz J. Three-dimensional ultrasound in the evaluation of fetal head and spine anomalies. *Ultrasound Obstet Gynecol* 1996;88(3):372.

29. Timor-Tritsch, I, Monteagudo A, Mayberry P. Three-dimensional ultrasound evaluation of the fetal brain: the three horn view. *Ultrasound Obstet Gynecol* 2000;16:302–306.

30. Monteagudo A, Timor-Tritsch I, Mayberry P. Three-dimensional transvaginal neurosonography of the fetal brain: "navigating" in the volume scan. *Ultrasound Obstet Gynecol* 2000;16:307–313.

31. Pretorius D, Nelson T. Prenatal utilization of cranial sutures and fontanelles with three-dimensional ultrasonography. *J Ultrasound Med* 1994;13:871–876.

32. Benacerraf B, Spiro R, Mitchell A. Using three-dimensional ultrasound to detect craniosynostosis in a fetus with Pfeiffer syndrome. *Ultrasound Obstet Gynecol* 2000;16:391–394.

33. Johnson DD, Pretorius DH, Riccabona M, Budorick NE, Nelson TR. Three-dimensional ultrasound of the fetal spine. *Obstet Gynecol* 1997;89:434–438.

34. Zosmer N, Jurkovic D, Jauniaux E, Grubaeck K, Lees C, et al. Selection and identification of standard cardiac views from three-dimensional volume scans of the fetal thorax. *J Ultrasound Med* 1996;15:25–32.

35. Leventhal M, Pretorius DH, Sklansky MS, Budorick NE, Nelson TR, et al. Three-dimensional ultrasonography of normal fetal heart: comparison with two-dimensional imaging. *J Ultrasound Med* 1998;17(6):341–348.

36. Nelson TR, Pretorius DH, Sklansky M, Hagen-Ansert S. Three-dimensional echocardiographic evaluation of fetal heart anatomy and function: acquisition, analysis and display. *J Ultrasound Med* 1996;158:1–9.

37. Deng J, Gardener JE, Rodeck CH, Lees W. Fetal echocardiography in three and four dimensions. *Ultrasound Med Biol* 1996;22(8):979–986.

38. Kwon J, Shaffer E, Shandas R, et al. Acquisition of three dimensional fetal echocardiograms using an external trigger source. *J Am Soc Echocardiog* 1996;9(3):389.

39. Sklansky MS, Nelson TR, Pretorius DH. Usefulness of gated three-dimensional fetal echocardiography to reconstruct and display structures not visualized with two-dimensional imaging. *Am J Cardiol* 1997;80(5):665–668.

40. Nelson TR. Three-dimensional fetal echocardiography. *Prog Biophys Mol Biol* 1998;69:257–272.

41. Chang FM, Hsu KF, Ko HC, Yao BL, Chang CH, et al. Fetal heart volume assessment by three-dimensional ultrasound. *Ultrasound Obstet Gynecol* 1997;9(1):42–48.

42. Meyer-Wittkopf M, Cook A, McLennan A, Summers P, Sharland GK, et al. Evaluation of three-dimensional ultrasonography and magnetic resonance imaging in assessment of congenital heart anomalies in fetal cardiac specimens. *Ultrasound Obstet Gynecol* 1996;8(5):303–308.

43. Sklansky MS, Nelson TR, Strachan VM, Pretorius DH. Real-time three-dimensional fetal echocardiography: initial feasibility study. *J Ultrasound Med* 1999;18:745–752.

44. Hata T, Aoki S, Manabe A, Hata K, Miyazaki K. Visualization of fetal genitalia by three-dimensional ultrasonography in the second and third trimesters. *J Ultrasound Med* 1998;17(2):137–139.

45. Lee A, Deutinger J, Bernaschek G. "Volvision": three-dimensional ultrasonography of fetal malformations. *Am J Obstet Gynecol* 1994;170:1312–1314.

46. Lev-Toaff A, Ozhan S, Pretorius D, Bega G, Kurtz A, et al. Three-dimensional multiplanar ultrasound for fetal gender assignment: value of the mid-sagittal plane. *Ultrasound Obstet Gynecol* 2000;16:345–350.

47. Budorick NE, Pretorius DH, Johnson DD, Nelson TR, Tartar MK, et al. Three-dimensional ultrasonography of the fetal distal lower extremity: normal and abnormal. *J Ultrasound Med* 1998;17:649–660.

48. Budorick NE, Pretorius DH, Johnson DD, Tartas MK, Lou KV, et al. Three-dimensional ultrasound examination of the fetal hands: normal and abnormal. *Ultrasound Obstet Gynecol* 1998;12:227.

49. Ploeckinger-Ulm B, Ulm MR, Lee A, Kratochwil A, Bernaschek G. Antenatal depiction of fetal digits with three-dimensional ultrasonography. *Am J Obstet Gynecol* 1996;175:571–574.

50. Hull AD, Pretorius DH, Lev-Toaff AS, Budorick NE, Salerno CC, et al. Artifacts and the visualization of fetal distal extremities using three dimensional ultrasound. *Ultrasound Obstet Gynecol* 2000;16:341–344.

51. Lee A, Kratochwil A, Deutinger J, Bernaschek G. 3D ultrasound in diagnosing phocomelia. *Ultrasound Obstet Gynecol* 1995;5:238–240.

52. Steiner H, Spitzer D, Weiss-Wichert PH, Graf AH, Staudack A. Three-dimensional ultrasound in prenatal diagnosis of skeletal dysplasia. *Prenat Diagn* 1995;15(4):373–377.

53. Brinkley JF, McCallum WD, Muramatsu SK. Fetal weight estimation from length and volumes found by 3D ultrasonic measurements. *J Ultrasound Med* 1984;3:162–169.

54. Lee W, Comstock CH, Kirk JS, Smith RS, Monck JW, et al. Birthweight predictions by three-dimensional ultrasono-

graphic volumes of the fetal thighs and abdomen. *J Ultrasound Med* 1997;161(12):799–805.

55. Chang FM, Hsu KF, Ko HC, Yao BL, Chang CH, et al. Three-dimensional ultrasound–assessed fetal thigh volumetry in predicting birth weight. *Obstet Gynecol* 1997;90:331–339.

56. Favre R, Bader AM, Nisand G. Prospective study on fetal weight estimation using limb circumferences obtained by three-dimensional ultrasound. *Ultrasound Obstet Gynecol* 1995;6(2):140–144.

57. Liang RI, Chang FM, Yao BL, Chang CH, Yu CH, et al. Predicting birth weight by fetal upper-arm volume with use of three-dimensional ultrasonography. *Am J Obstet Gynecol* 1997;177:632–638.

58. Song TB, Moore TR, Lee JI, Kim YH, Kim EK. Fetal weight prediction by thigh volume measurement with three-dimensional ultrasonography. *Obstet Gynecol* 2000; 96:157–161.

59. Schild RL. Can 3D volumetric analysis of the fetal upper arm and thigh improve conventional 2D weight estimates? *Ultraschall Med* 1999;20(1):31–37.

60. Laudy JAM, Janssen MMM, Struyk PC, Stijnen T, Wallenburg HCS, et al. Fetal liver volume measurement by three-dimensional ultrasonography: a preliminary study. *Ultrasound Obstet Gynecol* 1998;12:93–96.

61. Chang FM, Hsu KF, Ko HC, Yao BL, Chang CH, et al. Three-dimensional ultrasound assessment of fetal liver volume in normal pregnancy: a comparison of reproducibility with two-dimensional ultrasound and a search for a volume constant. *Ultrasound Med Biol* 1997;23(3):381.

62. Lee A, Kratochwil A, Stumpflen I, Deutinger J, Bernaschek G. Fetal lung volume determination by three-dimensional ultrasonography. *Am J Obstet Gynecol* 1996;175(3 Pt 1):588–592.

63. D'Arcy TJ, Hughes SW, Chiu WS, Clark T, Milner AD, et al. Estimation of fetal lung volume using enhanced 3-dimensional ultrasound: a new method and first result [see comments]. *Br J Obstet Gynaecol* 1996;103(10):1015–1020.

64. Bega G, Lev-Toaff A, Kuhlman K, Berghella V, Parker L, et al. Three-dimensional multiplanar transvaginal ultrasound of the cervix in pregnancy. *Ultrasound Obstet Gynecol* 2000;16:351–358.

65. Pretorius DH, Nelson TR, Baergen RN, Pai E, Cantrell C. Imaging of placental vasculature using three-dimensional ultrasound and color power Doppler: a preliminary study. *Ultrasound Obstet Gynecol* 1998;12:45–49.

66. Hull AD, Salerno CC, Saenz CC, Pretorius DH. Three-dimensional ultrasound (3DUS) and the diagnosis of placenta percreta with bladder involvement. *J Ultrasound Med* 1999;18:853–856.

67. Pretorius DH, Hull AD, Daneshmand S, James G, Nelson TR. Assessment of placental accreta/percreta, vasa previa and fetal vascularity using 3DUS power Doppler. *Radiology* 2000;217:255.

68. Lee W, Kirk J, Comstock C, Romero R. Vasa previa: prenatal detection by three-dimensional ultrasonography. *Ultrasound Obstet Gynecol* 2000;16:384–387.

69. Osborne N, Bonilla-Musoles F, Raga F, Bonilla F. Umbilical cord cysts: color Doppler and three-dimensional ultrasound evaluation. *Ultrasound Quarterly* 2000;16:133–139.

70. Heling K, Chaoui R, Bollmann R. Prenatal diagnosis of an aneurysm of the vein of Galen with three-dimensional color power angiography. *Ultrasound Obstet Gynecol* 2000;15:333–336.

71. Lee T, Shih S, Peng F, Lee C, Shyu M, et al. Prenatal depiction of angioarchitecture of an aneurysm of the vein of Galen with three-dimensional color power angiography. *Ultrasound Obstet Gynecol* 2000;15:337–340.

72. Bahlmann F. Three-dimensional color power angiography of an aneurysm of the vein of Galen. *Ultrasound Obstet Gynecol* 2000;15:341–344.

73. Pooh R. New application of B-flow sono-angiography in perinatology. *Ultrasound Obstet Gynecol* 2000;15:163.

74. Maier B, Steiner H, Wieneroither H, Staudach A. The psychological impact of three-dimensional fetal imaging on the fetomaternal relationship. In: Baba K, Jurkovic D, eds. *Three-dimensional ultrasound in obstetrics and gynecology.* New York: Parthenon Publishing Group 1997:67–74.

75. Pretorius DH. *Maternal smoking habit modification via fetal visualization.* University of California Tobacco Related Disease Research Program. Annual report to the California State Legislature 1996:76.

76. Baba K, Ishiihara O, Hayashi N, Saitoh M, Taya J, et al. Three-dimensional ultrasound in embryo transfer. *Ultrasound Obstet Gynecol* 2000;16:372–373.

77. Feichtinger W. Follicle aspiration with interactive three-dimensional digital imaging (Voluson): a step toward real-time puncturing under three-dimensional. *Fertil Steril* 1998;70:374–377.

FETAL MAGNETIC RESONANCE IMAGING*

The advent of fast magnetic resonance imaging (MRI) sequences has revolutionized the ability to visualize fetal anatomy and pathology. Whereas ultrasonography continues to be the primary screening modality for obstetric imaging, when additional information regarding fetal anatomy or pathology is needed for decision making in prenatal diagnosis, MRI can be extremely helpful. Because MRI provides excellent contrast resolution, uses no ionizing radiation, permits imaging in more than one plane, and has a large field of view, it allows for visualization of fetal anatomy in a manner not possible with sonography, and thus can add information in cases in which sonography is insufficient to provide an adequate diagnosis.

In the past, pelvic MRI was used during pregnancy to evaluate maternal anatomy and abnormalities such as adnexal masses. Although adnexal structures can be visualized with conventional techniques, fetal anatomy typically cannot be adequately assessed with conventional sequences because of degradation of image quality by fetal motion during the relatively long acquisition times.[1–3] New fast scan techniques allow for imaging without maternal or fetal sedation and have led to markedly increased enthusiasm for use of this imaging tool to evaluate the fetus.

SAFETY OF MAGNETIC RESONANCE IN PREGNANCY

There are no known biologic risks from MRI. No delayed sequelae from magnetic resonance examination have been encountered, and it is expected that the potential risk for any delayed sequelae is extremely small or nonexistent.[4–8] In a survey of female magnetic resonance workers, no substantial increase in adverse pregnancy outcomes was found.[7] In a study by Myers, no increased incidence of growth retardation was visualized in pregnancies undergoing MRI.[9] In a study of pregnant pigs measuring temperature of amniotic fluid, fetal brain, and fetal abdomen no temperature changes were noted using fast MRI techniques.[10] According to the Safety Committee of the Society for Magnetic Resonance Imaging,[11] magnetic resonance procedures are indicated for use in pregnant women if other nonionizing forms of diagnostic imaging are inadequate, or if the examination provides important information that would otherwise require exposure to ionizing radiation (i.e., x-ray computed tomography). It is required that pregnant patients be informed that, to date, although there is no indication that the use of clinical magnetic resonance procedures during pregnancy produces deleterious effects, according to the Food and Drug Administration, the safety of magnetic resonance procedures during pregnancy has not been definitively proven.[8] Because the greatest theoretic risk is at the time of organogenesis, and because the small fetal size makes evaluation of fetal anatomy difficult, early on in pregnancy, magnetic resonance in the first trimester is avoided whenever feasible.

As for all patients, there are absolute contraindications to MRI in pregnant patients (e.g., a ferromagnetic cerebral aneurysm clip), and some patients are too claustrophobic to undergo the examination. Use of short bore magnets should make claustrophobia less of a concern. However, an additional problem is that pregnant patients may have difficulty lying on their backs, especially in the third trimester.

FAST MAGNETIC RESONANCE IMAGING

The magnetic resonance images in this chapter were obtained with a 1.5 T superconducting system (Siemens Vision or Symphony, Erlangen, Germany), with a four element phased-array surface coil. The minimum gradient rise time is 600 μs (for a 25 mT peak gradient amplitude). The whole body specific absorption rate is less than 3.0 W/kg. Patients are positioned supine and feet first in the magnet to minimize claustrophobia. Because fetal motion generally occurs throughout the examination we have each acquisition serve as the scout for the subsequent

*The studies of magnetic resonance of fetal central nervous system in this chapter were supported by a National Institutes of Health grant, NS 37945.

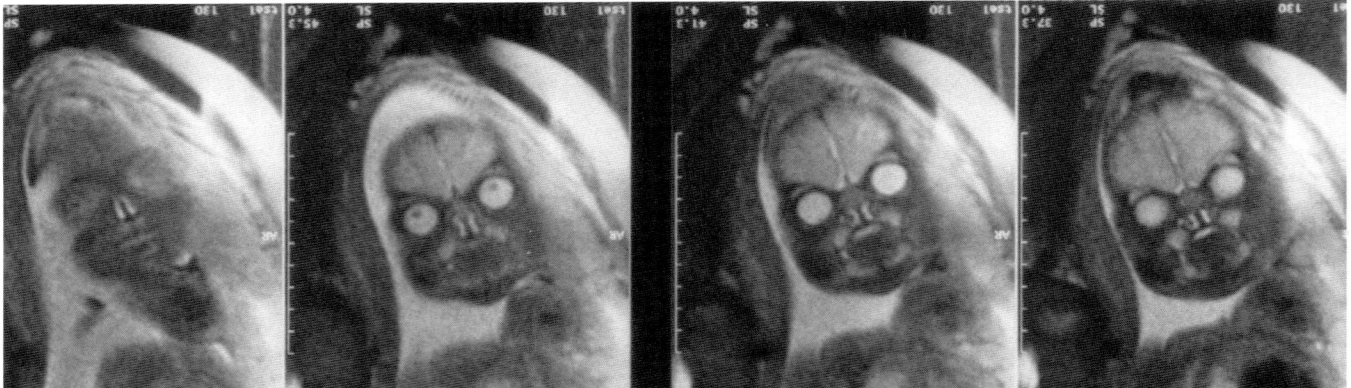

FIGURE 1. Normal fetal face. Four consecutive coronal images of the fetal face at 33 weeks' gestational age demonstrate the normal appearance of the facial structures. [Reproduced with permission from Trop I, Levine D. Normal fetal anatomy as visualized with fast magnetic resonance imaging. *Top Magn Reson Imaging* 2001;12(1):3–17.]

acquisition to obtain images in the fetal axial, coronal, and sagittal planes.

T2-WEIGHTED IMAGING

Half Fourier single-shot rapid acquisition with relaxation enhancement technique is used to obtain T2-weighted images. A typical sequence for fetal imaging uses an echo spacing of 4.2 milliseconds, an echo time of 60 milliseconds, an echo train length of 72, 1 acquisition, 4-mm section thickness, 24 × 24 cm field of view, and 192 × 256 acquisition matrix. A 130-degree refocusing pulse (instead of 180 degrees) is used to minimize the amount of radiofrequency power deposition.

The acquisition time per image is only 430 milliseconds. A 1-second delay between image acquisitions minimizes the specific absorption rate. Thus, the scan time for 13 slices acquired in a single sequence is 17 seconds. The highly T2-weighted rapid acquisition with relaxation enhancement images provide excellent contrast resolution of the fetal tissues (Fig. 1).[12–15]

T1-WEIGHTED IMAGING

T1-weighted imaging of the fetus is achieved using a fast low angle shot technique. The fast low angle shot sequence is a gradient-echo sequence that uses a spoiler gradient to disperse residual transverse magnetization. A typical sequence is performed during a maternal breath-hold using repetition time/echo time 126/4, 80-degree flip angle, 24 cm × 32 cm field of view, 96 × 256 acquisition matrix, 5 mm slice thickness, and one signal acquisition for an acquisition time of 17 seconds. While the images are degraded by motion that occurs during the breath-hold, gradient-echo T1-weighted images are useful for confirming hemorrhage or fat (Fig. 2C).

FETAL CENTRAL NERVOUS SYSTEM ANOMALIES

One area in which MRI has proven to be particularly beneficial is in evaluation of the fetal central nervous system (CNS). Sonographic evaluation of the fetal CNS is limited by the nonspecific appearance of some anomalies, by technical factors that limit resolution of the side of the brain near the transducer, by ossification that obscures visualization of posterior fossa structures, by low position of the fetal head in the third trimester, and by subtle parenchymal abnormalities that frequently cannot be visualized with ultrasound.[15,16] Multiplanar views of the CNS are difficult to obtain with sonography due to skull ossification and fetal position, however these factors do not limit magnetic resonance evaluation of the CNS. MRI allows for direct visualization of the brain parenchyma and thus allows for detailed evaluation of the CNS anatomy in a manner not possible with sonography. In an ongoing study evaluating fetal CNS abnormalities with ultrasound and MRI we have found that in more than 50% of cases with sonographically documented CNS abnormalities, the information provided by MRI is of the type that warrants changes in patient counseling or management. Magnetic resonance findings not visualized by ultrasound include porencephaly (Fig. 2B), hemorrhage (Fig. 2C), partial or complete agenesis of the corpus callosum (Figs. 3A and 3C), cortical gyral abnormality (Fig. 3D), tethered cord (Fig. 4), cortical clefts, midbrain abnormalities, partial or complete agenesis of the septi pellucidi, holoprosencephaly, cerebellar hypoplasia, subependymal (Fig. 5) and cortical tubers, vascular malformation, and vermian cysts.

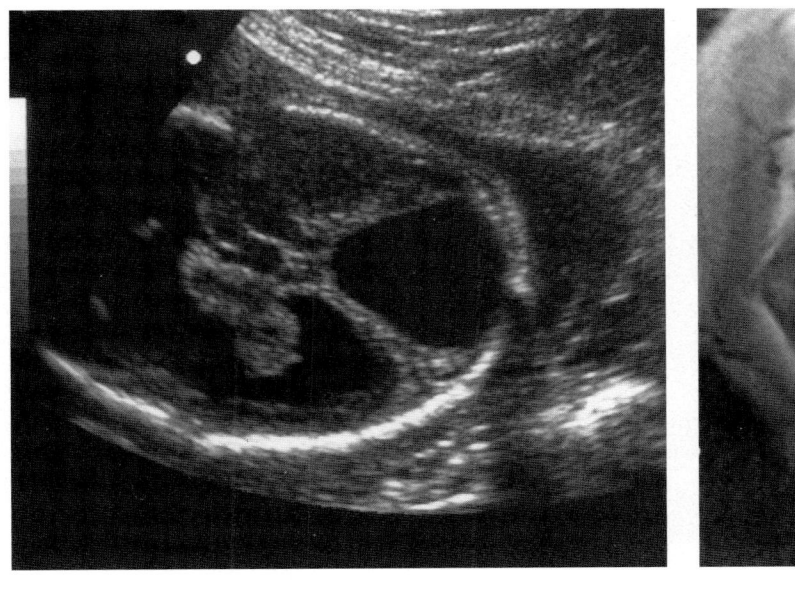

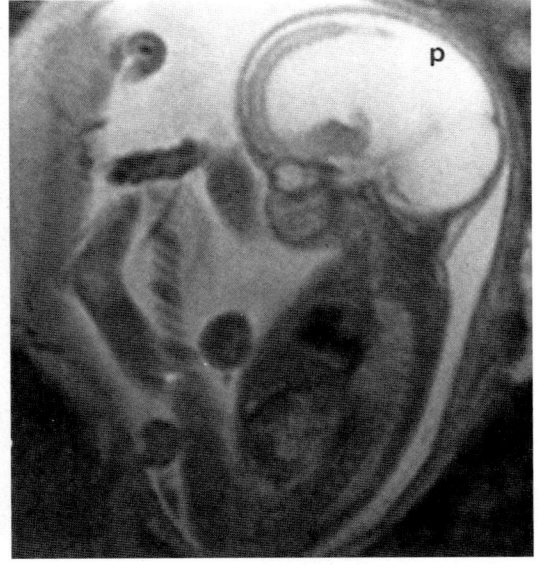

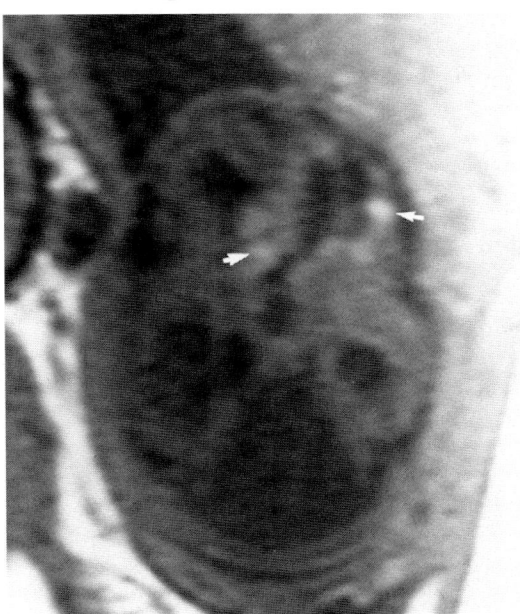

FIGURE 2. Dandy-Walker malformation and porencephaly. **A:** Axial sonogram at 25 weeks' gestation demonstrates a Dandy-Walker malformation and ventriculomegaly. The choroid plexus is prominent and irregular, suggestive of intraventricular hemorrhage. **B:** Sagittal half-Fourier acquisition single-shot turbo-spin echo image in same patient confirms the Dandy-Walker malformation and ventriculomegaly but also shows a large area of porencephaly (*p*). **C:** Axial T1-weighted magnetic resonance imaging shows areas of increased signal intensity (*arrows*) consistent with hemorrhage or mineralization. (Reproduced with permission from Levine D, Barnes PD, Madsen JR, Abbott J, Mehta T, et al. Central nervous system abnormalities assessed with prenatal magnetic resonance imaging. *Obstet Gynecol* 1999;94:1011–1019.)

Abnormalities better defined by MRI than ultrasound include encephaloceles (Fig. 6), arteriovenous malformations, distal neural tube defects, and the mass effect of arachnoid cysts (Fig. 7).[13,17,18]

The information provided by magnetic resonance allows for improved patient counseling, which may be used to assist patients in the decision to continue or discontinue a pregnancy (Fig. 6), or may be used to facilitate planning the mode of delivery and perinatal care. At times magnetic resonance in the third trimester can obviate the need for postnatal MRI (which may require neonatal sedation and its associated risks). MRI has facilitated counseling in patients with nonspecific sonograms (e.g., a large cisterna magna, for which an amniocentesis is performed for infe-

rior vermian agenesis but not for the normal variant of mega cisterna magna).

We have found MRI to be especially useful in fetuses with ventriculomegaly. The degree of ventriculomegaly, the cause of ventriculomegaly, and any associated findings are important in providing a management plan and prognosis for the fetus.[19–22] MRI has been beneficial in establishing the presence of a normal corpus callosum in fetuses with suspected callosal agenesis by directly visualizing the entire corpus callosum. Magnetic resonance also has been helpful in diagnosing callosal agenesis in fetuses when ultrasound findings are inconclusive (Fig. 3).[13,18]

Evaluation of neural tube defects can also be performed with MRI. Magnetic resonance examination is very helpful

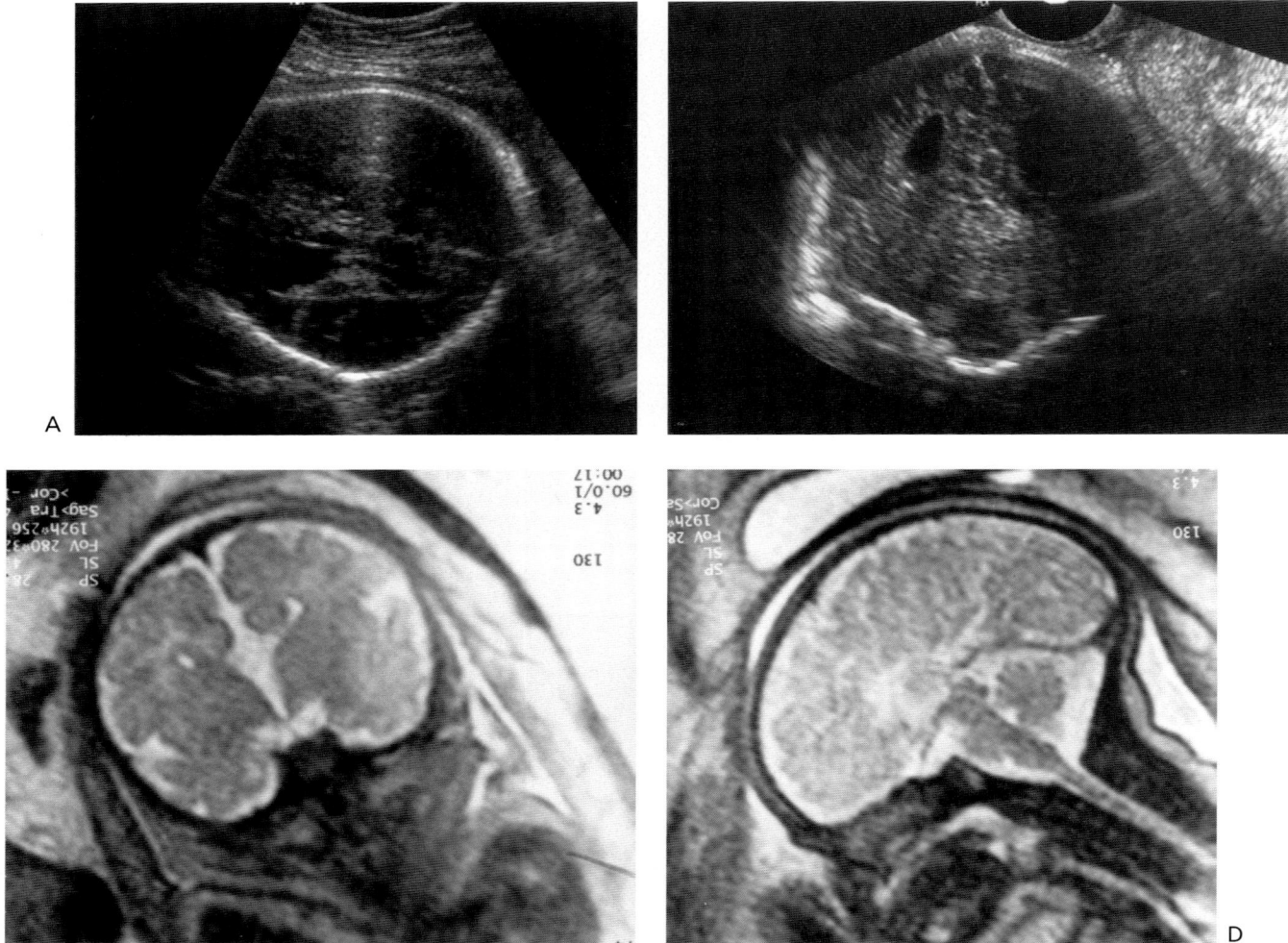

FIGURE 3. Unilateral ventriculomegaly, seen on ultrasound, with agenesis of the corpus callosum on magnetic resonance imaging in a fetus at 36 weeks' gestation. **A:** Transabdominal sonogram demonstrates moderate ventriculomegaly of the side away from the transducer. Artifact from the calvaria limits evaluation of the side near the transducer. **B:** Transvaginal ultrasound shows asymmetric ventriculomegaly. However, the anterior portion of the cortex and ventricles cannot be imaged due to fetal position. **C:** Coronal magnetic resonance imaging demonstrates agenesis of the corpus callosum. **D:** Sagittal midline view demonstrates polymicrogyria. (**A, C, D:** Reproduced with permission from Levine D, Barnes PD, Madsen J, Hulka C, Mehta T, et al. Fetal CNS anomalies depicted with ultrafast MR imaging. *AJR Am J Roentgenol* 1999;172:813–818.)

in visualizing caudal neural tube defects that may be difficult to visualize with ultrasound. MRI is also useful in visualizing posterior fossa structures in cases of Chiari's malformation type II malformation. This is helpful in the *in utero* assessment of fetuses after surgery for neural tube defects.[23] However, for the majority of well-visualized spinal neural tube defects in which fetal surgery is not being performed, magnetic resonance has limited potential to influence care.[18]

Magnetic resonance can also be used to assess normal and abnormal fetal cerebral cortical development. We found that cortical development by MRI follows a predictable course and lags slightly when compared to that described in anatomic specimens.[24] Cortical development is often further delayed in fetuses with mild ventriculomegaly or other CNS

abnormalities.[24] The time course of the appearance of normal cortical landmarks is important in screening for fetuses with suspected migrational disorders such as lissencephaly. In addition, if the cortical development is markedly delayed compared to the gestational age and the fetus has an otherwise normal-appearing brain, these neonates may benefit from early intervention postnatally.

FETAL NON–CENTRAL NERVOUS SYSTEM ANOMALIES

A rapidly expanding area for magnetic resonance is the evaluation of fetuses that potentially will undergo *in utero*

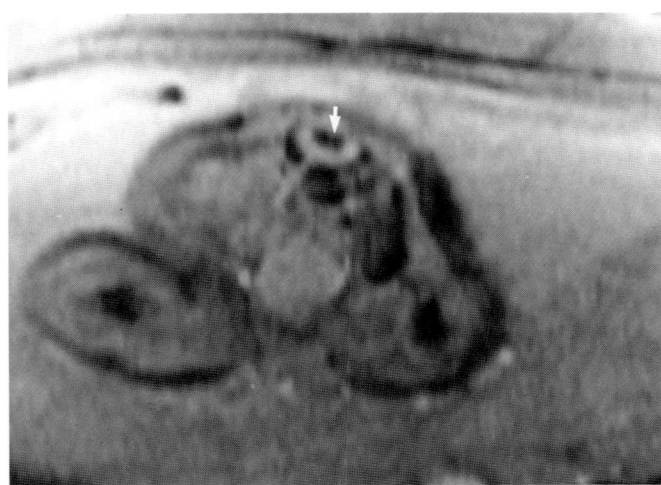

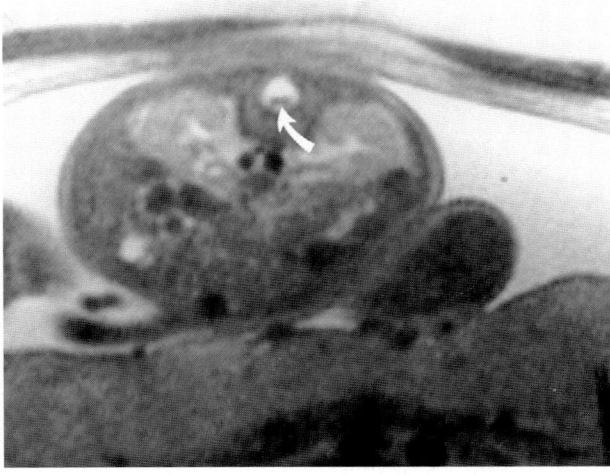

FIGURE 4. Diastematomyelia at 31 weeks' gestational age. **A:** Coronal spectral spatial water excitation image shows a widened spinal canal in the lumbosacral region with a fibrous or bony mass (*arrow*) inferiorly. **B:** Axial half-Fourier acquisition single-shot turbo-spin echo image shows the split cord (*curved arrow*). Although the diastematomyelia was evident on ultrasound, magnetic resonance imaging allowed for visualization of the split cord and tethered cord. Because tethered cord was expected in a diastematomyelia at this level, this is an example of the type of additional information provided by magnetic resonance imaging that does not change patient counseling or management. [Reproduced with permission from Levine D. Ultrasound versus magnetic resonance imaging in fetal evaluation. *Top Magn Reson Imaging* 2001;12(1):25–38.]

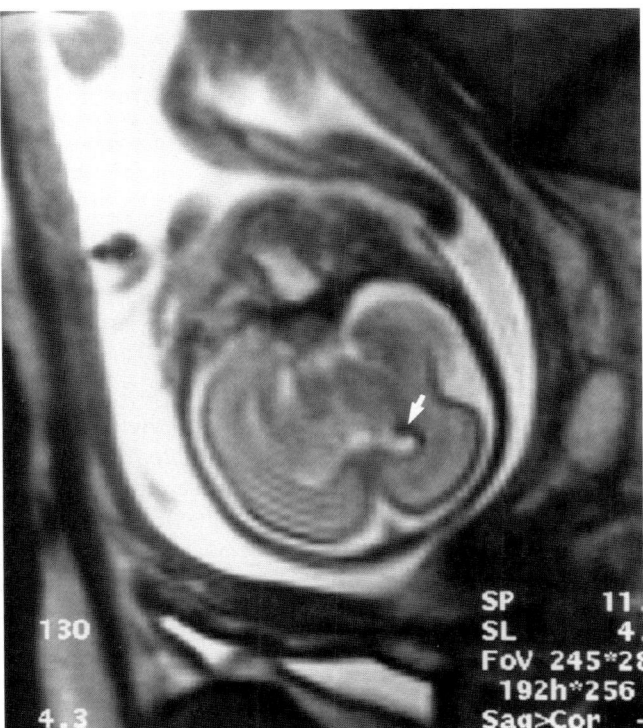

FIGURE 5. Subependymal tuber at 21 weeks. This fetus was at 50% risk for tuberous sclerosis because the patient's husband and their previous child were affected. The scan shows a low signal intensity nodule (*arrow*) impressing on the ventricle. This was seen in orthogonal planes. Follow-up scan at 32 weeks showed additional subependymal and cortical tubers. The diagnosis was confirmed at birth. (Reproduced with permission from Levine D, Barnes P, Korf B, Edelman R. Tuberous sclerosis: second trimester diagnosis of subependymal tubers with fast MRI. *AJR Am J Roentgenol* 2000;175:1067–1069.)

surgery. Fetal magnetic resonance has been shown to be helpful in evaluation of neck and chest masses that potentially obstruct the airway.[25,26] This type of information is critical for planning fetal interventional surgery. In addition, magnetic resonance is helpful in the documentation of liver position in fetuses with congenital diaphragmatic hernia.[27,28] The liver position is important for prognosis because isolated *liver-up* and *liver-down* congenital diaphragmatic hernias have a respective mortality of 5% and 7%.[27,29,30] Magnetic resonance is also helpful in fetuses with congenital diaphragmatic hernia in the assessment of the amount of normal-appearing lung remaining because the lung is poorly visualized with sonography but is well-depicted with MRI (Fig. 8).[27]

MRI is contributive in defining fetal abdominal, lung, and pelvic masses.[15,25] This can be especially helpful when differing opinions exist as to the etiology of a mass (Fig. 9). Further studies will be needed to assess how additional information from MRI affects patient management and outcome.

COMPARING ULTRASOUND TO MAGNETIC RESONANCE: ALLOWING FOR COUNSELING BY INDIVIDUALS UNFAMILIAR WITH ULTRASOUND

Prenatal counseling is frequently performed by pediatric specialists, such as pediatric neurosurgeons, who have experience reading magnetic resonance examinations but have limited ability to interpret sonograms. At times, the benefit of performing a fetal magnetic resonance is that a

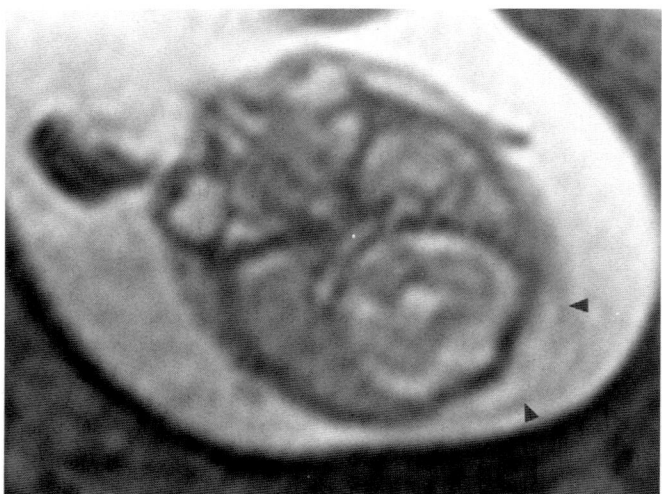

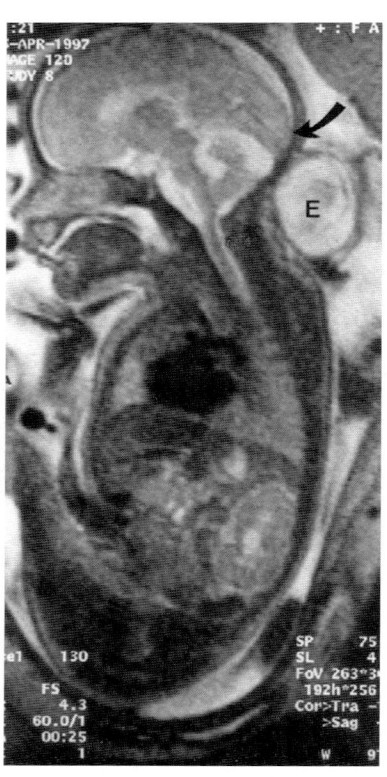

FIGURE 6. Posterior encephalocele in a fetus at 20 weeks' gestational age **(A)** and at 32 weeks' gestational age **(B)**. **A:** Axial magnetic resonance imaging shows a posterior encephalocele (*arrowheads*). The structures of the posterior fossa appear normal. The information that the majority of the brain appeared normal was helpful to the patient in deciding to continue the pregnancy. **B:** In the same fetus at 32 weeks' gestational age, sagittal image demonstrates that only a small portion of posterior cortex (*curved arrow*) is tented toward the encephalocele (*E*). At surgery, the encephalocele was removed, and a small portion of cortex was pushed back into the cranial vault without difficulty. Postnatally, a meningocele sac was excised and the neural content returned to the posterior fossa. **(A:** Reproduced with permission from Levine D, Barnes PD, Edelman RR. State of the art: obstetric MR imaging. *Radiology* 1999;211:609–617. **B:** Reproduced with permission Levine D, Barnes PD, Madsen J, Hulka C, Mehta T, et al. Fetal CNS anomalies depicted with ultrafast MR imaging. *AJR Am J Roentgenol* 1999;172:813–818.)

specialist can feel more confident about a specific diagnosis, and can therefore better counsel the patient.

One question that remains to be evaluated with respect to fetal counseling is how the magnetic resonance findings *in utero* correlate with magnetic resonance findings postnatally. For example, it is known that the degree of hydrocephalus is a less important factor than the intrinsic parenchymal damage.[31] However, it is possible that the consequences of parenchymal damage *in utero* may not be the same as parenchymal damage postnatally. Just as it is difficult to assess the amount of residual normal cortex in fetuses with severe ventriculomegaly before shunting, the same may be true in the assessment of porencephaly. Whereas there is no doubt that the visualization of parenchymal damage portends worse for the outcome than nonvisualization of cortical destruction, counseling of patients must be tempered because the knowledge of the natural history of prenatally diagnosed porencephaly with postnatal correlation is still limited. Similarly, counseling of patients with large arachnoid cysts must be tempered, because the knowledge of the natural history of these lesions is also limited (Fig. 7).

SCREENING FOR ANOMALIES FOR WHICH PRENATAL SCREENING WITH ULTRASOUND OR LABORATORY TESTS IS LIMITED

Magnetic resonance also has the potential to aid in genetic counseling and screening for a disease process for which limited prenatal diagnosis is available. Examples of this are tuberous sclerosis (Fig. 5)[32] in which subependymal tubers have been visualized with magnetic resonance as early as 21 weeks' gestational age, hemochromatosis,[33] and polymicrogyria or lissencephaly.[18] The sensitivity and specificity of prenatal magnetic resonance for evaluation of these anomalies remain to be determined.

POTENTIAL PITFALLS IN FETAL MAGNETIC RESONANCE IMAGING

Although artifacts from fetal motion are minimized using fast scan techniques, if the fetus moves continuously during a sequence, reduced image quality is inevitable. Ours is not currently a real-time technique, although real-time fast MRI acquisition methods using spiral or gradient-echo pulse

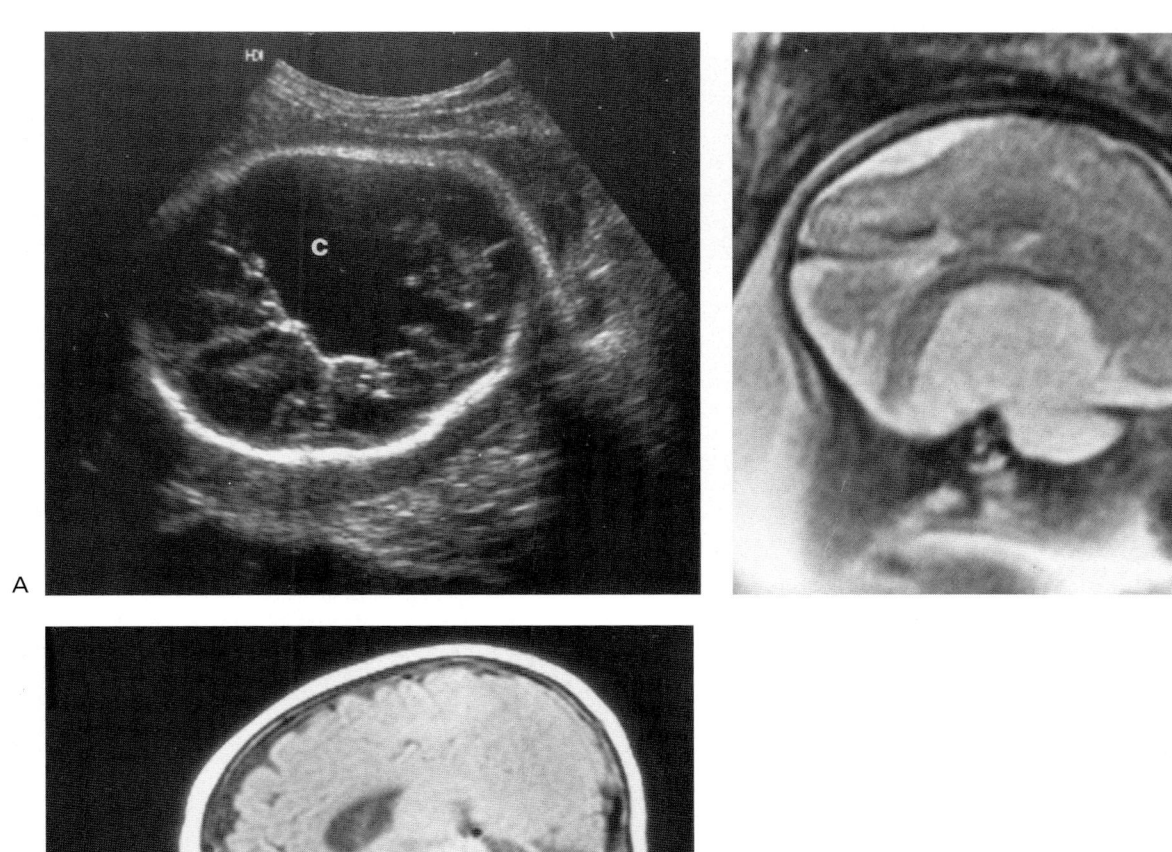

FIGURE 7. Arachnoid cyst in a fetus at 27 weeks' gestational age. **A:** Axial sonogram demonstrates an extraaxial collection (*C*), but it is difficult to assess involvement of the ventricular system. **B:** Sagittal magnetic resonance imaging clearly demonstrates the extraaxial nature of this extensive arachnoid cyst with mass effect on the surrounding structures. **C:** Postnatal magnetic resonance imaging demonstrates the arachnoid cyst, but with less mass effect than that seen prenatally, because the cyst has grown relatively less than the surrounding brain. The toddler has not yet been operated on because of a lack of symptoms. (**A, B:** Reproduced with permission from Levine D, Barnes PD, Edelman RR. State of the art: obstetric MR imaging. *Radiology* 1999;211:609–617.)

sequences are being developed. Motion commonly limits evaluation of the distal extremities. When motion is not a problem, sequential images allow for assessment of the hands and feet. However, even small amounts of motion limit viewing of the extremities in their entirety. Motion that occurs between imaging sequences makes it difficult to obtain images orthogonal to the fetus. When the entire fetus moves, the region of interest may not be in the image plane at all.

Another problem is that because of signal-to-noise limitations, small fetal structures may be difficult to identify and evaluate. Thin structures surrounded by fluid can be difficult to visualize due to partial volume averaging occurring over the thickness of the slice. Examples include the membranous

sac of a neural tube defect, the wall of an arachnoid cyst, and the forming corpus callosum in the second trimester.

Whereas magnetic resonance allows for excellent depiction of fetal anatomy, it is still important to have a high-quality sonogram performed before the MRI. This is important for research purposes, to assess the incremental benefit of magnetic resonance, and is also important for clinical care in the tailoring of the examination to assess a specific problem. In is important to realize that there are anomalies for which magnetic resonance performs less well than ultrasound. For example, because magnetic resonance scans are not gated for fetal cardiac motion, the chambers of the heart are not adequately assessed.[14] In addition, small encephaloceles, the sacs

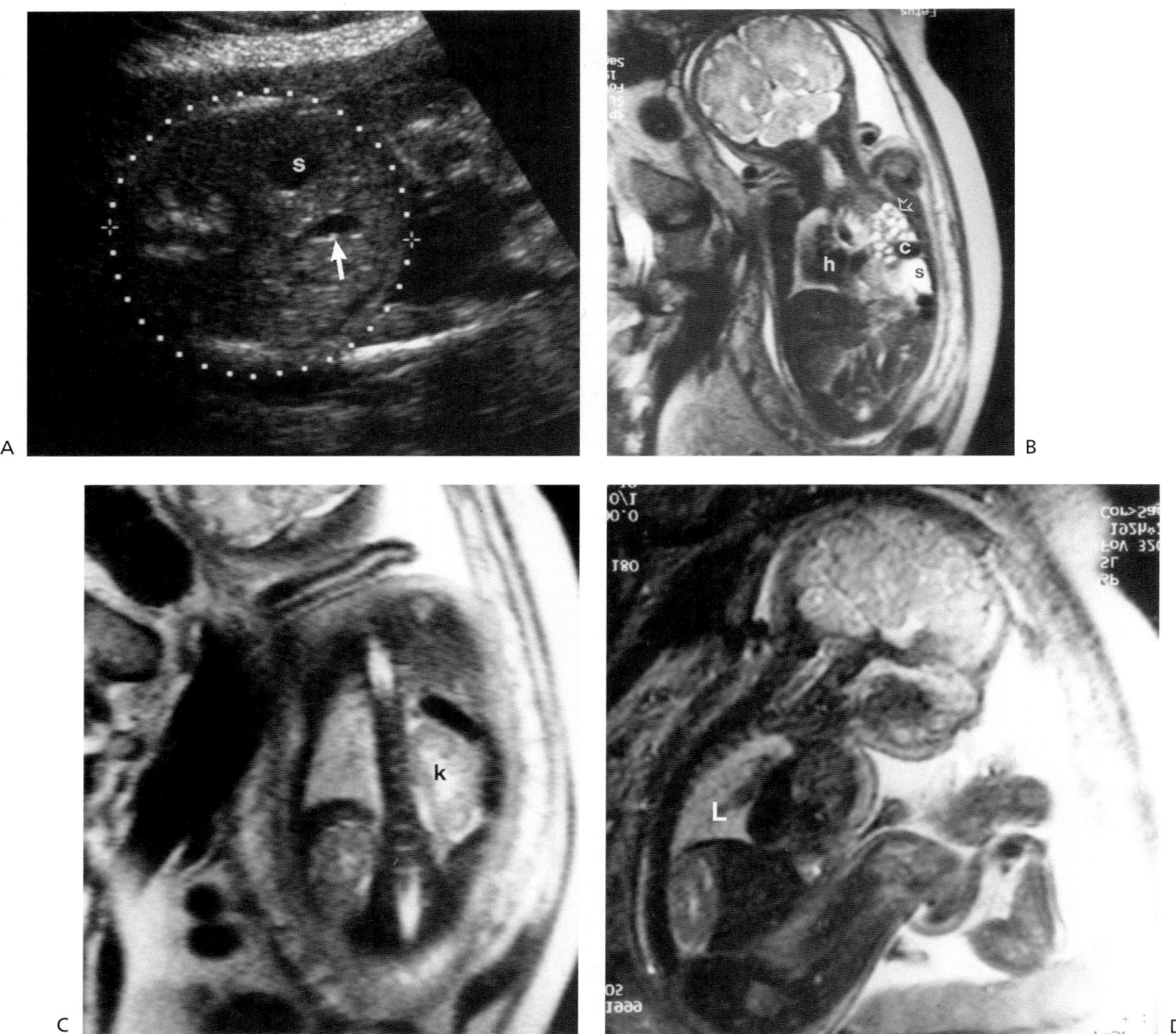

FIGURE 8. A: Axial sonogram of the fetal abdomen shows stomach (*s*) at the level of the portal vein (*arrow*). **B, C:** Coronal magnetic resonance image 41 days later shows the stomach (*s*), colon (*c*), small bowel (*open arrow*), and kidney (*k*) in the chest with mediastinal shift of the heart (*h*) to the right. **D:** Sagittal magnetic resonance image shows normal lung (*L*) that can be seen in the posterior right chest. This figure demonstrates the need for an ultrasound to be performed at the same time as the magnetic resonance image if diagnostic capabilities of the two modalities are going to be compared. [Reproduced with permission from Levine D. Ultrasound versus magnetic resonance imaging in fetal evaluation. *Top Magn Reson Imaging* 2001;12(1):25–38.]

of neural tube defects, and small arachnoid cysts also may be difficult to visualize with magnetic resonance due to partial volume averaging of the thin-walled structure surrounded by cerebrospinal or amniotic fluid (Fig. 6).[13]

Another reason a confirmatory sonogram is helpful is for proper placement of the surface coil. Given the relatively large size of the fetus in the third trimester, and the shape of the maternal abdomen, it is frequently not possible to optimally image the entire fetus with a surface coil. If the intracranial contents are of clinical concern and the fetal head is located low in the maternal pelvis, the surface coil should be centered over the region of interest. This decision can be made before placing the patient in the magnet. This decreases the need for repositioning of the patient. Simi-

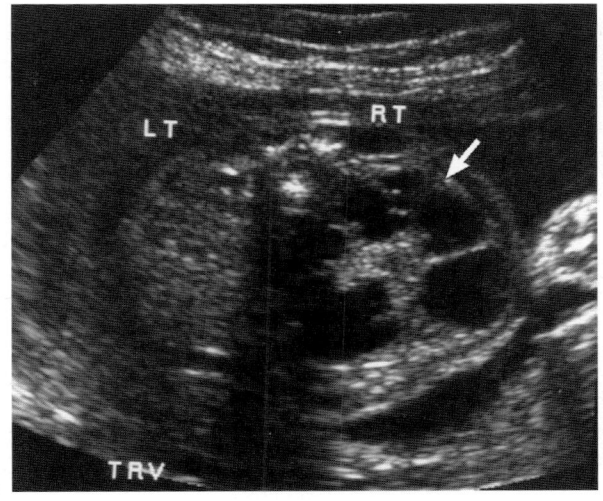

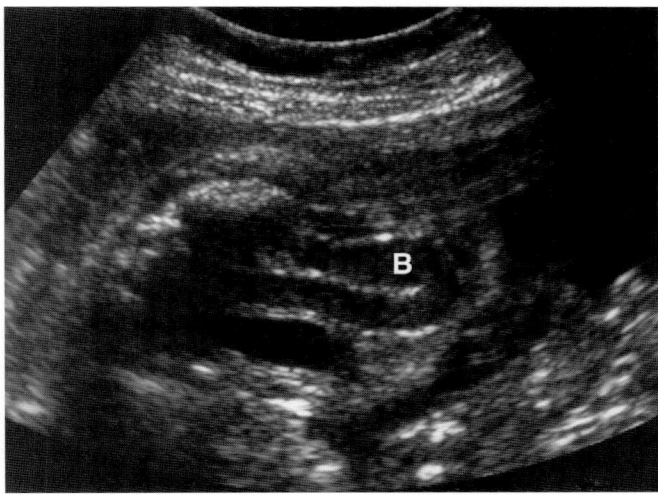

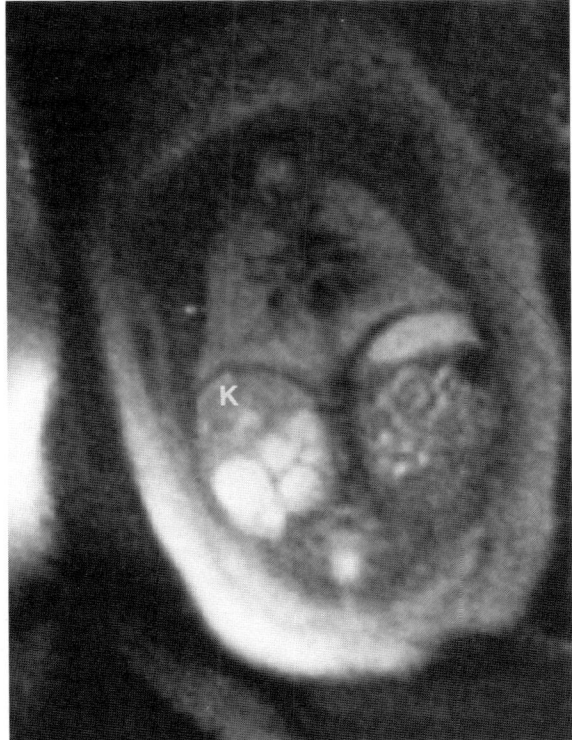

FIGURE 9. Crossed-fused multicystic dysplastic kidney in a fetus at 28 weeks' gestational age. **A:** Axial sonogram in abdomen shows a multiseptated mass of unclear origin (*arrow*). A portion of the right kidney was visualized (not shown), but this was the only normal-appearing renal tissue. LT, left; RT, right; TRV, transverse. **B:** Axial sonogram in the pelvis shows prominent loops of bowel (*B*). **C:** Coronal magnetic resonance imaging shows the multiseptated cyst arising from the lower pole of the right kidney (*K*), indicating a renal origin of the mass. There was no renal tissue in the left renal fossa. In this case, two sonologists had differing opinions as to the etiology of the mass at the time of the sonogram. One sonologist believed the mass was of bowel origin (i.e., a distal small bowel obstruction), and another sonologist believed that the mass was of renal origin (a duplex kidney with multicystic dysplastic kidney being the inferior moiety). The magnetic resonance image clearly showed the renal origin of this mass in this patient with a crossed fused ectopia, with the lower moiety being multicystic dysplastic. [Reproduced with permission from Levine D. Ultrasound versus magnetic resonance imaging in fetal evaluation. *Top Magn Reson Imaging* 2001;12(1):25–38.]

larly with multiple gestations, elucidation of the position of the abnormal gestation aids in placement of the surface coil and interpretation of the images.

HIDDEN RISKS OF MAGNETIC RESONANCE COMPARED WITH ULTRASOUND

When addressing the issue of using magnetic resonance in prenatal diagnosis, a hidden risk of magnetic resonance arises. Visualization of anatomy is possible in a manner not possible with ultrasound. Because of this,

incidental findings in the fetus are inevitably encountered, which will not change management and are unrelated to the referral diagnosis but increase patient anxiety. Additionally, findings of uncertain significance are discovered, which again increase patient anxiety. Examples of this are shown from a study in our laboratory in which normal sonograms were followed by magnetic resonance incidental findings of an enlarged subtemporal vein, a subependymal bleed (Fig. 10), and focal thoracic diastematomyelia.[17,18] An incidental finding is relatively less important when evaluating a fetus with a previously diagnosed sonographic abnormality

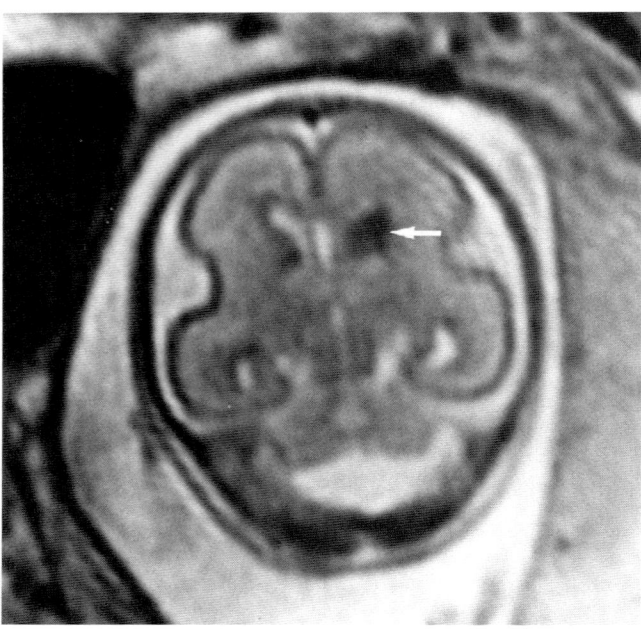

FIGURE 10. Fetus at 18 weeks with incidental finding of subependymal bleed. Coronal magnetic resonance imaging shows low-signal intensity (*arrow*) in the subependymal region on the left consistent with a bleed. [Reproduced with permission from Levine D. Ultrasound versus magnetic resonance imaging in fetal evaluation. *Top Magn Reson Imaging* 2001;12(1):25–38.]

because the patient already realizes that there is a congenital anomaly. However, incidental findings are of crucial importance when using magnetic resonance as a screening modality in otherwise normal fetuses. Patients enter into a screening program with the hope that the fetus will be normal. Even a minor abnormality, with no apparent consequence to the outcome of the pregnancy, can increase patient anxiety.

CONCLUSION

Ultrasound continues to be the screening modality of choice in the evaluation of the fetus due to its relatively low cost and real-time capability. The information provided by ultrasound is useful not only for screening but also as a guide for tailoring the magnetic resonance examination. Proper use and interpretation of ultrasound limits the cases in which magnetic resonance is necessitated. However, there are many cases in which alternative imaging is useful as an adjunct to ultrasound. As experience with fast magnetic resonance techniques increases, patients in whom MRI contributes to patient evaluation will continue to be identified.

REFERENCES

1. Weinreb JC, Lowe T, Cohen JM, Kutler M. Human fetal anatomy: MR imaging. *Radiology* 1985;157:715–720.
2. Antuaco TL, Shah HR, Mattison DR, Quirk JG Jr. MR imaging in high-risk obstetric patients: a valuable complement to US. *Radiographics* 1992;12:91–109.
3. Powell MC, Worthington BS, Buckley JM, Symonds EM. Magnetic resonance imaging (MRI) in obstetrics. II. Fetal anatomy. *Br J Obstet Gynaecol* 1988;95:38–46.
4. Schwartz JL, Crooks LE. NMR imaging produces no observable mutations or cytotoxicity in mammalian cells. *AJR Am J Roentgenol* 1982;139:583–585.
5. Wolff S, Crooks LE, Brown P, Howard R, Painter RB. Tests for DNA and chromosomal damage induced by nuclear magnetic resonance imaging. *Radiology* 1980;136:707–710.
6. Baker PN, Johnson IR, Harvey PR, Gowland PA, Mansfield P. A three-year follow-up of children imaged in utero using echo planar magnetic resonance. *Am J Obstet Gynecol* 1994;170:32–33.
7. Kanal E, Gillen J, Evans JA, Savitz DA, Shellock FG. Survey of reproductive health among female MR workers. *Radiology* 1993;187:395–399.
8. U.S. Food and Drug Administration. *Guidance for content and review of a magnetic resonance diagnostic device 510 (k) application.* Washington, D.C., August 2, 1988.
9. Myers C, Duncan KR, Gowland PA, Johnson IR, Baker PN. Failure to detect intrauterine growth restriction following in utero exposure to MRI. *Br J Radiol* 1998;71:549–551.
10. Levine D, Zuo C, Faro CB, Chen Q. Potential heating effect in the gravid uterus during MR HASTE imaging. *J Magn Reson Imaging* 2001;13(6):856–861.
11. Shellock FG, Kanal E. Policies, guidelines, and recommendations for MR imaging safety and patient management. SMRI Safety Committee. *J Magn Reson Imaging* 1991;1:97–101.
12. Yamashita Y, Namimoto T, Abe Y, et al. MR imaging of the fetus by a HASTE sequence. *AJR Am J Roentgenol* 1997;168:513–519.
13. Levine D, Barnes PD, Madsen JR, Li W, Edelman RR. Fetal central nervous system anomalies: MR imaging augments sonographic diagnosis. *Radiology* 1997;204:635–642.
14. Levine D, Barnes P, Sher S, et al. Fetal fast MR imaging: reproducibility, technical quality, and conspicuity of anatomy. *Radiology* 1998;206:549–554.
15. Levine D, Barnes PD, Edelman RR. State of the art: obstetric MR imaging. *Radiology* 1999;211:609–617.
16. Filly RA, Goldstein RB, Callen PW. Fetal ventricle: importance in routine obstetric sonography. *Radiology* 1991;181:1–7.
17. Levine D, Mehta T, Trop I, Barnes P. Fast MRI of fetal CNS anomalies with prenatal MRI: results of 149 cases. *Radiology* 2000;(RSNA program book):101.
18. Levine D, Barnes PD, Madsen JR, Abbott J, Mehta T, et al. Central nervous system abnormalities assessed with prenatal magnetic resonance imaging. *Obstet Gynecol* 1999;94:1011–1019.
19. Vergani P, Locatelli A, Strobelt N, et al. Clinical outcome of mild fetal ventriculomegaly. *Am J Obstet Gynecol* 1998;178:218–222.

20. Patel MD, Filly AL, Hersh DR, Goldstein RB. Isolated mild fetal cerebral ventriculomegaly: clinical course and outcome. *Radiology* 1994;192:759–764.

21. Bloom SL, Bloom DD, Dellanebbia C, Martin LB, Lucas MJ, et al. The developmental outcome of children with antenatal mild isolated ventriculomegaly. *Obstet Gynecol* 1997;90:93–97.

22. Nicolaides KH, Berry S, Snijders RJ, Thorpe-Beeston JG, Gosden C. Fetal lateral cerebral ventriculomegaly: associated malformations and chromosomal defects. *Fetal Diagn Ther* 1990;5:5–14.

23. Sutton LN, Adzick NS, Bilaniuk LT, Johnson MP, Crombleholme TM, et al. Improvement in hindbrain herniation demonstrated by serial fetal magnetic resonance imaging following fetal surgery for myelomeningocele [see comments]. *JAMA* 1999;282:1826–1831.

24. Levine D, Barnes PD. Cortical maturation in normal and abnormal fetuses as assessed with prenatal MRI. *Radiology* 1999;210:751–758.

25. Quinn TM, Hubbard AM, Adzick NS. Prenatal magnetic resonance imaging enhances fetal diagnosis. *J Pediatr Surg* 1998;33:553–558.

26. Levine D, Jennings R, Barnewolt C, Mehta T, Wilson J, et al. Progressive fetal bronchial obstruction caused by a bronchogenic cyst diagnosed by prenatal MR imaging. *AJR Am J Roentgenol* 2001;176(1):49–52.

27. Leung JWT, Coakley FV, Hricak H, et al. Prenatal MR imaging of congenital diaphragmatic hernia. *AJR Am J Roentgenol* 2000;174:1607–1612.

28. Hubbard AM, Adzick NS, Crombleholme TM, Haselgrove JC. Left-sided congenital diaphragmatic hernia: value of prenatal MR imaging in preparation for fetal surgery. *Radiology* 1997;203:636–640.

29. Metkus AP, Filly RA, Stringer MD, et al. Sonographic predictors of survival in fetal diaphragmatic hernia. *J Pediatr Surg* 1996:148–152.

30. Adzick SN, Harrison MR, Glick PL, Nakayama DK, Manning FA, et al. Diaphragmatic hernia in the fetus: prenatal diagnosis and outcome in 94 cases. *J Pediatr Surg* 1985;20:357–361.

31. Giudetti B, Occhipinti E, Riccio A. Ventriculo-atrial shunt in 200 cases of non-tumsoural hydrocephalus in children: remarks on the diagnostic criteria, postoperative complications and long-term results. *Acta Neurochir* 1969;21:295–308.

32. Levine D, Barnes P, Korf B, Edelman R. Tuberous sclerosis: second trimester diagnosis of subependymal tubers with fast MRI. *AJR Am J Roentgenol* 2000;175:1067–1069.

33. Coakley FV, Hricak H, Filly RA, Barkovich AJ, Harrison MR. Complex fetal disorders: effect of MR imaging on management—preliminary clinical experience. *Radiology* 1999;213:691–696.

SURGICAL MANAGEMENT OF PRENATALLY DIAGNOSED MALFORMATIONS

Routine obstetric sonography has changed the surgical management of many congenital anomalies. The widespread use of prenatal ultrasound has contributed immensely to the understanding of the natural history and pathophysiology of many diseases previously considered for only postnatal therapy. In some cases, prenatal diagnosis simply permits appropriate guidance and counseling. This may influence the timing (Table 1) or mode (Table 2) of delivery and in some cases lead to elective termination of the pregnancy. In others, various forms of *in utero* therapy may be possible either now or in the future (Table 3). This chapter discusses the current approach to the management of congenital diaphragmatic hernia (CDH), abdominal wall defects, hydronephrosis (HN), giant neck masses, sacrococcygeal teratoma (SCT), and myelomeningocele (MMC). Further discussion of the characteristic appearance of these anomalies on prenatal ultrasound may be found in their respective chapters. We have also found that ultrafast fetal magnetic resonance imaging (MRI) is a very useful adjunct to prenatal ultrasound for accurate diagnosis of various fetal anomalies and use this frequently in the prenatal evaluations.[1]

The finding of a significant anomaly on routine prenatal ultrasound should prompt a referral to a fetal diagnosis and treatment center for a full multidisciplinary evaluation. This usually involves a high definition ultrasound, fetal echocardiogram, ultrafast fetal MRI, as well as consultations with the fetal surgery team. The perinatal management of these patients involves many different medical disciplines, including obstetricians, sonographers, neonatologists, geneticists, pediatric surgeons, and pediatricians. It is essential that the affected family be managed using a team approach and that information and experience be exchanged freely.

CONGENITAL DIAPHRAGMATIC HERNIA

CDH occurs most commonly due to the failure of the pleuroperitoneal folds to fuse normally. It is more common on the left side and has a frequent association with other major congenital defects, especially cardiac and chromosomal anomalies. On prenatal ultrasound, it is possible to detect the herniated abdominal viscera, as well as possible mediastinal shift and polyhydramnios. To distinguish this lesion from other abnormalities, it is necessary to visualize abdominal contents on a transverse view at the level of the four-chamber view of the heart. In fetuses in which the liver has also herniated into the chest, it may be possible to see the hepatic veins coursing superiorly, although MRI is superior in visualizing the position of the liver.[2,3]

The main physiologic derangement in CDH is pulmonary hypoplasia secondary to mass effect from the herniated abdominal viscera. The size of the defect and the timing of herniation contribute to the severity of pulmonary hypoplasia. The physiologic basis for *in utero* treatment of CDH has been shown in lamb models of the disease, in which fetal tracheal occlusion has led to decreased lung liquid egress and ultimately resulted in compensatory lung growth.[4,5] The current strategy for fetal tracheal occlusion is to use a tracheal clip or a balloon; the latter may be deployed fetoscopically (Fig. 1).[6]

The most important prognostic indicator in fetuses with CDH is the ratio of the right lung to the head circumference (LHR), which is defined as the right lung area (measured at the level of the transverse four-chamber view of the heart) divided by the head circumference.[7] A prospective study has shown that fetuses with LHR less than 1 rarely survive, those with LHR greater than 1.4 nearly always survive, and those with LHR 1.0 to 1.4 have a 38% survival rate.[8] Also, patients who have liver herniation have lower survival rates and require extracorporeal membrane oxygenation more frequently.[9] Thus, fetuses with a poor prognosis based on these criteria are more likely to benefit from fetal intervention.[10] Our current algorithm for fetal intervention is only for fetuses who have an isolated CDH diagnosed before 26 weeks with liver herniation and LHR less than 0.9.

We have reviewed our experience with fetal tracheal occlusion in 15 fetuses who had isolated CDH, with LHR less

TABLE 1. DEFECTS THAT MAY LEAD TO PRETERM DELIVERY

Obstructive hydronephrosis
Gastroschisis or ruptured omphalocele
Intestinal ischemia and necrosis secondary to volvulus, meconium ileus, and such
Sacrococcygeal teratoma with hydrops

TABLE 2. DEFECTS THAT MAY REQUIRE CESAREAN DELIVERY

Myelomeningocele
Gastroschisis
Large sacrococcygeal teratoma
Giant neck masses (*ex utero* intrapartum treatment procedure)

than 1 and liver herniation.[11] There were five survivors (33%) and ten deaths, including two immediate postoperative deaths and eight postnatal deaths. In contrast, there were no survivors in a similar group that did not have fetal surgery, although the series is too small to form definitive conclusions. Interestingly, although animal models have shown consistent lung growth after fetal tracheal occlusion, there was variable lung growth seen in this series even after early occlusion, and patients with lung growth did not necessarily have improved lung function. These observations support a randomized clinical trial for rigorous testing of the fetal surgery strategy for CDH, which is currently under way.

NECK MASSES

Airway obstruction in a fetus may be caused by large neck masses such as cervical teratoma or cystic hygroma, or by intrinsic defects in the airway such as congenital high airway obstruction syndrome.[12] Cystic hygroma is a lymphatic abnormality that may be complicated by polyhydramnios and chromosomal abnormalities (most often Turner syndrome).[13] Prenatal diagnosis has defined two groups of patients with differing prognoses: those diagnosed early in gestation often have coexisting anomalies and more commonly develop hydrops, whereas those diagnosed later in gestation tend to have isolated lesions.[14] It is, therefore, important to obtain serial ultrasounds to evaluate for the development of hydrops. Prenatal MRI has also been used to determine the relationship of the mass to the airway in preparation for delivery.[15]

The fetus with a giant neck mass has an enormous perinatal mortality due to airway obstruction at the time of birth.[16] The *ex utero* intrapartum treatment procedure has

been life-saving for many such patients by converting a neonatal emergency into a controlled operation at delivery.[17] The *ex utero* intrapartum treatment procedure, originally developed for the removal of tracheal clips at the time of birth,[18] involves maternal hysterotomy and control of the airway while still on placental support (Fig. 2). It differs importantly from a cesarean section in that deep maternal anesthesia and only partial delivery of the fetus during the procedure prevent uterine contractions while the airway is being secured. After delivery of the head and shoulders, direct laryngoscopy and endotracheal intubation are performed. If this is not possible, a tracheostomy is done, which sometimes requires partial resection of the mass due to distortion of the normal anatomy. Our recent review showed an 80% survival rate in ten fetuses with giant neck masses with this strategy, with successful endotracheal intubation in six patients and tracheostomy in three patients.[12] One patient died because of parental refusal for a tracheostomy, and one patient died postnatally due to pulmonary hypoplasia.

We advocate that this procedure be performed by an experienced team anytime there is concern that a neck mass may cause respiratory compromise at the time of birth. Further, the *ex utero* intrapartum treatment procedure may be used for a variety of other abnormalities in which there is a danger of hemodynamic compromise at the time of birth, because it allows time for obtaining control of the airway and circulation while still on placental support.

ABDOMINAL WALL DEFECTS

An omphalocele is a midline defect containing herniated abdominal contents with a sac composed of amnion and

TABLE 3. DISEASES AMENABLE TO FETAL SURGICAL INTERVENTION IN SELECTED CASES

Malformation	Effect on development	*In utero* treatment
Congenital diaphragmatic hernia	Pulmonary hypoplasia, respiratory failure	Tracheal occlusion using a clip or balloon catheter
CCAM or BPS	Pulmonary hypoplasia, hydrops	Thoracoamniotic shunting, lobectomy
Sacrococcygeal teratoma	Massive arteriovenous shunting, placentomegaly, hydrops	Excision
Urethral obstruction	Hydronephrosis, lung hypoplasia	Vesicoamniotic shunting, fetoscopic ablation of posterior urethral valves
Myelomeningocele	Damage to spinal cord, paralysis, hydrocephalus	Closure of defect

BPS, bronchopulmonary sequestration; CCAM, congenital cystic adenomatoid malformation.

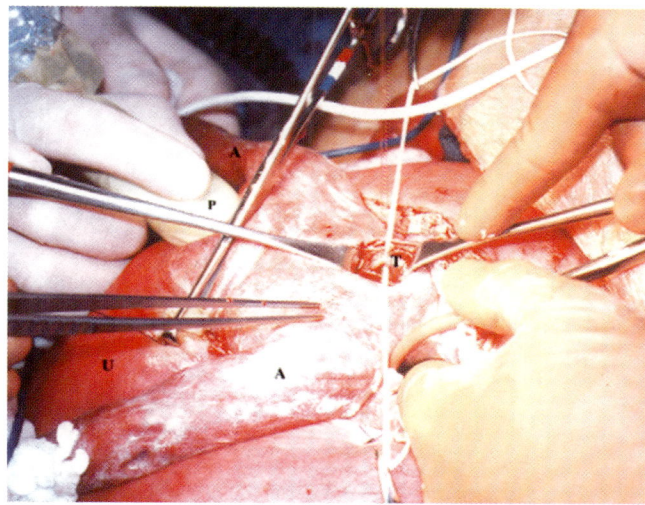

FIGURE 1. Intraoperative photograph before application of a tracheal clip. The head and arms (*A*) of the fetus have been delivered from the uterus (*U*), and the trachea (*T*) has been exposed. The ultrasound probe (*P*) provides continuous intraoperative monitoring of the fetal heart.

peritoneum, probably secondary to failure of the abdominal viscera to return to the abdomen in the tenth week of gestation.[19] It is commonly associated with major chromosomal anomalies such as Beckwith-Wiedemann syndrome, pentalogy of Cantrell, and renal and cardiac anomalies.[20] On ultrasound, it is possible to visualize the abdominal viscera as well as the liver, if present, in the hernia sac. The umbilical cord insertion is into the membrane covering the defect, which distinguishes it from gastroschisis.

Gastroschisis is usually a right paraumbilical defect with no membrane covering the exposed bowel. Although there is less association with other congenital anomalies, gastroschisis

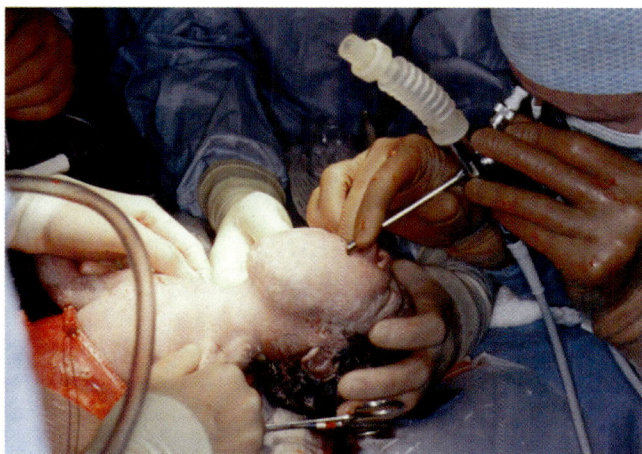

FIGURE 2. Photograph of an *ex utero* intrapartum treatment procedure for a large cervical teratoma, demonstrating rigid bronchoscopy before intubation. Note that only the head and shoulders of the fetus are delivered out of the uterus at this stage.

may be complicated by intestinal atresias or obstruction, leading to polyhydramnios. Animal models suggest that intestinal damage is secondary to amniotic fluid exposure as well as bowel constriction at the level of the defect, which leads to ischemia and venous obstruction.[21,22] On ultrasound, the bowel may appear thickened due to the formation of a fibrous peel from prolonged exposure to amniotic fluid. Serial ultrasounds are necessary to look for bowel dilatation that may be a sign of obstruction or intestinal atresia,[23] as well as bowel thickening and signs of increased peristalsis. Early delivery may be indicated in fetuses who show severe signs of bowel damage, although this must be weighed against the risks of prematurity.

There are conflicting views regarding the mode of delivery in patients with abdominal wall defects. Several series have indicated that there is no difference in outcome between vaginal and cesarean delivery in babies with abdominal wall defects.[24,25] However, other series indicate that cesarean delivery with immediate repair may lead to easier fascial closure, shorter time to enteral feeding, and shorter hospital stay.[26,27] Our current algorithm is to perform serial ultrasound measurements to monitor for the development of obstruction and to perform an immediate repair after a planned cesarean section.

HYDRONEPHROSIS

Prenatal HN is a relatively common diagnosis that may be secondary to ureteropelvic junction obstruction, multicystic kidney disease, primary obstructive megaureter, ureterocele, ectopic ureter, or posterior urethral valves.[28] In patients with unilateral obstruction[29] and renal pelvic diameter of less than 10 mm,[30] the prognosis is excellent. Ureteropelvic junction obstruction is the most common cause and carries the best prognosis, with one series showing normal renal function in 17% of patients at birth and in 80% of patients at 3 years.[31] However, because approximately 20% of patients need surgical intervention after birth (those with persistent marked HN, poor renal function, and recurrent infections), it is important to follow up prenatally diagnosed HN with ultrasound at birth and at 1 month.[32]

HN secondary to lower urinary tract obstruction is a more serious abnormality, which occurs most commonly due to posterior urethral valves in male fetuses (in female fetuses, it is usually part of a cloacal anomaly). On ultrasound, the fetus has bilateral HN, oligohydramnios, and a dilated bladder. Mortality and morbidity from this disease are secondary to pulmonary hypoplasia due to long-standing oligohydramnios *in utero*.[33] The most important prognostic indicator in these patients is serial fetal urine analysis after drainage of the bladder three times at 48- to 72-hour intervals. Fetuses with decreasing electrolytes, proteins, and tonicity have a favorable outcome after prenatal vesicoamniotic shunting.[34]

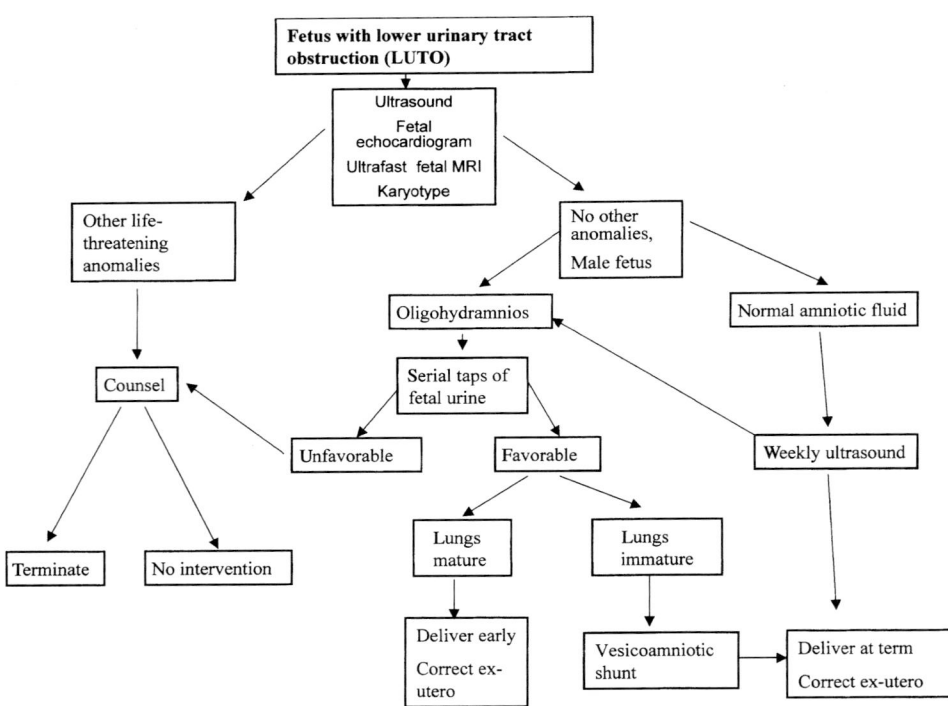

FIGURE 3. Algorithm for the management of a fetus with lower urinary tract obstruction. MRI, magnetic resonance imaging.

Sheep models of the disease have shown that prenatal correction of HN can improve the pulmonary hypoplasia.[35,36] Currently, this is achieved by vesicoamniotic shunting or fetal cystoscopic ablation of posterior urethral valves.[37] The patient population that benefits most from this procedure is male fetuses with bilateral HN, oligohydramnios, and bladder distension with favorable urine profiles after serial drainage.[38] In this carefully selected population, antenatal intervention leads to normal renal function in 43% of patients at 2 years after birth.[39] Figure 3 outlines our current algorithm for managing prenatally diagnosed lower urinary tract obstruction.

CONGENITAL CHEST LESIONS

The two most common pulmonary lesions detected on prenatal ultrasound are congenital cystic adenomatoid malformation (CCAM) and bronchopulmonary sequestration. CCAM is characterized by abnormal overgrowth of bronchioles in one lobe of lung, leading to disorganized cysts.[40] For prenatally diagnosed lesions, a distinction is made between macrocystic lesions (with cysts larger than 5 cm) or microcystic lesions, which contain multiple smaller cysts.[41] Bronchopulmonary sequestrations are nonfunctional masses of normal lung tissue that are not connected to the tracheobronchial tree and have a systemic blood supply. Hybrid lesions with CCAM-like histology and a systemic blood supply have also been described, illustrating the close embryologic association between congenital lung lesions.[42,43]

Although most of these lesions are detected by routine prenatal ultrasound, fetal MRI is useful in making a correct diagnosis when ultrasound is ambiguous. Lesions such as CDH, tracheal atresia, pulmonary agenesis, neurenteric cyst, and bronchopulmonary sequestration may be erroneously diagnosed as CCAM on ultrasound.[44] MRI is also useful in such cases to delineate normal from abnormal lungs. The location of systemic feeding vessels is best demonstrated by color-flow Doppler ultrasound.

We have learned that the size of the lesion and the resultant physiologic derangements secondary to compression and mediastinal shift are the most important predictors of outcome, rather than the histology of the mass. Pulmonary hypoplasia can occur secondary to compression of normal lung tissue by the mass. Polyhydramnios may result from esophageal compression. Most important, large chest masses may cause mediastinal shift and compression of the superior vena cava, leading to hydrops.[45] Because hydrops is an important harbinger of fetal demise, fetuses with these lesions should be followed closely with serial ultrasounds. The ratio of the size of the mass to the head circumference (CCAM volume ratio) correlates with prognosis in that patients with a CCAM volume ratio greater than 1.2 are more likely to develop hydrops.[46]

We reviewed our experience with 175 cases of prenatally diagnosed lung lesions.[47] There were 134 fetuses with CCAM, of which 101 were managed expectantly, with demise of all 25 fetuses who developed hydrops and were not treated *in utero*. In the fetal intervention category, 13 fetuses with hydrops underwent fetal lobectomy with eight survivors, whereas six fetuses with giant cysts underwent

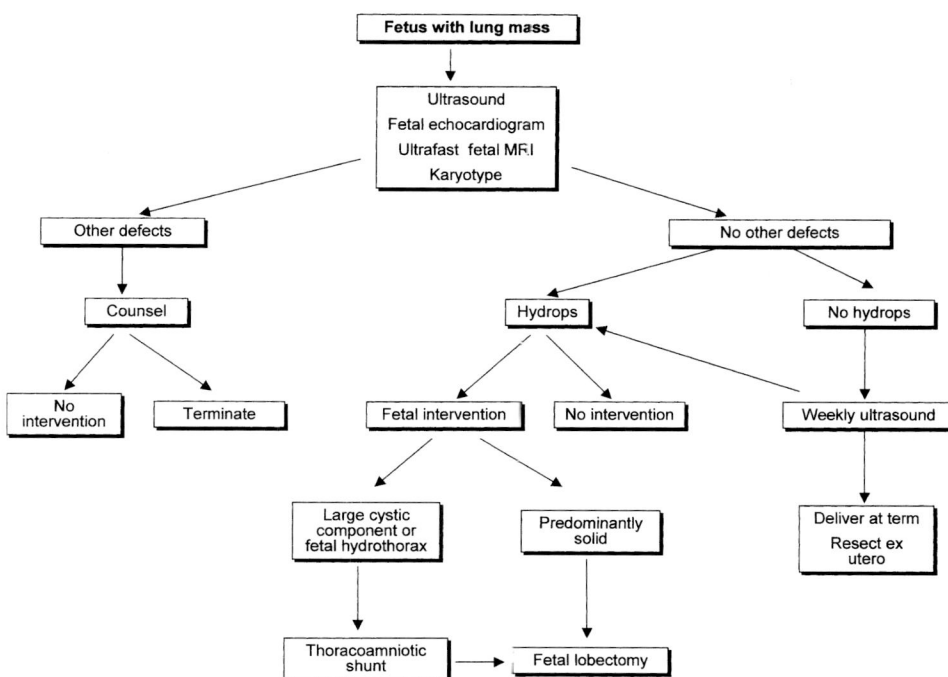

FIGURE 4. Algorithm for the management of a fetus with a lung mass. MRI, magnetic resonance imaging.

thoracoamniotic shunting, with five survivors. There were 41 prenatally diagnosed bronchopulmonary sequestrations, and three of these fetuses developed tension hydrothorax from fluid or lymph secretion by the mass and needed fetal treatment with thoracoamniotic shunt or thoracentesis. Seven patients underwent postnatal resection with good survival and one patient with hydrops died after delivery despite postnatal extracorporeal membrane oxygenation. Twenty-eight of 41 lesions regressed in size during gestation, and no resection was required postnatally. This experience highlights the benefits of fetal intervention (open lobectomy or thoracoamniotic shunting) in fetuses younger than 32 weeks who develop hydrops, while illustrating that fetuses with large chest masses without hydrops can be managed expectantly by planned delivery and postnatal resection (Fig. 4). Although some lesions may decrease in size during gestation,[48] a thorough postnatal evaluation must still be performed to detect residual lesions for resection.[49]

SACROCOCCYGEAL TERATOMA

SCT is the most common newborn tumor, occurring in 1 per 35,000 births.[50] Four subtypes are recognized, with varying degrees of internal and external components.[51] Overall, lesions that are entirely intrapelvic (type 4) have the worst prognosis because they are difficult to diagnose, less amenable to surgical resection, and frequently malignant at the time of postnatal diagnosis. Regardless of the subtype, prenatal diagnosis in general defines a group with a worse prognosis. As with other fetal anomalies, we have found fetal MRI to be a useful adjunct to ultrasound in the prenatal evaluation (Fig. 5).[52] MRI is superior to ultra-

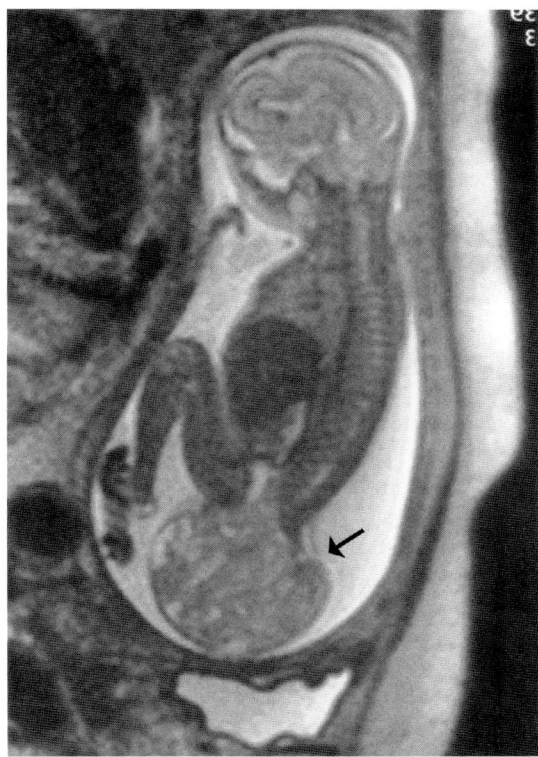

FIGURE 5. Ultrafast magnetic resonance imaging of a fetus with a large sacrococcygeal teratoma (*arrow*).

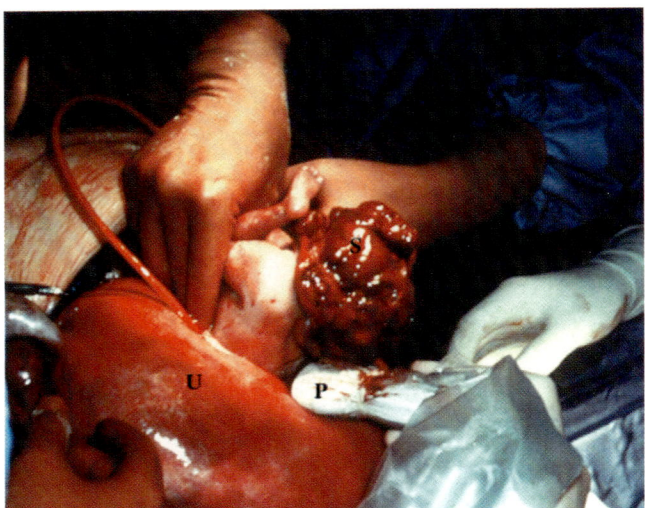

FIGURE 6. Intraoperative photograph of a fetal sacrococcygeal teratoma resection. The lower extremities and sacrococcygeal teratoma (*S*) have been delivered out of the uterus (*U*). Continuous intraoperative monitoring of the fetus is achieved by using a sterile ultrasound probe (*P*).

sound in mapping the intrapelvic portion of the tumor because it is not limited by acoustic shadowing from the pelvic bones.

The main physiologic derangement caused by the tumor is the shunting of blood to the tumor, as in a large arteriovenous fistula, causing high output cardiac failure.[53,54] Anemia from hemorrhage into the tumor compounds the stress on the fetal heart. Fetuses with a mainly solid and very vascular SCT have a higher risk of developing hydrops,[55,56] which carries a nearly 100% mortality without fetal intervention.[57]

Fetal resection of tumors with a large extrapelvic component may be lifesaving if hydrops is present or imminent. We reported the first successful case of a fetal SCT resection in a 26-week-old fetus who had a large SCT and accompanying polyhydramnios and early signs of hydrops (Fig. 6). Fetal resection of the mass reversed this pathophysiology and prevented the development of hydrops.[58] Our current algorithm for the management of prenatally diagnosed SCT is close monitoring by serial ultrasound for the development of placentomegaly and hydrops.[59] If these develop after pulmonary maturation, the fetus should be delivered by emergent cesarean section. If hydrops develops and the fetus is too young for immediate delivery, open fetal surgery may be considered.

MYELOMENINGOCELE

The repair of prenatally diagnosed MMC is an exciting new frontier in fetal surgery.[60] MMC is a neural tube defect affecting 1 in 2,000 births, characterized by the protrusion

of the spinal cord and meninges through open vertebral arches. MMC is usually first identified by abnormal maternal serum alpha-fetoprotein at 15 to 16 weeks and may be confirmed by amniocentesis and ultrasound.[61] The characteristics of this anomaly on ultrasound include frontal bone scalloping and abnormal anterior curvature of the cerebellar hemispheres (the *lemon* and *banana* signs, respectively).[62] Many fetuses also have an associated Arnold-Chiari malformation, consisting of caudal displacement of the vermis and cerebellum with midbrain herniation through the foramen magnum.

As in other fetal defects amenable to surgical repair, fetal lamb models have established a rationale for *in utero* intervention. The creation of MMC in fetal lambs leads to flaccid paraplegia, incontinence, and absent hind limb somatosensory potential, indicating that the spinal cord damage seen in MMC is secondary to prolonged exposure to amniotic fluid and the intrauterine environment. Experiments in which a fetal lamb MMC was created early in gestation and then repaired using a latissimus dorsi flap prevented neurologic damage in sheep.[63] Fetal repair may prevent chemical and mechanical trauma to the exposed spinal cord while altering the hemodynamics of CSF flow to allow resolution of hindbrain herniation. We reported the first successful case of open fetal repair of MMC in a 23-week-old fetus with a T11-S1 defect.[64] The fetus, delivered at 30 weeks, had improved neurologic function with resolution of the hindbrain herniation and did not require a ventriculoperitoneal shunt (Fig. 7).

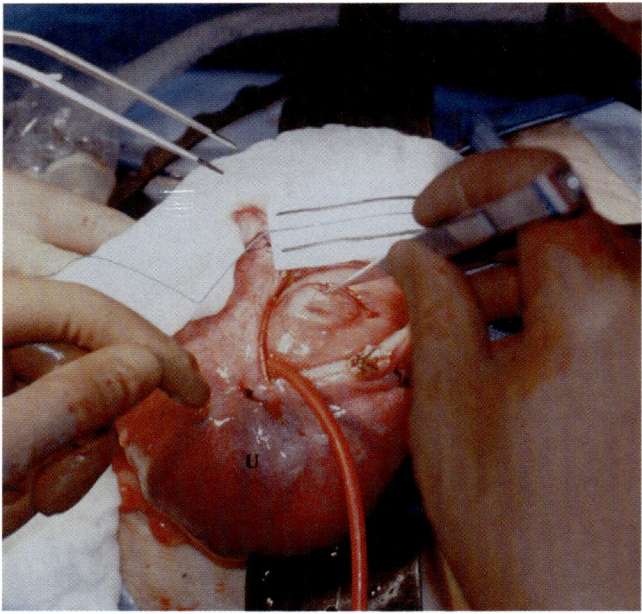

FIGURE 7. Intraoperative photograph of a fetal myelomeningocele repair showing the backside of the fetus with the myelomeningocele defect inside the stapled edge of the uterus (*U*).

The clinical experience since this initial report has been gratifying; fetuses who have undergone open fetal repair of MMC have resolution of the hindbrain herniation,[65,66] which is a significant achievement considering that much of the morbidity of this disease is secondary to the associated Arnold-Chiari malformation. There is also evidence to suggest that there is less incidence of shunting as well as improved neurologic function after *in utero* repair. The desire to repair the defect as early as possible (21 to 25 weeks) to avoid long-term exposure of the spinal cord to amniotic fluid must be weighed against the risks of preterm labor after fetal surgery. Therefore, we currently offer fetal intervention to patients who are less than 25 weeks' gestation with isolated MMC and an associated Arnold-Chiari malformation. A randomized clinical trial is being organized to compare outcomes in patients with and without fetal therapy. If fetal repair is not performed, we recommend delivery by cesarean section to avoid damage to the spinal cord during labor.[67,68]

CONCLUSION

Prenatal diagnosis and close follow-up of fetuses with congenital anomalies have been crucial in defining the pathophysiology and natural history of many lesions. In many cases, prenatal diagnosis has defined a *hidden mortality* in demonstrating that patients who are prenatally diagnosed have a poorer outcome than those who present later in life.[69] Careful evaluation of series of patients at fetal treatment centers has shown prognostic indicators for many congenital anomalies, which has been crucial for the prenatal management and counseling of these patients. The careful study of these lesions by fetal surgery teams, as well as the creation of similar lesions in large animal models, has also indicated very select groups of fetuses who may benefit from fetal intervention. In most cases, fetal surgery is advised only when the fetal demise is imminent but may also be considered for cases such as MMC in which there is promising evidence that fetal surgery may be superior to postnatal interventions for the ultimate outcome. Continued re-evaluation of prenatal and postnatal outcomes as well as the design of randomized controlled clinical trials, when feasible, is necessary to refine the management strategies outlined in this chapter.

REFERENCES

1. Quinn TM, Hubbard AM, Adzick NS. Prenatal magnetic resonance imaging enhances fetal diagnosis. *J Pediatr Surg* 1998;33:553–558.
2. Hubbard AM, Adzick NS, Crombleholme TM, Haselgrove JC. Left-sided congenital diaphragmatic hernia: value of prenatal MR imaging in preparation for fetal surgery. *Radiology* 1997;203:636–640.
3. Hubbard AM, Crombleholme TM, Adzick NS, et al. Prenatal MRI evaluation of congenital diaphragmatic hernia. *Am J Perinatol* 1999;16:407–413.
4. DiFiore JW, Fauza DO, Slavin R, Peters CA, Fackler JC, et al. Experimental fetal tracheal ligation reverses the structural and physiological effects of pulmonary hypoplasia in congenital diaphragmatic hernia. *J Pediatr Surg* 1994;29:248–56; discussion 256–257.
5. Davey MG, Hooper SB, Tester ML, Johns DP, Harding R. Respiratory function in lambs after in utero treatment of lung hypoplasia by tracheal obstruction. *J Appl Physiol* 1999;87:2296–2304.
6. VanderWall KJ, Bruch SW, Meuli M, et al. Fetal endoscopic ('Fetendo') tracheal clip. *J Pediatr Surg* 1996;31:1101–1103; discussion 1103–1104.
7. Metkus AP, Filly RA, Stringer MD, Harrison MR, Adzick NS. Sonographic predictors of survival in fetal diaphragmatic hernia. *J Pediatr Surg* 1996;31:148–151; discussion 151–152.
8. Lipshutz GS, Albanese CT, Feldstein VA, et al. Prospective analysis of lung-to-head ratio predicts survival for patients with prenatally diagnosed congenital diaphragmatic hernia. *J Pediatr Surg* 1997;32:1634–1636.
9. Albanese CT, Lopoo J, Goldstein RB, et al. Fetal liver position and perinatal outcome for congenital diaphragmatic hernia. *Prenat Diagn* 1998;18:1138–1142.
10. Harrison MR, Mychaliska GB, Albanese CT, et al. Correction of congenital diaphragmatic hernia in utero IX: fetuses with poor prognosis (liver herniation and low lung-to-head ratio) can be saved by fetoscopic temporary tracheal occlusion. *J Pediatr Surg* 1998;33:1017–1022; discussion 1022–1023.
11. Flake AW, Crombleholme TM, Johnson MP, Howell LJ, Adzick NS. Treatment of severe congenital diaphragmatic hernia by fetal tracheal occlusion: clinical experience with fifteen cases. *Am J Obstet Gynecol* 2000;183:1059–1066.
12. Liechty KW, Crombleholme TM. Management of fetal airway obstruction. *Semin Perinatol* 1999;23:496–506.
13. Descamps P, Jourdain O, Paillet C, et al. Etiology, prognosis and management of nuchal cystic hygroma: 25 new cases and literature review. *Eur J Obstet Gynecol Reprod Biol* 1997;71:3–10.
14. Gallagher PG, Mahoney MJ, Gosche JR. Cystic hygroma in the fetus and newborn. *Semin Perinatol* 1999;23:341–356.
15. Hubbard AM, Crombleholme TM, Adzick NS. Prenatal MRI evaluation of giant neck masses in preparation for the fetal EXIT procedure. *Am J Perinatol* 1998;15:253–257.
16. Langer JC, Fitzgerald PG, Desa D, et al. Cervical cystic hygroma in the fetus: clinical spectrum and outcome. *J Pediatr Surg* 1990;25:58–61; discussion 61–62.
17. Liechty KW, Crombleholme TM, Flake AW, et al. Intrapartum airway management for giant fetal neck masses: the EXIT (ex utero intrapartum treatment) procedure. *Am J Obstet Gynecol* 1997;177:870–874.
18. Mychaliska GB, Bealer JF, Graf JL, Rosen MA, Adzick NS, et al. Operating on placental support: the ex utero intrapartum treatment procedure. *J Pediatr Surg* 1997;32:227–30; discussion 230–231.
19. Langer JC. Gastroschisis and omphalocele. *Semin Pediatr Surg* 1996;5:124–128.
20. Dykes EH. Prenatal diagnosis and management of abdominal wall defects. *Semin Pediatr Surg* 1996;5:90–94.

21. Langer JC, Longaker MT, Crombleholme TM, et al. Etiology of intestinal damage in gastroschisis. I. Effects of amniotic fluid exposure and bowel constriction in a fetal lamb model. *J Pediatr Surg* 1989;24:992–997.

22. Langer JC, Bell JG, Castillo RO, et al. Etiology of intestinal damage in gastroschisis, II. Timing and reversibility of histological changes, mucosal function, and contractility. *J Pediatr Surg* 1990;25:1122–1126.

23. Brun M, Grignon A, Guibaud L, Garel L, Saint-Vil D. Gastroschisis: are prenatal ultrasonographic findings useful for assessing the prognosis? *Pediatr Radiol* 1996;26:723–726.

24. How HY, Harris BJ, Pietrantoni M, et al. Is vaginal delivery preferable to elective cesarean delivery in fetuses with a known ventral wall defect? *Am J Obstet Gynecol* 2000; 182:1527–1534.

25. Rinehart BK, Terrone DA, Isler CM, Larmon JE, Perry KG Jr, et al. Modern obstetric management and outcome of infants with gastroschisis [see comments]. *Obstet Gynecol* 1999;94:112–116.

26. Dunn JC, Fonkalsrud EW, Atkinson JB. The influence of gestational age and mode of delivery on infants with gastroschisis. *J Pediatr Surg* 1999;34:1393–1395.

27. Coughlin JP, Drucker DE, Jewell MR, Evans MJ, Klein MD. Delivery room repair of gastroschisis. *Surgery* 1993;114:822–826; discussion 826–827.

28. Elder JS. Antenatal hydronephrosis. Fetal and neonatal management. *Pediatr Clin North Am* 1997;44:1299–1321.

29. Coplen DE. Prenatal intervention for hydronephrosis. *J Urol* 1997;157:2270–2277.

30. Fasolato V, Poloniato A, Bianchi C, et al. Feto-neonatal ultrasonography to detect renal abnormalities: evaluation of 1-year screening program. *Am J Perinatol* 1998;15:161–164.

31. Kitagawa H, Pringle KC, Stone P, Flower J, Murakami N, et al. Postnatal follow-up of hydronephrosis detected by prenatal ultrasound: the natural history. *Fetal Diagn Ther* 1998;13:19–25.

32. Johnson MP, Freedman AL. Fetal uropathy. *Curr Opin Obstet Gynecol* 1999;11:185–194.

33. Nakayama DK, Harrison MR, de Lorimier AA. Prognosis of posterior urethral valves presenting at birth. *J Pediatr Surg* 1986;21:43–45.

34. Johnson MP, Corsi P, Bradfield W, et al. Sequential urinalysis improves evaluation of fetal renal function in obstructive uropathy [see comments]. *Am J Obstet Gynecol* 1995;173: 59–65.

35. Harrison MR, Ross N, Noall R, de Lorimier AA. Correction of congenital hydronephrosis in utero. I. The model: fetal urethral obstruction produces hydronephrosis and pulmonary hypoplasia in fetal lambs. *J Pediatr Surg* 1983;18: 247–256.

36. Harrison MR, Nakayama DK, Noall R, de Lorimier AA. Correction of congenital hydronephrosis in utero. II. Decompression reverses the effects of obstruction on the fetal lung and urinary tract. *J Pediatr Surg* 1982;17:965–974.

37. Quintero RA, Shukla AR, Homsy YL, Bukkapatnam R. Successful in utero endoscopic ablation of posterior urethral valves: a new dimension in fetal urology. *Urology* (Online) 2000;55:774.

38. Walsh DS, Johnson MP. Fetal interventions for obstructive uropathy. *Semin Perinatol* 1999;23:484–495.

39. Freedman AL, Johnson MP, Smith CA, Gonzalez R, Evans MI. Long-term outcome in children after antenatal intervention for obstructive uropathies [see comments]. *Lancet* 1999;354:374–377.

40. Stocker JT, Madewell JE, Drake RM. Congenital cystic adenomatoid malformation of the lung. Classification and morphologic spectrum. *Hum Pathol* 1977;8:155–171.

41. Adzick NS, Harrison MR, Glick PL, et al. Fetal cystic adenomatoid malformation: prenatal diagnosis and natural history. *J Pediatr Surg* 1985;20:483–488.

42. Cass DL, Crombleholme TM, Howell LJ, Stafford PW, Ruchelli ED, et al. Cystic lung lesions with systemic arterial blood supply: a hybrid of congenital cystic adenomatoid malformation and bronchopulmonary sequestration. *J Pediatr Surg* 1997;32:986–990.

43. Conran RM, Stocker JT. Extralobar sequestration with frequently associated congenital cystic adenomatoid malformation, type 2: report of 50 cases. *Pediatr Dev Pathol* 1999;2:454–463.

44. Hubbard AM, Adzick NS, Crombleholme TM, et al. Congenital chest lesions: diagnosis and characterization with prenatal MR imaging. *Radiology* 1999;212:43–48.

45. Rice HE, Estes JM, Hedrick MH, Bealer JF, Harrison MR, et al. Congenital cystic adenomatoid malformation: a sheep model of fetal hydrops. *J Pediatr Surg* 1994;29:692–696.

46. Liechty KW, Crombleholme TM, Coleman BG, Howell LJ, Flake AW, et al. Elevated cystic adenomatoid malformation volume ratio (CVR) is associated with development of hydrops. *Am J Obstet Gynecol* 1999;180:S165.

47. Adzick NS, Harrison MR, Crombleholme TM, Flake AW, Howell LJ. Fetal lung lesions: management and outcome. *Am J Obstet Gynecol* 1998;179:884–889.

48. MacGillivray TE, Harrison MR, Goldstein RB, Adzick NS. Disappearing fetal lung lesions. *J Pediatr Surg* 1993;28: 1321–1324; discussion 1324–1325.

49. Winters WD, Effmann EL, Nghiem HV, Nyberg DA. Disappearing fetal lung masses: importance of postnatal imaging studies. *Pediatr Radiol* 1997;27:535–539.

50. Flake AW. Fetal sacrococcygeal teratoma. *Semin Pediatr Surg* 1993;2:113–120.

51. Altman RP, Randolph JG, Lilly JR. Sacrococcygeal teratoma: American Academy of Pediatrics Surgical Section Survey—1973. *J Pediatr Surg* 1974;9:389–398.

52. Kirkinen P, Partanen K, Merikanto J, Ryynanen M, Haring P, et al. Ultrasonic and magnetic resonance imaging of fetal sacrococcygeal teratoma. *Acta Obstet Gynecol Scand* 1997; 76:917–922.

53. Bond SJ, Harrison MR, Schmidt KG, et al. Death due to high-output cardiac failure in fetal sacrococcygeal teratoma. *J Pediatr Surg* 1990;25:1287–1291.

54. Schmidt KG, Silverman NH, Harison MR, Callen PW. High-output cardiac failure in fetuses with large sacrococcygeal teratoma: diagnosis by echocardiography and Doppler ultrasound. *J Pediatr* 1989;114:1023–1028.

55. Holterman AX, Filiatrault D, Lallier M, Youssef S. The natural history of sacrococcygeal teratomas diagnosed through routine obstetric sonogram: a single institution experience. *J Pediatr Surg* 1998;33:899–903.

56. Westerburg B, Feldstein VA, Sandberg PL, Lopoo JB, Harrison MR, et al. Sonographic prognostic factors in fetuses

with sacrococcygeal teratoma. *J Pediatr Surg* 2000;35:322–325; discussion 325–326.

57. Chisholm CA, Heider AL, Kuller JA, von Allmen D, McMahon MJ, et al. Prenatal diagnosis and perinatal management of fetal sacrococcygeal teratoma. *Am J Perinatol* 1999;16:47–50.
58. Adzick NS, Crombleholme TM, Morgan MA, Quinn TM. A rapidly growing fetal teratoma. *Lancet* 1997;349:538.
59. Kitano Y, Flake AW, Crombleholme TM, Johnson MP, Adzick NS. Open fetal surgery for life-threatening fetal malformations. *Semin Perinatol* 1999;23:448–461.
60. Olutoye OO, Adzick NS. Fetal surgery for myelomeningocele. *Semin Perinatol* 1999;23:462–473.
61. Platt LD, Feuchtbaum L, Filly R, Lustig L, Simon M, et al. The California Maternal Serum Alpha-Fetoprotein Screening Program: the role of ultrasonography in the detection of spina bifida. *Am J Obstet Gynecol* 1992;166:1328–1329.
62. Van den Hof MC, Nicolaides KH, Campbell J, Campbell S. Evaluation of the lemon and banana signs in one hundred thirty fetuses with open spina bifida. *Am J Obstet Gynecol* 1990;162:322–327.
63. Meuli M, Meuli-Simmen C, Hutchins GM, et al. In utero surgery rescues neurological function at birth in sheep with spina bifida. *Nat Med* 1995;1:342–347.
64. Adzick NS, Sutton LN, Crombleholme TM, Flake AW. Successful fetal surgery for spina bifida [letter] [see comments]. *Lancet* 1998;352:1675–1676.
65. Sutton LN, Adzick NS, Bilaniuk LT, Johnson MP, Crombleholme TM, et al. Improvement in hindbrain herniation demonstrated by serial fetal magnetic resonance imaging following fetal surgery for myelomeningocele [see comments]. *JAMA* 1999;282:1826–1831.
66. Bruner JP, Tulipan N, Paschall RL, et al. Fetal surgery for myelomeningocele and the incidence of shunt-dependent hydrocephalus [see comments]. *JAMA* 1999;282:1819–1825.
67. Luthy DA. Maternal markers and complications of pregnancy [editorial; comment]. *N Engl J Med* 1999;341:2085–2087.
68. Scheller JM, Nelson KB. Does cesarean delivery prevent cerebral palsy or other neurologic problems of childhood? [See comments.] *Obstet Gynecol* 1994;83:624–630.
69. Harrison MR, Bjordal RI, Langmark F, Knutrud O. Congenital diaphragmatic hernia: the hidden mortality. *J Pediatr Surg* 1978;13:227–230.

APPENDICES

See also
    http://www.fetalultrasound.org
    http://www.perinatology.com/calculators/exbiometry.htm

Note: Most values expressed as fifth, fiftieth (mean), and ninety-fifth percentiles. The ninety-fifth percentile = mean + 1.6452 standard deviation and the fifth percentile = mean − 1.6452 standard deviation.

FIRST TRIMESTER VALUES

TABLE 1. COMBINED DATA COMPARING MENSTRUAL AGE WITH MEAN GESTATIONAL SAC DIAMETER, CROWN-RUMP LENGTH, AND HUMAN CHORIONIC GONADOTROPIN LEVELS

Menstrual age (d)	Menstrual age (wk)	Gestational sac size (mm)	Crown-rump length (mm)	Human chorionic gonadotropin level (first IRP), mean (U/L)	Human chorionic gonadotropin level (first IRP), range (U/L)
30	4.3	—	—	—	—
31	4.4	—	—	—	—
32	4.6	3	—	1,710	(1,050–2,800)
33	4.7	4	—	2,320	(140–3,760)
34	4.9	5	—	3,100	(1,940–4,980)
35	5	5.5	—	4,090	(2,580–6,330)
36	5.1	6	—	5,340	(3,400–8,450)
37	5.3	7	—	6,880	(4,420–10,810)
38	5.4	8	—	8,770	(5,680–13,660)
39	5.6	9	—	11,040	(7,220–17,050)
40	5.7	10	0.2	13,730	(9,050–21,040)
41	5.9	11	0.3	15,300	(10,140–23,340)
42	6	12	0.4	16,870	(11,230–25,640)
43	6.1	13	0.4	30,480	(13,750–30,880)
44	6.3	14	0.5	24,560	(16,650–36,750)
45	6.4	15	0.6	29,110	(19,910–43,220)
46	6.6	16	0.7	34,100	(25,530–50,210)
47	6.7	17	0.8	39,460	(27,470–57,640)
48	6.9	18	0.9	45,120	(31,700–65,380)
49	7	19	1.0	50,970	(36,130–73,280)
50	7.1	20	1.0	56,900	(40,700–81,150)
51	7.3	21	1.1	62,760	(45,300–88,790)
52	7.4	22	1.2	68,390	(49,810–95,990)
53	7.6	23	1.3	73,640	(54,120–102,540)
54	7.7	24	1.4	78,350	(58,100–108,230)
55	7.9	25	1.5	82,370	(61,640–112,870)
56	8	26	1.6	85,560	(64,600–116,310)
57	8.1	26.5	1.7	—	—
58	8.3	27	1.8	—	—
59	8.4	28	1.9	—	—
60	8.6	29	2.0	—	—
61	8.7	30	2.1	—	—
62	8.9	31	2.2	—	—
63	9	32	2.3	—	—
64	9.1	33	2.4	—	—
65	9.3	34	2.5	—	—
66	9.4	35	2.6	—	—
67	9.6	36	2.8	—	—
68	9.7	37	2.9	—	—
69	9.9	38	3.0	—	—
70	10	39	3.1	—	—
71	10.1	40	3.2	—	—
72	10.3	41	3.4	—	—
73	10.4	42	3.5	—	—
74	10.6	43	3.7	—	—
75	10.7	44	3.8	—	—
76	10.9	45	4.0	—	—
77	11	46	4.1	—	—
78	11.1	47	4.2	—	—
79	11.3	48	4.4	—	—
80	11.4	49	4.6	—	—
81	11.6	50	4.8	—	—
82	11.7	51	5.0	—	—
83	11.9	52	5.2	—	—
84	12	53	5.4	—	—

IRP, International Reference Preparation.
Reproduced with permission from Nyberg DA, Hill LM, Bohm-Velez M. *Transvaginal ultrasound*. St. Louis: Mosby–Year Book, 1992; Hadlock FP, Shah YP, Kanon DJ, et al. Crown-rump length: reevaluation of relation to menstrual age (5–18 weeks) with high-resolution real-time US. *Radiology* 1992;182:501; and Robinson HP. "Gestational sac" volumes as determined by sonar in the first trimester of pregnancy. *Br J Obstet Gynecol* 1975;82:100; and data from Daya S, Woods S. Transvaginal ultrasound scanning in early pregnancy and correlation with human chorionic gonadotropin levels. *J Clin Ultrasound* 1991;19:139.

TABLE 2. PREDICTED MENSTRUAL AGE FROM CROWN-RUMP LENGTH MEASUREMENTS

Crown-rump length (mm)	Menstrual age (wk)	Crown-rump length (mm)	Menstrual age (wk)
0.2	5.7	4.2	11.1
0.3	5.9	4.4	11.3
0.4	6.0	4.6	11.4
0.4	6.1	4.8	11.6
0.5	6.3	5.0	11.7
0.6	6.4	5.2	11.9
0.7	6.6	5.4	12.0
0.8	6.7	5.5	12.1
0.9	6.9	5.6	12.2
1.0	7.0	5.7	12.3
1.0	7.1	5.8	12.3
1.1	7.3	5.9	12.4
1.2	7.4	6.0	12.5
1.3	7.6	6.1	12.6
1.4	7.7	6.2	12.6
1.5	7.9	6.3	12.7
1.6	8.0	6.4	12.8
1.7	8.1	6.5	12.8
1.8	8.3	6.6	12.9
1.9	8.4	6.7	13.0
2.0	8.6	6.8	13.1
2.1	8.7	6.9	13.1
2.2	8.9	7.0	13.2
2.3	9.0	7.1	13.3
2.4	9.1	7.2	13.4
2.5	9.3	7.3	13.4
2.6	9.4	7.4	13.5
2.8	9.6	7.5	13.6
2.9	9.7	7.6	13.7
3.0	9.9	7.7	13.8
3.1	10.0	7.8	13.8
3.2	10.1	7.9	13.9
3.4	10.3	8.0	14.0
3.5	10.4	8.1	14.1
3.7	10.6	8.2	14.2
3.8	10.7	8.3	14.2
4.0	10.9	8.4	14.3
4.1	11.0	—	—

Reproduced with permission from Hadlock FP, Shah YP, Kanon DJ, Lindsey JV. Fetal crown-rump length: reevaluation of relation to menstrual age (5–18 weeks) with high-resolution real-time US. *Radiology* 1992;182:501–505.

TABLE 3. REFERENCE VALUES FOR CROWN-RUMP LENGTH COMPARED TO GESTATIONAL SAC SIZE

Gestational sac (mm)[b]	Crown-rump length (mm)[a]		
	Percentiles		
	5th	50th	95th
10	0	4	8
11	0	5	9
12	0	5	10
13	1	5	10
14	1	6	11
15	1	7	12
16	1	7	13
17	2	8	14
18	2	8	15
19	2	9	15
20	3	10	16
21	3	10	17
22	4	11	18
23	4	12	19
24	5	12	20
25	5	13	21
26	6	14	22
27	6	15	24
28	7	16	25
29	7	17	26
30	8	18	27
31	9	18	28
32	9	19	29
33	10	20	31
34	11	21	32
35	12	22	33
36	12	23	34
37	13	25	36
38	14	26	37
39	15	27	38
40	16	28	40
41	17	29	41
42	18	30	43
43	19	31	44
44	20	33	46
45	21	34	47
46	22	35	49
47	23	37	50
48	24	38	52
49	25	39	54
50	26	41	55

[a]Crown-rump length = $0.012 \times$ gestational sac size^2 + 0.9708 + $0.192 \times$ gestational sac size.
[b]Standard deviation = 0.9185 + $0.1599 \times$ gestational sac size.
Adapted from Grisolia G, Milano V, Pilu G, Banzi C, David C, et al. Biometry of early pregnancy with transvaginal sonography. *Ultrasound Obstet Gynecol* 1993;3:403–411.

AMNIOTIC FLUID INDEX

TABLE 4. REFERENCE VALUES FOR AMNIOTIC FLUID INDEX

Gestational age (wk)	Amniotic fluid index (mm)				
	Percentiles				
	2.5th	5th	50th	95th	97.5th
16	73	79	121	185	201
17	77	83	128	194	211
18	80	87	133	202	220
19	83	90	138	207	225
20	86	93	141	212	230
21	88	95	144	214	233
22	89	97	146	216	235
23	90	98	147	218	237
24	90	98	148	219	238
25	89	97	148	221	240
26	89	97	148	223	242
27	85	95	148	226	245
28	86	94	148	228	249
29	84	92	147	231	254
30	82	90	147	234	258
31	79	88	146	238	263
32	77	86	146	242	269
33	64	83	145	245	274
34	72	81	144	248	278
35	70	79	142	249	279
36	68	77	140	249	279
37	66	75	138	244	275
38	65	73	134	239	269
39	64	72	130	226	255
40	63	71	125	214	240
41	63	70	119	194	216
42	63	69	112	175	192

Note: Based on formula log (mean amniotic fluid index) = $0.2108 \pm 0.26599 \times$ gestational age $+ 0.01358 \times$ gestational age$^2 + 0.0003101 \times$ gestational age$^3 + 0.000002684 \times$ gestational age.^{4}

Modified from Moore TR, Gayle JE. The amniotic fluid index in normal human pregnancy. *Am J Obstet Gynecol* 1990;162:1168–1173.

BASIC BIOMETRY: HEAD CIRCUMFERENCE, BIPARIETAL DIAMETER, FEMUR LENGTH, AND ABDOMINAL CIRCUMFERENCE

TABLE 5. FORMULAS FOR PREDICTION OF GESTATIONAL AGE

Kurtz 1980[a]	$GA = 3.418 + 0.482\ BPD - 0.00457\ BPD^2 + 0.000037\ BPD^3$
Hadlock 1984[a]	$GA = 9.54 + 0.1482\ BPD + 0.001676\ BPD^2$
	$GA = 10.35 + 0.246\ FL + 0.0017\ FL^2$
	$GA = 10.61 + 0.00175\ BPD \times FL + 0.0297\ AC + 0.071\ FL$
Ott 1985[a]	$GA = 8.26128 + 0.206788\ BPD + 0.000012986\ BPD^3$
	$GA = 10.1438 + 0.215221\ FL + 0.0000265926\ FL^3$
Jeanty 1984[a]	$GA = 9.5411757 + 0.2977451\ FL + 0.0010388013\ FL^2$
Doubilet 1993[a]	$Ln(GA) = 2.27969 + 0.015091\ BPD$
	$Ln(GA) = 2.45132 + 0.016590\ FL$
	$Ln(GA) = 2.38631 + 0.0050012\ BPD + 0.0090476\ FL + 0.00048293\ AC$
	Truncated at 42 wk for each formula
Altman[b]	$Ln(GA) = 0.045575 - 0.0061838\ BPD \times log(BPD) + 1.985$
	$(SD = 0.0002531\ BPD + 0.02988)$
	$Ln(GA) = 0.01045\ HC - 0.000029919\ HC^2 + 0.43156 \times 10^{-7}\ HC^3 + 1.854$
	$(SD\ 0.00005945\ HC + 0.024261)$
	$Ln(GA) = 0.010611\ HC - 0.00003032\ HC^2 + 0.43498 \times 10^{-7}\ HC^3 + 1.848$
	$(SD = -0.00052635 + 0.000014204\ HC^2 + 0.08024)$

AC, abdominal circumference; BPD, biparietal diameter; FL, femur length; GA, gestational age; HC, head circumference; Ln(GA), natural log.
[a]Derived from Doubilet PM, Benson CB. Improved prediction of gestational age in the late third trimester. *J Ultrasound Med* 1993;12:647–653.
[b]Reproduced with permission from Altman DG, Chitty LS. New charts for ultrasound dating of pregnancy. *Ultrasound Obstet Gynecol* 1997;10(3):174–191.

TABLE 6. PREDICTED FETAL MEASUREMENTS AT SPECIFIC GESTATIONAL AGE (GA)

GA (wk)	Biparietal diameter (cm)[a]	Head circumference (cm)[b]	Femur length (cm)[c]	Abdominal circumference (cm)[d]
12	1.7	6.8	0.7	4.6
13	2.1	8.2	1.1	6.0
14	2.5	9.7	1.4	7.3
15	2.9	11.1	1.7	8.6
16	3.2	12.4	2.1	9.9
17	3.6	13.8	2.4	11.2
18	3.9	15.1	2.7	12.5
19	4.3	16.4	3.0	13.7
20	4.6	17.7	3.3	15.0
21	5.0	18.9	3.6	16.2
22	5.3	20.1	3.8	17.4
23	5.6	21.3	4.1	18.5
24	5.9	22.4	4.4	19.7
25	6.2	23.5	4.6	20.8
26	6.5	24.6	4.9	21.9
27	6.8	25.6	5.1	23.0
28	7.1	26.6	5.4	24.0
29	7.3	27.5	5.6	25.1
30	7.6	28.4	5.8	26.1
31	7.8	29.3	6.1	27.1
32	8.0	30.1	6.3	28.1
33	8.3	30.8	6.5	29.1
34	8.5	31.5	6.7	30.0
35	8.7	32.2	6.9	30.9
36	8.8	32.8	7.1	31.8
37	9.0	33.3	7.2	32.7
38	9.2	33.8	7.4	33.6
39	9.3	34.2	7.6	34.4
40	9.4	34.6	7.7	35.3

[a]Biparietal diameter = $-3.08 + 0.41 \times GA - 0.000061 \times GA^2$ (standard deviation, 3 mm).
[b]Head circumference = $-11.48 + 1.56 \times GA - 0.0002548 \times GA^2$ (standard deviation, 1 cm).
[c]Femur length = $-3.91 + 0.427 \times GA - 0.0034 \times GA^2$ (standard deviation, 3 mm).
[d]Abdominal circumference = $-13.3 + 1.61 \times GA - 0.00998 \times GA^2$ (standard deviation, 1.34 cm).
Data from Hadlock FP, Deter RL, Harrist RB, Park SK. Estimating fetal age: computer assisted analysis of multiple fetal growth parameters. *Radiology* 1984;152:497–501.

TABLE 7. REFERENCE VALUES FOR ABDOMINAL CIRCUMFERENCE

Menstrual age (wk)	Abdominal circumference (cm) Percentiles				
	3rd	10th	50th	90th	97th
14.0	6.4	6.7	7.3	7.9	8.3
15.0	7.5	7.9	8.6	9.3	9.7
16.0	8.6	9.1	9.9	10.7	11.2
17.0	9.7	10.3	11.2	12.1	12.7
18.0	10.9	11.5	12.5	13.5	14.1
19.0	11.9	12.6	13.7	14.8	15.5
20.0	13.1	13.8	15.0	16.3	17.0
21.0	14.1	14.9	16.2	17.6	18.3
22.0	15.1	16.0	17.4	18.8	19.7
23.0	16.1	17.0	18.5	20.0	20.9
24.0	17.1	18.1	19.7	21.3	22.3
25.0	18.1	19.1	20.8	22.5	23.5
26.0	19.1	20.1	21.9	23.7	24.8
27.0	20.0	21.1	23.0	24.9	26.0
28.0	20.9	22.0	24.0	26.0	27.1
29.0	21.8	23.0	25.1	27.2	28.4
30.0	22.7	23.9	26.1	28.3	29.5
31.0	23.6	24.9	27.1	29.4	30.6
32.0	24.5	25.8	28.1	30.4	31.8
33.0	25.3	26.7	29.1	31.5	32.9
34.0	26.1	27.5	30.0	32.5	33.9
35.0	26.9	28.3	30.9	33.5	34.9
36.0	27.7	29.2	31.8	34.4	35.9
37.0	28.5	30.0	32.7	35.4	37.0
38.0	29.2	30.8	33.6	36.4	38.0
39.0	29.9	31.6	34.4	37.3	38.9
40.0	30.7	32.4	35.3	38.2	39.9

Adapted from Hadlock FP, Deter RL, Harrist RB, Park SK. Estimating fetal age: computer-assisted analysis of multiple fetal growth parameters. *Radiology* 1984;152:497–501.

TABLE 8. PERCENTILE VALUES FOR HEAD CIRCUMFERENCE

Menstrual age (wk)	Head circumference (cm)				
	3rd	10th	50th	90th	97th
14.0	8.8	9.1	9.7	10.3	10.6
15.0	10.0	10.4	11.0	11.6	12.0
16.0	11.3	11.7	12.4	13.1	13.5
17.0	12.6	13.0	13.8	14.6	15.0
18.0	13.7	14.2	15.1	16.0	16.5
19.0	14.9	15.5	16.4	17.4	17.9
20.0	16.1	16.7	17.7	18.7	19.3
21.0	17.2	17.8	18.9	20.0	20.6
22.0	18.3	18.9	20.1	21.3	21.9
23.0	19.4	20.1	21.3	22.5	23.2
24.0	20.4	21.1	22.4	23.7	24.3
25.0	21.4	22.2	23.5	24.9	25.6
26.0	22.4	23.2	24.6	26.0	26.8
27.0	23.3	24.1	25.6	27.0	27.9
28.0	24.2	25.1	26.6	28.1	29.0
29.0	25.0	25.9	27.5	29.1	30.0
30.0	25.8	26.8	28.4	30.0	31.0
31.0	26.7	27.6	29.3	31.0	31.9
32.0	27.4	28.4	30.1	31.8	32.8
33.0	28.0	29.0	30.8	32.6	33.6
34.0	28.7	29.7	31.5	33.3	34.3
35.0	29.3	30.4	32.2	34.1	35.1
36.0	29.9	30.9	32.8	34.7	35.8
37.0	30.3	31.4	33.3	35.2	36.3
38.0	30.8	31.9	33.8	35.8	36.8
39.0	31.1	32.2	34.2	36.2	37.3
40.0	31.5	32.6	34.6	36.6	37.7

Adapted from Hadlock FP, Deter RL, Harrist RB, Park SK. Estimating fetal age: computer-assisted analysis of multiple fetal growth parameters. *Radiology* 1984;152:497–501.

TABLE 9. REFERENCE VALUES FOR FEMUR LENGTH

Menstrual age (wk)	Femur length (cm)				
	Percentiles				
	3rd	10th	50th	90th	97th
14.0	1.2	1.3	1.4	1.5	1.6
15.0	1.5	1.6	1.7	1.9	1.9
16.0	1.7	1.8	2.0	2.2	2.3
17.0	2.1	2.2	2.4	2.6	2.7
18.0	2.3	2.5	2.7	2.9	3.1
19.0	2.6	2.7	3.0	3.3	3.4
20.0	2.8	3.0	3.3	3.6	3.8
21.0	3.0	3.2	3.5	3.8	4.0
22.0	3.3	3.5	3.8	4.1	4.3
23.0	3.5	3.7	4.1	4.5	4.7
24.0	3.8	4.0	4.4	4.8	5.0
25.0	4.0	4.2	4.6	5.0	5.2
26.0	4.2	4.5	4.9	5.3	5.6
27.0	4.4	4.6	5.1	5.6	5.8
28.0	4.6	4.9	5.4	5.9	6.2
29.0	4.8	5.1	5.6	6.1	6.4
30.0	5.0	5.3	5.8	6.3	6.6
31.0	5.2	5.5	6.0	6.5	6.8
32.0	5.3	5.6	6.2	6.8	7.1
33.0	5.5	5.8	6.4	7.0	7.3
34.0	5.7	6.0	6.6	7.2	7.5
35.0	5.9	6.2	6.8	7.4	7.8
36.0	6.0	6.4	7.0	7.6	8.0
37.0	6.2	6.6	7.2	7.9	8.2
38.0	6.4	6.7	7.4	8.1	8.4
39.0	6.5	6.8	7.5	8.2	8.6
40.0	6.6	7.0	7.7	8.4	8.8

Adapted from Hadlock FP, Deter RL, Harrist RB, Park SK. Estimating fetal age: computer-assisted analysis of multiple fetal growth parameters. *Radiology* 1984;152:497–501.

TABLE 10. REFERENCE VALUES FOR ABDOMINAL CIRCUMFERENCE (AC), HEAD CIRCUMFERENCE (HC), BIPARIETAL DIAMETER (BPD), AND FEMUR LENGTH (FL)

GA (wk)	AC (mm) Percentiles			HC (mm) Percentiles			BPD (mm) Percentiles			FL (mm) Percentiles		
	5th	50th	95th	5th	50th	95th	5th	50th	95th	5th	50th	95th
14	76	86	97	97	105	113	27	30	32	13	16	18
15	84	95	107	106	115	123	30	32	35	16	18	21
16	92	104	117	116	125	134	32	35	38	18	21	23
17	100	113	127	126	135	146	35	38	41	20	23	26
18	109	123	138	136	146	157	38	41	45	23	26	29
19	118	133	150	146	157	170	41	44	48	25	28	32
20	127	144	162	157	169	182	44	48	52	28	31	35
21	137	155	174	168	181	195	47	51	55	30	34	37
22	147	166	187	179	192	207	50	54	59	33	36	40
23	157	178	200	190	204	220	53	57	62	35	39	43
24	168	189	213	201	216	233	56	61	66	38	42	46
25	178	201	226	212	228	246	59	64	69	41	44	49
26	189	213	239	222	240	258	62	67	73	43	47	51
27	199	225	253	233	251	270	65	70	76	45	50	54
28	210	237	266	243	262	282	67	73	80	48	52	57
29	220	248	279	253	272	293	70	76	83	50	55	59
30	230	260	292	262	282	304	73	79	86	52	57	61
31	240	271	305	270	291	314	75	82	89	54	59	64
32	250	282	317	278	300	323	78	84	92	56	61	66
33	259	292	329	285	308	331	80	87	94	58	63	68
34	268	302	340	292	314	339	82	89	97	60	65	70
35	276	312	350	297	320	345	84	91	99	62	67	72
36	284	320	360	302	325	350	85	93	101	64	68	74
37	291	328	369	305	329	354	86	94	102	65	70	75
38	297	336	377	307	331	357	88	95	103	66	71	77
39	303	342	384	309	333	358	88	96	105	67	73	78
40	307	347	390	309	333	359	89	97	105	69	74	79

GA, gestational age; MA, menstrual age.
Note: $\text{Log } 10 (AC + 9) = 1.3257977 + 0.0552337 \times GA - 0.0006146 \times GA^2$ (SD = .02947); $\text{Log } (HC + 1) = 1.3369692 + 0.0596493 \times GA - 0.0007494 \times GA^2$ (SD = 0.01887); $\text{Log } 10 (BPD + 5) = 0.9445108 + 0.0509883 \times MA - 0.0006097 \times GA^2$ (SD = .02056); and $FL^{.5} = -1.1132444 + 0.4263429 \times A33 - 0.0045992 \times GA^2$ (SD = .1852).
Reproduced with permission from Snijders RJM, Nicolaides KH. Fetal biometry at 14–40 weeks' gestation. *Ultrasound Obstet Gynecol* 1994;4:34–38.

TABLE 11. NORMAL BIOMETRIC RATIOS OF HEAD CIRCUMFERENCE (HC)/ABDOMINAL CIRCUMFERENCE (AC), AC/FEMUR LENGTH (FL), AND BIPARIETAL DIAMETER (BPD)/FL

GA (wk)	HC/AC[a]			AC/FL[b]			BPD/FL[c]		
	5th	50th	95th	5th	50th	95th	5th	50th	95th
14	1.13	1.23	1.34	4.93	5.51	6.16	1.75	1.92	2.11
15	1.12	1.22	1.33	4.73	5.29	5.92	1.66	1.82	2.00
16	1.11	1.21	1.32	4.57	5.11	5.71	1.58	1.74	1.91
17	1.10	1.20	1.31	4.43	4.95	5.54	1.52	1.67	1.83
18	1.09	1.19	1.30	4.32	4.83	5.40	1.47	1.61	1.77
19	1.08	1.18	1.29	4.23	4.73	5.29	1.42	1.56	1.71
20	1.07	1.17	1.28	4.16	4.65	5.20	1.39	1.52	1.67
21	1.06	1.17	1.27	4.11	4.59	5.13	1.36	1.49	1.64
22	1.05	1.16	1.26	4.07	4.55	5.08	1.34	1.47	1.61
23	1.04	1.15	1.25	4.04	4.52	5.05	1.32	1.45	1.59
24	1.03	1.14	1.24	4.03	4.50	5.03	1.30	1.43	1.57
25	1.02	1.13	1.23	4.02	4.50	5.03	1.29	1.42	1.56
26	1.01	1.12	1.22	4.03	4.50	5.03	1.29	1.41	1.55
27	1.00	1.11	1.21	4.04	4.51	5.04	1.28	1.41	1.54
28	0.99	1.10	1.20	4.05	4.53	5.06	1.28	1.40	1.54
29	0.98	1.09	1.19	4.07	4.55	5.09	1.28	1.40	1.54
30	0.97	1.08	1.18	4.10	4.58	5.12	1.27	1.40	1.53
31	0.96	1.07	1.17	4.12	4.61	5.15	1.27	1.40	1.53
32	0.95	1.06	1.16	4.15	4.64	5.18	1.27	1.39	1.53
33	0.94	1.05	1.16	4.17	4.67	5.22	1.27	1.39	1.52
34	0.94	1.04	1.15	4.20	4.69	5.24	1.26	1.38	1.52
35	0.93	1.03	1.14	4.21	4.71	5.27	1.25	1.37	1.51
36	0.92	1.02	1.13	4.23	4.73	5.28	1.24	1.36	1.50
37	0.91	1.01	1.12	4.23	4.73	5.29	1.23	1.35	1.48
38	0.90	1.00	1.11	4.23	4.73	5.29	1.21	1.33	1.46
39	0.89	0.99	1.10	4.22	4.71	5.27	1.19	1.30	1.43
40	0.88	0.98	1.09	4.19	4.69	5.24	1.16	1.28	1.40

GA, gestational age.
[a]HC/AC = $.3668952 - 0.0096 \times GA$ (SD = 0.064) (modified formula to fit published tabular data).
[b]Log (AC/FL) = $1.3260806 - 0.0693157 \times GA + 0.0023154 \times GA^2 - 0.0000248 \times GA^3$ (SD 0.02942).
[c]Log (BPD/FL) = $1.0205449 - 0.0865895 \times GA + 0.0028771 \times GA^2 - 0.0000321 \times GA^3$ (SD 0.02458).
Reproduced with permission from Snijders RJM, Nicolaides KH. Fetal biometry at 14–40 weeks' gestation. *Ultrasound Obstet Gynecol* 1994;4:34–38.

TABLE 12. VARIOUS FORMULAS USED TO ESTIMATE FETAL WEIGHT

Study	Formulas (in grams unless specified)
Warsof, 1977[a]: BPD, AC	Log_{10} (Wt in kg) = $-1.599 + (0.144 \times BPD) + (0.032 \times AC) - (0.000111 \times AC \times BPD^2)$
Shepard et al., 1982[b]: BPD, AC	Log_{10} (Wt in kg) = $-1.7492 + (0.166 \times BPD) + (0.046 \times AC) - (0.002646 \times AC \times BPD)$
Roberts, 1986[c]: BPD, HC, AC, FL	Log_{10} (Wt) = $1.6758 + (0.01707 \times AC) + (0.042478 \times BPD) + (0.05216 \times FL) + (0.01604 \times HC)$
Combs, 1993[d]: HC, AC, FL	Wt = $0.23718 \times AC^2 \times FL + (0.03312 \times HC^3)$
Hadlock, 1984[e]: FL, AC	Log_{10} (Wt) = $1.3598 + (0.051 \times AC) + (0.1844 \times FL) - (.0037 \times AC \times FL)$
Hadlock, 1984[e]: BPD, HC, FL, AC	Log_{10} (Wt) = $1.5115 + (0.0436 \times AC) + (0.1517 \times FL) - (0.00321 \times FL \times AC) + (0.0006923 \times BPD \times HC)$
Hadlock, 1985: BPD, HC, FL, AC	Log (Wt) = $1.3596 - 0.00386 \times FL \times AC + 0.0064 \times HC + 0.00061 \times BPD \times AC + 0.0424 \times AC + 0.174 \times FL$
Hadlock, 1985[f]: FL, AC	Log_{10} (Wt) = $1.304 + .05281 \times AC + 0.1938 \times FL - 0.004 \times AC \times FL$

AC, abdominal circumference; BPD, biparietal diameter; FL, femur length; HC, head circumference; Wt, weight.
[a]Reproduced with permission from Warsof SL, Gohari P, Berkowitz RL, et al. The estimation of fetal weight by computer-assisted analysis. *Am J Obstet Gynecol* 1977;128:881.
[b]Reproduced with permission from Shepard MJ, Richards VA, Berkowitz RL, et al. An evaluation of two equations for predicting fetal weight by ultrasound. *Am J Obstet Gynecol* 1982;142:47.
[c]Reproduced with permission from Roberts AB, Lee AJ, James AG. Ultrasonic estimation of fetal weight: a new predictive model incorporating femur length for the low-birth-weight fetus. *J Clin Ultrasound* 1986;13:555–559.
[d]Reproduced with permission from Combs CA, Jackle RK, Rosenn B, et al. Sonographic estimation of fetal weight based on a model of fetal volume. *Obstet Gynecol* 1993;82:365–370.
[e]Reproduced with permission from Hadlock FP, Harrist RB, Carpenter RJ, et al. Sonographic estimation of fetal weight. *Radiology* 1984;150:535–540.
[f]Reproduced with permission from Hadlock FP, Harrist RB, Sharman RS, Deter RL, Park SK. Estimation of fetal weight with the use of head, body and femur measurements: a prospective study. *Am J Obstet Gynecol* 1985;152:333–337.

TABLE 13. ESTIMATED FETAL WEIGHT (IN GRAMS) BASED ON FEMUR LENGTH (FL) AND ABDOMINAL CIRCUMFERENCE (AC)

FL (cm)	AC (cm)													
	15	15.5	16	16.5	17	17.5	18	18.5	19	19.5	20	20.5	21	21.5
3	325	340	356	373	390	409	428	448	469	491	514	538	563	590
3.1	334	350	366	383	401	420	440	460	481	504	527	552	578	604
3.2	345	360	377	394	413	432	452	472	494	517	541	566	592	619
3.3	355	371	388	406	424	444	464	485	507	531	555	580	607	634
3.4	366	382	399	418	436	456	477	498	521	544	569	595	622	650
3.5	377	394	411	430	449	469	490	512	535	559	584	610	637	666
3.6	388	405	423	442	462	482	503	526	549	573	599	625	653	682
3.7	400	417	436	455	475	495	517	540	564	588	614	641	669	699
3.8	412	430	448	468	488	509	531	555	579	604	630	657	686	716
3.9	424	442	461	481	502	524	546	570	594	620	646	674	703	733
4	437	456	475	495	516	538	561	585	610	636	663	691	720	751
4.1	450	469	489	509	531	553	576	601	626	652	680	709	738	769
4.2	464	483	503	524	546	569	592	617	643	504	697	726	757	788
4.3	478	497	518	539	561	585	609	634	660	504	715	745	776	808
4.4	492	512	533	555	577	601	625	651	677	504	734	764	795	827
4.5	507	527	549	571	594	618	643	668	695	504	753	783	815	847
4.6	522	543	565	587	611	635	660	687	714	504	772	803	835	868
4.7	538	559	581	604	628	653	678	705	733	504	792	823	856	889
4.8	554	576	598	621	646	671	697	724	752	504	812	844	877	911
4.9	571	593	616	639	664	690	716	744	772	504	833	865	899	933
5	588	610	634	658	683	709	736	764	793	504	855	887	921	956
5.1	606	628	652	677	702	729	756	785	814	504	877	910	944	980
5.2	624	647	671	696	722	749	777	806	836	504	899	933	967	1,003
5.3	643	666	691	716	743	770	798	828	858	504	922	956	992	1,028
5.4	662	686	711	737	764	791	820	850	881	504	946	981	1,016	1,053
5.5	682	706	732	758	785	814	843	873	904	504	970	1,005	1,041	1,079
5.6	702	727	753	780	808	836	866	897	928	504	995	1,031	1,067	1,105
5.7	724	749	775	802	831	860	890	921	953	504	1,021	1,057	1,094	1,132
5.8	745	771	798	826	854	884	914	946	979	504	1,047	1,084	1,121	1,160
5.9	768	794	821	849	878	908	939	971	1,005	504	1,074	1,111	1,149	1,188
6	791	818	845	874	903	934	965	998	1,031	504	1,102	1,139	1,178	1,217
6.1	815	842	870	899	929	960	992	1,025	1,059	504	1,130	1,168	1,207	1,247
6.2	839	867	895	925	955	987	1,019	1,052	1,087	504	1,160	1,198	1,237	1,278
6.3	865	893	922	951	982	1,014	1,047	1,081	1,116	504	1,189	1,228	1,268	1,309
6.4	891	919	949	979	1,010	1,042	1,076	1,110	1,146	504	1,220	1,259	1,299	1,341
6.5	918	946	976	1,007	1,039	1,072	1,105	1,140	1,176	504	1,251	1,291	1,332	1,373
6.6	945	975	1,005	1,036	1,068	1,101	1,136	1,171	1,207	504	1,284	1,323	1,365	1,407
6.7	974	1,004	1,034	1,066	1,099	1,132	1,167	1,203	1,240	504	1,317	1,357	1,399	1,441
6.8	1,003	1,033	1,065	1,097	1,130	1,164	1,199	1,235	1,273	504	1,351	1,391	1,433	1,477
6.9	1,033	1,064	1,096	1,128	1,162	1,196	1,232	1,269	1,306	504	1,385	1,427	1,469	1,513
7	1,064	1,096	1,128	1,161	1,195	1,230	1,266	1,303	1,341	504	1,421	1,463	1,506	1,550
7.1	1,096	1,128	1,161	1,194	1,229	1,264	1,301	1,338	1,377	504	1,458	1,500	1,543	1,588
7.2	1,129	1,162	1,195	1,229	1,264	1,299	1,336	1,374	1,414	504	1,495	1,538	1,581	1,626
7.3	1,163	1,196	1,230	1,264	1,299	1,336	1,373	1,412	1,451	504	1,534	1,577	1,621	1,666
7.4	1,199	1,232	1,266	1,300	1,336	1,373	1,411	1,450	1,490	504	1,573	1,616	1,661	1,707
7.5	1,235	1,268	1,303	1,338	1,374	1,411	1,450	1,489	1,529	504	1,614	1,657	1,702	1,749
7.6	1,272	1,306	1,341	1,376	1,413	1,451	1,490	1,529	1,570	504	1,655	1,699	1,745	1,791
7.7	1,310	1,345	1,380	1,416	1,453	1,491	1,531	1,571	1,612	504	1,698	1,742	1,788	1,835
7.8	1,350	1,384	1,420	1,457	1,494	1,533	1,573	1,613	1,655	504	1,741	1,786	1,833	1,880
7.9	1,390	1,426	1,462	1,499	1,537	1,576	1,616	1,657	1,699	504	1,786	1,832	1,878	1,926
8	1,432	1,468	1,505	1,542	1,580	1,620	1,660	1,702	1,744	504	1,832	1,878	1,925	1,973
8.1	1,475	1,511	1,549	1,586	1,625	1,665	1,706	1,748	1,791	504	1,879	1,926	1,973	2,021
8.2	1,520	1,556	1,594	1,632	1,671	1,712	1,753	1,795	1,838	504	1,928	1,974	2,022	2,070
8.3	1,566	1,603	1,640	1,679	1,719	1,759	1,801	1,844	1,887	504	1,977	2,024	2,072	2,121

						AC (cm)							
22	**22.5**	**23**	**23.5**	**24**	**24.5**	**25**	**25.5**	**26**	**26.5**	**27**	**27.5**	**28**	**28.5**
618	647	677	709	742	777	814	852	892	934	978	1,024	1,072	1,122
633	662	693	725	759	794	831	870	910	953	997	1,044	1,092	1,143
648	678	709	742	776	812	849	888	929	972	1,017	1,064	1,113	1,164
663	694	725	758	793	829	867	907	948	991	1,037	1,084	1,134	1,185
679	710	742	776	811	847	886	926	968	1,011	1,057	1,105	1,155	1,207
695	727	759	793	829	866	905	945	987	1,032	1,078	1,126	1,177	1,229
712	744	777	811	847	885	924	965	1,008	1,052	1,099	1,148	1,199	1,252
729	761	795	830	866	904	944	985	1,028	1,073	1,121	1,170	1,221	1,275
747	779	813	848	885	924	964	1,006	1,049	1,095	1,143	1,192	1,244	1,298
765	798	832	868	905	944	984	1,027	1,071	1,117	1,165	1,215	1,267	1,322
783	816	851	887	925	964	1,006	1,048	1,093	1,139	1,188	1,238	1,291	1,346
802	836	871	907	946	986	1,027	1,070	1,115	1,162	1,211	1,262	1,315	1,371
821	855	891	928	967	1,007	1,049	1,093	1,138	1,186	1,235	1,287	1,340	1,396
841	875	912	949	988	1,029	1,071	1,116	1,162	1,209	1,259	1,311	1,365	1,422
861	896	933	971	1,010	1,051	1,094	1,139	1,185	1,234	1,284	1,336	1,391	1,448
882	917	954	993	1,033	1,074	1,118	1,163	1,210	1,259	1,309	1,362	1,417	1,474
903	939	976	1,015	1,056	1,098	1,142	1,187	1,235	1,284	1,335	1,388	1,444	1,501
924	961	999	1,038	1,079	1,122	1,166	1,212	1,260	1,310	1,361	1,415	1,471	1,529
947	984	1,022	1,062	1,103	1,146	1,191	1,237	1,286	1,336	1,388	1,442	1,498	1,557
969	1,007	1,046	1,086	1,128	1,171	1,216	1,263	1,312	1,363	1,415	1,470	1,527	1,585
993	1,030	1,070	1,111	1,153	1,197	1,242	1,290	1,339	1,390	1,443	1,498	1,555	1,615
1,016	1,055	1,095	1,136	1,179	1,223	1,269	1,317	1,367	1,418	1,471	1,527	1,584	1,644
1,041	1,080	1,120	1,162	1,205	1,250	1,296	1,344	1,395	1,446	1,500	1,556	1,614	1,674
1,066	1,105	1,146	1,188	1,232	1,277	1,324	1,373	1,423	1,476	1,530	1,586	1,644	1,705
1,091	1,131	1,172	1,215	1,259	1,305	1,352	1,401	1,452	1,505	1,560	1,617	1,675	1,736
1,118	1,158	1,199	1,242	1,287	1,333	1,381	1,431	1,482	1,535	1,591	1,648	1,707	1,768
1,144	1,185	1,227	1,271	1,316	1,362	1,411	1,461	1,513	1,566	1,622	1,679	1,739	1,801
1,172	1,213	1,255	1,299	1,345	1,392	1,441	1,491	1,544	1,598	1,654	1,712	1,772	1,834
1,200	1,242	1,284	1,329	1,375	1,422	1,472	1,523	1,575	1,630	1,686	1,744	1,805	1,867
1,229	1,271	1,314	1,359	1,406	1,454	1,503	1,554	1,608	1,662	1,719	1,778	1,839	1,902
1,258	1,301	1,345	1,390	1,437	1,485	1,535	1,587	1,641	1,696	1,753	1,812	1,873	1,936
1,289	1,331	1,376	1,421	1,469	1,518	1,568	1,620	1,674	1,730	1,787	1,847	1,908	1,972
1,319	1,363	1,408	1,454	1,501	1,551	1,602	1,654	1,709	1,765	1,823	1,882	1,944	2,008
1,351	1,395	1,440	1,487	1,535	1,585	1,636	1,689	1,744	1,800	1,858	1,919	1,981	2,045
1,384	1,428	1,473	1,520	1,569	1,619	1,671	1,724	1,779	1,836	1,895	1,955	2,018	2,082
1,417	1,461	1,507	1,555	1,604	1,655	1,707	1,760	1,816	1,873	1,932	1,993	2,056	2,121
1,451	1,496	1,542	1,590	1,640	1,691	1,743	1,797	1,853	1,911	1,970	2,031	2,094	2,160
1,486	1,531	1,578	1,626	1,676	1,727	1,780	1,835	1,891	1,949	2,009	2,070	2,134	2,199
1,521	1,567	1,614	1,663	1,713	1,765	1,818	1,873	1,930	1,988	2,048	2,110	2,174	2,240
1,558	1,604	1,652	1,701	1,752	1,804	1,857	1,913	1,970	2,028	2,089	2,151	2,215	2,281
1,595	1,642	1,690	1,740	1,791	1,843	1,897	1,953	2,010	2,069	2,130	2,192	2,256	2,322
1,633	1,681	1,729	1,779	1,830	1,883	1,938	1,994	2,051	2,110	2,171	2,234	2,299	2,365
1,673	1,720	1,769	1,819	1,871	1,924	1,979	2,035	2,093	2,153	2,214	2,277	2,342	2,408
1,713	1,761	1,810	1,861	1,913	1,966	2,021	2,078	2,136	2,196	2,258	2,321	2,386	2,453
1,754	1,802	1,852	1,903	1,955	2,009	2,065	2,122	2,180	2,240	2,302	2,365	2,431	2,498
1,796	1,845	1,895	1,946	1,999	2,053	2,109	2,166	2,225	2,285	2,347	2,411	2,476	2,543
1,839	1,888	1,939	1,990	2,043	2,098	2,154	2,211	2,270	2,331	2,393	2,457	2,523	2,590
1,883	1,933	1,983	2,035	2,089	2,144	2,200	2,258	2,317	2,378	2,440	2,504	2,570	2,638
1,928	1,978	2,029	2,082	2,135	2,190	2,247	2,305	2,365	2,426	2,488	2,552	2,618	2,686
1,975	2,025	2,076	2,129	2,183	2,238	2,295	2,353	2,413	2,474	2,537	2,602	2,668	2,735
2,022	2,072	2,124	2,177	2,231	2,287	2,344	2,403	2,463	2,524	2,587	2,652	2,718	2,785
2,071	2,121	2,173	2,227	2,281	2,337	2,394	2,453	2,513	2,575	2,638	2,702	2,769	2,837
2,120	2,171	2,224	2,277	2,332	2,388	2,446	2,504	2,565	2,626	2,690	2,754	2,821	2,889
2,171	2,222	2,275	2,329	2,384	2,440	2,498	2,557	2,617	2,679	2,742	2,807	2,874	2,942

(continued)

TABLE 13. *CONTINUED*

FL (cm)	29	29.5	30	30.5	31	31.5	32	32.5	33	33.5	34	34.5	35	35.5
3	1,175	1,230	1,288	1,349	1,412	1,479	1,548	1,621	1,697	1,777	1,860	1,948	2,039	2,135
3.1	1,196	1,252	1,310	1,371	1,435	1,502	1,572	1,645	1,722	1,802	1,886	1,973	2,065	2,161
3.2	1,218	1,274	1,333	1,394	1,458	1,526	1,596	1,669	1,746	1,827	1,911	1,999	2,092	2,188
3.3	1,239	1,296	1,355	1,417	1,482	1,550	1,620	1,694	1,772	1,853	1,937	2,026	2,118	2,215
3.4	1,262	1,319	1,378	1,441	1,506	1,574	1,645	1,720	1,797	1,879	1,964	2,052	2,145	2,242
3.5	1,284	1,342	1,402	1,465	1,530	1,599	1,670	1,745	1,823	1,905	1,990	2,079	2,172	2,270
3.6	1,307	1,365	1,426	1,489	1,555	1,624	1,696	1,771	1,850	1,932	2,017	2,107	2,200	2,298
3.7	1,331	1,389	1,450	1,514	1,580	1,649	1,722	1,797	1,876	1,959	2,045	2,134	2,228	2,326
3.8	1,354	1,413	1,475	1,539	1,606	1,675	1,748	1,824	1,903	1,986	2,072	2,162	2,256	2,354
3.9	1,379	1,438	1,500	1,564	1,632	1,702	1,775	1,851	1,931	2,014	2,101	2,191	2,285	2,383
4	1,403	1,463	1,525	1,590	1,658	1,729	1,802	1,879	1,959	2,042	2,129	2,220	2,314	2,413
4.1	1,429	1,489	1,551	1,617	1,685	1,756	1,830	1,907	1,987	2,071	2,158	2,249	2,344	2,442
4.2	1,454	1,515	1,578	1,644	1,712	1,783	1,858	1,935	2,016	2,100	2,187	2,278	2,373	2,472
4.3	1,480	1,541	1,605	1,671	1,740	1,812	1,886	1,964	2,045	2,129	2,217	2,308	2,404	2,503
4.4	1,507	1,568	1,632	1,699	1,768	1,840	1,915	1,993	2,074	2,159	2,247	2,339	2,434	2,533
4.5	1,534	1,596	1,660	1,727	1,797	1,869	1,944	2,023	2,104	2,189	2,278	2,370	2,465	2,565
4.6	1,561	1,623	1,688	1,756	1,826	1,898	1,974	2,053	2,135	2,220	2,309	2,401	2,497	2,596
4.7	1,589	1,652	1,717	1,785	1,855	1,928	2,004	2,084	2,166	2,251	2,340	2,432	2,528	2,628
4.8	1,618	1,681	1,746	1,814	1,885	1,959	2,035	2,115	2,197	2,283	2,372	2,464	2,560	2,660
4.9	1,647	1,710	1,776	1,845	1,916	1,990	2,066	2,146	2,229	2,315	2,404	2,497	2,593	2,693
5	1,676	1,740	1,806	1,875	1,947	2,021	2,098	2,178	2,261	2,347	2,437	2,530	2,626	2,726
5.1	1,706	1,770	1,837	1,906	1,978	2,053	2,130	2,210	2,294	2,380	2,470	2,563	2,659	2,760
5.2	1,737	1,801	1,868	1,938	2,010	2,085	2,163	2,243	2,327	2,413	2,503	2,597	2,693	2,794
5.3	1,768	1,833	1,900	1,970	2,043	2,118	2,196	2,277	2,360	2,447	2,537	2,631	2,727	2,828
5.4	1,799	1,865	1,933	2,003	2,076	2,151	2,229	2,310	2,394	2,482	2,572	2,665	2,762	2,863
5.5	1,832	1,897	1,966	2,036	2,109	2,185	2,264	2,345	2,429	2,516	2,607	2,700	2,797	2,898
5.6	1,864	1,931	1,999	2,070	2,143	2,219	2,298	2,380	2,464	2,552	2,642	2,736	2,833	2,933
5.7	1,898	1,964	2,033	2,104	2,178	2,254	2,333	2,415	2,500	2,587	2,678	2,772	2,869	2,969
5.8	1,932	1,999	2,068	2,139	2,213	2,290	2,369	2,451	2,536	2,624	2,714	2,808	2,905	3,006
5.9	1,966	2,034	2,103	2,175	2,249	2,326	2,405	2,488	2,573	2,660	2,751	2,845	2,942	3,043
6	2,002	2,069	2,139	2,211	2,286	2,363	2,442	2,525	2,610	2,698	2,789	2,883	2,980	3,080
6.1	2,038	2,105	2,175	2,248	2,323	2,400	2,480	2,562	2,647	2,736	2,827	2,921	3,018	3,118
6.2	2,074	2,142	2,212	2,285	2,360	2,438	2,518	2,600	2,686	2,774	2,865	2,959	3,056	3,156
6.3	2,111	2,180	2,250	2323	2,398	2,476	2,556	2,639	2,724	2,813	2,904	2,998	3,095	3,195
6.4	2,149	2,218	2,289	2,362	2,437	2,515	2,595	2,678	2,764	2,852	2,943	3,037	3,134	3,235
6.5	2,187	2,256	2,328	2,401	2,477	2,555	2,635	2,718	2,804	2,892	2,983	3,077	3,174	3,274
6.6	2,227	2,296	2,367	2,441	2,517	2,595	2,675	2,759	2,844	2,933	3,024	3,118	3,215	3,315
6.7	2,267	2,336	2,408	2,481	2,557	2,636	2,716	2,800	2,885	2,974	3,065	3,159	3,256	3,355
6.8	2,307	2,377	2,449	2,523	2,599	2,677	2,758	2,841	2,927	3,015	3,107	3,200	3,297	3,397
6.9	2,348	2,418	2,490	2,564	2,641	2,719	2,800	2,884	2,969	3,058	3,149	3,242	3,339	3,438
7	2,391	2,461	2,533	2,607	2,683	2,762	2,843	2,926	3,012	3,101	3,191	3,285	3,381	3,481
7.1	2,433	2,504	2,576	2,650	2,727	2,806	2,887	2,970	3,056	3,144	3,235	3,328	3,424	3,523
7.2	2,477	2,547	2,620	2,694	2,771	2,850	2,931	3,014	3,100	3,188	3,279	3,372	3,468	3,567
7.3	2,521	2,592	2,664	2,739	2,816	2,895	2,976	3,059	3,145	3,233	3,323	3,416	3,512	3,610
7.4	2,566	2,637	2,710	2,785	2,861	2,940	3,021	3,105	3,190	3,278	3,368	3,461	3,557	3,655
7.5	2,612	2,683	2,756	2,831	2,908	2,987	3,068	3,151	3,236	3,324	3,414	3,507	3,602	3,700
7.6	2,659	2,730	2,803	2,878	2,955	3,034	3,115	3,198	3,283	3,371	3,461	3,553	3,648	3,745
7.7	2,707	2,778	2,851	2,926	3,002	3,081	3,162	3,245	3,330	3,418	3,508	3,600	3,694	3,791
7.8	2,755	2,826	2,899	2,974	3,051	3,130	3,211	3,294	3,379	3,466	3,555	3,647	3,741	3,838
7.9	2,805	2,876	2,949	3,024	3,100	3,179	3,260	3,343	3,427	3,514	3,604	3,695	3,789	3,885
8	2,855	2,926	2,999	3,074	3,151	3,229	3,310	3,392	3,477	3,564	3,653	3,744	3,837	3,933
8.1	2,906	2,977	3,050	3,125	3,202	3,280	3,360	3,443	3,527	3,614	3,702	3,793	3,886	3,981
8.2	2,958	3,029	3,102	3,177	3,253	3,332	3,412	3,494	3,578	3,664	3,752	3,843	3,935	4,030
8.3	3,011	3,082	3,155	3,230	3,306	3,384	3,464	3,546	3,630	3,716	3,803	3,893	3,985	4,080

Note: $Log_{10} = 1.3598 + (.051 \times AC) + (.1844 \times FL) - (.0037 \times AC \times FL)$.
Reproduced with permission from Hadlock FP, Harrist RB, Carpenter RJ, et al. Sonographic estimation of fetal weight. *Radiology* 1984;150:535–540.

AC (cm)														
36	36.5	37	37.5	38	38.5	39	39.5	40	40.5	41	41.5	42	42.5	43
2,236	2,341	2,451	2,566	2,687	2,813	2,945	3,083	3,228	3,380	3,539	3,705	3,880	4,062	4,253
2,262	2,367	2,478	2,593	2,714	2,840	2,972	3,111	3,256	3,407	3,566	3,732	3,906	4,087	4,278
2,289	2,394	2,505	2,620	2,741	2,868	3,000	3,138	3,283	3,434	3,593	3,758	3,932	4,113	4,303
2,316	2,422	2,532	2,648	2,769	2,896	3,028	3,166	3,311	3,462	3,620	3,785	3,958	4,139	4,328
2,344	2,450	2,560	2,676	2,797	2,924	3,056	3,194	3,339	3,489	3,647	3,812	3,985	4,165	4,353
2,371	2,478	2,588	2,704	2,825	2,952	3,084	3,222	3,367	3,517	3,675	3,839	4,011	4,191	4,379
2,399	2,506	2,617	2,733	2,854	2,981	3,113	3,251	3,395	3,545	3,703	3,867	4,038	4,217	4,404
2,428	2,534	2,646	2,762	2,883	3,010	3,142	3,280	3,424	3,574	3,731	3,894	4,065	4,244	4,430
2,457	2,563	2,675	2,791	2,912	3,039	3,171	3,309	3,452	3,602	3,759	3,922	4,093	4,270	4,456
2,486	2,593	2,704	2,821	2,942	3,068	3,200	3,338	3,481	3,631	3,787	3,950	4,120	4,297	4,482
2,515	2,622	2,734	2,850	2,972	3,098	3,230	3,367	3,511	3,660	3,816	3,978	4,148	4,324	4,508
2,545	2,652	2,764	2,880	3,002	3,128	3,260	3,397	3,540	3,689	3,845	4,007	4,175	4,351	4,534
2,575	2,683	2,794	2,911	3,032	3,159	3,290	3,427	3,570	3,719	3,874	4,035	4,203	4,378	4,561
2,606	2,713	2,825	2,942	3,063	3,189	3,321	3,458	3,600	3,748	3,903	4,064	4,231	4,406	4,588
2,637	2,744	2,856	2,973	3,094	3,220	3,351	3,488	3,630	3,778	3,933	4,093	4,260	4,434	4,614
2,668	2,776	2,888	3,004	3,125	3,251	3,383	3,519	3,661	3,809	3,962	4,122	4,288	4,461	4,641
2,700	2,807	2,919	3,036	3,157	3,283	3,414	3,550	3,692	3,839	3,992	4,151	4,317	4,489	4,668
2,732	2,839	2,951	3,068	3,189	3,315	3,446	3,582	3,723	3,870	4,022	4,181	4,346	4,517	4,696
2,764	2,872	2,984	3,100	3,221	3,347	3,478	3,613	3,754	3,901	4,053	4,211	4,375	4,546	4,723
2,797	2,905	3,017	3,133	3,254	3,379	3,510	3,645	3,786	3,932	4,083	4,241	4,404	4,574	4,751
2,830	2,938	3,050	3,166	3,287	3,412	3,542	3,677	3,818	3,963	4,114	4,271	4,434	4,603	4,779
2,864	2,972	3,083	3,200	3,320	3,445	3,575	3,710	3,850	3,995	4,145	4,302	4,464	4,632	4,806
2,898	3,005	3,117	3,233	3,354	3,479	3,608	3,743	3,882	4,027	4,177	4,332	4,494	4,661	4,835
2,932	3,040	3,152	3,268	3,388	3,513	3,642	3,776	3,915	4,059	4,208	4,363	4,524	4,690	4,863
2,967	3,075	3,186	3,302	3,422	3,547	3,676	3,809	3,948	4,091	4,240	4,394	4,554	4,720	4,891
3,002	3,110	3,221	3,337	3,457	3,581	3,710	3,843	3,981	4,124	4,272	4,426	4,584	4,749	4,920
3,037	3,145	3,257	3,372	3,492	3,616	3,744	3,877	4,015	4,157	4,304	4,457	4,615	4,779	4,948
3,073	3,181	3,293	3,408	3,527	3,651	3,779	3,911	4,048	4,190	4,337	4,489	4,646	4,809	4,977
3,110	3,218	3,329	3,444	3,563	3,686	3,814	3,946	4,082	4,224	4,370	4,521	4,677	4,839	5,006
3,147	3,254	3,365	3,480	3,599	3,722	3,849	3,981	4,117	4,257	4,403	4,553	4,709	4,869	5,036
3,184	3,291	3,402	3,517	3,636	3,758	3,885	4,016	4,151	4,291	4,436	4,586	4,740	4,900	5,065
3,222	3,329	3,440	3,554	3,673	3,795	3,921	4,052	4,186	4,326	4,470	4,618	4,772	4,931	5,095
3,260	3,367	3,478	3,592	3,710	3,832	3,957	4,087	4,222	4,360	4,503	4,651	4,804	4,962	5,125
3,299	3,406	3,516	3,630	3,747	3,869	3,994	4,124	4,257	4,395	4,537	4,684	4,836	4,993	5,154
3,338	3,445	3,555	3,668	3,785	3,906	4,031	4,160	4,293	4,430	4,572	4,718	4,868	5,024	5,185
3,377	3,484	3,594	3,707	3,824	3,944	4,069	4,197	4,329	4,465	4,606	4,751	4,901	5,056	5,215
3,418	3,524	3,633	3,746	3,863	3,983	4,106	4,234	4,365	4,501	4,641	4,785	4,934	5,087	5,245
3,458	3,564	3,673	3,786	3,902	4,021	4,144	4,271	4,402	4,537	4,676	4,819	4,967	5,119	5,276
3,499	3,605	3,714	3,826	3,941	4,060	4,183	4,309	4,439	4,573	4,711	4,854	5,000	5,151	5,307
3,541	3,646	3,754	3,866	3,981	4,100	4,222	4,347	4,477	4,610	4,747	4,888	5,034	5,184	5,338
3,583	3,688	3,796	3,907	4,022	4,139	4,261	4,386	4,514	4,647	4,783	4,923	5,067	5,216	5,369
3,625	3,730	3,837	3,948	4,062	4,180	4,300	4,425	4,552	4,684	4,819	4,958	5,101	5,249	5,400
3,668	3,772	3,880	3,990	4,103	4,220	4,340	4,464	4,591	4,721	4,855	4,994	5,136	5,282	5,432
3,712	3,815	3,922	4,032	4,145	4,261	4,380	4,503	4,629	4,759	4,892	5,029	5,170	5,315	5,464
3,756	3,859	3,965	4,075	4,187	4,303	4,421	4,543	4,668	4,797	4,929	5,065	5,205	5,348	5,496
3,800	3,903	4,009	4,118	4,230	4,344	4,462	4,583	4,708	4,835	4,966	5,101	5,240	5,382	5,528
3,845	3,948	4,053	4,161	4,272	4,386	4,504	4,624	4,747	4,874	5,004	5,137	5,275	5,415	5,560
3,891	3,993	4,098	4,205	4,316	4,429	4,545	4,665	4,787	4,913	5,042	5,174	5,310	5,449	5,592
3,937	4,039	4,143	4,250	4,359	4,472	4,587	4,706	4,827	4,952	5,080	5,211	5,346	5,484	5,625
3,984	4,085	4,188	4,295	4,404	4,515	4,630	4,748	4,868	4,992	5,118	5,248	5,381	5,518	5,658
4,031	4,131	4,234	4,340	4,448	4,559	4,673	4,790	4,909	5,031	5,157	5,286	5,417	5,553	5,691
4,079	4,179	4,281	4,386	4,493	4,603	4,716	4,832	4,950	5,072	5,196	5,323	5,454	5,587	5,724
4,127	4,226	4,328	4,432	4,539	4,648	4,760	4,875	4,992	5,112	5,235	5,361	5,490	5,622	5,758
4,176	4,275	4,376	4,479	4,585	4,693	4,804	4,918	5,034	5,153	5,275	5,399	5,527	5,658	5,791

TABLE 14. NEONATAL BIRTH WEIGHTS AND PERCENTILES BASED ON GESTATIONAL AGE (GA) DERIVED BY FIRST-TRIMESTER ULTRASOUND (MALES AND FEMALES COMBINED)

GA (wk)	Neonatal weight percentiles (g)						
	5th	10th	25th	50th	75th	90th	95th
25	450	489	564	660	772	890	968
26	523	568	652	760	885	1,016	1,103
27	609	659	754	875	1,015	1,160	1,257
28	707	764	870	1,005	1,161	1,323	1,430
29	820	884	1,003	1,153	1,327	1,505	1,623
30	947	1,019	1,152	1,319	1,511	1,707	1,836
31	1,090	1,170	1,317	1,502	1,713	1,928	2,070
32	1,249	1,337	1,499	1,702	1,933	2,167	2,321
33	1,422	1,519	1,696	1,918	2,168	2,422	2,588
34	1,607	1,713	1,906	2,146	2,416	2,688	2,865
35	1,804	1,918	2,126	2,383	2,671	2,960	3,148
36	2,006	2,128	2,350	2,622	2,927	3,231	3,428
37	2,210	2,339	2,572	2,859	3,177	3,493	3,698
38	2,409	2,544	2,786	3,083	3,412	3,737	3,947
39	2,595	2,734	2,984	3,288	3,622	3,952	4,164
40	2,762	2,903	3,156	3,462	3,798	4,128	4,340
41	2,900	3,041	3,293	3,597	3,929	4,255	4,462
42	3,002	3,141	3,388	3,685	4,008	4,323	4,523
43	3,060	3,195	3,433	3,717	4,026	4,325	4,515

Ln, natural log; Wt, weight.
Note: Ln (Wt) = $5.5952 - 0.16626 \times GA + 0.011973 \times GA^2 - 0.0001555 \times GA^3$; and SD of Ln (Wt) = $0.39269 - 0.0063838 \times GA$.
Data from Doubilet PM, Benson CB, Nadel AS, Ringer SA. Improved birth weight table for neonates developed from gestations dated by early ultrasonography. *J Ultrasound Med* 1997;16:241–249.

TABLE 15. GENDER-SPECIFIC REFERENCE VALUES FOR NEONATAL BIRTH WEIGHTS BASED ON GESTATIONAL AGE (GA) DERIVED BY FIRST-TRIMESTER ULTRASOUND

GA (wk)	Birth weights (g)													
	Males[a]							Females[b]						
	Percentiles							Percentiles						
	5th	10th	25th	50th	75th	90th	95th	5th	10th	25th	50th	75th	90th	95th
25	460	501	577	676	791	911	992	450	487	557	646	749	856	927
26	533	578	664	773	901	1,034	1,123	526	568	647	748	864	984	1,064
27	617	668	764	886	1,028	1,175	1,273	613	662	751	865	995	1,130	1,219
28	715	772	879	1,015	1,173	1,335	1,443	713	768	869	997	1,144	1,294	1,393
29	827	891	1,011	1,162	1,336	1,515	1,634	827	889	1,002	1,146	1,309	1,477	1,587
30	955	1,027	1,160	1,327	1,519	1,716	1,846	955	1,024	1,151	1,311	1,493	1,678	1,800
31	1,099	1,179	1,326	1,511	1,722	1,937	2,078	1,097	1,174	1,316	1,493	1,694	1,898	2,032
32	1,259	1,348	1,510	1,713	1,943	2,177	2,331	1,253	1,339	1,496	1,691	1,911	2,135	2,281
33	1,435	1,532	1,710	1,931	2,181	2,434	2,599	1,423	1,517	1,689	1,902	2,143	2,385	2,543
34	1,625	1,731	1,924	2,164	2,433	2,704	2,881	1,603	1,706	1,893	2,125	2,384	2,646	2,815
35	1,827	1,941	2,149	2,406	2,693	2,982	3,169	1,792	1,904	2,105	2,354	2,632	2,911	3,092
36	2,036	2,159	2,380	2,653	2,957	3,260	3,456	1,986	2,105	2,321	2,586	2,881	3,176	3,366
37	2,248	2,377	2,611	2,897	3,215	3,530	3,734	2,180	2,306	2,534	2,813	3,123	3,431	3,630
38	2,455	2,591	2,834	3,130	3,458	3,783	3,991	2,368	2,500	2,738	3,029	3,350	3,669	3,874
39	2,651	2,790	3,040	3,343	3,677	4,006	4,217	2,544	2,681	2,926	3,225	3,554	3,880	4,088
40	2,826	2,967	3,220	3,525	3,860	4,189	4,398	2,701	2,841	3,091	3,394	3,727	4,054	4,264
41	2,971	3,112	3,364	3,667	3,997	4,320	4,525	2,831	2,972	3,223	3,526	3,858	4,184	4,391
42	3,078	3,216	3,462	3,757	4,078	4,389	4,587	2,928	3,068	3,316	3,615	3,941	4,259	4,462
43	3,138	3,271	3,507	3,790	4,094	4,390	4,577	2,986	3,122	3,364	3,654	3,968	4,275	4,470

Ln, natural log; Wt, weight.
[a]Males: Ln (Wt) = $6.5464 - 0.24681 \times GA + 0.014222 \times GA^2 - 0.00017596 \times GA^3$; SD of Ln (Wt) = $0.39791 - 0.0065856 \times GA$.
[b]Females: Ln (Wt) = $4.4807 - 0.0689 \times GA + 0.0091683 \times GA^2 - 0.00012913 \times GA^3$; SD of Ln (Wt) = $0.35439 - 0.0053902 \times GA$.
Data from Doubilet PM, Benson CB, Nadel AS, Ringer SA. Improved birth weight table for neonates developed from gestations dated by early ultrasonography. *J Ultrasound Med* 1997;16:241–249.

TABLE 16. FETAL WEIGHT PERCENTILES BY GESTATIONAL AGE

Gestational age (wk)	Fetal weight percentiles (g)				
	3rd	10th	50th	90th	97th
10	26	29	35	41	44
11	34	37	45	53	56
12	43	48	58	68	73
13	54	61	73	85	92
14	69	77	93	109	117
15	87	97	117	137	147
16	109	121	146	171	183
17	135	150	181	212	227
18	166	185	223	261	280
19	204	227	273	319	342
20	247	275	331	387	415
21	298	331	399	467	500
22	357	397	478	559	599
23	424	472	568	664	712
24	500	556	670	784	840
25	586	652	785	918	984
26	681	758	913	1,068	1,145
27	787	876	1,055	1,234	1,323
28	903	1,005	1,210	1,415	1,517
29	1,029	1,145	1,379	1,613	1,729
30	1,163	1,294	1,559	1,824	1,955
31	1,306	1,454	1,751	2,048	2,196
32	1,457	1,621	1,953	2,285	2,449
33	1,613	1,795	2,162	2,529	2,711
34	1,773	1,973	2,377	2,781	2,981
35	1,936	2,154	2,595	3,036	3,254
36	2,098	2,335	2,813	3,291	3,528
37	2,259	2,514	3,028	3,542	3,797
38	2,414	2,687	3,236	3,785	4,058
39	2,563	2,852	3,435	4,018	4,307
40	2,700	3,004	3,619	4,234	4,538
41	2,825	3,144	3,787	4,430	4,749
42	2,935	3,266	3,934	4,602	4,933

Ln, natural log; MA, menstrual age; wt, weight.
Note: Ln (wt) = 0.578 + 0.332 MA − 0.00354 × MA^2; standard deviation = 12.7% of predicted weight.
Reproduced with permission from Hadlock FP, Harrist RB, Marinez-Poyer J. In utero analysis of fetal growth: a sonographic weight standard. *Radiology* 1991;181:129–133, extrapolated to 42 weeks from 40 weeks.

OTHER BONE AND EXTREMITY MEASUREMENTS

TABLE 17. REFERENCE VALUES OF MAJOR LONG BONES

GA (wk)	Femur (mm)[a]				Tibia (mm)[b]				Fibula (mm)[c]			
	Percentiles				Percentiles				Percentiles			
	5th	50th	95th	SD	5th	50th	95th	SD	5th	50th	95th	SD
12	3.9	8.1	12.3	2.5	3.3	7.2	11.2	2.4	1.7	5.7	9.6	2.4
13	6.8	11.0	15.2	2.5	5.6	9.6	13.6	2.4	4.7	8.7	12.7	2.4
14	9.7	13.9	18.1	2.6	8.1	12.0	16.0	2.4	7.7	11.7	15.6	2.4
15	12.6	16.8	21.0	2.6	10.6	14.6	18.6	2.4	10.6	14.6	18.6	2.4
16	15.4	19.7	23.9	2.6	13.1	17.1	21.2	2.5	13.3	17.4	21.4	2.5
17	18.3	22.5	26.8	2.6	15.6	19.7	23.8	2.5	16.1	20.1	24.2	2.5
18	21.1	25.4	29.7	2.6	18.2	22.3	26.4	2.5	18.7	22.8	26.9	2.5
19	23.9	28.2	32.6	2.6	20.8	24.9	29.0	2.5	21.3	25.4	29.5	2.5
20	26.7	31.0	35.4	2.7	23.3	27.5	31.6	2.5	23.8	27.9	32.0	2.5
21	29.4	33.8	38.2	2.7	25.8	30.0	34.2	2.5	26.2	30.3	34.5	2.5
22	32.1	36.5	40.9	2.7	28.3	32.5	36.7	2.5	28.5	32.7	36.9	2.5
23	34.7	39.2	43.6	2.7	30.7	34.9	39.1	2.6	30.8	35.0	39.2	2.6
24	37.4	41.8	46.3	2.7	33.1	37.3	41.6	2.6	33.0	37.2	41.5	2.6
25	39.9	44.4	48.9	2.7	35.4	39.7	43.9	2.6	35.1	39.4	43.6	2.6
26	42.4	46.9	51.4	2.7	37.6	41.9	46.2	2.6	37.2	41.5	45.7	2.6
27	44.9	49.4	53.9	2.8	39.8	44.1	48.4	2.6	39.2	43.5	47.8	2.6
28	47.3	51.8	56.4	2.8	41.9	46.2	50.5	2.6	41.1	45.4	49.7	2.6
29	49.6	54.2	58.7	2.8	43.9	48.2	52.6	2.6	42.9	47.2	51.6	2.6
30	51.8	56.4	61.0	2.8	45.8	50.1	54.5	2.7	44.7	49.0	53.4	2.7
31	54.0	58.6	63.2	2.8	47.6	52.0	56.4	2.7	46.3	50.7	55.1	2.7
32	56.1	60.7	65.4	2.8	49.4	53.8	58.2	2.7	47.9	52.4	56.8	2.7
33	58.1	62.7	67.4	2.8	51.1	55.5	60.0	2.7	49.5	53.9	58.4	2.7
34	60.0	64.7	69.4	2.9	52.7	57.2	61.6	2.7	50.9	55.4	59.9	2.7
35	61.8	66.5	71.2	2.9	54.2	58.7	63.2	2.7	52.3	56.8	61.3	2.7
36	63.5	68.3	73.0	2.9	55.8	60.3	64.8	2.8	53.6	58.2	62.7	2.8
37	65.1	69.9	74.7	2.9	57.2	61.8	66.3	2.8	54.9	59.4	64.0	2.8
38	66.6	71.4	76.2	2.9	58.7	63.2	67.8	2.8	56.0	60.6	65.2	2.8
39	68.0	72.8	77.7	2.9	60.1	64.7	69.3	2.8	57.1	61.7	66.3	2.8
40	69.3	74.2	79.0	3.0	61.5	66.1	70.7	2.8	58.1	62.8	67.4	2.8

GA (wk)	Humerus (mm)[d]				Radius (mm)[e]				Ulna (mm)[f]			
	Percentiles				Percentiles				Percentiles			
	5th	50th	95th	SD	5th	50th	95th	SD	5th	50th	95th	SD
12	4.8	8.6	12.3	2.3	3.0	6.9	10.8	2.4	2.9	6.8	10.7	2.4
13	7.6	11.4	15.1	2.3	5.6	9.5	13.4	2.4	5.8	9.7	13.7	2.4
14	10.3	14.1	17.9	2.3	8.1	12.0	16.0	2.4	8.6	12.6	16.6	2.4
15	13.1	16.9	20.7	2.3	10.5	14.5	18.5	2.4	11.4	15.4	19.4	2.4
16	15.8	19.7	23.5	2.3	12.9	16.9	20.9	2.4	14.1	18.1	22.1	2.4
17	18.5	22.4	26.3	2.4	15.2	19.3	23.3	2.5	16.7	20.8	24.8	2.5
18	21.2	25.1	29.0	2.4	17.5	21.5	25.6	2.5	19.3	23.3	27.4	2.5
19	23.8	27.7	31.6	2.4	19.7	23.8	27.9	2.5	21.8	25.8	29.9	2.5
20	26.3	30.3	34.2	2.4	21.8	25.9	30.0	2.5	24.2	28.3	32.4	2.5
21	28.8	32.8	36.7	2.4	23.9	28.0	32.2	2.5	26.5	30.6	34.8	2.5
22	31.2	35.2	39.2	2.4	25.9	30.1	34.2	2.5	28.7	32.9	37.1	2.5
23	33.5	37.5	41.6	2.4	27.9	32.0	36.2	2.5	30.9	35.1	39.3	2.5
24	35.7	39.8	43.8	2.5	29.7	34.0	38.2	2.6	33.0	37.2	41.5	2.6
25	37.9	41.9	46.0	2.5	31.6	35.8	40.0	2.6	35.1	39.3	43.5	2.6
26	39.9	44.0	48.1	2.5	33.3	37.6	41.9	2.6	37.0	41.3	45.6	2.6
27	41.9	46.0	50.1	2.5	35.0	39.3	43.6	2.6	38.9	43.2	47.5	2.6
28	43.7	47.9	52.0	2.5	36.7	41.0	45.3	2.6	40.7	45.0	49.3	2.6
29	45.5	49.7	53.9	2.5	38.3	42.6	46.9	2.6	42.5	46.8	51.1	2.6
30	47.2	51.4	55.6	2.6	39.8	44.1	48.5	2.7	44.1	48.5	52.8	2.7
31	48.9	53.1	57.3	2.6	41.2	45.6	50.0	2.7	45.7	50.1	54.5	2.7
32	50.4	54.7	58.9	2.6	42.6	47.0	51.4	2.7	47.2	51.6	56.1	2.7
33	52.0	56.2	60.5	2.6	44.0	48.4	52.8	2.7	48.7	53.1	57.5	2.7
34	53.4	57.7	62.0[i]	2.6	45.2	49.7	54.1	2.7	50.0	54.5	59.0	2.7
35	54.8	59.2	63.5	2.6	46.4	50.9	55.4	2.7	51.3	55.8	60.3	2.7
36	56.2	60.6	64.9	2.6	47.6	52.1	56.6	2.7	52.6	57.1	61.6	2.7
37	57.6	62.0	66.4	2.7	48.7	53.2	57.7	2.8	53.7	58.2	62.8	2.8
38	59.0	63.4	67.8	2.7	49.7	54.2	58.8	2.8	54.8	59.3	63.9	2.8
39	60.4	64.8	69.3	2.7	50.6	55.2	59.8	2.8	55.8	60.4	64.9	2.8
40	61.9	66.3	70.8	2.7	51.5	56.2	60.8	2.8	56.7	61.3	65.9	2.8

GA, gestational age.
[a]Femur (mean) = $-25.252 + 2.555 \times GA + 0.027566 \times GA^2 - 0.00073286 \times GA^3$ (Jeanty et al., 1984).
[b]Tibia (mean) = $5.555 + 0.915554 \times GA + 0.23359 \times GA^2 - 0.00638 \times GA^3 + 0.000055801 \times GA^4$ (Jeanty et al., 1984).
[c]Fibula (mean) = $-36.563 + 3.963 \times GA - 0.037 \times GA^2$ (Exacoustos et al., 1991).
[d]Humerus (mean) = $-16.24 + 0.76315 \times GA + 0.1683 \times GA^2 - 0.0056212 \times GA^3 + 0.000055666 \times GA^4$.
[e]Radius (mean) = $-29.09 + 3.371 \times GA - 0.031 \times GA^2$ (Exacoustos et al., 1991).
[f]Ulna (mean) = $-34.313 + 3.8685 \times GA - 0.036949 \times GA^2$ (Jeanty et al., 1984).
Derived from compilation of data: Jeanty P, Cousaert E, Cantraine F, Hobbins JC, Tack B, et al. A longitudinal study of fetal limb growth. *Am J Perinatol* 1984;1:136–144; Merz E, Grubner A, Kern F. Mathematical modeling of fetal limb growth. *J Clin Ultrasound* 1989;17:179–185; and Exacoustos C, Rosati P, Rizzo G, Arduini D. Ultrasound measurements of fetal limb bones. *Ultrasound Obstet Gynecol* 1991;1:325–330.

TABLE 18. REFERENCE VALUES FOR FOOT LENGTH

GA (wk)	Foot length (mm)		
	−2 SD	Mean	+2 SD
12	7	8	9
13	10	11	12
14	13	15	16
15	16	18	20
16	19	21	23
17	21	24	27
18	24	27	30
19	27	30	33
20	30	33	37
21	32	36	40
22	35	39	43
23	37	42	46
24	40	45	49
25	42	47	52
26	44	50	55
27	47	53	58
28	49	55	61
29	51	58	64
30	53	60	66
31	56	62	69
32	58	65	72
33	60	67	74
34	62	69	77
35	63	71	79
36	65	74	81
37	67	76	84
38	69	78	86
39	71	80	88
40	72	81	90

GA, gestational age.
Note: Modified formula to fit tabular data: foot length = $-0.02728 \times GA^2 + 4.045 \times GA - 36.74$ (range ± 11%).
Reproduced with permission from Mercer BM, Sklar S, Shariatmadar A, Gillieson MS, D'Alton ME. Fetal foot length as a predictor of gestational age. *Am J Obstet Gynecol* 1987;156:350–355.

TABLE 19. SCAPULAR LENGTH (±2 SD) COMPARED WITH GESTATIONAL AGE

Gestational age (wk)	Scapular length (mm)		
	−2 SD	Mean	+2 SD
14	10	10	10
15	11	11	11
16	12	12	12
17	13	13	13
18	14	14	14
19	14	15	15
20	15	16	16
21	16	17	17
22	17	18	18
23	18	19	19
24	19	20	20
25	20	21	21
26	21	22	22
27	22	23	23
28	23	23	24
29	24	24	25
30	25	25	26
31	26	26	27
32	27	27	28
33	28	28	29
34	29	29	30
35	30	30	31
36	31	31	32
37	32	32	32
38	33	33	33
39	34	34	34
40	35	35	35
41	35	36	36
42	36	37	37

Data from Sherer DM, Plessinger MA, Allen TA. Fetal scapular length in the ultrasonographic assessment of gestational age. *J Ultrasound Med* 1994;13:523–528.

TABLE 20. REFERENCE VALUES OF CLAVICLE LENGTH

GA (wk)	Jeanty[a]			Yarkoni[b]		
	Percentiles			Percentiles		
	5th	50th	95th	5th	50th	95th
12	8	13	18	—	—	—
13	10	15	20	—	—	—
14	11	16	21	—	—	—
15	12	17	22	11	16	21
16	13	18	23	12	17	22
17	14	19	24	13	18	23
18	15	20	25	14	19	24
19	16	21	26	15	20	25
20	17	22	27	16	21	26
21	18	23	28	17	22	27
22	20	25	30	18	23	28
23	21	26	31	19	24	29
24	22	27	32	20	25	30
25	23	28	33	21	26	31
26	24	29	34	22	27	32
27	25	30	35	23	28	33
28	26	31	36	24	29	34
29	27	32	37	25	30	35
30	29	34	39	26	31	36
31	30	35	40	27	32	37
32	31	36	41	28	33	38
33	32	37	42	29	34	39
34	33	38	43	30	35	40
35	34	39	44	31	36	41
36	35	40	45	32	37	42
37	36	41	46	33	38	43
38	37	42	47	34	39	44
39	39	44	49	35	40	45
40	40	45	50	36	41	46

GA, gestational age.
[a]From Jeanty, et al.
[b]Reproduced with permission from Yarkoni S, Schmidt W, Jeanty P, Reece EA, Hobbins JC. Clavicular measurement: a new biometric parameter for fetal evaluation. *J Ultrasound Med* 1985;4:467–470.
Note: Used modified formula to fit tabular data. Clavicle = 1.118303 + 0.988639 × GA (SD 2.920)

TABLE 21. REFERENCE VALUES FOR RIB LENGTH

GA (wk)	Rib length (mm)		
	Percentiles		
	5th	50th	95th
14	1.4	2.3	3.1
15	1.6	2.5	3.3
16	1.8	2.7	3.5
17	2.0	2.9	3.7
18	2.2	3.1	3.9
19	2.5	3.3	4.1
20	2.7	3.5	4.3
21	2.9	3.7	4.5
22	3.1	3.9	4.7
23	3.3	4.1	4.9
24	3.5	4.3	5.1
25	3.7	4.5	5.3
26	3.9	4.7	5.5
27	4.1	4.9	5.7
28	4.3	5.1	5.9
29	4.5	5.3	6.1
30	4.7	5.5	6.3
31	4.9	5.7	6.5
32	5.1	5.9	6.7
33	5.3	6.1	6.9
34	5.5	6.3	7.1
35	5.7	6.5	7.3
36	5.9	6.7	7.5
37	6.1	6.9	7.8
38	6.3	7.1	8.0
39	6.5	7.3	8.2
40	6.7	7.5	8.4

GA, gestational age.
Note: Rib length = −0.5834 + 0.203 × GA (SD = 0.5).
Adapted from Abuhamad AZ, Sedule-Murphy SJ, Kolm P, Youssef H, Warsof SL, et al. Prenatal ultrasonographic fetal rib length measurement: correlation with gestational age. *Ultrasound Obstet Gynecol* 1996;7:193–196.

OTHER STRUCTURES

TABLE 22. REFERENCE VALUES FOR TRANSVERSE CEREBELLAR DIAMETER (TCD) FROM THREE STUDIES

	TCD (mm)								
	Snijders[a]			Chang[b]			Goldstein[c]		
	Percentiles			Percentiles			Percentiles		
GA (wk)	5th	50th	95th	5th	50th	95th	10th	50th	90th
14	12	13	14	—	—	—	10	14	16
15	13	14	16	—	—	—	14	16	18
16	14	15	17	—	—	—	16	17	18
17	15	17	18	—	—	—	17	18	19
18	16	18	20	—	—	—	18	19	22
19	17	19	21	—	—	—	18	20	22
20	18	20	22	15	20	25	19	22	24
21	20	22	24	17	22	27	21	23	24
22	21	23	25	18	23	28	22	24	26
23	22	24	27	20	25	30	22	25	28
24	23	26	28	22	27	32	23	28	29
25	25	27	30	23	28	33	25	29	32
26	26	28	31	25	30	35	26	30	32
27	27	30	33	26	31	36	27	31	34
28	28	31	34	28	33	38	29	34	38
29	30	33	36	29	34	39	31	35	40
30	31	34	37	31	36	41	32	38	43
31	32	35	39	32	37	42	33	38	42
32	33	37	40	34	39	44	32	40	44
33	35	38	42	35	40	45	33	40	44
34	36	39	43	37	42	47	31	41	47
35	37	41	45	39	44	49	36	43	55
36	38	42	46	40	45	50	37	45	55
37	39	43	47	42	47	52	40	49	55
38	40	44	48	43	48	53	52	52	55
39	41	45	49	45	50	55	10	14	16
40	42	46	51	46	51	56	—	—	—

GA, gestational age.

Note: Log (TCD + 5) = 0.8129735 + 0.0367114 × GA − 0.000359 × GA² (SD 0.02504); TCD = −10.632 + 1.5486 × GA (SD = 3.03941).

[a]Reproduced with permission from Snijders RJM, Nicolaides KH. Fetal biometry at 14–40 weeks' gestation. *Ultrasound Obstet Gynecol* 1994;4:34–38.

[b]Reproduced with permission from Chang C-H, Chang F-M, Yu C-H, Ko Y-C, Chen H-Y. Three-dimensional ultrasound in the assessment of fetal cerebellar transverse and anterior-posterior diameters. *Ultrasound Med Biol* 2000;26:175–182.

[c]Reproduced with permission from Goldstein I, Reece A, Pilu G, Bovicelli L, Hobbins JC. Cerebellar measurements with ultrasonography in the evaluation of fetal growth and development. *Am J Obstet Gynecol* 1987;156:1065–1069.

TABLE 23. NORMAL VALUES (MEAN ± SD) OF THE CEREBELLAR VERMIS

Gestational age (wk)	Anteroposterior diameter (mm)	Superoinferior diameter (mm)	Circumference (mm)	Area (cm²)
21–22	10.6 ± 1.4	11.1 ± 1.1	43.8 ± 3.3	0.9 ± 0.2
23–24	12.9 ± 1.1	12.3 ± 1.4	47.5 ± 5.5	1.2 ± 0.2
25–26	13.5 ± 2.1	13.6 ± 0.9	50.9 ± 4.4	1.4 ± 0.2
27–28	16.3 ± 2.7	16.0 ± 1.6	58.9 ± 6.8	2.0 ± 0.5
29–30	17.5 ± 2.2	17.7 ± 2.1	64.7 ± 6.5	2.3 ± 0.4
31–32	19.0 ± 1.9	19.2 ± 1.1	70.7 ± 6.9	2.8 ± 0.4
33–34	19.2 ± 1.9	21.2 ± 2.3	72.7 ± 8.3	3.0 ± 0.8
35–36	21.4 ± 1.5	19.8 ± 1.0	77.6 ± 5.1	3.4 ± 0.3
37–38	22.1 ± 3.8	23.0 ± 4.6	80.7 ± 9.9	3.9 ± 1.4
39–40	25.7 ± 2.3	25.0 ± 2.6	86.7 ± 7.0	4.9 ± 0.7

Adapted from Malinger G, Ginath S, Lerman-Sagie T, Watemberg N, Lev D, et al. The fetal cerebellar vermis: normal development as shown by transvaginal ultrasound. *Prenat Diagn* 2001;21:687–692.

TABLE 24. REFERENCE VALUES FOR BINOCULAR DIAMETER, INTEROCULAR DIAMETER, AND OCULAR DIAMETER BY GESTATIONAL AGE

Gestational age (wk)	Binocular diameter (mm) Percentiles			Interocular diameter (mm) Percentiles			Ocular diameter (mm) Percentiles		
	5th	50th	95th	5th	50th	95th	5th	50th	95th
11	5	13	20	—	—	—	—	—	—
12	8	15	23	4	9	13	1	3	6
13	10	18	25	5	9	14	2	4	7
14	13	20	28	5	10	14	3	5	8
15	15	22	30	6	10	14	4	6	9
16	17	25	32	6	10	15	5	7	9
17	19	27	34	6	11	15	5	8	10
18	22	29	37	7	11	16	6	9	11
19	24	31	39	7	12	16	7	9	12
20	26	33	41	8	12	17	8	10	13
21	28	35	43	8	13	17	8	11	13
22	30	37	44	9	13	18	9	12	14
23	31	39	46	9	14	18	10	12	15
24	33	41	48	10	14	19	10	13	15
25	35	42	50	10	15	19	11	13	16
26	36	44	51	11	15	20	12	14	16
27	38	45	53	11	16	20	12	14	17
28	39	47	54	12	16	21	13	15	17
29	41	48	56	12	17	21	13	15	18
30	42	50	57	13	17	22	14	16	18
31	43	51	58	13	18	22	14	16	19
32	45	52	60	14	18	23	14	17	19
33	46	53	61	14	19	23	15	17	19
34	47	54	62	15	19	24	15	17	20
35	48	55	63	15	20	24	15	18	20
36	49	56	64	16	20	25	16	18	20
37	50	57	65	16	21	25	16	18	21
38	50	58	65	17	21	26	16	18	21

Reproduced with permission from Romero R, Pilu G, Jeanty F, et al. *Prenatal diagnosis of congenital anomalies.* Norwalk, CT: Appleton & Lange, 1988:83.

TABLE 25. PERCENTILE REFERENCE VALUES FOR EAR LENGTH

Gestational age (wk)	Ear length (mm)		
	Percentiles		
	5th	50th	95th
15	7	9	11
16	8	10	12
17	9	11	13
18	10	12	14
19	11	13	16
20	11	15	17
21	12	16	18
22	13	17	19
23	14	18	21
24	15	19	22
25	16	20	24
26	17	22	26
27	18	23	27
28	18	24	28
29	19	25	29
30	20	26	30
31	21	27	31
32	22	28	32
33	22	28	33
34	23	29	34
35	24	30	35
36	25	30	36
37	25	31	37
38	26	31	37
39	27	32	38
40	27	32	38

Note: Ratio biparietal diameter/ear length is 3.03 (SD, .29), independent of gestational age.
Modified data, smoothed and rounded to nearest millimeter, from Chitkara U, Lee L, El-Sayed YY, Holbrook RH Jr, Bloch DA, et al. Ultrasonographic ear length measurement in normal second- and third-trimester fetuses. *Am J Obstet Gynecol* 2000;183:230–234.
Reproduced with permission from Shimizu T, Salvador L, Allanson J, Hughes-Benzie R, Nimrod C. Ultrasonographic measurements of fetal ear. *Obstet Gynecol* 1992;80:381–384.

TABLE 26. REFERENCE VALUES FOR MANDIBLE LENGTH

MA (wk)	Mandible length (mm)		
	Percentiles		
	5th	50th	95th
15	11	14	18
16	13	17	20
17	15	19	22
18	17	21	24
19	19	23	26
20	21	25	28
21	23	26	30
22	25	28	32
23	27	30	33
24	28	32	35
25	30	33	37
26	31	35	38
27	33	36	40
28	34	38	41
29	36	39	43
30	37	41	44
31	39	42	45
32	40	43	47
33	41	45	48
34	42	46	49
35	43	47	50
36	44	48	51
37	45	49	52
38	46	50	53
39	47	51	54

GA, gestational age; MA, menstrual age.
Note: Mandible length (mm) = $-20.41 + 2.97 \times GA - 0.027 \times GA^2$ (SD, 2.077).
Reproduced with permission from Otto C, Platt LD. The fetal mandible measurement: an objective determination of fetal jaw size. *Ultrasound Obstet Gynecol* 1991;1:12–17.

TABLE 27. REFERENCE VALUES FOR LENGTH OF NASAL BONE

Gestational age (wk)	Length of nasal bone (mm)		
	–2 SD	Mean	+2 SD
14	3.3	4.2	5.0
16	3.1	5.2	7.3
18	5.0	6.3	7.6
20	5.7	7.6	9.5
22	6.0	8.2	10.4
24	6.8	9.4	12.0
26	7.2	9.7	12.3
28	7.8	10.7	13.6
30	8.3	11.3	14.4
32	8.0	11.6	15.2
34	7.5	12.3	17.0

Reproduced with permission from Guis F, Ville Y, Vincent Y, Doumerc S, Pons JC, et al. Ultrasound evaluation of the length of the fetal nasal bones throughout gestation. *Ultrasound Obstet Gynecol* 1995;5:304–307.

**TABLE 28. REFERENCE VALUES FOR
THYROID VOLUME**

GA (wk)	Thyroid volume (cm³)	
	Mean	Range
20–23	0.08	±.05
24–27	0.15	±.09
28–31	0.24	±.10
32–35	0.42	±.21
>35	0.63	±.22

EFW, estimated fetal weight; GA, gestational age.
Note: Volume = $0.38 - 0.02 \times$ GA $+ 0.3 \times$ EFW.
Reproduced with permission from Ho SSY, Metreweli C. Normal thyroid volume. *Ultrasound Obstet Gynecol* 1998;11:118–122.

TABLE 29. PERCENTILE REFERENCE VALUES FOR THORACIC CIRCUMFERENCE

Gestational age (wk)	Thoracic circumference (cm)								
	Percentiles								
	2.5th	5th	10th	25th	50th	75th	90th	95th	97.5th
16.0	5.9	6.4	7.0	8.0	9.1	10.3	11.3	11.9	12.4
17.0	6.8	7.3	7.9	8.9	10.0	11.2	12.2	12.8	13.3
18.0	7.7	8.2	8.8	9.8	11.0	12.1	13.1	13.7	14.2
19.0	8.6	9.1	9.7	10.7	11.9	13.0	14.0	14.6	15.1
20.0	9.5	10.0	10.6	11.7	12.9	13.9	15.0	15.5	16.0
21.0	10.4	11.0	11.6	12.6	13.7	14.8	15.8	16.4	16.9
22.0	11.3	11.9	12.5	13.5	14.6	15.7	16.7	17.3	17.8
23.0	12.2	12.8	13.4	14.4	15.5	16.6	17.6	18.2	18.8
24.0	13.2	13.7	14.3	15.3	16.4	17.5	18.5	19.1	19.7
25.0	14.1	14.6	15.2	16.2	17.3	18.4	19.4	20.0	20.6
26.0	15.0	15.5	16.1	17.1	18.2	19.3	20.3	21.0	21.5
27.0	15.9	16.4	17.0	18.0	19.1	20.2	21.3	21.9	22.4
28.0	16.8	17.3	17.9	18.9	20.0	21.2	22.2	22.8	23.3
29.0	17.7	18.2	18.8	19.8	21.0	22.1	23.1	23.7	24.2
30.0	18.6	19.1	19.7	20.7	21.9	23.0	24.0	24.6	25.1
31.0	19.5	20.0	20.6	21.6	22.8	23.9	24.9	25.5	26.0
32.0	20.4	20.9	21.5	22.6	23.7	24.8	25.8	26.4	26.9
33.0	21.3	21.8	22.5	23.5	24.6	25.7	26.7	27.3	27.8
34.0	22.2	22.8	23.4	24.4	25.5	26.6	27.6	28.2	28.7
35.0	23.1	23.7	24.3	25.3	26.4	27.5	28.5	29.1	29.6
36.0	24.0	24.6	25.2	26.2	27.3	28.4	29.4	30.0	30.6
37.0	24.9	25.5	26.1	27.1	28.2	29.3	30.3	30.9	31.5
38.0	25.9	26.4	27.0	28.0	29.1	30.2	31.2	31.9	32.4
39.0	26.8	27.3	27.9	28.9	30.0	31.1	32.2	32.8	33.3
40.0	27.7	28.2	28.8	29.8	30.9	32.1	33.1	33.7	34.2

Reproduced with permission from Chitkara U, Rosenberg J, Chervenak FA, et al. Prenatal sonographic assessment of the fetal thorax: normal values. *Am J Obstet Gynecol* 1987;156:1069.

TABLE 30. REFERENCE VALUES FOR LUNG VOLUMES CALCULATED BY THREE-DIMENSIONAL ULTRASOUND

GA (wk)	Lung volume (cm³)		
	Percentiles		
	5th	50th	95th
14	0.3	3.9	11.6
15	0.7	5.3	14.1
16	1.2	6.8	16.9
17	2.0	8.6	20.0
18	2.9	10.6	23.3
19	3.9	12.8	26.8
20	5.1	15.2	30.7
21	6.5	17.8	34.7
22	8.1	20.7	39.0
23	9.8	23.7	43.6
24	11.7	26.9	48.4
25	13.7	30.4	53.5
26	16.0	34.0	58.9
27	18.3	37.9	64.5
28	20.9	42.0	70.3
29	23.6	46.2	76.4
30	26.5	50.7	82.7
31	29.5	55.4	89.3
32	32.8	60.3	96.2
33	36.1	65.4	103.3
34	39.7	70.7	110.7
35	43.4	76.2	118.3
36	47.3	82.0	126.2
37	51.3	87.9	134.3
38	55.5	94.0	142.7
39	59.9	100.4	151.3
40	64.4	107.0	160.2

GA, gestational age.

Note: Mean volume$^{0.5}$ = −2.538094 + 0.322 × GA.

Reproduced with permission from Lee A, Kratochwil A, Stumpflen I, Deutinger J, Bernaschek G. Fetal lung volume determination by three-dimensional ultrasonography. *Am J Obstet Gynecol* 1996;175(3 Pt 1):588–592.

TABLE 31. REFERENCE VALUES FOR RENAL LENGTH AND VOLUME FROM 20 TO 38 WEEKS

Gestational age (wk)	Renal length (mm) Percentiles			Renal volume (cm³) Percentiles		
	5th	50th	95th	5th	50th	95th
20	16	21	29	1.1	1.7	2.5
22	20	25	33	1.6	2.6	3.9
24	24	29	36	2.4	3.8	5.7
26	27	32	40	3.4	5.3	7.9
28	30	35	42	4.5	7.1	10.6
30	32	38	45	5.8	9	13.5
32	34	40	47	7	10.9	16.4
34	36	41	48	8.1	12.7	19
36	37	42	50	9	14	21
38	38	43	50	9.5	14.8	22.2

Note: Volume can be estimated by length × height × width × 0.52.
Reproduced with permission from Gloor JM, Breckle RJ, Gehrking WC, Rosenquist RG, Mulholland TA, et al. Fetal renal growth evaluated by prenatal ultrasound examination. *Mayo Clin Proc* 1997;72:124–129.

TABLE 32. REFERENCE VALUES FOR RENAL VOLUMES BASED ON THREE-DIMENSIONAL ULTRASOUND

Gestational age (wk)	Renal volumes (cm³) Right kidney Percentiles					Left kidney Percentiles				
	5th	10th	50th	90th	95th	5th	10th	50th	90th	95th
20	0.3	0.6	1.5	2.4	2.7	0.6	0.9	1.8	2.7	3.0
21	0.8	1.1	2.2	3.3	3.6	1.2	1.5	2.6	3.6	4.0
22	1.4	1.7	3.0	4.2	4.6	1.7	2.1	3.3	4.6	4.9
23	1.9	2.3	3.7	5.1	5.5	2.3	2.7	4.1	5.5	5.9
24	2.4	2.9	4.5	6.0	6.5	2.8	3.3	4.8	6.4	6.9
25	3.0	3.5	5.2	6.9	7.4	3.4	3.9	5.6	7.3	7.8
26	3.5	4.0	5.9	7.8	8.4	4.0	4.6	6.5	8.4	9.0
27	4.0	4.6	6.7	8.7	9.3	4.5	5.1	7.1	9.2	9.8
28	4.5	5.2	7.4	9.7	10.3	5.0	5.6	7.9	10.1	10.8
29	5.1	5.8	8.2	10.6	11.2	5.6	6.3	8.7	11.0	11.7
30	5.6	6.3	8.9	11.5	12.2	6.1	6.9	9.4	12.0	12.7
31	6.1	6.9	9.6	12.4	13.1	6.7	7.4	10.2	12.9	13.7
32	6.7	7.5	10.4	13.3	14.1	7.2	8.0	10.9	13.8	14.6
33	7.2	8.1	11.1	14.2	15.0	7.8	8.6	11.7	14.7	15.6
34	7.7	8.6	11.9	15.1	16.0	8.3	9.2	12.5	15.7	16.6
35	8.3	9.2	12.6	16.0	16.9	8.9	9.8	13.2	16.6	17.6
36	8.8	9.8	13.3	16.9	17.9	9.4	10.4	14.0	17.5	18.5
37	9.3	10.4	14.1	17.8	18.9	10.0	11.0	14.7	18.4	19.5
38	9.8	11.0	14.8	18.7	19.8	10.5	11.6	15.5	19.4	20.5
39	10.4	11.5	15.6	19.6	20.7	11.1	12.2	16.3	20.3	21.4
40	10.9	12.1	16.3	20.5	21.7	11.8	13.0	17.2	21.4	21.7

Note: Volume can be estimated by length × height × width × 0.52.
Data adapted from Yu C, Chang F, Ko H, Chen H. Fetal renal volume in normal gestation: a three-dimensional ultrasound study. *Ultrasound Med Biol* 2000;26:1253–1256.

TABLE 33. REFERENCE VALUES OF FETAL LIVER VOLUME DETERMINED BY THREE-DIMENSIONAL ULTRASOUND COMPARED WITH ESTIMATED FETAL WEIGHT

Estimated fetal weight (g)	Liver volume (cm³) Percentiles		
	5th	50th	95th
400	5	17	29
500	9	21	33
600	12	24	37
700	16	28	40
800	19	32	44
900	23	35	47
1,000	27	39	51
1,100	30	42	55
1,200	34	46	58
1,300	37	50	62
1,400	41	53	65
1,500	45	57	69
1,600	48	60	73
1,700	52	64	76
1,800	55	68	80
1,900	59	71	83
2,000	63	75	87
2,100	66	78	91
2,200	70	82	94
2,300	73	86	98
2,400	77	89	101
2,500	81	93	105
2,600	84	96	109
2,700	88	100	112
2,800	91	104	116
2,900	95	107	119
3,000	99	111	123

GA, gestational age.
Note: Liver volume = 2.79 + .036 × GA (SD, 7.44).
Data from Laudy JAM, Janssen MMM, Struykk PC, Stijnen T, Wallenburg HCS, et al. Fetal liver volume measurement by three-dimensional ultrasonography: a preliminary study. *Ultrasound Obstet Gynecol* 1009;12:93–96.

TABLE 34. FETAL LIVER LENGTH[a] COMPARED WITH GESTATIONAL AGE

Gestational age (wk)	Liver length (mm) Percentiles		
	5th	50th	95th
13	10	13	16
14	11	14	18
15	13	16	19
16	13	17	21
17	14	19	23
18	16	20	25
19	18	22	28
20	18	24	30
21	20	26	32
22	22	28	34
23	23	29	36
24	25	31	38
25	26	33	41
26	28	35	43
27	29	37	45
28	30	39	47
29	32	40	50
30	33	42	52
31	34	43	53
32	35	45	55
33	36	46	56
34	37	47	58
35	38	48	60
36	38	49	62
37	39	50	63
38	39	50	63
39	40	51	64
40	40	51	64

[a]Values are approximate, based on graphic data only.
Reproduced with permission from Roberts AB, Mitchell JM, Pattison NS. Fetal liver length in normal and isoimmunized pregnancies. *Am J Obstet Gynecol* 1989;161:42–46.

TABLE 35. REFERENCE VALUES FOR SPLENIC LENGTH

Gestational age (wk)	Splenic length (mm)		
	Percentiles		
	5th	50th	95th
18	7	14	21
20	11	18	26
22	15	22	29
24	19	25	32
26	20	27	34
28	24	31	38
30	27	34	41
32	31	28	45
34	35	43	50
36	41	48	55
38	47	54	62
40	55	62	70

Reproduced with permission from Schmidt W, Yarkoni S, Jeanty P, et al. Sonographic measurement of the fetal spleen. Clinical implications. *J Ultrasound Med* 1985;4:667.

TABLE 36. REFERENCE VALUES FOR SPLENIC CIRCUMFERENCE BETWEEN 18 AND 37 WEEKS

Age (wk)	Splenic circumference	
	Percentiles	
	50th	95th
18	30.7	39.7
19	33.9	43.8
20	37.2	48.0
21	40.4	52.2
22	43.6	56.3
23	46.9	60.5
24	50.1	64.7
25	53.3	68.9
26	56.6	73.0
27	59.8	77.1
28	63.1	81.3
29	66.3	85.5
30	69.5	89.6
31	72.8	93.8
32	76.0	97.9
33	79.7	102.1
34	82.5	106.3
35	85.7	110.4
36	88.9	114.6
37	92.2	118.7

GA, gestational age.
Note: Splenic circumference = $-27.569 + 3.23654 \times GA$.
Reproduced with permission from Bahado-Singh R, Oz U, Mari G, Jones D, Paidas M, et al. Fetal splenic size in anemia due to Rh-alloimmunization. *Obstet Gynecol* 1998;92:828–832.

TABLE 37. NORMAL COLON DIAMETERS

Gestational age (wk)	Colon diameters (mm)		
	−2 SD	Mean	+2 SD
22	2	4	6
24	3	5	7
26	4	6	9
28	4	7	10
30	5	8	11
32	6	9	12
34	7	10	13
36	8	12	16
38	9	14	18
40	10	16	20

Data adapted from Harris RD, Nyberg DA, Mack LA, Weinberger E. Anorectal atresia: prenatal sonographic diagnosis. *AJR Am J Roentgenol* 1987;149:395–400.

CARDIAC MEASUREMENTS

TABLE 38. REFERENCE VALUES FOR AORTIC ROOT INTERNAL DIAMETER, PULMONARY ARTERY, LEFT VENTRICLE, RIGHT VENTRICLE, LEFT ATRIUM, AND RIGHT ATRIUM (VALUES ARE SHOWN FOR 5TH, 50TH, AND 95TH PERCENTILES)

GA (wk)	Aortic root (mm)[a]			Pulmonary artery (mm)[b]			Left ventricle (mm)[c]		
	5th	50th	95th	5th	50th	95th	5th	50th	95th
14.0	1.2	1.8	2.4	1.3	1.9	2.5	1.2	2.3	3.5
15.0	1.4	2.0	2.7	1.6	2.2	2.8	1.8	3.0	4.3
16.0	1.6	2.3	2.9	1.8	2.5	3.1	2.4	3.7	5.0
17.0	1.9	2.5	3.2	2.1	2.8	3.4	2.9	4.3	5.8
18.0	2.1	2.8	3.5	2.3	3.0	3.8	3.4	5.0	6.5
19.0	2.3	3.0	3.7	2.6	3.3	4.1	3.9	5.6	7.2
20.0	2.5	3.3	4.0	2.8	3.6	4.4	4.4	6.1	7.9
21.0	2.8	3.5	4.3	3.1	3.9	4.7	4.8	6.7	8.5
22.0	3.0	3.8	4.6	3.3	4.2	5.0	5.2	7.2	9.2
23.0	3.2	4.0	4.8	3.6	4.5	5.3	5.6	7.7	9.8
24.0	3.4	4.3	5.1	3.8	4.7	5.6	6.0	8.2	10.4
25.0	3.6	4.5	5.4	4.1	5.0	5.9	6.4	8.7	11.0
26.0	3.9	4.8	5.6	4.4	5.3	6.3	6.7	9.1	11.5
27.0	4.1	5.0	5.9	4.6	5.6	6.6	7.0	9.5	12.0
28.0	4.3	5.3	6.2	4.9	5.9	6.9	7.3	9.9	12.5
29.0	4.5	5.5	6.5	5.1	6.2	7.2	7.6	10.3	13.0
30.0	4.8	5.7	6.7	5.4	6.4	7.5	7.8	10.6	13.4
31.0	5.0	6.0	7.0	5.6	6.7	7.8	8.0	10.9	13.9
32.0	5.2	6.2	7.3	5.9	7.0	8.1	8.2	11.2	14.3
33.0	5.4	6.5	7.5	6.1	7.3	8.4	8.4	11.5	14.7
34.0	5.7	6.7	7.8	6.4	7.6	8.8	8.5	11.8	15.0
35.0	5.9	7.0	8.1	6.6	7.9	9.1	8.6	12.0	15.4
36.0	6.1	7.2	8.4	6.9	8.1	9.4	8.7	12.2	15.7
37.0	6.3	7.5	8.6	7.1	8.4	9.7	8.8	12.4	16.0
38.0	6.5	7.7	8.9	7.4	8.7	10.0	8.9	12.5	16.2
39.0	6.8	8.0	9.2	7.6	9.0	10.3	8.9	12.7	16.5
40.0	7.0	8.2	9.4	7.9	9.3	10.6	8.9	12.8	16.7

GA (wk)	Right ventricle (mm)[d]			Left atrium (mm)[e]			Right atrium (mm)[f]		
	5th	50th	95th	5th	50th	95th	5th	50th	95th
14.0	1.4	2.5	3.5	2.2	3.2	4.2	2.4	3.5	4.7
15.0	2.0	3.1	4.3	2.8	3.9	5.0	3.0	4.2	5.4
16.0	2.5	3.8	5.1	3.3	4.5	5.7	3.5	4.8	6.2
17.0	3.0	4.4	5.8	3.8	5.1	6.4	4.0	5.5	6.9
18.0	3.6	5.1	6.6	4.3	5.7	7.1	4.6	6.1	7.6
19.0	4.0	5.7	7.3	4.8	6.3	7.8	5.1	6.7	8.3
20.0	4.5	6.3	8.0	5.3	6.9	8.4	5.6	7.3	9.0
21.0	5.0	6.9	8.7	5.7	7.4	9.1	6.0	7.9	9.7
22.0	5.5	7.4	9.4	6.2	8.0	9.7	6.5	8.5	10.4
23.0	5.9	8.0	10.1	6.6	8.5	10.3	7.0	9.0	11.1
24.0	6.3	8.5	10.7	7.0	9.0	10.9	7.4	9.6	11.7
25.0	6.7	9.1	11.4	7.5	9.5	11.5	7.8	10.1	12.4
26.0	7.1	9.6	12.0	7.8	10.0	12.1	8.3	10.6	13.0
27.0	7.5	10.1	12.6	8.2	10.5	12.7	8.7	11.1	13.6
28.0	7.9	10.6	13.3	8.6	10.9	13.2	9.1	11.6	14.2
29.0	8.3	11.0	13.8	8.9	11.4	13.8	9.5	12.1	14.8
30.0	8.6	11.5	14.4	9.3	11.8	14.3	9.8	12.6	15.4
31.0	8.9	12.0	15.0	9.6	12.2	14.8	10.2	13.1	16.0
32.0	9.2	12.4	15.5	9.9	12.6	15.3	10.5	13.5	16.5
33.0	9.6	12.8	16.1	10.2	13.0	15.8	10.9	14.0	17.1
34.0	9.8	13.2	16.6	10.5	13.4	16.2	11.2	14.4	17.6
35.0	10.1	13.6	17.1	10.8	13.7	16.7	11.5	14.8	18.1
36.0	10.4	14.0	17.6	11.0	14.1	17.1	11.8	15.2	18.6
37.0	10.6	14.4	18.1	11.2	14.4	17.6	12.1	15.6	19.1
38.0	10.9	14.7	18.6	11.5	14.7	18.0	12.4	16.0	19.6
39.0	11.1	15.1	19.0	11.7	15.0	18.4	12.7	16.4	20.1
40.0	11.3	15.4	19.5	11.9	15.3	18.8	12.9	16.7	20.6

GA, gestational age.

[a]Aorta = $0.247 \times GA - 1.6638$ (SD = $0.0146 \times GA + 0.16$).
[b]Pulmonary artery = $0.283 \times GA - 2.055$ (SD = $0.018 \times GA + 0.11$).
[c]Left ventricle (end diastole) = $-0.01152 \times GA^2 + 1.024 \times GA - 9.735$ (SD = $0.065 \times GA - 0.234$).
[d]Right ventricle (end diastole) = $-0.006848 \times GA^2 + 0.866 \times GA - 8.306$ (SD = $0.071 \times GA - 0.359$).
[e]Left atrium = $-0.00698 \times GA^2 + 0.8422 \times GA - 7.2$ (SD = $0.05677 \times GA - 0.18$).
[f]Right atrium = $-0.00587 \times GA^2 + 0.8246 \times GA - 6.846$ (SD = $0.0634 \times GA - 0.21$).
Data adapted from Shapiro I, Degani S, Leibovitz Z, Ohel G, Tal Y, et al. Fetal cardiac measurements derived by transvaginal and transabdominal cross-sectional echocardiography from 14 weeks of gestation to term. *Ultrasound Obsetet Gynecol* 1998;12:404–418.

TABLE 39. REFERENCE VALUES FOR E/A RATIO OF MITRAL VALVE AND TRICUSPID VALVE

GA (wk)	Mitral valve[a]			Tricuspid valve[b]		
	Percentiles			Percentiles		
	5th	50th	95th	5th	50th	95th
20	0.47	0.59	0.71	0.51	0.62	0.74
21	0.48	0.60	0.72	0.52	0.63	0.75
22	0.48	0.61	0.73	0.53	0.64	0.76
23	0.49	0.62	0.74	0.54	0.65	0.77
24	0.50	0.63	0.76	0.55	0.66	0.78
25	0.51	0.64	0.77	0.56	0.67	0.79
26	0.52	0.65	0.78	0.57	0.68	0.80
27	0.53	0.66	0.79	0.58	0.69	0.81
28	0.53	0.67	0.81	0.59	0.70	0.82
29	0.54	0.68	0.82	0.60	0.71	0.83
30	0.55	0.69	0.83	0.61	0.72	0.84
31	0.56	0.70	0.85	0.62	0.73	0.84
32	0.57	0.71	0.86	0.63	0.74	0.85
33	0.58	0.73	0.87	0.64	0.75	0.86
34	0.59	0.74	0.89	0.65	0.76	0.87
35	0.60	0.75	0.90	0.66	0.77	0.88
36	0.61	0.76	0.92	0.67	0.78	0.89
37	0.62	0.77	0.93	0.68	0.79	0.90
38	0.63	0.79	0.95	0.69	0.80	0.91
39	0.64	0.80	0.96	0.70	0.81	0.92
40	0.65	0.81	0.98	0.71	0.82	0.93

GA, gestational age.
[a]Mitral valve log 10 (E/A ratio) = –0.3699 + 0.007 × GA (SD, 0.0687 transformed).
[b]Tricuspid valve E/A ratio = 0.428 + 0.0098 × A14 (SD, 0.0687).
Note: E/A ratio is equal to the peak velocity of E wave during early diastole/peak velocity with a wave during atrial contraction.
Data from Hecher K, Campbell S, Snijders R, Nicolaides K. Reference ranges for fetal venous and atrio-ventricular blood flow parameters. *Ultrasound Obstet Gynecol* 1994;4:381–390.

TABLE 40. NORMAL DOPPLER ECHOCARDIOGRAPHY IN THE FETUS

Valve	Tricuspid	Mitral	Pulmonary	Aorta
Maximal velocity (cm/sec)	51 ± 4	47 ± 4	60 ± 4	70 ± 3
Mean velocity (cm/sec)	12 ± 1	11 ± 1	16 ± 2	18 ± 2
Valve diameter (mm)[a]	8 ± 0.5	6.6 ± 0.4	7.6 ± 0.3	6.7 ± 0.2
Cardiac output (mL/kg/min)[a]	307 ± 30	232 ± 25	312 ± 11	250 ± 9
A/E ratio[a]	1.29 ± 0.04	1.35 ± 0.01	—	—
Deceleration time (msec)[a]	97 ± 29	110 ± 31	—	—
Acceleration time (msec)[a]	—	—	50.6 ± 12.0	46.7 ± 9.1

A/E, atrial contraction/early diastole.
[a]Varies with gestational age.
Reproduced with permission from Reed KL. Fetal Doppler echocardiography. *Clin Obstet Gynecol* 1989;32:728–737.

DOPPLER

TABLE 41. REFERENCE VALUES FOR UMBILICAL ARTERY DOPPLER RESISTIVE INDEX AND SYSTOLIC/DIASTOLIC RATIO

	Percentiles					
	5th		50th		95th	
GA (wk)	RI	Systolic/ diastolic ratio	Resistive index	Systolic/ diastolic ratio	Resistive index	Systolic/ diastolic ratio
16	0.70	3.39	0.80	5.12	0.90	10.50
17	0.69	3.27	0.79	4.86	0.89	9.46
18	0.68	3.16	0.78	4.63	0.88	8.61
19	0.67	3.06	0.77	4.41	0.87	7.90
20	0.66	2.97	0.76	4.22	0.86	7.30
21	0.65	2.88	0.75	4.04	0.85	6.78
22	0.64	2.79	0.74	3.88	0.84	6.33
23	0.63	2.71	0.73	3.73	0.83	5.94
24	0.62	2.64	0.72	3.59	0.82	5.59
25	0.61	2.57	0.71	3.46	0.81	5.28
26	0.60	2.50	0.70	3.34	0.80	5.01
27	0.59	2.44	0.69	3.22	0.79	4.76
28	0.58	2.38	0.68	3.12	0.78	4.53
29	0.57	2.32	0.67	3.02	0.77	4.33
30	0.56	2.26	0.66	2.93	0.76	4.14
31	0.55	2.21	0.65	2.84	0.75	3.97
32	0.54	2.16	0.64	2.76	0.74	3.81
33	0.53	2.11	0.63	2.68	0.73	3.66
34	0.52	2.07	0.62	2.61	0.72	3.53
35	0.51	2.03	0.61	2.54	0.71	3.40
36	0.50	1.98	0.60	2.47	0.70	3.29
37	0.49	1.94	0.59	2.41	0.69	3.18
38	0.47	1.90	0.57	2.35	0.67	3.08
39	0.46	1.87	0.56	2.30	0.66	2.98
40	0.45	1.83	0.55	2.24	0.65	2.89
41	0.44	1.80	0.54	2.19	0.64	2.81
42	0.43	1.76	0.53	2.14	0.63	2.73

GA, gestational age; RI, resistive index.
Note: $RI = 0.97199 - 0.01045 \times GA$ (SD = 0.06078); systolic/diastolic ratio = $1/(1 - RI)$.
Data from Kofinas AD, Espeland MA, Penry M, Swain M, Hatjis CG. Uteroplacental Doppler flow velocity waveform indices in normal pregnancy: a statistical exercise and the development of appropriate reference values. *Am J Perinatol* 1992;9:94–101.

TABLE 42. REFERENCE VALUES FOR PEAK SYSTOLIC VELOCITY OF THE MIDDLE CEREBRAL ARTERY

GA (wk)	Peak systolic velocity (cm/sec)				
	Multiples of the median				
	1	1.3	1.5	1.7	2
15	20	26	30	34	40
16	21	27	32	36	42
17	22	29	33	37	44
18	23	30	35	39	46
19	24	31	36	41	48
20	25	33	38	43	50
21	26	34	39	44	52
22	28	36	42	48	56
23	29	38	44	49	58
24	30	39	45	51	60
25	32	42	48	54	64
26	33	43	50	56	66
27	35	46	53	60	70
28	37	48	56	63	74
29	38	49	57	65	76
30	40	52	60	68	80
31	42	55	63	71	84
32	44	57	66	75	88
33	46	60	69	78	92
34	48	62	72	82	96
35	50	65	75	85	100
36	53	69	80	90	106
37	55	72	83	94	110
38	58	75	87	99	116
39	61	79	92	104	122
40	63	82	95	107	126

GA, gestational age.
Note: Peak systolic velocity (cm/sec) = $e^{(2.31 + 0.046 \times GA)}$.
Reproduced with permission from Mari G, Deter RL, Carpenter RL, Rahman F, Zimmerman R, et al. Noninvasive diagnosis by Doppler ultrasonography of fetal anemia due to maternal red-cell alloimmunization. Collaborative Group for Doppler Assessment of the Blood Velocity in Anemic Fetuses. *N Engl J Med* 2000;342:9–14.

TABLE 43. REFERENCE VALUES FOR PEAK SYSTOLIC VELOCITY AND PEAK VELOCITY INDEX FOR VEINS OF THE DUCTUS VENOSUS

GA (wk)	Peak systolic velocity			Peak velocity index for veins		
	Percentiles			Percentiles		
	5th	50th	95th	5th	50th	95th
20	47	66	84	0.40	0.61	0.81
21	50	68	87	0.39	0.60	0.80
22	52	70	89	0.38	0.59	0.79
23	54	72	91	0.37	0.58	0.78
24	56	74	93	0.36	0.57	0.77
25	57	76	94	0.35	0.56	0.76
26	59	77	96	0.34	0.55	0.75
27	60	78	97	0.33	0.54	0.74
28	61	79	98	0.32	0.53	0.73
29	62	80	99	0.31	0.52	0.72
30	62	81	99	0.30	0.51	0.71
31	62	81	100	0.29	0.50	0.70
32	63	81	100	0.28	0.49	0.69
33	62	81	100	0.27	0.48	0.68
34	62	81	99	0.26	0.47	0.67
35	62	80	99	0.25	0.46	0.66
36	61	79	98	0.24	0.45	0.65
37	60	78	97	0.23	0.44	0.64
38	59	77	96	0.22	0.43	0.63
39	57	76	95	0.22	0.42	0.62
40	56	74	93	0.21	0.41	0.61

GA, gestational age.
Note: Peak velocity = $-27.589 + 6.789 \times GA - 0.106 \times GA^2$ (SD, 11.295); peak velocity index for veins = (peak velocity or S wave – atrial contraction or a wave)/peak diastolic velocity or D wave = $0.805 - 0.0099 \times GA$ (SD, 0.1239).
Data from Hecher K, Campbell S, Snijders R, Nicolaides K. Reference ranges for fetal venous and atrioventricular blood flow parameters. *Ultrasound Obstet Gynecol* 1994;4:381–390.

ANEUPLOIDY TABLES

TABLE 44. ODDS (1:___) OF FETAL TRISOMY 21 VARYING WITH MATERNAL AGE AND GESTATIONAL AGE

Maternal age (wk)	Wk					
	10	12	14	16	20	40
20	983	1,068	1,140	1,200	1,295	1,527
25	870	946	1,009	1,062	1,147	1,352
30	576	626	668	703	759	895
31	500	543	580	610	658	776
32	424	461	492	518	559	659
33	352	383	409	430	464	547
34	287	312	333	350	378	446
35	229	249	266	280	302	356
36	180	296	209	220	238	280
37	140	152	163	171	185	218
38	108	117	125	131	142	167
39	82	89	95	100	108	128
40	62	68	72	76	82	97
41	47	51	54	57	62	73
42	35	38	41	43	46	55
43	26	29	30	32	35	41
44	20	21	23	24	26	30
45	15	16	17	16	19	23

Data from Snijders RJ, Sundberg K, Holzgreve W, Henry G, Nicolaides KH. Maternal age- and gestation-specific risk for trisomy 21. *Ultrasound Obstet Gynecol* 1999;13:167–170.

TABLE 45. COMPARISON OF LIKELIHOOD RATIOS REPORTED FOR SONOGRAPHIC MARKERS OF FETAL ANEUPLOIDY FROM TWO STUDIES AND FROM A METAANALYSIS STUDY

Sonographic marker	Nyberg et al.[a]	Bromley et al.[b]	Smith-Bindman et al.[c]
	Likelihood ratios (95% CI)	Likelihood ratios	Likelihood ratios (95% CI)
Nuchal thickening	11.0 (5.5–22.0)	12	17 (8–38)
Hyperechoic bowel	6.7 (2.7–16.8)	—	6.1 (3–12.6)
Short humerus	5.1 (1.6–16.5)	6	7.5 (4.7–12)
Short femur	1.5 (0.8–2.8)	1	2.7 (1.2–6)
Echogenic intracardiac focus	1.8 (1.0–3.0)	1.2	2.8 (1.5–5.5)
Pyelectasis	1.5 (0.6–3.6)	1.3	1.9 (0.7–5.1)
Normal ultrasound	0.36	0.2	—

CI, confidence interval.
[a]Reproduced with permission from Nyberg DA, Souter VL, El-Bastawissi A, Young S, Luthhardt F, et al. Isolated sonographic markers for detection of fetal Down syndrome in the second trimester of pregnancy. *J Ultrasound Med* 2001;20:1053–1063.
[b]Reproduced with permission from Bromley B, Lieberman E, Shipp T, Benacerraf BR. The genetic sonogram: a method of risk assessment for Down syndrome in the mid-trimester. *J Ultrasound Med* (*in press*).
[c]Reproduced with permission from Smith-Bindman R, Hosmer W, Feldstein VA, Deeks JJ, Goldberg JD. Second-trimester ultrasound to detect fetuses with Down syndrome: a meta-analysis. *JAMA* 2001;285:1044–1055.

TABLE 46. RISK OF FETAL DOWN SYNDROME, EXPRESSED AS ODDS (1:__) CATEGORIZED BY MATERNAL AGE AND PRESUMED SENSITIVITY OF ULTRASOUND

			Post-ultrasound risk								
		Sensitivity	10%	20%	30%	40%	50%	60%	70%	80%	90%
	A priori odds	False-positive rate	12%	12%	12%	12%	12%	12%	12%	12%	12%
Maternal age (wk)	(1:__)	LR[a]	1.0	0.91	0.80	0.68	0.57	0.45	0.34	0.23	0.11
20	1,176		1,150	1,294	1,478	1,724	2,069	2,586	3,448	5,171	10,341
21	1,160		1,134	1,276	1,458	1,701	2,041	2,551	3,401	5,101	10,200
22	1,136		1,111	1,250	1,428	1,666	1,999	2,498	3,330	4,995	9,989
23	1,114		1,089	1,225	1,400	1,633	1,960	2,450	3,266	4,898	9,795
24	1,087		1,063	1,196	1,366	1,594	1,912	2,390	3,187	4,779	9,558
25	1,040		1,017	1,144	1,307	1,525	1,830	2,287	3,049	4,573	9,144
26	990		968	1,089	1,244	1,452	1,742	2,177	2,902	4,353	8,704
27	928		907	1,021	1,166	1,361	1,633	2,040	2,720	4,080	8,159
28	855		836	940	1,075	1,254	1,504	1,880	2,506	3,759	7,516
29	760		743	836	955	1,114	1,337	1,671	2,227	3,341	6,680
30	690		675	759	867	1,012	1,214	1,517	2,022	3,033	6,064
31	597		584	657	750	875	1,050	1,312	1,749	2,623	5,246
32	508		497	559	638	745	893	1,116	1,488	2,232	4,463
33	421		412	463	529	617	740	925	1,233	1,849	3,697
34	342		334	376	430	501	601	751	1,001	1,501	3,002
35	274		268	301	344	401	481	602	802	1,202	2,403
36	216		211	238	271	316	379	474	632	947	1,893
37	168		164	185	211	246	295	368	491	736	1,471
38	129		126	142	162	189	226	283	376	564	1,127
39	98		96	108	123	143	172	214	286	428	855
40	74		72	81	93	108	129	162	215	322	643
41	56		55	62	70	82	98	122	162	243	485
42	42		41	46	53	61	73	91	121	181	362
43	31		30	34	39	45	54	67	89	133	265
44	23		23	25	29	33	40	49	66	98	195

Note: Reduction of risk varies markedly with sensitivity of ultrasound for a set false-positive rate.
[a]LR = likelihood ratio of normal ultrasound for identification of trisomy 21, calculated as false-negative rate/specificity. False-negative rate = (1 – sensitivity), specificity = (1 – false-positive rate). False-positive rate assumed to be 12% using multiple ultrasound markers.
Adapted from Nyberg DA, Luthy DA, Resta RG, Nyberg BC, Williams MA. Age-adjusted ultrasound risk assessment for fetal Down's syndrome during the second trimester: description of the method and analysis of 142 cases. *Ultrasound Obstet Gynecol* 1998;12:8–14.

TABLE 47. MATERNAL AGE–SPECIFIC ODDS (1:__) OF FETAL DOWN SYNDROME DURING THE SECOND TRIMESTER BASED ON SONOGRAPHIC MARKERS OF FETAL ANEUPLOIDY

Maternal age (wk)	Pre-ultrasound odds (1: _)	Normal ultrasound (1: _) LR .36	Nuchal thickness (1: _) LR 11.0	Hyperechoic bowel (1: _) LR 6.7	Short femur length (1: _) LR 1.5	Short humerus length (1: _) LR 5.1	Echogenic intracardiac focus (1: _) LR 1.8	Renal pelvis (1: _) LR 1.5
20	1,176	3,265	108	176	784	231	654	784
21	1,160	3,220	106	174	774	228	645	774
22	1,136	3,154	104	170	758	224	632	758
23	1,114	3,093	102	167	743	219	619	743
24	1,087	3,018	100	163	725	214	604	725
25	1,040	2,887	95	156	694	205	578	694
26	990	2,748	91	149	660	195	550	660
27	928	2,576	85	139	619	183	516	619
28	855	2,373	79	128	570	168	475	570
29	760	2,109	70	114	507	150	423	507
30	690	1,915	64	104	460	136	384	460
31	597	1,657	55	90	398	118	332	398
32	508	1,409	47	77	339	100	283	339
33	421	1,168	39	64	281	83	234	281
34	342	948	32	52	228	68	190	228
35	274	759	26	42	183	55	153	183
36	216	598	21	33	144	43	120	144
37	168	465	16	26	112	34	94	112
38	129	357	13	20	86	26	72	86
39	98	270	10	15	66	20	55	66
40	74	204	8	12	50	15	42	50
41	56	154	6	9	38	12	32	38
42	42	115	5	7	28	9	24	28
43	31	84	4	5	21	7	18	21
44	23	62	3	4	16	5	13	16

LR, likelihood ratio.
Note: Assuming LRs of Nyberg et al. in Table 45.
Note: Odds ratio (O) based on formula O (Down syndrome) = O (maternal age)/LR + 1 – 1/LR.
Reproduced with permission from Nyberg DA, Souter VL, El-Bastawissi A, Young S, Luthhardt F, et al. Isolated sonographic markers for detection of fetal Down syndrome in the second trimester of pregnancy. *J Ultrasound Med* 2001;20:1053–1063.

COMMONLY RECOGNIZED SYNDROMES

CHROMOSOME ABNORMALITIES

Down Syndrome

Also see Down Syndrome (Trisomy 21), in Chapter 5.

Inheritance/etiology: chromosomal abnormality; 95% nondisjunction trisomy 21 (increased incidence with advanced maternal age), 2% mosaicism (trisomy 21 normal), 3% translocation

Primary features: mental retardation, brachycephaly, upward-slanting palpebral fissures, hypotonia, cardiac defects, mildly shortened limbs (i.e., femur, humerus), nuchal fold thickening, pyelectasis, echogenic bowel, hypoplasia of middle phalanx of fifth finger, gastrointestinal obstruction

Trisomy 18 (Edwards Syndrome)

Also see Trisomy 18 (Edwards Syndrome), in Chapter 5.

Inheritance/etiology: chromosomal abnormality; nondisjunction (increased incidence with advancing maternal age), mosaicism, translocation, partial trisomy (variable phenotype)

Primary features: severe growth and mental deficiency, low-set ears, short palpebral fissures, micrognathia; clenched hands with index finger overlapping third, fifth overlapping fourth; cardiac defects, rocker-bottom feet, gastrointestinal obstruction

Trisomy 13 (Patau Syndrome)

Also see Trisomy 13, in Chapter 5.

Inheritance/etiology: chromosomal abnormality; nondisjunction (increased incidence with advancing maternal age), mosaicism, translocation, partial trisomy (variable phenotype)

Primary features: holoprosencephaly (varying degrees), severe mental retardation, microphthalmos, cleft lip with or without cleft palate, low-set ears, polydactyly, cardiac defects, cystic kidneys, omphalocele

Triploidy

Also see Triploidy and Tetraploidy, in Chapter 5.

Inheritance/etiology: chromosomal abnormality; 90% paternally derived (66% fertilization of a single ovum by two sperm; 24% fertilization by a diploid sperm); 10% maternally derived (fertilization of a diploid ovum); diploid/triploid mosaicism

Primary features: large, hydatidiform placenta with small fetus (paternally derived triploid), tiny placenta with larger fetus (maternally derived triploid); mental retardation, syndactyly, disproportionate growth deficiency, asymmetric skeletal growth (particularly in mosaics), cardiac defects, brain anomalies

4p– Syndrome (Wolf-Hirschhorn Syndrome)

Inheritance/etiology: chromosomal abnormality; partial deletion on the short arm of chromosome 4, usually *de novo*; parental balanced translocation is rarely involved; occasionally requires fluorescent *in situ* hybridization for detection

Primary features: mental retardation, microcephaly, prenatal growth deficiency, hypertelorism, beaked nose; low-set, large, "simple" ears; cleft lip with or without cleft palate

5p– Syndrome (Cri du Chat Syndrome)

Inheritance/etiology: chromosomal abnormality; partial deletion of the short arm of chromosome 5, usually *de novo*; parental balanced translocations account for 10% to 15% of cases

Primary features: mental retardation, growth delay, low birth weight, microcephaly, hypertelorism, epicanthal folds, downward-slanting palpebral fissures, cat-like cry

13q– Syndrome

Inheritance/etiology: chromosomal abnormality; partial deletion of the long arm of chromosome 13

Primary features: mental retardation, microcephaly, hypertelorism, prominent nasal bridge, large ears, absent or dysplastic thumbs

18p– Syndrome

Inheritance/etiology: chromosomal abnormality; partial deletion of the short arm of chromosome 18, occasionally due to a ring 18 chromosome, usually *de novo*; parental balanced translocation carriers and actual deletion carriers have been reported

Primary features: mild to severe mental retardation, growth deficiency; round, flat face; ptosis of eyelids, epicanthal folds, wide mouth; holoprosencephaly (12%)

18q– Syndrome

Inheritance/etiology: chromosomal abnormality; partial deletion of the long arm of chromosome 18, occasionally due to a ring 18 chromosome, usually *de novo*

Primary features: severe mental retardation, short stature, midfacial dysplasia, hypotonia, prominent and/or deformed ears, "carp-shaped" mouth

22q11 Deletion Syndrome (includes DiGeorge, Velocardiofacial, and Shprintzen Syndromes)

See also Velocardiofacial Syndrome, in Chapter 5.

Inheritance/etiology: chromosomal microdeletion syndrome; deletion on chromosome 22q11; may be vertically transmitted with variable expression; diagnosis requires fluorescent *in situ* hybridization

Primary features: conotruncal cardiac defects; overt or submucosal cleft of secondary palate; prominent nose; long, thin, hyperextensible hands/fingers; mild intellectual impairment; hypoparathyroidism with hypocalcemia; immunodeficiency

XYY Syndrome

Inheritance/etiology: chromosomal abnormality, presence of an extra Y chromosome

Primary features: tall stature, IQ 10 to 15 points below sibling controls, tendency toward behavior problems, poor fine motor coordination

XXY (Klinefelter) Syndrome

Inheritance/etiology: chromosomal abnormality, presence of an extra X chromosome, 22% mosaics

Primary features: IQ 10 to 15 points below sibling controls, tall stature, small penis/testes, infertility, tendency toward behavior problems

XO (Turner) Syndrome

Also see Turner Syndrome (45,X), in Chapter 5.

Inheritance/etiology: sporadic chromosomal abnormality, can occur as XX/XO or XY/XO mosaics

Primary features: small stature, ovarian dysgenesis, residual neck webbing due to prenatal cystic hygroma, broad chest with widely spaced nipples, horseshoe kidney, coarctation of the aorta; may have hydrops (skin thickening, pleural effusions, ascites) in prenatal period with extensive cystic hygroma

NONCHROMOSOMAL SYNDROMES

Achondrogenesis

Also see Achondrogenesis, in Chapter 15.

Inheritance/etiology: mendelian disorder; at least two distinct types exist based on radiographic findings and bone histopathology—type I, autosomal recessive (some cases due to mutation in *DTDST*), and type II, a new, dominant mutation in *COL2A1*

Primary features: skeletal dysplasia with severe limb shortening, often with decreased skeletal ossification, especially of the vertebral bodies, normal or decreased calvarial ossification

Achondroplasia

Also see Achondroplasia, in Chapter 15.

Inheritance/etiology: mendelian disorder, autosomal dominant with 80% new mutations in *FGFR3*

Primary features: moderate rhizomelia, relatively large calvaria with small skull base, absent nasal bridge, thoracolumbar kyphosis with lack of caudal increase in interpedicular distance, trident hands, squared iliac ala

Acrocallosal Syndrome

Inheritance/etiology: mendelian disorder, autosomal recessive

Primary features: macrocephaly, hypertelorism, polydactyly, mental retardation, agenesis of the corpus callosum, postaxial polydactyly of feet, hallucal duplication

Adams-Oliver Syndrome

Inheritance/etiology: mendelian disorder, autosomal dominant with variable expressivity

Primary features: mild growth deficiency, aplasia cutis congenita, terminal defects of limbs

Adrenogenital Syndrome

Inheritance/etiology: mendelian disorder, autosomal recessive

Primary features: 21-hydroxylase deficiency leading to virilization in affected females, ambiguous genitalia

Aicardi Syndrome

Inheritance/etiology: X-linked dominant with lethality in hemizygous males

Primary features: agenesis of the corpus callosum, vertebral anomalies, infantile spasms, mental delay, chorioretinopathy

Amniotic Band Syndrome

Also see Amniotic Band Syndrome, in Chapter 5.

Inheritance/etiology: sporadic; unknown etiology

Primary features: variable abnormalities, often including constriction rings, extremity amputations or lymphedema, bizarre facial clefts, large abdominal wall or chest wall defects, asymmetric encephaloceles

Amyoplasia Congenita Disruptive Sequence (Arthrogryposis Multiplex Congenita)

Also see Arthrogryposis/Akinesia Sequence, in Chapter 5.

Inheritance/etiology: sporadic; vascular disruptive defect, discordance for amyoplasia has been reported in a monozygotic twin pair

Primary features: flexion of hands and wrists with arms extended, internally rotated shoulders, dislocated hips, bilateral equinovarus; occasionally gastroschisis and/or intestinal atresia

Angelman Syndrome ("Happy Puppet")

Inheritance/etiology: majority sporadic; maternal chromosomal microdeletion, paternal disomy of chromosome 15 at band q11–13; 30% point mutations in *UBE3A*

Primary features: severe mental retardation, inappropriate laughter, ataxia, maxillary hypoplasia, prognathia, microcephaly

Apert Syndrome

Also see Apert Syndrome, in Chapter 5.

Inheritance/etiology: mendelian disorder, autosomal dominant; mutations in *FGFR2*, most cases represent new mutations

Primary features: craniosynostosis (usually coronal), acrocephaly, beaked nose, hypertelorism, hydrocephalus, syndactyly

Asphyxiating Thoracic Dysplasia (Jeune Syndrome)

Also see Asphyxiating Thoracic Dysplasia, in Chapter 15.

Inheritance/etiology: mendelian disorder, autosomal recessive

Primary features: skeletal dysplasia with marked thoracic hypoplasia, mild to moderate rhizomelic shortening, renal dysplasia, polydactyly (14%)

Ataxia-Telangiectasia Syndrome

Inheritance/etiology: mendelian disorder, autosomal recessive; most caused by mutations in *ATM*; chromosomal breakage is the cytogenetic marker

Primary features: growth deficiency, progressive ataxia, telangiectasia, immunodeficiency, increased risk for malignancy

Bardet-Biedl Syndrome

Inheritance/etiology: mendelian disorder, autosomal recessive; multiple genetic loci identified, one form allelic to McKusick-Kaufman syndrome

Primary features: obesity, polydactyly, retinitis pigmentosa, genital hypoplasia, mental deficiency, renal defects, cardiac defects

Basal Cell Nevus Syndrome

Inheritance/etiology: mendelian disorder, autosomal dominant; mutations in *PTCH* or *PTCH2*

Primary features: macrocephaly, facial cleft, calcification of falx cerebri, skin changes after birth, jaw cysts, basal cell carcinomas

Beckwith-Wiedemann Syndrome

Also see Beckwith-Wiedemann Syndrome, in Chapter 5.

Inheritance/etiology: usually sporadic; dosage imbalance of imprinted locus on chromosome 11 at band P 15.5 (multiple mechanisms)

Primary features: omphalocele or umbilical hernia, macroglossia, visceromegaly, neonatal hypoglycemia, ear crease, hemihypertrophy, Wilmss tumor

Bloom Syndrome

Inheritance/etiology: mendelian disorder, autosomal recessive; mutations in DNA helicase RecQ protein-like-2, increased rate of sister chromatid exchange is cytogenetic marker

Primary features: immunodeficiency, low birth weight, photosensitive rash

Branchiootorenal Dysplasia

Inheritance/etiology: mendelian disorder, autosomal dominant; mutations in *EYA1*

Primary features: hearing loss, preauricular pits, branchial fistulas/cysts, renal dysplasia

Camptomelic Dysplasia

Also see Camptomelic Dysplasia, in Chapter 15.

Inheritance/etiology: mendelian disorder, autosomal dominant; mutations in *SOX9*

Primary features: ventral bowing of the tibias and femora, talipes equinovarus, absent or hypoplastic fibulae and scapulae, sex reversal in chromosomally male fetuses

Carpenter Syndrome

Also see Craniosynostosis Syndromes (Fibroblast Growth Factor Receptor–Related), in Chapter 5.

Inheritance/etiology: mendelian disorder, autosomal recessive

Primary features: variable synostosis of coronal, sagittal, and lambdoid sutures leading to acrocephaly, polydactyly/syndactyly of feet

Caudal Regression Sequence

Also see Caudal Regression Syndrome, in Chapter 15.

Inheritance/etiology: sporadic, 16% of affected born to diabetic mothers

Primary features: incomplete development of the sacrum and lumbar vertebrae, absence of the body of the sacrum, flexion and abduction at hips, popliteal webs due to lack of movement, talipes equinovarus and calcaneovalgus deformities, disruption of distal spinal cord leading to neurologic impairment

Cerebro-Oculo-Facial-Skeletal (COFS) Syndrome

Inheritance/etiology: autosomal recessive

Primary features: micrognathia, microphthalmos, agenesis of the corpus callosum, cerebellar hypoplasia, mental retardation, contractures, scoliosis, death typically before age 5

CHARGE Association

Also see CHARGE Association, in Chapter 5.

Inheritance/etiology: mostly sporadic; unknown etiology

Primary features: colobomatous eye malformations, heart defects, atresia of the choanae, retarded growth or mental development, genital anomalies, ear anomalies, deafness

CHILD Syndrome

Inheritance/etiology: mendelian disorder; defect in cholesterol biosynthesis, X-linked dominant, mutations in *NSDHL* or *EBP*

Primary features: unilateral hypomelia and ichthyosis, cardiac septal defects, renal agenesis

Chondrodysplasia Punctata (Rhizomelic Type)

Also see Chondrodysplasia Punctata, in Chapter 15.

Inheritance/etiology: mendelian disorder, autosomal recessive; defect in peroxisomes, mutations in *PEX7*

Primary features: severe micromelia, especially of the humeri and femora with stippled epiphyses

Cleft Lip Sequence

Inheritance/etiology: heterogeneous; usually multifactorial

Primary features: failure of lip fusion, which may interfere with the closure of the palatal shelves as well (note: cleft palate alone is a different defect)

Cleidocranial Dysostosis

Also see Chapter 15.

Inheritance/etiology: mendelian disorder, autosomal dominant; mutations in *CBFA1*

Primary features: partial to complete aplasia of clavicle, late closure of fontanelles, brachycephaly, partial anodontia, short fingers

Coffin-Lowry Syndrome

Inheritance/etiology: mendelian disorder, X-linked; mutations in *RSK2*

Primary features: postnatal growth deficiency, severe mental retardation, hypotonia, coarse appearance with downward-slanting palpebral fissures; large, open mouth; vertebral defects, hypodontia, large hands with unusual epiphyses leading to a tapering appearance

Cornelia de Lange Syndrome

Also see Cornelia de Lange Syndrome, in Chapter 5.

Inheritance/etiology: mendelian disorder, autosomal dominant; vast majority of cases are new mutations

Primary features: microcephaly, low birth weight, characteristic facial features, cleft palate, micrognathia, dysplastic kidneys, cardiac malformations, genital anomalies, diaphragmatic hernia, ulnar limb defects

Crouzon Disease

Also see Craniosynostosis Syndromes (Fibroblast Growth Factor Receptor–Related), in Chapter 5.

Inheritance/etiology: mendelian disorder, autosomal dominant; most cases mutations in *FGFR2*

Primary features: craniosynostosis of coronal, lambdoid, and sagittal sutures; hypertelorism, shallow orbits leading to appearance of bulging eyes; conductive hearing loss; maxillary hypoplasia

Cystic Fibrosis

Inheritance/etiology: mendelian disorder, autosomal recessive; multiple mutations in *CFTR*

Primary features: meconium ileus (can present as echogenic bowel on prenatal ultrasound examination), pancreatic insufficiency, recurrent respiratory infections, increased chloride content in sweat, congenital bilateral absence of the vas deferens in males (98%)

de Lange Syndrome

See Cornelia de Lange Syndrome, earlier in this appendix.

Diastrophic Dysplasia

Inheritance/etiology: mendelian disorder, autosomal recessive, mutations in *DTDST*

Primary features: skeletal dysplasia with micromelia, "hitchhiker thumb," talipes, micrognathia, cleft palate, hypertrophic auricular cartilage in infancy, calcification of the pinnae

DiGeorge Sequence

See 22q11 Deletion Syndrome, earlier in this appendix.

Distal Arthrogryposis Type 1

Inheritance/etiology: mendelian disorder, autosomal dominant with extremely variable expressivity

Primary features: tightly clenched hands with adducted thumbs and medially overlapping fingers at birth (may resemble hand posturing in trisomy 18), distal contractures, positional deformities of feet

Early Urethral Obstruction Sequence

Inheritance/etiology: heterogeneous (may be sporadic or one feature of a pattern of malformations such as VATER association or persistent cloaca sequence)

Primary features: oligohydramnios deformation complex, bladder distention, bladder wall hypertrophy, hydroureter, renal dysplasia, abdominal distention, abdominal muscle deficiency, excess abdominal skin, cryptorchidism, persistent urachus, colon malrotation, iliac vessel compression, lower limb deficiency

Ectrodactyly-Ectodermal Dysplasia-Clefting Syndrome (EEC)

Inheritance/etiology: mendelian disorder, autosomal dominant; multiple gene loci; some cases result from mutations in p63

Primary features: ectodermal dysplasia (fair, thin skin; blue, photosensitive eyes; light, thin hair), cleft lip with or without cleft palate, defects in midhands and feet ranging from syndactyly to ectrodactyly, severe deficiency of middle rays

Ehlers-Danlos Syndrome

Inheritance/etiology: mendelian inheritance; Ehlers-Danlos syndrome encompasses a number of disorders of collagen (subclassified into "types") that are diverse in their phenotypes, severity, inheritance patterns, and clinical implications; autosomal dominant, autosomal, and X-linked forms

Primary features: clinical features depend on the type of EDS; features may include subluxation and dislocation of joints, kyphoscoliosis, poor wound healing, premature rupture of membranes, soft hyperextensible skin, bruising, periodontal disease, arterial rupture/rupture of pregnant uterus in third trimester (type IV)

Ellis-van Creveld Syndrome (Chondroectodermal Dysplasia)

Inheritance/etiology: mendelian disorder, autosomal recessive, mutations in the Ellis-van Creveld (EVC) gene

Primary features: short stature, heart defects (especially atrial septal defects), polydactyly, distal limb shortening, narrow chest

Exstrophy of Bladder Sequence

Inheritance/etiology: sporadic; unknown etiology

Primary features: breakdown of cloacal membrane, exposure of posterior wall of bladder, incomplete fusion of genital tubercles, epispadias, separated pubic rami, short lower abdominal wall, inguinal herniae

Exstrophy of Cloaca Sequence

Inheritance/etiology: sporadic; unknown etiology

Primary features: failure of cloacal separation with persistence of a common cloaca and breakdown of the cloacal membrane with exstrophy of the cloaca, failure of fusion of the genital tubercles and pubic rami, omphalocele, hydromyelia, imperforate anus, fused mullerian elements with bifid uterine horns and duplicated or atretic vaginas in affected females, cryptorchidism in affected males

Facioauriculovertebral Spectrum

See Goldenhar Syndrome.

Fanconi Anemia

Inheritance/etiology: mendelian disorder; autosomal recessive; multiple complementation groups, mutations known for most; chromosome breakage is cytogenetic marker

Primary features: low birthweight, short stature, abnormal skin pigmentation, abnormalities of thumb/radius, other congenital malformations, progressive bone marrow failure usually presenting in childhood

Fragile X Syndrome

Inheritance/etiology: mendelian disorder; X-linked; fragile site on X chromosome at Xq28 consisting of a trinucleotide repeat that tends to expand, particularly when passing through female meioses; females inheriting a full expansion can have varying degrees of mental retardation

Primary features: mental retardation, prominent jaw, large ears, macroorchidism, connective tissue involvement (hyperextensible fingers, joint laxity), autistic-like mannerisms, attention deficit, hyperactivity

Fraser Syndrome

Also see Fraser Syndrome, in Chapter 5.

Inheritance/etiology: mendelian disorder, autosomal recessive

Primary features: cryptophthalmos, commonly with eye defects; defect of the ear; mental retardation; cutaneous syndactyly; incomplete development of genitalia with clitoromegaly in females; renal agenesis; laryngeal atresia

Freeman-Sheldon Syndrome

Inheritance/etiology: mendelian disorder, autosomal dominant

Primary features: small, pursed mouth with "whistling" appearance, deep set eyes, broad nasal bridge, flexion of fingers, equinovarus with contracted toes, scoliosis

Frontonasal Dysplasia Sequence

Inheritance/etiology: heterogeneous

Primary features: hypertelorism, nasal deformity varying from notched, broad nasal tip to complete division of the nostrils with median cleft lip resulting from a primary defect in midline facial development

Fryns Syndrome

Also see Fryns Syndrome, in Chapter 5.

Inheritance/etiology: mendelian disorder, autosomal recessive

Primary features: central nervous system anomalies, microphthalmia, facial anomalies, pulmonary hypoplasia/abnormal lobation, diaphragmatic defects, kidney cysts, distal limb anomalies

Goldenhar Syndrome

Also see Goldenhar Syndrome, in Chapter 5.

Inheritance/etiology: usually sporadic; unknown etiology; minor features occasionally noted in relatives; defect in the morphogenesis of the first and second branchial arches

Primary features: asymmetric malar, maxillary, and/or mandibular hypoplasia; microtia; middle ear anomaly with variable deafness; cleft lip with or without cleft palate; anomalies in function or structure of tongue; hemivertebrae or hypoplasia of vertebrae; cardiac defects; renal anomaly; occasional mental deficiency

Grebe Syndrome

Inheritance/etiology: mendelian disorder, autosomal recessive, mutations in CDMP1

Primary features: severe distal limb reduction, short digits, polydactyly, normal facies and intelligence

Heterotaxy Syndrome

Inheritance/etiology: mostly sporadic; autosomal dominant, autosomal recessive, and X-linked forms have been reported

Primary features: asplenia syndrome (bilateral right sidedness) includes asplenia, situs inversus, complex heart defects, atrial isomerism, heart block, bilateral trilobed lungs; polysplenia syndrome (bilateral left sidedness) includes polysplenia, heart defects, bilateral bilobed lungs

Holoprosencephaly Sequence

Inheritance/etiology: heterogeneous; often one feature of a chromosome abnormality; increased frequency in infants of diabetics; multiple genetic loci; an autosomal dominant form results from mutations in SHH.

Primary features: incomplete cleavage and morphogenesis of forebrain, missing or incomplete midfacial development, hypotelorism to cyclopia, cleft lip and palate, single central incisor

Holt-Oram Syndrome

Also see Holt-Oram Syndrome, in Chapter 5.

Inheritance/etiology: mendelian disorder, autosomal dominant, mutations in TBX5

Primary features: cardiac malformations, defects of upper limb and shoulder girdle from thumb hypoplasia to phocomelia

Homocystinuria Syndrome

Inheritance/etiology: mendelian disorder; autosomal recessive; deficiency of cystathionine β-synthase

Primary features: tall, slim body habitus; arachnodactyly (features similar to those of Marfan syndrome); degeneration of aorta and arteries leading to thromboses; subluxation of lens leading to myopia; malar flush; osteoporosis; mental deficiency

Hydrocephalus, X-linked (Includes MASA Syndrome)

Inheritance/etiology: mendelian disorder, X-linked recessive, mutations in L1CAM

Primary features: mental retardation, aqueductal stenosis leading to hydrocephalus of varying severity (may not be present sonographically until the third trimester), adducted thumbs, aphasia, shuffling gait

Hydrolethalus Syndrome

Inheritance/etiology: mendelian disorder, autosomal recessive

Primary features: hydrocephalus, polyhydramnios, micrognathia, polydactyly (postaxial of hands, preaxial of feet), abnormal lobulation of lungs, cleft palate, heart defects, clubfoot

Hypochondroplasia

Inheritance/etiology: mendelian disorder, autosomal dominant, mutations in FGFR3

Primary features: short stature, short limbs, bowing of legs, caudal narrowing of spine, brachydactyly

Hypophosphatasia (Congenital)

Inheritance/etiology: mendelian disorder, autosomal recessive, mutations in ALPL gene

Primary features: moderate to severe extremity bone shortening, diffuse hypomineralization of bone

Infantile Polycystic Kidney Disease

Inheritance/etiology: mendelian disorder; autosomal recessive; mutations in the fibrocystin gene

Primary features: enlarged and echogenic kidneys, often with innumerable tiny cysts; oligohydramnios; hepatic fibrosis

Ivemark Syndrome

See Heterotaxy Syndrome.

Jarcho-Levin Syndrome

Inheritance/etiology: mendelian disorder, autosomal recessive, mutations in DLL3

Primary features: bone dysplasia with severe vertebral and rib anomalies, small thorax

Joubert Syndrome

See Joubert Syndrome, in Chapter 5.

Klippel-Feil Sequence

Inheritance/etiology: sporadic, unknown etiology

Primary features: fused cervical vertebrae, hemivertebrae, webbed neck, torticollis, facial asymmetry, neurologic deficits (paraplegia, hemiplegia)

Klippel-Trenaunay-Weber Syndrome

Also see Klippel-Trenaunay-Weber Syndrome, in Chapter 5.

Inheritance/etiology: sporadic, etiology unknown

Primary features: hemihypertrophy, asymmetric overgrowth of limbs, wide variety of vascular malformations

Kniest Dysplasia

Inheritance/etiology: mendelian disorder; autosomal dominant; mutations in COL2A1

Primary features: mild to moderate micromelia with metaphyseal and epiphyseal splaying, kyphoscoliosis, platyspondyly, cleft palate

Langer-Giedion Syndrome (Trichorhinophalangeal Syndrome Type II)

Inheritance/etiology: chromosomal microdeletion syndrome; deletion on chromosome 8q24.12-q24.13; vertical transmission has been reported

Primary features: growth deficiency, mental retardation, microcephaly, skin and joint laxity, multiple exostoses, bulbous nose, cupped ears

Larsen Syndrome

Inheritance/etiology: mendelian disorder with etiologic heterogeneity

Primary features: multiple joint dislocations, flat facies, long fingers with short metacarpals and fingernails

Laterality Sequence

See Heterotaxy Syndrome.

Lenz Microphthalmia Syndrome

Inheritance/etiology: mendelian disorder, X-linked
Primary features: microphthalmos or anophthalmos, microcephaly, renal dysgenesis, skeletal anomalies

Lethal Multiple Pterygium Syndrome

Inheritance/etiology: mendelian disorder, autosomal recessive
Primary features: prenatal onset of growth deficiency, flexion contractures of limbs, pterygia in multiple areas including ankles, knees, wrists, axillae, and neck

Limb-Body Wall Complex

Also see Limb-Body Wall Complex, in Chapters 5 and 12.
Inheritance/etiology: sporadic, unknown etiology
Primary features: severe kyphoscoliosis, thoracoabdominalschisis, neural tube defects, bizarre facial clefts, absent extremities, positional deformities, variable limb anomalies

Lowe Syndrome

Inheritance/etiology: mendelian disorder, X-linked, mutations in OCRL1
Primary features: moderate to severe mental retardation, cataract, renal tubular dysfunction

Marfan Syndrome

Inheritance/etiology: mendelian disorder, autosomal dominant, mutations in FBN1
Primary features: tall stature, high arched palate, aortic and mitral valve insufficiency after birth, lens dislocation

Marshall Syndrome

Inheritance/etiology: mendelian disorder, autosomal dominant, mutations in COL11A1
Primary features: short stature, flat nasal bridge, large-appearing eyes, myopia, cataracts, sensorineural deafness, calvarial thickening

McKusick-Kaufman Syndrome

McKusick-Kaufman syndrome includes one form of Bardet-Biedl syndrome.
Inheritance/etiology: mendelian disorder, autosomal recessive, mutations in MKKS

Primary features: vaginal atresia or duplication, hydrometrocolpos, genitourinary anomalies, anorectal atresia, cardiac defects, polydactyly

Meckel-Gruber Syndrome

Also see Meckel-Gruber Syndrome, in Chapter 5.
Inheritance/etiology: mendelian disorder, autosomal recessive, at least two genetic loci
Primary features: cystic kidneys, occipital encephalocele and/or polydactyly (postaxial), microcephaly, microphthalmia, cleft palate, genitourinary anomalies

Megacystis-Microcolon-Hypoperistalsis Syndrome

Inheritance/etiology: mendelian disorder; autosomal recessive; most common in females
Primary features: dilated bladder, hydronephrosis, microcolon, dilated proximal duodenum

Menkes Syndrome

Inheritance/etiology: mendelian disorder, X-linked recessive; mutations in Cu (2+) transporting adenosine triphosphatase
Primary features: copper deficiency leading to progressive neurologic deficit, growth deficiency, hypotonia, seizures, sparse "kinky" hair, wormian bones, and death usually by 3 years of age

Metatropic Dysplasia

Inheritance/etiology: mendelian disorder, autosomal recessive
Primary features: micromelia with marked metaphyseal flaring, narrow thorax but relatively long trunk, progressive kyphoscoliosis

Miller-Dieker Syndrome

Inheritance/etiology: chromosomal microdeletion syndrome; deletion on chromosome 17 at band pl 3.3 in most cases
Primary features: lissencephaly (incompletely developed brain with smooth surface), severe mental retardation, seizures, microcephaly, failure to thrive, cardiac defects

Miller Syndrome

Inheritance/etiology: mendelian disorder; presumed autosomal recessive
Primary features: Treacher Collins–like appearance (malar hypoplasia, eyelid colobomas), cleft lip with or without cleft palate; limb deficiencies, usually postaxial

Moebius Sequence

Inheritance/etiology: heterogeneous
Primary features: sixth and seventh nerve palsy giving an expressionless appearance, micrognathia, occasional mental deficiency

Multiple Exostoses Syndrome

Inheritance/etiology: mendelian disorder, autosomal dominant, several genetic loci, mutations in EXT1 or EXT2
Primary features: diaphyseal outgrowths leading to limb deformity

Multiple Pterygium Syndrome (Escobar Syndrome)

Inheritance/etiology: mendelian disorder, autosomal recessive
Primary features: small stature; multiple pterygia of neck, axillae, elbows, knees; micrognathia; camptodactyly; syndactyly

MURCS Association

Inheritance/etiology: sporadic; unknown etiology
Primary features: mullerian duct aplasia, renal aplasia, cervicothoracic somite dysplasia (sometimes referred to as the Klippel-Feil malformation sequence depending on severity)

Nager Syndrome

Also see Nager Syndrome (Acrofacial Dysostosis 1), in Chapter 5.
Inheritance/etiology: mendelian disorder, presumed autosomal dominant, most cases sporadic
Primary features: Treacher Collins–like appearance (malar hypoplasia, down-slanting palpebral fissures), conductive deafness, preauricular tags, cleft palate, radial limb hypoplasia

Neu-Laxova Syndrome

Inheritance/etiology: mendelian disorder, autosomal recessive
Primary features: central nervous system anomalies including agenesis of the corpus callosum and lissencephaly, microcephaly, sloped forehead, hypertelorism, micrognathia, flat nose, flexion deformities, overlapping fingers, scaling skin with edema, ichthyosis

Neural Tube Defects (Meningomyelocele, Anencephaly, Iniencephaly Sequences)

Inheritance/etiology: heterogenous; most cases multifactorial if isolated but may be seen with other defects as part of a single gene disorder; chromosome abnormality or other malformation complex
Primary features: failure of neural tube closure; spina bifida; hydrocephalus with varying degrees of mental retardation; clubfoot (meningomyelocele); incomplete development of brain with degeneration; incomplete development of calvarium; alteration in facies (anencephaly); abnormality of cervical vertebrae; defects of thoracic cage; hypoplasia of lung, heart, or both; short neck and trunk (iniencephaly)

Neurofibromatosis (Type I)

Inheritance/etiology: mendelian disorder, autosomal dominant, 50% of cases represent a new mutation, mutations in NF1 gene (chromosome 17)
Primary features: multiple neurofibromas, café au lait spots, osseous lesions, Lisch nodules, axillary freckling

Neurofibromatosis (Type II)

Inheritance/etiology: mendelian disorder, autosomal dominant, many cases represent a new mutation, mutations in NF2 gene (chromosome 22)
Primary features: eighth cranial nerve neurofibromas, particularly acoustic neuromas; schwannomas, neurofibromas, and other tumors of central nervous system; juvenile cataracts

Noonan Syndrome

Also see Noonan Syndrome, in Chapter 5.
Inheritance/etiology: mendelian disorder; presumed autosomal dominant
Primary features: short stature, webbed neck, lymphedema (including cystic hygromas, hydrops, and pulmonary lymphangiectasis), facial anomalies, congenital heart defects, cardiomyopathy, variable mental retardation

Oculodentodigital Syndrome

Inheritance/etiology: mendelian disorder, autosomal dominant
Primary features: microphthalmos, dental enamel hypoplasia, 4-5 syndactyly of fingers/toes, camptodactyly of fifth fingers

Omphalocele, Extrophy (of the Bladder), Imperforate (Anus), and Spinal Defects (OEIS) Complex

Inheritance/etiology: unknown; recurrence in siblings has been documented; may represent most severe manifestation of the extrophy of cloaca sequence

Primary features: omphalocele, extrophy of the cloaca, imperforate anus, spinal defect

Opitz Syndrome (G Syndrome)

Inheritance/etiology: mendelian disorder, autosomal dominant form at 22q11.2 and X-linked form at Xp22.3

Primary features: hypertelorism; micrognathia; cleft lip, palate, or both; esophageal dysfunction; hypospadias; laryngeal anomalies; cardiovascular anomalies (ventriculoseptal defect, atrial septal defect, coarctation of aorta), mild mental retardation

Orofaciodigital Syndrome I

Also see Oral-Facial-Digital Syndrome, in Chapter 5.

Inheritance/etiology: mendelian disorder, X-linked dominant with apparent lethality in males

Primary features: brain malformations including hydrocephalus and porencephaly, cleft palate, polydactyly of feet, buccal-alveolar webbing and facial milia, mental retardation

Orofaciodigital Syndrome II (Mohr Syndrome)

Inheritance/etiology: mendelian disorder, autosomal recessive

Primary features: cleft lip and palate, lobate tongue, dental abnormalities, hypoplasia of mandible, bilateral polydactyly of hands and feet (preaxial), conductive hearing deficit

Oromandibular-Limb Hypogenesis Spectrum

Inheritance/etiology: sporadic, etiology unknown

Primary features: limb hypoplasia, syndactyly, hypoglossia, micrognathia, variant clefting or aberrant attachments of tongue, cleft palate, cranial nerve palsies including Moebius sequence

Osteogenesis Imperfecta (Types I, III, IV)

Inheritance/etiology: mendelian disorder; autosomal dominant, mutations in COL1A1 or COL1A2, recurrences represent gonadal mosaicism in parent

Primary features: varying degrees of bone fragility and fractures, blue sclerae, hyperextensibility, hypoplasia of dentin with translucency of teeth (dentinogenesis imperfecta), hearing loss (features differ with each type)

Osteogenesis Imperfecta (Type II)

Also see Osteogenesis Imperfecta, in Chapter 15.

Inheritance/etiology: mendelian disorder; autosomal dominant; mutations in COL1A1 or COL1A2

Primary features: short, broad long bones; multiple fractures; soft calvarium; blue sclerae; lethal in perinatal period due to respiratory insufficiency

Osteopetrosis Congenita (Malignant Infantile)

Inheritance/etiology: mendelian disorder, autosomal recessive, mutations in TCIRG1 or CLCN7

Primary features: hepatosplenomegaly, anemia or pancytopenia, thick and dense bones

Otopalatodigital Syndrome (Type I)

Inheritance/etiology: mendelian disorder, X-linked semidominant with females expressing mild to complete features of the condition

Primary features: deafness, cleft palate, irregular length and form of distal phalanges, small stature, mild mental deficiency

Otopalatodigital Syndrome (Type II)

Inheritance/etiology: mendelian disorder, X-linked (may be allelic to type I)

Primary features: growth deficiency, cleft palate, hypertelorism, micrognathia; flexed, overlapping fingers with polydactyly/syndactyly; death commonly occurring in infancy most often due to respiratory failure

Pallister-Hall Syndrome

Inheritance/etiology: mendelian disorder, autosomal dominant, mutations in GLI3

Primary features: hypothalamic hamartoblastoma, insertional polydactyly, hypopituitarism, imperforate anus, endocardial cushion defect, renal defects

Pena-Shokeir Phenotype (Fetal Akinesia/ Hypokinesia Sequence)

Also see Arthrogryposis and Akinesia Sequence, in Chapter 5.

Inheritance/etiology: heterogeneous; mostly sporadic, some cases autosomal recessive; phenotype caused by various conditions leading to reduced fetal movement

Primary features: intrauterine growth retardation, craniofacial anomalies (hypertelorism, micrognathia, cleft palate, short neck), limb anomalies (contractures, hypoplasia, occasional pterygia), pulmonary hypoplasia, short umbilical cord, polyhydramnios

Pfeiffer Syndrome

See Craniosynostosis Syndromes (Fibroblast Growth Factor Receptor–Related), in Chapter 5.

Pierre Robin Sequence

Inheritance/etiology: heterogeneous
Primary features: micrognathia, cleft palate, glossoptosis

Poland Anomaly

Also see Poland Syndrome, in Chapter 15.
Inheritance/etiology: sporadic; possibly vascular in etiology
Primary features: hypoplasia to aplasia of pectoralis muscle with rib defects, syndactyly, brachydactyly

Polysplenia/Asplenia Syndrome

See Heterotaxy Syndromes (Cardiosplenic Syndromes, Polysplenia/Asplenia), in Chapter 5.

Popliteal Pterygium Syndrome

Inheritance/etiology: mendelian disorder, autosomal dominant
Primary features: contractures with webbing of popliteal regions, cleft lip and palate, syndactyly, talipes equinovarus

Potter Sequence (Oligohydramnios Sequence)

Inheritance/etiology: heterogeneous (depends on etiology of defect leading to oligohydramnios)
Primary features: oligohydramnios owing to defect of urinary output (renal agenesis, polycystic kidney disease or obstruction) or chronic leakage of amniotic fluid leading to growth deficiency, pulmonary hypoplasia, and fetal compression; "Potter facies," limb positioning defects, and breech presentation result from fetal compression

Prader-Willi Syndrome

Inheritance/etiology: paternal chromosomal microdeletion or maternal disomy of chromosome 15 at band q11-13; majority sporadic but occasional recurrence has been reported
Primary features: Obesity with bizarre eating habits, hypotonia, mental retardation, small hands and feet, marked neonatal hypotonia

Roberts-SC Phocomelia Syndrome

Also see Roberts Syndrome, in Chapter 5.
Inheritance/etiology: mendelian disorder; autosomal recessive; centromeric separation is cytogenetic marker
Primary features: limb abnormalities ranging from phocomelia to milder forms of limb reduction or hypoplasia (pseudothalidomide syndrome), cleft lip with or without cleft palate, cardiac defects, genitourinary anomalies, severe prenatal growth deficiency

Rubinstein-Taybi Syndrome

Inheritance/etiology: mutation or deletion of CREBBP gene on chromosome 16 at band p13; mostly sporadic
Primary features: microcephaly, beaked nose, glaucoma, mental retardation, cardiac defects, broad thumb, large nose

Russell-Silver Syndrome

Inheritance/etiology: unknown, evidence for heterogeneity
Primary features: prenatal onset of small stature that usually spares the head; asymmetry; café au lait spots

Saethre-Chotzen Syndrome

Inheritance/etiology: mendelian disorder, autosomal dominant, mutations in TWIST gene
Primary features: synostosis of coronal sutures, brachycephaly, hypertelorism, cutaneous syndactyly

Seckel Syndrome

Inheritance/etiology: autosomal recessive
Primary features: beaklike nose, narrow face; intrauterine growth restriction; chromosome instability, hematologic problems, or both; micrognathia, mental retardation, microcephaly

Short-Rib Polydactyly Syndrome

Inheritance/etiology: mendelian disorder, autosomal recessive
Primary features: micromelia, narrow thorax with short ribs, polydactyly, cardiac defects, renal dysplasia

Shprintzen Syndrome

See 22q11 Deletion Syndrome.

Sirenomelia Sequence

Also see Sirenomelia, in Chapter 15.
Inheritance/etiology: sporadic; alteration in early vascular development
Primary features: single lower extremity with posterior alignment of knees and feet, absence of sacrum, imperforate anus, absence of rectum, absence of external and internal genitalia, renal agenesis, absence of bladder

Smith-Lemli-Opitz Syndrome

Also see Smith-Lemli-Opitz Syndrome, in Chapter 5.
Inheritance/etiology: mendelian disorder, autosomal recessive, defect in cholesterol biosynthesis
Primary features: microcephaly; hydrocephalus; cerebellar hypoplasia; cardiac anomalies; genital anomalies; facial

anomalies, including cleft palate, facial capillary hemangioma, and micrognathia; polydactyly

Smith-Magenis Syndrome

Inheritance/etiology: chromosomal microdeletion syndrome; deletion on chromosome 17 at band 11.2
Primary features: mental retardation, sleep disturbances, failure to thrive, hypotonia, self-destructive behavior, brachycephaly, brachydactyly

Spondyloepiphyseal Dysplasia Congenita

Inheritance/etiology: mendelian disorder, autosomal dominant, mutations in COL2A1
Primary features: severe short stature, shortened and mildly bowed femora, short trunk, micrognathia, cleft palate

Stickler Syndrome

Inheritance/etiology: mendelian disorder, autosomal dominant with variable expressivity, mutations in COL2A1, COL11A1, COL11a2
Primary features: myopia, Robin-type cleft palate, hyperextensible joints, mild to moderate spondyloepiphyseal dysplasia, arthritis, sensorineural hearing loss

Thanatophoric Dysplasia

Inheritance/etiology: mendelian disorder; autosomal dominant; most cases result from a new mutation in FGFR3; recurrence due to gonadal mosaicism
Primary features: skeletal dysplasia with severe rhizomelic shortening of limbs, cloverleaf skull, platyspondyly, narrow spinal canal

Thrombocytopenia–Absent Radius Syndrome (TAR)

Also see Thrombocytopenia–Absent Radius Syndrome, in Chapter 5.
Inheritance/etiology: mendelian disorder, autosomal recessive
Primary features: radial aplasia with thumbs always present; lower extremity defects, thrombocytopenia, cardiac defects

Treacher Collins Syndrome

Also see Treacher Collins Syndrome, in Chapter 5.
Inheritance/etiology: mendelian disorder, autosomal dominant, mutations in TREACLE gene
Primary features: malar and mandibular hypoplasia, cleft palate, down-slanting palpebral fissures, lower eyelid coloboma, auricular malformations, conductive deafness

Trichorhinophalangeal Syndrome

Also see Langer-Giedion Syndrome.
Inheritance/etiology: chromosomal microdeletion syndrome, deletion on chromosome 8 at band q24
Primary features: mild growth deficiency, bulbous nose, large ears, epiphyseal coning, sparse hair

Tuberous Sclerosis

Also see Tuberous Sclerosis, in Chapter 5.
Inheritance/etiology: mendelian disorder, autosomal dominant, mutations in TCS1 or TCS2
Primary features: intracranial calcifications, mental retardation, seizures, renal cysts, renal tumors (angiomyolipomas), cardiac tumors (rhabdomyomas), depigmented skin lesions (ash-leaf spots), adenoma sebaceum

Twin-Twin Transfusion Sequence

Also see Twin-Twin Transfusion Syndrome, in Chapter 18.
Inheritance/etiology: sporadic, occurring only in monozygotic twins with placental vascular anastomoses
Primary features: growth-retarded twin with large, hydropic co-twin

VATER/VACTERL Association

Also see VATER/VACTERL Association, in Chapter 5.
Inheritance/etiology: sporadic; unknown etiology
Primary features: vertebral anomalies, anorectal atresia, cardiac defects, tracheoesophageal fistula, renal and limb anomalies, radial defects, single umbilical artery

Van der Woude Syndrome

Inheritance/etiology: mendelian disorder, autosomal dominant with variable expressivity
Primary features: lower lip pits, cleft lip with or without cleft palate, cleft palate alone, absent central and lateral incisors

Velocardiofacial Syndrome

See 22q11 Deletion Syndrome.

von Hippel-Lindau Syndrome

Inheritance/etiology: mendelian disorder, autosomal dominant, mutations in VHL
Primary features: ocular angiomas and cerebellar hemangioblastoma, tumors of kidneys and pancreas

Waardenburg Syndrome

Inheritance/etiology: mendelian disorder, autosomal dominant with variable expressivity, type I mutations in PAX3, type II mutations in MITF

Primary features: deafness, heterochromia of eyes, white forelock, broad nasal bridge and mandible

Walker-Warburg Syndrome

Also see Walker-Warburg Syndrome, in Chapter 5.
Inheritance/etiology: mendelian disorder, autosomal recessive
Primary features: encephalocele, agenesis of midline brain structures, type II lissencephaly, hydrocephalus, eye abnormalities

Williams Syndrome

Inheritance/etiology: chromosomal microdeletion syndrome encompassing elastin locus on chromosome 7 at band q11.2; usually sporadic
Primary features: mental retardation, characteristic facies, cardiac defects (especially supravalvular aortic stenosis)

Zellweger Syndrome

Inheritance/etiology: mendelian disorder, autosomal recessive, peroxisomal defect, mutations in PEX12
Primary features: hypotonicity; limb contractures; seizures; stippled epiphyses, especially patella; gross migrational defects in brain development

TERATOGENIC SYNDROMES

See Appendix 3.

Fetal Alcohol Effects (Fetal Alcohol Syndrome)

Etiology: prenatal ethanol exposure
Primary features: pre- and postnatal onset of growth deficiency, microcephaly, short palpebral fissures, thin and smooth upper lips, joint anomalies, cardiac defects (ventriculoseptal defect, atrial septal defect)

Fetal Carbamazepine Effects

Etiology: prenatal carbamazepine (Tegretol) exposure
Primary features: spina bifida (1%); variable development delay; pattern of minor malformations, including up-slanting palpebral fissures, hypertelorism, short and broad nose, long philtrum, epicanthal folds, hypoplastic fingernails

Fetal Cytomegalovirus Effects

Also see Chapter 17.
Etiology: prenatal infection with cytomegalovirus, particularly as a result of a primary maternal infection

Primary features: sensorineural hearing loss, variable mental retardation, chorioretinitis, hepatosplenomegaly

Fetal Hydantoin Effects

Etiology: prenatal phenytoin (Dilantin) exposure
Primary features: prenatal onset of growth deficiency, microcephaly, wide anterior fontanel, ocular hypertelorism, cleft lip and palate, hypoplasia of distal phalanges with small nails, dislocation of hip, short neck, rib anomalies, mild mental deficiency, cardiac defects

Fetal Lithium Effects

Etiology: prenatal exposure to lithium
Primary features: congenital defects of the cardiovascular system, particularly Ebstein anomaly

Fetal Parvovirus Effects

Etiology: fetal infection with parvovirus (Fifth disease)
Primary features: chronic hemolytic anemia, hydrops fetalis

Fetal Rubella Effects

Etiology: fetal infection with rubella virus
Primary features: growth deficiency, microcephaly, deafness, cataract, cardiac defects, myocardial disease

Fetal Toxoplasmosis Effects

Etiology: fetal infection with toxoplasmosis
Primary features: hydrocephalus, chorioretinitis, blindness, cerebral atrophy, intracranial calcifications, variable mental retardation

Fetal Valproate Effects

Etiology: prenatal valproic acid (Depakote) exposure
Primary features: meningomyelocele, cleft lip, cardiac defects, radial ray defects

Fetal Varicella Effects

Etiology: fetal infection with the varicella virus particularly during the first and second trimesters; frequency of fetal infection from mothers having the virus during pregnancy is 1% to 2%
Primary features: cicatricial skin lesions, limb hypoplasia, mental deficiency, seizures

Fetal Warfarin Effects

Etiology: prenatal warfarin (Coumadin) exposure

Primary features: nasal hypoplasia, stippled epiphyses, mental deficiency, occasional central nervous system defects including Dandy-Walker malformation and agenesis of corpus callosum

Retinoic Acid Embryopathy

Etiology: prenatal isotretinoin (Accutane) exposure

Primary features: central nervous system defects (hydrocephalus, microcephaly, posterior fossa abnormalities); bilateral microtia, anotia, or both; Robin-type cleft palate; cardiac defects; thymic abnormalities

SUGGESTED READINGS

GeneClinics: Clinical Genetic Information Resource [database online]. Copyright, University of Washington, Seattle. 1995. Updated weekly. Available at: http://www.geneclinics.org. Accessed October 16, 2002.

GeneTests [database online]. Copyright, Children's Health Care System, Seattle 1999. Available at: http://www.genetests.org. Accessed October 16, 2002.

Jones KL. *Smith's recognizable patterns of human malformation,* 5th ed. Philadelphia: WB Saunders, 1997.

McKusick VA, et al., eds. OMIM (Online Mendelian Inheritance in Man), National Center for Biotechnology Information, Johns Hopkins University. Available at: http://www.ncbi.nlm.nih.gov/omim/. Accessed January 2001.

Seashore MR, Wappner RS. *Genetics in primary care and clinical medicine.* Appleton & Lange, 1996.

View Dysmorphic Syndrome Features. Available at: http://www.hgmp.mrc.ac.uk/DHMHD/view_human.html. Accessed October 16, 2002; and http://www.fetalanomalies.com. Accessed October 16, 2002.

TERATOGENS AND MALFORMATIONS

These reference charts are intended for use as a general guideline for prenatal diagnosticians. They are not intended to be used to counsel patients regarding their risks with prenatal exposures. The agents and outcomes selected for these charts refer to the most commonly accepted major structural defects known to be associated with specific prenatal exposures. Not all associations reported in the literature are listed, and among those that are, the data supporting these associa-tions are of varying quantity and quality. A review of the lit-erature, reference to one of the available online databases such as TERIS (http://depts.washington.edu/~terisweb/teris/) or Reprotox (www.reprotox.org), and/or contact with a ter-atogen information service (www.otispregnancy.org)will pro-vide more comprehensive information on specific risks and timing of exposure that may be informative when planning, performing, or interpreting prenatal diagnostic procedures.

Teratogen: generic (trade name)	Indication/notes	Malformation
Acetaminophen (Tylenol)	—	Slight increased risk for gastroschisis
Alcohol	—	Microcephaly, short palpebral fissures, maxillary hypoplasia, short nose, smooth philtrum, thin upper lip; small distal phalanges, small fifth finger-nails; VSD; growth deficiency; occasionally—cleft lip and/or palate, micro-gnathia, TOF, coarctation of the aorta, meningomyelocele, hydrocephalus
Aminopterine	1–3 mg or more/qd—first trimester	Severe hypoplasia of frontal bone, parietal bones, temporal or occipital bones, wide fontanels, and synostosis of lambdoid or coronal sutures; upsweep of frontal scalp hair; broad nasal bridge, shallow supraorbital ridges, prominent eyes, micrognathia, low-set ears, maxillary hypoplasia, epicanthal folds, shortening of limbs (especially forearm), talipes equino-varus, hypodactyly, syndactyly, microcephaly, growth deficiency; occasion-ally—cleft palate, neural tube defects, dislocation of hip, retarded ossification of pubis and ischium, rib anomalies, dextroposition of the heart
Angiotensin-converting enzyme inhibitors (i.e., benazepril, captopril, enalapril, lisinopril) (Lotensin, Capoten, Vasotec, Zestril)	If used in second or third trimester	Hypocalvaria, oligohydramnios, neonatal renal failure, hypotension, pulmo-nary hypoplasia, joint contractures, IUGR, stillbirth
Aspirin (Bayer, St. Joseph)	At adult doses	Slight increased risk for gastroschisis; premature closure of the ductus arteri-osus; intracranial hemorrhage in premature or LBW infants
Carbon monoxide	Maternal CO poisoning	Stillbirth, neurologic deficits
Carbamazepine (Tegretol, Carbatrol, Epitol)	—	Myelomeningocele, heart defects, urinary tract defects, upward-slanting palpebral fissures, hypertelorism, short nose with long philtrum, epican-thal folds, hypoplastic fingernails
Cigarettes	—	Slight increased risk for oral clefts; IUGR
Cocaine	—	Vascular defects of genitourinary tract (hydronephrosis, hypospadias, prune belly), limb reduction defects, intercranial hemorrhage, cerebral infarcts
Corticosteroids (e.g., prednisone)	—	Slight increased risk for oral clefts

(continued)

Teratogen: generic (trade name)	Indication/notes	Malformation
Cyclophosphamide (Cytoxan, Neosar, Endoxan)	Antineoplastic, immuno-suppressant	Craniosynostosis, microcephaly, hypotelorism, blepharophimosis, microphthalmos, shallow orbits with proptosis, malformed ears, flat nasal bridge with bulbous nasal tip, cleft palate, radial anomalies, absent digits, hypoplasia of middle phalanx of fifth fingers, growth deficiency
Cytarabine (Cytosar-U)	Antineoplastic, antiviral	Very limited first-trimester information. Case reports: (1) bilateral microtia and atresia of external auditory canals, right hand lobster claw/3 digits, bilateral lower limb defects; (2) medial digits of both feet missing, distal phalanges of both thumbs missing with hypoplastic remnant of right thumb
Cytomegalovirus	—	Microcephaly, ventricular dilatation, cerebral calcification, ascites, hepato-splenomegaly, chorioretinitis, IUGR
Diethylstilbestrol (Stil-phostrol)	—	Structural abnormalities of the cervix, vagina, uterine cavity; epididymal cysts; hypoplastic testes; cryptorchidism
Fluconazole	At chronic, high doses	Brachycephaly, micrognathia, trigonocephaly, low ears, abnormal calvarial development, cleft palate, femoral bowing, thin ribs, humeral-radial fusion, arthrogryposis, heart defects
Hyperthermia	Fever of ≥102°F for ≥24 h	Neural tube defects, particularly anencephaly; microcephaly, small midface, microphthalmos, micrognathia, cleft uvula; digital anomalies; growth deficiency; stillbirth; occasionally—ear anomalies
Ibuprofen (Advil, Motrin)	—	Slight increased risk for gastroschisis; premature closure of ductus arteriosus
Lithium (Lithotabs, Eskalith, Lithobid)	—	Ebstein anomaly, heart rhythm disturbances
Lymphocytic choriomen-ingitis virus	—	Hydrocephalus, intracranial calcifications, chorioretinitis
Methotrexate (Rheu-matrex, Trexall)	—	See aminopterin information
Methylmercury	—	Microcephaly, cerebral palsy, spasticity, abnormal reflexes, involuntary movements, seizures, hearing loss, strabismus, growth deficiency
Misoprostol (Cytotec)	A vascular disruption mechanism has been proposed as the cause	Mobius' sequence: mask-like facies with sixth and seventh nerve palsy, usually bilateral, micrognathia, talipes equinovarus; terminal limb reduction defects
Oral contraceptives	If derived from androgens (i.e., ethisterone or norethindrone) and taken at high doses around the time of genital development	Masculinization of female genitalia (clitoral hypertrophy, labioscrotal fusion)
Parvovirus B19 (Fifth disease)	—	Hydrocephalus, myocarditis, hydrops; stillbirth
Penicillamine (Cuprimine, Depen)	At high doses, may be due to very low levels of copper	Cutis laxa
Phenobarbital (Luminal)	—	Hypoplastic fingernails, epicanthal folds, broad depressed nasal bridge, short nose with long philtrum; based on recent case-control study, increased risk for heart defects, oral clefts, urinary tract defects (including kidneys); hemorrhage
Phenylpropanolamine (Acutrim, Dexatrim, Phenyldrine)	—	Slight increased risk for gastroschisis; theoretic risk for bradycardia
Phenytoin (Dilantin, Phenytek)	—	Coarctation of aorta, cardiac septal defects; microcephaly, wide anterior fontanelle, ocular hypertelorism, broad depressed nasal bridge, short nose with bowed upper lip, short neck; cleft lip and palate; hypoplastic fingernails; growth deficiency
Primidone (Mysoline)	Structural analogue of phenobarbital	Brachycephaly, bilateral epicanthal folds, brachydactyly with small fingernails, hypertelorism; cleft lip and/or cleft palate; based on recent case-control study, increased risk for heart defects and defects of the urinary tract (including kidneys); hemorrhage
Pseudoephedrine (Sudafed)	—	Slightly increased risk for gastroschisis

(continued)

Teratogen: generic (trade name)	Indication/notes	Malformation
Quinine	At extremely high doses (generally those taken to induce abortion)	Hypoplasia of the auditory nerve, resulting in deafness; hypoplasia of the optic nerve
Radiation	Ionizing radiation; at levels greater than or equal to 10 rads	Microcephaly
Rubella	—	Microcephaly; cataract, glaucoma, corneal opacity, chorioretinitis, microphthalmos, strabismus; patent ductus arteriosus, pulmonic stenosis; septal defects; growth deficiency; occasionally—hypospadias, cryptorchidism
Sulfasalazine (Azulfidine)	Dihydrofolate reductase inhibitor	Slight increased risk for heart defects, oral clefts, and urinary tract defects
Tetracycline (Brodspec, Actisite)	If taken after 23 wk post-conception	Staining of teeth; depression of bone growth in premature babies
Thalidomide (Thalomid)	Critical period is 20–36 d from conception	Phocomelia, clubfeet and supernumerary toes; facial hemangioma, microtia, facial palsy, abnormalities of the pupil and external ocular muscles, colobomas, and/or microphthalmos; esophageal and duodenal atresia; TOF, VSD or ASD; renal agenesis
Thioguanine (6-TG)	Antineoplastic	Case reports: (1) missing distal phalanges of the thumbs and two missing toes on each foot, (2) craniosynostosis and radial aplasia, as well as digital defects
Thyroid medications (i.e. propylthiouracil, radioactive iodine)	—	Goiter, ablation of thyroid
Toluene	In cases of chronic abuse (i.e., sniffing one to four 16-oz cans of spray paint per day)	Microcephaly, small palpebral fissures, thin upper lip, midface hypoplasia, micrognathia, ear anomalies, down-turned corners of the mouth, large fontanelle; growth deficiency
Toxoplasmosis	—	Microcephaly, intracranial calcifications, encephalitis, hydrocephalus, hydrops, myocarditis, chorioretinitis, hepatosplenomegaly, glomerulitis, myositis, lymphadenopathy
Triamterene (Dyrenium)	Diuretic, antihypertensive	Slight increased risk for heart defects, oral clefts, and urinary tract defects
Trimethadione (Tridione)	—	Cleft lip and palate; septal defects, TOF; hypospadias, clitoral hypertrophy; micrognathia, hypoplastic midface, short up-turned nose with broad, low nasal bridge, prominent forehead, mild synophrys with unusual upward slant to eyebrows, strabismus, ptosis, epicanthal folds, rectangular or cupped and overlapping helix; growth deficiency
Trimethoprim (usually found in combination with sulfamethoxazole; e.g., in Bactrim, Septra)	Dihydrofolate reductase inhibitor	Slight increased risk for heart defects, oral clefts, urinary tract defects, and neural tube defects
Valproic acid (Depakote)	—	Myelomeningocele; cleft lip; coarctation of aorta, hypoplastic left heart Fetal valproate syndrome: epicanthal folds, broad, low nasal bridge with short nose and anteverted nostrils, long philtrum, thin vermilion border
Varicella (Chickenpox)	—	Microcephaly; chorioretinitis; limb hypoplasia with or without digits, clubfoot; cutaneous scars; growth deficiency
Vitamin A derivatives (Accutane, Etretinate)	—	Hydrocephalus, microcephaly; thymic and parathyroid abnormalities; conotruncal malformations; mild facial asymmetry, bilateral microtia, anotia, narrow sloping forehead, micrognathia, flat depressed nasal bridge, ocular hypertelorism; occasionally cleft palate
Warfarin (Coumadin)	Anticoagulant	Nasal hypoplasia, depressed nasal bridge, stippling of uncalcified epiphyses, mild hypoplasia of nails, shortened fingers
Other drugs for which concern has been raised		
Chloroquine (Aralen)	Chronic, high doses	Possible concern for retinal and ototoxicity; case report: cochleovestibular paresis
Ethosuximide (Zarontin)	Anticonvulsant	Very limited data; abnormalities reported include cleft lip and/or palate
Gabapentin (Neurontin)	In each case report, mother was also receiving other anticonvulsants	Case reports: (1) cyclopic holoprosencephaly, (2) absence of ear canal opening, (3) pyloric stenosis and inguinal hernias
Lamotrigine (Lamictal)	Newer antiepileptic	—
Levetiracetam (Keppra)	New antiepileptic	—

(continued)

Teratogen: generic (trade name)	Indication/notes	Malformation
Mifepristone (RU-486)	Antiprogesterone activity	—
Oxcarbazepine (Trileptal)	Derivative of carbamazepine	Possible carbamazepine-like effects
Paramethadione	Related to trimethadione	Possible trimethadione-like effects
Topiramate (Topamax)	—	Case report: prenatal onset growth deficiency, generalized hirsutism, a third fontanelle, short nose with anteverted nares, blunt distal phalanges and generalized blunting of the nails, with fifth nail hypoplasia
Nonteratogens associated with other complications		
Albuterol	Generally only at high, oral doses	Tachycardia
Azathioprine (Imuran)	Metabolized to mercaptopurine	Growth retardation
Beta blockers (i.e., atenolol, propranolol)	Hypertension	Bradycardia, growth retardation
Bromides	—	IUGR
Caffeine	At extremely high doses (>500 mg)	Cardiac arrhythmia
Phenylephrine	—	Possible bradycardia
Polychlorinated biphenyls	Maternal poisoning	Temporary gray-brown discoloration of the skin, gingiva, and nails, parchment-like skin with desquamation, conjunctivitis; low birth weight, IUGR

ASD, atrial septal defect; IUGR, intrauterine growth restriction; LBW, low birth weight; TOF, tetralogy of Fallot; VSD, ventricular septal defect.

INDEX

Page numbers followed by *f* refer to figures; those followed by *t* refer to tables.